Peripheral
Arterial
Disease

Notice

Medicine is an ever-changing science. As new research and clinical experience broaden our knowledge, changes in treatment and drug therapy are required. The authors and the publisher of this work have checked with sources believed to be reliable in their efforts to provide information that is complete and generally in accord with the standards accepted at the time of publication. However, in view of the possibility of human error or changes in medical sciences, neither the authors nor the publisher nor any other party who has been involved in the preparation or publication of this work warrants that the information contained herein is in every respect accurate or complete, and they disclaim all responsibility for any errors or omissions or for the results obtained from use of the information contained in this work. Readers are encouraged to confirm the information contained herein with other sources. For example and in particular, readers are advised to check the product information sheet included in the package of each drug they plan to administer to be certain that the information contained in this work is accurate and that changes have not been made in the recommended dose or in the contraindications for administration. This recommendation is of particular importance in connection with new or infrequently used drugs.

Peripheral Arterial Disease

Editors

Robert S. Dieter, MD, RVT
Assistant Professor of Medicine
Vascular and Endovascular Medicine
Cardiology
Loyola University
Maywood, Illinois

Raymond A. Dieter Jr., MD, MS
Past World President, International College of Surgeons
President, Center for Surgery
Glen Ellyn, Illinois

Raymond A. Dieter III, MD
Associate Professor of Surgery
Cardiothoracic Surgery
University of Tennessee Medical Center
Knoxville, Tennessee

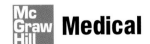

McGraw Hill Medical

New York   Chicago   San Francisco   Lisbon   London   Madrid   Mexico City   Milan
New Delhi   San Juan   Seoul   Singapore   Sydney   Toronto

The McGraw·Hill Companies

Peripheral Arterial Disease

1 2 3 4 5 6 7 8 9 0 CTP/CTP 12 11 10 9

ISBN 978-0-07-148179-3
MHID 0-07-148179-6

This book was set in Berling by Aptara®, Inc.
The editors were Ruth Weinberg, James F. Shanahan, and Peter J. Boyle.
The production supervisor was Sherri Souffrance.
Project management was provided by Satvinder Kaur, Aptara, Inc.
The interior and cover designer was Mary McKeon.
China Translation & Printing Services Ltd., was printer and binder.

This book is printed on acid-free paper.

Library of Congress Cataloging-in-Publication Data

Peripheral arterial disease / editors, Robert S. Dieter, Raymond A. Dieter Jr., Raymond A. Dieter III.
    p. ; cm.
  Includes index.
  ISBN-13: 978-0-07-148179-3 (hardcover : alk. paper)
  ISBN-10: 0-07-148179-6
  1. Peripheral vascular diseases. I. Dieter, Robert S., 1970- II. Dieter, Ray A., 1934- III. Dieter, Raymond A., 1962-
  [DNLM: 1. Peripheral Vascular Diseases. WG 500 P451 2009]
  RC694.P463 2009
  616.1'31–dc22

                                                          2008046346

To my wonderful wife who has been patient and supportive through all of my training and pursuits,
my children who bring a smile to my face every day,
my parents and family who taught me to always strive to do my best.
To God who makes it all possible.

Contents

Contributors

Victor Aboyans, MD, PhD
Department of Family and Preventive Medicine
University of California, San Diego
La Jolla, California
Department of Thoracic and Cardiovascular Surgery
  and Angiology
Dupuytren University Hospital
Limoges, France

M. Habeeb Ahmed, MD, RVT
Director, Center for Cardiovascular Care
San Jose, California

Daniel Alterman, MD
Department of Surgery
Graduate School of Medicine
University of Tennessee
Knoxville, Tennessee

Jose D. Amortegui, MD
Department of Surgery
Graduate School of Medicine
University of Tennessee
Knoxville, Tennessee

Brian H. Annex, MD
Division of Cardiology
Department of Medicine
Durham Veterans Affairs and
  Duke University Medical Center
Durham, North Carolina

Alex J. Auseon, DO
Division of Cardiovascular Medicine
Department of Internal Medicine
Ohio State University College of Medicine
Columbus, Ohio

J. Fernando Aycinena, MD
Department of Surgery
University of Tennessee Medical Center at Knoxville
Knoxville, Tennessee

Mamdouh Bakhos, MD
Professor and Chairman, Department of Thoracic
  and Cardiovascular Surgery
Loyola University Medical Center and Stritch
  School of Medicine
Maywood, Illinois

Robert J. Barnes, MD
Associate Clinical Professor of Ophthalmology
Loyola University Medical Center
Maywood, Illinois

Gerald J. Berry, MD
Professor of Pathology
Director of Cardiac Pathology
Stanford University Medical Center
Stanford, California

Rainer H. Böger, MD
Clinical Pharmacology Unit
Institute of Experimental and Clinical Pharmacology
University Hospital Hamburg-Eppendorf
Hamburg, Germany

Susan Bowes, RVT
Director
Non-Invasive Cardiology and Vascular Services
Washington Hospital Center
Washington, DC

Javed Butler, MD, MPH
Cardiology Division
Emory Crawford Long Hospital
Atlanta, Georgia

James C. Carr, MD
Department of Radiology
Feinberg School of Medicine
Northwestern University
Chicago, Illinois

David C. Cassada, MD
Division of Vascular/Transplant Surgery
University of Tennessee Medical Center
Knoxville, Tennessee

John B. Chang, MD
Professor of Clinical Surgery
Albert Einstein College of Medicine
Bronx, New York
Director
Long Island Vascular Center
Roslyn, New York

Robert W. Chang, MD
Department of Surgery
Division of Vascular Surgery
Dartmouth-Hitchcock Medical Center
Lebanon, New Hampshire

Leonardo Clavijo, MD, PhD
Assistant Professor of Clinical Medicine
Director of Vascular Medicine and
    Peripheral Interventions
University of Southern California
Los Angeles, California

Kevin P. Cohoon, DO
Cardiology
Loyola University Medical Center
Maywood, Illinois

Michael H. Criqui, MD, MPH
Department of Medicine
Department of Family and Preventive Medicine
University of California, San Diego
La Jolla, California

Brian J. Daley, MD
Department of Surgery
Graduate School of Medicine
University of Tennessee
Knoxville, Tennessee

Pranab Das, MD
Cardiology
Loyola University Stritch School of Medicine
Maywood, Illinois

Michael Davis, MD
Division of Cardiovascular Medicine
Ohio State University School of Medicine
Davis Heart and Lung Research Institute
Columbus, Ohio

John E. Deanfield, MB
BHF Vandervell Professor of Cardiology
Great Ormond Street Hospital and
    Institute of Child Health
University College London
London, England, United Kingdom

Terrence C. Demos, MD
Professor, Department of Radiology
Loyola University Medical Center and
    Stritch School of Medicine
Maywood, Illinois

Raymond A. Dieter Jr., MD, MS
Past World President
International College of Surgeons
President, Center for Surgery
Glen Ellyn, Illinois

Raymond A. Dieter III, MD
Associate Professor of Surgery
Cardiothoracic Surgery
University of Tennessee Medical Center
Knoxville, Tennessee

Robert S. Dieter, MD, RVT
Assistant Professor of Medicine
Cardiology
Loyola University
Maywood, Illinois

Ann E. Donald, AVS
Clinical Vascular Scientist (Research)
Department of Clinical Pharmacology
St. Thomas' Hospital
London, England, United Kingdom

Tina M. Dudney, MD
Pulmonary Disease Fellowship Program Director
Assistant Professor of Medicine
Graduate School of Medicine
University of Tennessee
Division Chief of Pulmonary/Critical Care and
    Section Chief of Pulmonary Medicine
University of Tennessee Medical Center
Knoxville, Tennessee

Michael L. Eng, MD
Assistant Professor
Department of Thoracic and Cardiovascular Surgery
Loyola University Medical Center
Maywood, Illinois

Esteban Escolar, MD
Washington Hospital Center and Georgetown University
Washington, DC

Ibrahim Fahsah, MD
Interventional Cardiology
University of Louisville
Louisville, Kentucky

Christopher Francois, MD
Department of Radiology
Feinberg School of Medicine
Northwestern University
Chicago, Illinois

Michael B. Freeman, MD
Professor of Surgery
Department of Surgery
Chief, Division of Vascular Surgery
Graduate School of Medicine
University of Tennessee
Knoxville, Tennessee

Jeffrey H. Freihage, MD
Cardiology
Loyola University Medical Center
Maywood, Illinois

Thomas E. Gaines, MD
Cardiothoracic Surgery
Graduate School of Medicine
University of Tennessee
Knoxville, Tennessee

Robert A. Gallino, MD
Washington Hospital Center and Georgetown University
Washington, DC

Lorena De Marco Garcia, MD
Department of Surgery
North Shore University Hospital
North Shore-Long Island Jewish Health System
Manhasset, New York

Parveen K. Garg, MD, MPH
Department of Medicine
New York University School of Medicine
New York, New York

Roberto Gedaly, MD
Department of Surgery
Transplant Division
University of Kentucky
Lexington, Kentucky

Giorgio Gimelli, MD
Director, Cardiac Catheterization Laboratory
Cardiovascular Medicine Division
University of Wisconsin School of Medicine and
    Public Health
Madison, Wisconsin

Jay Giri, MD, MPH
Department of Medicine
Massachusetts General Hospital
Harvard University
Boston, Massachusetts

John E. Gocke, MD, MPH, RVT, RPVI
Medical Director
Vascular Laboratory
Adventist La Grange Memorial Hospital
La Grange, Illinois

Mitchell H. Goldman, MD
Professor and Chairman
Department of Surgery
Graduate School of Medicine
University of Tennessee
Knoxville, Tennessee

Oscar Grandas, MD
Assistant Professor of Surgery
Department of Surgery
University of Tennessee
Knoxville, Tennessee

L. Michael Graver, MD
Clinical Professor of Surgery
Chairman
Department of Cardiothoracic Surgery
Long Island Jewish Medical Center
New Hyde Park, New York

Daniel R. Guerra, MD
Division of Cardiology
Department of Medicine
Durham Veterans Affairs and
    Duke University Medical Center
Durham, North Carolina

Brian Guttormsen, MD
Cardiovascular Medicine Division
University of Wisconsin School of Medicine and
    Public Health
Madison, Wisconsin

Julian P.J. Halcox, MA, MD
Professor of Cardiology
Cardiff University
Wales Heart Research Institute
Cardiff, Wales, United Kingdom

Kathryn L. Hassell, MD
Associate Professor of Medicine
Division of Hematology
University of Colorado Denver and Health Sciences Center
Denver, Colorado

José Hernández-Rodríguez, MD, PhD
Center for Vasculitis Care and Research
Department of Rheumatic and Immunologic Diseases
Cleveland Clinic
Cleveland, Ohio

Gary S. Hoffman, MD, MS
Center for Vasculitis Care and Research
Department of Rheumatic and Immunologic Diseases
Cleveland Clinic
Cleveland, Ohio

L. Nelson Hopkins, MD
Professor and Chairman of Neurosurgery, Professor of
    Radiology, and Director of Toshiba Stroke
    Research Center
State University of New York at Buffalo, New York
Chairman, Department of Neurosurgery
Millard Fillmore Gates Hospital
Kaleida Health
Buffalo, New York

Sohail Ikram, MD
Associate Professor of Medicine
Director of Peripheral Vascular Interventions
Associate Director of Interventional Cardiology
University of Louisville
Louisville, Kentucky

Salik Jahania, MD
Department of Surgery
Transplant Division
University of Kentucky
Lexington, Kentucky

Babak S. Jahromi, MD, PhD
Assistant Instructor of Clinical Neurosurgery and
    Endovascular Neurosurgery Fellow
Department of Neurosurgery and
    Toshiba Stroke Research Center
State University of New York at Buffalo, New York
Department of Neurosurgery
Millard Fillmore Gates Hospital
Kaleida Health
Buffalo, New York

Samuel L. Johnston, MD
Cardiology
Loyola University Medical Center and
    Stritch School of Medicine
Maywood, Illinois

Edward J. Keuer, MD
Department of Medicine (Dermatology) and
    Pediatrics
Loyola University Medical Center and
    Stritch School of Medicine
Maywood, Illinois

Ghazanfar Khadim, MD
Division of Cardiovascular Medicine
Medical College of Wisconsin
Milwaukee, Wisconsin

George B. Kuzycz, MD
Cardiothoracic and Vascular Surgery
Northern Illinois Center for Surgery
Naperville, Illinois

John R. Laird, MD
Medical Director
Vascular Center
University of California Davis Medical Center
Sacramento, California

Peter Langenstroer, MD, MS
Associate Professor of Urology
Department of Urology
Medical College of Wisconsin
Milwaukee, Wisconsin

Christy M. Lawson, MD
Department of Surgery
University of Tennessee
Knoxville, Tennessee

Michael H. Lebow, MD
Department of Surgery
Graduate School of Medicine
University of Tennessee
Knoxville, Tennessee

Massoud Leesar, MD
Professor of Medicine
Director of Cardiac Catheterization
    Laboratory
Director of Interventional Cardiology
University of Louisville
Louisville, Kentucky

Bruce E. Lewis, MD
Professor
Cardiology
Loyola University Medical Center
Maywood, Illinois

Ferdinand S. Leya, MD
Professor of Medicine and
    Cardiology
Medical Director
Cardiac Catheterization Laboratories
Loyola University Medical Center
Maywood, Illinois

David Liang, MD, PhD
Director
Stanford Center for Marfan Syndrome and
    Related Aortic Disorders
Associate Professor of Medicine
Division of Cardiovascular Medicine
Stanford University School of Medicine
Stanford, California

Dirk A. Loose, MD
European Centre for the Diagnosis and
    Treatment of Vascular Malformations
Hamburg, Germany

Robyn A. Macsata, MD
Department of Surgery
Washington Hospital Center
Washington, DC

Ali F. Mallat, MD
Department of Surgery
University of Michigan
Ann Arbor, Michigan

Michael T. McCormack, MD
Director of Basic Science and Research
Pulmonary Disease Fellowship Program
Clinical Assistant Professor of Medicine
Graduate School of Medicine
University of Tennessee
Staff Physician
University of Tennessee Medical Center
Knoxville, Tennessee

Raymond Q. Migrino, MD
Division of Cardiovascular Medicine
Medical College of Wisconsin
Milwaukee, Wisconsin

J. William Mix, MD
Department of Surgery
Division of Vascular Surgery
Graduate School of Medicine
University of Tennessee
Knoxville, Tennessee

Emile R. Mohler III, MD, MS
Cardiovascular Division
Vascular Medicine Section
University of Pennsylvania School of Medicine
Philadelphia, Pennsylvania

Eamonn S. Molloy, MD, MS
Center for Vasculitis Care and Research
Department of Rheumatic and Immunologic Diseases
Cleveland Clinic
Cleveland, Ohio

Karen Moncher, MD
Assistant Professor of Medicine
Division of Cardiovascular Medicine
University of Wisconsin School of Medicine
Madison, Wisconsin

Ali Morshedi-Meibodi, MD
Coast Cardiology Medical Associates
Los Angeles, California

Debabrata Mukherjee, MD
Gill Heart Institute and
    Division of Cardiovascular Medicine
University of Kentucky
Lexington, Kentucky

Aravinda Nanjundappa, MD, RVT
Associate Professor of Medicine and
    Surgery West Virginia University Charleston
West Virginia

Richard F. Neville, MD
Associate Professor
Department of Surgery
Chief, Division of Vascular Surgery
Georgetown University Hospital
Washington, DC

Gustavo Oderich, MD
Division of Vascular Surgery
Mayo Clinic
Rochester, Minnesota

John P. Pacanowski Jr., MD
Vascular Surgery
Agave Medical Associates
Tucson, Arizona

Ryan Payne, MD
Department of Urology
Medical College of Wisconsin
Milwaukee, Wisconsin

David Pitrak, MD
Professor of Medicine
Chief of Infectious Diseases
University of Chicago
Chicago, Illinois

Sridevi R. Pitta, MD
Cardiovascular Medicine
Mayo Clinic
Rochester, Minnesota

Kailash Prasad, MD, PhD
Professor Emeritus
Department of Physiology
College of Medicine
University of Saskatchewan
Saskatoon, Saskatchewan, Canada

Trent L. Prault, MD
Department of Vascular Surgery and
    Endovascular Interventions
Harbin Clinic
Rome, Georgia

Manu Rajachandran, MD
Director Comprehensive Vascular Program
Chair
Department of Endovascular Medicine
Deborah Heart and Lung Center
Clinical Associate
Professor of Medicine
UMDNJ-Robert Wood Johnson
    Medical School
New Brunswick, New Jersey

Sanjay Rajagopalan, MD
Division of Cardiovascular Medicine
Ohio State University School of Medicine
Davis Heart and Lung Research Institute
Columbus, Ohio

Ravi K. Ramana, DO
Cardiology
Division of Cardiology
Loyola University Medical Center
Maywood, Illinois

Charulata Ramaprasad, MD, MPH
Infectious Diseases
University of Chicago
Chicago, Illinois

Dinesh Ranjan, MD
Department of Surgery
Transplant Division
University of Kentucky
Lexington, Kentucky

Brian Reed, MD
Department of Surgery
Graduate School of Medicine
University of Tennessee
Knoxville, Tennessee

Arti Rupani, MD
Loyola University
Maywood, Illinois

James M. Scanlon, MD
George Washington University Medical Center
Washington, DC

Robert M. Schainfeld, DO
Associate Director
Vascular Medicine
Massachusetts General Hospital
Associate Physician
Harvard Medical School
Boston, Massachusetts

Michael J. Schneck, MD
Associate Professor of Neurology and
    Neurosurgery
Department of Neurology
Loyola University Stritch School of Medicine
Maywood, Illinois

Jeffrey P. Schwartz, MD
Cardiovascular and Thoracic Surgery
Loyola University Medical Center
Maywood, Illinois

Patrick Segers, PhD
Cardiovascular Mechanics and
    Biofluid Dynamics
Institute Biomedical Technology
Ghent University
Ghent, Belgium

Anton N. Sidawy, MD
Department of Surgery
Washington Hospital Center and
    Georgetown University Hospital
Washington, DC

Monica Simionescu, MD
Department of Neurology
Loyola University Chicago
Stritch School of Medicine
Maywood, Illinois

Madhurmeet Singh, DO
Loyola University Medical Center
Maywood, Illinois

David G. Stanley, MD
Medical Director
Wound Treatment Center
Methodist Medical Center
Oak Ridge, Tennessee

Lowell H. Steen, MD
Cardiology
Loyola University Stritch School of Medicine
Maywood, Illinois

Daniel H. Steinberg, MD
Washington Hospital Center and Georgetown University
Washington, DC

Scott L. Stevens, MD
Division of Vascular/Transplant Surgery
University of Tennessee Medical Center
Knoxville, Tennessee

Timothy M. Sullivan, MD
Vascular and Endovascular Surgery
North Central Heart Institute
Sioux Falls, South Dakota

Jessica A. Sutherland, MD
Division of Cardiology
Caritas St. Elizabeth's Medical Center
Boston, Massachusetts

Dana A. Taylor, MD
Department of Surgery
University of Tennessee Medical Center at Knoxville
Knoxville, Tennessee

J. Michael Tuchek, DO
Cardiac Surgery Associates
Loyola University Medical Center
Maywood, Illinois

Ramachandra P. Tummala, MD
Assistant Professor of Neurosurgery, Neurology, and
    Radiology
University of Minnesota Medical School
Minneapolis, Minnesota

Suneel M. Udani, MD, MPH
John H. Stroger Hospital of Cook County
Chicago, Illinois

Luc M. Van Bortel, MD, PhD
Heymans Institute of Pharmacology
Ghent University
Ghent, Belgium

Simona Velicu, MD
Department of Neurology
Loyola University Stritch School of Medicine
Maywood, Illinois

Pascal R. Verdonck, PhD
Cardiovascular Mechanics and Biofluid Dynamics
Institute Biomedical Technology
Ghent University
Ghent, Belgium

Ron Waksman, MD
Washington Hospital Center
Washington, DC

Neil J. Weissman, MD
Washington Hospital Center and
    Georgetown University
Washington, DC

Foreword

Vascular disease has affected mankind since at least the beginning of recorded history. Ancient Egyptian mummies show evidence of calcification, atheromatous lesions, and other degenerative changes in the aorta, coronary, and peripheral arteries. Only since the mid-twentieth century, however, has vascular care evolved into a distinct specialty. To a great extent, this specialty owes its existence to surgical experience gained during wartime. Other important advances include the development of synthetic grafts and, later, of angioplasty procedures. Today, owing to the advent of minimally invasive technologies, the endovascular approach is widely used in the repair of vascular lesions. As the average age of the population continues to rise and as obesity, diabetes, and other chronic conditions take a growing toll, the need for vascular treatment can only be expected to increase.

The present book, *Peripheral Arterial Disease*, edited by my colleague and friend Ray Dieter Jr. and his sons Ray Dieter III and Robert Dieter, is a welcome addition to the literature about vascular disorders. This comprehensive, multiauthored volume covers all the major organ systems involved in peripheral arterial disease. In addition to discussing the pathogenesis, diagnosis, treatment, and prevention of such disease, the authors cover various supporting services that are integral to vascular care. The text is enhanced by a generous array of references, figures, and tables, all presented in an eye-pleasing format.

I congratulate the editors for producing this excellent volume, which should be an outstanding reference book for clinicians, researchers, and other professionals concerned with the management of peripheral arterial disease.

Denton A. Cooley, MD
President Emeritus and Surgeon-in-Chief
Texas Heart Institute
Houston, Texas

Preface

Our goal with this textbook on peripheral arterial disease is to make it a reference which crosses disciplines. The comprehensive approach of this text and each outstanding chapter is truly a reflection of the efforts of all the contributing authors. We sincerely appreciate their hard work and contribution to this reference.

To many, peripheral arterial disease represents only diseases (mainly atherosclerotic) of the lower extremities. We have, however, decided to use a broader definition of peripheral arterial disease, to reflect extracardiac arterial diseases. This is a more encompassing definition, designed to allow a discussion of arterial diseases in multiple arterial beds. We recognize that some readers, including us at times, wish to restrict this term to the lower extremities.

We have intentionally not attempted to draw strict borders between chapters. Such distinctions are neither practical nor how we approach diseases and patients. The textbook attempts to regionalize arterial diseases, but we recognize the significant overlap of diseases and thus some chapters will cover topics that are also found in other chapters. Furthermore, although this book is centered around diseases of the arterial circulations, there are obviously areas and diseases that overlap with lymphatic, venous, and other diseases, and these are discussed when appropriate.

Finally, we hope that the reader, of any discipline, finds this textbook useful. We greatly appreciate the assistance of the staff at McGraw-Hill.

Robert S. Dieter, MD, RVT
Raymond A. Dieter Jr., MD, MS
Raymond A. Dieter III, MD

The Epidemiology of Peripheral Arterial Disease

Victor Aboyans, MD, PhD / *Michael H. Criqui, MD, MPH*

● INTRODUCTION

Peripheral arterial disease (PAD) is one of the several terms referring to a partial or complete obstruction of one or more arteries below the aortic bifurcation. Although the term PAD is sometimes inclusive of all peripheral arteries and/or any etiology, in this chapter PAD refers to atherosclerotic occlusive disease of lower extremity arteries. Other terms used for this affliction in the literature are peripheral vascular disease (PVD), peripheral arterial occlusive disease (PAOD), and lower extremity arterial disease (LEAD).

The epidemiologic data regarding this condition have evolved dramatically over the past three decades. Initially, only symptomatic PAD was studied. However, with the development of investigative methods applicable in epidemiology, several studies have suggested that during the natural course of this disease, symptomatic PAD is preceded by a long period of asymptomatic disease. These studies showed that asymptomatic PAD is not innocuous, since patients at this initial stage of the disease are already at a higher risk of cardiovascular events. Consequently, the more recent studies have used objective investigation methods and typically include both symptomatic and asymptomatic forms of the disease. This has led to better estimates of PAD prevalence and incidence. PAD that exhibits typical symptomatology, usually in the form of leg pain brought about by walking, has been conservatively estimated to reduce the quality of life in at least 2 million Americans and in some cases leads to revascularization or amputation.[1] Recent estimates place the total number of persons with PAD in the United States at more than 8 million.[2]

● SYMPTOMS AND MEASURES OF PAD IN EPIDEMIOLOGY

It was recognized as long ago as the 18th century that an insufficient blood supply to the legs could cause pain and dysfunction. This type of pain is known as intermittent claudication (IC) and is characterized as leg muscle pain occurring when walking and relieved at rest. IC is generally indicative of exercise-induced ischemic pain.

Early studies focused primarily on claudication as the chief symptomatic manifestation of PAD. A number of patient questionnaires have been developed to uniformly identify claudication and to distinguish it from other types of leg pain. The first of these was the Rose questionnaire, also referred to as the World Health Organization questionnaire.[3] However, despite initial good results of the questionnaire to accurately detect PAD, this questionnaire is known as to present a low sensitivity, from 68% down to 9% in different studies.[4] Two attempts have been made to improve the diagnostic performances. The Edinburgh Claudication Questionnaire[5] is a modification of the Rose questionnaire, presenting 47% to 91% sensitivity and 95% to 99% specificity in different studies.[5-7] The San Diego Claudication Questionnaire is another modified version of the Rose questionnaire and additionally captures information on the laterality of symptoms.[8] The interviewer administered form of the San Diego Claudication Questionnaire is presented in Table 1-1.

Although considered as typical, it should be emphasized that the classical IC is not the sole clinical pattern related to PAD. Besides rest pain, occurring at a more evolved stage of the disease, several patterns of atypical pain can be related

TABLE 1-1. The San Diego Claudication Questionnaire (Interviewer Administered Version)[8]

		Right	Left
1. Do you get pain or discomfort in either leg or either buttock on walking? (If no, stop)	No... Yes...	1 2	1 2
2. Does this pain ever begin when you are standing still or sitting?	No... Yes...	1 2	1 2
3. In what part of the leg or buttock do you feel it? a. Pain includes calf/calves b. Pain includes thigh/thighs c. Pain includes buttock/buttocks	No... Yes... No... Yes... No... Yes...	1 2 1 2 1	1 2 1 2 1
4. Do you get it when you walk uphill or hurry?	No... Yes... Never walks uphill/hurries...	2 1 2 3	2 1 2 3
5. Do you get it when you walk at an ordinary pace on the level?	No Yes...	1 2	1 2
6. Does the pain ever disappear while you are walking?	No... Yes...	1 2	1 2
7. What do you do if you get it when you are walking?	Stop or slow down... Continue on...	1 2	1 2
8. What happens to it if you stand still? (If unchanged, stop)	Lessened or relieved... Unchanged...	1 2	1 2
9. How soon?	10 minutes or less... More than 10 minutes...	1 2	1 2

(1) No pain – Q1 = 1.
(2) Pain at rest – Q1 = 2 and Q2 = 2.
(3) Noncalf – Q1 = 2 and Q2 = 1 and Q3a = 1 and Q3b = 2 or Q3c = 2.
(4) Non-Rose calf – Q1 = 2 and Q2 = 1 and Q3a = 2, and not Rose.
(5) Rose – Q1 = 2 and Q2 = 1 and Q3a = 2 and Q4 = 2 or 3 (and if Q4 = 3, then Q5 = 2), and Q6 = 1 and Q7 = 1 and Q8 = 1 and Q9 = 1.

to PAD. For example, in the PAD Awareness, Risk, and Treatment: New Resources for Survival (PARTNERS) program, more than half of the PAD patients reported symptoms, but few reported classic Rose claudication.[9] In another similar study in a large Dutch population, the typical "Rose" claudication was reported only in 1.6%, whereas overall 6.6% had different patterns of vascular claudication, including other localization than calves.[10] The definitional distinctions used to separate IC from other types of leg pain make the former more specific to arterial disease, but less sensitive to other types of pain that may in some cases be related to arterial disease. Spinal stenosis can cause leg pain during exercise that is similar to arterial IC. Neurogenic IC accounts for almost 5% to 10% of patients with claudication referred to vascular clinics,[11] but this ratio is unknown in general population.

Two attempts, both using the San Diego Claudication Questionnaire (Table 1-2), have been made to qualify different patterns of nontypical pain. In one report, five categories of symptoms have been proposed[8]: no pain, pain on exertion and rest, noncalf pain, atypical calf pain, and eventually classic claudication (Table 1-2). A respectively increasing prevalence of PAD was found in these five groups.

In another study, McDermott et al.[12] proposed a sixth category by splitting the "no pain" group according to whether people walk enough to experience exertional pain (Table 1-2). They also divided atypical leg pain according to whether the subject stops or carries on with this pain. The authors not only found different mean ABI values in different categories, but also found several concomitant disorders (i.e., neurological and articular), which can make symptoms ischemic muscle cramp less typical.[12]

Patients with PAD may present more severe clinical forms of PAD, with pain in the legs at rest, trophic lesions, or both. In this situation the vitality of the limb is threatened because of severe arterial insufficiency and the risk of limb loss in the absence of medical care is high. Consequently, this clinical pattern is defined as critical limb ischemia (CLI), grouping typical chronic ischemic rest pain and ischemic skin lesions, either ulcers or gangrene.[13]

● ANKLE–BRACHIAL INDEX

In addition to difficulties to define PAD according to different symptoms categories, it is now well established that

TABLE 1-2. Different Classifications of Typical/Atypical Pain in PAD Based on the San Diego Claudication Questionnaire

	Criqui et al.[8]		McDermott et al. [12]	
	Pain Category	*Definition*	*Pain Category*	*Definition*
Asymptomatic	No pain	No pain in either leg or buttock on walking	No exertional pain/active	No pain in either leg or buttock on walking. Subject walking >6 blocks.
			No exertional pain/inactive	No pain in either leg or buttock on walking. Subject not walking >6 blocks.
Atypical pain	Pain on exertion/rest	Pain in either leg or buttock on walking, can sometimes begin when standing still or sitting	Pain on exertion/rest	Pain in either leg or buttock on walking, can sometimes begin when standing still or sitting.
	Noncalf pain	Pain not in calf region but in thighs or buttocks, only when walking.	Atypical exertional leg pain/stop	Noncalf pain, starting only when walking, the subject stops walking.
	Atypical calf pain	Pain in calf region, starting only when walking, but different from classic claudication pain	Atypical exertional leg pain/carry on	Pain starting only when walking, the subject carries on walking.
Typical "Rose" pain	Classic claudication	Pain in calf region, starting only when walking, does not disappear during walk, causing subject to halt or slow down; pain is lessened or relieved within 10 min if walking halted	Intermittent claudication	Pain in calf region, starting only when walking, does not disappear during walk, causing subject to halt or slow down. Pain is lessened or relieved within 10 min if walking halted.

atherosclerosis may have been developing for many years before claudication begins, and the extent to which it occurs is influenced by factors other than disease per se, such as the patient's level of activity.[14] For all these reasons, another method of diagnosing PAD was needed.

Low blood pressure at the ankle was proposed as a test for PAD as early as 1950[15] and led to the development of a simple measure called the ankle–brachial index (ABI). Also sometimes called the ankle–brachial pressure index (ABPI)[16] or the ankle–arm index (AAI),[17] the ABI is the ratio of the systolic blood pressure at the ankle to that in the arm. An abnormally low value of ABI is indicative of atherosclerosis of the lower extremities. The ABI has been shown to have good receiver operating curve characteristics as a test for PAD. Although there is no clear-cut threshold to confirm or exclude the presence of PAD, an ABI less than or equal to 0.90 is commonly used in both clinical practice and epidemiologic research to define PAD. More recently, it has been suggested that an ABI between 0.90 and 1.00 is correlated to atherosclerotic disease in other vascular territories,[18] and is associated with higher rates of IC[19] and CV events than in subjects with ABI >1.00.[20–22] In a large German primary care cohort, compared to the reference group with an ABI ≥1.1, mortality rates were increased for ABI values within the 0.9 to 1.1 interval.[23] At least for the 0.9 to 1.0 ABI interval, it is suggested to

consider this situation as "borderline PAD." It is estimated that one out of four subjects with an ABI in the interval 0.90 to 1.00 actually have PAD.[2]

The major interest of ABI-defined PAD is in that it covers both symptomatic and asymptomatic PAD. In the Rotterdam study, 99.4% of subjects with ABI ≥0.9 did not have claudication, but only 6.3% of subjects with ABI <0.9 had claudication.[24] In a study of elderly women in the United States, these percentages were found to be 93.3% and 18.3%, respectively.[25] In the Wang et al. study, even in limbs with ABI ≤0.50, considered as severe PAD, 17% of limbs did not present any exertional pain.[19] In the general population, it is estimated that for every prevalent case of typical IC, two to five[10,14,26] other asymptomatic cases are generally found with the use of ABI. On this basis it may be said that PAD defined by ABI is much more common than claudication in the general population, and large numbers of patients without IC can be shown to have a low (<0.90) ABI.

To validate the ABI, early studies compared the ABI result to angiography, considered as the "gold standard" for the visualization of atherosclerosis in the legs. Two such studies are often cited, in which the sensitivity and specificity of the ABI were shown to be in the 97% to 100% range.[27,28] However, because angiography is an invasive investigative method with a potential risk of complication, it was not ethical to perform it on subjects who were not suspected to have PAD. Therefore, these studies involved comparisons of patients with angiographically confirmed PAD with young, healthy individuals assumed not to have PAD. The sensitivities and specificities calculated are therefore based on the ability of the ABI to discriminate between extremes of disease and health. Using also angiography as the gold standard, Lijmer et al. studied the verification bias, related to the fact that only highly suspect cases are deferred to angiography.[29] Even after correcting the diagnostic performance results by the estimation of this selection bias, they found an area under the ROC curve at 0.95 when using ABI to detect >50% stenosis at angiography.[29] In that study, the corrected sensitivity and specificity of an ABI <0.91 was estimated respectively at 79% and 96%. This lower sensitivity can be explained in part by some PAD patients with stiff peripheral arteries and false negative ABIs.[30–32] Another explanation can be different normal values in both sexes and different ethnic groups (see below).[33]

The ABI has been demonstrated to have a strong association with cardiovascular (CVD) risk factors and disease outcomes. In the Cardiovascular Health Study cohort, a dose–response relationship was demonstrated between ABI and cardiovascular disease risk factors, as well as a both clinical and subclinical cardiovascular disease.[26] In the Edinburgh Artery Study, asymptomatic patients with an ABI <0.9 were shown to have a higher risk of developing claudication and higher mortality.[34] In one clinical study, patients with ABI <0.9 and who did not have exertional leg pain were shown to have poorer lower extremity functioning, even after adjustment for traditional risk factors and comorbidities.[35] The ABI correlates with the ability to exercise as measured on an accelerometer,[36] and an ABI <0.6 is related to the development of walking impairment.[37] Thus, even aside from its association with claudication, the ABI is considered as a powerful marker for functional outcomes, risk factors, and associated diseases that one would expect of a measure of PAD. The ABI has also been shown to have high intra- and interrater reliability.[38]

In practice, the ABI is measured using a blood pressure cuff with a standard sphygmomanometer and a Doppler instrument to detect pulses. The pressure measurements are made after a rest in a supine position for 5 minutes. It is recommended to measure ankle pressure in both legs at the dorsalis pedis and posterior tibial arteries. The higher pressure measurement in each ankle has traditionally been used as the numerator of the ABI for that ankle. Using the lower or average pressure can substantially change estimates of PAD prevalence; one study reported 47% prevalence based on the higher pressure versus 59% based on the lower.[36] Results of two recent studies support the use of the average of dorsalis pedis and posterior tibial pressures as the ankle pressure for each leg, based on superior reproducibility in repeated tests and closer statistical association with leg function.[36,39] Recently, comparing to color Duplex used as the reference, Schröder et al. reported an improved diagnostic performance when the lower pressure was used to determine the ankle's pressure instead of the higher pressure, with sensitivities at 89% versus 68%

and specificities at 93% versus 99%, respectively.[40] Similar findings are reported by Niazi et al.,[41] who reviewed ABI results of 208 limbs versus digital substraction angiography and found that compared to the use of the higher pressure, the mode using the lower pressure as the ABI numerator was more sensitive (84% vs. 69%), although less specific (64% vs. 83%), but with a higher overall diagnostic accuracy (80% vs. 72%). However, the relative predictive value of the higher versus the average or the lower of the two ankle pressures for CVD risk factors or clinical events has not yet been evaluated in general population. Practice also differs as to the brachial pressure used as the denominator of the ABI; the same brachial pressure is usually used for both the left and right ABIs in the same patient, but that pressure maybe the right arm, the average of both arms, or the highest of both arms. A recent study supports the use of the average of the left and right arms, based on superior reproducibility,[39] but another study shows a strong correlation between PAD and subclavian stenosis, suggesting the highest arm pressure should be used in the ABI calculation.[42] A useful compromise is to average the brachial pressures if the absolute difference is <10 mm Hg.[35–37] Based on the numerators and denominators described, separate ABIs are calculated for the left and right legs of each subject. In epidemiologic analyses, the unit of analysis is either the leg, with appropriate statistical adjustments for intraindividual correlation, or the subject, with disease status classified based on the "worst" limb, that is, the limb with the lowest ABI.

The ABI has several limitations as a measure of PAD. Occlusive disease located in arteries distal to the site of pressure measurement is not detected by the ABI. Other measures, such as pressure ratios using pressures measured in the toe, are required for detecting such distal disease. It is suggested that ABI would also be sensitive to the subject's height, with taller patients having slight higher ABIs; but this is not constant in all studies.[43–45] Similarly, it has been noted in several studies that the ABI in the left foot are slightly lower on average than the ABI in the right foot.[43,44] It is unlikely these differences are related to real differences in PAD.

Arterial calcification (medial calcinosis) can make the arteries of the ankle incompressible and lead to artificially high values of the ABI. This is particularly common in patients with diabetes.[46,47] Values of the ABI above 1.5 are often excluded in epidemiologic analyses, and should be viewed with suspicion clinically.[25,26,48–50] In two large population-based studies in the United States, the proportion of patients with such elevated values was around one half of 1%.[26,50] Some investigators use the more conservative cutpoint of 1.3. New evidence suggests 1.4 maybe a good compromise.[18,19] A recent report suggests that in more than 80% of cases with an ABI >1.40, concomitant occlusive disease can be identified when using other diagnostic methods.[32] This can explain the similar rates of IC and association with subclinical disease in other vascular beds found in this ABI range, compared to an ABI <0.90.[18,19]

● INCIDENCE AND PREVALENCE OF PAD

Currently, the prevalence of PAD in North America and Europe is estimated at approximately 27 million people, with a majority of these subjects being unaware of their condition.[51] Recently, after pooling and adjusting the data of seven U.S. population studies, Allison et al. estimated that 6.8 million people aged ≥40 years in the year 2000 had PAD in this country, corresponding to 5.8% of this population.[2] This estimation includes both people with an abnormal (<0.90) ABI and those with normal ABI values after lower limb revascularization.

This prevalence is very low among younger people, but increases sharply after the age of 55 to 60 years. For example in the San Diego Population Study, the risk of PAD doubled for each decade, independent from other risk factors.[31] Almost 20% of individuals over the age of 70 years have this disease. Table 1-3 presents the prevalence of PAD in epidemiological studies using an ABI <0.90 for PAD definition. Figures 1-1 and 1-2 show prevalence estimates of ABI-based PAD in population studies by age in women and men. Although the estimates vary somewhat, prevalence appears to be well under 5% before age 50, around 10% by age 65, and in excess of 25% in patients 80 years of age or older. All studies show this curvilinear relationship of prevalence to age in both genders, although there is some variability in the age at which prevalence begins to increase most dramatically.

Estimates of PAD incidence are reported somewhat less frequently in the literature, with more data for claudication incidence than for ABI. Figure 1-3 presents the incidence of IC according to age in available studies. Data from the Framingham Study show IC in men rising from less than 0.4 per 1000 per year in men aged 35 to 45 years to over 6 per 1000 per year in men aged 65 years and older.[72] Incidence among women ranged from 40% to 60% lower by age, although estimates in men and women were similar by age 65 to 74. In a group of Israeli men, incidence of claudication ranged from 6.3 per 1000 per year at ages 40 to 49 to 10.5 per 1000 per year at age 60 and greater.[1] In a study of 4570 men from Quebec, claudication incidence rose from 0.7 per 1000 per year at ages 35 to 44, to 3 per 1000 per year at ages 45 to 54, 7 per 1000 per year at ages 55 to 63, and 9 per 1000 at age 65 and greater.[73] In the Speedwell study, which followed English men aged 45 to 63 years for 10 years, claudication incidence per 1000 per year ranged from 3.1 in the youngest to 4.9 in oldest age group based on age at baseline exam.[74] A higher incidence of 15.5 per 1000 per year was reported among men and women aged 55 to 74 in the Edinburgh Artery Study; however, this study did not apply strict Rose criteria for probable claudication.[20] Figure 1-3 shows incidence rates by age for various studies identifying PAD based on IC.[1,73–76] Of note, the greater variability for IC incidence compared to data obtained by ABI might reflect a less standardized assessment of the former.

There are very few ABI-based studies of PAD incidence, given the time and resources required to periodically retest study subjects for incident disease. In male participants of the Limburg PAOD Study, annual incidence of ABI <0.95 was 1.7 per 1000 at ages 40 to 54; 1.5 per 1000 at ages 55 to 64; and 17.8 per 1000 at ages >65 and greater.[77] Annual incidence in women was higher: 5.9, 9.1, and 22.9 per 1000 for the same age groups.[77]

Data on temporal changes in PAD incidence and prevalence are very scarce. In the Reykjavik Study, Ingolfsson and colleagues[75] used Poisson regression techniques to conclude that IC rates among Icelandic men dropped significantly between 1968 and 1986. Among 50-year-old men, the estimate of claudication rates dropped from 1.7 per 1000 per year in 1970 to 0.6 per 1000 per year in 1984, while in 70-year-old men it dropped from 6.0 to 2.0 per 1000 per year.[75] The authors attributed this to decreased smoking and cholesterol levels. In the Framingham Study, Murabito and colleagues presented a decrease of incident IC, from 282 per 100 000 person-years during the 1950–59 period to 225 per 100 000 person-years during the 1990–1999 period.[78]

Sex differences in the incidence and prevalence of PAD are less clear than those in other cardiovascular disease. Claudication incidence and prevalence have usually been found to be higher in men than in women. For example, in the Framingham Study, annual claudication incidence for all ages combined was 7.1 per 1000 in men versus 3.6 per 1000 in women, for a male/female ratio of 1.97.[72] In the Framingham Offspring Study,[50] claudication prevalence was 1.9% in men versus 0.8% in women (ratio = 2.38), while in the Rotterdam study it was 2.2% in men versus 1.2% in women (ratio = 1.83).[24]

The case for an excess of disease among male is even weaker for PAD diagnosed based on ABI. When using the usual 0.90 ABI threshold to define ABI (Table 1-3), the male/female ratio in population studies varies from 1.68 in the Hoorn and San Diego Population Studies[31,58] to 0.71 in the ARIC study.[60,71] This is true even in those studies finding clear male excess with respect to claudication. For example, in the Framingham Offspring Study, the male/female PAD prevalence ratio based on ABI <0.90 was of 1.18.[24] In the Cardiovascular Health Study, ABI <0.9 was somewhat more prevalent in men than women (13.8% vs. 11.4%, ratio = 1.21), but the association of disease with sex was not significant after adjustment for age and CVD status.[26] In the Atherosclerosis Risk in Communities (ARIC) study, this male/female ratio was similar in whites and blacks, at 0.71.[71] Interestingly, this sex ratio became inverted when using lower ABI thresholds,[71] suggesting more frequent cases of severe PAD among men. However, this can also be explained by potential different normal ABI values in both sexes. Recently, it has been suggested that women have a multiple risk factors adjusted 0.02 lower normal ABI values than men.[33] Consequently, the same threshold for both sexes would lead to PAD prevalence overestimation in women, which was estimated at +36% in the Multi-Ethnic Study on Atherosclerosis (MESA).[33]

The prevalence of chronic CLI ranges from 0.05% to 0.1% of the general population.[13,79]

TABLE 1-3. Prevalence of PAD (ABI <0.90) in Epidemiological Studies (Rates with 95% Interval Confidence)

Study, first author, Year	Country	n	Age	Total	Men	Women
Kornitzer et al. 1978[52]	Belgium	3179	40–55	—	5.1 (4.7–5.5)	—
DeBacker et al. 1979[53]	Belgium	1039	18–50	3.0 (2.5–3.5)	—	—
Schroll and Munck 1981[54]	Denmark	666	60	14.3 (12.9–15.7)	16.0 (14.1–17.9)	13.0 (11.1–14.9)
Jerusalem Lipid Research Clinic Study, Gofin 1987[55]	Israel	1592	40–60	4.6 (4.1–5.1)	4.2 (3.6–4.8)	5.4 (4.4–6.4)
Edinburgh Study, Fowkes 1992*[56]	U.K.	1592	55–74	18.3 (17.3–19.3)	18.3 (16.4–20.2)	18.3 (16.4–20.2)
Cardiovascular Health Study, Newman 1993[26]	U.S.	5084	≥65	12.4 (11.9–12.9)	13.8 (13.1–14.5)	11.4 (10.8–12.0)
Osteoporotic Fractures Multicenter Study, Vogt 1993[14]	U.S.	1492	65–93	—	—	5.5 (4.3–6.7)
Men Born in 1914, Ögren 1993[57]	Sweden	477	68	—	14.0 (12.4–15.6)	—
Hoorn Study, Beks 1995[58]	Netherlands	631	50–75	7.3 (6.3–8.3)	9.4 (7.7–11.1)	5.6 (4.3–6.9)
Honolulu Heart Program, Curb 1996[59]	U.S.	3450	45–68	—	13.6 (13.0–14.2)	—
ARIC Study, Zheng 1997, blacks[60]	U.S.	4082	45–64	3.7 (3.4–4.0)	3.1 (2.5–3.8)	4.4 (3.7–5.2)
ARIC Study, Zheng 1997, whites[60]	U.S.	8091	45–64	2.9 (2.7–3.1)	2.3 (1.9–2.7)	3.2 (2.8–3.7)
Strong Heart Study, Fabsitz 1999[61]	U.S.	4304	45–74	5.3 (5.0–5.6)	5.6 (5.0–6.2)	4.8 (4.4–5.2)
Rotterdam Study, Meijer 2000[17]	Netherlands	7715	>55	19 (18–20)	16.9 (15.4–18.3)	20.5 (19.2–21.8)
Chennai Urban Population Study, Premalatha 2000[62]	India	631	46	3.2 (1.9–4.9)	—	—
Framingham Offspring Study, Murabito 2002[50]	U.S.	3313	59	3.6 (3.3–4.0)	3.9 (3.4–4.4)	3.3 (2.9–3.7)
Cui et al. 2003[63]	Japan	1219	60–79	—	5.0 (4.4–5.62)	—
NHANES, Selvin and Gregg 2004[64,65]	U.S.	2873	≥40	4.5 (4.1–4.9)	4.5 (2.9–6.1)	4.2 (2.8–5.6)
San Diego Population Study, Criqui 2005[131]	U.S.	2343	29–91	4.4 (4.0–4.8)	6.1 (4.7–7.5)	3.6 (2.6–4.6)
Kweon et al. 2005[66]	South Korea	1943	45–74	2.0 (1.7–2.3)	2.2 (1.6–2.8)	1.8 (1.4–2.2)
Multi-Ethnic Study on Atherosclerosis, Allison 2006[67]	U.S.	6653	45–85	4.1 (3.9–4.3)	4.1 (3.7–4.4)	4.2 (3.9–4.5)
Heinz Nixdorf Recall, Kroger 2006[68]	Germany	4735	45–75	5.8 (5.5–6.2)	6.4 (5.9–6.9)	5.1 (4.7–5.6)
Copenhagen City, Eldrup 2006[69]	Denmark	4159	≥20	19.4 (18.8–20.0)	—	—
Albacete Study, Carbayo 2007[70]	Spain	784	≥40	10.5 (8.4–12.8)	11.4 (9.7–13.1)	9.7 (8.3–11.1)

*PAD defined according to ABI <0.90 and/or abnormal hyphemia reactive test. [†] PAD defined according to ABI <0.90 and/or abnormal posterior tibial artery Doppler waveform.

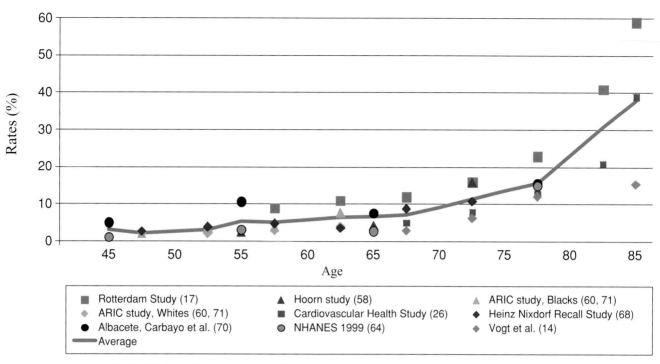

● **FIGURE 1-1.** Prevalence of PAD in women, according to age in epidemiological studies.

● PAD RISK FACTORS

Prior to the literature review, it should be kept in mind that PAD epidemiology encounters several methodological issues. First, as mentioned above, the definition of disease has evolved over time, with earlier studies focusing more on claudication, defined by Rose and other criteria, and later studies using the ABI, with a value less than or equal to 0.90 now widely used to define disease. Second, while the strongest epidemiological evidence for a causal relationship between disease and putative risk factors comes from

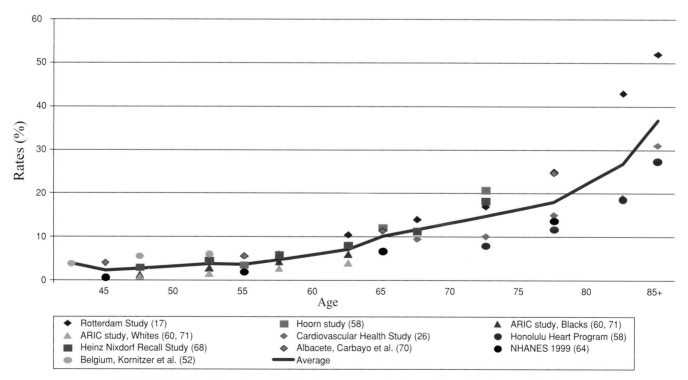

● **FIGURE 1-2.** Prevalence of PAD in men, according to age in epidemiological studies.

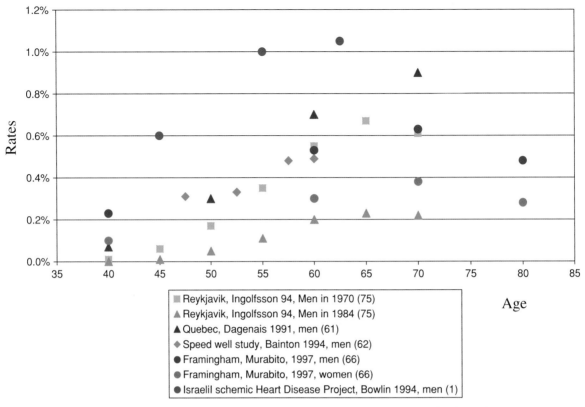

FIGURE 1-3. Incidence of intermittent claudication by age in population-based studies.

studies of incident disease, the great majority of the available epidemiological studies on PAD are cross-sectional. While such studies are informative, the reported associations are more subject to bias than prospective studies. Caution should therefore be exercised in reviewing the results of such cross-sectional studies, particularly where reverse causation is plausible. For example, low physical activity might cause claudication, but claudication might just as plausibly cause low physical activity. Third, since the potential risk factors for PAD are themselves interrelated in various ways, adjustments for multiple potential risk factors in a single statistical model is mandated, in order to estimate accurately the independent contribution of any single risk factor. The estimates presented below (Table 1-4) are based on such multiple adjustments for all traditional PAD risk factors, except as noted. Null findings may indicate the lack of a real association, but may also be based on insufficient sample size. Most of the null findings discussed below are based on failure of the risk factor of interest to remain statistically significant in stepwise regression models, which vary as to their algorithms for variable selection.

Smoking

Smoking is the single most important risk factor for PAD in virtually all studies. The relation was first identified by Erb in 1911, reporting a threefold risk excess of IC in smokers.[80] The population attributable risk for smoking and IC calculated in cross-sectional studies ranges from 14% to 53%.[81] For current smoking, this attributable risk was estimated at

18% to 26% when PAD was defined by the ABI.[14,17] Studies vary as to their measurement of smoking, often combining a categorical assessment of smoking status (current, past, or never) with some measure of current or historical volume of smoking; these multiple approaches to measurement make comparisons difficult (Table 1-4). However, even with some type of additional adjustment for volume of smoking, current smoking has been shown to at least double the odds of PAD versus nonsmoking, with some estimates as high as a six times greater risk than among nonsmokers. All large, population-based studies that were reviewed have found a significant, independent association between PAD and smoking (Table 1-4).

In several studies, an increasing risk of IC and PAD was found with the growing amount of cigarettes smoked, but smoking cessation was systematically followed by a consistent decrease of PAD occurrence or progression. Smoking cessation was followed by a rapid decline in the incidence of IC,[75] and the IC risk for ex-smokers 1 year after quitting approximates that for nonsmokers.[73,75] Cessation of smoking among patients with claudication has been shown to improve various functional and physiologic measures related to PAD as well as reduce mortality.[82–84] However, because symptomatic PAD patients have long been advised to quit smoking, it is possible that observational comparisons of patients who quit smoking with those who do not are confounded by other differences in compliance with other medical advice between the two groups. Randomized trials of this question would raise ethical issues. However,

TABLE 1-4. Major Traditional Cardiovascular Risk Factors Associated with PAD: Odds Ratios in Multivariable Models in Population Studies with Objective Methods of Disease Definition

Year, first author	Population	PAD Definition	Smoking	Diabetes	Hypertension	Dyslipidemia (definition)	Obesity	Adjusted for
1993 Newman[26]	5084 M & W, >65 y	ABI <0.90	1.01/p-y, Current: 2.55	4.05	1.51	TC = 1.10/10 mg/dL HDL-C = 0.99 mg/dL	0.94 kg/m²	Age, ethnicity, creatinine
1993 Vogt[14]	1601 W, >65 y	ABI <0.90	Current: 6.4	—	SBP = 1.4/10 mm Hg	—	1.0 kg/m²	Age, diuretics, coffee intake, arthritis, exercise, Waist/hip ratio
1995 Beks[58]	631 M & W, 50–74 y	ABI <0.90 or DW	Ever: 1.91	3.43	2.08	ns	0.93 kg/m²	Age
1996 Curb[59]	3450 M, >70 y	ABI <0.90	Current: 4.32 Past: 1.40	1.53	1.79	TC = 1.36 mg/dL HDL-C = 0.68 mg/dL	0.64 kg/m²	Age, fibrinogen, fasting glucose, alcohol, physical activity
1996 Stoffers[10]	3171 M & W, 45–74 y	ABI <0.95	Current: 3.2 Past: 1.9	1.9	1.4	1.2 (TC ≥6.5 mmol/L)	BMI >30 : 0.7	Age, sex, physical activity, familial CVD history
1999 Fabsitz[61]	4549 M & W, 45–74 y	ABI <0.90	Current: 1.99 1.10/10 p-y	—	SBP = 1.21/20 mm Hg	LDL = 1.19 30 mg/dL	—	Age, fibrinogen, alcohol, micro & macroalbuminuria
2000 Meijer[17]	6450 M & W, >55 y	ABI <0.90	Current: 2.64 Past: 1.15	1.89	1.32 SBP = 1.30/10 mm Hg	TC = 1.19 mmol/L HDL-C = 0.58 mmol/L	—	Age, sex, alcohol fibrinogen, leucocytes, homocysteine
2002 Murabito[50]	3313 M & W ≥40 y	ABI <0.90	Ever: 2.0 1.3/10 p-y	Ns	2.2	HDL-C: 0.90/5 mg/dL	ns	Age, fibrinogen, CAD
2003 Cui[63]	726 M, 60–79 y	ABI <0.90	Current: 3.8 Past: 2.6	1.0	2.7	TC = 1.2/0.88 mmol/L HDL-C = 0.6/0.44 mmol/L	0.4/3.1 kg/m²	Age, alcohol, ECG changes, Stroke history, CHD history

(continued)

TABLE 1-4. (Continued)

Year, first author	Population	PAD Definition	Smoking	Diabetes	Hypertension	Dyslipidemia (definition)	Obesity	Adjusted for
2004 Selvin[64]	2174 M & W, >40 y	ABI <0.90	Current: 4.23 Former: 1.28	2.08	1.75	Hchol = 1.67 (TC >240 mg/dL or history)	BMI >30 : 0.54	Age, sex, ethnicity, personal CVD history, GFR
2005 Criqui[31]	2343 M & W, 29–91 y	ABI <0.90 or posterior tibial DW	1.63/20p-y	6.9	1.85	TC/HDL = 1.17	0.88 kg/m^2	Age, sex, ethnicity, education, occupation, lipid and anti-hypertensive therapy, height, personal & parental CVD
2006 Allison[67]	6653 M & W, 45–84 y	ABI <0.90	Current: 3.42	2.12	1.63	1.58 (TC/HDL >5 or medication)	0.97 kg/m^2	Age, ethnicity, education
2007 Carbayo[70]	784 M & W, >40 y	ABI <0.90	1.48 /10p-y	1.83	1.95	1.65 (TC >6.5 mmol/L)	BMI ≥30: 0.75	Age, history of CVD, hyperfibrinogenemia

Note: Significant ($p < 0.05$) results are presented in bold. Abbreviations: DW, abnormal Doppler waveform; GFR, glomerular filtration rate; P-Y, pack-years; SBP, systolic blood pressure; TC, total cholesterol.

10

substantial bias is unlikely given the large effect size for cigarette smoking.

Because of the substantial decline of smoking in general population following smoking ban legislation in several western countries, the relative influence of smoking on incident PAD is changing. In a 50-year trend of IC in the Framingham Study, the proportion of smokers in incident cases dropped from 42% in the 1950s to 16% during the 1990s.[78]

Diabetes

Diabetes is strongly associated with elevated risk of PAD, although the evidence for an independent role in multivariable analysis is not entirely consistent (Table 1-4). IC was more frequently observed in case of diabetes in the Framingham,[85] Quebec,[73] Speedwell,[74] and Israeli civil servants[1] studies, whereas this association was not found in the Reykjavik Study.[75] In the Edinburgh Study, the association between diabetes and IC was nonsignificant, whereas a significant inverse relationship was found with the ABI.[56] In Table 1-4, only 2 out of 11 population studies including the ABI measurement in the disease definition did not find a significant association between diabetes and PAD in multivariate models.[24,63]

In positive studies, according to different models used, the adjusted-risk excess for PAD in patients with diabetes ranged from[59] +53% to almost[31] +700% (Table 1-4).

More severe and/or longstanding diabetes appears to be more strongly related to PAD. In the Hoorn Study, it was shown that known diabetes was associated with PAD in multivariable analysis, while newly diagnosed diabetes was only of borderline significance and impaired glucose tolerance was not associated with PAD.[58] In that study, after excluding known diabetics, none of the common glycemic indices that were tested was significantly associated with PAD based on ABI, although significant associations were observed when the PAD criteria were broadened to include patients with additional criteria. Studies conducted in patients with diabetes have shown that duration of diabetes and use of insulin are associated with PAD.[86–88]

Outcomes of PAD in patients with diabetes have been shown to be worse. In one study, diabetic patients with PAD were five times more likely to have an amputation than other patients with PAD, and also had over three times the odds of mortality.[89] There is also some evidence to support a somewhat different anatomic distribution of disease, with greater involvement of the profunda femoris and crural arteries in patients with diabetes.[89–92]

Because of the dramatic epidemic of diabetes in western countries, the proportion of diabetes-related PAD may increase dramatically. In the Framingham Study, the proportion of incident cases with diabetes increased from 5% in the 1950s to 11% in the 1990s.[78]

Hypertension and Blood Pressure

The association of hypertension with PAD has been demonstrated in most studies in which blood pressure was studied.

All major epidemiological studies reported a significant association between hypertension as a categorical variable and PAD (Table 1-4). The lowest reported odds ratio was 1.32 as reported in the Rotterdam Study; this is somewhat understated relative to the others, as it was based on a model that included both a categorical hypertension variable and an adjustment for systolic blood pressure level that was also significant.[17] Each time both systolic and diastolic pressure were considered, systolic pressure was usually found to be associated with PAD, while diastolic pressure was not significantly associated[17,26,93] or had a nonlinear relationship with PAD.[59]

Two studies did not find any association between hypertension and IC. In the Israeli Ischemic Heart Disease Project cohort, neither systolic nor diastolic blood pressure was associated with claudication,[1] while in the Reykjavik Study systolic and diastolic blood pressure were significantly associated with claudication in cross-sectional but not longitudinal models.[75] It has been speculated that elevated central perfusion pressure, as indicated by arm blood pressure, will sometimes delay the onset of claudication by increasing the blood pressure in the lower extremities, which if true would obscure the relationship of hypertension with underlying disease processes.[94] In line with this hypothesis, in the Framingham Study, Murabito et al. reported a lower prevalence of "high-normal" blood pressure in those with IC than the free of IC counterparts, whereas severe hypertension was more common in the former group.[76] Nevertheless, randomized trials of blood pressure lowering in patients with PAD do not report worsened claudication.

Although the relative risks associated with hypertension are modest in some studies, its high prevalence, particularly among older patients, makes it a significant contributor to the total burden of PAD in the population. For example, because of a high prevalence of hypertension in the elderly, the etiological fraction (attributable risk) of PAD related to this factor was at 17%, in the Rotterdam Study, which was second only to current smoking in this group.[17] In the Framingham study, 30% of the risk of claudication in the population was attributable to blood pressure in excess of 160/100 mm Hg.[76]

Lipids

As is the case in cardiovascular disease epidemiology, the challenge of defining the roles of the various lipid fractions in PAD lies in identifying the strongest independent risk factors from among multiple correlated measures. Results from population studies are presented in Table 1-4.

Total cholesterol has been the most widely studied lipid measure. Total cholesterol has been examined as a potential risk factor in several studies (Table 1-4), and was significantly associated with PAD in multivariable analysis in a majority of them. In two studies,[24,63] total cholesterol was found to be significant in univariate analysis, but dropped out of multivariable models in which other lipid measures were considered. Conversely, three studies presented null findings for total cholesterol as the sole lipid measure analyzed.[10,70,73]

High-density-lipoprotein cholesterol (HDL-C) has been shown to be protective against PAD in most studies where it was evaluated, usually in models that also considered total cholesterol (Table 1-4). In three studies both HDL-C and total cholesterol were significant in multivariable analysis,[17,26,59] while in two studies HDL-C (but not total cholesterol) was significant.[63]

Two measures that combine total and HDL cholesterol into a single number have been proposed. Bowlin and colleagues found that non-HDL cholesterol (total cholesterol minus HDL cholesterol) was significantly associated with incident claudication in a large cohort of Israeli men; neither total cholesterol nor HDL cholesterol was significantly associated with disease in models that included non-HDL cholesterol.[1] In a comparison of incident cases of claudication with healthy controls in the Physician's Health Study, Ridker and colleagues found that the ratio of total to HDL cholesterol was the lipid measure most strongly associated with disease, with patients in the highest quartile having 3.9 times the claudication risk of patients in the lowest quartile; screening for other lipid fractions was judged to have little clinical usefulness beyond measurement of this ratio.[95] In the San Diego Population Study, the total/HDL-cholesterol ratio was an independent significant risk factor of PAD (Table 1-4).[31]

The evidence for high triglycerides as an independent risk factor for PAD is fragmentary. Early case–control studies showed a very consistent relationship between triglycerides and PAD, suggesting a uniquely strong relationship with PAD. However, large, population-based cohort studies employing multivariable modeling later called this into question.[56,96] In the Cardiovascular Health Study and the Framingham Offspring Study, triglycerides were significant in univariate analysis, but dropped out of multivariable models derived based on stepwise logistic regression.[24,26] Similarly, in the Jerusalem Lipid Research Clinic Prevalence Study and the Edinburgh Artery Study cohort as well as in a large study of geriatric patients in the United States, triglycerides were not significantly associated with PAD after adjustment for other lipid measures.[55,56,97] However, other studies have shown triglycerides to be significantly and independently associated with PAD in multivariable analysis.[74,86,98] There are also conflicting findings regarding the relationship between elevated triglycerides and disease progression or more severe PAD.[45,99,100]

In summary, while total cholesterol, HDL-C, and triglycerides all appear to be associated with PAD on a univariate basis, in multivariable analysis triglycerides frequently drops out as an independent risk factor. Although it has been the most extensively studied, it is not clear whether total cholesterol is an independent risk factor for PAD; in one comparison of patients with PAD with healthy controls, it was found that mean total cholesterol did not differ significantly, while triglycerides, VLDL-cholesterol, LDL cholesterol, HDL cholesterol, and the total-to-HDL cholesterol ratio all did.[101] Total and HDL cholesterol seem to provide distinct information, although these may lend themselves to summarization in a single ratio or difference. Because many early studies considered only total cholesterol, the full resolution of the question of which lipid measures are the most strongly and independently related to PAD awaits the completion of additional large-scale studies that assess all of the relevant lipid risk factors. However, because of the increasing use of lipid-lowering drugs, especially statins, population studies will have to take into account these treatments when assessing the effects of lipids.

Finally, a growing amount of evidence suspects the plasma levels of Lipoprotein(a) as a determining risk factor or PAD. This has been observed in case of PAD occurring at a young age,[102] in patients with diabetes,[103] as well as a case–control study.[104] Recently Lp(a) was found as an independent factor of PAD progression.[45] However, large population-based studies are still required to confirm this hypothesis.

Obesity

Among the conditions known as being harmful for the cardiovascular system, obesity presents the most conflicting results regarding its association to PAD. To date, the preponderance of evidence fails to support a consistent, independent positive association between obesity and PAD. In one of the few large studies with a positive finding, Bowlin and colleagues estimated an odds ratio of 1.24 (95%, CI = 1.05–1.46) for incident claudication related to a 5.0 kg/m^2 difference in body mass index (BMI) in a study of 10 059 Israeli men.[1] A number of large, population-based studies have failed to find a significant association between obesity and PAD or claudication after multivariable adjustment (Table 1-4).[17,24,64,70] In a majority of studies using ABI, higher weight or BMI was actually shown to be protective against PAD.[10,26,31,58,59,63,67,105] In the Framingham Study, claudication was significantly inversely related to relative weight in men in multivariate analysis and appeared to have a "U-shaped" relationship with relative weight in women.[72] Conversely, in the Framingham Offspring Study, BMI was associated with ABI in females but not in males.[50]

Obesity has been implicated in the etiology of other risk factors for PAD, such as hypertension, type II diabetes, and dyslipidemia. In epidemiology, adjusting for factors that are on the causal pathway between a risk factor and disease is known to attenuate the observed strength of that risk factor. Therefore, the estimates of risks related to obesity in multivariable models are estimates of the risk of obesity that artificially ignore most of the mechanisms by which obesity might reasonably cause PAD. In a few cases, unadjusted models or models adjusted only for age and sex show a significant association with PAD, even though obesity was nonsignificant or protective after multivariable adjustment.[24,56,106] However, in other studies, obesity was found to be either protective or nonsignificant even in unadjusted models, or models adjusted only for age and sex.[17,26,59,70,72,74,107] Thus, the failure to find more cases of positive association between PAD and obesity is not simply an artifact of adjusting for factors on the causal pathway in multivariable modeling, but seems to suggest a real lack of consistent evidence that such a relationship exists at all.

Unaccounted for in the multivariate analyses cited above is possible residual confounding by cigarette smoking, which is strongly associated with both PAD and lower BMI. In addition, chronic illness in older persons, where PAD is most common, may lead to weight loss thus, allowing for a spurious inverse correlation between obesity and PAD. Recent studies suggest a relationship between osteoporosis and PAD (see below), and low bone mass can partially contribute to weight loss with aging. Similarly, muscular fiber loss was found in patients with PAD.[108] All these considerations concur to the fact that BMI estimating the body mass as a whole is not the most adequate variable since it cannot characterize the different components of body mass.

As in coronary heart disease epidemiology, there is some evidence to suggest that central adiposity, rather than obesity per se, maybe more closely related to an increased risk of PAD. Vogt and colleagues found that, after adjustment for BMI, higher waist/hip ratio (WHR) was associated with a significantly higher risk of PAD.[14] In a group of patients with diabetes, it was shown that WHR, but not BMI or body fat percentage, was associated with prevalent PAD.[86] This has also been confirmed prospectively in patients with diabetes of the ARIC study: incident PAD was associated to baseline WHR but not BMI.[109]

Alcohol Consumption

Evidence for a protective effect of light to moderate alcohol consumption, as seen in coronary heart disease, is less consistent for PAD. In the Rotterdam Study, moderate alcohol consumption was found protective in women but not in men,[110] whereas a protective effect of alcohol was seen in men but not women in the Edinburgh Artery Study, this association disappearing after adjustment for social class.[111] The most protective effect of moderate alcohol for PAD was found in the Strong Heart Study, which is exclusively focused on Native American Indians.[61] Conversely, in elderly Japanese American men, alcohol intake was found to increase rather than decrease the risk of incident PAD.[59] Data from the Physician's Health Study suggest that a protective effect related to moderate alcohol consumption may exist.[112] In that study, there was no univariate association between alcohol and claudication incidence, but further adjustment for cigarette smoking actually revealed a significant protective association, reflecting the positive correlation of alcohol consumption with smoking—a strong risk factor for PAD. Based on this, it seems possible that incomplete adjustment for smoking in other studies might allow residual confounding that would obscure any protective effect of alcohol despite multivariate adjustment.[110]

Race and Ethnicity

Data on the association of race with PAD are limited, because many of the large studies of PAD have been conducted in non-Hispanic white groups. Additionally, differences in PAD incidence and prevalence in different ethnic groups could be related to nongenetic factors, for example, social and nutritional factors, and these issues are only partially controlled when comparing different ethnic groups in a same country. For this case, fragmentary data are available only in the United States. Recently, pooled data of seven U.S. population-based cross-sectional studies reported different rates of PAD among five ethnic groups.[2] The prevalence of PAD in the >40-year-old population in 2000 was estimated, respectively, at 5.5%, 8.8%, 2.8%, 2.6%, and 6.1% in non-Hispanic whites, African Americans, Hispanics, Asians, and Native Americans. The higher prevalence of PAD in African Americans is consistent in all large American epidemiological studies.[26,31,35,60,67]

In the MESA, the odds for PAD remained significantly increased at 1.47 among blacks compared to whites, even after adjustments for traditional risk factors as well as for inflammatory markers, homocysteine, D-dimers, and levels of education and income.[67] However, in another study performed in a subset of the MESA population free of PAD and without any of the four traditional risk factors of PAD (smoking, hypertension, diabetes, and dyslipidemia), it has been argued that even after adjustments for a full range of anthropometric, biological, and social variables, black subjects would have a lower normal ABI of around 0.02.[33] This small difference affects the prevalence of low ABI, overestimating the PAD prevalence by about +10% in this ethnic group. Nonetheless, even taking this into account, there is still a higher prevalence of PAD in blacks compared to whites. Similar findings have been found in another cohort of siblings of subjects with premature atherosclerosis.[113] Interestingly, hospital-based studies suggest that the anatomic distribution of disease may differ in blacks, with a higher percentage of distal disease in black subjects, even after adjustment for diabetes and other cardiovascular risk factors.[114]

Data on other races and ethnic groups are even more fragmentary. One study showed, compared to non-Hispanic whites, a slightly lower prevalence of PAD in Hispanics and Asians after multivariable adjustment, although neither result achieved statistical significance.[31] In another study, Asians were reported to have lower PAD prevalence than comparable non-Hispanic whites subjects.[59] In the MESA population, the odds for PAD remained significantly lower in Asians and Hispanics compared to non-Hispanic whites, even after adjustments for a full range of confounding factors.[67] A study of Native Americans suggested PAD prevalence comparable to that in non-Hispanic whites.[61]

Homocysteine

The association of homocysteine with PAD has been examined in a number of studies, with conflicting results. A 1995 meta-analysis of early case–control studies suggested an odds ratio of 6.8 for every 5 mmol/L fasting homocysteine (tHcy) increase.[115] In this light, an odds ratio of 6.8 might make homocysteine the single most powerful risk factors for PAD, but to put this in perspective, the differences between the 25th and 75th percentiles of tHcy among controls in the Physician's Health Study and a study of women in the Netherlands were between 3.5 and 4.0 μmol/L.[95,116] Hence, the 5 μmol/L difference noted above is unreasonable as the difference between low and high tHcy in the population.

In contrast, more recent studies have produced much lower and even nonsignificant estimates of the PAD risk associated with homocysteine. In a large European case–control study, Graham and colleagues estimated an odds ratio of 1.7 for subjects in the top quintile of homocysteine for their control group versus all other subjects—a result of only borderline statistical significance.[117] A Dutch population-based study found a 1.44 odds ratio for every 5 μmol/L increase in fasting tHcy, based on an extreme definition of PAD involving surgery or an ABI <0.5.[118] Conversely, in an analysis of a subset of the Rotterdam Study cohort, Meijer et al. found no significant relationship between tHcy and PAD, based either on the conventional 0.9 ABI cut-off or on a 0.7 ABI cut-off for severe disease.[17] Similarly, a nested case–control study using the Physician's Health Study cohort failed to find any association between quartiles of fasting tHcy and claudication.[95] A recent case–control study of young women in the Netherlands also failed to find any significant association between tHcy and symptomatic PAD.[116]

Recently, in the National Health and Nutrition Examination Study (NHANES), Guallar et al. reported an odds ratio for PAD at 1.92 for the top quintile of homocysteine, corresponding to a mean difference of 4.5 μmol/L with the lowest quintile.[119] However, after controlling this association for smoking, renal failure, lead, and cadmium levels (all affecting blood homocysteine levels), this association was no more significant, suggesting that confounding factors could explain this association.

In the MESA, homocysteine showed a borderline association with PAD after multiple adjustments for age, sex, traditional risk factors, education, and income.[67]

The relationship between homocysteine and PAD has been even more tempered by the lack of improvement of the disease under vitamin B and folates supplementation. These substances are known as co-enzymes playing a key role in the homocysteine metabolism. In a clinical study, this supplementation was followed by a significant decrease of blood homocysteine concentration, without any change on the clinical course of PAD.[120] Similarly, another study[45] failed to evidence any association between blood homocysteine levels and PAD progression, defined by a substantial ABI decrease.

At this point, even though it is still plausible that homocysteine maybe an independent risk factor for PAD, it appears that the earlier results may have overestimated its importance. Further investigations are mandatory to elucidate specifically the association of homocysteine with incident PAD.

Inflammatory Markers

Fibrinogen and C-reactive protein are two inflammatory markers that have been shown to be associated with PAD in several studies. In an analysis from the Physician's Health Study, each was found to be significantly associated with IC in multivariable models, with odds ratios for the upper versus lower population quartiles of 2.2 for fibrinogen and 2.8 for C-reactive protein.[95] In studies using ABI, fibrinogen was significantly associated with PAD in multivariable analysis in six studies.[17,24,59,61,121,122] Only Carbayo et al.[70] reported a negative result, but conversely to other studies, their fibrinogen variable in the model was categorical (>vs. ≤400 mg/dL). Beyond a marker of inflammation, fibrinogen is a major determinant of blood viscosity. Hence, the relationship between PAD and fibrinogen can also be a result of rheological factors affecting distal limbs perfusion.[122] Other studies have also reported significant and independent associations of PAD with C-reactive protein.[112,121]

Chronic Kidney Disease

In patients at end-stage renal disease, the prevalence of PAD (ABI <0.90) is extremely high, estimated at 38% in a mono-center study, to which should be added 14% of cases with incompressible ankle arteries.[123] Chronic kidney disease (CKD) and PAD share several common risk factors, especially age, hypertension, and diabetes. Nevertheless, in the Cardiovascular Health Study, creatinine levels were independently associated with prevalent PAD, after adjusting for usual risk factors.[26] In the NHANES, CKD defined as GFR <60 mL/mn/1.73m^2 was an independent factor associated for PAD (OR = 2.17, 95% CI 1.10 to 4.30).[64] Recently, after following 14 280 middle-aged men for a mean period of 13 years in the ARIC study, CKD was shown to be significantly associated with incident PAD defined by an ABI <0.90, with a hazard ratio at 1.56 in a multivariable model including usual risk factors.[124] Further studies, especially longitudinal, are required to confirm and explain the relationship between CKD and PAD.

Other Risk Factors

A variety of other potential risk factors for PAD have been examined. In several studies, various measures of oral health have been shown to be independently associated with PAD.[125,126] During a follow-up of 1110 male veterans during 25 years, men with periodontal disease had a 2.3 times higher risk of incidence of PAD versus men without periodontal disease.[126] Similar findings were noted in the Health Professionals' Follow-up Study, with an excess risk for incident PAD in case of periodontal disease or tooth loss (OR = 1.40, $p < 0.05$), independent of age and traditional CVD risk factors. These findings are possibly explained by common inflammatory pathways. A study in young women found that self-reported history of various types of infectious diseases, such as chicken pox, shingles, mumps, pneumonia, chronic bronchitis, or peptic ulcer, was independently and significantly related to PAD.[116] Another study found that a history of arthritis was associated with PAD.[14] In one NHANES report, monocyte count—but not other white blood cell subtypes—was significantly and independently associated to higher prevalent PAD.[107] Psychosocial factors were found to be associated with PAD in one large cohort in Scotland,[127] while in a large study of Israeli men, anxiety, job-related stress, and manner of coping with job-related conflicts were all significantly related to incident claudication even after adjustment for traditional risk factors.[1] Among patients with PAD, depressive symptoms were found to be associated with poorer lower extremity functioning.[128] In the MESA study, a low level of education and income were both associated with PAD.[67]

Recent studies point out the role of genetic factors in the development of PAD, but data are still limited. In a study of fraternal and identical twins, Carmelli and colleagues[129] estimated that 48% of the variability in ABI could be explained by additive genetic effects, whereas only 21% of the interindividual variability was attributable to genetic effects in the Framingham Offspring Study.[130] Heritability might be more evident in the younger (premature PAD),[131] since traditional risk factors play a greater role in atherosclerotic disease as people age. Genetic conditions found to be associated with PAD are familial hypercholesterolemia[132] as well as apolipoprotein E, (130 fibrinogen,[133] CD-14,[134] and methylene-tetra-hydrofolate reductase[135] polymorphism, but additional data are necessary.

There is a growing amount of evidence for an association between osteoporosis and atherosclerosis, and this association is also found with PAD.[136–140] In the study of osteoporotic fractures,[138] cross-sectional and prospective data have shown that among elderly women, the mineral density measured in several bones was positively correlated with the ABI and the annual ABI decrease was positively correlated with bone loss rates. In the Rotterdam Study,[139] the risk of PAD (ABI < 0.90) was increased in women (but not in men) who had a low femoral neck bone mineral density (BMD), whereas no association was found between PAD and lumbar spine BMD. Similarly, in an Italian cross-sectional study, when BMD was assessed at the femoral neck, ABI levels were found to be lower in postmenopausal women with osteoporosis compared to osteoporosis-free counterparts.[137] This association remained significant even after multivariate analysis controlling PAD and osteoporosis risk factors. Again this study did not find any relationship between lumbar spine BMD and PAD.[137] However, further longitudinal studies are warranted to clarify pathways explaining this association. In the Vogt et al. study, ABI was also correlated with BMD assessed in the wrist, excluding the hypothesis of a direct role of obstructed arteries impeding the bone cells nutrient supply.[138] Several studies generated other hypotheses regarding mechanisms, such as the calcium transfer from bones to the atherosclerotic plaque, as well as potential roles for estrogen deficiency, a direct role of LDL oxydative products inhibiting osteoblastic differentiation, secondary hypoparathyroidism, vitamin D

excess and vitamin K deficiency, and the inflammatory process favoring the osteoclastic activity.

Other possible risk factors for which some supporting data exist include antiphospholipid antibodies,[141,142] hypothyroidism,[143] sedentary lifestyle,[144] and higher lead and cadmium blood levels.[119,145] Possible protective effects have been reported for antioxidants,[146,147] high dietary intake of vitamin E,[146,148] fibers,[148,149] and vegetable lipids[147] as well as hormone replacement therapy.[150] However, the Women's Health Initiative randomized clinical trial of combined estrogen/progestin therapy showed no beneficial effect on incident PAD.[151]

Interaction and Risk Factor Comparisons

Some research has been conducted into potential variations in the significance and strength of the various risk factors as they are estimated in different subgroups and for different PAD-related outcomes. Differences in the relative strength and significance of risk factors in men and women have been examined in several studies. Many of these studies have concluded that risk factors do not differ substantially in men and women.[17,24,76] In a study of Medicare beneficiaries in the United States (ages 65 and older), similar risk factor associations were found with ABI in men in women, except for total and LDL cholesterol, which were related to ABI in women but not men.[26]

Regarding potential interactions between ethnicity and cardiovascular risk factors, the San Diego Population Study showed no evidence that a greater sensitivity of blacks to traditional CVD risk factors explained ethnic differences in PAD.[31]

Meijer and colleagues looked at whether severe PAD, defined by an ABI <0.70, had different risk factors than ABI diagnosed based on the traditional cutpoint of 0.90.[17] In their analysis, the direction and magnitude of odds ratios were similar for most risk factors under the two criteria. The point estimates suggested that age and current smoking were greater risk factors for conventionally defined PAD, while diabetes was more important for severe PAD. However, the 95% confidence intervals overlapped in all cases.

● PROGRESSION OF PAD

The natural history of PAD can be drawn through studies performed several years ago, prior to the advent of revascularization techniques and medications improving the local and general prognosis. In a classical study of a cohort of 520 patients the diagnosis of "arteriosclerosis obliterans" managed between 1939 and 1948 in the Mayo Clinic, the diagnosis was limited to symptoms and clinical examination.[152] Two-third patients presented IC, while others presented pain at rest and/or trophic lesions. The survival rates at 5 and 10 years were around 75 and 50%, respectively. Three-fourth of deaths were related to cardiovascular causes. Amputation was required in 8.9% of cases (almost 15% of the survivors) during the 5-year follow-up, but this concerned only 3% of patients who initially had an IC. Importantly,

11.3% of patients who continued smoking experienced an amputation, but none who abstained smoking. In a Finnish series of patients with PAD (3/4 with IC, 1/4 with more progressed disease) followed approximately 10 years, one-half died. Among survivors, 1/4 clinically improved, 1/2 were clinically stable, and 1/4 experienced clinical worsening. In a population >65 years of age with IC, the 5-year clinical progression can be summarized as follows: symptoms deteriorated in 25% of patients, with claudication worsening in almost 15% of cases, while 5% to 10% progressed to CLI with approximately 5% requiring amputation.[153] In a study defining disease progression by the occurrence of rest pain or gangrene, PAD progressed in 2.5% of patients annually, with a progression rate approximately three times greater in the first year following diagnosis than in subsequent years.[154] Nowadays, the limb prognosis of patients with symptomatic PAD has not substantially improved, though direct comparisons are difficult, since the access to health care for PAD probably differs in different periods and different countries, and the patterns of risk factors, especially the prevalence of diabetic patients has changed, and the overall survival improved. In SMART study conducted in the Netherlands in this new century, during a mean follow-up of 5.5 years of patients with clinical PAD, 7.6% experienced amputation.[155] However, these results are related to cases referred to vascular centers, and it is well known that almost one half of patients with clinical symptoms, probably those at a less severe stage, are not addressed for specialized management. In two large epidemiological studies, only 1.6% and 1.8% of patients who developed claudication came to amputation.[72,156] In the Edinburgh Artery Study, 8.2% of claudicants at baseline had undergone vascular surgery or amputation.[34] It should, however, be emphasized that the clinical progression of PAD does not systematically follow the asymptomatic–exercise pain–rest pain–trophic lesions scheme, and a patient can directly switch from an asymptomatic PAD to chronic limb ischemia, especially in the elderly, when subjects might have walking limitations for other reasons masking exertional pain, and a minor trauma can have delayed healing and turn quickly the limb's clinical state into CLI. In one of the largest series of CLI, about 15% of cases did not present any prior IC.[157]

Little is known about the early natural history of PAD, particularly the progression of the disease during the asymptomatic period, and the transition from asymptomatic to early symptomatic disease. In the Edinburgh Artery Study, the 5 year incidence of IC was estimated at 3.2% in those who initially had no asymptomatic PAD (normal ABI and reactive hyperhemia test), while the same incidence rose to 9.3% when asymptomatic PAD was initially diagnosed.[34]

The average annual change in ABI has been estimated as −0.01 and −0.02 in various groups.[99,158] However, these figures maybe somewhat misleading, because average change in ABI masks a variety of changes of different directions and magnitudes. A more meaningful approach maybe to look at the percentage of the population achieving some categor-

ically defined measure of change. Nicoloff and colleagues found that in 5 years, 37% of patients experienced a significant (≥ 0.15) worsening of ABI, while 22% of patients experienced clinical progression of PAD based on a change in symptoms or a need for surgical intervention.[159] Among 415 English smokers with PAD referred for a surgical opinion, about half experienced a significant (≥ 0.14) drop in ABI over the following 48 months.[100] In a group of German patients with PAD, it was reported to progress in 18.6% of patients during an average follow-up of 64 months, based on a variety of criteria including change in ABI.[160] Bird and colleagues defined a ranked series of six categories of PAD defined based on ABI and other tests in a study of patients referred to a vascular laboratory, 30.2% of limbs progressed to a more serious category of PAD over an average follow-up time of 4.6 years, but 22.8% of limbs regressed to a less severe category during the same period.[159]

Recently, two studies addressed the epidemiology of PAD progression.[45,161–163] For approximately 5 years, the ABI change was at −0.06 in a clinical cohort[45] and −0.03 in a general population cohort.[161–163] In the clinical cohort composed of subjects with and without PAD having visited a vascular laboratory, active smoking, the TC/HDL-C ratio, Lp(a), and C-reactive protein were significant markers of substantial ABI decrease.[45] Interestingly, in this study, diabetes was not associated with ABI decline, but was the sole significant risk factor for small-vessels disease progression, defined by a substantial toe-brachial index drop without any noticeable ABI change. Inflammation markers were also found as independent and significant factors associated with ABI decline in the Edinburgh Artery Study, with fibrinogen and interleukin-6 as the most significant factors.[162,163]

In the Cardiovascular Health Study, cystatin C, a marker of renal function, was positively correlated with the rates of further interventions (revascularization/amputation) in patients with PAD.[164]

Additionally, it can be postulated that patients with a more progressive PAD might be at higher risk of CV death. In this case, the progression of PAD in longitudinal studies might be underestimated because of selective mortality in patients with greater progression.

● CO-PREVALENCE OF PAD AND OTHER ATHEROSCLEROTIC DISEASE

Given the common risk factors for PAD and other cardiovascular and cerebrovascular disease, it is not surprising that cross sectionally people with PAD are more likely to have these other disorders and vice versa. In patients with clinical PAD, 40% to 60% also have clinical CAD,[165,166] whereas in a series of 1000 PAD patients undergoing revascularization surgery, a systematic coronary angiography revealed that 90% of these had angiographic lesions.[167] Among 5084 Medicare recipients in the Cardiovascular Health Study, the prevalence of history of MI was 2.5 times as high in subjects with PAD (based on ABI <0.9) versus those without; for angina, congestive heart failure, stroke, and TIA, the prevalence was 1.9, 3.3, 3.1, and 2.3 times as high, respectively.[26] Conversely, the prevalence of PAD was 2.1 times as high in patients with a history of myocardial infarction versus those without. The corresponding ratios for angina, congestive heart failure, stroke, and TIA were 1.7, 2.6, 2.4, and 2.1, respectively.[26] Other cross-sectional studies have found similar correlation.[60,68,106,168] Subjects with PAD have also been shown to have an elevated prevalence of carotid artery stenosis[169,170] with a prevalence of >30% carotid stenosis estimated between 51% and 72% of cases[166] and a prevalence of >70% carotid stenosis up to 25% in a Chinese study.[171] A modest but significant correlation between the severity of the two diseases has been demonstrated.[172,173]

● PAD AS A PREDICTOR OF MORTALITY AND MORBIDITY

Beyond the cross-sectional associations discussed above, it has been shown that PAD is prospectively related to morbidity or mortality related to other types of atherosclerotic disease, even after adjustment for known common risk factors. Although few events and deaths are directly related to PAD, the presence of this condition has to be considered as a marker for underlying atherosclerotic processes affecting other vascular beds. These prospective relationships are of clinical importance, since the prognostic value of PAD is independent of other known risk factors.

The first studies on the cardiovascular prognosis of patients with clinical PAD started in the 1960s[152] and were followed in the 1970s and 1980s by the Framingham cohort, although this excess risk was markedly attenuated when subjects with baseline cerebrovascular and coronary heart disease were excluded.[72,174,175] Similarly, a Finnish study in 1982 failed to find an association between IC and total or cardiovascular mortality in men after adjustment for cardiovascular risk factors and baseline cardiovascular disease.[176] Other studies demonstrated increased mortality risk among claudicants, but did not fully adjust for the conventional cardiovascular risk factors.[34,73,154,177] However, in the largest and most methodologically rigorous study of its kind, data from the 18 403 men in the Whitehall cohort were used to show that after adjusting for cardiovascular risk factors, claudication was a significant predictor of cardiovascular disease mortality, even after excluding subjects with baseline disease.[178] Interestingly, in the Framingham Study, despite a 20% decline of IC incidence from the 1950s to 1990s, the vital prognosis of this condition remained unchanged.[78] The survival of PAD patients is dramatically poor in case of occurrence of CLI, since it is estimated that 20% to 25% of patients die during the first year of medical management.[13,157]

The development of the ABI and other noninvasive measures of PAD permitted further investigation of the association of PAD and cardiovascular disease. In 1985, it was first demonstrated that a combination of noninvasive measures including ABI were prospectively related to all-cause mortality, even after adjustment for cardiovascular risk factors and exclusion of subjects with baseline cardiovascular disease.[30] Relative risks in this study were in the range of 4 to 5. A later reanalysis of the same cohort with a longer follow-up period demonstrated elevated relative risks for cardiovascular disease and coronary heart disease in particular, with no significant increase in noncardiovascular death.[179]

Following this study, several other prospective studies confirmed that ABI was related to cardiovascular disease, based on either mortality or combined mortality and morbidity. This was found to be true in a variety of populations, including vascular laboratory patients,[48,180] elderly patients with hypertension,[181] elderly women,[25] an employment-based cohort from Belgium,[52] the population-based Edinburgh Artery Study,[20] and the Cardiovascular Health Study cohort.[49] Most of these studies controlled for various known cardiovascular disease risk factors and the presence of cardiovascular disease at baseline. The relative risks reported ranged approximately from 2 to 5. Many of these studies also found PAD to be significantly associated with incident coronary heart disease in particular, although the very large Cardiovascular Health Study failed to find such associations for either total myocardial infarction or angina.[49]

The data regarding the association of PAD with cerebrovascular disease are less conclusive. Data from the Cardiovascular Health Study failed to show a relationship between low ABI and incident stroke.[49] Data from the Edinburgh Artery Study also showed such an association based on ABI, although after multivariate adjustment the association persisted for nonfatal but not fatal stroke.[20] Another large study, the ARIC Study, showed a significant association between ABI as a continuous variable and ischemic stroke after multivariate adjustment, but failed to show such association when ABI was categorized based on a 0.80 cutpoint.[182]

Table 1-5 provides a summary of studies of the association of PAD with various mortality and morbidity outcomes. The table is limited to studies using a noninvasive measure of PAD (usually ABI) and logistic or proportional hazards regression models, with multivariate adjustment for conventional cardiovascular risk factors. The results are shown with multivariate adjustment and after exclusion of subjects with baseline cardiovascular disease where such exclusion was attempted. In a meta-analysis including nine of these studies (over 28 000 subjects), the likelihood of a low ABI (between 0.80 and 0.90) to predict all-cause mortality was around 4, rising to 5.6 when only cardiovascular deaths were considered.[183] These data emphasize the poorer prognosis of subjects affected by PAD.

● SUMMARY AND CONCLUSION

PAD corresponds to the obstruction of the arteries of the lower extremities because of the development of atherosclerosis. The most common symptom of PAD is IC, defined by pain in the leg(s) associated with walking and that is relieved by rest. However, noninvasive measures such as the ABI show that asymptomatic PAD is several

TABLE 1-5. Low-ABI Prognostic Value in Prospective Cohorts

First author	Population	Age	Follow-Up Duration (years)	ABI Thresholds	Relative Risk				
					Total Mortality	CV Death	Fatal CHD	Myocardial Infarction	Stroke
McKenna[48]	744 M & W*	66†	3.3	0.40–0.85 vs. >0.85	2.0	—	—	—	—
				<0.40 vs. >0.85	3.4				
Criqui[179]	565 M & W	66†	10	<0.8 vs. >0.8	3.1	5.9	6.6	—	—
Newman[26]	1537 M & W	75†	4	<0.9 vs. >0.9	3.8	3.7	3.2	—	—
Ögren[184,185]	477 M	68†	10	<0.9 vs. >0.9	2.3	—	2.6	2.3	2.0
Vogt[25]	1492 W§	≥65	4.3	<0.9 vs. >0.9	3.1	4.0	3.7	—	—
Leng[20]	1592 M & W	55–74	5	<0.9 vs. >0.9	1.8	2.3	2.2	1.4‡	1.9
Newman[49]	5888 M & W	≥65	6	<0.9 vs. >0.9	2.4	2.8	—	2.0	1.6
Vogt[186]	1930 M & W*	≥50	—	<0.9 vs. >0.9	—	—	2.2	—	—
Kornitzer[52]	1592 M	40–50	10	<0.9 vs. >0.9	—	3.6	—	—	—
Abbott[187]	2863 M	>70	3 to 6	<0.8 vs. >1.0	—	—	—	3.3	—
Abbott[188]	2767 M	>70	3 to 6	<0.9 vs. >0.9	—	—	—	—	2.0
Jönsson[189]	353 M & W	50–89	10	0.51–0.8 vs. >1	2.1	—	—	—	—
				≤0.51 vs. >1	3.4				
Tsai[182]	14 839 M & W	45–64	7	<0.8 vs. >1.2	—	—	—	—	5.7
Resnick[21]	4393 M & W	45–74	8.3	<0.9 vs. 0.9–1.40	2.1	3.8	—	—	—
				>1.40 vs. 0.9–1.40	2.2	2.7	—	—	—

* Patients addressed to a vascular center, † mean age, ‡ nonfatal MI, § all hypertensive, p = ns.

times more common in the population than IC. The prevalence of PAD is largely age-related, rising to over 10% after the sixth and seventh decades. This prevalence appears to be higher among men than women for moderate to severe disease. The major risk factors for PAD are similar to those for cardiovascular and cerebrovascular disease, with some differences in the relative importance of factors. Smoking is a particularly strong risk factor for PAD, but the contribution of diabetes and the metabolic syndrome in incident cases is currently increasing. In cross-sectional studies, PAD is associated with cardiovascular and cerebrovascular disease. In longitudinal studies, after adjustment for known cardiovascular disease risk factors, PAD is associated with an increased risk of cardiovascular and cerebrovascular disease morbidity and mortality.

With the general aging of the population, it seems likely that PAD will be increasingly common in the future. The diagnosis and treatment of PAD in its asymptomatic stage maybe highly beneficial, particularly with respect to interventions aimed at controlling risk factors common to atherosclerotic disease of the several vascular beds.

REFERENCES

1. Bowlin SJ, Medalie JH, Flocke SA, et al. Epidemiology of intermittent claudication in middle-aged men. *Am J Epidemiol.* 1994;140:418-430.

2. Allison MA, Ho E, Denenberg JO, et al. Ethnic-specific prevalence of peripheral arterial disease in the United States. *Am J Prev Med.* 2007;32:328-333.

3. Rose G. The diagnosis of ischaemic heart pain and intermittent claudication in field surveys. *Bull WHO.* 1962;27:645-658.

4. Leng GC. Questionnaire. In: Fowkes FGR, ed. *Epidemiology of Peripheral Vascular Disease.* London: Springer-Verlag; 1991:29-40.

5. Leng GC, Fowkes FG. The Edinburgh Claudication Questionnaire: an improved version of the WHO/Rose Questionnaire for use in epidemiological surveys. *J Clin Epidemiol.* 1992;45:1101-1109.

6. Aboyans V, Lacroix P, Waruingi W, et al. Traduction française et validation du questionnaire d'Edimbourg pour le dépistage de la claudication intermittente. *Arch Mal Cœur.* 2000;93:1173-1177.

7. Lacroix P, Aboyans V, Boissier C, Bressollette L, Leger P. Validation d'une traduction française du questionnaire d'Edimbourg au sein d'une population de consultants en médecine générale. *Arch Mal Cœur.* 2002;95:596-600.

8. Criqui MH, Denenberg JO, Bird CE, et al. The correlation between symptoms and non-invasive test results in patients referred for peripheral arterial disease testing. *Vasc Med.* 1996;1:65-71.

9. Hirsch AT, Criqui MH, Treat-Jacobson D, et al. Peripheral arterial disease detection, awarness and treatment in primary care. *JAMA.* 2001;286:1317-1324.

10. Stoffers HE, Rinkens PE, Kester AD, et al. The prevalence of asymptomatic and unrecognized peripheral arterial occlusive disease. *Int J Epidemiol.* 1996;25:282-290.

11. Neurospinous claudication. *Lancet.* 1985;ii:704.

12. McDermott MM, Greenland P, Liu K, et al. Leg symptoms in peripheral arterial disease. Associated clinical characteristics and functionnal impairment. *JAMA.* 2001;286:1599-1606.

13. Norgren L, Hiatt WR, Dormandy JA, et al. Inter-society consensus for the management of peripheral arterial disease (TASC II). *Eur J Vasc Endovasc Surg.* 2007;33:S1-S75.

14. Vogt MT, Cauley JA, Kuller LH, et al. Prevalence and correlates of lower extremity arterial disease in elderly women. *Am J Epidemiol.* 1993;137:559-568.

15. Winsor T. Influence of arterial disease on the systolic blood pressure gradients of the extremity. *Am J Med Sci.* 1950;220:117-126.

16. Hooi JD, Stoffers HE, Kester AD, et al. Peripheral arterial occlusive disease: prognostic value of signs, symptoms, and the ankle-brachial pressure index. *Med Decis Making.* 2002;22:99-107.

17. Meijer WT, Grobbee DE, Hunink MG, et al. Determinants of peripheral arterial disease in the elderly: the Rotterdam Study. *Arch Intern Med.* 2000;160:2934-2938.

18. McDermott MM, Liu K, Criqui MH, et al. Ankle-brachial index and subclinical cardiac and carotid disease. The Multi-Ethnic Study of Atherosclerosis. *Am J Epidemiol.* 2005;162:33-41.

19. Wang JC, Criqui MH, Denenberg JO, et al. Exertional leg pain in patients with and without peripheral arterial disease. *Circulation.* 2005;112:3501-3508.

20. Leng GC, Fowkes FG, Lee AJ, et al. Use of ankle brachial pressure index to predict cardiovascular events and death: a cohort study. *BMJ.* 1996;313:1440-1444.

21. Resnick HE, Lindsay RS, McDermott MM, et al. Relationship of high and low ankle brachial index to all-cause mortality. The Strong Heart Study. *Circulation.* 2004;109:733-739.

22. O'Hare AM, Katz R, Shilipak MG, et al. Mortality and cardiovascular risk accross ankle-arm index spectrum: results from the Cardiovascular Health Study. *Circulation.* 2006;113:388-393.

23. Diehm C, Lange S, Darius H, et al. Association of low ankle brachial index with high mortality in primary care. *Eur Heart J.* 2006;27:1743-1749.

24. Meijer WT, Hoes AW, Rutgers D, et al. Peripheral arterial disease in the elderly: the Rotterdam Study. *Arterioscler Thromb Vasc Biol.* 1998;18:185-192.

25. Vogt MT, Cauley JA, Newman AB, et al. Decreased ankle/arm blood pressure index and mortality in elderly women. *JAMA.* 1993;270:465-469.

26. Newman AB, Siscovick DS, Manolio TA, et al. Ankle-arm index as a marker of atherosclerosis in the Cardiovascular Health Study. Cardiovascular Heart Study (CHS) Collaborative Research Group. *Circulation.* 1993;88:837-845.

27. Yao ST, Hobbs JT, Irvine WT. Ankle systolic pressure measurements in arterial disease affecting the lower extremities. *Br J Surg.* 1969;56:676-679.

28. Ouriel K, McDonnell AE, Metz CE, et al. Critical evaluation of stress testing in the diagnosis of peripheral vascular disease. *Surgery.* 1982;91:686-693.

29. Lijmer JG, Hunink MG, van den Dungen JJ, et al. ROC analysis of noninvasive tests for peripheral arterial disease. *Ultrasound Med Biol.* 1996;22:391-398.

30. Criqui MH, Coughlin SS, Fronek A. Noninvasively diagnosed peripheral arterial disease as a predictor of mortality: results from a prospective study. *Circulation.* 1985;72:768-773.

31. Criqui MH, Vargas V, Denenberg JO, et al. Ethnicity and peripheral arterial disease. The San Diego Population Study. *Circulation.* 2005;112:2703-2707.

32. Aboyans V, Ho E, Deneberg JO, et al. The association between elevated ankle systolic pressures and peripheral occlusive arterial disease in diabetic and nondiabetic subjects. *J Vasc Surg.* 2008 (in press).

33. Aboyans V, Criqui MH, McClelland RL, et al. Intrinsic contribution of gender and ethnicity to normal ankle-brachial index values: The Multi-Ethnic Study of Atherosclerosis (MESA). *J Vasc Surg.* 2007;45:319-327.

34. Leng GC, Lee AJ, Fowkes FG, et al. Incidence, natural history and cardiovascular events in symptomatic and asymptomatic peripheral arterial disease in the general population. *Int J Epidemiol.* 1996 25:1172-1181.

35. McDermott MM, Fried L, Simonsick E, et al. Asymptomatic peripheral arterial disease is independently associated with impaired lower extremity functioning: the women's health and aging study. *Circulation.* 2000;101:1007-1012.

36. McDermott MM, Criqui MH, Liu K, et al. Lower ankle/brachial index, as calculated by averaging the dorsalis pedis and posterior tibial arterial pressures, and association with leg functioning in peripheral arterial disease. *J Vasc Surg.* 2000;32:1164-1171.

37. McDermott MM, Ferrucci L, Simonsick EM, et al. The ankle brachial index and change in lower extremity functioning over time: the Women's Health and Aging Study. *J Am Geriatr Soc.* 2002;50:238-246.

38. de Graaff JC, Ubbink DT, Legemate DA, et al. Interobserver and intraobserver reproducibility of peripheral blood and oxygen pressure measurements in the assessment of lower extremity arterial disease. *J Vasc Surg.* 2001;33:1033-1040.

39. Aboyans V, Lacroix P, Lebourdon A, et al. The intra- and interobserver variability of ankle-arm blood pressure index according to its mode of calculation. *J Clin Epidemiol.* 2003;56:215-220.

40. Schröder F, Diehm N, Kareem S, et al. A modified calculation of ankle-brachial pressure index is far more sensitive in the detection of peripheral arterial disease. *J Vasc Surg.* 2006;44:531-536.

41. Niazi K, Khan TH, Easley KA. Diagnostic utility of the two methods of ankle brachial index in the detection of peripheral arterial disease of lower extremities. *Catheter Cardiovasc Interv.* 2006;68:788-792.

42. Shadman R, Criqui MH, Bundens WP, et al. Subclavian stenosis: the prevalence, risk factors and association with other cardiovascular diseases. *J Am Coll Cardiol.* 2004;44:618-623.

43. Fowkes FG, Housley E, Cawood EH, et al. Edinburgh Artery Study: prevalence of asymptomatic and symptomatic peripheral arterial disease in the general population. *Int J Epidemiol.* 1991;20:384-392.

44. Hiatt WR, Hoag S, Hamman RF. Effect of diagnostic criteria on the prevalence of peripheral arterial disease. The San Luis Valley Diabetes Study. *Circulation.* 1995;91:1472-1479.

45. Aboyans V, Criqui MH, Denenberg JO, et al. Risk factors for progression of peripheral arterial disease in large and small vessels. *Circulation.* 2006;113:2623-2629.

46. Kreines K, Johnson E, Albrink M, et al. The course of peripheral vascular disease in non-insulin-dependent diabetes. *Diabetes Care.* 1985;8:235-243.

47. Orchard TJ, Strandness DE Jr. Assessment of peripheral vascular disease in diabetes. Report and recommendations of an international workshop sponsored by the American Heart Association and the American Diabetes Association 18–20 September 1992, New Orleans, Louisiana. *Diabetes Care.* 1993;16:1199-1209.

48. McKenna M, Wolfson S, Kuller L. The ratio of ankle and arm arterial pressure as an independent predictor of mortality. *Atherosclerosis.* 1991;87:119-128.

49. Newman AB, Shemanski L, Manolio TA, et al. Ankle-arm index as a predictor of cardiovascular disease and mortality in the Cardiovascular Health Study. The Cardiovascular Health Study Group. *Arterioscler Thromb Vasc Biol.* 1999;19:538-545.

50. Murabito JM, Evans JC, Nieto K, et al. Prevalence and clinical correlates of peripheral arterial disease in the Framingham Offspring Study. *Am Heart J.* 2002;143:961-965.

51. Belch JJF, Topol EJ, Agnelli G, et al. Critical issues in peripheral arterial disease detection and management. A call to action. *Arch Intern Med.* 2003;163:884-892.

52. Kornitzer M, Dramaix M, Sobolski J, et al. Ankle/arm pressure index in asymptomatic middle-aged males: an independent predictor of ten-year coronary heart disease mortality. *Angiology.* 1995;46:211-219.

53. De Backer G, Kornitzer M, Sobolski J, et al. Intermittent claudication - epidemiology and natural history. *Acta Cardiol.* 1979;125-132.

54. Schroll M, Munck O. Estimation of peripheral arteriosclerotic disease by ankle blood pressure measurements in a population study of 60-year-old-men and women. *J Chron Dis.* 1981;34:261-269.

55. Gofin R, Kark JD, Friedlander Y, et al. Peripheral vascular disease in a middle-aged population sample. The Jerusalem Lipid Research Clinic Prevalence Study. *Isr J Med Sci.* 1987;23:157-167.

56. Fowkes FG, Housley E, Riemersma RA, et al. Smoking, lipids, glucose intolerance, and blood pressure as risk factors for peripheral atherosclerosis compared with ischemic heart disease in the Edinburgh Artery Study. *Am J Epidemiol.* 1992;135:331-340.

57. Ogren M, Hedblad B, Jungquist G, et al. Low ankle-brachial pressure index in 68-year-old men: prevalence, risk factors and prognosis. Results from prospective population study

"Men born in 1914," Malmo, Sweden. *Eur J Vasc Surg.* 1993;7:500-506.

58. Beks PJ, Mackaay AJ, de Neeling JN, et al. Peripheral arterial disease in relation to glycaemic level in an elderly Caucasian population: the Hoorn Study. *Diabetologia.* 1995;38:86-96.

59. Curb JD, Masaki K, Rodriguez BL, et al. Peripheral artery disease and cardiovascular risk factors in the elderly. The Honolulu Heart Program. *Arterioscler Thromb Vasc Biol.* 1996;16: 1495-1500.

60. Zheng ZJ, Sharrett AR, Chambless LE, et al. Associations of ankle-brachial index with clinical coronary heart disease, stroke and preclinical carotid and popliteal atherosclerosis: The Atherosclerosis Risk in Communities (ARIC) Study. *Atherosclerosis.* 1997;131:115-125.

61. Fabsitz RR, Sidawy AN, Go O, et al. Prevalence of peripheral arterial disease and associated risk factors in American Indians: The Strong Heart Study. *Am J Epidemiol.* 1999;149:330-338.

62. Premalatha G, Shanthirani S, Deepa R, et al. Prevalence and risk factors of peripheral vascular disease in a selected South Indian population: The Chennai Urban Population Study. *Diabetes Care.* 2000;23:1295-1300.

63. Cui R, Iso H, Yamagishi K, et al. Ankle-arm blood pressure index and cardiovascular risk factors in elderly japanese men. *Hypertens Res.* 2003;26:377-382.

64. Selvin E, Erlinger TP. Prevalence of and Risk Factors for peripheral arterial disease in the United States results from the National Health and Nutrition Examination Survey, 1999–2000. *Circulation.* 2004;110:738-743.

65. Gregg EW, Sorlie P, Paulose-Ram R, et al. 1999–2000 national health and nutrition examination survey. Prevalence of lower-extremity disease in the US adult population ≥40 years of age with and without diabetes: 1999–2000 national health and nutrition examination survey. *Diabetes Care.* 2004;27:1591-1597.

66. Kweon SS, Shin MH, Park KS, et al. Distribution of the ankle-brachial index and associated cardiovascular risk factors in a population of middle-aged and elderly koreans. *J Korean Med Sci.* 2005;20:373-378.

67. Allison MA, Criqui MH, McClelland RL, et al. The effect of novel cardiovascular risk factors on the ethnic-specific odds for peripheral arterial disease in the Multi-Ethnic Study of Atherosclerosis (MESA). *J Am Coll Cardiol.* 2006;48:1190-1197.

68. Kröger K, Stang A, Kondratieva J, et al. Prevalence of peripheral arterial disease—results of the Heinz Nixdorf recall study. *Eur J Epidemiol.* 2006;21:279-285,

69. Eldrup N, Sillesen H, Prescott E, et al. Ankle brachial index, C-reactive protein, and central augmentation index to identify individuals with severe atherosclerosis. *Eur Heart J.* 2006;27:316-322.

70. Carbayo JA, Divison JA, Escribano J, et al. Using ankle-brachial index to detect peripheral arterial disease: prevalence and associated risk factors in a random population sample. *Nutr Metab Cardiovasc Dis.* 2007;17:41-49.

71. Zheng ZJ, Rosamond WD, Chambless LE, et al. Lower extremity arterial disease assessed by ankle–brachial index in a middle-ages population of African Americans and Whites. *Am J Prev Med.* 2005;29(5S1):42-49.

72. Kannel WB, McGee DL. Update on some epidemiologic features of intermittent claudication: the Framingham Study. *J Am Geriatr Soc.* 1985;33:13-18.

73. Dagenais GR, Maurice S, Robitaille NM, et al. Intermittent claudication in Quebec men from 1974–1986: The Quebec Cardiovascular Study. *Clin Invest Med.* 1991;14:93-100.

74. Bainton D, Sweetnam P, Baker I, et al. Peripheral vascular disease: consequence for survival and association with risk factors in the Speedwell prospective heart disease study. *Br Heart J.* 1994;72:128-132.

75. Ingolfsson IO, Sigurdsson G, Sigvaldason H, et al. A marked decline in the prevalence and incidence of intermittent claudication in Icelandic men 1968–1986: a strong relationship to smoking and serum cholesterol—The Reykjavik Study. *J Clin Epidemiol.* 1994;47:1237-1243.

76. Murabito JM, D'Agostino RB, Silbershatz H, et al. Intermittent claudication. A risk profile from The Framingham Heart Study. *Circulation.* 1997;96:44-49.

77. Hooi JD, Kester AD, Stoffers HE, et al. Incidence of and risk factors for asymptomatic peripheral arterial occlusive disease: a longitudinal study. *Am J Epidemiol.* 2001;153:666-672.

78. Murabito JM, Evans JC, D'Agostino RB, Wilson PWF, Kannel WB. Temporal trends in the incidence of intermittent claudication from 1950 to 1999. *Am J Epidemiol.* 2005;162:430-437.

79. Verhaeghe R. Epidemiology and prognosis of peripheral arteriophaty. *Drugs.* 1998;56(S3):1-10.

80. Erb W. Klinische Beiträge zur Pathologie des Intermittierenden Hinkens. *Munch Med Wochenschr.* 1911;2:2487.

81. Fowkes FG. Epidemiology of atherosclerotic arterial disease in the lower limbs. *Eur J Vasc Surg.* 1988;2:283-291.

82. Faulkner KW, House AK, Castleden WM. The effect of cessation of smoking on the accumulative survival rates of patients with symptomatic peripheral vascular disease. *Med J Aust.* 1983;1:217-219.

83. Jonason T, Bergstrom R. Cessation of smoking in patients with intermittent claudication. Effects on the risk of peripheral vascular complications, myocardial infarction and mortality. *Acta Med Scand.* 1987;221:253-260.

84. Quick CR, Cotton LT. The measured effect of stopping smoking on intermittent claudication. *Br J Surg.* 1982;69(suppl):S24-S26.

85. Brand FN, Abbott RD, Kannel WB. Diabetes intermittent claudication and risk of cardiovascular events in Framingham Study. *Diabetes.* 1989;38:504-509.

86. Katsilambros NL, Tsapogas PC, Arvanitis MP, et al. Risk factors for lower extremity arterial disease in non-insulin-dependent diabetic persons. *Diabet Med.* 1996;13:243-246.

87. Kallio M, Forsblom C, Groop PH, et al. Development of new peripheral arterial occlusive disease in patients with type 2 diabetes during a mean follow-up of 11 years. *Diabetes Care.* 2003;26:1241-1245.

88. Tseng CH. Prevalence and risk factors of peripheral arterial obstructive disease in Taiwanese type 2 diabetic patients. *Angiology.* 2003;54:331-338.

89. Jude EB, Oyibo SO, Chalmers N, et al. Peripheral arterial disease in diabetic and nondiabetic patients: a comparison

of severity and outcome. *Diabetes Care.* 2001;24:1433-1437.

90. Haltmayer M, Mueller T, Horvath W, et al. Impact of atherosclerotic risk factors on the anatomical distribution of peripheral arterial disease. *Int Angiol.* 2001;20:200-207.

91. King TA, DePalma RG, Rhodes RS. Diabetes mellitus and atherosclerotic involvment of the profunda femoris artery. *Surg Gynecol Obstet.* 1984;159:553-556.

92. Strandness DE Jr, Priest RR, Gibbons GE. Combined clinical and pathological study on non-diabetic and diabetic vascular disease. *Diabetes,* 1964;13:366-372.

93. Criqui MH, Deneberg JO, Langer RD, et al. Peripheral arterial disease and hypertension. In: Izzo JL, Black HR, eds. *Hypertension Primer.* Dallas: American Heart Association; 2003:250-252.

94. Dormandy J, Heeck L, Vig S. Predictors of early disease in the lower limbs. *Semin Vasc Surg.* 1999;12:109-117.

95. Ridker PM, Stampfer MJ, Rifai N. Novel risk factors for systemic atherosclerosis: a comparison of C-reactive protein, fibrinogen, homocysteine, lipoprotein(a), and standard cholesterol screening as predictors of peripheral arterial disease. *JAMA.* 2001;285:2481-2485.

96. Fowkes FGR. Epidemiology of atherosclerotic arterial disease in the lower limbs. *Eur J Vasc Surg.* 1988;2:283-291.

97. Ness J, Aronow WS, Ahn C. Risk factors for symptomatic peripheral arterial disease in older persons in an academic hospital-based geriatrics practice. *J Am Geriatr Soc.* 2000;48:312-314.

98. Cheng SW, Ting AC, Wong J. Lipoprotein(a) and its relationship to risk factors and severity of atherosclerotic peripheral vascular disease. *Eur J Vasc Endovasc Surg.* 1997;14:17-23.

99. Fowkes FG, Lowe GD, Housley E, et al. Cross-linked fibrin degradation products, progression of peripheral arterial disease, and risk of coronary heart disease. *Lancet.* 1993;342:84-86.

100. Smith I, Franks PJ, Greenhalgh RM, et al. The influence of smoking cessation and hypertriglyceridaemia on the progression of peripheral arterial disease and the onset of critical ischaemia. *Eur J Vasc Endovasc Surg.* 1996;11:402-428.

101. Mowat BF, Skinner ER, Wilson HM, et al. Alterations in plasma lipids, lipoproteins and high density lipoprotein subfractions in peripheral arterial disease. *Atherosclerosis.* 1997;131:161-166.

102. Valentine RJ, Grayburn PA, Vega DL, et al. Lp(a) lipoprotein is an independent discriminating risk factor for premature peripheral atherosclerosis among white men. *Arch Intern Med.* 1994;154:801-806.

103. Tseng CH. Lipoprotein(a) is an independent risk factor for peripheral arterial disease in chinese type 2 diabetic patients in Taiwan. *Diabetes Care.* 2004;27:517-521.

104. Cheng SW, Ting AC, Wong J. Fasting total plasma homocysteine and atherosclerotic peripheral vascular disease. *Ann Vasc Surg.* 1997;11:217-223.

105. Mangion DM, Howley MS, Norcliff D. Lower limb arterial disease: assessment of risk factors in an elderly population. *Atherosclerosis.* 1991;91:137-143.

106. Ness J, Aronow WS. Prevalence of coexistence of coronary artery disease, ischemic stroke, and peripheral arterial disease in older persons, mean age 80 years, in an academic hospital-based geriatrics practice. *J Am Geriatr Soc.* 1999;47:1255-1256.

107. Nasir K, Guallar E, Navas-Acien A, et al. Relationship of monocyte count and peripheral arterial disease: results from the National Health and Nutrition Examination Survey 1999–2002. *Atheroscler Thromb Vasc Biol.* 2005;25:1966-1971.

108. Askew CD, Green S, Walker PJ, et al. Skeletal muscle phenotype is associated with exercise tolerance in patients with peripheral arterial disease. *J Vasc Surg.* 2005;41:802-807.

109. Wattanakit K, Folsom AR, Selvin E, et al. Risk factors for peripheral arterial disease incidence in persons with diabetes: The Atherosclerosis Risk in Communities (ARIC) Study. *Atherosclerosis.* 2005;180:389-397.

110. Vliegenthart R, Geleijnse JM, Hofman A, et al. Alcohol consumption and risk of peripheral arterial disease: the Rotterdam Study. *Am J Epidemiol.* 2002;155:332-338.

111. Jepson RG, Fowkes FG, Donnan PT, et al. Alcohol intake as a risk factor for peripheral arterial disease in the general population in the Edinburgh Artery Study. *Eur J Epidemiol.* 1995;11:9-14.

112. Camargo CA Jr, Stampfer MJ, Glynn RJ, et al. Prospective study of moderate alcohol consumption and risk of peripheral arterial disease in U.S. male physicians. *Circulation.* 1997;95:577-580.

113. Danyi P, Yanel LR, Moy TF, et al. Ankle-brachial index is lower in asymptomatic African Americans independent of risk factors and body mass index in families at high risk of premature coronary disease. *Circulation.* 2007;115:e287.

114. Hobbs SD, Wilmink AB, Bradbury AW. Ethnicity and peripheral arterial disease. *Eur J Vasc Endovasc Surg.* 2003;25:505-512.

115. Boushey CJ, Beresford SA, Omenn GS, et al. A quantitative assessment of plasma homocysteine as a risk factor for vascular disease. Probable benefits of increasing folic acid intakes. *JAMA.* 1995;274:1049-1057.

116. Bloemenkamp DG, van den Bosch MA, Mali WP, et al. Novel risk factors for peripheral arterial disease in young women. *Am J Med.* 2002;113:462-467.

117. Graham IM, Daly LE, Refsum HM, et al. Plasma homocysteine as a risk factor for vascular disease. The European Concerted Action Project. *JAMA.* 1997;277:1775-1781.

118. Hoogeveen EK, Kostense PJ, Beks PJ, et al. Hyperhomocysteinemia is associated with an increased risk of cardiovascular disease, especially in non-insulin-dependent diabetes mellitus: a population-based study. *Arterioscler Thromb Vasc Biol.* 1998;18:133-138.

119. Guallar E, Silbergeld EK, Navas-Acien A, et al. Confounding of the relation between homocysteine and peripheral arterial disease by Lead, Cadmium, and Renal Function. *Am J Epidemiol.* 2006;163(8):700-708.

120. Taylor LM Jr, Moneta GL, Sexton GJ, et al. Prospective blinded study of the relationship between plasma homocysteine and progression of symptomatic peripheral arterial disease. *J Vasc Surg.* 1999;29:8-19.

121. Wildman RP, Muntner P, Chen J, et al. Relation of inflammation to peripheral arterial disease in the National Health and

Nutrition Examination Survey, 1999–2002. *Am J Cardiol.* 2005;96:1579-1583.

122. Lowe GD, Fowkes FG, Dawes J, et al. Blood viscosity, fibrinogen, and activation of coagulation and leukocytes in peripheral arterial disease and the normal population in the Edinburgh Artery Study. *Circulation.* 1993;87:1915-1920.

123. Fishbane S, Youn S, Kowalski EJ, et al. Ankle-arm blood pressure index as a marker for atherosclerotic vascular diseases in hemodialysis patients. *Am J Kidney Dis.* 1995;25:34-39.

124. Wattanakit K, Folsom AR, Selvin E, et al. Kidney function and risk of peripheral arterial disease: results from the Atherosclerosis Risk in Communities (ARIC) Study. *J Am Soc Nephrol.* 2007;18:629-636.

125. Hung HC, Willett W, Merchant A, et al. Oral health and peripheral arterial disease. *Circulation.* 2003;107:1152-1157.

126. Mendez MV, Scott T, LaMote W, et al. An association between perodontal disease and peripheral vascular disease. *Am J Surg.* 1998;176:153-157.

127. Whiteman MC, Deary IJ, Fowkes FG. Personality and social predictors of atherosclerotic progression: Edinburgh Artery Study. *Psychosom Med.* 2000;62:703-714.

128. McDermott MM, Greenland P, Guralnik JM, et al. Depressive symptoms and lower extremity functioning in men and women with peripheral arterial disease. *J Gen Intern Med.* 2003;18:461-467.

129. Carmelli D, Fabsitz RR, Swan GE, et al. Contribution of genetic and environmental influences to ankle-brachial blood pressure index in the NHLBI Twin Study. National Heart, Lung, and Blood Institute. *Am J Epidemiol.* 2000;151:452-458.

130. Murabito JM, Guo CY, Fox CS, et al. Heritability of the ankle-brachial index: the Framingham Offspring Study. *Am J Epidemiol,* 2006;164:963-968.

131. Valentine RJ, Guerra R, Stephan P, et al. Family history is a major determinant of subclinical peripheral arterial disease in young adults. *J Vasc Surg.* 2004;39:351-356.

132. Kroon AA, Ajubi N, van Asten WN, et al. The prevalence of peripheral vascular disease in familial hypercholesterolaemia. *J Intern Med.* 1995;238:451-459.

133. Lee AJ, Fowkes FG, Lowe GD, et al. Fibrinogen, factor VII and PAI-1 genotypes and the risk of cornary and peripheral atherosclerosis: the Edinburgh Artery Study. *Thromb Haemost.* 1999;81:553-560.

134. Vainas T, Stassen FR, Bruggeman CA, et al. Synergistic effect of Toll-like receptor 4 and CD 14 polymorphisms on the total atherosclerosis burden in patients with peripheral arterial disease. *J Vasc Surg.* 2006;44:326-332.

135. Sofi F, Lari B, Rogolino A, et al. Thrombophilic risk factors for symptomatic peripheral arterial disease. *J Vasc Surg.* 2005;41:255-260.

136. Laroche M, Pouilles JM, Ribot C, et al. Comparison of the bone mineral content of the lower limbs in men with ischaemic atherosclerotic disease. *Clin Rheumatol.* 1994;13:611-614.

137. Mangiafico RA, Russo E, Riccobene S, et al. Increased prevalence of peripheral arterial disease in osteoporotic postmenopausal women. *J Bone Miner Metab.* 2006;24:125-131.

138. Vogt MT, Cauley JA, Kuller LH, et al. Bone mineral density and blood flow to the lower extremities: the study of osteoporotic fractures. *J Bone Miner Res.* 1997;12:283-289.

139. van der Klift M, Pols HA, Hak AE, et al. Bone mineral density and the risk of peripheral arterial disease: the Rotterdam Study. *Calcif Tissue Int.* 2002;70:443-449.

140. Pennisi P, Signorelli SS, Riccobene S, et al. Low bone density and abnormal bone turnover in patients with atherosclerosis of peripheral vessels. *Osteoporos Int.* 2004;15:389-395.

141. Taylor LM Jr, Chitwood RW, Dalman RL, et al. Antiphospholipid antibodies in vascular surgery patients. A cross-sectional study. *Ann Surg.* 1994;220:544-550.

142. Lam EY, Taylor LM Jr, Landry GJ, et al. Relationship between antiphospholipid antibodies and progression of lower extremity arterial occlusive disease after lower extremity bypass operations. *J Vasc Surg.* 2001;33:976-982.

143. Mya MM, Aronow WS. Increased prevalence of peripheral arterial disease in older men and women with subclinical hypothyroidism. *J Gerontol A Biol Sci Med Sci.* 2003;58:68-69.

144. Asgeirsdottir LP, Agnarsson U, Jonsson GS. Lower extremity blood flow in healthy men: effect of smoking, cholesterol, and physical activity—a Doppler study. *Angiology.* 2001;52:437-445.

145. Navas-Acien A, Silbergeld EK, Sharrett AR, et al. Metals in urine and peripheral arterial disease. *Environ Health Perspect.* 2005;113:164-169.

146. Klipstein-Grobusch K, den Breeijen JH, Grobbee DE, et al. Dietary antioxidants and peripheral arterial disease: the Rotterdam Study. *Am J Epidemiol.* 2001;154:145-149.

147. Antonelli-Incalzi R, Pedone C, McDermott MM, et al. Association between nutrient intake and peripheral artery disease: Results from the InCHIANTI study. *Atherosclerosis.* 2006;186:200-206.

148. Donnan PT, Thomson M, Fowkes FG, et al. Diet as a risk factor for peripheral arterial disease in the general population: The Edinburgh Artery Study. *Am J Clin Nutr.* 1993;57:917-921.

149. Tornwall ME, Virtano J, Haukka JK, et al. Prospective study of diet, lifestyle, and intermittent claudication in male smokers. *Am J Epidemiol.* 2000;151:892-901.

150. Westendorp IC, in't Veld BA, Grobbee DE, et al. Hormone replacement therapy and peripheral arterial disease: the Rotterdam Study. *Arch Intern Med.* 2000;160:2498-2502.

151. Hsia J, Criqui MH, Rodabough R, et al. Estrogen plus progestin and the risk of peripheral arterial disease: The Women's Health Initiative. *Circulation.* 2004;109:620-626.

152. Juergens JE, Parker NW, Hines EA. Arteriosclerosis obliterans: review of 520 cases with special reference to pathogenic and prognostic factors. *Circulation.* 1960;21:188-195.

153. Meru AV, Mittra S, Thyagarajan B, et al. Intermittent claudication: an overview. *Atherosclerosis.* 2006;187:231-237.

154. Jelnes R, Gaardsting O, Hougaard Jensen K, et al. Fate in intermittent claudication: outcome and risk factors. *Br Med J (Clin Res Ed).* 1986;293:1137-1140.

155. Goessens BMB, van der Graaf Y, Olijhoek JK, et al. The course of vascular risk factors and the occurrence of vascular events in patients with symptomatic peripheral arterial disease. *J Vasc Surg.* 2007;45:47-54.

156. Widmer LK, Biland L, DaSilva A. Risk profile and occlusive peripheral arterial disease (OPAD). In proceedings of 13th International congress of Angiology, Athens 1985.

157. Bertele V, Roncaglioni MC, Pangrazzi J, et al. Clinical outcome and its predictors in 1560 patients with critical leg ischemia. *Eur J Vasc Endovasc Surg.* 1999;18:401-410.

158. Bird CE, Criqui MH, Fronek A, et al. Quantitative and qualitative progression of peripheral arterial disease by non-invasive testing. *Vasc Med.* 1999;4:15-21.

159. Nicoloff AD, Taylor LM Jr, Sexton GJ, et al. Relationship between site of initial symptoms and subsequent progression of disease in a prospective study of atherosclerosis progression in patients receiving long-term treatment for symptomatic peripheral arterial disease. *J Vasc Surg.* 2002;35:38-46.

160. Taute BM, Glaser C, Taute R, et al. Progression of atherosclerosis in patients with peripheral arterial disease as a function of angiotensin-converting enzyme gene insertion/deletion polymorphism. *Angiology.* 2002;53:375-382.

161. Smith FB, Lee AJ, Price JF, et al. Changes in ankle brachial index in symptomatic and asymptomatic subjects in the general population. *J Vasc Surg.* 2003;38:1323-1330.

162. Tzoulaki I, Murray GD, Lee AJ, et al. C-reactive protein, interleukin-6, and soluble adhesion molecules as predictors of progressive peripheral atherosclerosis in the general population. Edinburgh Artery Study. *Circulation.* 2005;112:976-983.

163. Tzoulaki I, Murray GD, Price JF, et al. Hemostatic factors, inflammatory markers, and progressive peripheral atherosclerosis. The Edinburgh Artery Study. *Am J Epidemiol.* 2006;163:334-341.

164. O'Hare AM, Newman AB, Katz R, et al. Cystatin C and incident peripheral arterial disease events in the elderly. Results from the Cardiovascular Health Study. *Arch Intern Med.* 2005;165:2666-2670.

165. Dormandy J, Mahir M, Ascady G, et al. Fate of a patient with chronic ischaemia. *J Cardiovasc Surg.* 1989;30:50-57.

166. Golomb BA, Dang TT, Criqui MH. Peripheral arterial disease. Morbidity and mortality implications. *Circulation.* 2006;114:688-699.

167. Hertzer NR, Beven EG, Young JR, et al. Coronary artery disease in peripheral vascular patients. Classification of 1000 coronary angiograms and results of surgical management. *Ann Surg.* 1984;199:223-233.

168. Criqui MH, Denenberg JO, Langer RD, et al. The epidemiology of peripheral arterial disease: importance of identifying the population at risk. *Vasc Med.* 1997;2:221-226.

169. Alexandrova NA, Gibson WC, Norris JW, et al. Carotid artery stenosis in peripheral vascular disease. *J Vasc Surg.* 1996;23: 645-649.

170. Pilcher JM, Danaher J, Khaw KT. The prevalence of asymptomatic carotid artery disease in patients with peripheral vascular disease. *Clin Radiol.* 2000;55:56-61.

171. Cheng SW, Wu LL, Lau H, et al. Prevalence of significant disease carotid stenosis in Chinese patients with peripheral

and coronary artery disease. *Aust N Z J Surg.* 1999;69:44-47.

172. Long TH, Criqui MH, Vasilevskis EE, et al. The correlation between the severity of peripheral arterial disease and carotid occlusive disease. *Vasc Med.* 1999;4:135-142.

173. Aboyans V, Lacroix P, Guilloux J, et al. A predictive model for screening cerebrovascular disease in patients undergoing coronary artery bypass grafting. *Interactive Cardiovasc Thor Surg.* 2005;4:90-95.

174. Kannel WB, Shurtleff D. The natural history of arteriosclerosis obliterans. *Cardiovasc Clin.* 1971;3:37-52.

175. Kannel WB, Skinner JJ Jr, Schwartz MJ, et al. Intermittent claudication. Incidence in the Framingham Study. *Circulation.* 1970;41:875-883.

176. Reunanen A, Takkunen H, Aromaa A. Prevalence of intermittent claudication and its effect on mortality. *Acta Med Scand.* 1982;211:249-256.

177. Kallero KS. Mortality and morbidity in patients with intermittent claudication as defined by venous occlusion plethysmography. A ten-year follow-up study. *J Chronic Dis.* 1981;34:455-462.

178. Smith GD, Shipley MJ, Rose G. Intermittent claudication, heart disease risk factors, and mortality. The Whitehall Study. *Circulation.* 1990;82:1925-1931.

179. Criqui MH, Langer RD, Fronek A, et al. Mortality over a period of 10 years in patients with peripheral arterial disease. *N Engl J Med.* 1992;326:381-386.

180. McDermott MM, Feinglass J, Slavensky R, et al. The ankle-brachial index as a predictor of survival in patients with peripheral vascular disease. *J Gen Intern Med.* 1994;9:445-449.

181. Newman AB, Sutton-Tyrrell K, Vogt MT, et al. Morbidity and mortality in hypertensive adults with a low ankle/arm blood pressure index. *JAMA.* 1993;270:487-489.

182. Tsai AW, Folsom AR, Rosamond WD, et al. Ankle-brachial index and 7-year ischemic stroke incidence: the ARIC Study. *Stroke.* 2001;32:1721-1724.

183. Doobay AV, Anand SS. A systematic review sensitivity and specificity of the Ankle–Brachial index to predict future cardiovascular outcomes. *Atheroscler Thromb Vasc Biol.* 2005;25:1463-1469.

184. Ögren M, Hedblad B, Isacsson SO, et al. Non-invasively detected carotid stenosis and ischaemic heart disease in men with leg arteriosclerosis. *Lancet.* 1993;342:1138-1141.

185. Ögren M, Hedblad B, Isacsson SO, et al. Ten year cerebrovascular morbidity and mortality in 68 year old men with asymptomatic carotid stenosis. *Br Med J.* 1995;310:1294-1298.

186. Vogt MT, McKenna M, Anderson SJ, et al. The relationship between ankle-arm index and mortality in older men and women. *J Am Geriatr Soc.* 1993;41:523-530.

187. Abbott RD, Petrovitch H, Rodriguez BL, et al. Ankle/brachial blood pressure in men >70 years of age and the risk of coronary heart disease. *Am J Cardiol.* 2000;86:280-284.

188. Abbott RD, Rodriguez BL, Petrovitch H, et al. Ankle-brachial blood pressure in elderly men and the risk of stroke: The Honolulu Heart Program. *J Clin Epidemiol.* 2001;54:973-978.

189. Jönsson B, Skau T. Ankle-Brachial index and mortality in a cohort of questionnaire recorded leg pain on walking. *Eur J Vasc Endovasc Surg.* 2002;24:405-410.

190. Pomrehn P, Duncan B, Weissfeld L, et al. The association of dyslipoproteinemia with symptoms and signs of peripheral arterial disease: The Lipid Research Clinic Program Prevalence Study. *Circulation.* 1986;73(suppl I):I-100-I-107.

191. Hughson WG, Mann JI, Garrod A. Intermittent claudication: prevalence and risk factors. *Br Med J.* 1978;1:1379-1381.

192. Resnick HE, Rodriguez B, Havlik R, et al. Apo E genotype, diabetes, and peripheral arterial disease in older men: the Honolulu–Asia Aging Study. *Genet Epidemiol.* 2000;19:52-63.

chapter 2

Gender Differences in the Epidemiology and Management of Vascular Disease

Parveen K. Garg, MD, MPH / *Suneel M. Udani, MD, MPH* / *Arti Rupani, MD* /
Karen Moncher, MD / *Robert S. Dieter MD, RVT*

● INTRODUCTION

Although gender-related differences in the diagnosis and management of cardiovascular disease have been well established, gender differences in noncoronary vascular disease have gained increasing awareness only in the recent years. Much of the known research has suggested delays in diagnosis, anatomic differences, and clinicians' underestimation of disease magnitude to contribute to gender-driven differences in disease prevalence and outcome.[1]

This chapter will review the available literature regarding gender differences in noncoronary vascular disease. Specifically, we will focus on peripheral arterial disease (PAD), cerebrovascular disease, carotid artery disease, renovascular disease, pulmonary vascular disease, mesenteric arterial disease, and the systemic vasculitides. Only with a continued effort into understanding these differences can solutions be offered to help enhance vascular disease recognition and outcomes in women.

● PERIPHERAL ARTERIAL DISEASE

PAD is a highly prevalent disease, affecting as much as 12 million people in the United States, and is a major cause of disability, loss of work, and lifestyle changes.[2–11] PAD can raise one's risk of death between two- and sixfold over a 10-year period.[11,12] The incidence of PAD dramatically increases with age and, considering the extended longevity in industrialized nations, this number is only expected to increase in the upcoming years.[13,14] More importantly, it is predicted that nearly two-thirds of those affected with PAD over the age of 65 would be females.[15]

Although less so recently, traditionally little attention has focused on gender differences in PAD or its epidemiology in women. Many studies cite no gender differences in PAD epidemiology, while others do.[16] It has become widely recognized, however, that the number of PAD cases has been underreported by clinicians especially among women, as symptoms of intermittent claudication on presentation only represent a small fraction of all cases.[3,17–19]

Epidemiology

Nearly 12% of men and women in the community and up to 16% to 19% of the elderly population are affected with PAD.[20–22] Although intermittent claudication is the most common presenting symptom for patients with PAD, it alone is an insufficient diagnostic indicator for PAD in women particularly.[1] In a study of PAD detection, only 7% of female participants reported symptoms of claudication.[23] In a large observational study of more than 3000 patients only one-quarter of those with PAD reporting symptoms of claudication were female.[18]

However, ankle–branchial index (ABI) has been found to detect at least four- to fivefold more PAD in women than intermittent claudication by history.[24] While only 7% of females reported symptoms of claudication in the above mentioned Chicago-based study of PAD detection including nearly 500 participants with significant PAD, more than

35% of female participants met diagnostic criteria using an ABI < 0.90. Among elderly women, 82% of those with PAD were asymptomatic.[24] Several studies have noted that the average resting ABI is lower in women than men.[5,25] When asymptomatic PAD prevalence is determined, women may comprise as many, if not more, cases as men.[4,18,26,27]

Although women with asymptomatic PAD may not present with classical symptoms of claudication, they have reported more difficulty with activities of daily living, are less active, have lower physical endurance, diminished leg strength, and have a slower cadence.[22,28,29] These functional impairments all contribute to masking symptoms of intermittent claudication. It has also been suggested that, like coronary heart disease, women may more frequently present with atypical symptoms of PAD.[4,28,30]

The true prevalence of PAD in women is likely much higher than has been reported and is comparable to that of men. More recent studies have demonstrated an equal prevalence of PAD in men and women when more sensitive and specific noninvasive measures of PAD such as ABI are taken into account.[5,17,31,32] Risk factor profiles are similar between men and women with PAD.[31] Among females, African American and Hispanic women were noted to have a nonsignificant trend toward increased PAD prevalence when compared with white women.[31]

Disease Course and Clinical Outcomes

Women with PAD were found to have similar percentages for comorbidities except for lower levels of cardiovascular disease in certain studies.[4,17,33] Additionally, women with PAD are also found to be more functionally impaired than men.[33] On measures of walking performance, women were found to be significantly worse for walking distance, walking speed, and stair climbing.[31,33] One prior study has demonstrated that variation in leg strength, with women having poorer leg strength than men, may at least partially explain the gender variation in walking impairment.[33] Women with PAD are also reported to have a lower quality of life as compared to men.[34] As mentioned before, women are known to have more difficulty carrying out daily living activities and have lower physical endurance.

Although more functionally impaired than men, women with PAD are found to have lower rates of lower extremity revascularization.[33,35] The lower prevalence of typical claudication symptoms in women and differences in types of activities performed based on gender may explain the lower revascularization rates.[33] Women who do undergo revascularization procedures are reported to have more adverse outcomes than men.[36–39] These include lower long-term patency rates following vascular bypass grafting and higher rates of graft occlusion.[36,38] Delayed diagnosis, decreased referrals, more postoperative complications, and possibly the effect of their smaller arteries have all been suggested in order to account for these gender-based differences in outcomes.[19,37,40] Mortality for women with PAD, however, has been shown to be similar to that of men.[16]

Hormonal Factors

An abundance of evidence has suggested an association between the hormones estrogen/progestin as protective agents and the development of PAD in postmenopausal women. However, considering more recent research findings, it remains unclear what role hormones play in the development and progression of PAD.

Total and low-density lipoprotein cholesterol levels become higher in the postmenopausal years.[16] Both of these cholesterol components increase the risk of developing PAD in women.[32] Through this mechanism, the loss of estrogen and progesterone may amplify the risk of PAD in women.

Intermittent claudication is less frequent in premenopausal women and only in the postmenopausal years begins to approach that of men, usually by the sixth or seventh decade of life.[41] Framingham data have found the incidence in women more than doubled from the ages 45–54 years to 55–64 years.[42] However, as more objective criteria such as the ABI have become prevalent, rather than symptom based, current data have shown that prevalence does not seem to be significantly different between genders.

Hormone replacement therapy (HRT) in the prevention of vascular disease has gained considerable attention over the past decade. While HRT has been clearly shown to have no benefit but rather potential harm in the prevention of cardiovascular disease, its role in peripheral vascular disease remains in question.[43] Several clinical trials have evaluated the effects of combined HRT on PAD as measured in the carotid and/or femoral artery (Table 2-1).[44–47] None of these studies showed any differences in arterial thickness or slowed progression of arterial atherosclerosis between the treatment and control groups. One observational study has proposed that study length maybe playing a role in these conflicting results. More than 50% reduction in PAD was documented in postmenopausal users.[48] No benefit was seen though in the subset of patients who used HRT for less than 1 year.

Estrogen, however, has been shown to improve endothelial function in postmenopausal women and may exert an independent protective effect in the development of PAD.[49,50] Trials of estrogen-only HRT have had more promising results showing decreased progression of carotid artery atherosclerosis (Table 2-1).[51,52] However, because of the overall deleterious cardiac outcomes, HRT is generally not recommended for women with PAD.

● CEREBROVASCULAR DISEASE

Stroke is the third leading cause of death in the developed world and is a major cause of chronic disability.[53] Seventy percent of strokes are a result of cerebral ischemia, while the rest are predominantly caused by cerebral hemorrhage.[53] The incidence of stroke has varied according to reports from different countries.[54] Annual stroke rates have ranged from 1.35 to 4 cases per 1000.[55–60] While attention to understanding cerebrovascular diseases is strong, relatively little

TABLE 2-1. Studies Comparing Hormone Replacement Therapy and Vascular Disease

Study	Type of Therapy	Outcomes
Angerer et al.[183] ($n = 321$)	Combined (HRT)	No change in distensibility of carotid artery
Hodis et al.[51] ($n = 222$)	Estrogen	Slowed progression of carotid artery atherosclerosis
Angerer et al.[45] ($n = 321$)	Combined (HRT)	HRT did not slow progression of carotid artery atherosclerosis
Angerer et al.[47] ($n = 321$)	Combined (HRT)	HRT did not slow progression of carotid artery atherosclerosis
Byington et al.[46] ($n = 362$)	Combined (HRT)	No change in carotid artery thickness in treatment group
Le Gal et al.[52] ($n = 166$)	Estrogen (transdermal)	Decreased progression of atherosclerotic carotid plaques
Hsia et al.[44] ($n = 16,608$)	Combined (HRT)	No change in carotid artery, lower extremity, or aortic disease

HRT, hormone replacement therapy.
*Adapted from Nguyen L, Liles DR, Lin PH, Bush RL. Hormone replacement therapy and peripheral vascular disease in women. Vasc Endovascular Surg. 2004;38(6):547–556.

of this has been focused on gender-specific aspects of the disease.

Although stroke maybe similar in both sexes with regard to presentation and management, gender differences are clearly present in the epidemiology, pathophysiology, and outcomes of stroke.

Epidemiology

Stroke incidence appears to be higher in men than women, but increases with age in both sexes, with a doubling of stroke rates for each decade after the age of 55.[61–64] Overall, however, nearly 40 000 more women than men suffer a stroke each year.[65] This is thought to be a result of greater average life expectancy in women. Stroke prevalence data are similar. Up to approximately age 80, the prevalence, like the incidence, is higher among men.[66–68] After the age of 80, the prevalence of stroke is significantly higher in women. Again, this finding is thought to be secondary to the greater long-term survival of women.[69] As a result, stroke occurs, on average, approximately 5 to 10 years later in women than in men.[63,65,70–72] In terms of stroke recurrence, 5-year recurrence rates were almost twice as high in men than women.[73]

Pathophysiology

The risk factor profile for stroke are well established and similar in both genders.[74,75] However, evidence suggests that smoking and diabetes may have stronger relative impacts in women compared to men.[76,77] The relative risk associated with smoking maybe approximately 20% higher in women.[76] Oral contraceptives have been found to be risk factor for stroke that is unique to women. Studies have consistently indicated an increased risk ratio of between 1.5 and 3 with the use of oral contraceptives.[78–81] Recent evidence has suggested, however, that the increased risk associated with oral contraceptives is attributed to risk factors such as smoking, hypertension, and perhaps even migraines.[78,80,82,83] Along similar lines, clinical trials have shown that postmenopausal hormone therapy actually increases the risk of stroke.[84,85] Additionally, atrial fibrillation

has been noted to be more frequent in female patients with stroke.[71,86]

Information on stroke subtypes are relatively limited but some differences have been noted. A higher proportion of hemorrhagic strokes have been found to occur in men; however, subarachnoid hemorrhages are distinctly more commonly observed in women.[87,88] Cardioembolic strokes have been reported to be twice as frequent among women compared with men.[89,90]

Gender variability has also been noted with respect to cerebrovascular occlusive disease distribution in patients with stroke. Extracranial larger artery disease, particularly the internal carotid artery, predominated in men, whereas intracranial medium artery disease was more common in women.[91,92] Finally, posterior circulation stroke is less likely to occur in female cohorts compared to male ones.[93]

Disease Course and Clinical Outcomes

Gender appears to play a role on outcomes after stroke.[72,90,94] Women suffer from greater functional disability in terms of motor function, cognitive function, and activities of daily living function.[72,86,95–100] Women are also more likely to be institutionalized or placed in nursing homes following strokes.[71] They also have higher rates of poststroke depression and risk for suicide compared to men.[101–103] It must be noted, however, that on average, women are older than men at the time of the stroke and most studies did not take into account various social and cultural aspects that may have explained these differences.[63]

Mortality data following stroke have been more conflicting and is still under exploration. According to the American Heart Association more than 60% of deaths caused by stroke in 2000 occurred in women.[65] However, when adjusted for age, reports have found an overall mortality risk that is higher in men.[104,105] Equivocal data have also been reported when specifically looking at short-term mortality as well. Case-fatality rate up to 6 months after the stroke event has been found to be higher in women in some reports but not significantly different in others.[71,72]

Stratified by age, death from ischemic stroke was lower for women younger than 65 years of age, but higher for those at least 65 years old when compared to men.[65,106] Similar to patterns of prevalence, mortality risk was lower in women for intracerebral hemorrhagic stroke at all ages studied, but higher for subarachnoid hemorrhage, with gender differences widening with age.[65,106]

● CAROTID ARTERY DISEASE

One risk factor for stroke, carotid artery stenosis (CAS), merits its own discussion. CAS > 50% is viewed as significant carotid artery disease.[107] The prevalence of CAS >50% and >80% is between 2%–8% and 1%–2%, respectively.[108] Prevalence is higher in males, and male gender has been found to be an independent predictor for the development of CAS.[109]

The outcome of patients with known CAS has been found to be affected by gender depending on the treatment strategy. With respect to conservative treatment of asymptomatic CAS, gender seems to be no risk factor for stroke.[107] Several reports have observed in women a significantly less benefit from carotid endarterectomy (CEA) and higher risk of perioperative stroke in asymptomatic as well as symptomatic disease compared to men.[110–117] Although some studies have reported no differences in perioperative neurologic events between men and women,[118,119] no reports have shown an increased risk in men. While the risk of perioperative stroke in women is low, there seems to be a tendency of a similar to twofold higher risk in women.[107]

This adverse effect of female gender on outcome in CEA is more pronounced in asymptomatic disease.[110,113,114] Research to understand these gender differences in outcome have helped to offer some answers as to why CEA is not as beneficial for women with asymptomatic CAS. The impact of hormones on atherosclerosis is becoming better known; however, no direct link has been found between hormones and carotid surgery outcomes.[120] Analyses of the carotid artery before surgery have demonstrated that women, compared to men, have more stable, less atheromatous, plaques (Figure 2-1). Plaque volume, a predictor of clinical outcome, is smaller in women at a comparable stenosis grade and the plaques have been found to contain less fat and macrophages and more smooth muscle cells and collagen fibers (Figure 2-1).[121,122]

● RENOVASCULAR DISEASE

Within the realm of PAD, as with other vascular beds, there has been limited investigation regarding gender differences in renal atherosclerotic disease. Nevertheless, there are some differences that emerge in the existing literature. The effect of conventional risk factors for atherosclerosis on atherosclerotic renal disease maybe attenuated in women. Further, while the overall epidemiology appears to be similar, the predisposition of fibromuscular dysplasia in the renal artery to affect women creates a small, but significant distinction. Data on therapy for renovascular disease as a whole are limited, and this holds true for differences in gender as well.

Epidemiology

The epidemiology of renal atherosclerotic disease in the general population is difficult to assess because of the lack of a standardized screening study. The existing data regarding the general population come from autopsy evaluation. Other evaluations of epidemiology have focused on select populations, primarily those with existing atherosclerotic disease elsewhere or underlying risk factors.

Whether or not differences in the prevalence of renal atherosclerotic disease according to gender are present appears to depend on the population selected and, perhaps, the diagnostic method used. In a Brazilian study where individuals undergoing coronary angiography were also evaluated for renal artery stenosis as diagnosed by digital subtraction angiography, Tumulero et al. found that women were more likely than men to have renal artery stenosis ≥50%. However, when evaluating the difference in prevalence among patients with renal artery stenosis ≥70%, no significant difference was found between men and women.[123] In a Japanese population evaluated with magnetic resonance angiography, where atherosclerotic renal artery disease was defined as ≥50% decrease in renal artery diameter (corresponding to a ≥75% decrease in cross-sectional area), no difference in prevalence was found according to gender.[124] The patient population differed from the Brazilian study. Individuals with known preexisting aortitis or renal artery disease were excluded and the inclusion criteria were individuals older than 40 years of age with one or more risk factor atherosclerotic renal disease (hypertension, DM or dyslipidemia). In a Canadian study by Buller et al., patients with risk factors for atherosclerotic disease undergoing renal angiography found female gender to be associated with the presence of severe renal artery stenosis (70%–99%) with an odds ratio of 1.9.[125]

The variable results of the above studies highlight the intrinsic difficulty in defining the epidemiology of renal artery stenosis. The overall prevalence and, thus, the epidemiological differences according to gender depend on the study population evaluated and the diagnostic criteria used. Therefore, while there are some suggestions that atherosclerotic disease maybe more prevalent and/or more severe in women, no definitive statement can be made.

Pathogenesis and Clinical Presentation

While the prevalence of renal atherosclerotic disease according to gender is variable, the general clinical experience is that progression of renal dysfunction is slower in women as compared to men.[126,127] The pathogenesis of renal atherosclerotic disease has been outlined extensively elsewhere, but the pathogenic mechanisms and their outcomes may have slight variation in women versus men and suggest a putative mechanism why female gender is protective. As previously described, endothelial dysfunction plays a role in both etiology and consequence of atherosclerotic progression.

Endothelial function and damage are linked with activity of nitric oxide and angiotensin II. Two separate animal

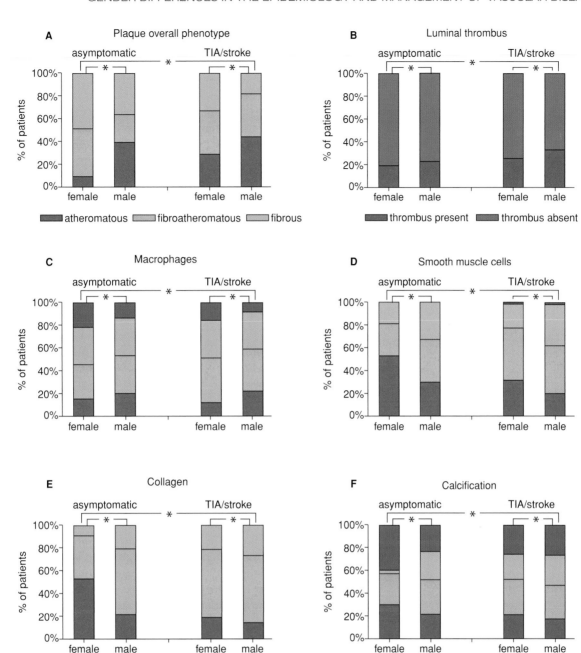

● **FIGURE 2-1.** Comparison of carotid plaque histology between men and women, subdivided by symptom status: asymptomatic versus transient ischemic attack/stroke (* $p < 0.05$.).

Adapted from Hellings WE, Pasterkamp G, Verhoeven BA, et al. Gender-associated differences in plaque phenotype of patients undergoing carotid endarterectomy. J Vasc Surg. 2007;45(2):289-296; discussion 296-287.

models support the theory that the renal response to hypertension, that is, endothelial damage, differs according to gender.[128] Ji et al. found that in the renal wrap model of hypertension, blood pressure increase was the same between genders. Nevertheless, the degree of renal damage in each gender was significantly different: more necrosis, tubular dilatation, and cellular proliferation were present in the male kidneys.[126] Therefore, for the same increase in blood pressure, more damage occurs in male kidneys. The

underlying reason for this difference is not clear. Ji et al. also found that the male kidneys upregulated eNOS more than do female kidneys.[126] Whether the upregulation represents a consequence of increased renal damage or highlights an increased sensitivity to nitric oxide with increased blood pressure is unclear.

Microvascular renal damage is also propagated by the effects of angiotensin II. It appears that the impact of angiotensin II on renal parenchyma varies according to gender as well. Animal models suggest that the presence of estradiol attenuates the deleterious effects of angiotensin II. In female rats lacking ovaries (and thus normal female levels of estrogen), the binding of angiotensin receptors is significantly increased. Estrogen replacement attenuated angiotensin binding equivalent to rats containing intact ovaries.[127] Therefore, through modification of the nitric oxide and angiotensin II pathways, it appears that female gender protects against progressive renal cellular damage. Nevertheless, despite these outlined cellular mechanisms and clinical experiences, there is a lack of large population-based data confirming the protective effect of female gender on progression of atherosclerosis in the renal circulation.

Fibromuscular Dysplasia

Fibromuscular dysplasia represents a unique peripheral artery pathology with an epidemiology, pathogenesis, and treatment distinct from atherosclerotic renovascular disease. While fibromuscular dysplasia can manifest in any vascular bed, it primarily affects the renal and carotid circulations. The underlying etiology of approximately 90% of renal artery stenosis is secondary to atherosclerosis. The remaining 10% is primarily caused by fibromuscular dysplasia. The epidemiology of fibromuscular dysplasia significantly differs according to gender. Rather than the minimal, if any, differences in the prevalence of atherosclerotic renal disease between genders, fibromuscular dysplasia affects women approximately 10 times more often than men and more often manifests at a younger age.[129,130] Because of the greater success in treating the refractory hypertension with revascularization, recognizing fibromuscular dysplasia as the underlying etiology for renal artery stenosis is of great importance.

Therapy

The therapy of renal atherosclerotic disease as a whole is clouded by a lack of clear, randomized data. The questions regarding therapy as related to gender are no different with respect to lack of clear guidelines. With regard to microvascular atherosclerotic renal disease, the studies evaluating the potential interventions of statins and agents active against the RAAS have included more men as a whole and have failed to find any significant difference in effect according to gender.[131,132]

While there is no extensive research experience with gender differences in outcomes of large vessel renal artery stenosis, prospective studies have examined whether gender predicts response to revascularization. Harjai et al. published a prospective study following men and women who underwent renal artery stenting for renovascular hypertension (defined as refractory hypertension in setting of ≥70% stenosis). The investigators observed no difference in outcome, that is, change in blood pressure or rate of restenosis.[133] Burket et al., in a separate prospective trial, evaluated 127 patients who underwent renal artery stenting based on angiographic stenosis ≥60% or translesional

gradient pressure ≥20 mm Hg (reasons for referral for renal artery angiography varied). Once again, gender was not associated with a change in outcome.[134] These findings have been confirmed by others in prospective evaluations attempting to identify factors that are predictive of successful renal artery stenting.[135,136] Zeller et al., however, found female gender to have an association with improved blood pressure after renal artery stenting. However, baseline blood pressure and indirect assessment of renal parenchymal damage were also associated with successful intervention.[137] Whether these factors were different in women was not outlined. Therefore from the existing data it appears that female gender is not associated with better outcomes after revascularization for atherosclerotic renal artery disease.

The treatment for fibromuscular dysplasia differs in that it is primarily focused on blood pressure control via revascularization. Individuals with fibromuscular dysplasia are less likely to have concomitant renal dysfunction or atherosclerotic disease. Success rates for blood pressure control are, overall, higher for fibromuscular dysplasia ranging from 70% to 80% versus 50% to 60% for renal atherosclerotic disease.[138,139] Thus, if the etiology of renal artery stenosis in women is fibromuscular dysplasia, they appear to have better response in blood pressure control after revascularization.

Overall, we still have limited data on gender differences in renovascular disease. The preponderance of fibromuscular dysplasia in women changes the epidemiology slightly; however, the most common cause of renovascular disease, atherosclerosis, appears to be similarly distributed among men and women. The progression of microvascualar renal atherosclerotic disease appears to be attenuated by the presence of estrogen, suggesting that premenopausal women are protected. After menopause, however, this protection is lost and the differences in gender blur. If fibromuscular dysplasia is identified as the cause for renal artery stenosis, the treatment and outcome of treatment is more favorable. For renal atherosclerotic disease, however, no clear difference in treatment for men and women can be found.

● PULMONARY VASCULAR DISEASE

In general, information regarding gender differences in pulmonary vascular disease processes is not well known. From the information that has been gathered, it is well established that pulmonary hypertension, both primary and those associated with autoimmune diseases, occurs more frequently in women. This section will concentrate on this specific pulmonary vascular disease.

Primary Pulmonary Hypertension

Primary pulmonary hypertension is relatively rare. Traditionally viewed as a vasoconstrictive disorder, it is a disease of the small pulmonary arteries manifested by concentric laminar intimal fibrosis, medial hypertrophy, and plexiform lesions.[140] In situ thrombi are also common in primary pulmonary hypertension. The prevalence is approximately one to two cases in a million; however, there is a female preponderance of approximately 2:1 in the global incidence of primary pulmonary hypertension.[141–143] The onset is usually in the third and fourth decades of life. The disease, however, is not restricted to this age group. In the United States, for example, 10% of patients were older than 60 years.[142] Onset of the disease is usually later in men than women.[144]

Some explanations exist to help account for the variation in incidence by gender. Primary pulmonary hypertension can be familial.[144] The familial form is an autosomal dominant disorder that make up at least 6% of cases, and possibly more.[142,143,145] More girls than boys are born to women who have the gene, identified as the bone morphogenetic protein receptor type 2 gene (BMPR2).[144,146,147] Primary pulmonary hypertension can also be anorexigenic in nature. Associations have been reported with aminorex fumarate and fenfluramine derivatives.[148,149] These drugs can carry a greater than 20-fold increased risk of developing primary pulmonary hypertension with long-term use.[144] As such drugs are used much more frequently by women, this also may explain the increased incidence of the disease in women.

Interestingly, no association has been found between oral contraceptive use and primary pulmonary hypertension, suggesting that hormonal differences, at least exogenous, unlikely explain the obvious differences in disease incidence.[144] Of note, although their significance is unknown, elevated titers of autoantibodies and antithyroid antibodies are more frequently present in primarily pulmonary hypertension.[144] These elevations occur more frequently in women.

Pulmonary Hypertension from Autoimmune Disease

Many autoimmune disorders are associated with pulmonary hypertension. These include, but are not restricted to, Hashimoto thyroiditis, Graves disease, dermatomyositis, systemic lupus erythematosis, scleroderma, and rheumatoid arthritis.[144] Except for dermatomyositis, all these diseases have a female preponderance.[144] Sex differences in autoimmune disease incidence can be caused by genetic, hormonal, or environmental triggers that may differ between men and women based on societal or anatomic routes to exposure.

● MESENTERIC ARTERIAL DISEASE

Information regarding gender differences in mesenteric arterial disease is scant as well. One relatively rare condition, however, has already been described. The median arcuate ligament syndrome, also labeled as celiac artery compression syndrome, typically occurs in young patients and is more common in thin, active women.[150] The median arcuate ligament is a fibrous arch that unites the diaphragmatic crura on either side of the aortic hiatus, usually passing superior to the celiac axis origin. In up to 25% of people, however, the ligament may cross anterior to the artery,

potentially resulting in compression of the celiac axis that compromises blood flow and causes symptoms.[151] The presenting symptoms are often postprandial epigastric pain and weight loss.[152,153]

● ABDOMINAL AORTIC ANEURYSMS

Some limited data are available for differences in incidence, progression, and management of abdominal aortic aneurysms (AAA). Among men and women aged 65 years or older approximately 9% have an AAA.[154] Male gender has been commonly recognized as one of the most powerful predictors with respect to the incidence of an AAA.[155,156] This becomes more apparent when looking only at the prevalence of an AAA 3 cm or greater—4% of men versus 1% of women.[157]

Although disease incidence is higher in men, disease progression and outcomes are poorer in women. Also women typically present with AAAs at an older age, but risk of aneurysm rupture is independently associated with female gender.[1,158] Mortality associated with ruptured AAAs for those who do not make it to the hospital as well as those who do but are not operated on are both higher in women.[159] In addition, women who are operated on, either electively or secondary to rupture, carry a significantly higher risk of death than do their male counterparts.[160]

The notion that an AAA of the same size may represent more advanced disease in women compared with men, resulting in referral for surgery at a later stage of disease among women, has been offered to explain the gender-related mortality differences.[160] Matching for age and body surface area, infrarenal aortic diameter was found to be smaller in women.[161,162] This has led many to advocate the use of other criteria rather than exclusive reliance on aortic diameter to characterize risk and need for surgery.

● SYSTEMIC VASCULITIDES

The vasculitides are a group of uncommon diseases whose hallmark is blood vessel inflammation and necrosis.[163] Many epidemiologic studies for these diseases have become available in recent years. Although the causes of most forms of vasculitis are unknown, gender does appear to at least partly account for differences in the incidence of these syndromes. This section will focus on known gender differences in both primary and secondary vasculitis.

Primary Vasculitis

Primary vasculitis can be subdivided into vasculitis affecting predominantly large-, medium-, and/or small-sized blood vessels.

Vasculitis Affecting Predominantly Large-, Medium-, and Small-Sized Blood Vessels. This category includes giant cell (temporal) arteritis (GCA) and Takayasu arteritis (TA). GCA is the most prevalent systemic vasculitis in western countries, associated with polymyalgia rheumatica in almost half of all cases.[164,165] GCA either associated or not associated with polymyalgia manifestations is generally more common in women.[163]

TA, most common in eastern countries, involves primarily large vessels such as the aorta in addition to the pulmonary and coronary arteries.[166–170] Most patients with TA are young women[171]; however, no female predominance has been reported in some series.[172,173] The disease occurs more commonly during a woman's childbearing years, and the peak onset of the disease occurs in the third decade of life.[171]

Vasculitis Affecting Predominantly Medium- and Small-Sized Blood Vessels. This group is composed of polyarteritis nodosa (PAN), Wegener granulomatosis (WG), and Churg–Strauss syndrome (CSS). The overall annual incidence of this group of conditions is more common in men (23.5 per million) than in women (16.4 per million), with a peak in the 65- to 74-year-old age group in both men and women.[174]

Trends are similar among the individual vasculitides. PAN is classically considered to affect twice as many men as women and to develop typically between the middle of the fifth and sixth decades of life.[175] Only in one series did men not predominate.[165] Likewise, the incidence rate of CSS has a male-to-female ratio ranging between 1.1 and 3.[176,177] Most studies on WG have shown that women and men are equally represented.[178,179] One study originating from Spain, however, observed a nonsignificantly higher frequency in women.[165]

Vasculitis Affecting Predominantly Small-Sized Blood Vessels. This class consists of diseases such as Henoch–Schonlein purpura, hypersensitivity vasculitis, cutaneous leukocytoclastic angiitis, and vasculitis secondary to essential mixed cryoglobulinemia.

Henoch–Schonlein purpura is classically associated with arthralgias, purpura, abdominal symptoms, and renal involvement and is the most common vasculitis in children although infrequent in adults. Reported incidence is higher in boys than in girls, with a male-to-female ratio of 3:2.[180] A higher incidence in men has been reported as well.[181]

Hypersensitivity vasculitis is a disease that includes prominent involvement of the skin and frequently seems to be precipitated by the use of drugs.[181] Reports on the incidence of hypersensitivity vasculitis have found conflicting data regarding whether it was more common in men or women.[181,182]

Secondary Vasculitis

Patients with secondary vasculitis generally have clinical or laboratory evidence of an underlying disease, most commonly rheumatoid arthritis or systemic lupus erythematosus systemic lupus erythematosus.[165] While rheumatoid vasculitis has been found to be more common in men, systemic lupus erythematosus vasculitis is almost four times more frequent in women than in men.

● CONCLUSION

In addition to the coronary circulation, gender differences exist across all vascular beds. It is important to continue exploring gender differences in the risk factor profile and management strategies in vascular disease. Only toward this end will we be able to adopt a more effective strategy of global vascular management for their patients, with a more complete evaluation, care, and intervention plan.

REFERENCES

1. Nguyen L, Liles DR, Lin PH, Bush RL. Hormone replacement therapy and peripheral vascular disease in women. *Vasc Endovascular Surg.* 2004;38(6):547-556.

2. Criqui MH, Fronek A, Barrett-Connor E, Klauber MR, Gabriel S, Goodman D. The prevalence of peripheral arterial disease in a defined population. *Circulation.* 1985;71(3):510-515.

3. Criqui MH, Denenberg JO, Langer RD, Fronek A. The epidemiology of peripheral arterial disease: importance of identifying the population at risk. *Vasc Med.* 1997;2(3):221-226.

4. Meijer WT, Hoes AW, Rutgers D, Bots ML, Hofman A, Grobbee DE. Peripheral arterial disease in the elderly: the Rotterdam Study. *Arterioscler Thromb Vasc Biol.* 1998;18(2):185-192.

5. Fowkes FG, Housley E, Cawood EH, Macintyre CC, Ruckley CV, Prescott RJ. Edinburgh Artery Study: prevalence of asymptomatic and symptomatic peripheral arterial disease in the general population. *Int J Epidemiol.* 1991;20(2):384-392.

6. Dormandy JA, Rutherford RB. Management of peripheral arterial disease (PAD). TASC Working Group. TransAtlantic Inter-Society Consensus (TASC). *J Vasc Surg.* Jan 2000;31 (1 Pt 2):S1-S296.

7. Pentecost MJ, Criqui MH, Dorros G, et al. Guidelines for peripheral percutaneous transluminal angioplasty of the abdominal aorta and lower extremity vessels. A statement for health professionals from a special writing group of the Councils on Cardiovascular Radiology, Arteriosclerosis, Cardio-Thoracic and Vascular Surgery, Clinical Cardiology, and Epidemiology and Prevention, the American Heart Association. *Circulation.* 1994;89(1):511-531.

8. Second European Consensus Document on chronic critical leg ischemia. *Circulation.* 1991;84(4 suppl):IV1-26.

9. Weitz JI, Byrne J, Clagett GP, et al. Diagnosis and treatment of chronic arterial insufficiency of the lower extremities: a critical review. *Circulation.* 1996;94(11):3026-3049.

10. Smith GD, Shipley MJ, Rose G. Intermittent claudication, heart disease risk factors, and mortality. The Whitehall Study. *Circulation.* 1990;82(6):1925-1931.

11. Criqui MH, Langer RD, Fronek A, et al. Mortality over a period of 10 years in patients with peripheral arterial disease. *N Engl J Med.* 1992;326(6):381-386.

12. McKenna M, Wolfson S, Kuller L. The ratio of ankle and arm arterial pressure as an independent predictor of mortality. *Atherosclerosis.* 1991;87(2–3):119-128.

13. Khaw KT. Healthy aging. *BMJ.* 1997;315(7115):1090-1096.

14. Butler RN. Population aging and health. *BMJ.* 25 1997;315 (7115):1082-1084.

15. Vogt MT, Wolfson SK, Kuller LH. Lower extremity arterial disease and the aging process: a review. *J Clin Epidemiol.* 1992;45(5):529-542.

16. Higgins JP, Higgins JA. Epidemiology of peripheral arterial disease in women. *J Epidemiol.* 2003;13(1):1-14.

17. Hirsch AT, Criqui MH, Treat-Jacobson D, et al. Peripheral arterial disease detection, awareness, and treatment in primary care. *JAMA.* 2001;286(11):1317-1324.

18. Stoffers HE, Rinkens PE, Kester AD, Kaiser V, Knottnerus JA. The prevalence of asymptomatic and unrecognized peripheral arterial occlusive disease. *Int J Epidemiol.* 1996;25 (2):282-290.

19. Cheng SW, Ting AC, Lau H, Wong J. Epidemiology of atherosclerotic peripheral arterial occlusive disease in Hong Kong. *World J Surg.* 1999;23(2):202-206.

20. McDermott MG, P. Clinical significance and functional implications of peripheral arterial disease. In: Olin J, ed. *Clinical Evaluation and Office-Based Detection of Peripheral Arterial Disease. An Office-Based Approach to the Diagnosis and Treatment of Peripheral Arterial Disease.* Manchester: Society for Vascular Medicine and Biology; 1998:20-26.

21. Newman AB, Sutton-Tyrrell K, Kuller LH. Lower-extremity arterial disease in older hypertensive adults. *Arterioscler Thromb.* 1993;13(4):555-562.

22. Newman AB. Peripheral arterial disease: insights from population studies of older adults. *J Am Geriatr Soc.* 2000;48(9): 1157-1162.

23. McDermott MM, Greenland P, Liu K, et al. The ankle brachial index is associated with leg function and physical activity: the Walking and Leg Circulation Study. *Ann Intern Med.* 2002;136(12):873-883.

24. Vogt MT, Cauley JA, Kuller LH, Hulley SB. Prevalence and correlates of lower extremity arterial disease in elderly women. *Am J Epidemiol.* 1993;137(5):559-568.

25. Hiatt WR, Hoag S, Hamman RF. Effect of diagnostic criteria on the prevalence of peripheral arterial disease. The San Luis Valley Diabetes Study. *Circulation.* 1995;91(5):1472-1479.

26. Ness J, Aronow WS, Ahn C. Risk factors for symptomatic peripheral arterial disease in older persons in an academic hospital-based geriatrics practice. *J Am Geriatr Soc.* 2000;48 (3):312-314.

27. Hooi JD, Kester AD, Stoffers HE, Overdijk MM, van Ree JW, Knottnerus JA. Incidence of and risk factors for asymptomatic peripheral arterial occlusive disease: a longitudinal study. *Am J Epidemiol.* 2001;153(7):666-672.

28. McDermott MM, Mehta S, Liu K, et al. Leg symptoms, the ankle-brachial index, and walking ability in patients with peripheral arterial disease. *J Gen Intern Med.* 1999;14(3):173-181.

29. Vogt MT, Cauley JA, Kuller LH, Nevitt MC. Functional status and mobility among elderly women with lower extremity

30. Jackson G. Coronary artery disease and women. *BMJ.* 1994;309(6954):555-557.

31. Collins TC, Suarez-Almazor M, Bush RL, Petersen NJ. Gender and peripheral arterial disease. *J Am Board Fam Med.* 2006;19(2):132-140.

32. Newman AB, Siscovick DS, Manolio TA, et al. Ankle-arm index as a marker of atherosclerosis in the Cardiovascular Health Study. Cardiovascular Heart Study (CHS) Collaborative Research Group. *Circulation.* 1993;88(3):837-845.

33. McDermott MM, Greenland P, Liu K, et al. Sex differences in peripheral arterial disease: leg symptoms and physical functioning. *J Am Geriatr Soc.* 2003;51(2):222-228.

34. Bloemenkamp DG, Mali WP, Tanis BC, et al. Functional health and well-being of relatively young women with peripheral arterial disease is decreased but stable after diagnosis. *J Vasc Surg.* 2003;38(1):104-110.

35. Feinglass J, McDermott MM, Foroohar M, Pearce WH. Gender differences in interventional management of peripheral vascular disease: evidence from a blood flow laboratory population. *Ann Vasc Surg.* 1994;8(4):343-349.

36. Enzler MA, Ruoss M, Seifert B, Berger M. The influence of gender on the outcome of arterial procedures in the lower extremity. *Eur J Vasc Endovasc Surg.* 1996;11(4):446-452.

37. Norman PE, Semmens JB, Lawrence-Brown M, Holman CD. The influence of gender on outcome following peripheral vascular surgery: a review. *Cardiovasc Surg.* 2000;8(2):111-115.

38. Magnant JG, Cronenwett JL, Walsh DB, Schneider JR, Besso SR, Zwolak RM. Surgical treatment of infrainguinal arterial occlusive disease in women. *J Vasc Surg.* 1993;17(1):67-76; discussion 76-68.

39. Gardner AW, Poehlman ET. Exercise rehabilitation programs for the treatment of claudication pain. A meta-analysis. *JAMA.* 1995;274(12):975-980.

40. Frangos SG, Karimi S, Kerstein MD, et al. Gender does not impact infrainguinal vein bypass graft outcome. *Surgery.* 2000;127(6):679-686.

41. Hale WE, Marks RG, May FE, Moore MT, Stewart RB. Epidemiology of intermittent claudication: evaluation of risk factors. *Age Ageing.* 1988;17(1):57-60.

42. Kannel WB, McGee DL. Update on some epidemiologic features of intermittent claudication: the Framingham Study. *J Am Geriatr Soc.* 1985;33(1):13-18.

43. Grady D, Herrington D, Bittner V, et al. Cardiovascular disease outcomes during 6.8 years of hormone therapy: heart and Estrogen/progestin Replacement Study follow-up (HERS II). *JAMA.* 2002;288(1):49-57.

44. Hsia J, Criqui MH, Rodabough RJ, et al. Estrogen plus progestin and the risk of peripheral arterial disease: the Women's Health Initiative. *Circulation.* 2004;109(5):620-626.

45. Angerer P, Stork S, Kothny W, Schmitt P, von Schacky C. Effect of oral postmenopausal hormone replacement on progression of atherosclerosis : a randomized, controlled trial. *Arterioscler Thromb Vasc Biol.* 2001;21(2):262-268.

46. Byington RP, Furberg CD, Herrington DM, et al. Effect of estrogen plus progestin on progression of carotid

arterial disease: the Study of Osteoporotic Fractures. *J Am Geriatr Soc.* 1994;42(9):923-929.

atherosclerosis in postmenopausal women with heart disease: HERS B-mode substudy. *Arterioscler Thromb Vasc Biol.* 2002;22(10):1692-1697.

47. Angerer P, Stork S, Kothny W, von Schacky C. Effect of postmenopausal hormone replacement on atherosclerosis in femoral arteries. *Maturitas.* 2002;41(1):51-60.

48. Westendorp IC, in't Veld BA, Grobbee DE, et al. Hormone replacement therapy and peripheral arterial disease: the Rotterdam study. *Arch Intern Med.* 2000;160(16):2498-2502.

49. Gerhard M, Walsh BW, Tawakol A, et al. Estradiol therapy combined with progesterone and endothelium-dependent vasodilation in postmenopausal women. *Circulation.* 1998; 98(12):1158-1163.

50. Lieberman EH, Gerhard MD, Uehata A, et al. Estrogen improves endothelium-dependent, flow-mediated vasodilation in postmenopausal women. *Ann Intern Med.* 1994;121(12): 936-941.

51. Hodis HN, Mack WJ, Lobo RA, et al. Estrogen in the prevention of atherosclerosis. A randomized, double-blind, placebo-controlled trial. *Ann Intern Med.* 2001;135(11): 939-953.

52. Le Gal G, Gourlet V, Hogrel P, Plu-Bureau G, Touboul PJ, Scarabin PY. Hormone replacement therapy use is associated with a lower occurrence of carotid atherosclerotic plaques but not with intima-media thickness progression among postmenopausal women. The vascular aging (EVA) study. *Atherosclerosis.* 2003;166(1):163-170.

53. Foulkes MA, Wolf PA, Price TR, Mohr JP, Hier DB. The Stroke Data Bank: design, methods, and baseline characteristics. *Stroke.* 1988;19(5):547-554.

54. Thorvaldsen P, Asplund K, Kuulasmaa K, Rajakangas AM, Schroll M. Stroke incidence, case fatality, and mortality in the WHO MONICA project. World Health Organization Monitoring Trends and Determinants in Cardiovascular Disease. *Stroke.* 1995;26(3):361-367.

55. Incidence of stroke in Oxfordshire: first year's experience of a community stroke register. *Br Med J (Clin Res Ed).* 1983;287(6394):713-717.

56. Gross CR, Kase CS, Mohr JP, Cunningham SC, Baker WE. Stroke in south Alabama: incidence and diagnostic features—a population based study. *Stroke.* 1984;15(2):249-255.

57. Reunanen A, Aho K, Aromaa A, Knekt P. Incidence of stroke in a Finnish prospective population study. *Stroke.* 1986; 17(4):675-681.

58. Boysen G, Nyboe J, Appleyard M, et al. Stroke incidence and risk factors for stroke in Copenhagen, Denmark. *Stroke.* 1988;19(11):1345-1353.

59. Ricci S, Celani MG, Guercini G, et al. First-year results of a community-based study of stroke incidence in Umbria, Italy. *Stroke.* 1989;20(7):853-857.

60. Lauria G, Gentile M, Fassetta G, et al. Incidence and prognosis of stroke in the Belluno province, Italy. First-year results of a community-based study. *Stroke.* 1995;26(10):1787-1793.

61. Stegmayr B, Asplund K, Kuulasmaa K, Rajakangas AM, Thorvaldsen P, Tuomilehto J. Stroke incidence and mortality correlated to stroke risk factors in the WHO MONICA Project. An ecological study of 18 populations. *Stroke.* 1997;28(7):1367-1374.

62. Sudlow CL, Warlow CP. Comparable studies of the incidence of stroke and its pathological types: results from an international collaboration. International Stroke Incidence Collaboration. *Stroke.* 1997;28(3):491-499.

63. Murphy SJ, McCullough LD, Smith JM. Stroke in the female: role of biological sex and estrogen. *Ilar J.* 2004;45(2):147-159.

64. Ellekjaer H, Holmen J, Indredavik B, Terent A. Epidemiology of stroke in Innherred, Norway, 1994 to 1996. Incidence and 30-day case-fatality rate. *Stroke.* 1997;28(11):2180-2184.

65. American Heart Association. 2002 Heart and Stroke Statistical Update. http://www.americanheart.org/statistics.

66. Wyller TB, Bautz-Holter E, Holmen J. Prevalence of stroke and stroke-related disability in North Trondelag county, Norway. *Cerebrovasc Dis.* 1994;4:421-427.

67. Geddes JM, Fear J, Tennant A, Pickering A, Hillman M, Chamberlain MA. Prevalence of self reported stroke in a population in northern England. *J Epidemiol Community Health.* 1996;50(2):140-143.

68. Bonita R, Solomon N, Broad JB. Prevalence of stroke and stroke-related disability. Estimates from the Auckland stroke studies. *Stroke.* 1997;28(10):1898-1902.

69. Wyller TB. Stroke and gender. *J Gend Specif Med.* 1999;2(3): 41-45.

70. Bonita R. Epidemiology of stroke. *Lancet.* 1992;339(8789): 342-344.

71. Niewada M, Kobayashi A, Sandercock PA, Kaminski B, Czlonkowska A. Influence of gender on baseline features and clinical outcomes among 17,370 patients with confirmed ischaemic stroke in the international stroke trial. *Neuroepidemiology.* 2005;24(3):123-128.

72. Di Carlo A, Lamassa M, Baldereschi M, et al. Sex differences in the clinical presentation, resource use, and 3-month outcome of acute stroke in Europe: data from a multicenter multinational hospital-based registry. *Stroke.* 2003;34(5): 1114-1119.

73. Sacco RL, Wolf PA, Kannel WB, McNamara PM. Survival and recurrence following stroke. The Framingham study. *Stroke.* 1982;13(3):290-295.

74. Bronner LL, Kanter DS, Manson JE. Primary prevention of stroke. *N Engl J Med.* 1995;333(21):1392-1400.

75. Khaw KT. Epidemiology of stroke. *J Neurol Neurosurg Psychiatry.* 1996;61(4):333-338.

76. Shinton R, Beevers G. Meta-analysis of relation between cigarette smoking and stroke. *BMJ.* 1989;298(6676):789-794.

77. Tuomilehto J, Rastenyte D, Jousilahti P, Sarti C, Vartiainen E. Diabetes mellitus as a risk factor for death from stroke. Prospective study of the middle-aged Finnish population. *Stroke.* 1996;27(2):210-215.

78. Heinemann LA, Lewis MA, Thorogood M, Spitzer WO, Guggenmoos-Holzmann I, Bruppacher R. Case-control study of oral contraceptives and risk of thromboembolic stroke: results from International Study on Oral Contraceptives and Health of Young Women. *BMJ.* 1997;315(7121): 1502-1504.

79. Beral V, Hermon C, Kay C, Hannaford P, Darby S, Reeves G. Mortality associated with oral contraceptive use: 25 year follow up of cohort of 46 000 women from Royal

College of General Practitioners' oral contraception study. *BMJ.* 1999;318(7176):96-100.

80. Ischaemic stroke and combined oral contraceptives: results of an international, multicentre, case-control study. WHO Collaborative Study of Cardiovascular Disease and Steroid Hormone Contraception. *Lancet.* 1996;348(9026):498-505.

81. Haemorrhagic stroke, overall stroke risk, and combined oral contraceptives: results of an international, multicentre, case-control study. WHO Collaborative Study of Cardiovascular Disease and Steroid Hormone Contraception. *Lancet.* 1996;348(9026):505-510.

82. Petitti DB, Sidney S, Bernstein A, Wolf S, Quesenberry C, Ziel HK. Stroke in users of low-dose oral contraceptives. *N Engl J Med.* 1996;335(1):8-15.

83. Schwartz SM, Petitti DB, Siscovick DS, et al. Stroke and use of low-dose oral contraceptives in young women: a pooled analysis of two US studies. *Stroke.* 1998;29(11):2277-2284.

84. Wassertheil-Smoller S, Hendrix SL, Limacher M, et al. Effect of estrogen plus progestin on stroke in postmenopausal women: the Women's Health Initiative: a randomized trial. *JAMA.* 2003;289(20):2673-2684.

85. Viscoli CM, Brass LM, Kernan WN, Sarrel PM, Suissa S, Horwitz RI. A clinical trial of estrogen-replacement therapy after ischemic stroke. *N Engl J Med.* 2001;345(17):1243-1249.

86. Holroyd-Leduc JM, Kapral MK, Austin PC, Tu JV. Sex differences and similarities in the management and outcome of stroke patients. *Stroke.* 2000;31(8):1833-1837.

87. Anderson CS, Jamrozik KD, Burvill PW, Chakera TM, Johnson GA, Stewart-Wynne EG. Determining the incidence of different subtypes of stroke: results from the Perth Community Stroke Study, 1989–1990. *Med J Aust.* 1993;158(2):85-89.

88. Davis P. Stroke in women. *Curr Opin Neurol.* 1994;7(1):36-40.

89. Cabin HS, Clubb KS, Hall C, Perlmutter RA, Feinstein AR. Risk for systemic embolization of atrial fibrillation without mitral stenosis. *Am J Cardiol.* 1990;65(16):1112-1116.

90. Roquer J, Campello AR, Gomis M. Sex differences in first-ever acute stroke. *Stroke.* 2003;34(7):1581-1585.

91. Caplan LR, Gorelick PB, Hier DB. Race, sex and occlusive cerebrovascular disease: a review. *Stroke.* 1986;17(4):648-655.

92. Patrick SJ, Concato J, Viscoli C, Chyatte D, Brass LM. Sex differences in the management of patients hospitalized with ischemic cerebrovascular disease. *Stroke.* 1995;26(4):577-580.

93. Libman RB, Kwiatkowski TG, Hansen MD, Clarke WR, Woolson RF, Adams HP. Differences between anterior and posterior circulation stroke in TOAST. *Cerebrovasc Dis.* 2001;11(4):311-316.

94. Glader EL, Stegmayr B, Norrving B, et al. Sex differences in management and outcome after stroke: a Swedish national perspective. *Stroke.* 2003;34(8):1970-1975.

95. Kelly-Hayes M, Wolf PA, Kannel WB, Sytkowski P, D'Agostino RB, Gresham GE. Factors influencing survival and need for institutionalization following stroke: the Framingham Study. *Arch Phys Med Rehabil.* 1988;69(6):415-418.

96. Leibson CL, Ransom JE, Brown RD, O'Fallon WM, Hass SL, Whisnant JP. Stroke-attributable nursing home use: a population-based study. *Neurology.* 1998;51(1):163-168.

97. Wyller TB, Sodring KM, Sveen U, Ljunggren AE, Bautz-Holter E. Are there gender differences in functional outcome after stroke? *Clin Rehabil.* 1997;11(2):171-179.

98. Sheikh K, Brennan PJ, Meade TW, Smith DS, Goldenberg E. Predictors of mortality and disability in stroke. *J Epidemiol Community Health.* 1983;37(1):70-74.

99. Tatemichi TK, Desmond DW, Stern Y, Paik M, Sano M, Bagiella E. Cognitive impairment after stroke: frequency, patterns, and relationship to functional abilities. *J Neurol Neurosurg Psychiatry.* 1994;57(2):202-207.

100. Lofgren B, Nyberg L, Osterlind PO, Gustafson Y. Inpatient rehabilitation after stroke: outcome and factors associated with improvement. *Disabil Rehabil.* 1998;20(2):55-61.

101. Kotila M, Numminen H, Waltimo O, Kaste M. Depression after stroke: results of the FINNSTROKE Study. *Stroke.* 1998;29(2):368-372.

102. Andersen G, Vestergaard K, Ingemann-Nielsen M, Lauritzen L. Risk factors for post-stroke depression. *Acta Psychiatr Scand.* 1995;92(3):193-198.

103. Stenager EN, Madsen C, Stenager E, Boldsen J. Suicide in patients with stroke: epidemiological study. *BMJ.* 18 1998;316(7139):1206.

104. Tuomilehto J, Rastenyte D, Sivenius J, et al. Ten-year trends in stroke incidence and mortality in the FINMONICA Stroke Study. *Stroke.* 1996;27(5):825-832.

105. Modan B, Wagener DK. Some epidemiological aspects of stroke: mortality/morbidity trends, age, sex, race, socioeconomic status. *Stroke.* 1992;23(9):1230-1236.

106. Ayala C, Croft JB, Greenlund KJ, et al. Sex differences in US mortality rates for stroke and stroke subtypes by race/ethnicity and age, 1995–1998. *Stroke.* 2002;33(5):1197-1201.

107. Rijbroek A, Wisselink W, Vriens EM, Barkhof F, Lammertsma AA, Rauwerda JA. Asymptomatic carotid artery stenosis: past, present and future. How to improve patient selection? *Eur Neurol.* 2006;56(3):139-154.

108. Hill AB. Should patients be screened for asymptomatic carotid artery stenosis? *Can J Surg.* 1998;41(3):208-213.

109. Mathiesen EB, Joakimsen O, Bonaa KH. Prevalence of and risk factors associated with carotid artery stenosis: the Tromso Study. *Cerebrovasc Dis.* 2001;12(1):44-51.

110. Halliday A, Mansfield A, Marro J, et al. Prevention of disabling and fatal strokes by successful carotid endarterectomy in patients without recent neurological symptoms: randomised controlled trial. *Lancet.* 8 2004;363(9420):1491-1502.

111. Goldstein LB, Samsa GP, Matchar DB, Oddone EZ. Multicenter review of preoperative risk factors for endarterectomy for asymptomatic carotid artery stenosis. *Stroke.* 1998;29(4):750-753.

112. Rothwell PM, Slattery J, Warlow CP. Clinical and angiographic predictors of stroke and death from carotid endarterectomy: systematic review. *BMJ.* 1997;315(7122):1571-1577.

113. Endarterectomy for asymptomatic carotid artery stenosis.

Executive Committee for the Asymptomatic Carotid Atherosclerosis Study. *JAMA.* 1995;273(18):1421-1428.

114. Rothwell PM. ACST: which subgroups will benefit most from carotid endarterectomy? *Lancet.* 2004;364(9440): 1122-1123; author reply 1125-1126.

115. Beneficial effect of carotid endarterectomy in symptomatic patients with high-grade carotid stenosis. North American Symptomatic Carotid Endarterectomy Trial Collaborators. *N Engl J Med.* 1991;325(7):445-453.

116. Barnett HJ, Taylor DW, Eliasziw M, et al. Benefit of carotid endarterectomy in patients with symptomatic moderate or severe stenosis. North American Symptomatic Carotid Endarterectomy Trial Collaborators. *N Engl J Med.* 1998;339(20):1415-1425.

117. Chambers BR, You RX, Donnan GA. Carotid endarterectomy for asymptomatic carotid stenosis. *Cochrane Database Syst Rev.* 2000(2):CD001923.

118. Akbari CM, Pulling MC, Pomposelli FB, Jr., Gibbons GW, Campbell DR, Logerfo FW. Gender and carotid endarterectomy: does it matter? *J Vasc Surg.* 2000;31(6):1103-1108; discussion 1108-1109.

119. Rockman CB, Castillo J, Adelman MA, et al. Carotid endarterectomy in female patients: are the concerns of the Asymptomatic Carotid Atherosclerosis Study valid? *J Vasc Surg.* 2001;33(2):236-240; discussion 240-231.

120. Mendelsohn ME, Karas RH. Molecular and cellular basis of cardiovascular gender differences. *Science.* 2005;308(5728): 1583-1587.

121. Iemolo F, Martiniuk A, Steinman DA, Spence JD. Sex differences in carotid plaque and stenosis. *Stroke.* 2004;35(2):477-481.

122. Hellings WE, Pasterkamp G, Verhoeven BA, et al. Gender-associated differences in plaque phenotype of patients undergoing carotid endarterectomy. *J Vasc Surg.* 2007;45(2):289-296; discussion 296-287.

123. Tumelero RT, Duda NT, Tognon AP, Thiesen M. Prevalence of renal artery stenosis in 1,656 patients who have undergone cardiac catheterization. *Arq Bras Cardiol.* 2006;87(3):248-253.

124. Tanemoto M, Saitoh H, Satoh F, Satoh H, Abe T, Ito S. Predictors of undiagnosed renal artery stenosis among Japanese patients with risk factors of atherosclerosis. *Hypertens Res.* 2005;28(3):237-242.

125. Buller CE, Nogareda JG, Ramanathan K, et al. The profile of cardiac patients with renal artery stenosis. *J Am Coll Cardiol.* 2004;43(9):1606-1613.

126. Ji H, Pesce C, Zheng W, et al. Sex differences in renal injury and nitric oxide production in renal wrap hypertension. *Am J Physiol Heart Circ Physiol.* 2005;288(1):H43-H47.

127. Rogers JL, Mitchell AR, Maric C, Sandberg K, Myers A, Mulroney SE. Effect of sex hormones on renal estrogen and angiotensin type 1 receptors in female and male rats. *Am J Physiol Regul Integr Comp Physiol.* 2007;292(2):R794-R799.

128. Ahmed SB, Fisher ND, Hollenberg NK. Gender and the renal nitric oxide synthase system in healthy humans. *Clin J Am Soc Nephrol.* 2007;2(5):926-931.

129. Olin JW. Recognizing and managing fibromuscular dysplasia. *Cleve Clin J Med.* 2007;74(4):273-274, 277-282.

130. Slovut DP, Olin JW. Fibromuscular dysplasia. *N Engl J Med.* 2004;350(18):1862-1871.

131. Chrysostomou A, Pedagogos E, MacGregor L, Becker GJ. Double-blind, placebo-controlled study on the effect of the aldosterone receptor antagonist spironolactone in patients who have persistent proteinuria and are on long-term angiotensin-converting enzyme inhibitor therapy, with or without an angiotensin II receptor blocker. *Clin J Am Soc Nephrol.* 2006;1(2):256-262.

132. Douglas K, O'Malley PG, Jackson JL. Meta-analysis: the effect of statins on albuminuria. *Ann Intern Med.* 2006;145(2): 117-124.

133. Harjai K, Khosla S, Shaw D, et al. Effect of gender on outcomes following renal artery stent placement for renovascular hypertension. *Cathet Cardiovasc Diagn.* 1997;42(4):381-386.

134. Burket MW, Cooper CJ, Kennedy DJ, et al. Renal artery angioplasty and stent placement: predictors of a favorable outcome. *Am Heart J.* 2000;139(1 Pt 1):64-71.

135. Chonchol M, Linas S. Diagnosis and management of ischemic nephropathy. *Clin J Am Soc Nephrol.* 2006;1(2):172-181.

136. Pearce JD, Craven BL, Craven TE, et al. Progression of atherosclerotic renovascular disease: a prospective population-based study. *J Vasc Surg.* 2006;44(5):955-962; discussion 962-953.

137. Zeller T, Frank U, Muller C, et al. Predictors of improved renal function after percutaneous stent-supported angioplasty of severe atherosclerotic ostial renal artery stenosis. *Circulation.* 2003;108(18):2244-2249.

138. Gill-Leertouwer TC, Gussenhoven EJ, Bosch JL, et al. Predictors for clinical success at one year following renal artery stent placement. *J Endovasc Ther.* 2002;9(4):495-502.

139. Surowiec SM, Sivamurthy N, Rhodes JM, et al. Percutaneous therapy for renal artery fibromuscular dysplasia. *Ann Vasc Surg.* 2003;17(6):650-655.

140. Bjornsson J, Edwards WD. Primary pulmonary hypertension: a histopathologic study of 80 cases. *Mayo Clin Proc.* 1985; 60(1):16-25.

141. Gaine SP, Rubin LJ. Primary pulmonary hypertension. *Lancet.* 1998;352(9129):719-725.

142. Rich S, Dantzker DR, Ayres SM, et al. Primary pulmonary hypertension. A national prospective study. *Ann Intern Med.* 1987;107(2):216-223.

143. Runo JR, Loyd JE. Primary pulmonary hypertension. *Lancet.* 2003;361(9368):1533-1544.

144. Robles AM, Shure D. Gender issues in pulmonary vascular disease. *Clin Chest Med.* 2004;25(2):373-377.

145. Loyd JE, Butler MG, Foroud TM, Conneally PM, Phillips JA, 3rd, Newman JH. Genetic anticipation and abnormal gender ratio at birth in familial primary pulmonary hypertension. *Am J Respir Crit Care Med.* 1995;152(1):93-97.

146. Deng Z, Morse JH, Slager SL, et al. Familial primary pulmonary hypertension (gene PPH1) is caused by mutations in the bone morphogenetic protein receptor-II gene. *Am J Hum Genet.* 2000;67(3):737-744.

147. Lane KB, Machado RD, Pauciulo MW, et al. Heterozygous germline mutations in BMPR2, encoding a TGF-beta receptor,

cause familial primary pulmonary hypertension. The International PPH Consortium. *Nat Genet*. 2000;26(1): 81-84.

148. Kay JM, Smith P, Heath D. Aminorex and the pulmonary circulation. *Thorax*. 1971;26(3):262-270.

149. Abenhaim L, Moride Y, Brenot F, et al. Appetite-suppressant drugs and the risk of primary pulmonary hypertension. International Primary Pulmonary Hypertension Study Group. *N Engl J Med*. 1996;335(9):609-616.

150. Horton KM, Talamini MA, Fishman EK. Median arcuate ligament syndrome: evaluation with CT angiography. *Radiographics*. 2005;25(5):1177-1182.

151. Lindner HH, Kemprud E. A clinicoanatomical study of the arcuate ligament of the diaphragm. *Arch Surg*. 1971;103(5): 600-605.

152. Sproat IA, Pozniak MA, Kennell TW. US case of the day. Median arcuate ligament syndrome (celiac artery compression syndrome). *Radiographics*. 1993;13(6):1400-1402.

153. Dunbar JD, Molnar W, Beman FF, Marable SA. Compression of the celiac trunk and abdominal angina. *Am J Roentgenol Radium Ther Nucl Med*. 1965;95(3):731-744.

154. Newman AB, Arnold AM, Burke GL, O'Leary DH, Manolio TA. Cardiovascular disease and mortality in older adults with small abdominal aortic aneurysms detected by ultrasonography: the cardiovascular health study. *Ann Intern Med*. 2001;134(3):182-190.

155. Lederle FA, Johnson GR, Wilson SE, et al. Prevalence and associations of abdominal aortic aneurysm detected through screening. Aneurysm Detection and Management (ADAM) Veterans Affairs Cooperative Study Group. *Ann Intern Med*. 1997;126(6):441-449.

156. Blanchard JF, Armenian HK, Friesen PP. Risk factors for abdominal aortic aneurysm: results of a case-control study. *Am J Epidemiol*. 2000;151(6):575-583.

157. Lederle FA, Johnson GR, Wilson SE. Abdominal aortic aneurysm in women. *J Vasc Surg*. 2001;34(1):122-126.

158. Brown LC, Powell JT. Risk factors for aneurysm rupture in patients kept under ultrasound surveillance. UK Small Aneurysm Trial Participants. *Ann Surg*. 1999;230(3):289-296; discussion 296-287.

159. Semmens JB, Norman PE, Lawrence-Brown MM, Holman CD. Influence of gender on outcome from ruptured abdominal aortic aneurysm. *Br J Surg*. 2000;87(2):191-194.

160. Katz DJ, Stanley JC, Zelenock GB. Gender differences in abdominal aortic aneurysm prevalence, treatment, and outcome. *J Vasc Surg*. 1997;25(3):561-568.

161. Sonesson B, Hansen F, Stale H, Lanne T. Compliance and diameter in the human abdominal aorta–the influence of age and sex. *Eur J Vasc Surg*. 1993;7(6):690-697.

162. Sonesson B, Lanne T, Hansen F, Sandgren T. Infrarenal aortic diameter in the healthy person. *Eur J Vasc Surg*. 1994;8(1):89-95.

163. Gonzalez-Gay MA, Garcia-Porrua C. Epidemiology of the vasculitides. *Rheum Dis Clin North Am*. 2001;27(4):729-749.

164. Gonzalez-Gay MA, Garcia-Porrua C, Salvarani C, Hunder GG. Diagnostic approach in a patient presenting with polymyalgia. *Clin Exp Rheumatol*. 1999;17(3):276-278.

165. Gonzalez-Gay MA, Garcia-Porrua C. Systemic vasculitis in

adults in northwestern Spain, 1988–1997. Clinical and epidemiologic aspects. *Medicine (Baltimore)*. 1999;78(5):292-308.

166. Numano F. Differences in clinical presentation and outcome in different countries for Takayasu's arteritis. *Curr Opin Rheumatol*. 1997;9(1):12-15.

167. Koide K. Takayasu arteritis in Japan. *Heart Vessels Suppl*. 1992;7:48-54.

168. Park YB, Hong SK, Choi KJ, et al. Takayasu arteritis in Korea: clinical and angiographic features. *Heart Vessels Suppl*. 1992; 7:55-59.

169. Subramanyan R, Joy J, Balakrishnan KG. Natural history of aortoarteritis (Takayasu's disease). *Circulation*. 1989;80(3):429-437.

170. Zheng D, Fan D, Liu L. Takayasu arteritis in China: a report of 530 cases. *Heart Vessels Suppl*. 1992;7:32-36.

171. Kerr GS. Takayasu's arteritis. *Rheum Dis Clin North Am*. 1995;21(4):1041-1058.

172. Chugh KS, Jain S, Sakhuja V, et al. Renovascular hypertension due to Takayasu's arteritis among Indian patients. *Q J Med*. 1992;85(307-308):833-843.

173. Deutsch V, Wexler L, Deutsch H. Takayasu's arteritis. An angiographic study with remarks on ethnic distribution in Israel. *Am J Roentgenol Radium Ther Nucl Med*. 1974;122(1):13-28.

174. Watts RA, Lane SE, Bentham G, Scott DG. Epidemiology of systemic vasculitis: a ten-year study in the United Kingdom. *Arthritis Rheum*. 2000;43(2):414-419.

175. Conn DL. Polyarteritis. *Rheum Dis Clin North Am*. 1990; 16(2):341-362.

176. Kurland LCTHG. The epidemiology of systemic arteritis. In: Shulman L, ed. *The Epidemiology of the Rheumatic Disease*. New York: Grover Publishing; 1984:196-205.

177. Lhote F, Guillevin L. Polyarteritis nodosa, microscopic polyangiitis, and Churg-Strauss syndrome. Clinical aspects and treatment. *Rheum Dis Clin North Am*. 1995;21(4):911-947.

178. Hoffman GS, Kerr GS, Leavitt RY, et al. Wegener granulomatosis: an analysis of 158 patients. *Ann Intern Med*. 15 1992;116(6):488-498.

179. Carruthers DM, Watts RA, Symmons DP, Scott DG. Wegener's granulomatosis–increased incidence or increased recognition? *Br J Rheumatol*. 1996;35(2):142-145.

180. Gonzalez-Gay MG-P, C. Henoch–Schonlein purpura. In: Ball GB, SL, ed. *Vasculitis Textbook*. Oxford: Oxford University Press; 2001.

181. Garcia-Porrua C, Gonzalez-Gay MA. Comparative clinical and epidemiological study of hypersensitivity vasculitis versus Henoch–Schonlein purpura in adults. *Semin Arthritis Rheum*. 1999;28(6):404-412.

182. Watts RA, Jolliffe VA, Grattan CE, Elliott J, Lockwood M, Scott DG. Cutaneous vasculitis in a defined population–clinical and epidemiological associations. *J Rheumatol*. 1998;25(5):920-924.

183. Angerer P, Kothny W, Störk S, von Schacky C. Hormone replacement therapy and distensibility of carotid arteries in postmenopausal women: a randomized, controlled trial. *J Am Coll Cardiol*. 2000;36(6):1789-1796.

chapter 3

Lipids in the Pathogenesis of Peripheral Arterial Disease

Jay Giri, MD, MPH / Emile R. Mohler III, MD, MS

Dyslipidemia is a risk factor for atherosclerosis and PAD. This chapter will address (1) the significance of dyslipidemia in the pathogenesis of PAD, (2) the evidence for dyslipidemia as a risk factor for existence and progression of PAD, and (3) the evidence regarding lipid-modifying therapy in PAD.

Dyslipidemia is a key pathogenic factor predisposing to atherosclerosis. Lipoproteins are instrumental in the initiation of atherosclerotic plaques and their progression to hemodynamically significant lesions that cause arterial insufficiency.

Low-density lipoprotein cholesterol (LDL) is a key driver of the atherosclerotic process. Fatty streaks, the earliest visible sign of atherosclerosis, consist mainly of macrophage-containing foam cells that are full of oxidized LDL.[1] Multiple factors including increased endothelial permeability, retention of lipoproteins in the intima, and sluggish removal of lipoproteins result in accumulation of LDL in the vessel wall.[2-4] Oxidized LDL and its products cause a vigorous inflammatory and proatherogenic response through chemotactic signaling for monocytes, smooth muscle cells, and T lymphocytes.[5,6] Oxidized LDL leads to increased expression of a host of inflammatory factors including vascular cell adhesion molecule-1, monocyte chemoattractant protein-1, intracellular adhesion molecule-1, and macrophage colony stimulating factor.[7-15] The net effect of this is to attract, trap, and tether leukocytes to the endothelium, initiate transformation of monocytes into macrophage foam cells, and enhance smooth muscle cell proliferation in the intima to form an atheroma. Oxidized modification of LDL may also contribute to so-called plaque vulnerability through induction of type 1 metalloproteinase expression and an increase in tissue factor activity.[5] The oxidation of LDL, then, is an initial insult that leads to a cascade of immunologic and vascular events that cause endothelial dysfunction as well as initiation and progression of atherosclerotic plaques (Figure 3-1).

Further supporting the pivotal role of LDL in atherosclerosis, atherosclerotic lesion formation in mice has been inhibited through immunization with products of oxidized LDL.[16-19] Not surprisingly, in numerous human trials, lowering LDL through pharmacological means has been shown to reduce progression of atherosclerosis as well as the incidence of cardiovascular events.[20-28]

Low levels of high-density lipoprotein cholesterol (HDL) also strongly predict cardiovascular events. Low levels of HDL are associated with insufficient reverse cholesterol transport.[29,30] When human ApoA-I, the major protein in HDL, was increased in mice by using liver-directed gene transfer, reverse cholesterol transport was promoted and regression of atherosclerotic lesions was seen.[31,32] Additionally, HDL has antioxidant properties at least partially mediated by paraoxonase—an enzyme associated with HDL that degrades oganophsosphates.[33,34] This presumably allows for protection against oxidation of LDL.

While the above information provides a framework for understanding the mechanisms of atherosclerosis in the vasculature in general, facets specific to the peripheral arteries have not been well studied. Unlike in the coronary arteries, in situ thrombosis in the peripheral arteries resulting in acute limb ischemia is a rare event. This maybe due to differences in the mechanical forces of blood flow through the peripheral arteries when compared to their coronary counterparts, vascular cell heterogeneity, and variation in plaque composition in distinct vascular beds.[35-42] Additionally, recent studies support different pathogenic mechanisms and risk factors for large-vessel, or proximal,

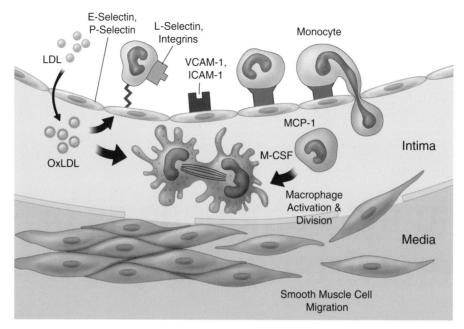

● **FIGURE 3-1.** Oxidized low-density lipoprotein (OxLDL) stimulates induction of inflammatory mediators and cellular adhesion molecules including selectins, vascular cell adhesion molecule-1 (VCAM-1), intracellular adhesion molecule-1 (ICAM-1), monocyte chemoattractant protein-1 (MCP-1), and macrophage colony stimulating factor (M-CSF). Selectins trap leukocytes while VCAM-1 and ICAM-1 promote firm attachment of these leukocytes to the endothelium. MCP-1 further attracts monocytes and also allows cellular flow into the intimal layer. M-CSF is integral in the transformation of monocytes to macrophage foam cells that internalize oxLDL. The early atheromatous lesion becomes a fibrous atheroma through smooth muscle migration into the intimal layer.

PAD versus small-vessel, or distal, PAD.[43,44] However, the latter has not been well studied to this point. For this reason, PAD atherosclerosis is currently hypothesized to be progressive stenosis of the larger peripheral arteries. This has been measured in various ways including symptom indices, Doppler wave forms, and angiography. The current accepted standard test for diagnosis of PAD is the easy, inexpensive ankle-brachial index (ABI). An ABI < 0.9 denotes PAD, and the ABI is a sensitive and specific marker for diagnosis and progression of the disease.[45]

It is important to note that vascular calcification is a common component of peripheral atherosclerotic plaques. The calcification of atherosclerotic plaque is localized to the intimal layer. However, calcification may also occur, especially in patients with diabetes mellitus, in the medial layer causing supranormal ABI. The pathophysiology of intimal vascular calcification is an active process involving extracellular bone matrix proteins in the setting of inflammatory cells.[46] A high calcification content relative to lipid content is indicative of a more stable plaque.[47] More research is needed to determine if plaque rupture or hemorrhage is a significant part of the progression of atherosclerotic lesions in the lower extremities.

● HDL, LDL, AND TRIGLYCERIDES AS RISK FACTORS FOR PAD

There is an abundance of data identifying elevated LDL levels and decreased HDL levels as independent risk factors for coronary atherosclerosis.[20–30] Hypertriglyceridemia has also been shown to confer a more modest amount of increased cardiovascular risk in large epidemiological studies.[48] However, in contrast to studies targeted to reducing LDL, substantial "proof-of-concept" data do not exist regarding treatment of hypertriglyceridemia as a means for decreasing cardiovascular events.

Early studies of patients with PAD revealed positive associations with triglycerides, mixed associations with LDL, and negative associations with HDL.[49–57] Unfortunately, these studies were limited by small sample sizes and inconsistency in the criteria used to define PAD. Large epidemiologic studies using more rigorous statistical methods, including multivariate regression, have helped better define the role of lipid moieties as independent risk factors for the presence of PAD.

An initial analysis of data from the Framingham cohort revealed that there was a 20% increase in risk of intermittent claudication seen for every 40-point increase in total cholesterol.[58] This study was limited by a lack of data on fractionated cholesterol and an insensitive measure of PAD, intermittent claudication. An analysis of data from the Systolic Hypertension in the Elderly Trial revealed univariate positive correlations between LDL, total cholesterol, and triglycerides with PAD as well as a negative correlation with HDL level and PAD.[59] Later studies continued to use the more sensitive measure of ABI <0.9 to define PAD and also used multivariate statistical models to more specifically identify independent risk factors for PAD. For example, a subsequent more detailed analysis of the Framingham Offspring cohort showed a 10% increase in PAD for every five-point decrease in HDL by using multivariate regression.[60] LDL, total cholesterol levels, and triglycerides were not significantly associated with the presence of PAD in this model. In a large epidemiological study of Asian men older than 70 years, multivariate regression revealed an odds ratio for PAD of 1.36 when comparing patients in the highest quintile of total cholesterol to those in the lowest quintile of total cholesterol.[61] With this method, HDL showed a significant inverse association with PAD with an odds ratio of 0.68 in this cohort. LDL and triglycerides were not specifically examined. In the Strong Heart Study examining a diverse population of American Indians, LDL was the only lipid moiety shown to be significantly associated with PAD.[62] A 19% increase in the risk of PAD was seen for every 30-point increase in LDL in this group. In data analyzed from the Cardiovascular Health Study, a population of more than 5000 patients older than 65 years, it was found that HDL decreased with decreasing ABI in all patients.[63] In this cohort, LDL and total cholesterol were significantly associated with PAD in women, but not in their male counterparts. Triglycerides were not shown to be significantly associated with ABI in multivariate analyses. In the Edinburgh Artery Study, multiple regressions of risk factors for PAD revealed inverse associations with HDL, but only univariate associations with triglycerides.[64] Finally, data from a large cohort of physicians showed total cholesterol/HDL ratio to be a stronger predictor of PAD than any individual lipid or inflammatory marker.[65]

In summary, existing data seem to most strongly support decreased HDL levels as an independent risk factor for PAD. Multiple studies also reveal an association between total cholesterol levels and PAD. The data on LDL as an independent PAD risk factor are mixed in large epidemiological studies. However, patients with Fredrickson class IIa dyslipidemia (familial hypercholesterolemia) with an LDL receptor deficiency have a dramatically increased incidence of PAD.[66] Also, patients with Fredrickson class III dyslipidemia, a genetic defect in apoE synthesis leading to increased LDL, have an increased risk of PAD.[67] Lastly, while multiple studies have shown univariate associations between increased triglyceride levels and the presence of PAD, these associations largely disappear with multivariate analysis decreasing the strength of the evidence for hypertriglyceridemia as an independent risk factor for PAD.

Most studies examining risk factors for the progression of PAD have not focused on lipids and instead examined more novel inflammatory markers. A study of 381 patients revealed baseline hypertriglyceridemia to be associated with the progression of PAD for more than 3-year follow-up.[68] Another study examining a group of elderly patients showed LDL levels greater than 147 mg/dL to be associated with declining ABI.[69] In this analysis, association with triglycerides and HDL was not significant. Overall, studies directly examining lipid levels and progression of PAD are scant. However, there have been a number of studies examining the effects of lipid-modifying therapy on functional outcomes in patients with PAD; these are detailed next.

● Lp(a) IN PAD

Lipoprotein(a), or Lp(a), is a modified form of LDL that has been implicated as an independent risk factor for coronary heart disease in patients with hypercholesterolemia.[70] There is also evidence that Lp(a) is associated with acute coronary syndromes and strokes.[71–73]

A number of studies have attempted to establish whether Lp(a) levels are significantly associated with PAD. In a small study comparing 17 patients younger than 45 years with PAD to a control group without PAD, the patients with PAD were 3.9 times more likely to have a high Lp(a) level (greater than 30 mg/dL) than those without PAD.[74] In a post-hoc analysis of the Systolic Hypertension in Elderly Trial, 36% of patients with Lp(a) > 20 mg/dL had an ABI < 0.9 versus only 14% with Lp(a) < 20 mg/dL.[75] In this analysis, levels of Lp(a) were also correlated with disease severity as measured by worsening ABI. A study of Chinese patients with diabetes confirmed these results and noted that diabetic patients with an Lp(a) level > 13.3 mg/dL had a 2.7-fold increased risk of PAD.[76] A study examining novel risk factors for PAD did not find an association between PAD and Lp(a) levels.[65] This study, however, used self-reported claudication as the measure of PAD. This is now known to be a quite insensitive marker for the disease. Finally, a recent trial has shown that baseline Lp(a) levels are correlated with progression of PAD.[43] Overall, existing data have established an inverse correlation between ABI and Lp(a) levels. Lp(a) may also be a risk factor for PAD progression.

● LIPID-MODIFYING THERAPY IN PAD

HMG-Co-A reductase inhibitors (statins) were initially noted as a promising treatment for vascular disease because of their effects on lipids. Statins are now recognized as having positive effects apart from modification of the lipid profile. The so-called pleiotropic effects of statins include stabilization of atheromatous plaques, elevation of endothelial nitric oxide concentration, and reduction of inflammation systemically.[77–79] Pleiotropic properties of statins maybe partially responsible for reductions in cardiovascular events in patients taking the drugs.[80–82]

The Adult Treatment Panel III Guidelines of The National Cholesterol Education Panel label PAD as a coronary heart disease equivalent. According to these recommendations, all patients with PAD should have aggressive management of their LDL with a goal LDL of less than 100.[83] This usually necessitates statin therapy. Large randomized trial data from the Heart Protection Study showed that patients with PAD near this goal and not on a statin received further protection from cardiovascular events with statin therapy.[23] Overall, there are significant data to suggest that treatment of PAD with statins confers protection against cardiac events.

There is also an emerging body of literature regarding the direct functional impact of statins on leg functioning in

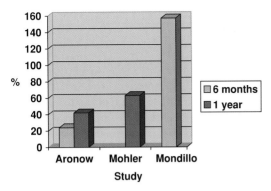

● **FIGURE 3-2.** Percentage improvement in treadmill walking among PAD patients on statins. The Aronow Trial[86] used 40 mg simvastatin and measured pain-free walking times. The Mohler (acronym TREADMILL) Trial[87] used 80 mg of atorvastatin and measured pain-free walking times. The Mondillo Trial[88] used 40 mg of simvastatin and measured pain-free walking distances.

PAD. A cross-sectional analysis showed that patients with PAD on statins had better objective measures of leg functioning (6-minute walk time and 4-m walking velocities) than their counterparts not on statins.[84] Three-year follow-up data of this cohort showed that PAD participants using statins had less annual decline in measures of lower extremity performance compared to nonusers.[85] Three placebo-controlled randomized trials have evaluated statin use in patients with PAD with intermittent claudication (Figure 3-2).[86–88] All showed improvements in pain-free walking time or distance in groups of patients with PAD on statins. However, two of the trials showed conflicting results regarding maximal walking capacity in these patients, with one demonstrating significant improvement in maximal treadmill walking distance and the other showing no significant improvement in maximal treadmill walking time.

In these trials, total cholesterol and LDL levels were predictably lower in patients on statins. However, ABI, when measured, did not show a significant change with statin therapy. This is not surprising as statins do not have dramatic effects on arterial plaque regression.[89] It is possible that anti-inflammatory effects of statins explained the association of statin use with decreased functional decline. Sarcopenia, an age-related decline in muscle strength and mass, maybe fueled by systemic inflammation.[90–92] Statins may help slow this process and improve endothelial function in peripheral arteries.[93] This beneficial effect may occur via mobilization of endothelial progenitor cells from the bone marrow. Exercise may also raise circulating bone marrow derived endothelial progenitor cells, but the clinical significance of this effect on exercise performance is unknown.[94]

Beyond statins, both fibrates and niacin have demonstrated favorable affects upon the lipid profile—particularly for hypertriglyceridemia and low HDL-c. In the Arterial Biology for the Investigation of the Treatment Effects of Reducing Cholesterol 3 Trial, patients receiving extended release niacin had a regression in the carotid intimal medial thickness measurements. In a multifactorial analysis, these changes were independently associated with increases in the HDL-c. Extended release niacin has been associated with 24% increases in HDL-c, 16% reduction in LDL-c, 25% reduction in Lp(a), and 32% reduction in triglyceride levels.[95]

In summary, there is a strong evidence to suggest that all patients with PAD should be prescribed statins for the benefits provided in symptomatic claudication and leg functioning. Additionally, statins provide important secondary prevention against future cardiovascular events in patients with PAD. The positive impact of statins in PAD is likely only partially related to effects on the lipid profile.

REFERENCES

1. Ross R. Atherosclerosis—an inflammatory disease [see comment]. *N Engl J Med.* 1999;340:115-126.

2. Schwenke DC. Comparison of aorta and pulmonary artery: II. LDL transport and metabolism correlate with susceptibility to atherosclerosis. *Circ Res.* 1997;81:346-354.

3. Schwenke DC. Comparison of aorta and pulmonary artery: I. Early cholesterol accumulation and relative susceptibility to atheromatous lesions. *Circ Res.* 1997;81:338-345.

4. Camejo G, Hurt-Camejo E, Wiklund O, Bondjers G. Association of apo B lipoproteins with arterial proteoglycans: pathological significance and molecular basis. *Atherosclerosis.* 1998;139:205-222.

5. Steinberg D. Atherogenesis in perspective: hypercholesterolemia and inflammation as partners in crime. *Nat Med.* 2002;8:1211-1217.

6. Navab M, Hama SY, Reddy ST, et al. Oxidized lipids as mediators of coronary heart disease [erratum appears in Curr Opin Lipidol. 2002 Oct;13(5):589 Note: Ready Srinu T [corrected to Reddy Srinu T]]. *Curr Opin Lipidol.* 2002;13:363-372.

7. Dansky HM, Barlow CB, Lominska C, et al. Adhesion of monocytes to arterial endothelium and initiation of atherosclerosis are critically dependent on vascular cell adhesion molecule-1 gene dosage. *Arterioscler Thromb Vasc Biol.* 2001;21:1662-1667.

8. Cybulsky MI, Gimbrone MA, Jr. Endothelial expression of a mononuclear leukocyte adhesion molecule during atherogenesis. *Science.* 1991;251:788-791.

9. Cybulsky MI, Iiyama K, Li H, et al. A major role for VCAM-1, but not ICAM-1, in early atherosclerosis [see comment]. *J Clin Invest.* 2001;107:1255-1262.

10. Collins RG, Velji R, Guevara NV, Hicks MJ, Chan L, Beaudet AL. P-Selectin or intercellular adhesion molecule (ICAM)-1 deficiency substantially protects against atherosclerosis in apolipoprotein E-deficient mice. *J Exp Med.* 2000;191:189-194.

11. Boring L, Gosling J, Cleary M, Charo IF. Decreased lesion formation in CCR2-/- mice reveals a role for chemokines in the initiation of atherosclerosis. *Nature.* 1998;394:894-897.

12. Gu L, Okada Y, Clinton SK, et al. Absence of monocyte chemoattractant protein-1 reduces atherosclerosis in low density lipoprotein receptor-deficient mice. *Mol Cell.* 1998;2:275-281.

13. Gosling J, Slaymaker S, Gu L, et al. MCP-1 deficiency reduces susceptibility to atherosclerosis in mice that overexpress human apolipoprotein B. *J Clin Invest.* 1999;103:773-778.

14. Smith JD, Trogan E, Ginsberg M, Grigaux C, Tian J, Miyata M. Decreased atherosclerosis in mice deficient in both macrophage colony-stimulating factor (op) and apolipoprotein E. *Proc Natl Acad Sci USA.* 1995;92:8264-8268.

15. Rajavashisth TB, Andalibi A, Territo MC, et al. Induction of endothelial cell expression of granulocyte and macrophage colony-stimulating factors by modified low-density lipoproteins. *Nature.* 1990;344:254-257.

16. Palinski W, Ord VA, Plump AS, Breslow JL, Steinberg D, Witztum JL. ApoE-deficient mice are a model of lipoprotein oxidation in atherogenesis. Demonstration of oxidation–specific epitopes in lesions and high titers of autoantibodies to malondialdehyde-lysine in serum. *Arterioscler Thromb.* 1994;14:605-616.

17. Ameli S, Hultgardh-Nilsson A, Regnstrom J, et al. Effect of immunization with homologous LDL and oxidized LDL on early atherosclerosis in hypercholesterolemic rabbits. *Arterioscler Thromb Vasc Biol.* 1996;16:1074-1079.

18. Freigang S, Horkko S, Miller E, Witztum JL, Palinski W. Immunization of LDL receptor-deficient mice with homologous malondialdehyde-modified and native LDL reduces progression of atherosclerosis by mechanisms other than induction of high titers of antibodies to oxidative neoepitopes. *Arterioscler Thromb Vasc Biol.* 1998;18:1972-1982.

19. Zhou X, Caligiuri G, Hamsten A, Lefvert AK, Hansson GK. LDL immunization induces T-cell-dependent antibody formation and protection against atherosclerosis. *Arterioscler Thromb Vasc Biol.* 2001;21:108-114.

20. Randomised trial of cholesterol lowering in 4444 patients with coronary heart disease: the Scandinavian Simvastatin Survival Study (4S) [see comment]. *Lancet.* 1994;344:1383-1389.

21. Sacks FM, Pfeffer MA, Moye LA, et al. The effect of pravastatin on coronary events after myocardial infarction in patients with average cholesterol levels. Cholesterol and Recurrent Events Trial investigators [see comment]. *N Engl J Med.* 1996;335:1001-1009.

22. Tonkin AM, Colquhoun D, Emberson J, et al. Effects of pravastatin in 3260 patients with unstable angina: results from the LIPID study [see comment]. *Lancet.* 2000;356:1871-1875.

23. Heart Protection Study Collaborative, Group. MRC/BHF Heart Protection Study of cholesterol lowering with simvastatin in 20,536 high-risk individuals: a randomised placebo-controlled trial [see comment] [summary for patients in Curr Cardiol Rep. 2002 Nov;4(6):486-7; PMID: 12379169]. *Lancet.* 2002;360:7-22.

24. Cannon CP, Braunwald E, McCabe CH, et al.; Pravastatin or atorvastatin evaluation and infection therapy—thrombolysis in myocardial infarction 22, investigators. Intensive versus moderate lipid lowering with statins after acute coronary syndromes [see comment] [erratum appears in N Engl J Med. 2006 Feb 16;354(7):778]. *N Engl J Med.* 2004;350:1495-1504.

25. Pedersen TR, Faergeman O, Kastelein JJ, et al.; Incremental Decrease in End Points Through Aggressive Lipid Lowering (IDEAL) Study Group. High-dose atorvastatin vs usual-dose simvastatin for secondary prevention after myocardial infarction: the IDEAL study: a randomized controlled trial [see comment]. *JAMA.* 2005;294:2437-2445.

26. LaRosa JC, Grundy SM, Waters DD, et al.; Treating to New Targets (TNT) Investigators. Intensive lipid lowering with atorvastatin in patients with stable coronary disease [see comment]. *N Engl J Med.* 2005;352:1425-1435.

27. de Lemos JA, Blazing MA, Wiviott SD, et al. Early intensive vs. a delayed conservative simvastatin strategy in patients with acute coronary syndromes: phase Z of the A to Z trial. [see comment]. *JAMA.* 2004;292:1307-1316.

28. Nissen SE, Tuzcu EM, Schoenhagen P, et al.; REVERSAL I. Effect of intensive compared with moderate lipid-lowering therapy on progression of coronary atherosclerosis: a randomized controlled trial [see comment]. *JAMA.* 2004;291:1071-1080.

29. Gordon T, Kannel WB, Castelli WP, Dawber TR. Lipoproteins, cardiovascular disease, and death. The Framingham study. *Arch Intern Med.* 1981;141:1128-1131.

30. Rader DJ. Regulation of reverse cholesterol transport and clinical implications. *Am J Cardiol.* 2003;92:42J-49J.

31. Tangirala RK, Tsukamoto K, Chun SH, Usher D, Pure E, Rader DJ. Regression of atherosclerosis induced by liver-directed gene transfer of apolipoprotein A-I in mice [see comment]. *Circulation.* 1999;100:1816-1822.

32. Zhang Y, Zanotti I, Reilly MP, Glick JM, Rothblat GH, Rader DJ. Overexpression of apolipoprotein A-I promotes reverse transport of cholesterol from macrophages to feces in vivo. *Circulation.* 2003;108:661-663.

33. Shih DM, Gu L, Xia YR, et al. Mice lacking serum paraoxonase are susceptible to organophosphate toxicity and atherosclerosis. *Nature.* 1998;394:284-287.

34. Mackness MI, Mackness B, Durrington PN, et al. Paraoxonase and coronary heart disease. *Curr Opin Lipidol.* 1998;9:319-324.

35. Smith EB. Fibrin deposition and fibrin degradation products in atherosclerotic plaques. *Thromb Res.* 1994;75:329-335.

36. Wootton DM, Ku DN. Fluid mechanics of vascular systems, diseases, and thrombosis. *Annu Rev Biomed Eng.* 1999;1:299-329.

37. He X, Ku DN. Pulsatile flow in the human left coronary artery bifurcation: average conditions. *J Biomech Eng.* 1996;118:74-82.

38. Ku DN, Giddens DP, Zarins CK, Glagov S. Pulsatile flow and atherosclerosis in the human carotid bifurcation. Positive correlation between plaque location and low oscillating shear stress. *Arteriosclerosis.* 1985;5:293-302.

39. Badimon JJ, Ortiz AF, Meyer B, et al. Different response to balloon angioplasty of carotid and coronary arteries: effects on acute platelet deposition and intimal thickening. *Atherosclerosis.* 1998;140:307-314.

40. Rosenberg RD. Vascular-bed-specific hemostasis and hypercoagulable states: clinical utility of activation peptide assays in predicting thrombotic events in different clinical populations. *Thromb Haemost.* 2001;86:41-50.

41. Aird WC. Endothelial cell heterogeneity. *Crit Care Med.* 2003;31:S221-S230.

42. Gittenberger-de Groot AC, DeRuiter MC, Bergwerff M, Poelmann RE. Smooth muscle cell origin and its relation to heterogeneity in development and disease. *Arterioscler Thromb Vasc Biol.* 1999;19:1589-1594.

43. Aboyans V, Criqui MH, Denenberg JO, Knoke JD, Ridker PM, Fronek A. Risk factors for progression of peripheral arterial disease in large and small vessels. *Circulation.* 2006;113:2623-2629.

44. Criqui MH, Browner D, Fronek A, et al. Peripheral arterial disease in large vessels is epidemiologically distinct from small vessel disease. An analysis of risk factors. *Am J Epidemiol.* 1989;129:1110-1119.

45. Mohler ER, 3rd. Peripheral arterial disease: identification and implications. *Arch Intern Med.* 2003;163:2306-2314.

46. Iyemere VP, Proudfoot D, Weissberg PL, Shanahan CM. Vascular smooth muscle cell phenotypic plasticity and the regulation of vascular calcification. *Journal of Internal Medicine.* 2006;260(3):192-210.

47. Hunt JL, Fairman R, Mitchell ME, et al. Bone formation in carotid plaques: a clinicopathological study. *Stroke.* 2002;33(5):1214-1219.

48. Austin MA, Hokanson JE, Edwards KL. Hypertriglyceridemia as a cardiovascular risk factor. *Am J Cardiol.* 1998;81:7B-12B.

49. Newall RG, Bliss BP. Lipoproteins and the relative importance of plasma cholesterol and triglycerides in peripheral arterial disease. *Angiology.* 1973;24:297-302.

50. Davignon J, Lussier-Cacan S, Ortin-George M, et al. Plasma lipids and lipoprotein patterns in angiographically graded atherosclerosis of the legs and in coronary heart disease. *Can Med Assoc J.* 1977;116:1245-1250.

51. Bradby GV, Valente AJ, Walton KW. Serum high-density lipoproteins in peripheral vascular disease. *Lancet.* 1978;2:1271-1274.

52. Greenhalgh RM, Rosengarten DS, Mervart I, Lewis B, Calnan JS, Martin P. Serum lipids and lipoproteins in peripheral vascular disease. *Lancet.* 1971;2:947-950.

53. Whayne TF, Alaupovic P, Curry MD, Lee ET, Anderson PS, Schechter E. Plasma apolipoprotein B and VLDL-, LDL-, and HDL-cholesterol as risk factors in the development of coronary artery disease in male patients examined by angiography. *Atherosclerosis.* 1981;39:411-424.

54. Pilger E, Pristautz H, Pfeiffer KP, Kostner G. Risk factors for peripheral atherosclerosis. Retrospective evaluation by stepwise discriminant analysis. *Arteriosclerosis.* 1983;3:57-63.

55. Pomrehn P, Duncan B, Weissfeld L, et al. The association of dyslipoproteinemia with symptoms and signs of peripheral arterial disease. The Lipid Research Clinics Program Prevalence Study. *Circulation.* 1986;73:100-107.

56. Vitale E, Zuliani G, Baroni L, et al. Lipoprotein abnormalities in patients with extra-coronary arteriosclerosis. *Atherosclerosis.* 1990;81:95-102.

57. Mowat BF, Skinner ER, Wilson HM, Leng GC, Fowkes FG, Horrobin D. Alterations in plasma lipids, lipoproteins and high density lipoprotein subfractions in peripheral arterial disease. *Atherosclerosis.* 1997;131:161-166.

58. Murabito JM, D'Agostino RB, Silbershatz H, Wilson WF. Intermittent claudication. A risk profile from The Framingham Heart Study. *Circulation.* 1997;96:44-49.

59. Newman AB, Tyrrell KS, Kuller LH. Mortality over four years in SHEP participants with a low ankle-arm index. *J Am Geriatr Soc.* 1997;45:1472-1478.

60. Murabito JM, Evans JC, Nieto K, Larson MG, Levy D, Wilson PW. Prevalence and clinical correlates of peripheral arterial disease in the Framingham Offspring Study. *Am Heart J.* 2002;143:961-965.

61. Curb JD, Masaki K, Rodriguez BL, et al. Peripheral artery disease and cardiovascular risk factors in the elderly. The Honolulu Heart Program. *Arterioscler Thromb Vasc Biol.* 1996;16:1495-1500.

62. Fabsitz RR, Sidawy AN, Go O, et al. Prevalence of peripheral arterial disease and associated risk factors in American Indians: the Strong Heart Study. *Am J Epidemiol.* 1999;149:330-338.

63. Newman AB, Siscovick DS, Manolio TA, et al. Ankle-arm index as a marker of atherosclerosis in the Cardiovascular Health Study. Cardiovascular Heart Study (CHS) Collaborative Research Group. *Circulation.* 1993;88:837-845.

64. Fowkes FG, Housley E, Riemersma RA, et al. Smoking, lipids, glucose intolerance, and blood pressure as risk factors for peripheral atherosclerosis compared with ischemic heart disease in the Edinburgh Artery Study. *Am J Epidemiol.* 1992;135:331-340.

65. Ridker PM, Stampfer MJ, Rifai N. Novel risk factors for systemic atherosclerosis: a comparison of C-reactive protein, fibrinogen, homocysteine, lipoprotein(a), and standard cholesterol screening as predictors of peripheral arterial disease [see comment]. *JAMA.* 2001;285:2481-2485.

66. Hutter CM, Austin MA, Humphries SE. Familial hypercholesterolemia, peripheral arterial disease, and stroke: a HuGE minireview.*American Journal of Epidemiology.* 2004;160(5):430-435.

67. Resnick HE, Rodriguez B, Havlik R, et al. Apo E genotype, diabetes, and peripheral arterial disease in older men: The Honolulu–Asia Aging Study. *Genet Epidemiol.* 2000;19:52-63.

68. Smith I, Franks PJ, Greenhalgh RM, Poulter NR, Powell JT. The influence of smoking cessation and hypertriglyceridaemia on the progression of peripheral arterial disease and the onset of critical ischaemia. *Eur J Vasc Endovasc Surg.* 1996;11:402-408.

69. Kennedy M, Solomon C, Manolio TA, et al. Risk factors for declining ankle-brachial index in men and women 65 years or older: the Cardiovascular Health Study. *Arch Intern Med.* 2005;165:1896-1902.

70. Danesh J, Collins R, Peto R. Lipoprotein(a) and coronary heart disease. Meta-analysis of prospective studies. *Circulation.* 2000;102:1082-1085.

71. Dangas G, Ambrose JA, D'Agate DJ, et al. Correlation of serum lipoprotein(a) with the angiographic and clinical presentation of coronary artery disease. *Am J Cardiol.* 1999;83:583-585.

72. Stubbs P, Seed M, Lane D, Collinson P, Kendall F, Noble M. Lipoprotein(a) as a risk predictor for cardiac mortality in patients with acute coronary syndromes. *Eur Heart J.* 1998;19:1355-1364.

73. Ariyo AA, Thach C, Tracy R, Cardiovascular Health Study I. Lp(a) lipoprotein, vascular disease, and mortality in the elderly [see comment]. *N Engl J Med.* 2003;349:2108-2115.

74. Valentine RJ, Grayburn PA, Vega GL, Grundy SM. Lp(a) lipoprotein is an independent, discriminating risk factor for premature peripheral atherosclerosis among white men. *Arch Intern Med.* 1994;154:801-806.

75. Sutton-Tyrrell K, Evans RW, Meilahn E, Alcorn HG. Lipoprotein(a) and peripheral atherosclerosis in older adults. *Atherosclerosis.* 1996;122:11-19.

76. Tseng CH. Lipoprotein(a) is an independent risk factor for peripheral arterial disease in Chinese type 2 diabetic patients in Taiwan. *Diabetes Care.* 2004;27:517-521.

77. Takemoto M, Liao JK. Pleiotropic effects of 3-hydroxy-3-methylglutaryl coenzyme a reductase inhibitors. *Arterioscler Thromb Vasc Biol.* 2001;21:1712-1719.

78. Hernandez-Perera O, Perez-Sala D, Navarro-Antolin J, et al. Effects of the 3-hydroxy-3-methylglutaryl-CoA reductase inhibitors, atorvastatin and simvastatin, on the expression of endothelin-1 and endothelial nitric oxide synthase in vascular endothelial cells. *J Clin Invest.* 1998;101:2711-2719.

79. Laufs U, La Fata V, Plutzky J, Liao JK. Upregulation of endothelial nitric oxide synthase by HMG CoA reductase inhibitors. *Circulation.* 1998;97:1129-1135.

80. O'Driscoll G, Green D, Taylor RR. Simvastatin, an HMG-coenzyme A reductase inhibitor, improves endothelial function within 1 month. *Circulation.* 1997;95:1126-1131.

81. Crisby M, Nordin-Fredriksson G, Shah PK, Yano J, Zhu J, Nilsson J. Pravastatin treatment increases collagen content and decreases lipid content, inflammation, metalloproteinases, and cell death in human carotid plaques: implications for plaque stabilization. *Circulation.* 2001;103:926-933.

82. Treasure CB, Klein JL, Weintraub WS, et al. Beneficial effects of cholesterol-lowering therapy on the coronary endothelium in patients with coronary artery disease [see comment]. *N Engl J Med.* 1995;332:481-487.

83. National Cholesterol Education Program (NCEP) Expert Panel on Detection, Evaluation,and Treatment of High Blood Cholesterol in Adults (Adult Treatment Panel III). Third Report of the National Cholesterol Education Program (NCEP) Expert Panel on Detection, Evaluation, and Treatment of High Blood Cholesterol in Adults (Adult Treatment Panel III) final report [see comment]. *Circulation.* 2002;106:3143-3421.

84. McDermott MM, Guralnik JM, Greenland P, et al. Statin use and leg functioning in patients with and without lower-extremity peripheral arterial disease. *Circulation.* 2003;107:757-761.

85. Giri J, McDermott MM, Greenland P, et al. Statin use and functional decline in patients with and without peripheral arterial disease. *J Am Coll Cardiol.* 2006;47:998-1004.

86. Aronow WS, Nayak D, Woodworth S, Ahn C. Effect of simvastatin versus placebo on treadmill exercise time until the onset of intermittent claudication in older patients with peripheral arterial disease at six months and at one year after treatment. *Am J Cardiol.* 2003;92:711-712.

87. Mohler ER, III, Hiatt WR, Creager MA. Cholesterol reduction with atorvastatin improves walking distance in patients with peripheral arterial disease. *Circulation.* 2003;108:1481-1486.

88. Mondillo S, Ballo P, Barbati R, et al. Effects of simvastatin on walking performance and symptoms of intermittent claudication in hypercholesterolemic patients with peripheral vascular disease. *Am J Med.* 2003;114:359-364.

89. Ross SD, Allen IE, Connelly JE, et al. Clinical outcomes in statin treatment trials: a meta-analysis. *Arch Intern Med.* 1999;159:1793-1802.

90. Griggs RC, Jozefowicz R, Kingston W, Nair KS, Herr BE, Halliday D. Mechanism of muscle wasting in myotonic dystrophy. *Ann Neurol.* 1990;27:505-512.

91. Goodman MN. Tumor necrosis factor induces skeletal muscle protein breakdown in rats. *Am J Physiol.* 1991;260:E727-E730.

92. Ferrucci L, Penninx BW, Volpato S, et al. Change in muscle strength explains accelerated decline of physical function in older women with high interleukin-6 serum levels. *J Am Geriatr Soc.* 2002;50:1947-1954.

93. Tousoulis D, Antoniades C, Bosinakou E, et al. Effects of atorvastatin on reactive hyperemia and inflammatory process in patients with congestive heart failure. *Atherosclerosis.* 2005;178:359-363.

94. Shaffer RG, Greene S, Arshi A, et al. Effect of acute exercise on endothelial progenitor cells in patients with peripheral arterial disease. *Vasc Med* 2006;11(4):219-261.

95. Taylor AJ, Lee HJ, Sullenberger LE. The effect of 24 months of combination statin and extended-release niacin on carotid intima-media thickness: ARBITER 3. *Curr Med Res Opin.* 2006;22:2243-2250.

chapter 4

Vulnerable Plaque and the Role of Inflammation in Arterial Disease

Ghazanfar Khadim, MD / *Javed Butler, MD, MPH* / *Raymond Q. Migrino, MD*

● INTRODUCTION

Atherothrombosis is a systemic arterial disease of large- and medium-sized arteries including the coronary, carotid, aorta, and peripheral arteries. The clinical manifestations depend on the size of the vessels and the regional circulation involved and include coronary artery disease, stroke, and peripheral vascular disease. A paradigm shift is occurring with a change in focus from the assessment and treatment of luminal narrowing toward greater understanding of the vascular biology in the arterial wall that leads to plaque vulnerability. Recent research has shown that inflammation plays a key role in the pathogenesis and progression of atherothrombosis. The basic concepts of evolution of atherothrombosis, and the role of inflammation leading to vulnerable plaque, will be discussed here.

● PLAQUE COMPOSITION

The main components of atherothrombotic plaques are[1-7] (1) connective tissue extracellular matrix, including collagen, proteoglycans, and fibronectin elastic fibers; (2) crystalline cholesterol, cholesteryl esters, and phospholipids; (3) cellular components such as macrophages, T lymphocytes, and smooth muscle cells; and (4) thrombotic material with platelets and fibrin deposition. The proportion of these components varies in different plaques, and explains the heterogeneity of lesions and potential vulnerability to plaque rupture.

● CLASSIFICATION OF ATHEROTHROMBOTIC LESIONS

According to a simplified modification of the criteria set forth by the American Heart Association Committee on Vascular Lesions,[3] plaque progression can be classified into five phases as shown in Figure 4-1.

Phase 1 (early): These lesions are small and commonly seen in individuals younger than 30 years. Based on their composition, these plaques are categorized into three types: type I lesions, consisting of macrophage-derived foam cells with intracellular lipid droplets; type II lesions, consisting of macrophages, smooth muscle cells, and extracellular lipid deposits; and type III lesions, consisting of smooth muscle cells surrounded by extracellular connective tissue, fibrils, and lipid deposits. It is possible for these early lesions to regress to normal.[8]

Phase 2 (advanced): These lesions, although not necessarily stenotic, may be prone to disruption because of their high lipid content, thin fibrous caps, and increased inflammation. They are categorized into two types: type IV lesions, which consist of confluent cellular lesions with a great deal of extracellular lipid intermixed with fibrous tissue, and type Va lesions, which possess an extracellular lipid core covered by a thin fibrous cap. Phase 2 plaques can evolve into the acute phases 3 and 4, and either of these can evolve into phase 5 plaques.

Phase 3: This phase consists of acute complicated type VI lesions, originating from disrupted type IV or Va lesions, and leading to mural, nonobstructive thrombosis. Although clinically silent, the process may occasionally lead to the onset of angina.[9]

Phase 4: This phase includes acute complicated type VI lesions, with fixed or repetitive occlusive

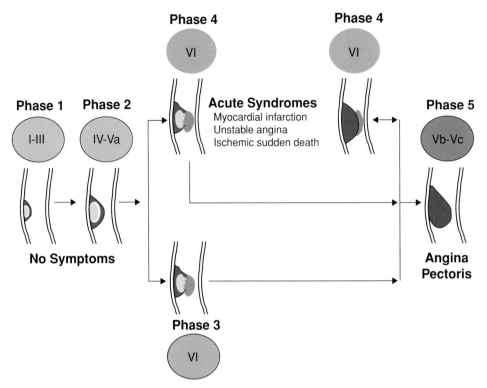

● **FIGURE 4-1.** Modified AHA classification of lesion morphology of coronary atherosclerosis according to gross pathological and clinical findings.

Reproduced with permission from Springer Science and Business Media. Corti R et al. Evolving concepts in the triad of atherosclerosis, inflammation and thrombosis. J Thromb Thrombolysis. 2004;17:35-44.

thrombosis. This process may be silent,[10,11] but usually leads to an acute coronary syndrome (ACS).

Phase 5: This phase includes type Vb (calcific) or Vc (fibrotic) lesions that may cause angina; however, if preceded by stenosis or occlusion with associated ischemia, the myocardium may be protected by collateral circulation, and such lesions may then be silent or clinically inapparent.[12,13]

● EARLY ATHEROTHROMBOSIS

Endothelial Dysfunction

Under basal conditions, the endothelium functions to maintain the vessel in a relatively dilated state. In response to various physical stimuli, such as shear stress, the blood vessels dilate by an endothelial dependent process called *flow-mediated dilation*. This response is principally regulated by release of nitric oxide (NO) from the endothelium. NO is synthesized from amino acid L-arginine by endothelial nitric oxide synthase (eNOS). By virtue of NO, the endothelium regulates anti-inflammatory, mitogenic, and contractile activities of the vessel wall as well as the hemostatic process within the vessel lumen[14] (Figure 4-2).

Endothelial dysfunction has been traditionally described as the earliest manifestation of atherosclerosis. It is often

the result of a disturbance in the physiologic pattern of blood flow at bending points and near bifurcations.[15,16] In addition, it is associated with biohumoral risk factors such as hypercholesterolemia, diabetes, hypertension, obesity, smoking, and advanced age[17–19] (Figure 4-3). A dysfunctional endothelium, characterized by decreased NO synthesis, facilitates vessel wall entry and oxidation of circulating lipoproteins, monocyte entry, smooth cell proliferation and extracellular matrix deposition, vasoconstriction, as well as a prothrombotic state within the vessel lumen.[20,21]

Extracellular Lipid Accumulation: Lipoprotein Transport and Modification

Low-density lipoproteins (LDLs) infiltrate through the arterial endothelium into the intima.[8] The binding of LDL to proteoglycan in the intima leads to the retention of these particles. The proteoglycan bound LDL particles have an increased susceptibility to oxidative and other chemical modifications, making them proinflammatory, chemotoxic, cytotoxic, and proatherogenic. The mechanisms responsible for the atherogenic modification of these LDL particles are not known, but may involve oxidation mediated by myeloperoxidase, 15-lipoxygenase, and nitric oxide synthase (NOS).[22]

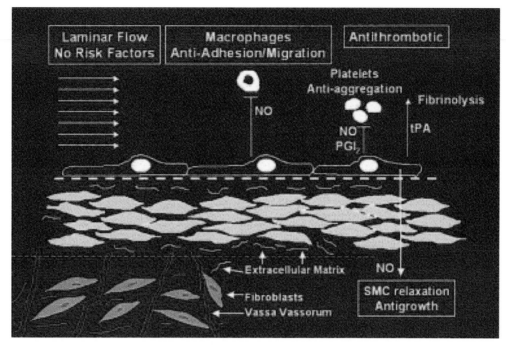

● **FIGURE 4-2.** Healthy endothelium under laminar flow conditions and no risk factors. A single molecule, nitric oxide (NO), is involved in multifactorial pathways preventing monocyte adhesion, platelet aggregation, and smooth muscle cell proliferation. PGI$_2$, prostacyclin 2; SMC, smooth muscle cell; tPA, tissue plasminogen activator.

Reproduced with permission from Elsevier Science. Fuster V et al. Atherothrombosis and high-risk plaque. J Am Coll Cardiol. 2005;46:937-954.

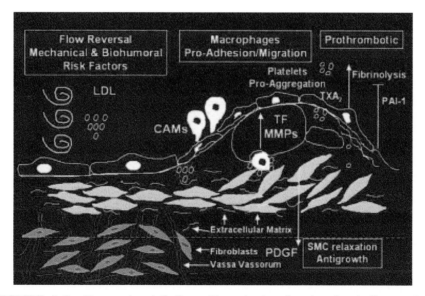

● **FIGURE 4-3.** Diseased endothelium with nonlaminar flow, low-density lipoprotein (LDL) deposition, cell adhesion molecule (CAM) expression, macrophage migration, tissue factor (TF), and matrix metalloproteinase (MMP) expression leading to smooth muscle cell (SMC) proliferation and vasa vasorum neovascularization. PDGF, platelet-derived growth factor; PAI-1, plasminogen activator inhibitor-1; TXA$_2$, thromboxane A2.

Reproduced with permission from Elsevier Science. Fuster V et al. Atherothrombosis and high-risk plaque. J Am Coll Cardiol. 2005;46:937-954.

Leukocyte Adhesion and Migration

Normal endothelium generally resists leukocyte adhesion. However, in response to atherogenic and proinflammatory stimuli, particularly oxidized LDL particles in the intima, the endothelial cells are activated. Activated endothelial cells express adhesion molecules, primarily vascular cell adhesion molecules-1 on their surface. These molecules regulate the interaction of monocytes and T cells with the endothelium. Besides vascular cell adhesion molecules-1, other adhesion molecules, such as intercellular adhesion molecule-1 , E selectin, and P selectin, likely contribute to recruitment of leukocytes to the atherosclerotic lesion.[23,24]

Once adherent to the endothelium, migration of leukocytes into the arterial wall involves the action of protein molecules known as chemotactic cytokines, or chemokines. Experimental studies indicate that the most important chemoattractants are oxidized LDL and monocyte chemotactic protein-1 (MCP-1). MCP-1 is a powerful chemokine and its receptor CCR2 on the monocyte/macrophages may be significantly upregulated during plaque progression. It attracts both monocytes and T cells, but not neutrophils and B cells, and likely plays a key role in the intimal recruitment of these cells. Endothelial cells, smooth muscle cells (SMCs), and macrophages all contribute to the overexpression of MCP-1 in atherosclerosis. Thus, monocyte-derived macrophages in the intima may recruit more monocytes into the intima by secreting MCP-1. Cytokines, such as interleukin-8, may also play a role in leukocyte migration.[22]

Intracellular Lipid Accumulation: Foam Cell Formation

Once within the intima, the monocytes differentiate into macrophages under the influence of macrophage colony-stimulating factor (M-CSF), produced by endothelial and SMCs. These macrophages internalize the oxidized LDL particles via the scavenger receptors, of which SR-A and CD36 have been shown to play a significant role in experimental atherosclerosis.[25] The development of lipid-laden macrophages, the foam cells, is the hallmark of both early and late atherosclerotic lesions. Aside from their scavenger function, macrophages also express matrix degrading proteolytic enzymes, matrix metalloproteinases (MMPs), and tissue factor (TF), which contribute to their significant destabilizing and thrombogenic properties.

Once macrophages have taken up residence in the intima and become foam cells, they not infrequently replicate. The factors that trigger macrophage cell division in the atherosclerotic plaque likely include M-CSF, interleukin-3, and granulocyte-macrophage colony stimulating factor.

Smooth Muscle Cell Migration, Proliferation, and Death

In the development of early and asymptomatic foam cell lesion, the fatty streak, the cells responsible are mostly endothelial cells, macrophages, and a few T cells. With plaque progression, the fibroproliferative response mediated by the SMCs plays a key role in the evolution of atheroma into more complex plaques. The SMCs are the principal connective tissue producing cells in the normal and atherosclerotic intima.[26] Some SMCs likely arrive in the arterial intima early in life, while others migrate into the intima from the underlying media. The chemoattractants for SMCs include molecules such as platelet-derived growth factor, secreted by activated macrophages and overexpressed in human atherosclerosis. These intimal SMCs are capable of multiplying by cell division.

While the repairing and protective capabilities of SMCs are considered beneficial, the impaired function or death of these cells is likely detrimental, suggested by the local loss of SMCs at the rupture site of plaques. The exact mechanism for SMC loss at rupture sites is not known, but apoptotic cell death may play a role.[27,28] Apoptosis can occur in response to inflammatory cytokines in the evolving atheroma or by elimination of some SMCs by the T cells.

Thus, SMC accumulation in the growing atherosclerotic plaque results from a balance between cell replication and cell death. In addition to SMCs, the endothelial and monocyte/macrophage foam cells are also subject to cell death by apoptosis, and this process contributes significantly to increased TF activity and thrombogenicity of the lipid-rich core.[29]

Innate and Adaptive Immune Response to Autoantigens

Over the past few years, basic and clinical research has demonstrated a fundamental role for inflammation in atherogenesis.[30,31] The macrophage foam cells not only serve as a reservoir for excess lipid but also provide a rich source of proinflammatory mediators, such as cytokines and chemokines and various eicosanoids and lipids such as platelet-activating factor. These phagocytic cells can elaborate significant amounts of oxidant species such as superoxide anion within the atherosclerotic plaque.[32] The inflammatory mediators promote inflammation in the plaque and thus contribute to the progression of lesions. This amplification of the inflammatory response, which is not dependent on antigenic stimulation, is referred to as *innate immunity*. The important receptors for innate immunity in atherothrombosis are the scavenger receptors and the toll-like receptors (TLRs).[33]

As described earlier, the scavenger receptors SR-A and CD-36 mediate the uptake of oxidized LDL and transform the macrophage into a foam cell.[34,35] Macrophage foam cells produce cytokines that promote monocyte migration, macrophage foam cell formation, and activation of neighboring smooth muscle cells.[7] Furthermore, this pathway activates the proinflammatory NF-κ-B nuclear transcriptional factor, which triggers a potent chemoattractant response involving MCP-1, leukotriene LTB_4, and M-CSF.[34–36] This leads to further monocyte migration and macrophage/foam cell formation.

The role of cytokine-mediated inflammation and the resulting plaque instability are being increasingly recognized.

The cytokine production is initiated by signaling through TLRs that recognize host-derived molecules released from injured tissue and cells. TLRs also activate the NF-κ-B pathway, resulting in production of cytokines that augment local inflammation.[37] TLR1, TLR2, and TLR4 are shown to be upregulated in the endothelium and in areas infiltrated with inflammatory cells. In addition, adventitial fibroblasts and dendritic cells express TLR4 receptors and are able to produce a variety of cytokines after TLR4 activation.[38]

In addition to innate immunity, evidence also supports a prominent role for adaptive or antigen-specific immunity in plaque progression.[30,31] In addition to the mononuclear phagocytes, dendritic cells in atherosclerotic lesion can present antigens to the T cells, including modified lipoproteins, heat shock proteins, beta-2 glycoprotein 1b, and infectious agents. The antigen-presenting cells (macrophages, dendritic cells, or endothelial cells) allow the antigen to interact with T cells, leading to their activation and subsequent release of large quantities of cytokines that modulate atherogenesis.

Arterial Extracellular Matrix

Extracellular matrix constitutes much of the volume of an advanced atherosclerotic plaque. The major extracellular matrix components of atheroma include interstitial collagens (types I and III), proteoglycans, and elastin,[39,40] produced primarily by SMCs. Stimuli for excessive collagen production by SMCs include platelet-derived growth factor and transforming growth factor-beta (TGF-β)—a constituent of platelet granules and a product of many cell types found in lesions.

The biosynthesis of the extracellular matrix molecules is balanced by breakdown catalyzed in part by catabolic enzymes known as MMPs. Dissolution of extracellular matrix macromolecules undoubtedly plays a role in the migration of SMCs as they penetrate into the intima from the media through a dense extracellular matrix, traversing the elastin-rich internal elastic lamina. Extracellular matrix dissolution also likely plays a role in the arterial remodeling that accompanies lesion growth.

Plaque Mineralization

Focal calcification in atherosclerotic plaques is common and increases with age.[41] Plaque calcification is considered an active process and resembles calcification in bone. The total amount of calcification, the coronary artery calcium score, is a marker of coronary plaque burden and provides prognostic information beyond that provided by traditional risk factors.[42] Coronary calcification is composed of both hydroxyapatite and organic matrix, including type I collagen and noncollagenous bone-associated proteins.[43] The most relevant noncollagenous bone-associated proteins associated with vascular calcification include osteopontin, osteonectin, osteoprotegerin, and matrix Gla protein. The most studied noncollagenous bone-associated protein in atherothrombosis is osteopontin, which is highly expressed by macrophages in the intima

of human arteries.[44] Clinical observations suggest that culprit lesions responsible for ACSs are generally less calcified than plaques responsible for stable angina, and the pattern of plaque calcification may be different in these two patient subsets.[45,46]

● ADVANCED ATHEROTHROMBOSIS

Continuous exposure to the systemic, proatherogenic milieu will increase chemotaxis of monocytes thus leading to lipid accumulation, development of necrotic core, and fibrous cap formation, evolving into advanced atherosclerosis. More recently, new structural and functional features of these lesions have been described, including vascular remodeling and vasa vasorum neovascularization.

Eccentric Vascular Remodeling

Described by Glagov et al. in 1987,[47] vascular remodeling involves eccentric and outward plaque growth with compensatory enlargement of the vessel wall (Figure 4-4). Luminal stenosis tends to occur only after the plaque burden exceeds some 40% of the cross-sectional area of the artery. This so-called positive remodeling or "compensatory enlargement" must involve turnover of extracellular matrix molecules to accommodate the circumferential growth of the artery. Several studies have shown increased macrophage-derived matrix metalloproteinases MMP-2 and -9 expression within the intima–media interface of remodeled plaques.[48] The increased activity of MMPs digests the internal elastic lamina, modulating the process of remodeling.

Plaques susceptible to rupture and those responsible for ACSs are more likely to exhibit expansive remodeling, while those that more likely lead to luminal narrowing and resulting stable angina exhibit "negative" or "constrictive remodeling."[49]

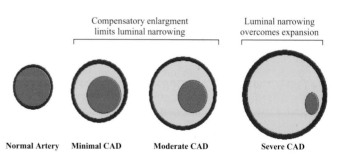

● **FIGURE 4-4.** Vascular remodeling. Early plaque accumulation in human coronary arteries is associated with compensatory enlargement of the vessel size (positive remodeling) to accommodate the growing plaque. Hence, lumen size is either unaffected or minimally reduced. As atherosclerosis becomes severe, enlargement is overcome by plaque progression (left to right) and luminal narrowing is no longer prevented.

Adapted from Glagov S et al. Compensatory enlargement of human atherosclerotic coronary arteries. N Engl J Med. 1987;316:1371-1375.

Neovascularization and Intraplaque Hemorrhage

Angiogenesis is common in advanced atherosclerosis and is associated closely with plaque progression.[50–53] Endothelial proliferation is predominantly thought to arise from the adventitia, where there is abundance of preexisting vasa vasorum. A breech in the medial wall likely facilitates the rapid in-growth of microvessels from the adventitia, and exposure to an inflammatory environment stimulates the development of immature endothelial tubes with leaky linings. This network of incompetent blood vessels is a viable source of intraplaque hemorrhage that may promote transition from a stable to an unstable lesion.

Angiogenesis depends on the interplay of various cytokines and growth factors released by the infiltrating inflammatory cells, including macrophages and T cells. Macrophages, attracted by oxidized LDL, are responsible for cytokine production, leading to neo-vessel growth.[54,55] In addition, varying degrees of T lymphocytes are present in areas of neovascularization, specifically in the deep intima around the base and shoulder region of the necrotic core. Activated T cells are a known source of angiogenic factors, including vascular endothelial growth factor, and can stimulate angiogenesis in association with early lymphocyte recruitment.[56]

● PLAQUE RUPTURE

Two mechanisms can trigger plaque rupture. The first is related to physical forces and occurs most frequently where the fibrous cap is weakest. This is most often the shoulder region between the plaque and the adjacent vessel wall,[57] where the cap is thinnest and is heavily infiltrated by foam cells with relative loss of SMCs.

The second mechanism involves an active process within the plaque leading to rupture. The macrophages and mast cells are capable of degrading extracellular matrix by phagocytosis or secretion of proteolytic enzymes. Thus enzymes such as plasminogen activators and MMPs, including collagenases, elastases, gelatinases, and stromelysins, degrade components of the extracellular matrix, may weaken the fibrous cap, and predispose it to rupture.[58,59]

● THROMBOTIC COMPLICATIONS

Acute Coronary Thrombosis

Rupture of a high-risk vulnerable plaque may result in mural thrombus without evident clinical symptoms, or acute occlusion or subocclusion with clinical manifestations of unstable angina or ACS.[60,61] A number of factors, including plaque-derived thrombogenic substrate, rheology, and systemic procoagulant activity, may influence the stability and magnitude of the resulting thrombus and, thus, the severity of the coronary syndrome.[62]

Plaque-Derived Thrombogenic Substrate. Exposure of the thrombogenic substrate within the plaque to the arterial circulation is the key factor in determining local thrombogenicity at the site of plaque rupture or erosion. The main thrombogenic components of the plaque are its lipid and TF content. Lipid-rich plaques are by far the most thrombogenic, which explains why their rupture is the most frequent cause of coronary thrombosis in ACS. In addition, thrombogenicity is also modulated by TF content, mostly located in macrophage-rich areas.[63–65] TF, a small-molecular-weight glycoprotein, initiates the extrinsic clotting cascade and is believed to be a major regulator of coagulation, hemostasis, and thrombosis.[66] It forms a high-affinity complex with coagulation factors VII/VIIa; TF/VIIa complex activates factors IX and X, which, in turn, leads to thrombin generation.

Rheology and Thrombosis. The degree of luminal narrowing caused by the ruptured plaque and the overlying mural thrombi are also important for determining thrombogenicity at the local arterial site. Specifically, shear rate is directly related to flow velocity and inversely related to the third power of the lumen diameter. Thus, acute platelet deposition after plaque rupture is highly modulated by the degree of narrowing after rupture. Furthermore, mural thrombus formation may contribute to vasoconstriction originated from platelets, serotonin, and thromboxane A2, increasing shear force-dependent platelet deposition.[67,68]

Systemic Procoagulant Activity. Two major pathways are involved in systemic procoagulant activity: coronary risk factors and circulating TF.

Abnormalities in lipid metabolism, cigarette smoking, and hyperglycemia are associated with increased blood thrombogenicity.[69–71] Recent observations indicate that the prothrombotic state associated with high LDL cholesterol, cigarette smoking, and diabetes may share a common biological pathway. That is, an activation of leukocyte-platelet interactions associated with release of TF and thrombin activation has been observed in these conditions.[72]

Circulating TF antigen has been associated with increased blood thrombogenicity in patients with ACS[73,74] and chronic coronary artery disease.[75] Atherosclerotic plaques have been shown to contain TF that is associated with macrophages within the lesion. It is now believed that circulating monocytes also supply TF that trigger and propagate acute thrombi overlying unstable atherosclerotic plaques, and monocyte infiltration of the thrombus has been shown to correlate with the presence of an occlusive thrombus.[76] Monocytes and neutrophils were identified in the fibrous cap by myeloperoxidase staining. The precise role of myeloperoxidase in triggering acute coronary thrombosis is unclear. In addition to providing a prooxidant milieu and increasing oxidized LDL cholesterol, there is evidence that macrophage myeloperoxidase might be responsible for the disruption of the fibrous cap owing to the production of hypochlorous acid.[77]

Thus, aside from macrophages in atherosclerotic plaques, activated monocytes in the circulating blood seem

TABLE 4-1. Atherothrombosis—Complicated Lesions

	Suggested Predominant Mechanisms Plaque Rupture		
	---	---	---
Location	Lipid Rich	Nonlipid Rich	Blood Thrombogenicity
Coronaries	+	±	+
Carotids	±	+	−
Thoracic aorta	+	−	−
Peripheral	−	−	+

+, Predominant; ±, nonpredominant; −, no mechanism.
Reproduced with permission from Elsevier Science. Fuster V et al. Atherothrombosis and high-risk plaque. J Am Coll Cardiol. 2005;46:937-954.

to be a source of TF and may represent the result of the activation by the cardiovascular risk factors, contributing to thrombotic events.[65,78] Indeed, the predictive value of C-reactive protein and CD40L may in part be a manifestation of such systemic phenomena. C-reactive protein, like fibrinogen, is a protein of the acute-phase response and a sensitive marker of low-grade inflammation. It is produced in the liver as a result of mediators such as interleukin-6 generated by inflammation in the vessel wall (i.e., macrophages) or extravascularly (i.e., circulating monocytes).[79] Increased levels of C-reactive protein (lower limit of normal is ≤3 mg/mL) have been reported to predict acute coronary events,[80] independent of lipid levels.[81,82]

Acute Thrombosis and Embolism of Noncoronary Arteries

Carotid atherothrombosis frequently results from dissection or rupture of heterogenous plaques. The likely mechanisms responsible include rupture of the vasa vasorum with resulting intraplaque hemorrhage and the impact of systemic high-velocity blood flow against the plaque

TABLE 4-2. Definitions for Terminology Commonly Used in Atherothrombosis and Acute Coronary Syndromes

Culprit lesion	A lesion in a coronary artery considered, on the basis of angiographic, autopsy, or other findings, to be responsible for the clinical event. In unstable angina, myocardial infarction, and sudden coronary death, the culprit lesion is often a plaque complicated by thrombosis extending into the lumen.
Eroded plaque	A plaque with loss and/or dysfunction of the luminal endothelial cells leading to thrombosis. There is usually no additional defect or gap in the plaque, which is often rich in smooth muscle cells and proteoglycans.
High-risk, vulnerable, and thrombosis-prone plaque	These terms can be used as synonyms to describe a plaque that is at increased risk of thrombosis and rapid stenosis progression.
Inflamed thin cap fibroatheroma	An inflamed plaque with a thin cap covering a lipid-rich, necrotic core. An inflamed thin cap fibroatheroma is suspected to be a high-risk/vulnerable plaque.
Plaque with a calcified nodule	A heavily calcified plaque with the loss and/or dysfunction of endothelial cells over a calcified nodule, resulting in loss of fibrous cap, that makes the plaque high-risk/vulnerable. This is the least common of the three types of suspected high-risk/vulnerable plaques.
Ruptured plaque	A plaque with deep injury with a real defect or gap in the fibrous cap that had separated its lipid-rich atheromatous core from the flowing blood, thereby exposing the thrombogenic core of the plaque. This is the most common cause of thrombosis.
Thrombosed plaque	A plaque with an overlying thrombus extending into the lumen of the vessel. The thrombus may be occlusive or nonocclusive.
Vulnerable patient	A patient at high risk (vulnerable, prone) for experiencing a cardiovascular ischemic event caused by a high atherosclerotic burden, high-risk vulnerable plaques, and/or thrombogenic blood.

Adapted with permission from Schaar JA et al. Terminology for high-risk and vulnerable coronary artery plaques. Eur Heart J. 2004;25:1077-1082.

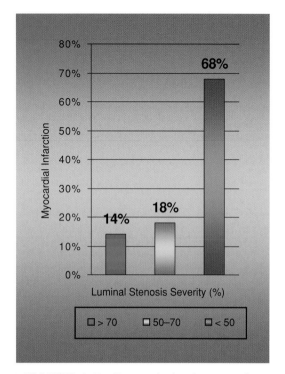

● **FIGURE 4-5.** Bar graph showing stenosis severity and associated risk of coronary occlusion and myocardial infarction (MI) as evaluated by serial angiographic examination. The more stenotic an individual coronary segment is at baseline, the more frequently it progresses to occlusion and/or gives rise to infarction. Because less obstructive plaques by far outnumber severely obstructive plaques, most occlusions and infarctions result from progression of the former plaques.

Modified from Falk E et al. Coronary plaque disruption. Circulation. 1995;92:657-671.

TABLE 4-3. Features Associated with Plaque Vulnerability

Structural
• Large and soft lipid-rich core
• Thin and collagen-poor fibrous cap
Cellular
• Lack of SMCs at rupture site
• Accumulation of MACRs at rupture site
Function
• Impaired matrix synthesis (SMC-related)
• Increased matrix breakdown (MACR-derived MMPs)
Remodeling
• Expansive (outward) vascular remodeling
Others
• Adventitial inflammation and neovascularization

MACR, macrophages; MMP, matrix metalloproteinase; SMC, smooth muscle cell.
Adapted with permission from Elsevier Science. Falk E. Pathogenesis of atherosclerosis. J Am Coll Cardiol. 2006;47:C7-C12.

surface.[83,84] Plaque rupture with exposure of the plaque-derived lipid core has been documented as a common form of stroke.[85–90] Atherothrombosis originating from the thoracic aorta is also a consequence of plaque rupture,[91–93] as described in approximately two-thirds of acute coronary thrombosis.[91] Thrombosis of the peripheral arteries, on the other hand, is most frequently observed on the surface of stenotic plaques, probably related to mechanisms

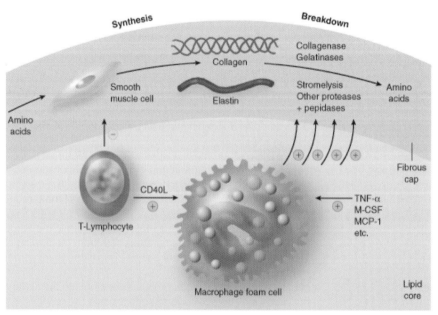

Copyright 2005 by Elsevier Science

● **FIGURE 4-6.** A schematic relating extracellular matrix metabolism to intimal inflammation during atherogenesis (see text for details).

Reproduced with permission from Lippincott, Williams, & Wilkins. Libby P. Molecular bases of the acute coronary syndromes. Circulation. 1995;91:2844-2850.

similar to those described in approximately one-third of acute coronary thrombosis.[94,95] In the peripheral vascular bed, atherothrombosis is predominantly the consequence of thrombogenic systemic blood in association with risk factors such as smoking, diabetes, and dyslipidemia.[94,96–98] Finally, acute occlusion of the peripheral vasculature frequently results from thromboemboli of cardiac or abdominal aortic origin[94,97,98] (Table 4-1).

● VULNERABLE PLAQUE

In the literature, the term "culprit plaque" is frequently used to describe the lesion responsible for acute vessel occlusion and the resulting cardiovascular event. Several terms, including high-risk plaque, vulnerable plaque, unstable plaque, and thin cap fibroatheroma (TCFA), have been used to describe lesions with a higher likelihood of becoming future culprit plaques. To properly define adequate terminology and avoid confusion, a written consensus from a group of experts properly standardized these terms thus providing definitions for proper implementation, as summarized in Table 4-2.

Characteristics of Vulnerable Plaque

Atherosclerosis is generally asymptomatic until plaque stenosis exceeds 70% to 80% of lumen diameter. These stenotic plaques can produce hemodynamically significant reduction in flow to the myocardium, resulting in angina pectoris. In contrast, acute coronary and cerebrovascular syndromes are often caused by rupture of plaques with less than 50% stenosis[99] (Figure 4-5). This is supported by studies of patients with an ACS who had a recent prior coronary angiogram; the artery involved in the subsequent acute event was only moderately diseased. In view of these observations, the main focus in understanding the pathophysiology of acute coronary, cerebrovascular, and peripheral events has been on lesion characteristics rather than luminal loss.

The stability of the plaque depends on the dynamic regulation of the fibrous cap. As shown in Figure 4-6, the integrity of the atheroma cap depends on the balance between synthesis and catabolism of the extracellular matrix proteins, collagen, and elastin. Using amino acids as the substrate, SMC synthesizes collagen and elastin. The macrophage foam cell, activated by inflammatory mediators within the plaque including TNFa, M-CSF, MCP-1, etc. as well as interferon gamma produced by the T lymphocyte, releases several proteases. These include collagen degrading MMPs, and elastolytic enzymes including certain nonmetalloenzymes, such as cathepsins S and K, which promote matrix catabolism. Interferon gamma, in addition, also inhibits SMC replication and their ability to synthesize collagen. The net effect is progressive fibrous cap weakening, which makes the plaque more susceptible to disruption and associated thrombotic complications. The features associated with plaque vulnerability are shown in Table 4-3.

Three different mechanisms, i.e., plaque rupture, plaque erosion, and calcified nodule, can give rise to arterial

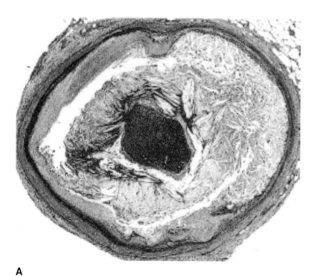

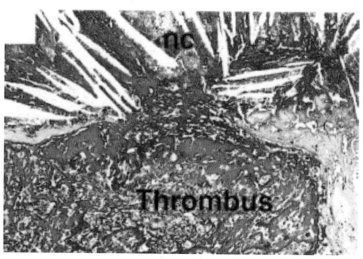

A   B

● **FIGURE 4-7.** Coronary plaque rupture. (A) Low-power view of a circumferential coronary plaque with fibrous cap rupture. Note the large necrotic core with numerous cholesterol clefts. There is a focal disruption of a thin fibrous cap (arrow) with an occlusive luminal thrombus (Movat Pentachrome, ×20). (B) High-power view of the rupture site showing fibrous cap disruption (arrows); the thrombus shows communication with the underlying necrotic core (Movat Pentachrome, ×400).

Reproduced with permission from Elsevier Science. Vermani R et al. Pathology of the vulnerable plaque. J Am Coll Cardiol. 2006;47:C13-C18.

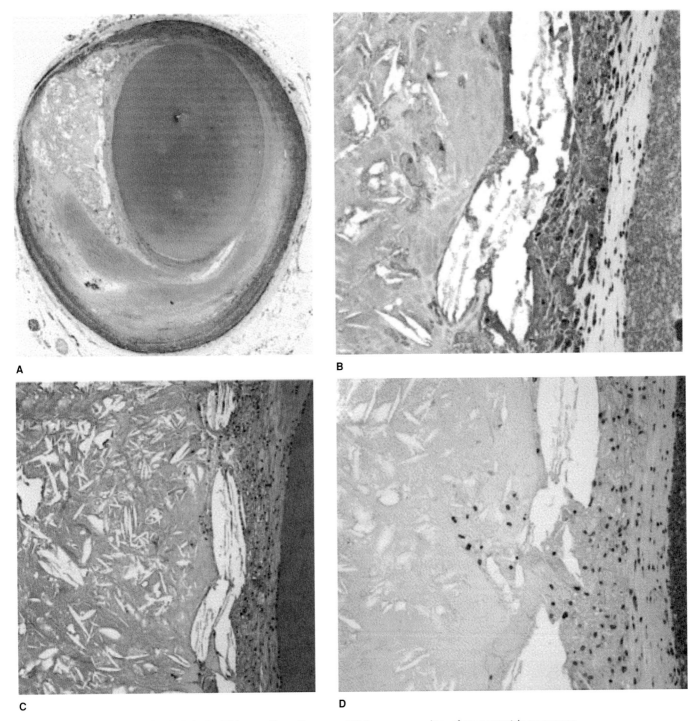

● **FIGURE 4-8.** Thin cap fibroatheroma. (A) Low-power view of an eccentric coronary plaque showing a thin fibrous cap overlying a relatively large necrotic core; the vessel was injected with barium (Movat Pentachrome, ×20). (B) Immunohistochemical staining reveals numerous CD68-positive macrophages within the fibrous cap (rose-red reaction product, ×400). (C) A cellular-rich thin fibrous cap with cholesterol clefts. (D) Staining for alpha-actin positive smooth muscle cells within the fibrous cap was virtually negative (×400).

Reproduced with permission from BMJ Publishing Group. Kolodgie FD et al. Pathologic assessment of the vulnerable human coronary plaque. Heart. 2004;90:1385-1391.

thrombosis. The frequency of thrombosis in sudden death is approximately 60%. The underlying mechanism related to thrombosis is plaque rupture in 55% to 60%, plaque erosion in 30% to 35%, and calcified nodule in 2% to 7% of cases.[100–105]

Plaque Rupture. A ruptured plaque is characterized by necrotic core with an overlying thin-ruptured cap infiltrated by macrophages (Figure 4-7). SMCs within the cap are a few or none. The thickness of the fibrous cap near the rupture site measures 23 ± 19 μm, with 95% of the caps

TABLE 4-4. Comparison of the Size of the Necrotic Core, Number of Cholesterol Clefts, Macrophage Infiltration, Number of Vasa Vasorum, and Hemosiderin-Laden Macrophages in Plaque Rupture, TCFAs, Erosion, and Stable Plaques

Plaque Type	Necrotic Core (%)	No. of Cholesterol Clefts (%)	Macrophage Infiltration, Fibrous Cap (%)	Mean Vasa Vasorum	Mean Hemosiderin-Laden Macrophages
Rupture ($n = 25$)	$34 \pm 17^{*\dagger}$	$12 \pm 12^{\ddagger\S}$	$26 \pm 20^{\|\|\P\#}$	$44 \pm 22^{**\dagger\dagger\ddagger\ddagger}$	$18.9 \pm 11^{\S\S\|\|\|\|\P\P}$
TCFA ($n = 15$)	24 ± 17	8 ± 9	$14 \pm 10^{\|\|}$	$26 \pm 23^{**}$	$4.4 \pm 3.6^{\S\S}$
Erosion ($n = 16$)	$14 \pm 14^{*}$	$2 \pm 5^{\ddagger}$	$10 \pm 12^{\P}$	$28 \pm 18^{\dagger\dagger}$	$4.3 \pm 4.7^{\|\|\|\|}$
Stable ($n = 19$)	$12 \pm 25^{\dagger}$	$4 \pm 6^{\S}$	$3 \pm 0.7^{\#}$	$13 \pm 9^{\ddagger\ddagger}$	$5.0 \pm 9.3^{\P\P}$

TCFA, thin cap fibroatheroma.

$^{*}p = 0.003$; $^{\dagger}p = 0.01$; $^{\ddagger}p = 0.002$; $^{\S}p = 0.04$; $^{\|\|}p = 0.005$; $^{\P}p < 0.0001$; $^{\#}p = 0.0001$; $^{**}p = 0.07$; $^{\dagger\dagger}p = 0.02$; $^{\ddagger\ddagger}p = 0.01$; $^{\S\S}p = 0.001$; $^{\|\|\|\|}p < 0.0001$; $^{\P\P}p = 0.03$.

Reproduced with permission from BMJ Publishing Group. Kolodgie FD et al. Pathologic assessment of the vulnerable human coronary plaque. Heart. 2004;90:1385-1391.

measuring <65 μm.[100] It has been observed that some plaques at other sites in the vascular tree resemble the ruptured plaque, but lack a luminal thrombus: these lesions have been designated as TCFA or vulnerable plaques.[103]

The TCFAs differ from ruptured plaques (Figure 4-8) by having a smaller necrotic core, less macrophage infiltration of the fibrous cap, and less calcification. Virmani and colleagues have quantitated, in cross-sections of coronary arteries with various types of plaques, the size of the necrotic core, the proportion of the lesion composed of cholesterol clefts, the percent macrophage infiltration of the fibrous cap, the number of vasa vasorum within the atherosclerotic plaque, and the number of hemosiderin-laden macrophages[106] (Table 4-4). The numbers of cholesterol clefts in the necrotic core, vasa vasorum, and hemosiderin-laden macrophages were significantly greater in the ruptured plaques than in erosion or stable plaques with >75% cross-sectional luminal narrowing. Significant differences between rupture and TCFAs were only seen for necrotic core size, macrophages, and hemosiderin infiltration.

Plaque Erosion. Plaque erosion is characterized by acute thrombus in direct contact with the intima, in an area of absent endothelium (Figure 4-9). These plaques are rich in SMCs and proteoglycan matrix,[107] with relatively a few or none macrophages and lymphocytes. The most frequent location for both erosion and rupture is the proximal left anterior descending artery (66%) followed by the right (18%) and the left circumflex (14%). Single-vessel disease (56%) is twice as frequent as double-vessel disease (26%). Plaque erosions tend to embolize more frequently than plaque rupture (74% vs. 40%, respectively).[108]

Plaque erosion accounts for greater than 80% of thrombi occurring in women younger than 50 years. It is frequently associated with smoking, especially in women. In a study by Farb et al.,[109] eroded plaques were more frequently seen in premenopausal women, were less stenotic, and had a much lower incidence of calcification. Coronary vasospasm has been implicated in the pathophysiology of plaque erosion

based on increased medial thickening and endothelial loss at the site of plaque erosion compared with plaque rupture.[110]

Calcified Nodule. The least frequent lesion of thrombosis shows a plaque that is heavily calcified consisting of calcified plates and surrounding area of fibrosis in the presence or absence of a necrotic core (Figure 4-10). The luminal region of the plaque shows presence of breaks in the calcified plate, bone formation, and interspersed fibrin with a disrupted surface fibrous cap and an overlying thrombus. There is often fibrin present in between the bony spicules along with osteoblasts, osteoclasts, and inflammatory cells.[103] It is more common in older men than women. It is believed that these lesions are commoner in the carotid arteries than the coronary and might be related to the frequent occurrence of plaque hemorrhage.

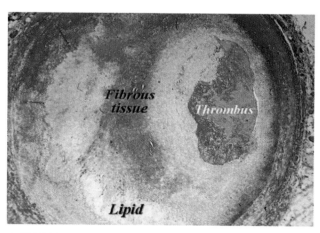

● **FIGURE 4-9.** Plaque erosion. Cross section of a coronary artery containing a stenotic atherosclerotic plaque with an occlusive thrombosis superimposed. The endothelium is missing at the plaque–thrombus interface, but the plaque surface is otherwise intact. Trichrome stain, rendering thrombus *red*, collagen *blue*, and lipid *colorless*.

Reproduced with permission from Elsevier Science. Fuster V et al. Atherothrombosis and high-risk plaque. J Am Coll Cardiol. 2005;46:937-954.

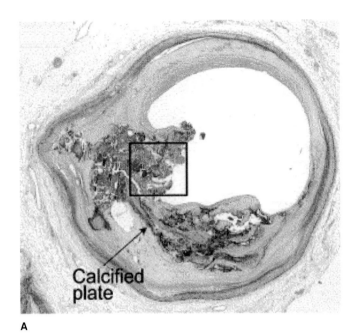

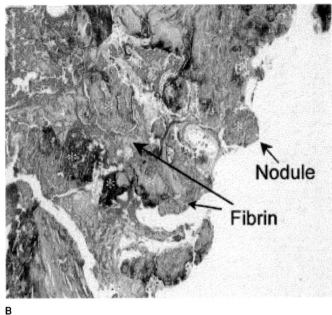

A

B

● **FIGURE 4-10.** Calcified nodule. (A) Low-power view coronary artery showing a heavily calcified eccentric plaque with eruptive calcified nodules (Movat Pentachrome, ×20). (B) Higher power view of the plaque surface of the lesion in (A), showing eruptive nodules with accumulated fibrin (×400).

Reproduced with permission from Elsevier Science. Vermani R et al. Pathology of the vulnerable plaque. J Am Coll Cardiol. 2006;47:C13-C18.

● CLINICAL PERSPECTIVE

The understanding of the biology of the vulnerable plaque necessarily leads to reassessment of current clinical approach. There is an emerging recognition that identifying a single vulnerable plaque and delivering targeted mechanical intervention is an inadequate approach to therapy. It is now known that vulnerable plaques are numerous and multiple disrupted plaques of varying local flow consequences may exist simultaneously with the culprit lesion. In patients presenting with ACS, intravascular ultrasound studies demonstrate multiple disrupted plaques proximal to the culprit lesion[111] as well as in other major coronary arteries.[112] Furthermore in patients with myocardial infarction or un-

stable angina, the elevation of inflammatory markers such as CD68 (macrophage), CD3 (lymphocytes), and HLA-DR were comparable between infarct- and noninfarct-related arteries[113,114] and between ischemic and nonischemic coronary microvasculature.[115] Atherosclerosis is a systemic disease, and plaque vulnerability also exists in multiple vascular beds. The complex interactions among the inflamed plaque, systemic procoagulant activity ("vulnerable blood"), local rheologic factors, and overall plaque burden ultimately define the vulnerable patient. Primary prevention, local mechanical therapy as needed, and, more importantly, systemic therapy that addresses the inflammatory burden underlying the vulnerable plaque are necessary to address the tremendous burden of this disease.

REFERENCES

1. Stary HC. Composition and classification of human atherosclerotic lesions. *Virchows Arch.* 1992;421:277-290.

2. Stary HC, Chandler AB, Glagov S, et al. A definition of initial, fatty streak, and intermediate lesions of atherosclerosis. A report from the Committee on Vascular Lesions of the Council on Arteriosclerosis, American Heart Association. *Circulation.* 1994;89:2462-2478.

3. Stary HC, Chandler AB, Dinsmore RE, et al. A definition of advanced types of atherosclerotic lesions and a histologic classification of atherosclerosis. A report from the Committee on Vascular Lesions of the Council on Arteriosclerosis, American Heart Association. *Circulation.* 1995;92:1355-1374.

4. Schwartz SM, deBlois D, O'Brien ER. The intima. Soil for atherosclerosis and restenosis. *Circ Res.* 1995;77:445-465.

5. Daugherty A, Pure E, Delfel-Butteiger D, et al. The effects of total lymphocyte deficiency on the extent of atherosclerosis in apolipoprotein E/mice. *J Clin Invest.* 1997;100:1575-1580.

6. Daugherty A, Rateri DL. T lymphocytes in atherosclerosis: the yin–yang of Th1 and Th2 influence on lesion formation. *Circ Res.* 2002;90:1039-1040.

7. Libby P, Ridker PM, Maseri A. Inflammation and atherosclerosis. *Circulation.* 2002;105:1135-1143.

8. Steinberg DPS, Carew TE, Khoo JC, Witztum JL. Beyond cholesterol. Modifications of low-density lipoprotein that

increase its atherogenicity. *N Engl J Med*. 1989;320:915-924.

9. Davies MJ. Stability and instability: two faces of coronary atherosclerosis. The Paul Dudley White Lecture 1995. *Circulation*. 1996;94:2013-2020.

10. Canto JG, Shlipak MG, Rogers WJ, et al. Prevalence, clinical characteristics, and mortality among patients with myocardial infarction presenting without chest pain. *JAMA*. 2000;283:3223-3229.

11. Sheifer SE, Manolio TA, Gersh BJ. Unrecognized myocardial infarction. *Ann Intern Med*. 2001;135:801-811.

12. Pohl T, Seiler C, Billinger M, et al. Frequency distribution of collateral flow and factors influencing collateral channel development. Functional collateral channel measurement in 450 patients with coronary artery disease. *J Am Coll Cardiol*. 2001;38:1872-1878.

13. Werner GS, Ferrari M, Betge S, Gastmann O, Richartz BM, Figulla HR. Collateral function in chronic total coronary occlusions is related to regional myocardial function and duration of occlusion. *Circulation*. 2001;104:2784-2790.

14. Bonetti PO, Lerman LO, Lerman A. Endothelial dysfunction: a marker of atherosclerotic risk. *Arterioscler Thromb Vasc Biol*. 2003;23:168-175.

15. Ravensbergen J, Ravensbergen JW, Krijger JK, Hillen B, Hoogstraten HW. Localizing role of hemodynamics in atherosclerosis in several human vertebrobasilar junction geometries. *Arterioscler Thromb Vasc Biol*. 1998;18:708-716.

16. Nerem RM. Vascular fluid mechanics, the arterial wall, and atherosclerosis. *J Biomech Eng*. 1992;114:274-282.

17. Traub O, Ishida T, Ishida M, Tupper JC, Berk BC. Shear stressmediated extracellular signal-regulated kinase activation is regulated by sodium in endothelial cells. Potential role for a voltage-dependent sodium channel. *J Biol Chem*. 1999;274:20144-20150.

18. Kunsch C, Medford RM. Oxidative stress as a regulator of gene expression in the vasculature. *Circ Res*. 1999;85:753-766.

19. Cai H, Harrison DG. Endothelial dysfunction in cardiovascular diseases: the role of oxidant stress. *Circ Res*. 2000;87:840-844.

20. Ignarro LJ, Napoli C. Novel features of nitric oxide, endothelial nitric oxide synthase, and atherosclerosis. *Curr Atheroscler Rep*. 2004;6:281-287.

21. Voetsch B, Jin RC, Loscalzo J. Nitric oxide insufficiency and atherothrombosis. *Histochem Cell Biol*. 2004;122:353-367.

22. Glass CK, Witztum JL. Atherosclerosis. The road ahead. *Cell*. 2001;104:503-516.

23. Libby P. Inflammation in atherosclerosis. *Nature*. 2002;420:868-874.

24. Hansson GK. Inflammation, atherosclerosis, and coronary artery disease. *N Engl J Med*. 2005;352:1685-1695.

25. Falk E. Pathogenesis of atherosclerosis. *J Am Coll Cardiol*. 2006;47:C7-C12.

26. Schwartz SM, Virmani R, Rosenfeld ME. The good smooth muscle cells in atherosclerosis. *Curr Atheroscler Rep*. 2000;2:422-429.

27. Geng YJ, Libby P. Progression of atheroma: a struggle between death and procreation. *Arterioscler Thromb Vasc Biol*. 2002;22:1370-1380.

28. Kolodgie FD, Petrov A, Virmani R, et al. Targeting of apoptotic macrophages and experimental atheroma with radiolabeled annexin V: a technique with potential for noninvasive imaging of vulnerable plaque. *Circulation*. 2003;108:3134-3139.

29. Tedgui A, Mallat Z. Apoptosis as a determinant of atherothrombosis. *Thromb Haemost*. 2001;86:420-426.

30. Hansson GK, Libby P, Schonbeck U, et al. Innate and adaptive immunity in the pathogenesis of atherosclerosis. *Circ Res*. 2002;91:281-291.

31. Binder CJ, Chang MK, Shaw PX, et al. Innate and acquired immunity in atherogenesis. *Nat Med*. 2002;8:1218-1226.

32. Griendling KK, Harrison DG. Out, damned dot: studies of the NADPH oxidase in atherosclerosis. *J Clin Invest*. 2001;108:1423-1424.

33. Andersen HO, Holm P, Stender S, Hansen BF, Nordestgaard BG. Dose-dependent suppression of transplant arteriosclerosis in aortaallografted, cholesterol-clamped rabbits. Suppression not eliminated by the cholesterol-raising effect of cyclosporine. *Arterioscler Thromb Vasc Biol*. 1997;17:2515-2523.

34. Steinberg D, Witztum JL. Is the oxidative modification hypothesis relevant to human atherosclerosis? Do the antioxidant trials conducted to date refute the hypothesis? *Circulation*. 2002;105:2107-2111.

35. Hansson GK. Immune mechanisms in atherosclerosis. *Arterioscler Thromb Vasc Biol*. 2001;21:1876-1890.

36. Rosenfeld ME. Leukocyte recruitment into developing atherosclerotic lesions: the complex interaction between multiple molecules keeps getting more complex. *Arterioscler Thromb Vasc Biol*. 2002;22:361-363.

37. Virmani R, Kolodgie FD, Burke AP, et al. Atherosclerotic plaque progression and vulnerability to rupture: angiogenesis as a source of intraplaque hemorrhage. *Arterioscler Thromb Vasc Biol*. 2005;25:2054-2061.

38. Vink A, Schoneveld AH, van der Meer JJ, et al. In vivo evidence for a role of toll-like receptor 4 in the development of intimal lesions. *Circulation*. 2002;106:1985-1990.

39. Wight TN. Versican: a versatile extracellular matrix proteoglycan in cell biology. *Curr Opin Cell Biol*. 2002;14:617-623.

40. Williams KJ. Arterial wall chondroitin sulfate proteoglycans: diverse molecules with distinct roles in lipoprotein retention and atherogenesis. *Curr Opin Lipidol* 2001;12:477-487.

41. Hoffmann U, Brady TJ, Muller J. Cardiology patient page. Use of new imaging techniques to screen for coronary artery disease. *Circulation*. 2003;108:e50-e53.

42. Pletcher MJ, Tice JA, Pignone M, Browner WS. Using the coronary artery calcium score to predict coronary heart disease events: a systematic review and meta-analysis. *Arch Intern Med*. 2004;164:1285-1292.

43. Fitzpatrick LA, Severson A, Edwards WD, Ingram RT. Diffuse calcification in human coronary arteries. Association of osteopontin with atherosclerosis. *J Clin Invest*. 1994;94:1597-1604.

44. Ikeda T, Shirasawa T, Esaki Y, Yoshiki S, Hirokawa K. Osteopontin mRNA is expressed by smooth muscle-derived foam

cells in human atherosclerotic lesions of the aorta. *J Clin Invest.* 1993;92:2814-2820.

45. Beckman JA, Ganz J, Creager MA, Ganz P, Kinlay S. Relationship of clinical presentation and calcification of culprit coronary artery stenoses. *Arterioscler Thromb Vasc Biol.* 2001;21:1618-1622.

46. Ehara S, Kobayashi Y, Yoshiyama M, et al. Spotty calcification typifies the culprit plaque in patients with acute myocardial infarction: an intravascular ultrasound study. *Circulation.* 2004;110:3424-3429.

47. Glagov S, Weisenberg E, Zarins CK, Stankunavicius R, Kolettis GJ. Compensatory enlargement of human atherosclerotic coronary arteries. *N Engl J Med.* 1987;316:1371-1375.

48. Tronc F, Mallat Z, Lehoux S, Wassef M, Esposito B, Tedgui A. Role of matrix metalloproteinases in blood flow-induced arterial enlargement: interaction with NO. *Arterioscler Thromb Vasc Biol.* 2000;20:E120-E126.

49. Vink A, Schoneveld AH, Richard W, et al. Plaque burden, arterial remodeling and plaque vulnerability: determined by systemic factors? *J Am Coll Cardiol.* 2001;38:718-723.

50. Barger AC, Beeuwkes R III, Lainey LL, Silverman KJ. Hypothesis: vasa vasorum and neovascularization of human coronary arteries. A possible role in the pathophysiology of atherosclerosis. *N Engl J Med.* 1984;310:175-177.

51. Kolodgie FD, Gold HK, Burke AP, et al. Intraplaque hemorrhage and progression of coronary atheroma. *N Engl J Med.* 2003;349:2316-2325.

52. Virmani R, Kolodgie FD, Burke AP, et al. Atherosclerotic plaque progression and vulnerability to rupture angiogenesis as a source of intraplaque hemorrhage. *Arterioscler Thromb Vasc Biol.* 2005;25:2054-2061.

53. Casscells W, Hassan K, Vaseghi MF, et al. Plaque blush, branch location, and calcification are angiographic predictors of progression of mild to moderate coronary stenoses. *Am Heart J.* 2003;145:813-820.

54. Polverini PJ, Cotran PS, Gimbrone MA Jr, Unanue ER. Activated macrophages induce vascular proliferation. *Nature.* 1977;269:804-806.

55. Lee WS, Jain MK, Arkonac BM, et al. Thy-1, a novel marker for angiogenesis upregulated by inflammatory cytokines. *Circ Res.* 1998;82:845-851.

56. Hansson GK. Immune mechanisms in atherosclerosis. *ArteriosclerThromb Vasc Biol.* 2001;21:1876-1890.

57. Davies MJ, Richardson PD, Woolf N, Katz DR, Mann J. Risk of thrombosis in human atherosclerotic plaques: role of extracellular lipid, macrophage, and smooth muscle cell content. *Br Heart J.* 1993;69:377-381.

58. Shah PK, Falk E, Badimon JJ, et al. Human monocyte-derived macrophages induce collagen breakdown in fibrous caps of atherosclerotic plaques. Potential role of matrix-degrading metalloproteinases and implications for plaque rupture. *Circulation.* 1995;92:1565-1569.

59. Shah PK, Galis ZS. Matrix metalloproteinase hypothesis of plaque rupture: players keep piling up but questions remain. *Circulation.* 2001;104:1878-1880.

60. Fuster V, Badimon L, Badimon JJ, Chesebro JH. The pathogenesis of coronary artery disease and the acute coronary syndromes. Parts 1 and 2. *N Engl J Med.* 1992;326:242-250 and 310-318.

61. Theroux P, Fuster V. Acute coronary syndromes: unstable angina and non–Q-wave myocardial infarction. *Circulation.* 1998;97:1195-1206.

62. Fuster V. Mechanisms leading to myocardial infarction: insights from studies of vascular biology. *Circulation.* 1994;90:2126-2146.

63. Toschi V, Gallo R, Lettino M, et al. Tissue factor modulates the thrombogenicity of human atherosclerotic plaques. *Circulation.* 1997;95:594-599.

64. Fernandez-Ortiz A, Badimon JJ, Falk E, et al. Characterization of the relative thrombogenicity of atherosclerotic plaque components:implications for consequences of plaque rupture. *J Am Coll Cardiol.* 1994;23:1562-1569.

65. Marmur JD, Thiruvikraman SV, Fyfe BS, et al. Identification of active tissue factor in human coronary atheroma. *Circulation.* 1996;94:1226-1232.

66. Nemerson Y. Tissue factor and hemostasis. *Blood.* 1988;71:1-8.

67. Maseri A, L'Abbate A, Baroldi G, et al. Coronary vasospasm as a possible cause of myocardial infarction. A conclusion derived from the study of "preinfarction" angina. *N Engl J Med.* 1978;299:1271-1277.

68. Kullo IJ, Edwards WD, Schwartz RS. Vulnerable plaque: pathobiology and clinical implications. *Ann Intern Med.* 1998;129:1050-1060.

69. Salomaa V, Rasi V, Kulathinal S, et al. Hemostatic factors as predictors of coronary events and total mortality: the FINRISK '92 Hemostasis study. *Arterioscler Thromb Vasc Biol.* 2002;22:353-358.

70. Edelberg JM, Christie PD, Rosenberg RD. Regulation of vascular bed-specific prothrombotic potential. *Circ Res.* 2001;89:117-124.

71. Edgington TS. So what is critically lacking with coronary atherosclerotic plaques? Perhaps the antithrombotic control. *Am J Pathol.* 2001;159:795-796.

72. Sambola A, Osende J, Hathcock J, et al. Role of risk factors in the modulation of tissue factor activity and blood thrombogenicity. *Circulation.* 2003;107:973-977.

73. Soejima H, Ogawa H, Yasue H, et al. Heightened tissue factor associated with tissue factor pathway inhibitor and prognosis in patients with unstable angina. *Circulation.* 1999;99:2908-2913.

74. Soejima H, Ogawa H, Yasue H, et al. Angiotensin-converting enzyme inhibition reduces monocyte chemoattractant protein-1 and tissue factor levels in patients with myocardial infarction. *J Am Coll Cardiol.* 1999;34:983-988.

75. Saito Y, Wada H, Yamamuro M, et al. Changes of plasma hemostatic markers during percutaneous transluminal coronary angioplasty in patients with chronic coronary artery disease. *Am J Hematol.* 1999;61:238-242.

76. Burke AP, Kolodgie FD, Farb A, Weber D, Virmani R. Role of circulating myeloperoxidase positive monocytes and neutrophils in occlusive coronary thrombi. *J Am Coll Cardiol.* 2002;39:256A.

77. Sugiyama S, Okada Y, Sukhova GK, et al. Macrophage myeloperoxidase regulation by granulocyte macrophage

colony-stimulating factor in human atherosclerosis and implications in acute coronary syndromes. *Am J Pathol.* 2001;158:879-891.

78. Rauch U, Osende JI, Fuster V, Badimon JJ, Fayad Z, Chesebro JH. Thrombus formation on atherosclerotic plaques: pathogenesis and clinical consequences. *Ann Intern Med.* 2001;134:224-238.

79. Munford RS. Statins and the acute-phase response. *N Engl J Med.* 2001;344:2016-2018.

80. Blake GJ, Ridker PM. Novel clinical markers of vascular wall inflammation. *Circ Res.* 2001;89:763-771.

81. Ridker PM, Rifai N, Clearfield M, et al. Measurement of C-reactive protein for the targeting of statin therapy in the primary prevention of acute coronary events. *N Engl J Med.* 2001;344:1959-1965.

82. Bickel C, Rupprecht HJ, Blankenberg S, et al. Relation of markers of inflammation (C-reactive protein, fibrinogen, von Willebrand factor, and leukocyte count) and statin therapy to long-term mortality in patients with angiographically proven coronary artery disease. *Am J Cardiol.* 2002;89:901-908.

83. Glagov S, Zarins C, Giddens DP, Ku DN. Hemodynamics and atherosclerosis. Insights and perspectives gained from studies of human arteries. *Arch Pathol Lab Med.* 1988;112:1018-1031.

84. Toussaint JF, LaMuraglia GM, Southern JF, Fuster V, Kantor HL. Magnetic resonance images lipid, fibrous, calcified, hemorrhagic, and thrombotic components of human atherosclerosis in vivo. *Circulation.* 1996;94:932-938.

85. Carr S, Farb A, Pearce WH, Virmani R, Yao JS. Atherosclerotic plaque rupture in symptomatic carotid artery stenosis. *J Vasc Surg.* 1996;23:755-765.

86. Virmani R, Narula J, Farb A. When neoangiogenesis ricochets. *Am Heart J.* 1998;136:937-939.

87. Yuan C, Mitsumori LM, Ferguson MS, et al. In vivo accuracy of multispectral magnetic resonance imaging for identifying lipid-rich necrotic cores and intraplaque hemorrhage in advanced human carotid plaques. *Circulation.* 2001;104:2051-2056.

88. Yuan C, Zhang SH, Polissar NL, et al. Identification of fibrous cap rupture with magnetic resonance imaging is highly associated with recent transient ischemic attack or stroke. *Circulation.* 2002;105:181-185.

89. Milei J, Parodi JC, Alonso GF, Barone A, Grana D, Matturri L. Carotid rupture and intraplaque hemorrhage: immunophenotype and role of cells involved. *Am Heart J.* 1998;136:1096-1105.

90. Spagnoli LG, Mauriello A, Sangiorgi G, et al. Extracranial thrombotically active carotid plaque as a risk factor for ischemic stroke. *JAMA.* 2004;292:1845-1852.

91. Davies MJ, Richardson PD, Woolf N, Katz DR, Mann J. Risk of thrombosis in human atherosclerotic plaques: role of extracellular lipid, macrophage, and smooth muscle cell content. *Br Heart J.* 1993;69:377-381.

92. Meyer BJ, Badimon JJ, Mailhac A, et al. Inhibition of growth of thrombus on fresh mural thrombus. Targeting optimal therapy. *Circulation.* 1994;90:2432-2438.

93. Meyer BJ, Badimon JJ, Chesebro JH, Fallon JT, Fuster V, Badimon L. Dissolution of mural thrombus by specific thrombin inhibition with r-hirudin: comparison with heparin and aspirin. *Circulation.* 1998;97:681-685.

94. Ouriel K. Peripheral arterial disease. *Lancet.* 2001;358:1257-1264.

95. Jackson MR, Clagett GP. Antithrombotic therapy in peripheral arterial occlusive disease. *Chest.* 2001;119:283S-299S.

96. Schmieder FA, Comerota AJ. Intermittent claudication: magnitude of the problem, patient evaluation, and therapeutic strategies. *Am J Cardiol.* 2001;87:3D-13D.

97. Dieter RS, Chu WW, Pacanowski JP Jr, McBride PE, Tanke TE. The significance of lower extremity peripheral arterial disease. *Clin Cardiol.* 2002;25:3-10.

98. Faxon DP, Fuster V, Libby P, et al. Atherosclerotic Vascular Disease Conference: Writing Group III: pathophysiology. *Circulation.* 2004;109:2617-2625.

99. Falk E, Shah PK, Fuster V. Coronary plaque disruption. *Circulation.* 1995;92:657-671.

100. Burke AP, Farb A, Malcom GT, et al. Coronary risk factors and plaque morphology in men with coronary disease who died suddenly. *N Engl J Med.* 1997;336:1276-1282.

101. Burke AP, Farb A, Malcom GT, et al. Effect of risk factors on the mechanism of acute thrombosis and sudden coronary death in women. *Circulation.* 1998;97:2110-2116.

102. Farb A, Tang AL, Burke AP, et al. Sudden coronary death. Frequency of active coronary lesions, inactive coronary lesions, and myocardial infarction. *Circulation.* 1995;92:1701-1709.

103. Virmani R, Kolodgie FD, Burke AP, Farb A, Schwartz SM. Lessons from sudden coronary death: a comprehensive morphological classification scheme for atherosclerotic lesions. *Arterioscler Thromb Vasc Biol.* 2000;20:1262-1275.

104. Kolodgie FD, Burke AP, Farb A, et al. The thin-cap fibroatheroma: a type of vulnerable plaque: the major precursor lesion to acute coronary syndromes. *Curr Opin Cardiol.* 2001;16:285-292.

105. Virmani R, Burke AP, Kolodgie FD, Farb A. Vulnerable plaque: the pathology of unstable coronary lesions. *J Interv Cardiol.* 2002;15:439-446.

106. Virmani R, Burke AP, Farb A, Kolodgie FD. Pathology of Vulnerable Plaque. *J Am Coll Cardiol.* 2006;47:C13-C18.

107. Farb A, Burke AP, Tang AL, et al. Coronary plaque erosion without rupture into a lipid core. A frequent cause of coronary thrombosis in sudden coronary death. *Circulation.* 1996;93:1354-1363.

108. Farb A, Burke AP, Kolodgie FD, et al. Platelet-rich intramyocardial thromboemboli are frequent in acute coronary thrombosis, especially plaque erosions. *Circulation.* 2000;102:II774.

109. Farb A, Burke AP, Tang AL, et al. Coronary plaque erosion without rupture into a lipid core. A frequent cause of coronary thrombosis in sudden coronary death. *Circulation.* 1996;93:1354-1363.

110. Hao H, Gabbiani G, Camenzind E, Bacchetta M, Virmani R, Bochaton-Piallatt ML. Phenotypic modulation of intima and medial smooth muscle cells in fatal cases of coronary artery lesions. *Arterioscler Thromb Vasc Biol.* 2006;26:326-332.

111. Schoenhagen P, Stone GW, Nissen SE, et al. Coronary plaque morphology and frequency of ulceration distant from culprit

lesions in patients with unstable and stable presentation. *Arterioscler Thromb Vasc Biol.* 2003;23:1895-1900.

112. Rioufol G, Finet G, Ginon I, et al. Multiple atherosclerotic plaque rupture in acute coronary syndrome: a three-vessel intravascular ultrasound study. *Circulation.* 2002;106:804-808.

113. Spagnoli LG, Bonanno E, Mauriello A, et al. Multicentric inflammation in epicardial coronary arteries of patients dying of acute myocardial infarction. *J Am Coll Cardiol.* 2002;40:1579-1588.

114. Libby P. Atherosclerosis: disease biology affecting the coronary vasculature. *Am J Cardiol.* 2006;98:3Q-9Q.

115. Neri Serneri GG, Boddi M, Modesti PA, et al. Immunomediated and ischemia-independent inflammation of coronary microvessels in unstable angina. *Circ Res.* 2003;92:1359-1366.

chapter 5

The Endothelium in Health and Disease

Rainer H. Böger, MD

● INTRODUCTION

Each and every blood vessel throughout the body is covered, at its inner, luminal surface, by a monolayer of specialized cells, i.e., the vascular endothelial cells. This monolayer represents the primary anatomical site that separates the compartment of the flowing blood from the body's interstitium. Although spread throughout the body and thus not easily discernible, all endothelial cells together cover a surface that has been estimated as 350 m^2 (see Ref. 1) and may count as many as 60 trillion (6×10^{13}) cells.[2] The total weight of all endothelial cells has been estimated to be between 110 g[3] and 750 g, or as much as the liver.[4] Recent scientific evidence has made clear that the endothelium may not be less metabolically active than the liver. It was 25 years ago when the ground-breaking experimental studies discovered the crucial role of the endothelium in regulating vascular smooth muscle tone and coagulation and it was concluded that the endothelium is not merely a passive barrier.[5–7]

Endothelial cells are polygonal in shape and generally orientated along the long axis of the vessels, thereby responding to the forces that the shear of the flowing blood exerts on their surface. Endothelial cells are polarized cells, with an apical (luminal) membrane facing the blood stream and an abluminal membrane facing the intercellular space. This polarity is manifested by a distinct protein composition of the two membranes and the controlled transport of molecules along either of these membranes. Intercellular tight junctions impede intercellular diffusion of molecules between the apical and abluminal membrane.

Because of its position, the endothelium is permanently exposed to hemodynamic forces exerted by blood flow, blood pressure, and vascular wall distension. In addition to these mechanical stimuli, the endothelium receives a plethora of chemical signals, both blood-borne and tissue-derived, which may elicit endothelial responses acting on the vessel wall itself or on more distant target sites. Some of these signals play an important role in modifying the primary function of the endothelium, that is, the precise control of the passage of solutes, macromolecules, and blood cells across the vascular wall.

● ANATOMICAL FEATURES OF THE ENDOTHELIUM IN DIFFERENT VASCULAR SEGMENTS

Morphologically, endothelial cells are flat cells that usually spread out broadly on the inner surface of a blood vessel; the nucleus can be prominently seen on microscopic images, protruding into the lumen (Figure 5-1). However, endothelial cells from different vascular beds vary considerably in phenotype. Thus, in different areas of the circulatory system, the endothelium is characterized by anatomically distinct features, which allow it to adapt to the varying regulatory functions of different organs. Depending on the presence of intercellular junctions, endothelia can be classified as "continuous," "fenestrated," or "discontinuous." For example, in the brain a continuous endothelial monolayer is part of the blood–brain barrier,[8] whereas in the renal glomerulus, fenestrated endothelia aid in maintaing the kindey's functions in filtration, secretion, and reabsorption of small and large molecules.[9] Discontinuous endothelia can be found mainly in the liver, bone marrow, and spleen, where many cells migrate from the blood stream into the tissue and back physiologically (Figure 5-2). Moreover, endothelia from arterial and venous blood vessels also vary both in phenotype and in function. Adapting to high shear

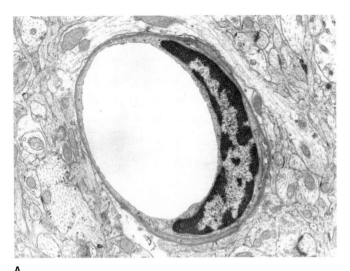

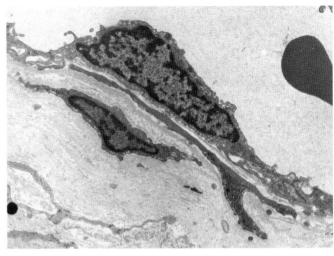

A

B

● **FIGURE 5-1.** (A) Electron microscopic image of a small arteriolar vessel with an endothelial cells spanning the complete inner surface of the arteriole. The endothelial cells are spread out so thinly at the vessels inner, luminal lining that the vessel wall is significantly thicker where the endothelial cell nucleus is located. Original magnification 1:25 000. (B) Another example of an endothelial cell lining the inner lumen of a blood vessel. The protrusion of the nucleus into the lumen and the many vesicles and pits that line the endothelial cell membrane are clearly seen, exemplifying this cell type as one of major metabolic activity. Original magnification 1:20 000.

The microphographs were kindly provided by Prof. Udo Schumacher, Institute of Anatomy and Experimental Morphology, University Medical Center Hamburg-Eppendorf, Germany.

stress in the arterial vascular bed, endothelial cells from arterioles are generally elongated in the axis of the blood flow, reaching a width-to-length ratio of 1:7 in rat tracheal mucosa, whereas capillary (1:5) and particularly venous (1:2.4) endothelial cells are rounder.[10] Also, endothelium-dependent vasorelaxation—one of the most important features by which the endothelium actively controls locoregionary blood flow—are generally more pronounced in arteries than in corresponding veins (see later).[11] However, when venous vessels are transplanted into the arterial system (like it happens in venous coronary bypass grafts), the endothelium in these bypass vessels is flexible enough to rapidly adapt its phenotype to the novel microenvironment.

The endothelium is far from being an inert, wallpaper-like inner lining of the vessel surface: quite in contrast, many regulatory functions that critically influence the vascular homeostasis are regulated in the endothelium. Some of the most potent vasoconstrictors and vasodilators interact with each other in the fine tuning of vascular tone. The hemostatic and fibrinolytic systems are controlled by endothelium-based mechanisms. Hormonal and paracrine systems such as the renin–angiotensin–aldosterone system, the eicosanoid pathways, the coagulation and fibrinolytic systems, and the nitric oxide (NO) pathway are tuned at the endothelial level. Finally (and by these biochemical means), the endothelium critically steers the activation, adhesion, and aggregation of blood platelets and the interaction of specific subtypes of leukocytes with the endothelium.

Thus, the delicate balance between the two functions as a transducing surface and as a barrier between blood and interstitium critically depends upon the structural and functional integrity of the endothelial monolayer, which must be able to adapt to changing hemodynamic situations and tolerate to a certain degree a variety of adverse conditions such as ischemia, hypoxia, and exposure to oxidants. Interaction of endothelial signalling pathways with such changes in the environment are crucial in the prevention or progression of vascular disease in a way that many vascular diseases actually start as an endothelial dysfunction. Moreover, the endothelium is able to respond to injury with specific repair mechanisms including angiogenesis and reendothelialization of a denuded vascular intima.

● **MECHANICAL PROPERTIES OF THE ENDOTHELIUM AND REGULATION OF ENDOTHELIAL PERMEABILITY**

With a few exceptions, such as the liver, the kidney, the adrenals, the chemoreceptor trigger zone in the brain, and the bone marrow sinusoids, endothelial cells form a selective barrier between blood and tissue. This barrier function can be altered under specific conditions, such as inflammation and neovascularization. Thus, the concept of endothelial permeability is not uniform and depends on the vascular area and the (patho-)physiological context.

Why, for example, do large molecules penetrate poorly into a tumor which is otherwise characterized by leaky blood vessels?[12]

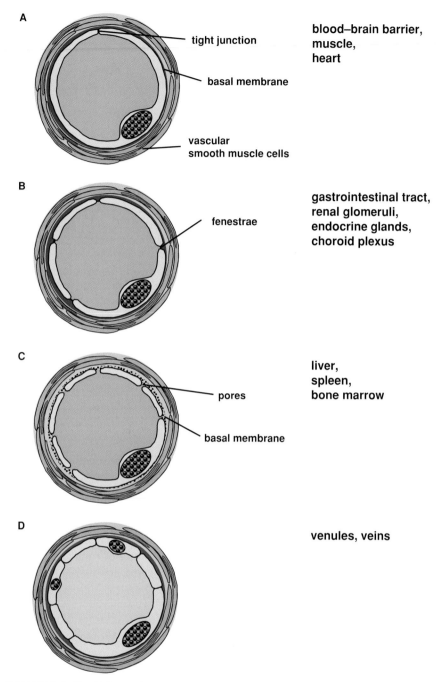

A
tight junction
basal membrane
vascular
smooth muscle cells

blood–brain barrier,
muscle,
heart

B
fenestrae

gastrointestinal tract,
renal glomeruli,
endocrine glands,
choroid plexus

C
pores
basal membrane

liver,
spleen,
bone marrow

D

venules, veins

● FIGURE 5-2. Schematic representation of different types of endothelial cells and their function and distribution throughout various organs.

Why are postcapillary venules the major location of extravasation of macromolecules during inflammation,[13] if it is the capillaries that are the part of the vascular tree where tubular structures aid in the exchange of macromolecules?[14]

And further, what is the mechanism by which even capillary microvessels become leaky in angiogenesis?

The diverse functional properties of the endothelium require active changes in cellular shape and at the same time require the generation of internal isometric forces appropriate to counteract changing hemodynamic loads acting on the monolayer.

It has been long since the discovery that the endothelial monolayer is covered by a coat of membrane-bound molecules, including glycolipids, glycoproteins, and proteoglycans, which in their totality have been named the endothelial glycocalix (Figure 5-3A). The glycocalix shows an average thickness of approximately 60 to 110 nm, which is in line with the assumed length of typical glycoproteins and proteoglycans.[15] Prominent examples of molecular components of the glycocalix are components of the coagulation and fibrinolytic system like tissue factor and plasminogen, and cell adhesion molecules such as selectins and integrins, which are involved in cell–cell interactions during

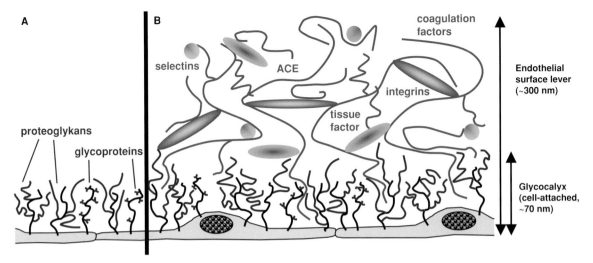

● **FIGURE 5-3.** The endothelial glycocalyx and surface layer. This thick stationary layer is composed of the endothelial glycocalyx and an additional layer of macromolecules that are not tightly fixed in the endothelial cell membrane. (A) The glycocalyx consists of glycoproteins and heparan sulfate proteoglycans. Glycoproteins (like integrins, selectins, and members of the immunoglobulin superfamily) are characterized by short and branched carbohydrate side chains, while proteoglykans exhibit long unbranched side chains. (B) A compex three-dimensional array of soluble plasma components including a variety of proteins, glycosaminoglycans, and hyaluronan forms a thick layer attached to the glycocalyx at the luminal side. Components of this layer dynamically exchange with the flowing plasma, but are relatively decelerated by adhesion to this layer.

immune reactions and inflammatory processes. Experimental data suggest that besides this layer of large molecules that are anchored in the endothelial plasma membrane, an additional layer of macromolecules covers the endothelial surface which are not tightly fixed in the membrane of endothelial cells, but which are kept in place by molecular interactions with the glycocalix. This thick stationary layer is called the endothelial surface layer (Figure 5-3B).[1] In their entirety, the glycocalix and the endothelial surface layer constitute the first line of the blood–tissue interface and are thus involved in a substantial number of physiological processes regulated by the endothelium: among these are the impact of mechanical stress on endothelial cell physiology and endothelial regulation of vascular tone, regulation of coagulation and fibrinolysis, blood cell–endothelial cell interactions during inflammation and atherogenesis, angiogenesis, and others.[3]

● ENDOTHELIUM-DERIVED FACTORS IN THE CONTROL OF VASCULAR TONE

Endothelium-Derived Vasorelaxing Factors

The endothelium plays a crucial role in the vasodilator response to a large variety of physiological situations as well as numerous vasoactive drugs. In 1980 Furchgott and coworkers discovered that the presence of an intact endothelium is mandatory for the relaxation of isolated blood vessels by acetylcholine in vitro, whereas acetylcholine induced contractions in arterial preparations in which the endothelium

had been injured or mechanically removed.[6] It was soon discovered that endothelial cells release an unknown soluble relaxing factor, which was named endothelium-derived relaxing factor[7] and was shown to be virtually identical with NO in 1987,[16] in response to a variety of pharmacological and physiological stimuli (Figure 5-4). NO is involved in a wide variety of regulatory mechanisms of the cardiovascular system, including vascular tone. In fact, it is regarded by many as the major mediator of endothelium-dependent vasodilation. It also regulates vascular structure (inhibition of smooth muscle cell proliferation) and cell–cell interactions in blood vessels (inhibition of platelet adhesion and aggregation; inhibition of monocyte adhesion). Thus, NO plays a crucial role in the endothelium-mediated regulation of vascular homeostasis (Figure 5-5).[17] Dysfunction of the endothelial NO pathway is a common mechanism by which several cardiovascular risk factors mediate certain deleterious effects on the vascular wall. Among these are hypercholesterolemia, hypertension, smoking, diabetes mellitus, homocysteine, and vascular inflammation.[18–20]

NO activates vascular smooth muscle soluble guanylate cyclase, increasing cyclic GMP and decreasing intracellular Ca^{2+} concentrations. The enzyme converting L-arginine to NO was purified and cloned in 1991 and was named nitric oxide synthase (NOS).[21] This enzyme releases NO from the terminal guanidino nitrogen group of L-arginine, producing L-citrulline as a by-product; it is inhibited by analogs of L-arginine that are substituted at the terminal guanidino group, like N^ω-monomethyl-L-arginine (L-NMMA),

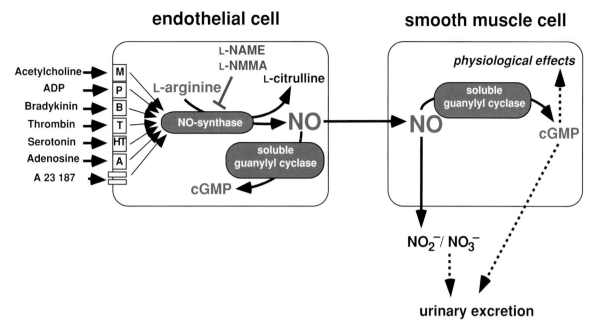

● **FIGURE 5-4.** Schematic representation of the L-arginine–nitric oxide pathway in the vascular wall. ADP, adenosine diphosphate; A 23187, calcium ionophore A 23187; L-NAME, N^{ω}-nitro-L-arginine-methyl ester; L-NMMA, N^{ω}-monomethyl-L-arginine; cGMP, cyclic 3′, 5′-guanosine monophosphate.

Reproduced with permission from Böger RH. Asymmetric dimethylarginine (ADMA): a novel risk marker in cardiovascular medicine and beyond. Ann Med. 2006;38:126-136.

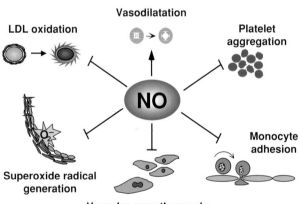

● **FIGURE 5-5.** Nitric oxide (NO) exerts pleiotropic effects on the cardiovascular system. NO has been shown to induce endothelium-dependent vasodilation, and to inhibit platelet aggregation, leukocyte adhesion, and smooth muscle cell proliferation. NO also exerts antioxidant effects, resulting in reduced superoxide radical generation and diminished oxidation of LDL cholesterol. As all of these mechanisms are known to contribute to the pathogenesis of atherosclerosis. NO is called an "endogenous anti-atherogenic molecule." Any condition that will reduce endothelial NO production may therefore promote atherosclerosis.

Reproduced with permission from Böger RH. The emerging role of ADMA as a novel cardiovascular risk factor. Cardiovasc Res. 2003;59:824-833.

N^{ω}-nitro-L-arginine (L-NNA), or N^{ω}-nitro-L-arginine methyl ester (L-NAME). NOS is present in at least three isoforms mainly in three types of tissues: in central and peripheral nervous tissues a constitutive isoform was isolated (NOS I), in activated macrophages an inducible NOS (NOS II) participates in unspecific host defence, and an endothelial isoform (NOS III) that constitutively releases NO is involved in the regulation of vascular tone and blood pressure. The characteristics of the three isoenzymes have been reviewed in detail by Förstermann et al.[22] NO has a very short half-life, which has been determined in experimental settings to be approximately 3 to 5 seconds.[23] Because of its chemical nature as a radical, it reacts with a variety of other chemical entities.[24]

The basal release of NO from endothelial cells produces a constant, active vasodilator tone that antagonizes a variety of vasoconstrictor mediators.[25] This basal NOS activity is maintained mainly by flow-induced shear stress that is exerted by the force the viscous blood exerts on the endothelial lining while it is flowing past this monolayer.[26] As any luminal narrowing of arterial vessels locally increases blood flow velocity, this may in turn induce the release of NO and contribute to poststenotic vasodilation—a phenomenon well known in the clinical setting. Flow-induced vasodilatation also occurs during physical exercise, and NO has been shown to mediate exercise-induced vasodilatation. Acute physical exercise is also a potent stimulus for systemic NO production in humans, as indicated by the observation that the urinary excretion rates of the NO metabolite, nitrate, and its second messenger, cyclic

GMP, are doubled after a 30-minute submaximal exercise in healthy subjects.[27] Moreover, chronic exercise has been shown to induce endothelial NOS gene expression in dogs. The molecular mechanism behind the shear stress-induced release of NO is the phosphorylation of several serine and threonine residues in the NOS protein. Phosphorylation of Ser^{1177} occurs in response to endothelial cell activation as well as hemodynamic stimulation. This serine is located in the reductase domain of the enzyme. By contrast, Thr^{495}, which is located in a site that binds an essential cofactor, calmodulin, is constitutively phsophorylated and becomes dephosphorylated upon endothelial stimulation. The dephosphorylation of this threonine residue facilitates the Ca^{2+}-dependent association of calmodulin with endothelial NOS, which is regarded as one important mechanism of NOS activation (for review, cf. Fleming and Busse[28]).

Besides fluid shear stress, a number of chemical entities can also activate endothelial NOS. Among them are acetylcholine (which, when the endothelial cells are dysfunctional, may alternatively bind to muscarinergic receptors on the vascular smooth muscle cell membrane and thereby induce vasoconstriction), thrombin, serotonin, adenosine diphosphate, and bradykinin. The common mechanism by which these chemical stimuli activate NOS is the increasing intracellular Ca^{2+} concentration.

NO is not the only vasodilator mediator that is actively secreted by the endothelium into the circulation and into the adjacent tissue, preferably the vascular smooth muscle cell layer; shear stress and cyclic stretch of the vessel wall are also known to stimulate the formation of the vasodilator autacoids, prostacyclin, and the endothelium-derived hyperpolarizing factor (EDHF). Prostacyclin is the major product of cyclooxygenase activity in endothelial cells. Like NO, it not only vasodilates vascular smooth muscle but also exerts an inhibitory effect on thrombocytes, thereby acting as an antithrombotic autacoid. Recent research has shown that the main isoform of cyclooxygenase that is expressed in endothelial cells even under noninflammatory conditions is COX-2—an observation that may help to explain the prothrombotic effects of the so-called selective COX-2 inhibitors and possibly also the classical nonsteroidal antiinflammatory drugs.[29]

EDHF is a term that applies not just to a single factor but rather to a variety of mechanisms inducing vasodilation via hyperpolarization of the endothelial cell membrane.[30] Currently four molecular mechanisms are discussed to account for EDHF-mediated responses: (a) the efflux of K^+ from endothelial cells that activates either the Na^+K^+ATPase or inwardly rectifies K^+ channels on smooth muscle cells; (b) generation of hydrogen peroxide (H_2O_2); (c) generation of a vasodilator epoxyeicosatrienoic acid by a cytochrome P450 epoxygenase; or (d) transmission of an electrical signal via gap junctions and the formation of intracellular cyclic AMP. Most of these potential mechanisms accounting for EDHF activity are difficult to study, and they may occur in parallel in the same or in different segments of the vascular tree and, so their relative contributions to the regulation of vascular tone are still not entirely clear.

Endothelium-Derived Vasoconstricting Factors

The major vasocontrictor mediator of endothelial origin is endothelin-1 (ET-1), a peptide belonging to a family of 21-amino acid peptides that are synthesized in various cell types. The production and release of ET-1 is stimulated by many hormonal and metabolic factors, by hypoxia, and by shear stress and cyclic stretch of the endothelium. Once released, ET-1 binds to two subtypes of endothelin receptors, i.e., ET_A and ET_B receptors. The ET_A receptors are located mainly on vascular smooth muscle cells and mediate vasoconstriction, whereas ET_B receptors on the endothelium are linked to NO and prostacyclin release. There is evidence that the production and action of ET-1 and NO are interrelated in multiple ways.[31]

Oxygen-derived free radicals are another important vasoconstrictor stimulus under certain (patho-)physiological conditions. Free radical production within the vascular wall is of crucial importance for the regulation of vascular tone not only by determining the bioactivity of NO but also by regulating the formation of hydrogen peroxide and peroxynitrite, which are two very important radical-type vasoactive compounds (Figure 5-6). Free radicals in the vascular wall are tonically produced, as evidenced by the improvement in vasodilatation that can be observed after the addition of superoxide dismutase to vascular tissues. NADPH oxidases have been regarded as a major enzymatic source of superoxide radicals; however, many other enzymes can release oxygen-derived free radical species during their principal enzymatic activity. Among them are cyclooxygenase, enzymes of the mitochondrial respiratory chain, cytochrome P450 monooxygenases, and xanthine oxidase. NADPH oxidases have been recognized to play a central role in the induction of what is often called "vascular oxidative stress," referring to a state of pathological oxidative burden in the vascular wall that may trigger or accelerate atherosclerosis (see later). NADPH oxidases can be activated by angiotensin II—an observation that may relate an atherogenic risk factor (hypertension) with vascular oxidative stress and might thereby suggest a molecular mechanism for the relationship between this risk factor and vascular atherosclerotic disease. Superoxide radicals released from NADPH oxidase may, in turn, trigger the release of oxygen-derived free radicals from other enzymatic sources and thus induce a self-enhancing process of oxidative stress and vascular inflammation.

Under pathophysiological conditions, other sources of oxygen-derived free radicals may come into play. Central among them is endothelial NOS, which—under conditions of substrate or cofactor deficiency—may produce superoxide instead of NO. This state is known as "eNOS uncoupling" and means the conversion of NOS from an atheroprotective into a pro-atherogenic enzymatic entity.[32,33]

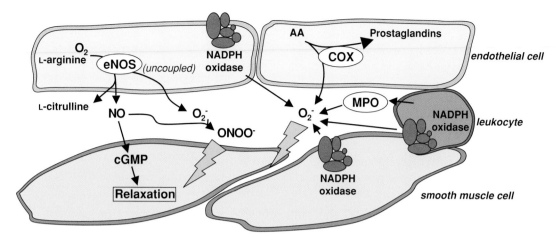

● **FIGURE 5-6.** Interaction between nitric ocide (NO) and oxygen-derived free radicals in the vascular wall. While NO is normally formed by NO synthase, certain pathophysiological conditions may lead to uncoupling of this enzyme, meaning that the NO synthase is unable to generate NO. Instead, it will produce superoxide radicals (O_2^-) under these conditions, making it a generator of cellular toxins instead of a cell-protecting molecule. Examples for other important sources of superoxide in the vascular wall are NADPH oxidases (a family of enzymes consisting of several catalytic and regulatory subunits), myeloperoxidase (the main enzyme responsible for cytotoxic activity of leukocytes), and cyclooxygenase. eNOS, endothelial nitric oxide synthase; NADPH, nicotinamide adenine dinucleotide phosphate; COX, cyclooxygenase; NO, nitric oxide; MPO, myeloperoxidase; O_2^-, superoxide radical; $ONOO^-$, peroxynitrite; cGMP, cyclic guanosine monophosphaste.

● CAVEOLAE: A MICROENVIRONMENT FOR TIGHT BIOCHEMICAL REGULATION OF ENDOTHELIAL FUNCTION

The endothelial plasma membrane exhibits membrane-associated microdomains, among which are vesicles, fenestrae, coated pits, and transendothelial channels. Among these, caveolae are the most characteristic structure of endothelial cells; they have first been described by Palade as spherical vesicles of 60- to 70-nm diameter and are in direct continuity of the endothelial cell plasma membrane and open to the extracellular space through a narrow neck.[34] Caveolae have long been understood as dynamic structures that have their main role in enabling transcytosis, frequently undergoing fission and fusion with the membrane.[35] However, caveolae have recently been identified as chemically and functionally distinct microdomains of the endothelial cell surface. The marker protein of endothelial vesicles, caveolin-1, is highly abundant in caveolae and plays an important role in signal transduction processes.[36] A plethora of receptors involved in numerous signal transduction pathways have also been shown to colocalize with caveolin-1, such as the epidermal growth factor receptor, the platelet-derived growth factor receptor, the endothelin B receptor, the interleukin (IL)-1 receptor, eNOS, and many others.

Ultrastructural analysis of microvessels from caveolin-1 knockout mice has revealed the absence of caveolae, but the presence of fenestrae and larger vesicular structures, which apparently are not dependent on caveolin-1 for their assembly. This may explain why homozygous knockout of the CAV-1 gene is not lethal, suggesting that other plasmalemmal vesicles and compensatory mechanisms like increased permeability of tight junctions may compensate for the lack of caveolae. As a functional phenotype, caveolin-1 knockout mice show uncontrolled endothelial cell proliferation, lung fibrosis, defective calcium signalling, and impaired endocytosis of macromolecules like albumin. The most striking finding, however, was that caveolin-1 knockout mice also present a severalfold higher plasma NO level.[37] This finding supports the hypothesis that caveolin-1 plays a role in regulating eNOS activity,[38] suggesting that eNOS becomes hyperactive in the absence of caveolin-1.

● ENDOTHELIAL CONTROL OF HEMOSTASIS AND FIBRINOLYSIS

When the continuity of the endothelium is disrupted, platelets and fibrin are activated to seal off the vascular defect. The process of hemostasis is subdivided into primary (involving mainly platelet activation) and secondary hemostasis (mainly related to blood coagulation and fibrin formation). When the defect is healed and the blood clot is no longer needed, the fibrinolytic system will dissolve it. The endothelial cells synthesize and release activators and inhibitors of platelet aggregation, blood coagulation, and fibrinolysis, and thereby play a pivotal role in the local regulation of these systems and the fine tuning of their interplay by providing both procoagulant and anticoagulant substances.

Primary hemostasis is activated when subendothelial matrix and collagen fibres are exposed to flowing blood after an injury to the vessel wall has occurred. Circulating platelets adhere to these structures by specific collagen receptors on the platelets' surface, such as glycoprotein (GP)

VI and GP $\alpha_2\beta_1$. Platelets also adhere to subendothelial von Willebrand factor by GP Ib. Adhering platelets undergo shape change and, by releasing vasoactive mediators like serotonin, thromboxane A_2, ADP, and platelet-derived growth factor, induce both vasoconstriction and the activation of secondary amplification loops in other platelets, resulting in the recruitment of additional platelets to the site, which finally initiates arrest of blood flow. Moreover, platelets activate the coagulation cascade by exposing tissue factor and delivering the first trace amounts of activated factor V. Once critical amounts of factor Xa, which is required for the initiation of thrombin generation, have been formed, the extrinsic pathway of caogulation is turned off by tissue factor pathway inhibitor. Further formation of thrombin is maintained by positive feedback loops involving thrombin-induced activation of factors V, VIII, and XI. Thrombin converts soluble fibrinogen to insoluble fibrin, which stabilizes the blood clot by tightly binding to platelet GP IIb/IIIa receptors. Excess thrombin is efficiently inhibited by its physiological inhibitor antithrombin III and also via downregulation of its own formation by activation of the protein C pathway.

Endothelial cells promote coagulation by several mechanisms: They synthesize and bind coagulation factors like factors V and VIII. Expression of these factors on the endothelial surface is enhanced by mechanical injury, as is the release of von Willebrand factor. This is remarkable, as most coagulation factors (with the exception of fibrinogen and prothrombin) are trace proteins that, for efficient interaction with each other and their receptors, must be concentrated on a cell surface. Phosphatidylserine residues, which normally are sequestered in the inner leaflet of a cellular phospholipid bilayer, may become exposed upon activation or mechanical injury of cells, serving as a catalytic site.[39] Other coagulation factors are bound to platelet membranes, and secondary to platelet adhesion also crowd into the endothelial microenvironment.

On quiescent endothelial cells, the formation of thrombin and the deposition of fibrin are antagonized by tissue factor pathway inhibitor, a Kunitz type inhibitor, and by the serine protease inhibitor, antithrombin.[40] Both inhibitors neutralize factor VIIa when it is bound to tissue factor, but not when it is soluble. Another endothelial cell–dependent anticoagulant pathway involves the integral membrane GP thrombomodulin, which binds, neutralizes, and degrades thrombin and generates activated protein C. The zymogen protein C is a vitamin K–dependent protein. Its activation by thrombin is accelerated by up to 20 000-fold by thrombomodulin. Activated protein C has anticoagulant activity by inhibiting factors Va and VIIIa. This reaction is modulated at the endothelial cell surface by protein S, another vitamin K–dependent cofactor that binds to the endothelial cell membrane and to protein C, thereby forming a cell surface–bound protein complex.[41]

Finally, the fibrinolytic system is organized to activate an inactive proenzyme, i.e., plasminogen, by converting it to the active enzyme plasmin, which in turn degrades fibrin. Activation of plasmin occurs by two immunologically distinct plasminogen activators, tissue-type (t-PA) and urokinase-type (u-PA) plasminogen activator. Inhibition of this fibrinolytic system may occur either at the level of the plasminogen activators, by specific plasminogen activator inhibitors (PAI-1 and PAI-2),[42] or at the level of plasmin, mainly by α_2-antiplasmin.

● THE ENDOTHELIUM IN INFLAMMATION AND TUMORS

A common mechanism that links tumor growth, inflammatory diseases, and the healing of injured tissues has recently been identified: it is the outgrowth of new blood and lymph vessels that occurs not only during embryonic development but also in each of these diseases. Endothelial cells play a key role in neovascularization. At the beginning, new blood and lymph capillaries consist of thin-walled tubular structures that are composed of nothing but a single layer of endothelial cells. These endothelial cells originate either from the minute fraction of 0.01% of mature endothelial cells in established blood vessels that undergo cell division or from circulating or bone marrow–derived endothelial progenitor cells (EPCs).[43] Quiescent vascular and lymphatic endothelial cells are activated by angiogenic factors such as vascular endothelial growth factor (VEGF), which promote new vessel formation by stimulating endothelial cell proliferation and migration. Circulating EPCs have recently attracted much attention as a cell type that is involved in the continuous repair of the endothelial monolayer.[44] While there is now evidence that therapeutic administration of reconstituted EPCs or their recruitment from bone marrow may stipulate beneficial effects in ischemic heart disease,[45] the molecular mechanism by which these cells act is still controversial because there is no clear evidence so far that progenitor cells can integrate into ischemic myocardium in humans. Some investigators argue that progenitor cells induce an inflammatory reaction that leads to the release of inflammatory cytokines, and in turn mediate the functional changes observed in clinical trials.

EPCs also significantly contribute to de novo vessel formation during wound healing, limb ischemia, recovery after myocardial infarction, and endothelialization of vascular grafts. However, besides these beneficial effects, excessive proliferation of mature differentiated endothelial cells or EPCs contributes to numerous malignant and nonmalignant diseases. With respect to therapeutic administration or stimulation of such cells in ischemic diseases, this marks the dark side of potential induction of malignancies. On the other hand, pharmacological inhibitors of endothelial proliferation and migration as well as inhibitors of EPC activation have been successfully developed for cancer chemotherapy, for the treatment of ocular neovascularization as it occurs in certain forms of macula degeneration, and other diseases.[46]

Blood vessels can grow in several ways: angiogenesis and arteriogenesis refer to the sprouting of preexisting vessels and subsequent stabilization of these sprouts by mural cells, whereas vasculogenesis refers to the development of new blood vessels by EPCs. Collateral growth depicts the expansive growth and largening of preexisting vessels.[46] In cancer, either of these mechanisms, plus the co-option of normal vessels by the tumor, contributes importantly to tumor survival. Excessive angiogenesis occurs in cancer to meet the ever-increasing demand of the tumor mass for nutrient and oxygen supply. Hence, it is no surprise that hypoxia is a strong stimulus for angiogenesis. Hypoxia is a frequent feature of the microenvironment of solid tumors.[47] Cells in tumors become hypoxic when they are too distant from nearby vessels, which happens as a result of cell division and tumor growth. Hypoxia activates hypoxia-inducible transcription factors (HIFs), which stimulate a large array of pro-angiogenic factors, including VEGF, NOS, adrenomedullin, Ang-2, placenta-derived growth factor, and others, in tumor and inflammatory cells. Under normal conditions, the von Hippel-Lindau gene product acts as a tumor suppressor by targeting HIF for ubiquitination and subsequent degradation under normoxic conditions.[48] However, when gene mutations inactivating the von Hippel-Lindau tumor suppressor gene occur, HIFs can exert their stimulatory action on neovascularization unrestrictedly. For example, inactivating von Hippel-Lindau gene mutations occur in approximately 50% of renal cell carcinomas, where particularly high levels of VEGF-A expression have been found.[49]

Maintenance of new blood vessels largely depends on the homeostasis between de novo formation and survival of endothelial cells. Therefore, endothelial apoptosis is another important regulator of neovascularization. It is stimulated by deprivation of nutrients or survival signals.[50] Endothelial apoptosis can be induced not only by VEGF pathway inhibitors but also by NO, oxygen-derived free radicals, and interferon-γ. Most angiogenesis inhibitors that are under development for therapeutic use cause endothelial apoptosis by directly interfering with cell surface molecules on endothelial cells.

● THE ENDOTHELIUM IN VASCULAR DISEASE, HYPERLIPIDEMIA, AND DIABETES MELLITUS

Dysfunction of the endothelium is a common mechanism by which several cardiovascular risk factors mediate their deleterious effects on the vascular wall. Among them are hypercholesterolemia, hypertension, smoking, diabetes mellitus, homocysteine, and vascular inflammation.[18–20,51] The endothelial L-arginine/NO pathway is thought to be the major effector of endothelial control of vascular homoeostasis because NO is involved in a wide variety of regulatory mechanisms of the cardiovascular system, including endothelium-dependent vasodilation, inhibition of smooth muscle cell proliferation, inhibition of platelet adhesion and aggregation, and inhibition of monocyte adhesion. It therefore plays a crucial role in the endothelium-mediated regulation of vascular homeostasis and acts as an endogenous anti-atherogenic molecule. Endothelium-dependent relaxation is impaired in animals with experimentally induced atherosclerosis, in isolated atherosclerotic human coronary arteries in vitro, and in the coronary microcirculation of patients with coronary artery disease in vivo. In these patients, the degree of impairment of acetylcholine-induced coronary vasodilatation has been correlated to the number of atherosclerotic risk factors present and to the progression of atherosclerosis. This defect extends beyond the coronary circulation in patients with coronary artery disease, pointing to the presence of a systemic endothelial defect in these patients. Further evidence suggests that the biological activity of NO is also decreased in early hypercholesterolemia, which may suggest that this biochemical defect is a cause, and not a consequence, of atherosclerotic disease.

Endothelial dysfunction is thus a state of endothelial cell activation and decreased levels of bioactive NO. The presence of endothelial dysfunction can best be measured in terms of impaired or lacking endothelium-mediated vasodilation in response to stimuli like intra-arterial acetylcholine (which activates eNOS via endothelial muscarinergic receptors when this enzyme is functional, but which induces vasoconstriction when the endothelial NOS pathway is dysfunctional via stimulation of muscarinergic receptors on vascular smooth muscle cells). Acetylcholine-induced vascular responses can be visualized by angiography or by venous occlusion plethysmography in the forearm (Figure 5-7A). Moreover, NO is also critically involved in the vasodilator response to increased flow (i.e., shear stress, see earlier in the chapter). When vascular occlusion is maintained by a blood pressure cuff inflated to suprasystolic pressure levels during several minutes and rapidly deflated thereafter, a hyperemic reaction is induced in the forearm microcirculation secondary to the accumulation of ischemic metabolites in the tissues. The high demand leads to an increased flow velocity in the brachial artery, which—via increased shear stress—results in upstream vasodilation of conducting vessels like the brachial artery itself. This vasodilation can be blocked by the infusion of an inhibitor of NOS. Thus, hyperemia-induced brachial artery vasodilation (or flow-mediated vasodilation, FMD, as it is commonly called) is a measure of the functional integrity of the endothelial NOS pathway (Figure 5-7B). This method has the advantage that it can be assessed by using the non-invasive method of high-resolution ultrasound. Consensus has been reached to methodological standards for investigators using this latter method.[52]

When endothelium-dependent vasodilation is measured either by quantitative coronary angiography after intracoronary infusion of acetylcholine or by brachial artery FMD, endothelial dysfunction is highly suggestive of a patient who is at an increased risk of experiencing major adverse cardiovascular events in the near future. Several prospective clinical trials have independently proven that endothelial dysfunction is of prognostic relevance for the occurrence of major cardiovascular events in a given patient.[53] This evidence was later reproduced and extended for patients with coronary artery disease by showing that oxidative stress plays a major role in reducing endothelium-dependent

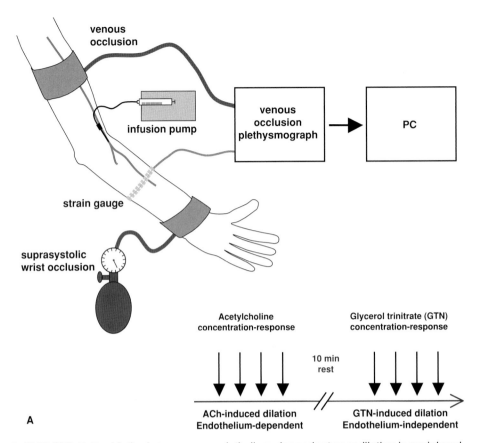

● FIGURE 5-7. Methods to assess endothelium-dependent vasodilation in peripheral arteries. (A) Noninvasive determination of flow-mediated vasodilation by high-resolution ultrasound. A high-resolution ultrasound probe is used to measure the longitudinal diameter of the brachial artery proximal to the antecubital fossa in a resting patient. Reliability of this method requires that the ultrasound image be recorded and analyzed using an image analysis software after digitalization of the images and transfer to a computer. After the baseline measurement, a blood pressure cuff is inflated to suprasystolic pressure in order to induce ischemia of the arm that is maintained during 5 minutes. The pressure in the cuff is to be controlled repeatedly in order to ensure complete stasis of blood, which can be controlled and documented by using the Doppler function of the ultrasound probe. After 5 minutes, the cuff is released rapidly. Accumulated ischemic metabolites in the forearm (like lactate, ADP, hypoxia, etc.) lead to peripheral vasodilation of resistance vessels in the forearm—the phenomenon well known as hyperemia. Hyperemia causes increased flow velocity in the brachial artery in order to compensate the increased demand for oxygen and nutrients in the arm; this increase in flow results in shear stress at the brachial artery endothelium, which in turn causes the release of nitric oxide (NO) and results in endothelium-dependent vasodilation of the brachial artery. The maximum dilation during hyperemia usually occurs at 60 seconds after cuff release; brachial artery diameter is recorded again at this time, and the difference between basal and hyperemic diameter is expressed as percent flow-mediated vasodilation (FMD). After 30 minutes of rest, another baseline diameter is recorded, and 0.8 μg of glycerol trinitrate (GTN) is applied sublingually. At 3 minutes after GTN maximal vasodilation is usually reached, arterial diameter is measured once again. The difference between the second baseline diameter recording and the GTN-induced diameter is called the endothelium-independent vasodilation. This is an important control feature, as GTN-induced vasodilation is also mediated via NO, but it does not test the endothelial capacity to release biologically active NO. Thus, changes in smooth muscle responsiveness to NO can be identified, which may blur interpretation of FMD when this test is repeatedly performed, like before and after pharmacotherapeutic intervention with some kind of vasoactive medication. (*continued*)

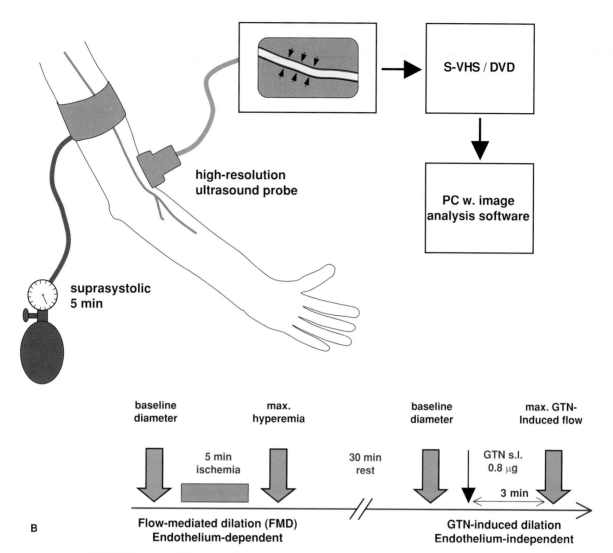

high-resolution ultrasound probe

S-VHS / DVD

PC w. image analysis software

suprasystolic 5 min

baseline diameter

max. hyperemia

baseline diameter

max. GTN-Induced flow

5 min ischemia

30 min rest

GTN s.l. 0.8 μg

3 min

Flow-mediated dilation (FMD) Endothelium-dependent

GTN-induced dilation Endothelium-independent

B

● FIGURE 5-7. (*Continued*) (B) Venous occlusion plethysmographic determination of acetylcholine-induced forearm vasodilation. An indwelling needle is placed into the brachialartery under local anesthesia for the infusion of acetylcholine, GTN, and potentially other drugs. A cuff around the wrist cuts off perfusion of the hand during the measurement period. Acetylcholine induces endothelial activation of NO synthase; release of NO leads to vasodilation of small arterioles in the forearm. The venous occlusion plethysmograph detects the dilation of an elastic strain gauge placed around the forearm during occlusion of venous blood flow at the upper arm. Occlusion pressure is increased to supravenous, but infradiastolic pressure transiently and repeatedly; the dilation of the strain gauge is continuously recorded; the slope of the resulting curve is a measure of forearm vasodilation. This method is more invasive than the method described in (A); however, it has the advantage that inhibitors of NO synthase, antioxidants, or other pharmacologically active substances can be co-infused thus allowing to gain a more detailed insight into the pathophysiological mechanisms underlying endothelial dysfunction.

vasodilation and prognosis in this disese.[54] Furthermore, similar data were also found for patients with peripheral arterial disease,[55] where the finding of impaired endothelium-dependent vasodilation was found to add diagnostic value to the measurement of ankle–brachial index.[56] Moreover, endothelial dysfunction was also shown to be of prognostic relevance in hypertensive patients[57] and in those patients with the most advanced chronic cardiac disease, congestive heart failure.[58]

The clinical phenomenon of endothelial dysfunction has been described in patients with overt atherosclerotic disease—in such patients, endothelial dysfunction extends to those areas of the vascular tree that are not affected by atherosclerotic plaques. More importantly, however, even patients with preclinical disease, such as asymptomatic young patients with isolated hypercholesterolemia, hypertension, smokers, diabetes mellitus, even impaired glucose tolerance, and several other preclinical medium- or high-risk situations, endothelial dysfunction has been observed. On the basis of such experimental and clinical evidence, there is agreement that endothelial dysfunction is an early common denominator by which several (if not all) cardiovascular risk factors initiate the process of atherogenesis. There is, however, debate on the nature of the primary molecular defect that causes such endothelial dysfunction. While reduced expression of eNOS has been excluded as a cause quite early, enhanced oxidative inactivation of NO on

one hand and reduced production of NO on the other hand have for long been the two poles between which discussion extended. The potential sources of oxygen-derived free radical species that may inactivate NO have already been described in the chapter; under pathological conditions they maybe joined by enzymes, e.g., myeloperoxidase (a major enzyme present in leukocytes that invade the hypercholesterolemic vascular wall), oxidants derived from cigarette smoke, or uncoupling of eNOS itself. Oxygen-derived radicals may impair NOS activity by uncoupling this enzyme and so the clear discrimination of these antipodes maybe difficult.

On the other hand, reduced enzymatic activity of NOS maybe brought about by the presence of increased levels of endogenous NOS inhibitors like monomethyl-L-arginine (L-NMMA) or asymmetric dimethylarginine (ADMA)—two arginine derivatives that have been shown to be present endogenously.[59] While L-NMMA circulates in human plasma only in trace amounts, ADMA is present in concentrations that are clearly sufficient to regulate NO activity; it has been shown to induce great changes in NO production even when only tiny changes in its plasma levels can be detected. Intensive clinical and experimental research in recent years has significantly advanced our understanding of the role of this molecule for regulating NO production in vivo (Figure 5-8).[60,61] In prospective clinical trials, ADMA has been identified as a reliable and

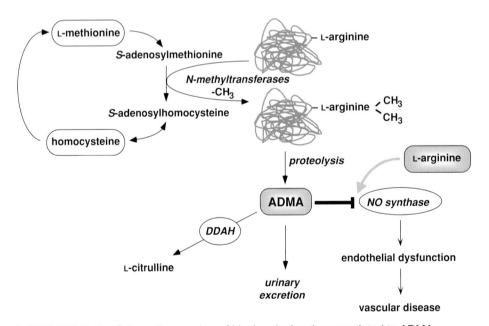

● FIGURE 5-8. Schematic overview of biochemical pathways related to ADMA. Methylation of arginine residues within proteins or polypeptides occurs through *N*-methyltransferases, which utilize *S*-adenosylmethionine as a methyl group donor. After proteolytic breakdown of proteins, free ADMA is present in cytoplasm. It can also be detected circulating in human blood plasma. ADMA acts as an inhibitor of NO synthase by competing with the substrate of this enzyme, L-arginine, and causes endothelial dysfunction and, subsequently, atherosclerosis. ADMA is eliminated from the body in part via urinary excretion and, more importantly, via metabolism by the enzyme dimethylarginine dimethylaminohydrolase (DDAH) to citrulline and dimethylamine.

Reproduced with permission from Böger RH. The emerging role of ADMA as a novel cardiovascular risk factor. Cardiovasc Res. 2003;59:824-833.

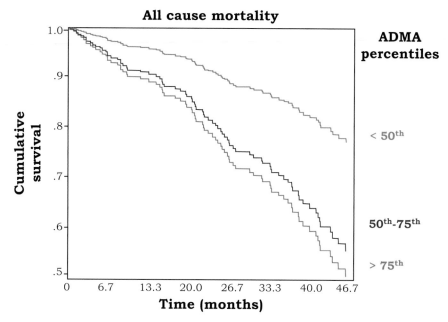

FIGURE 5-9. Kaplan–Meier plot of all-cause mortality in patients with chronic renal failure. Patients were stratified according to percentiles of ADMA plasma concentration at baseline and were followed for a mean of 33.4 months. The risk of dying of any cause was significantly higher in patients with elevated ADMA concentration.

Data are taken from Böger RH. Asymmetric dimethylarginine (ADMA): a novel risk marker in cardiovascular medicine and beyond. Ann Med. 2006;38:126-136.

independent cardiovascular risk marker[61,62] (Figure 5-9). Its diagnostic use is currently being evaluated in large clinical studies using a validated immunoassay method developed in our laboratory[63]. Inhibition of eNOS by ADMA may cause uncoupling of this enzyme[64] and may induce vascular oxidative stress and upregulation of redox-regulated endothelial genes, leading to leukocyte accumulation in the subendothelial space and vascular inflammation.[65] Again, reduced NO production and increased oxidative inactivation of NO may hardly be discernible as the primary cause of the disease.

In fact, the primary cause of the endothelial dysfunction that was found in various cardiovascular diseases or in the presence of various cardiovascular risk factors may differ and be multifactorial. The sequence of events outlined above makes it clear that either of the two primary defects will lead to both reduced NO production by eNOS and enhanced superoxide radical release into the vascular wall. Taken together, this clearly is a major impetus for vascular inflammation, leukocyte invasion, oxidation of LDL cholesterol, upregulation of the expression of genes contributing to plaque formation of destabilization, and thereby, complete vascular occlusion and death. The endothelium has therefore become a major target for pharmacotherapeutic intervention, gene therapy, and nonpharmacological measures of primary prevention.

REFERENCES

1. Pries AR, Secomb TW, Gaehtgens P. The endothelial surface layer. *Pflugers Arch.* 2000;440:653-666.

2. Simionescu M, Antohe F. Functional ultrastructure of the vascular endothelium: changes in vascular pathologies. In: Moncada S, Higgs EA, eds. *The Vascular Endothelium. Handbook of Experimental Pharmacology.* Vol 176/I.Heidelberg: Springer; 2006:41-69..

3. Pries AR, Kuebler WM. Normal endothelium. In: Moncada S, Higgs EA, eds. *The Vascular Endothelium. Handbook of Experimental Pharmacology.* Vol 176/I. Heidelberg: Springer; 2006: 1-40.

4. van Hinsburgh VWM, van Nieuw Amerongen GP, Draijer R. Regulation of the permeability of human endothelial cell monolayers. In: Born GVR, Schwartz CJ, eds. *Vascular Endothelium.* Stuttgart: Schattauer; 1997:61-76.

5. Moncada S, Herman AG, Higgs EA, Vane JR. Differential formation of prostacyclin (PGX or PGI2) by layers of the arterial wall. An explanation for the anti-thrombotic properties of vascular endothelium. *Thromb Res.* 1977;11:323-344.

6. Furchgott RF, Zawadzki JV. The obligatory role of endothelial cells in the relaxation of arterial smooth muscle by acetylcholine. *Nature.* 1980;288:373-376.

7. Furchgott RF. Role of endothelium in responses of vascular smooth muscle. *Circ Res.* 1983;53:557-573.

8. Ballabh P, Braun A, Nedergaard M. The blood-brain barrier: an overview: structure, regulation, and clinical implications. *Neurobiol Dis.* 2004;16:1-13.

9. Adeagbo AS. Endothelium-derived hyperpolarizing factor: characterization as a cytochrome P450 1A-linked metabolite

of arachidonic acid in perfused rat mesenteric prearteriolar bed. *Am J Hypertens.* 1997;10:763-771.

10. McDonald DM. Endothelial gaps and permeability of venules in rat tracheas exposed to inflammatory stimuli. *Am J Physiol.* 1994;266:L61-L83.

11. Seidel CL, LaRochelle J. Venous and arteria endothelia: different dilator abilities in dog vessels. *Circ Res.* 1987;60:626-630.

12. Jain RK. Hemodynamic and transport barriers to the treatment of solid tumours. *Int J Radiat Biol.* 1991;60:85-100.

13. Joris I, Cuenoud HF, Doern GV, Underwood JM, Majno G. Capillary leakage in inflammation. A study by vascular labelling. *Am J Pathol.* 1990;137:1353-1363.

14. Dvorak HF. Tumors: wounds that do not heal. Similarities between tumor stroma generation and wound healing. *N Engl J Med.* 1986;315:1650-1659.

15. Hjalmarsson C, Johansson BR, Haraldsson B. Electron microscopic evaluation of the endothelial surface layer of glomerular capillaries. *Microvasc Res.* 2004;67:9-17.

16. Palmer RMJ, Ashton DS, Moncada S. Vascular endothelial cells synthesize nitric oxide from L-arginine. *Nature.* 1988;333:664-666.

17. Böger RH, Bode-Böger SM, Frölich JC. The L-arginine—nitric oxide pathway: role in atherosclerosis and therapeutic implications. *Atherosclerosis.* 1996;127:1-11.

18. Panza JA, Quyyumi AA, Brush JE Jr, Epstein SE. Abnormal endothelium-dependent vascular relaxation in patients with essential hypertension. *N Engl J Med.* 1990;323:22-27.

19. Böger RH, Bode-Böger SM, Szuba A, et al. ADMA: a novel risk factor for endothelial dysfunction. Its role in hypercholesterolemia. *Circulation.* 1998;98:1842-1847.

20. Hingorani AD, Cross J, Kharbanda RK, et al. Acute systemic inflammation impairs endothelium-dependent dilatation in humans. *Circulation.* 2000;102:994-999.

21. Pollock JS, Förstermann U, Mitchell JA, et al. Purification and characterization of particulate endothelium-derived relaxing factor synthase from cultured and native bovine aortic endothelial cells. *Proc Natl Acad Sci USA.* 1991;88:10480-10484.

22. Förstermann U, Closs EI, Pollock JS, et al. Nitric oxide synthase isoenzymes. Characterization, purification, molecular cloning, and functions. *Hypertension.* 1994;23:1121-1131.

23. Griffith TM, Edward DH, Lewis MJ, Newby AC, Henderson AH. The nature of the endothelium-derived vascular relaxant factor. *Nature.* 1984;308:645-647.

24. Ignarro LJ. Biosynthesis and metabolism of endothelium-derived nitric oxide. *Annu Rev Pharmaol Toxicol.* 1990;30:535-560.

25. Rees DD, Palmer RMJ, Moncada S. Role of endothelium-derived nitric oxide in the regulation of blood pressure. *Proc Natl Acad Sci USA.* 1989;86:3375-3378.

26. Pohl U, Holtz J, Busse R, Bassenge E. Crucial role of endothelium in the vasodilator response to increased flow in vivo. *Hypertension.* 1986;8:37-44.

27. Bode-Böger SM, Böger RH, Schröder EP, Frölich JC. Exercise increases systemic NO production in men. *J Cardiovasc Risk.* 1994;1:173-178.

28. Fleming I, Busse R. Molecular mechanisms involved in the regulation of the endothelial nitric oxide synthase. *Am J Physiol.* 2003;284:R1-R12.

29. Kearney PM, Baigent C, Godwin J, Halls H, Emberson JR, Patrono C. Do selective cyclo-oxygenase-2 inhibitors and traditional non-steroidal anti-inflammatory drugs increase the risk of atherothrombosis? Meta-analysis of randomised trials. *Br Med J.* 2006;332:1302-1308.

30. Busse R, Edwards G, Feletou M, Fleming I, Vanhoutte PM, Weston AH. EDHF: Bringing the concepts together. *Trends Pharmacol Sci.* 2002;23:374-380.

31. Lavallee M, Takamura M, Parent R, Thorin E. Crosstalk between endothelin and nitric oxide in the control of vascular tone. *Heart Fail Rev.* 2001;6:365-376.

32. Stuehr D, Pou S, Rosen GM. Oxygen reduction by nitric oxde synthases. *J Biol Chem.* 2001;276:14533-14536.

33. Landmesser U, Dikalov S, Price SR, et al. Oxidation of tetrahydrobiopterin leads to uncoupling of endothelial cell nitric oxide synthase in hypertension. *J Clin Invest.* 2003;111:1201-1209.

34. Palade GE. Fine structure of blood capillaries. *J Appl Physics.* 1953;24:1424.

35. Simionescu and Simionescu 1991

36. Rothberg KG, Heuser JE, Donzell WC, Ying YS, Glenney JR, Anderson RG. Caveolin, a protein component of caveolae membrane coats. *Cell.* 1992;68:673-682.

37. Zhao YY, Liu Y, Stan RV, et al. Defects in caveolin-1 cause dilated cardiomyopathy and pulmonary hypertension in knockout mice. *Proc Natl Acad Sci USA.* 2002;99:11375-11380.

38. Bucci M, Gratton JP, Rudic RD, et al. In vivo delivery of the caveolin-1 scaffolding domain inhibits nitric oxide synthesis and reduces inflammation. *Nat Med.* 2000;6:1362-1367.

39. Sims PJ, Wiedmer T. Unraveling the mysteries of phospholipid scrambling. *Thromb Haemost.* 2001;86:266-175.

40. Rapaport SI, Rao VM. The tissue factor pathway: how it has become a "Prima Ballerina." *Thromb Haemost.* 1995;74:7-17.

41. Esmon CT. Molecular events that control the protein C anticoagulant pathway. *Thromb Haemost.* 1993;70:29-35.

42. Kruithof EKO. Plasminogen activator inhibitors—a review. *Enzyme.* 1988;40:113-121.

43. Carmeliet P. Mechanisms of angiogenesis and arteriogenesis. *Nat Med.* 2000;6:389-395.

44. Seeger FH, Zeiher AM, Dimmeler S. Cell-enhancement strategies for the treatment of ischemic heart disease. *Nat Clin Pract Cardiovasc Med.* 2007;4(suppl 1):S110-S113.

45. Asahara T, Isner JM. Endothelial progenitor cells for vascular regeneration. *J Hematother Stem Cell Res.* 2002;11:171-178.

46. Carmeliet P. Angiogenesis in health and disease. *Nat Med.* 2003;9:653-660.

47. Harris AL. Hypoxia – a key regulatory factor in tumour growth. *Nat Rev Cancer.* 2002;2:38-47.

48. Safran M, Kaelin WG Jr. HIF hydroxylation and the mammalian oxygen-sensing pathway. *J. Clin. Invest.* 2003;111:779-783.

49. Seizinger BR, Rouleau GA, Ozelius LJ, et al. von Hippel-Lindau disease maps to the region of chromosome 3 associated with renal cell carcinoma. *Nature.* 1988;332:268-269.

50. Carmeliet P, Jain RK. Angiogenesis in cancer and other diseases. *Nature.* 2003;407:249-257.

51. Celermajer DS, Sorensen KE, Georgakopoulos D, et al. Cigarette smoking is associated with dose-related and potentially reversible impairment of endothelium-dependent dilation in healthy young adults. *Circulation.* 1993;88:2149-2155.

52. Corretti MC, Anderson TJ, Benjamin EJ, et al. Guidelines for the ultrasound assessment of endothelial-dependent flow-mediated vasodilation of the brachial artery. *J Am Coll Cardiol.* 2002;39:257-265.

53. Schächinger V, Britten MB, Zeiher AM. Prognostic impact of coronary vasodilator dysfunction on adverse long-term outcome of coronary heart disease. *Circulation.* 2000;101:1899-1906.

54. Heitzer T, Schlinzig T, Krohn K, Meinertz T, Munzel T. Endothelial dysfunction, oxidative stress, and risk of cardiovascular events in patients with coronary artery disease. *Circulation.* 2001;104:2673-2678.

55. Gokce N, Keaney JF Jr, Hunter LM, et al. Predictive value of noninvasively determined endothelial dysfunction for long-term cardiovascular events in patients with peripheral vascular disease. *J Am Coll Cardiol.* 2003;41:1769-1775.

56. Brevetti G, Silvestro A, Schiano V, Chiariello M. Endothelial dysfunction and cardiovascular risk prediction in peripheral arterial disease: additive value of flow-mediated dilation to ankle–brachial pressure index. *Circulation.* 2003;108:2093-2098.

57. Perticone F, Ceravolo R, Pujia A, et al. Prognostic significance of endothelial dysfunction in hypertensive patients. *Circulation.* 2001;104:191-196.

58. Heitzer T, Baldus S, von Kodolitsch Y, Rudolph V, Meinertz T. Systemic endothelial dysfunction as an early predictor of adverse outcome in heart failure. *Arterioscler Thromb Vasc Biol.* 2005;25:1174-1179.

59. Vallance P, Leone A, Calver A, Collier J, Moncada S. Accumulation of an endogenous inhibitor of NO synthesis in chronic renal failure. *Lancet.* 1992;339:572-575.

60. Böger RH. The emerging role of ADMA as a novel cardiovascular risk factor. *Cardiovasc Res.* 2003;59:824-833.

61. Böger RH. Asymmetric dimethylarginine (ADMA): a novel risk marker in cardiovascular medicine and beyond. *Ann Med.* 2006;38:126-136.

62. Zoccali C, Bode-Böger SM, Mallamaci F, et al. Asymmetric dimethylarginine (ADMA): An endogenous inhibitor of nitric oxide synthase predicts mortality in end-stage renal disease (ESRD). *Lancet.* 2001;358:2113-2117.

63. Schulze F, Wesemann R, Schwedhelm E, et al. Determination of ADMA using a novel ELISA assay. *Clin Chem Lab Med.* 2004;42:1377-1383.

64. Sydow K, Münzel T. ADMA and oxidative stress. *Atherosclerosis.* 2003;4(suppl. 4):41-51.

65. Böger RH, Bode-Böger SM, Tsao PS, Lin PS, Chan JR, Cooke JP. An endogenous inhibitor of nitric oxide synthase regulates endothelial adhesiveness for monocytes. *J Am Coll Cardiol.* 2000;36:2287-2295.

chapter 6

Clinical Assessment of Endothelial Function

Julian P. J. Halcox, MA, MD / *Ann E. Donald, AVS* / *John E. Deanfield, MD*

It has become increasingly apparent that the atherosclerotic disease process begins early in life. Dynamic changes in vascular biology are involved in the initiation and progression of disease as well as in the destabilization of established plaques that gives rise to acute clinical events.[1] The vascular endothelium has been shown to be the central regulator of vascular health, accomplished through the production of a wide range of factors that affect vascular tone, cellular adhesion, thrombosis, smooth muscle cell proliferation, and vessel wall inflammation as described in Chapter 5. Because of its intimate interface between the circulating blood and the vessel wall, it is ideally placed to function as an active signal transducer for circulating modulators of vessel wall biology.[2] Alterations in endothelial function are the earliest pathological vascular changes that can be detected clinically. These typically precede the evolution of structural atherosclerotic disease, contributing mechanistically to lesion development and to later clinical complications.[1]

Appreciation of the central role of the endothelium throughout the atherosclerotic disease process has led to the development of a wide variety of tests to evaluate its various functional properties. These techniques have provided valuable insights into the role of the endothelium in the maintenance of a healthy circulation and the pathogenesis of arterial disease. These different methods will be discussed in this chapter in relation to the opportunities provided for the detection of preclinical disease, understanding the impact of risk factors, and the vascular response to interventions.

● PRINCIPLES OF ENDOTHELIAL FUNCTION TESTING

The importance of the endothelium was first recognized by its role in the regulation of vascular tone. This is achieved by production and release of vasoactive molecules (including nitric oxide [NO], prostacyclin and other vasoactive prostanoids, endothelium-derived hyperpolarizing factor [EDHF], endothelin-1 [ET-1], and free radicals) as well as the response to and modification of circulating vasoactive mediators (including angiotensin, bradykinin, and thrombin). These agents predominantly act locally, but may also have wider systemic influences acutely on vascular tone and chronically on arterial structure and remodeling. In addition to its vasodilator functions, NO has an important function in the maintenance of vascular health through its inhibitory effects on inflammation, thrombosis, and cell proliferation. When exposed to factors that "activate" the endothelium, a switch in the biology occurs from a NO-dominant quiescent phenotype to an activated phenotype in which "uncoupled" eNOS (endothelial Nitric Oxide Synthase) at generates reactive oxygen species in the absence of its cofactor tetrahydrobiopterin (superoxide) and or the substrate L-arginine (hydrogen peroxide). Indeed, most conventional and many novel risk factors activate common pathways within the endothelium thus resulting in the dysfunction of this system. This dual role of eNOS in both the maintenance of a basal quiescent status and activation of the endothelium places the enzyme at the center of endothelial and therefore arterial homeostasis. A number of changes occur with activation of the endothelium including expression of proinflammatory chemokines, cytokines, and adhesion molecules; alteration of production of factors that modulate the local thrombogenic balance; release of endothelial microparticles; and ultimately senescence and detachment of endothelial cells from the arterial wall.

An improved understanding of the vascular biology of the endothelium has permitted the development of clinical tests that evaluate several of the functional properties of normal and activated endothelium.[3] Ideally, such tests should be safe, noninvasive, reproducible, repeatable, cheap, and standardized between laboratories. The results should also reflect the dynamic biology of the endothelium throughout the natural history of atherosclerotic disease, define subclinical disease processes, as well as provide prognostic information for risk stratification in the later clinical phase. No single test currently fulfils all of these requirements, and a panel of several tests may therefore be needed to characterize these multiple facets of endothelial biology.

Clinical assessment of endothelial function can be split into two main areas: Firstly, evaluation of endothelium-dependent vasomotor function, which involves application of pharmacological and physiological techniques that can serve as functional "bioassays" of local NO bioavailability; secondly, development of assays for measurement of circulating biochemical and cellular markers of endothelial activation, damage, and repair capacity that can provide insight into systemic and regional changes in endothelial biology relevant to the pathogenesis of arterial disease.

● CLINICAL ASSESSMENT OF ENDOTHELIUM-DEPENDENT VASOMOTOR FUNCTION

Principles of Endothelial Vasomotor Function Testing

Endothelium-dependent vasomotion has been the most widely used clinical end point for the assessment of endothelial function because changes in arterial diameter and blood flow can be measured reliably in patients both invasively and noninvasively. Testing primarily involves pharmacological and/or physiological stimulation of net endothelial release of NO and other vasoactive compounds. NO activates guanylate cyclase in vascular smooth muscle leading to an increased production of cyclic guanosine monophosphate, a reduction in intracellular calcium leading to muscle relaxation, and vasodilatation. The magnitude of the induced vasodilatation typically reflects local bioavailability of NO and also the responsiveness of the vascular smooth muscle. Thus, in order to localize any observed defect to the endothelium, a comprehensive vascular function testing protocol will usually include assessment of the vasodilator response to an endothelium-independent dilator for comparison. These tests determine the effect of local endothelial NO bioavailability on vasomotor tone and also reflect its other important biological functions in health and disease.

Invasive Assessment of Vascular Function

Pharmacological assessment of vascular function is most commonly undertaken using intra-arterial infusions of acetylcholine (ACH) or bradykinin (BK) as endothelium-dependent agonists that mediate the release of NO, prostacyclin, and EDHF from endothelial cells. This is followed by infusion of an NO-donor such as sodium nitroprusside (NTP) or nitroglycerine (NTG) to assess endothelium-independent smooth muscle function. These studies are direct clinical analogs of Furchgott and Zawadski's pioneering experimental work.[4] These studies are invasive by nature. The original clinical investigations of endothelial function were undertaken in the coronary circulation, but brachial artery cannulation for pharmacological assessment of forearm vascular function is a useful alternative and commonly undertaken for clinical research purposes.

Assessment of Coronary Vasomotor Function. Direct assessment of coronary endothelial vasomotor function is undertaken at the time of cardiac catheterization and involves assessment of epicardial and microvascular responses to local infusion of endothelium-dependent pharmacologic probes, measured using quantitative coronary angiography and Doppler flow wire techniques. Inhibition of eNOS by intracoronary infusion of the L-arginine analog, L-N^{G-}monomethyl arginine (L-NMMA), increases coronary vascular resistance and constricts epicardial coronary arteries, confirming the importance of basal generation of NO in the maintenance of human coronary vasodilator tone.[5] This effect is diminished in subjects with atherosclerosis or its risk factors, suggesting reduced bioavailability of NO in these individuals. Most human coronary vascular studies have employed muscarinic agonists to test endothelial function. The integrity of the endothelium is defined by the presence of a preserved vasodilator response to intra-arterial ACH, whereas abnormal function is characterized by a constrictor response of coronary epicardial vessels and/or a depressed microvascular vasodilator response. This occurs as a result of the smooth muscle response to direct muscarinic receptor stimulation overwhelming the depressed or absent dilator effect when availability of endothelium-derived NO is diminished.[5,6] Doses of ACH that result in final blood concentrations in the range of 10^{-8} to 10^{-5} mol are the most appropriate for assessment of the physiological range of responses.[7] Co-infusion of L-NMMA almost completely abolishes the epicardial dilation and a significant proportion of the coronary microvascular dilation that is mediated by ACH, substance-P, and metabolic stress demonstrating the important contribution of NO release to the vasomotor responses provoked by these stimuli in vivo.[5,6,8,9]

A comprehensive assessment of coronary anatomy and physiology has been termed a "functional angiogram." The study should be performed after withholding cardioactive medications for at least 24 hours, and ideally for at least five half-lives. NTG should be withheld at least 4 hours prior to the study. After diagnostic cardiac catheterization, which will identify any important structural coronary lesions, the patient is anticoagulated with heparin and a guiding catheter is positioned in the left coronary ostium. A Doppler FloWire is then advanced into a straight, non-branching segment of the proximal mid left anterior descending artery, and a narrow-guage infusion catheter is advanced over this with its tip just distal to the tip of the wire. Coronary blood flow reserve may then be assessed using the Doppler wire with intracoronary boluses of adenosine to achieve maximal hyperemia (18–42 μg). Endothelium-dependent coronary function is then determined by infusing ACH at increasing doses to achieve intracoronary concentrations (10^{-7}–10^{-5} mol/L). The patient is closely monitored for symptoms, hemodynamic, and electrocardiographic changes. Intracoronary NTG (100–200 μg) is given to assess endothelium-independent vasomotor function, or a dose–response study to NTP maybe performed as an alternative. Quantitative coronary angiography for measuring epicardial diameter is performed at the end of each infusion and Doppler velocities are recorded. Coronary artery diameter (D) at the level of the Doppler wire and the average peak velocity (APV) from the Doppler signal are used to calculate coronary blood flow by means of the formula $D^2 \times$ APV/8.

Two to three straight, nonbranching segments of the study artery are also measured at baseline and following infusion of ACH and NTG and the epicardial endothelium-dependent and -independent vasomotor responses are determined by calculating the percentage change in arterial diameter from baseline[3] ($D_{\text{ACH or NTG}} - D_{\text{baseline}}/D_{\text{baseline}} \times 100\%$) (Figure 6-1).

Similarly, endothelial function can be assessed by determining the responses to other agents such as BK or substance-P, although dysfunctional vasoconstrictor responses are not typically seen with these agents. Physiological responses to cold-pressor testing and flow-mediated dilatation of proximal epicardial coronary arteries in response to a more distal infusion of adenosine have also been used to assess coronary vascular function. These studies have provided important insights into the effects of atherosclerosis and its risk factors on coronary regulatory physiology and risk stratification (Figure 6-2) as well as the potential reversibility in response to agents such as statins and ACE-inhibitors.[5,6,9–14]

These highly invasive studies are, of necessity, restricted to use in subjects with clinical indications for cardiac catheterization, limiting the research opportunities to the later more advanced stages of arterial disease using this methodology.

Invasive Assessment of Forearm Vascular Function

Assessment of endothelium-dependent vasodilatation in the forearm microcirculation uses similar methodology as used for coronary circulation. The brachial artery is cannulated and endothelium-dependent and -independent agonists and antagonists can be infused at doses that influence local physiology without systemic effects. Changes in forearm blood flow are measured using strain gauge venous occlusion plethysmography.[15]

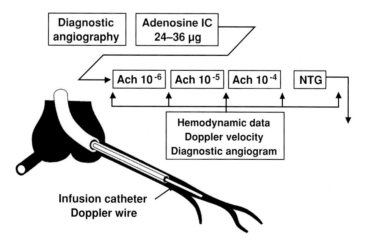

● FIGURE 6-1. Protocol for functional angiogram. ACH (acetylcholine) is administered intracoronary (IC) via the infusion catheter to assess endothelium-dependent responses; NTG (glyceryl trinitrate), also infused IC, is used to assess endothelium-independent smooth muscle responses for comparison. Adenosine is administered to assess coronary flow reserve as a marker of maximal microvascular dilator function. Coronary responses are measured using the Doppler FloWire to measure changes in coronary blood flow and vascular resistance and using quantitative coronary angiography to measure changes in epicardial arterial diameter.

Reproduced with permission from Deanfield J, Donald A, Ferri C, et al. Endothelial function and dysfunction. Part I: Methodological issues for assessment in the different vascular beds: a statement by the Working Group on Endothelin and Endothelial Factors of the European Society of Hypertension. J Hypertens. 2005;23(1):7-17.

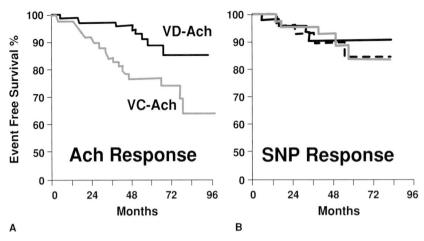

● **FIGURE 6-2.** Endothelial dysfunction and prognosis. A study of 308 patients (132 with and 176 without CAD) showing relationship between coronary vasodilator function and acute cardiovascular events. Kaplan–Meier analyses demonstrate proportion of patients surviving free from acute cardiovascular events during long-term follow-up. Study cohort is divided into those with epicardial vasoconstrictor or vasodilator responses with ACh (A) and into tertiles according to epicardial vasodilator response to SNP (B). Black line represents those with epicardial vasodilation in response to ACh (A) or tertile with greatest epicardial vasodilation with SNP (B); dashed line represents tertile with intermediate epicardial vasodilation with SNP (B); and gray line represents those with epicardial vasoconstriction with ACh (A) or tertile with least epicardial vasodilation with SNP (B).

Modified with permission from Halcox JP, Schenke WH, Zalos G, et al. Prognostic value of coronary vascular endothelial dysfunction. Circulation. 2002;106(6):653-658.

Although invasive, the methodology is generally considered to be reasonably safe and the technique is used in many research laboratories worldwide. Ideally, FBF must be measured in both forearms to adjust the stimulated changes in the experimental arm for minor systemic fluctuations in basal blood flow and blood pressure that may occur during the study.[15,16] The majority of studies measure the percentage differences in forearm blood flow and resistance between the experimental and control arms in response to increasing doses of endothelium-dependent (e.g., ACH or BK) and -independent (e.g., NTP or NTG) agonists. The contribution of NO can also be evaluated by assessment of changes in blood flow and resistance following eNOS antagonists (e.g., L-NMMA and L-NAME), with endothelium-independent vasoconstrictor responses to, for example, phenylephrine used as a comparison. More detailed assessment of the contribution of NO to the endothelium-dependent responses to ACH or BK can be studied in the presence of a NO-clamp. This involves co-administration of NTP to counteract the constrictor effect of L-NMMA, thus allowing appropriate comparison of the responses under control conditions and NO-synthase blockade without the confounding effect of different baseline blood flow rates.[3,17] As usual, testing of endothelium-independent responses by construction of a dose–response curve to NTG or NTP is also necessary to determine the endothelial specificity of any differences in the responses to ACH or BK. Endothelium-dependent vasodilator responses in the forearm microcirculation involve different pathways, and although responses to the commonly used agents predominantly reflect NO release, the contribution of other mediators such as EDHF increases when NO bioavailability is diminished.[18,19]

The main advantages of this technique are that, although invasive, it can be applied both to patients and healthy volunteers; it allows careful clinical pharmacological assessment of combinations of agonists and antagonists to test other pathways in addition to endothelial-derived and exogenous NO (e.g., indomethacin to block cyclooxygenase[20] and vitamin C to assess oxidative stress[21]). Furthermore, although forearm microcirculation is clearly not a target organ for atherosclerosis, the responses to ACH and modulation by vitamin C are predictive of cardiovascular outcome,[21] suggesting that systemic, as well as coronary endothelial function, is an important marker of global cardiovascular risk. Despite the detailed data that can be obtained, the invasive nature of this technique limits its repeatability and prohibits its use in larger studies. Results are also difficult to standardize because baseline resistance vessel tone is variable within and between subjects, and testing protocols and setup differ between research laboratories. Therefore noninvasive techniques are required with broader applicability to larger study populations including younger adults and children.

Noninvasive Assessment of Vascular Function

Flow-Mediated Vasodilatation. Endothelial cells release NO and other endothelium-derived relaxing factors in response to mechanical stress. The precise mechanisms for the acute detection of shear forces and subsequent signal

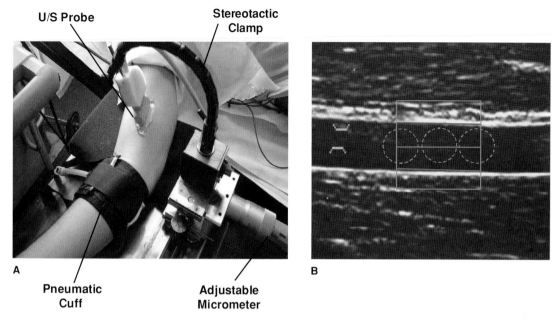

U/S Probe   Stereotactic Clamp

A   B

Pneumatic Cuff   Adjustable Micrometer

● **FIGURE 6-3.** Brachial artery vasomotor function testing. (A) Image illustrating the equipment setup to conduct a brachial artery vasomotor function study. The ultrasound probe is positioned over the brachial artery above the elbow and held in place by an adjustable clamp with a micrometer attachment for fine positional adjustment. A pneumatic cuff is positioned around the forearm just below the elbow and is attached to an automatic pump allowing rapid inflation and deflation. (B) A representative B-mode longitudinal image of brachial artery during analysis. The placement of the region of interest box and edge detection markers for measurement of the vessel diameter are shown.

transduction to modulate vasomotor tone are not fully understood, but probably involve calcium-activated potassium channel opening, membrane hyperpolarization, and calcium-mediated activation of eNOS. Thus, in vivo, the endothelium can respond dynamically to shear stresses mediated by increased flow, by releasing NO that mediates vasodilatation. Using these principles, we developed and refined a technique for assessment of flow-mediated endothelium-dependent dilatation (FMD).[22] This method involves measurement of the change in diameter of a conduit artery (most commonly the brachial artery) in response to increased flow, typically induced by a period of ischemia in the distal circulatory bed (Figures 6-3 and 6-4). FMD when performed under appropriate conditions is highly reproducible, is predominantly mediated by NO (Figures 6-5 and 6-6), and is depressed in subjects with atherosclerosis and its risk factors (Figure 6-7).[23–27] These measurements also correlate well with coronary vascular endothelial vasodilator function[28] (Figure 6-8) and serological markers of endothelial perturbation as well as predicting long-term cardiovascular outcome (Figure 6-9).[29,30]

This technique is well tolerated, noninvasive, and repeatable. As a result, it lends itself to studies investigating the impact of risk factors at an early preclinical phase of disease including children as young as 5 years of age. Response to lifestyle and pharmacological interventions can be studied in the young[31] at a stage when the arterial disease process is likely to be at its most reversible.

Equipment and Protocol for Assessment of FMD (Figure 6-3). Accurate assessment of FMD is technically challenging, and investigators should undergo appropriate training and validation prior to undertaking such studies.[3] The laboratory should be equipped with a high-resolution ultrasound machine with vascular and cardiac capabilities, a high-frequency (5–13 MHz) linear array probe, a super VHS video and printer, and an arm rest with stereotactic clamp. Computer image acquisition and analysis software for diameter measurements is also required. Studies should be carried out in a warm, temperature-controlled room. Subjects should be fasting or have had only a low-fat meal and caffeine should be avoided for at least 2 hours prior to the study. Cardiovascular risk factors, for example, diabetes, hypertension, smoking, family history, medications, and recent/current infections, along with the stage of menstrual cycle in women should be documented.

After ECG monitoring electrodes are attached, the participant should rest in a supine position for at least 10 minutes (to allow hemodynamic stabilization). The brachial artery is then imaged in longitudinal section, 5 to 10 cm proximal to placement of a blood pressure cuff, just below the ante cubital fossa (Figure 6-3A). It has been shown that the dilatation using this cuff and probe position can be blocked by infusion of LNMMA, confirming the NO dependence of this response[26,32] (Figures 6-5 and 6-6). The probe is held in a stereotactic clamp, preferably with a micrometer allowing fine adjustment. When the clearest

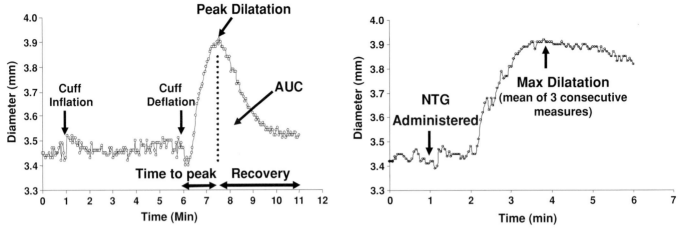

● **FIGURE 6-4.** Brachial artery vasomotor function response profiles. (A) Representative readout of the brachial diameter measurements obtained during the course of a brachial artery FMD study. A single diameter measurement (represented by a small circle) is made approximately every 3 seconds (acquired from the ECG R wave-triggered end-diastolic image). The baseline measurements are made between 0 and 1 minute. The cuff is inflated between 1 and 6 minutes. The cuff is then deflated resulting in flow-mediated dilatation of the artery that reaches its maximal value after approximately 1 minute. The time taken to achieve peak dilatation, the area under the dilatation versus time curve (AUC), and the maximal dilatation (expressed as a percent change or absolute change in millimeters from baseline) can be determined from this profile. (B) A representative readout of the brachial diameter measurements obtained during assessment of brachial artery dilator response to sublingual glyceryl trinitrate (NTG 25 mcg). The images are acquired and measured in the same way as during the FMD study, with baseline determined between 0 and 1 minute. The NTG is then administered sublingually and the data acquired over the subsequent 5 minutes. The maximal dilatation is then determined and is usually expressed as a percent change from baseline, but can also be expressed as an absolute change in millimeters.

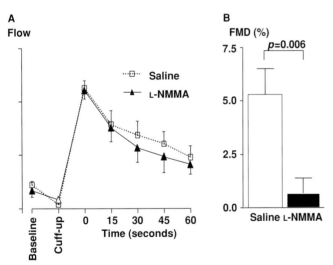

● **FIGURE 6-5.** Nitric oxide dependence of flow-mediated dilatation. L-NMMA (L-*N*-monomethyl arginine, a competitive antagonist of nitric oxide synthase) had no effect on radial artery blood flow at baseline or during cuff inflation or reactive hyperemia (A) but almost completely attenuated FMD in response to reactive hyperemia (B), suggesting that this response is almost entirely mediated by endothelial NO release.

Reproduced with permission from Mullen MJ, Kharbanda RK, Cross J, et al. Heterogenous nature of flow-mediated dilatation in human conduit arteries in vivo: relevance to endothelial dysfunction in hypercholesterolemia. Circ Res. 2001;88(2):145-151.

B-mode image through the center of the vessel is obtained with optimal contrast between the anterior and posterior vessel walls and the lumen of the vessel (Figure 6-3B), the stereotactic clamp is fixed in place. A Doppler signal is recorded from the center of the vessel with the range gate set at 1.5 mm. If possible, the B-mode should be set to update synchronously with the R-Wave of the ECG together with a continuous Doppler reading throughout. However, not all ultrasound machines have this capability.

Endothelium-Dependent (Flow-Mediated) Vasodilation. The baseline image and Doppler signal should be recorded for 30 seconds to 1 minute, following which the blood pressure cuff should be inflated to suprasystolic pressure for 5 minutes (Figure 6-4A). The cuff should then be rapidly deflated and the artery imaged and Doppler signal recorded for 2 to 5 minutes post-cuff deflation. Brachial artery FMD is calculated as the maximum change in diameter from baseline, expressed as a percentage. The degree of cuff inflation should be standardized to either (a) 300 mm Hg for adults, and 200 mm Hg for children or (b) 50 mm Hg above the study participant's systolic BP. On cuff deflation, the resultant reactive hyperemia is calculated from the Doppler signal as the change in blood flow from baseline, expressed as a percentage. While this

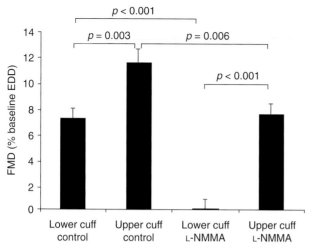

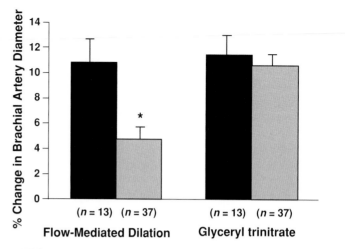

● **FIGURE 6-6.** Influence of cuff position on flow-mediated dilatation (FMD). The response is represented as a percentage change from baseline end-diastolic diameter (EDD). When the cuff is placed proximally to the probe on the upper arm (resulting in a larger volume of ischemic arm tissue and also producing ischemia of the study vessel), a greater degree of vasodilatation is induced than when the cuff is positioned distally to the vessel. However, the dilatation mediated by the upper arm occlusion protocol is only partially attenuated by inhibition of nitric oxide synthase with L-*N*-monomethyl arginine (L-NMMA), suggesting only partial NO dependence, whereas the response to the lower arm occlusion protocol is entirely NO dependent, illustrated by complete attenuation by L-NMMA.

Reproduced with permission from Doshi SN, Naka KK, Payne N, et al. Flow-mediated dilatation following wrist and upper arm occlusion in humans: the contribution of nitric oxide. Clin Sci (Lond). 2001;101(6):629-635.

● **FIGURE 6-8.** Relationship between endothelial vasomotor function responses in the brachial and coronary arteries. Black columns represent responses in subjects with preserved coronary endothelial function. Hatched columns represent responses in patients with coronary endothelial dysfunction, illustrating depressed endothelium-dependent brachial flow-mediated dilatation but similar endothelium-independent responses to glyceryl trinitrate.

does not give precise quantitative measures of forearm blood flow (as the angle of insonation is above 60 degrees), relative changes are accurate.

Endothelium-Independent (GTN Mediated) Dilatation. The effect of an endothelium-independent stimulation can be assessed by administration of a sublingual dose of GTN (Figure 6-4B). As with the assessment of FMD, the baseline image and Doppler signal should be recorded for 30 seconds to 1 minute. GTN is then administered sublingually, and the vessel image is recorded for a further 3 to 5 minutes. GTN-mediated brachial artery dilatation is also calculated as the maximum change from baseline, expressed as a percentage change in diameter.

Although many studies have used 200- to 400-μg doses of GTN, we typically use a 25-μg dose that results in a similar magnitude of dilatation as seen with FMD in healthy controls. This small dose also allows serial measures to be taken on the same day, as the blood vessels return to resting diameter within 20 minutes. This enables assessment of smooth muscle function in acute intervention studies and also minimizes potential side effects from larger doses of GTN.

Similar principles can also be applied to assessment of FMD in the radial artery, femoral artery, and posterior tibial artery in which case the blood pressure cuff is inflated at the wrist, just below the popliteal fossa, and at the ankle, respectively. Endothelium-independent dilation is measured using the same dose of sublingual GTN.

In summary, FMD of the brachial artery is the most commonly performed and best-validated technique for noninvasive assessment of conduit vessel function. When performed using these established techniques, FMD is NO

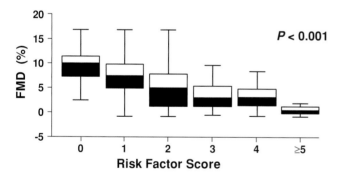

● **FIGURE 6-7.** Relationship of endothelial flow-mediated dilation (FMD) to risk factor burden in 500 asymptomatic subjects. This clearly illustrates diminishing FMD in association with increasing risk factor burden. Risk factors considered include age, hypercholesterolemia, smoking, hypertension, family history of premature cardiovascular disease, and male gender.

Reproduced with permission from Celermajer DS, Sorensen KE, Bull C, Robinson J, Deanfield JE. Endothelium-dependent dilation in the systemic arteries of asymptomatic subjects relates to coronary risk factors and their interaction. J Am Coll Cardiol. 1994;24(6):1468-1474.

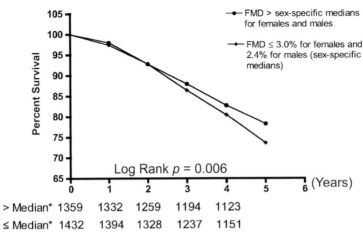

● **FIGURE 6-9.** Brachial artery endothelial function and prognosis. Life-table analysis of event-free survival for cardiovascular events of subjects above, below, or equal to sex-specific medians of flow-mediated dilatation (FMD percent). *Number at risk.

Reproduced with permission from Yeboah J, Crouse JR, Hsu FC, Burke GL, Herrington DM. Brachial flow-mediated dilation predicts incident cardiovascular events in older adults: the Cardiovascular Health Study. Circulation. 2007;115(18):2390-2397.

dependent, correlates well with coronary arterial endothelial function, may impart prognostic information, and is ideally suited for studies investigating factors and interventions that may influence endothelial function and vascular risk.

Emerging Noninvasive Techniques for Assessment of Endothelial Function.

There is a pressing need for more extensive assessment of the value of endothelial function testing in cardiovascular risk stratification and therapeutic decision making. This will require large, prospective, population-based studies. However, most of the available methodologies for assessing endothelial function are unsuitable for studying large populations. Measurement of endothelial function in the coronary circulation and forearm resistance vessels is invasive, and the most widely used noninvasive methodology, FMD, is technically specialized, time consuming, and requires relatively expensive ultrasound equipment. Therefore, a number of alternative noninvasive approaches have been developed recently to study vascular biology in the peripheral circulation. Several rely on the ability of the β2 agonist salbutamol to reduce arterial stiffness in an endothelial-derived, NO-dependent manner without a significant reduction in blood pressure when administered via inhaler at standard clinical doses.[33–35] The changes in arterial stiffness can be measured either using pulse wave analysis by radial artery tonometry or pulse contour analysis by digital photoplethysmography.[33–35] The changes in augmentation index and reflection index can be measured from the peripheral arterial waveform,[33,34] or changes in the central aortic waveform derived from pulse wave analysis data by a transfer function that has been validated in adults.[33–35] Alternatively, reactive hyperemia has been used to elicit changes in conduit artery pulse wave velocity and also digital pulse velocity that can be measured by oscillometry or digital pulse volume that can be digital pulse amplitude tonometry.[36–38]

Several of these methods have been validated as measures of NO bioavailability, have been shown to change with exposure to risk factors and with atherosclerotic disease, and may complement or even provide an alternative to FMD testing.[33,35,36,38] However, their relationship with and contribution to development of structural alterations in the vessel wall and endothelial-dependent biology is as yet unproven. We have recently demonstrated that the reproducibility of endothelial function testing using salbutamol-mediated changes in arterial stiffness parameters is less good than FMD, particularly in children, and these measures appear to be affected differently in response to an inflammatory stress.[24] The increase in skin blood flow in the distal forearm following 4.5 minutes of ischaemia, or iontophoretic application of endothelial agonists that can be measured using laser digital Doppler flowmetry, has also recently been proposed as a measure of endothelial function and may even be suitable for use in infancy. However, while responses are depressed in subjects with risk factors, the limited reproducibility of this method remains a concern as does the lack of data confirming wider relationships between skin responses and those in other more clinically relevant vascular beds.[3] Digital peripheral applanation tonometry assessment of the response to reactive hyperemia (EndoPAT, Itamar Medical, Israel) is currently emerging as the most promising alternative to FMD testing, largely because of the simplicity and low training requirement of the methodology. However, as with all these techniques, further validation is required that should involve wider studies of reproducibility in different age groups and stages of disease as well as broader comparisons of their relationships with other established measures of endothelial function (Table 6-1).

TABLE 6-1. Methods for Clinical Assessment of Endothelial Function

Technique (Outcome Measure)	Noninvasive	Repeatable	Reproducible*	Reflects Biology	Reversible	Predicts Outcome†
Cardiac catheterization (change in diameter, change in coronary blood flow)	−	−	+/−	+	+	+
Venous occlusion plethysmography (change in forearm blood flow)	−	+/−	+/−	+	+	+
Ultrasound FMD (change in brachial artery diameter)	+	+	+/−	+	+	+‡
PWA (change in augmentation index)	+	+	+/−	+	−	−
PCA (change in reflective index)	+	+	+/−	+	−	−
PAT (change in pulse amplitude)	+	+	+/−	+	−	−

+, Supportive evidence in literature; −, insufficient evidence; FMD, flow-mediated dilatation; PWA, pulse wave analysis; PCA, pulse contour analysis; and PAT, pulse amplitude tonometry.
*Reproducibility of PWA, PCA, and PAT has been less extensively investigated than FMD.
†Studies that link PWA, PCA, and PAT to outcome have not yet been reported.
Adapted with permission from Deanfield et al. Circulation 2007;115:1285-1295.

Circulating Biomarkers of Endothelial Function

Serological Factors. Measurement of circulating factors such as inflammatory cytokines and adhesion molecules released by activated endothelial cells is an alternative means of assessing endothelial status. Information provided by these assays maybe valuable complementary information to vascular physiological measures. Well-characterized molecules that can be measured in the circulation with commercial immunoassays include E-selectin, vascular cell adhesion molecule 1, intercellular adhesion molecule 1, and P-selectin.[39] These factors variously trigger important processes in the arterial wall including leukocyte homing, adhesion, and migration into the subendothelial space, fundamental to the initiation, progression, and destabilization of atherosclerotic lesions. Circulating levels typically increase in association with cardiovascular risk factors, reflect structural and functional measures of atherosclerotic disease, and predict adverse cardiovascular prognosis.[40,41] Although these molecules may arise from multiple sources, E-selectin has the greatest endothelial specificity. In addition, changes in the local thrombotic balance because of endothelial activation can be assessed by measuring levels of von Willebrand factor, tissue plasminogen activator, and its endogenous inhibitor, plasminogen activation inhibitor-1.[42,43]

Markers of Cellular Injury and Repair. Appreciation that endothelial function reflects the net balance between injury and repair has led to the development of assays to quantify the detached mature endothelial cells and activated endothelium-derived microparticles—to represent the degree of damage, as well as determination of the number and functional characteristics of circulating endothelial progenitor cells—to reflect the endogenous repair potential.

Detached mature circulating endothelial cells can be measured in the circulation using a combination of magnetic bead selection and fluorescent microscopy.[44] The increased levels of circulating endothelial cells seen in patients with atherosclerotic disease and vascular inflammation reflect the extent of endothelial injury. Similarly, levels of endothelial microparticles (EMPs—vesicles formed by the cell membrane after endothelial activation) are increased in a variety of conditions associated with endothelial activation or apoptosis.[45,46] The function of EMPs is unclear, but they may differ in composition depending on the activation state of the parent cell and maybe diffusible, proinflammatory, cell signalling mediators.[47] While these observations reflect interesting advances, clinical validation of the assays and a better understanding of the pathophysiological role of EMPs remain necessary before their measurement can be incorporated into routine practice.

Circulating endothelial progenitor cells can be characterized by the coexpression of a combination of progenitor (e.g., CD34 and CD133) and endothelial surface markers (e.g., KDR, CD144, CD31) that are detectable by flow cytometry. However, the specificity of these measurements remains controversial because of the intrinsic dynamic plasticity of leukocyte subparticles that appear to have the potential to develop along the endothelial lineage depending on local conditions.[48] Therefore, further methods to characterize circulating endothelial progenitor cell biology have been developed. These include quantification of the potential of peripheral blood mononuclear cells to differentiate into an endothelial cell phenotype as well as determination of their functional characteristics. These mononuclear cells have colony formation, migration toward a chemical stimulus (e.g., stromal cell–derived factor 1, vascular endothelial growth factor) adhesion, formation of vascular tubules, and the ability to attenuate ischemia in animal models.[49,50] Measurement of circulating endothelial cells, EMPs, and endothelial progenitor cells may therefore provide a novel and relevant means to follow the determinants and balance of endothelial injury and repair in clinical subjects. Although these measures have already been linked to other in vivo measures of endothelial function and future cardiovascular events, they still remain far from use in routine clinical practice. Nevertheless, important new mechanistic insights and potential therapeutic options for arterial disease are likely to emerge from this exciting and rapidly developing field.

● CONCLUSION

Noninvasive clinical testing strategies that refine risk assessment in individual subjects, and in particular identify those at high risk and measure responses to treatment, are of particular relevance to earlier stages of the disease process and most suitable for clinical use in younger subjects. Despite the promise shown by endothelial function testing, it is not yet suitable for widespread screening or use for specific clinical decision making in individual patients. Established measures of endothelial function reflect important vascular biological processes, are associated with disease burden and outcome, and respond to interventions. However, currently available tests have not been validated for routine clinical use. The technical complexity and physiological variability outside of carefully controlled laboratory conditions may well preclude routine clinical use. Furthermore, as with other biomarkers used in research, the incremental clinical value of measures of endothelial function over and above current clinical predictors needs to be established.[51] Nevertheless, our understanding of the evolution of atherosclerotic disease has been transformed by the ability to measure endothelial function noninvasively. We now have the opportunity to build on this previous work by incorporating a comprehensive portfolio of tests including measures of conventional risk factors, genetic markers, physiological and circulating measures of endothelial activation injury and repair, and structural arterial disease for assessment of risk and evaluation of new treatment strategies. This approach will likely be of particular importance during the early preclinical, more reversible stages of disease, during which improved treatment is likely to result in a greatly leveraged long-term risk reduction that should result in major public health benefits.

REFERENCES

1. Ross R. Atherosclerosis—an inflammatory disease. *N Engl J Med.* 1999;340(2):115-126.

2. Vita JA, Keaney JF Jr. Endothelial function: a barometer for cardiovascular risk? *Circulation.* 2002;106(6):640-642.

3. Deanfield J, Donald A, Ferri C, et al. Endothelial function and dysfunction. Part I: Methodological issues for assessment in the different vascular beds: a statement by the Working Group on Endothelin and Endothelial Factors of the European Society of Hypertension. *J Hypertens.* 2005;23(1): 7-17.

4. Furchgott RF, Zawadzki JV. The obligatory role of endothelial cells in the relaxation of arterial smooth muscle by acetylcholine. *Nature.* 1980;288(5789):373-376.

5. Quyyumi AA, Dakak N, Andrews NP, et al. Nitric oxide activity in the human coronary circulation. Impact of risk factors for coronary atherosclerosis. *J Clin Invest.* 1995;95(4):1747-1755.

6. Quyyumi AA, Dakak N, Mulcahy D, et al. Nitric oxide activity in the atherosclerotic human coronary circulation. *J Am Coll Cardiol.* 1997;29(2):308-317.

7. Okumura K, Yasue H, Matsuyama K, et al. Effect of acetylcholine on the highly stenotic coronary artery: difference between the constrictor response of the infarct-related coronary artery and that of the noninfarct-related artery. *J Am Coll Cardiol.* 1992;19(4):752-758.

8. Lefroy DC, Crake T, Uren NG, Davies GJ, Maseri A. Effect of inhibition of nitric oxide synthesis on epicardial coronary artery caliber and coronary blood flow in humans. *Circulation.* 1993;88(1):43-54.

9. Quyyumi AA, Dakak N, Andrews NP, Gilligan DM, Panza JA, Cannon RO III. Contribution of nitric oxide to metabolic coronary vasodilation in the human heart. *Circulation.* 1995;92(3):320-326.

10. Ludmer PL, Selwyn AP, Shook TL, et al. Paradoxical vasoconstriction induced by acetylcholine in atherosclerotic coronary arteries. *N Engl J Med.* 1986;315(17):1046-1051.

11. Vita JA, Treasure CB, Nabel EG, et al. Coronary vasomotor response to acetylcholine relates to risk factors for coronary artery disease. *Circulation.* 1990;81(2):491-497.

12. Halcox JP, Schenke WH, Zalos G, et al. Prognostic value of coronary vascular endothelial dysfunction. *Circulation.* 2002;106(6):653-658.

13. Mancini GB, Henry GC, Macaya C, et al. Angiotensin-converting enzyme inhibition with quinapril improves endothelial vasomotor dysfunction in patients with coronary artery disease. The TREND (Trial on Reversing ENdothelial Dysfunction) Study. *Circulation.* 1996;94(3):258-265.

14. Anderson TJ, Meredith IT, Yeung AC, Frei B, Selwyn AP, Ganz P. The effect of cholesterol-lowering and antioxidant therapy on endothelium-dependent coronary vasomotion. *N Engl J Med.* 1995;332(8):488-493.

15. Benjamin N, Calver A, Collier J, Robinson B, Vallance P, Webb D. Measuring forearm blood flow and interpreting the responses to drugs and mediators. *Hypertension.* 1995;25(5):918-923.

16. Petrie JR, Ueda S, Morris AD, Murray LS, Elliott HL, Connell JM. How reproducible is bilateral forearm plethysmography? *Br J Clin Pharmacol.* 1998;45(2):131-139.

17. Stroes ES, Luscher TF, de Groot FG, Koomans HA, Rabelink TJ. Cyclosporin A increases nitric oxide activity in vivo. *Hypertension.* 1997;29(2):570-575.

18. Halcox JP, Narayanan S, Cramer-Joyce L, Mincemoyer R, Quyyumi AA. Characterization of endothelium-derived hyperpolarizing factor in the human forearm microcirculation. *Am J Physiol Heart Circ Physiol.* 2001;280(6):H2470-H2477.

19. Taddei S, Ghiadoni L, Virdis A, Buralli S, Salvetti A. Vasodilation to bradykinin is mediated by an ouabain-sensitive pathway as a compensatory mechanism for impaired nitric oxide availability in essential hypertensive patients. *Circulation.* 1999;100(13):1400-1405.

20. Taddei S, Virdis A, Ghiadoni L, Magagna A, Salvetti A. Cyclooxygenase inhibition restores nitric oxide activity in essential hypertension. *Hypertension.* 1997;29(1,pt 2):274-279.

21. Heitzer T, Schlinzig T, Krohn K, Meinertz T, Munzel T. Endothelial dysfunction, oxidative stress, and risk of cardiovascular events in patients with coronary artery disease. *Circulation.* 2001;104(22):2673-2678.

22. Celermajer DS, Sorensen KE, Gooch VM, et al. Non-invasive detection of endothelial dysfunction in children and adults at risk of atherosclerosis. *Lancet.* 1992;340(8828):1111-1115.

23. Celermajer DS, Sorensen KE, Bull C, Robinson J, Deanfield JE. Endothelium-dependent dilation in the systemic arteries of asymptomatic subjects relates to coronary risk factors and their interaction. *J Am Coll Cardiol.* 1994;24(6):1468-1474.

24. Donald AE, Charakida M, Cole TJ, et al. Non-invasive assessment of endothelial function: which technique? *J Am Coll Cardiol.* 2006;48(9):1846-1850.

25. Joannides R, Haefeli WE, Linder L, et al. Nitric oxide is responsible for flow-dependent dilatation of human peripheral conduit arteries in vivo. *Circulation.* 1995;91(5):1314-1319.

26. Mullen MJ, Kharbanda RK, Cross J, et al. Heterogenous nature of flow-mediated dilatation in human conduit arteries in vivo: relevance to endothelial dysfunction in hypercholesterolemia. *Circ Res.* 2001;88(2):145-151.

27. Sorensen KE, Celermajer DS, Spiegelhalter DJ, et al. Non-invasive measurement of human endothelium dependent arterial responses: accuracy and reproducibility. *Br Heart J.* 1995;74(3):247-253.

28. Anderson TJ, Uehata A, Gerhard MD, et al. Close relation of endothelial function in the human coronary and peripheral circulations. *J Am Coll Cardiol.* 1995;26(5):1235-1241.

29. Boulanger CM, Amabile N, Tedgui A. Circulating microparticles—a potential prognostic marker for atherosclerotic vascular disease 2. *Hypertension.* 2006;48(2):180-186.

30. Yeboah J, Crouse JR, Hsu FC, Burke GL, Herrington DM. Brachial flow-mediated dilation predicts incident cardiovascular events in older adults: the Cardiovascular Health Study. *Circulation.* 2007;115(18):2390-2397.

31. Woo KS, Chook P, Yu CW, et al. Effects of diet and exercise on obesity-related vascular dysfunction in children. *Circulation.* 2004;109(16):1981-1986.

32. Doshi SN, Naka KK, Payne N, et al. Flow-mediated dilatation following wrist and upper arm occlusion in humans: the contribution of nitric oxide. *Clin Sci* (*Lond*). 2001;101(6):629-635.

33. Chowienczyk PJ, Kelly RP, MacCallum H, et al. Photoplethysmographic assessment of pulse wave reflection: blunted response to endothelium-dependent beta2-adrenergic vasodilation in type II diabetes mellitus. *J Am Coll Cardiol.* 1999;34(7):2007-2014.

34. Hayward CS, Kraidly M, Webb CM, Collins P. Assessment of endothelial function using peripheral waveform analysis: a clinical application. *J Am Coll Cardiol.* 2002;40(3):521-528.

35. Wilkinson IB, Hall IR, MacCallum H, et al. Pulse-wave analysis: clinical evaluation of a noninvasive, widely applicable method for assessing endothelial function. *Arterioscler Thromb Vasc Biol.* 2002;22(1):147-152.

36. Bonetti PO, Pumper GM, Higano ST, Holmes DR Jr, Kuvin JT, Lerman A. Noninvasive identification of patients with early coronary atherosclerosis by assessment of digital reactive hyperemia. *J Am Coll Cardiol.* 2004;44(11):2137-2141.

37. Naka KK, Tweddel AC, Doshi SN, Goodfellow J, Henderson AH. Flow-mediated changes in pulse wave velocity: a new clinical measure of endothelial function. *Eur Heart J.* 2006;27(3):302-309.

38. Nohria A, Gerhard-Herman M, Creager MA, Hurley S, Mitra D, Ganz P. Role of nitric oxide in the regulation of digital pulse volume amplitude in humans. *J Appl Physiol.* 2006;101(2):545-548.

39. Ridker PM, Brown NJ, Vaughan DE, Harrison DG, Mehta JL. Established and emerging plasma biomarkers in the prediction of first atherothrombotic events. *Circulation.* 2004;109(25)(suppl 1):IV6-IV19.

40. Hwang SJ, Ballantyne CM, Sharrett AR, et al. Circulating adhesion molecules VCAM-1, ICAM-1, and E-selectin in carotid atherosclerosis and incident coronary heart disease cases: the Atherosclerosis Risk in Communities (ARIC) study. *Circulation.* 1997;96(12):4219-4225.

41. Ridker PM, Hennekens CH, Roitman-Johnson B, Stampfer MJ, Allen J. Plasma concentration of soluble intercellular adhesion molecule 1 and risks of future myocardial infarction in apparently healthy men. *Lancet.* 1998;351(9096):88-92.

42. Mannucci PM. von Willebrand factor: a marker of endothelial damage? *Arterioscler Thromb Vasc Biol.* 1998;18(9):1359-1362.

43. Vaughan DE. PAI-1 and atherothrombosis. *J Thromb Haemost.* 2005;3(8):1879-1883.

44. Woywodt A, Blann AD, Kirsch T, et al. Isolation and enumeration of circulating endothelial cells by immunomagnetic isolation: proposal of a definition and a consensus protocol. *J Thromb Haemost.* 2006;4(3):671-677.

45. Diamant M, Tushuizen ME, Sturk A, Nieuwland R. Cellular microparticles: new players in the field of vascular disease? *Eur J Clin Invest.* 2004;34(6):392-401.

46. Werner N, Wassmann S, Ahlers P, Kosiol S, Nickenig G. Circulating CD31+/annexin V+ apoptotic microparticles correlate with coronary endothelial function in patients with coronary artery disease. *Arterioscler Thromb Vasc Biol.* 2006;26(1):112-116.

47. Boulanger CM, Scoazec A, Ebrahimian T, et al. Circulating microparticles from patients with myocardial infarction cause endothelial dysfunction. *Circulation.* 2001;104(22):2649-2652.

48. Urbich C, Heeschen C, Aicher A, Dernbach E, Zeiher AM, Dimmeler S. Relevance of monocytic features for neovascularization capacity of circulating endothelial progenitor cells. *Circulation.* 2003;108(20):2511-2516.

49. Heeschen C, Aicher A, Lehmann R, et al. Erythropoietin is a potent physiologic stimulus for endothelial progenitor cell mobilization. *Blood*. 2003;102(4):1340-1346.

50. Murohara T, Asahara T, Silver M, et al. Nitric oxide synthase modulates angiogenesis in response to tissue ischemia. *J Clin Invest*. 1998;101(11):2567-2578.

51. Tardif JC, Heinonen T, Orloff D, Libby P. Vascular biomarkers and surrogates in cardiovascular disease. *Circulation*. 2006;113(25):2936-2942.

chapter 7

Flow Dynamics and Arterial Physiology

Patrick Segers, PhD / Luc M. Van Bortel, MD, PhD / Pascal R. Verdonck, PhD

● INTRODUCTION

This chapter mainly deals with the physiology of the arterial system and the hemodynamic analysis of pressure and flow in the arterial tree. Although most of the topics covered are generic and applicable to the systemic and pulmonary circulation, there is no doubt that the main focus is on the systemic circulation because it is the most studied, and also the most accessible, certainly for noninvasive measurement technology.

Before tackling arterial system physiology, we first provide the reader with a concise overview of some elementary laws of flow dynamics that are frequently used and cited in clinical literature, but without going in detail on the mathematical derivation.

The chapter first provides the "classic" analysis of hemodynamic data in the frequency domain, which is based on the parallelism between flow dynamics and electric system analysis. Input and characteristic impedance are defined and discussed, and it is demonstrated how arterial wave reflection can be assessed and quantified from pressure and flow. In addition to this classic view, we also consider wave intensity analysis, which is an alternative method of analyzing arterial hemodynamic data and wave reflection, but in what is perhaps a more intuitive way in the time domain.

A subsequent section is dedicated to the analysis of "arterial function" and "arterial stiffness," which is a new emerging domain of clinical research. Different methods are described, ranging from local measurement of arterial properties to parameters describing the complete arterial tree, most of them emerging from an electrical analog representation of the arterial tree. The clinical applicability of the methods, their strong and weak points, and the relevance of measuring arterial stiffness in general are discussed.

● BLOOD FLOW IN ARTERIES—GENERAL FLUID DYNAMIC LAWS

Blood flow in the arterial tree is of a relatively complex nature, for many different reasons. First of all, blood in itself is a complex liquid.[1,2] As a suspension of biochemically active cells in plasma, it is a non-Newtonian liquid, which implies that it has a nonconstant viscosity. When not in motion, red blood cells coagulate and rouleaux formation occurs, increasing the viscosity of blood. Under the action of shear forces within the blood (see later in the chapter), these rouleaux break up when blood flows and the viscosity of the blood decreases. Blood is therefore known as a "shear thinning liquid," with viscosity at high shear rates in the order of 3 to 4 mPa s (or cPoise). Blood can be generally considered as a homogenous liquid, except at the level of the arterioles and capillaries, where the size of the red blood cells (8 μm) becomes relatively large with respect to the vessel diameter (100 μm and less). Here, more complex rheological models should be considered, or blood should be treated as a multiphase liquid.

To define "shear rate," we take the example of flow of a liquid in a long, straight cylindrical tube. When the liquid starts to flow, a velocity profile will be installed, with maximal flow at the center. Near the tube wall the velocity is zero, which means that over the cross section of the tube the velocity gradients exist. The slope to the velocity profile, that is, the derivative of velocity with respect to the radial coordinate, $\partial u/\partial r$, is the shear rate. One can visualize the flow as consisting of concentric cylindrical shells gliding over each other (thus exerting a shear force), with

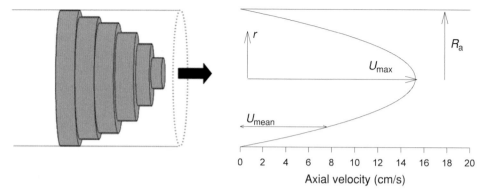

● **FIGURE 7-1.** Laminar, steady flow in a tube can be viewed as concentric layers gliding over each other, with zero velocity near the wall and maximal velocity at the center. Poiseuille flow is characterized by a parabolic profile. The slope of the velocity profile is the shear rate.

the outer shell standing still and the inner core having the highest velocity (Figure 7-1).

Steady Laminar Flow: Poiseuille Flow

It has been shown by Poiseuille[3] that for a Newtonian liquid in fully developed steady flow with "no-slip" boundary conditions (zero velocity near the wall) and up to a certain flow level, the velocity profile is parabolic, with the maximum velocity, U_{max}, at the center of the tube (Figure 7-1). With r the radial distance from the center and R_a the radius of the tube, the velocity at a given distance r is

$$U(r) = U_{max}\left(1 - \left(\frac{r}{R_a}\right)^2\right).$$

The mean velocity, U_{mean}, equals $U_{max}/2$. The absolute value of the shear rate (making abstraction of the sign of γ) is

$$\gamma = \frac{2r}{R_a^2}U_{max},$$

where γ is zero at the center of the blood vessel and maximal near the wall, where it becomes $2U_{max}/R_a$. The shear stress, τ, that is exerted on the wall by the blood flow is the product of dynamic blood viscosity (μ) and γ, and thus becomes $2\mu U_{max}/R_a$. Equilibrium of forces requires that the resultant of the shear stresses along the vessel lumen over a segment L is balanced by the pressure difference (ΔP) that exists over that segment, and this results in

$$\Delta P = \frac{8\mu U_{mean}L}{R^2} = \frac{8\mu QL}{\pi R^4},$$

where Q is the flow through the tube. The resistance of a blood vessel, $\Delta P/Q$, is thus proportional to the dynamic viscosity of the blood, the length of the vessel, and inversely proportional to the vessel radius to the fourth power! As such, it is mainly the small diameter vessels that generate the fluid dynamic resistance in the arterial tree.

The above relations apply only to highly structured, organized (laminar) steady flow in a straight tube. The dimensionless parameter that expresses whether a flow is laminar or not is the Reynolds (Re) number (with ρ the density of blood and D the vessel diameter)[4]:

$$Re = \frac{\rho U_{mean}D}{\mu}.$$

Flow is laminar for Reynolds numbers up to 2000. For higher values, the fluid loses its structure and turbulences will occur, introducing extra energy (pressure) losses and flattening the velocity profile. Note that the presence of a vortex does not necessarily imply that the flow is turbulent. In bends and branches, steady vortices may occur without losing the structured character of the flow. In that case, the flow is still laminar.

Oscillatory Laminar Flow: The Womersley Number

In the arterial tree, and then especially at the level of the large arteries, blood flow is not steady but pulsatile. Flow can still be perfectly laminar in these conditions. Oscillatory (sinusoidal), laminar flow in a tube has been studied by Womersley around 1940–1950; he developed a mathematical framework that allows to analytically calculate velocity profiles in these conditions.[5,6] Full elaboration of the Womersley theory is beyond the scope of this chapter, and can be found elsewhere. It suffices here to define the so-called Womersley number, often termed α:

$$\alpha = R\sqrt{\frac{\rho 2\pi f}{\mu}},$$

where f is the frequency of the oscillation. The Womersley parameter is, as the Reynolds number, a dimensionless parameter and it expresses the ratio of the inertial effects over the viscous friction effects. The higher the α, the more the inertia will play a role.

The effect of α on the velocity profiles is illustrated in Figure 7-2. For small α, the velocity profile is close to a parabola, with an amplitude that changes with time. The higher the α becomes, the more the inertia will become important, especially for the core flow at the center of the blood vessel. Near the wall the friction remains important

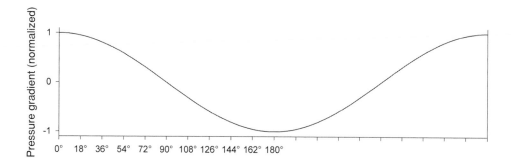

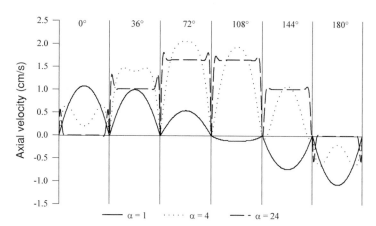

● **FIGURE 7-2.** Demonstration of the effect of the Womersley number on the flow profile. The top panel shows the sinusoidal variation of the pressure gradient over a tube segment. The bottom panel illustrates the velocity profiles at different moments in the cycle (from 0 to 180 degrees). When α is low, the flow is in phase with the pressure gradient, and the velocity profile maintains a parabolic shape. With increasing α, inertia dominates the flow at the center of the tube, which lags behind the pressure gradient. Near the wall, friction remains dominant and so the velocity profiles change completely in shape, with a more flat profile at the center and larger velocity gradients near the wall.

and the flow is in phase with the pressure gradient. In the core, phase lags will occur, with peak flow being reached 90 degrees out of phase with the pressure gradient that drives the blood flow. The velocity profile also becomes flatter.

In the systemic arterial tree, the highest Womersley numbers occur in the aorta (values in the order of 20) with flattened velocity profiles. In the small arteries, viscous effects dominate and velocity profiles will rather be parabolic.

Bernoulli's Law: Conservation of Energy

Finally, to conclude this section, it is worth mentioning Bernoulli's law,[7] which expresses the conservation of energy along a streamline in an incompressible, steady, isothermal flow, ignoring the effects of viscosity, the heat transfer, and the work done.[4] Along a stream line, it applies that

$$p + \rho g h + \frac{1}{2}\rho v^2 = \text{cst},$$

where p is the static pressure, g the gravitational constant, h the height of the point above a reference level, v the velocity in that point, and ρ the density. $p + \rho g h$ represents the potential energy of the liquid, with p the static pressure and $\rho g h$ the hydrostatic pressure. $\rho v^2/2$ represents the kinetic energy (dynamic pressure).

The Bernoulli's law can be extended with an extra term ΔF, which stands for extra losses that occur between points 1 and 2 (e.g., because of turbulences occurring as a consequence of a sudden expansion or narrowing).

$$p_1 + \rho g h_1 + \frac{1}{2}\rho v_1^2 = p_2 + \rho g h_2 + \frac{1}{2}\rho v_2^2 + \Delta F.$$

The Bernoulli equation, in a simplified form, is often used to calculate the pressure drop over a stenosis (Figure 7-3). In that case, neglecting ΔF, the blood is accelerated in the stenosis, with conversion of potential energy into kinetic energy. Assuming point 2 to be in the stenosis and v_1 negligible compared to v_2, ΔP over the stenosis approximates $\rho v_2^2/2$. With a blood density of 1050 kg/m^3 and accounting for a conversion factor 133.3 to convert pressure in Pa to pressure in mm Hg (1 mm Hg = 133.3 Pa), this equation is in the clinical setting often approximated as

$$\Delta P \approx 4v^2,$$

where v is the velocity in the stenosis, expressed in meters per second and ΔP is the pressure drop, expressed in millimeters of mercury. This expression is known as the "simplified Bernoulli equation" and generally overestimates the true pressure drop because v_1 is not totally zero and,

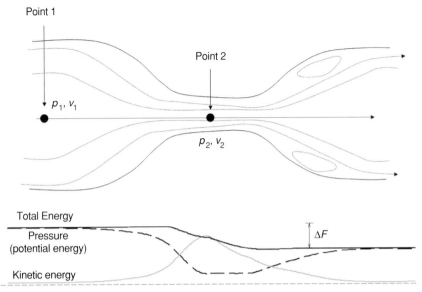

● **FIGURE 7-3.** The Bernoulli's law applied to flow through a stenosis. Flow accelerates, resulting in a decrease of pressure in the narrowing (conversion of potential into kinetic energy). Distal to the stenosis, flow velocity decreases, with only a partial recovery of pressure. In this case, the pressure drop over the stenosis is ΔF. The dashed line is the reference energy level.

more important, there is commonly a partial recovery of the pressure distal to the stenosis, with restoration of part of the kinetic energy into potential energy.

● THE ARTERIAL SYSTEM: AN ELASTIC RESERVOIR OR AN ELASTIC TUBE?

The blood pressure in the large arteries results from the interaction between the cyclic ejection of blood from the ventricle into the systemic or pulmonary circulation. It is forcing an open door when we state that the blood pressure is determined by both the function of the heart and by the properties of the arterial system.[8,9] In clinical terms, "blood pressure" is commonly interpreted as the upper (systolic; SBP) and lower (diastolic; DBP) value of pressure measured at the level of the brachial artery. Epidemiologic studies, the most famous one being the Framingham Heart Study, have demonstrated that normal ageing is associated with a gradual monotonic increase in SBP, while DBP rises up to the age of 60 and declines beyond that age[10] (Figure 7-4). The same "uncoupling" between systolic and diastolic blood pressure is also found in patients with so-called isolated systolic hypertension, i.e., those who have an elevated systolic blood pressure but normal-to-low diastolic blood pressure. Studies have demonstrated that an increased pulse pressure (PP), i.e., the difference between systolic and diastolic blood pressure, implies an increased cardiovascular risk and that PP has a higher prognostic power than SBP and/or DBP by themselves.[11]

The determining factors of arterial (pulse) pressure become immediately clear when considering the most simple mechanical equivalent of the cardiovascular system, that is, that of an antique fire hose (Figure 7-5), where the pulsatile action of the pump is attenuated by an air chamber, which

transforms the pulsatile flow into an almost steady outflow at the level of the nozzle.[8,12] The pump obviously stands for the heart, while the air chamber stands for the buffering function of the large elastic arteries (the "total arterial compliance," C). The nozzle represents the total vascular resistance (R), generated mainly in the arterioles and capillaries. This model was first suggested by reverend Stephen Hales (1733).[13] In 1899, Otto Frank translated this into a mathematical formulation,[14,15] and it was Frank who introduced the terminology "windkessel models," windkessel being the German word for air chamber, after the buffer chamber used in the antique fire hose. Assuming venous pressure to be negligible compared to arterial pressure, the

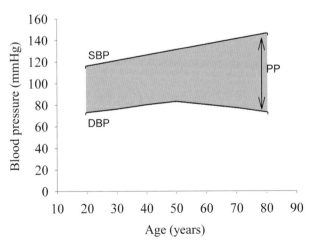

● **FIGURE 7-4.** Evolution of systolic (SBP) and diastolic (DBP) blood pressure with age. The difference between systolic and diastolic blood pressure is the pulse pressure, PP, which monotonically increases with age.

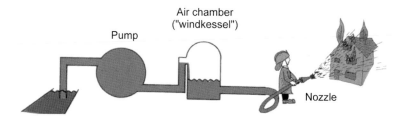

● **FIGURE 7-5.** Mechanical equivalent of the heart and the arterial tree: The heart is represented by a pump; the buffer function of the large elastic vessels is mimicked by the air chamber (windkessel), while the resistance of the arterioles and capillaries is represented by the nozzle. The system converts the pulsatile action of the pump into an almost steady, continuous flow at the nozzle. (*Courtsey of N. Westerhof.*)

arteriovenous pressure difference approximates mean arterial pressure (MAP), which can be deduced using the Ohm's law as the product of cardiac output (CO) and total vascular resistance: $MAP = CO \times R$. The PP is (mainly) determined by the capacity of the air chamber and the stroke volume[8] (SV): $PP \approx SV/C$. It is clear that a loss of arterial compliance gives rise to an increase in PP.

The windkessel model is, however, too simple an approximation of the arterial system. In physiological terms, it is much more accurate to consider it as a (complex topological) network of elastic arteries. When the left or right ventricle ejects its stroke volume into the systemic or pulmonary circulation, it generates pressure and flow waves that travel within the respective arterial networks. Measurements of pressure and flow in mammals and humans along the aorta and arterial tree in the second half of 20th century evidenced the existence of these waves. From the ascending to abdominal aorta, for instance, there is a measurable time delay between the onset of rise of pressure (or flow), and the wavefront (rising slope) of the pressure is steeper at the abdominal aorta. Furthermore, it was found that the peak of the pressure wave (systolic blood pressure) is higher at the abdominal than at the ascending aorta.[16] These observations can only be explained by wave reflection since in the absence of wave reflection the dissipation would lead to less steep wavefronts, attenuation of maximal pressure,

and one would also expect similarity of pressure and flow wave morphology, which is certainly not the case. The existence of wave reflection is, of course, not surprising given the complex anatomical structure of the arterial tree, with geometric and elastic tapering (the further away from the heart, the stiffer the vessel), its numerous bifurcations, and the arterioles and capillaries making the distal terminations.

As such, the blood pressure waveform measured at any location within the arterial tree is the result of the superposition of forward and backward running pressure waves. Besides the magnitude of the reflected waves, the timing of their arrival in the central aorta is a major determinant of the morphology and amplitude of the pressure wave (Figure 7-6). In young subjects, arteries are most elastic (deformable) and the pulse wave velocity (PWV—the speed with which a pressure or flow wave propagates through an artery) is much lower than in older subjects, or in patients with hypertension or diabetes. In the young, it takes more time for the forward wave to travel to the reflection site and for the reflected wave to arrive at the ascending aorta. Both interact only in late systole (late systolic inflection point), causing little extra load on the heart (this waveform was called a "C-type" waveform by Murgo et al.). In older subjects, on the other hand, PWV is much higher, and the inflection point shifts to early systole. The early arrival of the reflected wave literally boosts systolic pressure, causing

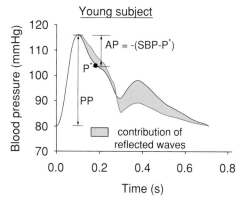

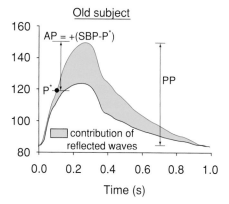

● **FIGURE 7-6.** Pressure waveforms measured at the level of the carotid artery in a young and old subject. In the young, the reflected wave arrives late in systole (late inflection point P^*), without augmenting systolic pressure. This waveform is called a C-type wave. In the older subject, early return of the reflected wave boosts systolic pressure. The waveform, characterized by an early inflection point, is of the so-called A-type.

an augmentation of systolic and PP.[17] Murgo et al. classified this waveform type as an "A-type" waveform.

Since the pulse wave velocity is directly related to the stiffness of the arterial tree, the overall conclusion is that, irrespective of the way the arterial tree is being studied (as a windkessel model or as an elastic tube system), an increase in arterial stiffness results in an increase in systolic blood pressure and PP. Given their association with an increased cardiovascular risk, there has been an increased interest in measuring arterial stiffness and wave reflection in the past two to three decades and also because an increase in arterial stiffness and/or wave reflection may be an early, intermediate phenotype of atherosclerosis.[18]

● "CLASSICAL" FREQUENCY DOMAIN VIEW ON HEMODYNAMICS AND THE ARTERIAL TREE

Pressure and Flow Waves as a "Series of Harmonics"

In the pioneering studies on arterial hemodynamics, the analysis of the arterial system and the (invasively measured) pressure and flow waveforms was based on parallelisms between hemodynamics and the electrical network and electrical transmission line theory. This also explains why models of the arterial system are often represented as an "electrical analog" model, consisting of resistors, inductors, and/or capacitance elements. The electrical analog of the basic windkessel model, for instance, is a parallel connection of a resistance (total vascular resistance, R) and a capacitance (total arterial compliance, C).

In these models, blood pressure is the analog of electrical voltage, and flow is the analog of electrical current. An electrical signal is generally considered as the superposition of a steady, direct current (the DC signal) and an alternating, oscillatory current (the AC signal), which is a pure sinusoidal wave (the mean value is zero) with a given frequency. Although arterial pressure and flow waves are approximately periodic (assuming a regularly beating heart), the flow is pulsatile and certainly not oscillatory.

Luckily, the Fourier theorem resolves this problem. Using this theorem, the pulsatile pressure and flow waves can be transformed into a "Fourier series," consisting of a steady component and sinusoidal waves with an incremental frequency ("harmonics") that, superimposed, yield the original pulsatile wave. In general, 10 to 15 harmonics are sufficient to describe hemodynamic variables such as pressure or flow. The frequency of the first (fundamental) harmonic is the cardiac frequency, and the higher harmonics have a frequency that is a natural multiple of the fundamental frequency. Assuming that the superposition principle is valid ("the sum of the effects of all individual harmonics is the same as the effect of the superimposed harmonics"), the hemodynamic analysis can be performed for a given harmonic with a given frequency. Thus, instead of considering the measured pressure and flow wave, individual harmon-

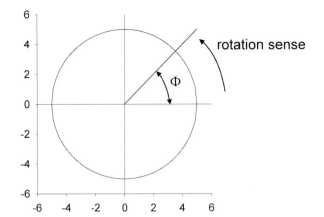

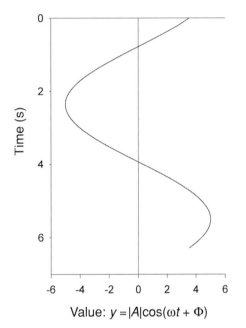

● **FIGURE 7-7.** Representation of an individual harmonic as a rotor rotating counterclockwise. The start position at $t = 0$ equals Φ. The value is the projection of the rotor on the horizontal axis, which equals $|A|\cos(\omega t + \Phi)$, with $|A|$ the amplitude of the harmonic.

ics are studied, and the properties of the arterial tree are displayed as a function of frequency.

The sinusoidal waves or harmonics can be described by their amplitude and their "phase angle," which can mathematically be represented using a complex formalism (Figure 7-7). For the nth harmonic, the pressure (P) and flow (Q) component can be written as

$$P_n = |P_n| e^{i(n\omega t + \Phi_{Pn})} \quad Q_n = |Q_n| e^{i(n\omega t + \Phi_{Qn})},$$

where $|P_n|$ and $|Q_n|$ are the amplitudes (or modulus) of the pressure and flow sine waves, having phase angles Φ_{Pn} and Φ_{Qn} (to allow for a phase lag in the harmonic), respectively. Time is indicated by t and ω is the fundamental angular frequency, given by $2\pi/T$ with T the duration of a heart cycle (RR interval). For a heart rate of 75 beats/min, T is 0.8 seconds. The fundamental frequency is 1.25 Hz, and ω becomes 7.85 rad/s.

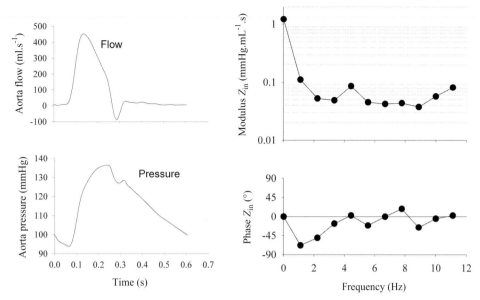

● **FIGURE 7-8.** Input impedance modulus (top right) and phase (bottom right) calculated from a measured aortic pressure and flow wave (left panel) in a human subject.

The Impedance of the Arterial Tree

Impedance is a general measure of the "resistance to flow" and is defined as the ratio of pressure and flow: $Z = P/Q$. As it also accounts for pulsatile flow, it surpasses the definition of systemic vascular resistance, which only accounts for mean pressure and flow. Z has the dimensions of mm Hg mL^{-1}s (kg m^{-4} s^{-1} in SI units; dyn cm^{-5}s in older units) if pressure is expressed in mm Hg and flow in mL s^{-1}. Z is calculated for each individual harmonic, and displayed as a function of frequency (Figure 7-8). Since both P and Q are complex numbers, Z is complex as well and also has a modulus and a phase angle, except for the steady ("DC") component at 0 Hz, which is nothing but the ratio of mean pressure and mean flow, that is, the value of total vascular resistance. For all higher harmonics, the modulus of the nth harmonic is given as $|Z_n| = |P_n|/|Q_n|$, and its phase Φ_{Zn} is given as $\Phi_{Pn} - \Phi_{Qn}$.

Arterial impedance requires simultaneous measurement of pressure and flow at the same location. Although it can be meaningfully calculated at any location along the arterial tree, it is most commonly measured at the entrance of the systemic or pulmonary circulation and is called "input" impedance, often denoted as Z_{in}. Z_{in} fully captures the relation between pressure and flow, and is determined by all downstream factors influencing this relation (arterial network topology, branching patterns, stiffness of the vessels, vasomotor tone, . . .). It provides a powerful description of the arterial circulation, since it captures all effects, but this is at the same time its greatest weakness, as Z_{in} is not very sensitive to local changes in arterial system properties, such as focal atherosclerotic lesions.

It is not always easy to give an interpretation to an impedance pattern. This is, however, facilitated when one considers the impedance of basic electrical or mechanical "building blocks"[19-21]:

- When a system behaves strictly resistive, there is a linear relation between the pressure (difference) and flow. Pressure and flow are always in phase, Z_n is a real number, and Φ_Z is zero.
- In case there is only inertia in a system, pressure is ahead of flow; for sine waves, the phase difference between both is a quarter of a wavelength, or +90 degrees in terms of phase angle.
- In the case that the system behaves like a capacitor, flow is leading pressure, again 90 degrees out of phase, so that Φ_Z is –90 degrees.

Figure 7-8 displays the input impedance calculated from a measured aorta pressure and flow waveform. The impedance modulus drops from the value of total systemic vascular resistance at 0 Hz to much lower values at higher frequencies. The phase angle is negative up until the fourth harmonic, showing that capacitive effects dominate at these low frequencies, although the phase angle never reaches –90 degrees, indicating that inertial effects are present as well. For higher harmonics, the phase angle is close to zero, or at least oscillating around the zero value. At the same time, the modulus of Z_{in} is nearly constant. For these high frequencies, the system seems to act as a pure resistance, and the impedance value, averaged over the higher harmonics (typically from the third to the 10th harmonic), has been termed the characteristic impedance (Z_0).

Input Impedance Explained from the Viewpoint of Wave Transmission and Reflection

The above-mentioned characteristic impedance, Z_0, is an important property of the arterial tree that deserves some further attention. In the hypothetical case that the arterial tree were an infinitely long and uniform tube, wave reflection would be totally absent. Under these conditions, the relation between pressure and flow harmonics would be solely dependent on the geometric and mechanical properties of the tube itself. The ratio of pressure and flow harmonics, Z, would be a constant—the characteristic impedance Z_0, which can be approximated as

$$Z_0 = \rho \times \text{PWV}/A,$$

where ρ is the density of blood (1050 kg/m³), PWV the pulse wave velocity of the tube, and A the cross-sectional area of the tube. In that hypothetical case, the input impedance thus equals the characteristic impedance. Later in the chapter we address how Z_0 can be assessed in vivo.

The arterial system, however, is not an infinitely long, uniform tube free of reflections, which is the reason the input impedance is more complex than a simple real constant. Despite the fact that it is difficult (and perhaps impossible) to fully pinpoint wave reflection in the arterial tree, the problem is often approached in a pragmatic and simple way, with the arterial tree being considered as a tube with an "effective length,"[22,23] and a single reflection site at the end. The input impedance of such a system can be calculated, as demonstrated in Figure 7-9. In that example, a uniform tube of diameter 1.5 cm and PWV of 6.2 m/s is assumed, yielding a value for Z_0 of 0.275 mm Hg mL^{-1} s. It is further assumed that the tube has a length of 50 cm, and

is ended by a (linear) resistance of 1 mm Hg mL^{-1} s. The impedance mismatch between the tube and its terminal resistance gives rise to wave reflections and oscillations in the input impedance pattern, and many features, observed in vivo,[24] can be explained on the basis of this model.

Assume there is a sinusoidal wave running in the system with a wavelength λ being four times the length of the tube. This means that the phase angle of the reflected wave, when arriving back at the entrance at the tube, will be 180 degrees out of phase with respect to the forward wave. The sum of the incident and reflected wave will be minimal, since they interfere in a maximally destructive way. If this wave is a pressure wave, measured pressure at the entrance of the tube will be minimal for waves with this particular wavelength. There is a relation between PWV, λ, and frequency f, that is, $\lambda = \text{PWV}/f$. Thus, in an input impedance spectrum, the frequency $f_{\min}$ where input impedance is minimal corresponds to a wave with a wavelength that is equal to four times the distance to the reflection site, L: $4L = \text{PWV}/f_{\min}$, or $L = \text{PWV}/4 f_{\min}$ and $f_{\min} = \text{PWV}/4L$. Applied to the example of the tube, $f_{\min}$ is expected at $6.2/2 = 3.1$ Hz. This equation is known as the "quarter wavelength" formula, and is used to estimate the effective length of the arterial system.

Linear Wave Separation Analysis

Although the wave reflection pattern in the arterial system is complex,[25] pressure (P) and flow (Q) are considered to be composed of only one forward running component, P_f (Q_f), and one backward running component, P_b (Q_b), where the single forward and backward running components are the resultant of all forward and backward traveling waves, including the forward waves that result from re-reflection at the aortic valve of backward running waves.[26]

At all times, it applies that

$$P = P_f + P_b \quad \text{and} \quad Q = Q_f + Q_b.$$

Furthermore, if the arterial tree is considered as a tube, defined by its characteristic impedance Z_0, the following relations also apply:

$$Z_0 = P_f/Q_f = -P_b/Q_b,$$

since Z_0 is the ratio of pressure and flow in the absence of wave reflection,[19–21] which is the case when only forward or backward running components are taken into consideration. The negative sign in the equation above appears because the flow is directional, considered positive in the direction away from the heart, and negative toward the heart, while the value of the pressure is insensitive to direction.

Combing these equations, $P = P_f - Z_0 Q_b = P_f - Z_0$ $(Q - Q_f) = 2P_f - Z_0 Q$, so that

$$P_f = (P + Z_0 Q)/2.$$

Similarly, it can be deduced that

$$P_b = (P - Z_0 Q)/2.$$

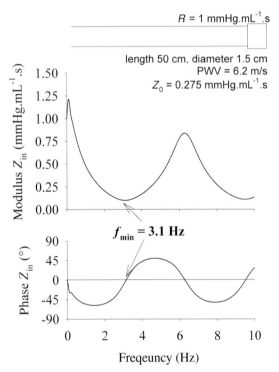

● **FIGURE 7-9.** Input impedance pattern of a tube of a length of 50 cm, a pulse wave velocity of 6.2 m/s, and characteristic impedance of 0.275 mm Hg mL^{-1} s. The top panel shows the impedance modulus; the bottom panel shows the impedance phase. The frequency at which the modulus of Z_{in} is minimal is coupled to the distance to the reflection site via the quarter-wavelength formula (see text).

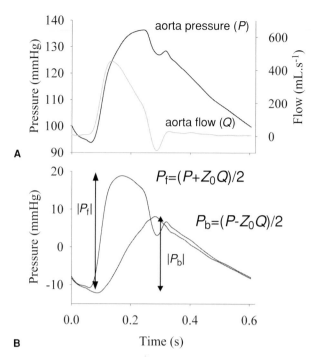

A

B

● **FIGURE 7-10.** Linear wave separation analysis applied to the measured aorta pressure and flow data from Figure 7-8. The ratio of the amplitude of the backward pressure wave ($|P_b|$) to the amplitude of the forward pressure wave ($|P_f|$) is a straightforward measure of wave reflection, also called the reflection magnitude.

These equations were first derived by Westerhof et al. and are known as the linear wave separation equations.[26] The linear wave separation analysis is demonstrated in Figure 7-10. In principle, the separation should be calculated on individual harmonics, and the net P_f and P_b wave then follows from summation of all forward and backward harmonics. In practice, however, the equations are often used in the time domain, using measured pressure and flow as input. Note, however, that wave reflection applies only to the pulsatile part of pressure and flow, and mean pressure and flow should be subtracted from measured pressure and flow before applying the equations.

Quantifying Wave Reflection

From the analysis above, it follows that the ratio of the amplitude of the backward and forward pressure wave, $|P_b|/|P_f|$, adequately quantifies pressure wave reflection. This parameter has been termed the reflection magnitude.[27]

From the equations above, one can also deduce the reflection coefficient (Γ) as

$$\Gamma = \frac{P_b}{P_f} = \frac{P - QZ_0}{P + QZ_0} = \frac{Z_{in} - Z_0}{Z_{in} + Z_0}.$$

In this equation, Γ is a complex frequency-dependent property, with a modulus and a phase angle, and thus more difficult to interpret than $|P_b|/|P_f|$. One therefore often uses the amplitude or real part of Γ at the fundamental frequency to quantify wave reflection.

Estimating Characteristic Impedance

As clear from the above, wave separation analysis requires knowledge of characteristic impedance, which can be estimated both in the frequency and time domain.[28] It was already noted that for the higher harmonics (>third harmonic), Z_{in} fluctuates around a constant value, Z_0, and with a phase angle approaching zero. Assuming wave speed to be approximately 5 m/s, the wavelength λ for these higher harmonics (e.g., the fifth harmonic for a heart rate of 60 beats/min), being the product of the wave speed and wave period (0.2 seconds), becomes shorter (1 m) than the average arterial path length. Waves reflect at distant locations throughout the arterial tree (with distal ends of vascular beds less than 50 cm to approximately 2 m away from the heart in humans), return to the heart with different phase angles, and interfere with each other in a destructive manner, so that the net effect of the reflected waves appears inexistent. For these higher harmonics, the arterial system thus appears reflectionless, and under these conditions, the ratio of pressure and flow is, by definition, the characteristic impedance. Therefore, averaging the input impedance modulus of the higher harmonics, where the phase angle is approximately zero, yields an estimate of the characteristic impedance (Figure 7-11).[19-21]

Characteristic impedance can also be estimated in the time domain. In early systole, the reflected waves did not yet reach the ascending aorta, and in the early systolic ejection period, the relation between pressure and flow is linear (Figure 7-11), as can be observed when plotting P as a function of Q.[28,29] The slope of the Q–P relationship

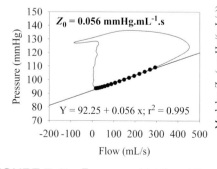

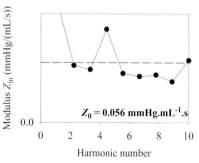

● **FIGURE 7-11.** Frequency (right) and time-domain (left) estimate of characteristic impedance using the pressure and flow data also used in Figure 7-8.

during early systole is the time domain estimate of Z_0, and is generally in good agreement with the frequency domain estimate.[28]

Both the time and frequency domain approach, however, are sensitive to subjective criteria such as the selection of the early systolic ejection period, or the selection of the harmonic range that is used for averaging. Both techniques are illustrated in Figure 7-11, where they are applied to the data earlier shown in Figure 7-8.

● "TIME DOMAIN" APPROACH OF ARTERIAL HEMODYNAMICS: WAVE INTENSITY ANALYSIS

With its origin in electrical network theory, much of the arterial hemodynamic analysis, including wave reflection, is done in the frequency domain. Besides the fact that this analysis is, strictly speaking, applicable only to linear systems with periodic signal changes, the analysis is quite complex because of the necessity of Fourier decomposition and is not intuitively comprehensible. An alternative method of analysis, performed in the time domain and not requiring linearity and periodicity, is the analysis of the wave intensity, elaborated by Parker and Jones in the late 1980s.[30]

Disturbances to the flow lead to changes in pressure (dP) and flow velocity (dU), "wavelets," which propagate along the vessels with a wave speed (PWV), as defined above. There is, however, a relation between the magnitude of these dP and dU wavelets. Accounting for conservation of mass and momentum, it can be shown that

$$dP_\pm = \pm \text{PWV} \rho \, dU_\pm,$$

where "+" denotes a forward traveling wavelet (for a defined positive direction), while "−" denotes a backward traveling wavelet. This equation is also known as the waterhammer equation. Waves characterized by a $dP > 0$, that is, a rise in pressure, are called compression waves, while waves with $dP < 0$ are expansion waves. Note that this terminology still reflects the origin of the theory in gas dynamics.

Considering a tube, with left-to-right as the positive direction, four possible types of waves can be discerned:

(1) Blowing on the left side of the tube—pressure rises ($dP > 0$) and velocity increases ($dU > 0$). This is a *forward compression wave*.

(2) Blowing on the right side of the tube—pressure increases ($dP > 0$), but velocity decreases ($dU < 0$) with our convention. This is a *backward compression wave*.

(3) Sucking on the left side of the tube—pressure decreases ($dP < 0$) as well as the velocity ($dU < 0$) decreases, but the wavefront propagates from left to right. This wave type is a *forward expansion wave*.

(4) Finally, sucking on the right side of the tube—pressure ($dP < 0$) decreases, but velocity ($dU > 0$) increases. This is a *backward expansion wave*.

The nature of a wave is most easily comprehended by analyzing the wave intensity, dI, which is defined as the

product of dU and dP, and is the energy flux carried by the wavelet:

$$dI = dU \, dP.$$

It can be deduced from the above that dI is always positive for forward running waves and always negative for backward waves, irrespective of the fact that it is a compression or expansion wave. When dI is positive, forward waves are dominant; otherwise, backward waves are dominant. Analysis of dP reveals whether the wave is a compression or an expansion wave.

These wavelets are easily calculated from a measured pressure and flow velocity signal; dP (dU) is simply the difference between pressure (flow velocity) measured at instant n minus the value at instant $n - 1$: $dP = P(n) - P(n-1)$. Since the absolute value of the difference depends on the sampling rate of the signal, one can also calculate a so-called normalized value, which is $dP/dt = [P(n) - P(n-1)]/[t(n) - t(n-1)]$ with t the time. Similar equations apply to the flow velocity.

Figure 7-12 shows the wave intensity calculated from the data displayed in Figure 7-8, showing a typical aortic wave intensity pattern characterized by three major peaks. The first peak is a forward compression wave, associated with the ejection of blood from the ventricle. The second positive peak is associated with a forward running wave, but $dP < 0$, and is therefore a forward running expansion wave because of ventricular relaxation, slowing down the ejection from the heart. During systole, reflected waves are dominant, resulting in a negative wave intensity but with, in this case, positive dP. The negative peak is thus a backward compression wave, resulting from the peripheral wave reflections.

It can further be mentioned that, similar to the Westerhof work,[26] here also, the wavelets dP and dU can be decomposed into their forward and backward components.[29] It can be derived that

$$dP_\pm = \frac{1}{2}(dP \pm \rho \text{PWV} \, dU)$$

and

$$dU_\pm = \pm \frac{1}{2}\left(\frac{dP}{\rho \text{PWV}} \pm dU\right).$$

The total forward and backward pressure and flow wave can be obtained as $P_+ = P_\text{d} + \sum_{t=0}^{t} dP_+$, with P_d the diastolic blood pressure, which is added to the forward wave, and $P_- = \sum_{t=0}^{t} dP_-$.[29] Similarly, for the forward and backward velocity wave, it applies that $U_+ = \sum_{t=0}^{t} dU_+$ and $U_- = \sum_{t=0}^{t} dU_-$. Wave intensity in itself, dI, can also be separated in a net forward and backward wave intensity: $dI_+ = dP_+ dU_+$ and $dI_- = dP_- dU_-$, with $dI = dI_+ + dI_-$.

Wave intensity is certainly an appealing method to gain insight into complex wave (reflection) patterns, as in the arterial system, and the method is increasingly being used.[31–33] The drawback of the method is the fact that dI is calculated as the product of two derivatives dP and dU,

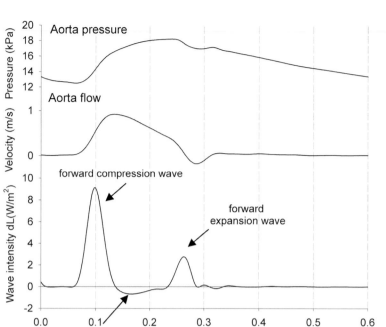

Wave intensity pattern obtained from the aorta pressure and flow from Figure 7-8. Pressures were converted to kPa; flow velocity was derived from the flow assuming the aortic diameter to be 2.5 cm. The typical pattern with the forward compression wave (ventricular ejection), backward compression wave (wave reflection in the periphery), and forward expansion wave (ventricular relaxation) are retrieved.

and thus highly sensitive to noise in the signal. Adequate filtering of basic signals and derivatives is mandatory. As for the more "classic" impedance analysis, it is also required that pressure and flow be—preferably simultaneously—measured at the exact same location.

● (CLINICAL) APPROACH TO MEASURE ARTERIAL PROPERTIES

One of the main obstacles impeding the clinical implementation of "textbook" hemodynamics and impedance analysis is the practical applicability of the methodology. The above-mentioned analysis is based on simultaneous measurement of central pressure and flow waveforms, which is often not doable in a clinical setting that requires noninvasive measurements. Although it is feasible to noninvasively measure aortic flow (using Doppler ultrasound technology), and carotid or subclavian pressure tracings (by applanation tonometry) as surrogate for central aortic pressure, the processing of the data is complex and time consuming and provides only an estimate of arterial properties because of the assumptions underlying the data. In addition to the complex measurement, the interpretation of impedance patterns remains complex and, as mentioned before, it is a gross measure of arterial function, which is not likely to provide a measure that is sensitive to subtle changes in arterial properties.

As such, in the past few years, several "clinically applicable" methods have emerged in the literature, all claiming to measure (aspects of) the function of the arterial system and/or wave reflection. In an attempt to provide some sort of classification, we have categorized the methods as to whether they measure arterial properties at one specific location (local measurements), over an arterial segment, or whether they provide a measure of the entire (systemic) circulation.

Measuring Local Arterial Stiffness: DC and CC

These measurements are based on local measurements of arterial pressure and vessel diameter, and are applied to superficial arteries such as the radial, brachial, carotid, and femoral artery, with the carotid artery considered representative for the large, central elastic arteries, and the radial, brachial, and femoral artery for the more peripheral, muscular arteries.

When measuring local arterial stiffness, it is important that pressures are being measured at the same anatomical location as where the diameter measurements are being exerted. We have developed a tonometry-based measurement platform for that purpose. Applanation tonometry yields the *profile* of the pressure wave, but it does not provide reliable values of pressure. The tonometry curves therefore require calibration. The method that we commonly use starts from tonometry measurements at the level of the brachial artery (see also Figure 7-13). This is the only location in the body where the peak and trough of the measured pressure waveform equal the sphygmomanomer systolic and diastolic blood pressure. As such, this curve can be perfectly scaled. With this calibrated curve, it is possible to accurately determine mean arterial blood pressure as the average of that curve. Others have shown that diastolic and mean blood pressure remain as good as constant over the larger arteries (but not systolic blood pressure that is amplified toward the periphery, at least up to the level of large- and mid-sized arteries). With the knowledge of diastolic and mean blood pressure from the brachial

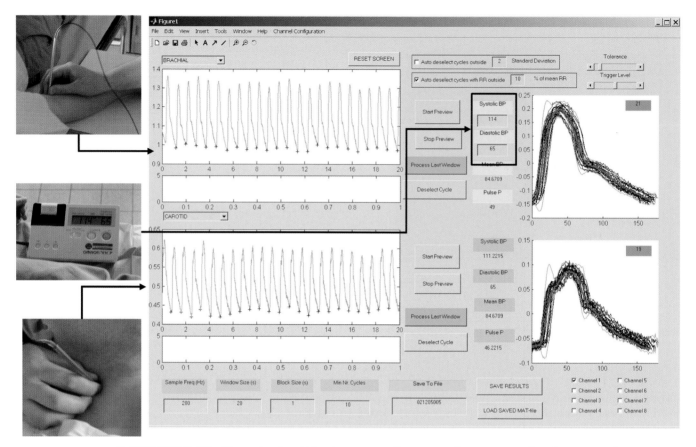

● **FIGURE 7-13.** Measuring local blood pressures: Sequence of measurement and calibration when applying tonometry at the carotid artery. The pressure wave is first measured and calibrated at the level of the brachial artery (two upper graphs). The left panel shows a sequence of 20 seconds with indication of the cycles that are used to calculate an average curve (in red) and the rejected cycles (in cyan). The right panel shows the averaged wave (dark blue line). Next, waveforms are measured at another location (here the carotid artery; lower graphs). After averaging, the averaged waveform is calibrated using the mean and diastolic blood pressure determined at the brachial artery. The pictures on the left show the measuring platform and the pen-type Millar tonometer (SPT301, Millar, Houston, TX) that was used.

artery, one can calibrate tonometry curves at other locations and obtain an estimate of local systolic and PP[34–36] (Figure 7-13).

For measurement of the arterial diameter (or, better, the cyclic change of diameter, also called the distension), there are several commercially available systems, all based on ultrasound. Some systems, such as the Wall Track or ART.LAB system (Easote Europe, Maastricht, The Netherlands), automatically detect the vessel wall from the measured radiofrequency ultrasound data, and track the displacement of the vessel wall as a function of time using algorithms based on cross- or autocorrelation methods. As we have demonstrated using a prototype wall tracking system (Vivid7, GE Vingmed Ultrasoud, Horten, Norway), knowledge of which point in the vessel wall is being tracked, is important.[37] Irrespective of eventual inhomogeneities in the vessel wall, tracking the inside of the blood vessel (e.g., the transition between the lumen and vessel intimal layer) will yield substantially larger displacements than when tracking the outside of the vessel (e.g., the transition

between the media layer and the adventitia).[37] This simply follows from the law of conservation of mass. Commercial systems most frequently detect and track the easy-to-find media-adventitia transition.

The information that one minimally obtains from these measurements are the local distensibility (DC) and compliance coefficient (CC), defined as

$$DC = (\Delta A / A) / \Delta P \quad (\text{in mm Hg}^{-1} \text{ or Pa}^{-1})$$

$$CC = \Delta A / \Delta P \quad (\text{in mm}^2 \cdot \text{mm Hg}^{-1} \text{ or mm}^2 \cdot \text{Pa}^{-1}),$$

where A is the cross-sectional area of the artery in diastole, ΔA the systolic–diastolic difference in cross-sectional area, and ΔP the locally assessed PP.[38] DC describes the intrinsic stiffness of the vessel that is studied, while CC reflects the local buffer capacity. Ideally, it is also possible to construct pressure–diameter curves that allow us to calculate CC or DC at different blood pressure levels, or to assess other parameters obtained from fitting a prescribed pressure–diameter law, such as an exponential or the arc-tangent relation of Langewouters et al., through the data.[39,40] Note that these indices describe the function of the vessel; they do not provide any intrinsic insight into the properties of the wall material in itself.

Regional Measurements: Pulse Wave Velocity

An often applied method to assess the stiffness of an arterial segment is to measure the velocity by which a "perturbation" propagates over that arterial segment.[41] This perturbation can be a pressure wave, but also a diameter distension or flow velocity wave. What is required are measurements of pressure/diameter/flow velocity at two locations, a distance Δx of each other (Figure 7-14).[42,43] Because of the elasticity of the vessel, it will take an instant (ΔT) before the perturbation has propagated from location 1 to location 2. The ratio $\Delta x/\Delta T$ is the propagation speed of the wave (pulse wave velocity). For a uniform, straight cylindrical tube, PWV is directly related to the aforementioned DC[9,38]:

$$PWV = 1/\sqrt{\rho DC},$$

with ρ the density of blood. Although the arterial system is not a uniform tube with continuous changes in vessel diameter and stiffness and numerous branches, PWV is still generally considered as one of the most pure (and certainly one of the easiest to measure) indices of arterial stiffness.[44] Ideally, PWV is derived from simultaneous measurements at the two locations. If this is practically impossible, sequential measurements can be performed using, for instance, the time delay between the R-top of the ECG signal and the foot of the wave on these two locations. A bigger problem is the measurement of the distance Δx. One often calculates PWV from measurements on the carotid and femoral artery. In that case, one should compensate for the fact that

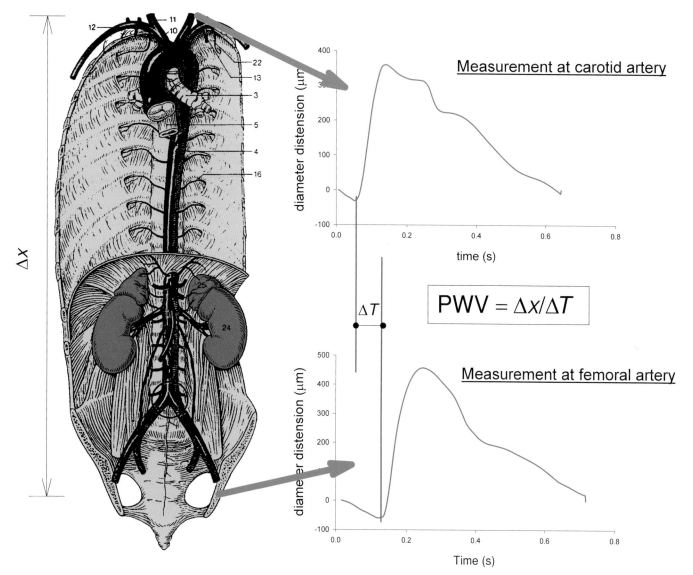

● **FIGURE 7-14.** Principle of measuring pulse wave velocity (PWV). The propagation of a "perturbation" in the arterial tree is measured, illustrated here using measurements of the distension of the carotid and femoral artery, a distance Δx apart.

while traveling up the carotid (a proximal branch of the aorta) the pulse has also already traveled further down the aorta. In older people, and in patients with aortic pathologies, the aorta may be tortuous, complicating the reliable measurement of Δx.

It appears that especially carotid-femoral PWV, which best approximates the stiffness of the aorta, carries important prognostic information. Increased PWV implies an increased risk of cardiovascular incidents in high-risk patients (diabetes, hypertension, etc.), but recent studies have shown that, also in the general population, PWV has added prognostic value, on top of all known classical risk factors, including systolic blood pressure and PP.[45–47]

Global Measures of the Complete (Systemic) Circulation: Total Arterial Compliance

As mentioned above, it is not totally impossible to measure central pressure and flow in a clinical setting using noninvasive technology. Aortic flow can be measured with Doppler ultrasound, while carotid or subclavian applanation tonometry yields a surrogate for central blood pressure. From these data, the arterial input impedance as well as, probably more useful, the number of indices or parameters that describe the properties of the complete arterial tree, such as the total arterial compliance, can be assessed.[8] A disadvantage of these global indices is that they are strongly determined by height and weight of the individual, introducing considerable variability in these measurements. The necessity of measurement of pressure and flow also impedes the clinical use of these measures.

The assessment of total arterial compliance from pressure and flow is generally based on an approximation of the arterial tree by a simple, lumped parameter windkessel model. In the following section, the two-element windkessel model and some of the more complex models, as well as how they can be used to estimate total arterial compliance, are discussed. The procedures commonly include a curve fitting part. A generic methodology for all models described is to use the measured flow (or pressure) as input into the model and to calculate the pressure (or flow) response predicted by the model with an initial set of parameter values. By optimizing the parameter set, one can minimize the difference between the measured pressure (or flow) and the output predicted by the model. The parameter set that yields the closest agreement between the measured and predicted signal is then considered as the optimal representation of the arterial system.

The Two-Element Windkessel Model. While there are many different windkessel models in use,[8,48] the two basic components contained within each model are a compliance element, C (mL mm Hg^{-1}), and a resistor element, R (mm Hg mL^{-1} s). C represents the volume change associated with a unit change in pressure; R represents the pressure drop over the resistor associated with a unit flow.

In diastole, when there is no new inflow of blood into the windkessel, the arterial pressure decays exponentially following $P(t) = P_0 e^{-t/RC}$. RC is the product of R and C and is called the arterial decay time. The higher the RC time, the slower the pressure decay. It is the time required to reduce P_0 to 37% of its initial value (note that the 37% is a theoretical value, usually not reached in vivo because the next beat impedes a full pressure decay). One can make use of this property to estimate the arterial compliance: Fitting an exponential curve to the diastolic decaying pressure, RC is obtained and thus, when R is known, so is C.[8,49–51] This method is known as the decay time (or time decay) method.

The question how well a windkessel model represents the actual arterial system can be answered by studying the input impedance of both. In the complex formulation, the input impedance of a two-element windkessel model is given as

$$Z_{i-\text{WK2}} = \frac{R}{1 + i\omega RC},$$

where i is the complex constant, $\omega = 2\pi f$, and f is the frequency. The DC value (0 Hz) of Z_{in} is thus R; at high frequencies, it becomes zero. The phase angle is 0 at 0 Hz, and –90 degrees for all other frequencies. Compared to input impedance as measured in mammals, the behavior of a two-element windkessel model reasonably represents the behavior of the arterial system for the low frequencies (up to third harmonic), but not for higher frequencies[8,19,52] (Figure 7-15). This means that it is justified to use the model for predicting the low-frequency behavior of the arterial system, that is, the low-frequency response to a flow input. This property is used in the so-called pulse pressure method—an iterative method to estimate arterial compliance: With R assumed known, the PP response of the two-element windkessel model to a (measured) flow stimulus is calculated with varying values of C. The value of C yielding the PP response matching the one measured in vivo is considered to be the correct one.[53] In Comparison to the decay time method the pulse pressure method is insensitive to deviations of the decaying pressure from the true exponential decay.[51]

The Three-Element and Higher-Order Windkessel Models. The major shortcoming of the two-element windkessel model is the inadequate high-frequency behavior.[8,12,19] Westerhof et al. resolved this problem by adding a third resistive element proximal to the windkessel, accounting for the resistive-like behavior of the arterial system in the high-frequency range.[12] This model yields markedly improved fitting between measured and model predicted data (Figure 7-15). The third element represents the characteristic impedance of the proximal part of the ascending aorta and integrates the effects of inertia and compliance. Adding the element, the input impedance of the three-element windkessel model becomes

$$Z_{i-\text{WK3}} = Z_0 + \frac{R}{1 + i\omega RC}.$$

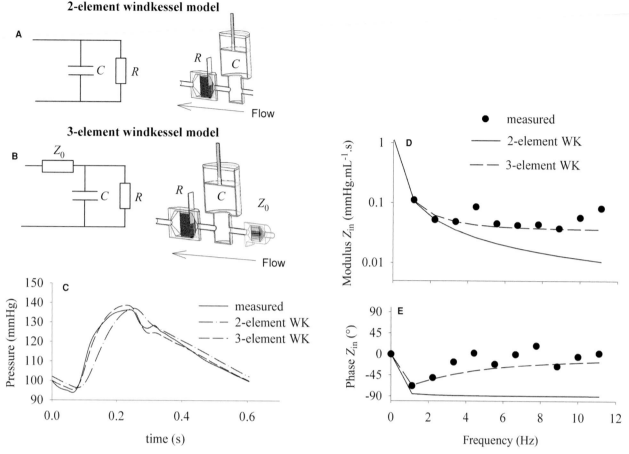

● **FIGURE 7-15.** Windkessel model fittings. Measured flow (from Figure 7-8) is used as input into the two- and three-element windkessel model, and the model parameters are adjusted until the difference between the measured and estimated pressure is minimal. Panels A and B show the electrical and mechanical analogs, panel C shows the comparison between measured pressure and optimized model response, and panels D and E illustrate the comparison in modulus and phase of the measured input impedance and the impedance obtained for the two- and three-element windkessel model after parameter optimization.

The effect is that the phase angle is negative for lower harmonics, but returns to zero for higher harmonics, where the impedance modulus asymptotically reaches the value of Z_0. For the systemic circulation, the ratio of Z_0 and R is 0.05:0.1.[54]

The major disadvantage of the three-element windkessel model is that Z_0, which should represent the high-frequency behavior of the arterial system, plays a role at all frequencies, including at 0 Hz. This has as a negative consequence: When the three-element windkessel model is used to fit data measured in the arterial system, the compliance is systematically overestimated.[51,55] The only way to "neutralize" the contribution of Z_0 at the low frequencies is to artificially increase the compliance of the model.

The "ideal" model would incorporate both the low-frequency behavior of the two-element windkessel model and the high frequency Z_0, though without interference of the latter at the low frequencies. This can be achieved by adding an inertial element in parallel to the characteristic impedance, as demonstrated by Stergiopulos et al.,[56] elab-orating on a model first introduced by Burattini et al.[57] For the DC component and low frequencies, Z_0 is bypassed through the inertial element. For the high frequencies, Z_0 takes over. It has been demonstrated, fitting the four-element windkessel model to data generated using an extended arterial network model, that L effectively represents the total inertia present in the model.[56]

Obviously, by adding more elements, it is possible to develop models that are able to further enhance the matching between model and arterial system behavior,[8,48] but the uniqueness of the model may not be guaranteed, and the physiological interpretation of the model elements is not always clear.

Although lumped parameter models cannot explain all aspects of hemodynamics, they are very useful as a concise representation of the arterial system. Mechanical versions are frequently used in hydraulic bench experiments, or as highly controllable afterload systems for in vivo experiments. An important field of application of the mathematical version is of parameter identification: Fitting arterial pressure and flow data measured in vivo to these models, the arterial system can be characterized and quantified (e.g., the total arterial compliance) through the model parameter values.[8,19]

It is important to stress that these lumped models represent the behavior of the arterial system as a whole and that there is no relation between model components and anatomical parts of the arterial tree.[19] For instance, although Z_0 represents the properties of the proximal aorta, there is no drop in mean pressure along the aorta, which one would expect if the three-element windkessel model were to be interpreted in a strict anatomical way. The combination of elements simply yields a model that represents the behavior of the arterial system as it is seen by the heart.

The Goldwyn and Watt Four-Element Windkessel Model.

Finally, it is worth to mention a windkessel model that is the backbone of an arterial system analysis method promoted by Dr. Cohn and coworkers. This four-element windkessel model was described in 1967 and contains, apart from the obligatory total arterial compliance (C_1) and total vascular resistance (R), two extra components: a second, smaller compliance (C_2) and an inductance (L) that reflects the inertia of the blood in the vasculature.[58] This model is used to describe the diastolic part of the pressure curve measured at the level of the radial artery (Figure 7-16). The shape of this curve is an exponentially decaying pressure, on which a sinusoidally varying part can be superimposed.[58] The model contains enough parameters to adequately describe this shape, and curve fitting techniques generally provide excellent fittings of the model to the data. The problem, however, is the obscure physical/physiological meaning of the model parameters C_2 and L,[59,60] which is reflected in the changing nomenclature for the parameter C_2 and has earlier been termed "distal," "oscillatory," or "re-

flective" compliance. The theoretical basis of the method has also been questioned, and the methodology has a very high black box character with strong assumptions regarding the cardiac output (which is required in the parameter estimation process). Nevertheless, there are several studies that have reported a decrease especially in C_2 in high-risk patient populations such as patients with hypertension or diabetes.[61,62] In our opinion, the method is sensitive to changes in radial pressure wave morphology—and hence yields changes in the value of model parameters[59]—but the physiological foundation of the model and the method are debatable,[63] and the parameter C_2 is not likely to relate to arterial stiffness at any level.

Ratio of Stroke Volume and PP. Irrespective of the models and methods that have been discussed in the preceding sections, a simple approximation of total arterial compliance (C) is the ratio of stroke volume (SV) and central PP:

$$C \approx SV/PP.$$

For typical hemodynamic conditions in humans at rest (systolic/diastolic pressure of 120/80 mm Hg, respectively, stroke volume 80 mL), SV/PP is 2 mL mm Hg^{-1}. This value is considered as an overestimation of the actual arterial compliance[8,52] as it is assumed that the total SV is buffered during systole, which is not the case.

● CLINICAL APPROACH TO WAVE REFLECTION: THE AUGMENTATION INDEX

As mentioned before, the pressure wave is the superposition of a forward running, incident component, and a backward running, reflected component. The contour of the pressure wave depends on the magnitude and timing of these components (Figure 7-17). The gold standard quantification of wave reflection is through the reflection coefficient or the ratio of the amplitude of the backward to forward wave ($|P_b|/|P_f|$). Because of the requirement of simultaneous pressure and flow measurement, it is not always possible to assess this index in a clinical environment.

To resolve this problem, the so-called augmentation index (AIx) has been proposed. AIx aims to quantify the contribution of the reflected pressure wave to the total PP (Figure 7-17).[64] Measurement of AIx requires only the contour of the pressure wave, and the identification of a "characteristic point" on the curve (P^*, Figure 7-17) that identifies the instant in time when the reflected wave starts to contribute to the total pressure. Once this point is known, one can calculate the augmented pressure (AP, augmented pressure) as well as the AIx itself[9]:

$$AIx = 100 \times AP/PP.$$

For an A-type wave with early return of the reflected pressure wave, AP equals SBP − P^* and yields a positive value (SBP is the systolic blood pressure). The AIx will therefore be positive in older and in short subjects. For C-type waves (young, tall subjects) with a late inflection point,

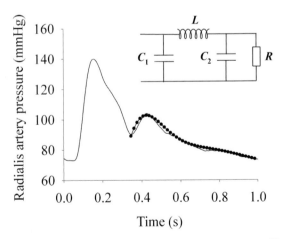

● **FIGURE 7-16.** Illustration of the system identification method based on the four-element windkessel model of Goldwyn and Watt. The diastolic part of a pressure waveform measured at the radial artery is selected, and the model is fitted to the data. Resulting parameters are RC_1, RC_2, and L/R. When cardiac output is known, resistance R can be calculated and model parameters can be derived.

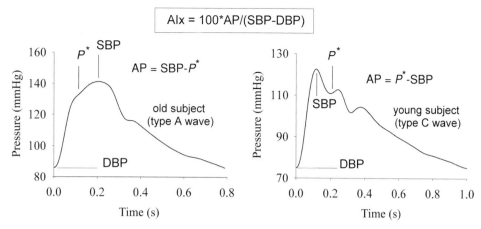

$$AIx = 100*AP/(SBP-DBP)$$

● FIGURE 7-17. Definition of the augmentation index in case of an A-type wave (old subject; left figure) or C-type wave (young subject; right figure). The characteristic point is first defined to identify the nature of the wave. Then, augmented pressure is calculated. AIx is the ratio of augmented pressure to pulse pressure, expressed as a percentage.

the augmented pressure is negative (P^*- SBP), as will be AIx.

In these days, AIx is frequently assessed in clinical studies, in part thanks to the work of O'Rourke and colleagues who were also the driving force behind the development of a commercial system (Sphygmocor©, Atcor Medical, Sydney, Australia). In that system, central blood pressure is mathematically calculated from a pressure wave, measured noninvasively at the level of the radial artery by use of a so-called generalized pressure transfer function that expresses the mathematical relation between the radial and aortic blood pressure.[65,66] The arteries in the arm are here considered as a type of catheter with its tip ending in the aorta. The pressure transfer function describes the characteristics of this "catheter." This approach certainly raises some questions. The transfer function used is a generalized one, measured in a relatively low number of patients, despite the fact that one might expect some interindividual variability in the transfer function.[67] Another concern relates to the observation that there is a very strong correlation between AIx values that are derived directly from the radial pressure waveform and those derived from the mathematically transformed central pressure waveform,[34,68] with correlation coefficients exceeding 0.9. There is little doubt that this is because of the assumption of a generalized transfer function, which implies that the information contents carried by the radial pressure wave is essentially the same as the information contents carried by the transformed curve. The added value of transforming the radial pressure waveform is then indeed debatable. Finally, it has also been observed that the value of AIx (from the central pressure) reaches a plateau level from the age of 55 to 60 onward, with an upper limit of about 50%.[69] As such, one cannot expect AIx to be a sensitive and specific index for assessing cardiovascular risk in older patient populations; from that perspective, the augmented pressure in itself might be a better marker. Although there are some studies suggesting an association between AIx and cardiovascular risk in

specific patient populations,[70] the extra prognostic value of AIx remains to be demonstrated in the general population. Furthermore, the interpretation of AIx is also not always straightforward, as there are many factors that affect the relative timing of the interaction between the forward and backward running pressure waves, such as the height of a subject, the distance to the effective reflection site, but also the heart rate and the pattern of left ventricular ejection. It is therefore unclear whether AIx is an appropriate measure of pressure wave reflection, and it should certainly not be used as a measure of arterial stiffness.[71]

● **WHAT TO MEASURE IN CLINICAL PRACTICE AND WHY SHOULD ONE CARE FOR ARTERIAL STIFFNESS?**

Of all above-mentioned methods to assess the (elastic) properties of the arterial tree, there is little doubt that PWV is, at present, the most widely investigated and applied method. It is probably also the most promising method, as PWV is the only measure that appears to have prognostic value that adds to the classical risk factors.[46] For the other methods, data are less conclusive. Nevertheless, at present, one seems to live to the principle that, while awaiting conclusive data, it does not harm to measure several parameters of arterial function.[72] A number of researchers, predominantly based in Europe, have assembled consensus documents with guidelines for measurement of central blood pressure and arterial stiffness.[44] These documents provide some structure in this highly unstructured research domain, but the documents largely remain inconclusive with respect to which arterial property should be measured. Large-scale longitudinal studies, with comparison of the different methodologies, are awaited to assess the prognostic value of each of these indices.

What is certainly important to stress is the relevance of measuring central blood pressure. Blood pressure in the upper arm is not an exact replica of blood pressure in the aorta, and thus of the blood pressure faced by the heart during ventricular ejection. It is well known that there is central-to-peripheral amplification of the pressure pulse, and it has been demonstrated that certain drugs have a different effect on central and peripheral blood pressure, especially those drugs affecting heart rate, e.g., β-blockers.[73] When addressing arterial physiology, it is advisable to measure central blood pressure (as well as aortic flow), whenever possible, with a preference for the earlier described method of applanation tonometry at the brachial and carotid artery.[34,35] Nevertheless, from a clinical standpoint, it is acknowledged that, until now, there is no scientific evidence showing that central blood pressure would have a higher prognostic value than the blood pressure value measured at the brachial artery.

Although there is a growing interest in measuring arterial properties, it remains a fairly small field of research with mainly the interest of angiologists, nephrologists, and intensivists treating patients with hypertension. There are, however, many reasons cardiologists in general should show interest in this matter. Studies focussing on ventriculoarterial coupling and interaction clearly demonstrate that arterial stiffening is paralleled by "ventricular stiffening,"[74] with an increase in the end-systolic elastance. Arterial stiffness also leads to the so-called isolated systolic hypertension, where systolic blood pressure is elevated while diastolic blood pressure is normal or even low. This condition is unfavorable to the heart for many reasons:

- Because of the high systolic blood pressure, the energy expenditure of the heart increases, and the heart often responds through the development of ventricular hypertrophy.
- The diastolic passive properties of hypertrophic hearts change, with an increase in diastolic ventricular stiffness and less optimal filling of the ventricles.
- The perfusion of the endocardium may be hampered by the increase in thickness of the myocardium.
- Hearts with elevated end-systolic elastance become sensitive to blood volume shifts, and small changes in filling pressures have large effects in the pressure generated by these ventricles.
- An increased afterload of the heart directly affects its diastolic function via a reduction in the active relaxation of the ventricle, which may further increase the diastolic dysfunction of the heart.
- The lower diastolic blood pressure in the circulation also reduces the coronary perfusion pressure with potential consequences for myocardial perfusion.

Given these arguments, it is no surprise that an increase in arterial stiffness is associated with a reduction of the exercise capacity of patients.[74]

As a general conclusion, it is therefore safe to state that (also for cardiologists), it is most relevant to look beyond the coronary arteries, and we plead for more attention for the (systemic) arterial circulation. It is, however, the task of researchers active in the domain of arterial function and stiffness to come to a general consensus on which parameters to measure, how they should be measured, and to provide standardization of measurement techniques.

REFERENCES

1. Skalak R, Keller SR, Secomb TW. Mechanics of blood flow. *J Biomech Eng.* 1981;103(2):102-115.

2. Cokelet GR. Rheology and hemodynamics. *Annu Rev Physiol.* 1980;42:311-324.

3. Poiseuille J. Recherches expérimentales sur le mouvement des liquides dans les tubes de très petits diamètres. *Mémoire Savants Etrangers.* 1846;9:463-544.

4. Welty J, Wicks C, Wilson R, Rorrer G. *Fundamentals of Momentum, Heat and Mass Transfer.* 4th ed. New York: John Wiley and Sons; 2001.

5. Womersley J. *The Mathematical Analysis of the Arterial Circulation in a State of Oscillatory Motion.* Wright Air Development Center; 1957. WADC-TR56-614.

6. Womersley JR. Mathematical theory of oscillating flow in an elastic tube. *J Physiol.* 1955;127(2):37P-38P.

7. Bernoulli D. *Hydrodynamica.* 1738.

8. Segers P, Verdonck P. Principles of vascular physiology. In: Lanzer P, Topol EJ, eds. *Pan Vascular Medicine. Integrated Clinical Management.* Heidelberg: Springer-Verlag; 2002.

9. Nichols W, O'Rourke M. *McDonald's Blood Flow in Arteries. Theoretical, Experimental and Clinical Principles.* 5th ed. London: Hodder Arnold–Oxford University Press; 2005.

10. Franklin SS, Gustin WT, Wong ND, et al. Hemodynamic patterns of age-related changes in blood pressure. The Framingham Heart Study. *Circulation.* 1997;96:308-315.

11. Haider AW, Larson MG, Franklin SS, Levy D. Systolic blood pressure, diastolic blood pressure, and pulse pressure as predictors of risk for congestive heart failure in the Framingham Heart Study. *Ann Intern Med.* 2003;138(1):10-16.

12. Westerhof N, Elzinga G, Sipkema P. An artificial arterial system for pumping hearts. *J Appl Physiol.* 1971;31(5):776-781.

13. Hales S. *Statical Essays: Containing Haemostatics (reprint 1964).* New York: Hafner Publishing; 1733.

14. Frank O. Die Grundfurm des arteriellen Pulses. Erste Abhandlung. Mathematische analyse. *Z Biol.* 1899;37:483-526.

15. Frank O. Der Puls in den Arterien. *Z Biol.* 1905;46:441-553.

16. Asmar RG, London GM, O'Rourke ME, Safar ME. Improvement in blood pressure, arterial stiffness and wave reflections with a very-low-dose perindopril/indapamide combination in hypertensive patient: a comparison with atenolol. *Hypertension.* 2001;38(4):922-926.

17. O'Rourke MF. Mechanical principles. Arterial stiffness and wave reflection. *Pathol Biol (Paris).* 1999;47(6):623-633.

18. Laurent S, Cockcroft J, Van Bortel L, et al. Expert consensus document on arterial stiffness: methodological issues and clinical applications. *Eur Heart J.* 2006;27(21):2588-2605.

19. Westerhof N, Stergiopulos N, Noble M. *Snapshots of Hemodynamics. An Aid for Clinical Research and Graduate Education.* New York: Springer Science + Business Media; 2004.

20. Nichols WW, O'Rourke MF. *McDonald's Blood Flow in Arteries.* 3rd ed. London: Edward Arnold; 1990.

21. Milnor WR. *Hemodynamics.* 2nd ed. Baltimore, MD: Williams & Wilkins; 1989.

22. Wang DM, Tarbell JM. Nonlinear analysis of oscillatory flow, with a nonzero mean, in an elastic tube (artery). *J Biomech Eng.* 1995;117(1):127-135.

23. Campbell K, Lee CL, Frasch HF, Noordergraaf A. Pulse reflection sites and effective length of the arterial system. *Am J Physiol.* 1989;256:H1684-H1689.

24. Latham R, Westerhof N, Sipkema P, Rubal B, Reuderink P, Murgo J. Regional wave travel and reflections along the human aorta: a study with six simultaneous micromanometric pressures. *Circulation.* 1985;72:1257-1269.

25. Berger D, Li J, Laskey W, Noordergraaf A. Repeated reflection of waves in the systemic arterial system. *Am J Physiol.* 1993;264:H269-H281.

26. Westerhof N, Sipkema P, van den Bos CG, Elzinga G. Forward and backward waves in the arterial system. *Cardiovasc Res.* 1972;6:648-656.

27. Westerhof BE, Guelen I, Westerhof N, Karemaker JM, Avolio A. Quantification of wave reflection in the human aorta from pressure alone: a proof of principle. *Hypertension.* 2006;48(4):595-601.

28. Dujardin J, Stone D. Characteristic impedance of the proximal aorta determined in the time and frequency domain: a comparison. *Med Biol Eng Comput.* 1981;19:565-568.

29. Khir AW, O'Brien A, Gibbs JS, Parker KH. Determination of wave speed and wave separation in the arteries. *J Biomech.* 2001;34(9):1145-1155.

30. Parker KH, Jones CJ. Forward and backward running waves in the arteries: analysis using the method of characteristics. *J Biomech Eng.* 1990;112(3):322-326.

31. Bleasdale RA, Mumford CE, Campbell RI, Fraser AG, Jones CJ, Frenneaux MP. Wave intensity analysis from the common carotid artery: a new noninvasive index of cerebral vasomotor tone. *Heart Vessels.* 2003;18(4):202-206.

32. Wang Z, Jalali F, Sun YH, Wang JJ, Parker KH, Tyberg JV. Assessment of left ventricular diastolic suction in dogs using wave-intensity analysis. *Am J Physiol Heart Circ Physiol.* 2004;24.

33. Sun YH, Anderson TJ, Parker KH, Tyberg JV. Effects of left ventricular contractility and coronary vascular resistance on coronary dynamics. *Am J Physiol Heart Circ Physiol.* 2004;286(4):H1590-H1595.

34. Segers P, Rietzschel E, Heireman S, et al. Carotid tonometry versus synthesized aorta pressure waves for the estimation of central systolic blood pressure and augmentation index. *Am J Hypertens.* 2005;18(9, pt 1):1168-1173.

35. Verbeke F, Segers P, Heireman S, Vanholder R, Verdonck P, Van Bortel LM. Noninvasive assessment of local pulse pressure: importance of brachial-to-radial pressure amplification. *Hypertension.* 2005;46(1):244-248.

36. Van Bortel LM, Balkestein EJ, van der Heijden-Spek JJ, et al. Non-invasive assessment of local arterial pulse pressure: comparison of applanation tonometry and echo-tracking. *J Hypertens.* 2001;19(6):1037-1044.

37. Segers P, Rabben SI, De Backer J, et al. Functional analysis of the common carotid artery: relative distension differences over the vessel wall measured in vivo. *J Hypertens.* 2004;22(5):973-981.

38. Van Bortel L, Segers P. Direct measurement of local arterial stiffness and pulse pressure. In: Safar M, MF OR, eds. *Handbook of Hypertension—Arterial Stiffness in Hypertension*: Amsterdam: Elsevier; 2006:35-51.

39. Meinders JM, Hoeks AP. Simultaneous assessment of diameter and pressure waveforms in the carotid artery. *Ultrasound Med Biol.* 2004;30(2):147-154.

40. Hayashi K. Experimental approaches on measuring the mechanical properties and constitutive laws of arterial walls. *J Biomech Eng.* 1993;115:481-488.

41. Bramwell CJ, Hill A. The velocity of the pulse wave in man. *Proc R Soc Lond [Biol].*1922;93:298-306.

42. Avolio A, Chen S, Wang R, Zhang C, Li M, O'Rourke M. Effects of aging on changing arterial compliance and left ventricular load in a northern Chinese urban community. *Circulation.* 1983;68:50-58.

43. Lehmann E, Gosling R, Fatemi-Langroudi B, Taylor M. Noninvasive Doppler ultrasound technique for the in vivo assessment of aortic compliance. *J Biomed Eng.* 1992;14:250-256.

44. Van Bortel LM, Duprez D, Starmans-Kool MJ, et al. Clinical applications of arterial stiffness, Task Force III: recommendations for user procedures. *Am J Hypertens.* 2002;15(5):445-452.

45. Laurent S, Boutouyrie P, Asmar R, et al. Aortic stiffness is an independent predictor of all-cause and cardiovascular mortality in hypertensive patients. *Hypertension.* 2001;37(5):1236-1241.

46. Willum-Hansen T, Staessen JA, Torp-Pedersen C, et al. Prognostic value of aortic pulse wave velocity as index of arterial stiffness in the general population. *Circulation.* 2006;113(5):664-670.

47. Mattace-Raso FU, van der Cammen TJ, Hofman A, et al. Arterial stiffness and risk of coronary heart disease and stroke: the Rotterdam Study. *Circulation.* 2006;113(5):657-663.

48. Toy SM, Melbin J, Noordergraaf A. Reduced models of arterial systems. *IEEE Trans Biomed Eng.* 1985;32:174-176.

49. Liu Z, Brin K, Yin F. Estimation of total arterial compliance: an improved method and evaluation of current methods. *Am J Physiol.* 1986;251:H588-H600.

50. Simon A, Safar L, London G, Levy B, Chau N. An evaluation of large arteries compliance in man. *Am J Physiol.* 1979;237:H550-H554.

51. Stergiopulos N, Meister JJ, Westerhof N. Evaluation of methods for the estimation of total arterial compliance. *Am J Physiol.* 1995;268:H1540-H1548.

52. Chemla D, Hébert J-L, Coirault C, et al. Total arterial compliance estimated by stroke volume-to-aortic pulse pressure ratio in humans. *Am J Physiol.* 1998;274:H500-H505.

53. Stergiopulos N, Segers P, Westerhof N. Use of pulse pressure method for estimating total arterial compliance in vivo. *Am J Physiol.* 1999;276:H424-H428.

54. Westerhof N, Elzinga G. Normalized input impedance and arterial decay time over heart period are independent of animal size. *Am J Physiol.* 1991;261(1, pt 2):R126-R133.

55. Segers P, Brimioulle S, Stergiopulos N, et al. Pulmonary arterial compliance in dogs and pigs: the three-element windkessel model revisited. *Am J Physiol.* 1999;277:H725-H731.

56. Stergiopulos N, Westerhof B, Westerhof N. Total arterial inertance as the fourth element of the windkessel model. *Am J Physiol.* 1999;276:H81-H88.

57. Burattini R, Gnudi G. Computer identification of models for the arterial tree input impedance: comparison between two new simple models and first experimental results. *Med Biol Eng Comput.* 1982;20:134-144.

58. Goldwyn R, Watt T. Arterial pressure pulse contour analysis via a mathematical model for the clinical quantification of human vascular properties. *IEEE Trans Biomed Eng.* 1967;14:11-17.

59. Segers P, Qasem A, De Backer T, Carlier S, Verdonck P, Avolio A. Peripheral "oscillatory" compliance is associated with aortic augmentation index. *Hypertension.* 2001;37(6):1434-1439.

60. Segers P, Verdonck P, Verhoeven R. Evaluation of the non-invasive determination of arterial compliance with the Goldwynn–Watt model. *J Cardiov Diagn Proc.* 1997;14(1):3-8.

61. McVeigh G, Finkelstein S, Cohn J. Assessment of arterial compliance in hypertension. *Curr Opin Nephrol Hypertens.* 1993;2:82-86.

62. McVeigh GE, Bratteli CW, Morgan DJ, et al. Age-related abnormalities in arterial compliance identified by pressure pulse contour analysis: aging and arterial compliance. *Hypertension.* 1999;33(6):1392-1398.

63. Fogliardi R, Burattini R, Shroff SG, Campbell KB. Fit to diastolic arterial pressure by third-order lumped model yields unreliable estimates of arterial compliance. *Med Eng Phys.* 1996;18:225-233.

64. Kelly R, Hayward C, Avolio A, O'Rourke M. Noninvasive determination of age-related changes in the human arterial pulse. *Circulation.* 1989;80(6):1652-1659.

65. Chen CH, Nevo E, Fetics B, et al. Estimation of central aortic pressure waveform by mathematical transformation of radial tonometry pressure. Validation of generalized transfer function. *Circulation.* 1997;95(7):1827-1836.

66. Karamanoglu M, O'Rourke M, Avolio A, Kelly R. An analysis of the relationship between central aortic and peripheral upper limb pressure waves in man. *Eur Heart J.* 1993;14:160-167.

67. Segers P, Carlier S, Pasquet A, et al. Individualizing the aorto-radial pressure transfer function: feasibility of a model-based approach. *Am J Physiol.* 2000;279:H542-H549.

68. Millasseau SC, Patel SJ, Redwood SR, Ritter JM, Chowienczyk PJ. Pressure wave reflection assessed from the peripheral pulse: is a transfer function necessary? *Hypertension.* 2003;41(5):1016-1020.

69. McEniery CM, Yasmin, Hall IR, Qasem A, Wilkinson IB, Cockcroft JR. Normal vascular aging: differential effects on wave reflection and aortic pulse wave velocity: the Anglo-Cardiff Collaborative Trial (ACCT). *J Am Coll Cardiol.* 2005;46(9):1753-1760.

70. Weber T, Auer J, O'Rourke MF, et al. Arterial stiffness, wave reflections, and the risk of coronary artery disease. *Circulation.* 2004;109(2):184-189.

71. Segers P, De Backer JF, Devos D, et al. Aortic reflection coefficients and their association with global indices of wave reflection in healthy controls and patients with Marfan disease. *Am J Physiol Heart Circ Physiol.* 2006;290(6):H2385-H2392.

72. Woodman RJ, Kingwell BA, Beilin LJ, Hamilton SE, Dart AM, Watts GF. Assessment of central and peripheral arterial stiffness: studies indicating the need to use a combination of techniques. *Am J Hypertens.* 2005;18(2, pt 1):249-260.

73. Takazawa K, Tanaka N, Takeda K, Kurosu F, Ibukiyama C. Underestimation of vasodilator effects of nitroglycerin by upper limb blood pressure. *Hypertension.* 1995;26(3):520-523.

74. Kass DA. Ventricular arterial stiffening: integrating the pathophysiology. *Hypertension.* 2005;46(1):185-193.

chapter 8

Blood Pressure Regulation

Kailash Prasad, MD, PhD

● ARTERIAL PRESSURE

Definition

Lateral pressure exerted by the column of blood against the arterial wall is called the arterial pressure (blood pressure), and this pressure is referred to as the height of the column of blood supported by the force within a blood vessel. In a cardiac cycle, the highest pressure attained is the systolic pressure and the lowest pressure is the diastolic pressure. The equation "MAP – RAP = CO × TPR" is used to derive mean arterial pressure (MAP), where RAP is right arterial pressure, CO is cardiac output, and TPR is total peripheral resistance. Since RAP is very small, MAP (mm Hg) is the product of CO (liters per minute) and total peripheral resistance (mm Hg/liter/minute). The MAP is the geometric mean, and the calculation of MAP requires integration of pressure pulse.

An approximate estimate of MAP can be derived from the following equations:

$$MAP = (systolic\ pressure + 2\ diastolic\ pressure)/3$$

$$MAP = diastolic\ pressure + 1/3\ of\ pulse\ pressure.$$

Normal Arterial Pressure

Normal arterial pressure varies with age. It is approximately 70/50 mm Hg on the first day after birth, and gradually increases during the next several months to approximately 90/60 mm Hg. During subsequent years the rise is very slow and reaches 115/70 mm Hg at adolescence. There is a progressive increase in the pressure with age in the average population. The systolic pressure rises approximately 1 mm Hg/yr from 110 mm Hg at the age of 15 years. This probably reflects progressive reduction in arterial compliance. Diastolic pressure increases approximately 0.4 mm Hg/yr from 70 mm Hg at the age of 15 years. This rise probably reflects an increase in total peripheral resistance. The progressive increase in arterial pressure with age could also result from the effects of aging on the long-term blood pressure control mechanisms. Although average pressure in a population rises with age, the pressure never rises with age in certain people. MAP for a population is composed of individuals whose blood pressure does not change with advancing age and of individuals whose pressure increases with advancing age. There is no dividing line between normal and high blood pressure. An arbitrary level of normal blood pressure has been established to define those who have an increased risk of developing morbid cardiovascular events and/or clearly benefit from medical therapy. Arterial pressure is somewhat damaging. Life expectancy is inversely proportional to arterial pressures. The logic is to define hypertension at levels where treatment can provide benefits that outweigh risks. Males with normal diastolic pressure but elevated systolic pressure (> 158 mm Hg) have a 2.5-fold increase in cardiovascular mortality rates when compared to individuals with similar diastolic pressure but normal systolic pressure.

Arterial pressure is slightly higher in the right arm than in the left arm. Simultaneous measurement of blood pressure in both arms shows a difference of 10 mm Hg (both systolic and diastolic) in approximately 3% of normotensive and 6% of hypertensive subjects. However, when the measurements are not made simultaneously a difference of 10 mm Hg or more in systolic pressure is observed in 20% of normotensive and 30% of hypertensive individuals, and a difference in diastolic pressure of 10 mm Hg or more is observed in 10% of normotensive and 15% of hypertensive subjects. Although diastolic pressure is similar in the arms and thighs, systolic pressure is 10 to 40 mm Hg higher in thighs than in arms. The Joint National Committee on Prevention, Detection, Evaluation and Treatment of High Blood Pressure defines systolic and diastolic pressures less than 120 and 80 mm Hg, respectively, as normal.[1] The guideline committee of the European Society of Hypertension—European Society of Cardiology defines systolic and diastolic pressures <120 mm Hg and <80 mm Hg, respectively as optimal; systolic pressure of 120 to 129, and diastolic pressure of 80 to 84 mm Hg as normal; and systolic pressure, 130 to 139, and diastolic pressure 85 to 89 mm Hg as high normal.[2] Both guidelines consider a patient as hypertensive when the systolic and diastolic pressures are ≥140 mm Hg and ≥90 mm Hg, respectively.

Factors That Determine Systolic, Diastolic and Pulse Pressure, and Clinical Implications

Factors that determine systolic pressure include stroke volume, peak systolic rate of cardiac ejection, and arterial compliance (distensability of arterial wall). Systolic pressure increases with increases in stroke volume and peak systolic ejection rate, and a decrease in arterial compliance. Decreases in systolic pressure are associated with decreases in stroke volume and peak systolic ejection rate, and an increase in arterial compliance. Diastolic pressure is determined by total peripheral vascular resistance, heart rate, systolic pressure, and arterial elastic recoil. Increases in these parameters increase the diastolic pressure and vice versa. Loss of elastic recoil in the arterial wall that occurs with aging decreases the diastolic pressure.

Pulse pressure (PP) describes the oscillation around the MAP and is the difference between systolic and diastolic pressure. PP is influenced by the velocity of ventricular ejection, elastic properties of the arterial wall, the timing of the reflected waves, and the total peripheral vascular resistance. PP is approximately one-half of the diastolic pressure and is affected by various clinical situations (Table 8-1). A wide PP reflects systolic hypertension and increased central arterial stiffness. In hypertensives a wide PP is a reasonable surrogate for increased arterial stiffness. PP has both diagnostic and prognostic values. The mechanism underlying the prognostic effect of PP may be because of the fact that cardiovascular risk is strictly related to the pulsatile stress caused by large artery stiffness during systole. Arterial stiffness has two consequences: (a) It increases systolic blood pressure which in turn increases left ventricular afterload and mass and (b) it lowers diastolic pressure resulting in decreased coronary artery perfusion.

Increased PP elevates left ventricular systolic wall stress, decreases coronary flow reserve, impairs left ventricular relaxation, and may lead to diastolic dysfunction. Increased PP is the major factor in the development of left ventricular hypertrophy with increased requirement for coronary flow. A decrease in diastolic pressure compromises oxygen supply by reducing coronary flow. Wide PP also leads to endothelial dysfunction with greater propensity for coronary atherosclerosis and rupture of unstable atherosclerotic plaques. Wide PP may simply serve as a marker for diffuse atherosclerosis. There is an independent relationship among PP, left ventricular mass index, carotid intima-media thickness, and carotid cross-sectional area. Elevated PP is an effective predictor of cardiovascular risk in hypertensive

TABLE 8-1. Clinical Conditions Affecting Pulse Pressure

Increased	Decreased
1. Decreased total peripheral resistance • Anxiety • Exercise • Fever • Hyperthyroidism • Anemia • Paget disease of bone • A–V fistula 2. Decreased arterial compliance • Atherosclerosis • Hypertension 3. Increased stroke volume • Bradycardia • Complete heart block • Aortic regurgitation • Thyrotoxicosis • Anemia • Vitamin deficiency • Arteriovenous malformation	1. Mechanical obstruction • Aortic stenosis • Mitral stenosis • Mitral regurgitation 2. Decreased stroke volume • Heart Failure • Shock • Tachycardia • Cardiac tamponade

subjects.[3] Wide PP is a powerful predictor of myocardial infarction in patients with hypertension. It is associated with aging, high left ventricular stroke volume, abnormal left ventricular function, cardiovascular mortality, and stroke. Wide PP has been identified as an independent predictor of coronary events[4,5] and is independently associated with total mortality in the Balloon Angioplasty Revascularization Investigation.[6] Systolic blood pressure is superior to diastolic blood pressure as a predictor of coronary artery disease risk after the age of 50 years. PP is a better predictor than systolic or diastolic blood pressure. Pulse wave velocity is a clinical surrogate for large arterial stiffness. Increased pulse wave reflections are associated with the presence and extent of coronary artery disease.[7] Increased wave reflections are independently associated with increased risk for cardiovascular events in patients undergoing PCI.[8]

● COMMON CAUSES OF BLOOD PRESSURE VARIATION

Blood pressure varies throughout the day and with various activities.

- Diurnal variation—Blood pressure changes are associated with levels of arousal. On the onset of sleep, blood pressure falls gradually and reaches the lowest level (decrease of 15%–20%) after 2 hours. The blood pressure is higher between 10 AM and 6 PM, and lower at night with a dip between midnight and 3 AM. There is a slow and steady rise in blood pressure between 3 AM and 6 AM, and there is a sudden and steep rise shortly after awakening. The early morning blood pressure surge continues for approximately 4 to 6 hours.[9] The early morning surge in blood pressure probably is because of an increase in sympathetic activity, and a rise in plasma renin and cortisol. The increase during the early hours of the morning could contribute to the high incidence of cerebral hemorrhage and myocardial infarction in these hours.[10] Diurnal variation may be because of morning diurnal peaks in total blood volume, central blood volume, sympathetic activity, and plasma renin activity.[11]

Circadian rhythm in arterial pressure of patients with hypertension is similar to that of patients with normotension except that the entire blood pressure profile is shifted upward. Circadian rhythm for blood pressure is lost following an acute stroke. There is a paradoxical elevation of pressure during the first part of the night and the lowest pressure of the day in the morning in patients with idiopathic orthostatic hypotension.

- Physical activity—Physical activity raises blood pressure. The type of activity determines the amount of rise in blood pressure. Talking raises blood pressure. Severe physical activity can raise arterial pressure to a level of 240 mm Hg.
- Meals—There is an increase in the heart rate, a decrease in the diastolic pressure, and a little change in systolic pressure for 3 hours after a meal.[12] There is a marked fall in both systolic and diastolic pressure in older individuals following a meal.
- Seasonal variation—Blood pressure is approximately 5 to 9 mm Hg higher in winter than in summer in temperate climates. Possibly cold stimulates the vasoconstrictor area. Warmer climates are vasodilative. The systemic response to cold is vasoconstriction through a reflex mechanism.
- Mental activity—Mental activity elevates blood pressure.
- Sex—Systolic and diastolic pressures are lower in women than in men younger than 40 to 50 years, and are higher in women than in men older than 50 years. This difference could be because of the hormonal changes in women that take place at menopause.
- Weight—Systolic and diastolic pressures are directly related to the weight of the individual.
- Posture—In the erect position, cardiac output and thoracic arterial pressure decrease because of a decrease in venous return. There is a reflex increase in the heart rate and systemic vascular resistance resulting in an increase in both systolic and diastolic pressure, the increase being greater in the latter.

- Pain—Headache and other types of chronic pain elevate arterial pressure.
- Hypoglycemia—A rapid decrease in blood sugar stimulates the sympathoadrenal system and blood pressure rises. In some cases it might reach the range of 250/150 mm Hg.
- Race and socioeconomic status—Blood pressures are higher in blacks than in whites, across all ages and for both sexes. Genetic and environmental factors, particularly socioeconomic, may be involved in this difference.

● PRESSURE CONTROL MECHANISMS

Arterial pressure moves blood throughout the body to provide nutrients to the tissue. Regulation of arterial pressure is essential to maintain tissue perfusion during various pathophysiologic conditions. Arterial pressure is regulated essentially by three mechanisms: (a) a rapidly acting pressure control mechanism, (b) an intermediate time-period pressure control mechanism, and (c) a long-term pressure control mechanism.

Neural Control

A brief review of the autonomic control of the cardiovascular system is described below.[13–15] The organization of the vasomotor center and autonomic nervous system is shown in Figure 8-1. The vasomotor center is situated bilaterally in the medulla and lower third of the pons. It comprises three regions namely, vasoconstrictor, vasodilator, and sensory nucleus tractus solitarius (NTS). The vasoconstrictor region is located in the dorsolateral part of the medulla. Fibers from the vasoconstrictor regions descend and synapse in the intermediolateral gray matter of the spinal cord at different levels of the thoracolumbar region (T_1 to L_2 or L_3). The fibers (preganglionic) then leave the cord to synapse with paravertebral sympathetic ganglia. Postganglionic sympathetic fibers from various ganglia innervate the arteries, veins, and heart. Norepinephrine released at the postganglionic nerve endings binds to alpha-adrenergic receptors on vascular smooth muscle cells to cause vasoconstriction.

Sympathetic nerve fibers innervate all the vessels except precapillary sphinctors, capillaries, and meta-arterioles. Sympathetic stimulation constricts the resistance vessels (arterioles) thus increasing the total vascular resistance. Constriction of capacitance vessels (venules and small veins) pushes the blood into the heart resulting in increased stroke volume. Sympathetic stimulation to the heart increases the heart rate and contraction, resulting in an increase in cardiac output. It should be pointed out that an increase in peripheral resistance raises blood pressure but decreases the organ perfusion. Acting on the heart, norepinephrine increases the heart rate, force of contraction, and conduction in the heart. The adrenergic receptors in the nodal regions and in the myocardium are predominantly of the beta types. The vasoconstrictor region is tonically

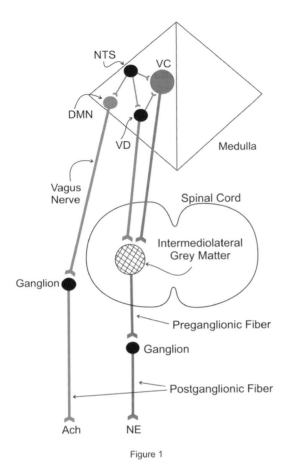

Figure 1

● **FIGURE 8-1.** Schematic diagram of the neural control of the arterial pressure. NTS, nucleus tractus solitarius; VC, vasoconstrictor area; VD, vasodilator area; DMN, dorsal motor nucleus of vagus; Ach, acetylcholine; NE, norepinephrine.

medulla controls autonomic functions such as peripheral arterial pressure, heart rate, and myocardial contractility.

The parasympathetic nervous system has two divisions: cranial (III, VII, IX, and X nerves) and sacral (second through fourth sacral nerves). Approximately 75% of all parasympathetic nerve fibers are in the vagus nerve that arises in the dorsal vagal nucleus in the medulla lateral to the hypoglossal nuclei. These fibers synapse with ganglia close to the organs. At the postganglionic nerve ending, acetylcholine is released. Acetylcholine relaxes blood vessels and decreases the heart rate, myocardial contractility, and conduction in the atrioventricular node. The cranial division of parasympathetic fibers supply blood vessels of the heart and viscera, while fibers from the sacral division supply blood vessels of the genitalia, bladder, and large intestine.

Factors Affecting the Vasomotor Center

The vasomotor center is affected by stimuli from other areas of the brain. The hypothalamus plays a crucial role in the control of blood pressure and cardiac function through behavioral and emotional changes. Stimulation of the anterior portion of the hypothalamus causes mild excitation of inhibition depending upon which part of the anterior portion of the hypothalamus is stimulated. In general, stimulation of the anterior portion of the hypothalamus produces hypotension and bradycardia, whereas stimulation of the posterolateral region of the hypothalamus produces a rise in arterial pressure and tachycardia. The hypothalamus contains a temperature-regulating center. Stimulation by cold application to the skin or cold blood reaching the hypothalamus results in constriction of skin vessels, while a warm stimulus causes cutaneous vasculation.

Stimulation of the motor cortex and premotor area can excite or inhibit the vasomotor center through the hypothalamus. Stimulation results in a vasopressor effect. Vasodilation and vasodepressor responses may occur as blushing or fainting in response to emotional stimuli.

Painful stimuli may result in pressor or repressor responses depending upon the magnitude and location of the stimuli. Distension of the abdominal viscera often evokes a vasodepressor response, while a painful stimulus on the body surface usually evokes a pressor response.

● RAPIDLY ACTING PRESSURE CONTROL MECHANISMS

Baroreceptor Mechanism

Baroreceptors (pressoreceptors) are stretch receptors and are sensitive to pressure changes.[16,17] They are located in the carotid sinus and aortic arch. The carotid sinus is a slight dilation of the internal carotid artery located near its origin above the bifurcation of the common carotid artery (Figure 8-2). Aortic baroreceptors are located in the wall of the arch of the aorta. Impulses arising from the carotid sinus travel via the sinus nerve through the glossopharyngeal nerve to the NTS in the medulla. Impulses from the aortic arch travel to the NTS through the aortic nerve via

active, fires continuously at a rate of one-half to two impulses per second, and maintains basal tone in the blood vessels. Stimulation of the vasoconstrictor region increases tonic activity and hence increases the frequency of impulse formation in the sympathetic nerves, resulting in vasoconstriction and increases in heart rate and force of cardiac contraction. On the other hand, inhibition of the vasoconstrictor region will have opposite effects. The vasoconstrictor region may show rhythmic changes in tonic activity resulting in oscillation of arterial pressure. Traube–Hering waves occur at the frequency of respiration and are caused by an increase in sympathetic activity during inspiration. Myer waves, on the other hand, are caused by oscillation of baroreceptor and chemoreceptor reflexes, and central nervous system (CNS) ischemic response.

The vasodepressor region is located caudal and ventromedial to the vasoconstrictor region, and produces decreases in blood pressure, heart rate, and myocardial contractility when stimulated.

The NTS in the medulla is the sensory termination of both vagal and glossopharyngeal nerves that transmit sensory signals from chemoreceptors, baroreceptors, and several other peripheral receptors. All the signals from the peripheral areas help control blood pressure. The NTS in the

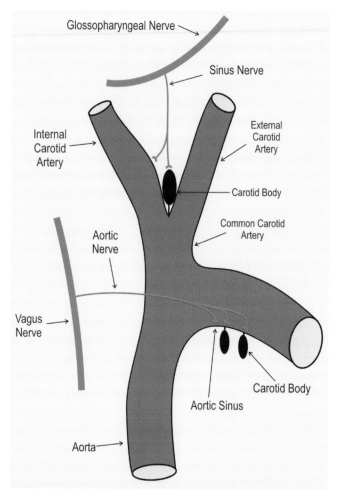

● **FIGURE 8-2.** Diagram showing aortic and carotid sinuses and bodies and their innervation by various efferent nerves. The nerves are shown in green, the aortic and sinus bodies in black, and blood vessels in red.

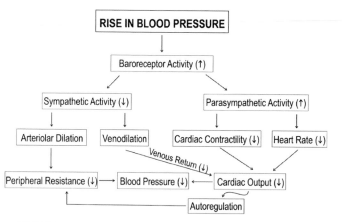

● **FIGURE 8-3.** Baroreceptor pressure control mechanism with rise in the arterial pressure. ↓, Decrease; ↑, increase.

the vagus nerve. An increase in arterial pressure stretches the baroreceptors in the carotid sinus and aortic arch, and therefore increases their firing frequency. These impulses stimulate the NTS, which in turn inhibits the vasoconstrictor area to decrease sympathetic activity to the heart and blood vessels, and stimulate the vagal center to decrease the heart rate and contractility. Stimulation of NTS also depresses the vasodepressor area. These changes in neural activity result in decreases in cardiac output and vascular resistance, and hence, a decrease in arterial pressure. Thus stimulation of the baroreceptors decreases arterial pressure by decreasing vasoconstrictor activity and increasing vagal and vasodepressor activity (Figure 8-3). The reverse occurs when the arterial pressure falls (Figure 8-4). The fall in arterial pressure decreases the number of impulses reaching the NTS and hence there is less inhibition of the vasoconstrictor area, resulting in increased sympathetic activity. Decreases in impulses arising from baroreceptors also decrease the activity of the vasodepressor area and dorsal nucleus of the vagus. These changes result in an increase in sympathetic and a decrease in parasympathetic activity, and hence an increase in the heart rate, stroke volume, and systemic vas-

cular resistance culminating in return of the blood pressure to control levels. The effect of increased baroreceptor activity on the arteries of the brain and heart is less compared to those of skeletal muscle, splanchnic area, and skin. Blood flow to the brain decreases slightly but that to the heart increases because of increased metabolic activity.

The baroreceptor system is a potent regulator of arterial pressure when the pressure is in the normal range but it becomes useless as a pressure regulator once the pressure falls below 60 to 70 mm Hg. The effective range of the arterial baroreceptor mechanism is approximately 60 to 180 mm Hg. The blood pressure threshold for impulse formation in the sinus nerve is 50 mm Hg and a maximum sustained firing is attained at around 200 mm Hg. The firing rate of the baroreceptor increases with PP for a given MAP. The receptor in the carotid sinus is more sensitive than that in the aortic sinus. Aortic baroreceptors do not fire until a pressure of approximately 100 mm Hg is attained. Carotid sinus receptors are very sensitive in certain individuals. Tight collars or other forms of external pressure over the carotid sinus area in such individuals may result in hypotension and fainting. On the other hand, baroreceptor sensitivity decreases in hypertensive subjects when

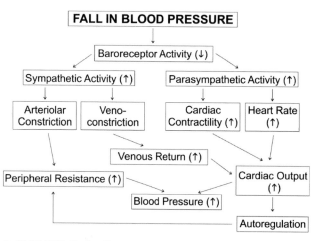

● **FIGURE 8-4.** Baroreceptor pressure control mechanism with fall in the arterial pressure. ↓, Decrease; ↑, increase.

the carotid sinus becomes stiffer and less deformable. Feedback gain (amount of correction of abnormality divided by the remaining degree of abnormality, i.e., effectiveness of the control system) for baroreceptors is less than that for the CNS ischemic response, but greater than the gain for the chemoreceptor mechanism.

The baroreceptor, chemoreceptor, and CNS ischemic response mechanisms respond in seconds, which is important for keeping the arterial pressure on an even keel when a person changes posture, bleeds rapidly, or is centrifuged by a tight turn of an airplane. The baroreceptor mechanism adapts quickly and works for 1 to 2 days.

Cardiopulmonary Baroreceptors

The atria, ventricles, and pulmonary arteries have baroreceptors (low pressure receptors). Stimulation of these receptors by an increase in volume elicits reflexes that would depress the vasoconstrictor area and decreases the arterial pressure.[17]

Chemoreceptor Mechanism

Chemoreceptors are highly vascular bodies located at the bifurcation of the carotid artery (carotid body) and in the region of the aortic arch (aortic body) (Figure 8-2). They are very sensitive to changes in blood pO_2, pCO_2, and pH, the sensitivity being less to pCO_2 and pH than to pO_2.[18] The chemoreceptors are stimulated when (a) pO_2 of the arterial blood is low, (b) pCO_2 is high, (c) pH is low, (d) the blood flow through the bodies is very low or stopped, or (e) a chemical is present that blocks oxidative metabolism in chemoreceptor cells. Impulses from the chemoreceptors reach the vasoconstrictor area resulting in an increased vascular resistance as well as an increase in heart rate and stroke volume through increased sympathetic activity. These changes lead to an increase in arterial pressure.

The chemoreceptor reflex mechanism is not a powerful regulator of arterial pressure in the normal range because the receptors are stimulated only when the arterial pressure falls below approximately 80 mm Hg. It is effective until the pressure falls to 40 mm Hg. It responds in seconds, is effective for an hour or so, and its feedback gain is smallest among nervous system control mechanisms (baroreceptor, chemoreceptor, and CNS ischemic response).

CNS Ischemic Response

The chemosensitive areas of the medulla (vasoconstrictor zone) are very sensitive to changes in pCO_2 and pH.[19] Increases in pCO_2 and decreases in pH stimulate the vasoconstrictor area resulting in an increase in sympathetic activity leading to increased total peripheral resistance and cardiac output. These changes lead to an increase in arterial pressure. On the other hand, decreases in pCO_2 and increases in pH have opposite effects. pO_2 has a relatively small effect on the vasoconstrictor area. A moderate reduction in pO_2 stimulates the vasoconstrictor area, while a severe reduction produces depression of the area. CNS ischemic response is very powerful and can raise the arterial pressure to as high as 250 mm Hg. This system works best in the arterial pressure range of approximately 20 to 40 mm Hg. When the arterial pressure falls below 20 mm Hg, the CNS ischemic response becomes ineffective. This is called the "last ditch stand" pressure control mechanism. Cushing's response is a type of CNS ischemic response that results from increased intracranial pressure. The response time for this reflex mechanism of pressure control is in seconds and the feedback gain for this response is the largest among the neural control mechanisms.

● INTERMEDIATE TIME-PERIOD PRESSURE CONTROL MECHANISM

The intermediate mechanism includes the renin–angiotensin system, stress relaxation, capillary fluid shift, aldosterone, and antidiuretic hormone (ADH) and becomes activated within minutes to several hours. This mechanism is effective for long periods of time (days if necessary) and is important because by this time the nervous mechanisms are less active. This mechanism plays an important role especially in slow hemorrhage or overtransfusion. The feedback gain of the intermediate pressure control mechanism is very small and is the smallest of all the pressure control mechanisms.

Renin–Angiotensin System

Renin is synthesized and stored in an inactive form called prorenin in the juxtaglomerular (JG) cells. The JG cells are located in the walls of the afferent arterioles proximal to the glomeruli. A fall in the arterial pressure below 100 mm Hg leads to an increase in synthesis and release of angiotensin, which in turn increases arterial pressure. There are three hypotheses of renin release in the kidney:

(A) According to the baroreceptor hypothesis the JG cells are stimulated in response to decreases in stretch as a result of reduced pressure and renal blood flow. (B) Because of a reduction in glomerular filtration caused by reduced pressure, the sodium load reaching the distal tubules is reduced, which is sensed by the macula densa. The macula densa is in close proximity to the JG cells, and possibly through the action of a local hormone renin is released from the JG cells. (C) According to the adrenergic hypothesis, a fall in the arterial pressure increases sympathetic activity and causes an increase in the release of norepinephrine. JG cells are innervated by the sympathetic nerve, and are stimulated by norepinephrine to release renin. Elevated plasma levels of norepinephrine during hypotension also stimulate JG cells. Catecholamines and prostaglandins stimulate, whereas angiotensin and potassium inhibit the release of renin from JG cells.

Synthesis of angiotensin II (Ang II)[20,21] is shown in Figure 8-5. Renin acts on a plasma globulin—a renin substrate (angiotensinogen) that is formed in the liver. Synthesis of angiotensinogen is increased by estrogens such as oral contraceptives. Renin activity in the blood lasts for 30 to

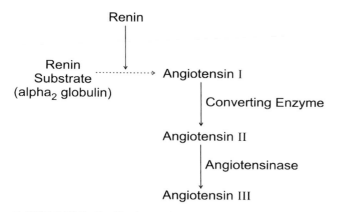

● **FIGURE 8-5.** Renin–angiotensin system.

60 minutes. Renin acts on angiotensinogen to produce angiotensin I (Ang I).

Ang I is converted into Ang II by angiotensin converting enzyme present in the endothelium of the lung blood vessels. Angiotensinase converts Ang II to angiotensin III (Ang III) and also metabolizes the vasodilator bradykinin. Angiotensin-converting enzyme inhibitors therefore reduce blood pressure by decreasing the formation of Ang II and sparing the destruction of bradykinin. Ang III is almost as powerful a vasoconstrictor as Ang II. Ang II persists in the blood only for 1 or 2 minutes because it is rapidly inactivated by angiotensinases.

A schematic diagram showing the mechanisms through which Ang II raises arterial pressure is shown in Figure 8-6. Ang II raises blood pressure in two major ways: through increases in total peripheral resistance and cardiac output. Ang II produces vasoconstriction directly through the release of norepinephrine from the sympathetic nerve endings. The increase in the release of norepinephrine is primarily because of stimulation of the vasomotor center, adrenal medulla, and sympathetic nerve endings. Ang II increases the blood volume through an increase in thirst, sodium, and water reabsorption. Ang II stimulates the zona glomerulosa of the adrenal cortex to release aldosterone that increases reabsorption of sodium in the renal distal tubules. The increase in sodium causes water retention. Ang II increases the release of ADH, which increases water reabsorption in

the renal tubules. The direct effect of Ang II on the kidney and its effects acting through aldosterone and ADH increase the fluid volume, which in turn increases the cardiac output. An increase in the cardiac output through autoregulation increases total peripheral resistance. Thus both direct vasoconstriction and cardiac output-induced autoregulation increase the total vascular resistance. The renin–angiotensin mechanism is most effective in the pressure range of 60 to 110 mm Hg and begins acting within a few minutes. The feedback gain is smaller than that of the neural mechanisms.

Ang II increases production of oxygen radicals through stimulation of nicotinamide adenine dinucleotide phosphate (NADPH)-oxidase.[22] Oxygen radicals are known to increase vascular tone and peripheral vascular resistance.[23] Ang II activation of Ang II type 1 (AT_1) receptors upregulates NADPH-oxidase. There is evidence that Ang II–induced hypertension is mediated by oxygen radicals.[24] It appears that oxygen radicals may also play a role in the regulation of arterial pressure.

Activation of the cardiopulmonary receptors because of an increase in arterial pressure inhibits the release of angiotensin, aldosterone, and ADH. These changes will reduce cardiac output and total peripheral resistance and hence lower the arterial pressure. The effects are opposite when the arterial pressure falls. The arterial baroreceptor stimulation has similar effects on ADH release. The aldosterone mechanism works best in the pressure range of 40 to 150 mm Hg. The feedback gain is not well determined but appears to be similar to that of the stress–relaxation mechanism.

Stress–Relaxation

Stretch–relaxation is the phenomenon in which an increase in arterial pressure stretches the blood vessels slowly allowing the pressure to fall toward the control value. Reverse stress–relaxation causes the blood vessels to contract around the diminished blood volume that occurs in hypovolemic shock. This mechanism serves as an intermediate-term pressure "buffer." The stress–relaxation mechanism is effective at all values of arterial pressure and works quickly, within a few minutes of a change in pressure.

Capillary Fluid Shift

Capillary structure, and filtration and reabsorption in the capillaries have been described in detail.[25–27] Capillary hydrostatic pressure varies from tissue to tissue but averages approximately 32 mm Hg at the arteriolar end of the capillaries and 15 mm Hg at the venular end. The oncotic pressure is the osmotic pressure exerted by the plasma protein and is approximately 25 to 28 mm Hg. The point of intersection of hydrostatic pressure and oncotic pressure is the equilibrium point at which there is no flux of fluid (Figure 8-7A). To the left of the equilibrium point there is filtration, whereas to the right of the equilibrium there is absorption. Normally 85% of filtered plasma is reabsorbed into the capillaries and the remaining is returned to the

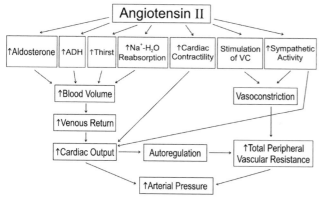

● **FIGURE 8-6.** Mechanisms involved in the control of arterial pressure with angiotensin II. ADH, antidiuretic hormone; Na^+, sodium; H_2O, water; VC, vasoconstrictor area.

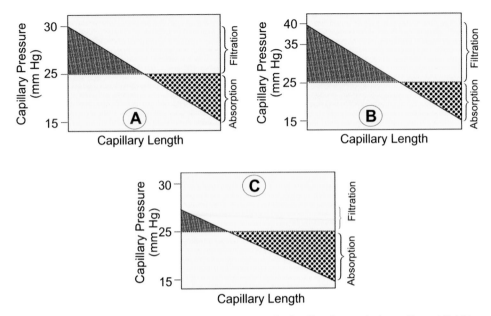

● **FIGURE 8-7.** Diagram showing the changes in the filtration and absorption of fluid in the capillaries in normal condition (A), with increased hydrostatic pressure (B), and with decreased hydrostatic pressure (C). Note that an increase in hydrostatic pressure increases filtration and decreases reabsorption, while a decrease in the arterial pressure has opposite effects.

vascular system through the lymphatic system. A rise in arterial pressure increases the hydrostatic pressure in the arterial end of the capillaries and the equilibrium point is shifted to the right and so filtration is greater and absorption is less (Figure 8-7B). These changes lead to decreases in blood volume and cardiac output, resulting in lowering of blood pressure toward control levels. On the other hand, during a fall in the arterial pressure below normal, as in hemorrhagic shock, the equilibrium point is shifted to the left (Figure 8-7C) thus resulting in increased absorption. These changes increase blood volume and cardiac output, raising arterial pressure toward normal levels.

In summary, this mechanism involves the filtration and absorption of fluid in the capillaries based on the hydrostatic and oncotic pressures in the capillaries. Elevation of arterial pressure increases capillary hydrostatic pressure leading to transudation of the fluid from the capillaries, resulting in decreased blood volume and a decrease in arterial pressure. Conversely, with a fall in the arterial pressure, there is a decrease in the hydrostatic pressure and the extracellular fluid is reabsorbed. This leads to an increase in the circulating blood volume and hence an increase in arterial pressure. This mechanism gets activated within 30 minutes to several hours. It works at all values of arterial pressure but the feedback gain is very small, and less than in the neural control mechanisms.

● LONG-TERM PRESSURE CONTROL MECHANISM

Renal Body Fluid Pressure Control

The renal body–fluid system for arterial pressure control is the fundamental basis for long-term arterial pressure control.[28–30] The renal body–fluid system for control of arterial pressures is dependent upon two factors: (A) The renal urinary output curve (renal function curve) for water and salt in response to changing arterial pressure and (B) the net water and salt intake (Figure 8-8). The net intake is defined as intake minus nonrenal output such as loss through the gut or/and by sweating. Over a long period of time the net intake equals renal output, and the arterial pressure is determined by the point at which the two curves intersect, the equilibrium point at 100 mm Hg (see point A in Figure 8-8). When the arterial pressure falls to approximately 50 mm Hg, urinary output is zero (Figure 8-8). However, when the arterial pressure rises from the normal value of 100 mm Hg to 200 mm Hg, the urinary output of salt and water increases six- to eightfold[25,26] (Figure 8-8). This curve, shown in Figure 8-6, is called the renal output curve. A rise in arterial pressure increases sodium output (pressure natriuresis) as well as urinary output. When the arterial pressure rises to 150 mm Hg, urinary output of salt and water increases to approximately three times normal when the net intake remains unchanged. In such circumstances the fluid is lost, causing a decrease in blood volume and leading to a decrease in cardiac output and the arterial pressure. The decrease in arterial pressure is also caused by a decrease in total peripheral resistance because of autoregulation. The arterial pressure gradually reaches 100 mm Hg where the renal output and net intake become equal again, and the arterial pressure stabilizes at that point. This negative balance of fluid will not cease until the pressure falls back to reach the equilibrium point.

When the arterial pressure decreases below the equilibrium point at 100 mm Hg, and the net intake of salt and water remains unchanged, renal output decreases.

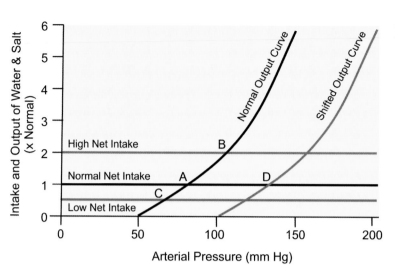

● **FIGURE 8-8.** Changes in the arterial pressures with changes in net intake and the renal urinary output curve. Normal net intake and renal output curve are depicted in black; shift in urinary renal output curve and high net intake of salt and water are depicted in red; and low intake is shown in green. Points A, B, C, and D are equilibrium points, where output equals intake and determines the arterial pressure.

Therefore, at low pressure the net intake will be greater than the renal output. As a consequence, salt and water will accumulate, increasing blood volume and cardiac output and resulting in increased arterial pressure, until the pressure reaches the equilibrium point (Figure 8-8).

When the net intake of salt and water vastly increases, the arterial pressure rises to the equilibrium point B (Figure 8-8) at a pressure level of approximately 140 mm Hg, which is 40 mm Hg greater than normal. On the other hand, when the net intake of salt and water decreases, arterial pressure decreases to an equilibrium point C (Figure 8-8), which is lower than the normal arterial pressure of 100 mm Hg. An increase in salt intake is far more likely to raise arterial pressure than is an increase in water intake. Pure water is excreted rapidly by the kidneys, while salt is not. An accumulation of salt increases fluid volume through an increase in fluid osmolality and increased release of ADH. Accumulation of salt increases osmolality of extracellular fluid. Osmolality is known to increase thirst by stimulating the thirst center in the brain. Increased thirst will cause the person to drink more water, which in turn will increase extracellular fluid in the body. Increased osmolality stimulates the osmorecepters in the posterior pituitary gland to secrete ADH and in turn increases reabsorption of water in the renal tubules. An increase in both osmolality and ADH increases the extracellular fluid accumulation, resulting in increased cardiac output and arterial pressure. However, one has to remember that increasing plasma volume by decreasing oncotic pressure and sympathetic activity, and by increasing atrial natriuretic factor, could decrease sodium reabsorption in the proximal renal tubes and the collecting ducts leading to increased Na^+ excretion.[30] This might be the reason that normal salt intake does not produce hypertension.

A shift in the renal output curve caused by an abnormality in the kidneys could also affect the arterial pressure. If the renal output curve is shifted to the right with net intake remaining unaltered, the equilibrium point moves to D (Figure 8-8), which is 50 mm Hg higher than normal.

The renal body–fluid mechanism for pressure control is effective in all ranges of blood pressure. This mechanism for arterial pressure control is useless for regulation of arterial pressure over a period of minutes or hours. This mechanism starts later than other mechanisms, but works until the pressure is returned to normal. Feedback gain for this mechanism is infinite. The other arterial pressure control systems all have finite gain. It is important to note that two other conditions must be satisfied to qualify the infinite gain principle. These two conditions are (a) intake of water and salt and (b) functional capabilities of kidney.

Feedback Loop Mechanism

The mechanisms involved in the renal body–fluid pressure control system are shown in Figure 8-9. The rate of change of extracellular fluid volume is determined by the difference between net intake of salt and water, and renal output of salt and water. A positive rate of change increases extracellular volume, while a negative change has the opposite effect. With a fall in the arterial pressure below normal in the presence of unaltered net intake, the renal output becomes less than intake, increasing the extracellular volume. Increases in the extracellular volume in turn increase the blood volume, circulatory filling pressure, venous return, and cardiac output. An increase in cardiac output increases arterial pressure in two separate ways. Firstly, cardiac output directly affects blood pressure that is the product of cardiac output and total peripheral resistance. Secondly, an increase in cardiac output through autoregulation increases total peripheral resistance. Most of the increase in arterial pressure occurs initially because of the direct effect of cardiac output. The autoregulatory increase in peripheral resistance occurs over several days.

● OXYGEN RADICALS AND REGULATION OF BLOOD PRESSURE

Oxyradicals may play a role in the regulation of blood pressure. Oxygen radicals, specifically superoxide anion and hydrogen peroxide, are vasoconstrictors.[31,32] Oxygen radicals

● **FIGURE 8-9.** Feedback loop of the renal body–fluid arterial pressure control mechanism.

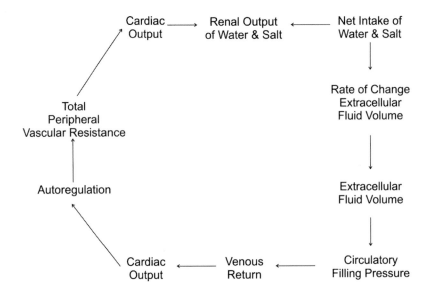

are generated by polymorphonuclear leukocytes, and administration of oxygen radicals increase peripheral vascular resistance.[23,33]

Various pressure control mechanisms such as baroreceptors, chemoreceptors, and the renin–angiotensin system regulate blood pressure through release of epinephrine, norepinephrine, and angiotensin. Epinephrine through autooxidation[34] and Ang II through stimulation of NADPH-oxidase[22] increase the synthesis of oxygen radicals.

● IMPLICATIONS OF COMPLEX PRESSURE CONTROL SYSTEMS

Advantages

There are some advantages to having numerous pressure control systems:

(1) Cooperation of pressure-regulating systems allows rapid and definite responses to emergencies.

(2) Fine-tuning capabilities.

(3) Fail-safe and backup systems enable removal of entire components without loss of pressure control (i.e., adrenalectomy, nephrectomy).

(4) Complexity allows local changes to supersede systemic control in vital organs such as the heart and brain.

Disadvantages

(1) Absolute levels of pressure are not sensed by pressure control systems.

(2) There is a potential danger in having sensors independent of each other. Renal ischemia can overdrive the system because local conditions near one sensor may not reflect the status of the body as a whole.

(3) The system fails to sense the capacity of the effectors to perform.

(4) There is a lack of ability on part of the pressure control systems to sense total fluid volume.

● ACKNOWLEDGMENTS

I am very thankful to Ms. Barbara Raney and Ms. Gladys Wiebe for their assistance in the preparation of this chapter.

REFERENCES

1. The seventh of the Joint National Committee on Prevention, Detection, Evaluation, and Treatment of High Blood Pressure. National Heart, Lung and Blood Institute, National Institutes of Health; May 2003. NIH Publication No. 03-5233.

2. Guideline Committee of the European Society of Hypertension—European Society of Cardiology. 2003 European Society of Hypertension—European Society of Cardiology guidelines for management of arterial hypertension. *J Hypertens.* 2003;21:1011.

3. Rizzo V, de Maio F, Petretto F, et al. Ambulatory pulse pressure, left ventricular hypertrophy and function in arterial hypertension. *Echocardiography.* 2004;21:11.

4. Casiglia E, Tikhonoff V, Mazza A, et al. Pulse pressure and coronary mortality in elderly men and women from general population. *J Hum Hypertension.* 2002;16:611.

5. Safar ME, Smulyan H. Coronary ischemic disease, arterial stiffness, and pulse pressure. *Am J Hypertens.* 2004;17: 724.

6. Domanski MJ, Sutton-Tyrrell K, Mitchell GF, et al. Determinants and prognostic information provided by pulse pressure in patients with coronary artery disease undergoing revascularization. The Balloon Angioplasty Revascularizaton Investigation (BARI). *Am J Cardiol.* 2001;87:675.

7. Weber T, Auer J, O'Rourke MF, et al. Arterial stiffness, wave

reflections, and the risk of coronary artery disease. *Circulation.* 2004;109:184.

8. Weber T, Auer J, O'Rourke MF, et al. Increased arterial wave reflections predict severe cardiovascular events in patients undergoing percutaneous coronary interventions. *Eur Heart J.* 2005;26:2657.

9. Redon J. The normal circadian pattern of blood pressure; implications for treatment. *Int J Clin Pract.* 2004;58(suppl 145):3.

10. Giles TD. Circadian rhythm of blood pressure and the relation to cardiovascular events. *J Hypertens Suppl.* 2006;24: S11.

11. Prasad K. Blood pressure and its control mechanism. In: Chang JB, Olsen ER, Prasad K, Sumpio BE, eds. *Textbook of Angiology.* New York: Springer-Verlag; 2000:46.

12. Fagan TC, Conrad KA, Mar JH, et al. Effects of meals on hemodynamics: implications for antihypertensive drug studies. *Clin Pharmacol Ther.* 1986;39:255.

13. Dampney RA, Horiuchi J, Tagawa T, et al. Medullary and supramedullary mechanisms regulating sympathetic vasomotor tone. *Acta Physiol Scand.* 2003;177:209.

14. Cao WH, Fan W, Morrison SF. Medullary pathways mediating specific sympathetic responses to activation of dorsomedial hypothalamus. *Neuroscience.* 2004;126:229.

15. Guyton AC, Coleman TG, Granger HJ. Circulation: overall regulation. *Annu Rev Physiol.* 1972;34:13.

16. Persson PB. Modulation of cardiovascular control mechanisms and their interaction. *Physiol Rev.* 1996;76:193.

17. Floras JS. Arterial baroreceptor and cardiopulmonary reflex control of sympathetic outflow in human heart failure. *Ann N Y Acad Sci.* 2001;940:500.

18. Kara T, Narkiewicz K, Somers VK. Chemoreflexes – physiology and clinical implications. *Acta Physiol Scand.* 2003; 177:377.

19. Sagawa K, Taylor AE, Guyton AC. Dynamic performance and stability of cerebral ischemic pressor response. *Am J Physiol.* 1961;201:1164.

20. DiBona GF. Peripheral and central interactions between the renin–angiotensin system and the renal smpathetic nerves in control of renal function. *Ann N Y Acad Sci.* 2001;940: 395.

21. Mazzolai L, Nussberger J. The renin–angiotensin-aldosterone system. In: Battegay E, Lip GYH, Bakris GL, eds. *Hypertension—Principles and Practice.* Boca Raton: Taylor & Francis; 2005:143.

22. Griendling KK, Minieri CA, Ollerenshaw JD, et al. Angiotensin II stimulates NADH and NADPH oxidase activity in cultured vascular smooth muscle cells. *Circ Res.* 1994; 74:1141.

23. Prasad K, Kalra J, Chaudhary AK, et al. Effect of polymorphonuclear leukocyte—derived oxygen free radicals and hypochlorous acid on cardiac function and some biochemical parameters. *Am Heart J.* 1990;119:538.

24. Prasad K. Oxyradicals as a mechanism of angiotensin-induced hypertension. *Int J Angiol.* 2004;13:59.

25. Taylor AE. Capillary fluid filtration. Starling forces and lymph flow. *Circ Res.* 1981;49:557.

26. Levick JR, Mortimer PS. Fluid "balance" between microcirculation and interstitium in skin and other tissues: revision of the classical filtration—reabsorption scheme. *Prog Appl Microcirc.* 1999;23:42.

27. Michel CC. Microvascular permeability, ultrafiltration, and restricted diffusion. *Am J Physiol Heart Circ Physiol.* 2004;287: H1887.

28. Guyton AC. Dominant role of the kidney in long-term regulation of arterial pressure and in hypertension: the integrated system for pressure control. In: Guyton AC, Hall JE, eds. *Textbook of Medical Physiology.* 11th ed. Philadelphia: WB Saunders; 2006:216.

29. Cowley AW Jr. Long-term control of arterial blood pressure. *Physiol Rev.* 1992;72:231.

30. Best CH. Regulation of volume and abnormality of body fluids. In: West JB, ed. *Best and Taylor's Physiological Basis of Medical Practice.* 12th ed. Baltimore: Williams & Wilkins Co; 1991:478.

31. Bharadwaj L, Prasad K. Mediation of H_2O_2-induced vascular relaxation by endothelium-derived relaxing factor. *Mol Cell Biochem.* 1995;149/150:267.

32. Bharadwaj L, Prasad K. Mechanism of superoxide anion-induced modulation of vascular tone. *Int J Angiol.* 2002;11:23.

33. Prasad K, Kalra J, Chan WP, et al. Effect of oxygen free radicals on cardiovascular function at organ and cellular levels. *Am Heart J.* 1989;117:1196.

34. Singal PK, Kapur N, Dhillon KS, et al. Role of free radicals in catecholamine-induced cardiomyopathy. *Can J Physiol Pharmacol.* 1982;60:1390.

chapter 9

Hypertension

Kailash Prasad, MD, PhD

● INTRODUCTION

Hypertension accounts for 6% of deaths worldwide. In Canada, the overall prevalence of hypertension was 22% and was higher in men (26%) than in women (18%) in a survey done between 1986 and 1992.[1] Hypertension prevalence increases progressively with age, being lower in women than men aged 18 to 34 years (2% vs.11%) and aged 35 to 64 years (21% vs. 31%).[1,2] However, in the group aged 65 to 74, women had a higher prevalence than men (58% vs. 56%). The overall prevalence of hypertension in the United States in 2004 was 72 000 000 (33 000 000 males; 39 000 000 females). A higher percentage of men than women have hypertension until age 45 years. The percentage of hypertension is similar in men and women between the ages of 45 and 54. After the age of 54, a higher percentage of women have hypertension than men. It is estimated that middle-aged North Americans have a 90% life-time risk of developing hypertension. The prevalence of hypertension is higher in southeastern United States as compared to other regions.[3] Hypertension in black men and women in the southern states is higher (35–34%) as compared to other parts of the United States (27–33%). The prevalence of hypertension in white men and women in the southern United States is slightly higher (21.5% to 26.5%) as compared to other parts of the United States (21% to 24.3%). When Canadian survey data were compared to similar data from the United States, hypertension prevalence was similar between the two countries (20.1% vs. 21.1%, Canadian vs. American), but awareness of the diagnosis (69% vs. 57%), and treatment of hypertension (52% vs. 34%) were substantially higher in the United States than in Canada.[1] Recent data from the United States show a further improvement in treatment and control rates. There was a large increase in diagnosis (51%) and treatment (66%) of hypertension between 1994 and 2003.[4] There is substantial evidence that the patient management guidelines are not followed frequently, and the current practice patterns present a major barrier to treatment and control of hypertension.[5] It is not only the treatment practice but also the pathophysiology of the disease that affects the outcome. There has been advancement in understanding the mechanism of the disease and in diagnostic and treatment modalities. This chapter will deal with the definition of hypertension, measurement of blood pressure, epidemiology, pathophysiology, complications, and treatment.

● DEFINITION AND CLASSIFICATION OF HYPERTENSION

The higher the pressure, the worse the prognosis. The prognosis is based not on whether hypertension is thought to be present, but on the actual recorded pressure. However the question is "At what pressure level should treatment be instituted?" The dividing line between normotension and hypertension is arbitrary. The decision to treat should be based on the evaluation of risk. The reason for a dividing line is to initiate treatment. The risk associated with blood pressure increases monotonocally with blood pressure, hence the benefit of treatment is progressively higher at higher levels of blood pressure. Blood pressure has been classified into four groups (Table 9-1) by the Joint National Committee on Prevention, Detection, Evaluation and Treatment of High Blood Pressure (JNC-7).[6] Normal blood pressure is systolic <120 mm Hg and diastolic <80 mm Hg. Hypertension is classified into three groups: prehypertension, stage 1 and stage 2 hypertension. The European Society of Hypertension—European Society of Cardiology guidelines in 2003 classified blood pressure into seven categories (Table 9-1): optimal, normal, high normal, Grade 1 hypertension (mild), Grade 2 hypertension (moderate), Grade 3 hypertension (severe), and isolated systolic hypertension (ISH).[7] According to the Framingham criteria, the terms low, moderate, high, and very high added risk indicate a

TABLE 9-1. Classification of Blood Pressure

JNC-7 Guidelines Class	Systolic (mm Hg)	Diastolic (mm Hg)
Normal	<120	<80
Prehypertension	120–139	80–89
Hypertension (stage 1)	140–159	90–99
Hypertension (stage 2)	≥160	≥100
European Societies of Hypertension and Cardiology Guidelines*		
Optimal	<120	<80
Normal	120–129	80–84
High normal	130–139	85–89
Hypertension Grade 1 (mild)	140–159	90–99
Hypertension Grade 2 (moderate)	160–179	100–109
Hypertension Grade 3 (severe)	≥180	≥110
Isolated systolic hypertension	≥140	≥90

*Reprinted with permission from the 2003 European Society of Hypertension—European Society of Cardiology Guidelines for management of arterial hypertension. J Hypertens. 2003;21:1011.

10 year risk of cardiovascular disease of <15%, 15% to 20%, 20% to 30%, and >30%, respectively.

ISH is a separate class in itself. It can be graded as 1, 2, and 3 according to the systolic pressure ranges indicated in Table 9-1. Systolic pressure rises almost linearly between the ages of 30 and 84 years, while diastolic pressure rises until age 50 years, levels off, and then declines. More than 90% of untreated hypertensive subjects in the United States have ISH by the time they reach 70 to 75 years of age.[8] ISH accounts for 57.4% of all hypertension in men and 65% in women aged 65 to 89 years. ISH is associated with increased risks of all cardiovascular disease complications and is an independent risk factor. For every 1 mm Hg elevation in systolic blood pressure there is a 1% increase in all causes of mortality. Pulse pressure indicates stiffening of the aorta and is an accurate predictor of cardiovascular risk in normotensive subjects, and a predictor of recurring events in patients with impaired left ventricular function after myocardial infarction.

● BLOOD PRESSURE MEASUREMENT

Accurate measurement of blood pressure is of utmost importance for the diagnosis of hypertension. Presently, blood pressures are being measured by (a) physicians in office (office measurement or auscultatory method), (b) self (self-measurement), and (c) 24 hour measurement (ambulatory measurement).

Auscultatory Method

The gold standard for clinical blood pressure measurement is by the sphygmomanometer and the Korotkoff sound technique. However, the auscultatory office blood pressure measurement has shortcomings such as (a) inaccuracy in methods, which includes mechanical defects and noncompliance of official guidelines for their use; (b) inherent variability of blood pressure; and (c) the white-coat effect (WCE).[6,9]

Mercury Sphygmomanometer

The inaccuracy in blood pressure measurement is related to cuff size. The ideal cuff should have a bladder length that is 80% and a width that is at least 40% of the arm circumference (a length-to-width ratio of 2:1). The cuff should be at the level of the right atrium. Diastolic pressure is approximately 5 mm Hg higher in the sitting position than in the supine position, while systolic pressure is 8 mm Hg higher in the supine than in the sitting position. Crossing of the legs raises systolic pressure by 2 to 8 mm Hg. The blood pressure is high when the arm is below the level of the right atrium, and low when the arm is above the level of right atrium. For every inch below or above the heart level, there is a change of 2 mm Hg. If the arm is held up by the individual the isometric exercise will raise the pressure. The mercury column should be deflated at 2 to 3 mm/s. Neither patient nor the physician should talk during the measurement. Blood pressure should be checked in both arms. The first reading is the highest. A minimum of two measurements should be made at intervals of 1 minute, and the average should be recorded. If the difference between the first and second readings is more than 5 mm Hg, an additional one or two readings should be taken to calculate the average.

White-Coat Effect. WCE is defined as a transient rise in blood pressure and sometimes in heart rate, in the presence of the health professional, that disappears when the patient has left the office. This phenomenon occurs in both normotensive and hypertensive subjects irrespective of medications. In many cases it diminishes or disappears with repeated measurements. As a result of the WCE, an individual has elevated blood pressure in the physician's office but a normal blood pressure outside the office, a phenomenon called white-coat hypertension (WCHT).[10] Office blood pressure values equal to or higher than 140 mm Hg systolic and/or 90 mm Hg diastolic, with self-measured or daytime ambulatory blood pressure lower than 135 mm Hg systolic and 85 mm Hg diastolic, is defined as WCHT. The prevalence of WCHT varies from 15% to over 50% in patients with mildly elevated blood pressure, 25% to 35% in patients with diagnosed hypertension and around 10% in the population at large and in clinical practice. The study of Verberk el al[10] showed that 33% of the patients having mild-to-moderate hypertension consistently had a substantial WCE and 14% had WCHT. WCHT has been associated with a significantly lower incidence of cardiovascular events than sustained hypertension. However, some studies suggest that the rate of cardiovascular events is higher in individuals with WCHT than in normotensives. Subjects with WCHT have a more marked morning blood pressure surge and greater daytime blood pressure variability compared to normotensives, although significantly lower than hypertensives. The cardiovascular risk of individuals with WCHT and normotensives is fairly similar and WCHT is benign compared to hypertension.

The aneroid sphygmomanometer measures blood pressure by a mechanical system of metal bellows that expand as the cuff pressure increases, and a series of levers that register the pressure on a circular scale. The stability of this system over time deteriorates and requires calibration. The inaccuracy of the aneroid devices varies between 1% and 44%.

Self-Measurement of Blood Pressure

Recently, automated oscillometric blood pressure devices are being used for office, home, and ambulatory pressure measurements. The advantages of automated methods include elimination of observer error, minimizing WCE, and increasing the number of readings. However, this method has a few disadvantages, that is, inherent error in the oscillometric method and epidemiologic data are based on the auscultatory method. The devices should be validated before the reading is accepted. The validation requires comparison of the device measurements (four measurements) alternating with five mercury sphygmomanometer measurements. Validation requires that both systolic and diastolic pressures are within 5 mm Hg of each other for at least 50% of the readings.

Several types of blood pressure monitoring devices are available for home use. Self-monitored blood pressure may be more representative of 24 hour blood pressure. The reproducibility of self-measurement is twice as good as the clinic blood pressure. The advantages of self-monitoring blood pressure are that it (i) distinguishes sustained hypertension from WCHT, (ii) improves patient adherence to treatment, and (iii) reduces management costs.

Ambulatory Blood Pressure Measurement

Ambulatory blood pressure measurement (ABPM), a noninvasive fully automated method, measures blood pressure during daily activities and sleep every 15 to 30 minutes. The devices measure blood pressure commonly by oscillometry or the auscultation method. The oscillometric measurement depends upon detection of pulsatile oscillations of the brachial artery in the cuff. The oscillometric technique is accurate for midrange blood pressure, but is less accurate in older patients or in patients with low or high blood pressure. Blood pressure has a reproducible circadian rhythm with higher values while awake, and mentally and physically active, and much lower values during sleep, and an early morning surge. The suggested daytime optimal, normal, and abnormal systolic and diastolic pressures are <130/80, <135/85, and >140/90 mm Hg, respectively, night time values are <115/65, <120/70, and >125/75 mm Hg, respectively and 24 hour averages are <125/75, <130/80 and >135/85 mm Hg, respectively. In most individuals the blood pressure drops by 10% to 20% during the night. Individuals with a nondipping pattern (<10%) are at increased risk of cardiovascular events. Individuals whose 24 hour blood pressure is greater than 135/85 mm Hg are nearly twice as likely to have a cardiovascular event as those with 24 hour mean blood pressure of <135/85 mm Hg, irrespective of office blood pressure level.[6] ABPM is helpful in the following clinical situations; WCHT, hypertension with or without target organ involvement, antihypertensive drug resistance, episodic hypertension, automomic dysfunction, and hypotensive symptoms with antihypertensive medication.

● PATHOPHYSIOLOGY OF HYPERTENSION

Hypertension is of two types: (I) essential or primary hypertension where the etiology is unknown. This type of hypertension accounts for approximately 90% to 95% of all hypertension, and (II) secondary hypertension where the etiology is known. The prevalence of this type of hypertension is 5% to 10%.

Essential Hypertension

Essential hypertension, also called primary or idiopathic hypertension, is hypertension of unknown etiology. The mechanism(s) responsible for essential hypertension is complex because of the numerous factors involved in the regulation of blood pressure and their complex interactions. Hypertension seems to be a reflection of separate disease processes. Essential hypertension may likely have a number of discrete etiologies.

Heredity and Genomics. Approximately 50% of hypertension is genetically controlled and the other 50% environmentally controlled. First degree relatives of patients with hypertension have a twofold greater risk of hypertension and this risk increases to fourfold when more family members are hypertensive. A family history of hypertension in blacks increases the risk of hypertension ninefold. A family history of hypertension at an early age increases the risk. Essential hypertension is a polygenic disorder. More than 60 genes have been studied and the genetic variants associated with hypertension in different ethnicities have been identified. These variants are genes from the renin—angiotensin (Ang)–aldosterone system, adrenergic receptor system, renal kallikrein–kinin system, α-adducin, and epithelial sodium channel. Some of the genes, such as Ang-converting enzyme, angiotensinogen, Ang II type 1 receptor, aldosterone synthase, glucocorticoid receptor, α-adducin, α-2 adrenergic receptor, β-2 adrenergic receptor, epithelial sodium channel, kallikrein, G-protein β-3 subunit, and WNK4, have either familial aggregation and linkage or an association to essential hypertension.[11–13] Many of these genes encode proteins that are directly or indirectly involved with renal ion transport. The genes encode angiotensinogen, Ang-converting enzyme, α-adducin, G-protein β3 subunit, sodium epithelial channel and WNK kinases. Gene-by-environment interactions between genetic variations and environmental factors contribute to the development of essential hypertension.

Salt Sensitivity. Salt sensitive individuals respond to high salt intake with an increase in blood pressure, while salt resistant individuals do not. Fifty-one percent of hypertensives and 26% of normotensive are salt sensitive. The subjects whose blood pressure rises with high salt diet and falls with salt restriction are salt sensitive individuals. The hypertension in salt sensitive hypertensives may be because of changes in renin activity, increased activity of the sympathetic nervous system, and chloride ions. Genetic marker candidates for salt sensitivity may be angiotensinogen and α-adducin. α-adducin induces signal transduction in renal tubular cells and regulates sodium reabsorption. With unaltered sodium intake, the incidence of hypertension in the AA genotype of angiotensinogen is more than in the GG genotype. Increased insulin resistance and abnormalities in glucose disposal are observed in normotensive salt sensitive individuals and salt sensitive subjects with essential hypertension.[14] Insulin resistance could also be involved in hypertension through accumulation of aldehydes.[15]

Insulin Resistance. Insulin resistance and hyperinsulinemia are associated with hypertension. The mechanism of hypertension in individuals with insulin resistance could be multifactorial. Insulin increases the activity of the sympathetic nervous system leading to increases in cardiac output and peripheral vascular resistance.[16] Insulin is known to increase sodium and water retention through its effect on renal tubules. Insulin-induced hypertension may be mediated through its effect at the cellular level. It has been shown that in insulin resistance, glucose metabolism through the glycolytic pathway is impaired, resulting in accumulation of glyceraldehyde and glyceraldehyde-3-phosphate. These metabolites are further metabolized to the highly reactive aldehyde, methylglyoxal. Methyloglyoxal binds with free sulfhydryl (SH) and amino groups of membrane proteins forming aldehyde conjugates, leading to altered cellular structure and function.[17] Excess aldehyde binds SH groups of the calcium channel leading to increased cytosolic $[Ca^{2+}]_i$ and hence increased vascular resistance.[15,18] Aldehydes may also alter the function of enzymes, including antioxidant enzymes and nitric oxide synthase, and vascular tissue proteins that play a role in hypertension.[15,19] Chronic dietary administration of methylglyoxal to rats increases tissue aldehyde conjugate, cytosolic $[Ca^{2+}]_i$ and blood pressure, and decreases plasma levels of nitric oxide.[15] Elevated levels of $[Ca^{2+}]_i$ and decreased levels of $[Mg^{2+}]_i$ have been reported in patients with essential hypertension, and insulin resistance.

Cellular and Plasma Ions. It is generally accepted that sodium ions play a major role in hypertension. However suggestions have been made that chloride ions may also play a role in hypertension. In support of this, it has been shown that feeding of chloride ion-free sodium salts to salt sensitive rats does not produce hypertension. As mentioned in the preceding section, $[Ca^{2+}]_i$ levels are high in patients with hypertension. Intracellular calcium is influenced by the extracellular environment. Low renin hypertensive subjects have lower serum ionized Ca^{2+} and calcitonin levels, and higher serum Mg^{2+}, parathormone and 1,25-dihydroxycholecalciferol as compared to normotensive individuals. Intracellular calcium is elevated in all types of hypertension. However, there are variations (lower/higher) in the levels of extracellular Ca^{2+} and Mg^{2+}.

Obesity. Obesity and recent weight gain account for 70% of new onset hypertension. The mechanism of hypertension in obese subjects is not definitely known. Increased sodium intake does not explain the etiology of hypertension in obese individuals because continued salt intake with weight loss lowers blood pressure. Obesity is associated with insulin resistance, hyperinsulinemia, salt-sensitivity, and hyperleptinemia. Insulin and leptin increase sympathetic activity that would increase blood pressure. Increased renal sympathetic activity would cause salt retention via the reabsorption of sodium in the renal tubules.

Renin. Renin has been implicated in essential hypertension. There are three types of essential hypertension based on plasma renin levels: low renin, high renin, and nonmodulating.

The prevalence of low renin essential hypertension is 20%. These patients have increased extracellular fluid possibly because of sodium retention, and renin suppression because of increased levels of unidentified mineralocorticoids. The adrenal cortex may be more sensitive to Ang II. However, altered sensitivity to Ang II has been observed in patients with normal renin hypertension.

The prevalence of high renin essential hypertension is approximately 15%. The high renin levels may be secondary to increased sympathetic activity.

The prevalence of nonmodulating hypertension is 25% to 30%. In nonmodulating essential hypertension, the adrenal response to sodium reduction is reduced. Sodium intake does not modulate adrenal or renal vascular responses to Ang II, and this has been termed nonmodulating hypertension. These individuals have high or normal levels of plasma renin activity (PRA).

Oxygen Radicals. Recently, oxygen radicals (ORs) have been implicated in the pathophysiology of hypertension. Sources of ORs have been described in detail earlier.[20] Exogenously generated ORs have been shown to increase systemic and pulmonary vascular resistance.[21,22] Superoxide anion (O_2^-)[23] and hydrogen peroxide (H_2O_2)[24] induce increased vascular tone in rabbit aorta. ORs have been implicated in the pathophysiology of human essential hypertension.[25-27] Antioxidant status is decreased in essential hypertension.[28] Although there are various sources of ORs, NADPH oxidase seems to be the most important in the causation of hypertension. NADPH oxidase is present in the vascular endothelial cells, vascular smooth muscle cells, polymorphonuclear leukocytes, and adventitial fibroblasts.[29] The role of vascular NADPH oxidase in the development and progression of hypertension in numerous animals has been established.[30,31] Ang II induced hypertension is associated with oxidative stress.[29] Ang II upregulates NADPH oxidase.[29] Genetic factors, including polymorphism in the genes encoding the NADPH oxidase subunits, modulate O_2^- production, influencing hypertension.[32] ORs could contribute to development of hypertension in some other ways besides direct vasoconstriction. Superoxide anions combine with nitric oxide to form peroxynitrite thereby reducing the bioavailability of nitric oxide, a vasodilator. Peroxynitrite is a weak vasodilator compared to nitric oxide. Critical imbalances between superoxide anions and nitric oxide could lead to the development of hypertension. Superoxide anion is destroyed by superoxide dismutase. However, the reaction between superoxide anion and nitric oxide is three times faster than the reaction between superoxide anion and superoxide dismutase. ORs produce endothelial dysfunction, thus reducing the release of vasodilator substances such as prostanoids and nitric oxide. In such circumstances, there is unopposed action of circulating vasoconstrictors resulting in a rise in blood pressure.

C-Reactive Protein.

C-reactive protein (CRP) is an inflammatory marker synthesized and secreted mainly by hepatocytes in response to the cytokines interleukin-6 and tumor necrosis factor-alpha. It is markedly increased in inflammatory diseases, acute or chronic.[33] Hypertension is associated with increased CRP.[34] Higher levels of high sensitive CRP in patients with hypertension as compared to normotensive individuals have been reported.[35] A cross-sectional study has correlated CRP with blood pressure. CRP directly stimulates polymorphonuclear leukocytes to produce ORs.[36] ORs could produce hypertension through direct vasoconstriction and endothelial cell dysfunction. There are, however, no longitudinal data to support the role of CRP in the development of hypertension.

Soluble Receptor for Advanced Glycation End Products.

Advanced glycation end products (AGEs) are a heterogeneous group of adducts resulting from nonenzymatic glycation and oxidation of proteins, lipids, and nucleic acids. Glucose and other reducing sugars produce AGEs. AGE formation proceeds slowly under normal glycemic conditions, but is accelerated in the presence of hyperglycemia and oxidative stress. There are mainly two receptors for AGE (RAGE): full length (RAGE) and soluble receptor for AGEs (sRAGE). Binding of AGE with full length receptor results in activation of nuclear factor-kappaB (NF-kB), increased expression of cytokines, adhesion molecules and tissue factor, and induction of oxidative stress. sRAGE acts as a decoy for RAGE ligands. This occurs by sequestering circulating AGEs or competing with full length RAGE. The interaction of AGE and RAGE has been implicated in the pathogenesis of hypertension, atherosclerosis, coronary artery disease, diabetic complications, and restenosis, as reviewed earlier.[37] Several studies suggest a role of AGE in the progression and maintenance of hypertension. AGE and RAGE interaction may produce hypertension through oxygen radical generation and expression of vascular cell growth factor. ORs are known to increase vascular tone.[21–24] sRAGE levels in the plasma are lower in patients with hypertension compared to normotensive individuals.[38,39] sRAGE levels are inversely correlated with systolic blood pressure and pulse pressure. It appears that sRAGE is a marker for essential hypertension.

Homocysteine.

Homocysteine (Hcy) is a sulfur-containing amino acid derived from methionine and is essential for a number of biochemical processes including the metabolism of nucleic acids, fats, and high energy bonds. The synthesis and metabolism of Hcy involve three processes: demethylation, transmethylation, and transsulfuration, and are reviewed in detail elsewhere.[40] There are various ways by which Hcy is elevated in plasma and tissue: (i) methionine-rich protein diets, (ii) enzyme deficiency, (iii) vitamin deficiency, (iv) drugs, and (v) certain diseases.[40] Hyperhomocysteinemia is commonly associated with vitamin B12 and folic acid deficiency, the heterozyous/homozygous trait for β synthase, and polymorphism of methylenetetrahydrofolate reductase C677T.

Recently hyperhomocysteinemia has been implicated in the pathophysiology of hypertension.[41–44] Hcy, through various mechanisms could lead to endothelial cell dysfunction. Endothelial cell injury could be caused by generation of ORs by Hcy.[40] Autooxidation of Hcy generates superoxide anions and H_2O_2. Hcy also reduces antioxidant status. Endothelial dysfunction would reduce the formation of vasodilatory prostanoids and nitric oxide, and circulating vasoconstrictors in the blood would then have unopposed action on the vessels, resulting in hypertension.[40]

Hcy combines with nitric oxide to form s-nitrosohomocysteine, which is a weak vasodilator. ORs generated by Hcy would also destroy nitric oxide. These effects would reduce the bioavailability of nitric oxide resulting in the development of hypertension.[40] Nitric oxide combines with superoxide anion to form peroxynitrite in the mitrochondria. Peroxynitrite in the presence of thiol causes nitration of tyrosine, forming nitrotyrosine. Hcy thus could reduce the bioavailability of nitric oxide.[45]

Hcy breaks downs elastin through activation of matrix metalloproteinases (MMPs), which could lead to vascular stiffness.[45] Hcy proliferates vascular smooth muscle cells[46] and elicits calcium-dependent vascular contraction. These structural changes with Hcy lead to an increase in vascular resistance resulting in hypertension.

In summary, Hcy causes hypertension by (i) increasing ORs, (ii) decreasing bioavailability of nitric oxide and other vasodilator metabolites, (iii) increasing matrix metalloproteinase activity causing collagenolysis and increasing resistance, and (iv) altering the vascular matrix resulting in a decrease in the vascular lumen.

TABLE 9-2. Causes of Secondary Hypertension

A. Renal Disease
   Renovascular: renal artery stenosis, intrarenal
      vasculitis
   Renal parenchymal: acute glomerulonephritis,
      chronic nephritis, polycystic disease,
      diabetic nephropathy, hydronephrosis
   Renin-producing tumors
B. Endocrine
   Hyperthyroidism
   Hypothyroidism
   Hyperparathyroidism
   Acromegaly
   Adrenal cortex
     (i) Cushing's syndrome
     (ii) Primary aldosteronism
     (iii) Congenital adrenal hyperplasia
   Adrenal medulla
     (i) Pheochromocytoma
     (ii) Extra-adrenal chromaffin tumors
C. Heart and blood vessels
   Coarctation of aorta, aortic valvular insufficiency,
      A–V fistula, Paget's disease of bone, patent
      ductus arteriosus
D. Preeclampsia
E. Neurologic disorders
   Increased intracranial pressure: brain tumor,
      encephalitis, respiratory acidosis
   Quadriplegia
   Acute porphyria
   Guillain-Barré syndrome
   Sleep apnea
F. Exogenous substances
   Oral contraceptive pills
   Glucocorticoids
   Nonsteroidal anti-inflammatory drugs
   Cyclosporine
   Glycyrrhizinic acid (licorice)
   Sympathomimetics
   Tyramine-containing food
   Monoamine oxidase inhibitors
   Acute alcohol

Secondary Hypertension

There are numerous causes of secondary hypertension. Some of the important causes are shown in Table 9-2. The mechanism of hypertension and the diagnosis criteria are described briefly in the following section.

Renal Disease

Renovascular Hypertension. Pathophysiology of renovascular hypertension has been reviewed earlier.[47] Renal artery stenosis is responsible for 0.2% to 5% of all hypertension. Ninety percent of renovascular hypertension is caused by renal atherosclerosis and 10% is caused by fibromuscular dysplasia. There are two main mechanisms of this hypertension: (a) renin–Ang activation and (b) salt and water retention. Decrease in the renal perfusion pressure as a result of stenosis leads to hypertension. Renin is released as a result of decreased perfusion pressure at the juxtaglomerular cells, and decreased sodium and chloride delivery to macula densa cells in the ascending loop of Henle. Renin leads to the formation of Ang I and Ang II. As discussed in the blood pressure regulation section of this book, Ang II increases the peripheral vascular resistance and extracellular fluid.

Reduced renal arterial pressure reduces sodium excretion and minimizes the sodium excretory responses to natriuretic stimuli activated by volume expansion. Increased Ang II constricts vessels, stimulates net sodium reabsorption, and increases sodium retention through increased aldosterone. Thus the combination of renin and inadequate excretion of sodium induces hypertension. The management of this type of hypertension includes (a) medical therapy with Ang-converting enzyme inhibitor with or without a diuretic or calcium antagonist, (b) percutaneous transluminal renal angioplasty with or without stenting, and (c) surgery. Antihypertensive therapy should be used carefully as renal failure may ensue because of an excessive fall in pressure.

Renal Parenchymal Hypertension. Renal parenchymal hypertension is associated with glomerulonephritis, polycystic kidney, chronic pyelonephritis, and tubulointerstitial disease. Several factors are involved in the causation of renal parenchymal hypertension. There is an increase in intravascular sodium and volume, activation of the renin–Ang system (RAS), and increased sympathetic activity that could lead to hypertension in renal parenchymal disease. An endogenous compound, asymmetrical dimethylarginine (ADMA) is elevated in patients with uremia on chronic dialysis.[48] ADMA is an inhibitor of nitric oxide synthase, and hence it could contribute to hypertension. Oxidative stress, erythropoietin, parathyroid hormone, and divalent ions have also been implicated in this type of hypertension. The best tests of the relative role of the RAS in renal hypertension are the measurement of renal vein renin levels and testing the pressure change after administration of ACE inhibitors. Peripheral PRA is not very specific for renal disease. Changes in PRA in various conditions are given in Table 9-3. It is important to note that a high level of potassium lowers PRA. Potassium acts directly on the juxtaglomerular cells to inhibit renin release. Potassium also increases aldosterone secretion which in turn causes a loss of potassium. Since there is no need of vasoconstriction, there is no need of renin release.

Endocrine

Hyperthyroidism/Hypothyroidism[49–51]. The prevalence of hypertension in hyperthyroidism is between 20% and 30%. There is systolic hypertension in this case because of increased stroke volume, cardiac output, heart rate, and contractility. Because of decreased peripheral resistance,

TABLE 9-3. Changes in Plasma Renin Activity (PRA) in Various States

Increased PRA	*Decreased PRA*
• Renal vascular hypertension (renal vein)	• Low renin essential hypertension
• Renal secreting tumor	• Adrenal hyperplasia
• Parenchymal renal disease	• Aldosterone-secretive tumor
• Nephrotic syndrome	• Antisympathomimetic drugs
• Pregnancy or estrogen therapy	• Inhibitor of prostaglandin synthesis (nonsteroidal anti-inflammatory drugs)
• Adrenal insufficiency	• Hyperkalemia
• Cirrhosis of liver with ascites	• Hypernatremia
• Heart failure	
• Bartter's syndrome	
• Dehydration	
• Diuretics	
• Hemorrhage	
• Salt depletion	
• Vasodilators	
• Malignant hypertension	
• Standing	
• Exercise	
• Stress	
• Prostaglandin	
• ACE inhibitor and AngII blocker	
• Sympathomimetics	

diastolic pressure may even decrease. Patients with hyperthyroidism have normal or low levels of plasma norepinephrine. There might be increased density of β-adrenergic receptors. Pro-renin activity is increased in hyperthyroidism and that may activate the RAS to produce hypertension. An increase in PRA may be related to thyroid hormone-induced hepatic synthesis of renin substrate. However, administration of ACE inhibitors does not lower blood pressure in these patients suggesting no role of the RAS in hypertension in hyperthyroidism.

The prevalence of hypertension in hypothyroidism varies between 0% and 48%. The diastolic pressure is elevated, which is associated with increased peripheral vascular resistance. There is an increase in the levels of catecholamines and decreases in the levels of aldosterone and PRA, and density of β-adrenergic receptors.

Parathyroid. The prevalence of hypertension in primary hyperparathyroidism is between 10% and 60%, and in pseudohypoparathyroidism between 40% and 50%. Hypertension in hyperparathyroidism may be multifactorial because of a high prevalence of essential hypertension and hyperparathyroidism in the elderly population. Hypercalcemia in hyperparathyroidism may be responsible for hypertension. However hypocalcemia has also been shown to be associated with hypertension. Patients with both primary hyperparathyroidism and pseudohypoparathyroidism have high levels of parathyroid hormone and hypertension.

There are increased levels of PRA and aldosterone in hyperparathyroidism. Hypertension in hyperparathyroidism may be caused by increased levels of parathormone, PRA, and aldosterone. Parathyroidectomy normalizes the blood pressure.

Acromegaly. Fifty percent of patients with acromegaly develop hypertension. Hypertension may be caused by growth hormone-induced sodium retention, an increased sympathetic tone, and impaired endothelial cell-mediated vasodilation.

Adrenal Cortical Hormones

Primary Hyperaldosteronism[52,53]. Two-thirds of primary hyperaldosteronism is caused by an adrenal adenoma of the glomerulosa zone (Conn's syndrome) of usually one gland. Adrenal hyperplasia involving the glomerulosa zone of both glands is the second most common cause of primary hyperaldosteronism. Adrenal carcinomas are a rare cause (<2%) of primary hyperaldosteronism. Clinical features of primary hyperaldosteronism are nondistinctive.

Primary hyperaldosteronism is caused by high levels of aldosterone or compounds with mineralocorticoid action such as deoxycorticosterone. These hormones induce hypertension by increasing sodium and water reabsorption by the kidney, and hence increasing extracellular fluid volume. There is also increased peripheral vascular resistance. Aldosterone increases excretion of potassium.

Most symptoms are related to hypokalemia or water and salt retention and include tiredness, muscle weakness, thirst, polyuria, and nycturia. There is no edema in primary hyperaldosteronism. Hypertension that is present rarely reaches as high as 280/140 mm Hg. This condition is characterized by wide QT intervals with U waves in the ECG, myocardial fibrosis and left ventricular hypertrophy, impaired insulin secretion, diminished glucose tolerance, and blunted circulatory reflex responses with postural hypotension. Primary hyperaldosteronism is characterized by (a) High levels of aldosterone in blood (>10 ng/100 mL) and in urine (>20 μg/day). The best test for diagnosis is the measurement of 24 hour urinary aldosterone excretion during salt loading.[54] Twenty-four hour urinary aldosterone excretion rate >54 nmol with high sodium diet (>4 to 5 g sodium/d) distinguishes primary hyperaldosteronism from essential hypertension. (b) Low plasma renin levels. (c) Hypokalemia in most patients; however some patients are normokalemic. Severe hypokalemia is observed more in adrenal adenoma than in adrenal hyperplasia. (d) High urine potassium excretion because of the high level of aldosterone that increases reabsorption of sodium and excretion of potassium. A urinary excretion of potassium greater than 30 mmol/L daily in the presence of serum potassium lower than 3.5 mmol/L reflects renal potassium wasting. (e) Hypokalemic alkalosis because of loss of potassium along with hydrogen ions (H^+). H^+ enters the cells to replace potassium, which then lowers the H^+ concentration in the blood leading to alkalosis. (f) Mild hypomagnesemia.

A simultaneous measurement of plasma aldosterone concentration (PAC) and active plasma renin (aPR) is used to calculate the PAC/aPR ratio in pmol/L:mU/L, a sensitive screening test for primary hyperaldosteronism. This ratio is >80 in patients with primary hyperaldosteronism and <25 in patients with essential hypertension.

TESTS

(1) Imaging with CT and MRI are radiological procedures of choice that would be done after establishing a biochemical diagnosis as stated above. The CT scan does not detect adenoma.

(2) Sampling of adrenal venous blood with corticotrophin stimulation for measurement of aldosterone, and cortisol is considered the gold standard test for diagnosis but is risky.

(3) Nuclear scanning with 131_I-6 β-idiomethyl-19-norcholesterol in dexamethasone-suppressed patients with suspected adrenal hyperplasia is useful.

TREATMENT. Surgery is the best treatment for solitary tumors, with a success rate of 70%. The surgical success rate for bilateral hyperplasia is 20%. Medical treatment in patients who cannot be operated on includes diuretics and spironolactone, a competitive inhibitor of aldosterone.

Glucocorticoid Hypertension. Cortisol is a weak mineralocorticoid and has 1/400th the potency of aldosterone.

Its concentration is 1000 times higher than aldosterone. It can exert mineralocorticoid effects in high concentrations. It acts on the proximal tubules of the kidney to increase reabsorption of sodium and water.

Cushing's Syndrome. Hypertension (80%) and hypokalemia are presenting clinical features in Cushing's syndrome. The causes of Cushing's syndrome include Cushing's disease (68%), ectopic adrenocorticotrophic hormone excess (12%), adrenal adenoma (10%), adrenal carcinoma (8%), and adrenal hyperplasia (2%). Cushing's syndrome is characterized by an increased production of cortisol. The clinical presentations include truncal obesity, diabetes, hypertension, moon facies, plethora, easy bruising, muscle weakness and fatigue, amenorrhoea, libido, and osteoporosis. The mechanisms of hypertension in Cushing's syndrome are increased production of angiotensinogen in the liver, increased sensitivity of peripheral blood vessels to adrenergic drugs, and activation of the renal tubular mineralocorticoid receptors.

Adrenal Medullary Hormone

Pheochromocytoma[55]. Pheochromocytoma is a rare catecholamine-secreting tumor that produces hypertension (systolic and diastolic) in approximately 0.05% of patients with hypertension. Pheochromocytomas are tumors of chromaffin cells of the sympathetic nervous system. Two-thirds of pheochromocytomas develop in the adrenal medulla, one-third in the abdominal sympathetic chain, and a few arise in the bladder, neck, chest, ear, and eye. Most pheochromocytomas (90%) are benign, but 10% are malignant. Pheochromocytomas are familial in 10% of the cases. Adrenal pheochromocytomas arise bilaterally in 10% of cases, while 90% are unilateral.

CLINICAL FEATURES. Clinical features are primarily because of the release of norepinephrine and epinephrine and, to a lesser extent, to the cosecretion of other substances. Typical signs and symptoms include:

(1) Hypertension, primarily systolic in epinephrine secretors (adrenal medulla), and systolic plus diastolic pressures in norepinephrine secretors (non adrenal medulla origin). Fifty percent have sustained hypertension, 45% have paroxysmal hypertension, and 5% remain normotensive, especially those with familial tumors.

(2) Severe headache.

(3) Sweating.

(4) Palpitation with tachycardia, but rarely reflex bradycardia.

(5) Perspiration/pallor.

(6) Nervousness.

(7) Nausea and vomiting.

The classical triad of symptoms consists of headache, perspiration/pallor, and palpitation, has an episodic character, and occurs in up to 95% of persons. Hypertension is also paroxysmal in 50% of cases and sustained in the other 50%. Hyperepinephrinemia and hypernorepinephrinemia may cause hyperglycemia, triglyceridemia and hyperreninemia, weight loss, constipation, and, rarely, ischemic enterocolitis. Paroxysms of these signs and symptoms can be provoked by a variety of stimuli, such as smoking, drugs, exercise, fear, anesthetics, food, and micturition.

DIAGNOSTIC TESTS

(1) Measurement of plasma free metanephrine and normetanephrine. These metabolites of epinephrine and norepinephrine are continuously produced within the pheochromocytoma cells and circulate in the blood. Plasma free metanephrine and normetanephrine are less influenced by physiologic activation. The sensitivity of free metanephrine and normetanephrine in the diagnosis of pheochromocytoma is 100% and 97%, respectively.

(2) Measurement of 24 hour urinary metanephrine and normetanephrine is considered to be the preferred diagnostic test. The upper limit of normal for metanephrine is 200 nmol/mmol creatine (<1500 nmol/24 h) and for normetanephrine is 250 nmol/mmol creatine (<4500 nmol/24 h).

(3) Measurement of plasma and urinary catecholamines may be useful when clinical symptoms are highly suggestive of pheochromocytoma.

(4) A clonidine-suppression test should be done if catecholamine levels are elevated. A positive clonidine-suppression test is indicated by failure of the plasma catecholamines to fall at least 40% from baseline after a single oral dose of 0.3 mg clonidine.

(5) The glucagon stimulation test is a provocative test and stimulates secretion of catecholamines by adrenal tumors but not by normal adrenal glands. Pheochromocytomas have receptors for glucagon. The glucagon stimulation test is positive when the plasma catecholamine level rises to threefold 2 minutes after a bolus intravenous administration of 1 mg glucagon.

(6) Measurement of urinary vanillylmandelic acid, the end product of catecholamine metabolism, provides the sum of all catecholamines. However, this test is imprecise and the sensitivity is only 46%. Drugs and foods that can interfere with levels of catecholamines and metabolites include:
  • Vanilla, which interferes with measurement of catecholamines based on vanillylmandelic acid.
  • Foods such as banana, coffee, or chocolate.
  • Drugs such as methyldopa, levadopa, labetalol, sotalol, tricyclic antidepressants, and antipsychotic drugs that contain catecholamines, benzodiazepines, acetaminophen, phenoxybenzamine, and ethanol.
  • Major physical stress.

(7) CT scan and MRI should be used to locate the tumor after biochemical tests have confirmed the diagnosis of pheochromocytoma.

TREATMENT. Surgical removal of the tumor is the definitive therapy.

Heart and Blood Vessels

Coarctation of Aorta[56,57]. Coarctation, narrowing of the aorta, produces hypertension. The incidence of adult hypertension is 75% in patients 20 to 30 years after surgery. Of these approximately 3% to 26% have recurrence of coarctation. Repair after the age of 10 is associated with increased hypertension in adult life. Hypertension related to coarctation of the aorta can be classified into three categories: prerepair hypertension, postrepair paradoxical hypertension, and late postrepair hypertension. The mechanism of hypertension in these three types seems to be different.

Prerepair hypertension may be caused by mechanical obstruction to left ventricular output, leading to hypertension proximal to the obstruction, readjustment of aortic baroreceptors to provide adequate blood supply to organs distal to the obstruction, and stimulation of the RAS. Obstruction (constriction) in the aorta produces renal hypoperfusion, which leads to activation of the RAS. When patients with coarctation of the aorta become volume depleted, PRA is increased and blood pressure becomes responsive to ACE inhibitors and Ang II blockers.

Postrepair paradoxical hypertension occurs during the first week after surgery. There are two mechanisms of this hypertension: the sympathetic nervous system and the RAS. Damage of the afferent sympathetic nerve during surgery may cause an imbalance between excitatory and inhibitory sympathetic mechanoreceptors leading to an increase in sympathetic activity, which in turn could activate the RAS.

Late postrepair hypertension may be caused by increased vascular reactivity to norepinephrine in the arm and normal vascular reactivity in the legs.

Several studies have implicated the RAS and the sympathetic nervous system in the development of hypertension in patients with coarctation of the aorta. However, the results are not conclusive. After repair of the coarctation of the aorta, changes in the vascular bed and hemodynamics occur in the prestenotic vessels despite normal circulating levels of renin and catecholamines at rest. An increase in pressure in the prestenotic aortic arch could lead to left ventricular hypertrophy and hyperkinesis, increased aortic stiffness, structural changes in the arterial wall and exaggerated vascular responses, depletion of vasodilatory mediators, abnormal baroreceptor responses, and an increased release of catecholamines and renin in response to stimuli. These changes could ultimately lead to sustained hypertension and exercise-induced hypertension.

CLINICAL SIGNS AND SYMPTOMS

  • Arterial pressure is higher in the arms than in the legs or in one arm compared to the other. There is a systolic pressure gradient between the right arm and the legs. Normally thigh pressure is slightly higher than pressure in the arms.

- Diminished femoral pulses.
- Systolic murmur over the chest, best heard in the posterior left interscapular area.
- Occasional pain and weakness in the legs during exercise.
- Abnormal responses to exercise. There is an excessive increase in the systolic pressure with delay in recovery.

DIAGNOSTIC TESTS

- CT or MRI.
- Echocardiography.
- Chest X-ray showing a dent along the right-hand edge of the profile of the aorta, and notching of the ribs.

TREATMENT. Treatment includes surgical correction of the coarctation of the aorta, balloon angioplasty, and stenting.

Sleep Apnea[58]. Sleep apnea is a sleep disorder in breathing characterized by more than five apneas or hypopneas per hour of sleep, and daytime hypersomnolence. Its prevalence in adults is 2% for women and 4% for men. Fifty to ninety percent of individuals with sleep apnea have hypertension. The evidence suggests that there is a causal relationship between sleep apnea and hypertension. There are marked fluctuations in systolic and diastolic pressure associated with moderate to severe sleep apnea.

There are at least three factors that may be involved in the development of hypertension in patients with sleep apnea.

(1) Activation of the sympathetic nervous system.
(2) Activation of the RAS. PRA is reduced in individuals with sleep apnea. Sleep apnea and hypoxia raise plasma levels of atrial natriuretic peptide, which inhibits release of plasma renin.
(3) Endothelial dysfunction. There is an increase in the levels of endothelin and a decrease in the levels of nitric oxide in the blood of subjects with sleep apnea. Endothelin is a vasoconstrictor and nitric oxide is a vasodilator.

Preeclampsia[59,60]. Preeclampsia is characterized by hypertension, proteinuria, edema, consumptive coagulopathy, sodium retention, and hyperreflexia during pregnancy. The incidence of preeclampsia is over 3% of all pregnancies, 7% in nulliparous, and 20% to 25% in high risk populations such as patients with diabetes, renal disease, or those carrying twins. The underlying mechanism of hypertension is not well understood. Despite sodium retention, intravascular volume is contracted. The hypertension may be caused by increased vascular reactivity, sympathetic activity, and activity of the renin–Ang–aldosterone system.

Increased vascular reactivity has been postulated to be caused by an imbalance between vasodilator prostaglandins and nitric acid, and vasoconstrictors such as endothelin, Ang II, and their receptor density. Endothelial dysfunction may be present because of oxidative stress and increased levels of cytokines. There is an imbalance between oxidants and antioxidants during preeclampsia. Insulin resistance is associated with hyperinsulinemia, which may increase sympathetic activity. Patients with preeclampsia have lower levels of circulating renin, Ang II, and aldosterone. However there is upregulation of Ang II receptor. An increased sensitivity to Ang II is the basis for the "roll-over test." In the supine position the reduction in venous return because of compression by gravid uterus increases circulating Ang II resulting in hypertensive responses.

Neurologic Disorders. Many neurologic disorders cause hypertension. They will be discussed briefly in the following section.

Intracranial tumors are associated with hypertension because of increased intracranial pressure, increased catecholamine production, and direct stimulation or inhibition of cardiovascular centers in the medulla.

In spinal cord injury, acute hypertension is a result of sympathetic activation caused by a spinal reflex mechanism called autonomic dysreflexia. Autonomic dysreflexia occurs with spinal cord injury at level-T6 or higher. Bladder distension below the level of the lesion generates spinal cord-mediated sympathetic activation.

Hypertension after brain injury is caused by increased intracranial pressure via Cushing response, which is defined as hypertension caused by increased intracranial pressure. Injury to blood pressure regulatory centers in the medulla and increased levels of circulating catecholamines may also contribute to hypertension.

Exogenous Substances

Oral Contraceptives[61]. Approximately 5% of women using oral contraceptives develop arterial hypertension in the first year and some become severely hypertensive. The incidence of hypertension with use of estrogen increases with time and goes up to 15% after 5 year use. Obesity and a family history of hypertension increase the odds for development of hypertension.

The following factors are involved in estrogen-induced hypertension:

(1) Estrogen increases the synthesis of the renin substrate angiotensinogen in the liver. Increased amounts of Ang I and Ang II are generated in the presence of increased angiotensinogen and renin. Ang II increases production of aldosterone. As a result of increased Ang II, renin release is inhibited resulting in a decrease in its concentration in blood. However, PRA is elevated despite a decrease in plasma renin concentration. The rise in blood pressure would thus be caused by increased plasma

volume as a result of sodium retention and by Ang II induced vasoconstriction.

(2) Estrogen potentiates the actions of catecholamines by inducing an increase in the number of catecholamine receptors. Postmenopausal estrogen use may induce hypertension but not as much as the use of estrogen for contraception.

Alcohol. Several epidemiological and clinical studies have established a clear association between alcohol consumption and hypertension. In contrast to the immediate vasodilator effect of alcohol, chronic consumption, even of moderate quantities, may raise the blood pressure. In larger quantities alcohol may be responsible for significant hypertension. More than 6 units of alcohol/d increases the prevalence of hypertension twofold to threefold as compared to a nondrinker.

There are numerous possible mechanisms of alcohol-induced hypertension.

(1) Stimulation of the sympathetic nervous system.[62]

(2) Insulin resistance with subsequent hyperinsulinemia. Low blood pressure in a low alcohol consumer may be related to improved insulin sensitivity.[63]

(3) Increased cortisol secretion.

(4) Alcohol induces diuresis, which can decrease plasma volume resulting in activation of the renin–Ang–aldosterone system.

(5) Alteration in cell membrane function resulting in increased intracellular calcium. Alcohol oxidation in the body results in the production of acetaldehyde. A low concentration of acetaldehyde is vasoconstrictive. Acetaldehyde binds with calmodulin and may inhibit the calmodulin-dependent calcium pump that pumps calcium out of the cell. This effect of acetaldehyde would increase intracellular calcium. Acetaldehyde may affect the calcium channel by binding to the sulfhydryl group of calcium channel proteins. Disruption of the vascular calcium channel by acetaldehyde could increase intracellular calcium resulting in increased vascular tone and hence hypertension. Vasdev et al.[64] have reported that alcohol increases the uptake of calcium in aortic tissue and platelets.

● COMPLICATIONS OF HYPERTENSION

There are two types of pathology associated with hypertension: (a) hypertensive vascular disease and (b) target organ pathology.

Hypertensive Vascular Disease

Hypertension increases arterial wall tension as well as tissue and plasma mediators of endothelial cell injury, which leads to arterial smooth muscle hyperplasia and hypertrophy, and increased endothelial permeability to plasma electrolytes, H_2O_2, and protein. Tissue and plasma mediators may include catecholamines, renin, endothelin, CRP, Hcy, growth factors, cytokines, etc. Some of these mediators increase the synthesis of DNA, RNA, protein, collagen, elastin, and acid mucopolysaccharides resulting in fibromuscular thickening of the intima and the media of large and small arteries. Fibromuscular thickening of the arteries would lead to hypertensive vascular disease resulting in increased peripheral vascular resistance and acceleration of atherosclerotic disease. Increased peripheral resistance would further increase the blood pressure. Hypertension begets hypertension. Most of the premature morbidity and mortality associated with hypertension is related to atherosclerosis. In the response-to-injury hypothesis of atherosclerosis, endothelial cell injury leads to a cascade of events resulting in atherosclerosis.[65,66]

Target Organ Pathology

Heart Failure and Ischemic Heart Disease. The sequence of heart failure and ischemic heart disease is shown in Figure 9-1. Hypertension increases left ventricular systolic pressure leading to an increase in intramyocardial wall tension. Increased wall tension induces left ventricular hypertrophy and a decrease in myocardial contractility resulting in heart failure. Increased myocardial wall tension and left ventricular hypertrophy increase myocardial oxygen demand. Oxygen supply is compromised because vascular growth does not parallel myocardial growth. Oxygen supply is also compromised because of hypertensive vascular changes in the coronary arteries that would lead to narrowing of coronary arteries. Thus there is an imbalance between myocardial oxygen supply and demand, which leads to myocardial ischemia (angina) and myocardial infarct, which also contribute to heart failure. Cardiac arrhythmia that occurs in ischemia/infarction could also lead to the development of heart failure.

Cerebrovascular Disease and Stroke. The mechanism of cerebrovascular disease and stroke in hypertensives is schematically represented in Figure 9-2. Hypertension via increased cerebral arterial wall tension produces fibromuscular thickening of cerebral arteries, both small and large. Narrowing of small vessels produces hypertensive microvascular disease including cerebral ischemia, intracerebral microaneurysm, and microthrombi. Cerebral ischemia causes ischemic attack. Microthrombi cause microinfarcts leading to thrombotic stroke. A rupture of a microaneurysm leads to cerebral hemorrhage resulting in hemorrhagic stroke. Hypertensive stroke includes both hemorrhagic and thrombotic strokes.

Fibromuscular thickening of large and small vessels leads to hypertensive and atherosclerotic vascular disease. Hypertensive and atherosclerotic disease of the cerebral arteries may cause cerebral thrombosis leading to an atherothrombotic stroke. Narrowing of the large and small vessels could produce cerebral ischemia resulting in transient ischemic attacks. Hypertension predisposes to stroke in three different ways:

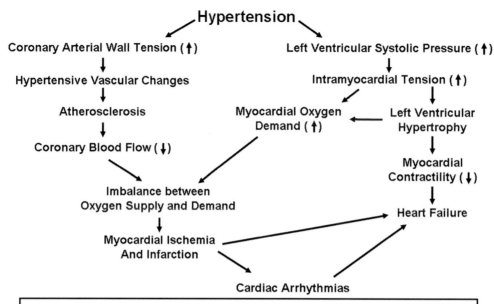

Adverse Effects of Hypertension on Heart

● FIGURE 9-1. Cardiovascular complications in hypertension: (↑), increase; (↓), decrease.

Modified from Hollander W. Role of hypertension in atherosclerosis and cardiovascular disease. Am J Cardiol. 1976;38:786, used with permission.

(1) Accelerated atherosclerosis, with thrombosis of large arteries, causes cerebral infarction. The intimal plaques and narrowing of the lumen predispose to thrombi. This mechanism accounts for 80% of all strokes.

(2) Rupture of berry aneurysms of the circle of Willis with subarachnoid hemorrhage accounts for 10% of all strokes.

(3) Rupture of tiny microaneurysms in small vessels (Charcot–Bouchard aneurysms) with hemorrhage

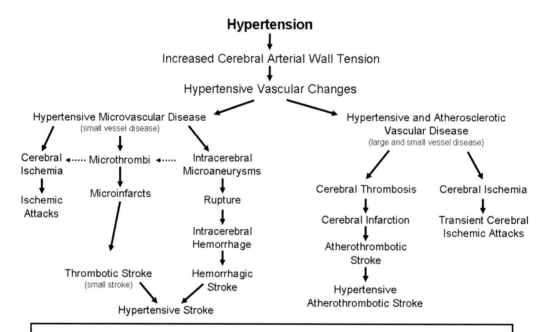

Hypertension and Cerebrovascular Disease and Stroke

● FIGURE 9-2. Cerebrovascular complications in hypertension.

Modified from Hollander W. Role of hypertension in atherosclerosis and cardiovascular disease. Am J Cardiol. 1976;38:786, used with permission.

in the brain parenchyma accounts for 10% of all strokes.

Hypertensive Retinopathy. Microscopic changes in the retinal arterioles in hypertension are:

(1) Thickening of the arterial wall presses on the soft veins where they criss-cross. This causes the "A–V nicking" seen on retinal examination.

(2) Hemorrhages into the retina from ruptured arterioles.

(3) Exudates, composed of partially reabsorbed hemorrhages, seen as cottony or waxy spots.

Grades I and II hypertensive retinopathy comprises changes in retinal arterioles showing generalized narrowing. Grades III and IV hypertensive retinopathy comprises changes that involve the retina, optic disc, and choroid plexus. These changes include microaneurysms, intraretinal hemorrhages, cotton–wool spots, hard exudates or macular stars, and papilloedema. A flame-shaped hemorrhage is the hallmark of hypertension.

Renal Dysfunction. Hypertension causes structural and functional renal dysfunction. There is hyalinization and sclerosis of the afferent arteriolar walls. Renal involvement is usually asymptomatic. Nocturia may be the first indication. Microalbuminuria is the first sign and serves as a marker for impaired kidney function. Microalbuminuria is not only a predictor of progressive renal damage but also a predictor of cardiovascular morbidity.

● CAUSES OF MORTALITY IN HYPERTENSIVES

The mortality rates in hypertensives are as follows:

(1) Congestive heart failure: 45%

(2) Ischemic heart disease: 35%

(3) Cerebrovasuclar accidents: 15%

(4) Renal failure: 5%

● MANAGEMENT OF HYPERTENSION

This chapter reviews the general guidelines recommended for management of hypertension by the Seventh Joint National Committee on Prevention, Detection, Evaluation and Treatment of High Blood Pressure (JNC-7),[6] the American Diabetic Association, the National Kidney Foundation, and the Canadian Guideline.[67] This is a guideline only and details for therapeutic drugs and their doses will be given. Other sources should be examined for therapeutic agents, their mechanisms of action, doses, and side effects.

The goal of the management of hypertension is to reduce cardiovascular and renal morbidity and mortality. The aim is to reduce blood pressure to <140/90 mm Hg. In hypertensive patients with diabetes and/or renal disease, the goal is <130/80 mm Hg. Lowering blood pressure has three benefits: (i) reduction in incidence of stroke by 35% to 40%; (ii) reduction in myocardial infarction by 20% to 25%, and (iii) reduction in heart failure by more than 50%. A healthy lifestyle prevents the development of hypertension and is an important part of the management of hypertension. Prehypertensive individuals (systolic pressure between 120 and 140 mm Hg) would benefit from lifestyle changes. However if those patients have diabetes or kidney disease, pharmacological agents should be instituted as well as lifestyle changes. The management of hypertension is therefore divided into two parts: (a) lifestyle modifications and (b) Therapeutic approaches.

Lifestyle Modifications

Lifestyle modifications can lower blood pressure, reduce incidence of diabetes, reduce lipid levels, and improve quality of life. Modification in lifestyle is expected to reduce systolic blood pressure by 5 mm Hg and hence reduce the mortality of stroke by 14%, coronary artery disease by 9%, and mortality by all causes by 7% in the general population. Lifestyle modification is the first-line treatment for prevention and management of hypertension. Lifestyle modifications include the following:

Weight Reduction

The ideal weight is calculated as body mass index and should be between 18.5 to 24.9 kg/m^2, and waist circumference less than 102 cm for men and 88 cm for women. Weight loss as little as 4.5 kg (10 lbs) reduces blood pressure and/or prevents hypertension. Weight reduction reduces the systolic blood pressure by approximately 5 to 20 mm Hg /10 kg.

Physical Exercise

For both hypertensives and nonhypertensives 30 to 60 minutes of moderate exercise (walking, jogging, cycling, or swimming) for 4 to 7 days a week is recommended. Higher intensities of exercise are not more effective. An intensity of 50% to 69% of maximum heart rate is considered moderate, and an intensity greater than 70% of maximum heart rate is vigorous exercise. Maximum heart rate is calculated by subtracting age from 220. An approximate reduction in systolic blood pressure is 4 to 9 mm Hg.

Dietary Approach

Dietary approaches to stop hypertension, termed the DASH diet, includes fruits, vegetables, low fat dairy products, whole grains, poultry, fish and nuts, small amounts of red meat and sugar, with low amounts of dietary cholesterol, total fat, and saturated fat. This diet reduces systolic blood pressure by approximately 8 to 14 mm Hg. The therapeutic effects of the DASH diet approach the level of pharmacologic treatment with a single drug.

Dietary Sodium. Dietary sodium should be reduced to 100 mmol per day, that is, 2.4 g sodium or 6 g sodium choride daily, for normotensive individuals at increased risk of developing hypertension and considered salt sensitive (Canadians of African descent, persons older than 45 years, and persons with chronic kidney disease or diabetes). Sodium intake in patients with hypertension should be reduced to 65 mmol/d (1.56 g). This diet reduces systolic blood pressure by 2 to 8 mm Hg.

Potassium, Calcium, and Magnesium. Patients with hypertension, or normotensives at risk of developing hypertension and considered salt sensitive, should have an adequate intake of potassium, calcium, and magnesium from their diet. At least 80 mmol of potassium per day should be taken.

Alcohol. Alcohol consumption should be limited to no more than two drinks per day in most men and no more than one drink per day in women and light weight persons. One drink is considered 13.6 g or 17.2 mL of ethanol, 1.5 ounces of 80 proof whisky, 12 oz of 5% beer, or 5 ounces of 12% wine. Moderate alcohol consumption reduces systolic blood pressure by 2 to 4 mm Hg.

Flaxseed Diet. Flaxseed slightly lowers blood pressure. However the lignan (secoisolariciresinol diglucoside) isolated from flaxseed has a potent hypotensive effect in animal studies.[68] Secoisolariciresinol diglucoside also lowers blood cholesterol and blood glucose. This compound is beneficial for metabolic syndrome. FDA-approved flax lignan complex, which contains 35% secoisolariciresinol diglucoside, reduces serum cholesterol and atherosclerosis.[69] It is available on the market as Beneflax as a dietary supplement.

Stress Management

Stress management should be considered as an adjunct therapy for treatment of hypertension: stress includes socioeconomic status, job stress, etc.

Therapeutic Approaches

A large number of drugs are available for reducing blood pressure. Details of commonly used drugs, their usual dose range, and frequency of administration can be obtained from the JNC-7 report.[6] Commonly used antihypertensive drugs are: diuretics (thiazide, loop, potassium-sparing), aldosterone receptor blockers, beta adrenergic blockers (BBs), alpha-1 blockers, central alpha-2 agonists, combined alpha and BBs (Carvedilol), Ang-converting enzyme inhibitors (ACEIs), Ang II antagonists, calcium channel blockers (CCBs) (dihydropyridines and nondihydropyridines), and direct vasodilators.

Indications for Treatment of Adult Hypertension Without Compelling Indications for Specific Agents

(1) Therapy is indicated in individuals with systolic pressure ≥160 mm Hg and diastolic pressure ≥100 mm Hg in patients without macrovascular target organ damage or other risk factors.

(2) Individuals with diastolic pressure ≥90 mm Hg in the presence of target organ damage or other cardiovascular risk factors.

(3) Individuals with systolic pressure ≥140 mm Hg.

Therapeutic Algorithm

Therapy should start with lifestyle modification. If the blood pressure goal (<140/90 mm Hg or <130/80 mm Hg for patients with diabetes or chronic kidney disease) is not achieved, the drug choices depend upon the compelling or noncompelling indications. Compelling indications are hypertensive patients with heart failure, postmyocardial infarction, coronary artery disease, chronic renal disease or diabetes, or the need to prevent recurrent stroke.

Initial drug choices for stage I hypertension without compelling indications are monotherapy with thiazide diuretics, ACEIs, Ang receptor blockers (ARBs), BBs, CCBs, or a combination. For stage II hypertension without compelling indications the therapeutic choices are combinations of thiazide diuretics and ACEIs or ARBs, BBs, or CCBs. For additional hypotensive effect in dual therapy a drug combination from group A (thiazide diuretic or long acting CCB) and group B (CCBs or ACEIs) should be considered.

Initial therapy with more than one drug increases the likelihood of achieving the blood pressure goal. Combination therapy produces greater reduction in blood pressure at lower doses, resulting in fewer side effects.

More than 66% of individuals with hypertension cannot be controlled with one drug and will require two or more drugs selected from different classes of drugs. Low dose aspirin should be considered only when the blood pressure is controlled because of an increased risk of hemorrhagic stroke when hypertension is not controlled.

Recommended therapy for hypertension with compelling indications are as follows:

(1) Hypertension with heart failure: diuretics, BB, ACEI, ARB, CCB.

(2) Hypertension with postmyocardial infarction: BB, ACEI.

(3) Hypertension with high coronary disease risk: diuretics, BB, ACEI, CCB.

(4) Hypertension with diabetes: diuretics, BB, ACEI, ARB, CCB.

(5) Hypertension with chronic renal disease: ACEI, ARB.

(6) Hypertension and recurrent stroke prevention: diuretics, ACEI.

If blood pressure target is not achieved after use of combination of three of more drugs, one should consider reasons for not achieving the target. Some of the reasons may include, secondary hypertension, nonadherence, interfering substances, WCHT, or other causes of resistant hypertension.

● ACKNOWLEDGEMENTS

The author is very thankful to Ms. Barbara Raney and Ms. Gladys Wiebe for their valuable assistance in the preparation of this manuscript for the book.

REFERENCES

1. Joffres MR, Ghadirian P, Fodor JG, et al. Awareness, treatment, and control of hypertension in Canada. *Am J Hypertens.* 1997;10:1097.

2. Calhoun DA, Oparil S. Gender and blood pressure. In: Izzo JL Jr, Black HR, eds. *Hypertension Primer.* 3rd ed. Philadelphia: Lippincott Williams & Wilkins; 2003:253.

3. Burt VL, Whelton P, Roccella EJ, et al. Prevalence of hypertension in the US adult population: results from the Third National Health and Nutrition Examination Survey, 1988–1991. *Hypertension.* 1995;25:305.

4. Onysko J, Maxwell C, Eliasziw M, et al. Canadian Hypertension Education Program. Large increases in hypertension diagnosis and treatment in Canada after a healthcare professional education program. *Hypertension.* 2006;48:853.

5. Hyman DJ, Pavlik VN. Self-reported hypertension treatment practices among primary care physicians: blood pressure thresholds, drug choices, and the role of guidelines and evidence-based medicine. *Arch Intern Med.* 2000;160: 2281.

6. The Seventh Report of the Joint National Committee on Prevention, Detection, Evaluation, and Treatment of High Blood Pressure. National Heart, Lung, and Blood Institute, National Institutes of Health, August 2004; NIH publication no. 04-5230.

7. Guidelines Committee of the European Society of Hypertension—European Society of Cardiology. 2003 European Society of Hypertension—-European Society of Cardiology guidelines for the management of arterial hypertension. *J Hypertens.* 2003;21:1011.

8. Black HR, Kuller LH, O'Rourke MF, et al. The first report of the Systolic and Pulse Pressure (SYPP) Working Group. *J Hypertens.* 1999;17(suppl 5):S3.

9. Rabbia F, Del Colle S, Testa E, et al. Accuracy of the blood pressure measurement. *Minerva Cardioangiol.* 2006;54:399.

10. Verberk WJ, Kroon AA, Thient T, et al. Prevalence of the white-coat effect at multiple visits before and during treatment. *J Hypertens.* 2006;24:2357.

11. Binder A. Identification of genes for a complex trait: examples from hypertension. *Curr Pharm Biotechnol.* 2006;7:1.

12. Zhu H, Wang X, Lu Y, et al. Update on G-protein polymorphisms in hypertension. *Curr Hypertens Rep.* 2006;8:23.

13. Casas JP, Cavalleri GL, Bautista LE, et al. Endothelial nitric oxide synthase gene polymorphisms and cardiovascular disease: a HuGE review. *Am J Epidemiol.* 2006;164:921.

14. Sharma AM, Schorr U, Distler A. Insulin resistance in young salt-sensitive normotensive subjects. *Hypertension.* 1993;21:273.

15. Vasdev S, Ford CA, Longerich L, et al. Aldehyde induced hypertension in rats: prevention by N-acetyl cysteine. *Artery.* 1998;23:10.

16. Baron AD. Hemodynamic actions of insulin. *Am J Physiol.* 1994;267:E187.

17. Alt N, Carson JA, Alderson NL, et al. Chemical modification of muscle protein in diabetes. *Arch Biochem Biophys.* 2004;425:200.

18. Vasdev S, Gill V, Parai S, et al. Dietary vitamin E supplementation attenuates hypertension in Dahl salt-sensitive rats. *J Cardiovasc Pharmacol Ther.* 2005;10:103.

19. Wu L, Juurlink BH. Increased methylglyoxal and oxidative stress in hypertensive rat vascular smooth muscle cells. *Hypertension.* 2002;39:809.

20. Prasad K. Oxygen free radicals and peripheral vascular disease. In: Chang JB, Olson ER, Prasad K, Sumpio BE, eds. *Textbook of Angiology.* New York: Springer Verlag; 2000:427.

21. Prasad K, Kalra J, Chan WP, et al. Effect of oxygen free radicals on cardiovascular function at organ and cellular levels. *Am Heart J.* 1989;117:1196.

22. Prasad K, Kalra J, Chaudhary AK, et al. Effect of polymorphonuclear leukocyte-derived oxygen free radicals and hypochlorous acid on cardiac function and some biochemical parameters. *Am Heart J.* 1990;119:538.

23. Bharadwaj LA, Prasad K. Mechanisms of superoxide anion-induced modulation of vascular tone. *Int J Angiol.* 2002;11:23.

24. Bharadwaj LA, Prasad K. Mediation of H_2O_2-induced vascular relaxation by endothelium-derived relaxing factor. *Mol Cell Biochem.* 1995;149/150:267.

25. Sagar S, Kallo IJ, Kaul N, et al. Oxygen free radicals in essential hypertension. *Mol Cell Biochem.* 1992;111:103.

26. Kumar KV, Das UN. Are free radicals involved in the pathobiology of human essential hypertension? *Free Radic Res Commun.* 1993;19:59.

27. Lassegue B, Griendling KK. Reactive oxygen species in hypertension, an update. *Am J Hypertens.* 2004;17:852.

28. Rahman I, Nath N. Glutathione and its redox system, superoxide anion and superoxide dismutases of polymorphonuclear leukocytes in essential hypertension. *Indian J Med Res.* 1988;88:64.

29. Prasad K. Oxyradicals as a mechanism of angiotensin-induced hypertension. *Int J Angiol.* 2004;13:59.

30. Beswick RA, Dorrance AM, Leite R, et al. NADH/NADPH oxidase and enhanced superoxide production in the mineralocorticoid hypertensive rat. *Hypertension.* 2001;38:1107.

31. Zalba G, Beaumont FJ, San Jose G, et al. Vascular NADH/NADPH oxidase is involved in enhanced superoxide production in spontaneously hypertensive rats. *Hypertension.* 2000;35:1055.

32. Zalba G, San Jose G, Moreno MU, et al. NADPH oxidase-mediated oxidative stress: genetic studies of the p22 (phox) gene in hypertension. *Antioxid Redox Signal.* 2005;7:1327.

33. Prasad K. C-reactive protein and cardiovascular diseases. *Int J Angiol.* 2003;12:1.

34. Yasunari K, Maeda K, Nakamura M, et al. Oxidative stress in leukocytes is a possible link between blood pressure, blood glucose and C-reacting protein. *Hypertension.* 2002;39:777.

35. Fadl YY, Zareba W, Moss AJ, et al. History of hypertension and enhanced thrombogenic activity in postinfarction patients. *Hypertension.* 2003;41:943.

36. Prasad K. C-reactive protein increases oxygen radical generation by neutrophils. *J Cardiovasc Pharmacol Ther.* 2004;9:203.

37. Prasad K. Soluble receptor for advanced glycation end products (sRAGE) and cardiovascular disease. *Int J Angiol* 2006;15:57.

38. Geroldi D, Falcone C, Emanuele E, et al. Decreased plasma levels of soluble receptor for advanced glycation end-products in patients with essential hypertension. *J Hypertens.* 2005;23:1725.

39. Nakamura K, Yamagishi S, Nakamura Y, et al. Telmisartan inhibits expression of a receptor for advanced glycation end products (RAGE) in angiotensin II-exposed endothelial cells and decreases serum levels of soluble RAGE in patients with essential hypertension. *Microvasc Res.* 2005;70:137.

40. Prasad K. Homocysteine, a risk factor for cardiovascular disease. *Int J Angiol.* 1999;8:76.

41. Malinow MR, Levenson J, Giral P, et al. Role of blood pressure, uric acid, and hemorheological parameters on plasma homocyst(e)ine concentration. *Atherosclerosis.* 1995;114:175.

42. Sutton-Tyrrell K, Bostom A, Selhub J, et al. High homocysteine levels are independently related to isolated systolic hypertension in older adults. *Circulation.* 1997;96:1745.

43. Levenson J, Malinow MR, Giral P, et al. Increased plasma homocysteine levels in human hypertension. *J Hypertens.* 1994;12:S74.

44. Ustundag S, Arikan E, Sens S, et al. The relationship between the levels of plasma total homocysteine and insulin resistance in uncomplicated mild-to-moderate primary hypertension. *J Hum Hypertens.* 2006;20:379.

45. Tyagi N, Moshal KS, Ovechkin AV, et al. Mitochondrial mechanism of oxidative stress and systemic hypertension in hyperhomocysteinemia. *J Cell Biochem.* 2005;96:665.

46. Tsai JC, Perrella MA, Yoshizumi M, et al. Promotion of vascular smooth muscle cell growth by homocysteine: a link to atherosclerosis. *Proc Natl Acad Sci USA.* 1994;91:6369.

47. Martinez-Maldonado M. Pathophysiology of renovascular hypertension. *Hypertension.* 1991;17:707.

48. Kielstein JT, Boger RH, Bode-Boger SM, et al. Marked increase of asymmetric dimethylarginine in patients with incipient primary chronic renal disease. *J Am Soc Nephrol.* 2002;13:170.

49. Akpunonu BE, Mulrow PJ, Hoffman EA. Secondary hypertension: evaluation and treatment. *Dis Mon.* 1996;42:609.

50. Saito I, Ito K, Saruta T. Hypothyroidism as a cause of hypertension. *Hypertension.* 1983;5:112.

51. Bergus GR, Mold JW, Barton ED, et al. The lack of association between hypertension and hypothyroidism in a primary care setting. *J Hum Hypertens.* 1999;13:231.

52. Fardella CE, Mosso L, Gomez-Sanchez C, et al. Primary hyperaldosteronism in essential hypertensives: prevalence, biochemical profile, and molecular biology. *J Clin Endocrinol Metab.* 2000;85:1863.

53. Ganguly A. Prevalence of primary aldosteronism in unselected hypertensive populations: screening and definitive diagnosis. *J Clin Endocrinol Metab.* 2001;86:4002.

54. Bravo EL, Tarazi RC, Dustan HP, et al. The changing clinical spectrum of primary aldosteronism. *Am J Med.* 1983;74:641.

55. Manger WM, Gifford RW. Pheochromocytoma. *J Clin Hypertens* (*Greenwich*). 2002;4:62.

56. Mullen MJ. Coarctation of the aorta in adults: do we need surgeons? *Heart.* 2003;89:3.

57. Barton CH, Ni Z, Vaziri ND. Enhanced nitric oxide inactivation in aortic coarctation-induced hypertension. *Kidney Int.* 2001;60:1083.

58. Nieto FJ, Young TB, Lind BK, et al. Association of sleep-disordered breathing, sleep apnea, and hypertension in a large community based study. Sleep Heart and Health Study. *JAMA.* 2000;283:1829.

59. Walker JJ. Pre-eclampsia. *Lancet.* 2000;356:1260.

60. Schobel HP, Fischer T, Heuszer K, et al. Preeclampsia – a state of sympathetic overactivity. *N Eng J Med.* 1996;335:1480.

61. Lubianca JN, Faccin CS, Fuchs FD. Oral contraceptives: a risk factor for uncontrolled blood pressure among hypertensive women. *Contraception.* 2003;67:19.

62. Randin D, Vollenweider P, Tappy L, et al. Suppression of alcohol-induced hypertension by dexamethasone. *N Eng J Med.* 1995;332:1733.

63. Kiechl S, Willeit J, Poewe W, et al. Insulin sensitivity and regular alcohol consumption: large, prospective, cross sectional populaton study (Bruneck Study). *Br Med J.* 1996;313:1040.

64. Vasdev S, Whalen M, Ford CA, et al. Ethanol- and threonine-induced hypertension in rats: a common mechanism. *Can J Cardiol.* 1995;11:807.

65. Prasad K. Pathophysiology of atherosclerosis. In: Chang JB, Olsen ER, Prasad K, Sumpio BE, eds. *Textbook of Angiology.* New York: Springer Verlag; 2000:85.

66. Ross R. Atherosclerosis—an inflammatory disease. *N Eng J Med.* 1999;340:115.

67. Khan NA, McAlister FA, Lewanczuk RZ, et al. The 2005 Canadian Hypertension Education Program recommendations for the management of hypertension: Part II—Therapy. *Can J Cardiol.* 2005;21:657.

68. Prasad K. Antihypertensive activity of secoisolariciresinol diglucoside (SDG) isolated from flaxseed: role of guanylate cyclase. *Int J Angiol.* 2004;13:7.

69. Prasad K. Hypocholesterolemic and antiatherosclerotic effect of flax lignan complex isolated from flaxseed. *Atherosclerosis.* 2005;179:269.

chapter 10

Hypercoagulability and Peripheral Arterial Disease

Kathryn L. Hassell, MD

● INTRODUCTION

Hemostasis is the physiologic response to bleeding that occurs when a vessel wall is disrupted and is regulated through several processes. In the arterial hemostatic system, the first response is the activation, adhesion, and aggregation of platelets. The platelet plug that forms is stabilized by the deposition of fibrin, which is generated on the surface of the platelet membrane and on nearby disrupted vessel surfaces. The extent of thrombosis is limited by endogenous anticoagulant systems and by the fibrinolytic system, which preclude the development of thrombosis beyond the site of injury.[1]

Thrombosis is a pathologic process characterized by an inappropriate or exaggerated generation of clot. It may occur if there is vessel wall injury without disruption (i.e., no bleeding), or in the setting of excess activation of platelets or coagulation factors. Inadequate endogenous anticoagulant or fibrinolytic function may also contribute to the development of thrombosis.

In the arterial circulation, hemostasis and thrombosis are platelet dependent, where high shear stresses and potentially turbulent flow stimulate this mechanism and where the fibrinolytic system regulates secondary fibrin formation.[2,3] By contrast, the venous system is characterized by low flow and stasis, permitting the development of hemostasis and thrombosis through activation of the coagulation cascade and regulation by endogenous anticoagulant proteins.[1] This distinction is important when considering defined hypercoagulable states and the role they may play in peripheral arterial disease.

● MECHANISM OF ARTERIAL HEMOSTASIS AND THROMBOSIS

The initiation of hemostasis or thrombosis in the arterial system is dependent on the platelet, with stabilization of the platelet plug with fibrin. The basic pathway and contributing factors are depicted in Figure 10-1.

Platelet-Dependent Thrombosis

Platelet Adhesion. Under normal conditions, platelets do not adhere to the normal endothelial surface of the arterial wall. If there is a disruption of the endothelial surface, platelets will spontaneously adhere to the exposed subendothelial matrix, medial wall, or adventitial layers. This adhesion is mediated by integrin receptors on the platelet surface, including glycoprotein (GP) Ia/IIa, which binds to collagen.[2,3] Collagen may be the most important component of the subendothelial matrix for the initiation of platelet adhesion.[4] von Willebrand factor (vWF) is also embedded in the subendothelial matrix,[5] which is preferentially recognized over circulating plasma vWF by GP Ib/IX, another key integrin receptor on the platelet surface, creating platelet adhesion.[2,5]

Disruption of the smooth endothelial surface creates turbulent flow and, if the vessel becomes narrowed by vasospasm or irregularities on the endovascular surface, shear stress on the platelet may increase. Platelet binding to subendothelial matrix appears to be significantly augmented at higher sheer stress.[6] Platelet receptor–ligand interactions result not only in platelet adhesion but also

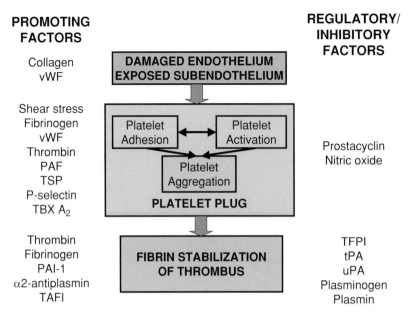

PROMOTING FACTORS

Collagen
vWF

Shear stress
Fibrinogen
vWF
Thrombin
PAF
TSP
P-selectin
TBX A$_2$

Thrombin
Fibrinogen
PAI-1
α2-antiplasmin
TAFI

DAMAGED ENDOTHELIUM EXPOSED SUBENDOTHELIUM

Platelet Adhesion ↔ Platelet Activation

Platelet Aggregation

PLATELET PLUG

FIBRIN STABILIZATION OF THROMBUS

REGULATORY/ INHIBITORY FACTORS

Prostacyclin
Nitric oxide

TFPI
tPA
uPA
Plasminogen
Plasmin

● **FIGURE 10-1.** Basic steps in arterial hemostasis. vWF, von Willebrand factor; PAF, platelet activation factor; TSP, thrombospondin; TBX A$_2$, thromboxane A$_2$; PAI-1, plasminogen activator inhibitor-1; TAFI, thrombin-activated fibrinolytic inhibitor; TFPI, tissue factor pathway inhibitor; tPA, tissue plaminogen activator; uPA, urokinase-like plaminogen activator.

in platelet activation. When activated, intracellular signaling results in activation of GP IIb/IIIa receptors on the platelet surface.[7] Multiple ligands bind to this receptor, including vWF, fibrinogen, fibronectin, vitronectin, and other proteins with the amino acid sequence arginine-glycine-aspartate (RGD) present in subendothelial matrix and augment platelet adhesion.[8] Platelets taken from patients with peripheral arterial disease demonstrate increased adhesivity in vitro under flow conditions.[9]

Platelet Activation. Adhesion of platelets induces platelet activation, which results flattening and pseudopod extension of the platelet membrane.[10] Activated platelets also release platelet aggregation agents from storage pool granules, including adenosine diphosphate (ADP), fibrinogen, collagen, fibronectin, thrombospondin, epinephrine, platelet-activation factor (PAF), serotonin, and vWF.[2,3,10] Thromboxane A$_2$ production and release are stimulated.[1,10] Each of these factors promotes platelet aggregation. P-selectin is found on the membrane of alpha granules and is rapidly elaborated on the platelet surface when platelets are activated, which serves as a receptor for white cell adhesion.[11] Increased platelet activation, indicated by P-selectin expression, platelet fibrinogen binding, and activated microparticle formation, has been demonstrated in peripheral vascular disease.[12,13]

Platelet Aggregation. With the release of potent mediators, platelet aggregation rapidly follows platelet adhesion and activation, covering the exposed subendothelial surface or area of vessel injury with a platelete-rich thrombus. Collagen, fibrinogen, and vWF mediate platelet aggregation by

serving as bridging ligands between platelets via GP IIb/IIIa receptors.[7,14] Thrombin is a potent platelet agonist, causing both platelet activation and aggregation.[15] However, during arterial hemostasis and thrombosis, platelet adhesion, aggregation, and accumulation occur within milliseconds, leading some authors to argue that there is insufficient time for thrombin formation to play a significant role in the initial formation of the platelet-rich thrombus.[2,16] In experimental models, however, platelet deposition in the thrombus formation has been attenuated by treatment with direct thrombin inhibitors.[3,17] Initiation of arterial thrombosis may thus be dependent on small amounts of thrombin as a platelet agonist for hemostasis. Pathological platelet-dependent thrombosis may occur more readily in the setting of arterial vascular disease, where stenosis may increase shear stresses and atherosclerotic plaque rupture releases adhesive, activating, and aggregatory platelet ligands.[18] Increased spontaneous platelet aggregation has been demonstrated in blood taken from patients with peripheral artery disease as compare to controls.[9,19]

Fibrin Formation. Histopathological and experimental observations demonstrate that formation of a fibrin-rich thrombus is an important second phase of arterial hemostasis and thrombosis.[4] Activated platelets more readily bind fibrin and fibrinogen through GPIIb/IIIa receptors.[7,14] In arterial thrombosis, fibrin generation occurs on the phospholipid membrane of platelets, the site of activation and effective propagation of thrombin generation.[1]

Initiation and Activation of Coagulation. When activated, the phospholipid component of the platelet membrane is altered, and phosphotidylserine flipped to the external surface, which promotes and supports coagulation.[20] Initiation of the coagulation cascade on these procoagulant surfaces begins when tissue factor (TF) binds to factor VIIa.[21] There are several potential sources for TF in arterial hemostasis and thrombosis, some of which are dependent on the presence of activated platelets. Damage to the endothelial surface of the vessel may expose flowing blood to the smooth muscle cells in the media. TF is elaborated by these cells when stimulated by agonists such as platelet-derived growth factor, which is stored in platelet granules and released with platelet activation.[22] With deeper vessel wall injury, the adventitial layer is exposed, where TF is present in normal vessels.[23] Increased elaboration of TF by the smooth muscle cells and monocytes/macrophages involved in the development of the atherosclerotic plaque, especially when stimulated by inflammatory markers, likely enhance the risk for thrombosis in peripheral arterial disease.[3]

Thrombin and Fibrin Generation. TF/activated factor VII (factor VIIa) complexes form on procoagulant surfaces (platelet membrane, media, and adventitia), initiating coagulation by the extrinsic pathway[21] (Figure 10-2). TF/VIIa complexes in turn activate factor X. Factor V, released from platelet granules, and factor VIII are activated by thrombin. Factor Xa/Va complexes form and convert prothrombin into thrombin. The generation of thrombin results in a multitude of effects, including recruitment and activation of additional platelets.[24] Feedback activation of factor Va and VIIIa by thrombin contributes to the sustained and amplified activation of the coagulation cascade through the intrinsic pathway and to further thrombin

generation.[25] Thrombin cleaves fibrinogen into fibrin and activates factor XIII, which cross-links and stabilizes the fibrin mesh. In arterial hemostasis, the generation of thrombin is thought to occur predominately on the phospholipid surface of the accumulated platelets and is highly dependent on the presence of platelet deposition.[1,24,26]

Regulation by Fibrinolysis. Hemostasis is regulated by the fibrinolytic system, which is activated when plasminogen binds to the fibrin present in a thrombus. Endothelial cells secrete plasminogen activators when stimulated by the fibrin, thrombin, and by the altered flow or absence of flow created by the thrombus.[27] Tissue plaminogen activator (tPA) binds to fibrin and to the plasminogen bound there, cleaving the plasminogen to plasmin.[28] Plasmin lyses both the cross-linked and uncross-linked fibrin to which it is bound.[27,28] This process opens additional binding sites for plasminogen, extending thrombolysis. Plasmin also cleaves tPA into a two-chain molecule that has a greater affinity for fibrinogen, which further limits the thrombus propagation by reducing the amount of fibrinogen locally available for clot building.[27,28] Adjacent to the area of injury and thrombus, intact endothelial cells with surface receptors for tPA, urokinase-like plasminogen activator (uPA), and plasminogen facilitate the generation of plasmin and limit the propagation of thrombus beyond the area of injury.[29]

Excess fibrinolysis at the site of injury is regulated by fibrinolytic inhibitors. Major vascular physiologic inhibitors of fibrinolysis include α_2-antiplasmin and plasminogen activator inhibitor-1 (PAI-1).[27–29] α_2-Antiplasmin is a plasma protein that binds and inhibits plasminogen, reducing the amount of substrate available for plasmin generation. PAI-1 binds and inhibits tPA and uPA, which reduces the activation of plasminogen to plasmin. PAI-1 is made in endothelial cells, smooth muscle cells, adipose tissue, hepatocytes, and platelets.[30] PAI-1 is released from platelet granules during platelet aggregation[31] and is present in the subendothelial matrix,[32] which limits fibrinolytic activity at the site of injury, permitting stabilization of the thrombus.

The overall net effect of the fibrinolytic system in response to vascular injury is to limit thrombolysis at the site of injury (subendothelial matrix) but facilitate thrombolysis to limit the extent of thrombosis at the surface of the clot (on fibrin) and on the surface of intact endothelial cells adjacent to the site of injury.

The inadequate release of fibrinolytic activators or excessive release of fibrinolytic inhibitors can result in reduced fibrinolytic activity and permit the pathologic propagation of thrombosis.[27] Some reports note an increase in tPA antigen in plasma[33] and vessel walls,[34] which is thought to represent a compensatory physiological activation of the fibrinolytic system in response to the pathologic changes in atherosclerosis. However, significant reductions in circulating tPA activity and increased activity of PAI-1 have been reported in peripheral arterial disease, resulting in a loss of fibrinolytic potential activity[33] and diminished capacity to limit thrombus propagation.

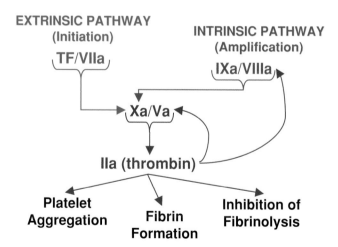

● **FIGURE 10-2.** Simplified coagulation cascade. Hemostasis is initiated by tissue factor (TF)/factor VIIa complexes through the extrinsic pathway, which generates factor Xa. Factor Xa/Va complexes convert prothrombin (factor II) into thrombin (IIa). Thrombin has multiple effects, including platelet aggregation, fibrin formation, and inhibition of fibrinolysis. Thrombin also provides feedback amplification of the coagulation cascade through the intrinsic pathway, activating factors Va and VIIIa, which contribute to further generation of factor Xa.

Regulation by Endogenous Anticoagulants. Regulation of thrombin generation is mediated by endogenous anticoagulant proteins, including tissue factor pathway inhibitor (TFPI), antithrombin (AT, formerly known as antithrombin III), protein C, and protein S. TFPI is produced by endothelial cells and binds to factor Xa.[35] TFPI/Xa complexes then bind with TF/VIIa complexes, forming a quaternary structure that renders all these factors inactive, which inhibits the extrinsic pathway of coagulation necessary for initiation of thrombosis.[35] Antithrombin binds and inactivates activated clotting factors, especially factors Xa and IIa (thrombin), in the presence of glycosaminoglycans on the surface of the endothelium.[36] Protein C is activated by thrombin/thrombomodulin complexes on the surface of endothelial cells.[37] Activated protein C (aPC) then binds to protein S on a phospholipid surface; this aPC/PS complex inactivates factors Va and VIIIa.[37] Resistance to the activity of aPC, most commonly conferred by the presence of the factor V Leiden (FVL) mutation, results in a modest reduction of endogenous anticoagulant activity.[38]

Although abnormalities in these endogenous anticoagulant pathways may limit thrombin generation and fibrin deposition, there is little consistent evidence that deficiencies of or resistance to these anticoagulant factors increases the risk of arterial thrombosis.[2]

Role of Abnormal Vessel Wall

The balance of pro- and antithombotic factors in normal hemostasis is heavily influenced by the vascular endothelium. The vascular endothelium produces and releases antithrombotic factors, including prostacyclin, nitric oxide, tissue plasminogen activator (tPA), and TFPI.[39] Elaboration of surface-bound factors, including thrombomodulin, heparin sulfate proteogycans, and ecto-ADPase, enhances endogenous anticoagulant activity and further limit unwanted thrombosis.[39] Processes intrinsic to peripheral arterial disease significantly alter these regulatory factors and create and increase potential for thrombosis.

Disturbed Flow. Blood flow through normal arteries is laminar, applying minimal shear stress to platelets as well as to the endothelial surface. In contrast, arteriovascular disease, especially atherosclerosis, creates vessel wall abnormalities and endovascular remodeling creating abnormal turbulent flow[40] through stenotic and irregular areas that may increase platelet activation, adhesion, and aggregation. The correlation demonstrated between peripheral arterial disease severity and markers of platelet activation and aggregation[12,13,19] supports the concept that disturbed flow may contribute to platelet abnormalities. Correlation between platelet microparticle formation with ankle brachial index[41] and evidence of increased platelet activation in the common femoral vein in proportion to degree of stenosis by angiography[42] suggest abnormal vasculature contributes to platelet abnormalities. Other reports note that while markers of platelet activation are elevated in peripheral artery disease, there is limited correlation with the severity of disease.[43] The diminished capacity of platelets from patients with very severe peripheral arterial disease to be activated in vitro[12,44] suggests that perhaps platelets may be affected and ultimately "exhausted" by in the atherosclerotic circulation.

In addition to effects on platelets, disturbed flow and shear forces may activate or damage endothelial cells.[45,46] Initially, healthy endothelial cells respond to shear stress by increasing synthesis of nitric oxide and prostacyclin, which inhibit platelet aggregation[39] and upregulate TFPI,[39] functionally reducing available TF.[47] Release of tPA enhances fibrinolysis.[39] However, continued shear stress may lead to endothelial injury and dysfunction, resulting in loss of these antithrombotic properties, upregulation of TF,[48] adhesion molecules,[49] release of vWF,[50] and PAI-1.[39] Attenuation of vasodilation caused by decreased production of nitric oxide by endothelial cells may further compromise blood flow, though most of observations of this phenomenon have been made in coronary arteries.[51]

Inflammation, Oxidative, and Lipid-Mediated Injury. Atherosclerosis in peripheral arterial disease involves several processes, including inflammation and oxidative injury.[51] In addition to the shear stress created by endovascular remodeling, the inflammatory response to atherosclerotic plaque development leads to endothelial dysfunction, abnormal subendothelial matrix, and smooth muscle proliferation and migration.[51] Endothelial stimulation by cytokines leads to increased expression of adhesion molecules, including P-selectin[52] and release of vWF.[39] Altered or decreased expression of surface receptors for plasmin(ogen), tPA, and uPA[53,54] related to these processes may limit fibrinolytic capacity. Functional impairment of the fibrinolytic system, with impaired release of tPA, has been demonstrated in various disease states, including hypertension, chronic kidney disease,[55] and increased PAI capacity noted in patients with arterial vascular disease.[56] High levels of plasma lipoproteins, especially very low density lipoprotein, modulate endothelial production and release of tPA and PAI-1,[57] and increased fibrinogen deposition has been noted in arterial segments from patients undergoing arterial surgery.[58] Lipoprotein(a) is composed of a low-density lipoprotein particle linked to apliliprotein B-100, which is highly homologous to plasminogen and inhibits fibrinolysis through plasminogen competition.[59] Inflammatory mediators downregulate concentrations of heparin-like molecules and the expression of thrombomodulin and endothelial protein C receptor on the endothelial cell surface, diminishing endogenous regulation of thrombin.[54] Decreased activity of the thrombomodulin/protein C system has been associated with increased fibrin deposition on cell surfaces.[60] The net effect of these inflammatory, oxidative, and lipid-mediated changes is a loss of fibrinolytic capacity with increased fibrin deposition.

Abnormal Cellular Elements, Matrix, and Plaque Formation. If the normal vascular endothelium is denuded, normal subendothelial matrix containing vonWillebrand factor, collagen, vitronectin, and PAI-1 is exposed to flowing blood, promoting platelet adhesion and thrombosis.[61] The source of these factors is the medial smooth muscle cell, which is activated by injury and growth factors released in the process of atherogenesis.[34] During atherogenesis, smooth muscle cells increase production and elaboration of extracellular matrix proteins,[51] which promote platelet adhesion and aggregation. These cells also elaborate increased amounts of TF[62] and PAI-1 in excess of tPA.[30,34] In advanced atherosclerosis, all of these factors are concentrated in the atherosclerotic plaque, which can rapidly promote local thrombosis in the event of plaque rupture.[18]

Implications of Abnormal Hemostatic Markers

The impact of the vascular changes induced by atherosclerosis would be predicted to produce measurable changes in hemostatic factors. Table 10-1 lists changes in hemostatic factors that have been demonstrated in patients with peripheral arterial disease (see also Refs. 9, 12, 13, 19, 33–35, 37, 42–44, 56, 58, 63–77.) As noted in Table 10-1, several changes are independently characteristics of patients with peripheral arterial disease. However, there is often a significant interaction between these hemostatic changes, traditional vascular risk factors, and inflammation.[65,68] For example, factor VII activity is correlated with lipid levels[45] and markers of inflammation,[68] but is not consistently independently associated with peripheral arterial disease.[67,71] Claudicants with diabetes have significantly higher levels of vWF, fibrinogen, and thrombin–antithrombin complexes, as compared to nondiabetic cluadicants; coronary and cerebrovascular diseases have also been found to be more common in these patients.[78] Thus, both the metabolic changes of diabetes and the presence of other affected vascular bed may impact hemostatic factors. The fibrinolytic system in particular may be differentially affected by diabetes.[79] Factor VIII and vWF are released from damage endothelium, often in response to inflammatory mediators.[39,49,53] Since most data are collected from patients with known peripheral arterial disease, which can induce the changes in the coagulation system, it is not clear whether the hemostatic changes are a cause or a consequence of the vascular injury underlying the disease process.

The presence of the hypercoagulability associated with peripheral arterial disease, even if secondary to the process itself, may predict future thrombotic events. Increased platelet aggregability,[76] markers of coagulation activation,[71,76] and impaired fibrinolysis[71] have been associated with an increased risk of vascular events in peripheral arterial disease. Increased markers of inflammation, platelet, and coagulation activation have been observed after angioplasty,[80] though the correlation of these changes with postprocedure stenosis or occlusion has been inconsistent.[80,81] Postoperative markers of increased coagulation are also seen after surgical revascularization, despite aspirin and heparin,[82] but subsequent restenosis may be more related to cellular activation and inflammation.[83]

In contrast to the multiple hemostatic abnormalities described in patients with recognized peripheral artery disease, the Edinburgh Artery Study demonstrated that only fibrinogen and lipoprotein(a) uniquely predicted for the subsequent development of symptomatic peripheral arterial disease.[84]

● ROLE OF DEFINED HYPERCOAGULABLE STATES

Specific inherited and acquired hypercoagulable states can be identified by laboratory testing; common disorders are listed in Table 10-2.[85] Inherited and long-standing acquired hypercoagulable states have the potential to augment the hypercoagulability induced by pathophysiologic processes and traditional vascular risk factors in peripheral arterial disease. However, the extent to which the presence of these conditions changes the risk of the development of peripheral arterial disease or its complications remains unclear despite ongoing investigation.

Platelet Disorders

Thrombocythemia. Thrombocytosis that develops in response to inflammation, iron deficiency, or other processes is not thought to contribute significantly to a risk of arterial thrombosis, even when platelet numbers exceed $1 000 000/mm^3$.[86] However, there are a few data assessing the impact of elevated platelet count in patients with peripheral arterial disease. In a single report, modest elevation in platelet counts correlated with severity of peripheral arterial disease in diabetic patients with end-stage renal disease.[87] However, this could occur as a secondary response reflecting underlying chronic inflammation or other pathological processes. Myeloproliferative disorders including polycythemia vera and essential thrombocythemia that may be characterized by marked elevation in platelet count are associated with macro- and microvascular arterial events in 20% to 30% of patients, especially in those with platelet counts $>500 000/mm^3$.[88,89] In this subset of patients, platelets produced in myeloproliferative disorders may be hypersensitive and more readily activated.[88] Thrombocytosis has been associated with spontaneous peripheral arterial microembolization from established arterial lesions.[90] The elevated red blood cell mass in polycythemia vera, in conjunction with elevated platelet count, may contribute to increased blood viscosity that may impact flow through diseased circulation.[61] Adequate therapy of the myeloproliferative state, in addition to antiplatelet therapy, is associated with a reduction in risk of vascular events.[88]

Platelet Hyperaggregability

Genetic variation in the platelet receptor GP IIIa locus may impact platelet aggregation. Some studies attribute an increased risk of cardiovascular disease and myocardial infarction to the presence of the Pl^{A2} allele,[91] though meta-analysis of available studies concluded there was no

TABLE 10-1. Hemostatis Changes in Patients with Peripheral Arterial Disease

Hemostatic Factor	Change	Correlation with Disease Severity	References
Platelet function			
P-selectin	Increased expression on intact platelet	Yes/no	12, 43, 63
	Increased expression on platelet microparticles	ND	13
	Decreased quantity in alpha granules	Yes	12
Platelet aggregation	Spontaneous aggregation in vitro	Yes	9, 19
	Presence of microaggregates	No	41, 44
CD40-L	Increased levels of soluble CD40L	Yes	43
Procoagulant factors			
von Willebrand factor	Increased plasma levels of antigen and activity	Yes	63–68
Factor VII	Increased, correlated with triglycerides	ND	65
	Increased, correlated with markers of inflammation	ND	68
Factor VIII	Increased antigen, activity if history of myocardial infarction	ND	64, 65
	Increased, correlated with fibrinogen	ND	65
Fibrinogen	Increased plasma levels of antigen and activity	Yes	9, 58, 63, 66, 67, 69, 70
	Increased if history of myocardial infarction	ND	64, 65
	Increased, correlated with markers of inflammation	Yes	68, 69
	Does not predict for vascular complications	ND	69, 71
Fibrinolytic factors			
Tissue plaminogen activator (tPA)	Increased antigen	Yes	37
	Decreased activity	Yes	33
	Diminished expression in vessel walls	ND	58
	Increased expression in vessel walls in advanced disease	Yes	34
Plasminogen activator inhibitor-1 (PAI-1)	Increased activity	No	33, 67, 72
	Increased antigen, predicts for vascular complications	ND	69, 71, 73
	Increased PAI-1 capacity	No	56
	Diminished expression in vessel walls	No	58
	Increased expression in vessel walls	Yes	34
	Decreased PAI-1/tPA ratio	Yes	63
A$_2$-antiplasmin	Increased antigen if cerebral vascular disease	Yes	64
Markers of coagulation activation			
D-dimer	Increased	Yes	9, 56, 70, 72–74
	Increased if history of cardiac or cerebrovascular events	Yes	69
	Increased in arterial but not venous samples	ND	75
	Increased, may predict thrombotic events	ND	71
Prothrombin fragment 1 + 2	Increased if history of cardiac or cerebrovascular events	Yes	69
	Increased, correlated with D-dimer	No	74
Thrombin—antithrombin complexes (TAT)	Increased	ND	9, 56, 73
	Increased, correlated with D-dimer	ND	74
	Increased, predictive of vascular events	ND	71
Whole blood clotting	Hypercoagulable changes by thromboelastography (TEG)	ND	42
	Shortened endotoxin-induced recalcification time	ND	77
Endogenous anticoagulants			
Antithrombin (III)	Modest decreased activity	Yes	63
Protein C	Decreased activity levels	ND	73
	Levels correlated with factor VII	ND	65
Thrombomodulin	Increased soluble TM plasma levels	ND	72

TABLE 10-2. Defined Clinical Hypercoagulable States[85]

Condition	Type of Thrombosis	Screening Test(s)	Abnormal Result
Myeloproliferative disorders (polycythemia vera, essential thrombocythemia)	Arterial or venous	CBC	Elevated platelet
Dysfibrinogenemia	Arterial or venous	Euglobulin lysis time	Prolonged
		Thrombin time	Shortened
Hyperhomocysteinemia	Arterial or venous	Plasma homocysteine	Above upper limit of normal (usually >14 μmol/L)
Antiphospholipid antibody syndrome	Arterial or venous	Anticardiolipin antibody (IgG, IgM)	Moderate-strong positive titer (usually >40 GPL)
		Anti-β2glycoprotein antibody (IgG, IgM)	Moderate-strong positive titer (usually >20 units)
		Lupus anticoagulant test (e.g., dilute Russell viper venom time)	Present
Antithrombin deficiency	Venous	AT activity	<50%
Protein C deficiency	Venous	Protein C activity	<40%
Protein S deficiency	Venous	Free protein S antigen	<40%
Activated protein C resistance	Venous	aPCR assay	Low ratio (usually <1.6)
Factor V Leiden	Venous	DNA analysis	Presence of mutation
Prothrombin G20210A mutation	Venous	DNA analysis	Presence of mutation

association.[92] A single study in patients with claudication noted a lower incidence of the Pl[A2] allele as compared to controls; this association of Pl[A2] with a lower risk of peripheral vascular disease was lost when adjustment was made for lifetime smoking and fibrinogen levels.[93] Congenital platelet hyperactivity, termed "sticky platelet syndrome," has been described in families with early arterial thrombotic events as well as in case series of patients with arterial and venous thrombosis.[89] Diagnosis is made by the demonstration of hyperaggregability with ADP and/or epinephrine agonists.[94] The detection of this phenomenon appears to be highly variable and susceptible to operator technique, limiting reproducibility and applicability in larger studies and populations.[94] The role of antecedent or underlying platelet hyperaggregability, as distinct from changes potentially induced by vascular disease itself, has not be explored in peripheral arterial disease.

Dysfibrinogenemia

Inherited and acquired abnormalities in the fibrinogen molecule generally lead to an increased risk of hemorrhage, but can also result in an increased risk of arterial and venous thrombosis.[91,95] These very rare disorders can be difficult to diagnose, especially since plasma fibrinogen values are affected by pathophysiological processes, including inflammation and vascular injury, and there is a lack of laboratory measurement standardization.[96] Although a case report identified a novel fibrinogen mutation in a patient with peripheral arterial disease,[97] investigation for dysfibrinogenemia is generally not necessary or recommended in patients with peripheral arterial disease.

Abnormal Fibrinolysis

Inherited defects in the fibrinolytic system, including reduced production of plasminogen, diminished release of activators (tPA, uPA), or increased production or release of inhibitors (PAI-1, TAFI) have been described, but are rare.[98] Genetic polymorphisms in the PAI-1 gene, specifically 4G/4G, have been associated with increased basal PAI-1 transcription rate.[98] The Edinburg Artery Study did not demonstrate a correlation between these polymorphisms and peripheral arterial disease.[99] There was no correlation between PAI-1 plasma levels or late postangioplasty restenosis and the PAI-1 4G allele, though there was a higher frequency of early thrombotic reocclusion in patients with the PAI-4G allele undergoing percutaneous angioplasty.[100] Polymorphisms of the lipoprotein(a) gene may result in increased production,[101] potentially inhibiting fibrinolysis through competition with plasminogen for activators. The impact of these polymorphisms on peripheral arterial disease has not been carefully studied. While some reports note that elevated plasma lipoprotein(a) levels are associated with symptomatic peripheral arterial disease,[81,102] the strength of this association is diminished in the setting of other lipid abnormalities and risk factors.[70,84]

Hyperhomocysteinemia

Methionine, a critical amino acid for protein synthesis, is catabolized to homocysteine, which in turn is catabolized to cysthathionine using vitamin B6 as a cofactor.[103] Homocysteine is also converted back to methionine by methionine synthase, which requires vitamin B12 as a cofactor and methylenetetrahydrofolate as a substrate. Elevated homocysteine levels develop with vitamin B6 deficiency, which reduces catabolism of homocysteine, and folic acid and vitamin B12 deficiencies, which interrupt homocysteine conversion back to methionine.[103] Methylenetetrahydrofolate reductase is also necessary in the cycle through which homocysteine is converted back to methionine. This enzyme has two common polymorphisms that potentially impact the efficiency of metabolism and may result in accumulation of homocysteine.[104] Elevation of homocysteine also occurs with even very mild renal insufficiency or with the administration of drugs that interfere with folic acid metabolism.[103]

Homocysteine, with its reactive sulfur group, oxidizes lipoproteins and affects the reduction-oxidation equilibrium of tissues, potentially contributing to atherosclerosis when it accumulates.[105] In the presence of modest elevations of plasma homocysteine (mean levels of 14.4 μmol/L), endothelial dysfunction as assessed by reduction in flow-dependent vasodilation was demonstrated in patients with peripheral arterial disease.[106] Platelets from patients with peripheral arterial disease and hyperhomocysteinemia have demonstrated increased platelet reactivity and decreased sensitivity to nitric oxide inhibition of aggregation as compared to platelets from patients with normal homocysteine plasma levels.[107]

Hyperhomocysteinemia, generally considered to be plasma values >14 μmol/L104, appears to be prevalent in patients with peripheral arterial disease, though the association was weak in large studies including the National Health and Nutrition Survey[108] and a large cross-sectional study of primary care patients.[109] Some studies suggest hyperhomocysteinemia may play a role in peripheral arterial vascular disease in young patients, particularly women, but the modest association is generally in the setting of traditional risk factors.[110–113] Other data suggest hyperhomocysteinemia is a marker of general atherosclerosis and may predict for cardiovascular morbidity and mortality in peripheral arterial disease patients.[114] There is no demonstrated relationship between vitamin levels[113,115] or the presence of the themolabile polymorphism of the methylenetetrahydrofolate reductase[103,104,113,115] and the presence or severity of peripheral arterial disease. Elevated homocysteine levels may impact the development of peripheral arterial disease[116] and predict for the occurrence of vascular events,[117] even though reduction in homocysteine levels with vitamin therapy does not correlate with reduced markers of inflammation or coagulation in patients with peripheral vascular disease.[118]

Antiphospholipid Antibodies

Antiphospholipid antibodies are a heterogenous set of antibodies associated with an increased risk of arterial and venous thrombosis. Initially described in lupus and other autoimmune disorders, these antibodies can occur in patients of all ages, both sexes, and in the absence of a defined autoimmune condition.[119] Antiphospholipid antibody syndrome is diagnosed when either the lupus anti-coagulant, anticardiolipin (ACA), or anti-β2glycoprotein-1 (β2GP-1) antibodies are identified on two occasions at least 3 months apart in a person who has experienced an arterial or venous thrombosis or a characteristic set of pregnancy losses.[120] These antibodies may contribute to atherogenesis[121] through various mechanisms, including oxidative modification of lipoproteins,[122] and may induce an endothelial proinflammatory phenotype by upregulation of E-selectin, intercellular adhesion molecule-1, and vascular cell adhesion molecule-1 as well as release of inflammatory cytokines.[123]

The development of arterial vascular events is associated with the presence of any of the three diagnostic antibodies in patients with lupus, independent of the predictive risk factors of smoking, age, and elevated C-reactive protein.[124] The presence of ACA and β2GP-1 antibodies has been associated with arterial thrombosis[119] and with the presence of peripheral arterial disease.[125,126] ACA antibodies were more prevalent and of higher titers in patients with critical limb ischemia as compared to stable claudicants and age-matched controls.[127] In one study, ACA antibodies were identified in 14% of young patients with severe premature atherosclerosis.[128] Patients with antibodies had a lower incidence of hyperlipidemia/dyslipidemia as compared to those without antibodies, suggesting that the antibodies contributed to the severity of atherosclerosis in those patients.[128] In one series, the lupus anticoagulant, determined by the dilute Russell viper venom time, was detected in 43% of patients of intermittent claudication, critical limb ischemia, or aortic aneurysm as compared to 0% of general surgery patients,[129] though other series report a much lower incidence (3%–8%).[130,131] The presence of ACA antibodies in patients with peripheral vascular disease has been associated with an increased risk of overall mortality, and is an independent risk factor for cardiovascular death.[132] Antiphospholipid antibodies are associated with restenosis and reduced graft patency in some reports,[131,133] but a lack of correlation has also been reported.[134]

Endogenous Anticoagulant Deficiencies

A number of studies have been conducted to screen for the presence of endogenous anticoagulant deficiencies in patients with peripheral arterial disease. Classical, inherited antithrombin, protein C, and protein S deficiencies are characterized by diminished activity levels of <50%, <40% to 50%, and 40% to 50%, respectively, and are not generally associated with arterial thrombosis.[135,136] Accurate diagnosis of these disorders is compromised when testing during an acute thrombotic episode, in the setting of severe medical illness or inflammation, in the presence of antiphospholipid antibodies or during anticoagulant therapy.[91] Old small case series report lower average antithrombin values in peripheral vascular patients as compared to controls,[63,64,137] but larger contemporary studies fail to demonstrate the presence of true antithrombin deficiency (activity levels <50%) in these patients.[129,138–140] Similarly, diminished levels of protein C and protein S (<60%–75%) are reported to occur in 1% to 17% in patients with peripheral arterial disease,[129,138–142] but the setting of testing and prevalence of classic genetic deficiency (activity levels <40%–50%) are poorly characterized in these studies. Other studies fail to demonstrate endogenous anticoagulant deficiencies or reduction in levels in patients with arterial thrombosis and peripheral arterial disease.[140,143]

Thrombophilic Genetic Polymorphisms

Activated Protein C Resistance/FVL. Resistance to aPC is characterized by reduced plasma protein C anticoagulant activity.[91] This is most commonly caused by FVL, a point mutation that renders factor V more resistance to cleavage, and inactivation by aPC92 FVL affects 5% to 6% of persons of Caucasian descent, and is associated with venous thrombosis, usually in high-risk settings. It is not a deficiency state, and more than 90% of heterozygous carriers will not experience thrombosis.[91,144]

The preponderance of available data fails to demonstrate a consistent relationship between FVL and peripheral arterial disease. An increased prevalence of aPC resistance was demonstrated in patients with peripheral arterial disease when measured before vascular surgery, which worsened after surgery[145]; this increase was associated with a tendency to graft re-occlusion and mortality.[146] More recent studies conducted in larger peripheral arterial disease populations fail to confirm an increase in aPC resistance, correlation with disease severity, or with the need for or failure of subsequent bypass grafting.[147,148] While most assays for aPC resistance correct for the interfering effect of elevated fibrinogen and factor[91] VIII, abnormal results may reflect acquired inflammatory and prothrombotic changes caused by atherosclerosis, rather than indicate an underlying cause of thrombosis.[145] When testing for FVL by DNA analysis, which is more specific for the underlying inherited aPC resistant state, a consistent relationship with peripheral arterial disease is not demonstrated. While case reports and some studies note the presence of FVL in peripheral arterial disease patients, lack of comparison with an appropriate control group precludes the identification of the background incidence of the gene in the general population.[138,149] Some series note an increased prevalence of FVL in peripheral arterial disease patients presenting for surgery[145] or with a history of vascular surgery.[150] However, in several large studies, the presence of the FVL mutation is not associated with the presence of severity symptomatic peripheral arterial disease[101,151,152] or bypass patency.[153] Systematic literature reviews and a meta-analysis of the available information do not support a strong or consistent association.[144,154] The clinical implications of a modest apparent increased risk of peripheral arterial disease associated with FVL observed some subgroups, including younger patients,[154] women,[154] and those with fewer traditional vascular risk factors[150,153,155] are unclear.

Prothrombin G20201A Mutation. This genetic polymorphism is created by a point mutation in an untranslated portion of the prothrombin or factor II gene, which results in a modest increase in basal levels of functionally normal prothrombin.[91] Between 2% and 5% of the Caucasian population carry the polymorphism in the heterozygous state, which imparts a modestly increased risk of venous thrombosis.[138] As for FVL, the relationship between prothrombin G20210A and arterial thrombosis is uncertain and inconsistently demonstrated. Case reports and series that link this mutation with increased arterial wall thickness and risk of recurrent ischemic events are limited by the absence of appropriate control groups, and they note increased cardiovascular events rather than peripheral vascular events in affected patients.[156–159] When adjusted for traditional vascular risk factors by multivariate analysis, the presence of the prothrombin G20210A mutation retains a modest association with the presence, but not severity, of peripheral arterial disease,[101] though subgroup analysis demonstrates potential synergistic effects between smoking, hypercholesterolemia, hypertension, diabetes, and the mutation.[152] However, another report notes that carriers of the prothrombin gene are less likely to have traditional risk factors.[157] Other series and meta-analysis fail to demonstrate a relationship between peripheral arterial disease and prothrombin G20210A mutation.[144,151,154]

Potential Implications of Hypercoagulable States

Role of Screening in Typical Peripheral Arterial Disease. The major pathophysiological factors in peripheral arterial disease create vascular injury, including endothelial dysfunction, vessel wall remodeling, and plaque formation. The process of thrombosis in this setting may be potentially exacerbated by the coexistence of hypercoagulable states associated with an increased risk of arterial thrombosis, including abnormalities of platelets and the fibrinolytic system. Acquired conditions that contribute to vascular injury, including antiphospholipid antibody syndrome and hyperhomocysteinemia, would also be expected to increase risk of peripheral arterial disease and its complications. However, hypercoabulable states that primarily impact thrombin generation through the coagulation cascade should have less impact, given the limited role of this aspect of coagulation in the pathophysiology of atherosclerotic vascular disease and arterial thrombosis. This is supported by clinical observations demonstrating consistent correlation between arterial hypercoagulable states and peripheral arterial disease, but a weak or absence association of venous hypercoagulable states with peripheral arterial disease.

Treatment for peripheral arterial disease is focused on modification of vascular risk factors (e.g., lipid-lowering therapy) and antiplatelet therapy, appropriately directed at the underlying pathophysiology of platelet-dependent thrombosis. Preliminary data suggest that this management may actually impact the hypercoagulable changes, such as decreasing circulating tissue factor, even though the therapy is not directed at the coagulation cascade itself.[158]

Reduction of hyperhomocysteinemia with vitamin therapy is often advocated,[101,103] especially in the setting of cardiovascular disease,[108,109] even though no benefit has been demonstrated.[118] There are no studies defining a role for oral anticoagulation instead of or in addition to antiplatelet therapy in patients with an apparent underlying hypercoagulable state.[139–141] Such a change from antiplatelet therapy to oral anticoagulation may actually be detrimental, as demonstrated by the example of persistent risk of occlusive vascular events in patients with thrombocythemia despite oral anticoagulation and in the absence of antiplatelet therapy.[88] In the absence of recognized venous thrombosis, and even in after an initial venous thrombotic event, sustained oral anticoagulation is not necessary in most hypercoagulable states.[91] Since no specific change in management is directed by the detection of an underlying hypercoagulable state, there is little justification for screening for these states in patients with typical peripheral arterial disease.[139,140,144,151,152]

Role of Screening in Predicting or Explaining Intervention Failures.

It might be expected that patients with an underlying hypercoagulable state who develop peripheral arterial disease would be at an increased risk of thrombosis and/or restenosis after angioplasty or bypass grafting. However, data addressing this hypothesis are conflicting, especially regarding aPC resistence[145,146,148] and hyperhomocysteinemia.[81,153] Retrospective case series, combining a variety of acquired and inherited hypercoagulable changes, note an increased rate of surgical intervention and risk of revascularization failures in patients with "a thrombophilic defect,"[141] but there is no consensus as to which defects are most predictive or associated with postintervention complications. Prospective data in patients with antiphospholipid antibodies and peripheral arterial disease suggest there is a higher risk of early graft thrombosis[129,131,133] and restenosis,[131] which is expected given the significant increased propensity for thrombosis in these patients. To date, however, there are no trials that demonstrate benefit of alternative management approach, or even consensus-driven recommended therapeutic approaches,[138–140] which would support a recommendation of routine preprocedure screening. Unexpected

early, severe, or repetitive graft thrombosis and/or stenosis may be indicative of an underlying hypercoagulable state. In that setting, testing for hypercoagulable states that are associated with an increased risk of arterial thrombosis is managed with oral anticoagulation in other settings, or can be modulated by unique interventions (e.g., vitamin therapy). This testing would include assessment for antiphospholipid antibody syndrome[139] and hyperhomocysteinemia, as outlined in Table 10-2.

There is no accepted screening test for dystibrinogenious associated with thrombosis, though a shortened thrombin time or prolonged euglobin lysis time may indicate the presence of a dysfibrinogenemia or an acquired prolongation of the ELT may be seen in acquired conditions, including obesity.[85] Abnormalities of tPA PAI-1 may be secondary to underlying PAD rather than diagnostic of a primary hypercoagulable state.

Role for Screening in Explaining Arterial Thrombosis in Absence of Atherosclerosis.

Arterial thrombosis in the absence of classical or severe vessel changes associated with typical peripheral arterial disease may be indicative of an underlying hypercoagulable state. Studies note that patients with underlying hypercoagulable states who present with arterial thrombosis tend to be younger and have fewer traditional vascular risk factors (see Refs. 128, 132, 138, 141, 150, 151, 154). As depicted in Table 10-2, only a small number of inherited and acquired hypercoagulable states are associated with arterial thrombosis. Although advocated in the vascular surgical literature,[134,138,141] broad screening for predominately venous hypercoagulable states, especially common genetic polymorphisms and rare deficiencies, may lead to confusion about causation of clinical arterial events and inappropriate use of oral anticoagulation. Screening for arterial disorders could be considered in individuals with a personal or family history of thrombotic events, early onset of disease, or in the absence of any of the usual risk factors for peripheral vascular disease, including a family history of atherosclerotic complications. This approach is advocated by at least one consensus document,[159] though the appropriate subsequent management of patients identified with a hypercoagulable state has not been standardized or well studied.

REFERENCES

1. Hoffman M, Monroe DM. Coagulation 2006: a modern view of hemostasis. *Hematol Oncol Clin North Am.* 2007;22:1.

2. Stormorken H, Sakariassen KS. Hemostatic risk factors in arterial thrombosis and atherosclerosis: the thrombin-fibin and platelet-vWF axis. *Thromb Res.* 1997;88:1.

3. Eisenberg PR, Ghigliotti G. Platelet-dependent and procoagulant mechanisms in arterial thrombosis. *Int J Cardiol.* 1998;68(suppl 1):S3.

4. Kirchhofer D, Tschopp TB, Steiner B, et al. Role of collagen-adherent platelets in mediating fibrin formation in flowing whole blood. *Blood.* 1995;86:3815.

5. Turitto VT, Weiss HJ, Zimmerman TS, et al. Factor VIII/von Willebrand factor in subendothelium mediates platelet adhesion. *Blood.* 1985;65:823.

6. Ruggeri ZM. The role of von Willebrand factor and fibrinogen in the initiation of platelet adhesion to thrombogenic surfaces. *Thromb Haemost.* 1995;74:460.

7. Cassar K, Bachoo P, Brittenden J. The role of platelets in peripheral vascular disease. *Eur J Vasc Endovasc Surg.* 2003; 24:6.

8. Hawiger J. Adhesive interaction of platelets and their blockade. *Ann N Y Acad Sci.* 1991;614:270.

9. Reininger CB, Graf J, Reininger AJ, et al. Increased platelet and coagulatory activity indicate ongoing thrombogenesis in peripheral artery disease. *Thromb Res.* 1996;82:523.

10. Zarbock A, Polanowska-Grawbowska RK, Ley K. Platelet-neutrophil interactions: linking hemostasis and inflammation. *Blood Rev.* 2006;21:99.

11. Palabrica T, Lobb R, Furic BC, et al. Leukocyte accumulation promoting fibrin deposition is mediated in vitro by P-selectin on adherent platelets. *Nature.* 1992;359:848.

12. Cassar K, Bachoo P, Ford I, et al. Platelet activation is increased in peripheral arterial disease. *J Vasc Surg.* 2003;38:99.

13. van der Zee P, Biro E, Ko Y, et al. P-selectin- and CD63-exposing platelet microparticles reflect platelet activation in peripheral arterial disease and myocardial infarction. *Clin Chem.* 2006;52:4.

14. Kulkarni S, Dopheide SM, Yap CL, et al. A revised model of platelet aggregation. *J Clin Invest.* 2006;105:6.

15. Eidt JF, Allison P, Noble S, et al. Thrombin is an important mediator of platelet aggregation in stenosed canine coronary arteries with endothelial injury. *J Clin Invest.* 1989;84:18.

16. Luscher EF, Weber S. The formation of the hemostatic plug—a special case of platelet aggregation. *Thromb Haemost.* 1993;70:234.

17. Harker LA, Hanson SR, Runge MS. Thrombin hypothesis of thrombin generation and vascular lesion formation. *Am J Cardiol.* 1995;75:1213.

18. Siegel-Axel DI, Gawan M. Platelets and endothelial cells. *Semin Thromb Hemost.* 2007;33:128.

19. Robless PA, Okonko D, Lintott P, et al. Increased platelet aggregation and activation in peripheral arterial disease. *Eur J Endovasc Surg.* 2003;25:16

20. Zwaal RFA, Schroit AJ. Pathophysiologic implications of membrane phospholipid asymmetry in blood cells. *Blood.* 1997;89:1121.

21. Schenone M, Furie GC, Furie B. The blood coagulation cascade. *Curr Opin Hematol.* 2004;11:272.

22. Schecter AD, Giesen PL, Taby O, et al. Tissue factor expression in human arterial smooth muscle cells. TF is present in three cellular pools after growth factor stimulation. *J Clin Invest.* 1997;100:2276.

23. Barstad RM, Hamers MJ, Kierulf P, et al. Procoagulant human monocytes mediate tissue factor/factor VIIa-dependent platelet-thrombus formation with exposed to flowing nonanticoagulated human blood. *Arteriscler Thromb Vasc Biol.* 1995;15:11.

24. Davie EW, Kulman JD. An overview of the structure and function of thrombin. *Semin Thromb Hemost.* 2006;32(suppl 2):3.

25. Ghighliotti G, Waissbluth AR, Speidel C, et al. Prolonged activation of prothombin on the vascular wall after arterial injury. *Arterisclor Thromb Vasc Biol.* 1998;18:250.

26. Eisenberg PR. Important of platelets in arterial clot-associated procoagulant activity. *Circulation.* 1995;92:803.

27. Francis, CW. *Hemostasis and Thrombosis.* Philadelphia: J.B. Lippincott; 1994:1085.

28. Cesarmon-Maus G, Hajjar K. Molecular mechanisms of fibrinolysis. *Br J Hematol.* 2005;129:307.

29. Plow E. *Thrombosis and Hemorrhage.* Baltimore: Williams and Wilkins, 1998; Chap 18.

30. Huber K. Plasminogen activator inhibitor type-1 (part one): basic mechanisms, regulation and role for thrombembolic disease. *J Thromb Thrombolys.* 2001;11:183.

31. Kruithof EK, Tran-Thang C, Bachmann F. Studies on the release of plaminogen activator inhibitor by human platelets. *Thromb Haemost.* 1986;55:201.

32. Mimuro J, schleef RR, Loskutoff DJ. Extracellular matrix of cultured bovine aortic endothelial cells contain functionally active type I plasminogen activator inhibitor. *Blood.* 1987;70:721.

33. Killewich LA, Gardner AW, Macko RF, et al. Progressive intermittent claudication is associated with impaired fibrinolysis. *J Vasc Surg.* 1998;27:645.

34. Schneider D J, Ricci MA, Taatjes DJ, et al. Changes in arterial expression of fibrinolytic system proteins in atherogenesis. *Arterioscler Thromb Vasc Biol.* 1997;17:3294.

35. Broze G J Jr, Warren LA, Novotny WF, et al. The lipoprotein associated coagulation inhibitor that inhibits factor VII-tissue factor complex also inhibits factor Xa: insight into its possible mechanism of action. *Blood.* 1988;73:335.

36. Marcum JA, Rosenberg RD. Anticoagulantly active heparin-like molecules from vascular tissue. *Biochemistry.* 1984;32:1730.

37. Esmon CT. The protein C anticoagulant pathway. *Atheroscler Thromb.* 1992;12:135.

38. Martinelly I, Botasso B, Duca F, et al. Heightened thrombin generation in individuals with resistance to activated protein C. *Thromb Haemost.* 1996;75:703.

39. Wu KK, Thiagarajan P. Role of endothelium in thrombosis and hemostasis. *Annu Rev Med.* 1996;47:315.

40. Warwick S, Mangin P, Salem HH, Jackson S. The impact of blood rheology on the molecular and cellular events underlying arterial thrombosis. *J Mol Med.* 2006;84:989-995.

41. Kudoh T, Sakamoto T, Miyamoto S, et al. Relation between platelet microaggregates and ankle brachial index in patients with peripheral arterial disease. *Thromb Res.* 2006;117:263.

42. Shankar VK, Chaudhury SR, Uthappa MC, et al. Changes in blood coagulability as it traverses the ischemic limb. *J Vasc Surg.* 2004;39:1033.

43. Blann AD, Tan KT, Tayebjee MH, Davagnanam I, et al. Soluble CD40L in peripheral artery disease. Relationship with disease severity, platelet markers and the effects of angioplasty. *Thromb Hasemost.* 2005;93:578.

44. McBane RD, Karnicki K, Miller R, Owen W. The impact of peripheral arterial disease on circulating platelets. *Thromb Res.* 2004;113:137.

45. Simpson JD, Doux JD, Lee PY, et al. Peripheral arterial disease: a manifestation of evolutionary dislocation and feedforward dysfunction. *Med Hypothesis.* 2006;67:947.

46. Davies PR, Spaan JA, Krams R. Shear stress biology of the endothelium. *Ann Biomed Eng.* 2005;33:1714.

47. Grabowski E P, Reininger AJ, Petteruti PG, et al. Shear stress decreases endothelial cell tissue factor activity by augmenting secretion of tissue factor pathway inhibitor. *Arterioscler Thromb Vasc Biol.* 2001;21:157.

48. Mazzolai L, Silacci P, Bouzourene K, Daniel F, et al. Tissue factor activity is upregulated in human endothelial cells exposed to oscillatory shear stress. *Thromb Haemost.* 2002;87:1062.

49. Tesfamariam B, DeFelice AF. Endothelial injury in the initiation and progression of vascular disorders. *Vasc Pharm.* 2007;46:229.

50. Goto S. Role of von Willebrand factor for the onset of arterial thrombosis. *Clin Lab.* 2001;47:327.

51. Faxon DP, Cochair VF, Cochair PL, et al. Atherosclerotic vascular disease conference writing group III: pathophysiology. *Circulation.* 2004;109:2617.

52. Merten M, Thiagarajan P. P-selectin in arterial thrombosis. *Z Kardiol.* 2004;93:855.

53. Strukova S. Blood coagulation-dependent inflammation. Coagulation-dependent inflammation and inflammation-dependent thrombosis. *Front Biosci.* 2006;11:59.

54. Esmon CT. The interactions between inflammation and coagulation. *Br J Haematol.* 2005;131:417.

55. Hrafnkelskotti T, Ottosson P, Gudnason T, et al. Impaired endothelial release of tissue-type plamsinogen activator in patients with chronic kidney disease and hypertension. *Hypertension.* 2004;44:300.

56. Speiser W, Speiser P, Minar E, et al. Activation of coagulation and fibrinolysis in patients with arteriosclerosis: relation to localization of vessel disease and risk factors. *Thromb Res.* 1990;59:77.

57. Badimon L, Martinez-Gonzalez J. Endothelium and vascular protection: an update. *Rev Esp Cardiol.* 2002;55(suppl 1):17.

58. Martin-Paredero V, Vadillo J, Diaz A, et al. Fibrinogen and fibrinolysis in blood and in the arterial wall: its role in advanced atherosclerotic disease. *Cardiovasc Surg.* 1998;6:457.

59. Hajjar KA, Nachman RL. The role of lipoprotein(a) in atherogenesis and thrombosis. *Annu Rev Med.* 1996;47:423.

60. Cadroy Y, Diquelon A, Dupouy D, et al. The thrombomoduline/protein C/protein S anticoagulant pathway modulates the thrombogenic properties of normal resting and stimulated endothelium. *Arterioscler Thromb Vasc Biol.* 1997;17:520.

61. Makin A, Silvrman SH, Lip GYH. Peripheral vascular disease and Virchow's triad for thrombogenesis. *Q J Med.* 2002;95:199.

62. Osterud B, Bjorklid E. Sources of tissue factor. *Semin Thromb Hemost.* 2006;32:11.

63. Koksch M, Zeiger F, Wittig K, et al. Haemostatic derangement in advanced peripheral occlusive arterial disease. *Int Angiol.* 1999;18:256.

64. Christe M, Delley A, Marbet GA, et al. Fibrinogen, factor VIII related antigen, antithrombin III and alpha 2-antiplasmin in peripheral arterial disease. *Thromb Haemost.* 1984;52:240.

65. Cortellaro M, Boschetti C, Cofrancesco E, et al. The PLAT study: a multidisciplinary study of hemostatic function and conventional risk factors in vascular disease patients. *Atherosclerosis.* 1991;90:109.

66. Smith FB, Lee AJ, Fowkes FG, et al. Smoking, haemostatic factors and the severity of aorto-iliac and femoro-popliteal disease. *Thromb Haemost.* 1996;75:19.

67. Philipp CS, Cisar LA, Kim HC, et al. Association of hemostatic factors with peripheral vascular disease. *Am Heart J.* 1997;134:978.

68. Tzoulaki I, Murray GD, Proce JF, et al. Hemostatic factors, inflammatory markers, and progressive peripheral atherosclerosis. The Edinburgh Artery Study. *Am J Epidemiol.* 2005;163:334.

69. McDermott MM, Green D, Greenland P, et al. Relation of levels of hemostatic factors and inflammatory markers to the ankle brachial index. *Am J Cardiol.* 2003;92:194.

70. Ridker PM, Stampfer MJ, Rifai N. Novel risk factors for systemic atherosclerosis: a comparison of C-reactive protein, fibrinogen, homocysteine, lipoprotein(a) and standard cholesterol screening as predictors of peripheral arterial disease. *JAMA.* 2001;285:2481.

71. Boneu B, Leger P, Arnaud C. Haemostatic system activation and prediction of vascular events in patients presenting with stable peripheral arterial disease of moderate severity. Royat Study Group. *Blood Coagulation Fibrinolysis.* 1998;9:129.

72. Trifiletti A, Barbera N, Pizzoleo MA, et al. Hemostatic disorders associated with arterial hypertension and peripheral arterial disease. *J Cardiovasc Surg (Torino).* 1995;36:483.

73. Hoppensteadt S, Walenga JM, Fareed J, et al. Plasma levels of the molecular markers of coagulation and fibrinolysis in patients with peripheral arterial disease. *Semin Thromb Hemost.* 1996;22(suppl 1):35.

74. van der Bom JG, Bots ML, Haverkate F, et al. Activation products of the haemostatic system in coronary, cerebrovascular and peripheral arterial disease. *Thromb Haemost.* 2001;85:234.

75. Woller T, Lawall H, Amann B, et al. Comparison of haemostatic parameters in arterial and venous blood from patients with peripheral arterial occlusive disease. *Vasa.* 1999;28:10.

76. Komarov AL, Panchenko EP, Dobrovolsky AB, et al. D-dimer and platelet aggregability are related to thrombotic events in patients with peripheral arterial occlusive disease. *Eur Heart J.* 2002;23:1309.

77. Spillert CR, Millazzo VJ, Suval WD, et al. Hypercoagulability in arterial disease. *Angiology.* 1989;40:886.

78. Gosk-Bierska T, Adamiec r, Alexewicz P, et al. Coagulation in diabetic and non-diabetic claudicants. *Int Angiol.* 2002;21:128.

79. Lapolla A, Piarulli F, Sartore G, et al. Peripheral artery disease in type 2 diabetes: the role of fibrinolysis. *Thromb Haemost.* 2003;89:91.

80. Wahlgren CM, Sten-Linder M, Egberg N, et al. The role of coagulation and inflammation after angioplasty in patients with peripheral arterial disease. *Cardiovasc Intervent Radiol.* 2006;29:530.

81. Roller RE, Schnedl WJ, Korninger C. Predicting the risk of restenosis after angioplasty in patients with peripheral arterial disease. *Clin Lab.* 2001;47:555.

82. Collins P, Ford I, Greaves M, et al. Surgical revascularization in patients with severe limb ischaemia induces a prothrombotic state. *Platelets.* 2006;17:311.

83. Esposito CJ, Popescu WM, Rinder HM, et al. Increased leukocyte-platelet adhesion in patients with graft occlusion after peripheral vascular surgery. *Thromb Haemost.* 2003;90:1128.

84. Tzoulaki I, Murray GD, Lee AJ, et al. Inflammatory, haemostatic, and rheological markers for incident peripheral arterial disease: Edinburgh Artery Study. *Eur Heart J.* 2007;28:354.

85. Van Cott EM, Lapiosata M, Prins MH. Laboratory evaluation of hypercoagulability with venous or arterial thrombosis. *Arch Path Lab Med.* 2002;126:1281.

86. Frenkel EP. The clinical spectrum of thrombocytosis and thrombocythemia. *Am J Med Sci.* 1991;301:69.

87. Sokunbi DO, Wadhwa NK, Suh H. Vascular disease outcome and thrombocytosis in diabetic and nondiabetic end-stage renal disease patients on peritoneal dialysis. *Adv Perit Dial.* 1994;10:77.

88. Michiels JJ, Berneman ZWI, Schroyens W, et al. Platelet-mediated erythromelalgic, cerebral, ocular and coronary microvascular ischemic and thrombotic manifestations in patients with essential thrombocythemia and polycythemia vera: a distinct aspirin-responsive and coumadin-resistant arterial thrombophilia. *Platelets.* 2006;17:528.

89. Frenkel EP, Mammen EF. Sticky platelet syndrome and thrombocythemia. *Hematol Oncol Clin N A.* 2003;17:63.

90. Katz SG, Kohl RD. Spontaneous peripheral arterial microembolization. *Ann Vasc Surg.* 1992;6:334.

91. Franchini M, Veneri D, Salvagno GL, et al. Inherited thrombophilia. *Crit Rev Clin Lab Sci.* 2006;43:249.

92. Zhu MM, Weedon J, Clark LT. Meta-analysis of the association of platelet glycoprotein IIIa PlA1/A2 polymorphism with myocardial infarction. *Am J Cardiol.* 2000;86:1000.

93. Smith FB, Connor JM, Lee AJ, et al. Relationship of the platelet glycoprotein PlA and fibrinogen T/G+1689 polymorphisms with peripheral arterial disease and ischaemic heart disease. *Thromb Res.* 2003;112:209.

94. Mammen EF. Ten years' experience with the "sticky platelet syndrome." *Clin Appl Thromb Haemost.* 1995;1:68.

95. Mosesson MW. Dysfibrinogenemia and thrombosis. *Semin Thromb Hemost.* 1999;25:311.

96. Golec DB. Fibrinogen and thrombophilia. *Clin Lab Sci.* 2001;14:269.

97. Song KS, Park NJ, Choi JR, et al. Fibrinogen Seoul (FGG Ala341Asp): a novel mutation associated with hyhpodysfibrinogenemia. *Clin Appl Thromb Hemost.* 2006;12:338.

98. Kwaan HC, Nabhan C. Hereditary and acquired defects in the fibrinolytic system associated with thrombosis. *Hematol Oncol Clin N A.* 2003;17:103.

99. Lee AJ, Fowkes FG, Lowe GD, et al. Fibrinogen, factor VII and PAI-1 genotypes and the risk of coronary and peripheral atherosclerosis: Edinburgh Artery Study. *Thromb Haemost.* 1999;81:553.

100. Mlekusch W, Schillinger M, Exner M, et al. Plasminogen activator inhibitor-1 and outcome after femoropoliteal angioplasty: analysis of genotype and plasma levels. *Thromb Haemost.* 2003;90:717.

101. Voetsch B, Loscalzo J. Genetics of thrombophilia: impact on atherogenesis. *Curr Opin Lipidol.* 2004;15:129.

102. Sofi F, Lari B, Rogolino A, et al. Thrombophilic risk factors for symptomatic peripheral arterial disease. *J Vasc Surg.* 2005;41:255.

103. Kuan Y, Dear AE, Grigg MJ. Homocysteine: an aetiological contributor to peripheral vascular disease. *ANZ J Surg.* 2002;72:668.

104. Fowkes FG, Lee AJ, Hau CM, et al. Methylene tetrahydrofolate reductase (MTHFR) and nitric oxide synthase (ecNOS) genes and risks of peripheral arterial disease: Edinburgh Artery Study. *Athereosclerosis.* 2000;150:179.

105. Langman LJ, Cole DEC. Homocysteine: cholesterol of the 90s? *Clin Chim Acta.* 1999;286:63.

106. Sydow K, Hornig B, Arakawa N, et al. Endothelial dysfunction in patients with peripheral arterial disease and chronic hyperhomocysteinemia: potential role of ADMA. *Vasc Med.* 2004;9:93.

107. Riba R, Nicolaou A, Troxler M, et al. Altered platelet reactivity in peripheral vascular disease complicated with elevated plasma homocysteine levels. *Atherosclerosis.* 2004;175:69.

108. Lane JS, Vittinghoff E, Lane KT, et al. Risk factors for premature peripheral vascular disease: results for the National Health and Nutritional Survey, 1999–2002. *J Vasc Surg.* 2006;44:319.

109. Darius H, Pittrow D, Habert R, et al. Are elevated homocysteine plasma levels related to peripheral artery disease? Results from a cross-sectional study of 6880 primary care patients. *Eur J Clin Invest.* 2003;33:751.

110. Bloemenkamp DG, van den Bosch, MA, Mali WP, et al. Novel risk factors for peripheral arterial disease in young women. *Am J Med.* 2002;113:462.

111. van don Bosch M, Bloemenkamo DG, Mali WP, et al. Hyperhomocysteinemia and risk for peripheral arterial occlusive disease in young women. *J Vasc Surg.* 2003;38:772.

112. de Jong SC, Stehouwer CD, Mackaay AJ, et al. High prevalence of hyperhomocysteinemia and asymptomatic vascular disease in siblings of young patients with vascular disease and hyperhomocysteinemia. *Arterioscler Thromb Vasc Biol.* 1997;17:2655.

113. Stricker H, Soldati G, Balmelli T, et al. Homocysteine, vitamins and gene mutations in peripheral arterial disease. *Blood Coag Fibrin.* 2001;12:469.

114. Taute BM, Taute R, Heins S, et al. Hyperhomocysteinemia: marker of systemic atherosclerosis in peripheral arterial disease. *Int Angiol.* 2004;23:35.

115. Ciccarone E, Castelnuovo AD, Assanelli D, et al. Homocysteine levels are associated with the severity of peripheral arterial disease in type 2 diabetic patients. *J Thromb Haemost.* 2003;1:2540.

116. Loncar R, Hrboka V, Tabakovic-Loncar V, et al. Screening of plasma homocysteine in peripheral arterial disease. *Ann Med.* 2001;33:48.

117. Bertine MB, Goessens B, van der Graaf Y, et al. The course of vascular risk factors and the occurrence of vascular events in patients with symptomatic peripheral arterial disease. *J Vasc Surg.* 2007;45:47.

118. Schernthanner GH, Plank C, Minar E, et al. No effect of homocysteine-lowering therapy on vascular inflammation and haemostasis in peripheral arterial occlusive disease. *Eur J Clin Invest.* 2006;36:333.

119. Soltesz P, Veres K, Lakos G, et al. Evaluation of clinical and laboratory features of antiphospholipid syndrome: a retrospective study of 637 patients. *Lupus.* 2003;12:302.

120. Miyakis S, Lockshin MD, Atsumi T, et al. International consensus statement on an update of the classification criteria for definite antiphospholipid syndrome (APS). *J Thromb Haemost.* 2006;4:295.

121. Jara LJ, Medina G, Vera-Lastra O, et al. Atherosclerosis and antiphospholipid antibody syndrome. *Clin Rev Allergy Immunol.* 2003;25:79.

122. George J, Harats D, Gilburd B, et al. Adoptive transfer of β2glycoprotein-1-reactive lymphocytes enhances early atherosclerosis in LDL receptor-deficient mice. *Circulation.* 2000;102:1822.

123. Armitage JD, Homer-Vanniasinkam SH, Lindsey NJ. The role of endothelial cell reactive antibodies in peripheral vascular disease. *Autoimmunity Rev.* 2004;3:39.

124. Toloza SM, Uribe AG, McGwin G, et al. Systemic lupus erythemastosus in a multiethnic U.S. cohort (LUMINA). *Arthritis Rheum.* 2004;50:3947.

125. Wang CR, Chou CC, Hsieh KH, et al. Lupus patients with peripheral vascular thrombosis: the significance of measuring anticardiolipin antibody. *Am J Emerg Med.* 1993;11:468.

126. Friehs I, Eber B, Fiehs G, et al. IgG-anticardiolipin-antibodies are markers for cerebral and peripheral artery disease. *Vasa.* 1992;21:158.

127. Armitage JD, Lindsey NJ, Homer-Vanniasinkam. The role of endothelial cell reactive antibodies in peripheral arterial disease. *Eur J Vasc Endovasc Surg.* 2006;31:170.

128. Nityanand S, Bergmark C, deFaire U, et al. Antibodies against endothelial cells and cardiolipin in young patients with peripheral artherosclerotic disease. *J Intern Med.* 1995;238:437.

129. Fligelstone LJ, Cachis PG, Ralis H, et al. Lupus anticoagulant in patients with peripheral vascular disease: a prospective study. *Eur J Vasc Endovasc Surg.* 1995;9:277.

130. Donaldson M, Weinberg DS, Belkin M, et al. Screening for hypercoagulable states in vascular surgical practice: a preliminary study. *J Vasc Surg.* 1990;11:825.

131. Taylor LM, Chitwood RW, Dalman RL, et al. Antiphospholipid antibodies in vascular surgery patients: a cross-sectional study. *Ann Surg.* 1994;4:544.

132. Puisieux F, de Groote P, Masy E, et al. Association between anticardiolipin antibodies and mortality in patients with peripheral arterial disease. *Am J Med.* 2000;109:633.

133. Nielsen TG, Nordestgaard BG, von Jessen F, et al. Antibodies to cardiolipin may increase risk of failure of peripheral vein bypasses. *Eur J Vasc Endovasc Surg.* 1997;14:177.

134. Tsakiris DA, Tschopl M, Jager K, et al. Anticardiolipin antibodies are not associated with restenosis or endothelial activation after percutaneous transluminal angioplasty. *Int Angiol.* 1997;16:88.

135. Betina RM. Factor V Leiden and other coagulation factor mutations affecting thrombotic risk. *Clin Chem.* 1998;44:1580.

136. Carraro P. European Communities Confederation of Clinical Chemistry and Laboratory Medicine, Working Group on Guidelines for Investigation of Disease: guidelines for the laboratory investigation of inherited thrombophilias. Recommendations for the first level clinical laboratories. *Clin Chem Lab Med.* 2003;42:382.

137. Collins GJ, Heymann RL, Zajtchuk R. Hypercoagulability in patients with peripheral vascular disease. *Am J Surg.* 1975;130:2.

138. Vig S, Chitolie A, Bevan D, et al. The prevalence of thrombophilia in patients with symptomatic peripheral vascular disease. *Br J Surg.* 2006;93:577.

139. Burns PJ, Mosquera DA, Bradbury AW. Prevalence and significance of thrombophilia in peripheral arterial disease. *Eur J Vasc Endovasc Surg.* 2001;22:98.

140. Walker ID. Masterclass series in peripheral arterial disease: inherited thrombophilia. *Vasc Med.* 2004;9:219.

141. Vig S, Chitolie A, Sieight S, et al. Prevalence and risk of thrombophilia defects in vascular patients. *Eur J Vasc Endovasc Surg.* 2004;28:12.

142. Cho YP, Kwon TW, Ahn JH, et al. Protein C and/or protein S deficiency presenting as peripheral arterial insufficiency. *Br J Radiol.* 2005;78:601.

143. Trifiletti A, Pizzoleo MA, Scamardi R, et al. Protein S in normal subjects and patients with peripheral arterial disease. *Panminerva Med.* 1997;39:263.

144. Bohm G, Al-Khaffaf H. Thrombophilia and arterial disease. An uo-to-date review of the literature for the vascular surgeon. *Int Angiol.* 2003;22:116.

145. Senanu E, Sampram K, Lindblad B, et al. Acitvated protein C resistance in patients with peripheral vascular disease. *J Vasc Surg.* 1998;28:624.

146. Fishert CM, Tew K, Appleberg M. Prevalence and outcome of activated protein C resistance in patients after peripheral arterial bypass grafts. *Cardiovasc Surg.* 1999;7:519.

147. Koppel H, Renner W, Krippl P, et al. Diminished response to activated protein C is not correlated with severity of peripheral arterial occlusive disease. *Clin Lab.* 2004;50:689.

148. Aleksci M, Jahn P, Heckenkamp J, et al. Comparison of the prevalence of APC-resistance in vascular patients and in a normal population cohort in Western Germany. *Eur J Vasc Endovasc Surg.* 2005;30:160.

149. Page C, Rubin LE, Gusberg RJ, et al. Arterial thrombosis associated with heterozygous factor V Leiden disorder, hyperhomocysteinemia, and peripheral arterial disease: importance of synergistic factors. *J Vasc Surg.* 2005;42:1014.

150. Sampram ESK, Lindblad B. The impact of factor V mutation on the risk of occlusion in patients undergoing peripheral vascular resconstructions. *Eur J Vasc Endovasc Surg.* 2001;22:134.

151. Mueller T, Marschon R, Dieplinger B, et al. Factor V Leiden, prothrombin G20210A, and methylenetetrahydrofolate reductase C677T mutations are not associated with chronic limb ischemia: the Linz Peripheral Arterial Disease (LIPAD) study. *J Vasc Surg.* 2005;41:808.

152. Reny JL, Alhenc-Gelas M, Fontana P, et al. The factor II G20210A gene polymorphism, but not factor V Arg506Gln, is associated with peripheral arterial disease: results of a case-control study. *J Thromb Haemost.* 2004;2:1334.

153. Kibbe MR, Cortese Hassett AL, McSherry F, et al. Can screening for genetic markers improve peripheral artery bypass patency? *J Vasc Surg.* 2006;36:1198.

154. Kim RJ, Becker RC. Association between factor V Leiden, prothrombin G20210A, and methylenetetrahydrofolate reductase C677T and events of the arterial circulatory system: a meta-analysis of published studies. *Am Heart J.* 2003;146: 948.

155. Nanas JN, Gougoulakis A, Kanakakis J. Acute coronary and peripheral arterial thrombosis following percutaneous coronary intervention in a patient with previously undiagnosed inherited thrombophilia. *Can J Cardiol.* 2003;19: 1063.

156. Gerdes VEA, cate HT, Groot ED, et al. Arterial wall thickness and the risk of recurrent ischemic events in carriers of the prothrombin G20210A mutation with clinical manifestation of atherosclerosis. *Atherosclerosis.* 2002;163: 135.

157. Arruda VR, Annichino-Bizzacchi JM, Goncalves MS, et al. Prevalence of the prothomobin gene variant (nt20210A) in venous thrombosis and arterial disease. *Thromb Haemost.* 1997;78:1430.

158. Rao AK, Vaidyula VR, Bagga S, et al. Effect of antiplatelet agents clopidogrel, aspirin, and cilostazol on circulating tissue factor procoagulant activity in patients with peripheral arterial disease. *Thromb Haemost.* 2006;96:738.

159. TransAtlantic Inter-Society Consensus (TASC) Working Group. Management of peripheral arterial disease. *Int Angiol.* 2000;19(suppl 1):65.

chapter 11

Infections of the Peripheral Arterial System

Charulata Ramaprasad, MD, MPH / David Pitrak, MD

● INTRODUCTION

Peripheral vascular disease can result in a number of serious infections complicating ischemia. However, infections as primary causes of peripheral vascular disease, although uncommon, are also very important clinically. Overall, the arterial vascular system is relatively resistant to infection, but infections do occur, often with terrible consequences. Although uncommon, arterial infections can be seen with a variety of microbial pathogens. Pyogenic bacterial infections are most frequently recognized, but infections with atypical bacterial pathogens, spirochetes, mycobacteria, fungi, parasites, helminths, and even viruses also occur. Diagnosis can be extremely difficult, and many times the infection is not diagnosed until the time of vascular surgery for arterial rupture or another catastrophic event, or at autopsy. Therapy can be just as challenging. Even with a combined medical and surgical approach, arterial infections can be very difficult to eradicate. These infections are associated with significant morbidity and mortality, even if microbiological cure can be achieved.

Not all the effects of infection on peripheral arteries are direct. In some cases, the infection incites a vasculitis. It is the resulting inflammation, with or without ongoing arterial infection, that leads to arterial disease. Finally, direct infection and indirect effects of chronic infections on the arterial system may be subclinical, but these asymptomatic infections may cause endothelial cell dysfunction or lead to pathologic changes, including accelerated atherosclerosis.

Peripheral arterial infections have been comprehensively reviewed in a number of books, chapters, and other reviews.[1,2] This chapter will attempt to review the subject with inclusion of new information and a discussion of contemporary management issues and controversies, as well as discuss the entire breadth of infectious agents that can directly or indirectly affect the peripheral vascular system.

● NATURALLY OCCURRING BACTERIAL AND FUNGAL INFECTIONS OF THE ARTERIAL VASCULATURE, I.E., INFECTIOUS ARTERITIS

Classification and Nomenclature

Although the term mycotic aneurysm is often used for any arterial infection, other terminology may be used that gives some insight into the pathogenesis. Wilson et al.[3] devised a commonly used classification of arterial infections: Mycotic aneurysms caused by septic embolization from endocarditis, secondarily infected atherosclerotic aneurysms, infectious arteritis without aneurysm formation or necrotizing arteritis, and finally infected pseudoaneurysms from trauma or a vascular procedure. Even this classification is not all encompassing, and does not include arterial infections caused by local spread from an adjacent site of infection.

Incidence and Epidemiology

Infections of the arterial system are relatively rare. In general, the ability of bacteria to bind and cause infection of the arterial endothelial surface is low, but the exact incidence of infectious arteritis is not well defined. Even autopsy data on the frequency of this type of infection is limited, and usually reports only focus on very large vessels, such as the aorta or, in some studies, the femoral arteries. Furthermore, many of the large autopsy studies that reference infectious arteritis were done decades ago, and the relative incidence of different types of arterial infections has dramatically changed over time. However, these earlier studies do highlight the rarity of these infections. For example, the frequency of aneurysms of the aorta in a frequently referenced autopsy study at the Boston City Hospital from 1902 to 1951 was very low, 1.5%, and only 2.6% of these were infectious.[4] The presence of an atherosclerotic plaque or aneurysm predisposes a patient to this type of infection, and this is the reason for the historic male predominance and older age, usually more than 65 years. The reported incidence of infected aneurysms at other sites, such as the iliac arteries, is also low. Data from examination of pathology samples indicate that abdominal aortic aneurysms may be infected relatively frequently compared to other arterial structures, but the majority of patients have no constitutional symptoms, signs, or laboratory evidence of infection premortem. Some studies have shown a high incidence of positive arterial cultures, even in cases of clean elective vascular repair.[5] This may indicate that the infection is very well localized or is just a bystander infection, but if a repair is performed in-situ, these infections can certainly have importance.[6] If these infections are not diagnosed until surgery is performed, then there is the risk of recurrent infection, especially if there has been a repair using a prosthetic device. Conversely, if a patient has fever, there is at least a clue that may indicate the presence of infection and allow diagnosis prior to local arterial complications such as rupture.

In the preantibiotic era, the vast majority of clinically apparent mycotic aneurysms were caused by septic embolization in patients with bacterial endocarditis.[3] Antibiotic therapy for endocarditis has greatly reduced the incidence of arterial infection. As the frequency of mycotic aneurysms from endocarditis has decreased, the proportion of infectious arteritis cases caused by seeding of an atherosclerotic aneurysm or plaque has increased, at least in the United States. Infectious arteritis is rare in childhood, except in the case of mycotic aneurysms from infective endocarditis or congenital cardiovascular malformations, such as coarctation of the aorta. Both the mode of arterial infection and the etiologic agent can vary geographically, and is quite different in the tropics as compared to developed countries. For example, cerebrovascular disease in the tropics may be attributable to one of a multitude of infectious etiologic agents, including cysticercosis, infective endocarditis, Chaga's disease, viral hemorrhagic fevers, gnathosomiasis, leptospirosis, cerebral malaria, and tuberculosis (TB)—infections that would for the most part be extremely unlikely in the United States.[7]

Pathogenesis

Several routes of infection have been recognized in the pathogenesis of infections of the peripheral arterial system. Infections of the arterial vasculature can result from septic embolization from the heart, seeding from bacteremia or fungemia, or local invasion from an adjacent infectious process. Penetrating injuries, accidental or related to drug use, or related to invasive medical procedures involving arteries, are another route of local invasion. The relative importance of each of these modes of infection has changed since the advent of antibiotic therapy.

Mycotic aneurysm is the term most often used for local arterial infection caused by septic embolization. Although mycotic is an adjective usually reserved for fungal infections, this term has now been adopted for local arteritis from embolization as a result of all types of pathogens, even when there is no actual dilation of the involved vessel. Mycotic aneurysms from septic embolization most often occur from occlusion of the lumen of a vessel, usually at the vessel's bifurcation, with a large and infected embolus. Small micromboli can also go the vaso vasorum of larger arteries, also leading to the formation of mycotic aneursysms. As already stated, mycotic aneursysms from embolization occur most frequently in patients with endocarditis. Although this complication is much less frequent today than in the antibiotic era, it is still associated with significant morbidity and mortality. In a recent study of patients with endocarditis, 18% developed mycotic aneurysms, and the morbidity and mortality from rupture was significant.[8] Most of the mycotic aneurysms complicating endocarditis involve the sinuses of Valsalva or the most proximal ascending aorta just above the heart valves. Less often, major intracranial, peripheral, and visceral arteries are involved. One of the most serious complications of septic embolization in infective endocarditis is cerebral artery embolization. When this occurs, the mortality rate from endocarditis greatly increases. Even if the patient survives the stroke, the risk of subsequent rupture remains. Anticoagulation, which is often necessary in patients who have required valve replacement after an episode of endocarditis, results in extremely high mortality if bleeding occurs. Although rupture and bleeding of mycotic aneurysms is usually caused by dilation and thinning of the vessel wall, bleeding from non-dilated infected vessels termed septic necrotic arteritis, can also occur.

Visceral aneurusysms are extremely rare, but are caused by either infective endocarditis or polyarteritis nodosa (PAN). These may involve the superior mesenteric artery, celiac artery, or hepatic artery, resulting in ischemia of visceral organs. Involvement of other visceral arteries is less common.

Cerebral infarction caused by infectious endarteritis can also be a complication of severe bacteremic infections other than endocarditis, including common infections such as community-acquired bacterial pneumonia. Septic emboli from non-cardiac sources, arteritis as a result of seeding during high grade bacteremia, and/or activation of the coagulation system can all result in cerebral infarction from infectious endarteritis.[9]

Mycotic anerusysms or necrotizing arteritis from seeding of an atherosclerotic vessel is found most often in the abdominal aorta. 70% of the time the ascending thoracic aorta is involved, and 15% of the time the descending thoracic aorta is involved. Infected aneurysms usually show neutrophilic infiltration, necrosis, abscess formation, and hemorrhage. Thoracic or lumbar vertebral osteomyelitis can sometimes be found. The contiguous spread may be in either direction, from the osteomyelitis to the aorta or from the aorta to the bone.

Although atherosclerosis is the most common preexisting arterial abnormality, other arterial diseases such as medial necrosis and vasculitis can also predispose a patient to arterial infection. Any organism causing transient bacteremia could do this, including transient bacteremia complicating invasive procedures. Infectious endarteritis in the absence of an aneurysm or preexisting atherosclerotic disease may occur, but this is extremely rare and often not identified premortem.

Local infection can result in arterial infection through direct extension. For example, cerebral arteritis and aneurysm formation may also complicate acute bacterial meningitis.[10] Cerebral artery angiitis from an adjacent subdural empyema has also been reported.[11] Carotid artery occlusion resulting in a stoke syndrome has occurred as a consequence of necrotizing fasciitis of the lateral neck space.[12] Actinomycosis has caused a severe vasculitis in arteries in the basilar meningeal region caused by direct intracranial spread from a local head and neck infection.[13] Arterial infection can also complicate sinusitis, complicated skin and soft tissue infections, vertebral osteomyelitis caused by pyogenic bacteria or tuberculosis, or any local infection with adjacent spread.

● ARTERIAL INFECTIONS CAUSED BY TRAUMA, PROCEDURES, AND DEVICES

Arterial Infections Caused by Trauma and Intravenous Drug Use

Any accidental trauma can result in an arterial infection, particularly if there is significant arterial damage, as is often seen with gun shot wounds and motor vehicle accidents.[14] This usually involves the extremities and in most cases, there is pseudoaneurysm formation. Injection drug use is one nonaccidental, nonmedical procedure that can cause arterial trauma and arterial infection. The incidence of infections of peripheral arteries caused by injection drug use is lower than one might expect, only 0.03% in one study.[15] When these infections do occur, they can be any artery that is injected, including the brachial, radial, carotid, femoral, or other lower extremity arteries. There is often an associated subcutaneous abscess or musculoskeletal infection such as septic arthritis.

Arterial Infections Caused by Medical Procedures

Given the relatively low rates of infections complicating injection drug use, it is not surprising that invasive procedures performed using standard sterile procedures are infrequently associated with arterial infection. Despite low rates, however, these infections occur in ever-increasing numbers because of the vast numbers of procedures performed, including vascular surgery, cardiac catheterization, angioplasty, stent placement, arterial chemotherapy catheters, and radial artery catheters for monitoring.

Arterial Infections Caused by Percutaneous Procedures. Even a one-time puncture of an artery for a procedure, or even an arterial puncture to obtain a blood gas

specimen, can result in inoculation and infection or intimal damage and subsequent seeding of the artery from transient bacteremia or fungemia. Although infection would be expected at the site of the arterial puncture, infection of an external iliac artery has occurred a distance from the insertion site, presumably from trauma caused by the tip of the catheter.[16] Infection of percutaneous suture closure devices can occur after catheter-based interventions. Infection is rare with only six infections in 822 cases (0.7%) in one study.[17] Resolution requires exploration, removal of the suture closure device, and in most cases, autologus repair. In some cases, even more extensive surgical management is needed for complications from these devices.[18]

Arterial Infections Caused by Indwelling Catheters. Some arterial manipulations are performed early in life, and newborn infants undergoing umbilical artery catheterization may develop staphylococcal mycotic aneurysms affecting the aorta, femoral arteries, or multiple sites.[19] Radial artery infections secondary to arterial lines are rare, but have serious complications. The incidence is only 0.2%, but bacteremia, radial artery mycotic aneurysms, and secondary sternal wound infections may occur.[20]

Arterial Infections Caused by Previously Operated Vessels. Arterial surgery can also lead to arterial infections, even without grafting. When arteritis complicates cardiac surgery, the results are often disastrous. The organisms most often involved are common nosocomial pathogens associated with wound infections, but more unusual organisms may be seen in immunocompromised hosts. A number of cases have resulted from *Listeria*, most often in the very young, very old, or immunosuppressed.[21] *Candida* spp. may also be involved, and interestingly has been seen in many renal transplant patients, with infection of the vascular pedicle. In one case, this pathogen was most likely carried over from the donor, as it was found in the conservation fluid from the graft.[22] Renal artery mycotic aneurysms in general are a particular problem for renal transplant recipients. A postoperative peripnephric infection can result in infection at the arterial anastomosis.[23] *Candida* infection of the graft used to vascularize the pancreas graft was seen in two recipients of pancreas–kidney transplants. This led to the loss of both pancreatic grafts.[24]

Arterial Stent Infections

Infected stents may lead to arterial infection, and this has resulted in subclavian arteritis and pseudoaneurysm formation.[25] Rupture of the iliac artery and anursysmal transformation of the abdominal aorta has been reported with infection of metallic iliac artery stent placement.[26] Renal artery stents have also become infected.[27]

Vascular Graft Infections.

Epidemiology. Prosthetic vascular grafts are even more susceptible to infection, and the rates vary between 1% and 6% depending on many factors.[28,29] Emergency surgery, reoperation, and diabetes are major risk factors. The site of the graft also contributes to the risk of infection, with lower rates for aortic grafts, intermediate rates for aortofemoral grafts, and the highest rates for femoro-popliteal grafts. All are associated with significant mortality, 17% to 24%, and an even higher rate of morbidity, usually limb amputation.[30]

Pathogenesis. Just as native arteries can be infected by a number of routes, prosthetic vascular grafts can also be infected by several routes. The grafts may be infected at the time of placement or after subsequent manipulations, including repair. Infection can also spread from a local area of infection or colonization, including the surgical wound. Other local infections, including cellulitis or other skin and soft tissue infections can lead to graft infection. Grafts can also be infected hematogenously. The risk of hematogenous seeding is greatest early after implantation, when the graft has not been endothelialized, but never disappears because graft coverage is never complete. Although early graft infection can occur, most infections present after many months.

● MICROBIOLOGY OF ARTERIAL INFECTIONS

The microbiology of arterial infections is quite varied. In mycotic aneurysms from septic embolization, the microbial etiology mirrors that of endocarditis, and all the organisms that are recognized as principal endocarditis agents may be involved. The agents listed in the revised Duke criteria for endocarditis include *Staphylococcus aureus*, viridans streptococci, Enterococci, *Streptococcus bovis*, and HACEK organisms (*Hemophilus* spp., *Actinobacillus*, *Cardiobacterium*, *Eikenella*, and *Kingella*, all gram-negative coccobacilli) are the usual culprits. These organisms are readily isolated from the blood in most circumstances.

In the preantibiotic era, infectious arteritis caused by bacteremia complicating common pyogenic infections involved pneumococcus, group A streptococcus, and gonococcus. These agents also commonly caused endocarditis in that era. In many instances, no underlying arterial disease was known to preexist. These infections are now rare, as are the cases of endocarditis caused by these agents, but some organisms can still infect normal arteries. Meningococcus frequently infects the walls of arteries, resulting in obstruction and infarction of the skin, and is one of the causes of purpura fulminans. Visceral organs such as the adrenals may also infarct from vascular occlusion. In one study,[31] 20 patients with peripheral arteritis presumed as a result of infection were studied to find out the etiology. Ten patients had meningococcal disease. Meningococci were found in the vessel walls of ischemic areas. Other patients did not have organisms in the vessel wall, but had vasculitis following streptococcal infection and measles, and these patients seemed to respond to anticoagulation with heparin. *Pseudomonas aeruginosa* can cause severe vascular disease and vascular occlusion in patients with neutropenia.[32] The characteristic necrotic lesions of ecthyma gangrenosum result from occlusion of cutaneous vessels by the organisms themselves.

Many bacterial pathogens can infect an atherosclerotic plaque or aneurysm. Gram-positives, *S. aureus*, different coagulase-negative staphylococcal species, viridans streptococci, and enterococci predominate, but a variety of enteric gram-negative rods have been implicated. *Listeria monocytogenes* is an uncommon cause of arterial infection but can occur in aneurysms of previously operated arteries in very young, very old, or immunocompromised patients.[21] Several anaerobes have also been involved. *Clostridium septicum* can cause aortitis in patients with an underlying gastrointestinal (GI) or hematologic malignancy, with mortality approaching 70%.[33] Although many organisms can cause arterial infection, certain organisms are preferentially associated with this type of infection. Although arterial infection with *Salmonella* is rare, it remains one of the most common causes of primary mycotic aneurysm.[34,35] Overall, *Salmonella* spp. are involved in up to 20% of the cases. Although bacteremias can occur from gastroenteritis with any species of *Salmonella*, when patients are older than 50 years of age, bacteremia is associated with an intravascular focus in up to 25% of cases. Forty percent of the *Salmonella* isolates are *Salmonella enteritidis* strains, which is similar to the proportion of cases causing gastroenteritis. Not all cases result from enteric infection, and *Salmonella* bacteremia can also complicate urinary tract infections with these species.[36] Other species, however, have an even greater propensity for vascular infection. *Salmonella choleraesuis*, the best example, may be involved in 30% of cases of aneurysms infected with *Salmonella*, a much higher percent than that for enteritis caused by this organism.[37] A retrospective study showed a gradual increase in bacteremia caused by *Salmonella* from 11 cases in 1984 to 58 cases in 1988.[38] *Arizona* spp. are closely related to *Salmonella*, and they have also been involved in aortic infection complicating atherosclerosis.[39]

Certain bacteria are not seen in cases of infectious arteritis in the United States, but have been implicated in endemic areas. *Burkhoderia pseudomallei* bacterial arteritits occurs in endemic areas in Southeast Asia.[40]

Syphillis can cause an arteritis. Classically this is an ascending aortitis in patients with longstanding infection. Syphilis can also cause central nervous system (CNS) disease resulting from an arteritis that can be demonstrated by conventional angiography or MRA.[41] Although this can occur in anyone with tertiary syphilis, it is more common in human immunodeficiency virus (HIV)-infected patients. Labauge et al.[42] reported on a HIV-infected patient with infarction of the pons caused by neurosyphilis. After the patient developed right hemiparesis, he recovered after two courses of IV penicillin.[42] Syphilis can also cause areas of vasculitis and obliterative arteritis in the placenta as a result of maternal infection.[43] Sometimes a spirochetal infection can mimic a non-infectious vasculitis.[44] A 71-year-old male developed vision loss and headache. Temporal artery biopsy showed giant cell arteritis (GCA), but corticosteroid therapy failed. A blood culture later grew spirochetes. The patient was subsequently treated with ceftriaxone and regained some sight. Leptospirosis can also be associated with cerebrovascular disease. Twelve cases caused by *Leptospirosis pomona* have been characterized, with cerebral panarteritis and infarctions.[45]

Fungi are much less common agents of mycotic aneurysms and septic arteritis, except in the chest. When infection with fungi occur, most are caused by *Candida* or certain molds, particularly *Aspergillus* and the agents of mucormycosis. These infections usually affect immunocompromised patients or result from nosocomial complications. A renal transplant patient developed a painless groin mass caused by a common femoral artery pseudoaneurysm and saccular aneurysm of the infrarenal aorta due to Candida that occurred a few weeks after a colonoscopy.[46] An infected abdominal aortic aneurysm occurred after a nosocomial catheter-related candidemia. These incidence of such secondary fungal infections may start to increase as the incidence of nosocomial fungemia increases.[47]

Aspergillus spp. and the zygomycetes, the agents of mucormycosis, have a propensity to invade blood vessels. This occurs most frequently with infections in the chest or sinuses.[48] Infection can spread from the sinuses to the orbital and CNS, and it may be the subsequent cerebrovascular involvement that predominates.[49,50] This may result in confusion with another non-infectious condition, and a case of orbital aspergillosis mimicking temporal arteritis (TA) has been described.[50] These species can also cause fungal arteritis with vascular occlusion at operative sites.[49,51-53] Intracranial aneurysms caused by *Aspergillus* have a tendency to rupture and bleed.[54,55]

The endemic fungi, such as histoplasmosis and coccidioidomycosis, may rarely cause vascular disease.[56] However, one fungal pathogen can cause a vasculitis, usually in the lower extremities, as a result of soft tissue infection. *Pythium insidiosum*, is the agent of pythiosis, a life-threatening infection of both humans and animals.[57,58] This infection is endemic in Thailand and presents as keratitis or arteritis. There can be vascular occlusion of the large vessels of the lower extremities caused by ascending artertis, often in patients with thalessemia or in patients on chelation therapy with deferoxamine. Infection may also be an occupational disease, as most of the affected individuals have been farmers. This serous infection often leads to limb amputation.[59]

The usual mycotic aneurysm from *Mycobacterium tuberculosis* is a pulmonary artery aneurysm from a cavitary lung infection. This is the classic Rasmussen's aneurysm, which can rupture and lead to death due to massive hemoptysis. Infection of peripheral arteries is much less frequently recognized. Bacteremia and dissemination occurs frequently in tuberculosis, but this is often asymptomatic and subclinical except in patients with the syndrome of miliary TB. Although arterial involvement can be a part of disseminated disease, this is extremely rare. More frequent is involvement of the aorta and formation of a mycotic aneruysm caused by reactivation from a granuloma in close proximity.

Arteritis from parasitic diseases is very uncommon and varies according to geographic location. In the United States, cysticercosis occurs fairly frequently, usually in immigrants or in those with a history of travel to endemic areas. Cerebral arteritis can occur with subarachnoid cysticercosis. This can be seen on angiography even in the absence of clinical symptoms. Most cases involve the middle and posterior cerebral arteries. When symptoms do occur, stroke is the most common syndrome.[60] Another infection seen in the United States is strongyloidasis. Patients with immune deficiencies can develop a hyperinfection syndrome from this usually less severe intestinal infection. One case report describes a patient with strongyloides hyperinfection and related *E. coli* sepsis, who also developed mesenteric thrombosis. The occluded vessel contained numerous filiform larvae.[61] In other countries, helminths may cause vascular occlusion in affected individuals.[62]

The aneurysms and arteritis associated with injection drug use are usually caused by *S. aureus* and *P. aeruginosa*, but other pathogens have been reported. Arterial infections caused by invasive arterial procedures and vascular surgery are similar to those seen in other nosocomial infections. Most are common noscomial bacterial pathogens. Nosocomial fungal pathogens, *Candida* and *Aspergillus*, and rapid-growing mycobacteria that can be involved in surgical infections, can also occur. Although unusual, endemic fungi and even *M. tuberculosis* have been involved in prosthetic vascular graft infections.[63,64]

Up to this point, the discussion has focused on macroscopic arteritis, but small arterial vessels may also be the target of infection. Lacunar infarcts in the CNS caused by small vessel disease can result from a number of etiologies. Infection with syphilis, cysticercosis, *Helicobacter pylori*, HIV, and other viruses have all been implicated.[65]

● CLINICAL MANIFESTATIONS

When arterial infections occur as a consequence of septic embolization, usually there is other evidence of the underlying infectious disease, such as endocarditis, in the majority of patients. However, complications from the septic embolization, including mycotic aneurysm, may be the clinical reason that a patient will present. Small intracranial mycotic aneurysms are often clinically silent, but patients will develop heachache and rapid alterations in the level of consciousness when hemorrhage or rupture occurs. Larger emboli may cause a stroke. This occurs in up to 21% of cases of infective endocarditis.[66] Focal neurologic deficits or seizures may occur first, allowing for imaging and diagnosis prior to rupture and bleeding. Rupture occurs anywhere from 0 to 35 days or longer after the initial diagnosis of infective endocarditis.

Clinical diagnosis of primary arterial infection is often difficult, and patients, unfortunately, may have symptoms for months before a diagnosis is made. Primary bacterial infections of the aorta are particularly difficult to diagnose. The diagnosis should be considered in the setting of fever of uncertain origin combined with pain in the abdomen or back, all fairly nonspecific findings.[67] Fever is not a universal finding by any means and is absent in up to 30% of cases. The nonspecific nature of many of the clinical symptoms and signs, however, results in late diagnosis, often after rupture of the aneruysm in approximately 70% of the cases. Rupture can occur with bleeding into the peritoneal cavity, retroperitoneum, pleural cavity, or mediastinum. Rupture may even occur in the absence of aneurysm formation.[68] Sometimes, an aortoenteric fistula, usually between the aorta and the third portion of the duodenum, will present with upper GI bleeding. Less frequent signs are an abdominal mass, ureteral obstruction caused by mass effect, or lower GI bleeding. Aneurysms of the iliac or femoral artery result in leg pain. When more peripheral arteries are involved, a painful swelling may be present as a result of a mycotic aneurysm or pseudoaneurysm. A pulsatile mass due to hematoma from hemorrhage may occur, without true dilation of the lumen.[69] A draining sinus is rare, but is very indicative of infective. A patient with continuing primary bacteremia (despite appropriate antibiotic therapy in patients without endocarditis on echocardiography) should be suspected of having an infected aneurysm.

The clinical presentation of arterial infections from instrumentation or involving a prosthetic graft is similar to that of primary arterial infection.[70] Patients with an aortofemoral graft infection often present with a painful mass in the groin, with or without fever. Patients with more peripheral graft infection usually have fever and a purulent wound infection. Pseudoaneuruysms will form at anastomotic sites. Distal septic emboli and graft occlusion may also occur. Pateints who develop an aortoenteric fistula between the graft and small bowel may present with GI bleeding.

● DIAGNOSIS OF ARTERIAL INFECTIONS

Microbiological Evaluation

There are no definitive routine laboratory tests that can be performed to make this diagnosis. Leukocytosis and elevations of acute phase reactants are frequent, but nonspecific. Microbiologic investigations are obviously necessary to determine the infectious etiology. Bacteremia is common, but the proportion of patients with positive blood cultures varies according to the type of aneurysm or arteritis, even though all these infections are intravascular and continuous bacteremia with multiple positive blood cultures over time would be expected. Blood cultures are positive in approximately 90% of the cases of aneurysms complicating infective endocarditis, while atherosclerotic anerusyms that are infected are associated with positive blood cultures in only 50% of cases. Fungal pathogens, most often *Candida* spp., can be isolated from blood, but others, such as *Aspergillus* spp., are almost never isolated from blood (Figure 11-1). Cultures of perigraft fluid can be helpful when obtained, but this requires a clinical suspicion and imaging of the involved vessel. In cases of arterial occlusion from an embolus that is managed by thrombectomy, the removed clot should be sent for smears, cultures, and histopathology. If infection is suspected and the patient undergoes surgery, it is extremely important to perform microbiologic evaluation of samples taken, in particular of the involved portion of the vessel that may be removed.

Many of the pathogens previously discussed do not readily grow in culture. They may be seen on pathologic examination, but other testing can be useful in the preoperative diagnosis. For example, serologic testing for syphilis is quite sensitive and specific.

Imaging Studies

Radiographic imaging is usually required to document or confirm the clinical diagnosis of an arterial infection (Figure 11-2). Plain films have rarely shown gas in the surrounding tissues with arterial infection, but in general are of little help. Aortic infections may be well demonstrated by helical CT.[71] For other vessels, particularly the cerebrovasculature, arteriography still remains the reference examination for stenosing arteriopathies.[72] MRA can show small aneurysms, 2 to 3 mm in diameter. False tests can occur, and nothing performs better than the four-vessel cerebral angiography. It is generally the best test for demonstrating other vascular pathology, pseudoaneurysm and the extent of vascular occlusion. Although CT imaging is often helpful, it may not be sensitive enough to show the aneurysmal dilatation of the involved vessel. Abdominal aortic aneurysms that have no calcification should be considered to be infected, since calcification is very common in bland atherosclerotic aneurysms. Ultrasound can show fluid collections around infected arteries and prosthetic vascular grafts, but it is difficult to determine a perigraft fluid collection is infected in the early postoperative periods, is due to infection or simply post-operative inflammation. Perianeurysmal fluid collections are another sign of infection, and a potential source of culture material. Echocardiographic findings are major criteria for the diagnosis of endocarditis, but can also be useful in detecting mycotic aneurysms in the ascending aorta.

Labeled white cell studies also have a role in the diagnosis of vascular graft infections, but false-negative tests occur (Figure 11-3). Williamson et al. performed 30 Indium-111-labeled white blood cells scan in 21 patients with suspected vascular graft infections and compared the results to CT[73]. The scans were 100% sensitive in identifying all grafts found to be infected at surgery. Indium scanning was found to be 88% specific; there was 15 true negatives and 2 false positives. CT was less sensitive (37%) when the criteria of fluid and/or gas surrounding the fluid was used as an indicator of infection. The labeled white cell scans also identified extragraft infections. The usefulness of white cell scans has been shown in other studies as well, but false-positive tests have been seen in the first 4 weeks after graft implantation, and antibiotic therapy prior to the examination can decrease sensitivity.[74] Tc-99m-labeled antigranulocyte antibodies (LeukoScan) are also being evaluated for detection of infection in different clinical settings, but specific data on vascular infections, although favorable, are limited.[75]

In those patients who develop GI bleeding as a consequence of an aortoenteric fistula, endoscopy may help with diagnosis, but this manifestation is very unusual.

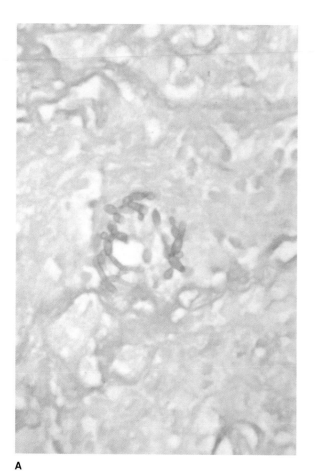
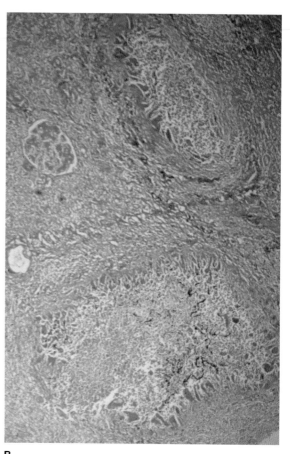

A **B**

● **FIGURE 11-1.** Microbiologic smears in the diagnosis of arterial infections. (A) A periodic-acid Schiff (PAS) stain demonstrating the pseudohyphae of a *Candida* spp. in the infected clot from a prosthetic arteriovenous fistula for hemodialysis. This confirmed that the graft was the source of candidemia in this patient. (B) A Gomori methenamine silver (GMS) stain demonstrating the uniform width, septate hyphae branching at 45-degree angles, which is characteristic of invasive aspergillosis. The hyphae are seen in a clot in the renal artery that extended from a prosthetic aortic graft. Blood cultures were negative, and the microbiologic studies of the material from the clot were the only specimens that identified the etiologic agent.

● THERAPY OF INFECTIOUS ARTERITIS

Despite comprehensive reviews of this topic, it is hard to be adamant about the management of arterial infections, since none of the approaches have been proven in controlled trials.[76,77] Management includes antimicrobial therapy with or without surgery, and the surgical approach can be debated. Often there will have to be a personalized treatment plan. The management of graft infections is particularly difficult, and the British Society for Antimicrobial Chemotherapy has set up a multidisciplinary working group to come up with a consensus statement that will make recommendations regarding diagnosis and therapy.[78] Some general principles, many shared with other types of prosthetic infections, can be followed.[79]

Antimicrobial Therapy

The antimicrobial therapy is probably most agreed upon course of action, with prolonged courses of intravenous antibiotics typically being recommended. In certain situations, such as cerebral artery mycotic aneurysms complicating septic embolization from infectious endocarditis, surgery is not a feasible option. Effective antimicrobial therapy alone, however, may result in reduction in size and complete resolution is not uncommon. Serial angiographic studies or other imaging may be useful in following mycotic aneurysms when a more expectant approach is taken.[80] In one series reported by Kovoor et al.,[81] complete resolution occurred in two-thirds of patients who were managed with antibiotics alone and repeat angiography. Mycotic aneurysms complicating septic embolization from infectious endocarditis are treated like endocarditis, with prolonged courses of parenteral, bactericidal antibiotics. Antibiotic therapy should be given for 4 to 6 weeks similar to the course recommended for infective endocarditis. In the case of device-related infections, prolonged courses of oral antibiotics have been used after a course of IV therapy when the device cannot be completely removed or in situ graft

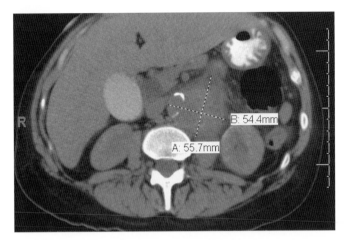

● **FIGURE 11-2.** Computed tomography (CT) in the diagnosis of an aortic mycotic aneurysm. The study shows a saccular aneurysm of the aorta at the level of the renal arteries. There is a large hematoma surrounding the aneurysm with extension into the retroperitoneum, indicating rupture of the aneurysm. Cultures from surgery grew *Streptococcus pneumoniae*.

replacement has been performed (see below). Even chronic suppressive therapy has been recommended in certain situations where device removal is contraindicated, and observational studies indicate this can be effective and safe.[82]

Antibiotic choices should be based on culture and susceptibility data when available, and if an infection is chronic, every attempt at making an etiologic diagnosis should be made prior to initiating therapy. Empiric therapy may be necessary for patients who are septic or having major complications.

Surgical Management

For extracranial sites, management of bacterial arteritis most often requires a combined medical and surgical approach.[77,83] Although morbidity and mortality is high when patients are treated with antibiotics alone, a combined surgical and medical approach to therapy is not necessarily any better, the exact approach is debatable, and amputation and mortality rates are high. When removal of the graft does not compromise arterial flow and limb or organ perfusion, such as with removal of infected hemodialysis catheters, good results can be expected.[84] However, grafts only often provide the arterial flow, removal presents greater challenges. The traditional approach has included surgical debridement, extra-anatomic bypass, and irrigation or other decontamination of the aneurysm cavity, in addition to systemic antibiotic therapy. Although the reasoning behind not placing a new graft into an infected site (in-situ grafting) appears obvious, the difficulties with

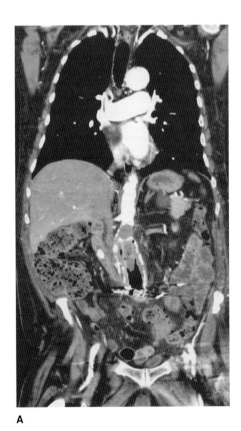

A

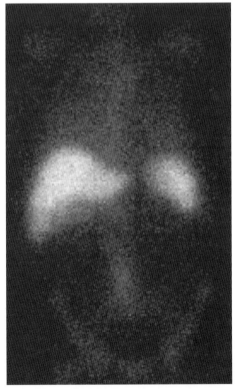

B

● **FIGURE 11-3.** Labeled white cell scanning in the radiographic evaluation of a mycotic aneurysm. (A) CT of the aorta with thrombosis of an aortic graft below the renal arteries. There is a gas/fluid level in the lumen. (B) Image from an Indium-labeled white cell scan after 6 weeks of intravenous, combination antibiotic therapy. There was still uptake in the same vicinity indicating persistent infection and resection of the involved graft was required for cure.

extra-anatomic bypass may make this approach preferable in some instances. Regardless of the approach, outcomes are often dismal. In one series of infected abdominal or iliac arteries (13 patients resulting in a 0.65% overall incidence of infection), treatment included resection, extra-anatomic bypass, in situ grafting, resection, and ligation; in this series, four patients died, three as a result of rupture.[85] Overall, only five (38%) patients had a good result. Organisms that were associated with poor outcomes were *S. aureus*, *Salmonella* spp., *Bacteroides fragilis*, and *Pseudomonas*.

The problems with arterial infection are further compounded in cases of prosthetic graft infections. It is even more difficult to sterilize a prosthesis compared to infected native arterial tissue, and in general, an infected prosthetic vascular graft must be removed for a satisfactory outcome. Similar to infective arteritis involving native vessels, the traditional approach to treating vascular graft infection has been the complete removal of the graft, extra-anatomic bypass, and antibiotics. However, other approaches may be taken, including graft removal with in situ replacement and graft preservation. Each of these approaches also have variations. Extra-anatomic bypass can be done before or simultaneously with excision of the infected graft. One study tried to determine the outcome if the extra-anatomic bypass occurred before or after the removal of the infected artery or prosthesis.[86] None of the 10 patients who had a bypass inserted first developed limb ischemic or infection of the remote graft. The mortality was only 26% if remote bypass was done first, whether or not enteric erosions or fistulas were present. A literature review of infected aortic grafts showed that if removal preceded remote bypass there was a mortality of 71%.

Although total aortic graft excision is still considered optimal by some vascular surgeons, partial excision and repair in situ using autologous vein, cryopreserved grafts, and antibiotic-impregnated or silver-coated protheses can be performed.[87,88] In situ replacement has some advantages, and in some series has been shown to have acceptable results. Extra-anatomic bypass often does not result in adequate perfusion. In situ replacement also avoids blowout of the stump, and multiple high-risk surgical procedures. Some authorities recommend the use of antibiotic-impregnated grafts, collagen-impregnated dacron grafts, or cryopreserved biografts to reduce the chance of infection of the new graft.[89] Antibiotic impregnated stents may have a role, but probably for patients with selected indications, that is, local infection, ruptured aneruysms, femoral–tibial stents, cases of axillofemoral revascularization, immunodeficient patients, reoperations, and postradiation arteritis, where the incidence of stent infection is higher.[90]

Decontamination of the field is important as well, and is most often accomplished with betadine irrigation or use of sulfamylon, or even antibiotic-coated methacrylate beads. Another important part of graft preservation or in situ grafting is coverage with muscle flaps, and the importance of plastic surgery has been stressed by several authors.[91]

One meta-analysis has questioned whether or not the traditional extra-anatomic bypass, graft removal should remain the preferred approach for treatment of aortic graft

infections.[92] Clinical events (mortality, conduit failure, amputation, reinfection, and mortality) were tallied for extra-anatomic bypass and in situ grafting with rifampin-bonded prostheses, cryopreserved allografts, or autologous veins. Overall, in situ grafting had superior outcomes in this analysis.

Zetrenne et al.[93] have devised an algorithm to help decide on the procedure of choice. Factors include Samson class, microbiology, and other anatomic considerations. The Samson classification looks at the depth of the infection. In groups 1 and 2, there is infection of the dermis or subcutaneous tissues over the graft, respectively, but the infection is not in contact with the graft. Group 3 involves infection of the graft itself, but no involvement of the anastomosis. Group 4 involves anastomosis, but without bleeding or bacteremia, while group 5 involves an anastomosis with bleeding and/or sepsis. In this schema, groups 3 to 5 require surgical intervention. This staging can be accomplished by imaging, most often CT. Exploration, however, may be necessary for accurate staging. Patients in group 3 are those who are most appropriate for graft or route salvage. As long as the involved portion of the graft is removed and surrounding tissue debrided, the wound can be sterilized and a plastic surgery procedure is performed to assure adequate wound coverage. The management of patients in group 4 is more difficult, and graft or route salvage may not be possible in all cases. The decision to even attempt this may hinge on the organisms involved. If the infection involves highly virulent organisms isolated from perigraft aspiration or wound cultures, such as *P. aeruginosa* or MRSA, graft or route preservation should be avoided. For Samson group 5 cases with anastomotic bleeding, graft occlusion, and/or sepsis, excision of the entire graft is necessary.

One important part of the management, regardless of the surgical procedure performed, is continued surveillance for recurrent infection. In addition to clinical evaluation, patients should have repeated ultrasounds or other imaging examinations on a regular basis.

● VIRAL INFECTIONS OF THE ARTERIAL SYSTEM

Some reviews of arterial infections state that viruses have not been shown to be a direct cause of infection, and infections with viruses only leads to an immune-mediated vasculitis. This view may not be entirely correct, and a number of observations suggest that active arterial infection with viruses does occur and can lead to vascular insufficiency or other vascular complications. To date, the most accumulated data is related to infection with the herpesviruses and human immunodeficiency virus (HIV). This is important since antiviral therapy may be part of the management of these infections.

Herpesvirus Infections

Of all the herpes viruses, varicella zoster virus (VZV) has most often been implicated in peripheral vascular disease. A rare case of cutaneous nodules and obliterative vasculitis with VZV detected in the vessel wall by polymerase chain reaction (PCR) has been reported.[94] Most often, however, VZV is associated with CNS manifestations and cerebrovascular disease. VZV can cause brain damage in a number of ways, including large/medium vessel vasculopathy with bland or hemorrhagic infarcts, small vessel vasculopathy with mixed ischemic and demyelinating lesions, and ventriculitis with periventriculitis.[95–97] VZV can also cause optic neuritis, acute retinal necrosis, and myelitis.[98,99] CNS arteritis can occur with primary infection, which is rare, or as a late complication of reactivation disease, herpes zoster. It is difficult to determine if the vascular disease is caused by active infection or is postinfectious in nature. Manifestations occur late, often up to 3 weeks after acute infection in the case of primary varicella.[100] Cases have also occurred after a very long period of time.[101] Kleinschmidt-DeMasters et al.[102] reported on ischemic stroke in previously healthy children occurring during recovery from chickenpox, but sometimes with a delay up to 4 years after the episode of varicella.

The onset of granulomatous angiitis of the CNS, weeks after herpes zoster ophthalmicus, is a recognized clinical syndrome. In some cases, there is both vasculitis and persistent infection. Although there is an immunologic component with granulomatous inflammation, the overall evidence suggests that VZV can infect the walls of CNS arteries and antigen has been found in the involved vessels at autopsy.[103,104] Another interesting presentation has been stroke secondary to granulmonatous angiitis which has been reported without the typical preceding contralateral episode of herpes zoster ophthalmicus in HIV-infected patients.[105] In one case, the CSF was positive for VZV by PCR. Another patient subsequently developed acute retinal necrosis, and both vitreous and CSF fluid were positive for VZV.

In some cases, VZV associated vasculitis can mimic a systemic vasculitis. A superficial granulomatous angiitis with deep PAN-like vasculitis has also been seen after herpes zoster infection.[106] Active herpes zoster vasculitis can mimic TA.[107]

Cytomegalovirus (CMV) can also cause a systemic vasculitis. Characteristic giant cells with owl-eyed intranuclear inclusions were seen in areas of occlusive arteritis in a patient with cerebral angiitis caused by CMV.[109] Active Epstein-Barr virus (EBV) infection has also been reported to cause peripheral vascular disease. An autopsy of a 10-year-old girl with chronic active EBV infection showed involvement of the coronary, carotid, subclavian, and common iliac arteries, as well as the abdominal aorta, with aneurysm formation.[110,111] Another autopsy report of a 61-year-old women with EBV showed a widespread granulomatous arteritis involving small arteries and arterioles.[112] There was also infiltration of many organs by hemophagocytic histiocytes. Active HHV-6 has also been reported to cause a chronic aortitis in a 9-month-old boy initially diagnosed with Kawasaki's disease.[113] Viral infection has even associated with other vascular manifestations. For example, herpes simplex virus-2 (HSV-2) infection has been associated with essential hypertension, even in the absence of otherwise clinically apparent arteritis, but how remains a mystery.[114]

There are also animal models of large-vessel vasculitis that indicate chronic viral infection rather than autoimmunity is the cause.[115] Immune mechanisms may be involved, as there is an interrelationship between herpesvirus latency, the immune system, and activation.[116] How these observations will change therapeutic approaches, including antiviral therapy, for vasculitis related to viral infection remains to be seen. Currently there is little data on the efficacy of antiviral agents for these infections, although they are often given because of desperation.

HIV Infection

HIV infection has been associated with peripheral vascular disease, but the pathogenesis is complicated.[117] The combination antiretroviral treatment regimens used for HIV have greatly decreased the morbidity and mortality caused by opportunistic infections and other AIDS-defining conditions, but these regimens also cause lipid abnormalities that may result in accelerated atherosclerosis (see following discussion of infections and atherosclerosis). In addition, there is substantial evidence that HIV infection itself, can cause endothelial cell dysfunction and vascular inflammation, even in patients who do not appear to have accelerated atherosclerosis. There can be macroscopic damage, including intracranial arteritis, arterial sclerosis, and fusiform aneurysm formation of the arteries of the circle of Willis apparently due to HIV itself.[118,119] This is most common in children but has occurred in adults as well. There can be catastrophic complications resulting. The aneurysms can become secondarily infected.[120] It is also quite possible that the excess number of unexplained seizures and cerebrovascular events in HIV patients are due to arteritis as well. In some of these cases, HAART has actually resulted in resolution as documented by repeat angiography.[121] MR can be helpful in diagnosis of cerebrovascular disease in these patients and its role in the etiology of neurolgoic or cognitive dysfunction.[122]

HIV can also cause occlusive arterial disease in the extremities. Twenty patients with peripheral arterial disease were identified in one vascular unit in a 3-year period. Pathologically the arterial disease was distinct from atherosclerosis, with microscopy demonstrating leukocytoclastic vasculitis.[123] A diffuse granulomatous vasculitis not restricted to the CNS has also been reported, and it can resolve with HAART.[124] HIV can cause a spontaneous AV which is otherwise rare.[125] Pathologic examination of these lesions shows changes similar to those seen in HIV-related large vessel aneurysms.

As with the herpes viruses, HIV patients have also been reported to develop a systemic vasculitis. A wide range of inflammatory vascular disease in these patients may occur, because of HIV itself, other infections agents, and/or drugs.[126] Corticosteroids may also be helpful with necrotizing vasculitis caused by HIV.[127]

● INFECTION AND THE VASCULITIDIES

The pathogenesis of vasculitis is extremely complex. In recent years, there have been many associations identified between infection and several of the vasculitides often in the setting of active infection. In other cases, the effect of infection in the pathognesis of vasculitis is more indirect, and many mechanisms have been proposed. This topic has recently been comprehensively reviewed.[128] Immune-mediated damage may result from immune complex deposition, molecular mimicry and induction of autoimmunity, inflammation secondary to super-antigens, and T-cell-mediated immune responses. In some cases, vasculitis occurs with specific markers of an autoimmune vasculitis, such as antineutrophil cytoplasmic antibodies (ANCA). It is proposed that infections not only up-regulate the surface expression of proteinase 3 (PR3) and myeloperoxidase (MPO), the antigenic targets of ANCA, but also proposed that certain infections may also induce these antibodies because of similar surface structure of microbial proteins to PR3 and MPO.

In some cases, an infectious etiology has been suggested by the epidemiology with seasonal variation or apparent outbreaks of vasculitis occurring from time to time. Giant cell artertis has been shown to follow a cyclic variation in incidence in some studies.[129] Epidemics of temporal arteritis and polymyalgia rheumatica have occurred in Denmark, with serologic evidence of infection with parvovirus B19, *Mycoplasma pneumoniae*, and *Chlamydia pneumoniae*.[130] Other studies have also suggested and association between parvovirus B19 infection and GCA.[131] *C. pneumoniae* infection has predated TA organism has been found in temporal artery biopsy in patients with GCA.[132] *Chlamydia psittaci* may also induce TA.[133] However, studies looking for *C. pneumoniae* and and parvovirus B19 these organisms in affected arteries have yielded conflicting results, and at least the majority of GCA cases as a result appear to be because of these organisms.[134] GCA and polymyalgia rheumatica can occur with *Borrelia burgdorferi*.[135,136] Lyme may cause a vascular inflammatory process, and anti-inflammatory therapy may be necessary even after adequate antibiotic therapy.[137] Several negative studies have excluded the herpesviruses as causes of GCA. More recently, techniques using PCR to detect any bacterial ribosomal RNA have been unable to detect any bacterial nucleic acid in temporal arteries. Although a number of infections have been reported to initiate GCA, in some cases, it may not be a particular pathogen. A matched case–control study was done with 100 patients with biopsy-proven CGA and 100 control patients who had surgery for hip fracture (who did not have GCA) were studied. The events in the months prior to diagnosis or surgery were reviewed, and infections were three times more likely in GCA patients.[138]

In other conditions, the association between infection and vasculitis has been demonstrated more convincingly. Systemic vasculitis may clearly occur as a consequence of viral hepatitis. PAN may occur after infection with hepatitis B, hepatitis C, and streptococcal infection.[139,140] Mixed cryoglobulinemia has also been clearly associated with hepatitis B and hepatitis C infection. A GI presentation may result, and a case of multiple colonic ulcers caused by PN in a patient with chronic hepatitis C infection has been reported.[141]

Again, *C. pneumoniae* has been proposed to induce vasculitis, and five patients who developed what was initially considered a noninfectious vasculitis had a preceding respiratory infection that was found to be caused by *C. pneumonia* serologically. The pattern of serological resonse indicated reinfection.[142] All required corticosteroids for recovery. Other studies, however, have failed to show an association between nonspecific arteritis and *C. pneumoniae* infection.[143]

Although Wegener's granulomatosis has been reported after viral infections, the strongest association is with *S. aureus*. The theory is that superantigens, particularly toxic shock syndrome toxin-1 toxin, induce a polyclonal immune response that includes an autoimmune response. Kawasaki's may be induced by human coronavirus. Other vasculitides, including Bechet's disease, Henoch–Schonlein Purpura, and Cogan's syndrome have also been associated with a wide variety of infections.[128]

Although bacterial and viral infections have most often been associated with systemic vasculitis, parasitic infections have also been implicated. One report of TA and renal involvement occurred in association with infection with *Toxocara canis*, an etiologic agent of visceral larva migrans.[144] The vasculitis was self-limited and resolved without steroids or other immunosuppressive therapy. During an outbreak of trichinosis, two men developed a systemic necrotizing vasculopathy that looked like PAN. A sustained remission occured with mebendazole, cyclophosphamide, and prednisone.[145]

In some instances, chronicity seems to be important in the pathogenesis. Two patients with longstanding chronic bronchitis and bronchial suppuration developed ANCA-positive Wegener's granulomatosis and polyarteritis.[146] This may be a nonspecific reaction as polyarteritis has occurred in the absence of ANCA as a result of a suppurative wound infection.[147]

In other cases, there definitely appears to be an immune cross-reaction rather than persistent infection that results in vasculitis. This is supported by cases of vasculitis that occur after vaccination.[148] Tuberculosis cannot only directly infect peripheral arterities in rare cases, but it has also been associated with large vessel vasculitis, including Takaysu's artertis.[149] TB produces autoimmune disease and vasculitis caused by induction of cross-reactive antibodies. The heat shock protein HSP-65 of *M. tuberculosis* can induce antibodies that react to its human homologue, HSP-60. This TB-induced autoimmunity can result in Takayasu's arteritis.[150] This autoimmunity may involve cellular immune responses as well.[151]

Although many associations have been made, the results of many studies are conflicting. Many studies are unable to identify an infectious etiology. Different animal models have been used to study large vessel vasculitis, including

C. pneumoniae, herpesviruses and RNA viruses.[152] Animal models have shown that microbes can induce autoimmunity and vasculitis, and this avenue of study may help reconcile discrepancies in clinical observations.

Infections and Atherosclerosis of the Peripheral Vasculature

Introduction. There are many links between atherosclerosis and infection. Links between viruses belonging to the Herpesvirus and Hepatitis virus families have long been proposed. Additionally, the relationship of Human Immunodeficiency Virus (HIV) and antiretroviral therapy to atherosclerosis is increasingly well recognized. Bacterial agents, especially the causative agents of periodontal disease, have also been associated with atherosclerosis. This section will review the links between atherosclerosis and infection and the evidence that supports these associations. Although many associations between infection and atherosclerosis have been found, much conflicting evidence exists. As will be seen, causality, in contrast to association, has often been difficult to prove. Although much of the information in the literature concerns coronary artery disease (CAD), it is relevant to the field of peripheral arterial disease.

Viruses.

Viral Hepatitis. Hepatitis A, B and C have all been studied with respect to their associations with atherosclerosis. Several large series have studied the association between CAD and Hepatitis A virus (HAV), with mixed results. A study by Zhu et al.[153] examined 391 patients undergoing coronary angiography. Anti-HAV-IgG and C-reactive protein (CRP) levels were measured to determine whether HAV-seropositivity predicts CAD and/or elevated CRP. The authors point out that unlike Hepatitis B virus (HBV) and Hepatitis C virus (HCV), HAV does not result in chronic liver disease. Two hundred and forty-eight (63%) of the 391 patients studied had evidence of CAD (>50% stenosis of 1 major coronary artery) and 205 (52%) were positive for HAV-IgG. 74% of the patients in the HAV-seropositive group had CAD as compared to 52% in the HAV-seronegative group ($p < 0.0001$). Additionally, mean CRP levels were found to be higher in the HAV-seropositive group than the HAV-seronegative group. Both of these associations held true after adjustment for other CAD risk factors and evidence of immunity against other infectious agents. Prasad et al.[154] also found an association between evidence of past infection with HAV and CAD assessed by angiography after adjusting for conventional CAD risk factors (OR 2.6, CI 1.4–5). They additionally found a relationship between severity of CAD and overall pathogen burden (a concept explored later in this chapter).

Other studies have failed to demonstrate an association between HAV serostatus and CAD. In contrast to the aforementioned coronary angiography studies, a study by Auer et al.[155] on 218 patients undergoing coronary an-

giography showed a CAD prevalence of 66.3% in HAV-seropositive individuals and 57.3% in HAV-seronegative individuals ($p = 0.385$). Examination of data from patients in the The Heart Outcomes Prevention Evaluation (HOPE) Study, a prospective study designed to examine ramipril and vitamin E in the secondary prevention of cardiovascular (CV) events, also found no association between HAV-IgG positivity and CV events. A study by Ongey et al.[156] found no association between HAV-seropositivity and cardiovascular disease (myocardial infarction [MI], stroke, coronary heart disease) in 365 diabetic patients from the German National Health Interview and Examination Survey.

The association of HBV and HCV-seropositivity with atherosclerosis has also been extensively studied. Hepatitis B and hepatitis C have known hepatic complications that arise from inflammatory effects in the liver. Proposed similar systemic inflammatory effects provide the basis for studying these viruses' association with atherosclerosis. In Shanghai, China, 434 patients underwent coronary angiography to assess for CAD. Patients were also tested for hepatitis B antigens (HBsAg and HBeAg) and antibodies (anti-HBs, anti-HBc, and anti-HBe).[157] No association between any of the HBV serologic markers and CAD was found. In fact, HBV-seropositivity was found to be negatively associated with CRP level, perhaps secondary to decreased expression of CRP by HBV induced liver dysfunction. Another study of 48 patients with chronic hepatitis (6 with HBV and 42 with HCV) found decreased carotid atherosclerosis in patients with chronic liver disease. Volzke et al.,[158] in a cross-sectional study of adults in Germany, also found no association between HBV or HCV seropositivity (as measured by anti-HBs and anti-HCV antibody) and the prevalence of MI, stroke and carotid disease. However, a cross-sectional study in Japan found that HBsAg positivity, a marker of hepatitis B virus carrier state, was associated with the presence of carotid plaque (intimal–medial layer focal thickening of ≥ 1.3 mm).[159] The same group of authors who demonstrated an association between the hepatitis B virus carrier state and presence of carotid plaque found that the same association with carotid disease exists for patients who have anti-HCV antibody as well as for those who are HCV core protein positive (a marker of viremia).[160,161] Another study of 491 patients with angiography-proven CAD found an HCV seropositivity rate of 6.3%, compared to 2% HCV seropositivity in the control group.[162] After adjusting for confounding variables, the odds ratio (OR) was still elevated at 4.2 (CI 1.4–13.0). However, a case–control study of some US military men aged 30 to 50 years on active duty who were hospitalized for first MI, failed to find an association between anti-HCV antibody and MI.[163]

Herpesviruses. The association between Herpesviruses and atherosclerosis has also been extensively researched. EBV, HSV-1, HSV-2, and CMV are most frequently studied. Much of the evidence for the role of herpesviruses in atherosclerosis comes from pathology data. Several studies have evaluated vascular specimens from surgery or autopsy. Using PCR, investigators have isolated EBV, HSV, and CMV DNA from atherosclerotic plaques at higher rates than from nonatherosclerotic blood vessels.[164,165]

There is some clinical data to support these associations as well. One study demonstrated that HSV-1 and CMV seropositivity was associated with the presence of the metabolic syndrome.[166] A cross-sectional study of 488 patients with hypertension (a known risk factor for atherosclerosis) and 756 patients without hypertension showed that hypertensive patients had a higher prevalence of HSV-2 IgG positivity than did nonhypertensive patients (38.3% vs. 29.8%, $p = 0.002$).[114] In another study, a group of 504 patients were followed for a period of more than 2.5 years to determine whether they had progressive carotid stenosis or increased intimal–medial thickness.[167] Testing for evidence of exposure to multiple prior pathogens, among them EBV, HSV-1, HSV-2, and CMV, demonstrated that elevated IgG antibodies against EBV and HSV-2 were associated with progression of carotid disease. However, as with viral hepatitis, there are also studies that found no evidence that HSV infection (HSV-1) is associated cardiac or vascular disease.[154] There are no studies investigating the impact of HSV therapy on vascular disease.

Exposure to CMV has been strongly associated with atherosclerosis. Recently, several theories about the pathogenesis of CMV in atherosclerosis have been put forth, implicating both direct viral effect and immune-mediated mechanisms.[168] One of the first such studies was a prospective study that sought to evaluate whether the presence of anti-CMV IgG in 75 patients undergoing coronary atherectomy was a risk factor for restenosis. Prior to this study, it was known that many restenosis lesions had evidence of CMV, and scientific papers postulated that viral proteins promoted proliferation of smooth muscle cells, leading to restenosis.[169] Evidence of previous CMV infection was found to be an independent risk factor for restenosis in this study. Subsequent studies examined renal and heart transplant patients and the role that CMV plays in cardiovascular mortality in these populations. CMV infection in cardiac transplant recipients is associated with increased graft atherosclerosis, in addition to increased rejection and death.[170] CMV infection in renal transplant patients is associated with increased cardiovascular mortality.[171]

Other Viruses. Studies like the ones that have found evidence of herpesviruses in atherosclerotic plaques have also found evidence of enterovirus (a nonherpesvirus) in such plaques.[172] Evidence of RNA from influenza viruses within atherosclerotic plaques has also been found, although influenza seropositivity is not associated with atherosclerotic disease.[173,174]

Bacteria.

Chlamydia. An association between *Chlamydia* and myocardial disease has been proposed since the 1960s. The presence of *C. pneumoniae* in atheromas has been documented.[175] However, the clinical significance of this remains unclear. In 1988, a paper in *The Lancet* examined

levels of antibodies to *Chlamydia* spp. and to a chlamydial lipopolysaccharide group antigen.[176] Levels of antibody in men with acute myocardial infarction (AMI), chronic coronary heart disease (CCHD) and matched controls were compared. Sixty-seven percent of men with AMI and 50% of men with CCHD had raised IgG and IgA levels, a significantly higher percentage than in the controls.

Subsequent investigations have yielded mixed results. Prospective studies of patients enrolled in the British Regional Heart Study were included in meta-analyses that were published in 2000 and 2002.[177,178] Examination of IgG and IgA levels in men who suffered fatal or nonfatal MI failed to show a strong association between *C. pneumoniae* titers and coronary heart disease after adjustments were made for other risk factors, including socioeconomic status. The OR for CHD with a positive IgG was 1.15 (CI 0.97–1.36); the OR for CHD with a positive IgA was 1.25 (CI 1.03–1.53). A nested case–control study of 300 active duty men in the United States Army who were hospitalized for first MI did show an association between elevated *C. pneumoniae* IgA level and MI (RR 1.67, CI 1.04–2.70).[179] Additionally, the relative risk for MI if the specimen had been collected in 1 to 5 years before the MI was 2.11 (CI 1.06–4.21); if the specimen was ≥5 years old, the relative risk was no longer significant (1.34, CI 0.67–2.65). The authors conclude that timing of infection may be important in determining risk for cardiovascular events.

There is no evidence that therapy of *C. pneumoniae* with macrolide antibiotics has a definitive role in primary or secondary prevention of CAD.[154]

H. pylori. Several studies have failed to show an association between antibodies to *H. pylori* and increased risk of cardiovascular disease or carotid disease.[180–182] There is evidence that eradication of *H. pylori* from the stool results in decreased CRP levels and increased high-density lipoprotein levels, and that the presence of *H. pylori* antibodies is associated with the metabolic syndrome.[183,184] However, in contrast to other pathogens, *H. pylori* DNA has not been successfully isolated from atherosclerotic plaques.[185,186]

Periodontal Disease. The relationship between dental and systemic health has been suspected since 1951. There is conflicting data about whether periodontal disease, by mediating a proinflammatory state, is an independent risk factor for coronary or cerebral arterial disease.[187] The literature favors an association, and controlling periodontal infections may improve inflammatory markers and endothelial dysfunction.[188,189] A study of monozygotic twins found that those with CHD had more evidence of periodontal disease as determined by bleeding, horizontal bone level, and pathologic pockets.[190] A meta-analysis of five studies yielded a relative risk for CHD of 1.24 (CI 1.10–1.38).[191]

The utility of therapeutic interventions remains to be seen.

Cumulative Infectious Burden. The association between microbes and atherosclerosis continues to be controversial, and studies are often contradictory. Several authors have proposed the concept of cumulative infectious burden as being a better method to quantify risk of atherosclerotic events. For instance, in the Heart Outcomes Prevention Evaluation Study, only one of four pathogens tested for was an independent risk factor for cardiovascular disease (CMV). However, total pathogen burden was also associated with cardiovascular disease (HR 1.41, CI 1.02–1.96).[192] Other studies also support this idea.[154]

HIV. Concerns about the effects of both HIV and its treatment on the cardiovascular system have been reported for the past decade. For patients who are receiving antiretroviral therapy, metabolic abnormalities, including those of insulin resistance, hyperlipidemia, fat maldistribution, and metabolic syndrome have been noted. However, there is uncertainty about the overall cardiovascular significance of the abnormalities, especially in light of the increasing overall survival of HIV-positive patients as compared to 10 years ago. In the case of the metabolic syndrome, it is unclear if the risk is any higher in HIV-positive versus HIV-negative Americans.[193]

AMI in patients with HIV was first reported in 1998. In 2003, *AIDS* published retrospective review of two cohorts in France that demonstrated the incidence of AMI in HIV-infected patients to be 5.0 to 5.5 per 1000 person-years, three times higher than the incidence in non-HIV-infected patients.[194] In contrast to those results, a retrospective study published the same year in *The New England Journal of Medicine* showed no relationship between the use of any class of HIV medicines and the hazard of cardiovascular or cerebrovascular events. As expected, the overall risk of death decreased with the use of these medications.[195]

As noted above, increased reporting of AMI started in 1998, two years after the introduction of protease inhibitors (PIs), one of the three major classes of medications used for the therapy of HIV. Given the timing of this increase, a link with increased PI use was suspected. Data from the HIV Outpatient Study, a prospective cohort study of patients from several major US cities, showed that the OR for AMI among patients taking PIs was 7.1 (CI 1.6–44.3). After adjusting for traditional risk factors, the OR was 6.5.[196] HIV-positive patients who are on PIs also have increased aortic stiffness, which is an early marker of arteriosclerosis.[197] Finally, on a genetic level, the APOA5-1131T C genotype (APOA5 is an apolipoprotein gene) predisposes HIV patients on a PI to hyperlipidemia.[198]

NNRTIs may also place patients at increased risk for atherosclerosis, although the risk may not be as high as with PIs. A cross-sectional analysis of patients enrolled in the DAD study (Data collection on Adverse events of anti-HIV Drugs) showed that the OR of hypercholesterolemia among patients on NNRTIs (without a PI) was 1.79 (CI 1.45–2.22). For patients on a PI (without an NNRTI), the OR was 2.35 (CT 1.92–2.87) and for patients on a PI + NNRI, the OR was 5.48 (CI 4.34–6.91).[199] AZT, an NRTI, has been found to induce endothelial dysfunction.[200]

HIV, in the absence of therapy, is also associated with metabolic changes that may lead to atherosclerosis. After infection with HIV, a decrease in high-density lipoprotein and increase in triglycerides is seen; after a period of time, a decrease in low-density lipoprotein takes place.[201] HIV may have direct inflammatory effects and may predispose to impaired endothelial function through abnormalities in adhesion molecule function.[202]

It is important to remember, however, that despite the metabolic abnormalities and ensuing risk of atherosclerosis that HAART may cause, the benefits of antiretroviral therapy far outweigh the absolute risk of adverse cardiovascular events.[203] Lifestyle modification and appropriate therapy with lipid lower medications should be instituted to help manage patients' cardiovascular risk.

REFERENCES

1. Baddour LM; IDSA Emerging Infections Network. Long-term suppressive antimicrobial therapy for intravascular device-related infections. *Am J Med Sci.* 2001;322(4):209-212.

2. Moore WS, Malone JM. Vascular infection. In: Howard RJ, Simmons RL, eds. *Surgical Infectious Diseases.* 2nd ed. East Norwalk, CT: Appleton & Lange; 1988:585.

3. Wilson SE, Van Wagenen P, Passaro E Jr. Arterial infection. *Curr Probl Surg.* 1978;15(9):1.

4. Parkhurst GF, Decker JP. Bacterial aortitis ad mycotic aneruysms of the aorta: a report of 12 cases. *Am J Pathol.* 1955;31:821.

5. MacBeth GA, Rubin JR, McIntrye RE, et al. The relevance of arterial wall microbiology to the treatment of prosthetic graft nfection: graft infection vs. arterial infection. *J Vasc Surg.* 1984;1:750.

6. Bandyk DF, Novotney ML, Back MR, et al. Expanded application of in situ replacement for prosthetic graft infection. *J Vasc Surg.* 2001;34:411-420.

7. Del Brutto OH. Cerebrovascular disease in the tropics. *Rev Neurol.* 2001;33(8):750-762.

8. Pelletier LL, Petersdorf RG. Infective endocarditis: a review of 125 cases from the University of Washington Hospitals. *Medicine.* 1977;56:287-313.

9. Syrjanen J. Infection as a risk factor for cerebral infarction. *Eur Heart J.* 1993;14(suppl K):17-19.

10. Mishima K, Watanabe T, Sasaki T, Saito I, Takakura K. An infected partially thrombosed giant aneurysm of the azygous anterior cerebral artery. *No Shinkei Geka.* 1990;18(5):475-481.

11. Horie N, Murakami R, Sato M, et al. Cerebral angiitis and cerebritis caused by subdural empyema: two cases report. *Brain Nerve.* 2001;53(9):881-885.

12. Bush JK, Givner LB, Whitaker SH, Anderson DC, Percy AK. Necrotiziing fasciitis of the parapharyngeal space with carotid artery occlusion and acutge hemiplegia. *Pediatrics.* 1984;73(3):343-347.

13. Koda Y, Seto Y, Takeichi S, Kimura H. Fatal subarachnoid hemorrhage complicating actinomycotic meningitis. *Forensic Sci Int.* 2003;134(2-3):169-171.

14. Engin C, Posacioglu H, Ayik F, Apaydin AZ. Management of vascular infection in the groin. *Tex Heart Inst J.* 2005;32(4):529-534.

15. Tsao JW, Marder SR, Goldstone J, et al. Presentation, diagnosis, and management of arterial mycotic pseudoaneurysms in injection drug users. *Ann Vasc Surg.* 2002;16:652-662.

16. Kardaras FG, Kardaras DF, Rontogiani DP, Mpourazanis IA, Flessas LP. Septic endarteritis following percutanous transpluminal coronary anigiopalsty. *Cathet Cardiovasc Diagn.* 1995;34(1):57-60.

17. Whitton HH Jr, Rehring TF. Femoral arteritis associated with the percutaneous suture closure: new technology, challenging complications. *J Vasc Surg.* 2003; 38(1):83-87.

18. Sprouse LR II, Botta DM Jr, Hamilton IN Jr. The management of peripheral vascular complications associated with the use of percutaneous suture-mediated closure devices. *J Vasc Surg.* 2001;33(4):688-693.

19. Cribari C, Meadors FA, Crawford ES, Coselli JS, Safi HJ, Svensson LG. Thoracoabdominal aortic aneurysm associated with umbilical artery catheterization: case report and review of the literature. *J Vasc Surg.* 1992;16:75-86.

20. El-Hamamsy I, Durrleman N, Stevens LM, et al. Incidence and outcome of radial artery infections following cardiac surgery. *Ann Thoracic Surg.* 2003;76(3):801-804.

21. Poli P, Riviere J, Watelet J, Testart J. A new case of arterial *Listeria* infection. *J Mal Vasc.* 1995;20(4):326-327.

22. Gari-Toussaint M, Ngoc LH, Gigante M, et al. Kidney transplant and *Candida albicans* arteritis. The importance of analyzing the transplant conservation fluid. *Presse Med.* 2004;33(13):866-868.

23. Fowler VG Jr, Scheld WM, Bayer AS. Endocarditis and intravascular infections. In: Mandell G, Bennett JE, Dolin P, eds. *Principles and Practice of Infectious Diseases.* 6th ed. Philadelphia, PA: Elsevier; 2005:975.

24. Cianco G, Burke GW, Viciana AL, et al. Destructive allograft fungal arteritis following simultaneous pancreas-kidney transplantation. *Transplantation.* 1996;61(8):1172-1175.

25. Malek AM, Higashida RT, Reilly LM, et al. Subclavian artertis and pseudoaneurysm formation secondary to stent infection. *Cardivasc Interv Radiol.* 2000;23(1):57-60.

26. Hoffman AI, Murphy TP. Septic arteritis causing iliac artery rupture and aneurysmal transformation of the distal aorta after iliac artery stent placement. *J Vasc Interv Radiol.* 1997; 8(2):215-219.

27. Gordon GI, Vogelzang RL, Curry RH, McCarthy WJ, Nemcek AA Jr. Endovascular infection after renal artery stent placement. *J Vasc Interv Radiol.* 1997;7(5):669-672.

28. Bunt TJ. *Vascular Graft Infections.* Armonk, NY: Futura Publishing Inc; 1994.

29. Seeger JM. Management of patients with prosthetic vascular graft infection. *Ann Surg.* 2000;66:166-177.

30. Pons VG, Wurtz R. Vascular graft infections: a 25-year experience of 170 cases. *J Vasc Surg.* 1991;13:751-752.

31. Junior C. Arteritis dependent on infective process: the convenience of heparin use. *Rev Hosp Clin Fac Med Sao Paulo.* 1991;46(1):1-8.

32. Somer T, Feingold SM. Vasculitides associated with infections, immunization, and antimicrobial drugs. *Clin Infect Dis.* 1995;20(4):1010-1036.

33. Sailors DM, Eidt JF, Gagne PJ, Barnes RW, Barone GW, McFarland DR. Primary *Clostridum septicum* aortitis: a rare caue of necrotizing suprarenal aortic infection. A case report and review of the literature. *J Vasc Surg.* 1996;23(4):714-718.

34. Flamand F, Harris KA, DeRose G, Karam B, Jamieson WG. Arteritis due to Salmonella with aneruysm formation: two cases. *Can J Surg.* 1992;35(3):248-252.

35. Cohen PS, O'Brien TF, Schoenbaum SC, Medeiros AA. The risk of endothelial infection in adults with *Salmonella* bacteremia. *Ann Intern Med.* 1978;89(6):931-932.

36. Lane GP, Cochrane AD, Fone DR. Salmonellal mycotic abdominal aortic aneurysm. *Med J Australia.* 1988;149(2):95-97.

37. Wilson SE, Gordon HE, Van Wagenen PB. *Salmonella* arteritis: a precursor of aortic rupture and pseudoanuerysm formation. *Arch Surg.* 1978;113(10):1163-1166.

38. Lester A, Eriksen NH, Nielsen H, et al. Bacteremia caused by zoonotic *Salmonella* types in greater Copenhagen in 1984-1988. *Ugeskr Laeger.* 1990;152(8):529-532.

39. McIntyre KE, Malone JM, Richards E, Axline SG. Mycotic aortic pseudoaneurysm with aortoenteric fistula cause by Arizona hinshawii. *Surgery.* 1982;91(2):173-177.

40. Azizi, ZA, Yahya M, Lee SK. Meliodosis and the vascular surgeon: hospital Kuala Lumpur experience. *Asian J Surg.* 2005;28(4):309-311.

41. Brightbill TC, Ihmeidan IH, Post MJ, Berger JR, Katz DA. Neurosyphilis in HIV-positive and HIV-negative patients: neurimaging findings. *Am J Neuradiol.* 1995;16(4):703-711.

42. Labauge R, Pages M, Tourniaire D, Blard JM. Infarction of the pons, neurosyphilis, and HIV infection. *Revue Neurologique.* 1991;147(5):406-408.

43. Lucas MJ, Theriot SK, Wendel GD Jr. Doppler systolic-diastoic ratios in preganancie scomplicated by syphilis. *Obstet Gynbe.* 1991;77(2):217-222.

44. Arello LD, MacDonald AB, Semlear R, DiLeo F, Berger B. Temporal arteritis associated with *Borrelia* infection. A case report. *J Clin Neuroophthalmol.* 1989;9(1):3-6.

45. Chen Y. A clinicopathologic anaylisis of 12 cases of cerebrovascular leptospirosis. *Chinese J Nuerol Psych.* 1990; 23(4):226-229.

46. Sailors DM, Barone GW, Gange PJ, Eidt JF, Ketel BL, Barnes BW. *Candida* arteritis: are GI endoscopic procedures a source of vascular infections? *Am Surgeon.* 1996;62(6):472-477.

47. Ikeda M, Kambayashi J, Kawasaki T. Contained rupture of infected abdominaol aortic aneurysm due to systemic candidiasis. *Cardiovasc Surg.* 1995;3(6):711-714.

48. Fernando SS, Lauer CS. *Aspergillus fumigatus* infection of the optic nerve with mycotic arteritis of cerebral vessels. *Histopathology.* 1982;6(2):227-234.

49. Calli C, Savas R, Parildar M, Pekindil G, Alper H, Yunten N. Pontine infarct due to basilar arteritis from rhinicerebral mucormycosis, seen on MRI. *Neuroradiology.* 1999;41(3):179-181.

50. Hutnik CM, Nicolle DA, Munoz DG. Orbital aspergillosis: a fatal maqueerader. *J Neuroophthalmol.* 1997;17(4):257-261.

51. Endo T, Tominaga T, Konno H, Yoshimoto T. Fatal subarachnoid hemorrhage, with brainstem and cerebellar infarction, caused by *Aspergillus* infection after cerebral artery aneurysm surgery: a case report. *Neurosurg.* 2002;50(5):1147-1150.

52. Piotrowrski WP, Pilz P. Postoperative fungal arteritis mimicking vasospasm—case report. *Neurol Med Chir (Tokyo).* 1994;34(5):315-318.

53. Sharma RR, Gurushinghe NT, Lynch PG. Cerebral infarction due to *Aspergillus* arteritis following glioma surgery. *Brit J Neursurg.* 1992;6(5):485-490.

54. Takahashi Y, Sugita Y, Maruiwa HH, Hirohata M, Tokutomi T, Shigemori M. Fatal hemorrhage from rupture of the intracranial internal carotid artery caused by *Aspergillus* arteritis. *Neurosurg Rev.* 1998;21(2-3):198-201.

55. Jamjoom AB, Hedaithy SA, Jamjoon ZA, et al. Intracranial mycotic infections in neurosurgical practice. *Acta Neurochir* (Wien). 1995;137(1-2):78-84.

56. Schwartz DN, Fihn SD, Miller RA. Infection of an arterial prosthesis as the presenting manifestation of disseminated coccidiomycosis: control of disease with fluconazole. *Clin Infect Dis.* 1993;16(4):486-488.

57. Krajaejun T, Kunakorn M, Prachartktam R, et al. Identification of a novel 74-kilodalton immunodominant antigen of ythium insidiosum by sera from human patients with pythiosis. *J Clin Micro.* 2006;44(5):1674-1680.

58. Wanachiwanawin W, Thianprasit M, Fucharoen S, et al. Fatal arteritis due to *Pythium insidiosum* in patients with thalassemia. *Trans R Soc Trop Med Hyg.* 1993;87:296-298.

59. Prasertwitayakij N, Louthrenoo W, Kasitanon N, Thamprasert K, Vanittanakom N. Human pythiosis, a rare cause of artertis: case report and literature review. *Semin Arthritis Rheum.* 2003;33(3):204-214.

60. Baringagarrementeria F, Cantu C. Frequency of cerebral arteritis in subarachnoid cysticercosis: an angiographic study. *Stroke.* 1998;29(1):123-125.

61. Ali-Kahn A, Seemayer TA. Fatal bowel obstruction and sepsis: an unusual complication of systemic strongyloidosis. *Trans Royal Soc Trop Med Hygiene.* 1975;69(5-6):473-476.

62. Siddorn JA. Schistosomiasis and anterior spinal artery occlusion. *Am J Trop Med Hygeine.* 1978;27(3):532-534.

63. Raffetto JD, Bernardo J, Menzoian JO. Aortobifemoral graft infection with *Mycobacterium tuberculosis*: treatment with abscess drainage, debridement, and long-term administration of antibiotic agents. *J Vascu Surg.* 2004;40(4):826-829.

64. Schwartz DN, Fihn SD, Miller RA. Infection of an arterial prosthesis as the presenting manifestation of disseminated coccidiomycosis: control of disease with fluconazole. *Clin Infect Dis.* 1993;16(4):486-488.

65. Arboix A, Marti-Vilalta JL. New concepts in lacunar stroke etiology: the constellation of small-vessel arterial disease. *Cerebrovasc Dis.* 2004;17(suppl 1):58-62.

66. Hart RG, Foster JW, Luther MF, Kanter MC. Stroke in infective endocarditis. *Stroke.* 1990;21(5):6950700.

67. Tiesenhausen K, Amann W, Thalhammer M. Die primar bakteriell infizierte arterie. *Chirurg.* 1999;70(10):1163-1167.

68. Stephens CT, Pounds LL, Killewich LA. Rupture of a nonaneurysmal aorta secondary to staphylococcus aortitis: a case report and review of the literature. *Angiology.* 2006;57(4):506-512.

69. Law NW, Parvin SD, Darke SG. Diagnostic features and management of bacterial arteritis with false aneruysm formation. *Eur J Vasc Surg.* 1994;8(2):199-204.

70. Baddour LM, Bettman MA, Bolger AF, et al. Nonvalvular cardiovascular device-related infections. *Circulation.* 2003;108:2015-2031.

71. Mesurolle B, Qanadli SD, Merad M, et al. Dual-slice helical CT of the thoracic aorta. *J Comp Assist Tomographty.* 2000;24(4):548-556.

72. Perot L, Chiras J, DeBussche-Depreister C, Dorman D, Bories J. Intracerebral stenosing arteriopathies, contribution of three radiographic techniques to the diagnosis. *J Neuroradiol.* 1991;18(1):32-48.

73. Williamson MR, Boyd CM, Read RC, et al. 111 In-labeled leukocytes in the detection of prosthetic vascular graft infections. *AJR.* 1986;147(1):173-176.

74. Dadparvar S, Kaufman CI, Krishna L, et al. Efficacy of 99mTc-wbc imaging in detection of prosthetic vascular graft infection. *Clin Nuc Med.* 1997;22(5):349.

75. Gratz S, Schipper ML, Dorner J, et al. LeukoScan for imaging infection in different clinical settings. A retrospective evaluation and extended review of the literature. *Clin Nuc Med.* 2003;28(4):267-276.

76. Dougherty SH. Prosthetic devices. Diagnosis and management of prosthesis infection. In: Meakins TL, ed. *Surgical Infections.* New York, NY: Scientific American, Inc; 1994:247.

77. Langsfield M, Weinstein ES. Prosthetic graft infection in vascular surgery. In: Fry DE, ed. *Surgical Infections.* 1st ed. Boston, MA: Little, Brown, and Co; 1995:551.

78. Fitzgerald SF, Kelly C, Humphreys H. Diagnosis and treatment of prosthetic aortic graft infections: confusion and inconsistency in the absence of evidence or consensus. *J Antimicrob Chemother.* 2005;56:996-999.

79. Baddour LM, Wilson WR. Infections of Prosthetic valves and other cardiovascular devices. In: Mandell G, Bennett JE, Dolin P, eds. *Principles and Practice of Infectious Diseases.* 6th ed. Philadelphia, PA: Elsevier; 2005:1022.

80. Tiesenhausen K, Amann W, Thalhammer M. Primary bacterial infection of an artery. *Chirurg.* 1999;70:1163-1167.

81. Kovoor JM, Jayakumar PN, Srikanth SG, Sampath S. Intracranial infective aneurysms: angiographic evaluation with treatment. *Neurology India.* 2001;49(3):262-266.

82. Baddour LM, Bettman MA, Bolger AF, et al. Nonvalvular cardiovascular device-related infections. *Circulation.* 2003;108:2015-2031.

83. Dougherty SH. Prosthetic devices. Diagnosis and management of prosthesis infection. In: Meakins TL, ed. *Surgical Infections.* New York, NY: Scientific American; 1994:247.

84. Ryan SV, Calligaro KD, Dougherty MJ. Management of hemodialysis access infections. *Semin Vasc Surg.* 2004;17(1):40-44.

85. Reddy DJ, Shepard AD, Evans JR, Wright DJ, Smith RF, Ernst CB. Management of infected aortoiliac aneurysms. *Arch Surg*. 1991;126(7):873-878.

86. Trout HH III, Kozloff L, Giordano JM. Priority of revascularization in patients with graft enteric fistulas, infection artertis or infected arterial protheses. *Ann Surg*. 1984;199(6):669-683.

87. Callaert JR, Fourneau I, Daenens K, Maleux G, Nevelsteen A. Endoprosthetic treatment of a mycotic superficial femoral artery aneurysm. *J Endovasc Surg*. 2003;10(4):843-845.

88. Swain TW III, Calligaro KD, Dougherty MD. Management of infected aortic prosthetic grafts. *Vasc Endovasc Surg*. 2004; 38(1):75-82.

89. Rowe NM, Impellizzeri P, Vaynblat M, et al. Studies in thoracic aortic graft infections: the development of a porcine model and a comparison of collagen-impregnated dacron grafts and cryopreserved allografts. *J Thorac Cardiovasc Surg*. 1999;118(5):857-865.

90. Melliere D, Zaouche S, Becquemin JP, et al. Antibiotic-impregnated prostheses: eclectic indications. *J Mal Vasc*. 1996;21(suppl A):139-145.

91. Seify H, Moyer HR, Jones GE, et al. The role of muscle flaps in wound salvage after vascular graft infections: the Emory experience. *Plast Reconstr Surg*. 2006;117(4):1325-1333.

92. O'Connor S, Andrew P, Batt M, Becquemin JP. A systematic review and meta-analysis of treatments for aortic graft infection. *J Vasc Surg*. 2006;44(1):38.

93. Zetrenne E, Wirth GA, McIntosh BC, Evenas GR, Narayan D. Managing extracavity prosthetic vascular graft infections: a pathway to success. *Ann Plast Surg*. 2006;57:677-682.

94. Aram G, Rohwedder A, Nazeer T, et al. Varciella zoster virus follicultis promoted cutanenous lymphoid hyperplasia. *Am J Dermatopath*. 2005;27(5):411-417.

95. Danchaivijitr N, Miravet E, Saunders DE, Cox T, Ganesan V. Post-varicella intracranial hemorrhage in a child. *Dev Med Child Neurol*. 2006;48(2):139-142.

96. Kramer LA, Villar-Cordova C, Wheless JW, Slopis J, Yeakley J. Magnetic resonance angiography of primary varicella vasculitis: report of two cases. *J Magn Reson Imaging*. 1999;9(3):491-496.

97. Martin JR, Mitchell WJ, and Henken DB. Neurotropic herpesviruses, neural mechanisms and arteritis. *Brain Pathol*. 1990;1(1):6-10.

98. Pina MA, Ara JA, Capablo JL, Omeneca M. Myelitis and optic neuritis caused by varicella. *Revista Neurologica*. 1997;25(146):1575-1576.

99. Culbertson WW, Blumenkranz MS, Pepose JS, Stewart JA, Curtin VT. Varicella zoster virus is a a cuase of the acute retinal necrosis syndrome. *Ophthalmol*. 1986;93(5):559-569.

100. Caruso JM, Tung GA, Brown WD. Central nervous system and renal vasculitis associated with primary varicella infection in a child. *Pediatrics*. 2001;107(1):E9.

101. Hausler MG, Ramaekers VT, Reul J, Meilicke R, Heimann G. Early and late onset manifestations of cerebral vascultis reatled to varicella zoster. *Neuropediatrics*. 1998;29(4):202-207.

102. Kleinschmidt-DeMasters BK, Amlie-LeFond C, Gilden GH. The patterns of varciella zoster virus encephalitis. *Human Pathol*. 1996;27(9):927-938.

103. Martin JR, Mitchell WJ, Henken DB. Neurotropic herpesviruses, neural mechanisms and arteritis. *Brain Pathol*. 1990;1(1):6-10.

104. Berger TM, Caduff JH, Gebbers J-O. Fatal varicella-zoster virus antigen-positive giant cell arteritis of the central nervous system. *Pediatr Infect Dis J*. 2000;19:653-656.

105. Picard O, Brunereau L, Pelosse B, Kerob D, Cabane J, Imbert JC. Cerebral infarction associated with vasculitis due to varicella zoster virus in patients infected with human deficiency virus. *Biomed Pharmacother*. 1997;51(10):449-454.

106. Rodriguez-Pereira C, Suarez-Penaranda JM, del Rio E, Forteza-Vila J. Cutaneous granulomatous vasculitis after herpes zoster infection showing polyarteritis-nodosa-like features. *Clin and Exp Dermatol*. 1997;22(6):274-276.

107. Al-Abdulla NA, Rismondo V, Minkowski JS, Miller NR. Herpes zoster vasculitis presenting as giant cell arteritis with bilateral ophthalmoplegia. *Am J Ophthalmol*. 2002; 134(6):912-914.

108. Koeppen AH, Lansing LS, Peng SK, Smith RS. Central nervous system vasculitis in cytomegalovirus infection. *J Neurol Sci*. 1981;51(3):395-410.

109. Duhaut P, Bosshard S, Ducroix JP. Is giant cell arteritis an infectious disease? Biological and epidemiological evidence. *Presse Med*. 2004;33(19, pt 2):1403-1408.

110. Murakami K, Ohsawa M, Hu SX, Kanno H, Aozasa K, Nose M. Large-vessel arteritis associated with chronic active Epstein-Barr virus infection. *Arthritis Rheum*. 1998;41(2):369-373.

111. Liozon E, Loustaud V, Ly K, Vidal E. Association between infection and the onset of giant cell arteritis: can seasonal patterns provide the answer? *J Rheumatol*. 2001;28(5):1197-1198.

112. Ban S, Goto Y, Kamada K, et al. Systemic granulomatous arteritis associated with Epstein-Barr virus infection. *Virchows Archiv*. 1999;434(3):249-254.

113. Toyable S, Harada W, Suzuki H, Hirokawa T, Uchiyama M. Large vessel arteritis associated with human herpsesvirus 6 infections. *Clin Rheum*. 2002;21(6):528-532.

114. Sun Y, Pei W, Wu Y, Jing Z, Zhang J, Wang G. Herpes simplex virus type 2 is a risk factor for hypertension. *Hypertens Res Clin Exp*. 2004;27(8):541-544.

115. Dal Canto AJD, Virgin HW. Animal models of infection-mediated vasculitis: implications for human disease. *Internatl J Cardiol*. 2000;27(suppl1):S37-S45.

116. Presti RM, Pollock JL, Dal Canto AJ, O'Guin AK, Virgin HW IV. Interferon gamma regulates acute na dlatent murine cytomegalovirus infection and chronic diasease of the great vessels. *J Exp Med*. 1998;188(3):577-588.

117. Fisher SD, Miller SL, Lipshultz SE. Impact of HIV and high active antiretroviral therapy on leukocyte adhesion molecules, arterial inflammation, dyslipidemia, and atherosclerosis. *Atherosclerosis*. 2006;185(1):1-11.

118. Ake JA, Erickson JC, Lowry KJ. Cerebral aneurysmal arteriopathy associated with HIV infection in an adult. *Clin Infect Dis*. 2006;43(5):e46-e50.

119. Shah SS, Zimmerman RA, Rorke LB, Vezina LG. Cerebrovascular complications of HIV in children. *Am J Neuroradiol*. 1996;17(10):1913-1917.

120. Sinzobahamvya N, Kalangu K, Hamel-Kalinowski W. Arterial aneuryssms asscoatied with human immunodeficiency

virus (HIV) infection. *Acta Chir Belg.* 1989;89(4):185-188.

121. Martinez-Longoria CA, Morales-Aguirre JJ, Villalobos-Acosta CP, Gomez-Barreto D, Cashat-Cruz M. Occurrence of intracerebral aneurysm in an HIV-infected child: a case report. *Ped Neurol.* 2004;31(2):130-132.

122. Patsalides AD, Wood LV, Atac GK, Sandifer E, Butman JA, Patronas NJ. Cerebrovascular disease in HIV-infected pediatric patients: neuroimaging findings. *AJR.* 2002;179(4):999-1003.

123. Nair R, Robbs JV, Chetty, R, Naidoo NG, Woolgar J. Occlusive arterial disease in HIV-infected patients: a preliminary report. *Eur J Vasc Endovasc Surg.* 2000;20(4):353-357.

124. Garcia-Garcia JA, Macias J, Castellanos V, et al. Necrotizing granulomatous vascultis in advanced HIV infection. *J Infection.* 2003;47(4):333-335.

125. Nair R, Chetty R, Woolgar J, Naido NG, Robbs, JV. Spontaneous arteriovenous fistula from HIV arteritis. *J Vasc Surg.* 2001;33(1):186-187.

126. Gherardi R, Belec L, Mhiri C, et al. The spectrum of vasculitis in human immunodeficiency virus-infected patients. A clinicopathoglic evaluation. *Arthritis Rheum.* 1993;36(8):1164-1174.

127. Chamouard JM, Smadja D, Chaunu MP, Bouceh P. Neuropathy caused by necrotizing vasculitis in HIV-1 infection. *Rev Neurol (Paris).* 1993;149(5):358-361.

128. Rodriguez-Pla A, Stone JH. Vasculitis and systemic infections. *Curr Opin Rheumatol.* 2006;18(1):39-47.

129. Lane SE, Watts R, Scott DG. Epidemiology of systemic vascultitis. *Curr Rheumatol Rep.* 2005;7(4):270-275.

130. Elling P, Olsen AT, Elling H. Synchronous variations in the incidence of termporal arteritis and polymyalgia rheumatica in Danish counties. Assocation with epidemics of Mycoplasma pneumonia. *J Rheumatol.* 1996;23(1):112-119.

131. Staud R, Corman LC. Association of parvovirus B 19 infection with giant cell arteritis. *Clin Infect Dis.* 1996;22(6):1123.

132. Rimenti G, Blasi F, Consentini R, et al. Temporal arteritis associated with *Chlamydia pneumoniae* DNA detected in an artery specimen. *J Rheumatol.* 2000;27(11):2718-2720.

133. Bonnet F, Morlat P, Delevaux I, et al. A possible association between Chamydia psittacci infection and temporal arteritis. *Joint Bone Spine.* 2000;67(6):550-552.

134. Helweg-Larsen J, Tarp B, Obel N, Baslund B. No evidence of parvovirus B19, *Chlamydia pneumoniae*, or human herpes virus infection in temporal artery biopsies in patients with giant cell arteritis. *Rheumatol.* 2002;41(4):445-449.

135. MacDonald AB. Giant cell arteritis and *Borrelia* infection. *J Clin Neuroophthalmol.* 1987;7(3):180-181.

136. Midgard JE, Gribble D. Unusual mainfestionatons of nervrous system *Borrelia burgdofferi* infection. *Arch Neurol.* 1987;44(7):781-783.

137. Delpla PA, Delisle MB, Arne-Bes MC, et al. Multipe mononeuritis and cerebral minigo-artertis. Wegner disase or Lyme disease? *Rev Neurol (Paris).* 1993;149(6-7):411-415.

138. Russo RG, Waxman J, Abdoh AA, Serebro LH. Corrleation between infection and the onset of giant cell (temporal) arteritis syndrome: a trigger mechanism? *Arthiritis Rheum.* 1995;38(3):374-380.

139. Canada R, Chaudry S, Gaber L, et al. Polyarteritis nodosa and cryoglobulinemic glomerulonephritis related to chronic hepatitis C. *Am J Med Sci.* 2006;331(6):329-333.

140. Stein RH, Phleps AG, Sapadin AN. Cutaenous polyarteritis nodosa after strpetococcal; necrtoziing fasciitis. *Mt Sinai J Med.* 2001;68(4-5):336-338.

141. Elias N, Sabo E, Naschitz JE, Yershurun D, Misselevich I, Boss JH. Colonic ulcers in a patient with hepatitis C virus-associated polyarteritis nodosa. *J Clin Gastroenterol.* 1998;26(3):212-215.

142. Ljungstrom L, Franzen C, Schlaug M, Elowson S, Viidas U. Reinfection with *Chlamydia pneumoniae* may induce isolated and systemic vasculitis in small and large vesssels. *Scand J Infect Dis Suppl.* 1997;104:37-40.

143. Bahl VK, Sengupta PP, Sathpathy G, et al. *Chlamydia pneumoniae* infection and nonspecific aortoarteritis: search for a link with a nonatherosclerotic inflammatory arterial disease. *Indian Heart J.* 2002;54(1):46-49.

144. Hamidou MA, Fradet G, Kadi AM, et al. Systemic vasculitis with lymphocytic temporal arteritis and *Toxocara canis* infection. *Arch Intern Med.* 2002;162(13):1521-1524.

145. Frayha RA. Trichinosis-related polyarteritis nodosa. *Am J Med.* 1981;71(2):307-312.

146. Sitara D, Hoffbrand BI. Chronic bronchial suppuration and antineutrophil cytoplasmic antibody (ANCA) positive systemic vasculitis. *Postgrad Med J.* 1990;66(778):669-671.

147. Branley P, Savige JA, Sinclair RA, Miach P. Microscopic polyarteritis following a suppurative wound infection. *Pathol.* 1997;29(4):403-405.

148. Saadoun D, Cacoub P, Mahoux D, et al. Postvaccine vasculitis: a report of three case. *Rev Med Interne.* 2001;22(2):172-176.

149. Morales MF, Ordway D, Oliveria L, et al. Cellular responses to *Mycobacterium tuberculosis* in a patient with Takayasu's arteritis. *Rev Port Cardiol.* 1999;18(4):359-367.

150. Hernandez-Pando R, Reyes P, Espitia C, et al. Raised a galactosyl IgG and antimycobacterial humoral immunity in Takayasu's arteritis. *J Rheumaotol.* 1994;21(10):1791-1795.

151. Kumar CS, Kumar TN, Sinha N, Singh M, Nityand S. Cellular and humoral immune responses to mycobacterial heat shock protein-65 and its human homologue in Takayasu's artertis. *Clin Exp Immunol.* 2004;138(3):547-553.

152. Dal Canto AJ, Virgin HW IV, Speck SH. Ongoing viral replication is required for gammagherpvirus 60-induced vascular damage. *J Virol.* 2000;74(23):11304-11310.

153. Zhu J, Quyyumi AA, Norman JE, Costello R, Csako G, Epstein S. The possible role of hepatitis A virus in the pathogenesis of atherosclerosis. *J Infect Dis.* 2000;192:1583.

154. Prasad A, Zhu J, Halcox JPJ, Waclawiw MA, Epstein SE, Quyyumi AA. Predisposition to atherosclerosis by infections. *Circulation.* 2002;106:184.

155. Auer J, Leitinger M, Berent R, et al. Hepatitis A IgG seropositivity and coronary atherosclerosis assessed by angiography. *Int J Cardiol.* 2003;90:175.

156. Ongey M, Brenner H, Thefeld W, Rothenbacher D. *Helicobacter pylori* and hepatitis A virus infections and the cardiovascular risk profile in patients with diabetes mellitus:

results of a population-based study. *Eur J Cardiovasc Pre Rehabil.* 2004;11:471.

157. Bilora F, Rinaldi R, Boccioletti V, Petrobelli F, Girolami A. Chronic viral hepatitis: a prospective factors against atherosclerosis. A study with echo-color Doppler of the carotid and femoral arteries and the abdominal aorta. *Gastroenterol Clin Biol.* 2002;26:1001.

158. Volzke H, Schwahn C, Wolff B, et al. Hepatitis B and C virus infection and the risk of atherosclerosis in a general population. *Ahterosclerosis.* 2004;174:99.

159. Ishizaka N, Ishizaka Y, Takahashi E, et al. Increased prevalence of carotid atherosclerosis in hepatitis B virus carriers. *Circulation.* 2002;105:1028.

160. Ishizaka N, Ishizaka Y, Takahashi E, et al. Association between hepatitis C virus seropositivity, carotid-artery plaque, and intima–media thickening. *Lancet.* 2002;359:133.

161. Ishizaka Y, Ishizaka N, Takahashi N, et al. Association between hepatitis C virus core protein and carotid atherosclerosis. *Circ J.* 2003;67:26.

162. Vassalle C, Masini S, Bianchi F, et al. Evidence for association between hepatitis C seropositivity and coronary artery disease. *Heart.* 2007;90:565.

163. Arcari CM, Nelson KE, Netski DM, Nieto FJ, Gaydos CA. No association between hepatitis C virus seropositivity and acute myocardial infarction. *Clin Infect Dis.* 2006;43:e53.

164. Ibrahim AI, Obeid MT, Jourma MJ, et al. Detection of herpes simplex virus, cytomegalovirus and Epstein-Barr virus DNA in atherosclerotic plaques and in unaffected bypass grafts. *J Clin Virol.* 2005;32:29.

165. Shi Y, Tokunaga O. Herpesvirus (HSV-1, EBV and CMV) infections in atherosclerotic compared with non-atherosclerotic aortic tissue. *Pathol Int.* 2002;52:31.

166. Nabipour I, Vahdat K, Jafari SM, Pazoki R, Sanjdideh Z. The association of metabolic syndrome and *Chlamydia pneumoniae, Helicobacter pylori*, cytomegalovirus, and herpes simplex virus type I: the Persian Gulf Healthy Heart Study. *Cardiovasc Diabetol.* 2006;5:25.

167. Espinola-Klein C, Rupprecht HJ, Blankenberg S, et al. Impact of infectious burden on progression of carotid atherosclerosis. *Stroke.* 2002;33:2581.

168. Stassen FR, Vega-Cordova X, Vliegen I, Bruggeman CA. Immune activation following cytomegalovirus infection: more important than direct viral effects in cardiovascular disease? *J Clin Virol.* 2006;35:349.

169. Zhou YF, Leon MB, Waclawiw MA, et al. Association between prior cytomegalovirus infection and the risk of restenosis after coronary atherectomy. *N Engl J Med.* 1996;335:624.

170. Grattan MT, Moreno-Cabral CE, Starnes VA, Oyer PE, Stinson EB, Shumway NE. Cytomegalovirus infection is associated with cardiac allograft rejection and atherosclerosis. *J Am Med Assoc.* 1989;261:3561.

171. Kalil RSN, Hudson SL, Gaston RS. Determinants of cardiovascular mortality after renal transplantation: a role for cytomegalovirus? *Am J Transplantat.* 2003;3:79.

172. Kwon TW, Kim DK, Ye JS, et al. Detection of enterovirus, cytomegalovirus, and *Chlamydia pneumoniae* in atheromas. *J Microbiol.* 2004;42:299.

173. Pleskov VM, Bannikov AI, Gurevich VS, Pleskova L. Influenza viruses and atherosclerosis: the role of atherosclerotic plaques in prolonging the persistent form of influenza infection [abstract]. *Vestn Ross Akad Med Nauk.* 2003;4:10.

174. Auer J, Leitinger M, Berent R, et al. Influenza A and B IgG seropositivity and coronary atherosclerosis assessed by angiography. *Heart Disease.* 2002;4:349.

175. Pislaru SV, deWerf FV. Antibiotic therapy for coronary artery disease. *J Am Med Assoc.* 2003;290:1515.

176. Saikku, Leinonen M, Mattila K, et al. Serological evidence of an association of a novel *Chlamydia*, TWAR, with chronic coronary heart disease and acute myocardial infarction. *Lancet.* 1988;2:983.

177. Danesh J, Whincup P, Walker M, et al. *Chlamydia pneumoniae* IgG titres and coronary heart disease: prospective study and meta-analysis. *Br Med J.* 2000;321:208.

178. Danesh J, Whincup P, Lewington S, et al. *Chlamydia pneumoniae* IgA titres and coronary heart disease. *Eur Heart J.* 2002;23:371.

179. Arcari CM, Gaydos CA, Nieto FJ, Krauss M, Nelson KE. Association between *Chlamydia pneumoniae* and acute mycoardial infarction in young men in the United States military: the importance of timing of exposure measurement. *Clin Infect Dis.* 2005;40:1123.

180. Ongey M, Brenner H, Thefeld W, Rothenbacher D. *Helicobacter pylori* and hepatitis A virus infections and the cardiovascular risk profile in patients with diabetes mellitus: results of a population-based study. *Eur J Cardiovasc Prev Rehabil.* 2004;11:471.

181. Smieja M, Gnarpe J, Lonn E, et al. Multiple infections and subsequent cardiovascular events in the heart outcomes prevention evaluation study. *Circulation.* 2003;107:251.

182. Koksal A, Ekmekci Y, Karadeniz Y, et al. *Helicobacter pylori* seropositivity and atherosclerosis risk factors. *Dig Dis.* 2004;22:386.

183. Kanbay M, Gur G, Yucel M, Yilmaz U, Boyacioglu S. Does eradication of *Helicobacter pylori* infecton help normalize serum lipid ad CRP levels? *Dig Dis Sci.* 2005;50:1228.

184. Nabipour I, Vahdat K, Jafari SM, Pazoki R, Sanjdideh Z. The association of metabolic syndrome and *Chlamydia pneumoniae, Helicobacter pylori*, cytomegalovirus, and herpes simplex virus type I: the Persian Gulf Healthy Heart Study. *Cardiovasc Diabetol.* 2006;5:25.

185. Weiss TW, Kvakan H, Kaun C, et al. No evidence for a direct role of *Helicobacter pylori* and *Mycoplasma pneumoniae* in carotid artery atherosclerosis. *J Clin Pathol.* 2006;59:1186.

186. Kaklikkaya I, Kaklikkaya N, Buruk K, et al. Investigation of *Chlamydia pneumoniae* dNA, chlamydial lipopolysaccharide antigens, and *Helicobacter pylori* DNA in atherosclerotic plaques of patients with aortoiliac occlusive disease. *Cardiovasc Pathol.* 2006;15:105.

187. Garfunkel AA. Recognizing the dental-medical symbiosis: back to basic sciences. *Compend Contin Educ Dent.* 2006;27(7):390-392.

188. Behle JH, Papapanou PN. Periodontal infections and atherosclerotic vascular disease: an update. *Int Dent J.* 2006;56:256.

189. Tonetti M, D'Aiuto F, Nibali L, et al. Treatment of periodontitis and endothelial function. *N Engl J Med.* 2007;356:911.

190. Tabrizi F, Buhlin K, Gustafsson A, Klinge B. Oral Health of monozygotic twins with and without coronary heart disease: a pilot study. *J Clin Periodontol.* 2007;34:220.

191. Danesh J. Coronary heart disease, *Helicobacter pylori*, dental disease, *Chlamydia pneumoniae*, and cytomegalovirus: meta-analyses of prospective studies. *Am Heart J.* 1999;138: S434.

192. Smieja M, Cinarpe J, Lonn E, et al. Multiple infections and subsequent cardiovascular events in the heart outcomes prevention evaluation study. *Circulation.* 2003;107:251.

193. Mondy K, Overton ET, Grubb J, et al. Metabolic syndrome in HIV-infected patients from an urban, midwestern US outpatient population. *Clin Infect Dis.* 2004;44:726.

194. Vittecoq D, Escaut L, Chironi G, et al. Coronary heart disease in HIV-infected patients in the highly active antiretroviral treatment era. *AIDS.* 2003;17:S70.

195. Bozzette SA, Ake CF, Tam HK, Chang SW, Louis TA. Cardiovascular and cerebrovascular events in patients treated for human immunodeficiency virus infection. *N Eng J Med.* 2003;348:702.

196. Holmsberg SD, Moorman AC, Williamson JM, et al. Protease inhibitors and cardiovascular outcomes in patients with HIV-1. *Lancet.* 2002;360:1747.

197. Schillaci G, De Socio GV, Pirro M, et al. Impact of treatment with protease inhibitors on aortic stiffness in adult patients with human immunodeficiency virus infection. *Arterioscler Thromb Vasc Biol.* 2005;25:2381.

198. Guardiolo M, Ferre R, Salazar J, et al. Proptease inhibitor-assocated dyslipidemia in HIV-infected patients is strongly influence by the APOA5-1131T→C gene variation. *Clin Chem.* 2006;52:1914.

199. Friis-Moller N, Weber R, Reiss P, et al. Cardiovascular disease risk factors in HIV patients: association with antiretroviral therapy. Results from the DAD study. *AIDS.* 2003;17:1179.

200. Jiang B, Hebert VY, Zavecz JH, Dugas TR. Antiretroviral induces direct endotheial dysfunction in vivo. *J Aquir Immune Defic Syndr.* 2006;24:391.

201. Sudano I, Spieker LE, Noll G, Corti R, Weber R. Cardiovascular disease in HIV infection. *Am Heart J.* 2006;151:1147.

202. deGaetano Donati K. HIV infection, HAART, and endothelial adhesion molecules: current perspectives. *Lancet Infect Dis.* 2004;4:213.

203. Friis-Moller N, Sabin CA, Weber R, et al. (The Data Collection on Adverse Events of Anti-HIV Drugs [DAD] Study Group). Combination antiretroviral therapy and the risk of myocardial infarction. *N Engl J Med.* 2003;349:1993.

chapter 12

Overlap of Atherosclerotic Disease

*Madhurmeet Singh, DO / Ali Morshedi-Meibodi, MD / Lowell H. Steen, MD /
Robert S. Dieter, MD, RVT*

● CORONARY ARTERY AND SYSTEMIC ARTERIAL DISEASE

According to the most recent data, currently there are approximately 71 million people in the United States with some form of cardiovascular disease (CVD).[1] The burden of CVD on the society is enormous. CVD has been the number one killer disease in the United States every year since 1900 except 1918.[1] It kills more Americans every year than the next four leading causes of death combined together (cancer, chronic lower respiratory tract disease, accidents, and diabetes).[1]

The spectrum of CVD includes hypertension (HTN), angina, myocardial infarction (MI), heart failure, cerebrovascular accidents, etc. Of this, the prevalence of coronary artery disease (CAD), which includes angina and MI, is estimated to be approximately 13 million.[1] Considering the diffuse nature of atherosclerotic vascular disease, it would be reasonable to expect patients with CAD to have a systemic distribution of arterial disease. In fact, it has been recognized since the middle of the 20th century that patients with atherosclerotic vascular disease in one vascular bed are likely to develop disease in other arteries as well and clinically manifest symptoms of such disease.[2]

When studying incidence of CAD, data suggest that the incidence of single and multiple vessel CAD (defined as >50% angiographic stenosis) is as high as 21% to 41%, respectively, regardless of the principal vascular diagnosis (AAA, PAD, carotid artery disease).[3] Manifestations of arterial disease frequently seen in patients with CAD include renal artery stenosis (RAS), peripheral arterial disease (PAD), carotid artery disease, and aneurysms of the aorta and its branches (subclavian artery, celiac trunk, superior mesenteric artery, and inferior mesenteric artery).

Recently, the REACH database, which included 67 888 patients from an international population, demonstrated that of patients with symptomatic atherothrombotic disease almost 16% had significant polyvascular disease.[4] It should be noted that the prevalence of polyvascular arterial disease would have been much higher had these patients also been screened for asymptomatic vascular disease.[4]

With this in mind, it should not be surprising that the risk of angiographically significant RAS increases with multivessel CAD.[5] Presence of significant CAD with more than two vessel involvement has been shown to be a predictor of RAS with a sensitivity of 0.84 and specificity of 0.77.[6] It has been further demonstrated that the risk of significant RAS (defined as >50% stenosis of a renal artery) ranges from 22% to 89% in patients with CAD.[7,8] In patients with prior history of percutaneous coronary intervention, the prevalence of significant RAS is around 39%[9] (Table 12-1).

Patients with CAD also tend to have a higher incidence of underlying carotid arterial occlusive disease and approximately 11% of patients with CAD have been reported to have significant carotid stenosis (defined as >70%).[10]

Along the same lines, it has been reported that individuals with CAD also tend to have a higher prevalence of PAD. One Finnish study reported that the relative risk of intermittent claudication (IC) in women and men with angina pectoris was 4 to 7 times higher, respectively, as compared to controls.[11] The Framingham heart study suggests that CAD confers almost a threefold increase in the risk of developing IC.[12] In a study that looked at patients hospitalized with medically stable CAD, Dieter et al.[13] found that as many as 40% of such patients had significant PAD (as defined by an ankle-brachial index [ABI] of <0.9 or history of revascularization for PAD).[13] Similarly, others have reported that one out of three patients aging 62 or older and with CAD also have underlying PAD.[14] The Cardiovascular Health Study demonstrated that there is a significant association between ABI and MI, congestive heart failure, and angina.[15] The TASC

TABLE 12-1. Risk of RAS in Patients with Known CAD

Authors	Year	Data (%)
Jean, et al.[8]	1994	22
Crowley, et al.[7]	1998	89
Charanjit, et al.[9]	2002	39

TABLE 12-3. Risk of CAD in Patients with RAS

Authors	Year	Data (%)
Tarazi, et al.[25]	1987	40
Valentine, et al.[23]	1993	58

II data suggest that as many as 10% to 30% of patients with ischemic heart disease will have underlying PAD[16] (Table 12-2).

● RENAL ARTERY STENOSIS

RAS is the most common cause of secondary HTN.[17] Until recently, estimating RAS in a population required invasive technique (e.g., angiography) and therefore a population-based study estimate of the prevalence of RAS had been difficult. Most of the estimates available were obtained either from necropsy reports or from angiographic evidence gathered during evaluation of other vascular regions. From a recent population-based study, the prevalence of RAS amongst the elderly Americans (65 years or older) was reported to be 6.8%.[18] In fact, atherosclerosis of the renal arteries is the most common disease to affect the renal arteries.[19]

RAS is much more common in patients who have clinical evidence of atherosclerotic arterial disease in vascular territory excluding the renal arteries (such as PAD, CAD, carotid occlusive disease, etc.). Various studies have demonstrated that once a diagnosis of arterial atherosclerotic disease has been made somewhere else in the arterial tree, the risk of having atherosclerotic RAS ranges from 26% to 50%.[5,9,20–23] It has been observed that approximately 31% of patients with mild atherosclerotic narrowing (<50% occlusion) of a renal artery have clinical evidence of symptomatic arterial disease in the coronary, cerebrovascular, or peripheral vascular circulation.[24] Moreover, in patients with moderate to severe stenosis of renal artery (>50%), 49% had clinical symptoms of extra-renal atherosclerotic arterial disease.[24] It has been observed that patients with RAS have a higher likelihood of having underlying CAD and more stenotic coronary segments have been observed in those with significant RAS as compared to those without RAS (3.8+ − 1.2 vs. 2.3 + −1.3; $p < 0.001$).[6] Further,

on average 58% of patients with 50% or greater RAS have been shown to have clinically overt CAD (ECG changes, symptoms, etc.)[23] It has been demonstrated that of patients with unilateral RAS requiring surgical intervention, as many as 14% of patients required myocardial revascularization when the coronary anatomy was evaluated after the diagnosis of RAS was made. This number was significantly worse in the bilateral RAS group which had as many as 40% of patients who needed myocardial revascularization or had advanced coronary disease[25] (Table 12-3).

As alluded to earlier, just as there is significant overlap between patients with RAS and CAD, there is also significant overlap between RAS, carotid artery disease, and PAD. In fact, it has been demonstrated that there is an association between the degree of RAS and the extent of disease in the extracranial carotids and lower extremity arteries.[26,27] It has been noted that among patients with renovascular HTN caused by occlusive renal arterial disease, as many as 83% had some degree of carotid arterial stenosis compared to 43% of patients with essential hypertension (EH). Hemodynamically significant carotid stenosis was seen in 10% of patients with renovascular HTN as compared to a 3% risk in patients with EH.[26] Further, it has also been demonstrated that 40% to 46% of patients with significant RAS tend to have moderate to severe occlusion of the carotid circulation[17,28] (Table 12-4). Carotid artery lesions are not only more common but also more severe and occur at a younger age in patients with renovascular HTN. Further exacerbating the situation, these plaques in patients with renovascular HTN tend to be more heavily calcified as compared to their counterpart with EH.[26] It has been observed that as the severity of RAS progresses from mild to severe, there is a fourfold increase in the prevalence of severe carotid artery disease.[27]

Similarly, patients are more likely to have moderate or severe lower extremity PAD in the presence of severe RAS.[27] In patients with moderate to severe RAS, as many as three out of four have been found to have PAD with

TABLE 12-2. Risk of PAD in Patients with CAD

Authors	Year	Data (%)
Aronow and Ahn[14]	1994	33
Dieter, et al.[13]	2003	40
Norgren, et al.[16]	2007	10–30

TABLE 12-4. Risk of CVD in Patients with RAS

Authors	Year	Data (%)
Rossi, et al.[26]	1992	83
Louie, et al.[17]	1994	40
Missouris, et al.[28]	1998	46

TABLE 12-5. Risk of PAD in Patients with RAS

Authors	Year	Data (%)
Tollefson, et al.[29]	1991	69
Louie, et al.[17]	1994	75

ABI less than 0.95.[17] Yet another study looked at patients with atherosclerotic RAS of variable degree and concluded that as many as 69% of these patients suffered from PAD[29] (Table 12-5).

MESENTERIC ARTERY ISCHEMIA

It is well known that the atherosclerotic disease of the celiac and mesenteric arteries is the most common cause for their obstruction.[30] Consequently, such patients present with the clinical symptomatology of postprandial abdominal pain (referred to as "intestinal angina"), which was first described in 1957 by Mikklesen.[31] The celiac, superior, and inferior mesenteric arteries are interconnected and the intestines are usually well perfused by a comprehensive network of collaterals. Therefore, an obstruction of one of the three vessels is usually well tolerated. It has been suggested that the classical symptoms of this disease process become evident when at least two of the three main intestinal arteries are obstructed, although cases of intestinal ischemia from obstruction of just the superior mesenteric artery have also been documented.[32] The clinical presentation of intestinal ischemia remains rare despite the relative commonness of this disease in the general population.[33] As a result, symptomatic mesenteric ischemia requiring surgical intervention or other diagnostic studies remains rare and therefore literature available for this disease process and overlap with other atheromatous disease processes remains sparse.

From unselected autopsy studies, it has been concluded that significant intestinal atherosclerotic obstruction is present in 6% to 10% of the population. This incidence has been reported to be as high as 14% to 24% in patients undergoing abdominal arteriography.[32] Coexistent arterial disease involving other arterial beds (cerebrovascular, renal, or lower extremity) has been seen in as many as 85% of patients with mesenteric ischemia requiring surgical intervention.[34] In patients with stenosis of both the celiac trunk and the superior mesenteric artery, as many as 71% have been reported to have RAS as well.[35]

Along the same lines, CAD has been seen in as many 33% to 50% of patients with chronic mesenteric occlusive disease.[34,35]

The prevalence of underlying PAD is also high in patients with mesenteric ischemia and is even more significant in those who have symptoms severe enough to require bypass graft. Underlying PAD has been observed in as many as 78% of patients undergoing surgical revascularization of the mesenteric vessels for history of ischemia[36] (Table 12-6).

PAD OF THE LOWER EXTREMITY

PAD is a common syndrome affecting 8 to 12 million Americans. It is estimated that symptomatic PAD has a negative impact on the quality of life of as many as 2 million adult Americans.[37] The burden of asymptomatic PAD is hard to ignore and is also associated with significant cardiovascular morbidity and mortality. The prevalence of PAD is expected to continue to increase as the population continues to grow and the average life expectancy increases.

The most common cause for PAD in the lower extremity is atherosclerosis. Any factor that contributes to atherosclerosis, such as HTN, dyslipidemia, cigarette smoking, diabetes, etc., increases the risk of development of lower extremity arterial disease. Based on data gathered from the Framingham Heart Study, it has been concluded that male sex and smoking are associated with a 1.5-fold increase in development of IC, DM, and SBP >160 or DBP >100 conferred a twofold increase in risk of IC and CAD conferred almost threefold increase in the risk of developing IC.[12] On the reverse side, many studies have demonstrated that the presence of PAD is associated with increased presence of CAD and related conditions, including angina, coronary artery bypass graft, MI, congestive heart failure, etc.

Compiled evidence from many studies, as reported by the TASC II working group, suggests that approximately 40% to 60% of patients with PAD will also have CAD and cerebrovascular disease and as many as 50% may have carotid artery disease.[16] The prevalence of CAD in patients with PAD ranges from 14% to 90%, with the wide range demonstrating the difference in sensitivity of the detection technique used for CAD.[38] The most sensitive means available to determine the extent of CAD, coronary angiography, has revealed CAD in as many as 90% of patients with PAD.[3] This has been further classified based on the degree of CAD and it has been reported that as many as 28% of patients with PAD may have severe three-vessel disease that requires revascularization or is already considered inoperable.[3]

Also, it is known that patients with symptomatic PAD (IC, a symptom classically attributed to PAD) are more likely to have angina as compared to patients with asymptomatic PAD.[39] In addition, more than half of patients with IC have coexisting overt CVD and IC is associated with a

TABLE 12-6. Overlap of Mesenteric Vascular Disease with CAD, RAS, and PAD

	CAD (%)	RAS (%)	PAD (%)	CVD, RAS, or PAD (%)
Mesenteric disease	33–50	71	81	85

TABLE 12-7. Risk of CAD in Patients with PAD

Authors	Year	Data (%)
Hertzer, et al.[3]	1984	90
Golomb, et al.[38]	2006	14–90
Norgren, et al.[16]	2007	40–60

TABLE 12-8. Risk of RAS in Patients with PAD

Authors	Year	Data (%)
Olin, et al.[21]	1990	39
Valentine, et al.[23]	1993	56
Missouris, et al.[49]	1994	16

two- to fourfold increase in mortality from CVD.[40] In addition, it is also known that that patients with both symptomatic and asymptomatic PAD have the same increased risk of cardiovascular events.[41] Subjects with ABI of less than 0.9 have an increased risk for nonfatal MI (RR 1.38), cardiovascular deaths (RR 1.85–4.16), and coronary mortality (RR 4.97).[42,43] Further analysis have demonstrated a 5- to 11-fold increase in death from CAD in patients with large vessel peripheral vascular disease with the relative risk varying based on the distribution of PAD (unilateral vs. bilateral), symptomatic vs. nonsymptomatic nature of PAD, and the severity of PAD (moderate vs. severe)[44] (Table 12-7).

It has also been observed that PAD is a stronger risk factor for death from cardiac causes even when compared to a previous MI.[45] For instance, in one study with almost 2300 patients with a history of PAD and who were followed for >10 years, it was observed that PAD was a stronger predictor of long-term risk of CAD with 19% greater likelihood of death at anytime during follow-up as compared to history of a previous MI. Based on this, it was suggested that PAD be considered an independent risk factor for the development of CAD and such patients should be managed aggressively (and treated as a coronary equivalent) to limit the morbidity and mortality associated with CAD.[45]

The Framingham data has shown that clinically evident occlusive PAD (femoral bruits or absent pedal pulses) puts one at increased risk for all CVD endpoints.[46] It has been known since the 1970s, from the Framingham data, that there exists an increased risk for cardiovascular morbidity and mortality in patients with IC.[39] In addition, patients with a low ABI tend to have a higher risk of strokes or TIA's.[47]

As mentioned earlier, there is a significant overlap in distribution of atherosclerotic occlusive arterial disease once a diagnosis in a certain region has been made. It has been observed that as many as 18% to 60% of patients with PAD also have atherosclerotic RAS (with this prevalence even higher in hypertensive patients) and significant RAS (>50% occlusion) has been observed in as many as 11% to 39% of such patients.[20–23,48–51] The incidence of RAS in patients with angiographically documented PAD has been reported to be as high as 31% to 60%, with significant RAS (>50% occlusion) observed in as many as 14% to 39% of such patients.[21,49–51] Further, as many as 3% to 14% of patients with AAA, aortoiliac occlusive disease, or lower extremity occlusive arterial disease have severe to totally occluded bilateral renal arteries[21] (Table 12-8).

In addition, the degree of RAS worsens as the extent of peripheral arterial involvement worsens. Disease in the femoral vessels alone is an independent predictor of RAS with 42% of such patients having RAS.[22] Furthermore, one out of two patients with aortic, bilateral iliac, femoral, and distal disease has been shown to have underlying RAS.[22] As the severity of PAD increases, the likelihood of having RAS increases as well.[49] It has been demonstrated that as PAD progresses to involve one or two vessels to involving more than five vessels, there is also an increase in the likelihood of having underlying RAS with the relative risk increasing from 3.97 to 6.97, respectively.[49]

Further, there is a higher prevalence of cerebrovascular disease in patients with PAD and has been observed to be approximately 25%.[38] One study of patients with peripheral arterial occlusive disease and who had no neurological symptoms reported the incidence of complete occlusion of an internal carotid artery to be 4.8% when evaluated by duplex scanning.[52] In addition, carotid artery stenosis (CAS) >50% was noted in as many as 33% of the patients. To further qualify the relationship between PAD and CAS, ABI was correlated with the degree of carotid stenosis and it was found that an ABI <0.8 was an independent risk factor for the development of CAS. Along the same lines, in patients who had an ABI <0.4 as many as 59% had carotid stenosis of >50%.[52] Similar studies done in younger patient populations (mean age 42 ± 0.5 at the time of onset of PAD symptoms) who had a low ABI (mean 0.49 ± 0.02) have shown as many as 11% to have internal carotid occlusion as demonstrated by duplex scanning. Of this young patient population, 18% had 60% to 99% occlusion and 21% had 40% to 59% occlusion. In this group of patients, of those with any degree of carotid stenosis, 27% were reported to have had suffered either a TIA or a cerebrovascular accident during the follow-up period[53] (Table 12-9).

Similarly, it has been reported that the elderly patients with an ABI <0.9 have a 6% increased a risk of a

TABLE 12-9. Risk of CVD in Patients with CAD

Authors	Year	Data (%)
Valentine, et al.[53]	1997	29
Cina, et al.[52]	2002	33
Golomb, et al.[38]	2006	25

stroke as compared to 3% risk in those with an ABI >0.9 (an age-adjusted twofold increase in risk) thereby establishing an inverse relationship between ABI and stroke risk.[54]

As one would expect, mesenteric artery stenosis also occurs at a rate higher than compared to the general population and has been observed in as many as 29% of patients with peripheral vascular disease of the lower extremity.[35] Also, as many as 1 out of 10 patients with peripheral vascular atherosclerotic disease have an underlying asymptomatic AAA.[55]

● ANEURYSMS OF THE ABDOMINAL AORTA

Aortic aneurysms pose the same threat of morbidity and mortality that is encountered with occlusive arterial disease because of the shared atherosclerotic risk factors and high cardiac event rate.[32] This holds true despite the fact that the etiologic factors underlying occlusive arterial disease and aortic aneurysms are different. The prevalence of abdominal aortic aneurysms (AAAs) varies with many demographic factors, including age, gender, family history, and cigarette smoking. Many studies have observed that the prevalence of AAA of dimension 2.9 to 4.9 cm in diameter is 1.3% for men between 45 to 54 years of age to 12.5% for men between 75 to 84 years of age. In contrast, the prevalence rate for AAA in women is much lower ranging from 0% to 5.2% in the same age group, respectively.[32]

It has been demonstrated that of patients undergoing elective AAA repair, as many as 48% to 60% have clinical or ECG evidence suggestive of CAD.[56,57] In such patients, the incidence of angiographically demonstrated severe CAD (amenable to coronary artery bypass graft or too advanced to be surgically corrected) ranges from 33% to 43%.[56,58] In patients with AAA but who were not considered surgical candidates, it has been reported that in as many as 17% to 41% of patients the eventual cause of death was CAD[59,60] (Table 12-10).

AAAs, like the other atherosclerotic arterial diseases, have significant overlap with RAS. It has been demonstrated that as many as 22% to 38% of patients with an AAA have a renal artery with significant stenosis causing occlusion of 50% or more.[21,23,35] In addition, approximately 22% of patients with AAA have been noted to have underlying RAS that was clinically asymptomatic at the time

TABLE 12-10. Risk of CAD in Patients with AAA

Authors	Year	Data (%)
Szilagyi, et al.[60]	1966	17
Szilagyi, et al.[59]	1972	41
Hertzer, et al.[56]	1979	60
Golden, et al.[57]	1990	48
Starr, et al.[58]	1996	33

TABLE 12-11. Risk of RAS in Patients with AAA

Authors	Year	Data (%)
Brewster, et al.[61]	1975	22
Olin, et al.[21]	1990	38
Valentine, et al.[35]	1991	22
Valentine, et al.[23]	1993	29

of diagnosis[61] (Table 12-11). Along the same lines, mesenteric artery stenosis has been observed in as many as 40% of patients with AAA.[35]

● CAROTID ARTERY DISEASE

Obstructive disease of the carotid arteries has long been linked to an increased risk of underlying CAD and increased risk of coronary events. Postmortem studies have suggested a close relationship between the degree of stenosis in the carotid and coronary arterial circulation.[2,62] It has been suggested that the risk of ischemic cardiac events is higher among patients who have asymptomatic carotid bruits or have documented stenosis of the carotid arteries as compared to those without CAS.[63–66] Although trials directly comparing and correlating the degree of carotid artery disease (as measured by ultrasound and other means) and CAD have yet to be conducted, many trials have been completed identifying the risk of developing CAD in patients with carotid artery disease by using surrogate markers for carotid artery occlusion (carotid bruits and history of ischemic strokes/TIAs.) On the basis of this data, it has been determined with a great degree of certainty that patients with carotid artery disease remain at high risk for underlying CAD and require intensive medical management and close follow-up for preventing associated morbidity and mortality. One such study identified patients with extracranial cerebrovascular disease (defined as asymptomatic bruits on clinical examination or prior history of neurologic symptoms) and performed coronary angiography on such patients in order to define the coronary anatomy. This study provided overwhelming evidence for suspecting CAD in patients with carotid arterial disease and demonstrated that 28% of the patients had severe but correctable CAD and 7% had severe inoperable CAD.[67] Overall, only 7% of the patients in this group were found to have normal coronaries.

Other studies have demonstrated a 32% prevalence of severe CAD (>70% stenosis of one or more coronary arteries) on angiography in patients who were scheduled to undergo carotid vascular surgical intervention because of asymptomatic carotid bruits or symptoms indicating neurological deficits.[3] To further develop an association between extracranial carotid artery disease and the likelihood of developing CAD, yet another study that followed patients with 40% to 100% extracranial carotid disease concluded that in such population, 26% of patients without a documented history of CAD developed silent ischemia at some point during ambulatory monitoring. In patients who developed silent ischemia, there was almost a fourfold increase in the risk of developing new coronary events in the future.[68] A similar study was undertaken to study the prevalence of asymptomatic CAD in patients who suffered from transient ischemic attack (TIA), reversible ischemic neurological deficit (RIND), or mild stroke and had angiographically documented carotid artery disease involving the internal carotid artery or the middle cerebral artery. As many as 28% of the patients with carotid artery occlusive disease were found to have evidence of underlying CAD on exercise ECG stress testing and exercise myocardial scintigraphy.[69] In a study looking specifically at patients older than 62 years of age, it was noted that 53% of such patients who had a history of atherothrombotic brain infarction also had evidence of CAD as suggested by ECG, angina, or previous history of MI.[14] There are other studies that have looked at the prevalence of CAD in patients with TIAs or mild neurological deficits but without objective evidence of CAS and have found the rate of CAD to be as high as 58% (diagnosed by radionuclide scan or angiography).[70] Essentially, depending on the age, clinical findings, and symptoms, the prevalence of CAD in patients

TABLE 12-12. Risk of CAD in Patients with CVD

Authors	Year	Data (%)
Hertzer, et al.[3]	1984	32
Rokey, et al.[70]	1984	58
Hertzer, et al.[67]	1985	35
Di Pasquale, et al.[69]	1986	28
Aronow, et al.[68]	1993	26
Aronow and Ahn[14]	1994	53

with carotid artery disease varies from approximately 26% to 53% (Table 12-12).

● CONCLUSION

As is evident from the above discussion, the ubiquitous distribution of atheromatous arterial disease in humans has very important implications. The burden of arterial disease is immense and risk stratification strategies need to take into account the widespread nature of atheromatous arterial disease to ensure that appropriate diagnostic and treatment options are pursued and implemented.

REFERENCES

1. American Heart Association. *Heart Disease and Stroke Statistics—2006 Update.* Dallas, TX: American Heart Association; 2006.

2. Mitchell J, Schwartz C. Relationship between arterial disease in different sites: a study of the aorta and coronary, carotid, and iliac arteries. *Br Med J.* 1962;1:1293-1301.

3. Hertzer N, Beven E, Young J, et al. Coronary artery disease in peripheral vascular patients: a classification of 1000 coronary angiograms and results of surgical management. *Ann Surg.* 1984;199:223-233.

4. Bhatt D, Steg P, Ohman E, et al. International prevalence, recognition, and treatment of cardiovascular risk factors in outpatients with atherothrombosis. *JAMA.* 2006;295:180-189.

5. Harding M, Smith L, Himmelstein S, et al. Renal artery stenosis: prevalence and associated risk factors in patients undergoing routine cardiac catheterization. *J Am Soc Nephrol.* 1992;2:1608-1616.

6. Weber-Mzell D, Kotanko P, Schumacher M, Klein W, Skrabala F. Coronary anatomy predicts presence or absence of renal artery stenosis: a prospective study in patients undergoing cardiac catheterization for suspected coronary artery disease. *Eur Heart J.* 2002;23:1684-1691.

7. Crowley J, Santos R, Peter R, et al. Progression of renal artery stenosis in patients undergoing cardiac catheterization. *Am Heart J.* 1998;136:913-918.

8. Jean W, Al-Bitar I, Zwicke D, Port S, Schmidt D, Bajwa T. High incidence of renal artery stenosis in patients with coronary artery disease. *Cathet Cardiovasc Diagn.* 1994;32:8-10.

9. Charanjit R, Textor S, Breen J. Incidental renal artery stenosis among a prospective cohort of hypertensive patients undergoing coronary angiography. *Mayo Clin Proc.* 2002;77:309-316.

10. Cheng S, Wu L, Lau H, Ting A, Wong J. Prevalence of significant carotid stenosis in Chinese patients with peripheral and coronary artery disease. *Aust N Z J Surg.* 1999;69:44-47.

11. Reunanen A, Takkunen H, Aromaa A. Prevalence of intermittent claudication and its effect on mortality. *Acta Med Scand.* 1982;211:249-256.

12. Murabito J, D'Agostino R, Silbershatz H, Wilson W. Intermittent Claudication: a risk profile from the Framingham heart study. *Circulation.* 1997;96:44-49.

13. Dieter R, Tomasson J, Gudjonsson T, et al. Lower extremity peripheral arterial disease in hospitalized patients with coronary artery disease. *Vasc Med.* 2003;4:233-236.

14. Aronow W, Ahn C. Prevalence of coexistence of coronary artery disease, peripheral arterial disease and atherothrombotic brain infarction in men and women ≥62 years of age. *Am J Cardiol.* 1994;74:64-65.

15. Newman A, Siscovick D, Manolio T, et al. Ankle-arm index as a marker of atherosclerosis in the Cardiovascular Health Study. *Circulation.* 1993;88:837-845.

16. Norgren L, Hiatt W, Dormandy J, et al. Inter-society consensus for the management of peripheral arterial disease (TASC II). *Eur J Vasc Endovasc Surg.* 2007;33(1 suppl):S1-S75.

17. Louie J, Isaacson J, Zierler R, Bergelin R, Strandness D. Prevalence of carotid and lower extremity arterial disease in patients with renal artery stenosis. *Am J Hypertens.* 1994;7:436-439.

18. Hansen K, Edwards M, Craven T, et al. Prevalence of renovascular disease in the elderly: a population-based study. *J Vasc Surg.* 2002;36:443-451.

19. Zoccali C, Mallamaci F, Finocchiaro P. Atherosclerotic renal artery stenosis: epidemiology, cardiovascular outcomes, and clinical prediction rules. *J Am So Nephrology.* 2002;13:s179-s183.

20. Wilms G, Marchal G, Peene P, Baert A. The angiographic incidence of renal artery stenosis in the arteriosclerotic population. *Eur J Radiol.* 1990;10:195-197.

21. Olin J, Melia M, Young J, Graor R, Risius B. Prevalence of atherosclerotic renal artery stenosis in patients with atherosclerosis elsewhere. *Am J Med.* 1990;88:46N-51N.

22. Metcalfe W, Reid A, Geddes C. Prevalence of angiographic atherosclerotic renal artery disease and its relationship to the anatomical extent of peripheral vascular atherosclerosis. *Nephrol Dial Transplant.* 1999;14:105-108.

23. Valentine R, Clagett G, Miller G, Myers S, Martin J, Chervu A. The coronary risk of unsuspected renal artery stenosis. *J Vasc Surg.* 1993;18:433-439.

24. Wollenweber J, Sheps S, Davis G. Clinical course of atherosclerotic renovascular disease. *Am J Cardiol* 1968;21:60-71.

25. Tarazi R, Hertzer N, Beven E, O'Hara P, Anton G, Krajewski L. Simultaneous aortic reconstruction and renal revascularization: risk factors and late results in eighty-nine patients. *J Vasc Surg.* 1987;5:707-714.

26. Rossi G, Rossi A, Zanin L, et al. Excess prevalence of extracranial carotid artery lesions in renovascular hypertension. *Am J Hypertens.* 1992;5:8-15.

27. Zierler R, Bergelin R, Polissar N, et al. Carotid and lower extremity arterial disease in patients with renal artery atherosclerosis. *Arch Intern Med.* 1998;158:761-767.

28. Missouris C, Papavassiliou M, Khaw K, et al. High prevalence of carotid artery disease in patients with atheromatous renal artery stenosis. *Nephrol Dial Transplant.* 1998;13:945-948.

29. Tollefson D, Ernst C. Natural history of atherosclerotic renal artery stenosis associated with aortic disease. *J Vasc Surg.* 1991;14:327-331.

30. Cunningham C, Reilly L, Rapp J, Schneider P, Stoney R. Chronic visceral ischemia: three decades of progress. *Ann Surg.* 1991;214:276-288.

31. Mikkelsen W. Intestinal angina: its surgical significance. *Surg Gynecol Obstet.* 1957;94:262-267.

32. Hirsch A, Haskal Z, Hertzer N, et al. ACC/AHA guidelines for the management of patients with peripheral arterial disease (lower extremity, renal, mesenteric, and abdominal aortic): executive summary: a collaborative report from the American Association for Vascular Surgery/Society for Vascular Surgery, Society for Vascular Medicine and Biology, Society of Interventional Radiology, and the ACC/AHA Task Force on Practice Guidelines (Writing Committee to Develop Guidelines for the Management of Patients With Peripheral Arterial Disease [Lower Extremity, Renal, Mesenteric, and Abdominal Aortic]). *J Am Coll Cardiol.* 2006;47:1239-1312.

33. Hollier L, Bernatz P, Pairolero P, Payne W, Osmundson P. Surgical management of chronic intestinal ischemia: a reappraisal. *Surgery.* 1981;90:940-946.

34. Mateo R, O'Hara P, Hertzer N, Mascha E, Beven E, Krajewski L. Elective surgical treatment of symptomatic chronic mesenteric occlusive disease early results and late outcomes. *J Vasc Surg.* 1999;29:821-831.

35. Valentine R, Martin J, Myers S, Rossi M, Clagett G. Asymptomatic celiac and superior mesenteric artery stenosis are more prevalent among patients with unsuspected renal artery stenosis. *J Vasc Surg.* 1991;14:195-199.

36. Johnston K, Lindsay T, Walker P, Kalman P. Mesenteric arterial bypass grafts: early and late results and suggested surgical approach for chronic and acute mesenteric ischemia. *Surgery.* 1995;118:1-7.

37. Marcoux R, Larrat E, Taubman A, Wilson J. Screening for peripheral arterial disease. *J Am Pharm Assoc (Wash).* 1996;NS36:370-373.

38. Golomb B, Dang T, Criqui M. Peripheral arterial disease: morbidity and mortality implications. *Circulation* 2006;114:688-699.

39. Kannel W, Skinner JJ, Schwartz M, Shurtleff D. Intermittent claudication. Incidence in the Framingham study. *Circulation.* 1970;41:875-883.

40. Kannel W, McGee D. Update on some epidemiologic features of intermittent claudication: the Framingham Study. *J Am Geriatr Soc.* 1985;33:13-18.

41. Leng G, Lee A, Fowkes F, et al. Incidence, natural history and cardiovascular events in symptomatic and asymptomatic peripheral arterial disease in the general population. *Int J Epidemiol.* 1996;25:1172-1181.

42. Leng G, Fowkes F, Lee A, Dunbar J, Housley E, Ruckley C. Use of ankle brachial pressure index to predict cardiovascular events and death: a cohort study. *BMJ.* 1996;313:1440-1444.

43. Kornitzer M, Dramaix M, Sobolski J, Degre S, De Backer G. Ankle/Arm pressure index in asymptomatic middle-aged males: an independent predictor of ten-year coronary heart disease mortality. *Angiology.* 1995;46:211-219.

44. Criqui M, Langer R, Fronek A, et al. Mortality over a period of 10 years in patients with peripheral arterial disease. *N Engl J Med.* 1992;326:381-386.

45. Eagle K, Rihal C, Foster E, Mickel M, Gersh B. Long-term survival in patients with coronary artery disease: importance of peripheral vascular disease. *J Am Coll Cardiol.* 1994;23:1091-1095.

46. Brand F, Kannel W, Evans J, Larson M, Wolf P. Glucose intolerance, physical signs of peripheral artery disease, and risk of cardiovascular events: the Framingham Study. *Am Heart J* 1998;136:919-927.

47. Murabito J, Evans J, Larson M, Nieto K, Levy D, Wilson P. The ankle-brachial index in the elderly and risk of stroke, coronary disease, and death: the Framingham Study. *Arch Intern Med.* 2003;163:1939-1942.

48. Swartbol P, Thorvinger B, Parsson H, Norgren L. Renal artery stenosis in patients with peripheral vascular disease and its correlation to hypertension: a retrospective study. *Int Angiol.* 1992;11:195-199.

49. Missouris C, Buckenham T, Cappuccio F, MacGregor G. Renal artery stenosis: a common and important problem in patients with peripheral vascular disease. *Am J Med.* 1994;96:10-14.

50. Salmon P, Brown M. Renal artery stenosis and peripheral vascular disease: implications for ACE inhibitor therapy. *Lancet.* 1990;336:321.

51. Choudhri A, Cleland J, Rowlands P, Tran T, McCarty M, al-Kutoubi M. Unsuspected renal artery stenosis in peripheral vascular disease. *Br Med J.* 1990;301:1197-1198.

52. Cina C, Safar H, Maggisano R, Bailey R, Clase C. Prevalence and progression of internal carotid artery stenosis in patients with peripheral arterial occlusive disease. *J Vasc Surg.* 2002;36:75-82.

53. Valentine R, Hagino R, Boyd P, Kakish H, Clagett G. Utility of carotid duplex in young adults with lower extremity atherosclerosis: how aggressive should we be in screening young patients? *Cardiovasc Surg.* 1997;5:408-413.

54. Abbott R, Rodriguez B, Petrovitch H, et al. Ankle-brachial blood pressure in elderly men and the risk of stroke: the Honolulu Heart Program. *J Clin Epidemiol.* 2001;54:971-972.

55. Cabellon S, Moncrief C, Pierre D, Cavanaugh D. Incidence of abdominal aortic aneurysms in patients with atheromatous arterial disease. *Am J Surg.* 1983;146:575-576.

56. Hertzer N, Young J, Kramer J, et al. Routine coronary angiography prior to elective aortic reconstruction: results of selective myocardial revascularization in patients with peripheral vascular disease. *Arch Surg.* 1979;114:1336-1344.

57. Golden M, Whittemore A, Donaldson M, Mannick J. Selective evaluation and management of coronary artery disease in patients undergoing repair of abdominal aortic aneurysms. A 16-year experience. *Ann Surg.* 1990;212:415-423.

58. Starr J, Hertzer N, Mascha E, et al. Influence of gender on cardiac risk and survival in patients with infrarenal aortic aneurysms. *J Vasc Surg.* 1996;23:870-880.

59. Szilagyi D, Elliott J, Smith R. Clinical fate of the patient with asymptomatic abdominal aortic aneurysm and unfit for surgical treatment. *Arch Surg.* 1972;104:600-606.

60. Szilagyi D, Smith R, DeRusso F, Elliott J, Sherrin F. Contribution of abdominal aortic aneurysmectomy to prolongation of life. *Ann Surg.* 1966;164:678-699.

61. Brewster D, Retana A, Waltman A. Angiography in the management of aneurysms of the abdominal aorta. Its value and safety. *N Engl J Med.* 1975;292:822-825.

62. Solberg L, McGarry P, Moossy J, Strong J, Tejada C, Löken A. Severity of atherosclerosis in cerebral arteries, coronary arteries, and aortas. *Ann NY Acad Sci.* 1968;149:956-973.

63. Chambers B, Norris J. Outcome in patients with asymptomatic neck bruits. *N Engl J Med.* 1986;315(14):860-865.

64. Wolf P, Kannel W, Sorlie P, McNamara P. Asymptomatic carotid bruit and risk of stroke: the Framingham study. *JAMA.* 1981;245:1442-1445.

65. Heyman A, Wilkinson W, Heyden S, et al. Risk of stroke in persons with cervical arterial bruits: a population study in Evans County, Georgia. *NEJM.* 1980;302:838-841.

66. Love B, Biller J, Grover-McKay M, Rezai K. Prevalence of coronary artery disease in patients with cerebrovascular disease. *Stroke.* 1991;22(1):126.

67. Hertzer N, Young J, Beven E, et al. Coronary angiography in 506 patients with extracranial cerebrovascular disease. *Arch Intern Med.* 1985;145:849-852.

68. Aronow W, Ahn C, Schoenfeld M, Mercando A, Epstein S. Prognostic significance of silent myocardial ischemia in patients >61 years of age with extracranial internal or common carotid arterial disease with and without previous myocardial infarction. *Am J Cardiol.* 1993;71:115-117.

69. Di Pasquale G, Andreoli A, Pinelli G, et al. Cerebral ischemia and asymptomatic coronary artery disease: a prospective study of 83 patients. *Stroke.* 1986;17:1098-1101.

70. Rokey R, Rolak L, Harati Y, Kutka N, Verani M. Coronary artery disease in patients with cerebrovascular disease: a prospective study. *Ann Neurol.* 1984;16:50-53.

chapter 13

Coronary Artery Disease in Patients with Peripheral Arterial Disease

Pranab Das, MD / Lowell H. Steen, MD / Debabrata Mukherjee, MD

● INTRODUCTION

Peripheral arterial disease (PAD) of the lower extremities affects nearly 8 to 12 million adults in the United States.[1] The age-adjusted prevalence of PAD is approximately 12% and accounts for significant morbidity and health care expenditure among the elderly. This disorder affects men and women equally.[2-5] Symptomatic PAD causes functional impairment and reduced mobility, and asymptomatic PAD may eventually progress to symptomatic PAD. Regardless of symptom status, PAD predicts future cardiovascular events such as myocardial infarction (MI), stroke, and death.

Diagnosis of Lower Extremity PAD

Although history suggestive of classic walking-induced lower extremity pain with resolution at rest and physical examination demonstrating absent or diminished pulses of lower extremities is sufficient to diagnose PAD, only 10% of patients with PAD may present with this classic presentation.[6,7] An ankle–brachial index (ABI), defined as the ratio of ankle to brachial systolic blood pressure, of ≤0.90 is 90% sensitive and 95% specific for the diagnosis of PAD.[8] Severe PAD is defined as ABI ≤ 0.40 and is associated with rest pain or ischemic ulceration.

Risk Factors of Lower Extremity PAD

A constellation of data from several studies[9-13] provides evidence that risk factors for PAD are essentially the same as those for coronary artery disease (CAD) with few exceptions. Therefore, age (>40 years), family history, diabetes, hyperlipidemia, cigarette smoking, and hypertension are the major risk factors for PAD. Cigarette smoking and diabetes are probably the most important of these

risk factors. The most common form of dyslipidemia causing PAD is the combination of elevated triglycerides and low high-density lipoprotein level (HDL)—a pattern most commonly seen among patients with uncontrolled diabetes ("metabolic dyslipidemia"). Female diabetic patients are more prone to develop PAD compared to male diabetic patients, and in women, it manifests as peroneal and tibial PAD. Smoking, on the other hand, causes mostly aortoiliac disease. Women with a history of heavy smoking often develop a distinct hypoplastic aortoiliac syndrome. In addition to these traditional risk factors, several other novel risk factors are found to be associated with increased risk of PAD. Elevated levels of lipoprotein (a), homocysteine, apolipoprotein (apo) A-1, apoB-100, high sensitive C-reactive protein, and fibrinogen predispose patients to PAD.[14] Impaired renal function has also been found to be a risk factor for developing PAD.[15]

Prevalence of Lower Extremity CAD in PAD

As the risk factors for PAD and CAD are very similar, there is a common association of these two disorders[16] (Table 13-1). However, depending on the methods used to diagnose and define CAD, the prevalence of CAD in PAD has been reported from 14% to 90%. When only clinical symptoms of angina and electrocardiograms were used to diagnose CAD among PAD patients, CAD prevalence was found to be from 19% to 47%. CAD prevalence increased to >60% when stress tests were used to diagnose CAD and to >90% when conventional angiograms were used to diagnose CAD.[17] In two separate reports, Hertzer[18] showed that by preoperative coronary angiogram, 36% of patients with abdominal aortic aneurysm and 28% of patients with lower extremity ischemia had severe CAD, 8% had normal

TABLE 13-1. Prevalence of PAD, Claudication, and Cardiovascular Disease*

Authors	No. of Subjects	Age (y)	Sex	Prevalence of PAD	Prevalence of Claudication (%)	Prevalence of Clinical Cardiovascular Disease
Schroll and Munck[69]	666	>60	M	16	6	—
			F	13	1	—
Meijer et al.[4]	7715	>55	M	17	2	48
			F	21	1	33
Fowkes et al.[70]	1592	55–74	Both	18	5	54
Newman et al.[71]	190	>60	Both	27	6	47
Newman et al.[22]	5084	≥65	M	14		56
			F	11	2	40
Zheng et al.[72]	15792	45–64	M	3	1	21
			F	3	1	5

*An ABI value of less than 0.90 was considered diagnostic of PAD in all the studies. Dashes indicate that no data were presented.
Reproduced with permission from Hiatt WR. Medical treatment of peripheral arterial disease and claudication. N Engl J Med. 2001;344:1608-1621.

coronaries, and 32% had mild to moderate CAD.[18,19] Thus, presence of PAD can be a surrogate marker of coexistent CAD (Table 13-1). Identification of these patients is of critical importance as primary and secondary prevention remains the key to minimizing cardiovascular mortality and morbidity among these high-risk patients.[20] In the PAD Awareness, Risk, and Treatment: New Resources for Survival (PARTNERS) program, a total of 6979 patients aged ≥70 years or aged 50 to 69 years and with a history of diabetes or smoking from primary care practice were screened for PAD by ABI. Although PAD was present in nearly 30% of the screened patients and these patients were at a high risk of cardiovascular morbidity and mortality, the patients had less intensive treatment for their concomitant cardiovascular risk factors.[21]

ABI and Cardiovascular Outcomes

The ABI is the ratio of the ankle to brachial systolic blood pressure and a value of <0.90 indicates the presence of significant arterial disease of the lower extremities. ABI can gauge the severity of PAD in symptomatic patients and at the same time can assess the cardiovascular risk in asymptomatic patients (Figure 13-1). The lower the ABI, the worse the cardiovascular outcome[22,23] (Figure 13-2). In a large meta-analysis of nine studies, the sensitivity and specificity of ABI to predict incident CAD were 16.5% and 92.7%, respectively.[24] Even in primary care settings, low ABI has been shown to be associated with premature death and vascular events.[25] Thus, ABI should be a part of an evaluation of any patient with suspected PAD and individuals with low or borderline ABI should be targeted for follow-up and aggressive risk factor modification and secondary prevention.

PAD and Cardiovascular Morbidity

Presence of any degree of PAD (symptomatic or asymptomatic) increases the risk of cardiovascular adverse out-

comes such as new angina, need for coronary artery bypass graft, nonfatal MI, congestive heart failure, and fatal MI or death.[26,27] The more severe the PAD, the more symptomatic the CAD and the worse the outcome of CAD (Figure 13-3). Symptomatic PAD is more likely to be associated with subsequent symptomatic angina (risk ratio 2.3) than is asymptomatic PAD.[17] Patients with PAD, even in the absence of MI, have the same risk of death from cardiovascular causes as do patients with a history of CAD.[16] PAD is thus considered to be CAD equivalent and denotes a heavy atherosclerotic burden. In addition, patients with symptomatic PAD are markedly impaired functionally and may thus limit their physical exercise, triggering weight gain and the associated comorbidities with obesity-related inactivity such as diabetes, hypertension, dyslipidemia, and metabolic syndrome. PAD has also been associated with endothelial dysfunction[28] as manifested by impaired endothelium-dependent vasodilatation and even by paradoxical vasoconstriction. Plasma levels of von Willebrand factors and thrombomodulin are increased in patients with PAD.[28] PAD patients thus have endothelial dysfunction and at the same time a heightened thrombophilic state that can be the trigger for a cardiovascular event.

PAD and Mortality

Patients with PAD, even in the absence of MI or cerebrovascular disease, have similar risk of death from cardiovascular causes as do patients with a history of CAD or cerebrovascular disease (Table 13-2). The all-cause mortality among PAD patients is similar between men and women. In a prospective cohort study of patients with PAD more than 10 years of follow-up, the relative risk of death from all causes among PAD patients was 3.1 (95% CI 1.9–4.9) compared to those with no PAD, 5.9 for all cardiovascular deaths (95% CI 3.0–11.4), and 6.6 (95% CI 2.9–14.9) for death from CAD.[26] The 10-year absolute mortality among patients with large vessel lower extremity arterial diseases

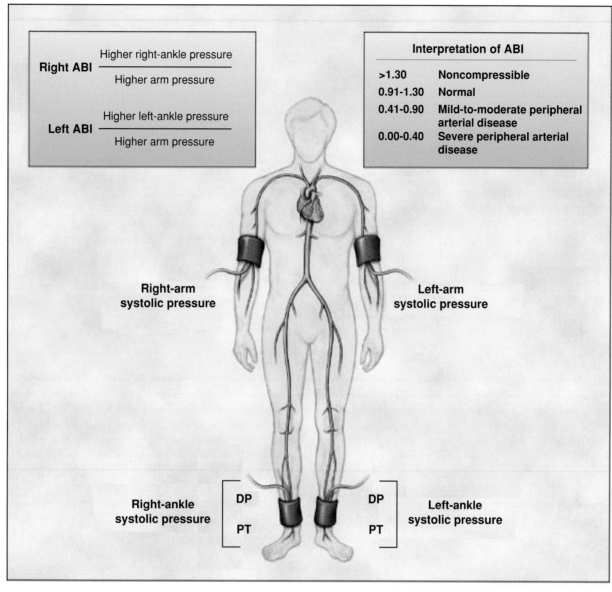

● **FIGURE 13-1.** Interpretation of ABI.

Reproduced with permission from Hiatt WR. Medical treatment of peripheral arterial disease and claudication. N Engl J Med. 2001;344:1610.

was 61.8% for men and 33.3% for women as compared to 16.9% and 11.6% among men and women respectively if they had no PAD.[26] Severe and symptomatic PAD can thus cause up to several-fold increase in cardiovascular mortality compared to patients with no PAD. Patients with severe PAD as manifested by critical limb ischemia have an annual mortality rate of 25%.[29]

Effects of PAD on the Outcomes of ACS Patients

One study reviewed the medical records of patients admitted for ACS and it was found that patients with prior PAD have low rates of prehospital use of ACE inhibitors, beta-blockers, aspirin, and lipid-lowering therapy.[30] Patients with PAD also have higher risk of adverse events and higher comorbidities. But they are again less likely to

receive aggressive treatment for reperfusion therapy, and less likely to undergo interventional procedures and revascularization during hospitalization for ACS. As such, the hospital outcomes of these patients in death, MI, stroke, and cardiogenic shock were also poorer compared to patients with no PAD.[30] In another study of acute coronary syndrome, the presence of extracardiac vascular disease appeared to portend a worse outcome and low likelihood of less aggressive treatment.[31] PAD has also been associated with lower long-term survival while recovering from acute MI.[32]

Outcome of Percutaneous Coronary Intervention Among Patients with PAD

The presence of PAD may lead to higher short- and long-term mortality and lower procedural success among

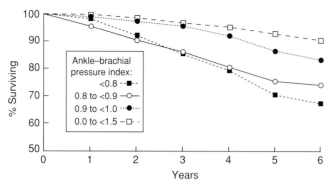

● **FIGURE 13-2.** Relation of cardiovascular events according to the ABI (Kaplan-Meier survival plot for 4268 patients at risk for incident cardiovascular disease, by level of ankle-brachial pressure index).

Reproduced with permission from Newman AB, Shemanski L, Manolio TA, et al. Ankle-arm index as a predictor of cardiovascular disease and mortality in the Cardiovascular Health Study. The Cardiovascular Health Study Group. Arterioscler Thromb Vasc Biol. 1999;19:543.

patients undergoing percutaneous coronary interventions (PCI). In a review of >10 000 patients undergoing PCI, PAD was identified in nearly one-fifth of patients and was associated with lower rates of procedural success, worse procedural, and in-hospital outcomes, and with higher rates of in-hospital and 1-year mortality. PAD was also an independent predictor of increased 1-year mortality.[33,34] In a pooled analysis of eight large randomized PCI trials of nearly 20 000 patients, PAD was present in 8% of patients. The presence of PAD was associated with higher incidences of death and MI as well as increased risk of bleeding.[35] PAD patients undergoing PCI thus remain to be a very high-risk group with higher post-PCI death and MI compared

to non-PAD subjects, and they may benefit from aggressive treatment strategy and closer monitoring.

Effects of PAD on CABG Outcomes

Patients with PAD are also at risk of adverse outcomes after undergoing CABG. Data from the Coronary Artery Surgery Study (CASS)[36] revealed that patients with PAD had a 25% greater likelihood of mortality than patients with no PAD (95% CI 1.15–1.36, $p < 0.001$). In another prospective analysis of 1022 patients[37] undergoing CABG, preoperative ABI were obtained. Among all enrolled patients, 14% had clinical PAD and 25% had subclinical PAD (ABI < 0.85 or incompressible arteries with ABI >1.5). Patients were prospectively followed up for 4.4 years. Besides having higher adverse cardiovascular events among PAD patients, clinical and subclinical PAD were independent predictors of overall and cardiovascular deaths.

Lower Extremity PAD and Preoperative Risk Stratification

As CAD is very highly prevalent among patients with PAD, optimal preoperative risk stratification is imperative in adequate management of these patients during their perioperative period. According to the current American College of Cardiology/American Heart Association guidelines,[38] peripheral vascular surgery is considered a high-risk surgery and patients should have their surgery deferred if they have any of the four major clinical predictors (acute coronary syndrome or Canadian Cardiovascular Class (CCS) III or IV angina, de-compensated heart failure, severe valvular disease, and significant ventricular or supraventricular arrhythmia). On the other hand, patients with any of the five intermediate clinical predictors (CCS I or II angina, previous

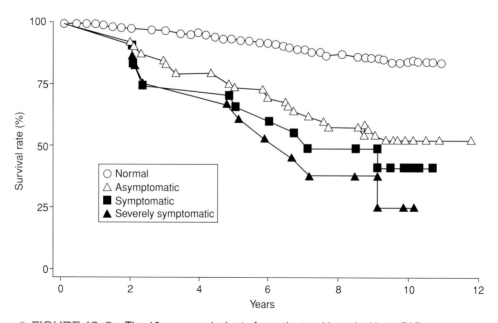

● **FIGURE 13-3.** The 10-year survival rate for patients with and without PAD.

Reproduced with permission from Criqui MH, Langer RD, Fronek A, et al. Mortality over a period of 10 years in patients with peripheral arterial disease. N Engl J Med. 1992;326:385.

TABLE 13-2. Risks of Death from all Causes and from Cardiovascular Causes in Patients with PAD*

Authors	Age (y)	Sex	No. of Subjects	Death from All Causes (% per year) Controls	Patients with PAD	RR (95%) CI	Death from Cardiovascular Disease — All Patients RR (95%) CI	Patients without Cardiovascular Disease at Entry RR (95%) CI
Criqui et al.[26]	38–82	M	256	1.7	6.2	3.3 (1.9–6.0)	5.1 (2.4–10.8)	3.9 (1.5–10.6)
		F	309	1.2	3.3	2.5 (1.2–5.3)	4.8 (1.6–14.7)	5.7 (1.4–23.2)
Vogt et al.[73]	≥65	F	1492	1.1	5.4	3.1 (1.7–5.5)	4.0 (1.3–8.5)	4.5 (1.5–6.7)
Leng et al.[74]	55–74	Both	1592	2.0	3.8 (with claudication)	1.6 (0.9–2.8)	2.7 (1.3–5.3)	—
				2.0	6.1 (without symptoms)	2.4 (1.6–3.7)	2.1 (1.1–3.8)	—
Newman et al.[23]	≥65	Both	5714	4.5	7.8	1.5 (1.2–1.9)	2.0 (1.1–2.8)	2.9 (1.8–4.6)
Newman et al.[75]	≥60	M	669	1.5	5.3	3.0 (2.8–5.3)	—	3.4 (1.3–8.9)
		F	868	1.3	3.8	2.7 (1.6–4.6)	—	3.3 (1.3–8.6)
Kornitzer et al.[76]	40–55	M	2023	0.4	1.0 (without symptoms)	2.8 (1.4–5.5)	—	4.2 (1.7–10.5)

RR, relative risk; CI, confidence interval.
* Dashes indicate that no data were presented.
Reproduced with permission from Hiatt WR. Medical treatment of peripheral arterial disease and claudication. N Engl J Med. 2001;344:1608-1621.

MI, compensated heart failure, renal insufficiency, and diabetes mellitus) or limited functional capacity should have perioperative noninvasive stress testing in addition to adequate perioperative beta blockade during this time. Guidelines recommend preoperative coronary angiography and revascularization preceding surgery for patients undergoing peripheral vascular surgery if noninvasive stress tests show high-risk results, unstable angina or medically refractory angina, or inconclusive noninvasive test results. These recommendations were adopted in the guidelines based mostly on consensus expert opinions and observational studies.

In their landmark Coronary Artery Revascularization before elective major vascular surgery (CARP) trial, McFalls et al.[39] randomly assigned a total of 510 patients undergoing a major vascular surgery to either preoperative coronary revascularization (41% surgical and 59% percutaneous) or no revascularization. The primary end point was long-term mortality. Only patients with stenosis of ≥70% in one or more vessel and amenable to revascularization were included in the study. Patients with left main stenosis of ≥50%, severe aortic stenosis, or low left ventricular ejection fraction of ≤20% were excluded from the study. At 2.7 years after randomization, mortality was 22% in the revascularization group and 23% in the no-revascularization group ($p = 0.92$). Within 30 days after the vascular surgery, postoperative MI occurred in 12% of revascularization group and 14% in the no-revascularization group ($p = 0.37$) (Figure 13-4). Thus, this study has shown that except for patients with significant left main disease, severe aortic stenosis, and severe left ventricular dysfunction, preoperative revascularization does not improve long-term mortality among high-risk surgical patients.

TREATMENT OF CAD AMONG PATIENTS WITH PAD

Reducing the Burden of Cardiovascular Events in PAD

Primary and secondary prevention of cardiovascular events in PAD are mostly based on the data extrapolated from observation studies of PAD patients and randomized trials in patients with CAD.

Smoking Cessation. Smoking remains to be the single most important risk factor of PAD and the survival benefit from cessation of smoking is unequivocal.[40,41] The association of smoking in PAD is twice as strong as that with CAD. In addition to accelerating the progression of PAD, smoking also enhances the progression of coronary atherosclerosis. Smoking cessation should be recommended to every patient with PAD as it will improve claudication symptoms, decrease the risk of amputation, and reduce the risk of coronary events.

Exercise and Weight Reduction. Weight reduction and regular exercise affords double protection against PAD and CAD as it improves the symptoms of claudication and also improves general cardiovascular health.[42,43] In two recent prospective, longitudinal studies of patients with PAD with several months to 7 years of follow-up,[44,45] higher physical activity resulted in a significant reduction in mortality and cardiovascular events compared to PAD patients with the lowest physical activity when adjusted for all confounders.

Treatment of Diabetes. Each 1% increase in glycosylated hemoglobin is associated with a 28% increased risk of

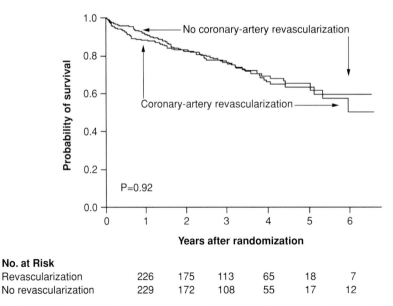

● FIGURE 13-4. Preoperative revascularization strategy before major vascular surgery and long-term outcome.

Reproduced with permission from McFalls EO, Ward HB, Moritz TE, et al. Coronary-artery revascularization before elective vascular surgery. N Engl J Med. 2004;351:2801.

incident PAD and a 28% increased risk of death, independent of other risk factors.[46,47] Although, data from randomized trials of intensive glucose control[46–48] have shown reduction in microvascular complications, macrovascular complications such as death, MI, stroke, or amputations were not significantly affected. Thus, treatment of PAD in diabetes should be based on a multipronged approach and should involve BP reduction <130/80, LDL-c <100, triglycerides <150, HDL-c >40, and glycosylated hemoglobin <7.[49]

Treatment of Hyperlipidemia. Lipid lowering with statins in patients with CAD is associated with reduction in intermittent claudication and also in major cardiovascular events.[50] The benefits of statins in improving overall survival among PAD patients are more exaggerated among those with elevated high sensitive C-reactive protein levels.[51] Current guidelines recommend a goal low-density lipoprotein of <100 and preferably <70 in patients with PAD.[52] Use of statins preoperatively reduces the risk of cardiac events such as death, MI, ischemia, congestive heart failure, and ventricular tachyarrhythmias (9.9% with statin use versus 16.5% without statin use, $p = 0.001$) during the index hospitalization among patients undergoing noncardiac vascular surgery (carotid, aortic, and lower extremity surgeries).[53]

Treatment of Hypertension

Angiotensin-converting enzyme inhibitors (ACEI) improve outcomes in patients with PAD as seen in the HOPE trial (Figure 13-5), and this benefit of reduced cardiovascular events is in addition to that of blood pressure lowering.[54] Patients with PAD and diabetes also benefit from intensive BP lowering as evidenced by reduced cardiovascular events.[55,56] Beta-blockers, contrary to the popular myth, can offer cardioprotective effects to patients with PAD and can improve long-term survival of these patients. In a prospective study of 2420 patients with PAD more than 8-year follow-up, statins (hazard ratio 0.46, 95% CI 0.36–0.58), beta-blockers (hazard ratio 0.68, 95% CI 0.58–0.80), aspirins (HR 0.71, 95% CI 0.61–0.84), and ACEI (HR 0.80, 95% CI 0.69–0.94) were associated with reduction in long-term mortality.[57]

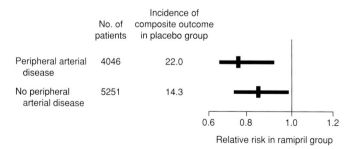

	No. of patients	Incidence of composite outcome in placebo group	
Peripheral arterial disease	4046	22.0	
No peripheral arterial disease	5251	14.3	

0.6   0.8   1.0   1.2
Relative risk in ramipril group

● **FIGURE 13-5.** Role of angiotensin converting enzyme inhibitors (ramipril) among patients with PAD in the HOPE trial.

Reproduced with permission from Hiatt WR. Medical treatment of peripheral arterial disease and claudication. N Engl J Med. 2001;344:1614.

Antiplatelet Therapy in PAD

Aspirin. Aspirin is by far the most common and cheapest antiplatelet agent proven to be effective in secondary prevention of stroke and MI. In the Antithrombotic Trialists' Collaborative meta-analysis,[58] aspirin use was associated with a 25% relative risk reduction in cardiovascular events among patients with atherosclerosis. In the Antiplatelet Trialists' Collaborative study,[59] aspirin has shown the similar effects of 34% relative risk reduction in cardiovascular events among atherosclerotic patients. Aspirin in doses of 75 to 160 mg daily is considered a class I therapy by the American College of Chest Physicians (ACCP)[60] in patients with PAD and concomitant coronary or cerebral arterial disease. Role of aspirin in isolated PAD without concomitant CAD or cerebrovascular disease remains less well studied. The ACCP also recommends aspirin as a class I therapy among patients undergoing endovascular therapy for PAD. It should also be used postoperatively following infrainguinal bypass surgery because it maintains graft potency in these patients.

Picotamide. Picotamide, a platelet thromboxane inhibitor, has similar antiplatelet effects to those of aspirin. In a large randomized trial of 1209 diabetic PAD patients,[61,62] picotamide showed a significant reduction in all-cause mortality compared to aspirin. Use of picotamide in PAD is awaiting further clinical evaluation.

Ticlopidine. Ticlopidine is a thienopyridine that blocks ADP receptors on platelets. Ticlopidine has been shown to improve claudication symptoms, walking distance, and ABI.[61,62] Its clinical use is limited because of the side effects such as neutropenia and thrombotic thrombocytopenic purpura (TTP). Incidence of TTP is 0.02% in ticlopidine-treated patients following coronary stenting while it occurs in 0.0004% in the general population, with a mortality rate exceeding 20%.[63]

Clopidogrel. Clopidogrel is another thienopyridine that acts on ADP receptors to block ADP-mediated platelet aggregation. It has minimal risk factors of TTP reported as an incidence of 1 case per 15 000 clopidogrel-treated patients.[64] In the Clopidogrel versus Aspirin in Patients at Risk of Ischemic Events (CAPRIE) trial,[65] 19 185 patients with atherosclerosis were randomized to aspirin 325 mg daily or clopidogrel 75 mg daily. Clopidogrel showed a significant 8.7% relative risk reduction in the composite of MI, ischemic stroke, and vascular death compared to aspirin (Figure 13-6). This benefit was even more profound with 23.8 % risk reduction in death, MI, and stroke among PAD patients. Another large, randomized trial of clopidogrel with aspirin versus clopidogrel alone was conducted with 7599 patients with ischemic stroke or transient ischemic attack within 3 months and all these patients had a concomitant history of coronary or PAD. The primary end point was a composite of ischemic stroke, MI, vascular death, or rehospitalization for acute

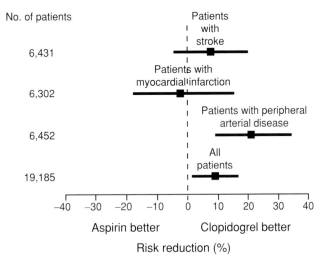

No. of patients

● FIGURE 13-6. Effects of clopidogrel in the reduction of cardiovascular events among patients with PAD.

Reproduced with permission from CAPRIE Steering Committee. A randomised, blinded, trial of clopidogrel versus aspirin in patients at risk of ischaemic events (CAPRIE). Lancet. 1996;348:1329-1339.

ischemia (including rehospitalization for transient ischemic attack, angina pectoris, or worsening of PAD). Although there was a nonsignificant 6% relative risk reduction in the vascular events favoring the combination, there was an associated increase in major bleeding with the combination therapy.[66] As in CAPRIE, the reduction in vascular events among the patients with PAD was markedly pronounced (19.1% with dual aspirin plus clopidogrel therapy versus 24% with clopidogrel alone). As these are reports of the subgroup analysis and the trial was not powered to address this specific question, the exact role of dual antiplatelet therapy with aspirin and clopidogrel in the treatment of PAD still remains controversial. In the recently published Clopidogrel and Aspirin versus Aspirin Alone for the Prevention of Atherothrombotic Events trial (CHARISMA),[67] dual antiplatelet therapy showed no benefit when compared with monotherpy of aspirin alone in reducing the events of MI, stroke, and overall cardiovascular deaths among asymptomatic patients with atherothrom-

bosis such as those with multiple risk factors. In contrast, a subgroup study of symptomatic, atherothrombotic patients showed that the combination of clopidogrel with aspirin caused a 12% relative risk reduction in cardiovascular death, MI, and stroke (6.9% with combination versus 7.9% with aspirin alone, relative risk 0.88; 95% CI 0.77–0.998; $p = 0.046$).

Warfarin. Adding warfarin to aspirin therapy in patients with PAD was evaluated in the Warfarin Antiplatelet Vascular Evaluation (WAVE) study, presented at the World Congress of Cardiology 2006,[68] and was found to yield no additive benefit. Approximately 2000 PAD patients were randomized to aspirin alone or aspirin plus warfarin with a goal INR of 1.8–3.5. The composite of cardiovascular death, MI, stroke, and severe ischemia in the coronary or peripheral arteries did not differ between the two groups. But the combination significantly increased the risk of moderate and life-threatening bleeds, including a 15-fold risk of hemorrhagic stroke among those taking both drugs compared with those receiving aspirin alone (HR 15.2; $p < 0.001$) (Table 13-3).

Conclusion

PAD is a marker of higher atherosclerotic burden as these patients are at markedly increased risk of cardiovascular morbidity and mortality. Early diagnosis and aggressive treatment of the accompanying risk factors are vital to reduce cardiovascular morbidity and mortality in PAD patients. Besides undertaking an elaborate history and thorough physical examination, evaluation of the patients at risk of developing PAD by measuring ABIs will facilitate early identification of this condition and guide appropriate therapy. A significant proportion of patients with PAD have concomitant CAD and a thorough history to assess for angina and comprehensive cardiac evaluation is indicated.

● ACKNOWLEDGMENT

We thank Ms. Donna Gilbreath for her excellent editorial support.

TABLE 13-3. Results of Warfarin Plus Aspirin versus Aspirin Alone in the Treatment of Peripheral Arterial Disease

End Point	Combination Group, n = 1080 (%)	Aspirin Only, n = 1081 (%)	Hazard Ratio	p
First primary end point*	12.2	13.3	0.92	0.49
Second primary end point[†]	15.9	17.4	0.91	0.38
Life-threatening bleeding	4	1.2	3.41	<0.001
Moderate bleeding	2.9	1.0	2.82	0.0018

*Composite of cardiovascular death, myocardial infarction, and stroke.
[†]Composite of cardiovascular death, myocardial infarction, stroke, and severe ischemia of limb or coronaries.

Reproduced with permission from theheart.org (Anand SS. Warfarin Antiplatelet Vascular Evaluation (WAVE) study, presented at the World Congress of Cardiology; September 5, 2006; Barcelona, Spain.)

REFERENCES

1. American Heart Association. PAD quick facts. Diseases and conditions. http://www.americanheart.org. Accessed June 26, 2008.

2. Criqui MH, Fronek A, Klauber MR, Barrett-Connor E, Gabriel S. The sensitivity, specificity, and predictive value of traditional clinical evaluation of peripheral arterial disease: results from noninvasive testing in a defined population. *Circulation.* 1985;71:516-522.

3. Criqui MH, Fronek A, Barrett-Connor E, Klauber MR, Gabriel S, Goodman D. The prevalence of peripheral arterial disease in a defined population. *Circulation.* 1985;71:510-515.

4. Meijer WT, Hoes AW, Rutgers D, Bots ML, Hofman A, Grobbee DE. Peripheral arterial disease in the elderly: the Rotterdam Study. *Arterioscler Thromb Vasc Biol.* 1998;18:185-192.

5. Hiatt WR, Hoag S, Hamman RF. Effect of diagnostic criteria on the prevalence of peripheral arterial disease. The San Luis Valley Diabetes Study. *Circulation.* 1995;91:1472-1479.

6. Hirsch AT, Criqui MH, Treat-Jacobson D, et al. Peripheral arterial disease detection, awareness, and treatment in primary care. *JAMA.* 2001;286:1317-1324.

7. Dieter RS, Biring T, Tomasson J, et al. Classic intermittent claudication is an uncommon manifestation of lower extremity peripheral arterial disease in hospitalized patients with coronary artery disease. *Angiology.* 2004;55:625-628.

8. Greenland P, Abrams J, Aurigemma GP, et al. Prevention Conference V: beyond secondary prevention: identifying the high-risk patient for primary prevention: noninvasive tests of atherosclerotic burden: writing Group III. *Circulation.* 2000;101:E16-E22.

9. Dieter RS, Tomasson J, Gudjonsson T, et al. Lower extremity peripheral arterial disease in hospitalized patients with coronary artery disease. *Vasc Med.* 2003;8:233-236.

10. Kannel WB, McGee D, Gordon T. A general cardiovascular risk profile: the Framingham Study. *Am J Cardiol.* 1976;38:46-51.

11. The ARIC investigators. The Atherosclerosis Risk in Communities (ARIC) Study: design and objectives. *Am J Epidemiol.* 1989;129:687-702.

12. Kagan A, Gordon T, Rhoads GG, et al. Some factors related to coronary heart disease incidence in Honolulu Japanese men: the Honolulu Heart Study. *Int J Epidemiol.* 1975;4:271-279.

13. Lee ET, Welty TK, Fabsitz R, et al. The Strong Heart Study: a study of cardiovascular disease in American Indians: design and methods. *Am J Epidemiol.* 1990;132:1141-1155.

14. Ridker PM, Stampfer MJ, Rifai N. Novel risk factors for systemic atherosclerosis: a comparison of C-reactive protein, fibrinogen, homocysteine, lipoprotein(a), and standard cholesterol screening as predictors of peripheral arterial disease. *JAMA.* 2001;285:2481-2485.

15. Selvin E, Erlinger TP. MPH prevalence of and risk factors for peripheral arterial disease in the United States. Results from the national health and nutrition examination survey, 1999–2000. *Circulation.* 2004;110:738-743.

16. Hiatt WR. Medical treatment of peripheral arterial disease and claudication. *N Engl J Med.* 2001;344:1608-1621.

17. Golomb BA, Dang TT, Criqui MH. Peripheral arterial disease: morbidity and mortality implications. *Circulation.* 2006; 114:688-699.

18. Hertzer NR. Clinical experience with preoperative coronary angiography. *J Vasc Surg.* 1985;2:510-514.

19. Hertzer NR, Beven EG, Young JR, et al. Coronary artery disease in peripheral vascular patients. A classification of 1000 coronary angiograms and results of surgical management. *Ann Surg.* 1984;199:223-233.

20. Dieter RS, Chu WW, Pacanowski JP, McBride PE, Tanke TE. The significance of lower extremity peripheral arterial disease. *Clin Cardiol.* 25:3-10.

21. Hirsch AT, Criqui MH, Treat-Jacobson D. Peripheral arterial disease detection, awareness, and treatment in primary care. *JAMA.* 2001;286:1317-1324.

22. Newman AB, Siscovick DS, Manolio TA, et al. Ankle-arm index as a marker of atherosclerosis in the Cardiovascular Health Study. Cardiovascular Heart Study (CHS) Collaborative Research Group. *Circulation.* 1993;88:837-845.

23. Newman AB, Shemanski L, Manolio TA, et al. Ankle-arm index as a predictor of cardiovascular disease and mortality in the Cardiovascular Health Study for The Cardiovascular Health Study Group. *Arterioscler Thromb Vasc Biol.* 1999;19: 538-545.

24. Doobay AV, Anand SS. Sensitivity and specificity of the ankle-brachial index to predict future cardiovascular outcomes: a systematic review. *Arterioscler Thromb Vasc Biol.* 2005;25: 1463-1469.

25. Diehm C, Lange S, Darius H, et al. Association of low ankle brachial index with high mortality in primary care. *Eur Heart J.* 2006;27:1743-1749.

26. Criqui MH, Langer RD, Fronek A, et al. Mortality over a period of 10 years in patients with peripheral arterial disease. *N Engl J Med.* 1992;326:381-386.

27. Hirsch AT, Haskal ZJ, Hertzer NR, et al. ACC/AHA 2005 guidelines for the management of patients with peripheral arterial disease (lower extremity, renal, mesenteric, and abdominal aortic): executive summary a collaborative report from the American Association for Vascular Surgery/Society for Vascular Surgery, Society for Cardiovascular Angiography and Interventions, Society for Vascular Medicine and Biology, Society of Interventional Radiology, and the ACC/AHA Task Force on Practice Guidelines (Writing Committee to Develop Guidelines for the Management of Patients With Peripheral Arterial Disease) endorsed by the American Association of Cardiovascular and Pulmonary Rehabilitation; National Heart, Lung, and Blood Institute; Society for Vascular Nursing; TransAtlantic Inter-Society Consensus; and Vascular Disease Foundation. *J Am Coll Cardiol.* 2006;47:1239-1312.

28. Silvestro A, Scopacasa F, Ruocco A, et al. Inflammatory status and endothelial function in asymptomatic and symptomatic peripheral arterial disease. *Vasc Med.* 2003;8:225-232.

29. Dormandy J, Heeck L, Vig S. The fate of patients with critical leg ischemia. *Semin Vasc Surg.* 1999;12:142-147.

30. Froehlich JB, Mukherjee D, Avezum A, et al. Association of peripheral artery disease with treatment and outcomes in acute coronary syndromes. The Global Registry of Acute

Coronary Events (GRACE). *Am Heart J.* 2006;151:1123-1128.

31. Cotter G, Cannon CP, McCabe CH, et al. Prior peripheral arterial disease and cerebrovascular disease are independent predictors of adverse outcome in patients with acute coronary syndromes: are we doing enough? Results from the Orbofiban in Patients with Unstable Coronary Syndromes-Thrombolysis In Myocardial Infarction (OPUS-TIMI) 16 study. *Am Heart J.* 2003;145:622-627.

32. Pardaens J, Lesaffre E, Willems JL, De Geest H. Multivariate survival analysis for the assessment of prognostic factors and risk categories after recovery from acute myocardial infarction: the Belgian situation. *Am J Epidemiol.* 1985;122:805-819.

33. Nikolsky E, Mehran R, Mintz GS, et al. Impact of symptomatic peripheral arterial disease on 1-year mortality in patients undergoing percutaneous coronary interventions. *J Endovasc Ther.* 2004;11:60-70.

34. Nikolsky E, Mehran R, Dangas G, et al. Prognostic significance of cerebrovascular and peripheral arterial disease in patients having percutaneous coronary interventions. *Am J Cardiol.* 2004;93:1536-1539.

35. Saw J, Bhatt DL, Moliterno DJ, et al. The influence of peripheral arterial disease on outcomes: a pooled analysis of mortality in eight large randomized percutaneous coronary intervention trials. *J Am Coll Cardiol.* 2006;48:1567-1572.

36. Eagle KA, Rihal CS, Foster ED, Mickel MC, Gersh BJ. Long-term survival in patients with coronary artery disease: importance of peripheral vascular disease. The Coronary Artery Surgery Study (CASS) Investigators. *J Am Coll Cardiol.* 1994;23:1091-1095.

37. Aboyans V, Lacroix P, Postil A, et al. Subclinical peripheral arterial disease and incompressible ankle arteries are both long-term prognostic factors in patients undergoing coronary artery bypass grafting. *J Am Coll Cardiol.* 2005;46:815-820.

38. Eagle KA, Berger PB, Calkins H, et al. ACC/AHA guideline update for perioperative cardiovascular evaluation for non-cardiac surgery: executive summary: a report of the American College of Cardiology/American Heart Association Task Force on Practice Guidelines (Committee to update the 1996 Guidelines on Perioperative Cardiovascular Evaluation for Noncardiac Surgery). *J Am Coll Cardiol.* 2002;39:542-553.

39. McFalls EO, Ward HB, Moritz TE, et al. Coronary-artery revascularization before elective vascular surgery. *N Engl J Med.* 2004;351:2795-2804.

40. Fowkes FG, Housley E, Riemersa RA, et al. Smoking, lipids, glucose intolerance, and blood pressure as risk factors for peripheral atherosclerosis compared with ischemic heart disease in the Edinburgh Artery Study. *Am J Epidemiol.* 1992;135;331-340.

41. Hobbs SD, Bradbury AW. Smoking cessation strategies in patients with peripheral arterial disease; an evidence-based approach. *Eur J Vasc Endovasc Surg.* 2003;26:341-347.

42. Fowler B, Jamrozik K, Norman P, Allen Y, Wilkinson E. Improving maximum walking distance in early peripheral arterial disease: randomized controlled trial. *Aust J Physiother.* 2002;48:269-275.

43. Garg PK, Tian Lu, Criqui MH, et al. Physical activity during daily life and mortality in patients with peripheral arterial disease. *Circulation* 2006;114:242-248.

44. Hooi JD, Kester AD, Stoffers HE, Overdijk MM, van Ree JW, Knottnerus JA. Incidence of and risk factors for asymptomatic peripheral arterial occlusive disease: a longitudinal study. *Am J Epidemiol.* 2001;153:666-672.

45. Hooi JD, Kester AD, Stoffers HE, Rinkens PE, Knottnerus JA, van Ree JW. Asymptomatic peripheral arterial occlusive disease predicted cardiovascular morbidity and mortality in a 7-year follow-up study. *J Clin Epidemiol.* 2004;57:294-300.

46. UK Prospective Diabetes Study (UKPDS) Group. Intensive blood glucose control with metformin on complications in overweight patients with type 2 Diabetes. *Lancet.* 1998;352:854-865.

47. Diabetes Control and Complications Trial (DCCT) Research Group. The effect of intensive treatment of diabetes on the development and progression of long-term complications in insulin-dependent diabetes mellitus. *N Engl J Med.* 1993;329:977-986.

48. UK Prospective Diabetes Study (UKPDS) Group. Intensive blood-glucose control with sulphonylurea or insulin compared with conventional treatment and risk of complications in patients with type 2 diabetes (UKPDS 33). *Lancet.* 1998;352:837-853.

49. Hankey GJ, Norman PE, Eikelboom JW. Medical treatment of peripheral arterial disease. *JAMA.* 2006;295:547-553.

50. Mohler PS, Hiatt W, Creager M, et al. MRC/BHF Heart Protection study of cholesterol lowering with simvastatin in 20,536 high-risk individuals: a randomized placebo-controlled trial. *Lancet.* 2002;360;7-22.

51. Schillinger M, Exner M, Mlekusch W, et al. Statin therapy improves cardiovascular outcome of patients with peripheral artery disease. *Eur Heart J.* 2004;25:742-748.

52. Grundy SM, Cleeman JI, Bairey-Merz CN, et al. Implications of recent clinical trials for the national cholesterol education program adult treatment panel III guidelines. *Circulation.* 2004;110:227-239.

53. O'Neil-Callahan K, Katsimaglis G, Tepper MR, et al. Statins decrease perioperative cardiac complications in patients undergoing noncardiac vascular surgery: the Statins for Risk Reduction in Surgery (StaRRS) study. *J Am Coll Cardiol.* 2005;45:336-342.

54. Yusuf S, Sleight P, Pogue J, Bosch J, Davies R, Dagenais G. Effects of an angiotensin-converting-enzyme inhibitor, ramipril, on cardiovascular events in high-risk patients. The Heart Outcomes Prevention Evaluation Study Investigators. *N Engl J Med.* 2000;342:145-153.

55. Ostergren J, Sleight P, Dagenais G, et al., HOPE Study Investigators. Impact of ramipril in patients with evidence of clinical or subclinical peripheral arterial disease. *Eur Heart J.* 2004;25:17-24.

56. Mehler PS, Coll JR, Estacio R, Esler A, Schrier RW, Hiatt WR. Intensive pressure control reduces the risk of cardiovascular events in patients with peripheral arterial disease and type 2 diabetes. *Circulation.* 2003;107:753-756.

57. Feringa HH, van Waning VH, Bax JJ, et al. Cardioprotective medication is associated with improved survival in patients with peripheral arterial disease. *J Am Coll Cardiol.* 2006;47:1182-1187.

58. Antithrombotic Trialists' Collaboration. Collaborative meta-analysis of randomised trials of antiplatelet therapy for

prevention of death, myocardial infarction, and stroke in high risk patients. *BMJ.* 2002;324:71-86.

59. Collaborative overview of randomised trials of antiplatelet therapy-III: Reduction in venous thrombosis and pulmonary embolism by antiplatelet prophylaxis among surgical and medical patients. Antiplatelet Trialists' Collaboration. *BMJ.* 1994;308:235-246.

60. Clagett GP, Sobel M, Jackson MR, Lip GY, Tangelder M, Verhaeghe R. Antithrombotic therapy in peripheral arterial occlusive disease: the Seventh ACCP Conference on Antithrombotic and Thrombolytic Therapy. *Chest.* 2004;126 (suppl):609S-626S.

61. Hiatt WR, Krantz MJ. Masterclass series in peripheral arterial disease. Antiplatelet therapy for peripheral arterial disease and claudication. *Vasc Med.* 2006;11:55-60.

62. Hiatt WR. Preventing atherothrombotic events in peripheral arterial disease: the use of antiplatelet therapy. *J Intern Med.* 2002;251:193-206.

63. Steinhubl SR, Tan WA, Foody JM, Topol EJ. Incidence and clinical course of thrombotic thrombocytopenic purpura due to ticlopidine following coronary stenting. *JAMA.* 1999;281:806-810.

64. Bennett CL, Connors JM, Moake JL. Clopidogrel and thrombotic thrombocytopenic purpura. *N Engl J Med.* 2000;343:1193-1194.

65. CAPRIE Steering Committee. A randomised, blinded, trial of clopidogrel versus aspirin in patients at risk of ischaemic events (CAPRIE). *Lancet.* 1996;348:1329-1339.

66. Diener HC, Bogousslavsky J, Brass LM, et al. Aspirin and clopidogrel compared with clopidogrel alone after recent ischaemic stroke or transient ischaemic attack in high-risk patients (MATCH): randomised, double-blind, placebo-controlled trial. *Lancet.* 2004;364:331-337.

67. Bhatt DL, Fox KAA, Hacke W, et al. Clopidogrel and aspirin versus aspirin alone for the prevention of atherothrombotic events. *N Engl J Med.* 2006;354:1706-1717.

68. Anand SS. Warfarin Antiplatelet Vascular Evaluation (WAVE) study. Paper presented at: the World Congress of Cardiology; September 5, 2006; Barcelona, Spain.

69. Schroll M, Munck O. Estimation of peripheral arteriosclerotic disease by ankle blood pressure measurements in a population study of 60-year-old men and women. *J Chronic Dis.* 1981;34:261-269.

70. Fowkes FGR, Housley E, Cawood EHH, Macintyre CCA, Ruckley CV, Prescott RJ. Edinburgh Artery Study: prevalence of asymptomatic and symptomatic peripheral arterial disease in the general population. *Int J Epidemiol.* 1991;20:384-392.

71. Newman AB, Sutton-Tyrrell K, Rutan GH, Locher J, Kuller LH. Lower extremity arterial disease in elderly subjects with systolic hypertension. *J Clin Epidemiol.* 1991;44:15-20.

72. Zheng ZJ, Sharrett AR, Chambless LE, et al. Associations of ankle-brachial index with clinical coronary heart disease, stroke and preclinical carotid and popliteal atherosclerosis: the Atherosclerosis Risk in Communities (ARIC) Study. *Atherosclerosis.* 1997;131:115-125.

73. Vogt MT, Cauley JA, Newman AB, Kuller LH, Hulley SB. Decreased ankle/arm blood pressure index and mortality in elderly women. *JAMA.* 1993;270:465-469.

74. Leng GC, Lee AJ, Fowkes FG, et al. Incidence, natural history and cardiovascular events in symptomatic and asymptomatic peripheral arterial disease in the general population. *Int J Epidemiol.* 1996;25:1172-1181.

75. Newman AB, Tyrrell KS, Kuller LH. Mortality over four years in SHEP participants with a low ankle-arm index. *J Am Geriatr Soc.* 1997;45:1472-1478.

76. Kornitzer M, Dramaix M, Sobolski J, Degre S, De Backer G. Ankle/arm pressure index in asymptomatic middle-aged males: an independent predictor of ten-year coronary heart disease mortality. *Angiology.* 1995;46:211-219.

chapter 14

Vasculitis

Eamonn S. Molloy, MD, MS / José Hernández-Rodríguez, MD, PhD / Gary S. Hoffman, MD, MS

● INTRODUCTION

The vasculitides are a heterogeneous group of systemic inflammatory disorders characterized by inflammation of blood vessels.[1] Vascular inflammation may cause vessel narrowing or occlusion leading to tissue ischemia or infarction, or may result in vessel rupture with subsequent hemorrhage. These effects underlie the significant morbidity and mortality associated with the vasculitides.

The various forms of vasculitis differ in regard to the size, type, and distribution of involved vessels. Vessel size alone is inadequate to distinguish between the vasculitides. Consequently, nomenclature and classification schemes also rely on the nature of the inflammatory lesion (e.g., granulomatous, leukocytoclastic, eosinophilic) and the organ systems that are most frequently affected (e.g., ear, nose, sinus, lung, kidney).[1] Inflammatory injury in these disorders may also occur in the absence of vasculitis.

Diagnostic Approach to Vasculitis

Even when a diagnosis of vasculitis has been clearly established on clinical and pathologic grounds, it must be determined whether the vasculitis is caused by a primary (idiopathic) vasculitic disorder or a secondary form of vasculitis. Secondary forms of vasculitis for which the etiology is known include: vasculities complicating a wide variety of viral, bacterial, mycobacterial, fungal, and other infectious agents; vasculitis caused by drug or toxin exposure; malignancies (paraneoplastic, embolic, invasive); and embolic (cholesterol) debris. Other secondary forms of vasculitis for which the etiology may lack details of factors such as vasculitis complicating other rheumatic disorders such as systemic lupus erythematosus (SLE), rheumatoid arthritis (RA), Sjogren's syndrome, and Behçet's disease (BD) that are secondary idiopathic forms of vasculitis.

The diagnosis of vasculitis stands challenging for a number of reasons. While vasculitis must be considered in the differential diagnosis of any patient with an unexplained multisystem illness or fever of unknown origin, most of the individual forms of vasculitis are uncommon. Early diagnosis of primary vasculitis is critical to ensure that when indicated, prompt and effective immunosuppressive treatment is instituted to minimize the significant morbidity and mortality associated with these disorders. In the diagnostic process, it is also essential to consider secondary forms of vasculitis and diseases that mimic vasculitis such as infectious (e.g., infective endocarditis), neoplastic and paraneoplastic, iatrogenic, genetic (e.g., Ehler-Danlos syndrome type IV, Marfan's syndrome), atheroembolic, vasospastic (e.g., caused by cocaine, amphetamine, and their derivatives), and other vascular disorders. Immunosuppressive therapy may have adverse and potentially fatal consequences in these disorders.

The diagnostic exercise combines information of several types: clinical phenotype, laboratory data, imaging abnormalities, and histopathologic characteristics. While histopathologic proof is often desirable, it may not be feasible as in the case of large vessel vasculitis (e.g., Takayasu's arteritis [TAK]), coronary vasculitis (e.g., Kawasaki's disease [KD]), or ischemic colitis in the absence of surgical indications (e.g., BD, polyarteritis nodosa [PAN], or vasculitis complicating inflammatory bowel disease).

When considering vasculitis in general, patients may present with impressive but nonspecific symptoms such as fatigue, weakness, malaise, fevers, sweats, anorexia, weight loss, arthralgias, and myalgias. More specific, although not diagnostic, features include palpable purpura, mononeuritis multiplex, and the pulmonary–renal syndrome, which raise suspicion of small–medium vessel vasculitides, and the presence of arterial tenderness (e.g., carotidynia) or asymmetry of pulses and blood pressure, which is suggestive of large vessel vasculitis. A thorough review of systems may reveal subtle but important symptoms that the patient may have overlooked. A history of drug or toxin exposure, prior illness (e.g., viral infection such as hepatitis, connective tissue disorder, remote malignancy), and family history (e.g., premature sudden death especially from vascular rupture) should also be sought. A careful physical examination is essential to assess the severity and extent of organ involvement and to help rule out other diseases. Urinalysis should be performed on all patients with evidence of a systemic inflammatory disorder, followed by careful urine microscopic examination if haematuria and/or proteinuria is detected; the presence of dysmorphic red blood cells and red blood cell casts in the urine is a sensitive indicator of glomerulonephritis and may be apparent before the onset of renal failure.

No currently available laboratory test is diagnostic for any form of vasculitis; however, some tests help to increase the degree of confidence in the presumed diagnosis. The most useful in this regard is finding an active urine sediment in the setting of multisystem disease that is not caused by sepsis. Other tests help determine the extent and severity of organ involvement. Therefore, at a minimum, complete blood count (CBC) and differential, serum creatinine, transaminases, and erythrocyte sedimentation rate (ESR) should be performed. An abnormal acute phase response is found in the majority of patients with vasculitis; however, this is not sufficiently sensitive or specific to either "rule-in" or "rule-out" a diagnosis of vasculitis. Culture of blood, tissue, and/or other specimens as indicated and serologic testing to exclude infection (especially hepatitis B and C) should be considered in most cases. Testing for antineutrophil cytoplasmic antibodies (ANCA) is useful if the pretest probability of Wegener's granulomatosis (WG), microscopic polyangiitis (MPA), or isolated renal vasculitis is moderate to high. If SLE, Sjogren's syndrome, or other related autoimmune disorders are suspected, antinuclear antibodies (ANA) can be helpful. Echocardiography and imaging of organs such as chest, sinuses, or central nervous system (CNS) are indicated if abnormalities are suspected in these sites.

Although biopsy proof of vasculitis in clinically involved organs or tissues provides visible evidence of vasculitis, false negatives may occur because of the small specimen size and the frequently patchy nature of the inflammation.[2–4] In addition, because the definitive diagnosis is the sum of clinical, laboratory, imaging, and pathologic information, biopsy alone may not be definitive in regards to final diagnosis. For patients with suspected large vessel or visceral involvement, biopsy is often not possible or may carry unacceptable risks. In such cases, angiography can be helpful. While invasive catheter-directed angiography is still the gold standard for imaging the aorta and its major branches, it is increasingly being supplanted by noninvasive angiographic techniques using magnetic resonance imaging (MRI), computed tomography (CT), and positron emission tomography (PET).[5–8] However, these noninvasive techniques do not currently provide sufficient resolution to visualize medium-sized visceral vessels; therefore, catheter-directed angiography is preferred to noninvasive

angiographic approaches to visualize vessels of the caliber of the mesenteric and/or renal arteries.[9]

Overview of the Management of Primary Vasculitis

The principles of management of primary vasculitis are the judicious use of immunosuppressive therapy when indicated, accurate assessment of disease activity, and careful monitoring for disease and treatment-related complications.

The choice and intensity of immunosuppressive therapy should be individualized for each patient. This choice will be influenced by the specific form of vasculitis and general knowledge of prognosis, the extent and severity of critical organ involvement, the rate of disease progression, previous immunosuppressive therapy, the presence of infection, or other comorbid illnesses. An inadequate clinical response to immunosuppressive therapy may indicate a requirement for more aggressive therapy; however, it may also be due to the presence of an unsuspected malignancy, infectious process, or vasculitis mimic (e.g., embolic disorders, atrial myxoma, vasoactive drug use). In addition, as immunosuppressive therapy confers an increased susceptibility to infection, and the clinical features of certain infections and malignancies may transiently improve with immunosuppressive therapy, ongoing vigilance is required in patients undergoing treatment for vasculitis.

Glucocorticoids (GC) are the cornerstone of pharmacologic therapy for vasculitis. Immediate life-threatening or critical organ-threatening disease is typically treated initially with intravenous GC, at doses of up to 1 g/d of methylprednisolone (or equivalent) for 3 days, followed by oral GC therapy. Standard doses of oral GC therapy for patients with moderate to severe disease activity are prednisone 1 mg/kg/d or equivalent, up to 60 to 80 mg/d.

Although a response to treatment is frequently seen within a week, this initial dose is continued for 1 month. Thereafter, the dose should be gradually tapered. There is no evidence-based GC tapering schedule, although alternate day tapering regimens have now fallen out of favor because of concerns regarding inadequate control of disease activity. A reasonable prednisone tapering schedule is by decrements of 5 mg every week until a dose of 20 mg/d is reached, followed by decrements of 2.5 mg every 1 to 2 weeks until a dose of 10 mg/d is reached; thereafter tapering should be individualized, by decrements of 1 mg every 1 to 4 weeks depending on the particular disease and the status of the patient. Tapering should be guided by clinical assessment and acute phase reactants, which are useful but imperfect markers of disease activity. Continued tapering of therapy is contraindicated in the setting of suspected relapse. The level of acute phase reactants should not be the sole basis for the diagnosis of a relapse in a patient without symptoms nor should normality of acute phase reactants be used to rule out relapse in a patient with suggestive clinical features. Some patients would be unable to maintain disease remission without continuation of GC therapy; in

TABLE 14-1. Main Adverse Effects of GC Therapy

Body changes
- Increased appetite and weight gain
- Redistribution of body fat (moon face, buffalo hump, and truncal obesity)
- Increased growth of body hair

Cardiovascular problems
- Peripheral edema
- Hypertension
- Dyslipidemia

Endocrine problems
- Hyperglycemia (impaired glucose tolerance and diabetes mellitus)
- Pituitary-adrenal axis suppression

Skin problems
- Increased risk of skin bacterial and fungal infections
- Skin thinning resulting in easy bruising (purpura), skin tearing after minor injury, slow healing, and stretch marks (striae)
- Acne/folliculitis

Skeletal complications
- Myopathy (weakness and atrophy specially in shoulders and thighs muscles)
- Osteoporosis and fractures (mostly spine, ribs, hips, and pelvis)
- Avascular necrosis of bone (femoral head most common)

Eye disease
- Blurred vision (caused by intraocular edema)
- Glaucoma
- Posterior subcapsular cataracts

Psychological effects
- Insomnia
- Mood changes (hypomania, irritability, and anxiety)
- Delirium or depression
- Psychosis
- Shakiness and tremor

Peptic ulceration (more common with concomitant NSAIDs)
Increased risk for serious infections

such patients the aim is to reduce the occurrence of adverse events by minimizing the GC dose, if possible below prednisone 7.5 mg/d or equivalent.[10–12] Adverse effects of GC are listed in Table 14-1.

Combination of GC with cyclophosphamide (CYC) remains the gold standard for the treatment of severe forms of vasculitis. The currently available evidence favors the use of daily oral rather than monthly pulse intravenous CYC for systemic vasculitis. Treatment with oral CYC is typically initiated at a dose of 2 mg/kg/d. This is continued until remission induction or marked improvement, typically for 3 to 6 months, during when CYC can be switched to an alternative immunosuppressive agent to maintain remission.

Dose reduction is required in the presence of renal failure. Other immunosuppressive agents such as methotrexate (MTX) and azathioprine (AZA) may also be used in the treatment of vasculitis. MTX is administered orally or parenterally once weekly; treatment is typically initiated at a dose of 15 mg and titrated upward to a maintenance dose of 20 to 25 mg as tolerated. MTX is relatively contraindicated in patients with serum creatinine >2.0 mg/dL, hepatic impairment, or bone marrow suppression. AZA is orally administered at a dose of 2 mg/kg, once or twice daily; dose reduction is required in renal failure. Adverse effects of CYC, MTX, and AZA are compared in Table 14-2.

There are some important considerations that apply to all patients undergoing immunosuppressive therapy. Because patients treated with more than 7.5 mg prednisone daily have two- to five-fold increased risk of bone fractures,[13] unless contraindicated, calcium, vitamin D supplementation, and bisphosphonate therapy should be given to minimize bone loss. A bone density scan is also recommended to assess the risk of fracture and to monitor bone density during follow-up.

All patients treated with high-dose GC in combination with CYC or other immunosuppressive drugs should receive prophylaxis against *Pneumocystis jivroveci* infection by using trimethoprim-sulfamethoxazole (T/S) as one single-strength tablet daily or one double strength tablet three times per week. Alternative strategies in sulfa-allergic patients include dapsone, atovaquone, and monthly inhaled pentamidine. Dosage of immunosuppressive drugs, and CYC in particular, should be titrated to maintain a white blood cell count greater than 4000×10^6/mL; induction of leukopenia is not a goal of therapy.

To reduce the risk of bladder toxicity in patients taking CYC, they should be advised to take the recommended dose once daily in the morning after liberal fluid intake, which is to continue throughout the day. These measures help minimize the duration of exposure of the bladder mucosa to acrolein—the toxic metabolite of CYC. Patients taking MTX should be advised to abstain from alcohol because of the risk of hepatotoxicity. Concurrent administration of folic acid (1 mg daily) or folinic acid (5 mg once weekly) reduces some of the adverse effects of MTX. When starting AZA, genotyping for the enzyme that metabolizes AZA (thiopurine methyltransferase) is appropriate, as individuals with deficient thiopurine methyltransferase activity are at an increased risk of AZA toxicity and therefore require a lower starting dose of AZA, and in the case of homozygous deficient patients, an alternative agent is required. Premenopausal female patients should use reliable contraceptive measures while taking immunosuppressive therapies such as CYC, MTX, and AZA. Both male and female patients taking these agents should be advised to avoid conception during and for at least 3 months after its discontinuation. Chronic immunosuppression increases the risk for serious infections and neoplasia.

Laboratory testing includes ESR, CBC, transaminases, creatinine, and urinalysis, and should be monitored

TABLE 14-2. Principal Adverse Events of the three Most Common Immunosuppressant Drugs, Other than Corticosteroids, Used for Treatment of Systemic Vasculitis

Adverse Effect/Immunosuppressant Drug	CYC	MTX	AZA
Fatigue	++	++	++
Loss of appetite/weight	++		++
Fever			+
Mucositis (mouth sores)	++	++	
Taste changes	+		
Hair loss or hair thinning	++	+	+
Nails and skin becoming dark	++		
Gastrointestinal involvement			
• Stomach ache		++	
• Nausea and vomiting	++		++
• Diarrhea			++
Hepatotoxicity	+	++	+
Bone marrow suppression			
• Leukopenia	++	+	+
• Anemia	+	+	+
• Thrombocytopenia	+	+	+
Hemorrhagic cystitis	++		
Reproductive organs			
• Amenorrhea	++		
• Loss of fertility*	++		
• Theratogenic	++	++	+
Interstitial pneumonitis	+	+	+
Fluid retention	+		
Skin rashes	+	+	+
Headache, dizziness	+	+	
Arthralgias/myalgias			+
Development of neoplastic diseases*			
• Bladder cancer	++		
• Lymphoma/Leukemia	++		+

* These are late complications that generally reflect the cumulative exposure to CYC.
Note: Well known associated (++) and sporadically communicated (+) adverse drug reactions.

regularly. While there is no systematic comparative risk–benefit data to guide the clinician in selecting particular intervals for laboratory monitoring, for the purposes of early detection of disease flares and of treatment-related toxicities, testing as outlined above is recommended no less than once per month, even when the patient is in remission. In addition, in patients receiving CYC, for which additive toxicity over time is most common, we recommend that the CBC and urinalysis should be monitored no less than every 1 to 2 weeks.

Endovascular and surgical techniques are also a critical element in the management of large- and medium-sized-vessel vasculitis. Such interventions are generally reserved for stenotic, occlusive, or aneurysmal lesions leading to organ- or life-threatening consequences. Assessment of vessel patency after vascular procedures requires careful clinical evaluation in combination with available imaging techniques. Interventional management of vascular lesions in the vasculitides will be discussed in greater detail below.

● LARGE VESSEL VASCULITIS

Primary vasculitides characterized by the involvement of aorta and its major branches include giant cell arteritis (GCA) and TAK. Other vasculitides that may involve large vessels include BD, sarcoidosis, Cogan's syndrome (CS), and KD. Less often aortitis may be a complication of rheumatic diseases such as RA, SLE, and the seronegative spondyloarthropathies as well as a number of infectious diseases, including syphilis and mycobacterial infection.

Giant Cell Arteritis

GCA is the most frequent form of vasculitis in people older than 50 years. Its annual incidence in North America and Europe ranges from 10 to 27 cases per 100 000 individuals older than 50 years.[12,14] Women are affected at least twice as often as men.[12]

Inflammatory cells in arteries of GCA patients reveal features of a delayed-type hypersensitivity reaction, with

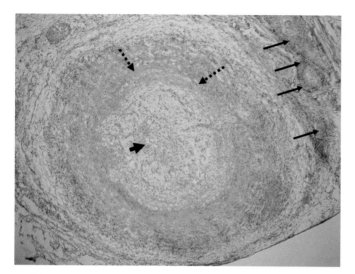

● **FIGURE 14-1.** Cross section of a temporal artery of a patient with GCA showing transmural inflammation. Although multinucleated giant cells are not clearly seen, intense inflammatory infiltrates surrounding the small adventitial vessels can be observed (long arrows). Disruption of the internal elastic lamina (dashed arrows) and severe intimal hyperplasia causing subtotal luminal occlusion (short arrow) are also seen.

a T-cell–mediated immune response that is presumed to be directed toward uncharacterized antigens in the arterial wall (Figure 14-1).[15–17] Cytokines such as tumor necrosis factor-α (TNF-α), interleukin-6 (IL-6), IL-1β and interferon-γ (IFN-γ), and a variety of chemokines and other proteins, such as matrix metalloproteinases, have been found in inflammatory lesions of GCA.[18–24]

Clinical Features. The most common symptoms of GCA relate to involvement of the extracranial branches of the carotid arteries.[11,12,25] Constitutional symptoms such as fever, anorexia, weight loss, malaise, and depression are also common features. The principal clinical characteristics in GCA are listed in Table 14-3. Ischemic manifestations (Table 14-3) constitute the most feared complications at disease onset. They are derived from the vascular occlusion of distal sites leading to organ dysfunction and are presented by 15% to 25% of GCA patients.[11,12,25] The occurrence of a transient ischemic event is a predictor of permanent ischemic lesions.[25] A lower systemic inflammatory response at diagnosis is also associated with a higher risk of developing ischemic events.[25,26]

Polymyalgia rheumatica (PMR), characterized by aching and stiffness in the neck and shoulder and hip girdles, is present in approximately 50% of GCA patients.[11,12] Polymyalgic symptoms can develop concomitantly with cranial symptoms of GCA or may precede for a number of years the appearance of clinically overt GCA. PMR can also exist as an isolated disease, without vascular involvement. When PMR occurs isolated, at least 10% of temporal artery biopsies of patients may demonstrate histologic evidence of GCA.[11,12]

TABLE 14-3. Clinical Findings in a Series of 250 GCA Patients (178 Females and 72 Males)

Clinical Features	Percentage
Cranial symptoms	86
Headache	77
Jaw claudication	44
Scalp tenderness	39
Facial pain/edema	18
Abnormal temporal arteries	74
Ocular pain	8
Tongue pain	5
Earache	18
Trismus	1
Carotidynia	5
Toothache	5
Odynophagia	12
Ischemics events	23
Amaurosis fugax	10
Established amaurosis	14
Transient diplopia	4
Permanent diplopia	2
Transient ischemic attack	1
Permanent ischemic attack	1
Other vascular territories	5
Systemic manifestations	74
Fever (>37°C)	47
Weight loss (≥10% or ≥4 kg)	61
PMR	48

Adapted from Cid MC, Hernández-Rodríguez J, Grau JM. Vascular manifestations in giant cell arteritis. In: Asherson RA, Cervera R, eds. Vascular Manifestations of Systemic Autoimmune Diseases. Boca Raton FL-London UK-New York NY,-Washington DC: CRC Press; 2001:37-249.

From 10% to 15% of GCA patients present with clinical features of large vessel involvement.[11,12] However, necropsy studies have suggested that large vessel vasculitis occurs in almost all cases.[27] Important findings on clinical examination include arterial tenderness, vascular bruits and diminished pulses, and asymmetry of blood pressure in the limbs. Careful physical examination is required to detect these findings since large-vessel involvement in GCA is frequently asymptomatic. When limb claudication occurs, it most commonly involves the upper extremities (Figure 14-2).[11,12] Compared with the normal population, patients with GCA have a 17- and 2.4-fold increased risk of developing thoracic and abdominal aortic aneurysms, respectively (Figure 14-2).[28] Several retrospective studies have described aortic aneurysms in 10% to 18% of GCA patients after a follow-up period of 2.5 months to 20 years. In half of these cases, death may occur from aortic rupture or dissection.[28–30] In a recent prospective study, aortic abnormalities (aneurysm or dilatation) developed in one-third of patients during a median follow-up period of 5.6 years (range 4–10.5 years).[31] These vascular complications tend to be apparent late over the course of the disease where such patients are usually in clinical remission.[31]

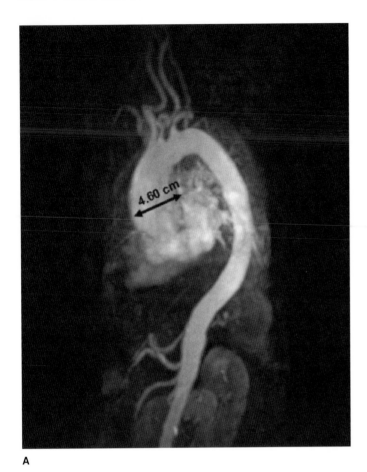

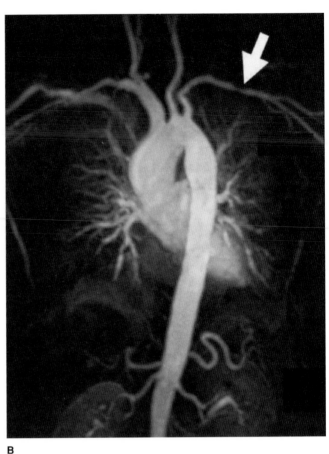

A

B

● **FIGURE 14-2.** Characteristic large vessel involvement in GCA includes aortic aneurysms and aortic arch branch vessel disease. Depicted above are magnetic resonance angiographic images demonstrating (A) an aneurysm of the aortic arch and (B) left subclavian artery stenosis.

Diagnosis. In the setting of a suspicious clinical picture, prominent acute phase laboratory findings play an important role in the diagnosis of GCA.[11,12] Classically the ESR is elevated, usually higher than 80 mm/h (Table 14-4). Proinflammatory cytokines, such as TNF-α and IL-6,[32] some soluble adhesion molecules, and other inflammatory proteins[33,34] are also increased in sera from GCA patients.

Histologic examination of the temporal artery biopsy may provide the definitive diagnosis of GCA. Preferably, 2 to 3 cm fragment of temporal artery has to be removed from a carefully selected site and different parts of the specimen should be histologically examined. Sensibility and specificity of the surgical procedure will depend on the pretest likelihood of GCA. The inflammatory infiltrate is constituted mainly by T lymphocytes, macrophages, and dendritic cells and is frequently organized in a granulomatous pattern. Multinucleated giant cells are observed in almost half of the cases, usually located near the internal elastic lamina which is often disrupted. Varying degrees of intimal hyperplasia may lead to partial or total luminal occlusion (Figure 14-1).[4,35]

If the pretest likelihood of GCA is high, a negative biopsy may still be obtained in 20% to 40% of cases. When this occurs, a contralateral temporal artery biopsy may increase

TABLE 14-4. Blood Chemistry and Hematological Values in a Series of 250 Patients with GCA

Parameter	Mean (Range)	Normal Values
ESR, mm/h	98 (15–147)	<20
CRP, mg/dL	9.5 (0.30–76)	<0.8
Haptoglobin, g/L	3.280 (0.079–7.490)	0.320–1.810
Hemoglobin, g/dL	11 (6.6–15.6)	12–16
Platelets, × 10⁹/L	362 (105–768)	150–350
Albumin, g/L	33 (20–49)	35–50
α₂-Globulin, g/L	9.7 (2.4–20.1)	0.6–1.0
Alkaline phosphatase, U/L	227 (63–1682)	95–235
Gamma glutamil transpeptidase, U/L	49 (2–383)	<40

Adapted from Cid MC, Hernández-Rodríguez J, Grau JM. Vascular manifestations in giant cell arteritis. In: Asherson RA, Cervera R, eds. Vascular Manifestations of Systemic Autoimmune Diseases. Boca Raton FL-London UK-New York NY,-Washington DC: CRC Press; 2001:37-249.

the sensitivity of diagnosis by 10% to 30%. A normal temporal artery biopsy does not exclude the diagnosis of vasculitis, given the patchy distributions of the inflammatory infiltrates.[11,12] For that reason, clinical and analytical criteria for the classification of GCA have been established.[36] Other systemic disorders can mimic GCA. These include infections or amyloidosis.[37–39] On the other hand, a temporal artery biopsy may occasionally demonstrate of distinct vasculitis caused by PAN, WG, Churg-Strauss Syndrome (CSS), cryoglobulinemic vasculitis, rheumatoid vasculitis, and thromboangiitis obliterans (TAO).[11,12,40–42]

If there is clinical suspicion of large vessel involvement, imaging of the aorta and major branch vessels should be undertaken. The use of newer angiographic techniques for detection of large vessel vasculitis is discussed under the following section on TAK. It has been proposed that ultrasonography (US) of the temporal artery may obviate the need for temporal artery biopsy for the diagnosis of GCA.[43] Proponents of US have claimed that the presence of a dark halo around the lumen of the temporal artery on color duplex US represent edema and inflammation in the vessel wall.[43,44] However, this remains an area of controversy.[12,41]

Treatment

Pharmacologic Therapy. GCs are the only proven useful anti-inflammatory for GCA. After initial doses of prednisone (or corticosteroid equivalent), which range between 40 and 60 mg/d, response to treatment is usually seen within a few days.[11,12] The dose should be gradually tapered as described above after the first month. Tapering is guided by clinical features and acute phase reactants. Therefore, the level of acute phase reactants should not be the sole basis for the diagnosis of a relapse in a patient without symptoms.[11,12] Total duration of therapy varies between patients. Withdrawal of steroid treatment is achieved in less than half of cases within 2 years. Most patients require GC therapy for several years, and some indefinitely.[11,12] Patients with a strong systemic inflammatory response at disease onset are those who typically require higher cumulative GC doses and more prolonged therapy.[32]

When GCA is suspected, the presence of ocular or neurologic disturbances should be considered a medical emergency necessitating immediate commencement of GC therapy. If visual loss is established, intravenous pulses of methylprednisolone of 1 g/d for 3 days are recommended by some authors.[26] In these situations, only the early administration of GC, within the 12 or 24 hours, appears to effect visual recovery.[26]

The efficacy of adjunctive therapy to GC with MTX has been examined in GCA patients, but its use remains controversial.[45,46] The potential role of infliximab, a chimeric monoclonal anti-TNF-α antibody, in the treatment of GCA has been recently investigated in a multicenter, randomized, double-blind, and placebo-controlled trial. Infliximab did not improve durability of remission or reduce cumulative GC doses in newly diagnosed GCA patients.[47] Low-dose aspirin taken daily has been shown,

in two retrospective studies, to reduce the risk of cranial ischemic complications in patients with GCA, without an increase of bleeding complications.[48,49] Statins have anti-inflammatory properties in cardiovascular disease; however, in one small study, statin use was not associated with clinically relevant GC-sparing effects in GCA patients.[50]

In patients with GCA and symptomatic involvement of large vessels, the addition of MTX to GC has been seldom reported.[51] However, this experience requires further validation in larger studies.

Endovascular and Surgical Considerations. Angioplasty or arterial bypass should be considered for symptomatic arterial stenoses. In a recent study, treatment with balloon angioplasty of arterial stenotic lesions of the upper extremities in 10 GCA patients led to a primary patency rate of 65% of the lesions. In spite of frequent restenosis, repetition of angioplasty up to three times showed an overall successful patency rate in almost 90% of vascular lesions during a mean follow-up of 2 years.[52] Bypass was necessary for the remaining patients. Surgical intervention of aortic aneurysms needs to be considered if the aneurysm becomes symptomatic or in any case when the aneurysm exceeds 5.5 cm in diameter in abdominal aorta, or 5 and 6 cm in ascending and descending thoracic aorta, respectively. Evidence of dissection or an accelerated growth rate, more than 5 mm in 6 months, and hemodynamically significant aortic regurgitation are other indications for surgical repair.[53]

Prognosis. Some studies have found that the overall mortality in patients with GCA is similar to that of age- and sex-matched controls.[54] However, there is no question that if GCA-related aneurysms contribute to death by dissection or rupture, in those patients mortality was increased because of GCA.[28,55]

Takayasu's Arteritis

TAK is a granulomatous vasculitis that has a predilection for the aorta and its primary branches. Sustained inflammation of involved vessels leads most often to stenotic or occlusive lesions, but may also result in aneurysm formation.[5] Although TAK has been described in patients of all races, it occurs most frequently in Asian patients. The estimated annual incidence in North America is only 2.6 cases per million population, approximately a 100-fold lower than that in Japan[5] females are affected up to 10 times more often than males, with the peak incidence occurring in the third decade of life.[5]

Macrophages and T lymphocytes, including cytotoxic and γ/δ T lymphocytes, are the constituents of inflammatory infiltrates in TAK.[18] A potential role for TNF-α in the pathogenesis of TAK is suggested by the efficacy of anti-TNF-α therapies in patients with refractory TAK.[56] Compared to normal controls, mRNA for TNF is increased in peripheral blood mononuclear cells.[22,57,58] Serum TNF-α is similarly increased in TAK patients compared to controls.[22,57,58]

TABLE 14-5. Clinical Characteristics at the Time of Onset of TAK in Five Large Series (Values Represent % of Patients)

Clinical Features at the Time of Disease Onset	CCF[59] n = 75	NIH[5] n = 60	Italian[60] n = 104	Mexican[61] n = 107	Indian[62] n = 106
Systemic manifestations					
Fatigue/Malaise	55	33	60	56	
Fever	35	22	40	18	
Weight loss (>10%)		12	20	22	
Arthralgias	25	11	30	53	5
Myalgias	18	3	25		
Cardiac and vascular involvement					
Diminishing or absence of pulse in extremities	57	22	72	96	
Blood pressure asymmetry of upper and lower limbs (>15 mm Hg)	53	13	66		
Vascular bruits	53	23	65	94	68
Carotid arteries	36				
Subclavian arteries	13				
Abdomen vasculature	15				
Femoral arteries	15				
Carotidynia	15	17	37		
Extremity claudication	48	36	43	29	
Hypertension (new onset)	28	17	40	72	52
Aortic valvular regurgitation	24	8			
Pericarditis	8				
Congestive heart failure	7	2			12
Angina pectoris	5				
Dyspnea				72	26
Neurovascular involvement					
Headache	52	18	29	57	44
Lightheadedness/dizziness	33				
Visual aberrations (blurring, scotoma, diplopia)	12	10			12
Amaurosis fugax	4				
Transient ischemic attack	3		1		
Stroke	5	5	2		10

Clinical Features. TAK presents with constitutional symptoms in approximately 50% of patients.[59] The most common symptoms and signs of TAK in different cohorts of patients (Americans, Italians, Mexicans, and Indians) are summarized in Table 14-5.[5,59–62] The most commonly affected arterial territories in an American cohort are indicated in Table 14-6. Stenotic vascular lesions (Figure 14-3) are found in >90% of patients; dilatation or aneurysm formation makes up approximately 25% of lesions.[59,60] The aortic root is the most frequent location of aneurysm formation. Root dilatation leads to valvular regurgitation in approximately 20% of patients. Aortic aneurysm rupture and congestive cardiac failure caused by aortic insufficiency are two of the main causes of death in TAK patients.[5,59,60]

Hypertension is a major source of disease-related morbidity, and although noted in up to 70% of patients from India, Japan, Mexico, and Korea, is present in approximately 40% of US and European patients.[59] Renal artery stenosis (Figure 14-3) occurs in 25% to 60% of patients and is the most common cause of hypertension.[59] Other

TABLE 14-6. Sites of Arterial Involvement Within 1 Year of Diagnosis in 75 Patients with Takayasu's Arteritis[59]

Arterial Territories	Percentage of Cases
Aorta	79
Subclavian	62
Carotid	43
Vertebral	14
Renal	25
Iliofemoral	26
Mesenteric	37
Coronary	11
Pulmonary	7

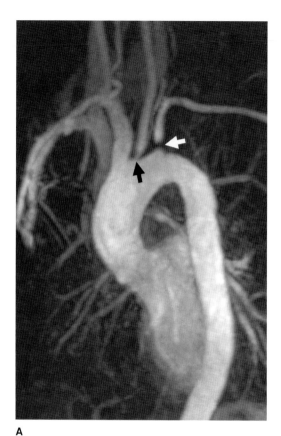

A

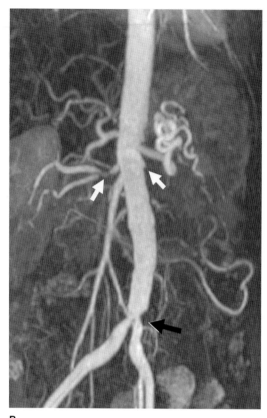

B

● FIGURE 14-3. Magnetic resonance angiography of arterial lesions in a patient with Takayasu's arteritis. (A) Stenotic lesions are observed at the origin of the left common carotid artery (black arrow) and left subclavian artery (white arrow). (B) Also evident is involvement of both renal arteries (white arrows), with total occlusion of the left renal artery, and abdominal aortic stenosis just proximal to the aortic bifurcation (black arrow).

causes include suprarenal aortic stenosis and diffuse aortic stiffening with loss of compliance.

Neurologic symptoms derived from stenoses of carotid or vertebral arteries are present in more than a half of patients (Table 14-5).[59] Visual disturbances, such as amaurosis fugax and permanent blindness, secondary to hypoperfusion retinopathy or derived from hypertension (hypertensive retinopathy) occur in up to 50% of TAK patients.[5,63]

Although pulmonary involvement may be asymptomatic in most patients, imaging abnormalities (e.g., perfusion scan) can be detected in more than half of TAK patients.[64,65] Visceral artery stenoses can occur in up to 60% of cases, but because of abundant anastomoses clinical symptoms are infrequent.[66] Dermatologic manifestations (erythema nodosum, erythema induratum, and pyoderma gangrenosum) have been noted in up to 28% of patients.[67]

Diagnosis. The diagnosis of TAK is based on clinical findings in the setting of compatible vascular imaging abnormalities. There are no serologic tests that are specific TAK diagnosis[68] and a large vessel biopsy is usually impractical. However, when a patient undergoes surgery for a vascular complication, it is recommended to obtain a specimen of an involved artery for histologic examination.[69] Distinct histopathologic patterns can be seen at different stages of

TAK. Active lesions may reveal granulomatous arteritis, with transmural inflammation, and patchy destruction of medial musculoelastic lamina. Cells within the infiltrate are mainly lymphoplasmacytic infiltrate, more prominent in the media, multinucleated giant cells, and cytotoxic and γ/δ T lymphocytes.[16,35,69] Both active and healing lesions include variable degrees of intimal and adventitial fibrosis and extensive scarring of the media.[35] The inflammatory process leads to myointimal proliferation with subsequent vessel wall thickening and luminal stenosis, resulting in reduction or abolition of blood supply and tissue ischemia.[16] Lesions that predominantly cause destruction of the muscularis and the elastica may result in vascular dilatation or aneurysms. The latter most commonly occurs in the aortic root and arch.[66]

Traditionally, the gold standard for diagnosis of TAK has been the combination of an appropriate clinical phenotype with catheter-directed angiography. Such study provides not only information about the vessel shape and luminal caliber, but also enable recording of intravascular blood pressure measurements. When indicated and disease is quiescent, it also provides opportunities for intervention (e.g., angioplasty).[5] Limitations of catheter-directed angiography include its inability to provide information about the vessel wall per se. It also carries risks related to arterial invasiveness, exposure to contrast agents (e.g., kidney toxicity), and high dose of ionizing radiation. Cardiovascular MRI with its two components, contrast-enhanced MRI and MRA (conventional or 3-D), is considered to have of similar diagnostic accuracy to catheter-directed angiography, and also the advantage of a better safety profile (nor radiation, risk of contrast, or vessel trauma). However, use of MRI does not allow measurement of intravascular pressure or the opportunity to carry out interventional procedures.[6] Although MRI can provide additional information regarding the appearance of the vessel wall, the value of this data regarding prediction of vascular anatomic change is uncertain.[7] FDG-PET has recently been demonstrated to be useful in identifying the presence or absence of inflammation within large vessels.[8] Combinations of some of these techniques are being used with promising results (Figure 14-9). Future studies will need to define more clearly the operating characteristics of these techniques, especially in regards to whether enhanced uptake (presumed inflammation) accurately predicts later vessel anatomic change (stenosis or aneurysm formation).

Disease Activity Assessment. Acute phase reactants may be helpful in assessing disease activity. However, in many patients, they may not correlate with systemic symptoms or progressive change on imaging studies, nor do normal acute phase reactants confirm disease remission.[59] Sequential imaging evaluations have revealed disease progression (as determined by the presence of new vascular lesions) in more than 50% of patients with clinically stable profiles and normal ESR.[59] Clinical evaluation also underestimates the presence of subclinical disease activity; almost a half of TAK patients with apparent clinically quiescent disease undergoing bypass have been noted to have histopathologic evidence of vascular inflammation.[5]

In 1994, Kerr et al.[5] defined active disease according to the existence of new or worsening of any two or more of the following parameters: (1) Signs or symptoms of vascular ischemia or inflammation; (2) Increase in sedimentation rate; (3) Angiographic features; and (4) Systemic symptoms not attributable to another disease.

These features have been demonstrated to be specific and helpful when present, but their absence does not insure disease remission. Studies that utilize these criteria in conjunction with sequential imaging modalities will better inform clinicians about the performance, characteristics of clinical features, laboratory surrogates of disease activity and enhancement per MRI or PET.

Treatment

Pharmacologic Therapy. GC therapy results in clinical improvement in almost all patients, and leads to remission in up to 90%. However, when prednisone is tapered, most patients suffer disease relapse.[59,70] Such patients require additional immunosuppressive therapy. Treatment with MTX may help achieve and maintain disease remission in patients with relapsing or GC-dependent disease.[69]

However, when GC discontinuation is attempted with the aid of MTX or other cytotoxic agents, relapses still occur in most patients. Hoffman et al. showed anti-TNF-α agents to be useful in sustaining GC-free remissions in more than 60% of patients with previously refractory TAK.[56] In an extended recently published study, the same authors have recently confirmed the sustainability of anti-TNF-α therapy in maintaining disease remission for a longer follow-up period (mean >2 years, range 2 months to 6.5 years).[71] Supporting these findings are several case reports of relapsing TAK that have been successfully treated with infliximab.[72] A randomized controlled study is required to establish the efficacy and safety of anti-TNF-α therapy in TAK.

Endovascular and Surgical Management. Indications for revascularization in TAK patients include symptomatic cervicocranial or coronary artery disease, renal artery stenosis leading to renovascular hypertension, aortic aneurysm with risk of dissection or rupture; sever extremity claudication and moderate-to-severe aortic valve regurgitation or coarctation of the aorta.[69] Procedures to re-establish flow in stenotic or occluded vessels include surgical placement of synthetic grafts or autologous vessel bypass and percutaneous transluminal angioplasty. Aortic root repair or replacement are employed for aortic insufficiency.[69] Kerr et al. found that 50% (30/60) patients followed more than a mean period of 5 years required intervention for either vessel stenosis or aortic regurgitation.[5] Revascularization procedures in TAK ideally should be performed during disease remission. Endarterectomy has been used in some cases of aortic branch vessel and coronary artery stenosis. However, this procedure is technically difficult or impossible to perform effectively, or may even be dangerous, because arterial lesions in TAK can be rigid and often involve the entire thickness of the vessel wall.[69]

A longitudinal study of 30 patients having 64 revascularization procedures was recently reported from the Cleveland Clinic. All patients were followed for a mean of 3 years and re-evaluated with sequential imaging studies, with there being a mean of 4.8 months between studies. One hundred percent of the patients had stenotic lesions. All but five cases were considered to have a quiescent disease activity at the time of the vascular procedure. Twenty angioplasty procedures were performed. Two were operative failures and in 14/18 (78%) longer-term follow-up revealed restenosis. Forty-four vascular bypass/reconstruction procedures were performed, 47% following previous intervention failures. Although surgical bypass was the most successful intervention, restenosis or occlusion occurred in 36%.

Percutaneous transluminal angioplasty and stenting used alone or as a combined treatment in TAK have been recently reviewed in a study that included 11 series of TAK patients and 224 vascular lesions. Patency rate was variable among series.[59] Bypass is especially successful when autologous donor vessels are used.[5,73]

Low mortality rates have been seen in American cohorts (3%–4%) more than a median follow-up periods of 3 to

5 years. However, chronic morbidity and disability is frequent in TAK.[5,59] Postoperative mortality, defined as death occurring during hospitalization, occurred in 11% of patients in a series of 106 patients with TAK.[74] Death occurred in most as a result of cardiovascular complications including congestive heart failure, aneurysm rupture, stroke, or hemorrhage.[69,75]

Prognosis. Satisfactory outcomes in TAK depend on achieving and sustaining suppression of disease activity, minimizing treatment toxicity, correcting severe anatomic lesions, and effectively controlling high blood pressure when present. Recognition of hypertension is often delayed because of the high frequency of stenoses of the branches of the aortic arch, which may result in misleading low peripheral blood pressure readings in reference to pressure in the aortic root. For that reason, blood pressure should be assessed in four extremities at the onset of the disease and during follow-up visits. Vascular imaging studies will inform the examiner of which extremities have unimpeded flow from the aortic root distally. When reliability of blood pressure recordings is questionable, an invasive angiogram with central aortic pressure measurements plus recordings across stenotic lesions will discern whether any extremity provides an accurate reflection of central aortic pressure. If hypertension is clearly related to renal artery stenosis, such lesions should be surgically corrected.

Morbidity and mortality in patients with TAK are directly correlated with the vascular territories involved and the extent of disease. Additional morbidity is because of the use of GC and other immunosuppressive therapies (e.g., infections, hypertension, diabetes, osteoporosis, or cataracts). Inadequately treated or unrecognized hypertension, aortic aneurysms, aortic valve insufficiency, and coronary artery disease carry a greater risk of premature death. Sudden death may result from myocardial infarction, stroke, or rupture or dissection of an aortic aneurysm. Despite these potential life-threatening complications, 5- to 10-year survival rates have been reported to be >90%.[59,69,76]

● MEDIUM-SIZED VESSEL VASCULITIS

By definition, medium vessels are those muscular arteries larger than arterioles and smaller than large arteries, sized from 50 μm to 1 cm in diameter.[3] Vasculitides that typically target medium-sized vessels include PAN, KD, and TAO. While PAN may affect individuals of any age, KD is seen in infants and small children. TAO is almost exclusively a disorder of adult smokers. Because chronic viral infections, especially hepatitis B, may cause a similar vasculitis to PAN, they have commonly been studied together, and will be discussed together below. It should also be appreciated that schemes based on vessel size are an over simplification. For example, illnesses that are considered "small vessel" vasculitides may also include medium-sized vessels (e.g., WG, CSS, MPA).

Polyarteritis Nodosa

PAN is a systemic necrotizing arteritis of medium-sized and small muscular arteries, and less commonly arterioles. No clear sex or race preference is observed in PAN; peak incidence is in the fifth to sixth decades. PAN is a rare disease with an annual incidence of 4.6 and 9 cases per million inhabitants in England and USA, respectively.[9]

Strictly speaking, PAN is not an immune-complex-mediated disease, making it distinct from similar disease phenotypes associated with viral infections or cryoglobulinemia.[77] A PAN-like presentation has been reported in chronic viral infections, particularly in association with hepatitis B virus (HBV). Before vaccination against HBV more than one third of cases presenting with features suggestive of PAN were associated with this viral infection, and since then, HBV- /PAN-like cases have decreased to 7%.[9] The mechanism of vascular inflammation implicated most commonly in HBV-vasculitis is an immune complex-induced lesion.[9]

In 1994, at the Chapel Hill International Consensus Conference, PAN was differentiated from MPA. MPA was defined as a systemic small to medium-sized vessel vasculitis that typically presents with rapidly progressive glomerulonephritis (RPGN) and pulmonary involvement.[1] The absence of pulmonary and glomerular capillary involvement in PAN has become useful in distinguishing this entity from WG, MPA, or CSS. Because of the low prevalence of PAN, many of the series in the medical literature combine discussion of PAN with MPA, CSS, and viral-associated vasculitis, thereby hindering clear characterization of PAN.

Clinical Features. PAN may be indolent and mild, or severe and rapidly progressive. Clinical features in PAN include constitutional symptoms such as malaise, weight loss, fever, and musculoskeletal symptoms in the majority of patients. Skin, peripheral nerve, gastrointestinal, and renal disease occur in most patients. The range of involvement of these and less commonly affected organs is noted in Table 14-7.

Renal failure in PAN is the consequence of multiple renal infarcts, complicated in some cases by malignant hypertension.[78,80] Renal infarctions may be clinically silent and renal insufficiency may develop over the course of months to years.[78,80] Renal hematomas caused by rupture of renal microaneurysms can also occur.[80]

It has traditionally been considered that patients with classic PAN rarely (<10%) suffer relapses,[81] in contrast to patients with WG or MPA.[82] However, a recent study of 10 PAN patients that strictly followed the Chapel Hill nomenclature for PAN has shown a relapse rate in PAN patients similar to that seen in those with MPA.[80]

Diagnosis. The diagnosis of PAN is often delayed because of the highly variable and sometimes indolent clinical presentation. There are no laboratory markers specific for PAN. Leukocytosis and elevated ESR and CRP are common. Occasionally hypereosinophilia (>1500/mm^3) is present.

TABLE 14-7. Principal Manifestations in Patients with PAN[78]

Territory Involved and Clinical Features	Prevalence of Finding (%)
Systemic manifestations	
Fever	31–69
Weight loss	16–66
Myalgias	30–54
Arthralgias	44–58
Cutaneous	28–58
Purpura, livedo reticularis, subcutaneous nodules, Raynaud phenomenon, distal digital ischemia	
Neurological	40–75
Mononeuritis multiplex	38–72
CNS	2–28
Palsies of cranial nerves	<2
Gastrointestinal tract	14–42
Abdominal pain*	100
Nausea/vomiting*	32
Diarrhea*	16
Hematochezia/melena*	13
Gastroduodenal ulcerations*	45
Colorectal ulcerations*	5
Surgical abdomen/Peritonitis*	45
Deaths*	18
Abnormal imaging studies*	
Abdominal angiogram*	74
Abdominal CT*	69
Renal	8–66
Cardiac	4–30
Vasculitis of coronary arteries	
Heart failure	
Hypertension	10–33
Eye	3–44
Retinal vasculitis, retinal detachment, cotton–wool spots	
Respiratory	5
Pleural effusion	
Testicles	218
Orchitis/epididymitis	

Gastrointestinal manifestations in a series of 17 patients with PAN.[79]

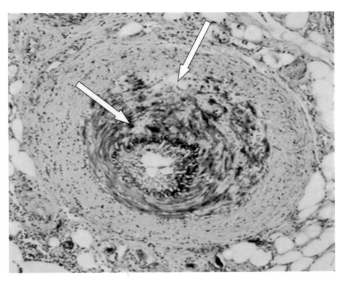

● **FIGURE 14-4.** Histopathologic evidence of medium vessel vasculitis in a patient with PAN. Lymphomononuclear infiltrate with fibrinoid necrosis and localized disruption are seen at the intimal–medial junction (arrows); such disruption is the precursor change of microaneurysm formation.

able number of neutrophils and eosinophils. Necrotizing vasculitis, proliferative and fibrotic or healed changes may coexist.[35,83]

Biopsies should be considered of symptomatic or clinically abnormal sites (e.g., muscle, sural nerve, testicle, or skin). In carefully selected individuals in whom systemic vasculitis is strongly suspected, muscular biopsies from clinically affected muscles and nerves may reveal vasculitis in approximately 70% of patients.[84] In cases where biopsies of muscle and nerve are blindly performed, vasculitis can be seen in less than one-third of patients.[85] While renal biopsy may reveal arteritis of medium-sized vessels (without glomerulonephritis),[85] the presence of renal microaneurysms increases the potential for hemorrhagic complications. Therefore, closed renal biopsy is not recommended to confirm the diagnosis of PAN, and if renal biopsy is considered necessary, an open procedure should be performed.

When the histologic diagnosis of vasculitis cannot be obtained, or patients are experiencing any symptoms suggestive of abdominal, cardiac, or renal involvement, an angiographic study should be performed. In these cases, if typical angiographic changes are found the diagnosis of PAN can be established. Microaneurysms and stenoses of medium-sized vessels are commonly present in PAN (Figure 14-4). Arterial saccular or fusiform 1 to 5 mm microaneurysms are predominantly seen in the kidneys, mesentery (Figure 14-5), and liver.[9]

Treatment. The main determinants of treatment for patients with PAN or a PAN-like illness are the presence of chronic viral infection, rate of disease progression and the distribution of involved organs.[42] In patients with PAN-like vasculitis associated with HBV infection, combination of GC with antiviral therapy, such as vidarabine,

Testing for chronic viral infection and ANCA should also be performed as positive results strongly suggest the alternative diagnoses of viral-associated vasculitis and either WG or MPA.

Ultimately, the diagnosis is clinical–angiographic or histologic. Biopsies of vascular lesions are characteristically patchy and segmental. Active histologic lesions include necrotizing vasculitis with fibrinoid necrosis, which is often associated with thrombosis. Severe vessel wall injury may result in the formation of typical microaneurysms (Figure 14-4). The inflammatory component of the infiltrate in PAN is formed by lymphomononuclear cells and vari-

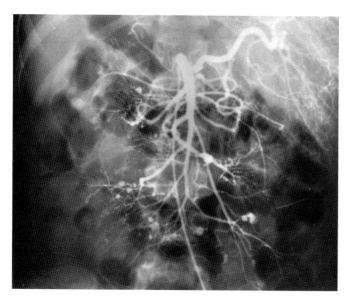

● **FIGURE 14-5.** Mesenteric angiogram in a patient with PAN demonstrating microaneurysms in the distal branches of the superior mesenteric artery.

interferon-α2a, or lamivudine, and in some cases plasma exchanges, may be effective in controlling the disease, and also in facilitating viral seroconversion and preventing the development of long-term hepatic complications of HBV infection. Relapses are rare in HBV-vasculitis and never occur when viral replication has stopped and seroconversion has been obtained.[79]

Milder forms of primary PAN may be treated with GC alone, typically at doses of 1 mg/kg/d. However, in the presence of critical organ- or life-threatening disease or in case of disease progression, intravenous methylprednisolone in pulses of 1000 mg/d for 1 to 3 days and cytotoxic therapy should be also initiated. CYC is used at doses of 2 mg/kg/d or as monthly intravenous doses of 0.6 g/m^2 for 6 to 12 months.[9,86,87] Following improvement, within 3 to 6 months, switching CYC to other maintenance immunosuppressive agents is preferred to continued use. This strategy helps to avoid long-term CYC toxicity. Initial methylprednisolone should be switched to prednisone at 1 mg/kg/d during 1 month with further tapering.[86,88] Surgical intervention may be required for complications such as bowel perforation, ischemia or hemorrhage, and hematoma or rupture of the kidney, or digital infarction.[89]

Prognosis. The prognosis of PAN depends of the severity and number of organs involved and may be estimated by the five factor score (FFS). The FFS is comprised of the following items: serum creatinine ≥1.58 mg/dL, proteinuria (≥1 g/d), presence of severe gastrointestinal tract disease (defined as bleeding, perforation, infarction, and/or pancreatitis), cardiac (infarction or heart failure), and CNS involvement; each factor is scored as 1 point.[80,89] The French Vasculitis Study Group has reported a 12% mortality at 5 years for PAN patients with FFS = 0, while mortality for FFS = 1 was 26%, and, 46% when FFS ≥2. Cardiac and CNS

involvement were found as independent factors predictive of early death in PAN and HBV-associated vasculitis.[81,90] The overall 7-year survival for PAN is 79%.[90]

Kawasaki's Disease

KD, also known as mucocutaneous lymph node syndrome, is an acute and self-limited vasculitis involving predominantly medium-sized vessels throughout the entire vascular tree. Larger arteries, small arterioles, capillaries, and veins are less commonly affected. This vasculitis affects infants and young children, usually younger than 5 years.[91] The annual incidence of KD in children of Japanese ancestry is approximately 150 per 100 000 children younger than 5 years. In the United States, KD affects from 9 to 32.5 per 100 000 of children depending on their descent, occurring more frequently in Americans of Asian and Pacific Island descent.[91] Since its first description in 1967, KD has surpassed acute rheumatic fever as the leading cause of acquired heart disease among children in developed countries.

Although the etiology of KD remains unknown, clinical, epidemiological, and immunologic features point to an infectious disease origin.[91] The oligoclonal immune response developed during active disease and the prominence of immunoglobulin A (IgA) plasma cells in the respiratory tract sharing similarities with that seen in some viral respiratory infections support the infectious hypothesis. However, no microbiological or environmental triggers have been identified to date. Macrophages, cytotoxic lymphocytes CD8+, and IgA appear to be involved in coronary arteritis. The strong systemic inflammatory response in KD is driven by inflammatory cascades and endothelial cell activation in which matrix metalloproteinases, growth factors, and chemokines and cytokines such as TNF-α seem to play a role in vascular inflammation and damage.[91,92]

Clinical Features. Typical clinical features of KD (Table 14-8) include fever, conjunctival injection, rash, erythema of the oral mucosa, erythema and swelling of the hands and feet, cervical adenopathy; aseptic meningitis, diarrhea, and hepatic dysfunction may also occur. The erythematosus rash and the eye involvement appear within the first 5 days of fever. Myocarditis and pericardial effusion may also occur. Coronary arteritis may be already present, but aneurysms are not generally detectable by echocardiography at this stage. The subacute phase begins when fever, rash, and lymphadenopathy abate after 1 to 2 weeks; typical symptoms include irritability, anorexia, conjunctival injection, and desquamation of the fingers and toes—this phase lasts usually until approximately 4 weeks after the onset of fever. Coronary aneurysms typically develop during this phase, and the risk for sudden death is highest at this time (Figure 14-6). The convalescence phase starts when clinical manifestations have resolved and last until the normalization of the ESR, usually at 6 to 8 weeks after the disease onset.[91,93]

Cardiac disease occurs in 20% to 25% of untreated patients and is the principal determinant of prognosis.

TABLE 14-8. Clinical and Analytical Features in KD. Diagnostic Criteria

1. Epidemiological case definition—classic clinical criteria

Fever persisting at least 5 days

Presence of at least four principal features:
  - Changes in extremities
    Acute: Erythema of palms, soles: edema of hands, feet
    Subacute: Periungueal peeling of fingers, toes in weeks 2 and 3
  - Polymorphous exanthema
  - Bilateral bulbar conjunctival injection without exudates
  - Changes in lips and oral cavitiy: Erythema, lips cracking, strawberry tongue, diffuse injection of oral and pharyngueal mucosae
  - Cervical lymphadenopathy (>1.5 cm diameter), usually unilateral.
  - Exclusion of other conditions with similar expression.

2. Other clinical findings

Cardiovascular findings
  Congestive heart failure, myocarditis, pericarditis, valvular regurgitation
  Coronary artery abnormalities
  Aneurysms of medium-size of noncoronary arteries
  Raynaud's phenomenon
  Peripheral gangrene
Musculoskeletal system
  Arthritis, arthralgia
Gastrointestinal tract
  Diarrhea, vomiting, abdominal pain
  Hepatic dysfunction
  Hydrops of gallbladder
CNS
  Extreme irritability
  Aseptic meningitis
  Sensorineural hearing loss
Genitourinary system
  Urethritis/meatitis
Other findings
  Erythema, induration at BCG inoculation site
  Anterior uveitis (mild)
  Desquamating rash in groin

3. Laboratory findings in acute phase
  Leukocytosis with neutrophilia and immature forms
  Elevated ESR
  Elevated CRP
  Anemia
  Abnormal plasma lipids
  Hypoalbuminemia
  Hyponatremia
  Thrombocytosis after week 1
  Sterile pyuria
  Elevated serum transaminases
  Elevated serum gamma glutamyl transpeptidase
  Pleocytosis of cerebrospinal fluid
  Leukocytosis in synovial fluid

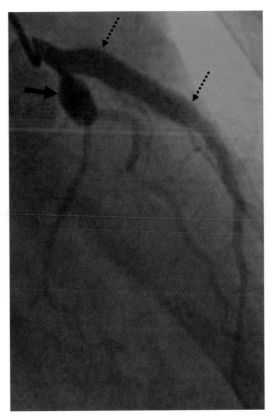

● **FIGURE 14-6.** Coronary angiogram in a patient with Kawasaki disease. Diffuse and irregular dilatation of the left main coronary artery (dashed arrows) and aneurysm of left circumflex coronary artery (arrow).

Echocardiographic abnormalities of coronary arteries may be appreciable as early as day 7 after onset of the illness. The pericardium, myocardium, endocardium and valves all may be involved.[91,94] Duration of fever has been confirmed as a powerful predictor of coronary artery aneurysms.[91] Mortality is more common in 2 to 12 weeks after the onset of symptoms and it has been estimated to be 2%—the main cause of death is myocardial infarction, typically resulting from thrombotic occlusion of a coronary aneurysm.[91,93]

Aneurysms in other noncoronary large and medium-sized arteries such as the aorta, axillary, iliac, and renal arteries have also been reported in approximately 2% of patients, typically occurring in patients that also have coronary artery aneurysms.[93] Recent reports also suggest that there may be a link with accelerated atherosclerosis in adulthood.[94]

Diagnosis. The diagnosis of KD is a clinical one, based on the presence of fever for 5 days or more, and at least 4 among the 6 manifestations listed in first section of Table 14-8. Patients with fever at least ≥ 5 days but without the 4 required criteria can be diagnosed with KD when coronary artery abnormalities are detected by 2-dimensional echocardiography or angiography.[91] An abnormal acute phase response is present in most cases, often with marked thrombocytosis. Biopsy is rarely necessary for the purposes of diagnosis, but pathologic specimens may be obtained in the rare cases where surgical intervention is necessary.

Typical laboratory findings include elevation of acute phase reactants, such as ESR, CRP, leukocytosis, thrombocytosis, and anemia (Table 14-8). Histopathology of KD in the early stages includes edema of endothelial cells with nuclear degeneration along with mild inflammatory infiltrates in the adventitial layer. Cells first arriving to inflammatory sites are neutrophils, followed by mononuclear cells with T lymphocytes (mainly CD8+) and IgA plasma cells. However, in severe disease the entire vascular wall can be affected. When the medial layer is involved, inflammation and necrosis of smooth muscle cells, with rupture of both elastic laminae usually occurs. This is the pathologic substrate for the development of aneurysms. Fibrous connective tissue replaces the inflammatory infiltrate 1 to 2 months after disease onset. Over time, the intima proliferates and becomes thickened, resulting in vascular stenosis or occlusion. Wall calcification and intraluminal organized and recanalized thrombi are late consequences of this process, reflected by the reports of accelerated atherosclerotic disease in young adults that had a history of KD in early childhood.[94] In addition, lymphadenopathy reveals postcapillary venules involvement during the acute phase of the disease, and eventually, thrombotic arteriolitis and severe lymphadenitis with necrosis can occur.[91,93]

Treatment and Prognosis

Pharmacologic Treatment. Treatment of acute KD in the first 10 days of illness with a single 2-g/kg dose of intravenous immunoglobulin (IVIG), given for more than 10 to 12 h, and with aspirin at 80 to 100 mg/kg/d reduces the prevalence of coronary artery abnormalities from approximately 20% in patients treated with aspirin alone to 4%.[93] Mortality is also decreased from 2% to 6% to less than 0.1% when treatment is given the first days.[91,93] IVIG also results in rapid defervescence and more rapid normalization of acute-phase reactants than is seen in patients treated with aspirin alone.[91,93] In addition, IVIG improves myocardial function in patients with acute KD.[91,93] The mechanism of action of IVIG in KD is not totally understood.[93] Aspirin has been used to treat KD patients for many years and is administered for both its anti-inflammatory and antithrombotic effects. During the acute phase of illness, aspirin is administered at 80 to 100 mg/kg/d every 6 h, in addition to IVIG. On day 14 of illness, when the fever has resolved, the dose of aspirin is reduced to antithrombotic doses of 3 to 5 mg/kg/d as a single daily dose. Approximately 10% of KD patients are "nonresponders" to this standard therapy and have persistent fever 48 h after IVIG infusion. These cases represent a significant clinical dilemma, since prolonged fever is a recognized risk factor for the development of more severe coronary disease. Limited uncontrolled data suggests that these patients may benefit from an additional infusion of IVIG.[91,93]

Controversy exists regarding the use of GC as initial treatment of KD. This issue was previously examined in a meta-analysis that included 862 patients from eight different studies; this analysis pointed to a significant reduction in the incidence of coronary aneurysms in patients initially treated with GC (OR 0.55).[95] Two recent multicenter-prospective and randomized trials using two different GC regimens had different results. A Japanese study of 178 patients with KD found that administration of GC in the acute phase of disease led to better coronary outcomes. Patients were assigned to IVIG (1 g/kg for 2 consecutive days) or IVIG plus prednisolone (2 mg/kg/d, 3 times daily). Prednisolone doses were tapered until discontinuation once CRP was normalized, with a median duration of 23 days (range 18 to 100). Patients receiving GC and IVIG had a significantly lower incidence of coronary artery abnormalities within the first month (2.2% vs. 11.4%), a shorter duration of fever, and a quicker CRP normalization than those that received IVIG alone. Initial treatment failure was also less frequent in patients receiving prednisolone.[96] The role of GC in the initial treatment of KD was also examined in a double-blind, placebo-controlled trial that enrolled 199 US patients. This study compared the addition of a single infusion of high-dose methylprednisolone (30 mg/kg) with placebo in infants with KD treated with conventional therapy (IVIG and aspirin). There was a trend toward a more rapid reduction in acute phase reactants in the steroid-treated group compared to the placebo group, but no differences were found in the duration of the febrile period, in the number of adverse events, or in coronary artery abnormalities at 5 weeks after randomization.[97] The differing outcomes of these two large trials may relate to the varying dosage and duration of GC therapy; these differences should be borne in mind when considering the use of GC in the initial treatment of KD patients.

With regards to the use of GC in refractory KD, a recent Canadian study analyzed the effects of GC in 26 patients with persistent fever despite treatment with IVIG and aspirin. Twenty-two of them had rapid and sustained resolution of fever after GC without serious adverse events. Seventeen patients developed coronary abnormalities (8 of them with aneurysm). Although 1 year later 46% of patients showed resolution of coronary arteries abnormalities, further prospective and randomized trials are need to prove the efficacy of GC in the late phase of KD.[98] The use of cyclosporine, CYC and infliximab has also been reported to be efficacious in small numbers of patients with refractory KD.[91]

Patients with KD should be carefully monitored for the recurrence of fever or other symptoms. A control echocardiogram should be obtained at 2 to 3 weeks, and again at 6 to 8 weeks following the onset of symptoms. If the ESR is back to normal after 6 to 8 weeks of the onset and the echocardiogram obtained at that time is also unremarkable, discontinuation of aspirin is recommended. In patients with coronary artery dilatation or aneurysm, aspirin is maintained indefinitely, even after apparent resolution of the abnormalities by echocardiogram.

Administration of live parenteral virus vaccines (measles–mumps–rubella and varicella vaccines) should be delayed for 6 to 11 months after administration of IVIG.[91] When a significant exposure to varicella virus occurs in an unvaccinated KD patient on chronic aspirin therapy, discontinuation of aspirin should be strongly considered to avoid the risk of Reye's syndrome. In these cases, if a high risk of thrombosis exists, another antiplatelet agent such as dipyridamole (2 to 3 mg/kg two or three times a day) should be temporarily added.[91]

Treatment of the Arterial Lesions. Management of KD patients with aneurysms is dependent upon the severity of coronary disease. Patients with a solitary small to medium-sized aneurysm should be maintained on long-term aspirin therapy but should not be restricted in activities except for avoidance of competitive contact athletics with endurance training. Stress testing, with dobutamine in cases of children unable to cooperate, may be suggested by the pediatric cardiologist for older children, and coronary angiography may be indicated if stress testing suggests the possibility of coronary artery stenosis. Patients with multiple small to medium-sized aneurysms or one or more giant coronary artery aneurysms should be maintained on aspirin therapy with or without coumadin anticoagulation. Physical activity in the first decade of life is unrestricted, but after that time a new cardiac evaluation is recommended (stress test with a myocardial perfusion scan) and coronary angiography is required when coronary disease is suspected. If coronary obstruction is confirmed, therapeutic options available will be needed such as bypass grafting, balloon angioplasty, or other procedures. When myocardial infarction occurs, acute thrombolytic therapy may be used. A Japanese study of 168 patients with KD, who underwent bypass grafting, the patency rate at 7 years after the procedure was 77% for arterial grafts compared to 46% for venous grafts.[93] There is little experience with heart transplantation in KD.[93]

Thromboangiitis Obliterans

TAO, also known as Buerger's disease, is a rare form of vasculitis that predominantly affects small and medium arteries and veins of the extremities.[99,100] Affected individuals are typically young, with onset in almost all cases of age less than 45 years; more than 95% are tobacco smokers, typically heavy smokers (>20 cigarettes per day). TAO was initially thought to almost exclusively affect males, but more recent reports suggest that 11% to 23% of TAO patients are female; this increased prevalence likely relates to higher rates of smoking among women. Although all races may be affected, there appears to be some geographic variability in prevalence, with higher rates reported in Southeast Asia and the Middle East.[101] The most distinguishing pathologic feature of the acute lesions of TAO is the apparent initiation of inflammation within the occlusive thrombus and not the vessel wall per se; however, the pathologic findings in more advanced lesions are less characteristic.

Clinical Features. The most common presenting symptoms of TAO are listed in Table 14-9. Claudication may initially be confined to the foot, leading to some diagnostic difficulty.[102] Even if patients present initially with

TABLE 14-9. Clinical Features of TAO[102]

Symptom	Frequency at Presentation (%)
Intermittent claudication	63
Rest pain	81
Ischemic ulcers	76
Superficial thrombophlebitis	38
Raynaud's phenomenon	44
Joint pain	12.5

symptoms in one extremity, angiography of all four limbs should be undertaken to detect asymptomatic lesions; all TAO patients will have involvement of a minimum of two limbs. Digital ischemia leads to ulceration in 76% of patients at presentation;[103] super-infection, necrosis, and digital gangrene can all occur. Superficial thrombophlebitis is common and is, typically recurrent and migratory;[102,103] however, deep venous thrombosis is rare and suggests an alternative diagnosis such as BD. Joint manifestations are common, consisting of transient episodes of a nonerosive, migratory, inflammatory monoarthritis, especially of the wrists or knees.[104] The joint symptoms may be present for an average of 10 years prior to the vascular symptoms, making diagnosis difficult. Systemic symptoms such as fever and weight loss are rare in patients with TAO. TAO may rarely be associated with visceral, coronary, renal, and CNS involvement.[103]

Diagnosis. The diagnosis of TAO can be difficult because of the lack of specific clinical, laboratory, or radiologic findings. Acute phase reactants are typically normal. Typical angiographic findings in TAO include segmental involvement of small and medium arteries (distal to the brachial and popliteal arteries); evidence of multiple vascular occlusions with associated corkscrew collateralization is common. While angiography is essential to diagnose TAO, identical findings may be found in any small vessel occlusive process. Important exclusions include atherosclerosis, exposure to drugs/toxins (e.g., cocaine, amphetamines), diabetes mellitus, hypercoagulable syndromes, embolic disease, hyperviscosity syndromes, systemic autoimmune diseases, cryoglobulinemia, and other primary systemic vasculitides. Although there are pathologic features that help distinguish TAO from other forms of vasculitis,[105] these are not specific. An occlusive thrombus is typically seen, with a nonspecific cellular infiltrate of the thrombus and intima, with relative sparing of the vessel wall, as reflected by the preservation of the internal elastic lamina and lack of fibrinoid necrosis. Linear deposition of immunoglobulin and complement may be found along the internal elastic lamina. Older lesions demonstrate organized thrombus, vessel occlusion with adventitial fibrosis.

Treatment and Prognosis

Physical and Pharmacologic Measures. The most important consideration in the management of patients with TAO is complete cessation of tobacco use. This increases the healing rates of existing ischemic lesions, prevents relapse of disease and can avoid amputation in patients in whom critical limb ischemia is not already present.[100,102] Assiduous wound care is important for management of digital ischemic lesions. Pain control may be difficult, requiring narcotic analgesics or epidural anesthesia in severe cases.

Prostacyclin analog infusions have demonstrated superiority to placebo infusions in controlled studies of TAO patients with ischemic ulcers, resulting in reduced pain, increased rates of healing and lower requirements for amputation.[106] In a randomized controlled trial, low-dose oral iloprost was moderately more effective in terms of pain control and ulcer healing, than either high-dose oral iloprost or placebo.[107] Other pharmacologic agents such as calcium channel blockers, cilostazol, anticoagulants, and plasma expanders have been used, although they are of unproven benefit. Short-term use of nonsteroidal anti-inflammatory drugs (NSAID) may be useful for the treatment of superficial thrombophlebitis. There is no established role for the use of GC or other immunosuppressive agents.

Surgical Management. Amputation is often required for patients with TAO; the 5 and 10 years risk of amputation is 25% and 45%, respectively. The risk of major amputation (above or below the knee, or above the hand) is 4% to 12%. The risk of amputation is 2.73-fold higher in patients that continue to smoke. Surgical procedures aimed at improving vascular flow include bypass procedures and sympathectomy. Because of the multifocal, diffuse and distal nature of the lesions in TAO, surgical revascularization procedures are rarely feasible. Where such procedures have been performed, long-term patency rates are poor, but short-term patency rates were sufficient to allow healing of TAO related ischemic ulcers and limb salvage rates were >90%.[108–110] Sympathectomy has been proposed as a safe and effective method of treatment for TAO;[111] however, a recent controlled study of 200 patients with TAO found that it was inferior to intravenous iloprost therapy for the relief of ischemic pain and ulcer healing.[112] The current role of sympathectomy in TAO is uncertain, but it may be considered as a last resort to avert amputation where other strategies have failed.

There have been reports of epidural spinal cord stimulator implantation in patients with TAO; in one study of 29 patients, marked improvement in regional perfusion was noted, with ulcer healing and good limb survival rates.[113] However, the utility of this approach in the management of patients with TAO is still unclear.

● SMALL VESSEL VASCULITIS

The primary systemic small vessel vasculitides include WG, CSS and MPA. As previously noted, the term small vessel vasculitis is potentially misleading, because each of these conditions can also involve medium-sized vessels. These conditions are also referred by some investigators as antineutrophil cytoplasmic antibody (ANCA)-associated vasculitides (AAV). This term emphasizes the similarities between these conditions including the predominant size of vessel involved, renal histology and association with ANCA. However, because these are usually easily distinguishable diseases, they are considered separately below.

Wegener's Granulomatosis

WG typically targets the upper and lower respiratory tracts and kidneys. It is characterized by granulomatous inflammation and vasculitis affecting small and medium-sized vessels. Estimates of disease prevalence range between 30 and 112 cases per million population; it may present at any age.[114–117]

Clinical Features. The most common initial features of WG are ear, nose, and throat (ENT) symptoms that are unresponsive to conventional therapies for allergy or infection. These may be associated with constitutional symptoms, migratory arthralgias, and myalgias. Over time, other manifestations commonly develop such as lung, renal, skin, neurologic, and cutaneous vasculitic features (Table 14-10).[118–121] However, essentially any organ in the body may be affected in WG; less common sites of disease include the parotid glands, pulmonary artery, breast, penis, urethra, cervix, and vagina.

WG is often referred to in the literature as "generalized" or "limited." The term "generalized" indicates the presence of glomerulonephritis. These are potentially misleading terms because they imply that such subclassification confers stability or clinical characteristics when, in fact, WG often changes and progresses. For example, approximately 20% of patients have glomerulonephritis at onset, but 70% to 80% will develop glomerulonephritis later in the disease course.[117] In addition, the term "limited" may be misleading by suggesting that the disease is mild when involvement of organs such as the CNS, lungs, heart, and gastrointestinal tract can be severe and life-threatening, even in the absence of glomerulonephritis. Therefore, these terms are best avoided.

Recent evidence suggests that there is an increased rate of venous thromboembolic events (VTE) in patients with WG, especially during periods of active disease.[122,123] A rate of seven symptomatic VTE (mainly deep venous thrombosis and pulmonary embolus) per 100 patient years of observation was recorded. This may be an underestimate, as ultrasound to detect asymptomatic thromboses was not performed. Nevertheless, it is significantly greater than the rates seen in patients with SLE, RA, or the general population.[122] These results were corroborated by another recent report that shows an increased rate of VTE in patients with WG, MPA, and renal-limited vasculitis.[123] No evidence of an underlying known thrombophilic disorder was found in patients tested. This has implications for the

TABLE 14-10. Clinical Features of WG[118-121]

Findings	At Diagnosis (%)	Over Disease Course (%)
Upper respiratory tract	73–93	92–99
Sinusitis		
Nasal obstruction, discharge, ulcers, septal perforation, saddle-nose deformity		
Otitis, vertigo, deafness, chondritis		
Oral ulcers, gingivitis, stomatitis		
SGS		
Lung	45–63	53–85
Focal or diffuse infiltrates		
Nodules (may cavitate)		
Pulmonary hemorrhage		
Endobronchial stenoses		
Pleurisy		
Kidney	18–60	70–77
Pauci-immune glomerulonephritis		
Musculoskeletal	20–61	67–77
Arthralgias, myalgias		
Arthritis, myositis		
Ocular	14–40	52–61
Conjunctivitis, uveitis, dacrocystitis, retinitis		
Orbital pseudotumor		
Cutaneous	13–25	33–46
Palpable purpura		
Nodules		
Digital infarcts, gangrene		
Cardiac	5–13	8–25
Pericarditis		
Cardiomyopathy		
Myocardial infarction		
Peripheral nerve	5–21	15–40
Mononeuritis multiplex		
Sensory polyneuropathy		
Cranial neuropathy		
CNS	6	8–11
Mass lesion		
Infarction, hemorrhage		
Meningitis		
Gastrointestinal	3	6–19

carotid intimal–medial thickness.[124,125] Further data is necessary to clearly delineate the magnitude of the risk of atherosclerotic disease in WG, but it is prudent that traditional cardiac risk factors be carefully addressed in WG patients.

Diagnosis. The diagnosis of WG is based on a combination of clinical, laboratory and, if necessary, pathologic features. If a typical clinical picture is associated with a positive ANCA finding with specificity for proteinase 3 (PR3), the diagnosis of WG can be presumed. It remains incumbent for the clinician to be certain that WG "mimics," especially granulomatous infection, are not present. In the setting of only a moderate suspicion of WG and a negative ANCA result, it would be judicious to pursue histologic support for the diagnosis. In the setting of nasal deformity and oral-sinus fistulae cocaine use should be considered, especially in the absence of systemic features of WG.

ANCAs have two distinct patterns: cANCA indicates cytoplasmic staining and refers to a coarse, granular, centrally accentuated, cytoplasmic fluorescence pattern, whereas pANCA refers to a perinuclear fluorescence pattern. The cANCA pattern is usually caused by antibodies against PR3. Antibodies to MPO are the most common cause for pANCA (MPO–ANCA). Approximately 80% to 90% of all ANCA found in WG are cANCA and PR3 specific. Approximately 10% to 20% of ANCA in WG may be pANCA and MPO specific. The sensitivity of PR3–ANCA in WG depends in part on disease severity and activity. Approximately 80% to 95% of patients with severe active disease and from 55% to 75% with milder limited active disease are ANCA-positive.[126] The combined use of indirect immunofluorescence and enzyme-linked immunosorbent assay for identification of antigen results in diagnostic specificity of up to 98%.[127] ANCA is a useful adjunct to clinical diagnosis; however, its presence per se is not diagnostic. ANCA, usually with other than PR3 targeting, may be present in various other diseases including inflammatory bowel disease, autoimmune liver disease, infections, malignancies, rheumatic diseases other than the vasculitides, and other illnesses.[126,127]

The differential diagnosis of WG depends on the clinical presentation. When pulmonary–renal syndrome is the presenting clinical feature, WG needs to be distinguished from antiglomerular basement membrane (GBM) disease, MPA, CSS, and SLE. These features plus a prior or persistent history of upper airway disease and PR3–ANCA positivity make the diagnosis of WG very likely. The presence within a biopsy of granulomatous inflammation, although not an absolute requirement for diagnosis in WG, represents an important distinction between that disease and MPA.[1] Pulmonary nodules are common in WG and can coexist with infiltrates, whereas nodules are almost always absent in anti-GBM disease, SLE, MPA, and CSS.

The renal lesion of WG is that of necrotizing crescentic glomerulonephritis with slight or no immune deposits by immunohistology, and slight or no electron-dense deposits by electron microscopy.[117,128,129] This lesion is clearly

differential diagnosis of pulmonary symptoms in WG patients and complicates the approach to treatment, particularly in the setting of pulmonary hemorrhage.

It has also been postulated that, similar to other rheumatic disorders such as RA and SLE, WG is associated with accelerated atherosclerosis.[124] WG has been associated with surrogate markers of coronary artery disease such as endothelial dysfunction, arterial stiffness, and distinct from immune complex-mediated glomerulonephritis and anti-GBM disease but is not distinguishable from the glomerular lesion of MPA or idiopathic rapidly progressive crescentic glomerulonephritis. The presence of red blood cell casts in the urine sediment can be used as a reliable surrogate marker for the diagnosis of glomerulonephritis and may eliminate the need for renal biopsy in some patients.

The diagnosis may be much less evident in patients with disease limited to ENT symptoms for a prolonged period. In this situation, the diagnosis is usually delayed until the onset of other organ involvement (e.g., lungs or kidneys), or the finding of biopsy features of WG from a surgical procedure. The differential diagnosis of granulomas in ENT biopsies includes chronic infections such as tuberculosis and syphilis, and sarcoidosis. The differential diagnosis of septal perforation is not very broad and includes infections, cocaine use, sarcoidosis, SLE, angiocentric lymphoma, and excessive use of intranasal GC.

Treatment and Prognosis. Untreated systemic WG follows a fulminant course, with a mean survival of 5 months.[130] The major breakthrough in the treatment of WG came with the introduction of a regimen combining daily oral CYC 2 mg/kg/d with prednisone 1 mg/kg/d.[131] In the original regimen developed by Fauci and Wolff, CYC treatment was continued for 12 months beyond remission, after which time it was tapered and discontinued.[132] This regimen dramatically altered the prognosis in WG, with 91% of patients improving significantly, 75% entering complete remission and an 80% survival rate with a mean follow-up of 8 years.[119] However, disease relapsed in 50% of cases that initially entered remission, serious morbidity from irreversible features of disease occurred in 86%, and treatment related toxicity developed in 42% of patients, including infection and cancer (in particular transitional cell carcinoma of the bladder).[120] These data stimulated the search for other treatment strategies that could combine comparable efficacy in remission induction with a lower risk of toxicity and a greater potential for sustained remission.

The use of intermittent intravenous CYC as an alternative to daily oral CYC has been proposed as a strategy to reduce the cumulative CYC dosage and thereby reduce the risk of treatment-related toxicity. Although bladder toxicity may be lessened by the use of intermittent administration, it remains unclear whether this lessens the risk of other CYC toxicities such as infection, infertility, or myelodysplasia. Data from open label studies and a few small randomized controlled trials have demonstrated conflicting findings, but concern remains that intermittent CYC is associated with a higher rate of relapse than daily oral administration.[90,133–135] A large, prospective, randomized, and controlled trial comparing daily oral and pulse intravenous CYC was established to overcome the difficulties in interpreting the existing data.[136] Pending further data, remission induction with daily oral CYC combined

with prednisone remains the approach for which there is the greatest body of evidence for efficacy.

The most recent therapeutic approaches in WG have separated treatment into two phases: induction of remission, followed by maintenance of remission. In most instances, remission induction occurs within 3 to 6 months. While daily CYC continues to be the first-line treatment for remission induction in patients with life- or organ-threatening WG, evidence is accruing to suggest that other agents, such as AZA and MTX, can effectively maintain remission. This facilitates a reduction in the cumulative dose of CYC, thereby limiting the incidence of CYC-induced toxicity. Thus, the option of CYC treatment remains available in the event of any future severe relapse. An unresolved question in the management of WG is the optimal duration of remission maintenance therapy. Given the significant risk of relapse for WG patients, it may be preferable to continue for a period of at least 2 years beyond induction of remission; the decision whether to continue maintenance therapy indefinitely depends on a number of factors such as tolerability, number of prior relapses and patient and physician preferences.

A randomized trial in 155 patients with WG and MPA that compared the use of AZA to daily CYC in the maintenance of remission[82] demonstrated that the relapse rates did not differ significantly between the two groups, and remission was sustained in approximately 85% of patients in each group over the 18-month duration of follow-up. MTX has been investigated as an alternative to CYC in the treatment of WG, both for initial therapy in selected patients[137–140] and for maintenance of disease remission.[141–143] These studies suggested that MTX can be safely and effectively used for remission maintenance in WG once remission has been induced with oral CYC and GC. In addition, MTX can induce remission in patients without life- or organ-threatening disease manifestations, thereby reducing the cumulative exposure to CYC. MTX is contraindicated in patients with significant hepatic, pulmonary or renal impairment, emphasizing the importance of other therapeutic options for such patients.

Other agents for which there is some evidence for efficacy from small studies include mycophenolate mofetil,[144,145] rituximab,[146–148] leflunomide,[149] and IVIG.[150] Larger studies will be needed to confirm the efficacy of these drugs in WG and determine their comparative efficacy against other, more established agents, such a trial is currently in progress for rituximab.

Trimethoprim/Sulfamethoxazole (T/S) monotherapy may have a role to play in the treatment of mild, isolated upper airways disease in WG, but it should not be used for the treatment of more severe disease manifestations. The most important use of T/S in WG is in the prophylaxis against *Pneumocystis carinii* in patients receiving immunosuppressive therapy.

Uncontrolled data have suggested that apheresis techniques may be of benefit for AAV patients with alveolar hemorrhage and/or RPGN.[151,152] As this subset of WG and MPA patients is likely to be at greater risk for complications of plasmapheresis, such as catheter-related sepsis, such techniques should be used with caution in selected patients, as an adjunct to other therapies.

Certain manifestations of WG, such as subglottic stenosis (SGS) and orbital pseudotumor are generally poorly responsive to systemic immunosuppressive therapy; in the absence of active disease affecting major organ sites, SGS is best managed using a combination of mechanical dilatation and intralesional GC injection.[127,153]

Microscopic Polyangiitis

Clinical Features. MPA is a systemic necrotizing small and medium vessel vasculitis in which involvement of pulmonary, renal, and peripheral nerve is the foremost clinical feature (Table 14-11).[154–158] Involvement of the ears, nose, and throat is unexpected, and when present, points instead to a diagnosis of WG.

Diagnosis. The diagnosis of MPA should be considered in any patient with the general features of a systemic vasculitis, such as prolonged unexplained fever, unexplained multisystem organ involvement (especially renal and pulmonary), and palpable purpura. MPA is prominent in the differential of pulmonary–renal syndrome, along with WG, SLE, and anti-GBM disease. MPO–ANCA is present in 60% to 85% of MPA patients, but occasionally, patients may be PR3–ANCA positive.[126] Although the diagnosis of MPA may at times be based on clinical and laboratory findings, it is preferable to obtain pathologic support for the diagnosis; the most common sites for biopsy are skin, kidney, and

TABLE 14-11. Clinical Features of MPA[154–158]

Findings	Prevalence of Finding (%)
Renal	79–100
Pauci-immune glomerulonephritis	
Constitutional	70–79
Fever, malaise, weight loss, fatigue	
Musculoskeletal	53–74
Arthralgias	28–65
Myalgias	25–51
Arthritis	6–32
Cutaneous	35–60
Palpable purpura	40–44
Other (digital infarction, splinter hemorrhages, livedo)	15–20
Pulmonary	25–55
Pulmonary hemorrhage	12–29
Infiltrates	10–30
Pleural effusion	6–19
Gastrointestinal	30–56
Ocular	24–30
Peripheral nerve	14–58
CNS	0–40
Cardiac	3–28

lung. It must be emphasized that in none of the organs is there a specific histopathologic picture of MPA. However, the presence of pulmonary capillaritis, necrotizing pauci-immune glomerulonephritis, or leukocytoclastic vasculitis (LCV) in skin can secure the diagnosis in the setting of a high clinical suspicion of MPA and the exclusion of alternative diagnoses.

The pulmonary histopathology of MPA is that of capillaritis. Characteristically, there is prominent neutrophilic leukocytosis of the alveolar septum, often accompanied by leucocytoclasia. The renal lesion is the same as that found in WG.[159,160]

MPA may be differentiated from classic PAN based on ANCA positivity, glomerular involvement and pulmonary capillary involvement, which are not features of PAN. MPA differs from WG in a number of aspects, including a lack of granuloma formation, absence of ENT involvement, and a predominance of MPO rather than PR3–ANCA antigen specificity.

Treatment and Prognosis. The treatment of MPA is based on the same therapeutic principles as those outlined for WG, not least because it has commonly been studied together with WG.[82] Although, the rate of relapse appears to be lower in MPA than in WG,[82] careful follow-up is critical, including serial monitoring of clinical symptoms and renal function with serial examination of the urinary sediment.

Churg-Strauss Syndrome

CSS is typified by the development of peripheral eosinophilia and eosinophil-rich and granulomatous inflammation involving the respiratory tract and small and medium vessel vasculitis, in patients with a prior history of allergic disease (usually asthma and/or allergic rhinitis).[77,161,162] A link between the use of leukotriene receptor antagonists and CSS has been suggested,[163] but the epidemiologic link between this class of drugs and vasculitis is not proven.[164] Some clinical and pathologic features of CSS are shared with WG and MPA, suggesting a possible pathogenic role for ANCA in CSS. Arguing against such a role is the fact that up to 60% of cases with CSS in some series may be ANCA negative.[165,166] At this point, it would be best to define CSS by its unique clinical and pathologic features, regardless of ANCA status.[167] CSS may involve a wide variety of target organs, including the respiratory tract, skin, heart, skeletal muscle, joints, eye, and GI tract.[162,168] The typical clinical features of CSS are listed in Table 14-12.[169–171]

Diagnosis. Peripheral eosinophilia at levels in excess of 1500 cells/mL^3 often occurs in the prodromal stages of CSS, associated with rhinitis and asthma. Occasionally patients have been described without significant blood eosinophilia but with prominent tissue eosinophilia.[172] There is no definite correlation between eosinophilia and disease activity, and eosinophils rapidly decrease on initiation of GC therapy. ANCA positivity (mostly MPO–ANCA) has been

TABLE 14-12. Clinical Features of CSS[169–171]

Findings	Prevalence of Finding (%)
Respiratory tract	>95
Asthma	>95
Infiltrates	33–72
Sinusitis/polyposis	52–74
Pulmonary hemorrhage	0–8
Nodules (do not cavitate)	Rare
Neurologic	
Peripheral	66–76
Mononeuritis multiplex > Sensory polyneuropathy	6–39
CNS	
Cutaneous	51–70
Palpable purpura, nodules	
Renal (usually mild)	25–58
Musculoskeletal	19–57
Gastrointestinal	13–59
Cardiac	10–49
Pericarditis, cardiomyopathy, myocardial infarction	

reported in approximately 40% of patients.[165,166] Clearly, a negative ANCA test should not dissuade the clinician from the diagnosis of CSS in the presence of typical clinical features.

The diagnosis of CSS should be based on the documentation of vasculitis with eosinophils occurring in a patient with adult-onset asthma or allergic rhinitis. The documentation of the presence of extravascular granulomas is of added specificity, although it is not essential. High-yield sites for biopsy include nerve and muscle if there is clinical evidence of their involvement. CSS shares the same renal lesion (i.e., necrotizing crescentic pauci-immune glomerulonephritis) with WG and MPA.

Treatment and Prognosis. Therapeutic trials in CSS have been limited, but have demonstrated that both GC alone and GC combined with CYC are efficacious.[173,174] The initial approach to treatment of most CSS patients consists of GC monotherapy,[175] a strategy not suitable for WG or MPA.[176,177] While the goal should remain reduction of GC to the lowest possible dose; asthma often limits the ability to stop GC therapy entirely. Daily CYC in combination with GC should be instituted in patients with severe CSS such as that involving the heart, CNS, GI tract, or kidney.[90,175] Uncontrolled studies have suggested benefit with the use of MTX and IVIG in CSS.[178,179] The outcome of patients with CSS is dependent on severity of the disease. In one series,[81] the overall 5-year survival rate for patients with CSS was 78.9%; poor outcomes were associated with the presence of azotemia (creatinine level > 1.58 mg/dL),

proteinuria (> 1 g/d), GI tract involvement, cardiomyopathy, and CNS involvement.

● SECONDARY FORMS OF VASCULITIS

Cutaneous LCV

The nomenclature of cutaneous vasculitis is confusing—various terms such as hypersensitivity vasculitis, allergic vasculitis, LCV, and cutaneous small vessel vasculitis have all been used. LCV refers to the typical underlying histologic findings of polymorphonuclear leucocyte infiltration of postcapillary venules and the presence of nuclear debris.

Clinical Features. The clinical hallmark of cutaneous LCV is palpable purpura—raised, red to violaceous, non-blanching skin lesions caused by extravasation of red blood cells from damaged cutaneous blood vessels (Figure 14-7). Lesions are more common in dependent areas or in areas subjected to mild trauma such as tight-fitting clothing. Lesions typically begin as minute macular petechiae, but may coalesce to form plaque like lesions. Other appearances such as nodules, urticaria, pustules, vesicles, and papules may be seen less frequently. Lesions are typically asymptomatic, but patients may describe pruritis or tenderness. Lesions typically change color from red to purple to brown and slowly resolve over days to weeks; however, postinflammatory hyperpigmentation is common. More severe manifestations such as necrosis and ulceration are unusual and may heal with scarring. Involvement of other organ systems, such as joint, renal, neurologic, or gastrointestinal involvement, mandates careful exclusion of an underlying systemic disorder (see below).

Diagnosis. The clinical and histopathologic features of LCV may be attributable to a wide variety of disorders or inciting agents that must be considered in all cases[180]; these include exposure to drugs or chemicals (10%–45%), infections (10%–36%), malignancy, and systemic inflammatory diseases (reviewed in Ref. 180). The presence of thrombocytopenia and other coagulopathies as a cause of noninflammatory purpura should be excluded also. No underlying etiology is found in more than half of all patients. Many drugs have been implicated, most notably antibiotics such as penicillins and sulfonamides, diuretics, NSAIDs, beta-blockers, allopurinol, propylthiouracil, and oral contraceptives. A careful history of all drug and chemical exposure including topical treatments (e.g., eye drops), nonprescription medication and herbal remedies should be sought. A wide variety of viral, bacterial, rickettsial, mycobacterial, fungal, and parasitic infections may trigger LCV. A recent history of upper respiratory tract infection is common. Myeloproliferative conditions, myelodysplasia, lymphoproliferative malignancies, and solid tumors may be associated with development of LCV and must also be considered in the work-up of such patients.[181] Clinical and laboratory evidence in support of an underlying diagnosis of a systemic

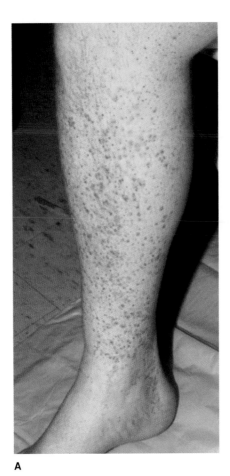

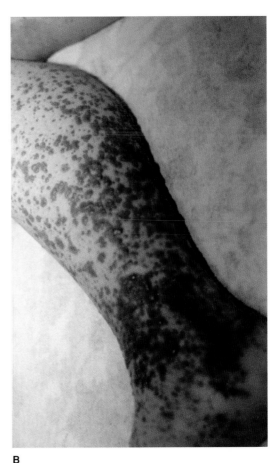

A   B

● **FIGURE 14-7.** Purpuric lesions in patients with cutaneous vasculitis in (A) a patient with lymphoma and (B) blistering lesions in adult onset Henoch-Schönlein purpura.

disorder such as connective tissue disorders and systemic vasculitides should also be sought (see above).

Treatment and Prognosis. The initial management of cutaneous vasculitis centers on the careful exclusion of an underlying trigger or systemic disorder. Where an inciting agent is identified, discontinuation, or avoidance may obviate the requirement for additional therapy. Other treatment options will vary depending on the presence of underlying infection, malignancy or systemic inflammatory diseases. In idiopathic LCV, the most important consideration is that the low morbidity generally associated with isolated cutaneous lesions, and the good long-term prognosis for these patients, should be balanced against the toxicities of potential treatments.[182] Nonpharmacologic strategies should be considered in all patients, including the use of support stockings and avoidance of aggravating factors such as trauma, edema and cold temperatures. There are no evidence-based strategies for the pharmacologic treatment of cutaneous LCV; therefore, for cases without necrotic or ulcerative lesions, treatment is initially attempted with agents with lower toxicity profiles, such as low-dose colchicine, a NSAID, pentoxifylline or hydroxychloroquine. If these agents are ineffective, other therapies such as dapsone or short-term low-dose GC may be considered. Long-term GC and immunosuppressive therapies such as MTX, AZA, and especially CYC, should be used with great reluctance for patients with isolated cutaneous vasculitis because of the unfavorable risk-benefit ratio; such aggressive therapy should be considered only for patients with ulcerative or gangrenous lesions that are severe and refractory to other therapies.[182]

Henoch-Schönlein Purpura

Henoch-Schönlein purpura (HSP) is the most common vasculitis in children, with 50% of cases occurring in children younger than 5 years and 75% in those less than 10 years of age; it can also occur in adulthood. It is generally a benign, self-limited disorder in children; outcomes are less favorable in adults. Up to 50% of cases have a documented history of infection in the days to weeks prior to the onset of HSP;[183,184] the large majority of these are upper respiratory tract infections. The organism most frequently isolated is Streptococcus pyogenes, although a wide variety of other organisms have also been implicated. Vaccination and certain drugs have also been reported to trigger HSP. Other possible associations include drug exposure and underlying malignancy, although these are less frequently observed with HSP as compared to cutaneous LCV. Typical clinical features of HSP are listed in Table 14-13.[185–188]

TABLE 14-13. Clinical Features of Henoch-Schonlein Purpura[185-188]

Findings	Prevalence of Findings (%)
Cutaneous	100
Purpura	
Musculoskeletal	74–82
Arthralgias, nondeforming arthritis	
Gastrointestinal	51–73
Abdominal pain	63
Abdominal bleeding (occult > gross)	18–33
Intestinal obstruction	1
Renal	40–54
Hematuria—microscopic	26–47
Hematuria—gross	<10
Proteinuria	24–42
Other	
Orchitis	4–13
Pulmonary	5
CNS	2–3

Diagnosis. The diagnosis of HSP is made on the basis of typical clinical features and compatible histologic findings of IgA deposition and LCV on skin biopsy.[189] Skin involvement in HSP is clinically and histologically indistinguishable from isolated cutaneous LCV (Figure 14-7); however, IgA deposition on immunofluorescence of skin biopsy specimens is an important means of differentiating these conditions,[77,190] and should prompt a search for occult hematuria and fecal blood in otherwise asymptomatic patients. Biopsy of other tissues (e.g., kidney, bowel) also typically reveals IgA deposition on immunofluorescence. Six grades of HSP glomerulonephritis have been defined on the basis of histologic findings; these correlate with clinical outcomes.[191,192] Elevation of acute phase reactants, leukocyte count and platelet count is common; reduced hematocrit points to the presence of gastrointestinal (or rarely pulmonary) hemorrhage. Elevated serum IgA may be found in a minority of patients.[193,194] Laboratory testing can be useful to differentiate HSP from other systemic autoimmune diseases; however, these distinctions are usually obvious based on clinical assessment. Serologic testing for ANA and ANCA should be negative, serum C3, C4, and CH50 are typically normal.

Treatment and Prognosis. In most cases, HSP is a self-limiting disease and supportive care only is required. Although recurrence of HSP is common, relapses tend to be less severe than the initial episode. NSAIDs may be used to treat joint pain, but should be avoided in patients with renal involvement. GCs are often used for more severe bowel, renal and rare pulmonary manifestations. The role of additional immunosuppressive therapies such as in IVIG, AZA, MTX, or CYC is unclear, these are generally reserved for severe or refractory disease. The prognosis of HSP depends largely on the degree of renal involvement; however, most patients have a full recovery of renal function.[195,196]

Cryoglobulinemic Vasculitis

Cryoglobulins are immunoglobulins that precipitate when maintained at reduced temperatures. The association of cryoglobulinemia with lymphoproliferative disorders and autoimmune diseases has long been recognized;[197,198] "essential mixed cryoglobulinemia" was the term used to refer to unexplained cases of cryoglobulinemia.[198] However, since the initial description of the association of HCV infection and cryoglobulinemia,[199] it has become apparent that HCV is the underlying cause of most cases of essential mixed cryoglobulinemia.[200,201] Many other infections have been also been sporadically associated with cryoglobulinemia.[200-202]

Three main types are described[203]—type I are monoclonal immunoglobulins, type II are monoclonal immunoglobulins with rheumatoid factor (RF) activity complexed to polyclonal immunoglobulins and type III are complexes of polyclonal immunoglobulins, some of which have RF activity. Type I (less commonly type II) cryoglobulins are associated with lymphoproliferative disorders such as multiple myeloma, lymphoma and Waldenstrom's macroglobulinemia; cryoglobulins associated with systemic autoimmune diseases (e.g., SLE, RA, Sjögren's syndrome) and chronic infections (e.g., HCV, subacute bacterial endocarditis, Epstein-Barr virus, cytomegalovirus) are either type II or type III.

The clinical manifestations of cryoglobulinemic vasculitis can vary depending on the underlying cause; the most common clinical features are listed in Table 14-14.[198,204-206] Cutaneous ulceration may be chronic; although ulcers typically develop around the malleoli, digital ulceration of upper and lower limbs may also occur. Renal involvement is typically mild, characterized by

TABLE 14-14. Clinical Features of Cryoglobulinemic Vasculitis[204-206]

Findings	Prevalence of Findings (%)
Cutaneous	
Purpura	73–95
Leg ulcers	4–8
Raynaud's phenomenon	7–31
Musculoskeletal	
Arthralgia/myalgia	33–90
Arthritis	10
Neurologic	12–69
Peripheral sensorimotor polyneuropathy	
Renal	8–33
Renal insufficiency	Rare
Others	
Cardiac, pulmonary, gastrointestinal	Rare

abnormalities of urinary sediment, without progression to renal insufficiency.[207] In a small percentage of patients, acute nephritic or nephrotic syndromes may occur and progress to renal failure, and rarely, death.[208]

Diagnosis. Diagnosis of cryoglobulinemia can readily be made, once clinical suspicion has led to the performance of appropriate laboratory testing. Detection of cryoglobulins requires collection, transport and storage of specimens at 37°C; if samples have cooled sufficiently to allow precipitation of cryoglobulins prior to centrifugation, a false-negative result will be obtained. However, the finding of elevated serum cryoglobulins alone is not sufficient to make the diagnosis of cryoglobulinemic vasculitis. Low C4 complement levels and a positive RF reflect ongoing immune complex activation. Pathologic specimens commonly show vasculitis, mainly affecting small, or less commonly medium sized vessels; skin biopsy of purpuric lesions most commonly reveals evidence of LCV. Immunofluorescence and electron microscopy can demonstrate immune deposits. Histologically, renal involvement is characterized by membrano-proliferative glomerulonephritis. The diagnosis of cryoglobulinemic vasculitis mandates a search for underlying causes, such as connective tissue disorders, lymphoproliferative syndromes and infectious causes, especially HCV and other chronic viral infections.

Treatment and Prognosis. There are no controlled therapeutic trials to guide the therapy of cryoglobulinemic vasculitis; key factors determining the approach to therapy include the severity of disease manifestations and the presence of an underlying disorder. Where an underlying condition can be identified, management is aimed at eliminating or controlling that underlying cause, for example, antiviral therapy for HCV. However, for patients in whom an underlying cause cannot be identified, or in whom efforts to control the underlying disease are unsuccessful, immunosuppressive therapy may be required, depending on the severity of clinical involvement.[207] GCs should be used judiciously, with higher doses being reserved for major disease complications, such as progressive renal disease, neuropathy, and refractory cutaneous ulcers. Other therapeutic options, such as IVIG and apheresis, may be of benefit based on uncontrolled studies; apheresis can provide temporary benefit, but must be combined with other strategies to provide more durable disease control. Rituximab, an anti-CD20 monoclonal antibody, has shown encouraging results in recent uncontrolled series.[209–211] Cytotoxic agents should be reserved for severe disease refractory to other agents.

● VASCULITIS ASSOCIATED WITH OTHER RHEUMATIC DISEASES

The occurrence of vasculitis is well described in rheumatic diseases such as RA, and other systemic autoimmune diseases[212] such as SLE, Sjögren's syndrome, idiopathic inflammatory myositis, systemic sclerosis, seronegative spondyloarthropathies, and relapsing polychondritis.[213] Vasculitis in these diseases may affect vessels of any size.[214,215] However, they rarely occur in the absence of characteristic features of the underlying rheumatic disorder, and therefore can usually be readily differentiated from primary vasculitic disorders on clinical grounds alone. Rheumatoid vasculitis is the best defined of these secondary vasculitides and is discussed below.

Rheumatoid Vasculitis

Rheumatoid vasculitis typically occurs in patients with longstanding, erosive RA that are strongly positive for RF, and have a high prevalence of rheumatoid nodules and other extra-articular manifestations.[216–218] The prevalence of rheumatoid vasculitis seems to have diminished in recent years;[219] this may reflect the more aggressive approach to treatment of RA. While any vessel size may be involved, small and/or medium vessel vasculitis are most common. Digital or nailfold infarcts are relatively benign, but more severe disease may be manifested by deep ulcerative lesions (usually on distal lower extremities) (Figure 14-8), gangrene, peripheral neuropathy, ocular, cardiac, and/or mesenteric vasculitis. Vasculitic involvement of lung and kidneys is rare. Constitutional symptoms, in particular weight loss and fatigue, are common, but may be multifactorial in patients with severe RA. The diagnosis is based on findings, in a patient with long-standing, severe RA, of typical clinical signs of vasculitis (e.g., unexplained cutaneous infarcts, palpable purpura, or neuropathy), with or without biopsy proof of vasculitis.

Minor degrees of vasculitis, such as isolated nailfold infarcts do not require specific therapy.[220] However, patients with visceral involvement, scleritis, or ulcerative keratitis, digital ischemia, severe cutaneous ulceration, or vasculitic neuropathy require combination therapy with high-dose GC and CYC.[221–223] AZA is an acceptable alternative for milder disease and for remission maintenance;[222] the successful use of anti-TNF agents has been reported in small numbers of refractory cases,[224,225] but their role remains to be clarified. Their use is complicated by anti-TNF agents having been implicated in producing autoimmune complications including positive ANAs, anti-dsDNA, polyarthritis and even vasculitis.

Behçet's Disease

BD is a multisystem disorder initially described as a triad of recurrent ulceration of the oral and genital mucosa and relapsing uveitis; however, it is now appreciated that BD may affect virtually any organ or tissue. Common clinical features of BD are listed in Table 14-15.[226–228]

Vasculitis is thought to be responsible for the clinical features of BD, which may affect arteries and/or veins of all sizes. While small vessel involvement predominates, large vessel vasculitis is seen in up to one third of BD patients.[229–233] Patients with involvement of large vessels in one area are more likely to have similar involvement in

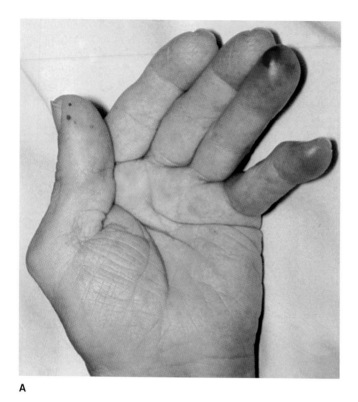

A

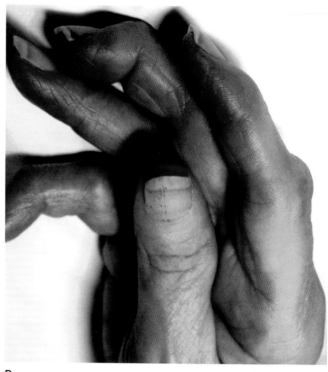

B

● **FIGURE 14-8.** Digital purpuric lesions in a patient with RA and subacute bacterial endocarditis (A). Digital ischemic and nailbed lesions in a patient with rheumatoid vasculitis (B).

other parts of the circulation (Figure 14-9). Aneurysm formation in BD occurs more often in the abdominal aorta, lower extremity vessels and pulmonary arteries, but any vessel may be affected.[232,234,235] Arterial obstruction may be caused by either thrombosis or stenosis. Thrombotic and inflammatory occlusion of large veins may include the vena cava. While large vessel vasculitis in BD can mimic TAK,[236] there appears to be a greater incidence of aneurysms in BD; other features to suggest BD rather than TAK include oral, genital and enteric mucosal ulcers, a strong predilection for young males and the presence of venous thromboses and/or migratory superficial thrombophlebitis.

The approach to treatment of large vessel vasculitis in BD is similar to that described above for TAK. Surgical intervention is frequently complicated by a "pathergic" response leading to exacerbations of disease, graft occlusion and/or anastomotic aneurysms.[235,237] This emphasizes the particular importance of controlling inflammation preoperatively in BD patients. Endovascular repair techniques have been used in an attempt to limit the morbidity and mortality associated with surgical procedures. A number of reports attest to the potential efficacy and safety of these techniques in BD patients;[238–242] however, more information is required regarding the long-term outcomes before such approaches can be routinely recommended for vascular lesions in BD.

Cogan's Syndrome

CS is a rare inflammatory disorder that predominantly affects young adults.[243] Onset of disease frequently occurs in the aftermath of an upper respiratory tract infection. It is characterized by the presence of ocular inflammation (classically interstitial keratitis) and audiovestibular dysfunction; in typical cases, these occur within a 2-year period of each other. While these two cardinal disease features are thought to be a consequence of nonvasculitic inflammation, they are accompanied by a systemic vasculitis in up to 15% of cases. While this is typically a large vessel vasculitis resembling TAK, small to medium vessel involvement has also been described.[244]

TABLE 14-15. Common Clinical Features of Behcet's Disease[226–228]

Findings	Prevalence of Findings (%)
Oral ulceration	96–100
Cutaneous lesions	73–94
Genital ulceration	72–79
Ocular involvement	48–75
Positive pathergy test	30–75
Arthritis	47–59
Large vessel vasculitis	7–38
Epididymitis	6–32
Gastrointestinal involvement	3–25
CNS involvement	8–20

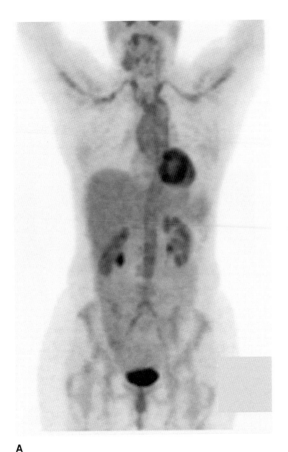

A

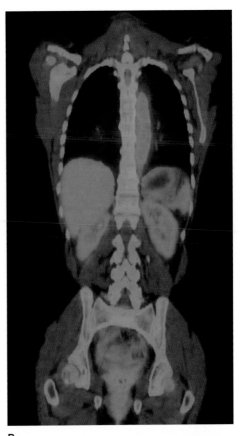

B

C

● **FIGURE 14-9.** Active large vessels vasculitis in a patient with BD assessed by (A) FDG-PET and (B and C) combined CT of the body with FDG-PET. (A) Increased isotope uptake can be seen in the aortic arch and both subclavian and axillary arteries. (B and C) Involvement of the entire aorta is evident on combined PET-CT imaging.

There are no controlled trials to guide treatment of CS. Eye disease, depending on severity, may be managed with topical or systemic GC.[245] Systemic therapy is required for audiovestibular and systemic manifestations and severe eye disease. Prompt treatment with GC may ameliorate hearing loss in addition to other clinical features.[246] Although additional immunosuppressive therapies such as CYC, MTX, AZA, and cyclosporine have been frequently employed, there is insufficient evidence to evaluate their efficacy. Cochlear implants may improve quality of life in patients with permanent hearing loss.

Sarcoidosis

Sarcoidosis is a multisystem disorder, the histologic hallmark of which is noncaseating granulomatous inflammation. Less often, patients may develop necrotizing granulomatous lesions. While pulmonary involvement is most frequent, any tissue in the body may be affected. Large, medium, and small vessel vasculitis have all been reported[247] in sarcoidosis (reviewed in Ref. 247). The diagnosis of sarcoidosis can generally be made on the basis of associated clinical findings such as hilar adenopathy, erythema nodosum, arthritis/periarthritis, and uveitis. Demonstration of well-formed noncaseating granulomata on histologic examination of extravascular tissue may be helpful. GC and cytotoxic therapies appear to be of benefit in sarcoid vasculitis, but relapses are common.[247] Surgical intervention may be required in selected cases.

● VASCULITIS ASSOCIATED WITH INFECTION

Infection is important in the differential diagnosis for all patients with suspected vasculitis, as many infections can mimic the presenting features of almost all forms of vasculitis. In addition, a wide variety of infectious organisms have been associated with the development of true vasculitis, making histologic interpretation difficult. In suspected cases of systemic vasculitis, infectious etiologies should be considered and ideally excluded prior to initiation of aggressive immunosuppressive therapy. Furthermore, as many systemic infections may improve transiently with immunosuppressive therapy, patients should be re-evaluated for possible underlying infection, if they develop early "relapse" of vasculitis, despite aggressive immunosuppression. In cases where the weight of evidence favors a primary vasculitis, or vasculitis caused by another rheumatic disease, severe illness often forces the use of aggressive immunosuppressive therapy; when such therapy is initiated, infection should concurrently be ruled out.

Chronic viral infections are an important exclusion for all patients with vasculitis.[248] HBV can cause small and/or medium vessel vasculitis that resembles MPA or PAN, as discussed above. HCV is a common cause of cryoglobulinemic vasculitis. Human immunodeficiency virus (HIV) may lead to small, medium or large vessel vasculitis;[249] potential mechanisms include opportunistic infection, malignancy, drug reactions or direct effects of the HIV virus itself. Many other viruses, including cytomegalovirus, Epstein-Barr virus, varicella-zoster virus and parvovirus B19 have all been associated with small or medium vessel vasculitis syndromes. Rickettsial infections may also be associated with vasculitis, most commonly small vessel cutaneous vasculitis.

Infective endocarditis can also result in a clinical picture resembling small-medium vessel vasculitis, caused by either embolic events and/or immune complex deposition (Figure 14-8A). Features include digital infarction, palpable purpura, cutaneous nodules or ulcers, glomerulonephritis and stroke.[250] Endocarditis may be particularly difficult to distinguish from systemic inflammatory disorders as it may be associated with positive tests for autoantibodies such as ANA and ANCA.

Acute infectious processes should be suspected in patients with aortic aneurysm and/or a cardiac murmur and fever; septicemia and endocarditis are important considerations in such settings. Bacterial infection may cause infection in pre-existing aortic aneurysms or be associated with mycotic aneurysm formation. In such cases blood cultures and echocardiography are essential. The presence of chronic infections such as syphilis, tuberculosis, fungal infections and HIV infection must also be considered in patients with aortitis;[248] diagnostic tests include blood cultures, serologic tests and tuberculin skin testing. However, it should be noted that serologic studies may be negative in tertiary syphilis. Appropriate staining and culture of aortic tissue should be undertaken if tissue is available. Other infectious causes such as leprosy should be considered in patients from endemic areas.

REFERENCES

1. Jennette JC, Falk RJ, Andrassy K, et al. Nomenclature of systemic vasculitides. Proposal of an international consensus conference. *Arthritis Rheum.* 1994;37:187-192.

2. Stone JH, Calabrese LH, Hoffman GS, et al. Vasculitis. A collection of pearls and myths. *Rheum Dis Clin North Am.* 2001;27:677-728.

3. Lie JT. Systemic and isolated vasculitis. A rational approach to classification and pathologic diagnosis. *Pathol Annu.* 1989;24(pt 1):25-114.

4. Lie JT, Brown AL Jr, Carter ET. Spectrum of aging changes in temporal arteries. Its significance, in interpretation of biopsy of temporal artery. *Arch Pathol.* 1970;90:278-285.

5. Kerr GS, Hallahan CW, Giordano J, et al. Takayasu arteritis. *Ann Intern Med.* 1994;120:919-929.

6. Steeds RP, Mohiaddin R. Takayasu arteritis: role of cardiovascular magnetic imaging. *Int J Cardiol.* 2006;109:1-6.

7. Tso E, Flamm SD, White RD, et al. Takayasu arteritis: utility and limitations of magnetic resonance imaging in

diagnosis and treatment. *Arthritis Rheum.* 2002;46:1634-1642.

8. Kobayashi Y, Ishii K, Oda K, et al. Aortic wall inflammation due to Takayasu arteritis imaged with 18F-FDG PET coregistered with enhanced CT. *J Nucl Med.* 2005;46:917-922.

9. Lhote F, Cohen P, Guillevin L. Polyarteritis nodosa, microscopic polyangiitis and Churg-Strauss syndrome. *Lupus.* 1998;7:238-258.

10. Koening CL, Langford CA. Novel therapeutic strategies for large vessel vasculitis. *Rheum Dis Clin North Am.* 2006;32:173-186.

11. Hunder GG. Giant cell arteritis and polymyalgia rheumatica. *Med Clin North Am.* 1997;81:195-219.

12. Salvarani C, Cantini F, Boiardi L, et al. Polymyalgia rheumatica and giant-cell arteritis. *N Engl J Med.* 2002;347:261-271.

13. Tamura Y, Okinaga H, Takami H. Glucocorticoid-induced osteoporosis. *Biomed Pharmacother.* 2004;58:500-504.

14. González-Gay MA, Miranda-Filloy JA, Lopez-Diaz MJ, et al. Giant cell arteritis in northwestern Spain: a 25-year epidemiologic study. *Medicine (Baltimore).* 2007;86:61-68.

15. Cid MC, Hernández-Rodríguez J, Grau JM. Vascular manifestations in giant-cell arteritis. In: Asherson RA, Cervera R, eds. *Vascular Manifestations of Systemic Autoimmune Diseases.* Boca Raton, FL: CRC Press; 2001:237-249.

16. Cid MC, Font C, Coll-Vinent B, et al. Large vessel vasculitides. *Curr Opin Rheumatol.* 1998;10:18-28.

17. Rodríguez-Pla A, Stone JH. Vasculitis and systemic infections. *Curr Opin Rheumatol.* 2006;18:39-47.

18. Arnaud L, Kahn JE, Girszyn N, et al. Takayasu's arteritis: an update on physiopathology. *Eur J Intern Med.* 2006;17:241-246.

19. Cid MC, Hoffman MP, Hernández-Rodríguez J, et al. Association between increased CCL2 (MCP-1) expression in lesions and persistence of disease activity in giant-cell arteritis. *Rheumatology (Oxford).* 2006;45:1356-1363.

20. Hernández-Rodríguez J, Segarra M, Vilardell C, et al. Tissue production of pro-inflammatory cytokines (IL-1beta, TNFalpha and IL-6) correlates with the intensity of the systemic inflammatory response and with corticosteroid requirements in giant-cell arteritis. *Rheumatology (Oxford).* 2004;43:294-301.

21. Segarra M, García-Martínez A, Sánchez M, et al. Leukocyte integrin alpha4 is associated with gelatinase (MMP2 and MMP9) and MMP14 expression and activity in giant-cell arteritis (GCA) lesions. *Arthritis Rheum.* 2006;54(suppl):S578.

22. Tripathy NK, Gupta PC, Nityanand S. High TNF-alpha and low IL-2 producing T cells characterize active disease in Takayasu's arteritis. *Clin Immunol.* 2006;118:154-158.

23. Wagner AD, Bjornsson J, Bartley GB, et al. Interferon-gamma-producing T cells in giant cell vasculitis represent a minority of tissue-infiltrating cells and are located distant from the site of pathology. *Am J Pathol.* 1996;148:1925-1933.

24. Weyand CM, Tetzlaff N, Bjornsson J, et al. Disease patterns and tissue cytokine profiles in giant cell arteritis. *Arthritis Rheum.* 1997;40:19-26.

25. Cid MC, Font C, Oristrell J, et al. Association between strong inflammatory response and low risk of developing visual loss and other cranial ischemic complications in giant cell (temporal) arteritis. *Arthritis Rheum.* 1998;41:26-32.

26. González-Gay MA, Blanco R, Rodríguez-Valverde V, et al. Permanent visual loss and cerebrovascular accidents in giant cell arteritis: predictors and response to treatment. *Arthritis Rheum.* 1998;41:1497-1504.

27. Ostberg G. Morphological changes in the large arteries in polymyalgia arteritica. *Acta Med Scand Suppl.* 1972;533:135-159.

28. Evans JM, Bowles CA, Bjornsson J, et al. Thoracic aortic aneurysm and rupture in giant cell arteritis. A descriptive study of 41 cases. *Arthritis Rheum.* 1994;37:1539-1547.

29. González-Gay MA, García-Porrua C, Pineiro A, et al. Aortic aneurysm and dissection in patients with biopsy-proven giant cell arteritis from northwestern Spain: a population-based study. *Medicine (Baltimore).* 2004;83:335-341.

30. Nuenninghoff DM, Hunder GG, Christianson TJ, et al. Incidence and predictors of large-artery complication (aortic aneurysm, aortic dissection, and/or large-artery stenosis) in patients with giant cell arteritis: a population-based study over 50 years. *Arthritis Rheum.* 2003;48:3522-3531.

31. García-Martínez A, Hernández-Rodríguez J, Arguis P, et al. Development of aortic aneurysm/dilatation during the followup of patients with giant cell arteritis: a cross-sectional screening of fifty-four prospectively followed patients. *Arthritis Rheum.* 2008;59:422-430.

32. Hernández-Rodríguez J, García-Martínez A, Casademont J, et al. A strong initial systemic inflammatory response is associated with higher corticosteroid requirements and longer duration of therapy in patients with giant-cell arteritis. *Arthritis Rheum.* 2002;47:29-35.

33. Coll-Vinent B, Vilardell C, Font C, et al. Circulating soluble adhesion molecules in patients with giant cell arteritis. Correlation between soluble intercellular adhesion molecule-1 (sICAM-1) concentrations and disease activity. *Ann Rheum Dis.* 1999;58:189-192.

34. Cid MC, Monteagudo J, Oristrell J, et al. Von Willebrand factor in the outcome of temporal arteritis. *Ann Rheum Dis.* 1996;55:927-930.

35. Lie JT. Illustrated histopathologic classification criteria for selected vasculitis syndromes. American College of rheumatology subcommittee on classification of vasculitis. *Arthritis Rheum.* 1990;33:1074-1087.

36. Hunder GG, Bloch DA, Michel BA, et al. The American college of rheumatology 1990 criteria for the classification of giant cell arteritis. *Arthritis Rheum.* 1990;33:1122-1128.

37. Auzary C, Le Thi Huong D, Delarbre X, et al. Subacute bacterial endocarditis presenting as polymyalgia rheumatica or giant cell arteritis. *Clin Exp Rheumatol.* 2006;24:S38-S40.

38. Salvarani C, Gabriel SE, Gertz MA, et al. Primary systemic amyloidosis presenting as giant cell arteritis and polymyalgia rheumatica. *Arthritis Rheum.* 1994;37:1621-1626.

39. Karahaliou M, Vaiopoulos G, Papaspyrou S, et al. Colour duplex sonography of temporal arteries before decision for biopsy: a prospective study in 55 patients with suspected giant cell arteritis. *Arthritis Res Ther.* 2006;8:R116.

40. Lie JT. When is arteritis of the temporal arteries not temporal arteritis? *J Rheumatol*. 1994;21:186-189.

41. Esteban MJ, Font C, Hernández-Rodríguez J, et al. Small-vessel vasculitis surrounding a spared temporal artery: clinical and pathological findings in a series of twenty-eight patients. *Arthritis Rheum*. 2001;44:1387-1395.

42. Genereau T, Lortholary O, Pottier MA, et al. Temporal artery biopsy: a diagnostic tool for systemic necrotizing vasculitis. French Vasculitis Study Group. *Arthritis Rheum*. 1999;42:2674-2681.

43. LeSar CJ, Meier GH, DeMasi RJ, et al. The utility of color duplex ultrasonography in the diagnosis of temporal arteritis. *J Vasc Surg*. 2002;36:1154-1160.

44. Nesher G, Shemesh D, Mates M, et al. The predictive value of the halo sign in color Doppler ultrasonography of the temporal arteries for diagnosing giant cell arteritis. *J Rheumatol*. 2002;29:1224-1226.

45. Hoffman GS, Cid MC, Hellmann DB, et al. A multicenter, randomized, double-blind, placebo-controlled trial of adjuvant methotrexate treatment for giant cell arteritis. *Arthritis Rheum*. 2002;46:1309-1318.

46. Jover JA, Hernández-García C, Morado IC, et al. Combined treatment of giant-cell arteritis with methotrexate and prednisone. A randomized, double-blind, placebo-controlled trial. *Ann Intern Med*. 2001;134:106-114.

47. Hoffman GS, Cid MC, Rendt-Zagar KE, et al. Infliximab for maintenance of glucocorticosteroid-induced remission of giant cell arteritis: a randomized trial. *Ann Intern Med*. 2007;146:621-630.

48. Lee MS, Smith SD, Galor A, et al. Antiplatelet and anticoagulant therapy in patients with giant cell arteritis. *Arthritis Rheum*. 2006;54:3306-3309.

49. Nesher G, Berkun Y, Mates M, et al. Low-dose aspirin and prevention of cranial ischemic complications in giant cell arteritis. *Arthritis Rheum*. 2004;50:1332-1337.

50. García-Martínez A, Hernández-Rodríguez J, Grau JM, et al. Treatment with statins does not exhibit a clinically relevant corticosteroid-sparing effect in patients with giant cell arteritis. *Arthritis Rheum*. 2004;51:674-678.

51. Scheel AK, Meller J, Vosshenrich R, et al. Diagnosis and follow up of aortitis in the elderly. *Ann Rheum Dis*. 2004;63:1507-1510.

52. Both M, Aries PM, Muller-Hulsbeck S, et al. Balloon angioplasty of arteries of the upper extremities in patients with extracranial giant-cell arteritis. *Ann Rheum Dis*. 2006;65:1124-1130.

53. Isselbacher EM. Thoracic and abdominal aortic aneurysms. *Circulation*. 2005;111:816-828.

54. González-Gay MA, Blanco R, Abraira V, et al. Giant cell arteritis in Lugo, Spain, is associated with low longterm mortality. *J Rheumatol*. 1997;24:2171-2176.

55. Uddhammar A, Eriksson AL, Nystrom L, et al. Increased mortality due to cardiovascular disease in patients with giant cell arteritis in northern Sweden. *J Rheumatol*. 2002;29:737-742.

56. Hoffman GS, Merkel PA, Brasington RD, et al. Anti-tumor necrosis factor therapy in patients with difficult to treat Takayasu arteritis. *Arthritis Rheum*. 2004;50:2296-2304.

57. Tripathy NK, Chauhan SK, Nityanand S. Cytokine mRNA repertoire of peripheral blood mononuclear cells in Takayasu's arteritis. *Clin Exp Immunol*. 2004;138:369-374.

58. Park MC, Lee SW, Park YB, et al. Serum cytokine profiles and their correlations with disease activity in Takayasu's arteritis. *Rheumatology (Oxford)*. 2006;45:545-548.

59. Maksimowicz-McKinnon K, Clark TM, Hoffman GS. Limitations of therapy and a guarded prognosis in an American cohort of Takayasu arteritis patients. *Arthritis Rheum*. 2007;56:1000-1009.

60. Vanoli M, Daina E, Salvarani C, et al. Takayasu's arteritis: a study of 104 Italian patients. *Arthritis Rheum*. 2005;53:100-107.

61. Lupi-Herrera E, Sanchez-Torres G, Marcushamer J, et al. Takayasu's arteritis. Clinical study of 107 cases. *Am Heart J*. 1977;93:94-103.

62. Jain S, Kumari S, Ganguly NK, et al. Current status of Takayasu arteritis in India. *Int J Cardiol*. 1996;54(suppl): S111-S116.

63. Chun YS, Park SJ, Park IK, et al. The clinical and ocular manifestations of Takayasu arteritis. *Retina*. 2001;21:132-140.

64. Manganelli P, Fietta P, Carotti M, et al. Respiratory system involvement in systemic vasculitides. *Clin Exp Rheumatol*. 2006;24:S48-S59.

65. Yamada I, Shibuya H, Matsubara O, et al. Pulmonary artery disease in Takayasu's arteritis: angiographic findings. *AJR Am J Roentgenol*. 1992;159:263-269.

66. Maksimowicz-McKinnon K, Hoffman GS. Large-vessel vasculitis. *Semin Respir Crit Care Med*. 2004;25:569-579.

67. Werfel T, Kuipers JG, Zeidler H, et al. Cutaneous manifestations of Takayasu arteritis. *Acta Derm Venereol*. 1996;76:496-497.

68. Hoffman GS, Ahmed AE. Surrogate markers of disease activity in patients with Takayasu arteritis. A preliminary report from The International Network for the Study of the Systemic Vasculitides (INSSYS). *Int J Cardiol*. 1998;66(suppl 1):S191-S194.

69. Liang P, Hoffman GS. Advances in the medical and surgical treatment of Takayasu arteritis. *Curr Opin Rheumatol*. 2005;17:16-24.

70. Hoffman GS. Takayasu arteritis: lessons from the American National Institutes of Health experience. *Int J Cardiol*. 1996;54(suppl):S99-S102.

71. Molloy ES, Langford CA, Clark TM, Gota CE, Hoffman GS. Antitumor necrosis factor therapy in patients with refractory Takayasu's arteritis: long-term follow-up. *Ann Rheum Dis*. 2008 [Epub ahead of print].

72. Tanaka F, Kawakami A, Iwanaga N, et al. Infliximab is effective for Takayasu arteritis refractory to glucocorticoid and methotrexate. *Intern Med*. 2006;45:313-316.

73. Liang P, Tan-Ong M, Hoffman GS. Takayasu's arteritis: vascular interventions and outcomes. *J Rheumatol*. 2004;31:102-106.

74. Miyata T, Sato O, Koyama H, et al. Long-term survival after surgical treatment of patients with Takayasu's arteritis. *Circulation*. 2003;108:1474-1480.

75. Lagneau P, Michel JB, Vuong PN. Surgical treatment of Takayasu's disease. *Ann Surg.* 1987;205:157-166.

76. Park MC, Lee SW, Park YB, et al. Clinical characteristics and outcomes of Takayasu's arteritis: analysis of 108 patients using standardized criteria for diagnosis, activity assessment, and angiographic classification. *Scand J Rheumatol.* 2005;34:284-292.

77. Jennette JC, Falk RJ, Andrassy K, et al. Nomenclature of systemic vasculitides. Proposal of an international consensus conference. *Arthritis Rheum* 1994;37:187-192.

78. Lhote F, Guillevin L. Polyarteritis nodosa, microscopic polyangiitis, and Churg-Strauss syndrome. Clinical aspects and treatment. *Rheum Dis Clin North Am.* 1995;21:911-947.

79. Pagnoux C, Mahr A, Cohen P, et al. Presentation and outcome of gastrointestinal involvement in systemic necrotizing vasculitides: analysis of 62 patients with polyarteritis nodosa, microscopic polyangiitis, Wegener granulomatosis, Churg-Strauss syndrome, or rheumatoid arthritis-associated vasculitis. *Medicine (Baltimore).* 2005;84:115-128.

80. Selga D, Mohammad A, Sturfelt G, et al. Polyarteritis nodosa when applying the Chapel Hill nomenclature—a descriptive study on ten patients. *Rheumatology (Oxford).* 2006;45:1276-1281.

81. Guillevin L, Lhote F, Gayraud M, et al. Prognostic factors in polyarteritis nodosa and Churg-Strauss syndrome. A prospective study in 342 patients. *Medicine (Baltimore).* 1996;75:17-28.

82. Jayne D, Rasmussen N, Andrassy K, et al. A randomized trial of maintenance therapy for vasculitis associated with antineutrophil cytoplasmic autoantibodies. *N Engl J Med.* 2003;349:36-44.

83. Coll-Vinent B, Cebrian M, Cid MC, et al. Dynamic pattern of endothelial cell adhesion molecule expression in muscle and perineural vessels from patients with classic polyarteritis nodosa. *Arthritis Rheum.* 1998;41:435-444.

84. Albert DA, Silverstein MD, Paunicka K, et al. The diagnosis of polyarteritis nodosa. II. Empirical verification of a decision analysis model. *Arthritis Rheum.* 1988;31:1128-1134.

85. Albert DA, Rimon D, Silverstein MD. The diagnosis of polyarteritis nodosa. I. A literature-based decision analysis approach. *Arthritis Rheum.* 1988;31:1117-1127.

86. Guillevin L. Treatment of classic polyarteritis nodosa in 1999. *Nephrol Dial Transplant.* 1999;14:2077-2079.

87. Guillevin L, Cohen P, Mahr A, et al. Treatment of polyarteritis nodosa and microscopic polyangiitis with poor prognosis factors: a prospective trial comparing glucocorticoids and six or twelve cyclophosphamide pulses in sixty-five patients. *Arthritis Rheum.* 2003;49:93-100.

88. Guillevin L, Lhote F, Jarrousse B, et al. Treatment of polyarteritis nodosa and Churg-Strauss syndrome. A meta-analysis of 3 prospective controlled trials including 182 patients over 12 years. *Ann Med Interne (Paris).* 1992;143:405-416.

89. Bourgarit A, Le Toumelin P, Pagnoux C, et al. Deaths occurring during the first year after treatment onset for polyarteritis nodosa, microscopic polyangiitis, and Churg-Strauss syndrome: a retrospective analysis of causes and factors predictive of mortality based on 595 patients. *Medicine (Baltimore).* 2005;84:323-330.

90. Gayraud M, Guillevin L, le Toumelin P, et al. Long-term followup of polyarteritis nodosa, microscopic polyangiitis, and Churg-Strauss syndrome: analysis of four prospective trials including 278 patients. *Arthritis Rheum.* 2001;44:666-675.

91. Newburger JW, Takahashi M, Gerber MA, et al. Diagnosis, treatment, and long-term management of Kawasaki disease: a statement for health professionals from the Committee on Rheumatic Fever, Endocarditis, and Kawasaki Disease, Council on Cardiovascular Disease in the Young, American Heart Association. *Pediatrics.* 2004;114:1708-1733.

92. Hui-Yuen JS, Duong TT, Yeung RS. TNF-alpha is necessary for induction of coronary artery inflammation and aneurysm formation in an animal model of Kawasaki disease. *J Immunol.* 2006;176:6294-6301.

93. Rowley AH, Shulman ST. Kawasaki syndrome. *Clin Microbiol Rev.* 1998;11:405-414.

94. Cheung YF, Ho MH, Tam SC, et al. Increased high sensitivity C reactive protein concentrations and increased arterial stiffness in children with a history of Kawasaki disease. *Heart.* 2004;90:1281-1285.

95. Wooditch AC, Aronoff SC. Effect of initial corticosteroid therapy on coronary artery aneurysm formation in Kawasaki disease: a meta-analysis of 862 children. *Pediatrics.* 2005;116:989-995.

96. Inoue Y, Okada Y, Shinohara M, et al. A multicenter prospective randomized trial of corticosteroids in primary therapy for Kawasaki disease: clinical course and coronary artery outcome. *J Pediatr.* 2006;149:336-341.

97. Newburger JW, Sleeper LA, McCrindle BW, et al. Randomized trial of pulsed corticosteroid therapy for primary treatment of Kawasaki disease. *N Engl J Med.* 2007;356:663-675.

98. Lang BA, Yeung RS, Oen KG, et al. Corticosteroid treatment of refractory Kawasaki disease. *J Rheumatol.* 2006;33:803-809.

99. Mills JL Sr. Buerger's disease in the 21st century: diagnosis, clinical features, and therapy. *Semin Vasc Surg.* 2003;16:179-189.

100. Olin JW. Thromboangiitis obliterans (Buerger's disease). *N Engl J Med.* 2000;343:864-869.

101. Olin JW, Shih A. Thromboangiitis obliterans (Buerger's disease). *Curr Opin Rheumatol.* 2006;18:18-24.

102. Olin JW, Young JR, Graor RA, et al. The changing clinical spectrum of thromboangiitis obliterans (Buerger's disease). *Circulation.* 1990;82:IV3-IV8.

103. Puechal X, Fiessinger JN. Thromboangiitis obliterans or Buerger's disease: challenges for the rheumatologist. *Rheumatology (Oxford).* 2007;46:192-199.

104. Puechal X, Fiessinger JN, Kahan A, et al. Rheumatic manifestations in patients with thromboangiitis obliterans (Buerger's disease). *J Rheumatol.* 1999;26:1764-1768.

105. Lie JT. Thromboangiitis obliterans (Buerger's disease) revisited. *Pathol Annu.* 1988;23(pt 2):257-291.

106. Fiessinger JN, Schafer M. Trial of iloprost versus aspirin treatment for critical limb ischaemia of thromboangiitis obliterans. The TAO Study. *Lancet.* 1990;335:555-557.

107. Oral iloprost in the treatment of thromboangiitis obliterans (Buerger's disease): a double-blind, randomised, placebo-controlled trial. The European TAO Study Group. *Eur J Vasc Endovasc Surg.* 1998;15:300-307.

108. Bozkurt AK, Besirli K, Koksal C, et al. Surgical treatment of Buerger's disease. *Vascular.* 2004;12:192-197.

109. Dilege S, Aksoy M, Kayabali M, et al. Vascular reconstruction in Buerger's disease: is it feasible? *Surg Today.* 2002;32:1042-1047.

110. Sayin A, Bozkurt AK, Tuzun H, et al. Surgical treatment of Buerger's disease: experience with 216 patients. *Cardiovasc Surg.* 1993;1:377-380.

111. Chander J, Singh L, Lal P, et al. Retroperitoneoscopic lumbar sympathectomy for Buerger's disease: a novel technique. *JSLS.* 2004;8:291-296.

112. Bozkurt AK, Koksal C, Demirbas MY, et al. A randomized trial of intravenous iloprost (a stable prostacyclin analogue) versus lumbar sympathectomy in the management of Buerger's disease. *Int Angiol.* 2006;25:162-168.

113. Donas KP, Schulte S, Ktenidis K, et al. The role of epidural spinal cord stimulation in the treatment of Buerger's disease. *J Vasc Surg.* 2005;41:830-836.

114. Cotch MF, Hoffman GS, Yerg DE, et al. The epidemiology of Wegener's granulomatosis. Estimates of the five-year period prevalence, annual mortality, and geographic disease distribution from population-based data sources. *Arthritis Rheum.* 1996;39:87-92.

115. Knight A, Ekbom A, Brandt L, et al. Increasing incidence of Wegener's granulomatosis in Sweden, 1975–2001. *J Rheumatol.* 2006;33:2060-2063.

116. Watts RA, Lane SE, Bentham G, et al. Epidemiology of systemic vasculitis: a ten-year study in the United Kingdom. *Arthritis Rheum.* 2000;43:414-419.

117. Hoffman GS, Kerr GS, Leavitt RY, et al. Wegener granulomatosis: an analysis of 158 patients [see comments]. *Ann Intern Med.* 1992;116:488-498.

118. Anderson G, Coles ET, Crane M, et al. Wegener's granuloma. A series of 265 British cases seen between 1975 and 1985. A report by a sub-committee of the British Thoracic Society Research Committee. *QJM.* 1992;83:427-438.

119. Hoffman GS, Kerr GS, Leavitt RY, et al. Wegener granulomatosis: an analysis of 158 patients. *Ann Intern Med.* 1992;116:488-498.

120. Matteson EL, Gold KN, Bloch DA, et al. Long-term survival of patients with Wegener's granulomatosis from the American college of rheumatology wegener's granulomatosis classification criteria cohort. *Am J Med.* 1996;101:129-134.

121. Reinhold-Keller E, Beuge N, Latza U, et al. An interdisciplinary approach to the care of patients with Wegener's granulomatosis: long-term outcome in 155 patients. *Arthritis Rheum.* 2000;43:1021-1032.

122. Merkel PA, Lo GH, Holbrook JT, et al. Brief communication: high incidence of venous thrombotic events among patients with Wegener granulomatosis: the Wegener's Clinical Occurrence of Thrombosis (WeCLOT) Study. *Ann Intern Med.* 2005;142:620-626.

123. Weidner S, Hafezi-Rachti S, Rupprecht HD. Thromboembolic events as a complication of antineutrophil cytoplasmic antibody-associated vasculitis. *Arthritis Rheum.* 2006;55:146-149.

124. Bacon PA. Endothelial cell dysfunction in systemic vasculitis: new developments and therapeutic prospects. *Curr Opin Rheumatol.* 2005;17:49-55.

125. de Leeuw K, Sanders JS, Stegeman C, et al. Accelerated atherosclerosis in patients with Wegener's granulomatosis. *Ann Rheum Dis.* 2005;64:753-759.

126. Hoffman GS, Specks U. Antineutrophil cytoplasmic antibodies. *Arthritis Rheum.* 1998;41:1521-1537.

127. Vassilopoulos D, Niles JL, Villa-Forte A, et al. Prevalence of antineutrophil cytoplasmic antibodies in patients with various pulmonary diseases or multiorgan dysfunction. *Arthritis Rheum.* 2003;49:151-155.

128. Anderson G, Coles ET, Crane M, et al. Wegener's granuloma. A series of 265 british cases seen between 1975 and 1985. A report by a sub–committee of the British thoracic society research committee. *QJM.* 1992;83:427.

129. Horn RG, Fauci AS, Rosenthal AS, et al. Renal biopsy pathology in Wegener's granulomatosis. *Am J Pathol.* 1974;74:423.

130. Walton EW. Giant-cell granuloma of the respiratory tract (Wegener's granulomatosis). *Br Med J.* 1958;2:265.

131. Fauci AS, Wolff SM. Wegener's granulomatosis: studies in eighteen patients and a review of the literature. *Medicine (Baltimore).* 1973;52:535.

132. Fauci AS, Haynes BF, Katz P, et al. Wegener's granulomatosis: prospective clinical and therapeutic experience with 85 patients for 21 years. *Ann Intern Med.* 1983;98:76.

133. Reinhold-Keller E, Kekow J, Schnabel A, et al. Influence of disease manifestation and antineutrophil cytoplasmic antibody titer on the response to pulse cyclophosphamide therapy in patients with Wegener's granulomatosis. *Arthritis Rheum.* 1994;37:919-924.

134. Hoffman GS, Leavitt RY, Fleisher TA, et al. Treatment of Wegener's granulomatosis with intermittent high-dose intravenous cyclophosphamide. *Am J Med.* 1990;89:403-410.

135. de Groot K, Adu D, Savage CO. The value of pulse cyclophosphamide in ANCA-associated vasculitis: meta-analysis and critical review. *Nephrol Dial Transplant.* 2001;16:2018-2027.

136. Watts R, Harper L, Jayne D, et al. Translational research in autoimmunity: aims of therapy in vasculitis. *Rheumatology (Oxford).* 2005;44:573-576.

137. Sneller MC, Hoffman GS, Talar-Williams C, et al. An analysis of forty-two Wegener's granulomatosis patients treated with methotrexate and prednisone. *Arthritis Rheum.* 1995;38:608-613.

138. Langford CA, Talar-Williams C, Sneller MC. Use of methotrexate and glucocorticoids in the treatment of Wegener's granulomatosis. Long-term renal outcome in patients with glomerulonephritis. *Arthritis Rheum.* 2000;43:1836-1840.

139. Hoffman GS, Leavitt RY, Kerr GS, et al. The treatment of Wegener's granulomatosis with glucocorticoids and methotrexate. *Arthritis Rheum.* 1992;35:1322-1329.

140. De Groot K, Rasmussen N, Bacon PA, et al. Randomized trial of cyclophosphamide versus methotrexate for induction of remission in early systemic antineutrophil

cytoplasmic antibody-associated vasculitis. *Arthritis Rheum.* 2005;52:2461-2469.

141. Langford CA, Talar-Williams C, Barron KS, et al. Use of a cyclophosphamide-induction methotrexate-maintenance regimen for the treatment of Wegener's granulomatosis: extended follow-up and rate of relapse. *Am J Med.* 2003;114: 463-469.

142. Langford CA, Talar-Williams C, Barron KS, et al. A staged approach to the treatment of Wegener's granulomatosis: induction of remission with glucocorticoids and daily cyclophosphamide switching to methotrexate for remission maintenance. *Arthritis Rheum.* 1999;42:2666-2673.

143. Reinhold-Keller E, Fink CO, Herlyn K, et al. High rate of renal relapse in 71 patients with Wegener's granulomatosis under maintenance of remission with low-dose methotrexate. *Arthritis Rheum.* 2002;47:326-332.

144. Langford CA, Talar-Williams C, Sneller MC. Mycophenolate mofetil for remission maintenance in the treatment of Wegener's granulomatosis. *Arthritis Rheum.* 2004;51:278-283.

145. Nowack R, Gobel U, Klooker P, et al. Mycophenolate mofetil for maintenance therapy of Wegener's granulomatosis and microscopic polyangiitis: a pilot study in 11 patients with renal involvement. *J Am Soc Nephrol.* 1999;10:1965-1971.

146. Eriksson P. Nine patients with anti-neutrophil cytoplasmic antibody-positive vasculitis successfully treated with rituximab. *J Intern Med.* 2005;257:540-548.

147. Keogh KA, Wylam ME, Stone JH, et al. Induction of remission by B lymphocyte depletion in eleven patients with refractory antineutrophil cytoplasmic antibody-associated vasculitis. *Arthritis Rheum.* 2005;52:262-268.

148. Keogh KA, Ytterberg SR, Fervenza FC, et al. Rituximab for refractory Wegener's granulomatosis: report of a prospective, open-label pilot trial. *Am J Respir Crit Care Med.* 2006; 173:180-187.

149. Metzler C, Fink C, Lamprecht P, et al. Maintenance of remission with leflunomide in Wegener's granulomatosis. *Rheumatology (Oxford).* 2004;43:315-320.

150. Jayne DR, Chapel H, Adu D, et al. Intravenous immunoglobulin for ANCA-associated systemic vasculitis with persistent disease activity. *QJM.* 2000;93:433-439.

151. Klemmer PJ, Chalermskulrat W, Reif MS, et al. Plasmapheresis therapy for diffuse alveolar hemorrhage in patients with small-vessel vasculitis. *Am J Kidney Dis.* 2003;42:1149-1153.

152. Hasegawa M, Kawamura N, Murase M, et al. Efficacy of granulocytapheresis and leukocytapheresis for the treatment of microscopic polyangiitis. *Ther Apher Dial.* 2004;8:212-216.

153. Langford CA, Sneller MC, Hallahan CW, et al. Clinical features and therapeutic management of subglottic stenosis in patients with Wegener's granulomatosis. *Arthritis Rheum.* 1996;39:1754-1760.

154. Adu D, Howie AJ, Scott DG, et al. Polyarteritis and the kidney. *QJM.* 1987;62:221-237.

155. D'Agati V, Chander P, Nash M, et al. Idiopathic microscopic polyarteritis nodosa: ultrastructural observations on the renal vascular and glomerular lesions. *Am J Kidney Dis.* 1986;7:95-110.

156. Savage CO, Winearls CG, Evans DJ, et al. Microscopic polyarteritis: presentation, pathology and prognosis. *QJM.* 1985;56:467-483.

157. Serra A, Cameron JS, Turner DR, et al. Vasculitis affecting the kidney: presentation, histopathology and long-term outcome. *QJM.* 1984;53:181-207.

158. Guillevin L, Durand-Gasselin B, Cevallos R, et al. Microscopic polyangiitis: clinical and laboratory findings in eighty-five patients. *Arthritis Rheum.* 1999;42:421-430.

159. Jennings CA, King TE Jr. Tuder R. Diffuse alveolar hemorrhage with underlying isolated pauci-immune pulmonary capillaritis. *Am J Respir Crit Care Med.* 1997;155:1101.

160. Schwarz MI. The nongranulomatous vasculitides of the lung. *Semin Respir Crit Care Med.* 1998;19:47.

161. Churg J, Strauss L. Allergic granulomatosis, allergic angiitis and periarteritis nodosa. *Am J Pathol.* 1951;27:277.

162. Lanham JG, Elkon KB, Pusey CD, et al. Systemic vasculitis with asthma and eosinophilia: a clinical approach to the Churg Strauss syndrome. *Medicine (Baltimore).* 1984;63:65.

163. Wechsler ME, Garpestad E, Flier SR, et al. Pulmonary infiltrates, eosinophilia and cardiomyopathy following corticosteroid withdrawal in patient with asthma receiving Zafirlukast. *JAMA.* 1998;279:455.

164. Keogh KA, Specks U. Churg-Strauss syndrome. *Semin Respir Crit Care Med.* 2006;27:148-157.

165. Sable-Fourtassou R, Cohen P, Mahr A, et al. Antineutrophil cytoplasmic antibodies and the Churg-Strauss syndrome. *Ann Intern Med.* 2005;143:632-638.

166. Sinico RA, Di Toma L, Maggiore U, et al. Prevalence and clinical significance of antineutrophil cytoplasmic antibodies in Churg-Strauss syndrome. *Arthritis Rheum.* 2005;52:2926-2935.

167. Hoffman GS, Langford CA. Are there different forms of life in the antineutrophil cytoplasmic antibody universe? *Ann Intern Med.* 2005;143:683-685.

168. Guillevin L, Lhote F, Amouroux J, et al. Antineutrophil cytoplasmic antibodies, abnormal angiograms and pathological findings in polyarteritis nodosa and Churg-Strauss syndrome: indications for the classification of vasculitides of the polyarteritis Nodosa Group. *Br J Rheumatol.* 1996;35:958-964.

169. Chumbley LC, Harrison EG Jr, DeRemee RA. Allergic granulomatosis and angiitis (Churg-Strauss syndrome). Report and analysis of 30 cases. *Mayo Clin Proc.* 1977;52:477-484.

170. Guillevin L, Cohen P, Gayraud M, et al. Churg-Strauss syndrome. Clinical study and long-term follow-up of 96 patients. *Medicine (Baltimore).* 1999;78:26-37.

171. Lanham JG, Elkon KB, Pusey CD, et al. Systemic vasculitis with asthma and eosinophilia: a clinical approach to the Churg-Strauss syndrome. *Medicine (Baltimore).* 1984;63:65-81.

172. Shields CL, Shields JA, Rozanski TI. Conjunctival involvement in Churg-Strauss syndrome. *Am J Ophthalmol.* 1986; 102:601.

173. Guillevin L, Gain O, Lhote F, et al. Lack of superiority of steroids plus plasma exchange to steroids alone in the treatment of polyarteritis nodosa and Churg-Strauss syndrome: a prospective, randomized trial in 78 patients. *Arthritis Rheum.* 1992;35:208.

174. Guillevin L, Jarrousse B, Lok C, et al. Longterm follow-up after treatment of polyarteritis nodosa and Churg-Strauss angiitis with comparison of steroids, plasma exchange and cyclophosphamide to steroids and plasma exchange: a prospective randomized trial of 71 patients. *J Rheumatol.* 1991;18:567.

175. Langford CA, Klippel JH, Balow JE, et al. Use of cytotoxic agents and cyclosporine in the treatment of autoimmune disease. Part 2: inflammatory bowel disease, systemic vasculitis, and therapeutic toxicity. *Ann Intern Med.* 1998;129:49-58.

176. Nachman PH, Hogan SL, Jennette JC, et al. Treatment response and relapse in antineutrophil cytoplasmic autoantibody-associated microscopic polyangiitis and glomerulonephritis. *J Am Soc Nephrol.* 1996;7:33-39.

177. Rottem M, Fauci AS, Hallahan CW, et al. Wegener granulomatosis in children and adolescents: clinical presentation and outcome. *J Pediatr.* 1993;122:26-31.

178. Tsurikisawa N, Taniguchi M, Saito H, et al. Treatment of Churg-Strauss syndrome with high-dose intravenous immunoglobulin. *Ann Allergy Asthma Immunol.* 2004;92:80-87.

179. Metzler C, Hellmich B, Gause A, et al. Churg Strauss syndrome—successful induction of remission with methotrexate and unexpected high cardiac and pulmonary relapse ratio during maintenance treatment. *Clin Exp Rheumatol.* 2004;22:S52-S61.

180. Carlson JA, Ng BT, Chen KR. Cutaneous vasculitis update: diagnostic criteria, classification, epidemiology, etiology, pathogenesis, evaluation and prognosis. *Am J Dermatopathol.* 2005;27:504-528.

181. Hutson TE, Hoffman GS. Temporal concurrence of vasculitis and cancer: a report of 12 cases. *Arthritis Care Res.* 2000;13:417-423.

182. Carlson JA, Cavaliere LF, Grant-Kels JM. Cutaneous vasculitis: diagnosis and management. *Clin Dermatol.* 2006;24:414-429.

183. Ballard HS, Eisinger RP, Gallo G. Renal manifestations of the Henoch-Schoenlein syndrome in adults. *Am J Med.* 1970;49:328-335.

184. Farley TA, Gillespie S, Rasoulpour M, et al. Epidemiology of a cluster of Henoch-Schonlein purpura. *Am J Dis Child.* 1989;143:798-803.

185. Calvino MC, Llorca J, García-Porrua C, et al. Henoch-Schonlein purpura in children from northwestern Spain: a 20-year epidemiologic and clinical study. *Medicine (Baltimore).* 2001;80:279-290.

186. Sano H, Izumida M, Shimizu H, et al. Risk factors of renal involvement and significant proteinuria in Henoch-Schonlein purpura. *Eur J Pediatr.* 2002;161:196-201.

187. Saulsbury FT. Henoch-Schonlein purpura in children. Report of 100 patients and review of the literature. *Medicine (Baltimore).* 1999;78:395-409.

188. Trapani S, Micheli A, Grisolia F, et al. Henoch Schonlein purpura in childhood: epidemiological and clinical analysis of 150 cases over a 5-year period and review of literature. *Semin Arthritis Rheum.* 2005;35:143-153.

189. Hene RJ, Velthuis P, van de Wiel A, et al. The relevance of IgA deposits in vessel walls of clinically normal skin. A prospective study. *Arch Intern Med.* 1986;146:745-749.

190. Giangiacomo J, Tsai CC. Dermal and glomerular deposition of IgA in anaphylactoid purpura. *Am J Dis Child.* 1977;131:981-983.

191. Counahan R, Winterborn MH, White RH, et al. Prognosis of Henoch-Schonlein nephritis in children. *Br Med J.* 1977;2:11-14.

192. Goldstein AR, White RH, Akuse R, et al. Long-term follow-up of childhood Henoch-Schonlein nephritis. *Lancet.* 1992;339:280-282.

193. Dillon MJ, Ansell BM. Vasculitis in children and adolescents. *Rheum Dis Clin North Am.* 1995;21:1115-1136.

194. García-Porrua C, González-Gay MA. Comparative clinical and epidemiological study of hypersensitivity vasculitis versus Henoch-Schonlein purpura in adults. *Semin Arthritis Rheum.* 1999;28:404-412.

195. Blanco R, Martínez-Taboada VM, Rodríguez-Valverde V, et al. Henoch-Schonlein purpura in adulthood and childhood: two different expressions of the same syndrome. *Arthritis Rheum.* 1997;40:859-864.

196. Kaku Y, Nohara K, Honda S. Renal involvement in Henoch-Schonlein purpura: a multivariate analysis of prognostic factors. *Kidney Int.* 1998;53:1755-1759.

197. Steinhardt MJ, Fisher GS. Essential cryoglobulinemia. *Ann Intern Med.* 1955;43:848-858.

198. Meltzer M, Franklin EC. Cryoglobulinemia—a study of twenty-nine patients. I. IgG and IgM cryoglobulins and factors affecting cryoprecipitability. *Am J Med.* 1966;40:828-836.

199. Pascual M, Perrin L, Giostra E, et al. Hepatitis C virus in patients with cryoglobulinemia type II. *J Infect Dis.* 1990;162:569-570.

200. Ferri C, La Civita L, Longombardo G, et al. Hepatitis C virus and mixed cryoglobulinaemia. *Eur J Clin Invest.* 1993;23:399-405.

201. Trejo O, Ramos-Casals M, García-Carrasco M, et al. Cryoglobulinemia: study of etiologic factors and clinical and immunologic features in 443 patients from a single center. *Medicine (Baltimore).* 2001;80:252-262.

202. Galli M, Invernizzi F, Chemotti M, et al. Cryoglobulins and infectious diseases. *Ric Clin Lab.* 1986;16:301-313.

203. Brouet JC, Clauvel JP, Danon F, et al. Biologic and clinical significance of cryoglobulins. A report of 86 cases. *Am J Med.* 1974;57:775-788.

204. Gorevic PD, Kassab HJ, Levo Y, et al. Mixed cryoglobulinemia: clinical aspects and long-term follow-up of 40 patients. *Am J Med.* 1980;69:287-308.

205. Meltzer M, Franklin EC, Elias K, et al. Cryoglobulinemia—a clinical and laboratory study. II. Cryoglobulins with rheumatoid factor activity. *Am J Med.* 1966;40:837-856.

206. Monti G, Saccardo F, Pioltelli P, et al. The natural history of cryoglobulinemia: symptoms at onset and during follow-up. A report by the Italian Group for the Study of Cryoglobulinemias (GISC). *Clin Exp Rheumatol.* 1995;13(suppl 13):S129-S133.

207. Braun GS, Horster S, Wagner KS, et al. Cryoglobulinaemic vasculitis: classification and clinical and therapeutic aspects. *Postgrad Med J.* 2007;83:87-94.

208. Tarantino A, De Vecchi A, Montagnino G, et al. Renal disease in essential mixed cryoglobulinaemia. Long-term follow-up of 44 patients. *QJM*. 1981;50:1-30.

209. Zaja F, De Vita S, Mazzaro C, et al. Efficacy and safety of rituximab in type II mixed cryoglobulinemia. *Blood*. 2003; 101:3827-3834.

210. Roccatello D, Baldovino S, Rossi D, et al. Long-term effects of anti-CD20 monoclonal antibody treatment of cryoglobulinaemic glomerulonephritis. *Nephrol Dial Transplant*. 2004;19:3054-3061.

211. Quartuccio L, Soardo G, Romano G, et al. Rituximab treatment for glomerulonephritis in HCV-associated mixed cryoglobulinaemia: efficacy and safety in the absence of steroids. *Rheumatology (Oxford)*. 2006;45:842-846.

212. Breedveld FC. Vasculitis associated with connective tissue disease. *Baillieres Clin Rheumatol*. 1997;11:315-334.

213. Del Rosso A, Petix NR, Pratesi M, et al. Cardiovascular involvement in relapsing polychondritis. *Semin Arthritis Rheum*. 1997;26:840-844.

214. Slobodin G, Naschitz JE, Zuckerman E, et al. Aortic involvement in rheumatic diseases. *Clin Exp Rheumatol*. 2006;24:S41-S47.

215. Uusimaa P, Krogerus ML, Airaksinen J, et al. Aortic valve insufficiency in patients with chronic rheumatic diseases. *Clin Rheumatol*. 2006;25:309-313.

216. Scott DG, Bacon PA, Tribe CR. Systemic rheumatoid vasculitis: a clinical and laboratory study of 50 cases. *Medicine (Baltimore)*. 1981;60:288-297.

217. Vollertsen RS, Conn DL, Ballard DJ, et al. Rheumatoid vasculitis: survival and associated risk factors. *Medicine (Baltimore)*. 1986;65:365-375.

218. Voskuyl AE, Zwinderman AH, Westedt ML, et al. Factors associated with the development of vasculitis in rheumatoid arthritis: results of a case-control study. *Ann Rheum Dis*. 1996;55:190-192.

219. Watts RA, Mooney J, Lane SE, et al. Rheumatoid vasculitis: becoming extinct? *Rheumatology (Oxford)*. 2004;43:920-923.

220. Watts RA, Carruthers DM, Scott DG. Isolated nail fold vasculitis in rheumatoid arthritis. *Ann Rheum Dis*. 1995;54:927-929.

221. Foster CS, Forstot SL, Wilson LA. Mortality rate in rheumatoid arthritis patients developing necrotizing scleritis or peripheral ulcerative keratitis. Effects of systemic immunosuppression. *Ophthalmology*. 1984;91:1253-1263.

222. Heurkens AH, Westedt ML, Breedveld FC. Prednisone plus azathioprine treatment in patients with rheumatoid arthritis complicated by vasculitis. *Arch Intern Med*. 1991;151:2249-2254.

223. Scott DG, Bacon PA. Intravenous cyclophosphamide plus methylprednisolone in treatment of systemic rheumatoid vasculitis. *Am J Med*. 1984;76:377-384.

224. Bartolucci P, Ramanoelina J, Cohen P, et al. Efficacy of the anti-TNF-alpha antibody infliximab against refractory systemic vasculitides: an open pilot study on 10 patients. *Rheumatology (Oxford)*. 2002;41:1126-1132.

225. Unger L, Kayser M, Nusslein HG. Successful treatment of severe rheumatoid vasculitis by infliximab. *Ann Rheum Dis*. 2003;62:587-588.

226. Kaklamani VG, Vaiopoulos G, Kaklamanis PG. Behcet's Disease. *Semin Arthritis Rheum*. 1998;27:197-217.

227. Sakane T, Takeno M, Suzuki N, et al. Behcet's disease. *N Engl J Med*. 1999;341:1284-1291.

228. Zouboulis CC, Kotter I, Djawari D, et al. Epidemiological features of Adamantiades-Behcet's disease in Germany and in Europe. *Yonsei Med J*. 1997;38:411-422.

229. Calamia KT, Schirmer M, Melikoglu M. Major vessel involvement in Behcet disease. *Curr Opin Rheumatol*. 2005;17:1-8.

230. Cooper AM, Naughton MN, Williams BD. Chronic arterial occlusion associated with Behcet's disease. *Br J Rheumatol*. 1994;33:170-172.

231. Gurler A, Boyvat A, Tursen U. Clinical manifestations of Behcet's disease: an analysis of 2147 patients. *Yonsei Med J*. 1997;38:423-427.

232. Hamza M. Large artery involvement in Behcet's disease. *J Rheumatol*. 1987;14:554-559.

233. Shahram F, Assadi K, Davatchi F, et al. Chronology of clinical manifestations in Behcet's disease. Analysis of 4024 cases. *Adv Exp Med Biol*. 2003;528:85-89.

234. Lakhanpal S, Tani K, Lie JT, et al. Pathologic features of Behcet's syndrome: a review of Japanese autopsy registry data. *Hum Pathol*. 1985;16:790-795.

235. Ceyran H, Akcali Y, Kahraman C. Surgical treatment of vasculo-Behcet's disease. A review of patients with concomitant multiple aneurysms and venous lesions. *Vasa*. 2003;32:149-153.

236. Matsumoto T, Uekusa T, Fukuda Y. Vasculo-Behcet's disease: a pathologic study of eight cases. *Hum Pathol*. 1991;22:45-51.

237. Saba D, Saricaoglu H, Bayram AS, et al. Arterial lesions in Behcet's disease. *Vasa*. 2003;32:75-81.

238. Kizilkilic O, Albayram S, Adaletli I, et al. Endovascular treatment of Behcet's disease-associated intracranial aneurysms: report of two cases and review of the literature. *Neuroradiology*. 2003;45:328-334.

239. Silistreli E, Karabay O, Erdal C, et al. Behcet's disease: treatment of popliteal pseudoaneurysm by an endovascular stent graft implantation. *Ann Vasc Surg*. 2004;18:118-120.

240. Bautista-Hernández V, Gutierrez F, Capel A, et al. Endovascular repair of concomitant celiac trunk and abdominal aortic aneurysms in a patient with Behcet's disease. *J Endovasc Ther*. 2004;11:222-225.

241. Robenshtok E, Krause I. Arterial involvement in Behcet's disease—the search for new treatment strategies. *Isr Med Assoc J*. 2004;6:162-163.

242. Nitecki SS, Ofer A, Karram T, et al. Abdominal aortic aneurysm in Behcet's disease: new treatment options for an old and challenging problem. *Isr Med Assoc J*. 2004;6:152-155.

243. St Clair EW, McCallum RM. Cogan's syndrome. *Curr Opin Rheumatol*. 1999;11:47-52.

244. Udayaraj UP, Hand MF, Shilliday IR, et al. Renal involvement in Cogan's syndrome. *Nephrol Dial Transplant*. 2004;19:2420-2421.

245. Chynn EW, Jakobiec FA. Cogan's syndrome: ophthalmic, audiovestibular, and systemic manifestations and therapy. *Int Ophthalmol Clin.* 1996;36:61-72.

246. Vollertsen RS, McDonald TJ, Younge BR, et al. Cogan's syndrome: 18 cases and a review of the literature. *Mayo Clin Proc.* 1986;61:344-361.

247. Fernandes SR, Singsen BH, Hoffman GS. Sarcoidosis and systemic vasculitis. *Semin Arthritis Rheum.* 2000;30:33-46.

248. Pagnoux C, Cohen P, Guillevin L. Vasculitides secondary to infections. *Clin Exp Rheumatol.* 2006;24:S71-S81.

249. Chetty R. Vasculitides associated with HIV infection. *J Clin Pathol.* 2001;54:275-278.

250. Conlon PJ, Jefferies F, Krigman HR, et al. Predictors of prognosis and risk of acute renal failure in bacterial endocarditis. *Clin Nephrol.* 1998;49:96-101.

chapter 15

Connective Tissue Disorders in Peripheral Arterial Disease

David Liang, MD, PhD / *Gerald J. Berry, MD*

The blood vessel is a complex organ with many mechanical and regulatory functions. Abnormalities in the structural characteristics of the extracellular matrix as well as the regulatory functions can results in significant dysfunction. This dysfunction can manifest itself as vascular fragility leading to aneurysms, dissections, and ruptures but it may also result in stenotic lesions.

Many of the conditions have their roots in mutations of the genes responsible for the constitutive proteins of the blood vessel wall, however, probably just as frequently the mutations result in disordered regulation of cell turnover and remodeling. In some cases the underlying abnormality has not been identified, however, the features of the conditions and when they should be suspected are shared with the more definitely identified connective tissue abnormalities and so are included in this chapter.

Beyond the underlying causal abnormality, the primary clinical feature shared by these conditions is the presence of vascular disease in a patient population typically not thought to be a risk: patients who are young and without usually precipitating causes such as hyperlipidemia, hypertension, and diabetes. Typically a familial clustering is also present which should raise concern for these diseases. In addition, the familial nature of these conditions even when a precise genetic syndrome cannot be identified should prompt an evaluation of first-degree relatives.

● EHLERS-DANLOS SYNDROME

Ehlers-Danlos Syndrome (EDS) is a collection of connective diseases characterized by hypermobility of the joints and hyperextensible joints. Following the initial description of the condition several subtypes have been identified with different underlying biochemical and genetic causes and different clinical presentations. Vascular manifestations of EDS are primarily limited to the vascular subtype,[1,2] which was known as EDS-IV or Sachs-Barabas syndrome in prior classifications.[3] Vascular fragility has been rarely described in other subtypes of EDS (kyphoscoliotic type [EDS-VI] and arthochalasis type [EDS-VII]) and collagen abnormalities, such as osteogenesis imperfecta, but the vast majority of vascular complications in EDS occur in the vascular subtype.[4-6] The principal clinical manifestations are vessel rupture and dissection with and without preceding blood vessel dilation. Internal organ rupture, uterus, and colon in particular, are also important causes of morbidity and mortality. Overall prevalence of EDS is estimated to be 1 in between 10 000 and 25 000, with vascular EDS constituting 4% of all EDS cases.[1,7]

Pathogenesis

Collagen III is the predominant type of collagen in blood vessel and visceral organ walls.[8] Abnormalities in collagen III synthesis were first identified by Pope et al.[9] in EDS-IV in 1975. Causative mutations in the COL3A1 gene coding for the procollagen proα1(III) chain of collagen III have been identified in the vast majority of cases. Over 114 different mutations involving the COL3A1 gene hve been documented in the most complete clinical series, with additional mutations described in smaller series and case reports.[10] The most common mutations aree point mutations leading to a substitution for a glycine within the triple-helical domain.

Procollagen III is formed as a homotripolymer of three identical chains, therefore abnormality of one of the allele results in normal procollagen polymers in only one-eighth of the procollagen polymers that are formed.[11] This results in a dominant negative mechanism for the autosomal dominant mode of inheritance seen clinically. With certain mutations, there are no abnormal procollagen strands available for formation of polymers; these mutations phenotypically present with clinical vascular EDS of similar severity. Haploinsuffciency therefore plays a role as well in the autosomal dominant mechanism.[12]

Reduction in the synthesis and deposition of collagen III leads to weakening of the vascular wall.

Clinical Manifestations

The vascular manifestations of EDS IV include dissection and rupture of blood vessels of all sizes from the level of the aorta down to arterioles. Fusiform aneurysms may form, but do not appear to precede dissections and ruptures in the majority of cases.[13] Thoracic and abdominal vessels appear to be most frequently involved with between 50% and 77% of vascular complications involving those vessels. Vessels of the head and neck are involved in between 10% and 16% of the cases.[10,13,14] Common central nervous system vascular complications are carotid–cavernous sinus fistula formation and vertebral and carotid artery dissections.

Age of presentation with vascular complications is typically in the early twenties, with median age of first vascular complication at 24.6 years. Presentation in childhood is unusual, but has been reported. In available retrospective series approximately 50% of affected individuals will develop a vascular manifestation. Approximately 30% will have a repeat event after first presentation.[10]

Rupture of internal organs is the other principal clinical complication of vascular EDS. Approximately 28% will have an internal organ perforation or rupture with the colon, spleen, and uterus most commonly involved.

Cause of mortality in EDS is vascular in 79% and because of organ and bowel complications in 18%. Ruptures of thoracic and abdominal vessels are responsible for more than 76% vascular deaths. Central nervous system hemorrhage is responsible for at least 9% of deaths. Life expectancy is 48 years, although individuals living to 73 years of age have been reported.[10]

Beyond the clinical complications of vascular EDS, there are several phenotypic features which may help with diagnosis. Joint hypermobility and skin hyperextensibility typical of the other EDS types is not a prominent feature of vascular EDS. Mild hyperextensibility of the small joints may be present. The skin rather than being hyperextensible is typically very thin and pale and in some cases can be translucent. As a result the subcutaneous veins become prominent, particularly over the chest and abdomen. Capillary fragility leads to easy bruisability. In extreme cases recurrent bruising can lead to subcutaneous hemosiderin deposits. The reduction in subcutaneous fat in some cases results in a characteristic delicate facial appearance with a pinch nose, sunken eyes and hollow cheeks.

Diagnosis

Although the phenotypic features are often cited in the diagnosis of vascular EDS, the sensitivity and specificity of these findings are not known and exclusion or diagnosis of vascular EDS based upon them solely is difficult. Of the clinical features bruisability is nearly uniformly present in affected individuals, however, other features such as translucent skin, typical facial features and joint hypermobility are not reliably present.[13] In most cases, the diagnosis of vascular EDS is made following an incident event or based upon family history.[10] Suspicion of vascular EDS should therefore be raised if an aneurysm, rupture or dissection occurs in a young person without obvious precipitating cause. The presence of abnormalities in multiple vascular beds should strongly raise the need to evaluate further for the diagnosis of vascular EDS (see Figure 15-1).

Screening of children and parents of the afflicted patient should always be performed. The need for screening of additional relatives depends upon the initial screening results, taking into account the autosomal dominant nature of inheritance.

Definitive diagnosis at this time relies upon identifying a disease-causing mutation in the COL3A1 gene or the identification of abnormal structure or quantity of collagen α1(III) chains in dermal fibroblast cell culture. Theoretically genetic analysis of the COL3A1 gene may miss some mutations in the promoter regions of the COL3A1 gene which lead to decreased transcription, since current sequencing techniques only sequence the exons of the COL3A1 gene. To date, there have been no proven cases of EDS IV caused by this type of mutation. Complete deletion of the COL3A1 gene in one allele leading to vascular EDS can usually be identified on genetic testing by the absence of variation in the typical polymorphism in the COL3A1 found during sequencing.

Pathological Findings

The macroscopic and microscopic vascular complications in vascular EDS are attributed to the qualitative and/or quantitative abnormalities of Collagen III. Medium and large vessels such as the branches of the aortic arch, descending thoracic aorta and abdominal aorta and its distal branches are commonly affected. The macroscopic changes include single or multiple tears, dissection, rupture with massive hemorrhage and/or pseudoaneurysm formation, aneurysms of peripheral, coronary and other muscular arteries, and tortuous arteries and varicose veins. Aortic tears and dissection with false channels are common but true aortic aneurysmal formation is less frequently observed.[15] In our experience, the pattern of vascular interruption is similar to other causes of aortic dissection (Figure 15-2). Complete transmural transverse tearing of the vessel can result in rupture; incomplete disruption can produce a dissection plane typically in outer third of the medial layer of the aorta. The microscopic findings are limited to a minimal degree of cystic medial degeneration (CMD) (Figure 15-2). CMD is characterized by loss of smooth muscle cells,

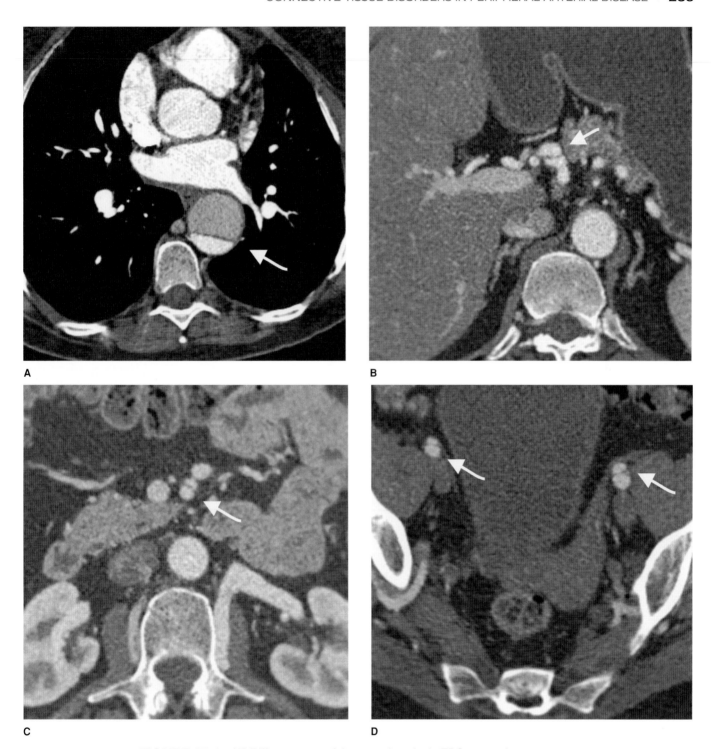

● **FIGURE 15-1.** (A) Diffuse nature of the vasculopathy in EDS—vascular type frequently results in multiple vessel dissections and aneurysms. In this example, the patient presented with an acute type B dissection. CT scan at the time of presentation also identified the presence of independent asymptomatic dissections of the (B) hepatic, (C) superior mesenteric, and (D) bilateral iliac arteries (arrow heads).

fragmentation, and loss of elastic fibers and accumulations of proteoglycans within the medial layer. A marked decrease in Type III collagen in the skin and the wall of the cerebral artery can be demonstrated by immunohistochemical staining techniques.[16] (Figure 15-2) At the ultrastructural level considerable variation in collagen fibril diameter

and an overall decrease in the cross sectional area of collagen fibrils in arterial walls has been reported.[17]

Management

There is no specific treatment for the underlying biochemical abnormality at this time. In the absence of complications

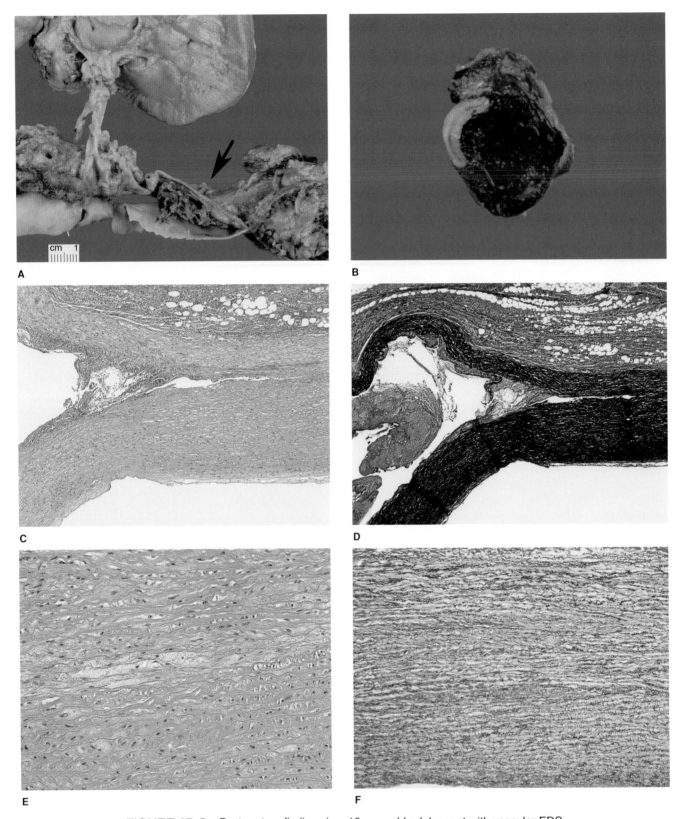

● FIGURE 15-2. Postmortem findings in a 16-year-old adolescent with vascular EDS who presented with acute type B dissection following an noncontact exertional activity. (A) The infrarenal portion of the abdominal aorta shows an acute dissection with thrombus filling the false lumen (arrow). (B) The acute dissection extended along the iliac artery. (C) Histopathological findings of acute aortic dissection with the dissection plane located in the outer third of the medial layer (H&E ×100). (D) The elastic von Gieson stain of the aorta highlighting the dissection (EVG ×100). (E) High power magnification of the aorta showing scattered collections of pale proteoglycans in the medial layer associated with a decrease in smooth muscle cells. These are some of the features of CMD (H&E × 400). (F) The colloidal iron stain renders the proteoglycans bright blue staining (Colloidal iron ×400). (*continued*)

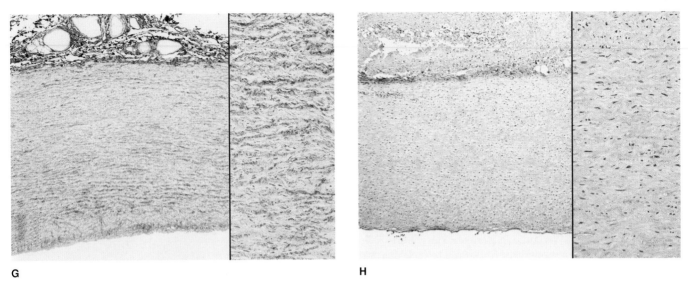

● **FIGURE 15-2.** (*Continued*) (G) Collagen III staining of a normal aorta. High power magnification shows linear arrangement of the fibers (×250; ×400). (H) Immunohistochemical staining of vascular EDS for collagen III showing marked decrease in fibers (×250; ×400).

the treatment is primarily targeted at reducing factors that may aggravate the known complications of vascular EDS. Vigilant control of blood pressure and the avoidance of activities that would tend to increase blood pressure excessively, for example, competitive sports and weightlifting are prudent, however, unproven. Activities that place the patient at risk for trauma, for example, contact sports, skiing, should also be avoided given the fragility of the blood vessels and organs. Avoidance of agents that impair hemostasis such aspirin and other nonsteroidal anti-inflammatory drugs is also typically recommended. Avoiding increased intraluminal pressure in the organs from straining may require the routine use of laxatives and stool softeners.

Because of the rarity of vascular EDS, there is no proven approach to the management of vascular complications. The marked fragility of the tissues and the high frequency of arterial tears and anastomotic breakdown that develops with surgical manipulation place all interventions at high risk. For this reason a conservative approach is generally recommended to manage non-life-threatening complications using compression and transfusions. Mortality rates associated with operative vascular intervention has been as high as 40% in retrospective series.[10] Surgical intervention can be performed successfully in some cases, so surgery should not be denied when conservative approaches are unlikely to work. The incidence of surgical complication remains high, with excessive bleeding being the most frequent complication. Late problems such as graft anastomosis aneurysms and anastomotic ruptures are very frequent affecting 40% of repairs.[13]

The use of percutaneous interventions with stents, covered stents and coils has also been performed with success in some patients with vascular EDS.[18–22] The precise role of such interventions is yet to be determined. Care must be taken with the vascular access in such cases, as there have been cases in which the procedure has been successful in treating the vascular complication, only to have the patient die from exsanguinations at the vascular entry site or other sites remote from the site of intervention.[23–25] Consideration of these complications should be made in planning any intervention[26,27] and wherever possible evaluation and planning should be undertaken by noninvasive means. Invasive angiography in a series of thirteen patients resulted in serious complication in three patients (23%).[13]

The role of surveillance imaging of the vasculature in patients with vascular EDS is uncertain. In many cases, the vascular complications are not preceded by aneurysm development or other features identifiable by noninvasive imaging. However, in a minority of cases, there is aneurysm or dissection before rupture. That combined with recent successes with percutaneous intervention suggests that routine surveillance imaging of the vasculature may have value.

● **MARFAN SYNDROME**

The elastic fibers also form an essential component of the blood vessel wall, particularly in the elastic arteries such as the aorta and its major branches.[28] Marfan syndrome (MFS) is caused by mutations on the FBN1 gene on chromosome 15.[29] Fibrillin is an important component of the microfibrils and is closely coupled to the extracellular elastic fibers.[30–32] Not surprisingly, most if not all of the vascular manifestations of MFS are therefore limited to the aorta and to much lesser degree the major branches of the aorta.

Pathogenesis

Shortly following the identification of fibrillin-1 in 1986, the FBN1 gene on chromosome 15 was identified as the causative mutation through linkage analysis and genetic sequencing. Subsequently, over 600 mutations of the fibrillin gene have been identified as causing MFS (http://www.umd.be:2030/). A MFS-2 locus has also been suggested on chromosome 3 involving the TGF-β receptor gene, however, the distinction between MFS-2 and Loeys-Dietz Syndrome (LDS) remains to be clarified and will be discussed later in this chapter.[33]

Genotype-to-phenotype correlation remains weak, with only mutations in the region of exons 24 to 32 appearing to result in the particularly severe neonatal form of MFS.[34,35] Beyond this finding the correlations are not strong enough to be useful in predicting clinical course.

Expression of MFS is an autosomal dominant pattern with some degree of variance in penetration. There have been no well documented cases of complete lack of phenotypic expression of a disease causing FBN1 mutation, although in some cases the penetrance can be very mild.

Because of the dominant nature of inheritance earlier proposals of disease mechanisms suggested a dominant negative mechanism with the belief that the abnormal transcript/protein interfered with translation and deposition of normal fibrillin.[36] More recent work, however, suggests that haploinsuffciency may also be an important mechanism of disease as well.[37,38]

The close association of the microfibrils to the elastic fibers suggested that abnormal microfibril synthesis leads to vascular weakness by causing disarrayed deposition of elastic fibers. However, the relatively normal nature of lung tissue at the time of birth suggested that the effects of the FBN1 mutation persisted beyond the time of elastogenesis. It is now thought that most if not all of the clinical manifestations are caused by loss of the regulatory role of extracellular matrix fibrillin on the signaling activity of TGF-β. Fibrillin is one of the principal extracellular binding sites for TGB-β either directly or through latent TGF-β binding protein. Reduction in the availability of extracellular matrix TGF-β binding sites by loss of FBN1 or alterations in the binding sites on mutant fibrillin results in excessive amounts of TGF-β available for interaction with cell surface receptors. The resulting biochemical changes seen in MFS match those seen with TGF-β over-activity. This underlying mechanism is supported by mouse models demonstrating the amelioration of the features of MFS with TGF-β binding antibodies.[39]

Clinical Manifestations

Because of the ubiquitous nature of fibrillin throughout the body the manifestations of MFS typically involve several organ systems. Although MFS is frequently associated with the musculoskeletal features of tall height, long limbs and flexibility, its most important manifestations from a diagnostic and prognostic standpoint are cardiovascular and ocular.

The cardiovascular complications of MFS are dominated by pathology of the aorta. Aortic root expansion is initiated at the sinuses of Valsalva and progressively enlarges in

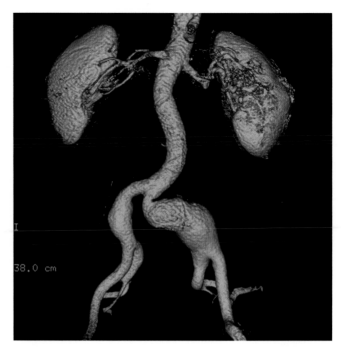

● **FIGURE 15-3.** Atypical presentation of spontaneous common iliac aneurysms on MRA in a patient with MFS who had previously undergone prophylactic aortic root replacement, but had no history of aortic dissection, hypertension, or atherosclerosis.

aneurysmal fashion to cause aortic dissection, aortic rupture and/or aortic regurgitation. Greater than 80% of patients with MFS will manifest some degrees of aortic enlargement or dissection with the aortic root most frequently involved.[40] Cardiovascular disease is the cause of death in untreated MFS in 71% of patients with median age of death of 41 years in men and 49 years in women.[41]

Vascular disease beyond the aorta is unusual in the absence of aortic dissection with extension into the branches of the aorta (Figure 15-3).[42–45] Independent involvement of the carotids and neck vessels has been suggested in some case reports, but whether the incidence in MFS exceeds that of the general population is uncertain.[46] Intracranial aneurysms have also been reported as case reports.[47] A population based study, however, showed no evidence of increased frequency.[48]

Diagnosis

Many of the features of MFS can be seen in the general population independent of any connective tissue disorder. Therefore, at this time the diagnosis currently depends upon a combination of the presence of the more specific findings such as aortic aneurysm, lens dislocation and family history. The formal diagnostic criteria in use currently were defined in 1996.[49] The presence of two major clinical features in separate organ systems and evidence of involvement in one additional organ system is required. The presence of a documented family history of MFS or genetic testing documenting a fibrillin mutation can be used to reduce the clinical findings needed to provide a definitive diagnosis. The Ghent criteria have proven to be very specific diagnostic criteria for MFS. In young patients and in patients without family history the criteria may be overly rigorous; therefore, care must be used in excluding the diagnosis of MFS in clinical practice using the Ghent criteria alone. Genetic testing is not definitive as FBN-1 mutations can also lead to other syndromes such as Weill-Marchesani and isolated ectopia lentis; these share some of the features of MFS, but have very different phenotypic features and prognostic implications. Correlation between the genetic findings and clinical features is necessary for determining the significance of DNA testing.

Other diagnoses to consider when presented with vascular findings associated with MFS include annuloaortic ectasia, FAA, and TAAD 1. The presence of features in other organ systems helps to exclude those diagnoses. LDS, which will be discussed in the next section, shares many features of MFS: the absence of lens dislocation and the presence of typical craniofacial abnormalities strongly favor the diagnosis of LDS. In the absence of these features, the diagnosis may require genetic testing. Other conditions such as Stickler syndrome, Schprintzen-Goldberg, and Homocystinuria may share the some of the musculoskeletal features that raise concern for MFS, but these conditions do not normally have the vascular manifestations of MFS.

Pathological Findings

The predominant cardiovascular abnormalities in MFS include mitral or tricuspid valve prolapse and aortic root and ascending aortic abnormalities.[50] The aortic changes include fusiform aneurysmal dilatation with or without aortic regurgitation and dissection. Dissections begin as a transverse tear in the ascending aorta within a few centimeters of the aortic valve annulus. The dissection plane is found within the outer third of the medial layer (as described above) and the false lumen propagates in an antegrade and/or retrograde direction as a hemorrhagic linear streak. The histologic hallmark is CMD. In comparison to vascular EDS and other disorders with CMD as a pathologic finding, CMD tends to be more pronounced in MFS. There is a wide range of severity, however, as some cases of aortic dissection exhibit minimal histologic findings. In some cases the false lumen of the initial dissection heals with whitish-tan granulation tissue and then fibrous tissue (Figure 15-4). A cross section of the aorta shows both the true lumen and the false lumen.

Management

Established management at this time focuses on avoiding activities that place additional stress on the aorta, for example, isometric exercise, competitive sports, contact sports and activities that will place the participant at risk for sudden acceleration and deceleration. Beta-blockers are currently the standard of care for decreasing the rate of growth of the aorta.[51] Dosing should be adjusted individually to achieve adequate blockade of the adrenergic receptors, for example, maintaining the heart rate below 100 bpm with moderate exertion such as climbing two flights of stairs briskly.

Regular monitoring of the aorta for aneurysms is an essential component of patient management. Typically annual or semi-annual imaging with echo, CT, or MRI is

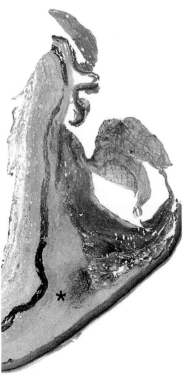
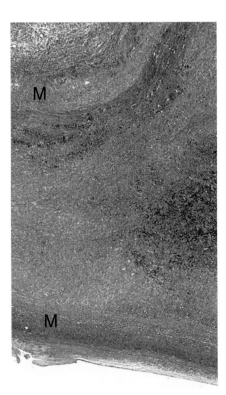

● **FIGURE 15-4.** Chronic aortic dissection in a patient with MFS. (A) EVG stain shows separation of the elastic fiber bundles of the media by collagenous fibroconnective tissue * (EVG ×60). (B) Trichrome stained slide from region marked by * showing the collagenous tissue interposed between the two portions of the medial layer (M) (Masson's trichrome ×400).

A   **B**

recommended with the frequency based upon the rate of growth of the aorta and the size of the aorta. The frequency should be increased when there is a significant chance that waiting longer between imaging studies would delay the time of prophylactic surgery. Imaging whether it be by echo, CT or MRI should include assessment of the aortic arch, the abdominal aorta and the descending thoracic aorta when possible. Regular imaging of the peripheral vessels is not currently recommended unless an aneurysm or dissection has been detected.

The success of prophylactic replacement of the aortic root has been well documented. Replacement of the aorta root, including the sinuses of Valsalva with a composite valve graft (modified Bentall procedure) remains the gold standard.[52] The desire to avoid lifelong anticoagulation has lead to valve sparing root replacement techniques.[53] The decreased morbidity of these strategies has lead to current recommendations to consider prophylactic aortic root replacement surgeries when the aortic root reaches between 4.5 and 5 cm.[54,55] The precise timing of intervention should take into account the degree to which the patient's aortic root deviates from the expected size, the rate of growth of the aorta, the presence of aortic dissections in affected relatives, symptoms, the patient's attitude toward their disease and the availability of an surgeon experienced in valve sparing techniques.

● LOEYS-DIETZ SYNDROME

LDS has been recently described and may overlap to some degrees with the previously described MFS-2.[56,57] It shares some of the vascular features of MFS and vascular EDS and may account for some of the more atypical cases that have previously been diagnosed with these conditions.[58] LDS is distinguished from MFS by a more aggressive and diffuse vascular involvement, characteristic craniofacial abnormalities and the absence of lens dislocation. The overlap with vascular EDS is perhaps even more pronounced. Patients previously thought to have vascular EDS but without confirmatory genetic or collagen analysis my have LDS instead.

Pathogenesis

LDS is caused by mutations of either the TGF-β receptor type I (TGFBR1) or II (TGFBR2) genes on chromosomes 9 and 3, respectively. The mutation results in overactivity of the TGF-β signaling pathway as documented by SMAD protein phosphorylation and thus shares a common biochemical pathway with MFS. The tissue specific occurrence of this over expression may account for the divergence of the clinical manifestations.

The inheritance is autosomal dominant with variable penetrance.

Clinical Manifestations

The vascular manifestation of LDS is marked vascular fragility resulting in vascular rupture and dissection. The aorta, and in particular the aortic root, is involved in 84%

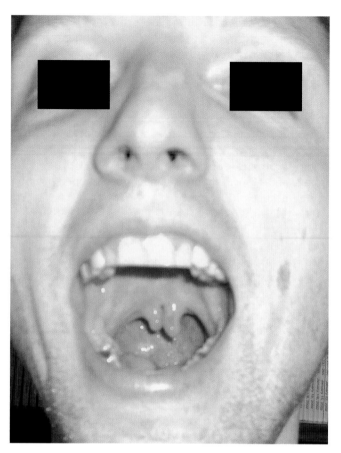

● **FIGURE 15-5.** Midline craniofacial features are a characteristic finding of Loeys-Dietz. This patient demonstrates a highly suggestive finding of a bifid uvula.

of cases. In contrast to MFS, involvement of other major arteries is also very frequent (57% prevalence). Intracranial aneurysms are also a feature of LDS. Approximately 80% of patients demonstrate vascular tortuosity, particularly of the cervical vessels as they approach the base of the skulls (see Figure 15-5). The tortuosity may also be seen in the iliac vessels. LDS shares with vascular EDS the risk of vessel rupture even when the vessel dilation is relatively limited, particularly when the craniofacial features of LDS are prominent.[59]

Extravascular manifestations of LDS are most notable for midline craniofacial features of hypertelorism, cleft palate and bifid uvula (see Figure 15-6). When present these features should raise concern for LDS. Congenital cardiac abnormalities such as atrial septal defect and patent ductus arteriosus are also frequently seen in LDS. Joint hypermobility and striae are also reported; however, unlike MFS the skeletal features caused by the long bone overgrowth occur less frequently. Similar to vascular EDS organ rupture occurs in LDS, with uterine and splenic rupture being the most common sites. The presence of instability of the cervical spine is also of significant clinical importance.

LDS can be subgrouped into LDS I and LDS II.[58] LDS I is marked by the presence of craniofacial features and whereas LDS II is characterized by the features suggestive of vascular EDS including organ rupture, easy bruisability,

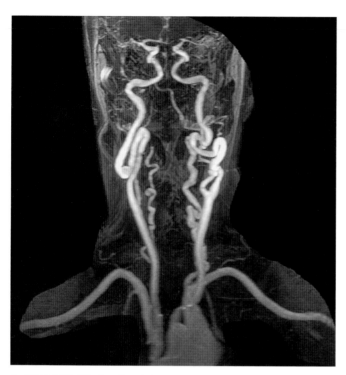

● **FIGURE 15-6.** Arterial tortuosity, particularly of the cervical vessels, is feature that should prompt suspicion of LDS. The degree of tortuosity as shown in this MR angiogram reconstruction is most apparent when 3-D reconstructions are created from MR angiograms or CT angiograms.

and translucent skin. The presence of craniofacial abnormalities correlates with earlier onset of vascular complication. The distinction between LDS I and II does not depend upon whether TGFBR1 or TGFBR2 are involved.

Median survival is 37 years. Mean age at first major event is 24.5 years in LDS I and 29.8 years in LDS II. Since LDS is a recently described condition the prognosis may evolve as additional cases are identified. The ominous prognosis as currently described may attenuate as less severely affected cases come to light. The prevalence of LDS is at this time unknown, but is probably less common than MFS.

Diagnosis

LDS should be considered as a potential cause of vascular complications in young patients presenting with aneurysms, dissections and vessel ruptures particularly if there is a family history of vascular or organ complications. Diagnosis at this time is based upon identification of a TGFB receptor mutation in the appropriate clinical context. Clues that LDS should be strongly considered are craniofacial abnormalities and the presence arterial tortuosity.

The clinical overlap with EDS IV and MFS suggests that cases, which have previously been ascribed to those conditions, should be assessed for the possibility of LDS if the diagnosis could not be confirmed genetically or if atypical features are present.[56,58]

Pathological Findings

The overlap of clinical findings of LDS with vascular EDS and MFS also extends to the pathological findings. Ascending aortic aneurysms and dissections are common vascular manifestations of LDS. Other abnormalities include generalized arterial tortuosity and aneurysms of other arteries such as nonaortic thoracic and head and neck arteries. There have been only a few reports of the histopathologic findings in LDS. In one report of a rapidly expanding acute Stanford type B aortic dissection, the aortic segment form the acute dissection region showed CMD.[59]

Management

The wide distribution of vascular abnormalities dictates the need to screen the entire vasculature for abnormalities. At this time this is most easily accomplished with CT angiography. The appropriate frequency for such screening is still unclear given the radiation exposure. Echocardiography also plays a role given that the aortic root remains the most frequent site of involvement.

The utility of these screening modalities comes from experience suggesting that prophylactic vascular intervention can be performed safely with relatively low risk in LDS in distinction to vascular EDS.[58]

In particular, the propensity toward aortic rupture and dissection at small aortic root sizes suggests prophylactic aortic root replacement surgery should be considered at aortic root sizes as small as 4 cm, if a valve-sparing aortic root replacement surgery is feasible. For patients with grave family histories root replacement surgery is advocated as soon as the aorta is shown to be definitively abnormal (>99th percentile) and an aortic graft large enough to accommodate adult blood flow can be used (~1.8 cm).[58]

Medical management has not been studied, however, the effects of blocking signaling at the angiotensin type II receptor on down regulating TGF-β signaling suggests that it may have a role to play in preventing the development of vascular complications.[39]

● ARTERIAL TORTUOSITY SYNDROME

Arterial tortuosity syndrome is a rare condition which manifests as extreme blood vessel tortuosity, particularly of the major branches of the aorta. Other clinical manifestations including joint laxity, contractures, hyperelastic skin, and arachnodactyly are also frequent and consistent with an underlying connective tissue abnormality.[60] The underlying genetic basis appears to be a mutation in the SLC2A10 gene on chromosome 20q13.1.[61] This gene encodes the GLUT10 glucose transporter. GLUT10 deficiency shares with MFS and LDS an increase in TGF-β signaling. Interestingly the manifestations are primarily of tortuosity, although aneurysm formation has been documented.[60] Histologically, the changes that have been described in the aorta include a wall thickness that was twice normal and an enlarged and fragmented elastic membrane.[62] The elastic and muscular arteries were elongated and spiraled in appearance. The walls of the muscular arteries were also thickened by intimal fibrosis, disruption of elastic fibers in the medial layer and fragmentation of the internal elastic membrane resulting in diminished luminal diameter.[63] Inheritance is autosomal recessive with most cases described in the literature from consanguineous families. It is likely that as more extensive imaging becomes available that additional cases will be identified.

● FIBROMUSCULAR DYSPLASIA

Fibromuscular dysplasia (FMD) is a noninflammatory nonatherosclerotic vascular disorder that typically presents with complications of stenotic lesions, however, aneurysms and dissection may also be part of more complex lesions. It is characterized by disorganization of the structural components of the wall of muscular arteries. The renal and the carotid arteries are the most common sites of involvement, however, it has been described in nearly every arterial bed.[64]

Pathogenesis

The clinical manifestations are the result of disordered organization of fibers within the vessel walls resulting in intermittent narrowing of the vascular lumen. An underlying genetic substrate for this abnormality has not yet been determined. Familial cases have been described suggesting an inheritable cause, although a putative gene has not been identified.[65–68] The majority of the cases, however, these appear to be sporadic. The inheritance pattern in familial cases suggests an autosomal dominant mechanism with variable inheritance.

Clinical Manifestations

FMD most frequently presents as occlusive and stenotic lesions of the medium sized arties. The renal and carotid arteries are most frequently involved with involvement in 89% and 26%, respectively. Other arteries include mesenteric arteries in 9%, subclavian arteries in 95 and iliac arteries in 5% of cases.[69] Age of presentation is typically between 15 and 50 years of age. There is a strong female predominance among afflicted individuals with female to male ratios between 5:1 and 9:1.[65,67] Aneurysms and dissections may also be manifestations of FMD.[70–72]

Involvement of the renal arteries is one of the major causes of secondary hypertension, particularly in patients under the age of 50, accounting for approximately 10% of all cases.[73] Occlusion of renal arteries, however, is uncommon.

Cerebrovascular involvement typically presents with symptoms of arterial insufficiency in the region supplied by the involved vessel. The symptoms may be nonspecific such as light-headedness or headache, but more specific neurological symptoms such as transient ischemic attacks, strokes or amaurosis fugax are reported.

Diagnosis

The beaded appearance of the affected blood vessels is the key diagnostic feature of FMD (see Figure 15-7A). This is most easily appreciated on angiography, but may also be visualized on CT[74] and MRI[75] (Figure 15-7B). Three-dimensional reconstructions or curved planar reconstructions of CT images may also be helpful in recognizing the characteristic appearance (Figures 15-7C and D). Medial hyperplasia is characterized by regions with thickened dysplastic media alternating with regions with thin media. Intimal, perimedial and adventitial are characterized by abnormal collagen deposition in the respective layers of the blood vessel wall.[64,76–79]

Pathological Findings

The beaded angiographic pattern reflects the alternating zones of luminal stenosis and normal vessel diameter and is confirmed at the time of surgical repair. In addition to fibrointimal proliferation the affected vessels show medial and adventitial changes and disorganization of elastic fibers in the medial layer. Three patterns have been described: medial, intimal and adventitial forms with the medial type accounting for the vast majority of cases. The medial form exhibits medial hyperplasia with replacement of some of the medial smooth muscle cells by fibrous connective tissue and fibroblastic cells and close spatial positioning of internal and external elastic membranes. In the intimal form, invaginating buds of fibrointimal tissue create luminal narrowing. Medial dissection and rupture have been reported in the medial type of FMD.

Management

Management is targeted at the vascular abnormalities. The stenotic lesions respond well to angioplasty and stenting with low risk of restenosis. In the renal arteries the initial success rate of angioplasty is between 82 and 100%.[73] Restenosis occurs in less than 11% to 23% of patients.[80,81] Revascularization of patients with hypertension caused by FMD results in amelioration or cure in nearly all cases.

Surgical intervention has also proven to be successful treatment modality. With the current success of percutaneous approaches it is usually reserved for cases where either percutaneous intervention has failed or is not feasible.

When the stenosis is not flow limiting, prophylactic antithrombotic treatment with aspirin is likely prudent, however, there are no clinical data as yet to support this approach.

● PSEUDOXANTHOMA ELASTICUM

Pseudoxanthoma elasticum (PXE) is an inherited condition characterized by premature vascular atherosclerosis, gastrointestinal bleeding as a result of vessel fragility in the gastrointestinal tract, angioid streaks in the eye and characteristic skin changes.

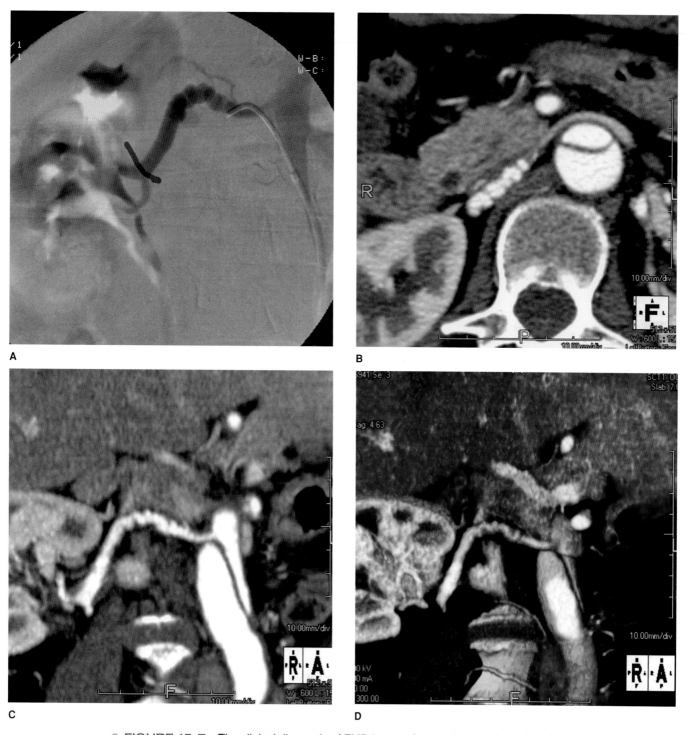

● **FIGURE 15-7.** The clinical diagnosis of FMD is most frequently made based on the characteristic beaded appearance of the affected vessels. It is most easily recognized on angiography as shown on the digital subtraction angiogram of (A) an affected renal artery. (B) The beaded appearance can also be seen on contrast CT scan axial images, however, full appreciation of the extent of the beaded appearance may be enhanced by (C) curved planar reconstructions or (D) 3-D reconstructions of the axial CT images.

Pathogenesis

The underlying genetic abnormality is caused by mutations in the *ABCC6* gene on chromosome 16p13.1, which belongs to the C subfamily of the ATP binding cassette (ABC) genes.[82–85] ABC proteins are transmembrane proteins that

act as active pumps for a variety of substrates. Interestingly, *ABCC6* is primarily expressed in the liver and kidney, with little expression in the tissues where PXE manifests itself clinically. This suggests that the mutation in *ABCC6* results in the lack of or accumulation of substances that interact with extracellular matrix synthesis and maintenance.[86] The altered extracellular metabolism results in the characteristic pathologic findings of elastic fiber fragmentation and mineralization.

Inheritance appears to be predominantly autosomal recessive, however, reports of autosomal dominant inheritance exist.[87]

Clinical Manifestations

The vascular manifestations of PXE include premature arterial narrowing and occlusion and mucosal bleeding.

The occlusive lesions typically involve small and medium sized arteries and may present with coronary artery disease, peripheral claudication or cerebrovascular disease.[88,89] Stenotic lesions develop slowly leading to extensive collateral formation. Histologically, the atheromatosis may be indistinguishable from that because of the traditional risk factors such as smoking and hypertension but occur at an earlier age and affect the arteries of the upper extremities.

Mucosal bleeding most frequently occurs in the gastrointestinal tract.[90] The precise mechanism of bleeding is unknown, but may relate to defective vasoconstriction. However, there is no evidence of vascular fragility.[91]

The skin manifestations of PXE are the clinical feature that typically leads to diagnosis, although it need not be uniformly present. The lesions typically consist of yellowish papules ranging in size from 1 to 5 mm. As they coalesce they may form patches that leads to the characteristic "plucked chicken skin" appearance. The lesions typically first become apparent on the lateral aspect of the neck and progress to involve the flexural regions, for example, the axillae, the antecubital, and popliteal fossa. The loss of elasticity of the tissue frequently results in redundant skin folds.

The disruption of the elastic fibers in Bruch's membrane within the eye leads to the characteristic angioid streaks on fundoscopic examination. Although the angioid streaks do not directly affect vision, the proliferation of brittle choroidal neovessels with subsequent retinal bleeding may lead to blindness.

Diagnosis

PXE should be suspected when the typical skin findings or unexplained vascular calcification is found. Confirmation by skin biopsy is easily available.

Inherited hemoglobinopathies, for example, β-thalassemia can mimic all of the findings of PXE, skin, cardiac, and ocular, however, they typically occur at an older age.[92] Therefore, exclusion of hemoglobinopathies is appropriate when considering the diagnosis of PXE.

Pathological Findings

The cardiovascular changes in PXE include endocardial plaques in the atria and occasionally on the leaflets of atrioventricular valves. The endomyocardial biopsy can be helpful in documenting the thickened endocardium composed of fragmented, thickened and calcified elastic fibers. The aorta is rarely affected; medium sized vessels are the primary site of involvement. These intimal changes produce luminal stenosis or aneurysmal dilatation and account for the accelerated atherosclerosis.[93]

Management

There is no specific treatment to prevent the vascular manifestations of PXE. Revascularization in the setting of coronary disease seems to be beneficial, however, the internal mammary artery should be used as a conduit only with care since it may also be involved in PXE.[94] Aggressive management of the usual risk factors for atherosclerosis such as hyperlipidemia, smoking, and diabetes also makes sense; however, there are no studies to support such an approach. The risk of mucosal bleeding makes the use of antithrombotic agents such as aspirin and clopidogrel somewhat problematic and the risk benefit ratio should be assessed individually.

REFERENCES

1. Barabas AP. Vascular complications in the Ehlers-Danlos syndrome, with special reference to the "arterial type" or Sack's syndrome. *J Cardiovasc Surg (Torino)*. 1972;13(2):160-167.

2. Beighton P, De Paepe A, Steinmann B, et al. Ehlers-Danlos syndromes: revised nosology, Villefranche, 1997. Ehlers-Danlos National Foundation (USA) and Ehlers-Danlos Support Group (UK). *Am J Med Genet*. 1998;77(1):31-37.

3. Beighton P, de Paepe A, Danks D, et al. International nosology of heritable disorders of connective tissue, Berlin, 1986. *Am J Med Genet*. 1988;29(3):581-594.

4. Malfait F, Symoens S, De Backer J, et al. Three arginine to cysteine substitutions in the pro-alpha (I)-collagen chain cause Ehlers-Danlos syndrome with a propensity to arterial rupture in early adulthood. *Hum Mutat*. 2007;28(4):387-395.

5. Plaisier E, Gribouval O, Alamowitch S, et al. COL4A1 mutations and hereditary angiopathy, nephropathy, aneurysms, and muscle cramps. *N Engl J Med*. 2007;357(26):2687-2695.

6. Wenstrup RJ, Murad S, Pinnell SR. Ehlers-Danlos syndrome type VI: clinical manifestations of collagen lysyl hydroxylase deficiency. *J Pediatr*. 1989;115(3):405-409.

7. Germain DP. Ehlers-Danlos syndrome type IV. *Orphanet J Rare Dis*. 2007;2:32.

8. Gelse K, Poschl E, Aigner T. Collagens—structure, function, and biosynthesis. *Adv Drug Deliv Rev*. 2003;55(12):1531-1546.

9. Pope FM, Martin GR, Lichtenstein JR, et al. Patients with Ehlers-Danlos syndrome type IV lack type III collagen. *Proc Natl Acad Sci U S A*. 1975;72(4):1314-1316.

10. Pepin M, Schwarze U, Superti-Furga A, et al. Clinical and genetic features of Ehlers-Danlos syndrome type IV, the vascular type. *N Engl J Med*. 2000;342(10):673-680.

11. Pyeritz RE. Ehlers-Danlos syndrome. *N Engl J Med*. 2000;342 (10):730-732.

12. Schwarze U, Schievink WI, Petty E, et al. Haploinsufficiency for one COL3A1 allele of type III procollagen results in a phenotype similar to the vascular form of Ehlers-Danlos syndrome, Ehlers-Danlos syndrome type IV. *Am J Hum Genet*. 2001;69(5):989-1001.

13. Oderich GS, Panneton JM, Bower TC, et al. The spectrum, management and clinical outcome of Ehlers-Danlos syndrome type IV: a 30-year experience. *J Vasc Surg*. 2005;42(1):98-106.

14. North KN, Whiteman DA, Pepin MG, et al. Cerebrovascular complications in Ehlers-Danlos syndrome type IV. *Ann Neurol*. 1995;38(6):960-964.

15. Barabas AP. Ehlers-Danlos syndrome type IV. *N Engl J Med*. 2000;343(5):366.

16. Nishiyama Y, Manabe N, Ooshima A, et al. A sporadic case of Ehlers-Danlos syndrome type IV: diagnosed by a morphometric study of collagen content. *Pathol Int*. 1995;45(7):524-529.

17. Crowther MA, Lach B, Dunmore PJ, et al. Vascular collagen fibril morphology in type IV Ehlers-Danlos syndrome. *Connect Tissue Res*. 1991;25(3-4):209-217.

18. Casana R, Nano G, Dalainas I, et al. Endovascular treatment of hepatic artery aneurysm in a patient with Ehlers-Danlos syndrome. Case report. *Int Angiol*. 2004;23(3):291-295.

19. Kurata A, Oka H, Ohmomo T, et al. Successful stent placement for cervical artery dissection associated with the Ehlers-Danlos syndrome. Case report and review of the literature. *J Neurosurg*. 2003;99(6):1077-1081.

20. Sugawara Y, Ban K, Imai K, et al. Successful coil embolization for spontaneous arterial rupture in association with Ehlers-Danlos syndrome type IV: report of a case. *Surg Today*. 2004;34(1):94-96.

21. Uchiyama D, Koganemaru M, Abe T, et al. Successful transcatheter arterial embolization for spontaneous rupture of the posterior tibial artery in a patient with Ehlers-Danlos syndrome type IV. *J Vasc Interv Radiol*. 2006;17(10):1716-1717.

22. Tonnessen BH, Sternbergh WC III, Mannava K, et al. Endovascular repair of an iliac artery aneurysm in a patient with Ehlers-Danlos syndrome type IV. *J Vasc Surg*. 2007;45(1):177-1779.

23. Schievink WI, Piepgras DG, Earnest FT, et al. Spontaneous carotid-cavernous fistulae in Ehlers-Danlos syndrome Type IV. Case report. *J Neurosurg*. 1991;74(6):991-998.

24. Horowitz MB, Purdy PD, Valentine RJ, et al. Remote vascular catastrophes after neurovascular interventional therapy for type 4 Ehlers-Danlos Syndrome. *AJNR Am J Neuroradiol*. 2000;21(5):974-976.

25. Freeman RK, Swegle J, Sise MJ. The surgical complications of Ehlers-Danlos syndrome. *Am Surg*. 1996;62(10):869-873.

26. Chuman H, Trobe JD, Petty EM, et al. Spontaneous direct carotid-cavernous fistula in Ehlers-Danlos syndrome type IV: two case reports and a review of the literature. *J Neuroophthalmol*. 2002;22(2):75-81.

27. Hollands JK, Santarius T, Kirkpatrick PJ, et al. Treatment of a direct carotid-cavernous fistula in a patient with type IV Ehlers-Danlos syndrome: a novel approach. *Neuroradiology*. 2006;48(7):491-494.

28. Vakonakis I, Campbell ID. Extracellular matrix: from atomic resolution to ultrastructure. *Curr Opin Cell Biol*. 2007;19(5): 578-583.

29. Dietz HC, Cutting GR, Pyeritz RE, et al. Marfan syndrome caused by a recurrent de novo missense mutation in the fibrillin gene. *Nature*. 1991;352(6333):337-339.

30. Sakai LY, Keene DR, Engvall E. Fibrillin, a new 350-kD glycoprotein, is a component of extracellular microfibrils. *J Cell Biol*. 1986;103(6, pt 1):2499-2509.

31. Reinhardt DP, Keene DR, Corson GM, et al. Fibrillin-1: organization in microfibrils and structural properties. *J Mol Biol*. 1996;258(1):104-116.

32. Ramirez F, Gayraud B, Pereira L. Marfan syndrome: new clues to genotype-phenotype correlations. *Ann Med*. 1999;31(3): 202-207.

33. Mizuguchi T, Collod-Beroud G, Akiyama T, et al. Heterozygous TGFBR2 mutations in Marfan syndrome. *Nat Genet*. 2004;36(8):855-860.

34. Kainulainen K, Karttunen L, Puhakka L, et al. Mutations in the fibrillin gene responsible for dominant ectopia lentis and neonatal Marfan syndrome. *Nat Genet*. 1994;6(1):64-69.

35. Faivre L, Collod-Beroud G, Loeys BL, et al. Effect of mutation type and location on clinical outcome in 1,013 probands with Marfan syndrome or related phenotypes and FBN1 mutations: an international study. *Am J Hum Genet*. 2007;81(3):454-466.

36. Aoyama T, Francke U, Dietz HC, et al. Quantitative differences in biosynthesis and extracellular deposition of fibrillin in cultured fibroblasts distinguish five groups of Marfan syndrome patients and suggest distinct pathogenetic mechanisms. *J Clin Invest*. 1994;94(1):130-137.

37. Judge DP, Biery NJ, Keene DR, et al. Evidence for a critical contribution of haploinsufficiency in the complex pathogenesis of Marfan syndrome. *J Clin Invest*. 2004;114(2):172-181.

38. Matyas G, Alonso S, Patrignani A, et al. Large genomic fibrillin-1 (FBN1) gene deletions provide evidence for true haploinsufficiency in Marfan syndrome. *Hum Genet*. 2007; 122(1):23-32.

39. Habashi JP, Judge DP, Holm TM, et al. Losartan, an AT1 antagonist, prevents aortic aneurysm in a mouse model of Marfan syndrome. *Science*. 2006;312(5770):117-121.

40. Aburawi EH, O'Sullivan J. Relation of aortic root dilatation and age in Marfan's syndrome. *Eur Heart J*. 2007;28(3):376-379.

41. Silverman DI, Burton KJ, Gray J, et al. Life expectancy in the Marfan syndrome. *Am J Cardiol*. 1995;75(2):157-160.

42. Nawa S, Ikeda E, Ichihara S, et al. A true aneurysm of axillary-subclavian artery with cystic medionecrosis: an unusual manifestation of Marfan syndrome. *Ann Vasc Surg*. 2003; 17(5):562-564.

43. Savolainen H, Savola J, Savolainen A. Aneurysm of the iliac artery in Marfan's syndrome. *Ann Chir Gynaecol*. 1993;82(3): 203-205.

44. Flanagan PV, Geoghegan J, Egan TJ. Iliac artery aneurysm in Marfan's syndrome. *Eur J Vasc Surg.* 1990;4(3):323-324.

45. de Virgilio C, Cherry KJ Jr, Schaff HV. Multiple aneurysms and aortic dissection: an unusual manifestation of Marfan's syndrome. *Ann Vasc Surg.* 1994;8(4):383-386.

46. Latter DA, Ricci MA, Forbes RD, et al. Internal carotid artery aneurysm and Marfan's syndrome. *Can J Surg.* 1989;32(6): 463-466.

47. Schievink WI, Parisi JE, Piepgras DG, et al. Intracranial aneurysms in Marfan's syndrome: an autopsy study. *Neurosurgery.* 1997;41(4):866-870; discussion 871.

48. Conway JE, Hutchins GM, Tamargo RJ. Marfan syndrome is not associated with intracranial aneurysms. *Stroke.* 1999;30 (8):1632-1636.

49. De Paepe A, Devereux RB, Dietz HC, et al. Revised diagnostic criteria for the Marfan syndrome. *Am J Med Genet.* 1996; 62(4):417-426.

50. Roberts WC, Honig HS. The spectrum of cardiovascular disease in the Marfan Syndrome: a clinico-morphologic study of 18 necropsy patients and comparison to 151 previously reported necropsy patients. *Am Heart J.* 1982;104:115-135.

51. Shores J, Berger KR, Murphy EA, et al. Progression of aortic dilatation and the benefit of long-term beta-adrenergic blockade in Marfan's syndrome. *N Engl J Med.* 1994;330(19):1335-1341.

52. Gott VL, Greene PS, Alejo DE, et al. Replacement of the aortic root in patients with Marfan's syndrome. *N Engl J Med.* 1999;340(17):1307-1313.

53. Tambeur L, David TE, Unger M, et al. Results of surgery for aortic root aneurysm in patients with the Marfan syndrome. *Eur J Cardiothorac Surg.* 2000;17(4):415-419.

54. Kim SY, Martin N, Hsia EC, et al. Management of aortic disease in Marfan Syndrome: a decision analysis. *Arch Intern Med.* 2005;165(7):749-755.

55. Milewicz DM, Dietz HC, Miller DC. Treatment of aortic disease in patients with Marfan syndrome. *Circulation.* 2005; 111(11):e150-e157.

56. Singh KK, Rommel K, Mishra A, et al. TGFBR1 and TGFBR2 mutations in patients with features of Marfan syndrome and Loeys-Dietz syndrome. *Hum Mutat.* 2006;27(8):770-777.

57. Loeys BL, Chen J, Neptune ER, et al. A syndrome of altered cardiovascular, craniofacial, neurocognitive and skeletal development caused by mutations in TGFBR1 or TGFBR2. *Nat Genet.* 2005;37(3):275-281.

58. Loeys BL, Schwarze U, Holm T, et al. Aneurysm syndromes caused by mutations in the TGF-beta receptor. *N Engl J Med.* 2006;355(8):788-798.

59. Lee RS, Fazel S, Schwarze U, et al. Rapid aneurysmal degeneration of a Stanford type B aortic dissection in a patient with Loeys-Dietz syndrome. *J Thorac Cardiovasc Surg.* 2007; 134(1):242-243.

60. Wessels MW, Catsman-Berrevoets CE, Mancini GM, et al. Three new families with arterial tortuosity syndrome. *Am J Med Genet A.* 2004;131(2):134-143.

61. Coucke PJ, Willaert A, Wessels MW, et al. Mutations in the facilitative glucose transporter GLUT10 alter angiogenesis and cause arterial tortuosity syndrome. *Nat Genet.* 2006;38(4): 452-457.

62. Beuren AJ, Hort W, Kalbfleisch H, et al. Dysplasia of the systemic and pulmonary arterial system with tortuosity and lengthening of the arteries. A new entity, diagnosed during life, and leading to coronary death in early childhood. *Circulation.* 1969;39(1):109-115.

63. Pletcher BA, Fox JE, Boxer RA, et al. Four sibs with arterial tortuosity: description and review of the literature. *Am J Med Genet.* 1996;66(2):121-128.

64. Stanley JC, Gewertz BL, Bove EL, et al. Arterial fibrodysplasia. Histopathologic character and current etiologic concepts. *Arch Surg.* 1975;110(5):561-566.

65. Grimbert P, Fiquer-Kempf B, Coudol P, et al. Genetic study of renal artery fibromuscular dysplasia. *Arch Mal Coeur Vaiss.* 1998;91(8):1069-1071.

66. Rushton AR. The genetics of fibromuscular dysplasia. *Arch Intern Med.* 1980;140(2):233-236.

67. Pannier-Moreau I, Grimbert P, Fiquet-Kempf B, et al. Possible familial origin of multifocal renal artery fibromuscular dysplasia. *J Hypertens.* 1997;15(12, pt 2):1797-1801.

68. Perdu J, Boutouyrie P, Bourgain C, et al. Inheritance of arterial lesions in renal fibromuscular dysplasia. *J Hum Hypertens.* 2007;21(5):393-400.

69. Luscher TF, Keller HM, Imhof HG, et al. Fibromuscular hyperplasia: extension of the disease and therapeutic outcome. Results of the University Hospital Zurich Cooperative Study on Fibromuscular Hyperplasia. *Nephron.* 1986;44(suppl 1): 109-114.

70. Bonardelli S, Vettoretto N, Tiberio GA, et al. Right subclavian artery aneurysms of fibrodysplastic origin: two case reports and review of literature. *J Vasc Surg.* 2001;33(1):174-177.

71. Kojima A, Shindo S, Kubota, K, et al. Successful surgical treatment of a patient with multiple visceral artery aneurysms due to fibromuscular dysplasia. *Cardiovasc Surg.* 2002;10(2):157-160.

72. Radhi JM, McKay R, Tyrrell MJ. Fibromuscular dysplasia of the aorta presenting as multiple recurrent thoracic aneurysms. *Int J Angiol.* 1998;7(3):215-218.

73. Safian RD, Textor SC. Renal-artery stenosis. *N Engl J Med.* 2001;344(6):431-442.

74. Sabharwal R, Vladica P, Coleman P. Multidetector spiral CT renal angiography in the diagnosis of renal artery fibromuscular dysplasia. *Eur J Radiol.* 2007;61(3):520-527.

75. Willoteaux S, Faivre-Pierret M, Moranne O, et al. Fibromuscular dysplasia of the main renal arteries: comparison of contrast-enhanced MR angiography with digital subtraction angiography. *Radiology.* 2006;241(3):922-929.

76. Harrison EG Jr, McCormack LJ. Pathologic classification of renal arterial disease in renovascular hypertension. *Mayo Clin Proc.* 1971;46(3):161-167.

77. Bragin MA, Cherkasov AP. Morphogenesis of fibromuscular dysplasia of the renal arteries (an ultrastructural study). *Arkh Patol.* 1979;41(2):46-52.

78. Begelman SM, Olin JW. Fibromuscular dysplasia. *Curr Opin Rheumatol.* 2000;12(1):41-47.

79. Vuong PN, Desoutter P, Mickley V, et al. Fibromuscular dysplasia of the renal artery responsible for renovascular hypertension: a histological presentation based on a series of 102 patients. *Vasa.* 2004;33(1):13-18.

80. Plouin PF, Darne B, Chatellier G, et al. Restenosis after a first percutaneous transluminal renal angioplasty. *Hypertension.* 1993;21(1):89-96.

81. Birrer M, Do DD, Mahler F, et al. Treatment of renal artery fibromuscular dysplasia with balloon angioplasty: a prospective follow-up study. *Eur J Vasc Endovasc Surg.* 2002;23(2):146-152.

82. Struk B, Cai L, Zach S, et al. Mutations of the gene encoding the transmembrane transporter protein ABC-C6 cause pseudoxanthoma elasticum. *J Mol Med.* 2000;78(5):282-286.

83. Bergen AA, Plomp AS, Schuurman EJ, et al. Mutations in ABCC6 cause pseudoxanthoma elasticum. *Nat Genet.* 2000;25(2):228-231.

84. Le Saux O, Urban Z, Tschuch C, et al. Mutations in a gene encoding an ABC transporter cause pseudoxanthoma elasticum. *Nat Genet.* 2000;25(2):223-227.

85. Ringpfeil F, Lebwohl MG, Christiano AM, et al. Pseudoxanthoma elasticum: mutations in the MRP6 gene encoding a transmembrane ATP-binding cassette (ABC) transporter. *Proc Natl Acad Sci USA.* 2000;97(11):6001-6006.

86. Le Saux O, Bunda S, VanWart CM, et al. Serum factors from pseudoxanthoma elasticum patients alter elastic fiber formation in vitro. *J Invest Dermatol.* 2006;126(7):1497-1505.

87. Plomp AS, Hu X, de Jong PT, et al. Does autosomal dominant pseudoxanthoma elasticum exist? *Am J Med Genet A.* 2004; 126(4):403-412.

88. Pavlovic AM, Zidverc-Trajkovic J, Milovic MM, et al. Cerebral small vessel disease in pseudoxanthoma elasticum: three cases. *Can J Neurol Sci.* 2005;32(1):115-118.

89. Khan MA, Beard J. Peripheral vascular disease in an individual with pseudoxanthoma elasticum. *Eur J Vasc Endovasc Surg.* 2007;34(5):590-591. Epub 2007 May 31.

90. McCreedy CA, Zimmerman TJ, Webster SF. Management of upper gastrointestinal hemorrhage in patients with pseudoxanthoma elasticum. *Surgery.* 1989;105(2, pt 1):170-174.

91. Chassaing N, Martin L, Calvas P, et al. Pseudoxanthoma elasticum: a clinical, pathophysiological and genetic update including 11 novel ABCC6 mutations. *J Med Genet.* 2005;42(12):881-892.

92. Aessopos A, Farmakis D, Loukopoulos D. Elastic tissue abnormalities resembling pseudoxanthoma elasticum in beta thalassemia and the sickling syndromes. *Blood.* 2002;99(1):30-35.

93. Mendelsohn G, Bulkley BH, Hutchins GM. Cardiovascular manifestations of Pseudoxanthoma elasticum. *Arch Pathol Lab Med.* 1978;102(6):298-302.

94. Iliopoulos J, Manganas C, Jepson N, et al. Pseudoxanthoma elasticum: is the left internal mammary artery a suitable conduit for coronary artery bypass grafting? *Ann Thorac Surg.* 2002;73(2):652-653.

chapter 16

History and Physical Examination

Jessica A. Sutherland, MD / Ferdinand S. Leya, MD / Robert S. Dieter, MD, RVT

● HISTORY TAKING

Importance of History Taking

A thorough history is essential in all fields of medicine. It has often been said that a majority of all diagnosis are suggested or made by the history, even more when aided by a careful physical examination. Although technology has greatly advanced and it is tempting to order a battery of tests to aid in diagnosis, the history remains the most valuable source of information concerning the patient's illness.

The history serves as the primary source for data gathering and should include both the patient's perspective and account of symptoms as well as information obtained from directed questioning by the examiner. The patient should be allowed to talk without interruption regarding their primary concern, and should also be able to voice an opinion about what he or she believes may be the underlying problem. When more information is needed, the examiner should use nonleading questions to collect further details and permit the patient to answer each question fully before moving on to the next. If the patient is acutely ill, however, it is reasonable for the examiner to limit the patient's time for response in order to allow for prompt evaluation and treatment. When possible, the examiner should speak with family members or close friends in order to better understand the extent of disability and the impact of illness not only on the patient but also on those around the patient.

Additionally, the time spent during the history allows the patient and examiner to develop a bond that will aid in future diagnosis and therapy. Maintaining eye contact and intent listening will demonstrate the clinician's compassion and understanding. Asking key questions in words the patient understands and using a nonjudgmental tone will enhance communication, instill confidence, and facilitate a trusting relationship that will lend support to acceptance of therapy and compliance with treatments.

Finally, the history serves as a way to organize the examiner's thoughts, maximize clinical reasoning, and create a comprehensive differential diagnosis. This in turn leads to a more proficient physical examination, appropriate use of diagnostic aids, and prioritization of therapeutic interventions.

Analysis of a Symptom

Often the patient will present with a main symptom or complaint for which they seek assistance. In accurately evaluating each symptom, it is important to recall the characteristics of symptom analysis (see Table 16-1). Using each attribute to further define an index symptom is fundamental in recognizing disease patterns and developing a detailed differential diagnosis.

Location. In determining location of a symptom, it is important to be as specific as possible. Patients will often include a location in their chief complaint such as "I have leg pain," etc., however, more precision is needed. For example, is the pain anterior, posterior, hip, thigh, calf, foot, left-sided, right-sided? In addition, does the pain radiate or change location? Some symptoms such as fatigue or weakness may not have a specific location, and this is valuable to document as well.

Quality. For some symptoms, more descriptive adjectives are easily applied. Regarding a chief complaint of pain, one could use words such as burning, pressure, heaviness, sharp, dull, or cramping for further qualification. With other symptoms, like dizziness, patients may have more difficulty expanding on their sensation without the examiner assisting with a question such as "Could you tell me more about what that was like for you?" Sometimes even the patient's inability to describe the symptom may be a clue in

TABLE 16-1. Characteristics of Symptom Analysis

Characteristic
Location
Quality
Quantity (severity)
Timing
Setting
Alleviating/aggravating factors
Associated manifestations

itself. Patient facial expressions and gestures can also be of support.

Quantity or Severity. Quantification of a symptom may use well-known units such as number of pillows for orthopnea, or teaspoons of sputum. An analogue scale from 0 to 10 can be used to evaluate severity for symptoms in which a numerical unit cannot be applied such as with pain. Occasionally quantification can be made in terms of how the symptom is affecting daily activities such as walking to the bathroom or carrying bags of groceries.

Timing. In evaluating the timing of a symptom, the examiner should note the onset, duration, and frequency. When was the symptom first appreciated or how long has it been taking place? In the case of an intermittent symptom, how long does it persist in terms of seconds, minutes, hours, or days when it does arise? Is the symptom a daily occurrence, twice a week, or maybe only once every few weeks?

Setting. Determining the setting of a symptom can be thought of as an expansion on its timing in that the examiner looks to identify *when* the symptom occurs. Using leg pain as an example, is it related to certain activities such as walking up stairs or prolonged periods of standing? Does it occur at specific times for example upon first waking and getting out of bed or during the night while sleeping? Were there any precipitating factors or events such a fall or car accident?

Alleviating and Aggravating Factors. Often the patient will have already made attempts to stop the symptom when it occurs or preempt it from happening altogether. Inquiries should be made as to anything the patient feels may help relieve the symptom including positional changes or medications, both over-the-counter and prescription. In addition, are there things that make the symptom worse or does the patient avoid certain actions in order to prevent the symptom from happening?

Associated Symptoms. Finally, the examiner should explore whether the patient's complaint is a lone symptom, or if there are other sensations that transpire along with

it. Patients may not even be aware of additional symptoms until questioned. Documentation of a lack of associated symptoms is helpful as well.

VASCULAR HISTORY

Peripheral arterial disease can involve the ascending aortic arch and its branches, the descending aorta and its branches, and all muscular arteries. Symptoms produced by peripheral arterial disease are often governed by the location of the lesion, the severity or chronicity of the lesion, and the status of collateral flow. Several questionnaires have been developed to assess the presence and severity of lower extremity peripheral arterial disease. The Rose Questionnaire was initially developed in 1962 to diagnose both angina and peripheral arterial disease in epidemiological surveys but was limited by low sensitivity. Modifications, including the Edinburgh Claudication Questionnaire and the San Diego Questionnaire, have been created and validated to be more sensitive and specific in comparison to a physician's diagnosis based on walking distance, walking speed, and nature of symptoms.[1-3] Most recently, the Walking Impairment Questionnaire has proven to be a validated instrument even after modification for self-administration (see Figure 16-1).[4]

In evaluating a patient's symptoms, the examiner must keep in mind risk factors that would yield a vascular etiology to be more likely and assess for them as well. Peripheral arterial disease may be a manifestation of systemic atherosclerosis and therefore shares similar risk factors. Major nonreversible risk factors for atherosclerosis consist of age, male sex, and family history of premature disease. Modifiable risk factors for the development and/or progression of atherosclerotic disease include tobacco smoking, dyslipidemia, diabetes mellitus, hypertension, hyperhomocysteinemia, and elevated C-reactive protein (see Table 16-2).[1,5]

Common Vascular Symptoms

Extremity Pain. The term *claudication* stems from the Latin verb *claudicare*, which means to limp. Intermittent claudication is one of the most common vascular complaints and is defined as a reproducible discomfort in a particular muscle group brought on by exercise and is relieved with rest (see Table 16-3). The actual muscle discomfort can vary from patient to patient, leading to variable descriptions of which the examiner must be aware including pain, cramping, tightness, burning, weakness, heaviness, or fatigue. The description offered by the patient may be helpful in quantifying the extent of ischemia; terms such as "heaviness" and "tiredness" typically represent minimal ischemic changes, but "pain" and "cramping" usually indicate more extensive disease.[6] The quantity of discomfort is proportional to the amount and vigorousness of exercise, so questions should be directed so as to determine not only the distance a patient can walk but also at what speed or incline. It is important to note that symptoms of joint or bone pain or those brought on by prolonged standing are

1. *Please place a* ✔ *in the box that best describes how much difficulty you have had walking due to pain, aches, or cramps during the last week. The response options range from "No Difficulty" to "Great Difficulty."*

During the last week, *how much difficulty have you had walking due to:*	**No Difficulty**	**Slight Difficulty**	**Some Difficulty**	**Much Difficulty**	**Great Difficulty**
a. Pain, aching, or cramps in your calves?	❑ 1	❑ 2	❑ 3	❑ 4	❑ 5
b. Pain, aching, or cramps in your buttocks?	❑ 1	❑ 2	❑ 3	❑ 4	❑ 5

For the following questions, the response options range from "No Difficulty" to "Unable to Do." If you **cannot physically perform** a specified activity, for example walk 2 blocks without stopping to rest because of symptoms such as leg pain or discomfort, please place a ✔ in the box labeled "Unable to Do."

However, if you **do not perform** an activity for reasons unrelated to your circulation problems, such as climbing a flight of stairs becuse your home is one level or your apartment has an elevator, please place a ✔ in the box labeled "Don't Do for Other Resons."

2. *Please place a* ✔ *in the box that best describes how hard it was for you to walk on level ground withot stopping to rest for each of the following distances during the last week.*

During the last week, *how difficult was it for you to:*	**No Difficulty**	**Slight Difficulty**	**Some Difficulty**	**Much Difficulty**	**Unable to Do**	**Did not Do for Other Reasons**
a. Walk indoors, such as around your home?	❑ 1	❑ 2	❑ 3	❑ 4	❑ 5	❑ 6
b. Walk 50 feet?	❑ 1	❑ 2	❑ 3	❑ 4	❑ 5	❑ 6
c. Walk 150 feet? (1/2 block)?	❑ 1	❑ 2	❑ 3	❑ 4	❑ 5	❑ 6
d. Walk 300 feet? (1 block)?	❑ 1	❑ 2	❑ 3	❑ 4	❑ 5	❑ 6
e. Walk 600 feet? (2 blocks)?	❑ 1	❑ 2	❑ 3	❑ 4	❑ 5	❑ 6
f. Walk 900 feet? (3 blocks)?	❑ 1	❑ 2	❑ 3	❑ 4	❑ 5	❑ 6
g. Walk 1500 feet? (5 blocks)?	❑ 1	❑ 2	❑ 3	❑ 4	❑ 5	❑ 6

● **FIGURE 16-1.** Walking Impairment Questionnaire modified for self-administration. (Continued)

Reproduced, with permission, from Coyne KS, Margolis MK, Gilchrist KA, et al. Evaluating effects of method of administration on walking impairment questionnaire. J Vasc Surg. 2003;38:296-304.

typically not claudication and another etiology should be sought (see Table 16-4).

The location of the discomfort gives clues to the arterial system compromised. Most often patients report calf pain which can be attributed to disease in the superficial femoral or popliteal artery; however, patients can also have foot pain from tibial–peroneal disease, gluteal, and thigh pain caused by aortoiliac disease, or arm pain secondary to subclavian involvement. While the occlusive process can be at multiple levels, the initial site of claudication usually reflects the most distal significant lesion or the area with the poorest collateral flow.[7] Occlusive arterial disease is often bilateral, although patients will frequently report only unilateral symptoms caused by varying degrees of hemodynamically significant obstruction.

Progression of arterial insufficiency can result in rest pain, especially at night when reclined. Often patients will provide a history of past claudication that had progressed, but will now deny claudication due to self-imposed sedentary lifestyle.[6] Rest pain is classically described as stabbing, burning, or stinging, and can be associated with coldness, numbness, or parasthesias of the toes. Patients will commonly relate that relief is only obtained by placing the feet on the floor, dangling them off the side of the bed, or sleeping in a seated position. This dependent posture permits gravity to assist with perfusion pressure and improve the transport of blood supply to the painful extremities.

Seventy to eighty percent of patients presenting with acute peripheral syndromes have suffered an embolic event, with acute thrombosis or mechanical compression

3. *Please place a ✔ in the box that best describes how hard it was for you to walk one city block on level ground at each of these speeds without stopping to rest during the last week. Please not 1 block is roughly equivalent to 300 feet.*

During the last week, *how difficult was it for you to:*	**No Difficulty**	**Slight Difficulty**	**Some Difficulty**	**Much Difficulty**	**Unable to Do**	**Did not Do for Other Reasons**
a. Walk 1 block slowly?	☐ 1	☐ 2	☐ 3	☐ 4	☐ 5	☐ 6
b. Walk 1 block at average speed?	☐ 1	☐ 2	☐ 3	☐ 4	☐ 5	☐ 6
c. Walk 1 block quickly?	☐ 1	☐ 2	☐ 3	☐ 4	☐ 5	☐ 6
d. Run or jog 1 block?	☐ 1	☐ 2	☐ 3	☐ 4	☐ 5	☐ 6

4. *Please place a ✔ in the box that best describes how hard it was for you to climb stairs withour stopping to rest durign the last week. Please note 1 flight of stairs is roughly equal to 14 steps.*

During the last week, *how difficult was it for you to:*	**No Difficulty**	**Slight Difficulty**	**Some Difficulty**	**Much Difficulty**	**Unable to Do**	**Did not Do for Other Reasons**
a. Climb 1 flight of stairs?	☐ 1	☐ 2	☐ 3	☐ 4	☐ 5	☐ 6
b. Climb 2 flights of stairs?	☐ 1	☐ 2	☐ 3	☐ 4	☐ 5	☐ 6
c. Climb 3 flights of stairs?	☐ 1	☐ 2	☐ 3	☐ 4	☐ 5	☐ 6

● **FIGURE 16-1.** (*Continued*)

occurring much less frequently.[8] The patient with acute arterial occlusion classically demonstrates the six p's: pain, pallor, pulselessness, parasthesias, poikilothermia, and paralysis. Acute arterial occlusion can cause sudden and severe pain that is continuous for the first few hours followed by a period of numbness as ischemic damage progresses. The often-excruciating pain is unrelated to physical exertion and is not relieved by rest or position changes.

Chest Pain. When a patient reports any form of chest pain, the heart is generally considered the most probable as well as the most worrisome source. Varying degrees of chest discomfort, however, can originate from several other noncardiac intrathoracic vascular sources and can be just as serious. The diagnosis and differentiation from myocardial ischemic pain requires careful symptom analysis, including location, radiation, quality, severity, timing, and aggravating or alleviating factors.

Sudden onset of severe chest pain is the single most common presenting symptom for acute aortic dissection, reported in 63% of type B dissections and 79% of type A dissections based on the International Registry of Acute Aortic Dissection (IRAD).[9] Patients will classically describe the quality of pain as "ripping," "stabbing," or "tearing" that often radiates to the back. The intensity of the pain is at its maximum at inception and is often unrelenting in na-

ture; it is not associated with physical activity nor is it relieved by rest or change in body position, although patients have been known to writhe in agony or pace relentlessly in an effort to find some relief. Location and radiation of the pain can be helpful in determining the origin and/or path of the dissection. Anterior chest pain with radiation to the neck, jaw, or face is strongly indicative of involvement of the ascending aorta and one or more arch vessels, whereas chest pain with radiation to the intrascapular or lower back correlates with descending aortic dissections.[10] Other clues to the diagnosis include a history of hypertension or connective tissue disorder such as Marfan's syndrome, and clinical manifestations depending on the branch arteries involved.

Noncardiac chest pain that is gradual in onset or of a more chronic nature can result from vascular etiologies such as aneurysms of the thoracic aorta (both ascending and arch) and pulmonary arterial hypertension. Although rare, pain secondary to nondissecting thoracic aneurysms is often related to mass effect on neighboring structures, the chest wall, or erosion into adjacent bones and has been described as a deep and steady, dull discomfort, unaffected by exertion or change in position. Substernal chest pain related to pulmonary hypertension, in contrast, is usually described as a pressure sensation, aggravated by effort and associated with dyspnea, cough, or wheeze.

TABLE 16-2. Modifiable Risk Factors for Peripheral Arterial Disease

Risk Factor	Estimated Relative Risk
Cigarette smoking	2.0–5.0
Diabetes mellitus	3.0–4.0
Hypertension	1.1–2.2
Hypercholesterolemia (per 40–50 mg/dL increase in total cholesterol)	1.2–1.4
Fibrinogen (per 0.7 g/L increase in fibrinogen)	1.35
C-reactive protein	2.1
Hyperhomocysteinemia	2.0–3.2

Reprinted with permission from Creager MA, Libby P. Peripheral arterial diseases. In: Zipes DP, Libby P, Bonow RO, Braunwald E, eds. Braunwald's Heart Disease: A Textbook of Cardiovascular Medicine. 7th ed. Philadelphia, PA: Elsevier Saunders; 2005:1437-1461.

Dyspnea. Dyspnea is the medical term for a range of patient complaints including shortness of breath, feelings of breathlessness, or difficulty breathing. As it is often a slowly progressive symptom over months or years, it may also represent a gradual decrease in exercise tolerance or the increasing need for "breaks" while completing daily activities. Most often dyspnea is related to cardiac decompensation or intrinsic pulmonary disease, however, vascular conditions such as pulmonary arterial hypertension, vascular compression of the left mainstem bronchus, or severe generalized vascular disease that limits oxygen delivery to metabolically active muscles can also result in difficulty breathing. Like cardiac dyspnea, vascular conditions may have associated symptoms such as cough, wheeze, or weakness and may be provoked by exertion. However, vascular dyspnea should not be initiated or made worse by change in body position.

Abdominal Pain. Vascular sources of abdominal pain, including aortic dissection, aneurysmal disease of the aorta and abdominal viscera, visceral ischemia, and celiac compression syndrome can have devastating consequences if not diagnosed quickly and accurately. While the majority of abdominal aortic aneurysms are asymptomatic and discovered incidentally, patients will occasionally complain of a steady, gnawing pain in the lower abdomen or back for hours or days at a time. Although movement does not usually affect aneurysm pain, some patients will note relief in certain positions, like lying supine with the legs drawn up. The development of new or worsening pain suggests expansion or impending rupture; it is classically described as severe and constant with possible radiation into the groin, buttocks, or legs. Actual rupture produces severe, diffuse abdominal pain and tenderness with hemodynamic compromise, although a rupture or leak contained by the retroperitoneum may localize the pain to the flank or groin.

Like aortic aneurysms, visceral aneurysms may remain asymptomatic until discovered by incidental imaging or they expand and impede upon nearby structures. When pain exists, it tends to be greatest over the region of the abdomen near the abdominal visera affected until rupture when it becomes more diffuse with associated tenderness.

The location of the pain induced by acute visceral ischemia may vary based on which arterial branch is occluded, however, symptoms are often nonspecific. With mesenteric disease, symptoms may begin with a very focal area of cramping pain or tenderness that progresses in severity as the duration of ischemia extends. Patients will report difficulty in finding a comfortable position to lie, and will frequently have associated bouts of nausea, vomiting, and bloody bowel movements. Typically, the abdominal examination will lag behind the patient's complaints of severe pain (i.e., pain out of proportion to the examination findings) which can delay diagnosis. Splenic artery occlusions may be accompanied by epigastric or left upper quadrant discomfort, whereas hepatic artery occlusions are either asymptomatic or present with right quadrant pain. Renal artery occlusions are most often silent, but may

TABLE 16-3. Classification of Peripheral Arterial Disease

Fontaine		Rutherford		
Stage	Clinical	Grade	Category	Clinical
I	Asymptomatic	0	0	Asymptomatic
IIa	Mild claudication	I	1	Mild claudication
IIb	Moderate-to-severe claudication	I	2	Moderate claudication
		I	3	Severe claudication
III	Ischemic rest pain	II	4	Ischemic rest pain
IV	Ulceration or gangrene	III	5	Minor tissue loss
		III	6	Major tissue loss

Reprinted with permission from Norgren L, Hiatt WR, Dormandy JA, Nehler MR, Harris KA, Fowkes FGR. Inter-society consensus for the management of peripheral arterial disease (TASC II). Eur J Vasc Endovasc Surg. 2007;33:S1-S75.

TABLE 16-4. Differential Diagnosis of Intermittent Claudication

Condition	Location	Symptoms	Effect of Exercise and Rest	Effect of Position
Calf claudication	Calf muscles	Cramping, aching	Reproducible onset; quickly relieved with rest	None
Thigh/buttock claudication	Buttocks, hip, thigh	Cramping, aching	Reproducible onset; quickly relieved with rest	None
Foot claudication	Foot arch	Severe pain	Reproducible onset; quickly relieved with rest	None
Chronic compartment syndrome	Calf muscles	Tight, bursting pain	After much exercise (jogging); subsides very slowly	Relief with elevation
Venous claudication	Entire leg, worse in calf	Tight, bursting pain	After walking; slowly subsides	Relief speeded by elevation
Nerve root compression	Radiates down leg	Sharp, lancinating pain	Induced by sitting, standing or walking; may be present at rest	Worse with sitting, improved by change in position or lying supine
Baker's cyst	Behind knee, down calf	Swelling, tenderness	Worse with exercise; often present at rest and not intermittent	None
Hip arthritis	Lateral hip, thigh	Aching discomfort	After variable degree of exercise; not quickly relieved with rest	Improved when not bearing weight
Spinal stenosis	Bilateral buttocks, posterior leg	Pain and weakness	May mimic claudication; variable relief, can take a long time to recover	Relief by lumbar spine flexion, worse with standing or extending spine

Modified from Norgren L, Hiatt WR, Dormandy JA, Nehler MR, Harris KA, Fowkes FGR. Inter-society consensus for the management of peripheral arterial disease (TASC II). Eur J Vasc Endovasc Surg. 2007;33:S1-S75.

eventually evolve into sharp back or flank pain associated with nausea, vomiting, and hematuria. Although all acute occlusions can incur without precipitating factors, the examiner's suspicion should be raised in patients with recent aortic instrumentation such as takes place with angiography.

Patients with chronic visceral ischemia may also complain of varying pain syndromes. Mesenteric disease again causes a cramping pain, although this pain usually only occurs 15 to 30 minutes after ingestion of a meal and may not be associated with a change in bowel habits. Over time, the pattern of colicky pain becomes so severe that the patient may shun eating altogether in an effort to diminish or avoid the expected abdominal discomfort. Consequently, significant weight loss may be reported by the patient as well.

Celiac compression syndrome (also referred to as median arcuate ligament syndrome, Dunbar syndrome, and celiac axis syndrome) produces abdominal pain through extrinsic compression of the vessels at the celiac axis origin by fibers of the median arcuate ligament of the diaphragm. Symptoms may include weight loss and postprandial pain, which is often augmented by full expiration. Despite many case reports, celiac compression syndrome's contribution to chronic abdominal pain and mesenteric ischemia remains uncertain given the rich supply of collaterals between the celiac axis and mesenteric arteries, the presence of compression in a significant proportion of asymptomatic patients, and the failure for surgical correction to reliably relieve symptoms. Other etiologies such as involvement of the splanchnic nerve plexus or delayed gastric emptying have been suggested, however, the diagnosis often remains one of exclusion.

Skin Changes. Because of its highly vascular nature, both acute and chronic occlusive arterial disease can lead to alterations in skin temperature, color, or integrity. A common office complaint is cold hands or feet and is often attributable to an individual's basic vasomotor tone; however, generalized coolness of an extremity can be related to more serious conditions. When temperature differences are asymmetric or involve only one limb, suspicion is higher for an occlusive process. Disease states resulting in an effective ischemia such as poor cardiac output, hemorrhage, or shock will lead to generalized coolness of all extremities.

Skin color varies with blood flow, and therefore can be affected by temperature, physical activity, and emotional

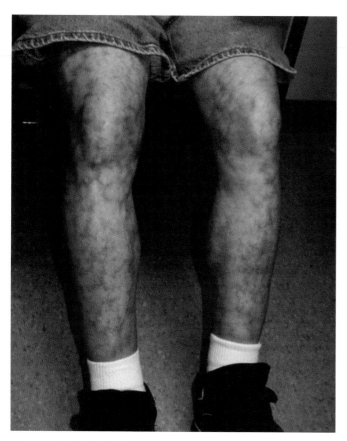

● **FIGURE 16-2.** Livedo reticularis.

Reprinted with permission from Beckman JA, Creager MA. The history and physical examination. In: Creager MA, Dzau VJ, Loscalzo J, eds. Vascular Medicine: A Companion to Braunwald's Heart Disease. 1st ed. Philadelphia, PA: Elsevier Saunders; 2006:135-145.

stimuli. Patients with Raynaud's phenomenon will note pale and often painful fingers or toes when exposed to cooler weather, and those with Chilblain lupus (also known as Pernio lupus) report reddish-blue skin nodules occurring in the cold. A violaceous discoloration or cyanosis of a digit or limb that may or may not blanch with pressure is indicative of ischemic disease. Vascultis or atheroembolic disease are common causes of livedo reticularis, a lace-like pattern in the skin consisting of reddish-blue superficial vessels surrounding a central area of clearing sometimes exacerbated by cold exposure (see Figure 16-2). Patients with ischemic rest pain who maintain their feet in a dependent position may develop persistent redness of the toes and feet known as dependent rubor.

In some cases of arterial occlusive disease or emboli, chronic ischemia contributes to hair loss and tissue breakdown. Nonhealing and tender ulcerations are often found in distal areas of limbs such as the toes, heel, or fingertips. Patients with peripheral neuropathy are especially at risk for formation of ulcers in areas of trauma. If ulcerations have developed, the patient often requires significant analgesia to combat the pain. Without proper treatment, ischemic ulcers may progress to tissue necrosis and gangrene, resulting in areas of dead tissue that blackens and sloughs.

Neurologic Manifestations. The majority of patients with significant stenoses of the carotid and vertebrobasilar arteries are asymptomatic; however, when symptoms do occur, they are mainly categorized by duration. Transient ischemic attacks (TIAs) are characteristically temporary episodes of spontaneous neurologic dysfunction, lasting from a few minutes to less than 4 hours (though, by definition up to 24 hours). When multiple attacks occur within a short period of time, the syndrome is known as crescendo TIAs. Reversible ischemic neurologic deficits are those that require greater than 24 hours for full recovery. Symptoms that persist for longer periods are generally related to cerebral infarction and are diagnosed as a stroke in evolution or a complete stroke.[11] In addition to duration of symptoms, the examiner should note location, setting, quality, and degree of disability when evaluating neurologic complaints to ascertain the affected vascular bed (see Table 16-5). In many instances, it is helpful to have family or friends provide the details of any neurologic manifestation associated with vascular events as confusion or sometimes even loss of consciousness may be a prominent feature.

A range of both motor and sensory symptoms might result from embolization of carotid or proximal aortic disease. Amaurosis fugax, or fleeting blindness, occurs when a plaque travels from the proximal aorta or internal carotid artery to the ipsilateral ophthalmic artery. Patients will frequently report monocular vision loss that begins as haziness in the upper fields and progresses downward, like "a veil" or "a shade being drawn." The vision loss is painless, often without a precipitating factor and usually only lasts for a few seconds or minutes. If both eyes are involved, the cause is rarely carotid artery disease although a vascular etiology should not be completely ruled out.

Embolic showers from the proximal aorta or an atheromatous carotid artery to the ipsilateral cerebral hemisphere result in deficits on the side opposite the involved area of the brain. Symptoms will differ based on the area of cerebral cortex supplied by the occluded vessel and can vary from a minor problem, as with a focal parasthesia, to more profound deficits such as aphasia or hemiparesis (see Figures 16-3 and 16-4). The larger the vascular territory, the more widespread is the dysfunction which may occur.

Vertebrobasilar disease can also produce parasthesias, dysarthria, or hemiparesis; however, the more likely expressions of ischemia for this arterial system include complaints of confusion, nausea, vomiting, vertigo, dizziness, and ataxia. One of the most frightening symptoms may be "drop attacks" in which patients relate suddenly finding themselves on the floor as a result of an unexpected loss of lower extremity motor function. Because of the anatomic pattern of the vertebral, basilar, subclavian, and innominate arteries, symptoms rarely arise when only one side is occluded. Even when significant bilateral disease is present, patients may remain asymptomatic as a result of the maintainance of adequate blood flow by the communicating arteries in the posterior circulation.

Vascultis of the cranial branches of the arteries arising from the aortic arch may also cause neurologic symptoms.

TABLE 16-5. Carotid Versus Vertebral-Basilar Symptoms

Symptoms and Signs Symptoms (attacks of)	Carotid System	Vertebral-Basilar System
Weakness	One side of face or limbs	Limbs in any combination
Numbness	One side, usually limbs	One or both sides of body
Aphasia	If dominant hemisphere is involved	No
Loss of Vision	In one eye on side of ischemia (amaurosis fugax)	Homonymous or bilateral hemianopsia
Diplopia	No	Yes
Other	—	Dysarthria, dysphagia, vertigo, ataxia of gait, or limbs
Physical signs (inconsistent)		
Diminished pulsation	In involved carotid artery	In subclavian artery
Change of pressure in ophthalmic artery	Decreased on involved side	—
Retinal emboli	Retinal arterioles on involved side	No
Bruits	Over involved carotid artery bifurcation or over globe of eye on involved side, occasionally over opposite carotid artery	Over subclavian artery or back of neck

Reprinted with permission from Siekert RG, Whisnant JP, Sundt TM Jr. Ischemic cerebrovascular disease. In: Juergens JL, Spittell JA Jr, Fairbairn JF, eds. Peripheral Vascular Diseases. 5th ed. Philadelphia, PA: W.B. Saunders Company; 1980:351-380.

Temporal arteritis, also known as giant-cell arteritis, is characterized by a myriad of symptoms which may be gradual or abrupt in onset. The development of a new headache, especially over one or both temporal regions with associated temporal artery tenderness, is the most common complaint reported in almost two-thirds of patients. Jaw pain secondary to claudication occurs in up to one-half of patients diagnosed with temporal arteritis. Patients may also report impaired vision as an early manifestation of the disease with the most common visual complaints being diplopia or

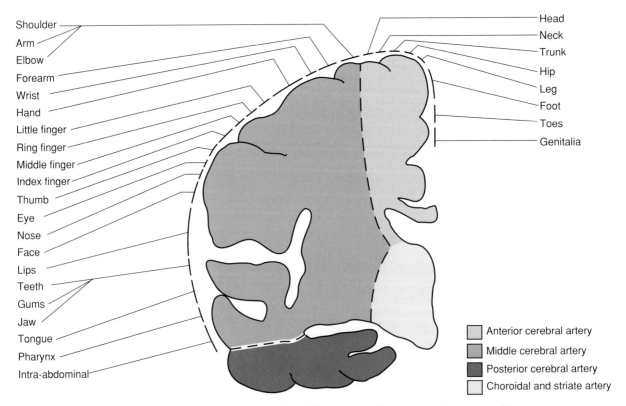

● FIGURE 16-3. Sensory homunculus with approximated vascular territories of the main cerebral arteries in the coronal section. The block line stemming from each body part roughly corresponds to the proportion of the sensory cortex devoted to it.

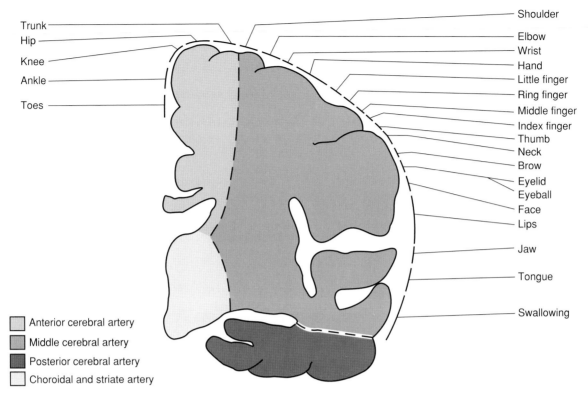

Trunk
Hip
Knee
Ankle
Toes

Shoulder
Elbow
Wrist
Hand
Little finger
Ring finger
Middle finger
Index finger
Thumb
Neck
Brow
Eyelid
Eyeball
Face
Lips
Jaw
Tongue
Swallowing

Anterior cerebral artery
Middle cerebral artery
Posterior cerebral artery
Choroidal and striate artery

● **FIGURE 16-4.** Motor homunculus with approximated vascular territories of the main cerebral arteries in the coronal section. Again, the block line stemming from each body part roughly corresponds to the proportion of the motor cortex devoted to it.

sudden monocular vision loss. Although complete vision loss in both eyes is rare—if left untreated approximately 15% to 20% of patients will progress to partial or complete vision loss in one or both eyes—sometimes in as quickly as a few days.[12]

Syncope. Syncope, described as transient and complete loss of consciousness, and its less complete variants presyncope, lightheadedness, and dizziness, have multiple etiologies and require careful symptom analysis to distinguish vascular from nonvascular causes. Details relating to the setting, duration, aggravating factors, and associated symptoms are important to identify; in addition, eyewitness accounts from family and friends can also lend important clues. Common nonvascular causes to exclude are cardiogenic syncope, epilepsy, hypoglycemia, or reflex syncope. Vasomotor syncope, although associated with vascular events such as bradycardia and peripheral vasodilatation, is not truly related to cardiac or vascular disease. Patients often described this type of syncope as being predictable, recurrent, and precipitated by features like pain, visually shocking sights (i.e., the sight of blood or a needle), fatigue, warm environments, prolonged standing, fasting, fear, or anxiety.

Vascular sources, namely cerebrovascular arterial insufficiency, are often part of a larger pattern of neurologic manifestations of arterial disease and can be attributed to occlusive embolic and thrombotic events or vasospasm within the cerebral or arch vessels. Stenosis of the subclavian artery by atherosclerosis or thoracic outlet obstruction can also lead to subclavian steal syndrome, in which retrograde flow of the vertebral artery to supply the ipsilateral subclavian artery leads to symptoms of vertebrobasliar insufficiency including syncope and presyncope.

Peripheral Edema. Edema, the accumulation of interstitial fluid, is often described by patients as "swelling" or "stiffness" in the legs or arms, however, it can also occur around the eyes, face, and sacrum. Patients may relate more subtle symptoms like the inability to fit in their shoes by the end of the day, or that their rings or watch no longer fit comfortably. Although edema is most often related to cardiac dysfunction, renal failure, or abnormalities of the peripheral venous circulation, it may also be a secondary manifestation of peripheral arterial disease. Patients with extremity pain caused by ischemia will often develop lower extremity edema as a result of maintenance of their feet in a dependent position in an attempt to find relief for their discomfort. Important clues to help distinguish between these causes may lie in how the patient tries to alleviate the edema.

Cough and Dysphagia. Although the complaint of cough is more often related to respiratory conditions, it may also be associated with vascular diseases including aortic aneurysms and pulmonary arterial hypertension. As a vascular symptom, cough is typically described as dry, nonproductive, and most often occurring at night. Vascular etiologies are mainly mechanical in nature. Thus, a dilated

---

TABLE 16-6. Vascular Rings

Name	Description
Complete vascular rings	
Double aortic arch	Paired dorsal embryonic aortic arches persist forming a ring around both the trachea and esophagus, with the right arch usually being larger and more cephalad in its course. The left arch distal to the left subclavian may become atretic and there is commonly a left ligamentum arteriosum or a ductus arteriosus present.
Right aortic arch	Right aortic arch with a left ductus or ligamentum arteriosum connecting the left pulmonary artery and the upper part of the descending aorta. May have an aberrant left subclavian artery arising from a structure known as the diverticulum of Kommerrell, causing compression of the airway.
Retroesophageal descending aorta	Presence of either a left aortic arch with a right descending aorta and right ductus, or a right aortic arch with a left descending aorta and left ductus.
Aberrant right subclavian artery (arteria lusoria)	Artery runs posterior to the esophagus, but only forms a ring if there is an associated right-sided ductus or ligamentum present.
Incomplete vascular rings	
Pulmonary artery sling	Left pulmonary artery arises from the right pulmonary artery and passes between the trachea and the esophagus prior to entering the left lung.
Innominate artery compression syndrome	Innominate or brachiocephalic artery originates later along the course of the transverse arch, resulting in a more leftward takeoff than normal. Tracheal compression may occur if the aberrant artery passes anterior to the trachea.

---

ascending aorta exerting pressure on the trachea and bronchi may stimulate a cough reflex. Hoarseness or a cough response may also result from irritation of the recurrent laryngeal nerve by an aortic arch aneurysm. Additional complaints of hemoptysis, dyspnea, and/or chest pain are the most commonly associated symptoms and frequently suggest increased pulmonary arterial pressures as the underlying pathology.

Peripheral arterial disease is a rare cause of dysphagia, however, several vascular abnormalities have been described in the literature. The term *vascular ring* encompasses several aortic arch or pulmonary artery malformations that exhibit an abnormal relation with the esophagus and trachea. The most common vascular ring is produced by a double aortic arch, in which both the right and left fourth embryonic aortic arches persist. Other vascular rings include a right aortic arch with a left ductus or ligamentum arteriosum, an anomalous origin of the right subclavian artery (arteria lusoria), retroesophageal descending aorta, and pulmonary artery sling (see Table 16-6).[13] Although patients may remain asymptomatic, complaints of dysphagia, stridor, and cyanosis, especially while eating, are not uncommon. The severity of symptoms produced by vascular rings depends upon the tightness of the anatomical constriction, which may explain why some patients are not diagnosed until much later in life.

● PHYSICAL EXAMINATION

General Considerations

A thorough history can establish a basis for presumptive arterial disease, and when followed by a precise physical examination, the accurate detection of a number of vascular processes is remarkably improved. Both efficiency and effectiveness of the examination are enhanced by the sequence of assessment techniques as well as the implications each technique has for the others. It is with this in mind that the examiner should minimize deviations from the planned approach and maintain proper examination procedures. When done carefully, a detailed examination will lead to the more appropriate application of diagnostic techniques, imaging, and therapeutic interventions.

The arterial vascular examination essentially consists of three parts: inspection, palpation, and auscultation. The inspection serves as more than a simple "once-over," but as a careful screen for both overt and subtle physical manifestations of vascular disease. Palpation of arterial and venous pulsations, pulsatile masses, heaves, thrills, edema, and surface temperature offers a mechanism for obtaining valuable information regarding adequacy of perfusion, the size, movements and functioning of several cardiac structures, and the hemodynamics of blood flow. Auscultation of the heart, peripheral arteries, and veins may confirm previous findings and offer additional insights into cardiac function, arterial pressures, and blood flow hemodynamics.

Palpation. To maximize detection, it is essential that proper palpation technique be employed. An examiner should use the pad of the fingertips to evaluate pulsations and edema, the palmar aspect overlying the distal metacarpals to detect vibrations, and the dorsal aspects of the fingers to recognize temperature variations. When palpating arterial pulses, the method for accurate palpation involves several key steps[3]:

1. Both the patient and the examiner should maintain a relaxed posture.

2. Use the surface area of three or four fingers when possible.

3. Control and relax the nearby joint with the other hand.

4. Begin with light pressure; increasing or varying pressure as needed.

5. Avoid the use of the thumb to prevent transmission of the examiner's own pulse.

When in doubt, Doppler signals should be used to determine whether a pulse is absent or merely obscured. Several methods are commonly used to describe a pulse. For example, the examiner's recording of a pulse may be simply as "present" or "absent." More specific portrayals utilizing qualitative grading scales of either 0 to 2 or 0 to 4, however, will enhance the clinical usefulness of the examination (see Table 16-7). Detection of a vibration, or thrill, may indicate some degree of vascular stenosis or the presence of a fistula. Size of the pulse should also be noted, as a dilated or expansive pulse may suggest ectatic or aneurysmal changes. When feasible, bilateral pulses should be assessed simultaneously for detection in delay or amplitude that may suggest some type of occlusion in the affected extremity.

Auscultation. Complete auscultation is a technically demanding skill requiring significant practice and focus. For arterial blood pressure determination, accuracy is dependent on proper equipment and technique. When recording blood pressure measurements, it is important to recall that readings can be affected by a multitude of factors: patient position, limb position, cuff size and placement, stethoscope placement, the length of time the artery is occluded, and the rate of cuff deflation.[6] As with palpation, bilateral readings should be obtained to assess for asymmetry, using a Doppler device if necessary.

The bell of the stethoscope should be used in auscultation of arterial blood flow for the detection of bruits representing turbulent blood flow caused by occlusive disease or vessel tortuosity. All bruits should be characterized as to location, pitch, timing (systolic, diastolic, or both), intensity, and configuration. Low-pitched bruits are common to larger vessels such as the aorta and the carotid or proximal limb arteries, while bruits generated by smaller vessels or a high-grade stensosis are higher-pitched. Low-grade stenoses typically produce early systolic bruits, whereas high-grade stenoses create holosystolic or systolic/diastolic bruits. Once a critical narrowing has been reached, however, an audible bruit may disappear. Pancyclic murmurs may also indicate arteriovenous malformations or shunts. Arterial bruits are located at the site of arterial narrowing, but can be audible for several centimeters downstream; therefore, it is important to listen proximal to the initial place of detection to try to pinpoint the actual site of narrowing.

When auscultating, care must be taken to exert minimal pressure with the stethoscope to avoid vessel compression and the creation of an artificial bruit in an otherwise normal vessel. In addition, bruits may also be detected in normal vessels during high-flow states such as anemia, severe aortic insufficiency, and hypothyroidism. Auscultation can also be used to evaluate the hemodynamics of blood flow in peripheral veins. Like its arterial counterpart, a venous hum should be evaluated for location, pitch, and timing. A typical venous hum is a low-pitched, continuous sound heard throughout the cardiac cycle. Although most are physiological in nature with no clinical significance, their presence should still be documented.

General Appearance

Assessment and recording of the patient's vital signs, including blood pressure, heart rate, and respiratory rate comprise the initial step in any comprehensive physical examination. Ideally, the blood pressure should be recorded in both arms, preferably in the supine, seated and standing positions. Height and weight should be recorded and the individual's body mass index calculated. The patient's general appearance is then appraised; observations of body habitus and conformations, posture, gait, nourishment, demeanor, and vocalizations can provide important clues that will further guide the examination.

Head and Neck

Inspection of the head and neck should commence with the possible observation of head bobbing, also known as de Mosset's sign, which can indicate aortic regurgitation or a widened pulse pressure that may be associated with an ascending aortic aneurysm or dissection. Facial asymmetries should also be noted, as they can be a sign of cranial nerve paralysis secondary to cerebrovascular disease in the form of a TIA, stroke in evolution, or completed stroke. Evidence of temporal wasting can be used to assess overall nutritional status. Observations of telangiectasias on the lips are

---

TABLE 16-7. Qualitative Grading of Arterial Pulse by Palpation

Grade	Pulse Character
0–2 Scale	
0	Pulse absent
1	Pulse diminished
2	Normal pulse
0–4 Scale	
0	Pulse absent
1	Pulse markedly diminished
2	Pulse moderately diminished
3	Pulse slightly diminished
4	Normal pulse

Adapted from Lanzer P. Peripheral vascular disease. In: Lanzer P, Topol EJ, eds. Panvascular Medicine: Integrated Clinical Management. 1st ed. New York, NY: Springer-Verlag Berlin Heidelberg; 2002:388-396, with kind permission of Springer Science and Business Media.

associated with pulmonary arteriovenous fistulae, whereas blue-tinged lips suggest central cyanosis and the presence of intrapulmonary or intracardiac right-to-left shunting. Inspection of oral mucous membranes may aid with the determination of a patient's fluid status.

External inspection of the eyes should note the presence or absence of lid xanthelsmae or a corneal arcus as possible manifestations of atherosclerotic disease. Corneal arcus is also known as arcus senilis because of its association with aging. When seen in men younger than 50 years, however, it is referred to as arcus juvenilis and has been linked to increased plasma cholesterol and low-density lipoprotein cholesterol levels as well as increased risk for having type IIa dyslipoproteinemia.[14,15] Blue sclera and dislocation of the lens are common features of Marfan's syndrome, and exophthalmia may indicate thyrotoxicosis and its associated cardiovascular manifestations. Fundoscopic examination is useful as a visualization of the arteriolar changes caused by hypertension (arteriovenous nicking, cotton wool patches, flame hemorrhages, papilledema), diabetes mellitus (neovascularization, microaneurysms), atherosclerosis (exudates, beading of the retinal artery), and atheromatous embolization (Hollenhorst plaques) (see Figure 16-5).

Inspection of the neck should include observations of both carotid arterial and jugular venous characteristics. Three features should be noted for carotid arterial pulsations: intensity (or amplitude), rate, and cadence. Intensity, when decreased, may reflect low-cardiac-output states, occlusive disease of the aortic arch, carotid arterial occlusions,

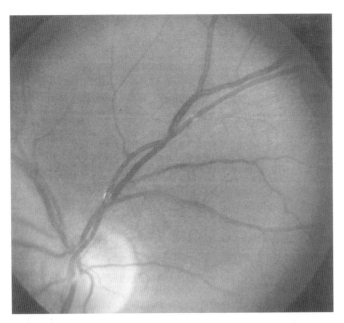

● FIGURE 16-5. Cholesterol emboli in the retinal arterioles of a patient with atherosclerotic disease of the ipsilateral carotid artery.

Reprinted with permission from Spittell JA Jr. Occlusive peripheral arterial disease. In: Spittell JA, ed. Peripheral Vascular Disease for Cardiologists: A Clinical Approach. 1st ed. New York, NY: Blackwell Publishing, Inc./Futura Division; 2004:1-29.

or hypotension. Variable amplitudes may signify arrhythmias or congestive heart failure. Rate and cadence, as timing characteristics of the pulsations, may reveal other abnormal electrical patterns that can be further defined later in the examination or with additional diagnostic testing.

Although jugular venous analysis is considered more predictive of cardiac than peripheral arterial disease, assessment of jugular venous filling as well as notation of the pattern of venous waveforms is part of a complete vascular examination. These observations are best made using the right internal jugular vein with the patient in the supine position on the examination table, their neck slightly extended and rotated to the left. The examiner should gradually raise the head of the table until he or she observes pulsations. In patients with normal central venous pressure, maximal visibility of venous pulsations should be observed just above the medial end of the clavicle with a 30- to 40-degree elevation of trunk. At this level, the amplitude of both the "a" and "v" waves and also the depths of the "x" and "y" troughs following these waves should be noted. Further elevation of the table to 90 degrees allows for measurement of the degree of venous distension. In normal patients, both the internal and external jugular veins are collapsed with no visible distension or pulsation. Dilated jugular veins may suggest arteriovenous fistulae, congestive heart failure, or proximal venous occlusion (e.g., superior vena cava syndrome).

Pulse palpation should begin with the temporal artery, located just anterior to the tragus of the ear. The strength of the pulse should be assessed, and the artery should be examined for thickening or dilatation, which may be signs of inflammation found with temporal arteritis or possible aneurysm. Palpation of the carotid artery should be low in the neck by hooking the fingers around in front of the sternocleidomastoid muscles. Care should be taken not to palpate the bifurcation of the artery higher in the neck, as this is the most common area for dislodgement of an atheromatous emboli or induction of marked bradycardia and/or asystole caused by a hypersensitive carotid sinus reflex. For the latter reason it is also not advisable to palpate both carotid arteries simultaneously. The carotid pulse provides the most accurate representation of the central aortic pulse.[16–18] Its classification by volume and contour can help identify changes in left ventricular stroke volume and ejection velocity (see Table 16-8). The subclavian pulse is most readily palpated just behind the clavicle in the anterior medial corner of the supraclavicular fossa. Unlike palpation of other arteries, it may be helpful for the examiner to use his or her thumb to reach the vessel, with the remaining fingers braced behind the neck. Prominent systolic pulsations in this region may be secondary to sublcavian or aortic root aneurysms.

A bruit heard with the bell over the globe of the eye suggests a possible intracranial carotid artery stenosis. The examination for carotid artery bruits should begin as high in the neck as possible, getting up under the mandible then slowly progressing down the course of the common carotid artery to the base of the neck. The sensitivity and specificity

TABLE 16-8. Carotid Pulse Contours

Name	Description	Example
Normal pulse	Feels smooth and rounded, and the notch on the descending slope of the pulse wave is not palpable.	
Bounding pulse	Feels strong or exaggerated with a rapid rise, brief peak, and rapid fall. Causes include high cardiac output states (anemia, hyperthyroidism, fever, pregnancy, patent ductus, A-V fistulas), bradycardia, and decreased compliance of arterial walls because of age and atherosclerosis.	
Pulsus alternans	Rhythm feels regular with alternating strong and weak pulses. Indicative of left ventricular failure.	
Bisferiens Pulse	Two systolic peaks (percussion and tidal waves) separated by a distinct mid-systolic dip. Most commonly caused by aortic regurgitation or the combination of aortic regurgitation and stenosis. Can also be felt with hypertrophic cardiomyopathy, but this is less likely to be palpable.	
Pulsus bigeminus	Alternating strong and weak pulses in an irregular rhythm, where the weak beat always follows a shorter interval. Caused by a normal beat alternating with a premature contraction.	
Dicrotic pulse	Two peaks, with the second being in diastole as an exaggerated wave following aortic valve closure. Usually seen in cases of cardiac tamponade, severe heart failure, or hypovolemic shock	
Corrigan pulse (water-hammer pulse)	Abrupt upstroke (percussion wave) followed by a rapid collapse later in systole. Suggests aortic regurgitation.	
Pulsus parvus et tardus	Initial upstroke feels slow and peak is late in systole. Seen with a fixed left ventricular outflow obstruction such as aortic stenosis.	
Pulsus paradoxus	Reduction in strength of the pulse during quiet inspiration. It is a characteristic finding with pericardial tamponade, but also occurs with chronic constrictive pericarditis, chronic lung disease (emphysema and bronchial asthma), pulmonary embolus, and hypovolemic shock.	I-----Expiration-----I-----Inspiration-----I

of a carotid bruit for the presence of a stenosis varies widely, ranging from 50% to 79% and 61% to 91% accordingly.[3,19] In addition, the presence or absence of a bruit has been shown to be unreliable in determining the significance of carotid artery disease, with several studies reporting only half of all patients with a carotid artery stenosis of at least 50% as having a detectable bruit on examination, and numerous cases of patients found to have a bruit despite the absence of any identifiable stenotic disease.[19,20] Vertebral artery bruits are best appreciated in the area posterior to the sternocleidomastoid muscles, while bruits of arteriovenous malformations may be loudest posteriorly in the neck and occipital areas. Bruits originating from the subclavian artery are best detected in the supraclavicular fossa. It should be noted that patients undergoing hemodialysis typically have supraclavicular bruits ipsilateral to their dialysis access. Using transient brachial artery occlusion while auscultating can differentiate a true stenosis from a dialysis-induced murmur—manual pressure on the brachial artery for less than 5 seconds will cause the latter to disappear.[21] When auscultating the vessels of the neck, the examiner should ask the patient to take short breath holds so the breath sounds will not obscure the vascular sounds.

In cases where the origin of a bruit may not be clear, a few simple maneuvers can assist the examiner. If a subclavian artery bruit is transmitted to the carotid artery area, it will disappear upon digital compression of the subclavian artery. Similarly, the bruit of a venous hum will disappear with light compression of the external jugular vein. Ausculation at the aortic and pulmonic areas of the chest will help determine whether or not neck bruits might be transmitted from the heart; usually the murmur of aortic stenosis or sclerosis will be transmitted equally to all the neck vessels and will decrease in intensity as the stethoscope is moved up the neck.

Chest

The examiner should evaluate the chest with the patient in the upright and supine positions, noting general contour, sternal, and spinal deformities, and anterior chest motions. Patients with coarctation of the aorta may exhibit a heavy muscular thorax with collateral arteries visible in the axillae and lateral chest wall contrasting to less developed lower extremities. Both pectus excavatum, posterior displacement of the sternum, and pectus carinatum, in which the sternum is displaced anteriorly, are common manifestations of Ehlers-Danlos syndrome and Marfan's syndrome. Lack of normal of kyphosis of the thoracic spine should be noted, as this may be associated with pulmonary artery prominence.

Cutaneous abnormalities, such as dilated veins on the anterior chest wall, suggest obstruction of the superior or inferior vena cava. Observations of pulsations throughout the precordium should be noted using a tangential light source. Usually only the point of maximal impulse (PMI) can be seen as a single impulse during systole at the apex of the heart. Prominent pulsations of the supraclavicular region are often associated with a dilated or dissecting ascending aorta, tortuous innominate artery, or right-sided aorta. Visible pulsations in the right second intercostal space (aortic area) may suggest aortic regurgitation, poststenotic dilatation of the ascending aorta, or ascending aortic aneurysms. Diseases associated with pulsations in the left second intercostal space (pulmonic region) include conditions causing pulmonary artery dilatation such as pulmonary arterial hypertension and pulmonary embolus. Enlargement of one or more cardiac of the chambers is suggested by pulsations over the left parasternum or a laterally displaced cardiac apex. A subxiphoid or epigastric pulsation may occur with right ventricular enlargement or a descending aortic aneurysm. Severe valvular regurgitation or large left-to-right shunts, especially a patent ductus arteriosus, can cause "shaking" of the entire precordium.

Palpation of the chest should take place with the examination table elevated at 30 degrees, with the patient both supine and in the partial left lateral decubitus position. The cardiac apex should be identified by palpation of the PMI, noting location, size, and duration of thrust. Left ventricular enlargement is suggested by an enlarged and laterally-displaced PMI, whereas hypertrophy causes a persistant thrust also known as a heave or lift. Anterior systolic movement over the left parasternal and/or subxiphoid region usually represents right ventricular enlargement or hypertrophy. This, combined with a prominent palpable pulsation of the pulmonary trunk in the second left intercostal space, reflects increased pulmonary arterial hypertension. The suprasternal notch should be palpated, as aneurysms of the ascending aorta or aortic arch may cause palpable systolic impulses in this area. In addition, the examiner should use the flat of the hand to identify any thrills, which are the palpable manifestations of severe valvular stenosis.

While the full cardiac auscultory examination is beyond the scope of this chapter, there are several key components that will aid in the diagnosis of peripheral arterial disease. When auscultating the chest, the examiner should be sure to place both the diaphragm and bell of the stethoscope at each of the four basic topographical areas: right second intercostal space (aortic area), left second intercostal space (pulmonic area), left lower sternal border (tricuspid area), and cardiac apex (mitral area). Each area should be examined while the patient is seated upright, supine, and in the left lateral decubitus position. The basic heart sounds, S1 (mitral valve closure) and S2 (aortic valve closure), are identified, making note of intensity and normal versus abnormal splitting. Next is the detection of any "extra" heart sounds such as an S3, S4, opening snap, click, or rub. Finally, if a murmur is appreciated, it should be characterized by location, intensity, pitch, configuration, quality, timing, and direction of radiation.

Several abnormal cardiac findings may be related to underlying peripheral arterial disease. The intensity of the A2 component is increased when the aorta is closer to the anterior chest wall, which may occur with aortic root dilation, transposition of the great vessels, or pulmonary atresia. A narrow yet fixed splitting of S2 and a loud P2 component are both associated with pulmonary arterial hypertension.

Paradoxical splitting of S2 can be heard with left-to-right shunts such as a patent ductus arteriosus.

Heart murmurs are generally classified by timing into three categories: systolic, diastolic, or continuous. Aortic systolic murmurs associated with peripheral arterial disease include those caused by supravalvular obstruction such as coarctation of the aorta, and those caused by dilatation of the ascending aorta and root, including aneurysm, atheroma, and aortitis. Early diastolic murmurs such as new onset aortic regurgitation are worrisome for aortic dissection, while pulmonic regurgitation caused by dilatation of the valve ring may be secondary to Marfan's syndrome. Increased flow across a nonstenotic mitral valve caused by a patent ductus arteriosus may cause a mid-diastolic murmur. Continuous murmurs, generated by flow from a vascular bed of higher resistance to one of lower resistance without phasic interruption between systole and diastole, are generally of four types: an aortopulmonary connection, (patent ductus arteriosus), an arteriovenous connection (coronary arteriovenous fistulas, bronchial collaterals), a disturbance of flow patterns in arteries (coarctation, systemic-to-pulmonary arterial collaterals), and a disturbance of flow patterns in veins (cervical venous hum).

Abdomen

Examination of the abdomen is performed as the patient lies supine on the examination table with legs outstretched. Visual inspection of the abdomen should identify any engorged superficial veins which may suggest obstruction of the inferior vena cava. In addition, prominent pulsations may be associated with dilated or aneurysmal vessels such as the descending aorta, renal and iliac arteries. Although difficult in obese patients, palpation of the descending and abdominal aorta should be attempted in all patients to assess the intensity of aortic pulsation as well as the diameter. Using the fingers of both hands, the examiner should identify each side of the aorta by its pulsation, starting superficial and gradually increasing pressure to achieve deepest palpation. Diminished pulsations may be associated with atherosclerotic disease or possible coarctation of the aorta. Pulsations that seem laterally expansile (in addition to physiologic anterior motion) or those that can be identified to the right of midline are suspicious for a dilated aorta or possible aortic aneurysm. In addition, palpation of pulsations below the normal position of the umbilicus suggests extension of the process into the common iliac arteries. Some mild patient discomfort is to be expected during deepest palpation, however, significant tenderness should suggest recent expansion or even contained rupture.

All four quadrants of the abdomen should be auscultated for the presence of bruits. A venous hum may be audible in the epigatric or right upper quadrant in cases of hepatic cirrhosis. Anterior bruits found by pressing the bell of the stethoscope deep into the abdomen at or just above the level of the umbilicus are suggestive of aortic, mesenteric, or renal artery disease. The three can usually be differentiated by utilizing a combination of pitch and radiation. As the abdominal aorta is a large and central vessel, aortic bruits are low-pitched and nonradiating. In contrast, the smaller mesenteric and renal arteries will have bruits of higher pitch, yet only true renal vascular bruits will radiate laterally to the flanks. Murmurs auscultated over either of the lower abdominal quadrants suggest iliac artery disease.

Extremities

The upper extremity examination should begin with inspection of the fingers for signs of impaired perfusion. Transient or patchy findings like successive pallor, cyanosis, or rubor may be apparent with Raynaud's phenomenon, especially if there are fluctuations of color with ambient temperature. Careful study may also reveal evidence of chronic occlusive or microembolic disease such as shiny or atrophic skin, ulcerations, and other localized gangrenous changes at the fingertips and edges of nail beds. Other abnormalities to recognize include the arachnodactyly associated with Marfan's syndrome, clubbing secondary to chronic hypoxemia, and capillary pulsations in the nail beds suggestive of significant aortic regurgitation or a widened pulse pressure. On the dorsal aspect of the hand, the examiner should make note of any extensor tendon xanthomas which may be linked to systemic atherosclerotic disease. Finally, the limbs should be examined for symmetry, evidence of venous distension, edema, traumatic injuries, and iatrogenic scars such as those representing the creation of an arteriovenous fistula for hemodialysis.

Lower extremity examination should include both static and dynamic inspection. Static inspection begins after the patient has dangled both lower extremities over the side of the examination table for several minutes. Color variations, specifically cyanosis and pallor should be noted, as well as distribution of hair growth and the general condition of the skin. If need be the room temperature should be adjusted to avoid induction of cyanosis from peripheral vasoconstriction. Taught, shiny skin, thickened nail plates, the absence of hair growth, and atrophy of underlying soft tissue and muscle all indicate arterial insufficiency. Careful attention should be paid to the "pressure points" of the feet and ankles, as these are the areas most prone to develop arterial ulcerations. Ulcers in these areas, the tips of the toes, dorsum of the feet, metatarsal heads, heel, and malleoli, tend to be painful, have sharp borders and flat, pale bases which may be covered by an eschar. These differ from venous ulcerations, which are usually found on the medial aspect of the lower calf and have poorly demarcated edematous borders and hyperpigmented bases often covered with purulent inflammatory secretions. As with the upper extremities, the lower limbs should also be examined for edema, venous distension, traumatic injuries, and iatrogenic scars such as those secondary to saphenous vein harvest for bypass surgery.

Dynamic inspection requires the patient to lie supine for at least 10 minutes with both legs exposed to room temperature. After noting the color of the extremities, the examiner then passively elevates both legs at a level above the heart (approximately 60 degrees) for 1 minute, and again notes the color for grading of elevation pallor. Although it is normal to have slight pallor upon elevation, occlusive arterial disease is present if there is significant elevation pallor within 30 seconds or less. If elevation pallor is observed, the legs are then lowered to the flat position and the time to return to baseline color is measured. In normal individuals, color should return within 10 seconds; those with significant arterial insufficiency will have a reperfusion time of greater than 45 seconds. If elevation pallor is not observed, the maneuver should be repeated after the patient actively exercises the legs by flexing and extending the feet for up to 1 minute.

Another variation involves the patient quickly sitting-up after determination of elevation pallor so that his or her legs dangle over the edge of the examination table. The length of time it takes the first vein to fill on the dorsum of the foot is then recorded, known as the venous filling time. With normal arterial circulation, the first veins should fill within 15 seconds. Venous filling times of 20 to 30 seconds suggest moderate ischemia, and those greater than 40 seconds indicate the presence of severe ischemia. Further observation for the development of dependent rubor should follow with more significant disease producing more significant rubor. Confirmation of poor arterial perfusion can be accomplished by assessment of capillary refill, in which the examiner induces blanching of the toes or distal feet by compression of the skin for a few seconds and then measures the time for return of color. Normal capillary refilling time is generally considered to be less than 2 seconds.

Palpation of the peripheral vasculature should proceed in stepwise fashion, minimizing patient movement, exposure, and discomfort. Using the fingertips, the examiner should grade the strength of the pulse and identify the presence or absence of aneurysmal dilatation. Subtle differences may be more easily detected by palpating symmetrical pulses simultaneously. When possible, the vessel should also be assessed for deformability as a vessel that is stiff, noncompressible, or rolls away from the examiner's fingertips suggests the presence of sclerosis. In addition, the presence of a radial-femoral delay, an examination finding highly indicative for coarctation of the aorta, should be ruled out by concurrent palpation of the ipsilateral radial and femoral pulses. Finally, the examiner should palpate the skin to evaluate for temperature differences, especially over symptomatic areas. Although coolness is an insensitive sign for ischemia, asymmetry between limbs may suggest chronic arterial insufficiency.

Palpation usually begins with examination of the pulses of the upper extremities with the patient sitting in the upright position. The radial artery is often the easiest to locate, while the ulnar artery may be obscured by a well-developed wrist. In both cases, the examiner's second hand should be used to relax the patient's flexor tendons by cupping the patient's wrist or using the "handshake position" to induce partial flexion. The brachial artery is found in the antecu-bital fossa while the elbow is partially flexed and the examiner's free hand supports the forearm. The patient should then be asked to lay supine with the arm stretched outward and elbow bent so the hand is behind the head. In this position, the axillary artery should be more easily accessible although deep palpation is still required.

For examination of the lower extremities, the patient should remain supine with the legs outstretched and uncrossed to avoid interference by tense muscles. The distal portion of the external iliac artery and the common femoral artery can be palpated just above and below the inguinal ligament. To palpate the popliteal artery, the examiner should cradle a slightly flexed knee in both hands so that all eight fingers may explore the popliteal crevice. The pulse should be felt directly below the lateral aspect of the patella, and often deep pressure is needed. The posterior tibial artery is found beneath and behind the medial malleolus and may be easier to palpate if the examiner uses the contralateral fingertips (i.e., use the left hand to examine the patient's right foot and right hand to examine the patient's left foot) and applies passive dorsiflexion with the free hand. On the dorsum of the foot in line with the second metatarsal bone approximately 2 to 3 inches distal to the joint crevice is where the dorsalis pedis artery pulse should be found, although it may not be palpable in up to 10% of the population because of an abherant course or being congenitally absent.[3,16,22]

If any color changes, edema or complaints of diffuse arm or hand pain are present, thoracic outlet maneuvers should be done to assess the arterial flow patterns of the proximal vasculature. Although the sensitivity and specificity of these tests are relatively low, between 46% and 62%, they can be helpful if they reproduce the patient's symptoms in addition to a diminished pulse or bruit.[23,24] For the hyperabduction maneuver to assess for subclavian artery compression, the patient sits upright with the head looking forward. The examiner braces the patient's shoulder with one hand as the other hand continuously palpates the radial pulse while abducting and externally rotating the patient's arm. Alternatively, the examiner may use the first hand to auscultate the supraclavicular area for development of a subclavian artery bruit during the same maneuver. If the pulse is not diminished, a bruit is not induced, or symptoms are not produced in this position, the patient should then be asked to look to both the ipsilateral followed by the contralateral side with the chin extended (Adson's maneuver). If the test is still negative, the patient's arm or neck should be passively moved and the pulse amplitude assessed to evaluate for positional compression of the axillary or subclavian arteries on the affected side. Finally, the costoclavicular maneuver evaluates for compression of the neurovascular bundle between the clavicle and first rib by having the patient stand at exaggerated military attention with the shoulders thrust backward and downward. Because many asymptomatic patients can have positive results, interpretation of all these tests must be made cautiously.

If occlusion of the vasculature distal to the wrist is suspected, an Allen test should be done to assess the patency

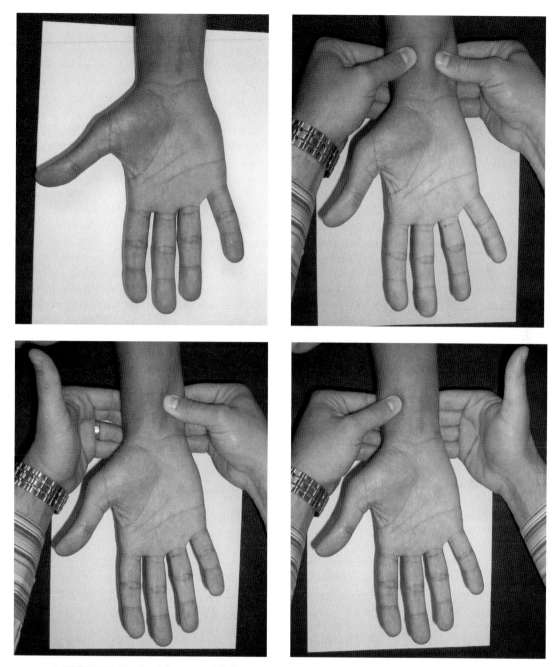

● **FIGURE 16-6.** Allen test. (A) Open hand at baseline. The patient should then make a fist while the examiner compresses the radial and ulnar arteries. (B) After making a fist, the open hand remains blanched with both arteries occluded. (C) Checking patency of the radial artery. (D) Checking patency of the ulnar artery.

of the radial, ulnar, palmar arch, and digital arteries (see Figure 16-6). As the patient tightly clenches his or her fist, the examiner simultaneously compresses both the radial and ulnar arteries using firm pressure of one or two fingers. Once the fist blanches, the patient opens the hand, taking care to maintain a relaxed posture. The examiner then releases one of the arteries and evaluates the rate of color return. If the hand returns to normal color within a few seconds, the released artery is patent and the test is considered negative. If the hand remains pale, however, occlusion

of the released artery is confirmed. The maneuver is then repeated for evaluation of the opposite vessel. When only part of the palm or certain digits fail to return to normal color, occlusion, or spasm of the palmar arch or a digital vessel is diagnosed. It is important to note a false-positive test may be induced by overextension of the fingers or wrist, as tense ligamentous structures compress an otherwise normal artery. However, even when done properly, the Allen test can have variable diagnostic accuracy, therefore should only be used for screening purposes.[25,26]

Auscultation for altered blood flow in the extremities should be attempted for the brachial, iliac, femoral, and popliteal arteries. One should not have difficulty identifying the affected vessel when a bruit is heard over the brachial or popliteal area, however, as a bruit detected in the inguinal region can have several sources, the examiner should attempt to localize the obstruction using a few simple techniques. First, the examiner should listen both proximal and distal to the area where the bruit is first auscultated. An iliac artery bruit should decrease in intensity as the examiner moves distally into the femoral region. On the other hand, a bruit that is louder in the femoral area and softer in the iliac fossa is likely secondary to disease of the common femoral artery, the superficial femoral artery and/or the profunda femoral artery. Further distinction among these sources can be made by compressing the superficial femoral artery near the apex of the femoral triangle. If the bruit disappears or decreases in intensity, a stenosis is more likely to be present in the common or superficial femoral artery. A bruit caused by a lesion in the profunda femoral artery will instead become louder with compression.

One last bedside maneuver that is helpful in assessing severity of presumed lower limb arterial ischemia is the determination of the ankle-brachial index (ABI). In this vertical assessment of arterial blood flow, the Doppler systolic pressure of either the dorsalis pedis or posterior tibial artery (whichever is higher among the two) is divided by the highest Doppler systolic pressure of the brachial arteries. In normal vessels, the Doppler systolic pressures at both sites should be nearly equal, resulting in an ABI of greater than or equal to 1.0. In order to allow for any intra- and interobserver variability, however, the normal range for an ABI is often extended down to 0.90. An ABI of less than 0.90 is usually indicative of some degree of arterial occlusive disease within the iliac, the femoral, or the popliteal artery. The lower the ABI, the greater is the severity of arterial insufficiency present. It is important to note that in order for an ABI measurement to be valid, the arteries must be compressible. Patients with heavily calcified or hardened vessel walls can often have a normal, near normal, or supranormal (>1.3) ABI despite the presence of severe occlusive disease. In addition, patients with bilateral subcalvian artery stenosis may also have false elevation of their ABI because of lower than normal brachial artery pressures.

● ACKNOWLEDGMENTS

The authors would like to thank Joshua Liberman, MD and Ravi K. Ramana, DO for their assistance in the completion of this chapter.

REFERENCES

1. Creager MA, Libby P. Peripheral arterial diseases. In: Zipes DP, Libby P, Bonow RO, Braunwald E, eds. *Braunwald's Heart Disease: A Textbook of Cardiovascular Medicine*. 7th ed. Philadelphia, PA: Elsevier Saunders; 2005:1437–1461.

2. Caralis DG. Claudication: clinical diagnosis and differential diagnosis. In: Caralis DG, Bakris GL, eds. *Lower Extremity Arterial Disease*. 1st ed. Totowa, NJ: Humana Press; 2005:1–21.

3. Beckman JA, Creager MA. The history and physical examination. In: Creager MA, Dzau VJ, Loscalzo J, eds. *Vascular Medicine: A Companion to Braunwald's Heart Disease*. 1st ed. Philadelphia, PA: Elsevier Saunders; 2006:135–145.

4. Coyne KS, Margolis MK, Gilchrist KA, et al. Evaluating effects of method of administration on walking impairment questionnaire. *J Vasc Surg*. 2003;38:296–304.

5. Bordeaux LM, Reich LM, Hirsch AT. The epidemiology and natural history of peripheral arterial disease. In: Coffman JD, Eberhardt RT, eds. *Peripheral Arterial Disease: Diagnosis and Treatment*. 1st ed. Totowa, NJ: Humana Press; 2003:21–34.

6. Arnold GJ. Peripheral vascular assessment: history taking and physical examination of the arterial and venous systems. In: Abela GS, ed. *Peripheral Vascular Disease: Basic Diagnostic and Therapeutic Approaches*. 1st ed. Philadelphia, PA: Lippincott William and Wilkins; 2004:37–52.

7. Joyce JW. Examination of the patient with vascular disease. In: Loscalzo J, Creager MA, Dzau VJ, eds. *Vascular Medicine: A Textbook of Vascular Biology and Diseases*. 2nd ed. New York, NY: Little, Brown and Company; 1996:397–413.

8. Lanzer P. Peripheral vascular disease. In: Lanzer P, Topol EJ, eds. *Panvascular Medicine: Integrated Clinical Management*. 1st ed. New York, NY: Springer-Verlag Berlin Heidelberg; 2002: 388–396.

9. Tsai TT, Nienaber CA, Eagles KA. Acute aortic syndromes. *Circulation*. 2005;112:3802–3813.

10. Spittell JA Jr. Occlusive peripheral arterial disease. In: Spittell JA, ed. *Peripheral Vascular Disease for Cardiologists: A Clinical Approach*. 1st ed. New York, NY: Blackwell Publishing/Futura Division; 2004:1–29.

11. Dilley RB. The history and physical examination in vascular disease. In: Berstein EF, ed. *Vascular Diagnosis*. 4th ed. Chicago, IL: Mosby-Year Book; 1993:7–13.

12. Aiello PD, Trautmann JC, McPhee TJ, Kunselman AR, Hunder GG. Visual prognosis in giant cell arteritis. *Ophthalmology*. 1993;100:550–555.

13. Pifarre R, Dieter RA Jr, Niedballa RG. Definitive surgical treatment of the aberrant retroesophageal right subclavian artery in the adult. *J Thorac Cardiovasc Surg*. 1971;61:154–159.

14. Farjo QA, Sugar A. Conjunctival and corneal degenerations. In: Yanoff M, Duker JS, Augsburger JJ, et al., eds. *Ophthalmology*. 2nd ed. St. Louis, MO: Mosby; 2004:446–453.

15. Segal P, Insull W, Chambless LE, et al. The association of corneal dyslipoproteinemia with corneal arcus and xanthelasma. The Lipid Research Clinics Program Prevalence Study. *Circulation*. 1986;73:I108–I118.

16. Braunwald E, Perloff JK. Physical examination of the heart and circulation. In: Zipes DP, Libby P, Bonow RO, Braunwald E, eds. *Braunwald's Heart Disease: A Textbook of Cardiovascular*

Medicine. 7th ed. Philadelphia, PA: Elsevier Saunders; 2005: 77–106.

17. Vlachopoulos C, O'Rourke M. Genesis of the normal and abnormal pulse. *Curr Prob Cardiol*. 2000;25:303–367.

18. Perloff JK. The physiologic mechanisms of cardiac and vascular physical signs. *J Am Coll Cardiol*. 1983;1:184–189.

19. Magyar MT, Nam E, Csiba L, Ritter MA, Ringelstein EB, Droste DW. Carotid artery auscultation – anachronism or useful screening procedure? *Neurol Res*. 2002;24:705–708.

20. Sauve JS, Thorpe KE, Sackett DL, et al. Can bruits distinguish high-grade from moderate symptomatic carotid stenosis? The North American symptomatic carotid endarterectomy trial (NASCET). *Ann Intern Med*. 1994;120:633–637.

21. Sapira JD. Arteries. In: Orient JM, ed. *The Art and Science of Bedside Diagnosis*, Philadelphia, PA: William and Wilkins; 1990:331–354.

22. Barnhorst DA, Barner HB. Prevalence of congenitally absent pedal pulses. *N Engl J Med*. 1968;278:264–265.

23. Dale WA, Lewis MR. Management of thoracic outlet syndrome. *Ann Surg*. 1975;181:575–585.

24. Conn J Jr. Thoracic outlet syndromes. *Surg Clin North Am*. 1974;54:155–164.

25. Jarvis MA, Jarvis CL, Jones PR, Spyt TJ. Reliability of Allen's test in selection of patients for radial artery harvest. *Ann Thorac Surg*. 2000;70:1362–1365.

26. Levinsohn DG, Gordon L, Sessler DI. The Allen's test: analysis of four methods. *J Hand Surg*. 1991;16:279–282.

chapter 17

Noninvasive Arterial Imaging

Kevin P. Cohoon, DO / John E. Gocke, MD, RVT / Susan Bowes, RVT / Robert S. Dieter, MD, RVT

● FUNCTIONAL MECHANICS OF NORMAL AND ABNORMAL VASCULAR FLOW

Describing pulsatile fluid systems mathematically is very complex. Hemodynamics can be defined as the physical factors that influence blood flow which is based on fundamental laws of physics, namely Ohm's law: Voltage (ΔV) equals the product of current (I) and resistance (R), i.e.,

$$\Delta V = I \times R.$$

In relating Ohm's law to fluid flow, the voltage is the pressure difference between two points (ΔP), the resistance is the resistance to flow (R), and the current is the blood flow (F):

$$F = \frac{\Delta P}{R}.$$

Resistance to blood flow within a vascular network is determined by the length and diameter of individual vessels, the physical characteristics of the blood (viscosity, laminar flow versus turbulent flow), the series and parallel arrangements of vascular network, and extravascular mechanical forces acting upon the vasculature. This is expressed in Poiseuille's law:

$$Q = (\pi \Delta P r^4)/(8\eta L).$$

Poiseuille's Law relates the rate at which blood flows through a small blood vessel (Q) with the difference in blood pressure at the two ends (ΔP), the radius (r) and the length (L) of the artery, and the viscosity (η) of the blood.

Of the above factors, changes in vessel diameter are most important quantitatively for regulating blood flow as well as arterial pressure within an organ. Changes in vessel diameter, either by constriction or dilatation, enable organs to adjust their own blood flow to meet the metabolic requirements of the tissue. Flow velocity increases as the pressure gradient increases and flow volumes are relatively preserved, only to a point though.

Osborne Reynolds determined how viscosity, vessel radius, and pressure/volume relations influenced the stability of flow through a vessel:

Reynolds number = [2(velocity)(density)(diameter)]/ viscosity

Density and viscosity are relatively constant, therefore the development of turbulence depends mainly on the velocity and size of the vessel. Density is defined as mass per unit volume and viscosity is defined as a measure of the resistance of a fluid to being deformed by either shear stress or extensional stress. A Reynolds number >2000 causes turbulence and vessel wall vibration producing a bruit. High velocities cause turbulence and hinder volumes flow, creating eddies.

● TYPES OF VASCULAR ULTRASOUND

Basics of Vascular Ultrasound

Ultrasonic waves entering human tissue are absorbed, reflected, and scattered to produce images of anatomic structures. The transmission properties of the sound waves depend on the density and elasticity of the tissues. Density and speed of propagation of ultrasound waves determine a tissue's acoustic impedance. The larger the differences in acoustic impedance between tissues, the more ultrasound waves are reflected. The reflection further depends on the angle of insonation. Strong reflective interfaces, such as air or bone, prevent imaging of weaker echoes from deeper tissue and cast shadows behind them. Tissues that strongly reflect ultrasound are termed hyperechoic, whereas poorly reflective tissues are termed hypoechoic.

The transducer repeatedly emits pulses of sound at a fixed repetition frequency. A detector records echoes originating from interfaces and scatterers in the sound beam. Echo signals are then amplified and processed into a format for display. If ultrasound is continuously transmitted along a particular path, the energy will also be continuously reflected back from any source in the path of the beam, making it difficult to predict the depth of the returning echoes. With pulse-echo techniques, it is possible to predict the distance of a reflecting surface from the transducer if the time between the transmission and reception of the pulse is measured and the velocity of the ultrasound along the path are known.

When the ultrasound pulse returns to the transducer, it causes the transducer to vibrate and will generate a voltage across the piezoelectric element. The amplitude of the returning pulse depends on several factors, including the proportion of the ultrasound reflected to the transducer and by which the signal has been reflected along its path. The amplitude of the pulse received back to the transducer can be displayed (A-mode) against time and then can be calibrated to time, thus showing the depth of the boundary in the tissue. The varying amplitude of the signal can be displayed as a spot of varying brightness. This type of display is known as a B-mode scan.

B-Mode Imaging

Structures imaged by B-mode, or brightness mode, are displayed proportionally to the intensity of returning echoes. The ultrasonic beam scanning through a tissue plane produces a two-dimensional gray-scale image. In clinical practice, the beam is swept quickly through the field of view, and the image is continuously renewed, allowing visualization of the underlying tissue anatomy.

B-mode ultrasound takes reflected signals and converts them to a series of dots on a display. A transducer, whose resonant frequency is between roughly 2 and 10 MHz, is used to transmit a short pulse of sound into a patient. The sound is reflected from a tissue interface where there are differences in acoustic impedance. The reflected pulse is received by the ultrasound instrument and the pulse amplitude is encoded as brightness and depth on a monitor. The time that is required for the pulse to travel from the transducer to the interface and back is directly proportional to its depth. The acoustic velocity is 1540 m/s. As the sound pulse propagates through tissue, it is attenuated and this would darken the parts of the image that correspond to regions further from the probe. In order to compensate for this attenuation, echoes originating from deeper tissues are amplified more than echoes originating near the probe. Because different tissues have different attenuation coefficients, the amplification can be varied as a function of depth. The exact manner in which the amplification depends on depth is usually displayed on the ultrasound instruments monitor as a depth-gain curve or time-gain curve. Usually, 100 to 200 separate ultrasound beam lines are used to construct each image.

Doppler Display Modes

Doppler ultrasound is a technique for recording noninvasive velocity measurements. The difference in frequency between emitted and returning ultrasonic echoes is the Doppler frequency shift.[1] As the blood is moving, the sound undergoes a frequency (Doppler) shift that is described by the Doppler equation[2,3]:

$$F = 2[(F_0)(v)(\cos \theta)]/c,$$

where c is the acoustic velocity in blood, 1540 m/s; F_0 is the transmitted frequency; θ is the Doppler angle; v is the velocity of the blood. The shift is measured only for the component of motion occurring along the ultrasound beam. Therefore, absolute velocity measurements require that a correction be made for the angle (θ) between the vessel and the beam as follows:

$$v = (\Delta F \times c)/(2F_0 \cos \theta).$$

Color Doppler Imaging

Color Doppler ultrasound is a technique for visualizing the velocity of blood within an image plane. Color is superimposed on a conventional gray-scale image to enhance the image of the Doppler frequency shift. A color Doppler instrument measures the Doppler shifts in a few thousand sample volumes located in an image plane. For each sample volume, the average Doppler shift is encoded as a color and displayed on top of the B-mode image. The way in which the frequency shifts are encoded is defined by the color bar located to the side of the image. By convention, positive Doppler shifts, caused by blood moving toward the transducer, are encoded as red and negative shifts are encoded as blue. Color Doppler images are updated several times per second, thus allowing the flowing blood to be easily visualized.

In healthy individuals, arterial flow is pulsatile and laminar, whereas stenoses, angles, or elevated velocities may cause the laminar flow pattern to be distrupted.[4] Additionally, turbulence at the stenosis and distal to the area causes an increase in the rage of flow velocities known as spectral broadening.[2] As the degree of stenosis progresses, flow velocities increase at the point of maximum narrowing. In very stenotic areas, marked reductions in the residual lumen cause flow velocities to fall, leading to flow cessation with complete lumen obliteration. Doppler insonation proximal to an occluded vessel assumes a stump flow pattern.

Continuous Wave Doppler

Continuous wave Doppler uses two piezoelectric crystal transducers where one crystal continuously emits toward the region of interest and the other continuously receives reflected echoes. Flow toward the transducer produces an increase in the received frequency, whereas flow away from the transducer causes a drop. Continuous Doppler does not provide information about the depth of the tissue.

Power Doppler

Power Doppler ultrasonography emphasizes the display of amplitude information rather than the relative velocity or direction of flow. This method of display has some advantages in that the power Doppler display is not dependent on the angle of insonation and has better sensitivity when compared with conventional Doppler frequency. Advantages of power Doppler include independence from the angle of insonation, absence of aliasing, and the ability to detect very low flows.

● NONINVASIVE DIAGNOSTIC IMAGING OF LOWER EXTREMITY PERIPHERAL ARTERIAL DISEASE

Lower extremity peripheral arterial disease (PAD) is associated with an amplified risk of cerebrovascular and cardiovascular morbidity and mortality, including stroke, myocardial infarction, and even death. The prevalence of PAD in North America and Europe is currently estimated to affect approximately 27 million people.[5]

Noninvasive tests are preformed to confirm and define the extent of obstruction in patients with suspected lower extremity PAD based upon the history (e.g., symptoms of intermittent claudication) or in patients with risks factors for vascular disease (e.g., older age, smoking, diabetes mellitus).[6] The establishment of successful patient stratification in vascular medicine is through a thorough clinical evaluation and accurate noninvasive testing. In this chapter, the focus is on the functional mechanics of normal and abnormal vascular flow, types of noninvasive imaging, limitations of noninvasive imaging, and recommendations and guidelines in lower extremity, carotid, renal artery, cerebral, mesenteric, upper extremity, and vertebral vascular diseases.

A variety of noninvasive examinations are available to provide an objective diagnostic tool to assess the presence and degree of PAD. The noninvasive vascular evaluation includes ankle and toe brachial index, exercise treadmill test, segmental limb pressures (SLPs), segmental volume plethysmography, and color duplex imaging. These examinations allow the clinician to objectively determine the presence of disease, localize lesions, and establish the severity of disease to determine the progression or its response to therapeutics. This section will review the evidence-based benefits, limitations, quality assurance, and guidelines of each of these vascular diagnostic techniques.

● LOWER EXTREMITY ARTERIAL VASCULAR TESTING

Patients should be evaluated for PAD if they are at increased risk from their age, presence of atherosclerotic risk factors, have leg pain suggestive of ischemia, or have distal limb ulceration (Table 17-1).

Many vascular practices use various algorithms for the diagnosis of PAD; however a thorough historical review of symptoms and atherosclerotic risks factors, physical ex-

---

TABLE 17-1. Indications for Noninvasive Physiologic Testing

- Exercise-related limb pain
- Abnormal ratio of ankle-to-brachial arterial systolic blood pressure
- Extremity ulcer/gangrene
- Assessment of healing potential
- Cold sensitivity
- Arterial trauma and aneurysms
- Absent peripheral pulses
- Digital cyanosis or limb pain at rest

This material was originally published in Guidelines for noninvasive vascular laboratory testing: a report from the American Society of Echocardiography and the Society of Vascular Medicine and Biology. J Am Soc Echocardiogr. 2006;19:955-972 and is reproduced with the permission of the copyright holder, the American Society of Echocardiog raphy www.asecho.org. Inclusion of this information does not necessarily imply endorsement of this product.

---

amination, and the use of noninvasive vascular tests are paramount in diagnosing PAD. The most cost-effective tool for lower extremity PAD detection is the ankle-brachial index (ABI) and should be performed in every patient suspected of having lower extremity PAD (Figure 17-1).[8]

Many vascular practices simultaneously obtain ABIs, SLPs, and pulse volume recordings (PVRs) in patients with suspected PAD as initial diagnostic tests.

● ANKLE-BRACHIAL INDEX

The ABI is a relatively simple, inexpensive, and reproducible method to confirm the clinical suspicion of arterial occlusive disease. Despite the increasing use of more sophisticated diagnostic tests, the ABI has been shown through epidemiology studies to predict future cardiovascular ischemic events. This has led to increasing use of the ABI examination in office practice. The sensitivity and specificity associated with an ABI threshold of 0.90 or less have ranged from a sensitivity of 79% to 95% and specificity of 96% to 100% compared with contrast angiography. Fowkes et al.[9] demonstrated that with an ABI diagnostic threshold of 0.90, the sensitivity of the ABI was 95% and specificity was 100% compared with angiography. Feigelson et al.[10] demonstrated using only posterior tibial measurements in assessing the ABI, that with an ABI diagnostic threshold of 0.8, the sensitivity of the ABI was 89% and specificity was 99% with a overall accuracy of 98% compared with angiography. Lijmer et al.[11] evaluated the ABI by using a receiver operating characteristic (ROC) to determine its diagnostic accuracy depending on the localization of the disease. This study demonstrated patients with significant PAD (lesions ≥50%), that with an ABI diagnostic threshold of 0.91, the sensitivity of the ABI was 79%, and specificity was 96%. Multiple investigations have also evaluated the interobserver variability of the ABI measurement. Endres et al.[12] tested the variability of a measured ABI with six angiologists, six primary care physicians, and six trained medical

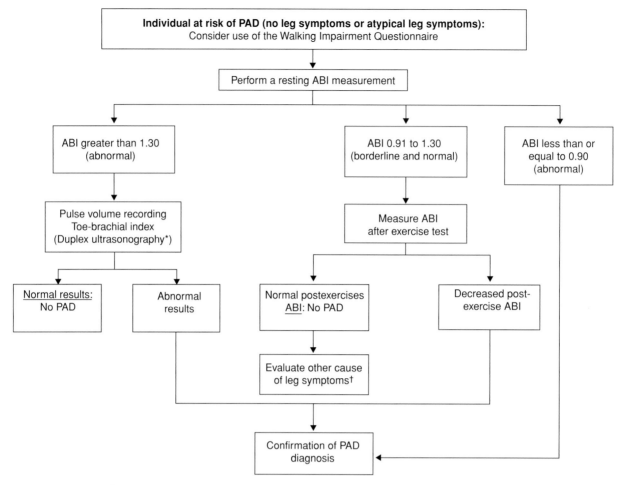

● **FIGURE 17-1.** Diagnosis of asymptomatic PAD and atypical leg pain. ABI, ankle-brachial index.

*Duplex ultrasonography should generally be reserved for use in symptomatic patients in whom anatomic diagnostic data is required for care.

†Other causes of leg pain may include lumbar disk disease, sciatica, radiculopathy; muscle strain; neuropathy; compartment syndrome.

It is not yet proven that treatment of diabetes mellitus will significantly reduce PAD-specific (limb ischemic) endpoints. Primary treatment of diabetes mellitus should be continued according to established guidelines.

Adapted with permission from Hiatt WR. Medical treatment of peripheral arterial disease and claudication. N Engl J Med. 2001;344:1608-1621 (179a).

office assistants. They performed two ABI measurements: each measurement on six individuals from a group of 36 unselected subjects aged 65 to 70 years and found mean differences between the ABI measurements very close to zero.[12]

Several studies have shown that the ABI is associated with functional capacity, even in asymptomatic patients. The Women's Health and Aging Study evaluated disabled women 65 years or older and used the ABI as a measure of lower extremity function. The results showed that decreasing ABI values were associated with worsening functional scores, even after adjustment for age, race, smoking status, and comorbidities.[13] Even lower ABI scores in the asymptomatic women in this study correlated with slower walking velocities, poorer standing balance scores, slower time to rise, and fewer blocks walked per week.[13] In the Study of Osteoporotic Fractures, 1492 women 65 years or older

were evaluated to compare the relationship between ABI (≤0.90) and extremity function.[14] This study showed patients with an ABI greater than 0.90 had significantly higher hip abduction force, knee extension force, walking velocity, and number of blocks walked than those with ABI of less than 0.90.

Studies have also shown that an abnormal ABI is predictive of both cardiovascular and cerebrovascular disease. Newman et al.[15] has shown an inverse relation between cardiovascular disease and ABI. For example, participants with an ABI <0.8 were more than twice as likely as those with an ABI of 1.0 to 1.5 to have a history of myocardial infarction, congestive heart failure, stroke, angina, or a transient ischemic attack in a cohort of 5084 participants. Mortality and morbidity in patients with lower extremity PAD has been quantitated by McKenna et al.,[16] who demonstrated

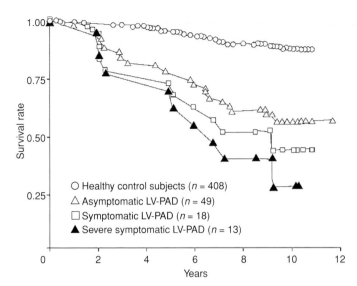

● FIGURE 17-2. Kaplan–Meier survival curves based on mortality from all causes among healthy control subjects and subjects with symptomatic or asymptomatic large-vessel PAD.

Reprinted with permission from Criqui MH, Langer RD, Fronek A, et al. Mortality over a period of 10 years in patients with peripheral arterial disease. N Engl J Med. 326:381-386, 1992.

a 5-year mortality of 50% and 30% in patients with an ABI of 0.40 and 0.70, respectively. It also has been shown that those with an ABI less than 0.50 demonstrated a 5-year mortality of 37%, 29% for patients with an ABI between 0.50 and 0.69, and 9% for patients with an ABI between 0.70 and 0.89.[17] Resnick et al.[18] demonstrated that patients with an ABI of less than 0.90 had an all cause mortality of 1.69 and cardiovascular mortality of 2.52, while patients with an ABI of 1.40 or greater had a all-cause mortality of 1.77 and cardiovascular mortality of 2.09.

Multiple studies have shown the importance of the ABI as a predictor of cardiovascular or all-cause mortality in asymptomatic patients. Criqui et al.[19] has evaluated a 10-year follow up of 67 patients with a diagnosis of PAD and a ABI of 0.80 or less, showing a dramatic increase in rate of mortality in both men (61.8%) and women (33.3%) when compared with men (16.9) and women (11.6%) without disease (Figure 17-2).

Thus, the accuracy in establishing the diagnosis and 5-year survival in patients with lower extremity PAD is well predicted by the ABI value. The American Diabetes Association and American Heart Association have long endorsed the ABI, suggesting that the procedure be preformed in all individuals with diabetes who are aged 50 years and older, in individuals with diabetes who are younger than 50 years of age and have other atherosclerosis risk factors, and in individuals with diabetes of more than 10 years duration.[20,21]

Assessing the ABI

The ABI is performed after the patient has been at rest in the supine position for 10 minutes. The systolic blood pressure should then be measured with appropriately sized cuffs from both brachial arteries and from both the poste-

rior tibial arteries and the dorsalis pedis with a handheld Doppler instrument (Figure 17-3).[8]

The cuff is then rapidly inflated above systolic pressures, thereby obliterating flow to the part under study. As the pressure in the cuff is gradually deflated, the point at which flow is resumed is taken as the opening or systolic pressure at that level. The ABI is calculated by dividing the highest systolic ankle pressure by the higher of the two systolic brachial pressures. Calculated values should be recorded to two decimal places. The average time required to perform the ABI is approximately 5 to 10 minutes. With increasing degrees of arterial stenosis, there is a progressive fall in systolic blood pressure distal to the sites of involvement. This extent to which the pressure falls is dependent on the extent of involvement. The interarm systolic pressure gradient during a routine examination should be less than 12 mm Hg in a normal individual. The ankle pressure in healthy individuals is usually 10 to 15 mm Hg higher than the brachial arterial systolic pressure caused by pulse wave reflections. Subclavian or axillary arterial stenosis is presumed to be present if the blood pressures in the arms are not equal, and the higher blood pressure should then be used for ratio calculations.

ABI values have been categorized to determine the presence and the severity of PAD. The National Heart, Lung, and Blood Institute initiated The Multi-Ethnic Study of Atherosclerosis (MESA) to further understand the pathogenesis of atherosclerosis by providing quantifiable measures of cardiovascular disease, characterization of cardiovascular disease to disrupt its natural course, and to optimize study of the progression of subclinical disease. The MESA cohort consists of 6814 men and women aged 45 to 84 years (38% whites, 28% African Americans, 23% Hispanics, 11% Asians, and approximately 50% females) who were enrolled at six US field centers. They all were free of clinically evident cardiovascular disease at the time of enrollment. Five ABI categories were defined: <0.90 (definite PAD), 0.90 to 0.99 (borderline ABI), 1.00 to 1.09 (low-normal ABI), 1.10 to 1.29 (normal ABI), and 1.30 (high ABI) (Table 17-2).[22]

Previous studies showed that an ABI less than 0.90 is 94% sensitive and 99% specific for angiographically diagnosed PAD.[23] Some studies have used ABI 1.50 to define the upper limit of normal, but generally an ABI of 1.3 is indicative of medial arterial calcinosis and noncompressible arteries.[24–27] Mild claudication or obstruction occurs with an ABI <0.9–0.75. Moderate to severe claudication occurs with an ABI <0.75–0.4. Jelnes et al.[28] demonstrated that an ABI value <0.50 suggests that progression to critical leg ischemia is likely in the subsequent 6.5 years of follow-up (Table 17-2). Thus, patients with severely decreased ABIs are at particularly high risk for the development of rest pain, ischemic ulceration, and gangrene. Absolute levels of tissue ischemia are typically associated with ankle blood pressure recordings of 35 mm Hg or less in nondiabetic subjects, and of less than 55 mm Hg in diabetic subjects.[29]

Additional noninvasive vascular studies can be preformed in patients with abnormal ABIs. Patients with leg

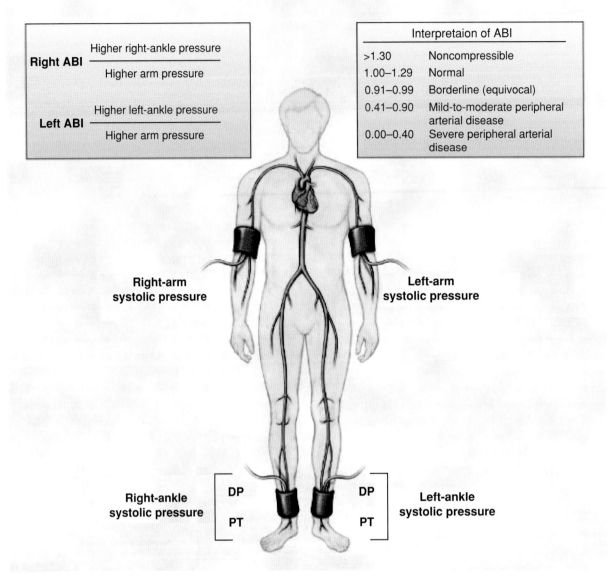

FIGURE 17-3. Ankle-brachial index. DP, dorsalis pedis; PT, posterior tibial artery.

Adapted with permission from Hiatt WR. Medical treatment of peripheral arterial disease and claudication. N Engl J Med. 2002;344:1608-1621.

pain on exertion who have ABI values of 0.91 to 1.30 should be considered for an exercise test, while patients less than 0.90 at rest needs no additional tests for the diagnosis of PAD (though maybe performed to assess functional limitations). If a patient's ABI value is above 1.30, then one should perform additional test such as pulse-volume recording, measurement of a toe-brachial index (TBI), or duplex ultrasonography to determine whether PAD exists (Figure 17-4).[8]

Toe blood pressure analysis is useful to screen for PAD in diabetic patients who may have medial calcinosis of medium-sized arteries or to evaluate for the presence of pedal and digital arterial disease in patients with nonhealing ulcers, rest pain, and gangrene. Patients with unaffected arteries to the level of the ankle but severe PAD in the ar-

teries of the feet and digits may have normal ABIs but a depressed TBI. TBIs less than 0.7 are abnormal, claudication indexes range from 0.35 to 0.69, and those with rest ischemia have indexes ranging from 0.11 to 0.24.[30–32] A toe blood pressure less than 30 mm Hg has 80% sensitivity for detecting limbs with rest ischemia.[31]

Transcutaneous oxygen and carbon dioxide pressure (PO_2 and PCO_2) foot monitoring has been compared with ankle Doppler-derived systolic pressure regarding their abilities to discriminate the severity of limb ischemia before vascular reconstruction and to predict surgical outcome early in the postoperative period. Transcutaneous PO_2 ($TcPCO_2$), foot-chest $TcPO_2$ index, transcutaneous PCO_2 ($TcPCO_2$), foot $TcPO_2/TcPCO_2$ index ($TcPO_2/TcPCO_2$), ankle Doppler systolic pressure (AP), and ABI have been

TABLE 17-2. Criteria for Abnormal ABI

- A normal ABI range is $\geq$1–1.3
- Borderline ABI 0.90–0.99
- Definite PAD <0.90
- Mild claudication or obstruction occurs with an ABI <0.9–0.75
- Moderate to severe claudication occurs with an ABI <0.75–0.4
- Ischemic rest pain and multilevel disease is present with an ABI <0.4
- Tissue loss may occur with an ABI <0.5

This material was originally published in Guidelines for noninvasive vascular laboratory testing: a report from the American Society of Echocardiography and the Society of Vascular Medicine and Biology. J Am Soc Echocardiogr. 2006;19:955-972 and is reproduced with the permission of the copyright holder, the American Society of Echocardiography www.asecho.org. Inclusion of this information does not necessarily imply endorsement of this product.

Limitations of the ABI

The ABI is an effective diagnostic tool, however it does not measure the effectiveness of preventive treatment. The ABI also may not be accurate in individuals whom have noncompressible arteries. The incidence of noncompressible arteries is higher in individuals with diabetes, those with renal insufficiency, and elderly patients as a result of calcified arteries that prevent occlusion of blood flow by the blood pressure cuff. This may result in an unusually high ABI reading, thus, for patients in whom symptoms strongly suggest PAD, the presence of a normal or high ABI should not be resumed to rule out the diagnosis. Also, patients with occlusions or severely stenotic iliofemoral arteries may also occasionally present with a normal ABI at rest because of the presence of collateral arterial networks. In these cases, an alternative diagnostic test (e.g., toe-brachial pressure, Doppler waveform analysis, PVR, exercise ABI test, or duplex ultrasound) should be performed.

ABI and Exercise Treadmill Testing

When the resting ABI is normal, but there is a high clinical suspicion for arterial disease, measurement of ABI coupled with exercise testing can be used to determine whether a patient's symptoms are caused by PAD (Table 17-3).[33,34]

When the patient exercises, this produces significant peripheral vasodilatation in the presence of arterial stenosis, resulting in significant blood pressure gradients. These blood pressure gradients cause the ABI to drop in patients with PAD, whereas in individuals without stenosis will have a slight increase or no change in the ABI.

When performing the test, a baseline ABI is obtained, then the patient is placed on a treadmill using a constant speed and grade until the patient has walked to maximal discomfort or a predefined end point. The patient's leg symptoms, location of symptoms, and their intensity should be recorded at symptom onset and at the time of maximal discomfort. Immediately after exercise, the patient is

evaluated with revascularized limbs. The measurement of $TcPO_2$ and foot-chest $TcPO_2$ has been found to be more sensitive to the degrees of severity of limb ischemia and more closely associated with the outcome of revascularization than AP and ABI. $TcPCO_2$ and $TcPO_2/TcPCO_2$ have not been useful in the assessment of the vascular patient undergoing reconstructive surgery. Before operation, $TcPO_2$ less than or equal to 22 torr and foot-chest $TcPO_2$ index less than or equal to 0.46 indicate severe limb ischemia requiring urgent revascularization. After operation, $TcPO_2$ less than or equal to 22 torr and foot-chest $TcPO_2$ index less than or equal to 0.53 indicate that revascularization is likely to fail.

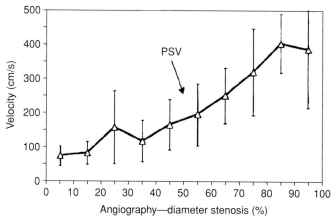

● **FIGURE 17-4.** The relationship between mean PSV and percentage of stenosis as measured arteriographically. PSV increases with increasing severity of stenosis. Note the marked overlap in adjacent categories of stenosis. Error bars = 1 SD about the mean.

Reprinted with permission from Grant EG, Duerinckx AJ, El Saden SM, et al. Ability to use duplex US to quantify internal carotid arterial stenoses: fact or fiction? Radiology. 214:247-252, 2000.

TABLE 17-3. Indications for Stress Testing of the Lower Extremities

- Normal resting lower extremity arterial SLPs and PVRs at rest, in the context of a history of intermittent claudication
- Resting lower extremity SLPs and PVR amplitudes mildly abnormal at rest (i.e., ABI >0.80 but <0.96) in a patient with a history of intermittent claudication

ABI, Ankle-brachial index.
This material was originally published in Guidelines for noninvasive vascular laboratory testing: a report from the American Society of Echocardiography and the Society of Vascular Medicine and Biology. J Am Soc Echocardiogr. 2006;19:955-972 and is reproduced with the permission of the copyright holder, the American Society of Echocardiography www.asecho.org. Inclusion of this information does not necessarily imply endorsement of this product.

ACC–AHA GUIDELINES FOR THE USE OF THE ABI[6]

● DIAGNOSTIC METHODS

Recommendations

Class I

1. The resting ABI should be used to establish the lower extremity PAD diagnosis in patients with suspected lower extremity PAD, defined as individuals with exertional leg symptoms, with nonhealing wounds, who are 70 years and older or who are 50 years and older with a history of smoking or diabetes. *(Level of Evidence: C)*

2. The ABI should be measured in both legs in all new patients with PAD of any severity to confirm the diagnosis of lower extremity PAD and establish a baseline. *(Level of Evidence: B)*

● FOLLOW-UP AFTER VASCULAR SURGICAL PROCEDURES

Recommendations

Class I

1. Patients who have undergone placement of aortobifemoral bypass grafts should be followed up with periodic evaluations that record any return or progression of claudication symptoms, the presence of femoral pulses, and ABIs at rest and after exercise. *(Level of Evidence: C)*

2. Patients who have undergone placement of a synthetic lower extremity bypass graft should, for at least 2 years after implantation, undergo periodic evaluations that record any return or progression of claudication symptoms; a pulse examination of the proximal, graft, and outflow vessels; and assessment of ABIs at rest and after exercise. *(Level of Evidence: C)*

● POSTSURGICAL CARE

Recommendations

Class I

1. Patients who have undergone placement of aortobifemoral bypass grafts should be followed up with periodic evaluations that record any return or progression of ischemic symptoms, the presence of femoral pulses, and ABIs. *(Level of Evidence: B)*

2. If infection, ischemic ulcers, or gangrenous lesions persist and the ABI is less than 0.8 after correction of inflow, an outflow procedure should be performed that bypasses all major distal stenoses and occlusions. *(Level of Evidence: A)*

3. Patients who have undergone placement of a synthetic lower extremity bypass graft should undergo periodic examinations that record any return of ischemic symptoms; a pulse examination of the proximal, graft, and outflow vessels; and assessment of ABIs at rest and after exercise for at least 2 years after implantation. *(Level of Evidence: A)*

Reprinted with permission of ACC/AHA 2005 practice guidelines for the management of patients with peripheral arterial disease (lower extremity, renal, mesenteric, and abdominal aortic): executive summary: a collaborative report from the American Association for Vascular Surgery/Society for Vascular Surgery, Society for Cardiovascular Angiography and Interventions, Society for Vascular Medicine and Biology, Society of Interventional Radiology, and the ACC/AHA Task Force on Practice Guidelines (Writing Committee to Develop Guidelines for the Management of Patients with Peripheral Arterial Disease). Circulation. 2006;113:1474-1547. © 2006, American Heart Association, Inc.

asked to lie in a supine position and the ABI should be measured at 1-minute intervals until the preexercise baseline is reached. ABI <0.90 at 1 minute after exercise indicates hemodynamically significant PAD (Table 17-4).

PAD is not the cause of the symptoms if the exercise produces discomfort or pain and the ABI remains unchanged or normal. Exercise treadmill tests should not be preformed in patients with lower extremity rest pain, noncompressible vessels on a resting study, acute deep venous thrombosis, shortness of breath at rest or with minimal exertion, uncontrolled angina, or a physical disability that limits the patient's ability to ambulate on a treadmill.

An alternative form of exercise testing is active pedal plantar flexion. The patients raise their heels as high as possible and then immediately lower them, repeating the cycle for up to 50 consecutive repetitions. ABIs are measured immediately after completing the exercise with the patient

TABLE 17-4. Interpretation of Postexercise ABI

• ABI <0.90 at 1 min after exercise indicates hemodynamically significant PAD

This material was originally published in Guidelines for noninvasive vascular laboratory testing: a report from the American Society of Echocardiography and the Society of Vascular Medicine and Biology. J Am Soc Echocardiogr. 2006;19:955-972 and is reproduced with the permission of the copyright holder, the American Society of Echocardiogr aphy www.asecho.org. Inclusion of th is information does not necessarily imply endorsement of this product.

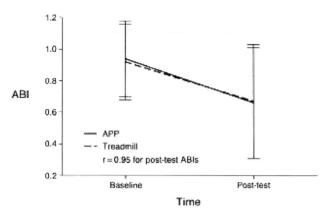

● **FIGURE 17-5.** Mean baseline and posttest ABIs ± 1 standard deviation for all subjects' APP and treadmill exercise results. ABI, ankle-brachial index; APP, active pedal plantarflexion.

Reprinted with permission of J Am Coll Cardiol, Ian R. McPhail, MD, Peter C. Spittell, MD, Susan A. Weston, MS and Kent R. Bailey, PhD, Intermittent claudication: an objective office-based assessment, vol 37, 1381-1385, Copyright Elsevier 2001.

in a supine position. McPhail et al.[35] compared the active pedal plantarflexion technique with the standard lower extremity vascular laboratory treadmill exercise. This study demonstrated an excellent correlation ($r = 0.95$, 95% confidence interval 0.93 to 0.97) between mean postexercise ankle-brachial systolic blood pressure indices for treadmill exercise and active pedal plantar flexion, while producing zero symptoms of angina or dyspnea (Figure 17-5).

The reactive hyperemia test is an alternative to the baseline ABI or treadmill test. If one is unable to walk on a treadmill, the reactive hyperemia test can be performed to diagnose PAD. Standard blood pressure cuffs are placed around the thighs and ankles. The thigh cuffs will be inflated above the patient's normal systolic blood pressure for 3 to 5 minutes. Once the thigh cuffs are deflated, the ankle cuffs are inflated briefly above the patient's systolic blood pressure, so that using the Doppler instrument, blood pressure measurements can be immediately taken at both ankles. A significant (50% or greater) decrease in ankle blood pressure indicates that there is a blockage in the leg arteries and thus is a diagnosis of PAD.

● SLP MEASUREMENT

When further detection, localization, or characterization of PAD is necessary, the measurement of segmental pressures and PVRs can be used. The ABI cannot determine the location of proximal arterial lesions or the relative significance of lesions at multiple levels. In contrast to ABI studies, the segmental pressure analysis is able to make measurement of systolic blood pressure along selected segments of each extremity and accurately determine the presence and severity of stenosis in the peripheral arteries. When SLP measurements are used in combination with PVRs, a 97% diagnostic accuracy is demonstrated when compared with angiography.[36]

Assessing SLP

The SLPs are preformed after the patient has been at rest in the supine position for 20 minutes. A series of pneumatic cuffs are placed on the upper and lower portions of

---

ACC–AHA GUIDELINES FOR THE USE OF THE TREADMILL EXERCISE TESTING[6]

Recommendations

Class I

1. Exercise treadmill tests are recommended to provide the most objective evidence of the magnitude of the functional limitation of claudication and to measure the response to therapy. (*Level of Evidence: B*)

2. A standardized exercise protocol (either fixed or graded) with a motorized treadmill should be used to ensure reproducibility of measurements of pain-free walking distance and maximal walking distance. (*Level of Evidence: B*)

3. Exercise treadmill tests with measurement of preexercise and postexercise ABI values are recommended to provide diagnostic data useful in differentiating arterial claudication from nonarterial claudication ("pseudoclaudication"). (*Level of Evidence: B*)

4. Exercise treadmill tests should be performed in individuals with claudication who are to undergo exercise training (lower extremity PAD rehabilitation) so as to determine functional capacity, assess nonvascular exercise limitations, and demonstrate the safety of exercise. (*Level of Evidence: B*)

Class IIb

1. A 6-minute walk test may be reasonable to provide an objective assessment of the functional limitation of claudication and response to therapy in elderly individuals or others not amenable to treadmill testing. (*Level of Evidence: B*)

Reprinted with permission of ACC/AHA 2005 practice guidelines for the management of patients with peripheral arterial disease (lower extremity, renal, mesenteric, and abdominal aortic): executive summary: a collaborative report from the American Association for Vascular Surgery/Society for Vascular Surgery, Society for Cardiovascular Angiography and Interventions, Society for Vascular Medicine and Biology, Society of Interventional Radiology, and the ACC/AHA Task Force on Practice Guidelines (Writing Committee to Develop Guidelines for the Management of Patients with Peripheral Arterial Disease). Circulation. 2006;113:1474-1547. © 2006, American Heart Association, Inc.

the thigh, the calf, above the ankle, and often over the metatarsal area of the foot and great toe. Likewise, in the upper extremity, pneumatic cuffs are placed on the upper arm over the biceps, on the forearm below the elbow, and at the wrist. Systolic pressure is determined at each level using a continuous-wave Doppler probe. In the upper extremities, the Doppler probe can be placed over the brachial artery in the antecubital fossa or over the radial and ulnar arteries at the wrist. The ABI is calculated, and then the pressure is sequentially inflated in each cuff to 20 to 30 mm Hg above the systolic pressure, or beyond the last audible Doppler arterial signal. The systolic pressure is recorded as the pressure at which the first audible Doppler arterial signal returns. If pressure measurements need to be repeated, the cuff should be fully deflated for about 1 minute prior to repeat inflation. The average time required to perform SLP is approximately 15 to 20 minutes.

In normal individuals, the difference in systolic pressure between any two adjacent levels (vertical) in the leg should be less than 20 mm Hg. A blood pressure gradient in excess of 20 mm Hg between successive cuffs usually signifies significant occlusive disease between the cuffs. The horizontal gradients between corresponding segments of the two legs may also indicate the presence of occlusive lesions. As the limb girth decreases from the thigh to the ankle, pressure measurements also decrease. The high-thigh pressure in the average sized limb is normally at least 20 to 30 mm Hg greater than the highest brachial pressure. If this difference is less than this amount from the high-thigh to brachial, then this would suggest an aortoiliac obstruction (or, CFA stenosis/CFA equivalent). In further determining the level at which there may be stenosis or occlusion, a thigh pressure index (ratio of high thigh systolic pressure to brachial systolic) can be calculated. The thigh pressure index is normally greater than 1.2, however an index between 0.8 and 1.2 suggests aortoiliac stenosis (Table 17-5). A complete iliac occlusion is consistent with a thigh pressure index less than 0.8.[37]

Significant reduction in blood pressure cuff positions[38]

- between the brachial artery and the upper thigh reflects aortoiliac, common femoral or both proximal superficial femoral artery and profunda disease,
- between the upper and lower thigh reflects femoral artery disease,
- between the lower thigh and upper calf reflects distal femoral artery or popliteal disease, and
- between the upper and lower calf reflects tibial disease.

● PULSE VOLUME RECORDINGS

PVR provide a method to evaluate the arterial pressure waveform with the use of pneumoplethysmograph. This allows one the ability to assess the change in limb volume between diastole and systole in a segmental manner from the thigh to the ankle. The magnitude of the

TABLE 17-5. Criteria for Abnormal Segmental Pressure Study

Level of disease	Findings
Aortoiliac	High thigh/brachial index <0.9 bilaterally
Iliac	High thigh/brachial index <0.9
Femoral disease	Gradient between high and low thigh cuffs
Distal SFA/popliteal	Gradient between thigh cuff and calf cuff
Infrapopliteal	Gradient between calf and ankle cuffs

Pressure gradient between 20 and 30 mm Hg is borderline, ≥30 mm Hg is abnormal.
SFA, Superficial femoral artery.
This material was originally published in Guidelines for noninvasive vascular laboratory testing: a report from the American Society of Echocardiography and the Society of Vascular Medicine and Biology. J Am Soc Echocardiogr. 2996;19:955-972 and is reproduced with the permission of the copyright holder, the American Society of Echocardiography www.asecho.org. Inclusion of this information does not necessarily imply endorsement of this product.

pulse volume correlates with blood flow and provides an index of large vessel patency. The device uses a large thigh cuff placed proximally and a calf and ankle cuffs used distally. A brachial cuff is also placed and PVR tracings are recorded to provide an index of normal pulsatility in a normal limb. The magnitude of the pulse amplitude and pulse upstroke provides a global physiological measurement of large-vessel patency and correlates with blood flow. Any deviation in the amplitude or upstroke signifies the presence of a flow limiting stenosis in the more proximal segment (Figure 17-6).[39,40]

Measurement of low PVR amplitude has been shown to correlate with arterial segmental pressure gradients of 10 mm Hg at rest or gradients of 20 mm Hg by injection with papaverine.[41] The accuracy of the combined PVR and segmental pressure measurements has been assessed by comparison to the angiographic gold standard in a prospective study of 50 patients with lower extremity PAD.[42] The overall accuracy ranged from 90% to 95% and the PVR-segmental pressure technique accurately predicted the severity of iliac and superficial femoral artery obstruction, distinguishing iliac from proximal superficial femoral artery disease (Figure 17-7).

PVR has been evaluated for its ability to predict limb prognosis and have correlated well with ankle systolic blood pressure. Kaufman et al.[43] evaluated the relationship of PVR tracings to limb outcome in 517 patients with lower extremity PAD and demonstrated 41.9% of patients with minimal symptoms with nearly flat recordings required surgical intervention, 85.7% of patients with nearly flat tracings with jeopardized limbs underwent surgery, and 97.9% of patients with jeopardized limbs and flat tracings underwent limb salvage surgery. Makisalo et al.[44] evaluated the

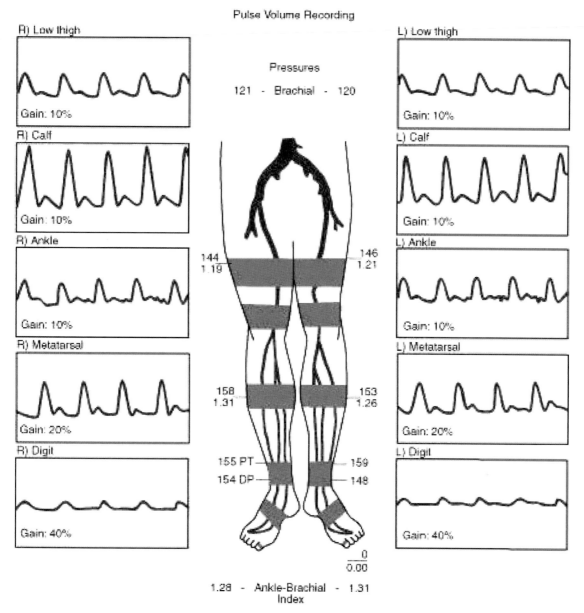

Pulse Volume Recording

R) Low thigh Gain: 10%
L) Low thigh Gain: 10%

Pressures
121 - Brachial - 120

R) Calf Gain: 10%
L) Calf Gain: 10%

R) Ankle Gain: 10%
L) Ankle Gain: 10%

144 1.19
146 1.21

R) Metatarsal Gain: 20%
L) Metatarsal Gain: 20%

158 1.31
163 1.26

R) Digit Gain: 40%
L) Digit Gain: 40%

155 PT 154 DP
159 148

0 0.00

1.28 - Ankle-Brachial - 1.31
Index

● **FIGURE 17-6.** SLPs, PVRs, and the ABI are often obtained in a single examination. All SLPs are systolic blood pressure measurements and recorded in millimeters of mercury (mm Hg). Cuffs at the brachial arteries (not shown in illustration) and ankles are used to record the systolic pressure for calculation of the ABI. PT, posterior tibial; DP, dorsalis pedis.

prognostic value of PVR tracings in predicting risk of amputation in 129 diabetics and nondiabetic renal transplant patients and took noninvasive measurements on lower limb amputations and found a low PVR amplitude prior to transplantation in 82% of the diabetic patients and 36% of the nondiabetic patients. The 5-year follow-up demonstrated that abnormal PVR values and TBI were the greatest predictors for proximal foot amputations.

PVR is a useful diagnostic test for patients with suspected lower extremity PAD and assesses limb perfusion after revascularization procedures. It also can predict limb ischemia and the risk of amputation. PVR can provide information regarding small-vessel disease when applied to the feet and is also useful in patients with noncompressible

vessiles in whom ABIs and segmental pressures are spuriously elevated.

Limitations of SLPs and PVR

Segmental limb pressure measurements have the same limitations as the ABI in individuals whom have noncompressible arteries, resulting in erroneously high indices. The incidence of noncompressible arteries is higher in individuals with diabetes and elderly patients as a result of calcified arteries that prevent occlusion of blood flow by the blood pressure cuff. Another limitation is that one cannot distinguish occlusions with collaterals from stenosis. Also, the true brachial pressure cannot be measured in patients with

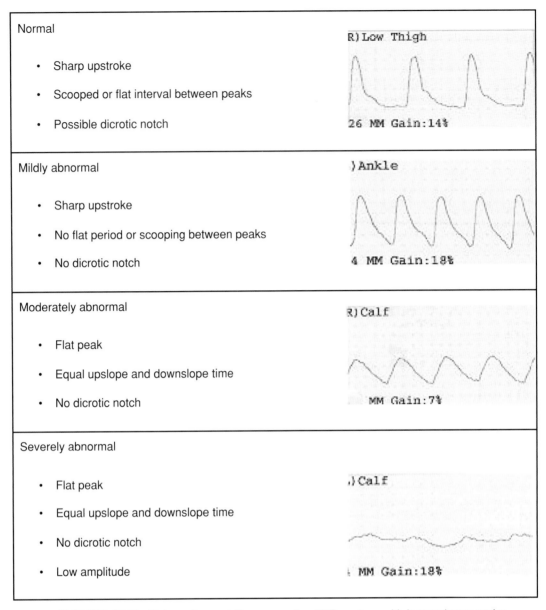

Normal	R) Low Thigh
• Sharp upstroke	
• Scooped or flat interval between peaks	
• Possible dicrotic notch	26 MM Gain:14%
Mildly abnormal	) Ankle
• Sharp upstroke	
• No flat period or scooping between peaks	
• No dicrotic notch	4 MM Gain:18%
Moderately abnormal	R) Calf
• Flat peak	
• Equal upslope and downslope time	
• No dicrotic notch	MM Gain:7%
Severely abnormal	.) Calf
• Flat peak	
• Equal upslope and downslope time	
• No dicrotic notch	
• Low amplitude	MM Gain:18%

● **FIGURE 17-7.** Pulse volume plethysmography: PVR contour with increasing vascular disease severity.

Guidelines for noninvasive vascular laboratory testing: a report from the American Society of Echocardiography and the Society for Vascular Medicine and Biology. Vasc Med. 2006;19:955-972 and is reproduced with the permission of the copyright holder, the American Society of Echocardiography www.asecho.org.

bilateral subclavian artery stenosis, making this a major limitation of the SLP, and the ABI.

● DUPLEX ULTRASONOGRAPHY OF THE LOWER EXTREMITIES

Arterial duplex ultrasonographic examination of the lower extremities can be used to noninvasively diagnose the anatomic location and degree of occlusions.[45] Duplex ultrasound also can be used to evaluate aneurysms, arterial dissection, AV fistulas, popliteal artery entrapment syndrome, evaluation of lymphoceles, and assessment of soft tissue masses in individuals with vascular disease. Gauthier and

Dieter demonstrated a case of a pseudoaneurysm, mimicking the presentation of a deep venous thrombosis by causing extrinsic compression of the venous system. The patient had complete resolution of the pseudoaneurysm and his symptoms following treatment with ultrasound-guided percutaneous thrombin injection.[46] Duplex ultrasound can determine artery wall thickness, degree of flow turbulence, vessel morphologic characteristics, and changes in blood flow velocity in areas of stenosis. The specificity of the duplex ultrasound ranges from 92% to 98% and its sensitivity ranges from 92% to 95%.[47] A meta-analysis comparison of the accuracy of the duplex Doppler performed with or without color imaging guidance demonstrated a sensitivity

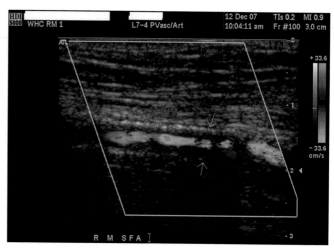

● **FIGURE 17-8.** Mid-superficial femoral artery stenosis.

of 93% using a color-guided duplex technique compared with 83% for noncolor duplex.[48] Peripheral arterial ultrasound is indicated in patients with claudication, leg pain, ulcers, and lower extremity revascularization.

Duplex ultrasound can predict if a patient's anatomy is suitable for angioplasty with an accuracy of 84% to 94%.[49,50] It has been used as a substitute for arteriography for infrainguinal bypass grafting to select the most appropriate tibial vessel for anastomosis.[51–53] Proia et al.[51] demonstrated no difference in patency of infrapopliteal bypass grafts in patients evaluated by preoperative duplex versus angiographic methods. However, Larch et al. demonstrated that color duplex sonography is inferior to angiography for evaluation of tibial arteries for distal bypass.[54] Even though there are discrepancies between studies, duplex ultrasonography can be used for prerevascularization decision making.

In patients who have undergone surgical bypass graft revascularization, especially with saphenous vein, failure may recur because of the development of stenoses. These stenoses develop at the anastomosis site, within the body of the graft, or proximal or distal from the graft in the native artery. Duplex ultrasound surveillance allows detection of these stenoses before the graft becomes thrombosed. Figure 17-8 represents a mid-SFA stenosis.

Most studies demonstrate that 80% of grafts can be salvaged if the stenosis is detected and repaired prior to graft thrombosis. Mattos et al.[55] showed that vein grafts that were revised secondary to positive findings on duplex ultrasound had a 90% 1-year patency rate. Graft stenoses that had not been revised despite the presence on duplex ultrasound had a 1-year patency rate of only 66%. Lundell et al.[56] reported a 3-year patency rate of vein grafts monitored with duplex ultrasound of 78% compared to a 53%

patency rate for those followed up with the ABI. Vein bypass grafts should be studied within 4 to 6 weeks after graft placement, then 3, 6, 9, 12 months, and annually for venous conduits. Other studies have found no improvement in the patency of *synthetic* grafts when using surveillance intervals with duplex ultrasound.[50,57,58]

Assessing Duplex Ultrasonography

Peripheral arterial stenosis is characterized using a 5 to 7.5 MHz transducer. The vessels are studied in the sagittal plane and Doppler velocities are obtained using a 60-degree angle. Angles above 60 degrees can result in significant overestimation of the velocity and should be avoided. Vessels are classified into one of five categories[59] (Table 17-6): Graft surveillance is preformed in manner identical to their use in native vessel arterial duplex ultrasonography (Figure 17-9).

TABLE 17-6. Diagnostic Criteria for Peripheral Arterial Diameter Reduction

- Normal: (no stenosis)
- 1% to 19% stenosis: when flow disturbances result in changes in the waveform but not in the PSV. PSV ratio <1.4 and <125 cm/s
- 20% to 49% stenosis: when the PSV increases by 30% to 100% relative to the proximal normal segment PSV ratio of 1.5 to 2.4 and a PSV <180 cm/s
- 50% to 99% stenosis: when the PSV increases by greater than 100% relative to the proximal normal segment; typically there is a loss of flow reversal
- Occlusion: if no flow is identified in the artery

This material was originally published in Guidelines for noninvasive vascular laboratory testing: a report from the American Society of Echocardiography and the Society of Vascular Medicine and Biology. J Am Soc Echocardiogr. 2006;19;955-972 and is reproduced with the permission of the copyright holder, the American Society of Echocardiography www.asecho.org. Inclusion of this information does not necessarily imply endorsement of this product.

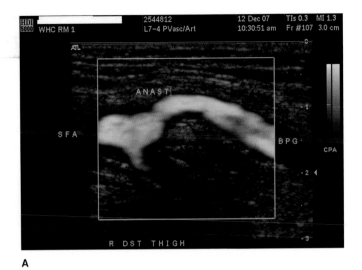

A

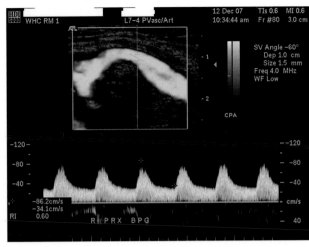

B

● **FIGURE 17-9.** (A and B) Duplex of lower extremity bypass graft and proximal anastomosis.

Peak systolic velocities and end-diastolic velocities are determined at each segment and compared to the segment of graft proximal to it. Doubling of the peak systolic velocity (PSV) within a stenotic segment relative to the normal segment indicates significant graft stenosis of greater than 50%, with a sensitivity of 95% and specificity of 100%.[60] Also, low-flow states (peak systolic velocities <45 cm/s) within a graft indicates an increased propensity for graft failure.[61]

Limitations of Duplex Ultrasonography

Although duplex ultrasonography is an accurate test, accuracy of the duplex examination depends on the ability of the technique to image the vessel. Difficulties in imaging can be attributed to body habitus, bowel gas, calcified vessels, and stenosis in the presence of tandem lesions. Stenoses in tandem lesions decrease the sensitivity range from 92% to 95% to approximately 60% to 65%.[62,63]

● **NONINVASIVE DIAGNOSTIC IMAGING OF UPPER EXTREMITY PAD**

Symptomatic arterial disease of the upper extremity accounts for approximately 5% of all cases of extremity ischemia.[64] In contrast to lower extremity ischemia, ischemia in the upper extremity may be caused by a variety of

---

ACC–AHA GUIDELINES FOR THE USE OF DUPLEX ULTRASOUND[6]

Recommendations

Class I

1. Duplex ultrasound of the extremities is useful to diagnose anatomic location and degree of stenosis of PAD. (*Level of Evidence: A*)

2. Duplex ultrasound is recommended for routine surveillance after femoral-popliteal or femoral-tibial pedal bypass with a venous conduit. Minimum surveillance intervals are approximately 3, 6, and 12 months, and then yearly after graft placement. (*Level of Evidence: A*)

Class II

1. Duplex ultrasound of the extremities can be useful to select patients as candidates for endovascular intervention. (*Level of Evidence: B*)

2. Duplex ultrasound can be useful to select patients as candidates for surgical bypass and to select the sites of surgical anastomosis. (*Level of Evidence: B*)

Class IIb

1. The use of duplex ultrasound is not well established to assess long-term patency of percutaneous transluminal angioplasty. (*Level of Evidence: B*)

2. Duplex ultrasound may be considered for routine surveillance after femoral-popliteal bypass with a synthetic conduit. (*Level of Evidence: B*)

Reprinted with permission of ACC/AHA 2005 practice guidelines for the management of patients with peripheral arterial disease (lower extremity, renal, mesenteric, and abdominal aortic): executive summary: a collaborative report from the American Association for Vascular Surgery/Society for Vascular Surgery, Society for Cardiovascular Angiology and Interventions, Society for Vascular Medicine and Biology, Society of Interventional Radiology, and the ACC/AHA Task Force on Practice Guidelines (Writing Committee to Develop Guidelines for the Management of Patients with Peripheral Arterial Disease). Circulation. 113:1474-1547, 2006. © 2006, American Heart Association, Inc.

TABLE 17-7. Causes of Large Artery
Disease in the Upper Extremity

TABLE 17-7. Causes of Large Artery
Disease in the Upper Extremity

Fibromuscular dysplasia
Arterial thoracic outlet syndrome
Atherosclerosis
Aneurysmal disease
Giant cell arteritis
Takayasu's arteritis
Cardiac emboli
Radiation arteritis

systemic diseases (Tables 17-7 and 17-8). Upper extremity disease can often be diagnosed using noninvasive diagnostic tests.

SEGMENTAL BLOOD PRESSURE RECORDINGS IN UPPER EXTERMITIES

Upper extremity segmental blood pressure recordings are performed similar to those of lower extremity. The equipment required for the upper extremity arterial examination includes 10- to 12-cm diameter pneumatic cuffs, which are placed around the proximal upper arm and around the forearm, and pulse volume waveforms are recorded at both levels. The systolic blood pressure is measured at both levels using the audible Doppler signal as an indication of systolic pressure.

When thoracic outlet obstruction is suspected, continuous wave Doppler should be used to monitor ulnar and radial artery flow patterns while the patient is guided through maneuvers that induce obstruction. The blood pressure cuffs are left on the arms to monitor the pulse volume waveforms during arm abduction and externally rotated position changes. If the patient has a thoracic outlet impingement, the PVR waveform tracing will show diminished amplitude or total flattening of the waveform, accompanied by dampening or total loss of the Doppler signal. If the signal recovers when the arm is moved out of position, the test is positive and indicates thoracic outlet impingement. This

TABLE 17-8. Causes of Small Artery
Disease in the Upper Extremity

Connective tissue disease
Vibration injury
Idiopathic vasospasm
Undifferentiated connective tissue disease
Hypercoagulable states
Neoplasm
Hypersensitivity angiitis
Frostbite
Emboli
Buerger disease
Chemical exposure

arm position should be repeated after recovery of the signal to ensure that the patient has an impingement.

A unilateral decrease in upper brachial pressures that are at least 10 to 20 mm Hg lower than the contralateral upper arm pressure is evident of occlusive disease.[65,66] Normal upper extremities have a difference in blood pressure from one side-to-another of 5 to 10 mm Hg while the difference between the upper arm, forearm, and wrist pressure generally differs by 5 mm Hg.[67] Indices should exceed 0.85 to 0.90 when comparing the ipsilateral arm pressure to the forearm or wrist blood pressure. An excessive drop in blood pressure between two contiguous levels indicates occlusive arterial disease of the intervening segment. In a study by Sumner, occlusive disease of the distal brachial, radial, or ulnar arteries documented angiographically has been found to cause a mean decrease in the distal upper extremity blood pressure of 42 mm Hg.[68]

The systolic pressures at the digit level are necessary if the patient is being evaluated for cold sensitivity or vasculitis. The systolic pressures are evaluated using a photoplethysmograph and a strip chart recorder to evaluate the shape of the waveform. The photocell is attached to the fingertips with tape or small gauges are placed around the fingertip. Blood pressure cuffs are placed around the proximal phalanx and waveforms are recorded at rest and again when cessation of blood flow occurs. Resting finger blood pressures should be obtained in a warm room to minimize cold-induced vasospasms.

A finger blood pressure normally should approximate the blood pressure of the ipsilateral wrist and upper arm and should be <10 mm Hg from adjacent digits.[60,69,70] A normal digital waveform has a rapid upstroke, a downstroke that bows toward the baseline, a dicrotic notch, and good amplitude. With cold challenge, Raynaud disease shows a mildly damped waveform with unusually high dicrotic notches while Raynaud's phenomenon shows severely damped waveforms. When the digital arteries are occluded, waveforms will be rounded, flat, or nearly flat and no amount of warming will restore the waveform contour to normal. A pressure difference between ipsilateral digits exceeding 15 mm Hg, a pressure difference between ipsilateral wrist and digits greater than 30 mm Hg, an absolute digital blood pressure less than 70 mm Hg, or an arm-finger pressure difference ≥20 in patients younger than 50 years of age is indicative of small-vessel arterial occlusive disease.[60–62,71] Arterial disease proximal to the wrist is likely if the wrist blood pressure is decreased without significant further decrement in the finger blood pressure.

Duplex ultrasound is an additional modality which can be used whenever the indirect tests suggest arterial obstruction. It can also be used to suggest if the occlusion is caused by atherosclerotic plaques or thrombus.

UPPER EXTREMITY DUPLEX SCANNING

Upper extremity duplex scanning is used to identify and grade the severity of arterial disease. It is carried out in a manner similar to arterial examination done elsewhere in the body. No patient preparation is required for examining the upper extremities. Examine the patient from the head of the bed, with the patient lying supine and the head of the bed flat. It may be easiest to scan from the side of the patient's bed in order to more easily adjust the patient's arm for best results.

The transducer should course each major artery including the subclavian, axillary, brachial, radial, ulnar, deep palmar arch, superficial palmar arch, and digital arteries. Transducer frequencies of 8 to 15 MHz should be used to assess most arm arteries because of their superficial locality while 3 to 8 MHz transducers evaluate areas near the clavicle.

Imaging of hand arteries requires higher frequencies because the vessels are extremely small. Duplex ultrasound imaging begins with short-axis view of the subclavian artery obtained above the clavicle. In the short-axis view, the artery and vein are identified side by side and compression with the transducer can be used to identify the artery and vein. Visualization of the subclavian artery is difficult because of interference from the clavicle. An alternative approach is to visualize the subclavian artery from an infraclavicular transducer position. This allows the artery and vein to be seen through the pectoral muscle in either the short or long axis views. Once the subclavian artery is identified, rotate the tranducer to visualize the artery in the long-axis view and examine proximally and distally as far as possible. At its distal end, the subclavian artery dives deeply and the operator should raise the patient's arm, repositioning the probe in the axilla to examine the axillary artery. After identifying the axillary artery, a long-axis view should be obtained and follow the axillary and brachial arteries down the medial side of the groove between the biceps and triceps muscles. The axillary artery becomes the brachial artery where it crosses the lower margin of the tendon of the teres major muscle. Roughly 1 cm below the elbow, the brachial artery divides into the ulnar and radial arteries. The radial artery is examined with long-axis views throughout its course along the radial side of the volar aspect of the forearm. At the wrist, the radial artery divides into the volar and connects with the superficial palmar arch. The arch should be followed as it loops around and connects with the ulnar artery. Two branches of the deep palmar arch are examined, the first (princes pollicis) beginning at the radial side, which is followed by another small branch called the radialis indicis. These two vessels occasionally share a common trunk. Flow and Doppler signals in these small vessels typically are quite weak. After evaluating the radial artery and deep palmar arch, the operator returns to the antecubital fossa to inspect the ulnar artery. The ulnar artery can be followed along the volar aspect of the medial side of the forearm. The interpretation of duplex findings in the upper extremity is similar to B-mode and Doppler signals gathered in other arterial systems with stenosis, resulting in high-velocity jets, dampened distal waveforms, and poststenotic turbulence. At present, there are no specific velocity or frequency criteria with which to gauge the severity of stenosis in the upper extremity; however, a doubling of the PSV across a stenosis compared with the proximal normal

adjacent segment is used to indicate an occlusion greater than 50%.

The normal appearance of upper extremity arteries is similar to duplex scanning of lower limb arteries. Spectral Doppler waveform is normally triphasic at rest and after exercise becomes hyperemic with a high diastolic flow. Changes in temperature can have distinct effects on the observed flow in the distal arteries. With cooling of the limb, the amplitude of the velocity waveform decreases dramatically with triphasic preservation. Vasoconstriction increases peripheral resistance that produces a decrease in flow and causes the waveform to become biphasic. Peripheral vasodilation will also cause the waveform in the radial and ulnar arteries to become hyperemic. The normal range of PSV in the subclavian artery is 80 to 120 cm/s.[72] The diagnosis of arterial occlusion is made by imaging the artery and using Doppler to show no flow within the lumen.

Continuous wave or pulsed wave Doppler can be used to evaluate blood flow velocity characteristics in the subclavian, axillary, brachial, radial, ulnar, and digital arteries. The arterial waveform should be evaluated for tardus-parvus changes and absence of early diastolic flow reversal to assess for peripheral arterial occlusive disease in the upper extremities. Also, if the direction of blood flow is reversed or ceases in either the ulnar or radial artery when the other is compressed, occlusive disease in the interrogated artery can be inferred in the proximal site to the Doppler sampling. The sonographic Allen test is performed by compressing both the radial and ulnar arteries and sequentially releasing only one of the two arteries, assessing the flow characteristics of the palmar arches in the midpalmar aspect of the hand. The Doppler signal should revert to normal if the feeding artery communicates with the palmar arch, however if it does not, direct continuity is absent, indicating occlusive disease. Taneja et al.[73] found that the absence of the axillary or subclavian artery normal flow reversal in early diastole was the most sensitive finding of hemodynamically significant peripheral arterial occlusive disease. This finding in subclavian steal is explained when the perfusion pressure and blood flow in the arm drops, the ipsilateral vertebral artery acts as a collateral vessel, channeling blood distal to the obstruction, ultimately reversing the blood flow direction in the vertebral artery. Cardiac disease can affect proximal aortic arch vessel waveforms.

Duplex Assessment of Hemodialysis Grafts and Fistulas

Duplex ultrasound is the most commonly used modality in identifying hemodialysis access dysfunction although angiography is the gold standard. The accuracy, sensitivity, and specificity of ultrasound are reported to be 86%, 92%, and 84% compared to angiography for the detection of stenosis. An ultrasound study includes a B-mode assessment of the access, venous run-off vessels and measurement of blood flow velocities, and inflow. Interrogating grafts for stenoses should include velocities and flow measurements at the arterial anastomosis, throughout the length of the access, at

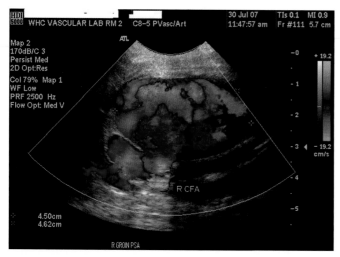

● **FIGURE 17-10.** A postcatheterization. PSA, psedoaneurysm.

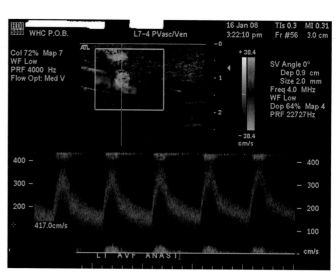

● **FIGURE 17-11.** Stenotic left AV fistula anastomosis.

the venous anastomosis, and at the venous run-off. If low-volume flow is detected in the absence of a stenosis, then arterial inflow must be imaged to evaluate if a stenosis is proximal to the graft. Venous outflow stenosis has 96% accuracy, 95% sensitivity, and 97% specificity. The NKF-K DOQI Clinical Practice Guidelines for Vascular Access recommend prospective surveillance of AV grafts and AV fistulas.

AV grafts have low rates of primary and cumulative patency, while most graft failures are associated with stenosis resulting from neointimal hyperplasia at the venous outflow anastomosis of the graft. Ultrasound techniques, Doppler flow, magnetic resonance have all been used to assess intra-access blood flow. Grafts with access flow less than 800 cc/min on ultrasound were shown to have a 92.9% incidence of thrombosis over 6 months, whereas those with higher access flows had a 25% to 28% incidence of thrombous. Ultrasound surveillance has shown patency rates to increase at 6, 12, 24, and 36 months after elective revisions of grafts for greater than 50% stenosis when compared to physical examination alone. Thus, ultrasound of hemodialysis grafts should be incorporated into access management programs to prevent and manage graft stenoses (Figures 17-10 and 17-11).[74]

NONINVASIVE DIAGNOSTIC IMAGING OF THE RENAL ARTERIES

Renal artery stenosis (RAS) is a progressive and common disease in patients with atherosclerosis and is a relatively common cause of secondary hypertension. Atherosclerotic RAS has become increasingly recognized as a contributor to resistant hypertension and deterioration in renal function.[75] Patients with atherosclerotic RAS requiring dialysis have a decreased long-term survival.[76] Patients at risk for the development of end-stage renal disease requiring dialysis are those with severe bilateral RAS, or stenosis to a solitary kidney.[77] Direct imaging modalities such as duplex ultrasonography, computed tomographic angiography (CTA),

and magnetic resonance angiography (MRA) are the best suited noninvasive methods used to diagnose renal artery stenosis. The choice of which diagnostic tool used depends on the availability, the experience of the technician, and characteristics or contraindications associated with the patient being tested.

RENAL ARTERY DUPLEX ULTRASOUND

Duplex ultrasonography is an ideal imaging modality in patients with RAS (Table 17-9).[78] Hansen et al.[79] demonstrated a prevalence rate of significant renal arterial disease

TABLE 17-9. Indications for Renal Duplex Ultrasound

- Sudden exacerbation of previously well-controlled hypertension
- New onset hypertension at a young age
- Malignant hypertension
- Unexplained azotemia
- An atrophic kidney
- Hypertension and aortoiliac or infrainguinal atherosclerosis
- Azotemia after administration of an angiotensin-converting enzyme inhibitor
- Recurrent flash pulmonary edema without cardiac explanation
- Evaluation of adequacy of renal artery revascularization
- Sudden exacerbation of previously well-controlled hypertension

This material was originally published in Guidelines for noninvasive vascular laboratory testing: a report from the American Society of Echocardiography and the Society of Vascular Medicine and Biology. J Am Soc Echocardiogr. 2006;19:955-972 and is reproduced with the permission of the copyright holder, the American Society of Echocardiog raphy www.asecho.org. Inclusion of this information does not necessarily imply endorsement of this product.

in 5.5% of women, 9.1% of men, 6.9% of white participants, and 6.7% of black participants in a study of 834 participants whom underwent renal artery duplex ultrasonography. Duplex ultrasound has a sensitivity range of 84% to 98% and a specificity range of 62% to 99% for detecting RAS when compared with angiography.[80–86]

Assessing Renal Artery Duplex Ultrasonography

Renal artery duplex ultrasonography requires an experienced vascular technologist. Patients are instructed to fast the night prior to the examination. A low-frequency 2.25- to 3.5-MHz pulsed Doppler transducer is required for adequate deep abdominal imaging, however if significant bowel gas is identified on examination, the study should be terminated and the patient should be rescheduled. The examination is started with the patient lying in the supine position in reverse Trendelenburg as the aorta is scanned in the longitudinal view while noting the presence of atherosclerotic plaque and aneurysms. The origin of the celiac, superior mesenteric, and inferior mesenteric arteries should be defined while aortic Doppler velocity at the level of the superior mesenteric artery is obtained at a 60-degree angle in the center of the artery. This velocity will be used for the renal to aortic ratio velocity calculation. The vascular technologist then reorients the transducer into the transverse plane to visualize the celiac and superior mesenteric arteries arising from the anterior aspect of the aorta. The left renal vein in 75% of patients crosses anterior to the abdominal aorta as it enters the inferior vena cava. The origin of the superior mesenteric artery and the left renal vein crossing anterior to the aorta are used to help identify the right renal artery. The right renal artery arises in an anterior fashion from the aorta and courses in a posterior fashion as it enters the hilum of the kidney, while the left renal artery arises inferior to the right and takes a posterior course. The Doppler cursor should be at a 60-degree angle or less. Peak systolic velocities and peak end-diastolic velocities should be obtained in the kidney's origin, proximal, mid, and most distal portion. It is important that the entire renal artery is visualized so that a stenosis of fibromuscular dysplastic kidney is not overlooked. The patient is then placed in the left and right lateral decubitus position to allow the visualization of both kidneys from the flank. Doppler velocities are then recorded at a 0-degree angle in the cortex, medulla, and hilum of the kidney to assess for RAS (Figure 17-12).

The renal duplex examination includes spectral Doppler velocities from the renal arteries, renal parenchyma, and abdominal aorta where peak systolic velocities and peak end-diastolic velocities obtained at the level of the renal medulla are used to calculate the renal resistive index (RRI) (Table 17-10).

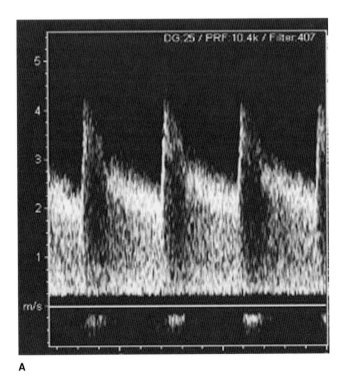

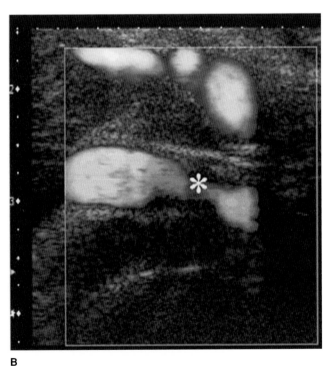

A   B

● **FIGURE 17-12.** (A) RAS. Doppler spectral waveform demonstrates turbulence with marked elevation in peak systolic and end-diastolic velocities. (B) Power Doppler indicating luminal narrowing (*) at site of stenosis.

Guidelines for noninvasive vascular laboratory testing: a report from the American Society of Echocardiography and the Society for Vascular Medicine and Biology. Vasc Med. 2006;19:955-972 and is reproduced with the permission of the copyright holder, the American Society of Echocardiography www.asecho.org.

TABLE 17-10. Diagnostic Criteria for Significant Renal Artery Stenosis

Renal artery to aorta PSV ratio is >3.5; >3.0 for a transplanted kidney

PSV >200 cm/s with evidence of poststenotic turbulence

EDV >150 cm/s (>80% RAS)

RI >0.7 is abnormal

RI >0.8 may predict failure to respond with intervention

An occluded renal artery demonstrates no flow in the affected vessel

---

EDV, end-diastolic velocity; PSV, peak systolic velocity; RI, resistive index (1 − [EDV/maximum systolic velocity] × 100).
This material was originally published in Guidelines for noninvasive vascular laboratory testing: a report from the American Society of Echocardiography and the Society of Vascular Medicine and Biology. J Am Soc Echocardiogr. 2006;19:955-972 and is reproduced with the permission of the copyright holder, the American Society of Echocardiography www.asecho.org. Inclusion of this information does not necessarily imply endorsement of this product.

Several criteria have been studied in predicting the severity of RAS. A diagnosis of RAS greater than 80% can be ascertained if the end-diastolic velocity is more than 150 cm per second.[87] Numerous Doppler velocity criteria are used that correlate with a 60% stenotic lesion. These include a direct PSV greater than 3.5, an acceleration index less than 300, a renal to aortic ratio grater than 3.5, and the difference in renal or segmental resistive index greater than 0.15 (Table 17-8). The most universally accepted Doppler criteria are a renal to aortic ratio exceeding 3.3 to 3.5 or a PSV in the stenosis of 180 to 200 cm/s or greater.[69,72,73,77,88–91] The PSV in normal renal arteries ranges from 74 to 127 cm/s.[53,81,92,93] The RRI is also used to evaluate the renal arteries and is calculated by using the following equation: 1 − [EDV/PSV] × 100, which reflects total renal flow, including the health of the renal parenchyma. Nephrosclerosis and glomerulosclerosis has been documented with an increased RRI in the context of longstanding hypertension.[94] However, there have been conflicting reports regarding the usefulness of the RRI in predicting individual response to revascularization. Radermacher et al.[95] demonstrated that an RRI greater than 0.80 predicted a lack of improvement in blood pressure and renal function after revascularization. However, this study has been criticized for the use of patients receiving balloon angioplasty instead of renal angioplasty with stent, thus the outcomes in response to renal revascularization therapy may have been underestimated in that report. Zeller et al.[96] demonstrated that patients with an elevated RRI had a favorable blood pressure response to renal artery stenting. They also demonstrated a 15% to 23% improvement in serum creatinine in patients with mild to moderate (RRI 0.7 to 0.8) and severe (RRI >0.80) nephrosclerosis. In addition, the examination

should include the interrogation of the entire renal artery from the ostium to the hilum.

Renal artery duplex ultrasonography is useful in monitoring renal artery patency after endovascular treatment or surgical revascularization of RAS.[97,98] Imaging the entire renal artery can detect early or late restenosis by documenting an increase in the PSV or the renal to aortic ratio within the stented segment.

In comparison, CTA can produce exceptional anatomical 3D images of the renal arteries while supplying images of the aorta and visceral arteries. CTA of the renal arteries has a sensitivity range from 59% to 96% and a specificity range from 82% to 99% compared with catheter-based contrast angiography.[99–105] Current CTA techniques using multidetector-row scanners have demonstrated sensitivities for detecting renal artery stenoses of 92% and specificities of 99%.[106]

Furthermore, contrast-enhanced magnetic resonance angiography (CEMRA) is performed with gadolinium, a less-nephrotoxic contrast agent, and provides high-resolution 3D data sets of the renal arteries in a single breath hold.[107–109] CEMRA can display detailed renal anatomy while reducing artifacts. If the patient is unable to hold breath, acquisition of images can be done over several minutes by slowing the infusion of contrast agent, however branch vessel images may be slightly degraded by their respiratory motion. CEMRA of the renal arteries has a sensitivity range from 90% to 100% and a specificity range from 76% to 94% for detecting RAS compared with catheter-based contrast angiography. Hany et al.[110] compared CEMRA relative to digital subtraction X-ray angiography and demonstrated a sensitivity of 93% and a specificity of 98% for identifying stenotic renal lesions greater than 50%. Snidow et al.[111] examined 32 patients using CEMRA compared to conventional X-ray angiography and demonstrated a sensitivity of 100% and a specificity of 62% in accessory renal artery occlusive disease. The lower specificity may have been related to the image selection, which were chosen to ensure the evaluation of the aorta and iliac inflow vessels with inadequate resolution depicting small accessory renal arteries.[101]

In an effort to move beyond correlating studies between MRA with conventional X-ray angiography, Prince et al.[112] demonstrated that MRA studies could be used to calculate the likelihood of success after revascularization. The investigators found that signal loss distal to a stenosis on the phase-contrast MRA examinations was significantly more prominent in those with hemodynamically significant stenosis. They also demonstrated that patients had better outcomes after revascularization if they had reduced renal lengths, poststenotic arterial dilatation, and reductions in parenchymal renal thickness.[102] This method demonstrates a more reliable image of the renal artery than noncontrast MRA techniques. The development of contrast-enhanced MRA of the renal arteries has led to significant improvements in the technical success rate and diagnostic accuracy, while providing a more reliable depiction of renal artery morphology.

Leung et al.[113] compared contrast-enhanced MRA with duplex ultrasonography for the detection of RAS using catheter angiography as the standard of reference. Eighty-nine patients with clinically suspected renovascular disease underwent contrast-enhanced MRA and duplex renal scanning. Sixty of these also underwent catheter angiography.[113] The sensitivity and specificity for hemodynamically significant (≥60% diameter reduction) main RAS were 90% and 86%, respectively, for MRA and 81% and 87% for duplex sonography.[113] When patients were excluded because of the presence of fibromuscular dysplasia, the sensitivity of MRA increased to 97%, with a negative predictive value of 98%. MRA detected 96% while duplex 5% of accessory renal arteries seen at catheter angiography.[113]

Limitations of Renal Artery Duplex Ultrasonography

Limitations of renal artery duplex ultrasonography include the difficulty or inability to image obese patients or patients with intervening bowel gas, the technical skill of the operator, and the diminished ability to visualize accessory renal arteries.[98] Other limitations when using renal hilar scanning includes the inability to discriminate between stenosis and occlusions, the inability to adequately determine the accessory renal arteries, and low sensitivity when compared to interrogating the entire renal artery from the ostium to the hilum.

● RENAL SCINTIGRAPHY

Captopril renal scanning is an indirect noninvasive method that provides information about renal size, perfusion, and the detection of RAS. The examination is performed by the administration of captopril 50 mg taken 60 minutes before the renal scintigraphic imaging with technetium-99m mercaptoacetyltriglycine or technetium-99 m diethylenetriaminepentaacetic acid. This examination relies on a decrease in renal blood flow and glomerular filtration rate after the administration of the captopril. The criteria to diagnose RAS includes a delayed time to maximal activity (greater than or equal to 11 minutes after captopril administration), significant asymmetry of peak activity of each kidney, marked cortical retention of the radionuclide after captopril administration, and marked reduction in calculated glomerular filtration rate of the ipsilateral kidney after captopril.[114] The reported sensitivity ranges from 45% to 94% while the specificity ranges from 81% to 100%.[114–125] The sensitivity and specificity decline substantially in patients with azotemia (serum creatinine greater than 2.0 mg/dL), RAS of a solitary functioning kidney, or bilateral RAS. Fommei et al.[126] demonstrated that patients with a serum creatinine of 1.5 mg per dL had a reduction in their positive predictive value (88% to 57%) with a minimal reduction in sensitivity and specificity.

When captopril renography was compared with catheter angiography, the sensitivity was only 74%, and the specificity was only 59%.[127] Thus, as other imaging modalities

---

ACC–AHA GUIDELINES FOR THE DIAGNOSIS OF RENAL ARTERY STENOSIS[6]

● DIAGNOSTIC METHODS

Recommendations

Class I

1. Duplex ultrasonography is recommended as a screening test to establish the diagnosis of RAS. (*Level of Evidence: B*)

2. Computed tomographic angiography (in individuals with normal renal function) is recommended as a screening test to establish the diagnosis of RAS. (*Level of Evidence: B*)

3. Magnetic resonance angiography is recommended as a screening test to establish the diagnosis of RAS. (*Level of Evidence: B*)

4. When the clinical index of suspicion is high and the results of noninvasive tests are inconclusive, catheter angiography is recommended as a diagnostic test to establish the diagnosis of RAS. (*Level of Evidence: B*)

Class III

1. Captopril renal scintigraphy is not recommended as a screening test to establish the diagnosis of RAS. (*Level of Evidence: C*)

2. Selective renal vein renin measurements are not recommended as a useful screening test to establish the diagnosis of RAS. (*Level of Evidence: B*)

3. Plasma renin activity is not recommended as a useful screening test to establish the diagnosis of RAS. (*Level of Evidence: B*)

4. The captopril test (measurement of plasma rennin activity after captopril administration) is not recommended as a useful screening test to establish the diagnosis of RAS. (*Level of Evidence: B*)

---

are so accurate, captopril renography should not be used as initial screening in patients with presumed RAS. It may however retain some value in the assessment of renal artery stenoses of borderline angiographic studies for which the physiological functional significance is unclear.

● NONINVASIVE DIAGNOSTIC IMAGING OF CAROTID ARTERIES

Barnett et al.[128] estimates that approximately 2 million individuals living in Europe and North America have asymptomatic extracranial carotid artery stenosis. The goal of noninvasive testing for carotid artery disease is to decrease the risk for transient neurologic events, permanent neurologic events, coronary atherosclerosis, myocardial infarction, and cardiovascular death. Noninvasive duplex ultrasonography provides a safe and accurate method of identifying significant stenosis of the extracranial carotid arteries.

● CAROTID ARTERY ULTRASOUND

The carotid duplex examination identifies plaque, stenoses, and occlusions in the common carotid artery, internal carotid artery, external carotid artery, and vertebral artery. This examination is indicated for patient with a history of transient ischemic attacks, stroke, cervical bruits, amaurosis fugax, and after surgical or endovascular revascularization (Table 17-11).

TABLE 17-11. Indications for Carotid Artery Ultrasound

- Cervical bruits
- Hemispheric stroke
- Amaurosis fugax
- Focal cerebral or ocular transient ischemic attacks (which demonstrate localizing symptoms such as weakness of one side of the face, slurred speech, weakness of a limb, retinal or hemispheric visual field deficits)
- Vasculitis involving extracranial arteries
- Pulsatile mass in the neck
- Trauma to neck
- Drop attacks or syncope (rare indications primarily seen in vertebrovascular insufficiency or bilateral carotid artery disease)
- Follow-up of carotid artery atherosclerosis not requiring revascularization
- Follow-up surveillance after carotid revascularization, a baseline ultrasound is recommended within 30 days after carotid stenting

---

This material was originally published in Guidelines for noninvasive vascular laboratory testing: a report from the American Society of Echocardiography and the Society of Vascular Medicine and Biology. J Am Soc Echocardiogr. 2006;19:955-972 and is reproduced with the permission of the copyright holder, the American Society of Echocardiography www.asecho.org. Inclusion of this information does not necessarily imply endorsement of this product.

The accuracy for detecting a 50% to 90% diameter stenosis is 93%, whereas the sensitivity is 99% and the specificity is 84% when compared to angiography.[129] Data from the NASCET trial showed that a carotid index (peak ICA velocity/CCA velocity) greater than 4 provided the highest accuracy (sensitivity 91%, specificity 87%, overall accuracy 88%) for predicting a high-grade (70% to 99%) stenosis.[130]

Carotid duplex utilizes B-mode (gray-scale), spectral Doppler, and color-flow to identify focal increases in blood flow velocity indicative of high-grade carotid stenosis from their supraclavicular origin to their retromandibular entrance into the skull base.

When angle-corrected velocities are unattainable, color-encoded and power Doppler imaging can assist in assessing the severity of stenosis and may allow detection of residual flow in patients with subtotal occlusions or calcification (Figure 17-13).[131,132]

Technical Considerations of Carotid Artery Ultrasound

The carotid arteries should be examined with the patient in the supine position and with the sonographer seated at the patient's head. This allows easy access to the neck and enables the operator to rest the arm on the examination table while performing the scan. The patient's head should be turned contralateral to the side being tested and the patient should drop the ipsilateral shoulder as far as possible to get maximal exposure of the patient's neck. The examination should be performed with a medium- to high-frequency flat linear array transducer (e.g., broad band 4 to 7 or 5 to 12 mHz transducer). The carotid arteries are best visualized through the sternocleidomastoid muscle, which can be done using a lateral rather than anterior approach. A Doppler angle of 45 to 60 degrees should be maintained to obtain consistent results in velocity measurements.

A carotid duplex ultrasound examination involves a complete survey of the extracranial carotid arteries in longitudinal and transverse views. This allows an assessment of the anatomy and identifies the presence or absence of disease and its location. The internal carotid arteries are usually located posterior and lateral in the neck, whereas the external carotid artery is more anterior and medial. The internal carotid artery signal is identified by the absence of flow reversal and the presence of forward flow during diastole (i.e, low resistance), while the external carotid signal is recognized by the presence of flow reversal (i.e, high resistance) and by the "temporal tap." Temporal tap refers to tapping the temporal region (artery), which is then reflected back to the external carotid artery (ECA) as "taps," making it useful in identifying the ECA. The common carotid artery is located lateral to the thyroid gland and medial to the internal jugular vein. The common carotid artery is less compressible than the internal jugular vein in most patients. However, it is important not to apply too much transducer pressure when scanning the carotid arteries as there is possibility of dislodging plaque from the vessel wall or stimulating the carotid bulb. As the common carotid artery

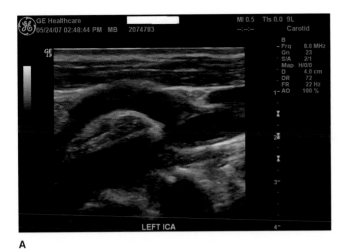 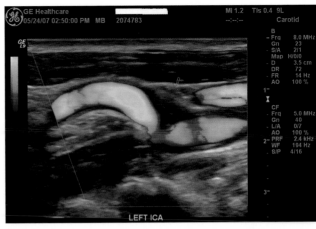

A **B**

● **FIGURE 17-13.** (A) Grayscale of internal carotid artery. (B) Color power angio of internal carotid artery.

and the subclavian artery branch from the brachiocephalic artery, they should be easily accessible to scan if the transducer is in a slight caudal angle. Survey of the bifurcation of the common carotid artery with color-flow imaging is preformed, beginning at the clavicle with longitudinal images, proceed to the bifurcation usually found at the level of the cricoid cartilage, and then continue into the external carotid artery and internal carotid artery. This will allow the sonographer to confirm the patency of the arteries while identifying plaque-laden areas. The internal carotid artery and external carotid artery are confirmed by their anatomic features (Table 17-12) and by their Doppler spectral signatures.

The proper identification of the branch vessels is essential because stenotic external carotid arteries are usually not treated invasively. This process is repeated with transverse images. With the survey completed and the identity of the internal carotid artery and external carotid artery confirmed, significant areas of plaque formation with notation of its thickness, the degree of lumen reduction, and its morphology are noted. Transverse images of the vessel are essential to assess the plaque thickness and its general degree of luminal narrowing. In areas of stenosis, it is important to report the angle-corrected velocity spectra. The vertebral artery flow and direction are also noted. Major elevations in peak frequency are characteristics of high-grade orifice stenosis. Finally, the subclavian arteries are evaluated.

Using Doppler spectral waveforms imaged from a long-axis perspective, low resistance or a damped pattern and lack of pulsatility suggests a stenotic lesion or an occlusion *proximal* to the point of Doppler examination.

Assessing Carotid Plaque and Surface Character with B-Mode Imaging

B-mode ultrasound provides information on the degree of carotid stenosis and on the characteristics of the arterial wall including the consistency and size of atherosclerotic plaques. Normal vessel walls, typically best visualized in the common carotid artery using B-mode, will often appear as a double layer structure when imaged in longitudinal view with a high-frequency transducer. The double line represents the thickness of the intima and media and is best seen when the vessels lie at right angles to the ultrasound beam.

TABLE 17-12. Differentiation of Internal and External Carotid Arteries

Internal carotid artery	External carotid artery
• Usually larger	• Usually smaller
• Usually lateral and posterior	• Usually medial and anterior
• Usually incorporates carotid bulb	• Usually does not incorporate carotid bulb
• No branches in the neck	• Eight branches in the neck
• Low resistance spectral waveform	• High resistance spectral waveform at rest
• Usually no oscillations in Doppler on temporal tap test	• Visible and audible oscillations on Doppler signal waveform on temporal tap test

This material was originally published in Guidelines for noninvasive vascular laboratory testing: a report from the American Society of Echocardiography and the Society of Vascular Medicine and Biology. J Am Soc Echocardiogr. 2006;19:955-972 and is reproduced with the permission of the copyright holder, the American Society of Echocardiography www.asecho.org. Inclusion of this information does not necessarily imply endorsement of this product.

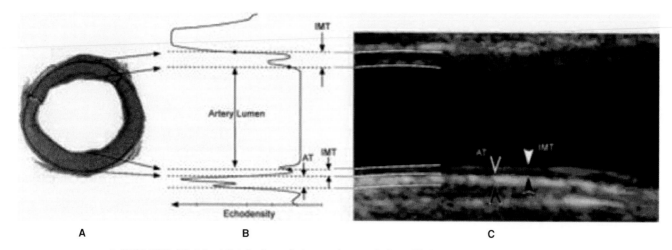

● **FIGURE 17-14.** Histologic and ultrasonic correlation of intima-media thickness (IMT). (A) The sets of two arrows at the top and bottom outline the IMT between the luminal border of the intima and the junction of the media and adventitia (AT). (B) Graph depicting the echogenicity profiles of the AT, media, intima, and arterial lumen. (C) The IMT and AT are respectively outlined by the closed and open arrowheads.

Reproduced with permission from Babikian VL, Wechsler LR, Higashida RT (eds): Imaging Cerebrovascular Disease. Philadelphia: Butterworth-Heinemann, 2003.

The first line represents the boundary between the blood and the intimal surface. The brighter second line represents the border between the intima and media and the adventitia (Figure 17-14).

Pignoli et al.[133] demonstrated that the normal thickness of this intima-media layer is ≤0.5 mm. It is often difficult to appreciate the double layer in the internal carotid artery because of the difficulty in obtaining perpendicular angles to the curved wall and thus is best visualized in the common carotid artery. In the early stages of carotid artery disease, the intima-media thickens and the double layer appears more widely separated with more echoes in the region between the lines. As the disease progresses, more substantial areas of atheroma can be visualized and the lines become indistinguishable, especially at the carotid bifurcation.

Many studies have been performed comparing the ultrasound appearance of atheromatous plaque with histological investigation to predict which plaques are more likely to be the source of emboli. Geroulakos et al.[134] introduced a modified version of the Gray–Weales classification using five different plaque types and by using a 50% area cutoff point instead of 75%: Type 1 (anechogenic with echogenic fibrous cap), Type 2 (predominantly anechogenic but with echogenic areas representing less than 25% of the plaque), Type 3 (predominantly hyperechogenic but with anechogenic areas representing less than 25% of the plaque), Type 4 (echogenic and homogeneous plaque), and Type 5 (unclassified plaque reflecting calcified plaques) (Figure 17-15).[134] Types 1 and 2 were seen significantly more frequently in symptomatic patients, whereas plaque types 3 and 4 were more commonly found in asymptomatic patients.[134]

The European Carotid Plaque Study Group showed that the echogenicity on the B-mode image was directly related to the presence of calcification and inversely related to the content of soft tissue.[135] The study further classified the plaque as either being homogenous or heterogeneous and described the plaque by using scales to represent the echogenicity (white) of the areas. Homogeneous plaques were described as having a uniform echogenicity and texture throughout while a heterogeneous plaque has mixed areas of brightness and textures.[135] The most brightly echogenic areas in the plaque are usually associated with calcium and may obstruct or dampen the Doppler signal making it difficult to obtain signals through important areas of stenosis. Some plaques are so densely calcified that Doppler signals are impossible to obtain, so assessing the flow velocity for the presence of poststenotic turbulence in a more distal segment maybe the only indication of a high stenotic lesion. In addition to brightly echogenic areas of plaque, there are areas of little or no ultrasonic signal that have been associated with hemorrhage, necrotic tissue, or lipids. Merrit and Bluth demonstrated an association between plaques that contained hemorrhage or lipid pools and transient ischemic attacks.[136] It is extremely difficult to distinguish these types of tissues with ultrasound.[136] Several classifications of plaque echogenicity have been described in the literature, often using very different classification systems and definitions yielding poor intra- and interobserver reproducibility. According to De Bray et al.[137] echogenicity should be standardized against blood (anechoic), mastoid muscle (isoechogenic), or bone (hyperechogenic) to avoid discrepancies in interpretation.

Most of these studies agree that anechogenic or heterogeneous plaques have a higher risk of subsequent neurological symptoms in comparison with echogenic or homogeneous plaques.[135,138–140] Johnson and associates were the first to indicate that the ultrasonic character of the plaque correlated with the risk of developing stroke. This study, at the end of the 3-year follow-up, demonstrated the

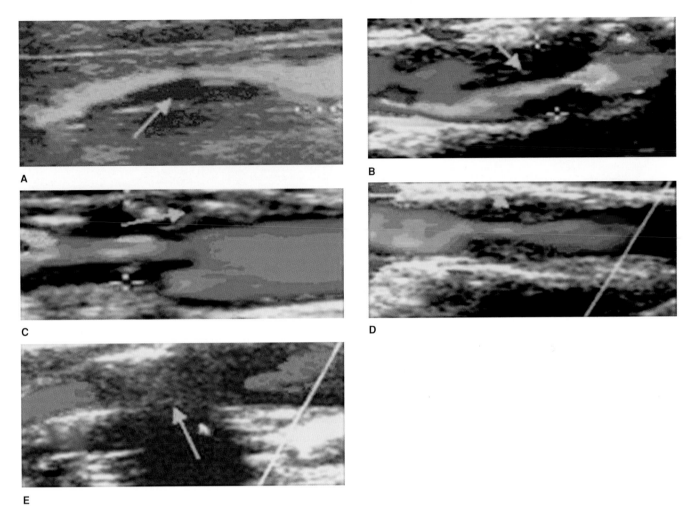

● FIGURE 17-15. Five different types of plaque according to Geroulakos et al.[134]. (A) Type 1, uniformly echolucent, (B) type 2, predominantly echolucent, (C) type 3, predominantly echogenic, (D) type 4, uniformly echogenic, and (E) type 5, unclassified plaques.

Reprinted with permission from Sztajzel R. Ultrasonographic assessment of the morphological characteristics of the carotid plaque. Swiss Med Wkly. 2005;135:635-643.

incidence of TIAs and stroke was twice as high in patients with soft plaques with more than 75% stenosis than those with dense plaques with the same degree of stenosis.[141] Langsfeld et al.[142] studied 419 patients with asymptomatic plaques for 22 months and found anechogenic plaques to be at increased risk of becoming symptomatic when compared with dense echorich plaques (p <0.02). Similarly, O'Holleran et al.[143] studied 293 patients for an average of 46 months and demonstrated that 100% of the patients with a soft lesion involving >75% stenosis became symptomatic as compared with only 60% of those with a dense plaque (p >0.05). In another study, Bock et al.[144] showed that echolucent plaques were associated with a 5.7% incidence of TIAs whereas echogenic plaques were associated with a 2.4% rate (p <0.01). In the Tromso study, a total of 223 patients with carotid stenosis were compared with 215 patients without stenosis to determine whether plaque morphology was associated with an increased risk of ischemic stroke or other cerebrovascular events.[145] They

assessed the echogenicity of the plaque by ultrasound at baseline and was scored as echolucent, predominantly echolucent, predominantly echogenic, or echogenic.[145] The results of the study demonstrated echolucent plaques had an increased risk of ischemic cerebrovascular events independently of the degree of stenosis, however many of the ischemic events occurred in a vascular territory different from that supplied by the artery with the plaque.[145] AbuRahma et al.[147] and Sterpetti et al.[146] found that heterogeneous plaques were significantly associated with an increased risk of stroke or TIA in comparison with homogeneous plaques. This holds true for risk stratification of lesion precarotid artery stenting.

Carotid plaque surface ulceration or irregularity has been shown to play an important role in ischemic stroke risk. The NASCET trial demonstrated patients with irregular plaques angiographically had a higher risk of stroke in comparison with patients presenting with smooth plaques.[148] The ECST trial showed that stroke risk was also increased among patients with irregular plaques independent of the degrees of stenosis.[149] The NASCET found an association between stroke and angiographic evidence of a plaque ulcer, showing patients with nonulcerated carotid stenosis had a risk of ipsilateral stroke at 24 months of 21.3% compared with 43.9% in patients with ulcerated stenosis.[150] Steinke et al.[151] showed that ulcerated plaques on ultrasound were less frequently found among asymptomatic patients (23%) than symptomatic patients (43%) in 63 patients with 80% or greater stenosis. Lusby et al.[152] suggested that ulcers may heal after the neurological events and cannot be found on ultrasound when performed after the occurrence of symptoms after demonstrating on B-mode a 77% sensitivity in plaques with less than 50% stenosis compared to 41% in plaques with >50% with similarity in angiography (77% and 48% respectively).

Assessing the Carotids with Color Imaging

The normal carotid arteries have a characteristic pulsatile forward flow on ultrasound when using color. Generally, the external carotid artery flow appears more pulsatile than the internal carotid artery and common carotid artery. The appropriate color pulse repetition frequency (PRF) should be adjusted to the expected velocity in the examined vessel so color continually fills the vessel lumen up to the walls. The scale in normal vessels should be adjusted to avoid diastolic flow gaps or systolic aliasing (low RPF), which would otherwise be interpreted as abnormal. The lack of color filling to the vessel wall may indicate the presence of stenosis or thrombous. It is important that color boxes cover the entire vessel diameter and are 1 to 2 cm of its length to ensure that filling defects are not caused by a poor Doppler angle, inappropriately high PRF, or to the presence of an image artifact of color bleeding ("blooming") into the adjacent tissues. Adjustments in the PRF are generally needed throughout the examination to allow for changes in velocity, which may occur in stenotic areas. The PRF range should be adjusted higher to detect increased velocities in the presence of stenosis, such as "color turbulence" is suggestive of a stenosis. The color PRF should be decreased in the poststenotic zone to observe lower velocities and flow direction changes in turbulent areas just beyond the stenosis. A decreased PRF should also be used in the presence of a carotid bruit to detect lower frequencies, high resistant signal associated with tight stenosis, and to confirm absence of color filling during diastolic flow from an occlusion or tight stenosis distally. Spectral Doppler should be used to confirm the absence of color filling during diastolic flow and both spectral Doppler and color should be used to carefully examine the distal vessels.

Assessing the Carotids with Spectral Doppler Waveforms

Spectral Doppler can be used to investigate the absence of diastolic flow in the distal carotid vessels indicating an occlusion or tight stenosis. The Doppler spectral waveform analysis is a signal processing technique that displays the amplitude and frequency content of the Doppler signal. This frequency is directly proportional to the blood cell velocity and the amplitude depends on the number of cells moving through the sample volume with a given frequency.

Normally, spectral Doppler recordings obtained from the external carotid artery show a high-resistance flow pattern with a pulsatile waveform and low diastolic flow. The center stream flow pattern in a normal artery is laminar. The presence of a narrowing within the carotid arteries will lead to an increase in the velocity of the blood across the stenosis. Significant changes in the velocity within and distally to the stenosis will be detected once the vessel becomes narrowed by >50%. The increase in velocity is related to the degree of narrowing and these changes can be used to grade the degree of stenosis. High resistant waveforms with low or absent flow during diastole may indicate a severe internal carotid artery stenosis or occlusion when obtained from the common carotid artery ("externalization"). Low velocities across the vessel can indicate the presence of disease proximal or distal to the site in which it is being examined. Reversal of flow also can be seen in patients with heart disease such as aortic valve regurgitation, causing abnormal reversals in both the right and left carotids. Doppler spectral waveform analysis is a valuable adjunct to B-mode imaging, allowing the examiner to detect changes in vessels that would not otherwise be apparent with a continuous wave device.

● GRADING CAROTID ARTERY STENOSIS

B-mode imaging is used for multiple purposes when evaluating carotid arteries. It provides information regarding plaque-laden areas predictive of stroke risk, evaluating cross-sectional narrowing of the artery, and is useful in measuring intima-media thickness, a marker of systemic atherosclerotic burden and cardiovascular risk used predominantly in trials assessing primary risk intervention strategies.[153–155] B-mode imaging is the most appropriate method to evaluate the degree of narrowing when the degree of lumen diameter reduction is less than 50%. A normal carotid artery is derived from a PSV of less than 125 cm/s in the internal carotid artery, a normal spectral window, and no visible plaque seen in B-mode image (Table 17-13).

Diagnostic criteria for carotid duplex rely on PSV, spectral Doppler patterns, end-diastolic velocities, and velocity ratios between the internal carotid artery and the common carotid artery. The PSV is the most frequently used measurement and the single most accurate duplex parameter to determine the severity of the stenosis though EDV may be more specific.[156–158] Several criteria have been published to detect the presence and severity of carotid artery disease and Table 17-13 summarizes useful absolute velocities and velocity ratios to diagnose carotid artery stenosis. These include PSV, end-diastolic velocity (EDV), and the ratio of PSVs in the ICA to the mid-common carotid artery (CCA) (ICA:CCA PSV ratio) (Table 17-14). Many laboratories also use the EDV or the ICA:CCA PSV ratio for

TABLE 17-13. Normal Reference Values for Blood Flow Velocities (in cm/s) in the Carotid and Vertebral Arteries in Different Age Groups*

Blood flow velocity	All (n = 182)	20–40 years (n = 71)	41–60 years (n = 64)	>60 years (n = 47)
Common carotid artery				
Peak systolic	80 (34–126)	96 (55–135)	75 (39–110)	61 (29–93)
End diastolic	21 (9–33)	23 (12–34)	21 (10–31)	16 (6–26)
Internal carotid artery				
Peak systolic	61 (27–94)	65 (40–92)	61 (24–97)	51 (21–81)
End diastolic	24 (9–39)	27 (15–38)	25 (9–50)	18 (7–30)
Vertebral artery				
Peak systolic	48 (26–69)	49 (29–69)	48 (23–73)	45 (26–63)
End diastolic	16 (10–23)	17 (11–23)	17 (10–27)	14 (8–20)

*Range of velocities (calculated as mean ± 2 standard deviations) is given in parentheses. Data from 182 healthy volunteers.
Source: Reproduced with permission from Babikian VL, Wechsler LR, Higashida RT (eds): Imaging Cerebrovascular Disease. Philadelphia: Butterworth-Heinemann, 2003.

improved diagnostic accuracy and to correct for factors that may alter the carotid blood flow, i.e., low cardiac output, valvular disease, acute elevations in blood pressure, anemia, and abnormal collateral flow.[159,160]

Any of these conditions can lead to alterations in the flow across a carotid plaque and may lead to either under- or overestimation of the true degree of stenosis.[161] In these circumstances, the ICA:CCA PSV ratio often helps in correcting hemodynamic disturbances.[162]

Patients with severe carotid artery stenosis or occlusion may have compensatory increases in their contralateral artery, resulting in spuriously high velocities. A better determinant of stenosis in these situations would be to use the velocity ratio between the peak systolic flow velocity in the proximal ICA and the distal common carotid artery.[163–165]

Limitations of Carotid Artery Ultrasound

Carotid artery ultrasound may underestimate disease in the presence of long smooth plaque that does not have the accelerated turbulent flow patterns associated with significant lesions, making it difficult to differentiate slow-velocity "trickle flow" from complete occlusions.[166] Carotid duplex ultrasound is less precise in determining stenotic lesions that are below 50% and may be less accurate in lesions that range from 50% to 60% when compared to a stenosis greater than 70%. Carotid duplex ultrasound has also been shown to overestimate the degree of stenosis.[167] This limitation may result in a significant number of unnecessary interventions and illustrates that carotid endarterectomy on the basis of carotid duplex ultrasound alone should be used with caution. Also, carotid duplex ultrasound may be limited in the presence of high and low cardiac states, extensive arterial calcifications, and when carotid bifurcations are high in the neck. These limitations are one reason why carotid ultrasound relies upon the experience and expertise of the ultrasonographer. When carotid duplex results are unclear, diagnostic accuracy may increase to 90% or greater when it is used in conjunction with CTA and/or MRA. Low velocities may also reflect proximal (intrathoracic) CCA stenosis.

TABLE 17-14. Criteria for Classification of Internal Carotid Artery Disease by Duplex Scanning with Spectral Waveform Analysis of Pulsed Doppler Signals

Degree of stenosis (%)	ICA/PSV (cm/s)	Plaque estimate (%)	ICA EDV (cm/s)	ICA CCA PSV ratio
Normal	<125	0	<40	<2
<50	<125	<50	<40	<2
50–69	125–230	>50	40–100	2–4
>70	>230	>50	>100	>4
Subtotal occlusion	Variable	>50 Narrow lumen	0	Variable
Total occlusion	0	>50	0	<1

CCA, Common carotid artery; EDV, end-diastolic velocity; ICA, internal carotid artery; PSV, peak systolic velocity.
This material was originally published in Guidelines for noninvasive vascular laboratory testing: a report from the American Society of Echocardiography and the Society of Vascular Medicine and Biology. J Am Soc Echocardiogr. 2006;19;955-972 and is reproduced with the permission of the copyright holder, the American Society of Echocardiography www.asecho.org. Inclusion of this information does not necessarily imply endorsement of this product.

NONINVASIVE DIAGNOSTIC IMAGING OF MESENTERIC CIRCULATION

Arterial occlusive disease of the mesenteric arteries is infrequent, however, the clinical manifestations of mesenteric lesions range from asymptomatic to catastrophic. Acute occlusions of a mesenteric artery secondary to embolism or thrombosis can produce irreversible gut ischemia, and mortality remains among the highest of all vascular diseases. Rapid restoration of the blood flow is mandatory in these situations and arteriography or surgery should be preformed without delay. If chronic mesenteric angina is suspected, duplex scanning can be of great value.

MESENTERIC DUPLEX SCAN

The Duplex examination of the mesenteric arteries should include the evaluation of the proximal abdominal aorta, celiac artery, superior mesenteric artery, as well as the inferior mesenteric artery. The distal segments of the mesenteric arteries cannot be visualized with ultrasound, however most atherosclerotic lesions occur at the ostia of these vessels. This feature makes the diagnosis of these lesions suitable for the use of duplex ultrasound.

Mesenteric duplex scanning is performed with the patient supine in reverse Trendelenburg, allowing the bowels and any bowel gas to shift to the lower abdomen, providing a better acoustic window for examination. A 12-hour fast should be stressed as fasting reduces the amount of scatter and attenuation from intra-abdominal bowel gas and avoids elevated velocities noted in the post prandial state, which can be confused with stenotic flow. A midline subxiphoid approach should be used with low-frequency transducers in the 2- to 5-MHz range. An anterior–posterior midline approach is used to obtain a sagittal scan of the aorta to document the presence of narrowing and aneurismal disease that might encroach on the orifices of the celiac and mesenteric arteries. The celiac artery and superior mesenteric artery are visualized as they course ventrally from the aorta above the left renal vein with the celiac lying cephalad to the origin of the superior mesenteric artery (Figure 17-16).

One variant to note is the presence of a common origin of the celiac artery and superior mesenteric artery. The inferior mesenteric artery originates from the left side of the infrarenal aorta just above the aortic bifurcation.

Pulsed Doppler examinations are obtained with a small sample volume (1.5 to 3 mm) to ensure that velocity information is derived from the vessel of interest. Most studies are performed at 60-degree angles to provide consistency in Doppler measurements, however, the angle correction may be necessary for evaluating the celiac artery because the artery projects toward the probe at a 0- to 30-degree angle. PSV, end-diastolic velocity (EDV), waveform configuration, and direction of flow should be evaluated and recorded.

The celiac trunk may be challenging to image, however, it is possible to trace the vessel to its branches, the splenic, common hepatic, and left gastric arteries. The celiac artery typically is no longer than 1 to 2 cm in length and its branches (splenic, left gastric, and common hepatic) may be variable. Increased velocities in the celiac artery (and occasionally, the SMA) can be caused by compression by the median arcuate ligament and if suspected, the patient should be asked to take a deep breath to evaluate for normalization of the velocity. Median arcuate ligament syndrome is regarded as a benign condition with little risk of intestinal ischemia; however, it has been reported to produce gastrointestional symptoms. The first 1 to 2 cm of the superior mesenteric artery generally has no branches but a right hepatic artery may originate from it in up to 20% of patients.

The inferior mesenteric artery can be identified by scanning down the infrarenal aorta toward the bifurcation where it originates from the left side of the aorta. Large collaterals in patients with aortoiliac occlusions may be mistaken for the inferior mesenteric artery on duplex scanning.

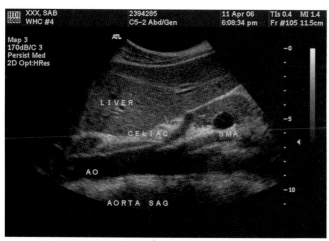

A

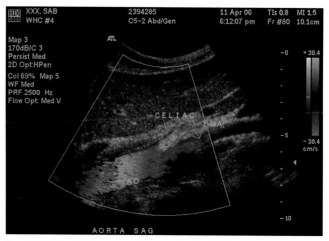

B

● **FIGURE 17-16.** (A) Grayscale of aorta demonstrating celiac artery and superior mesenteric artery. (B) Color duplex of aorta and mesenteric artery.

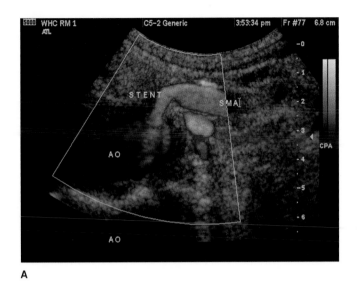

A

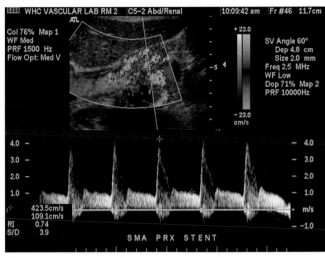

B

• **FIGURE 17-17.** (A and B) Duplex of superior mesenteric artery stent.

Another source of potential error in an attempt to scan the inferior mesenteric artery is the presence of an accessory lower pole of the renal artery originating from the left side of the infrarenal aorta. In most cases, the examination of occlusive lesions at the ostia of the celiac artery and superior mesenteric artery is sufficient, as the majority of involvement is within these areas.

Many different velocity criteria have been proposed for the diagnosis of significant mesenteric artery stenosis and no consensus has been reached regarding the optimal Doppler criteria. Moneta et al.[168] compared the results of mesenteric duplex scanning to arteriography with known atherosclerosis and showed that PSV greater than or equal to 200 cm/s in the celiac artery and greater than or equal to 275 cm/s (normal = 125 to 163 cm/s) in the superior mesenteric artery were predictive of stenosis of 70% or more. This study showed the sensitivity, specificity, and positive predictive value in the superior mesenteric artery to be 89%, 92%, and 80%, while they were 75%, 89%, and 85% in the celiac artery. They demonstrated that mesenteric duplex scanning was indeed sufficiently accurate to be clinically useful as a screening tool in patients with suspected celiac artery or superior mesenteric artery occlusive disease.[169] Lim et al.[170] confirmed the criteria Moneta et al.[168] demonstrated for the detection of mesenteric stenosis with an overall sensitivity of 100% and specificity of 87% for the celiac artery and 98% specificity for the superior mesenteric artery. Bowersox et al.[171] demonstrated that end-diastolic velocity greater than 45 cm/s was the best indicator of superior mesenteric stenosis and an elevated PSV was more specific and less sensitive for superior mesenteric artery stenosis. Zwolak et al.[172] also showed that the end-diastolic velocity was more accurate for the detection of significant mesenteric artery occlusion then PSV.

Adequate Doppler waveforms can be obtained to allow calculations of the PSV, end-diastolic, and resistive index in the inferior mesenteric artery. Erden et al.[173] demonstrated that the PSV varies with the degree of collateral flow through the inferior mesenteric artery when occlusive disease of the abdominal aorta is present. These patients with occlusion of the celiac, superior mesenteric artery, and common iliac arteries had PSV measurements up to 190 cm/s.[173] Mesenteric duplex scanning can become a routine noninvasive diagnostic testing modality for the evaluation of patients with suspected visceral ischemia and mesenteric artery stents (Figure 17-17).

However, newer modalities such as CTA and MRA, have demonstrated high accuracies in the noninvasive evaluation of the mesenteric arteries. The key to success in the detection of mesenteric occlusions relies less upon velocity criteria and more in accurate anatomic identification of the vessels.

● **NONINVASIVE DIAGNOSTIC IMAGING OF ABDOMINAL AORTIC ANEURYSMS**

Duplex ultrasound scanning is the preferred modality for initial screening of population for abdominal aortic aneurysms (AAA) (Figure 17-18).

Scanning has been used for screening and surveillance for both screening and follow-up of small infrarenal aneurysms. Multiple studies have demonstrated that ultrasound is an appropriate means to determine the presence or absence of an infrarenal aortic aneurysm in more than 95% of patients.[174–176] The specificity for the presence of an aneurysm is close to 100%, whereas the sensitivity ranges from 92% to 99%.[179–181] Ultrasound measurements are similar to those for computed tomographic scanning, making it an excellent tool for screening and surveillance (Figure 17-19). Computed tomographic imaging or MRA scanning is usually reserved for anatomic mapping prior to aneurysm repair.

Duplex ultrasound for suprarenal aortic and iliac aneurysms usually does not provide dependable imaging of aneurysms that extend close to the ostia of the renal arteries or into the suprarenal segment of the abdominal aorta. Lamah et al.[181] demonstrated accurately the upper and lower limits of AAA in only 47% and 41% of cases. Furthermore, ultrasound scanning is able to detect iliac artery involvement only about 50% of the time whereas a computed tomographic scan or MRA of the abdomen and pelvis is superior.[181]

The technique for performing AAA scan involves using low-frequency transducers after an overnight fast. The patient is examined in the supine, reverse Trendelenburg position, and the aorta is identified at the level of the diaphragm in the sagittal plane throughout its entire length. The probe is then oriented in the coronal plane and transverse measurements are obtained in the suprarenal, juxtarenal, and infrarenal positions. The normal infrarenal abdominal aortic diameter varies by age and sex with the aortic diameter in the transverse plane being 1.73 ± 0.30 cm. Limitations of screening include obesity and overlying bowel gas.

● NONINVASIVE DIAGNOSTIC IMAGING OF CEREBRAL VASCULAR DISEASES

Transcranial Doppler is a noninvasive method used for evaluating cerebral hemodynamics with color flow duplex and pulsed Doppler. It requires a technologist with intricate knowledge of the structural anatomy, course of the cerebral vessels, and normal and abnormal cerebral hemodynamics. The operator may scan from the head of the bed in a manner similar to that preferred by many users for a standard carotid examination. The examination typically takes 90 minutes and the patient should be positioned in a supine position to obtain transtemporal and transorbital images. After these views have been attained, the patient should be turned onto one side for the transoccipital approach. The transtemporal approach is used to evaluate the middle cerebral artery, posterior cerebral artery, anterior cerebral artery, and terminal internal carotid artery. The anterior and posterior communicating arteries are not usually seen unless they are large collaterals. Transcranial Doppler mostly uses a 2 MHz pulsed, ranged-gated Doppler device with

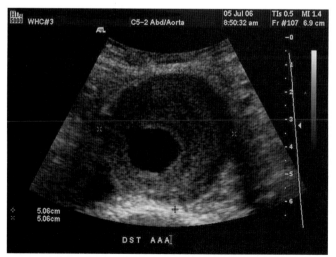

A

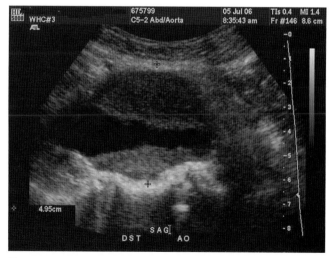

B

● FIGURE 17-18. (A and B) Grayscale of an AAA.

good directional resolution. Transcranial color-coded duplex sonography is performed with 1.8- to 3.6-MHz phased array sector transducer.

Four main ultrasound approaches have been described to evaluate the intracranial arteries: transtemporal, transorbital, transoccipital, and submandibular. In the transtemporal approach, the probe is placed on the temporal aspect of the head just cephalad to the zygomatic arch. The anterior orientation of the ultrasound beam allows for the visualization of the M_1 and M_2 segments of the middle cerebral arteries (depth of 35–55 mm), the C1 segment of the carotid siphon, the A1 segment of the anterior cerebral artery, and the anterior-communicating artery. The posterior orientation of the ultrasound beam allows visualization of the first and second segments of the posterior cerebral artery (depth of 65–70 mm), the basilar artery (75 mm), and the posterior-communicating arteries. It is most convenient to start with this approach to identify the middle cerebral artery and then to track the arterial network to obtain most views. The average mean velocity for the middle cerebral artery is 60 cm/s. The average mean velocity for the anterior cerebral artery is 50 cm/s and 40 cm/s for the posterior cerebral artery. In a normal patient, the middle cerebral artery mean velocity should always be greater than the anterior cerebral artery mean velocity, which is greater than the posterior cerebral artery (Table 17-15).

In the transorbital approach, the anterior cerebral circulation may be evaluated by placing the transducer on the closed eyelid. The power of the ultrasound should be reduced to avoid damage to the lenses of the eyes. The opthalamic artery can be visualized at depths of 45 to 50 mm, the C3 segment of the carotid siphon is seen at depths of 60 to 65 mm, and the C2 and C4 segment can be visualized at depths of 70 to 75 mm. The flow direction of the C2 segment is usually away from the probe, whereas the flow of the C4 segment shows flow toward the probe. This approach is much less validated than the transtemporal or transoccipital approach.

The transoccipital approach allows the visualization of the vertebral artery and the basilar artery throughout their entire lengths. The Doppler probe is aimed at the bridge of the nose between the spinous process of the first cervical vertebra and the posterior margin of the foramen magnum. The depth of the vertebral artery ranges from 35 mm to its deepest point set at 65 mm. The basilar artery is reached at a depth of approximately 95 to 125 mm. Doppler flow in the vertebral artery is toward the transducer, whereas the flow in the basilar artery is directed away from the probe.

The submandibular approach completes the examination with the detection of the internal carotid artery. This examination allows visualization and detection of internal carotid artery dissection and chronic occlusion. The carotid siphon connects to the internal carotid artery, which is usually visualized at a Doppler depth of 80 to 85 mm. The internal carotid artery can be traced from depths of 25 to 80 mm.

The detection of stenosis using transcranial Doppler was first reported in 1986 by Spencer and Whisler,[174] who used similar criteria to those used for evaluating carotid bifurcation disease. Many authors have reported similar findings to Spencer's and Whisler's and have extended these applications to other brain arteries.[1,183–186] Felberg et al.[185] demonstrated that detecting intracranial stenosis with a diameter of 50% or greater, has a mean velocity value of 100 cm/s with a sensitivity of 100% and specificity of 97.9%. Many authors concur that when comparing the contralateral vessel segment, a relative increase in PSV of more than 30% is suspect for hemodynamically significant stenosis and an increase of more than 50% indicates a definite intracranial artery stenosis.

The detection of occlusions using transcranial Doppler has showed a sensitivity of 83% and a specificity of 94%, with an overall accuracy of 91.6%.[1] The absence of arterial signals at an expected depth with altered flow in communicating vessels can confirm cerebral artery occlusions. Demchuk et al.[1] has developed the Thombolysis in Brain Ischemia (TIBI) criteria for the classification of the middle cerebral artery recanalization during and after thrombolytic therapy. The TIBI criteria was developed after evaluating 109 short-term stroke patients who underwent thrombolytic therapy, which was found to be accurate in the prediction of the clinical outcome. The scale ranges from 0 (MCA occlusion) to 5 (normal MCA) (Table 17-16).[187]

TABLE 17-15. Normal Reference Values for Blood Flow Velocities (cm/s) in the Basal Cerebral Arteries in Different Age Groups

Blood flow velocity	N	All	20–40 y	41–60 y	>60 y
Anterior cerebral artery	313				
Peak systolic		79 (37–121)	82 (40–124)	80 (36–124)	72 (52–102)
Mean (TAMAX)		53 (33–83)	56 (42–84)	53 (37–85)	44 (22–66)
End diastolic		35 (13–57)	38 (16–60)	35 (13–57)	28 (12–44)
Middle cerebral artery	335				
Peak systolic		110 (54–166)	120 (64–176)	109 (65–175)	92 (58–126)
Mean (TAMAX)		73 (33–133)	81 (41–121)	73 (35–111)	59 (37–81)
End diastolic		49 (21–77)	55 (29–81)	49 (23–75)	37 (21–53)
Posterior cerebral artery	336				
Peak systolic		71 (39–103)	75 (43–107)	74 (40–108)	62 (38–86)
Mean (TAMAX)		49 (25–73)	52 (28—-76)	51 (25–75)	40 (22–58)
End diastolic		33 (15–51)	36 (20–52)	34 (18–50)	26 (14–38)

TAMAX, time-averaged maximum velocity.
Range of velocities (calculated as mean ± 2 standard deviations) is given in parentheses.
Source: Adapted from J Krejza, Z Mariak, J Walecki, et al. Transcranial color Doppler sonography of basal cerebral arteries in 182 healthy subjects: age and sex variability and normal reference values for blood parameters. AJR Am J Roentgenol 1999;172:213-218.

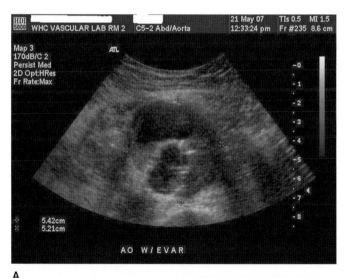

A

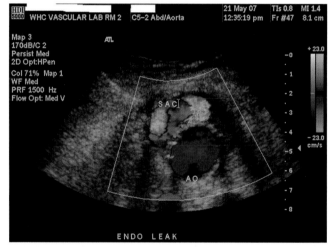

B

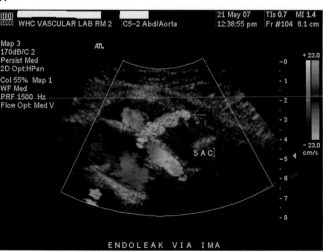

C

● FIGURE 17-19. (A) Grayscale of an AAA with endograft. (B) Color Doppler of an AAA endoleak. (C) Color Doppler of an AAA endoleak via internal mesenteric artery.

TABLE 17-16. Thombolysis in Brain Ischemia Criteria for Transcranial Doppler Monitoring During/After Thrombolytic Therapy

TIBI score	Status of the MCA flow	TCD criteria
0	Occlusion	No flow signal
1	Near occlusion	Early systolic low flow signal
		No diastolic flow signal
2	Strongly reduce	Reduced systolic/diastolic velocity
		Pulsatility index <1.2
		Flattened early systolic increment
3	Moderately reduced	Normal systolic increment
		Pulsatility index >1.2
		Relative reduction of blood flow velocity of >30% as compared with the contralateral side
4	Stenotic signal	Detection of turbulent flow
		Mean blood flow velocity >80 cm/s or relative increase of velocity >30% as compared to contralateral side
5	Normal signal	Side to side difference of blood flow velocity <30%

Detection of intracranial stenosis and occlusion with transcranial color-coded duplex sonography usually is diagnosed using the angle-corrected peak velocity. Baumgartner et al.[188] demonstrated that cutoff peak systolic values ranging from 220 cm/s for the middle cerebral artery to 120 cm/s for the verterbral artery had a sensitivity and specificity of 100%.[188] The accuracy in the detection of stenosis between 30% and 50% showed a moderate positive predictive value (73% to 100%) but had a high negative predictive value of 100%.[188]

Limitations of Cerebral Vascular Ultrasound

Noninvasive examination of intracranial arterial stenosis and occlusion is a valuable clinical tool, but various sources of error can occur. Common sources of error include misinterpretation of potential collateral pathways, displacement of arteries because of a space-occupying lesion, misdiagnosis of vasospasm as stenosis, and not able to recognize the possible physiologic variables in the circle of Willis.[189] Diagnostic accuracy within the verterbral artery and basilar artery system remains problematic. These difficulties result from highly variable flow patterns in the vessels, the location of the arteries and course are sometimes unpredictable, often the junction of the vertebral arteries cannot reliably be identified, the vertebral artery flow signal may be absent on one side, which may not represent disease and occlusion of one vertebral artery does not always lead to flow abnormalities.[190]

Quality Assurance and Vascular Laboratory Accreditation

The Intersocietal Commission for Accreditation of Vascular Laboratories (www.icavl.org) serves as an intersocietal, peer review organization that provides a mechanism for facilities to maintain the quality assurance of noninvasive vascular laboratory techniques. The "Essentials and Standards for Accreditation of Vascular Laboratories" defines a vascular laboratory as a unit performing noninvasive vascular diagnostic testing under the overall direction of a medical director. The medical director interprets and reports on all noninvasive vascular examinations. Reporting must be standardized and include the date of the examination, clinical indications, description of the test performed, results including the localization and quantification of abnormal findings and comparison with available previous studies, and the name of the sonographer performing the examination along with their signature. The director must have interpreted under the supervision of an experienced mentor, a minimum of 100 cases in each of the areas for which they will be interpreting studies and must interpret 75 visceral vascular duplex ultrasound cases.[191] Specific recommendations from Intersocietal Commission for Accreditation of Vascular Laboratories regarding vacular operations are available for visceral vascular testing, peripheral venous testing, peripheral arterial, intracranial cerebrovascular, and extracranial cerebrovascular testing.[76,192–195] Every module includes information on essentials and standards for instrumentation, indications, techniques, diagnostic criteria, and quality assurance.

REFERENCES

1. Demchuk AM, Christou I, Wein TH, et al. Accuracy and criteria for localizing arterial occlusion with transcranial Doppler. *J Neuroimaging.* 2000;10(1):1-12.

2. Nelson TR, Pretorius DH. The Doppler signal: where does it come from and what does it mean? *AJR Am J Roentgenol.* 1991;151:439-447.

3. Hoeks APG, Reneman SR. Biophysical principles of vascular diagnosis. *J Clin Ultrasound.* 1995;23:71-79.

4. McDonald DA. *Blood Flow in Arteries.* Baltimore: Williams & Wilkins; 1974.

5. American Heart Association. *Heart Disease and Stroke Statistics-2004 Update.* Dallas, TX: American Heart Association; 2003.

6. Hirsch AT, Haskal ZJ, Hertzer NR, et al. ACC/AHA 2005 practice guidelines for the management of patients with peripheral arterial disease (lower extremity, renal, mesenteric,

and abdominal aortic): executive summary: a collaborative report from the American Association for Vascular Surgery/Society for Vascular Surgery, Society for Cardiovascular Angiography and Interventions, Society for Vascular Medicine and Biology, Society of Interventional Radiology, and the ACC/AHA Task Force on Practice Guidelines (Writing Committee to Develop Guidelines for the Management of Patients with Peripheral Arterial Disease). *Circulation.* 2006;113:1474-1547.

7. Marie G-H, Julius MG, Michael J, Emile M, Mary R, Tasneem ZN. Guidelines for noninvasive vascular laboratory testing: a report from the American Society of Echocardiography and the Society of Vascular Medicine and Biology. *J Am Soc Echocardiogr.* 2006;19:955-972.

8. Hiatt WR. Medical treatment of peripheral arterial disease and claudication. *N Engl J Med.* 2001;344:1608-1621.

9. Fowkes FG. The measurement of atherosclerotic peripheral arterial disease in epidemiological surveys. *Int J Epidemiol.* 1988;17:248-254.

10. Feigelson HS, Criqui MH, Fronek A, et al. Screening for peripheral arterial disease: the sensitivity, specificity, and predictive value of noninvasive tests in a defined population. *Am J Epidemiol.* 1994;140:526-534.

11. Lijmer JG, Hunink MG, van den Dungen JJ, et al. ROC analysis of noninvasive tests for peripheral arterial disease. *Ultrasound Med Biol.* 1996;22:391-398.

12. Endres HG, Hucke C, Holland-Letz T, Trampisch HJ. A new efficient trial design for assessing reliability of ankle-brachial index measures by three different observer groups. *BMC Cardiovasc Disord.* 2006;6:33.

13. McDermott MM, Fried L, Simonsick E, Ling S, Guralnik JM. Asymptomatic peripheral arterial disease is independently associated with impaired lower extremity functioning: the Women's Health and Aging Study. *Circulation.* 2000;101:1007-1012.

14. Vogt MT, Cauley JA, Kuller LH, Nevitt MC. Functional status and mobility among elderly women with lower extremity arterial disease: the Study of Osteoporotic Fractures. *J Am Geriatr Soc.* 1994;42:923-929.

15. Newman AB, Siscovick DS, Manolio TA, et al. Ankle-arm index as a marker of atherosclerosis in the Cardiovascular Health Study. Cardiovascular Heart Study (CHS) Collaborative Research Group. *Circulation.* 1993;88:837-845.

16. McKenna M, Wolfson S, Kuller L. The ratio of ankle and arm arterial pressure as an independent predictor of mortality. *Atherosclerosis.* 1991;87:119-128.

17. Sikkink CJ, van Asten WN, van't Hof MA, et al. Decreased ankle/brachial indices in relation to morbidity and mortality in patients with peripheral arterial disease. *Vasc Med.* 1997;2:169-173.

18. Resnick HE, Lindsay RS, McDermott MM, et al. Relationship of high and low ankle brachial index to all-cause and cardiovascular disease mortality. The Strong Heart Study. *Circulation.* 2004;109:733-739.

19. Criqui MH, Langer RD, Fronek A, et al. Mortality over a period of 10 years in patients with peripheral arterial disease. *N Engl J Med.* 1992;326:381-386.

20. Orchard TJ, Strandness DE Jr. Assessment of peripheral vascular disease in diabetes: report and recommendations of an international workshop sponsored by the American Diabetes Association and the American Heart Association September 18-20, 1992 New Orleans, Louisiana. *Circulation.* 1993;88:819-828.

21. American Diabetes Association. Peripheral arterial disease in people with diabetes. *Diabetes Care.* 2003;26:3333-3341.

22. McDermott MM, Liu K, Criqui, MH, et al. Ankle-brachial index and subclinical cardiac and carotid disease. The Multi-Ethnic Study of Atherosclerosis. *Am J Epidemiol.* 2005; 162(1):33-41.

23. Ouriel K, Zarins CK. Doppler ankle pressure: an evaluation of three methods of expression. *Arch Surg.* 1982;117:1297-1300.

24. Newman AB, Sutton-Tyrrell K, Vogt MT, et al. Morbidity and mortality in hypertensive adults with a low ankle/arm blood pressure index. *JAMA.* 1993;270:487-489.

25. Vogt MT, McKenna M, Anderson SJ, et al. The relationship between ankle-arm index and mortality in older men and women. *J Am Geriatr Soc.* 1993;41:523-530.

26. McDermott MM, Greenland P, Liu K, et al. The ankle brachial index is associated with leg function and physical activity: the Walking and Leg Circulation Study. *Ann Intern Med.* 2002;136:873-883.

27. Newman A, Siscovick D, Manolio T, et al. Ankle-arm index as a marker of atherosclerosis in the Cardiovascular Health Study. Cardiovascular Health Study (CHS) Collaborative Research Group. *Circulation.* 1993;88:837-845.

28. Jelnes R, Gaardsting O, Hougaard Jensen K, et al. Fate in intermittent claudication: outcome and risk factors. *Br Med J (Clin Res Ed).* 1986;293:1137-1140.

29. Raines JK, Darling RG, Buth J, Brewster DC, Austen WG. Vascular laboratory criteria for the management of peripheral vascular disease of the lower extremities. *Surgery.* 1976;79:21-29.

30. Carter SA, Lezack JD. Digital systolic pressures in the lower limb in arterial disease. *Circulation.* 1971;43:905-914.

31. Vollrath KD, Salles-Cunha SX, Vincent D, Towne JB, Bernhard VM. Noninvasive measurement of toe systolic pressures. *Bruit.* 1980;4:27-30.

32. Ramsey DE, Manke DA, Sumner DS. Toe blood pressure: a valuable adjunct to ankle pressure measurement for assessing peripheral arterial disease. *J Cardiovasc Surg.* 1983;24: 43-48.

33. Pascarelli EF, Bertrand CA. Comparison of blood pressures in the arms and legs. *N Engl J Med.* 1964;270:693-698.

34. Yao ST, Hobbs JT, Irvine WT. Ankle systolic pressure measurements in arterial disease affecting the lower extremities. *Br J Surg.* 1969;56:676-679.

35. McPhail IR, Spittell PC, Weston SA, Bailey KR. Intermittent claudication: an objective office-based assessment. *J Am Coll Cardiol.* 2001;37(5):1381-1385.

36. Rutherford RB, Lowenstein DH, Klein MF. Combining segmental systolic pressures and plethysmography to diagnose arterial occlusive disease of the legs. *Am J Surg.* 1979;138:211-218.

37. Cutajar CL, Marston A, Newcombe JF. Value of cuff occlusion pressures in assessment of peripheral vascular disease. *Br J Med.* 1973;2:392-395.

38. Heintz SE, Bone GE, Slaymaker EE, et al. Value of arterial pressure measurements in the proximal and distal part of the thigh in arterial occlusive disease. *Surg Gynecol Obstet.* 1978;146:337.

39. Rutherford RB, Lowenstein DH, Klein MF. Combining segmental systolic pressures and plethysmography to diagnose arterial occlusive disease of the legs. *Am J Surg.* 1979;138:211-218.

40. Raines JK. The pulse volume recorder in peripheral arterial disease. In: Bernstein EF, ed. *Noninvasive Diagnostic Techniques in Vascular Disease.* St. Louis, MO: Mosby; 1985:513-544.

41. Jorgensen JJ, Stranden E, Gjolberg T. Measurements of common femoral artery flow velocity in the evaluation of aortoiliac atherosclerosis: comparisons between pulsatility index, pressures measurements and pulse-volume recordings. *Acta Chir Scand.* 1988;154:261-266.

42. Symes JF, Graham AM, Mousseau M. Doppler waveform analysis versus segmental pressure and pulse-volume recording: assessment of occlusive disease in the lower extremity. *Can J Surg.* 1984;27:345-347.

43. Kaufman JL, Fitzgerald KM, Shah DM, et al. The fate of extremities with flat lower calf pulse volume recordings. *J Cardiovasc Surg (Torino).* 1989;30:216-219.

44. Makisalo H, Lepantalo M, Halme L, et al. Peripheral arterial disease as a predictor of outcome after renal transplantation. *Transplant Int.* 1998;11(suppl 1):S140-S143.

45. Dormandy JA, Rutherford RB. Management of peripheral arterial disease (PAD): TransAtlantic Inter-Society Consensus (TASC). *J Vasc Surg.* 2000;31(suppl 1, pt 2):S1-S296.

46. Gauthier GM, Dieter RS. Successful treatment of a femoral artery pseudoaneurysm mimicking a deep venous thrombosis following cardiac catheterization. *Catheter Cardiovasc Interv.* 2002;57(1):75-78.

47. Papamichael CM, Lekakis JP, Stamatelopoulos KS, et al. Ankle-brachial index as a predictor of the extent of coronary atherosclerosis and cardiovascular events in patients with coronary artery disease. *Am J Cardiol.* 2000;86:615-618.

48. de Vries SO, Hunink MG, Polak JF. Summary receiver operating characteristic curves as a technique for meta-analysis of the diagnostic performance of duplex ultrasonography in peripheral arterial disease. *Acad Radiol.* 1996;3:361-369.

49. van der Heijden FH, Legemate DA, van Leeuwen MS, et al. Value of duplex scanning in the selection of patients for percutaneous transluminal angioplasty. *Eur J Vasc Surg.* 1993;7:71-76.

50. Edwards JM, Coldwell DM, Goldman ML, et al. The role of duplex scanning in the selection of patients for transluminal angioplasty. *J Vasc Surg.* 1991;13:69-74.

51. Proia RR, Walsh DB, Nelson PR, et al. Early results of infragenicular revascularization based solely on duplex arteriography. *J Vasc Surg.* 2001;33:1165-1170.

52. Ligush J Jr, Reavis SW, Preisser JS, et al. Duplex ultrasound scanning defines operative strategies for patients with limb-threatening ischemia. *J Vasc Surg.* 1998;28:482-490; discussion 490-491.

53. Ascher E, Mazzariol F, Hingorani A, et al. The use of duplex ultrasound arterial mapping as an alternative to conventional arteriography for primary and secondary infrapopliteal bypasses. *Surg Gynecol Obstet.* 1999;178:162-165.

54. Larch E, Minar E, Ahmadi R, et al. Value of color duplex sonography for evaluation of tibioperoneal arteries in patients with femoropopliteal obstruction: a prospective comparison with anterograde intraarterial digital subtraction angiography. *J Vasc Surg.* 1997;25:629-636.

55. Mattos MA, van Bemmelen PS, Hodgson KJ, et al. Does correction of stenoses identified with color duplex scanning improve infrainguinal graft patency? *J Vasc Surg* 1993;17:54-64; discussion 64-66.

56. Lundell A, Lindblad B, Bergqvist D, et al. Femoropopliteal-crural graft patency is improved by an intensive surveillance program: a prospective randomized study. *J Vasc Surg.* 1995;21:26-33; discussion 33-34.

57. Lalak NJ, Hanel KC, Hunt J, et al. Duplex scan surveillance of infrainguinal prosthetic bypass grafts. *J Vasc Surg.* 1994;20:637-641.

58. Dunlop P, Sayers RD, Naylor AR, et al. The effect of a surveillance programme on the patency of synthetic infrainguinal bypass grafts. *Eur J Vasc Endovasc Surg.* 1996;11:441-445.

59. Strandness DE Jr. Peripheral arterial system. In: Strandness DE Jr, ed. *Duplex Scanning in Vascular Disorders.* 3rd ed. Philadelphia, PA: Lippincott Williams & Wilkins; 2002:118-143.

60. Bandyk D. Nature and management of duplex abnormalities encountered during infrainguinal vein bypass grafting. *J Vasc Surg.* 1996;24:430-438.

61. Bandyk D, Cato R, Towne J. A low velocity predicts failure of femoropopliteal and femorotibial bypass grafts. *Surgery.* 1985;98:799-809.

62. Sacks D, Robinson ML, Marinelli DL, et al. Peripheral arterial Doppler ultrasonography: diagnostic criteria. *J Ultrasound Med.* 1992;11:95-103.

63. Allard L, Cloutier G, Durand LG, et al. Limitations of ultrasonic duplex scanning for diagnosing lower limb arterial stenoses in the presence of adjacent segment disease. *J Vasc Surg.* 1994;19:650-657.

64. Abou-Zamzam AM Jr, Edwards JM, Porter JM. Noninvasive diagnosis of upper extremity disease. In: AbuRahma AF, Bergan JJ, eds. *Noninvasive Vascular Diagnosis.* London, UK: Springer; 2000:269.

65. Mathiesen EB, Bonaa KH, Joakimsen O. Echolucent plaques are associated with high risk of ischemic cerebrovascular events in carotid stenosis: the Tromso Study. *Circulation* 2001;103:2171-2175.

66. De Bray JM, Baud JM, Dauzat M. Consensus concerning the morphology and the risk of carotid plaques. *Cerebrovasc Dis.* 1996;7:289-296.

67. Gross WS, Flanigan DP, Kraft RO, Stanley JC. Chronic upper extremity arterial insufficiency: etiology, manifestations, and operative measurement. *Arch Surg.* 1978;113:419-423.

68. Sumner DS. Evaluation of acute and chronic ischemia of the upper extremity. In: Rutherford RB, ed. *Vascular Surgery.* 4th ed. Philadelphia, PA: WB Saunders; 1995:918-935.

69. Nielson PE, Bell G, Lassen NA. The measurement of digital systolic blood pressure by stain gauge technique. *Scand J Clin Lab Invest.* 1972;29:371-379.

70. Downs AR, Gaskell P, Morrow I, Munson CL. Assessment of arterial obstruction in vessels supplying the fingers by measurement of local blood pressures and the skin temperature response test: correlation with angiographic evidence. *Surgery.* 1975;77:530-539.

71. Hirai M. Arterial insufficiency of the hands evaluated by digital blood pressure and arteriographic findings. *Circulation.* 1978;58:902-908.

72. Edwards JM, Zierler RE. Duplex ultrasound assessment of upper extremity arteries. In: Zwiebel WJ, ed. *Introduction to Vascular Ultrasonography.* 3rd ed. Philadelphia, PA: WB Saunders, Harcourt Brace Jovanovich; 1992:228.

73. Taneja K, Jain R, Sawhney S, Rajani M. Occlusive arterial disease of the upper extremity: colour Doppler as a screening technique and for assessment of distal circulation. *Australas Radiol.* 1996;40:226-229.

74. NKF-DOQI Clinical practice guidelines for vascular access: Update 2000. *Am J Kidney Dis* 2001;37(suppl 1): S137-S161.

75. Hollenberg NK. Medical therapy for renovascular hypertension: a review. *Am J Hypertens.* 1988;1:338S-343S.

76. Scoble JE, Maher ER, Hamilton G, Dick R, Swenty P, Moorhead JF. Atherosclerotic renovascular disease causing renal impairment—a case for treatment. *Clin Nephrol.* 1989;31: 119-122.

77. Mailloux LU, Napolitano B, Bellucci AG. Renal vascular disease causing end-stage renal disease, incidence, clinical correlates, and outcomes: a 20-year clinical experience. *Am J Kidney Dis.* 1994;24:622-629.

78. Gray BH, Olin JW, Childs MB, Sullivan TM, Bacharach JM. Clinical benefit of renal artery angioplasty with stenting for the control of recurrent and refractory congestive heart failure. *Vasc Med.* 2002;7:275-279.

79. Hansen KJ, Edwards MS, Craven TE, et al. Prevalence of renovascular disease in the elderly: a population-based study. *J Vasc Surg.* 2002;36:443-451.

80. Carman TL, Olin JW. Diagnosis of renal artery stenosis: what is the optimal diagnostic test? *Curr Interv Cardiol Rep.* 2000;2:111-118.

81. Olin JW. Role of duplex ultrasonography in screening for significant renal artery disease. *Urol Clin North Am.* 1994; 21:215-226.

82. Hoffmann U, Edwards JM, Carter S, et al. Role of duplex scanning for the detection of atherosclerotic renal artery disease. *Kidney Int.* 1991;39:1232-1239.

83. Kohler TR, Zierler RE, Martin RL, et al. Noninvasive diagnosis of renal artery stenosis by ultrasonic duplex scanning. *J Vasc Surg.* 1986;4:450-456.

84. Taylor DC, Kettler MD, Moneta GL, et al. Duplex ultrasound scanning in the diagnosis of renal artery stenosis: a prospective evaluation. *J Vasc Surg.* 1988;7:363-369.

85. Wilcox CS. Ischemic nephropathy: noninvasive testing. *Semin Nephrol.* 1996;16:43-52.

86. Carman TL, Olin JW, Czum J. Noninvasive imaging of the renal arteries. *Urol Clin North Am.* 2001;28:815-826.

87. Olin JW, Piedmonte MR, Young JR, et al. The utility of duplex ultrasound scanning of the renal arteries for diagnosing significant renal artery stenosis. *Ann Intern Med.* 1995;122: 833-838.

88. Dawson DL. Noninvasive assessment of renal artery stenosis. *Semin Vasc Surg.* 1996;9(3):172-181.

89. Baxter GM, Aitchison F, Sheppard D, et al. Colour Doppler ultrasound in renal artery stenosis: intrarenal waveform analysis. *Br J Radiol.* 1996;69(825):810-815.

90. Miralles M, Cairols M, Cotillas J, Giménez A, Santiso A. Value of doppler parameters in the diagnosis of renal artery stenosis. *J Vasc Surg.* 1996;23(3):428-435.

91. Brun P, Kchouk H, Mouchet B, et al. Value of Doppler ultrasound for the diagnosis of renal artery stenosis in children. *Pediatr Nephrol.* 1997;11(1):27-30.

92. Strandness DE Jr. Duplex scanning in diagnosis of renovascular hypertension. *Surg Clin North Am.* 1990;70:109-117.

93. Stanely JC. Renal vascular disease and renovascular hypertension in children. *Urol Clin North Am.* 1984;11:451-463.

94. Kim SH, Kim WH, Choi BI, et al. Duplex Doppler US in patients with medical renal disease: resistive index vs serum creatinine level. *Clin Radiol.* 1992;45:85-87.

95. Radermacher J, Chavan A, Bleck J, et al. Use of Doppler ultrasonography to predict the outcome of therapy for renal-artery stenosis. *N Engl J Med.* 2001;344:410-417.

96. Zeller T, Muller C, Frank U, et al. Stent angioplasty of severe atherosclerotic ostial renal artery stenosis in patients with diabetes mellitus and nephrosclerosis. *Catheter Cardiovasc Interv.* 2003;58:510-515.

97. Hudspeth DA, Hansen KJ, Reavis SW, et al. Renal duplex sonography after treatment of renovascular disease. *J Vasc Surg.* 1993;18:381-388; discussion 389-390.

98. Hansen KJ, Tribble RW, Reavis SW, et al. Renal duplex sonography: evaluation of clinical utility. *J Vasc Surg.* 1990;12:227-236.

99. Beregi JP, Elkohen M, Deklunder G, et al. Helical CT angiography compared with arteriography in the detection of renal artery stenosis. *AJR Am J Roentgenol.* 1996;167:495-501.

100. Halpern EJ, Rutter CM, Gardiner GA Jr, et al. Comparison of Doppler US and CT angiography for evaluation of renal artery stenosis. *Acad Radiol.* 1998;5:524-532.

101. Johnson PT, Halpern EJ, Kuszyk BS, et al. Renal artery stenosis: CT angiography—comparison of real-time volume-rendering and hypertenmaximum intensity projection algorithms. *Radiology.* 1999;211:337-343.

102. Kim TS, Chung JW, Park JH, et al. Renal artery evaluation: comparison of spiral CT angiography to intra-arterial DSA. *J Vasc Interv Radiol.* 1998;9:553-559.

103. Rubin GD, Dake MD, Napel S, et al. Spiral CT of renal artery stenosis: comparison of three-dimensional rendering techniques. *Radiology.* 1994;190:181-189.

104. Kawashima A, Sandler CM, Ernst RD, et al. CT evaluation of renovascular disease. *Radiographics.* 2000;20:1321-1340.

105. Lufft V, Hoogestraat-Lufft L, Fels LM, et al. Contrast media nephropathy: intravenous CT angiography versus intraarterial digital subtraction angiography in renal artery stenosis: a prospective randomized trial. *Am J Kidney Dis.* 2002;40:236-242.

106. Willmann JK, Wildermuth S, Pfammatter T, et al. Aortoiliac and renal arteries: prospective intraindividual comparison of contrastenhanced three-dimensional MR

angiography and multi-detector row CT angiography. *Radiology*. 2003;226:798-811.

107. Earls JP, Rofsky NM, DeCorato DR, Krinsky GA, Weinreb JC. Breath-hold single-dose gadolinium-enhanced three-dimensional MR aortography: usefulness of a timing examination and MR power injector. *Radiology*. 1996;201:705-710.

108. Leung DA, McKinnon GC, Davis CP, Pfammatter T, Krestin GP, Debatin JF. Breath-hold, contrast-enhanced, three-dimensional MR angiography. *Radiology*. 1996;200:569-571.

109. Siegelman ES, Gilfeather M, Holland GA, et al. Breath-hold ultrafast three-dimensional gadolinium-enhanced MR angiography of the renovascular system. *AJR Am J Roentgenol*. 1997;168:1035-1040.

110. Hany TF, Debatin JF, Leung DA, Pfammater T. Evaluation of the aortoiliac and renal arteries: comparison of breath hold, contrast enhanced three dimensional MR angiography with conventional catheter angiography. *Radiology*. 1997;204:357-362.

111. Snidow JJ, Johnson MS, Harris VJ, et al. Three-dimensional gadolinium-enhanced MR angiography for aortoiliac inflow assessment plus renal artery screening in a single breath hold. *Radiology*. 1996;198:725-732.

112. Prince MR, Schoenberg SO, Ward JS, Londy FJ, Wakefield TW, Stanley JC. Hemodynamically significant atherosclerotic renal artery stenosis: MR angiographic features. *Radiology*. 1997;205:128-136.

113. Leung DA, Hoffmann U, Pfammatter T, et al. Magnetic resonance angiography versus duplex sonography for diagnosing renovascular disease. *Hypertension*. 1999;33(2):726-731.

114. Prigent A, Cosgriff P, Gates GF, et al. Consensus report on quality control of quantitative measurements of renal function obtained from the renogram: international consensus committee from the scientific committee of radionuclides in nephrourology. *Semin Nucl Med*. 1999;29:146-159.

115. Nally JV Jr, Clarke HS Jr, Grecos GP, et al. Effect of captopril on 99mTc-diethylenetriaminepentaacetic acid renograms in two-kidney, one clip hypertension. *Hypertension*. 1986;8:685-693.

116. Setaro JF, Saddler MC, Chen CC, et al. Simplified captopril renography in diagnosis and treatment of renal artery stenosis. *Hypertension*. 1991;18:289-298.

117. Dondi M. Captopril renal scintigraphy with 99mTc-mercaptoacetyltriglycine (99mTc-MAG3) for detecting renal artery stenosis. *Am J Hypertens*. 1991;4(12, pt 2):737S-740S.

118. Fommei E, Ghione S, Hilson AJ, et al. Captopril radionuclide test in renovascular hypertension: a European multicentre study. European multicentre study group. *Eur J Nucl Med*. 1993;20:617-623.

119. Geyskes GG, Oei HY, Puylaert CB, et al. Renography with captopril. Changes in a patient with hypertension and unilateral renal artery stenosis. *Arch Intern Med*. 1986;146:1705-1708.

120. Sfakianakis GN, Bourgoignie JJ, Jaffe D, et al. Single-dose captopril scintigraphy in the diagnosis of renovascular hypertension. *J Nucl Med*. 1987;28:1383-1392.

121. Erbsloh-Moller B, Dumas A, Roth D, et al. Furosemide-131I-hippuran renography after angiotensin-converting enzyme inhibition for the diagnosis of renovascular hypertension. *Am J Med*. 1991;90:23-29.

122. Mann SJ, Pickering TG, Sos TA, et al. Captopril renography in the diagnosis of renal artery stenosis: accuracy and limitations. *Am J Med*. 1991;90:30-40.

123. Elliott WJ, Martin WB, Murphy MB. Comparison of two noninvasive screening tests for renovascular hypertension. *Arch Intern Med*. 1993;153:755-764.

124. van Jaarsveld BC, Krijnen P, Derkx FH, et al. The place of renal scintigraphy in the diagnosis of renal artery stenosis: fifteen years of clinical experience. *Arch Intern Med*. 1997;157:1226-1234.

125. Mittal BR, Kumar P, Arora P, et al. Role of captopril renography in the diagnosis of renovascular hypertension. *Am J Kidney Dis*. 1996;28:209-213.

126. Fommei E, Ghione S, Hilson AJ, et al. Captopril radionuclide test in renovascular hypertension: a European multicentre study. *Eur J Nucl Med*. 1993;20:617-623.

127. Huot SJ, Hansson JH, Dey H, et al. Utility of captopril renal scans for detecting renal artery stenosis. *Arch Intern Med*. 2002;162:1981-1984.

128. Barnett HJ, Eliasziw M, Meldrum HE, Taylor DW. Do the facts and figures warrant a 10-fold increase in the performance of carotid endarterectomy on asymptomatic patients? *Neurology*. 1996;46:603-608.

129. Cejna M. PTA versus Palmaz stent placement in femoropopliteal artery obstructions: a multicenter prospective randomized study. *J Vasc Interv Radiol*. 2001;12:23-31.

130. Moneta GL, Edwards JM, Chitwood RW, et al. Correlation of North American Symptomatic Carotid Endarterectomy Trial (NASCET) angiographic definition of 70 percent to 99 percent internal carotid artery stenosis with duplex scanning. *J Vasc Surg*. 1993;17:152.

131. Bray JM, Galland F, Lhoste P, et al. Colour Doppler and duplex sonography and angiography of the carotid artery bifurcations. Prospective, double-blind study. *Neuroradiology*. 1995;37:219-224.

132. Bluth EI, Sunshine JH, Lyons JB, et al. Power Doppler imaging: initial evaluation as a screening examination for carotid artery stenosis. *Radiology*. 2000;215:791-800.

133. Pignoli P, Tremoli E, Poli A, Oreste P, Paoletti R. Intimal plus medi thickness of the arterial wall: a direct measurement with ultrasound imaging. *Circulation*. 1986;74:1399-1409.

134. Geroulakos G, Ramaswami G, Nicolaides A. Characterisation of symptomatic and asymptomatic carotid plaques using high resolution real time ultrasound. *Br J Surg*. 1993;80:1274-1277.

135. European Carotid Plaque Study Group. Carotid artery plaque composition and relationship to clinical presentation and ultrasound B-mode imaging. *Eur J Vasc Surg*. 1995;10:23-30.

136. Merritt CRB, Bluth EI. Ultrasonographic characterization of carotid plaque. In: Labs KH, Jaeger KA, Fitzgerald DE, eds. *Diagnostic Vascular Ultrasound*. London, UK: Edward Arnold; 1992:213-224.

137. De Bray JM, Baud JM, Dauzat M. Consensus concerning the morphology and the risk of carotid plaques. *Cerebrovasc Dis*. 1996;7:289-296.

138. Mathiesen EB, Bonaa KH, Joakimsen O. Echolucent plaques are associated with high risk of ischemic cerebrovascular events in carotid stenosis: the Tromso Study. *Circulation.* 2001;103:2171-2175.

139. Polak JF, Shemanski L, O'Leary DH, et al. Hypoechoic plaque at US of the carotid artery: an independent risk factor for incident stroke in adults aged 65 years or older. Cardiovascular Health Study. *Radiology.* 1998;208:649-654.

140. Golledge J, Cuming R, Ellis M, Davies AH, Greenhalgh RM. Carotid plaque characteristics and presenting symptom. *Br J Surg.* 1997;84:1697-1701.

141. Johnson JM, Kennely M, Decesale D, Morgan S, Sparrow S. Natural history of asymptomatic plaque. *Arch Surg.* 1985; 120:1010-1012.

142. Langsfeld M, Gray-Weale AC, Lusby RJ. The role of plaque morphology and diameter reduction in the development of new symptoms in asymptomatic carotid arteries. *J Vasc Surg.* 1989;9:548-557.

143. O'Holleran LW, Kennelly MM, McClurken M, Johnson JM. Natural history of asymptomatic carotid plaque. Five year follow up study. *Am J Surg.* 1987;154:659-662.

144. Bock W, Lusby RJ. Carotid plaque morphology and interpretation of the echolucent lesion. In: Labs KH, Jäger KA, Fitzgerald DE, Woodcock JP, Neuerburg-Heusler D, eds. *Diagnostic Vascular Imaging.* London, UK: Arnold; 1992:225-236.

145. Mathiesen EB, Bonaa KH, Joakimsen O. Echolucent plaques are associated with high risk of ischemic cerebrovascular events in carotid stenosis: the Tromso Study. *Circulation* 2001;103:2171-2175.

146. Sterpetti AV, Schultz RD, Feldhaus RJ. Ultrasonographic features of carotid plaque and the risk of subsequent neurologic deficits. *Surgery.* 1988;104:652-660.

147. AbuRahma AF, Thiele SP, Wulu JT. Prospective study of the natural history of asymptomatic 60% to 69% carotid stenosis according to ultrasonic plaque morphology. *J Vasc Surg.* 2002;36:437-442.

148. North American Symptomatic Carotid Endartrectomy trial collaborators. Beneficial effect of carotid endarterectomy in symptomatic patients with high-grade carotid stenosis. *N Eng J Med.* 1991;325:445-453.

149. Rothwell PM. Carotid artery disease and the risk of ischemic stroke and coronary vascular events. *Cerebrovasc Dis.* 2000;10:21-33.

150. Eliassziw M, Streifler JY, Fox AJ, Hachinski VC, Ferguson GG, Barnett HJM for the North American Symptomatic Carotid Endarterectomy Trial. Significance of plaque ulceration in symptomatic patients with high-grade carotid stenosis. *Stroke.* 1994;25:304-308.

151. Steinke W, Hennerici M, Rautenberg W, Mohr JP. Symptomatic and asymptomatic high-grade carotid stenoses in Doppler color-flow imaging. *Neurology.* 1992;42:131-138.

152. Lusby RJ, Ferrell LD, Ehrenfeld WK, Stoney RJ, Wylie EJ. Carotid plaque hemorrhage: its role in production of cerebral ischemia. *Arch Surg.* 1982;117:1479-1488.

153. Lovett JK, Redgrave JN, Rothwell PM. A critical appraisal of the performance, reporting, and interpretation of studies comparing carotid plaque imaging with histology. *Stroke.* 2005;36:1091-1097.

154. Kastelein JJ, de Groot E, Sankatsing R. Atherosclerosis measured by B-mode ultrasonography: effect of statin therapy on disease progression. *Am J Med.* 2004;116(suppl 6A):31S-36S.

155. Hodis HN, Mack WJ, LaBree L, et al. The role of carotid arterial intima-media thickness in predicting clinical coronary events. *Ann Intern Med.* 1998;128:262-269.

156. Blakeley DD, Oddone EZ, Hasselblad V, et al. Noninvasive carotid artery testing. A meta-analytic review. *Ann Intern Med.* 1995;122:360-367.

157. Grant EG, Benson CB, Moneta GL, et al. Carotid artery stenosis: gray-scale and Doppler US diagnosis—Society of Radiologists in Ultrasound Consensus Conference. *Radiology.* 2003;229:340-346.

158. Randomised trial of endarterectomy for recently symptomatic carotid stenosis: final results of the MRC European Carotid Surgery Trial (ECST). *Lancet.* 1998;351:1379-1387.

159. O'Boyle MK, Vibhakar NI, Chung J, et al. Duplex sonography of the carotid arteries in patients with isolated aortic stenosis: imaging findings and relation to the severity of stenosis. *AJR Am J Roentgenol.* 1996;166:197-202.

160. Perret RS, Sloop GD. Increased peak blood velocity in association with elevated blood pressure. *Ultrasound Med Biol.* 2000;26:1387-1391.

161. Hayes AC, Johnston KW, Baker WH, et al. The effect of contralateral disease on carotid Doppler frequency. *Surgery.* 1988;103:19-23.

162. Ray SA, Lockhart SJ, Dourado R, et al. Effect of contralateral disease on duplex measurements of internal carotid artery stenosis. *Br J Surg.* 2000;87:1057-1062.

163. AbuRahma AF, Robinson PA, Strickler DL, et al. Proposed new duplex classification for threshold stenoses used in various symptomatic and asymptomatic carotid endarterectomy trials. *Ann Vasc Surg.* 1998;12:349-358.

164. Busuttil SJ, Franklin DP, Youkey JR, Elmore JR. Carotid duplex overestimation of stenosis due to severe contralateral disease. *Am J Surg.* 1996;172:144-147.

165. Fujitani RM, Kafie F. Screening and preoperative imaging of candidates for carotid endarterectomy. *Semin Vasc Surg.* 1999;12:261-274.

166. Paivansalo M, Leinonen S, Turunen J, et al. Quantification of carotid artery stenosis with various Doppler velocity parameters. *Rofo Fortschr Geb Rontgenstr Neuen Bildgeb Verfahr.* 1996;164:108-113.

167. Sabeti S, Schillinger M, Mlekusch W, et al. Quantification of internal carotid artery stenosis with duplex US: comparative analysis of different flow velocity criteria. *Radiology.* 2004;232(2):431-439.

168. Moneta GL, Yeager RA, Dalman R, et al. Duplex ultrasound criteria for diagnosis of splanchnic artery stenosis or occlusion. *J Vasc Surg.* 1991;14:511-520.

169. Moneta GL, Lee RW, Yeager RA, et al. Mesenteric duplex scanning: a blinded prospective study. *J Vasc Technol.* 1991;15:37.

170. Lim HK, Lee WJ, Kim SH, et al. Splanchnic arterial stenosis or occlusion: diagnosis at Doppler US. *Radiology.* 1999; 211:405-410.

171. Bowersox JC, Zwolak RM, Walsh DB, et al. Duplex ultrasonography in the diagnosis of celiac and mesenteric artery occlusive disease. *J Vasc Surg.* 1991;14:780-788.

172. Zwolak RM. Can duplex ultrasound replace arteriography in screening for mesenteric ischemia? *Semin Vasc Surg.* 1999;12(4):252-260.

173. Erden A, Yurdakul M, Cumhur T. Doppler waveforms of the normal and collateralized inferior mesenteric artery. *Am J Roentgenol.* 1998;171(3):619-627.

174. Spencer MP, Whisler D. Transorbital Doppler diagnosis of intracranial arterial stenosis. *Stroke.* 1986;17:916.

175. Lederle FA, Johnson GR, Wilson SE, et al. The aneurysm detection and management study screening program: validation cohort and final results. Aneurysm Detection and Management Veterans Affairs Cooperative Study Investigators. *Arch Intern Med.* 2000;160:1425-1430.

176. Lindholt JS, Henneberg EW, Fasting H, et al. Hospital based screening of 65-73 year old men for abdominal aortic aneurysms in the county of Viborg, Denmark. *J Med Screen.* 1996;3:43-46.

177. Pleumeekers HJ, Hoes AW, Hofman A, et al. Selecting subjects for ultrasonographic screening for aneurysms of the abdominal aorta: four different strategies. *Int J Epidemiol.* 1999;28:682-686.

178. Ebaugh JL, Garcia ND, Matsumura JS. Screening and surveillance for abdominal aortic aneurysms: who needs it and when. *Semin Vasc Surg.* 2001;14:193-199.

179. Vazquez C, Sakalihasan N, D'Harcour JB, et al. Routine ultrasound screening for abdominal aortic aneurysm among 65- and 75-year-old men in a city of 200,000 inhabitants. *Ann Vasc Surg.* 1998;12:544-549.

180. Lindholt JS, Vammen S, Juul S, et al. The validity of ultrasonographic scanning as screening method for abdominal aortic aneurysm. *Eur J Vasc Endovasc Surg.* 1999;17:472-475.

181. Lamah M, Darke S. Value of routine computed tomography in the preoperative assessment of abdominal aneurysm replacement. *World J Surg.* 1999;23:1076-1080; discussion 1080-1081.

182. Fillinger MF. Imaging of the thoracic and thoracoabdominal aorta. *Semin Vasc Surg.* 2000;13:247-263.

183. Niederkorn K, Neumayer K. Transcranial Doppler sonography: a new approach in the non-invasive diagnosis of intracranial brain artery disease. *Eur Neurol.* 1987;26(2):65-68.

184. de Bray JM, Missoum A, Dubas F, Emile J, Lhoste P. Detection of vertebrobasilar intracranial stenoses: transcranial Doppler sonography versus angiography. *J Ultrasound Med.* 1997;16(3):213-218.

185. Felberg RA, Christou I, Demchuk AM, Malkoff M, Alexandrov AV. Screening for intracranial stenosis with transcranial Doppler: the accuracy of mean flow velocity thresholds. *J Neuroimaging.* 2002;12(1):9-14.

186. Rorick MB, Nichols FT, Adams RJ. Transcranial Doppler correlation with angiography in detection of intracranial stenosis. *Stroke.* 1994;25(10):1931-1934.

187. Demchuk AM, Burgin WS, Christou I, et al. Thrombolysis in brain ischemia (TIBI) transcranial Doppler flow grades predict clinical severity, early recovery, and mortality in patients treated with intravenous tissue plasminogen activator. *Stroke.* 2001;32(1):89-93.

188. Baumgartner RW, Mattle HP, Schroth G. Assessment of ≥50% and <50% intracranial stenoses by transcranial color-coded duplex sonography. *Stroke.* 1999;30(1):87-92.

189. Ringelstein EB, Kahlscheuer B, Niggemeyer E, Otis SM. Transcranial Doppler sonography: anatomical landmarks and normal velocity values. *Ultrasound Med Biol.* 1990;16(8):745-761.

190. Brandt T, Knauth M, Wildermuth S, et al. CT angiography and Doppler sonography for emergency assessment in acute basilar artery ischemia. *Stroke.* 1999;30(3):606-612.

191. Mattos MA, Hodgson KJ, Faught W. Carotid endarterectomy without angiography: is color-flow duplex scanning sufficient? *Surgery.* 1994;116:776-783.

192. Dawson D, Zierler R, Strandess DJ. The role of duplex scanning and arteriography before endarterectomy: a prospective study. *J Vasc Surg.* 1993;18:673-683.

193. Hollenberg NK. Medical therapy for renovascular hypertension: a review. *Am J Hypertens.* 1988;1:338S-343S.

194. Mailloux LU, Napolitano B, Bellucci AG. Renal vascular disease causing end-stage renal disease, incidence, clinical correlates, and outcomes: a 20-year clinical experience. *Am J Kidney Dis.* 1994;24:622-629.

195. Eidt J, Fry R, Clagett G. Postoperative follow-up of renal artery reconstruction with duplex ultrasound. *J Vasc Surg.* 1988;8:667-673.

chapter 18

Magnetic Resonance Imaging in Peripheral Arterial Disease

Christopher Francois, MD / James C. Carr, MD / Alex J. Auseon, DO

● INTRODUCTION

Basic Principles and Physics

Magnetic resonance imaging (MRI) in clinical use relies on two fundamental principles: the excess of hydrogen molecules in water contained in the tissues of the human body (a) and (b) the phenomenon of magnetic resonance, specifically the magnetlike behavior of these protons that causes them to align and spin at a predictable frequency within an external magnetic field. This alignment occurs when a stationary field is applied by the superconducting magnet as the patient lies within the bore. For each imaging sequence, a smaller secondary set of coils within the bore produce rapid bursts of gradient magnetic fields that cause protons to transiently tilt off-axis. As these protons relax from their high-energy state to their original alignment within the static magnetic field, a radiofrequency signal is emitted from the patient and absorbed by the receiving coils strapped directly to the patient in the anatomic area being imaged (Figure 18-1). The characteristics of this signal are deciphered by the computer using complex algorithms to generate an image.

Although MRI has an excellent signal-to-noise ratio (SNR) allowing for superb tissue differentiation, additional clinical information is commonly obtained by using intravenous contrast agents. While several classes have been developed, only gadolinium-based agents are in clinical use in peripheral arterial imaging. Gadolinium is a toxic element, requiring a chelating agent before it can be employed in medical use. Once injected intravenously, it specifically shortens the T1 relaxation period of protons, resulting in an increased signal seen as a brightened structure on the MR image. Consequently, it has become an indispensable tool for imaging the vascular system. Compared with iodinated x-ray contrast, gadolinium-based agents are relatively benign and adverse reactions are rare. A relatively new manifestation of gadolinium-associated adverse reactions, nephrogenic systemic fibrosis (NSF), has been observed in patients with renal disease who receive contrast for MRI studies. Patients primarily experience thickening and tightening of the skin, but reports also describe involvement of the liver, lungs, muscles, and heart. Thus far, only 57 cases have been reported to the Food and Drug Administration, but these have prompted recommendations to minimize the use of gadolinium contrast agents in patients with advanced kidney disease as much as possible.[1,2]

While the lack of ionizing radiation in MRI compares favorably to x-ray methods, it does carry its own specific safety concerns. The large, superconducting magnet has potential to attract and/or interfere with all ferromagnetic objects within a sufficient distance. These include equipment within the MRI suite (oxygen canisters, IV poles, etc.) and devices implanted within the patient (pacemakers, defibrillators, TENS units, etc). It has been established that most types of cardiovascular stents, prosthetic heart valves, orthopedic implants, and surgical clips are safe, although in all instances, physician discretion is required to insure patient safety. While recent data have demonstrated that patients with pacemakers and defibrillators can be scanned safely with specific monitoring safeguards, these devices remain a strong relative contraindication to MRI.

The application of MRI to the peripheral arterial system has evolved significantly because of improvements in hardware and scanning techniques. In particular, high-performance magnetic field gradients allow very rapid image acquisition, and contrast-enhanced (CE) imaging

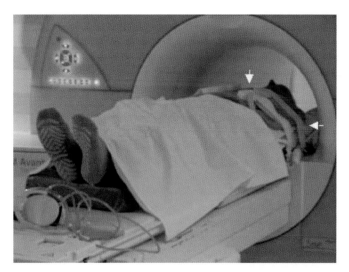

● **FIGURE 18-1.** Patient being placed into MRI scanner with receiving coils placed over the chest (arrows) for MRA of the thoracic aorta.

techniques have dramatically increased spatial resolution and the amount of data that can be acquired. Magnetic resonance angiography (MRA), in particular, offers several advantages when compared to conventional x-ray angiography or computed tomography angiography (CTA). MRA is minimally or noninvasive, acquires three-dimensional (3D) information, allows evaluation of structures outside of the vessel lumen, and perhaps most importantly, requires no radiation exposure or nephrotoxic, iodinated contrast.

There are several techniques used to perform an MR examination of the peripheral arterial system. These include time-of-flight (TOF), phase contrast (PC), black-blood, and contrast-enhanced MRA (CE-MRA) techniques. While these techniques are vastly different, all can be used to create MR images of the vasculature and use gradient-recalled echo (GRE) sequences. More recently, single-shot balanced, steady-state free precession techniques (SSFP) have been employed as a rapid means of evaluating the vasculature.

Techniques

Time-of-Flight MRA. Of the three MRA techniques, TOF has been in clinical use the longest and is still frequently used to image the intracranial vasculature.[3–5] TOF imaging requires both suppression of background signal and generation of signal from flowing blood. Rapid slice-selective radiofrequency excitation pulses are used to saturate the signal from stationary tissue, making them appear dark. Blood flowing into the imaging slice appears bright because it has not been exposed to the saturation pulse. The signal intensity of blood in TOF imaging increases as the flow velocity in the vessel increases. Problems can arise in TOF imaging when blood flow is so slow that blood exposed to the saturation pulse does not exit the imaging volume. TOF can

also be difficult when imaging tortuous vessels or vessels that are in the same plane as the imaging volume because of signal from the remaining suppressed blood.

Because arteries and veins usually travel together, signal from veins can obscure visualization of the adjacent arteries. To suppress the signal in the veins, a saturation pulse is applied above the desired imaging volume such that blood in veins will travel into the imaging volume without signal.[3,4] Similar techniques can be used to suppress unwanted signal because of motion of the diaphragm during respiration or the heart during the cardiac cycle.

TOF can be performed as either a two-dimensional (2D) or 3D acquisition. Where 3D acquisition is best performed in areas with relatively high flowing blood, 2D acquisitions are best in areas of slow flowing blood or areas that could be affected by respiratory motion. 3D TOF is higher resolution than 2D TOF and is less susceptible to signal loss in areas of turbulent flow.

Phase-Contrast MR. Phase contrast MR (PC-MR) uses the differences in speed, or phase shift, between magnetic spins moving in blood and spins in stationary tissue.[6,7] In contrast to TOF and CE-MRA techniques, PC-MR can be used to quantify flow velocities in addition to being used to generate angiographic images. Quantification of flow velocities with PC-MRA can be performed because the phase shift between mobile and stationary magnetic spins is linearly dependent on the flow velocity.

PC-MR is predominantly used to identify direction of flow and to quantify flow velocities and volumes through a specified area (Figure 18-2). It also has the advantage, compared to TOF, of improved background suppression, allowing imaging of smaller vessels and larger volumes, in addition to improved imaging of vascular structures with slow flow, such as vascular malformations and veins. However, PC-MR sequences usually have longer acquisition times and are more sensitive to magnetic field heterogeneities.

Dark-Blood Imaging. Dark-blood MR imaging techniques are used to image the vessel wall because of the high-contrast resolution of these sequences (Figure 18-3). Presaturation bands are used to null the signal of flowing blood within a vessel. As a result, high-velocity flowing blood will appear black because of the lack of signal as the blood flows into the imaging volume. Because of this, dark-blood techniques can suffer from artifacts when blood flow is slow, such as in a large aneurysm, when a patient has a very low cardiac output, or in the false lumen of a dissection. In these cases, slow flowing blood may mimic thrombosis or other pathologic findings.

Contrast-Enhanced MRA. With the development of CE-MRA techniques, MR angiography has significantly improved in quality and clinical acceptance.[8,9] CE-MRA sequences exploit the effect of gadolinium-based contrast agents on the T1 relaxation time of blood, greatly increasing the intensity of the detected signal compared to

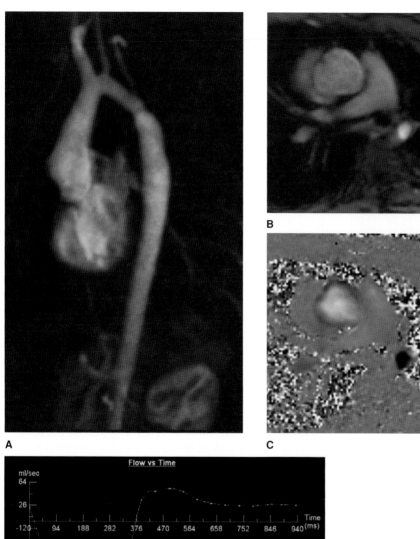

● **FIGURE 18-2.** MIP image (A) from a contrast-enhanced MRA performed in a patient with a history of repaired coarctation of the aorta. Magnitude (B) and phase contrast (C) images obtained at the level of the coarctation repair (line on image A). By placing regions of interest over the vessel on the images throughout the cardiac cycle and measuring the velocity at each phase, one can generate velocity-time or flow-time curves (D).

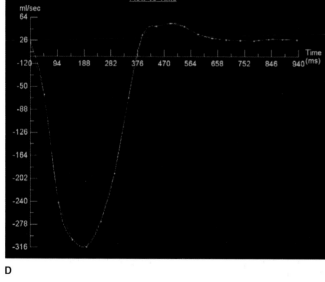

surrounding structures. Successful CE-MRA requires synchronization of image acquisition to the first pass of contrast material through the vessels of interest. As a result, extremely fast imaging sequences are used to acquire a 3D volume data set.

Several strategies have been implemented for timing of image acquisition. Test bolus injection of a small volume (2–3 mL) of contrast allows calculation of the delay from the time of injection to the time of contrast arrival in the region of interest. Another technique uses rapid, thin-slice acquisition to automatically detect the arrival of contrast prior to initiation of 3D CE-MRA acquisition.[10,11] More recently, dynamic, time-resolved CE-MRA techniques have been developed that allow one to obtain multiple 3D volumes, similar to conventional angiography[12–14] (Figure 18-4). After acquiring the images, one can select the 3D volume

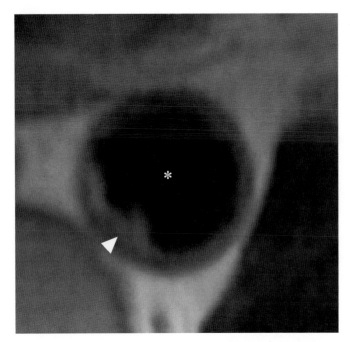

● **FIGURE 18-3.** Dark-blood image of the descending thoracic aorta. The vessel wall is clearly delineated against the nulled blood signal in the lumen (asterisk), and a moderate amount of atheroslcerotic plaque is present (arrow).

Steady-State Free Precession. SSFP is a noncontrast, bright-blood cine imaging technique utilized to view tissue morphology and blood flow through vascular structures. It is most commonly employed as an adjunct to dark-blood, PC-MR, and CE-MRA techniques and is an improvement from earlier forms of cine imaging using gradient-recalled echo sequences. Areas of high-velocity flow may produce some artifact, but it is a relatively simple and reproducible technique yielding quality motion images.

Postprocessing and Image Interpretation. Because multiple image sets are usually acquired during an MRA study, several methods have been developed to present the data in a manner more familiar to the clinician. However, any finding detected on these manipulated images needs to be confirmed on the original source images. Methods used to reconstruct the images include multiplanar reformatted (MPR) (Figure 18-5), maximum intensity projection (MIP), and volume rendered (VR) methods[18] (Figure 18-6). MPR involves reconstruction of the 3D data set on a computer workstation in any imaging plane, permitting the viewer to display the vessel along its longitudinal axis. Because vessels often curve in and out of a given plane, MIP methods combine data from multiple planes to produce images resembling those of conventional angiography. A limitation of MIP images is related to the fact that low-signal-intensity pixels at the edge of a vessel are lost because of automatic thresholds used in the image reconstruction. Therefore, the lumen diameter will appear smaller than in actuality, contributing to the overestimation of the degree of stenosis often noted in MRA. VR, or surface rendered, reconstructions are most useful for viewing the surface of vessels and for evaluating the 3D relationships of vessels and their surrounding structures.

that best demonstrates the vessel of interest. This last technique is useful when flow is asymmetric or to assess vessels at different points in time.[15]

While CE-MRA techniques are less susceptible to artifacts than other MRA sequences, artifacts do occur.[16,17] As with all MR sequences, CE-MRA is prone to susceptibility artifacts from metallic devices i.e., clips, stents, and prostheses. The degree of artifact depends on the ferromagnetic content of the material used to make the device. Incorrect timing of image acquisition can lead to opacification of veins in addition to arteries. If too many veins are opacified, evaluation of the arteries can be more difficult. Wraparound artifact occurs when the imaged volume does not include the entire volume of the patient's body at that level. If not enough contrast material is used, the SNR may be insufficient to accurately evaluate vascular anatomy.

● **CEREBROVASCULAR APPLICATIONS**

TOF, PC, and CE-MRA techniques are used to evaluate the intracranial and cervical vasculature. TOF-MRA can be performed as a 2D or 3D acquisition. 2D TOF-MRA involves the acquisition of multiple thin, contiguous, or overlapping slices, which are then combined to create a volume of MRA data. The images can then be viewed in an axial

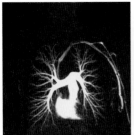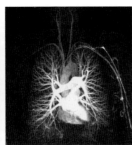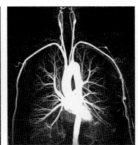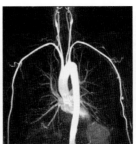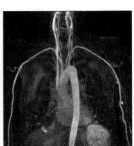

● **FIGURE 18-4.** Coronal MIP images from a time-resolved, dynamic, contrast-enhanced MRA of the chest. Each image took 3 seconds to acquire.

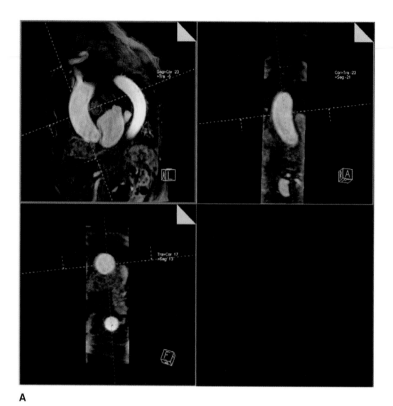

A

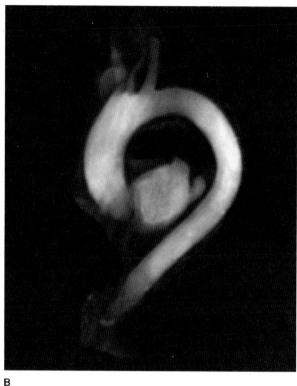

B

● **FIGURE 18-5.** Image from computer workstation demonstrating how multiplanar reformatted images are created from a 3D contrast-enhanced MRA data set (A). Sagittal-oblique MPR image of the thoracic aorta (B).

plane or by using image projection techniques mentioned previously, such as MIP, MPR, or VR. While 2D TOF is very sensitive to slow flowing blood, it can be very time consuming to perform. 3D TOF-MRA is faster than 2D TOF and has higher spatial resolution and more optimal SNR. However, 3D TOF is less sensitive to slow flowing blood. Another TOF technique, known as multiple overlapping thin-slab TOF combines aspects of both 2D and 3D methods. Multiple thick slabs are acquired contiguously and combined to create the full volume.

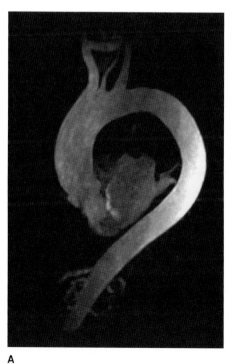

A

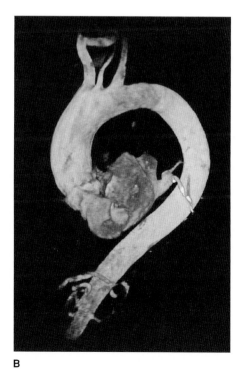

B

● **FIGURE 18-6.** MIP (A) and VR (B) images from a contrast-enhanced MRA of the thoracic aorta.

PC-MRA can produce cross-sectional images superior to those produced with TOF imaging because of the superior background suppression with PC imaging. In addition, PC-MRA allows one to calculate flow velocities through stenoses. However, these sequences are more susceptible to patient motion and artifacts related to turbulent flow than TOF sequences and take longer to acquire than comparable TOF-MRA sequences.

CE-MRA is predominantly used to evaluate the aortic arch and cervical vessels.[19] Bolus-timing or time-resolved CE-MRA techniques can be used for cervical and intracranial CE-MRA. Newer, stronger magnetic field gradients permit more rapid MRA acquisition, permitting imaging of exclusively arterial phase studies.

Intracranial Circulation

Atherosclerotic Disease. MRA is frequently performed at the same time as MRI of the brain in patients who have had a stroke or transient ischemic attack (TIA) to evaluate for the presence of occlusive atherosclerotic disease. A combination of TOF and CE-MRA techniques are used to visualize the intracranial vasculature[20] (Figures 18-7 and 18-8). MRA has a reported sensitivity of 80% to 100% and specificity of 80% to 99% for detecting stenoses of 50% or

greater in the proximal intracranial circulation. As in other areas of the body, MRA of the intracranial arteries tends to overestimate the degree of stenosis. In areas of focally severe stenosis, TOF-MRA can make a vessel appear occluded because of spin dephasing and acceleration in the area of stenosis.

Aneurysms. Although MRA is an attractive modality for identifying intracranial aneurysms because it is relatively noninvasive and does not use ionizing radiation,[21,22] it is somewhat limited by slightly lower-spatial resolution than conventional angiography and CTA. The spatial resolution of 3D TOF-MRA techniques is approximately 0.8 mm. It is commonly used to image the circle of Willis and to detect small (3–5 mm) intracranial aneurysms. The ability of MRA to detect aneurysms smaller than 3 mm is still limited, although studies have shown that these rarely rupture. MRA is also limited in its ability to accurately detect and define small branch vessels that can arise from or near intracranial aneurysms. However, evaluation of giant saccular aneurysms is an area where MRA may be superior to digital subtraction angiography (DSA).

Despite the previously mentioned limitations, MRI of the head and MRA of the head and neck are crucial in

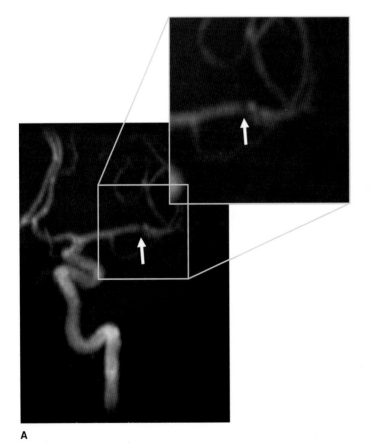
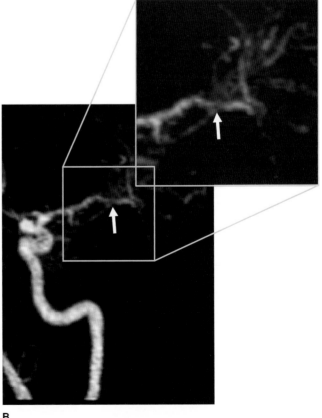

A

B

● **FIGURE 18-7.** (A) Time-of-flight and (B) contrast-enhanced MIP images from an MRA study in a patient with a left middle cerebral artery (MCA) territory stroke caused by focal severe stenosis in the distal MCA (arrows).

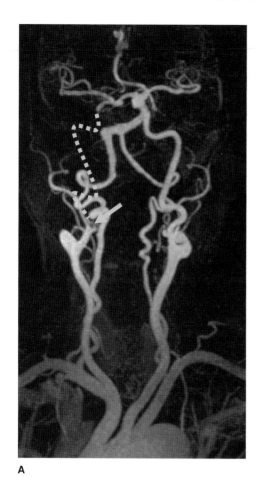

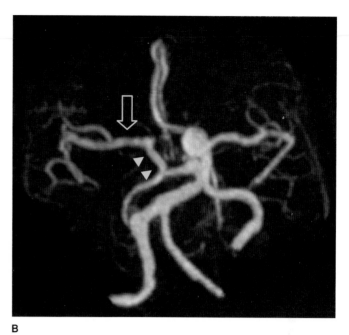

● **FIGURE 18-8.** (A) Contrast-enhanced MRA of the cervical and intracranial circulation in a patient with an occluded right internal carotid artery, just distal to the carotid artery bifurcation (arrow). The dashed line represents the expected location of the occluded right internal carotid artery. (B) The right middle cerebral artery (open arrow) fills via flow from the right posterior communicating artery (arrowheads).

the preintervention evaluation of patients with intracranial aneurysms (Figure 18-9). MRA has also been used to screen patients with an increased risk of intracranial aneurysms: patients with polycystic kidney disease, cerebral arteriovenous malformations (AVM), fibromuscular dysplasia, aortic coarctation, connective tissue disorders, and a family history of subarachnoid hemorrhage or aneurysms. Previous retrospective and prospective studies evaluating the sensitivity and specificity of MRI and MRA for the detection of intracranial aneurysms have found sensitivities of 69% to 99% and a specificity of 100%.[22] Sensitivies are lower for smaller aneurysms. Newer, faster CE-MRA techniques can image the intracranial circulation with contrast opacification of the arteries without venous contamination. Also, MRA at 3.0 T may be more sensitive at detecting small aneurysms than MRA at 1.5 T.[23,24]

MRI and MRA are routinely used to follow patients who have had surgical or percutaneous interventions for intracranial aneurysms.[25,26] Because the clips and endovascular coils used to treat aneurysms are not ferromagnetic, MR imaging is not affected by artifact as is seen with CT scan angiography in these patients.

Vascular Malformations. 3D TOF and CE-MRA techniques can be used to diagnose and characterize intracranial vascular malformations. In the case of AVM, MRA is used to identify feeding arteries, AVM nidus, and draining veins and to accurately measure the size of the lesion. MRI most accurately depicts the relationship of the AVM to the adjacent cerebral anatomy and the best 3D representation of the malformation. Limitations of MRA in evaluating AVMs include imaging flow in tortuous feeding arteries, differentiating blood flow from methemoglobin in a subacute hematoma, and poor conspicuity of slower flowing venous blood distal to the AVM. Despite these limitations, MRA is the preferred imaging modality for the pretreatment evaluation of patients with AVMs.

Carotid Arterial Disease

MRA of the carotid arteries was initially performed using 2D and 3D TOF sequences. These techniques have been largely replaced with CE-MRA techniques, which have short image acquisition times and are less prone to overestimation of stenosis. Both timing-bolus and time-resolved

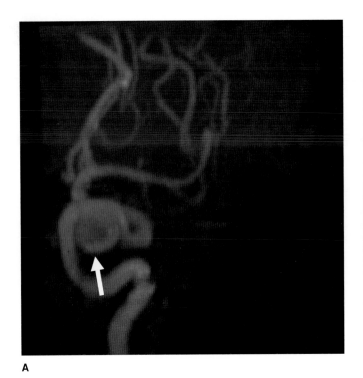

A

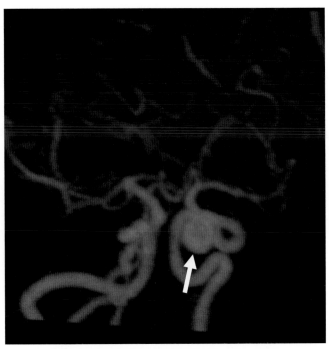

B

● **FIGURE 18-9.** MIP images from (A) time-of-flight and (B) contrast-enhanced MRA studies in a patient with a left internal carotid artery aneurysm.

techniques of performing CE-MRA have been evaluated for the detection and grading of carotid artery stenosis. These techniques are attractive because of their ability to image the carotid arteries without venous contamination. The sensitivity and specificity of MRA for carotid artery atherosclerotic disease are above 90%.[27–30] In addition to atherosclerotic disease, CE-MRA plays a significant role in the diagnosis of extracranial arterial dissections, allowing accurate visualization of intimal flaps and luminal flow[31] (Figure 18-10).

● **THORACIC APPLICATIONS**

Thoracic Aorta

Outside of the head and neck, the most commonly imaged vessel is the aorta. MRA is particularly useful when imaging the thoracic aorta to evaluate for the presence of aneurysms or acute aortic syndromes (AAS).[31,33] Typically, non-CE-MR techniques are acquired initially to obtain a quick assessment of the vasculature.[34] Non-CE cine MR imaging using SSFP can also be used to diagnose aortic pathology. Black-blood imaging reveals details of the vessel wall that may be useful in selected cases where inflammatory disease, atherosclerosis, or intramural hematoma (IMH) are suspected. CE-MRA techniques are then performed at the end of the examination. Because of the effects of cardiac motion on the thoracic aorta, especially in the root and ascending aorta, images are usually acquired using cardiac gating—a technique that requires image acquisition during the same phase of the cardiac cycle.

High resolution CE-MRA images of the aorta are obtained in a sagittal oblique orientation, allowing image acquisition in a single breath-hold. Because 3D techniques are used, resolution is isotropic and images can be reconstructed in any plane. As a result, highly accurate orthogonal measurements of the size of the aorta can be made at any level.

Aneurysms. MR angiography is often used in the initial work-up of patients with dilated thoracic aortas because it can accurately quantify the size and morphology of the aorta,[32–34] which is necessary in planning either surgical or endovascular repair (Figure 18-11). In addition, CE-MRA can accurately demonstrate the relationship of an aneurysm to major branch vessels, which is critical in deciding the therapeutic alternatives. Because patients with thoracic aortic aneurysms often require close follow-up to monitor progression, MRA is an ideal imaging modality because it does not require the use of iodinated contrast material and does not expose the patient to unnecessary ionizing radiation. Studies have shown that MRA can be used as the only imaging study prior to surgical or endovascular repair. Nonangiographic MR sequences (black-blood or SSFP) play a complementary role in the evaluation of aortic aneurysms because of the ability to detect thrombus within the aneurysm and perianeurysmal fluid that might suggest infection or rupture.[32,33]

Aneurysm morphology can also be characterized with MRI. Atherosclerotic aneurysms are typically fusiform and occur in the arch and descending thoracic aorta. Fusiform aneurysms isolated to the ascending aorta are most

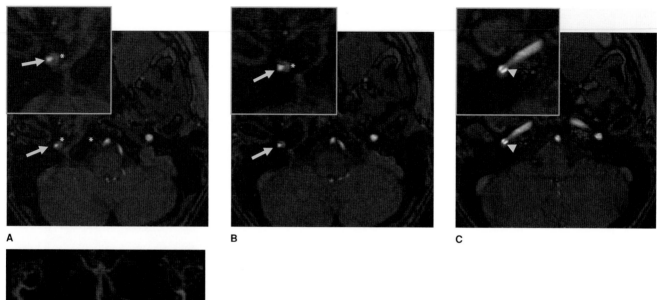

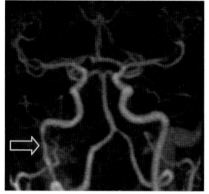

● FIGURE 18-10. Axial source images from a 3D time-of-flight MRA (A-C) in a patient with a right internal carotid artery (ICA) dissection demonstrate asymmetry in the caliber of right and left ICAs, right smaller than left (arrows); crescent-shaped hypointense signal surrounding the true lumen of the right ICA (A,B, asterisks) corresponding to slow flow in the false lumen; and a linear signal void within the right ICA (C, arrowhead), corresponding to the intimal flap. Contrast-enhanced MRA in the same patient reveal irregularity in the caliber of the right ICA (D) as a result of the dissection (open arrow).

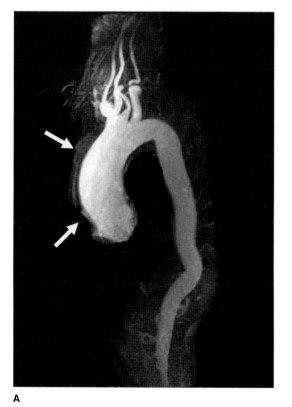

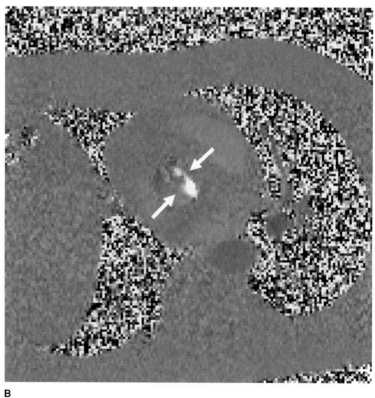

● FIGURE 18-11. (A) MIP image from a contrast-enhanced MRA study in a patient with an ascending aortic aneurysm and stenotic bicuspid aortic valve which can be further evaluated with phase-contrast imaging (B).

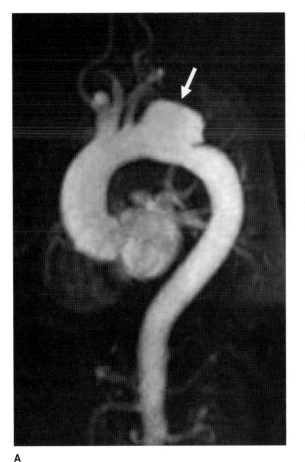
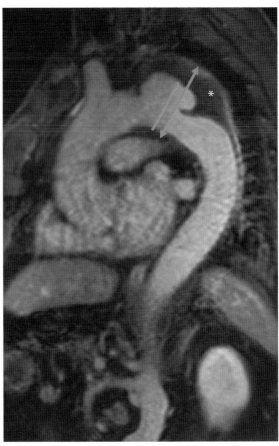

A   B

● **FIGURE 18-12.** (A) Sagittal-oblique MMIP image from a contrast-enhanced MRA study in a patient with a saccular aneurysm of the distal aortic arch (arrow). (B) Sagittal-oblique T1-weighted gradient-echo image obtained after the administration of intravenous contrast demonstrates a large amount of intra-aneurysmal thrombus (asterisk) and the true size of the aneurysm (double arrow) compared to the size that would be measured from the MRA (line).

commonly caused by cystic medial necrosis associated with syphilis or aortic valve disease. Saccular aneurysms arise at the site of a previous penetrating atherosclerotic ulcer and pseudoaneurysms are secondary to trauma, infection, or surgery (Figure 18-12).

Acute Aortic Syndromes. Patients with suspected AAS such as IMH, penetrating ulcer, or dissection, can be accurately evaluated with MRA (Figure 18-13). IMH will appear as crescent-shaped mural thickening on MR imaging.[35] The signal intensity of the hematoma will vary depending on the age of type of hemoglobin present. In the acute phase, an IMH will appear hyperintense on both T1- and T2-weighted sequences. To distinguish the increased signal in the aortic wall because of hemorrhage from the adjacent periaortic fat, dark-blood fat suppression techniques must be used. The normal thickness of the aortic wall by MR is approximately 3 mm. In the appropriate clinical setting, a mural thickness greater than 5 mm should suggest the diagnosis of IMH.

Penetrating ulcers are radiographically defined as a focal contour abnormality of the vessel wall containing contrast

in communication with the lumen. They occur at the site of an atherosclerotic plaque and usually in the descending aorta. Penetrating ulcers can be equally evaluated with noncontrast enhanced MR techniques and CE-MRA.[32] In addition to the focal ulceration, a variable degree of intramural hemorrhage may be present.

The role of MRA in patients with aortic dissections includes determining the location and extent, distinguishing between the true and false lumens, and assessing branch vessel involvement. In evaluating patients with suspected AAS, the sensitivity and specificity of MRA is >95%.[32,33] The diagnosis of a dissection is made when an intimal flap can be visualized between the true and false lumens. Because the appearance of an intimal flap varies considerably, it is important to review the raw data, MPR images, and MIP images. Time resolved CE-MRA can be used to show differences in flow between the two lumens, with delayed contrast opacification of the false lumen compared to the true lumen. Occasionally, the entry and exit points of the dissection can be visualized with MRA.

MRA has also been shown to be highly accurate in following patients for complications following surgical or

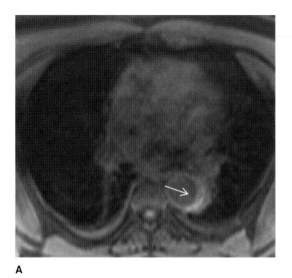
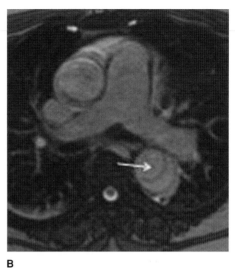
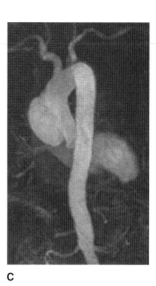

A   B   C

● **FIGURE 18-13.** (A) MRI in a patient with an intramural hematoma (IMH) in the descending thoracic aorta. The IMH is hyperintense on this precontrast, fat-suppressed T1-weighted image (arrow). (B) MRI in a patient with a dissection of the descending thoracic aorta. The intimal flap separating the true and false lumens is seen as a curved hypointense line on this axial balanced-SSFP image (arrow). (C) CE-MRA in a patient with a dissection of the ascending thoracic aorta.

endovascular therapy.[36,37] MRA is often preferred over CTA in patients who are likely to have frequent follow-up examinations, such as young adults, and in patients with renal insufficiency. Complications following surgical repair can occur in or near the graft, hematoma, pseudoaneurysm, or anastamotic stenosis, or in the native aorta and its branch vessels, leading to extension of a dissection proximally or distally, true lumen collapse, false lumen thrombosis, or pseudoaneurysm. Accurate measurements of luminal diameters on follow-up MRAs are necessary to detect anastamotic stenoses before they become symptomatic. Following aortic repair, it is normal to have concentric thickening around the graft. This is in contrast to a pathologic hematoma which may be asymmetric and heterogeneous in signal intensity. Studies have shown that the thickness of the periprosthetic hematoma on the first postoperative examination has prognostic significance. A hematoma that is greater than 15 mm in thickness has a higher probability of becoming a pseudoaneurysm, usually occurring in an area of suture dehiscence. This is demonstrated on CE-MRA images as a focal, saccular collection of contrast material outside of the graft lumen.

Coarctation. Both non-CE and CE-MRA techniques are used to assess aortic coarctations.[38,39] Because of the high spatial resolution of 3D CE-MRA, this technique is used for accurate morphologic assessment (Figure 18-14). Using a computer workstation, orthogonal measurements of the aorta can be made at multiple locations proximal and distal to the coarctation. PC-MRA can be used to quantify flow rates and flow velocities proximal and distal to the coarctation as well. Recently, the minimal cross-sectional area and the mean deceleration of flow in the descending aorta

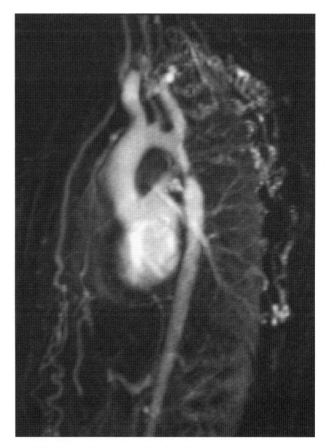

● **FIGURE 18-14.** Contrast-enhanced MRA in a 26-year-old patient with a history of unrepaired aortic coarctation. Numerous dilated collateral arteries are visualized.

have been found to be highly predictive of a moderate or severe coarctation gradient (≥20 mm Hg), when compared to pressure measurements made with catheter angiography. These measurements can then be used to follow patients prior to and after treatment. PC-MRA, when performed at the level of the aortic valve, can also be used to detect a bicuspid aortic valve, a relatively commonly associated finding in patients with aortic coarctation.

Vasculitis

Newer MRI and CE-MRA techniques allow higher spatial and contrast resolution imaging of the aorta, including the aortic wall. As a result, MR imaging is routinely utilized during diagnostic testing of patients with vasculitides, particularly in those affecting larger vessels, such as giant cell arteritis and Takayasu's arteritis.[31,32,40,41] MRA and dark-blood sequences of patients with Takayasu's arteritis, in addition to demonstrating the degree of luminal narrowing, will detail segmental thickening of the vessel wall, mural thrombus, inflammatory changes in the periaortic fat, vascular dilatation, and stenoses (Figure 18-15). Recently, delayed CE-MRI techniques, similar to those used to assess myocardial viability in the heart, have been used to characterize the degree of inflammation in the aortic wall of patients with Takayasu's arteritis. MRI with cine imaging of the heart can also be used to evaluate the effect of the disease on cardiovascular function. In addition to imaging at

the time of presentation, MRA can be used to assess patient response to therapy.

● ABDOMINAL APPLICATIONS

Abdominal Aorta

CE-MRA of the abdominal aorta is ideally performed in the coronal plane so that all of the aorta and its major branch vessels are included in the imaged volume. Because the abdominal aorta is not oriented straight in the craniocaudal direction, it is important to ensure that the imaging volume will not inadvertently exclude any portion of the aorta or branch vessels of interest. In addition to acquiring CE-MRA images of the abdominal aorta, a complete MR examination will also include other sequences to evaluate the characteristics of the vessel wall, the periaortic soft tissues, and the visceral organs.

Aneurysms. CE-MRA is sufficient to evaluate the abdominal aorta for the presence of abdominal aortic aneurysms (AAA).[8,9,42] Preprocedural planning for endovascular repair of abdominal aortic aneurysms requires accurate and reproducible angiographic images. CE-MRA has been shown to be a viable alternative to CTA or DSA as the sole imaging technique prior to endovascular stent-graft treatment. Postcontrast, T1-weighted images will demonstrate a thickened, enhancing aneurysmal wall with infiltration

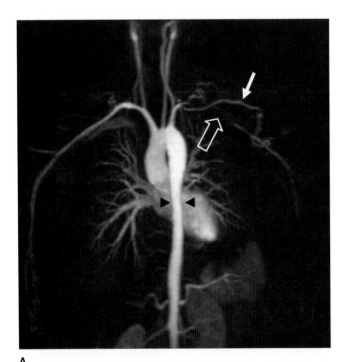

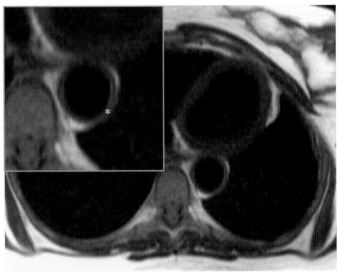

A

B

● **FIGURE 18-15.** (A) Contrast-enhanced MRA in a young woman with a history of Takayasu's arteritis. The mid-descending thoracic aorta is narrowed (black arrowheads) and the left subclavian artery is occluded (open arrow). Large collateral arteries have developed to provide flow to the left upper extremity (arrow). (B) An axial T1-weighted, dark-blood image in another patient with Takayasu's aortitis demonstrates circumferential thickening of the aortic wall (asterisk).

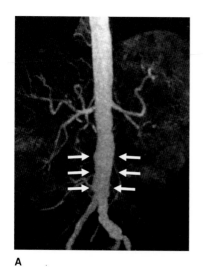
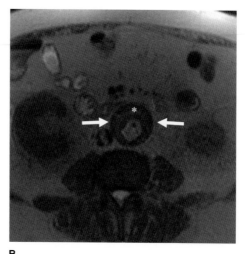
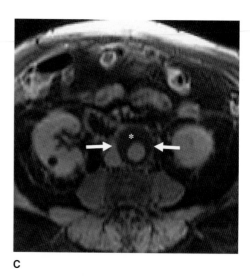

A   B   C

● **FIGURE 18-16.** (A) MIP image from a contrast-enhanced MRA study in a patient with a 49 mm × 47 mm abdominal aortic aneurysm (AAA). The true size of the AAA (arrows) is underestimated on the MIP when compared to the diameter based on the axial T2-weighted, precontrast (B) and T1-weighted, postcontrast (C) images because of the large amount of mural thrombus in the aneurysm (asterisk).

of the perianeurysmal fat. CE-MRA is used to accurately measure the maximum diameter, the length, the angulation, and the involvement of branch vessels (Figure 18-16).

MRA is also used to follow patients after endovascular stent-graft placement to ensure that the aneurysm continues to decrease in size and to detect complications.[43–46] Several studies have indicated that MRA may be more sensitive than CTA at detecting endoleaks in patients that have received nonferromagnetic stents. MRA is used to follow patients after surgical repair as well because of its ability to accurately document the presence of hematomas, pseudoaneurysms, infection, or fistulas between the aorta and surrounding structures.

Atherosclerotic Disease. The evaluation of the abdominal aorta and the visceral arteries for atherosclerotic disease is accurately performed using CE-MRA techniques[47,48] (Figures 18-17 and 18-18). Because the arterial access necessary for invasive angiography can be difficult in patients with arterial occlusive disease, CE-MRA is an ideal imaging modality to evaluate these patients. CE-MRA is used to determine the extent of occlusion and to identify collateral flow to the lower extremities. Occlusion usually occurs at the level of the bifurcation and occurs over an extended period of time so that extensive collateral vessels have time to develop. CE-MRA is also used in these situations to identify and characterize appropriate target vessels prior to revascularization. Further characterization of vessel wall atheroma burden and remodeling can be obtained with dark-blood imaging.

Renal Arteries

MRA is an accurate and safe technique for evaluating the main renal artery. High sensitivities (85%–100%) and speci-

ficities (86%–100%) have been reported for the detection of hemodynamically significant (>50%) renal artery stenosis when compared to DSA.[49–51] Because of the smaller size of the renal arteries, grading of renal artery stenosis with MRA is typically done using qualitative (normal, mild, moderate, severe) descriptors rather than quantitative measures. The accuracy of CE-MRA is greater for stenoses located in the proximal renal artery, where its diameter is largest. Because of the effects of respiratory motion, CE-MRA techniques are preferred over TOF and PC techniques. Although CE-MRA provides an accurate morphologic image of the renal vasculature, it cannot provide physiologic or hemodynamic information. Using dynamic, time-resolved CE-MRA one can evaluate asymmetry in the timing of renal enhancement suggesting a physiologically significant renal artery stenosis.

MRA is also a widely accepted modality for evaluating renal arterial anatomy prior to kidney transplantation.[52] Because no ionizing radiation or iodinated contrast are used, MRA is preferred over DSA or CTA when imaging renal donors prior to surgery. There is evidence that MRA may demonstrate a greater number of vascular anomalies than DSA. In addition, MR imaging can demonstrate other renal abnormalities (cysts, masses, etc.) that may not be as clearly evident on DSA.

Because of the lower spatial resolution of MRA compared with DSA and CTA, evaluation of patients with suspected fibromuscular dysplasia has been less reliable, especially in evaluating the distal renal arteries. 3D techniques permit accurate assessment of size, location, and anatomic relationships of AVM and renal artery aneurysms. Because of the rapid flow from renal artery to renal vein in AVMs and AVFs, CE-MRA will demonstrate early filling of the draining vein.

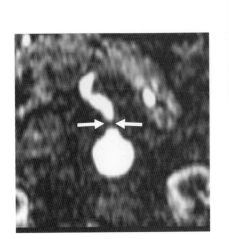
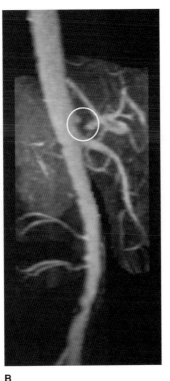
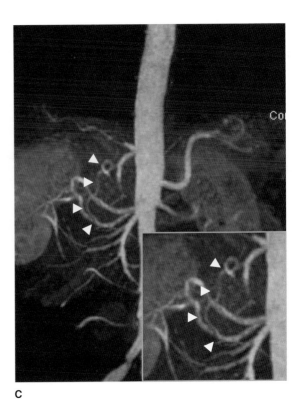

A

B

C

● **FIGURE 18-17.** (A) Axial source image from a contrast-enhanced (CE) MRA study in a patient with celiac artery occlusion (arrows). MIP images from the same study confirm occlusion of the celiac artery (B, circle) and filling of the celiac artery via superior mesenteric artery collaterals (C, arrowheads and inset).

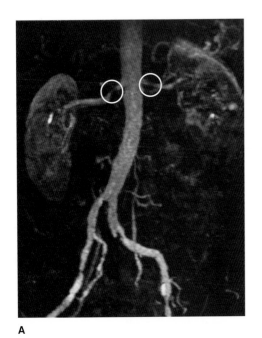
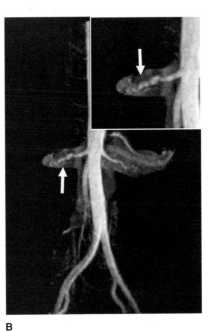
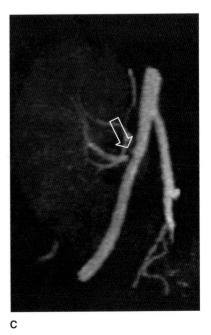

A

B

C

● **FIGURE 18-18.** (A) Contrast-enhanced (CE) MRA in a patient with atherosclerosis involving the renal and iliac arteries. Severe stenoses are present in both renal arteries (circles). (B) CE-MRA in a patient with uncontrollable hypertension caused by fibromuscular dysplasia, as noted by the serpiginous contour of the right renal artery (arrows, inset). (C) CE-MRA in a patient with a right iliac fossa renal transplant, uncontrollable hypertension, and rising serum creatinine levels demonstrates a focal severe stenosis at the anastamosis of the renal transplant artery to the right common iliac artery (open arrow).

Mesenteric Arteries

The most common indication for the evaluation of the mesenteric arteries with MRA is for mesenteric ischemia caused by atherosclerotic disease, although MRA is also used to evaluate for tumor encasement in patients prior to liver transplantation, and anatomic assessment prior to surgical shunt creation. CE-MRA is the most widely utilized MRA technique in the abdomen because of the effects of respiratory and bowel motion. Multiple CE-MRA data sets are acquired to visualize both the arterial and venous anatomy.

Because of the longer imaging times required with MRA, CTA is usually preferred for the evaluation of patients with suspected acute mesenteric ischemia. However, in patients with chronic mesenteric ischemia, either CTA or MRA can be used.[53,54] Studies suggest MRA may have sensitivities and specificities greater than 90% when diagnosing chronic mesenteric ischemia. MRA may be less accurate at diagnosing inferior mesenteric artery disease because of its smaller size.

● EXTREMITY APPLICATIONS

Atherosclerosis dominates disease in the arteries of the upper and lower extremities. In the peripheral arterial system, a stenosis is commonly considered hemodynamically significant if luminal obstruction exceeds 50%. Currently, CE-MRA techniques are preferred for imaging the peripheral vessels because of fewer artifacts and more reliable diagnostic images (Figure 18-19).

Because the length of coverage required to visualize the entire peripheral vasculature is greater than the anatomic coverage capable with most MR systems (40–55 cm), MRA protocols usually require acquisitions at multiple stations, i.e., abdomen/pelvis, thighs, and calves. To maintain high, near-isotropic resolution from the renal arteries to the pedal arch requires separate acquisitions for each anatomic area with 3D MRA techniques and dedicated peripheral vascular coils.

Originally, CE-MRA studies were performed sequentially from the abdomen and pelvis to thighs to calves. This was done with either separate contrast injections at each station or by rapid image acquisition following a single, prolonged injection while the table moved and the contrast material flowed distally, i.e., bolus-chase methods.[55,56] The bolus-chase method is similar to the approach used in conventional DSA and is popular because of its ability to scan a large anatomic area with a single injection (Figure 18-20). However, this approach is susceptible to significant venous contamination and special hardware and software are required. In addition, this method assumes that blood flow through both extremities is equal, which is often not the case in patients with atherosclerotic peripheral arterial disease.

More recently, hybrid or time-resolved techniques have been advocated to overcome the deficiencies of previous protocols. A hybrid MRA technique using separate test-bolus timing acquisitions in the pelvis and calves followed

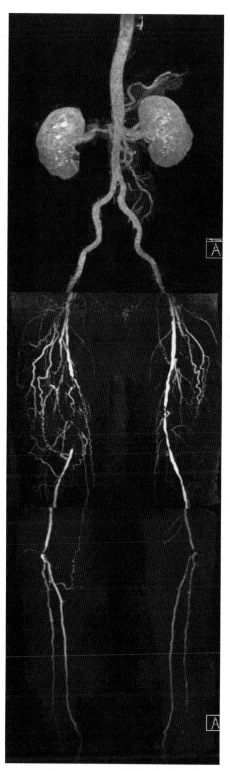

● **FIGURE 18-19.** Contrast-enhanced MRA in a patient with an occluded right superficial femoral artery with reconstitution of the distal SFA and popliteal arteries via profundus artery collaterals.

by two separate contrast material injections to first image the calves and then the pelvis and thighs (Figure 18-21), has recently been shown to provide diagnostic studies with less venous contamination than bolus chase MRA methods.[56,57] Time-resolved techniques[13,14,59–61] solve the issue of

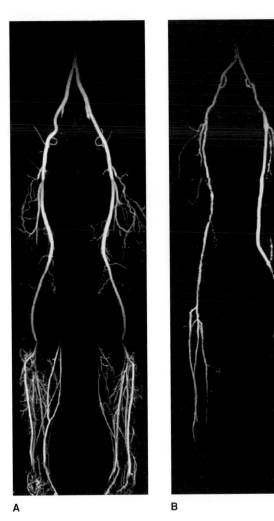

A   **B**

● **FIGURE 18-20.** (A) Bolus-chase MRA demonstrating pure arterial-phase images in the pelvis and thighs. Because of rapid distal runoff, severe venous contamination (arrows) limits the evaluation of the calves. (B) Bolus-chase MRA in a different patient demonstrating multifocal peripheral vascular disease in both thighs and incomplete opacification of the arteries in both calves, worse on the left.

sequence timing by rapidly acquiring multiple 3D volumes of data. This allows for multiple vascular phases of contrast flow (purely arterial, mixed arterial-venous, purely venous). The operator then selects the best phase to display the vessels of interest for image reconstruction. As with CE-MRA in the chest and neck, time-resolved techniques are extremely useful in the calves because of the rapid transit from arterial to venous phases. Time resolved MRA is also useful in diagnosing arteriovenous fistulas and malformations because it can demonstrate abnormal asymmetric filling of the affected veins. To be able to perform time-resolved CE-MRA, multiple acceleration techniques are employed; decreasing imaging volume, decreasing in-plane and through-plane resolution, decreasing repetition time, or using parallel imaging techniques.

Studies have shown that MRA has a high sensitivity, specificity, and accuracy (all >90%) for detection of peripheral stenoses greater than 50%.[58] In addition, more re-

cent studies have shown that hybrid or time-resolved MRA techniques are highly accurate with a higher degree of confidence and less venous contamination.[57–61] Other data have shown that CE-MRA has a higher interobserver agreement than CTA for evaluating peripheral atherosclerotic disease, especially in the presence of calcifications.[62,63]

Peripheral arterial aneurysms commonly occur in the femoral or popliteal arteries and MRA is used to determine their precise location, size, and extent.[64] In contrast to DSA, MRA can also detect the amount of thrombus present within an aneurysm, which is important in determining the likelihood of complications. In addition, MRI provides superior anatomic information, such as the course of the popliteal arteries, which is important in evaluating patients with popliteal artery entrapment syndrome. MRA of thromboangiitis obliterans will have a similar appearance to conventional angiography, demonstrating tapering, or abrupt occlusion of medium-sized peripheral arteries with enlarged collateral arteries and a corkscrew appearance.[65,66]

● **FUTURE ADVANCES IN PERIPHERAL MAGNETIC RESONANCE**

The majority of clinical MRI discussed above is performed using scanners that generate a static magnetic field with a field strength of 1.5 T, which is the equivalent of 15 000 gauss. By comparison, the earth's magnetic field measures 0.5 gauss, and open MRI machines typically generate less than 1 T. A strength of 1.5 T balances a strong SNR and excellent spatial resolution with a well-tolerated specific absorption ratio (SAR), a measure of a radiofrequency signal's effect on biologic tissue. MRI magnet strength can be as high as 8 T, which is employed only in research at select institutions. Over the next several years, clinical MRI of peripheral arterial disease will likely be increasingly performed using 3 T MRI systems. This increased field strength nearly doubles the SNR of 1.5 T without corresponding biologic effects.[67] Data already exist detailing its utility in neurologic, supraaortic, renal and lower extremity arterial imaging.[68–72]

Initial investigations of peripheral arterial MRI have begun to establish its utility as an invasive imaging and interventional tool. Traditional surface MRI can image deeper arterial beds, but a decreased SNR compromises its ability to accurately determine the structure of an atheromatous lesion. When compared with intravascular ultrasound (IVUS), intravascular MRI (IVMRI) performed utilizing specialized coil-containing catheters consistently characterized components of vessel wall plaque in diseased iliac arteries both ex and in vivo.[73] The field of interventional MRI has potential to avoid radiation exposure to both physician and patient during prolonged catheter-based diagnostic and therapeutic procedures. Dedicated catheters that produce a high-intensity signal seen well on MR imaging have allowed investigation of the placement of percutaneous valves, atrial septal defect occluder devices, coronary stents, caval filters, and aortic stents. The majority of literature published is in

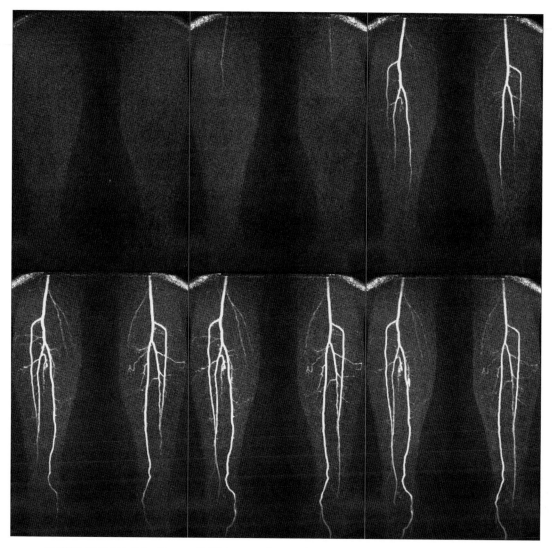

● **FIGURE 18-21.** Coronal MIP images from a time-resolved, dynamic contrast-enhanced MRA of the calves. Each image took 5 seconds to acquire.

animal models, but preliminary data exists detailing peripheral revascularization procedures in humans.[74]

In addition to advances in magnet technology, our understanding of the pathophysiology responsible for arterial disease, namely, atherosclerosis, continues to evolve. Plaque imaging and molecular characterization have become central to research seeking to identify high-risk lesions potentially leading to significant morbidity and mortality.[75] Current publications have focused on using targeted contrast agents to detect and quantify known elements of atherosclerotic lesions, such as fibrin and macrophages, in animal models.[76–78] In the future, these agents may help to add valuable information about peripheral arterial disease to the current array of MRI techniques.

REFERENCES

1. Mitka M. MRI contrast agents may pose risk for patients with kidney disease. *JAMA*. 2007;297:252-253.

2. CDC. Nephrogenic fibrosing dermopathy associated with exposure to gadolinium-containing contrast agents. *MMWR Morb Mortal Wkly Rep*. 2007;56:137-141.

3. Lewin JS, Laub G, Hausmann R. Three-dimensional time-of-flight MR angiography: applications in the abdomen and thorax. *Radiology*. 1991;179:261-264.

4. Edelman RR, Ahn SS, Chien D, et al. Improved time-of-flight MR angiography of the brain with magnetization transfer contrast. *Radiology*. 1992;184:395-399.

5. Willinek WA, Born M, Simon B, et al. Time-of-flight MR angiography: comparison of 3.0-T imaging and 1.5-T imaging—initial experience. *Radiology*. 2003;229:913-920.

6. Swan JS, Weber DM, Grist TM, et al. Peripheral MR angiography with variable velocity encoding: work in progress. *Radiology*. 1992;184:813-817.

7. Swan JS, Grist TM, Weber DM, et al. MR angiography of the

pelvis with variable velocity encoding and a phased-array coil. *Radiology*. 1994;190:363-369.

8. Prince MR, Yucel EK, Kaufman JA, et al. Dynamic gadolinium-enhanced three-dimensional abdominal MR arteriography. *J Magn Reson Imaging*. 1993;3:877-881.

9. Prince MR. Gadolinium-enhanced MR aortography. *Radiology*. 1994;191:155-164.

10. Foo TKF, Saranathan M, Prince MR, et al. Automated detection of bolus arrival and initiation of data acquisition in fast, three-dimensional, gadolinium-enhanced MR angiography. *Radiology*. 1997;203:275-280.

11. Pandharipande PV, Lee VS, Reuss PM, et al. Two-station bolus-chase MR angiography with a stationary table: a simple alternative to automated-table techniques. *AJR*. 2002;179:1583-1589.

12. Finn JP, Baskaran V, Carr JC, et al. Thorax: low-dose contrast-enhanced three-dimensional MR angiography with subsecond temporal resolution—initial results. *Radiology*. 2002;224:896-904.

13. Du J, Carroll TJ, Brodsky E, et al. Contrast-enhanced peripheral magnetic resonance angiography using time-resolved vastly undersampled isotropic projection reconstruction. *J Magn Reson Imaging*. 2004;20:894-900.

14. Swan JS, Carroll TJ, Kennell TW, et al. Time-resolved three-dimensional contrast-enhanced MR angiography of the peripheral vessels. *Radiology*. 2002;225:42-52.

15. Prince MR, Chabra SG, Watts R, et al. Contrast material travel times in patients undergoing peripheral MR angiography. *Radiology*. 2002;224:55-61.

16. Townsend TC, Saloner D, Pan XM, et al. CE MRA overestimates severity of carotid stenosis compared to 3D TOF MRA. *J Vasc Surg*. 2003;38:36-40.

17. Patel MR, Klufas RA, Kim D, et al. MR angiography of the carotid bifurcation: artifacts and limitations. *AJR*. 1994;162:1431-1437.

18. Baskaran V, Pereles FS, Nemcek AA, et al. Gadolinium-enhanced 3D MR angiography of renal artery stenosis: a pilot comparison of maximum intensity projection, multiplanar reformatting, and 3D volume-rendering postprocessing algorithms. *Acad Radiol*. 2002;9:50-59.

19. Yang CW, Carr JC, Futterer SF, et al. Contrast-enhanced MR angiography of the carotid and vertebrobasilar circulations. *AJNR Am J Neuroradiol*. 2005;26:2095-2101.

20. Bash S, Villablanca JP, Jahan R, et al. Intracranial vascular stenosis and occlusive disease: evaluation with CT angiography, MR angiography, and digital subtraction angiography. *AJNR*. 2005;26:1012-1021.

21. Mallouhi A, Felber S, Chemelli A, et al. Detection and characterization of intracranial aneurysms with MR angiography: comparison of volume rendering and maximum-intensity projection algorithms. *AJR*. 2003;180:55-64.

22. Brisman JL, Song JK, Newell DW. Cerebral aneurysms. *N Engl J Med*. 2006;355:928-939.

23. Cashen TA, Carr JC, Shin W, et al. Intracranial time-resolved contrast-enhanced MR angiography at 3 T. *AJNR Am J Neuroradiol*. 2006;27:822-829.

24. Frydrychowicz A, Bley TA, Winterer JT, et al. Accelerated time-resolved 3D contrast-enhanced MR angiography at 3 T: clinical experience in 31 patients. *MAGMA*. 2006;19:187-195.

25. Boulin A, Pierot L. Follow-up of intracranial aneurysms treated with detachable coils: comparison of gadolinium-enhanced 3D time-of-flight MR angiography and digital subtraction angiography. *Radiology*. 2001;219:108-113.

26. Pierot L, Delcourt C, Bouguigny F, et al. Follow-up of intracranial aneurysms selectively treated with coils: prospective evaluation of contrast-enhanced angiography. *AJNR Am J Neuroradiol*. 2006;27:744-749.

27. Alvarez-Linera J, Benito-Leon J, Escribano J, et al. Prospective evaluation of carotid artery stenosis: elliptic centric contrast-enhanced MR angiography and spiral CT angiography compared with digital subtraction angiography. *ANJR Am J Neuroradiol*. 2003;24:1012-1019.

28. Randoux B, Marro B, Koskas F, et al. Carotid artery stenosis: prospective comparison of CT, three-dimensional gadolinium-enhanced MR, and conventional angiography. *Radiology*. 2001;220:179-185.

29. Lenhart M, Framme N, Volk M, et al. Time-resolved contrast-enhanced magnetic resonance angiography of the carotid arteries: diagnostic accuracy and inter-observer variability compared with selective catheter angiography. *Invest Radiol*. 2002;37:535-541.

30. Nederkoorn PJ, van der Graaf Y, Hunink M. Duplex ultrasound and magnetic resonance angiography compared with digital subtraction angiography in carotid artery stenosis: a systematic review. *Stroke*. 2003;34:1324-1332.

31. Flis CM, Jager HR, Sidhu PS. Carotid and vertebral artery dissections: clinical aspects, imaging features and endovascular treatment. *Eur Radiol*. 2007;17(3):820-834.

32. Carr JC, Finn JP. MR imaging of the thoracic aorta. *Magn Reson Imaging Clin N Am*. 2003;11:135-148.

33. Ho VB, Prince MR. Thoracic MR aortography: imaging techniques and strategies. *Radiographics*. 1998;18:287-309.

34. Pereles FS, McCarthy RM, Baskaran V, et al. Thoracic aortic dissection and aneurysm: evaluation with nonenhanced true FISP MR angiography in less than 4 minutes. *Radiology*. 2002;223:270-274.

35. Song J-K. Diagnosis of aortic intramural haematoma. *Heart*. 2004;90:368-371.

36. Mesana TG, Caus T, Gaubert J, et al. Late complications after prosthetic replacement of the ascending aorta: what did we learn from routine magnetic resonance imaging follow-up? *Eur J Cardiothorac Surg*. 2000;18:313-320.

37. Garcia A, Ferreiros J, Santamaria M, et al. MR angiographic evaluation of complications in surgically treated Type A aortic dissection. *Radiographics*. 2006;26:981-992.

38. Nielsen JC, Powell AJ, Gauvreau K, et al. Magnetic resonance imaging predictors of coarctation severity. *Circulation*. 2005;111:622-628.

39. Riquelme C, Laissy J, Menagazzo D, et al. MR imaging of coarctation of the aorta and its postoperative complications in adults: assessment with spin-echo and cine-MR imaging. *Magn Reson Imaging*. 1999;17:37-46.

40. Gotway MB, Araoz PA, Macedo TA, et al. Imaging findings in Takayasu's arteritis. *AJR*. 2005;184:1945-1950.

41. Desai MY, Stone JH, Foo TKF, et al. Delayed contrast-enhanced MRI of the aortic wall in Takayasu's arteritis: initial experience. *AJR.* 2005;184:1427-1431.

42. Atar E, Belenky A, Hadad M, et al. MR angiography for abdominal and thoracic aortic aneurysms: assessment before endovascular repair in patients with impaired renal function. *AJR.* 2006;186:386-393.

43. van der Laan MJ, Bartels LW, Viergever MR, et al. Computed tomography versus magnetic resonance imaging of endoleaks after EVAR. *Eur J Vasc Endovasc Surg.* 2006;32:361-365.

44. Lookstein RA, Goldman J, Pukin L, et al. Time-resolved magnetic resonance angiography as a noninvasive method to characterize endoleaks: initial results compared with conventional angiography. *J Vasc Surg.* 2004;39:27-33.

45. Insko EK, Kulzer LM, Fairman RM, et al. MR imaging for the detection of endoleaks in recipients of abdominal aortic stent-grafts with low magnetic susceptibility. *Acad Radiol.* 2003;10:509-513.

46. van der Laan MJ, Bakker CJ, Blankensteijn JD, et al. Dynamic CE-MRA for endoleak classification after endovascular aneurysm repair. *Eur J vasc Endovasc Surg.* 2006;31:130-135.

47. Ruehm SG, Weishaupt D, Debatin JF. Contrast-enhanced MR angiography in patients with aortic occlusion (Leriche Syndrome) *J Magnet Reson Imaging.* 2000;11:401-410.

48. Pereles FS, Baskaran V. Abdominal magnetic resonance angiography: principles and practical applications. *Top Magn Reson Imaging.* 2001;12:317-326.

49. Prince MR, Schoenberg SO, Ward JS, et al. Hemodynamically significant atherosclerotic renal artery stenosis: MR angiographic features. *Radiology.* 1997;205:128-136.

50. Willmann JK, Wildermuth S, Pfammatter T, et al. Aortoiliac and renal arteries: prospective intraindividual comparison of contrast-enhanced three-dimensional MR angiography on multi-detector row CT angiography. *Radiology.* 2003;226:798-811.

51. Vasbinder GB, Nelemans PJ, Kessels AG, et al. Accuracy of computed tomographic angiography and magnetic resonance angiography for diagnosing renal artery stenosis. *Ann Intern Med.* 2004;141:674-682.

52. Kock MCJM, Ijzermans JNM, Visser K, et al. Contrast-enhanced MR angiography and digital subtraction angiography in living renal donors: diagnostic agreement, impact on decision making, and costs. *AJR.* 2005;185:448-456.

53. Meany JF, Prince MR, Nostrant TT, et al. Gadolinium-enhanced MR angiography of visceral arteries in patients with suspected chronic mesenteric ischemia. *J Magn Reson Imaging.* 1997;7:171-176.

54. Carlos RC, Stanley JC, Stafford-Johnson D, et al. Interobserver variability in the evaluation of chronic mesenteric ischemia with gadolinium-enhanced MR angiography. *Acad Radiol.* 2001;8:879-887.

55. Wang Y, Lee HM, Khilnani NM, et al. Bolus-chase MR digital subtraction angiography in the lower extremity. *Radiology.* 1998;207:263-269.

56. Schoenberg SO, Londy FJ, Licato P, et al. Multiphase-multistep gadolinium-enhanced MR angiography of the abdominal aorta and runoff vessels. *Invest Radiol.* 2001;36:283-291.

57. Pereles FS, Collins JD, Carr JC, et al. Accuracy of stepping-table lower extremity MR angiography with dual-level bolus timing and separate calf acquisition: hybrid peripheral MR angiography. *Radiology.* 2006;240:283-290.

58. Morasch MD, Collins J, Pereles FS, et al. Lower extremity stepping-table magnetic resonance angiography with multi-level contrast timing and segmented contrast infusion. *J Vasc Surg.* 2003;37:62-71.

59. Du J, Korosec FR, Thornton FJ, et al. High resolution peripheral MR angiography using undersampled projection reconstruction imaging. *Magn Reson Med.* 2004;52:204-208.

60. Hany TF, Carroll TJ, Omary RA, et al. Aorta and runoff vessels: single-injection MR angiography with automated table movement compared with multiinjection time-resolved MR angiography—initial results. *Radiology.* 2001;221:266-272.

61. Thornton FJ, Du J, Suleiman SA, et al. High-resolution, time-resolved MRA provides superior definition of lower-extremity arterial segments compared to 2D time-of-flight imaging. *J Magn Reson Imaging.* 2006;24:362-370.

62. Ouwendijk R, Kock MCJM, Visser K, et al. Interobserver agreement for the interpretation of contrast-enhanced 3D MR angiography and MDCT angiography in peripheral arterial disease. *AJR.* 2005;185:1261-1267.

63. Ouwendijk R, de Vries M, van Sambeek MRHM, et al. Imaging peripheral arterial disease: a randomized controlled trial comparing contrast-enhanced MR angiography and multi-detector row CT angiography. *Radiology.* 2005;236:1094-1103.

64. Sueyoshi E, Sakamoto I, Nakashima K, et al. Visceral and peripheral arterial pseudoaneurysms. *AJR.* 2005;185:741-749.

65. Olin JW, Shih A. Thromboangiitis obliterans (Buerger's disease). *Curr Opin Rheumatol.* 2006;18:18-24.

66. Olin JW. Thromboangiitis obliterans (Buerger's disease). *N Engl J Med.* 2000;343:864-869.

67. Fukatsu H. 3T for clinical use: update. *Magn Reson Med Sci.* 2003;2:37-45.

68. Nael K, Michaely HF, Villablanca P, et al. Time-resolved contrast enhanced magnetic resonance angiography of the head and neck at 3.0 tesla: initial results. *Invest Radiol.* 2006;41:116-124.

69. Nael K, Villablanca JP, Pope WB, et al. Supraaortic arteries: contrast-enhanced MR angiography at 3.0 T—highly accelerated parallel acquisition for improved spatial resolution over and extended field of view. *Radiology.* 2007;242:600-609.

70. Fenchel M, Nael K, Deshpande VS, et al. Renal magnetic resonance angiography at 3.0 tesla using a 32-element phased-array coil system and parallel imaging in 2 directions. *Invest Radiol.* 2006;41:697-703.

71. Leiner T, de Vries M, Hoogeveen R, et al. Contrast-enhanced peripheral MR angiography at 3.0 tesla: initial experience with a whole-body scanner in healthy volunteers. *J Magn Reson Imaging.* 2003;17:609-614.

72. Tongdee R, Narra VR, McNeal G, et al. Hybrid peripheral 3D contrast-enhanced MR angiography of calf and foot vasculature. *AJR.* 2006;186:1746-1753.

73. Larose E, Yeghiazarians Y, Libby P, et al. Characterization of human atherosclerotic plaques by intravascular magnetic resonance imaging. *Circulation.* 2005;112:2324-2331.

74. Lederman R. Cardiovascular interventional magnetic resonance imaging. *Circulation.* 2005;112:3009-3017.

75. Sirol M, Fuster V, Fayad ZA. Plaque imaging and characterization using magnetic resonance imaging: towards molecular assessment. *Curr Mol Med.* 2006;6:541-548.

76. Artemov D. Molecular magnetic resonance imaging with targeted contrast agents. *J Cell Biochem.* 2003;90:518-524.

77. Sirol M, Fuster V, Badimon JJ, et al. Chronic thrombus detection with in vivo magnetic resonance imaging and a fibrin-targeted contrast agent. *Circulation.* 2005;112:1594-1600.

78. Amierbekian V, Lipinski MJ, Briley-Saebo KC, et al. Detecting and assessing macrophages in vivo to evaluate atherosclerosis noninvasively using molecular MRI. *Proc Natl Acad Sci U S A.* 2007;104:961-966.

chapter 19

CT Angiography

Michael Davis, MD / *Sanjay Rajagopalan, MD*

● INTRODUCTION

Imaging modalities for peripheral arterial disease (PAD) cover the gamut from to noninvasive approaches to invasive digital subtraction angiography (DSA), which historically has been the reference standard. The advent of percutaneous revascularization has seen shift in imaging strategies to predominantly noninvasive approaches that can provide adequate visualization of arterial stenoses to allow accurate treatment planning. Because of the arterial puncture, DSA requires postprocedural monitoring and has a 2% to 3% major complication rate.[1,2] The advent of computed tomography (CT) and magnetic resonance angiography (MRA) has relegated DSA to an adjunctive role that may occasionally be required in some patients at the time of percutaneous revascularization. In this chapter, we will discuss the application of CT technology for the diagnosis of vascular disease in the specific vascular beds (extremities, extracranial vasculature, and thoracic and abdominal aorta).

● BASICS OF CT TECHNOLOGY

Current generation CT scanners employ the so-called "rotate/rotate" geometry, in which both x-ray source and detector are mounted onto a rotating gantry and rotate around the patient (Figure 19-1). Key requirement for the mechanical design of the gantry is the stability of both the x-ray source and detector position during rotation, in particular with regard to the rapidly increasing rotational speeds of modern CT systems (0.33 s for 64 slice systems). In a multidetector CT system (MDCT), the detector comprises several rows of 700 and more detector elements, which cover a scan field of view of usually 50 cm. The x-ray attenuation of the object is measured by the individual detector elements. Each detector element consists of a radiation-sensitive solid-state material (such as cadmium tungstate, gadolinium oxide, or gadolinium oxisulfide with suitable dopings), which converts the absorbed x-rays into visible light. The light is then detected by a silicone photodiode. The resulting electrical current is amplified and converted into a digital signal. The detectors laid out in the z-axis are an important determinant of volume coverage (along with other factors, see factors below). The "volume concept" pursued by GE, Philips, and Toshiba aims at a further increase in volume coverage by increasing the number of detectors (256 and beyond) without changing the physical parameters of the scanner compared to the 16-slice version. The "resolution concept" pursued by Siemens uses a set number of physical detector rows in combination with a oscillating x-ray source, enabled by a periodic motion of the focal spot in the z-direction, to simultaneously acquire twice the number of overlapping slices as the number of detectors using an overlapping approach (Figure 19-2).

State-of-the-art x-ray tube/generator combinations provide a peak power of 60 to 100 kW, usually at various user-selectable voltages, e.g., 80, 100, 120, and 140 kV. The two basic modes of MDCT data acquisition are axial and spiral (also called helical) scanning. Spiral/helical scanning is characterized by continuous gantry rotation and continuous data acquisition while the patient table is moving at constant speed into the scanner. Axial scanning has no role in computed tomographic angiography (CTA) applications.

Scanner Parameters

The selection of the specific acquisition parameters depends on the employed scanner model. In general, acquisition parameters for peripheral CTA are not significantly different from the ones used for abdominal MRA. A tube voltage of 120 kV with amperage of 200 to 250 mA s (adjustable based on the patient's body size) are generally used. Tube current may need to be increased in the obese patient to counter attenuation by fat and thoracic wall structures (causes for low signal to noise ratio).

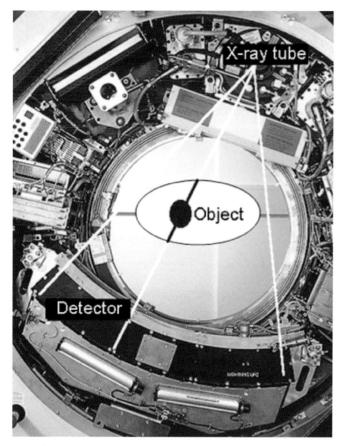

● **FIGURE 19-1.** Crossectional view of the inside of a modern CT gantry.

Reproduced with permission from Debabrata M, Rajagopalan S, eds. CT and MR Angiogrpahy of the Peripheral Circulation: Practical Approach With Clinical Protocols. 1st ed. Boca Raton, FL: Informa Healthcare, Taylor and Francis; 2007.

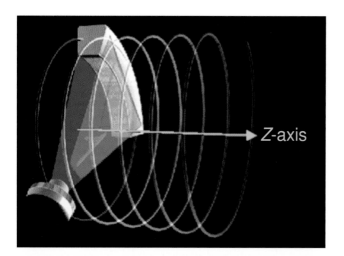

● **FIGURE 19-2.** Principle of spiral/helical CT-scanning: the patient table is continuously translated while multiple rotations of scan data are acquired. The path of x-ray tube and detector relative to the patient is a helix.

Reproduced with permission from Debabrata M, Rajagopalan S, eds. CT and MR Angiogrpahy of the Peripheral Circulation: Practical Approach With Clinical Protocols. 1st ed. Boca Raton, FL: Informa Healthcare, Taylor and Francis; 2007.

In multidetector CT spiral scans, the volume coverage speed (v, cm/s) can be estimated by the following formula:

$$v = \frac{M s_{\text{coll}} p}{t_{\text{rot}}}$$

The length of table feed per second in relationship to the width of the collimation define the pitch p. The pitch value indicates the degree of gaps in the acquisition ($p > 1$) or the extent of data overlap ($p < 1$).

By considering the formula reported above, it is evident that volume coverage can be increased by singularly or concomitantly changing the various scanner parameters (i.e., wider s_{coll}, shorter t_{rot}, higher p, and larger M). With current multislice CT, volume coverage speed may be too fast for an adequate visualization of contrast in the entire lower extremity vascular tree, especially in patients with significant stenotic lesions. For instance, a 64-slice scanner ($M = 64$), with 0.625 mm collimation, pitch of 1.375, and gantry rotation time of 0.5 second can be as fast as 110 mm/s. Such a coverage speed poses a considerable danger of "outrunning" the bolus when the table moves faster than the contrast medium bolus. It has been shown that consistently good results in peripheral CTA can be achieved if maximum acquisition speed does not exceed 30 mm/s. With a 4-slice scanner, a beam collimation of 4×2.5 mm, a pitch of 1.5 and 0.5-second gantry rotation time, would provide a volume coverage speed of 30 mm/s. With a 16-slice scanner, a volume coverage speed of 28.8 mm/s is obtained with 16×0.75 mm beam collimation at 0.5-second gantry rotation time and pitch of 1.2. The 64-slice scanners (64×0.6 mm detector configuration with Siemens scanners) have to be even more slowed down by choosing longer rotation times or reducing the pitch to values below 1. A suitable protocol for a 64-slice CT scanner includes 0.5-second gantry rotation time and pitch 0.8 for a volume coverage speed of 30.7 mm/s. A system with 64×0.625 mm collimation (GE scanners) has to be operated at a slower gantry rotation time of 0.7 second and pitch 0.5625 to achieve a volume coverage speed of 32 mm/s.

Scan Volume and Direction of Scanning

The prescribed scan volume depends on the vascular bed being examined. The direction of scanning can be switched from either a craniocaudal direction to a caudocranial direction depending on the application.

Acquisition Slice Thickness (Detector or Slice Collimation)

For most peripheral applications, detectors with submillimeter detector collimation (0.6–0.75 mm) are preferable in view of the size of the anatomic structures that may need to be characterized (e.g., small aneurysms, dissections, etc.). Table 19-1 lists the advantages and disadvantages of CT while Table 19-2 contrasts CT with MRA.

TABLE 19-1. Imaging Characteristics (Advantages and Disadvantages) of CT

Isotropic voxels (0.4 × 0.4 × 0.4)

MSCTA robust for PAD (PPV > 90%, NPV 99%, SENS 97%, SPEC 96% for popliteal-crural vessels)

High agreement for occlusion vs. nonocclusion assessment of distal vessels better with MSCTA vs. x-ray DSA

Calcified segments significant predictor of need for additional imaging and interobserver variability

Less expensive than MRA

● GENERAL PRINCIPLES OF CONTRAST ADMINISTRATION

Radiocontrast injection is perhaps the single most important factor in achieving consistently good results. The goal is to achieve homogeneous "pure arterial" (without venous or tissue contamination) enhancement synchronized with image acquisition.[3] Radiocontrast is injected through an appropriately sized (20 G or lower) antecubital vein with the attached IV tubing free of kinks. Saline flushing (30–50 cc) is routinely used after contrast media injection to transport the contrast media from the venous circulation into the arterial system. This saline chaser increases the amount of delivered iodine, contributing to arterial opacification, and reducing the overall amount of contrast media needed.[4] The usage of automated dual injectors that provide high flow rates followed by a saline bolus to compact the contrast bolus and to flush it from the peripheral to the central circulation. The imaging process must be timed with peak opacification of the arteries being studied using either by a test-bolus or an automatic bolus triggering in the abdominal aorta.[5] Factors that affect transit time such as low cardiac output states and severe PAD can alter filling of the arterial tree. Low osmolality, nonionic contrast agents are generally preferable (350–400 mg of iodine/mL). A volume of 60 to 100 mL (depending on the flow rate and the scan duration) at a flow rate of 4 to 5 mL/s is typically used. The length of the bolus at the very least should correspond to the acquisition time. In the event a "care of tracking bolus" approach is being used, an additional delay before the machine switches to the high-resolution mode (4–5 seconds) may be required.

Test Bolus

A test bolus of 10 mL of contrast is administered at the same flow rate as being planned for the CTA. A premonitoring slice with 5mm collimation may be obtained in a large vessel in proximity to the vascular bed that needs to be imaged. Repeated scans are obtained with lowest possible kV after a scan delay of 6 to 10 seconds (total duration being 30 seconds). The time to peak enhancement is evaluated from the scans. The scan delay for the CTA is calculated using the time to peak enhancement to which another 2 to 5 seconds are added; the longer the time to peak enhancement, the longer the time delay for contrast infusion.

Bolus Triggering Protocol

A region of interest is placed in a large vessel in proximity to the vascular bed of interest, with a predefined threshold of 50 to 70 Hounsfield units (HU) to initiate the CTA acquisition. The contrast medium infusion and the scanner are activated at the same time with monitoring scans starting after a scan delay of 6 to 10 seconds in order to allow contrast to travel from the peripheral circulation to the central circulatory system. The CTA acquisition mode is automatically activated from the bolus-tracking algorithm after a short pause (5–6 seconds depending on the CT scanner). Breathing instructions are given to the patient during this pause (4–5 seconds) if indicated (as may be case for thoracic or abdominal imaging).

TABLE 19-2. Relative Advantages and Disadvantages of CTA and MR Angiography (MRA) for the Evaluation of Peripheral Arteries

CTA	*MRA*
Advantages:	*Advantages:*
• Short scanning time	• Good contrast safety profile
• Low operator dependency	• Optimal delineation of vessel wall
• Widespread availability	• Dynamic flow information (phase-contrast, time-resolved imaging)
Disadvantages:	*Disadvantages:*
• Radiation exposure	• Technical challenging
• Contrast nephrotoxicity	• Contraindication in pts. with metallic implants
• Reduced accuracy in calcified vessels	• Tendency to overestimate stenosis severity

Prevention of Radiocontrast Nephropathy

All radiocontrast medias are intrinsically nephrotoxic with low or isoosmolar agents being least offensive. Risk factors for contrast nephropathy including prior renal dysfunction, concurrent use of nephrotoxic drugs, chronic heart failure, diabetes mellitus, low body mass, and advanced age should be identified a priori including estimation of the glomerular filtration rate (GFR) using the modified diet and renal disease (MDRD) equation. Patients at risk (GFR < 40 mL/min) may benefit from an alternate imaging modality or radiocontrast media prophylaxis.[6]

There are a variety of treatment strategies to prevent contrast-mediated nephrotoxicity. Most treatment regimens require the use of IV hydration, which constitutes the single most efficacious intervention.[7] At least 1 L of 0.9% NaCl solution starting several hours precontrast and continued postdye load to facilitate urine output is recommended with repeat chemistry analysis being performed in high-risk patients. Hydration with sodium bicarbonate versus sodium chloride solution was proven superior in preventing kidney dysfunction in a previously published study.[8] Another prophylactic strategy is administration of the thiol-containing antioxidant, *N*-acetylcysteine.[9] In contrast, recent statistical reviews have demonstrated mixed results regarding the beneficial effect of acetylcysteine in prevention of contrast-induced kidney injury with results yielding no statistical advantage.[10,11] Other adverse effects to contrast media include systemic adverse reactions such as nausea and vomiting, a metallic taste in the mouth, and generalized warmth or flushing. These reactions are usually non–life-threatening, self-limited problems, which require no intervention except adequate communication with patients prior to the procedure.[12] On rare occasions, iodinated contrast media can cause anaphylaxis (itching, urticaria, angioedema, and bronchospasm, or arterial hypotension and shock) within minutes after administration.[13] Although the incidence of severe anaphylaxis reaction is low, an epidemiological study of severe anaphylactic/anaphylactoid reactions among hospital patients found intermediate risk for anaphylaxis with contrast media. The incidence of anaphylaxis/anaphylactoid reactions due to contrast media in this report was 71 with high-osmolar contrast media and 35 with low-osmolar contrast media per 100 000 procedures.[14] To prevent such reactions, patients should have a meticulous allergy history taken, which elicits details from previous contrast exposure. Isoosmolar agents should be given preference if available. Some institutions will give prophylactic agents to retard against an allergic response. Recommendations for high-risk patients who must receive radiographic contrast media include use of a lower osmolar agent, pretreatment with a corticosteroid, and an H1-antagonist, discontinuation of beta-blockers if the patient is taking any, and bedside availability of appropriate medications and equipment to treat anaphylaxis.[15] After the test, the patient is reminded to drink sufficient fluids. Observation for a period of 20 to 30 minutes postprocedure is required for patients with known allergies or symptoms during the scan.

● CTA FOR PERIPHERAL ARTERIAL DISEASE

PAD is a manifestation of atherosclerosis in the arteries of the lower extremities. PAD affects 8 million Americans and is associated with significant morbidity and mortality.[16,17] The presence of PAD implies vascular disease at other sites including the cardiovascular and cerebral vascular beds. High-risk groups such as those with traditional cardiac risk factors, which include smoking, hyperlipidemia, and diabetes as well as end-stage renal disease (ESRD), should be evaluated for PAD to prevent associated vascular events. Early diagnosis and treatment of PAD is necessary principally to prevent adverse cardiovascular outcomes including death, myocardial infarction, amputations, and stroke and secondarily to reduce adverse limb outcomes including functional consequences of disabling claudication. The diagnosis of PAD is based in most cases on a careful history and physical examination, supplemented by determination of ankle brachial index. In some cases additional testing is required for the diagnosis and may include a variety of noninvasive modalities. Noninvasive imaging with CTA and magnetic resonance angiography are useful for the diagnosis but in most cases are invaluable in the treatment planning of patients with PAD.[18]

● RECONSTRUCTION AND POSTPROCESSING

Reconstruction of Peripheral Data Sets

In general, approaches for reconstruction of peripheral non-gated CTA images follow a similar protocol irrespective of the circulatory bed and will be expounded here. When reconstructing axial images from a CTA, a smooth convolution kernel (filter) is preferable (B25f or B30f). The kernel is an important parameter as the image resolution is mainly determined by the convolution kernel chosen for image reconstruction and not by the in-plane voxel size. Typical convolution kernels used for peripheral CTA studies provide a resolution of 8–10 line-pairs/cm, corresponding to 0.5 to 0.6 mm object size in the scan plane that can be resolved. All relevant information will be displayed as soon as the image voxel size is smaller than the minimum object size that can be resolved with the selected convolution kernel. For peripheral CTAs, this is usually achieved when the field-of-view (FOV) for image reconstruction is not larger than 250 to 300 mm. Further reducing the FOV will reduce the in-plane voxel size, but will not increase image resolution. Only in special cases, such as high-resolution thorax imaging with a large FOV of 350 to 400 mm, will the in-plane voxel size be the limiting factor for in-plane resolution. Reconstruction increment defines the overlap of the axial images during reconstruction. Overlap of 20% to 50% (reconstruction increment of 0.5–0.8) has been recommended for peripheral angiographic applications.

Postprocessing

The evaluation of a peripheral angiographic data set usually begins by quickly reviewing the axial source images to detect gross anatomic abnormalities or angiographic variations to evaluate the quality of acquisition (timing of contrast, signal-to-noise ratio) and to recognize any accompanying artifacts or source of misinterpretation (motion, metal, streaking, poor contrast opacification, calcium, etc.). The same data set may be then evaluated also by using an MIP format (with a variable thickness depending on the vessel bed) in traditional projections such as anterior-posterior, sagittal, and coronal views as well as in oblique projections. Using the three orientations, the operator attempts to orient the views to the anatomic axis of the vessel of structure of interest. If the workstation allows it, the entire 3-D data set can be manipulated in nonconventional views to define stenosis or other abnormalities. Rapid review of the data set in such a fashion can help rule out abnormalities. If an abnormality is detected, the segment is magnified and viewed as an multiplanar reformation (MPR) image to characterize the abnormality and to make measurements. The abnormality should always be viewed in multiple planes often orthogonal to each other. Scrolling through an MPR data set in a plane along the axis of the lumen will allow one to define the anatomic degree of stenosis and characterize other abnormalities including the performance of measurements. 3-D techniques such as volume rendering may be generated either in the beginning or at the end of the evaluation to define anatomic course and to evaluate anatomic variations if needed. These should not be used for diagnostic purposes.

CTA FOR DIAGNOSIS AND MANAGEMENT OF PAD

Indications

CTA has several advantages over other noninvasive diagnostic modalities such as ultrasonography when evaluating for PAD. Unlike ultrasonography, CTA of the extremities is relatively technician-independent with reproducible results. In patients with multilevel disease as is often the case in PAD, ultrasonography has poor specificity for anatomic localization of the culprit lesion and furthermore performance of a complete survey of the pelvis, and lower extremities is time-consuming and impractical in a busy clinical context.[19] CTA is useful for surgical or percutaneous planning as it can define proximal and distal anastamotic sites, concomitant disease processes (e.g., aneurysm, dissection, etc.), and proper sizing of prostheses/stents (Figures 19-3–19-5).

CTA is a useful modality for the evaluation of vascular trauma with sensitivity and specificity of 95% and 87%, respectively, for the diagnosis of vascular injury.[20] CTA can also be employed in the emergency setting of acute lower extremity ischemia. With the speed and availability of CTA in diagnosing acute arterial thrombosis, initiation of timely therapy is feasible. Aneurysm detection and follow-up are

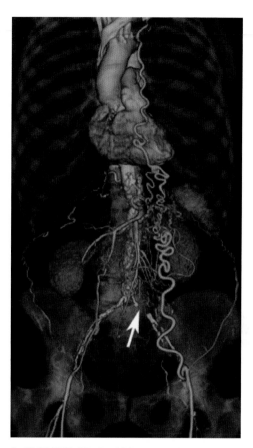

● **FIGURE 19-3.** Volume rendered image of a CTA evaluation of the thoracic and abdominal aorta including the pelvic vessels. The arrow indicated severe sequential stenosis/occlusion of the common iliac artery with evidence of extensive collaterals from the intraabdominal branches.

Reproduced with permission from Debabrata M and Rajagopalan S, eds. CT and MR Angiogrpahy of the Peripheral Circulation: Practical Approach With Clinical Protocols. 1st ed. Inform Healthcare; Boca Raton, FL: Taylor and Francis; 2007.

important indications for CTA. Image quality allows precise measurement of aneurysm dimensions and in the diagnosis of involvement of adjacent vessels and structures. CTA is the gold standard for endovascular aneurysm repair. CTA also allows bypass graft surveillance. Compared to DSA, CTA also has the advantage of evaluating for extraluminal processes such as atheroma and inflammatory disorders affecting the periarterial tissues.

Technique

The technical aspects of a CTA evaluation for lower extremity arterial disease are broadly similar across the vendor platforms. Typically, the patient is placed feet-first and supine on the scanner table, with feet and ankle joints in neutral position. The knees and ankles are restrained together in a comfortable position to restrict motion. The typical FOV for a "run-off" evaluation extends from the lower thorax (diaphragm) to the toes with an average scan length of 110 to 130 cm (Figure 19-6). A limited amount of breath-holding time is needed, which averages between

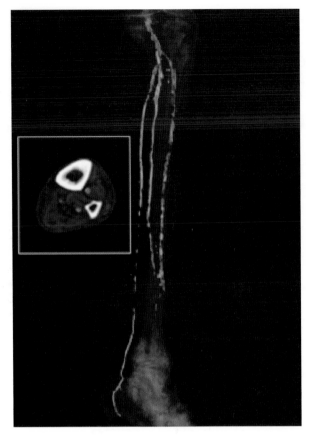

● **FIGURE 19-4.** Lower extremity atherosclerotic disease. Three dimensional CTA volume-rendered image (right anterior oblique) shows severe three vessel atherosclerotic disease of the leg. Axial CTA image (*inset*) shows calcification within the walls of the anterior tibial, posterior tibial, and peroneal arteries with poor luminal visualization.

Reproduced with permission from Debabrata M and Rajagopalan S, eds. CT and MR Angiogrpahy of the Peripheral Circulation: Practical Approach With Clinical Protocols. 1st ed. Inform Healthcare; Boca Raton, FL: Taylor and Francis; 2007.

12 and 15 seconds principally to allow motion-free imaging of the abdominal portion of the scan. An entire peripheral CTA study can easily performed in 10 to 15 minutes.

In our institute, we utilize a protocol in which the patient is scanned from the dome of the diaphragm to the feet, with the scan parameters being adjusted so that the scan duration is approximately 35 seconds. Obviously, the use of a 64-detector scanner should be preferred whenever possible to achieve submillimeter isotropic spatial resolution. Both test bolus and bolus tracking methodolgies are acceptable. In our experience, an automated bolus detection algorithm, with the region of interest located in the aorta immediately below the level of the diaphragm, works very well as it does not require additional injections. A repetitive monitor acquisition (120 kV, 10 mA s, 1-second interscan delay) is started 10 seconds after contrast injection begins. The actual peripheral CTA acquisition is then started when the contrast enhancement reaches a prespecified level (typically set between 150 and 200 HU). In general, the use of 370 mg/mL contrast agents yields excellent results. Several authors have utilized lower iodine concentrations (320

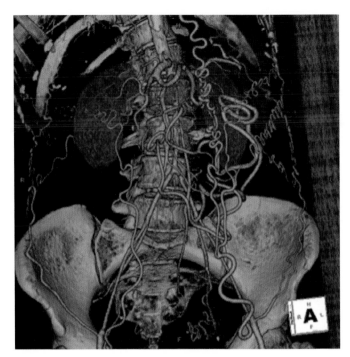

● **FIGURE 19-5.** Three-dimensional CTA volume-rendered image (anteroposterior view) shows circumferential severe narrowing of the distal abdominal aorta (*arrowhead*), common iliac, and external iliac arteries bilaterally (*arrows*). Multiple collateral vessels can be appreciated.

mg/mL) with equally good results, but this may warrant a higher flow rate (5–6 mL/s) to compensate for the lower iodine concentration. Breath-holding is requested only for the first segment (abdomen/pelvis) of the image acquisition.

Diagnostic Performance of CTA for PAD

The diagnostic accuracy of CTA in PAD when compared with historic standards such as DSA is excellent. CTA has excellent specificity in revealing severe (>75%) stenosis and arterial occlusion (97% and 98%, respectively), with excellent sensitivity (92% and 89%, respectively).[21] Other studies have reported CTA sensitivity at 72% to 99% and specificity at 92% to 99% relative to DSA for detection of ≥50% stenosis.[22–27]

● CTA FOR CAROTID DISEASE

Indications

The main indications for CTA of the extracranial circulation include atherosclerosis, fibromuscular dysplasia, aneurysms/pseudoaneurysms, and dissection involving the carotid, subclavian, vertebrobasilar system, and aorta. Additional indications include cervical tumors (carotid body) and follow-up after carotid stenting.

Technique

When scanning cervicocranial arteries, the patient is in supine position with upper arms along the body. The right

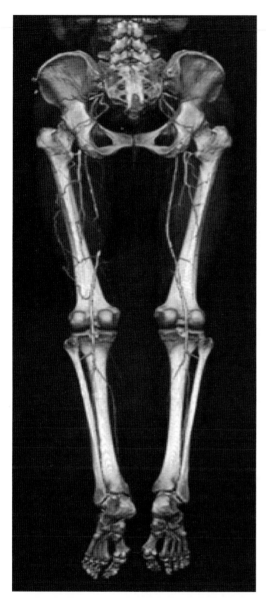

● **FIGURE 19-6.** Volume rendered 3-D image of a peripheral run-off study for the evaluation of PAD demonstrating multilevel disease. A total occlusion of the mid right SFA is noted.

antecubital vein is the preferred site for the venous access and contrast infusion to avoid "streak artifacts" related to high concentration of contrast media in the left subclavian vein. The imaging volume is planned based on the topogram, with the duration of scan determining the contrast medium bolus duration. The use of thin collimation (0.5–1 mm) is preferable when imaging the cervicocranial arteries to assure high spatial resolution. For imaging the cervicocranial vessels, pitch values of <1 are important when using fast scanners (≥16 detector scanners). A smooth convolution kernel is preferable (B25f or B30f). The use of high iodine concentrations (350 mg I/mL or greater) of contrast material for carotid CTA is supported by practical considerations and published data. Higher concentrations enable rapid infusion of the contrast bolus for an early arterial phase acquisition, and the results from multiple studies

reveal improved arterial enhancement or visualization using concentrations of 350–400 mg I/mL when compared with both disparate and equal iodine loads using 300 mg I/mL, infused at the same rate. Breath-holding of the patient should be used as the scan typically covers the aortic arch, which moves with respiration.

Diagnostic Performance of CTA for Carotid Disease

Early studies with 4-slice CT have demonstrated a high rate of accuracy for total occlusions and severe stenosis when compared with DSA. In addition, MDCT was helpful in distinguishing the underlying pathology such as dissection, thrombosis, and calcification (Figure 19-7). The diagnostic performance of CTA using modern 64-slice scanners has not been prospectively evaluated in the context of a large clinical trial comparing this to state of the art MR methodologies or 3-D DSA techniques. The limitations of CTA include the inability to assess luminal patency in arteries with extensive calcification. CTA can be used in the stented patient to assess restenosis. The caliber of the stent and the stent material determine the ability to assess lumen.

● CTA FOR THORACIC AORTIC DISEASE

Indications

CT and MRI are the preferred modalities for comprehensive evaluation of the aorta. Acute aortic syndromes (dissection, penetrating ulcer, and intramural hematoma), atherosclerotic disease, aneurysmal disease (diagnosis, follow-up, postsurgical or intervention (endoleak assessment), assessment of inflammatory aortic disease (immune, infectious), collagen vascular disease (Marfans and Ehlers Danlos syndromes), and congenital abnormalities (coarctation) are common indications (Figures 19-8 and 19-9).

Technique

An unenhanced CT may be performed prior to a contrast-enhanced CTA especially if acute aortic injury is present, to evaluate for intramural hematoma. This can be done using relatively thick (5 mm) collimation. A wide FOV (50 cm) is typical to allow coverage of all thoracic and subclavian. A useful landmark to set the FOV is outer rib to outer rib at the widest portion of the thorax. The superior extent of coverage is variable but should always include the thoracic inlet and extend to the aortic bifurcation, especially if one is evaluating for aneurysmal disease or aortic dissection. Electrocardiographic (ECG/EKG) gating is only required for thoracic aortic evaluations that include simultaneous assessment of the coronary arteries and to rule out subtle abnormalities (focal dissection flaps and intramural hematoma [IMH]) involving the proximal ascending aorta. The latter area in contrast to the distal ascending aorta and arch is prone to excessive pulsatility artifact. The entire thoracic aorta including the abdominal aorta can be covered in <10 seconds without EKG gating. For comprehensive

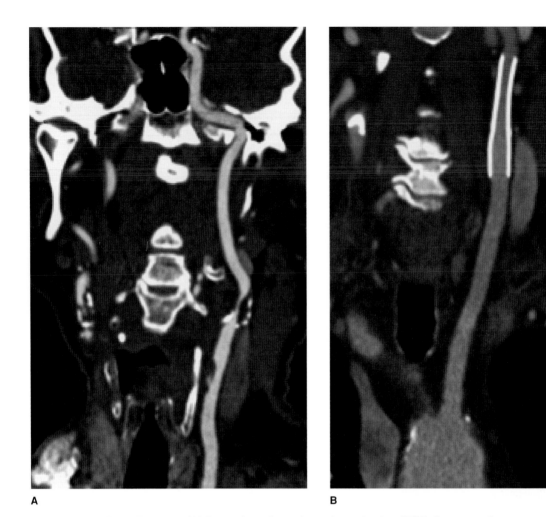

A   B

● **FIGURE 19-7.** (A) Coronal maximum intensity projection (MIP) demonstrating severe stenosis of the left internal carotid artery at the level of the buld with calcification. (B) MIP projection demonstrating a stented ICA.

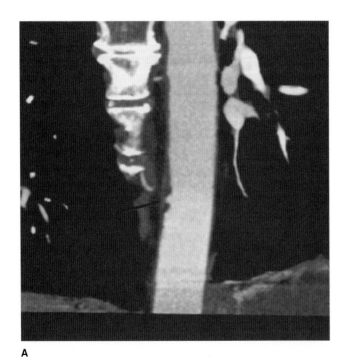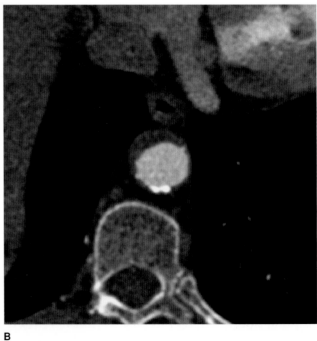

A   B

● **FIGURE 19-8.** (A) Coronal maximum intensity projection (MIP) of the descending thoracic aorta demonstrating moderate to severe atherosclerosis. (B) Axial MIP image demonstrates plaque with evidence of focal aortic wall calcification in another patient.

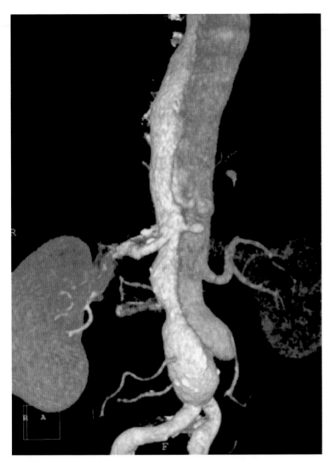

● **FIGURE 19-9.** Volume rendered image of a thoracoabdominal dissecting aneurysm. The true lumen has higher contrast content and therefore is seen as being brighter compared to the false lumen.

evaluation of the thoracic and abdominal aorta (non-EKG-gated), timing may be performed in the proximal descending aorta.

Clinical Applications

Acute Aortic Syndromes. The objectives during the CTA imaging evaluation of acute aortic syndromes are (i) identification of the dissection flap, ulcer, or hematoma, (ii) confirmation of diagnosis, (iii) assessment of the extent and the size of the aortic abnormality, (iv) assessment of the patency of the false lumen (if present) and degree of true lumen compression, and (v) evaluation for evidence of end-organ ischemia, branch vessel involvement (great vessels, mesenteric and renal arteries), and complications such as pericardial effusions or pleural effusion that may indicate rupture or imminent rupture. The most reliable criterion for the diagnosis of aortic dissection on CTA studies is the demonstration of an intimal flap separating the true and false lumen. In cases when an intimal flap is not seen, the diagnosis of aortic dissection must be made on the basis of ancillary criteria, such as distortion of the aortic contour, intramural high attenuation, periaortic hematoma, or displaced intimal calcifications. The false lumen is often larger than the true lumen and the intimal flap may be flat or

curved toward the true lumen although not always. Another indicator of the false lumen is the presence of aortic "cobwebs," which are irregular strands that represent fragments of sheared media and can be seen attached to the wall and projecting to the lumen. The angle between the false lumen and the intimal flap is usually acute ("beak sign") and is felt by some to be specific for identifying it. A false lumen with a convex orientation toward the true lumen is indicative of high pressure within the false lumen, which may in turn, be associated with increased incidence of complications. Outer wall calcification is seen only in the true lumen and never in the false lumen in acute dissection; however in chronic dissection, outer wall calcification may be seen in false lumens. Intraluminal thrombus is much more common in the false lumen and only rarely in the true lumen in both acute and chronic dissection. IMH appears as a focal thickening of the aortic wall that has high attenuation, and may be better appreciated in noncontrast images if these have been obtained. If there is adjoining calcium, this may often be displaced. Differentiation of IMH from intraluminal thrombus on a contrast-enhanced CT may be difficult. Intraluminal thrombus is often localized, and within a dilated aorta, whereas IMH may extend over a longer distance within a nondilated aorta. In some studies, IMH involved an 8.5 ± 5 cm length of the aorta.

Thoracic Aneurysms. CTA can clearly delineate the size, spatial extent, tortuosity, and morphological features of the aneurysm including the presence of calcification and thrombus in the aneurysm. The involvement of branch vessels and the effect on surrounding structures is clearly seen owing to the excellent spatial resolution. CTA findings of thoracic aortic aneurysm rupture or impending rupture include high-attenuation fluid in the pleural or pericardial spaces. When evaluating an aneurysm, it is important to assess its size along the long axis of the vessel. The maximal diameter, superior–inferior extent, and involvement of the branch vessels should be commented on.

CTA allows reliable assessment of size of the aneurysm and the status of the aortic branches as well as evaluation of the iliac and femoral arteries (diameter, tortuosity) for vascular access prior to endovascular abdominal aortic aneurysm repair of the thoracic aorta. Stent graft diameter is currently determined on the basis of CT findings rather than MR findings. Postprocedure, CTA is performed at the time of discharge, 3, 6, and 12 months after stent-graft insertion and annually thereafter. Chest radiographs are obtained at the same time intervals to assess for metallic failure of the stent-graft. The protocol for endoleak detection typically involves acquiring a CTA during the arterial phase and repeating a delayed phase after a few minutes. Endoleak is defined as the extravasation of contrast material outside of the graft during the delayed phase. Type 1 endoleaks result from incomplete sealing of the stent-graft at the proximal or distal attachment site and these along with type 3 are far more common than type 2 endoleaks (more common in the infrarenal aorta). Many type 1 and type 3 endoleaks may be treated with insertion of a longer stent-graft. There is some data to suggest that MR techniques maybe more sensitive than CT in detecting endoleaks, but less specific in precisely locating the site of the leak.

Performance of CTA

CTA of the thoracic aorta is currently the new reference standard for the diagnosis of aortic disease. Although MRA is advantageous in certain settings, the widespread availability of CT scanners, superior spatial resolution, and ease of performance have led to widespread acceptance. In the IRAD study, CT was the most commonly utilized imaging modality (93%) followed by transesophageal echocardiogram and MRI. In this study, which utilized predominantly single detector technology, the overall sensitivity of CT for dissection was 93% compared with 100% for MR (included very few patients).[28] A comparison of spiral CT, transesophageal echocardiography, and MR imaging in 49 patients who had clinically suspected aortic dissection showed 100% sensitivity for aortic dissection for all three techniques, specificity of 100% for CT, and 94% for both transesophageal echocardiography and MR imaging. In the diagnosis of aortic arch vessel involvement, CT was clearly superior with sensitivity and specificity of 93% and 97% compared with transesophageal echocardiography (60% and 85%) and MR imaging (67% and 88%).[29] A recent meta-analysis involving 1139 patients with suspected thoracic dissection demonstrated that helical CT yielded a sensitivity of 100% and a specificity of 98% in ruling out aortic dissection and all three imaging techniques, i.e., transesophageal echocardiogram, helical CT, and MRI, yield equally reliable diagnostic values for confirming or ruling out thoracic aortic dissection.[30] Large studies detailing the accuracy of multislice CTA ($\geq$16 detectors) for aortic disease and other aortic disorders are not yet available. Disadvantages of CTA for aortic disease include the inability to evaluate the aortic valve and assess stenotic or regurgitant involvement.

● CTA FOR ABDOMINAL/PELVIC AORTIC DISEASE

Indications

The indications for CT for the evaluation of abdominal aortic disease are mostly similar to the thoracic aorta but also include assessment of aortic visceral branch assessment. CTA of the abdomen/pelvis may be performed alone or in conjunction with comprehensive evaluation of the aorta.

Technique

Abdominal/pelvic CTA does not generally require specific patient preparation that differs from other contrast-enhanced CT examinations. If the bowel is to be evaluated within the same test, 500 to 1000 mL of oral water just prior to procedure helps with its delineation. Barium contrast should not be used. An intravenous access is placed in the arm (either side is acceptable), ideally with an 18–20 G cannula. In general, positioning the arms above the head is preferred to avoid streak artifacts arising from the arm bones or for remnant contrast in the arm with the intravenous access. For care bolus or bolus track, a region of interest (ROI) is placed in the diaphragmatic or supraceliac aorta. A trigger value of approximately 150 HU can be used for most patients, although 125 HU may provide more reliable triggering when used in obese patients with the contrast bolus duration covering the scan duration. The scanning volume is set so that the upper limit is the 12th rib and the caudal limit reaches the upper femoral heads (to include the iliac arteries) or the iliac crest (for limited renal or mesenteric segments only). If aortic pathology is known or suspected to extend to the intrathoracic segments, the scanning volume is modified accordingly. Scanning is performed in the craniocaudal direction. Cardiac gating is not generally needed unless the ascending thoracic aorta or the arch is included. In patients with isolated abdominal/pelvic studies, diagnostic images can generally be obtained even without breath-hold using a 16-detector CT scanner. Improved quality is seen with a breath-hold. A repeat (delayed) scan after the contrast can also be useful to evaluate venous anatomy, organ perfusion (i.e., kidneys), or slow bleeding.

Clinical Applications

Acute Aortic Syndromes. Acute aortic syndromes at the level of the abdominal aorta occur more commonly as a consequence of a ruptured abdominal aortic aneurysm (AAA), or due to the extension of a dissection involving the descending thoracic aorta. When assessing the abdominal aorta, either in cases of dissection or of AAA, the relation between aortic branches and a diseased aortic segment should be noted, particularly the presence of an occluded branch. This can have a significant impact on patient management, including the decision for surgery versus medical management. Other anatomic features that need to be identified are detailed in the previous section on thoracic aorta.

Diagnosis and Surveillance of Abdominal Aneurysmal Disease. It is important to realize that while CTA is nearly 100% sensitive for detecting AAAs, differentiation of acutely ruptured from nonruptured aneurysms has a sensitivity that is substantially lower. In a clinical study comparing CTA with open surgery, CTA had only 79% sensitivity in patients with known AAA and suspected rupture on clinical grounds. Thus, clinical presentation should be strongly considered despite a negative CT study in a patient with suspicion of impending rupture of an abdominal aneurysm. CTA is highly reproducible for the quantification of AAA dimensions. Surgical intervention and endovascular abdominal aortic aneurysm repair are planned on the basis of CTA findings. Some workstations incorporate dedicated 3-D software packages, which can assist in aortic stent planning, and it has been demonstrated that CTA is sufficient for successful repair of aneurysms without the use of prior

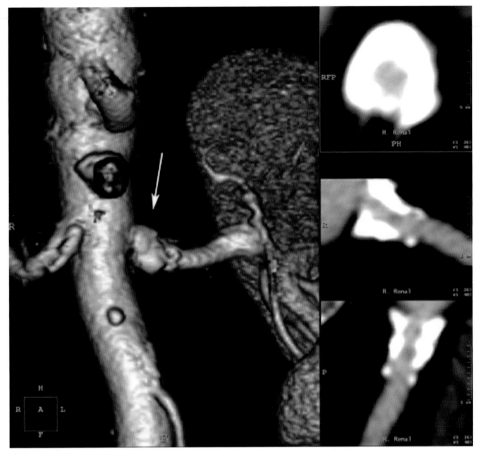

● **FIGURE 19-10.** Circumferential calcium (*arrow*) of the left renal ostium in a volume rendered image (*left*) of the left renal artery obscures visualization of the lumen of the vessel. Orthogonal curved planar reconstructions (*right*) demonstrate a patent lumen.

standard angiography. Morphologic features of AAAs that need to be reported for this purpose include the following:

- The proximal neck diameter and length relative to the renal artery origins and superior mesenteric artery.
- The diameter and configuration of the aneurysm body.
- The distal neck length and diameter relative to the aortic bifurcation.
- Common iliac artery involvement and length.
- Relation of the hypogastric (internal iliac) arteries to a point of potential distal fixation.
- Angulation and diameter of the iliac arteries and common femoral arteries.

Renal Artery Stenosis. In general terms, the clinical utility and diagnostic ability of CTA in the evaluation of renal artery disease is well documented and offers the benefits of being a noninvasive study. CTA has also proven to be useful in other clinical scenarios, such as fibromuscular dysplasia, renal artery aneurysms, or dissection, although the comparative accuracy to other imaging modalities has not been fully investigated. In addition, CTA can be useful in the follow-up of patients after renal artery intervention. In practice, CTA may be problematic in patients with

concomitant renal dysfunction. The presence of calcified plaques may obscure lumen visualization, although this is occasionally overcome with the use of thin, high-resolution reconstructions (Figure 19-10).

Mesenteric Ischemia. Branches of the celiac and superior mesenteric vessels are difficult to assess on axial or transverse sections due to their oblique course. However, slab-maximum intensity projections (slab-MIPS) in the frontal or coronal plane often give excellent visualization of the first- and second-order celiac artery and superior mesenteric artery branches. CTA is useful in acute and chronic mesenteric arterial disorders.

Diagnostic Performance of CTA for Abdominal Disease

CTA rivals DSA in the evaluation of renal arterial disease with prospective studies demonstrating very high agreement between studies mostly in studies involving atherosclerotic arterial disease. In a prospective multicenter triple imaging study examining CTA (including both single- and multidetector row systems), MRA, and DSA, Vasbinder et al. published sensitivity for both CTA and MRA as being 65% as compared to DSA.[31] In this study, a significant proportion of the patients with renal artery stenosis had fibromuscular dysplasia, a disorder more prevalent in children and young adults. Fibromuscular dysplasia is associated with more distal stenoses that are therefore more difficult to detect, whereas most cases of stenosis secondary to atherosclerotic disease are located proximally. There have been comparative studies examining CTA versus ultrasound as a means of identifying endoleaks. Although duplex ultrasound is safe and easily performed, it has relatively poor sensitivity for the detection of endoleaks and its routine use is not advocated. In general, CTA is also more sensitive than DSA because branch vessels are imaged simultaneously with the aneurysm sac in CTA, whereas a time delay may occur between maximum aortic opacification and branch vessel opacification for DSA. Aneurysm volume after stent repair as measured on CTA has also been demonstrated to be useful in evaluating endoleaks. Lack of volume decrease in the aneurysm of at least 0.3% at 6 months follow-up indicates the need for closer surveillance, and has a higher predictive accuracy for an endoleak than changes in maximum diameter.

● ARTIFACTS

Streak Artifacts

Streak artifact results from dense, highly concentrated contrast, causing beam hardening and obscuring photon transmission. Streak artifact commonly affects the left brachiocephalic vein and superior vena cava, potentially obscuring the aortic arch and ascending aorta, respectively. Streak artifacts also may result from pacemakers, surgical staples, external monitoring devices, or positioning the patient's arms at their sides during the scan. These artifacts are readily recognized by identifying their source. Streak artifacts may be reduced by injecting by the right upper extremity, using a compact bolus by injecting a saline chaser, and sometimes by using dilute contrast mixtures.

Motion Artifact

Motion artifacts can occasionally be problematic, particularly at the base of the heart surrounding the ascending aorta. Motion artifacts may simulate the appearance of aortic dissection. EKG gating is a good way to prevent artifacts and should be incorporated if one is interested in high-resolution, cardiac motion minimized imaging of the heart and great vessels.

● CONCLUSIONS

CTA is an accurate and an exceptionally efficient means for imaging the peripheral arterial circulation. The diagnostic usefulness is continually expanding with newer clinical applications currently being studied.

REFERENCES

1. Hessel SJ, Adams DF, Abrams HL. Complications of angiography. *Radiology.* 1981;138:273–281.

2. Egglin TKP, O'Moore PV, Feinstein AR, Waltman AC. Complications of peripheral arteriography: a new system to identify patients at increased risk. *J Vasc Surg.* 1995;22:787–794.

3. Duddalwar VA. Multislice CT angiography: a practical guide to CT angiography in vascular imaging and intervention. *Br J Radiol.* 2004;77(Spec No 1):S27–S38.

4. Jakobs TF, Wintersperger BJ, Becker CR. MDCT-imaging of peripheral arterial disease. *Semin Ultrasound CT MR.* 2004; 25:145–155.

5. Fleischmann D. Use of high concentration contrast media: principles and rationale-vascular district. *Eur J Radiol.* 2003; 45(suppl 1):S88–S93.

6. Stacul F. Managing the risk associated with use of contrast media for computed tomography. *Eur J Radiol.* 2007;62(suppl): 33–37.

7. Mueller C. Prevention of contrast-induced nephropathy with volume supplementation. *Kidney Int Suppl.* 2006:S16–S19.

8. Merten GJ, Burgess WP, Gray LV, et al. Prevention of contrast-induced nephropathy with sodium bicarbonate: a randomized controlled trial. *JAMA.* 2004;291:2328–2334.

9. Kay J, Chow WH, Chan TM, et al. Acetylcysteine for prevention of acute deterioration of renal function following elective coronary angiography and intervention: a randomized controlled trial. *JAMA.* 2003;289:553–558.

10. Zagler A, Azadpour M, Mercado C, Hennekens CH. *N*-acetylcysteine and contrast-induced nephropathy: a meta-analysis of 13 randomized trials. *Am Heart J.* 2006;151:140–145.

11. Van Praet JT, De Vriese AS. Prevention of contrast-induced nephropathy: a critical review. *Curr Opin Nephrol Hypertens.* 2007;16:336–347.

12. Maddox TG. Adverse reactions to contrast material: recognition, prevention, and treatment. *Am Fam Physician.* 2002;66: 1229–1234.

13. Tramer MR, von Elm E, Loubeyre P, Hauser C. Pharmacological prevention of serious anaphylactic reactions due to iodinated contrast media: systematic review. *BMJ.* 2006;333:675.

14. Risk of anaphylaxis in a hospital population in relation to the use of various drugs: an international study. *Pharmacoepidemiol Drug Saf.* 2003;12:195–202.

15. Wittbrodt ET, Spinler SA. Prevention of anaphylactoid reactions in high-risk patients receiving radiographic contrast media. *Ann Pharmacother.* 1994;28:236–241.

16. Hirsch AT, Criqui MH, Treat-Jacobson D, et al. Peripheral arterial disease detection, awareness, and treatment in primary care 10.1001/jama.286.11.1317. *JAMA.* 2001;286:1317–1324.

17. Hirsch AT, Haskal ZJ, Hertzer NR, et al. ACC/AHA 2005 Practice Guidelines for the management of patients with peripheral arterial disease (lower extremity, renal, mesenteric,

and abdominal aortic): a collaborative report from the American Association for Vascular Surgery/Society for Vascular Surgery, Society for Cardiovascular Angiography and Interventions, Society for Vascular Medicine and Biology, Society of Interventional Radiology, and the ACC/AHA Task Force on Practice Guidelines (Writing Committee to Develop Guidelines for the Management of Patients With Peripheral Arterial Disease): endorsed by the American Association of Cardiovascular and Pulmonary Rehabilitation; National Heart, Lung, and Blood Institute; Society for Vascular Nursing; TransAtlantic Inter-Society Consensus; and Vascular Disease Foundation. *Circulation.* 2006;113:e463–e654.

18. Kock MC, Adriaensen ME, Pattynama PM, et al. DSA versus multi-detector row CT angiography in peripheral arterial disease: randomized controlled trial. *Radiology.* 2005;237:727–737.

19. Lookstein RA. Impact of CT angiography on endovascular therapy. *Mt Sinai J Med.* 2003;70:367–374.

20. Rieger M, Mallouhi A, Tauscher T, Lutz M, Jaschke WR. Traumatic arterial injuries of the extremities: initial evaluation with MDCT angiography. *AJR Am J Roentgenol.* 2006;186:656–664.

21. Martin ML, Tay KH, Flak B, et al. Multidetector CT angiography of the aortoiliac system and lower extremities: a prospective comparison with digital subtraction angiography. *AJR Am J Roentgenol.* 2003;180:1085–1091.

22. Ofer A, Nitecki SS, Linn S, et al. Multidetector CT angiography of peripheral vascular disease: a prospective comparison with intraarterial digital subtraction angiography. *AJR Am J Roentgenol.* 2003;180:719–724.

23. Catalano C, Fraioli F, Laghi A, et al. Infrarenal aortic and lower-extremity arterial disease: diagnostic performance of multi-detector row CT angiography. *Radiology.* 2004;231:555–563.

24. Romano M, Mainenti PP, Imbriaco M, et al. Multidetector row CT angiography of the abdominal aorta and lower extremities in patients with peripheral arterial occlusive disease: diagnostic accuracy and interobserver agreement. *Eur J Radiol.* 2004;50:303–308.

25. Ota H, Takase K, Igarashi K, et al. MDCT compared with digital subtraction angiography for assessment of lower extremity arterial occlusive disease: importance of reviewing cross-sectional images. *AJR Am J Roentgenol.* 2004;182:201–209.

26. Edwards AJ, Wells IP, Roobottom CA. Multidetector row CT angiography of the lower limb arteries: a prospective comparison of volume-rendered techniques and intra-arterial digital subtraction angiography. *Clin Radiol.* 2005;60:85–95.

27. Willmann JK, Mayer D, Banyai M, et al. Evaluation of peripheral arterial bypass grafts with multi-detector row CT angiography: comparison with duplex US and digital subtraction angiography. *Radiology.* 2003;229:465–474.

28. Suzuki T, Mehta RH, Ince H, et al. Clinical profiles and outcomes of acute type B aortic dissection in the current era: lessons from the international registry of aortic dissection (IRAD) 10.1161/01.cir.0000087386.07204.09. *Circulation.* 2003;108:II-312–317.

29. Sommer T, Fehske W, Holzknecht N, et al. Aortic dissection: a comparative study of diagnosis with spiral CT, multiplanar transesophageal echocardiography, and MR imaging. *Radiology.* 1996;199:347–352.

30. Shiga T, Wajima Zi, Apfel CC, Inoue T, Ohe Y. Diagnostic accuracy of transesophageal echocardiography, helical computed tomography, and magnetic resonance imaging for suspected thoracic aortic dissection: systematic review and meta-analysis 10.1001/archinte.166.13.1350. *Arch Intern Med.* 2006;166:1350–1356.

31. Vasbinder GBC, Nelemans PJ, Kessels AGH, et al. Accuracy of computed tomographic angiography and magnetic resonance angiography for diagnosing renal artery stenosis. *Ann Intern Med.* 2004;141:674–682.

chapter 20

Peripheral Angiography

Sohail Ikram, MD / Massoud Leesar, MD / Ibrahim Fahsah, MD

● PERIPHERAL ANGIOGRAPHY

Peripheral arterial disease (PAD) comprises a host of non-coronary arterial syndromes due to various pathophysiological mechanisms resulting in stenosis or aneurysms in various vascular beds. Atherosclerosis (AS) remains by far the most common cause of this disease process. According to the recently released ACC/AHA guidelines for the management of patients with PAD, it is a major cause of decrement of functional capacity, quality of life, limb amputation, and increased risk of death.[1]

Millions of people worldwide are afflicted with this syndrome.[2,3] While awareness for coronary artery disease (CAD) has significantly increased in the last decade, the awareness, diagnosis, and treatment of PAD remain much underappreciated. With improvement in catheter-based and imaging technology, it was only natural that all specialties involved in the management of vascular disease would involve endovascular therapy of this potentially disabling and lethal disorder.[4–6]

Excellent reviews on PAD are already available in the literature. The ACC/AHA guidelines, Trans Atlantic Society Conference (TASC) Working Group document,[7] the ACC COCATS-2 Paper,[8] provide the basic fundamental material for a physician interested in the management of patients suffering from PAD. Based on literature review and our own experience at the Washington Hospital Center, Washington, DC, and University of Louisville, Louisville, KY, we have tried to focus in this chapter on the general principles of performing invasive peripheral angiography. We have also briefly described noninvasive imaging modalities of computed tomographic angiography (CTA), magnetic resonance angiography (MRA), and carbon dioxide (CO_2) angiography as their utility relates to each vascular bed. The full details of these other modalities are, however, out of the scope of this chapter. We hope that this chapter will provide the basic understanding in catheter angiography to an operator interested in treating patients with PAD.

Training Requirements

There are considerable differences of opinion that exist among various specialties regarding the optimal training required before certifying operators to safely perform peripheral vascular procedures.[9–16] Specialties including interventional cardiology, interventional radiology, vascular surgery, interventional neuroradiology, interventional nephrology, and interventional neurosurgery all possess basic and unique knowledge that positions them to advance their skills into peripheral angiography and interventions. The ACC COCATS-2 (Tables 20-1 and 20-2) provides guidelines for a cardiovascular trainee who wishes to be certified in the performance of such procedures.

A minimum of 12 months of training is required. Completion of 100 diagnostic angiograms and 50 peripheral vascular interventions has been recommended for unrestricted certification. Fifty percent of such procedures should be performed as "primary operator" under the guidance of a mentor who is certified in peripheral vascular interventions. Prior to the performance of invasive procedures, this physician should be knowledgeable in vascular medicine and noninvasive modalities in the diagnosis of peripheral vascular disorders. Before signing off the certificate, the mentor should require the trainee to have exposure in the angiography of various vascular beds. This should also include cases of vascular thromboses and their treatment. Carotid and vertebral artery angiography is excluded from most general guidelines and added skills are required in this vascular territory. The ACC/ACP/SCAI/SVMB/SVS Clinical Competent Statement outlines these requirements (Tables 20-3 and 20-4).

Restricted certificates can be awarded to physicians who achieve satisfactory skills in only certain vascular territories.

TABLE 20-1. Training in Diagnostic Cardiac Catheterization and Interventional Cardiology

Level 1—Trainees who will practice noninvasive cardiology and whose invasive activities will be confined to critical care unit procedures.
Level 2—Trainees who will practice diagnostic but not interventional cardiac catheterization.
Level 3—Trainees who will practice diagnostic and interventional cardiac catheterization.

Maintenance of certification is also required by continuous medical education and performance of 25 peripheral vascular interventions per year. For full details, the reader may refer consensus conference guidelines.[17]

● NONINVASIVE IMAGING

Noninvasive imaging is improving at a rapid pace and is replacing routine catheter angiography in many cases.

Magnetic Resonance Angiography

According to the ACC/AHA guidelines, MRA with gadolinium contrast is now a Class I indication (conditions for which there is evidence for and/or general agreement that a given procedure or treatment is beneficial, useful, and effective) and level of evidence A (data derived from multiple randomized trials or meta-analysis) to diagnose the anatomic location and degree of stenosis in the lower extremity PAD; and to select patients who are candidates for endovascular or surgical revascularization. MRA has Type IIb indication (conditions for which there is conflicting evidence and/or divergence of opinion about the usefulness/efficacy of a procedure or treatment. Weight of evidence/opinion is in favor of usefulness/efficacy) and level of evidence B (data derived from a single randomized trial or nonrandomized trials) in patients with PAD to select surgical sites for surgical bypass and for postsurgical and postendovascular revascularization surveillance. Gadolinium is less nephrotoxic and there is no exposure to

TABLE 20-3. Formal Training to Achieve Competence in Peripheral Catheter-Based Interventions

Training requirements for cardiovascular physicians
• Duration of training*—12 months
• Diagnostic coronary angiograms†—300 cases (200 as the primary operator)
• Diagnostic peripheral angiograms—100 cases (50 as primary operator)
• Peripheral interventional cases§—50 cases (25 as primary operator)

Training requirements for interventional radiologists
• Duration of training‡—12 months
• Diagnostic peripheral angiograms—100 cases (50 as primary operator)
• Peripheral interventional cases§—50 cases (25 as primary operator)

Training requirements for vascular surgeons
• Duration of training—12 months||
• Diagnostic peripheral angiograms¶—100 cases (50 as primary operator)
• Peripheral interventional cases§—50 cases (25 as primary operator)
• Aortic aneurysm endografts—10 cases (5 as primary operator)

This table is consistent with current Residency Review Committee requirements.
After completing 24 months of core cardiovascular training and 8 months of cardiac catheterization
†*Coronary catheterization procedures should be completed prior to interventional training.*
‡*After completing general radiology training.*
§*The case mix should be evenly distributed among the different vascular beds. Supervised cases of thrombus management for limb ischemia and venous thrombosis, utilizing percutaneous thrombolysis or thrombectomy should be included.*
||*In addition to 12 months of core vascular surgery training.*
¶*In addition to experience gained during open surgical procedures.*

ionizing radiation. Currently utilized techniques of MRA include time of flight (TOF), three-dimensional imaging, contrast enhancement with gadolinium subtraction, cardiac gating and bolus chase.[18] With the contrast-enhanced MRA (CE MRA), the sensitivity is 90% and specificity 97% in

TABLE 20-2. Summary of Training Requirements for Diagnostic and Interventional Cardiac Catheterization

Level	Duration of Training (mo)	Cumulative Duration of Training (mo)	Minimum no. of Procedures Diagnostic	Interventional	Cumulative no. of Examinations Diagnostic	Interventional
1	4	4	100	0	100	0
2	4	8	200	0	300	0
3	12	20	0	250	300	250

Only one level 1, 2, or 3 trainee may claim credit for a procedure. See text for explanation.

TABLE 20-4. Alternative Routes to Achieving Competence in Peripheral Catheter-Based Intervention*

1. Common requirements
   a. Completion of required training within 24-month period
   b. Training under proctorship of formally trained vascular interventionalist competent to perform full range of procedures described in this document
   c. Written curriculum with goals and objectives
   d. Regular written evaluations by proctor
   e. Documentation of procedures and outcomes
   f. Supervised experience in inpatient and outpatient vascular consultation settings
   g. Supervised experience in a noninvasive vascular laboratory
2. Procedural requirements for competency in all areas
   a. Diagnostic peripheral angiograms—100 cases (50 as primary operator)
   b. Peripheral interventions—50 cases (25 as primary operator)
   c. No fewer than 20 diagnostic/10 interventional cases in each area, excluding extracranial cerebral arteries[†]
   d. Extracranial cerebral (carotid/vertebral) arteries—30 diagnostic (15 as primary operator)/25 interventional (13 as primary operator)
   e. Percutaneous thrombolysis/thrombectomy—5 cases
3. Requirements for competency in subset of areas (up to 3, excluding carotid/vertebral arteries)
   a. Diagnostic peripheral angiograms per area—30 cases (15 as primary operator)
   b. Peripheral interventions per area—15 cases (8 as primary operator)
   c. Must include aortoiliac arteries as initial area of competency

---

*The fulfillment of requirements via an alternative pathway is only appropriate if the candidate physician has the cognitive and technical skills outlined in Table 20-4 and is competent to perform either coronary intervention, interventional radiology, or vascular surgery. These alternative routes for achieving competency are available for up to 5 years following publication of this document.

[†]Vascular areas are (1) aortoiliac and brachiocephalic arteries, (2) abdominal visceral and renal arteries, and (3) infrainguinal arteries.

Reproduced, with permission, from Creager MA, Goldstone J, Hirshfeld JW Jr, et al. ACC/ACP/SCAI/SVMB/SVS clinical competence statement on vascular medicine and catheter-based peripheral vascular interventions: a report of the American College of Cardiology/American Heart Association/American College of Physician Task Force on Clinical Competence (ACC/ACP/SCAI/SVMB/SVS Writing Committee to develop a clinical competence statement on peripheral vascular disease. J Am Coll Cardiol. 2004;44(4):941-957.

---

lower extremities PAD as compared to digital subtraction angiography (DSA).[19–21] Runoff vessels may, in fact, be better visualized with MRA than DSA.[22,23] In the patients diagnosed with critical limb ischemia (CLI), with intraoperative angiography as the standard, MRA had comparable accuracy to standard catheter angiography. Sensitivity and specificity for patent vessels was 81% and 85%, respectively. For the identification of segments suitable for bypass grafting, the sensitivity of contrast angiography was less than MRA (77% vs. 82%), but the specificity was better (92% vs. 84%).[24] A meta-analysis of MRA compared to catheter angiography for stenoses >50% showed that the sensitivity and specificity were 90% to 100%, especially when gadolinium was used.[25] Recent studies also show an agreement of 91% to 97% between MRA and catheter angiography.[26]

MRA, however, tends to overestimate the degree of stenosis and occlusions. It might also be inaccurate in assessing lesions with stents. Another limitation is in patients who have been implanted with automatic defibrillators, permanent pacemakers or who have intracranial coils or clips.[27,28] In these patients, MRA is generally contraindicated. Gadolinium is generally considered nonnephrotoxic, but one study reported nephrotoxicity in patients with baseline renal dysfunction.[29] A significant number of patients are also severely claustrophobic during imaging and require alternative testing.

Computed Tomographic Angiography

CTA is considered by ACC-AHA guideline committee to merit a Type IIb indication (usefulness/efficacy is less well established by evidence/opinion) and level of evidence B for diagnosing the anatomic location and presence of stenoses in patients with lower extremity PAD. It is considered as a substitute for MRA in patients who have contraindication to MRA.[30–34]

This technique was first started in 1992. Image acquisition is very rapid. Images can be rotated in three dimensions, thus bringing into view eccentric lesions that might be missed by two-dimensional catheter angiography. Older scanners had a single detector that acquired one cross-sectional image at a time and was very time-consuming. It also required more contrast load and there was overheating of the X-ray tube. The currently available multidetector CT (MDCT) scanners can acquire 64 slices simultaneously.[34–39] Abdominal aorta and the entire lower extremity can be imaged in less than 1 minute.[40] One hundred to one hundred eighty milliliters of iodinated contrast is injected at 1 to 3 mL per minute via a peripheral venous line. The radiation exposure is typically one-quarter of that in catheter angiography.

With the single detector scanners, the sensitivity for occlusions was 94% and specificity was 100%. For stenoses greater than 75%, the sensitivity and specificity dropped significantly to 36% and 58%, respectively, when maximum intensity projection was used and improved to 73% to 88% when each slice was individually analyzed. With the MDCT, the sensitivity for stenoses greater than 50% was 89% to 100% and the specificity was 92% to 100%.

CTA is useful in selecting patients who are candidates for endovascular or surgical revascularization. It also provides useful information about associated soft tissue structures that may affect decision making in the optimal endovascular treatment of PAD, e.g., vascular aneurysms. In one study, it showed that popliteal artery stenosis and occlusions occurred because of aneurysms, cystic adventitial disease, or entrapment.[41] Other advantages are patient comfort, and compared to DSA, it is noninvasive, less expensive, delivers less radiation (approximately one-fourth) and has better contrast resolution.[42]

The major limitation of CTA is the risk of contrast-induced nephropathy (CIN). Other drawbacks include lack of accuracy with single detector scanners, lower spatial resolution than DSA, venous filling obscuring arterial imaging, decreased accuracy in calcified vessels, and asymmetrical opacification of legs. The accuracy and effectiveness of CTA is not as well delineated as that of an MRA. Treatment plans based on CTA have not been compared with those of contrast angiography in lower extremity PAD.

Carbon Dioxide Angiography

CO_2 angiography is not available in most centers and generally reserved for patients with history of contrast allergy or renal dysfunction with creatinine clearance less than 20 mL per minute. The use is generally limited to arteries below the diaphragm to minimize the risk of cerebral embolism. DSA equipment is required for CO_2 angiography.[43–50]

● CONTRAST ANGIOGRAPHY

In spite of tremendous improvements in noninvasive imaging, catheter-based invasive iodine contrast catheter angiography remains the gold standard for the diagnosis of PAD in patients considered for endovascular intervention. It is the most widely available modality for the imaging of the vasculature. It is the only universally accepted technology for guiding percutaneous peripheral vascular interventions. Millions of angiographic procedures have been performed worldwide since William Forssman in 1929 passed a catheter from his own arm vein into his right atrium.[51] In the early period, direct punctures of the vessels of interest were performed.[52] This technique has essentially been abandoned and replaced by percutaneous needle access. Safe and good quality angiography requires adequate equipment, well-trained team of staff, and strict adherence to well-established principles.

Catheter angiography has a Class I ACC/AHA indication for delineating the anatomy in patients who require revascularization. Modern technology has permitted the use of smaller diameter sheaths and catheters, less toxic contrast agents, better imaging equipment in angiographic suites requiring less contrast load, thus decreasing the risks to the patient for adverse effects. Invasive angiography procedures, however, are still associated with rare but potentially devastating complications. The risk of severe contrast induced reaction is 0.1%.[53,54] There is significant risk of CIN in patients with baseline renal dysfunction, patients with diabetes mellitus, those with low cardiac output states or those who are dehydrated. Any combination of these is more adverse than an individual risk factor.

Informed consents should be obtained prior to the procedure from all patients after fully explaining all the risks, benefits, and alternatives. History of contrast-related allergic reactions should be documented and appropriate pretreatment should be administered. Decisions regarding revascularization should be made with complete anatomic assessment of the affected arterial territory including imaging of the occlusive lesion as well as of the inflow and outflow vessels. Noninvasive imaging techniques should be combined with vascular imaging for the information. DSA should be used to eliminate dense background tissues. Selective and superselective catheter placement should be done for better enhancement of vasculature and to reduce the contrast load and radiation exposure. Imaging should be done in multiple angulations to uncover vessel overlap, and transstenotic pressure gradients be measured in ambiguous lesions. In patients with renal dysfunction, appropriate hydration should be given prior to the procedure. Patients should be followed up within 2 weeks of the procedure to assess their renal function, the access site, and to make sure that they have not suffered adverse effects like atheroembolism.

Radiological Equipment

Peripheral angiography frequently requires imaging of large areas, which in the absence of a large field of view, will require multiple injections and significant contrast load. A 14-inches (36-cm) image intensifier is recommended (Figure 20-1). Cineangiography at 15 to 30 frames per second (FPS) is excellent for imaging of the moving beating heart.[55] Imaging of static structures with radioopaque bones in the background, e.g., blood vessels, especially the smaller branches will be suboptimal with this technique. Therefore, the technique of DSA should be utilized for peripheral angiography. In this technique, the patient is required to stay motionless during images; otherwise the image will be distorted. In carotid angiography, the patient should also be instructed not to swallow to prevent motion. In modern angiographic suites, ability to acquire DSA images has cut down on the contrast and radiation exposure. In DSA, a precontrast "mask" image is first obtained. Following contrast injection, subtraction of this image allows enhanced filling of the vasculature with masking of nonvascular structures like bones, air, and calcium.

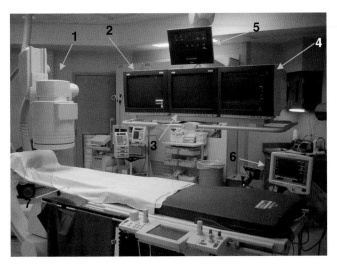

● FIGURE 20-1. Peripheral angiography suite at University of Louisville, Louisville, KY. (1) Fifteen-inch image intensifier; (2) live monitor; (3) reference monitor; (4) hemodynamic monitor; (5) equipment adjustment monitor; (6) fractional flow reserve (FFR) (RADI Sweden) monitor; (7) long patient bed.

Gadolinium or CO_2 angiography should be done in laboratories equipped with DSA; otherwise, the image quality is likely to be poor. "Road mapping," also called "trace subtract fluoroscopy," is usually available in catheter laboratories equipped with DSA capability. This is a very useful technique during interventional procedures. This can be conceptualized as fluoroscopy without the radioopaque background. A small amount of contrast is first injected to fill the vessel and the image is stored in memory as a mask. When the catheter is advanced under normal fluoroscopy, this mask is subtracted, thus allowing visualization of both the moving catheter and the vessel. The image in road mapping will appear white in contrast to DSA, where it will be black. Additional software, enabling quantitative angiography to measure lesion length and diameter should also be ideally available in current angiographic suites.

Examination Console

Highest kilovoltage peak (KVP) is required for cerebral and abdominal angiography, lowest for the extremities, and intermediate for the thorax. Frame rate is generally 2 to 3 FPS for arterial imaging. It is decreased for venous imaging due to long cine runs. Frame rate is increased for cases requiring gadolinium contrast. Newer laboratories will typically have the settings on the console that can be adjusted to optimize adequate imaging of each vascular bed.

In the imaging of the legs 12- to 15-inch image intensifier is required. A longer table is also desirable. Where these are not available, the patient can be positioned in reverse with feet facing the head end of the table. Multiple injections maybe required in the legs to image all the arteries. Depending on the operator and the staff experience, either a "stepped mode" method, which requires contrast bolus at each imaging site, or an "interactive" method where a single bolus of contrast is given in the abdominal aorta and

the table is automatically set to "chase" down the bolus all the way to the feet are utilized for angiography. In our own experience, the stepped mode technique produces better images with the flexibility of changing the amount of contrast and angles during imaging. It may however require slightly larger contrast load and exposes operators to more radiation.

In the "interactive" method, after the bolus is given, a DSA run of both the lower extremities is obtained followed by a "dry run" used for subtraction. This technique is sometimes limited by unequal visualization of both legs in larger patients or in the patients who have flow-limiting lesions in a segment of the vessel causing delayed filling distally. Patients may also be unable to lie motionless or hold their breath for the entire duration of the time required for imaging of all the segments. If free movement of the table is not confirmed prior to the automatic runs, there is a danger of pulling out of the imaging catheter and the sheath. We recommend suturing the sheath if using this method.

Radiation Exposure

Peripheral angiography procedures are typically more time consuming than coronary procedures. Frustration can easily set in during a difficult case especially if the staff is not completely familiar with the equipment and trouble shooting of the modalities commonly used, e.g., DSA, road mapping, bolus chase etc. Also, many laboratories have trainee fellows and less experienced operators trying to learn this increasingly popular skill. Basic principles to prevent radiation exposure can thus be overlooked.

Maximizing distance from the X-ray source is the best way to reduce exposure. Most procedures by the right-handed individuals are done from the right side of the table. Right anterior oblique (RAO) angulation moves the X-ray tube away from the operators, thus exposing them to less radiation than left anterior oblique (LAO) angles. Protective lead shields, good-quality lightweight aprons, thyroid collars, and leaded eyeglasses should be used as a habit. Use of DSA and road mapping will further cut down on flouro-time. Radiation badges should monitor radiation exposure of each operator and staff.

Intravenous Contrast Agents

All current contrast agents are iodine-based. The high atomic number and chemical versatility of iodine makes it ideal for vessel opacification.[56] They are classified as ionic or nonionic and further differentiated into high-osmolar, iso-osmolar, and low-osmolar based on their osmolality. Low- and iso-osmolar agents cause fewer side effects, e.g., hypotension, bradycardia, angina, nausea, and vomiting. They also cause less heat sensation and are better tolerated in peripheral angiography. The nonionic agents cause less allergic side-effects and may also be less nephrotoxic. The nonionic, hypo-osmolar and iso-osmolar agents are more expensive.[57–60] Some patients maybe intolerant to pain and heat sensation even with the iso-osmolar agents. A 50:50 mixture with saline using DSA imaging can be used in such cases. Many agents are commercially available in the market based on their ratio of iodine to ions and concentration of sodium (that determines their osmolality).

High-osmolar ionic ratio 1.5 agents contain three atoms of iodine for every two ions, e.g., Renografin (Bracco), Hypaque (Nycomed), and Angiovist (Berlex). Their sodium concentration is roughly equal to that of blood, making their osmolality very high (>1500 mosm/kg). They cause significant pain and are generally not tolerated well by patients undergoing peripheral angiography.

Low-osmolar ionic ratio-3 agents have three atoms of iodine for every one ion and are low osmolality agents. Their osmolality is roughly twice that of blood, e.g., Ioxaglate (Hexabrix, Mallinckrodt).

Low-osmolar nonionic ratio-3 agents are water-soluble and do not have any ions, e.g., Iopamidol (Isovue, Bracco), Iohexol (Omnipaque, Nycomed), Ioversol (optiray, Mallinckrodt). Their osmolality is also twice that of blood and cause burning in many patients.

Iso-osmolar nonionic ratio-6 agents have osmolality equal to that of blood (290 mosm/kg). They are very well tolerated by patients. Most commonly used is Iodixinol (Visipaque, Nycomed). It has fewer incidences of allergic

reactions than Ioxaglate and has shown no major increase in adverse coronary events like intravascular thrombosis, vessel closure, or perioperative myocardial infarction.[61] There is also some data suggesting less nephrotoxicity with them.

In all patients with renal dysfunction, intravenous hydration with normal saline at 1 mL/kg/h along with N-acetylcysteine (mucomyst) 600 mg orally twice a day should ideally be started 12 to 24 hours prior to the procedure. Gadolinium contrast or CO_2 angiography is another option in such patients.

Diagnostic Catheters and Guide Wires

Vascular access is commonly obtained with an 18-gauge needle that will accommodate most 0.038 inch or smaller wires. A smaller 21-gauge needle with a 0.018-inch wire is available in "micropuncture kit" (Cook, Bloomington, IN) that can be used for difficult femoral, brachial, radial, or antegrade femoral approaches (Figure 20-2). For a nonpalpable pulse Doppler, integrated needle (smart needle) can be used. Wires are available in 0.012 to 0.052 inch in diameter. Most commonly used are wires of 0.035 and 0.038 inch. In a standard guide wire, a stainless steel coil surrounds

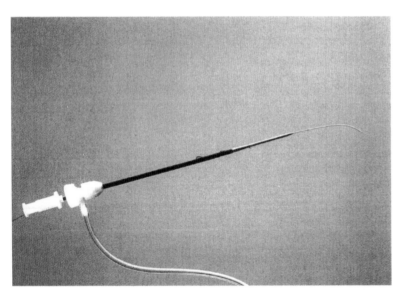

- Uniquely fabricated sheath design to provide maximum flexibility without kinking or compression.

- Initial access is gained using a 21-gauge entry needle.

- 0.018 inch nitinol wire guide with platinum tip is advanced through the needle and the needle removed.

- Introducer dilator incorporates a van Andel taper to facilitate placement into the vessel.

- Check-Flo® hemostasis valve accepts a broad range of sizes while preventing blood reflux and air aspiration.

- AQ® hydrophilic coating, when wet, provides an extremely low coefficient of friction, easing introduction into the vascular system.

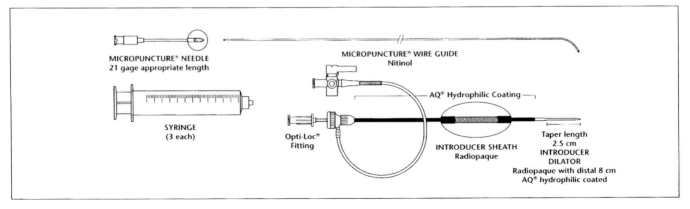

● **FIGURE 20-2.** Micropuncture kit.

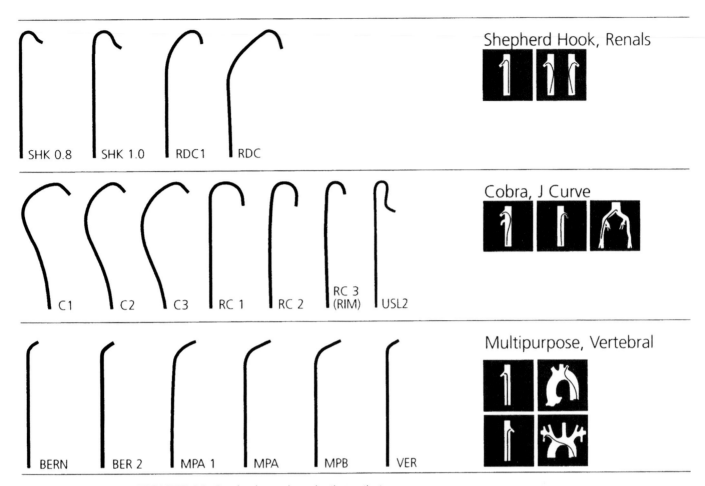

● FIGURE 20-3. Angiography selective catheters.

a tapered inner core. A central safety wire filament is incorporated to prevent separation in case of fracture. Typically they are 100 to 120 cm in length but can also be 260 to 300 cm. Wires are available when wire position needs to be maintained for catheter exchanges. Long wires are frequently required in peripheral angiography, more so than in coronary angiography and their use is encouraged when in doubt.

The tip of the wires can be straight, angled, or J-shaped. Some wires have the capability of increasing their floppy tip by having a movable inner core. Varying degrees of shaft stiffness, e.g., extra support, to provide a strong rail to advance catheters in tortuous anatomy versus extremely slick hydrophilic with low friction for complex anatomy have made peripheral vascular angiography and interventions a viable and many times a preferred treatment of PAD.

Every angiographic suite should have an inventory of such wires. The 0.035-inch wires used in our laboratory are standard J-shaped, Wholey, Straight and Angled Glide, Amplatz Super Stiff, and Supracore. Among the 0.018-inch wires inventory are the Steel Core and V18 Control. In addition to 0.014-inch coronary wires, we frequently use Sparta Core wire in renal and other peripheral vascular interventions. Glide wire (Terumo wire) is very useful in tracking most vessels but carries the risks of vessel dissection and perforation. It should not be used to traverse needles because of the potential of shearing.

Numerous catheters are available (Figures 20-3 to 20-5) and every operator should develop his own skill and "feel" of catheters he uses in peripheral angiography. An "ideal catheter" should be able to sustain high-pressure injections, to track well, be nonthrombogenic, have good memory, and should torque well.[62] Catheters are made of polyurethane, polyethylene, Teflon or nylon. They have a wire braid in the wall to impart torquibility and strength. They are available in different diameters and lengths. They can have an end hole, side holes, or both end and side holes. When using the femoral approach, short-length catheters (60–80 cm) are adequate for angiography of the structures below the diaphragm, whereas long catheters (100–120 cm) are needed for carotid artery, subclavian artery, or arm angiography. Five- to six-French catherter (1-F catheter = 0.333 mm) diameter catheters are most commonly used. Three- to four-French catheters are used for smaller vessels. Side-hole catheters are safe and allow large volume of contrast at a rapid rate with power injectors, e.g. pigtail, Omniflush, Grollman. They are commonly used for angiography of ascending aorta, aortic arch, and abdominal aorta.

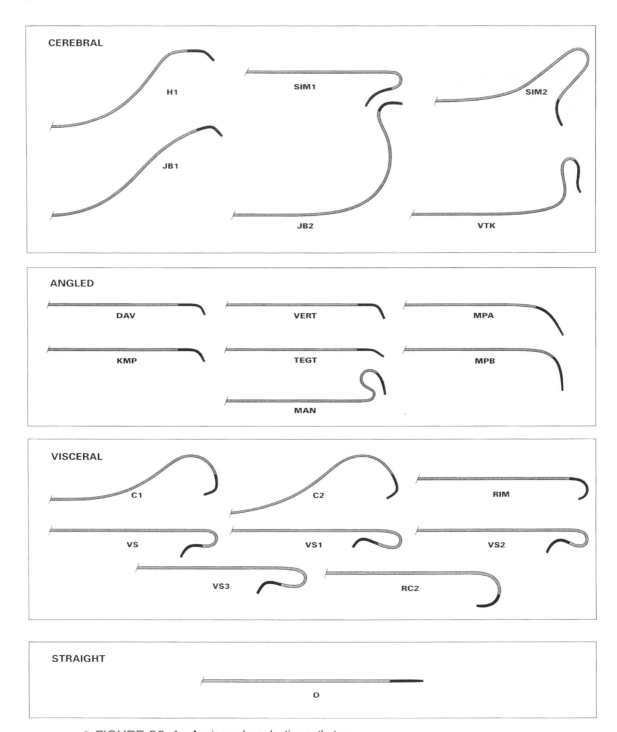

● FIGURE 20-4. Angiography selective catheters.

End-hole catheters are very useful in selective angiography using manual hand injections. For DSA, 5-F catheters are sufficient.

Omniflush catheter can be advanced over the wire beyond the aortic bifurcation and then pulled back to engage the contralateral common iliac artery for selective angiography of the leg. For type-1 aortic arch, a 5 F JR4 will be adequate for carotid, vertebral, subclavian artery angiography, and for nonangulated renal arteries. Simmons, Vitek, SOS, and Amplatz catheters are very useful in certain situations but require added skills and careful manipu-

lation. Heparin should be used with the use of these latter catheters. Simple curved catheters, e.g., Berenstein, Cobra, and Headhunter, are also useful in angulated renal arteries and vertebrals.

Vascular Access

Meticulous technique to achieve vascular access is essential for a successful angiographic procedure. In patients with PAD, the success or failure of a procedure will significantly depend on the correct choice of access site. Every effort

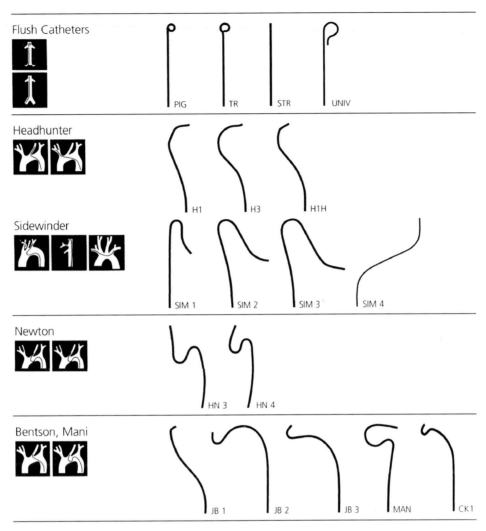

Flush Catheters

PIG   TR   STR   UNIV

Headhunter

H1   H3   H1H

Sidewinder

SIM 1   SIM 2   SIM 3   SIM 4

Newton

HN 3   HN 4

Bentson, Mani

JB 1   JB 2   JB 3   MAN   CK1

● **FIGURE 20-5.** Angiography selective catheters.

should be made to learn the vascular anatomy and direction of blood flow if the patient had previous bypass graft. Prior noninvasive studies like MRA, CTA, and Duplex ultrasonography (US) should be reviewed prior to the angiography. Peripheral bypass grafts in general should not be punctured for 6 to 12 months after surgery.

Most common vascular sites are common femoral artery (CFA) and brachial artery (BA).[63,64] Fluoroscopy should be routinely used to identify bony landmarks to avoid puncturing the artery too low or too high.

Femoral Approach

CFA is ideally suited because of its large caliber that can accommodate up to 14-F sheaths percutaneously and its central location, enabling access to all vascular territories. When compared to the arm approach, there is less radiation exposure but more incidence of bleeding and delayed ambulation. Both retrograde (toward the abdomen) and antegrade (toward the feet) CFA punctures are routinely done. For the antegrade approach, micropuncture technique using 21-gauge needle with 0.018-inch wire is recommended. It should always be done under fluoroscopy and should not

be done in very obese patients. It limits arteriography to the ipsilateral leg, but provides a better platform for interventions if needed. Patients are typically placed in reverse with the feet facing the head-end of the table, allowing maximum mobility of the image intensifier around the limbs. The skin puncture is made at the top of the femoral head. A less acute, less than 45-degree angle is usually required for smooth insertion of the sheath and catheters. Long tapered introducer-sheath instruments are sometimes needed. A short 4- to 5-F sheath should be introduced first and a cine angiogram performed to confirm access in the CFA, and wire position in the superficial femoral artery (SFA) before inserting the larger and longer sheaths and initiation of anticoagulation[65] (Figure 20-6). An ipsilateral 30 to 50 degrees angulation will open up the superficial and deep femoral artery (DFA) bifurcation. Anticoagulation can be reversed at the end of the procedure for early removal of sheath and to decrease the incidence of bleeding.

Brachial and Radial Approach

For radial artery (RA) and 5- to 6-F sheaths and for brachial artery 5- to 7-F sheaths can be used. The biggest

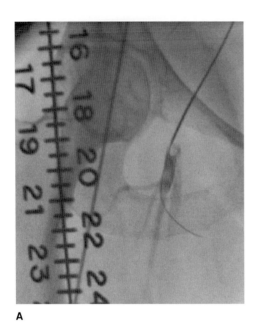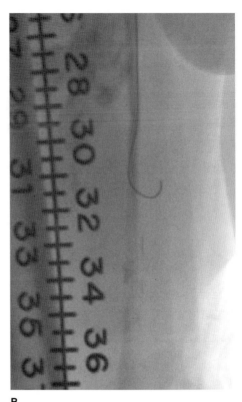

A   B

● FIGURE 20-6. (A) Antegrade femoral artery access technique under direct flouroscopy using micro puncture needle and wire. The wire is in the deep femoral artery. (B) The wire is directed under flouroscopy into the superficial femoral artery.

advantage with these approaches is less bleeding and early ambulation.[66–68] There are however more ischemic complications.[69] These approaches require crossing the great vessels of aorta and great care should be exercised to avoid causing embolic strokes.

For BA approach, the arm is abducted and the puncture is made at the site of maximum pulsation. Micropuncture technique is recommended. When using this approach, one should be aware of the need for longer length catheters if angiography and intervention of the lower extremities is anticipated. Left brachial approach has approximately 100 mm greater reach than the right brachial approach. Wholey wire, glide wire, and other soft wires should be used with these approaches to minimize trauma and spasm of the vessels.

For RA approach,[70] more skill is required. RA is superficial and lies against the bone. It has no major veins or nerves in the vicinity. Its smaller size, however, limits the use of some devices and larger stents. Hydrophilic sheaths and guiding catheters of upto 6- to 7-F are now available and can be used with this approach. They can accommodate most current balloons and stents. There is approximately a 3% incidence of RA occlusion postprocedure. Allen's test[71] should be performed prior to cannulating RA to confirm the ulnar artery patency (Figure 20-7). There is, however, some controversy regarding the absolute value of Allen's test. The success rate of this approach is 95%.[72] The

wrist is extended and the arm abducted in supine position. Using micropuncture technique, puncture is made 1 to 2 cm proximal to the wrist crease. After sheath insertion, the arm is brought back in the adducted neutral position. Right arm is preferred to preserve left RA for future bypass surgery if needed. Minimal local anesthesia is administered. Five F long hydrophilic sheath is a good choice. Heparin 2500 to 5000 units should be given directly in the sheath. Radial arteries are very prone to spasm and vasodilators should be used. Nitroglycerin 100 to 200 mg and Verapamil 1 to 2 mg is directly given through the sheath. A short cineangiogram should be performed to look for any

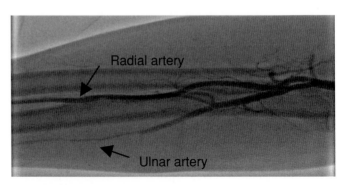

● FIGURE 20-7. Atretic ulnar artery in a patient with equivocal Allen's test.

anomalous arteries. One should look for radial recurrent artery. The sheath should be removed immediately after the procedure. Activated clotting time (ACT) check is not necessary. Compression straps, e.g., Hemoband (Hemoband Corp., Portland, OR) are placed directly over the puncture site. Pressure is maintained for approximately 90 minutes for diagnostic and 180 minutes for interventional procedures. Access site complications are very uncommon.

Other Vascular Access Sites

PA is uncommonly accessed. The patient has to lie prone. Puncture is performed under fluoroscopy and micropuncture technique is recommended. Axillary approach is more popular among interventional radiologists. Left axillary artery is preferred. The patient needs very close monitoring for bleeding after axillary artery puncture because even a medium-sized hematoma can cause nerve compression. BA cut down is very uncommon now. It is used in less than 10% of cases and should be performed only by experienced operators. Lumbar aortic punctures are again sometimes used by radiologists in patients who have extensive PAD.[73] Patient is placed prone. This site is only used as a last resort because in case of bleeding complications direct pressure cannot be applied and patient will likely require open surgical repair of the bleeding vessel.

Local Vascular Complications

Society for Cardiac Angiography and Interventions (SCAI) has reported an incidence of 0.5% to 0.6% local vascular complications. These complications comprise vessel thrombosis, dissection (Figure 20-8), bleeding, which can be free hemorrhage, retroperitoneal bleeding, or access site hematoma, arteriovenous fistula (Figure 20-9), distal embolization, or false aneurysm (pseudo aneurysm).

The operator should be well versed in the diagnosis and management of these complications. Adequate specialty care should be readily available at the facility where such procedures are performed.

Thoracic Aorta and Aortic Arch Angiography

Noninvasive modalities like MRA and three-dimensional CTA should be performed if available prior to invasive imaging. Angiography provides 2D imaging and may underestimate the tortuosity of various vessels (Figure 20-10). CTA and MRA will also provide information about the type of aortic arch, and anomalous origin of any vessel from the arch (Figure 20-11).

Thoracic Aorta

Commonly approached via right CFA utilizing 4- to 6-F sheath and diagnostic catheters. Pigtail or tennis racquet catheter is advanced over a soft J-tip guidewire under fluoroscopy. In cases of coarctation of the aorta, anteroposterior and lateral views are obtained with the contrast

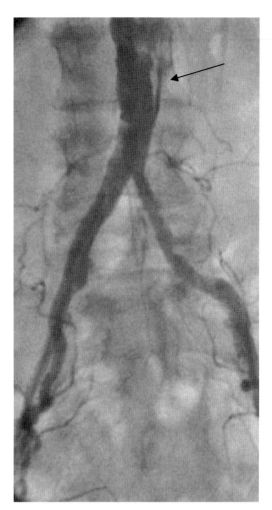

● **FIGURE 20-8.** Catheter-induced abdominal aortic dissection.

injected proximal to the coarctation. For cases of patent ductus arteriosus, selective aortic angiography is very sensitive in demonstrating small shunts and supercedes the sensitivity of right heart catheterization with stepwise oximetry. In cases of thoracic aortic aneurysms (TAA), MRA and CTA are again very useful initial tools (Figure 20-12), but catheter angiography is still considered essential to delineate the aneurysm and its relationship to the branches in the chest and abdomen. If endovascular thoracic aneurysm repair (ETAR) or open surgical repair is planned, then coronary, brachiocephalic, visceral, and renal arteriography should also be performed. For the diagnosis of thoracic aneurysms, angiography is performed in the ascending thoracic aorta above the aortic valve using 30 to 40 mL of iodinated contrast at 15 to 20 mL/s using power injection. TAA is less common than abdominal aortic aneurysm (AAA) but the incidence is increasing as the median age of the population is also increasing. It also has a higher incidence of rupture than AAA. Untreated, the mortality is greater than 70% within 5 years of diagnosis.[74] Open surgical repair has a mortality of 10% to 30%, spinal cord injury 5% to 15%, respiratory failure 25% to 45%, myocardial infarction 7% to

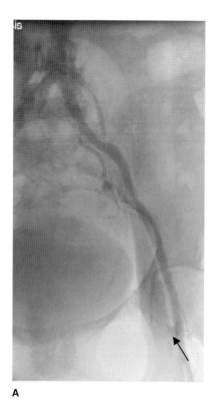

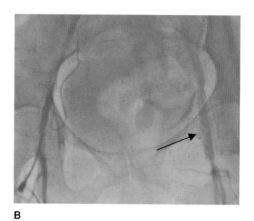

A   B

● **FIGURE 20-9.** (A) Arteriovenous fistula between left CFA and vein. (B) Repair of arteriovenous fistula with a covered stent.

20%, and renal dysfunction 8% to 30%.[75] Chronic obstructive pulmonary disease (COPD) and renal failure are strong predictors of rupture. In one series,[76] the rupture rate was high for aneurysms greater than 6 cm. In another series, no rupture was reported in aneurysms less than 5 cm. Mean size for rupture was 5.8 cm. With ETAR, the mortality and the morbidity has been reported to be much less.[77]

In cases of thoracic aortic dissection, angiography has a sensitivity of 80% and specificity of 95%. Noninvasive modalities like CTA, MRA, and transesophageal echocardiography have taken over as the initial diagnostic tools; however, cardiothoracic surgeons will still require an angiogram for additional information about coronary and branch vessel involvement and the competence of the aortic valve prior to aortic repair. A pigtail or tennis racquet catheter is advanced over a soft wire typically via the right CFA approach. Most of the aortic tears are at the greater (outer) curve and to avoid entry into the false lumen, the catheter is used to direct the wire toward the inner curve. Frequent contrast injections should be utilized to check the catheter position. Entry into the false lumen is not uncommon and if that occurs, the catheter should be gently retracted and advanced into the true lumen.

Aortic Arch

Catheter angiography is still considered the gold standard, but 3D CTA and MRA are excellent for imaging the aortic arch and should be considered prior to considering arch angiography. CFA is the most common access site. Brachial or radial approaches can be used in cases of suspected aortic dissection and in patients with severe ileofemoral or abdominal aortic atherosclerotic disease. A pigtail catheter is positioned above the sinus of valsalva and 40 to 60 mL of nonionic iso-osmolar contrast at the rate of 20 cc/s is injected with a power injector. Both cine and DSA imaging can be used. For a cine angiogram, 30 FPS and for DSA, 4 to 6 FPS are commonly used. LAO at 45 degrees angle opens up the aortic arch and the great vessels in most cases. DSA allows a lower contrast load of 30 mL injected at 20 cc/s.

Carotid and Cerebrovascular Angiography

Catheter angiography is the gold standard for aortic arch, cervical, and cerebral angiography. A major drawback for angiography in this territory has been the risk of strokes. There was 1.2% incidence of stroke in the hands of radiologists in the ACAS[78] trial. In a later study[79] performed by cardiologists, the risk was 0.5%. Proper patient selection and the procedural volumes and the technical skill of the operator are important predictors of this risk.

Carotid Artery

Many patients with carotid artery disease are asymptomatic. History and physical examination are therefore not very sensitive in detecting carotid artery disease. Carotid duplex ultrasound, CTA, and MRA should be utilized as the initial diagnostic tools (Figure 20-13). Invasive angiography

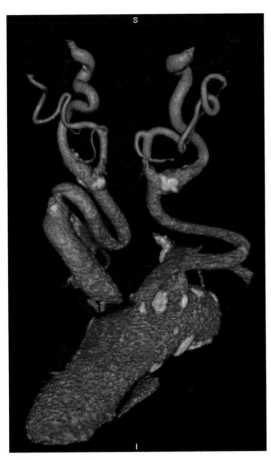

● FIGURE 20-10. CTA showing extremely tortuous carotid arteries making endovascular intervention an undesirable option in such cases.

Courtesy: Robert Falk MD, 3-DR Louisville, KY.

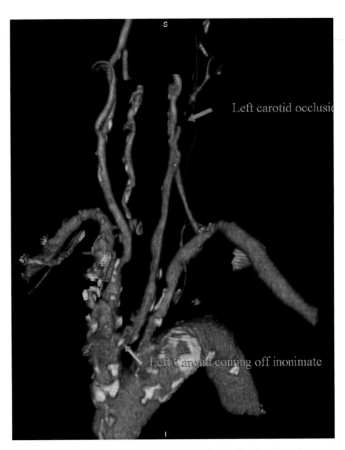

● FIGURE 20-11. CTA nicely showing a "bovine" aortic arch. There is also severe stenosis of the left internal carotid artery and the aortic arch is also "type 3" making carotid artery stenting an unsuitable option in this case.

Courtesy: Robert Falk MD, 3-DR Louisville, KY.

remains the gold standard in patients considered for carotid artery stenting (CAS). The landmark North American Symptomatic Carotid Endarterectomy Trial (NASCET), European Carotid Artery Surgery (ECAS), and Asymptomatic Carotid Artery Stenosis (ACAS)[78,80,81] trials were all based on angiography.

Brachiocephalic (BC) artery arises as the first great vessel from the aortic arch and divides into right subclavian (RSC) and right common carotid arteries (RCCA). RCCA almost always arises from the BC and rarely as a separate branch from the aorta. It may come from a single common carotid trunk that also gives rise to left common carotid artery (LCCA). RCCA further divides into right internal carotid artery (RICA) and right external carotid artery (RECA) at the fourth cervical vertebra. The angle of the mandible is a good bony landmark for the bifurcation of the CCA. ECA gives numerous branches (Figure 20-10). LCCA arises 75% of the time as a separate branch from aorta, 10% to 15% of the time as a common origin with the BC, and approximately 10% of the times from the BC (bovine origin) (Figure 20-11). ICA can be divided into four segments[82] (Figure 20-11).

a. *Prepetrous* (*cervical*). Between the CCA bifurcation and the petrous bone. This segment does not give rise to any

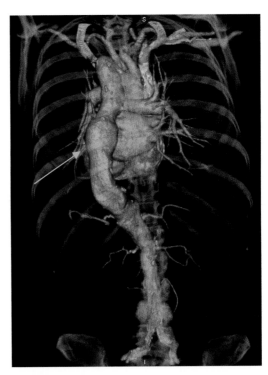

● FIGURE 20-12. CTA showing thoracic aortic aneurysm.

Courtesy: Robert Falk MD, 3-DR Louisville, KY.

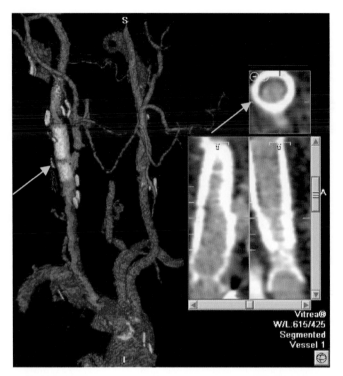

● **FIGURE 20-13.** CTA of carotid arteries showing patent stent in the right common and internal carotid arteries (*arrows*).

Courtesy: Robert Falk MD, 3-DR Louisville, KY.

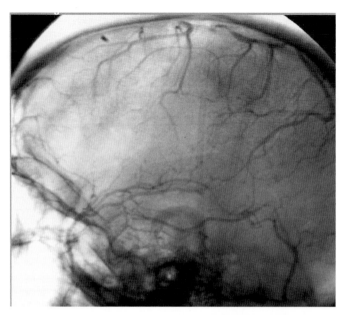

● **FIGURE 20-14.** Venous phase of cerebral angiogram.

major branches and is the most common site of carotid stenosis involving the ostial and the proximal portion of the artery.

b. *Petrous.* This segment courses through the petrous bone and makes a 90-degree L-shaped angle on angiogram.

c. *Cavernous.* This is the part through the cavernous sinus.

d. *Supraclinoid.* This segment gives ophthalmic, posterior communicating, and anterior choroidal branches before terminating as the middle and anterior cerebral arteries. Ophthalmic artery supplies the ipsilateral retina and optic nerve and is a source of important collateral route between ICA and ECA. Posterior communicating branch connects ICA with posterior cerebral artery to provide communication between the anterior and posterior circulation. The area supplied by ACA and MCA is referred to as "carotid territory of the brain."

Angiography

Angiography is considered to be the gold standard for the diagnosis of extracranial and intracranial carotid artery disease. For complete cerebrovascular circulation, carotid angiography should be done in conjunction with aortic arch and selective vertebral angiography. Knowledge of arch anatomy and presence of proximal AS and tortuosity are crucial in the appropriate selection of the catheters for selective angiography. For Type-I or Type-II arch, 5 F JR4, Davis, HH (Meditech Watertown, MA), or Berenstein catheters are adequate. In patients with bovine arch Vitek catheter is often needed. For Type-III arch (elon-

gated), reverse curve catheters like Simmons (Angiodynamics, Queensbury, NY) or Vitek are often required. Simmons catheter can be very useful as it "travels up" the carotid artery and does not get dislodged. Its use, however, requires more skill.

Meticulous technique and double flushing is recommended once the catheter is beyond the aortic arch. Diluted low- or iso-osmolar contrast is injected at 4 to 6 mL/s for a total of 8 mL for CCA angiography using DSA at 4 to 6 FPS.

Cerebral circulation imaging should be continued into the venous phase to rule out any venous anomaly (Figure 20-14). Multiple projections and angulation are sometimes needed for optimal visualization. In most cases, a straight AP and lateral or 30 to 40 degrees ipsilateral angle will open up the bifurcation to assess the lesion (Figures 20-15 and 20-16). RAO projection opens up the bifurcation of the BC artery. In patients who are undergoing carotid or vertebral interventions, cerebral angiography should be performed before and after the intervention, for comparison, in the event of suspected embolic stroke. It also provides information about intracranial aneurysms and atherosclerotic disease. A straight PA cranial view to bring the petrous bone at the base of the orbit (Towne's view) will nicely outline the cerebral circulation in most cases (Figure 20-17).

For assessment of the severity of carotid stenosis, the methodology used by NASCET investigators is most popular. This method compares the stenotic area with the most normal appearing artery distal to the stenosis.

Vertebral Artery

Left vertebral artery originates as the first branch of subclavian artery. In 3% to 5% of cases, it may arise directly from the aorta between LCCA and LSCA. Very rarely, it may originate distal to LSCA. Right vertebral artery can

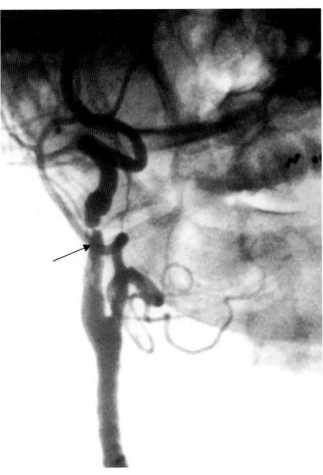

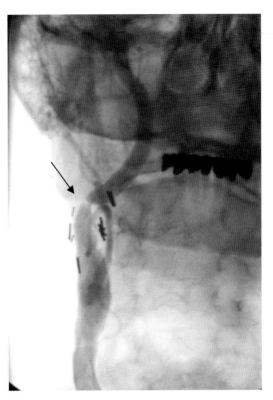

● FIGURE 20-16. Severe right carotid artery stenosis in a patient with previous carotid endarterectomy.

Courtesy: John Laird MD, Washington Hospital Center, Washington, DC.

● FIGURE 20-15. Severe stenosis of right internal carotid artery.

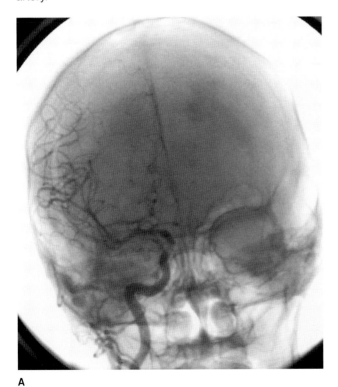

A

B

● FIGURE 20-17. (A) Right and (B) and lateral view of cerebral angiography in AP (Towne's view).

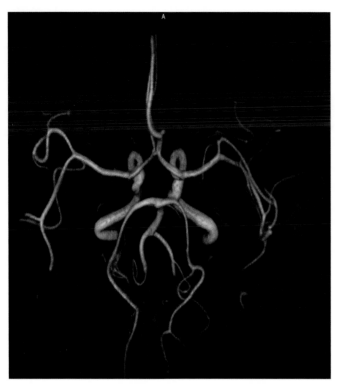

● **FIGURE 20-18.** CTA showing "Circle of Willis."

Courtesy: Robert Falk MD, 3-DR Louisville, KY.

Angiography

Subclavian and vertebral artery angiography is commonly performed from the CFA approach. For patients with severe lower extremity PAD with no femoral access or who have Type-III aortic arch ipsilateral brachial approach can also be used. Unfractionated heparin (3000–5000 units) are given when using the brachial approach. RA can also be used for angiography and in addition to heparin vasodilators should also be given with this approach. AP, RAO, and LAO projections will open up the SCA and VA. RAO cranial angle will show the origin of internal memory artery (IMA). JR4 catheter is usually adequate for straight aortic arch. For elongated aortic arch, Vitek, Head Hunter, or Simmons 1 or 2 are used (Figure 20-19). For vertebral artery, 3 to 4 mL/s for a total of 6 mL of contrast is generally sufficient. Nonselective angiography with a blood pressure cuff inflated on the ipsilateral arm will improve the visualization of ostial disease. Ostia are also better seen in the contralateral oblique projections and V2 and V3 segments are better seen in PA and lateral views or ipsilateral oblique views. Intracranial segments are best seen in steep 40 degrees PA cranial (Towne's) view and crosstable view.

originate from RCCA and duplication of vertebrals can occur at any level. It originates from the superior and posterior aspect of the RSCA. The two vertebrals converge to form the basilar artery at the base of the pons (Figure 20-18).

It can be divided into four segments[83]:

V-1: From the origin to the transverse foramen of the fifth and sixth cervical vertebrae.

V-2: Its course within the vertebra until it exits at C2 level.

V-3: Extracranial course between the transverse foramen of C2 and base of skull where it enters foramen magnum.

V-4: Intracranial course as it pierces the dura and arachnoid maters at the base of skull and ends as it meets the opposite vertebral artery (Figure 20-14).

Intracranial part gives anterior and posterior spinal branches; penetrating branches and posterior inferior cerebellar artery (PICA), which gives supply to dorsal medulla and cerebellum. Left vertebral artery is usually dominant and stenosis of the dominant vertebral is likely to cause symptoms.

AS is the dominant pathology involving the ostium and proximal extracranial segment of the VA. Surgical revascularization carries significant mortality and morbidity approaching 20%.[84] With rapidly improving skills and technology, endovascular revascularization is becoming a very attractive option for these patients.

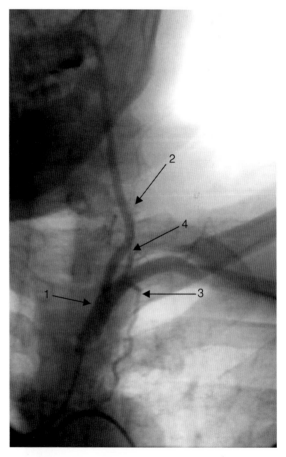

● **FIGURE 20-19.** Selective angiography of left subclavian artery (1) using a Simmons catheter. (2) A normal left vertebral artery, (3) a small internal mammary artery, and (4) thyrocervical trunk are also seen.

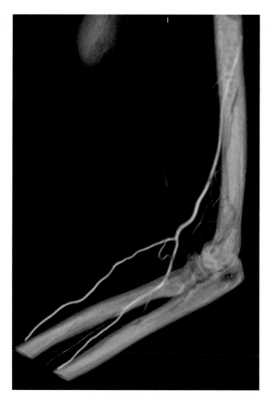

● **FIGURE 20-20.** CTA of brachial, radial, and ulnar arteries.

Courtesy: Robert Falk MD, 3-DR Louisville, KY.

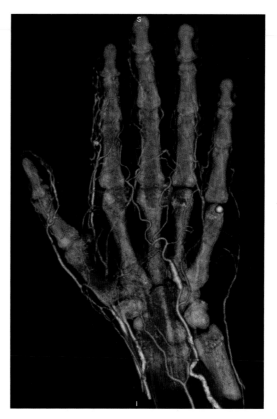

● **FIGURE 20-21.** CTA of hand arteries.

Courtesy: Robert Falk MD, 3-DR Louisville, KY.

Subclavian, Brachiocephalic, and Upper Extremity

This vascular bed constitutes approximately 15% of symptomatic extracranial cerebrovascular disease. Right subclavian artery (RSCA) arises from BCA on the right and LSCA is the last major branch from the aorta on the left. In 0.5% population, RSCA arises as the terminal branch from the descending thoracic aorta and courses over to the right toward its normal distribution to the right upper extremity. Rarely, RSCA and RCCA may have separate origins from the aorta instead of a BCA. It gives vertebral, IMA, and thyrocervical trunk (TCT) from its first segment. TCT gives inferior thyroid, suprascapular, and transverse cervical branches. SCA becomes axillary artery at the lateral margin of the first rib that in turn becomes BA at the anatomic neck of the humerus. Opposite to the neck of radius, BA divides into ulnar and radial arteries (Figure 20-20). In approximately 1.3% of cases, RA originates from the axillary artery and in 15% to 20% of cases from the upper BA. Ulnar artery helps to form the superficial palmar arch and the RA the deep palmar arch (Figure 20-21).

Angiography

Angiography is generally needed in patients presenting with arm claudication, and in other causes of arm ischemia, e.g., blue digit syndrome, severe digital ischemia, and blunt and penetrating trauma with vascular injury to these vessels. CTA and MRA are useful to delineate arch anatomy. Step-

wise angiography with iso-osmolar contrast is preferred. Contrast of 5 to 10 mL with hand injection using DSA will give good visualization of these vessels. JR4 catheter is routinely used (Figures 20-22 and 20-23). Vitek or Simmons catheter maybe required depending on the take off of SCA or BCA. Vitek catheter is advanced under fluoroscopy and positioned in the descending thoracic aorta with the curve facing the right side of the arch and the tip facing north. Catheter is gently advanced and each great vessel is selectively engaged. After completion of the angiogram, the catheter is removed over a wire. Simmons catheter is reshaped in the ascending thoracic aorta and is gently withdrawn to engage each vessel selectively. It is also removed after straightening with a wire.

Orthogonal oblique views will visualize SCA and its branches. LAO for RSCA and RAO for LSCA will give good views of these vessels (Figures 20-24 and 20-25). Patient's arm should be adducted to the neutral position during angiography. For axillary artery and BA angiography, catheter is advanced into distal SCA. Usually a long 300 cm Wholey, Magic Torque or a Stiff Shaft Angled Glide wire is used to exchange the JR4, Vitek, or Simmons catheter for a straight 4- to 5-F Glide catheter or a multipurpose catheter. Axillary artery is angiographed in adducted arm position and BA in an abducted position with forearm supine. For the forearm and hand angiogram, the diagnostic catheter is further advanced into the distal BA. Forearm should be supine, fingers splayed and thumb abducted. PA projection

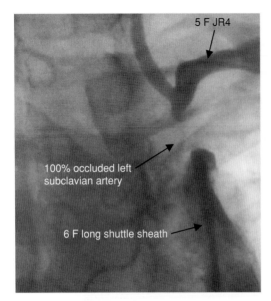

● **FIGURE 20-22.** Hundred percent occluded left subclavian artery. Dual injection technique is demonstrated with 5-F JR4 catheter in the subclavian artery and 6-F long shuttle sheath in the ascending aorta.

Courtesy: John Laird MD, Washington Hospital Center, Washington, DC.

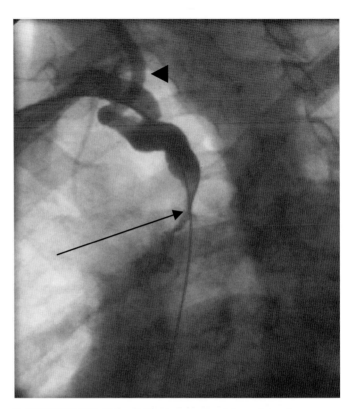

● **FIGURE 20-24.** Critical stenosis of the origin of innominate artery seen on angiogram performed via right radial artery. Aortic arch is not clearly opacified due to the stenosis. Right common carotid artery is patent (*arrow head*).

Courtesy: John Laird MD, Washington Hospital Center, Washington, DC.

is adequate. Vasodilators are given intraarterially due to the spasmodic nature of these arteries. For borderline lesions a translesional gradient can be measured using a 0.014-inch pressure wire or simultaneous measurement of pressure between 4- and 5-F catheter tip placed distal to the lesion and the side port of a long 6-F sheath positioned in the distal aorta. Vasodilators can be used to augment the gradient. A gradient greater than or equal to 15 mm Hg in SCA and BCA is considered significant.

Abdominal Aorta

Atherosclerotic disease is very common with more involvement of the infrarenal abdominal aorta. Abdominal aorta starts at the level of the diaphragm (T12) and continues anterior to the spine and to the left of inferior vena cava. It bifurcates at L4 level into the right and left common iliac artery.[85] AA is 15 to 25 mm in diameter and larger in males and older populations.[86] It gives rise to the celiac trunk at T12–L1, superior mesenteric artery (SMA) at L1–L2, and inferior mesenteric artery (IMA) at L3–L4 level. Renal arteries originate posterolaterally at L1–L2 level below the origin of the SMA. Four pairs of lumbar arteries originate below the renals.

Abdominal aorta is considered to be aneurysmal when the anteroposterior diameter is 3 cm. Diagnosis is based

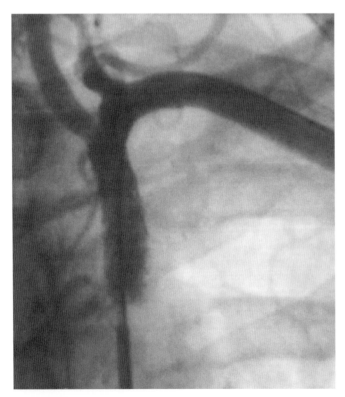

● **FIGURE 20-23.** Left subclavian artery widely patent after stenting.

Courtesy: John Laird MD, Washington Hospital Center, Washington, DC.

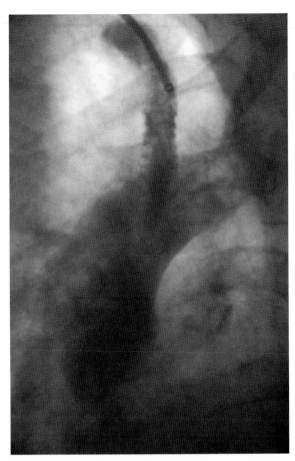

● **FIGURE 20-25.** Innonimate artery is widely patent after stenting with opacification of aortic arch.

Courtesy: John Laird MD, Washington Hospital Center, Washington, DC.

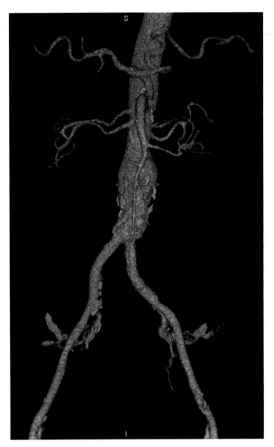

● **FIGURE 20-26.** CTA of abdominal aorta and iliac arteries showing infrarenal abdominal aortic aneurysm and accessory bilateral renal arteries.

Courtesy: Robert Falk MD, 3-DR Louisville, KY.

on formulas that adjust for age or body surface area or by calculating the ratio between the normal and dilated aortic segments.[87–90] The prevalence of AAA increases with age. In a necropsy study,[91] incidence was 5.9% in men aged 80 to 85 years and 4.5% in women who were older than 90 years of age. Based on U.S. studies, the prevalence for AAA 2.9 to 4.9 cm is 1.3% for men aged 45 to 54 years and up to 12.5% for men aged 75 to 84 years. Comparable prevalence for women is 0% to 5.2%.

Common iliac artery aneurysms are usually also found in association with AAA. One-third to one-half are bilateral and 50% to 85% are asymptomatic when diagnosed.[92,93] Rupture occurs when they are more than 5 cm.

For the diagnosis, a history of abdominal and back pain and presence of a pulsatile mass are important indicators of the presence of AAA. Plain X-ray film of the abdomen may show curvilinear aortic wall calcification as an incidental finding. US or nuclear scan of abdomen may show AAA as an incidental finding. Similarly, during unrelated arteriography, slow or turbulent flow in the aorta may suggest presence of AAA.

US has a specificity of nearly 100% and sensitivity of 92% to 99% for the diagnosis of infrarenal AAA.[87] For suprarenal AAA, the accuracy is much less. CTA and MRA are the current gold standard for the diagnosis of AAA.[94] Spiral contrast-enhanced CTA with 3D reconstruction is now the standard preop evaluation to look for vessel calcification, thrombus, and anatomy of the aneurysm for optimal stent graft placement (Figure 20-26). In addition to previously described limitations, CTA tends to overestimate the diameter of the neck and underestimate the length of the neck of the aneurysm. MRA is inferior to spiral contrast-enhanced CTA in spatial resolution and not very good for detecting vessel wall calcification. MRA is slower than CTA but not inferior in the diagnosis. It is considered superior to catheter angiography for defining the proximal extent of the AAA, venous anatomy, intraluminal thrombus and iliac aneurysms.[95] Renal arteries can also be imaged accurately with the new scanners. Standard MRA protocols for AAA are not available everywhere.

Catheter angiography is always done at the time of endovascular aneurysm repair (EVAR). Pelvic angiography is also done at the same time to visualize iliac arteries, which are also frequently involved with abdominal aortic aneurysm. It also helps in the optimal visualization of collateral or variant arterial anatomy.[96,97] Contrast angiography, however, is not accurate in estimating the diameter of the AAA due to presence of thrombus that is usually present in the aneurysms. CTA or MRA are thus needed

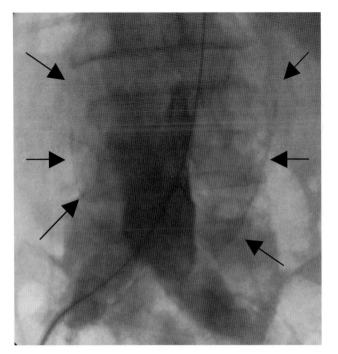

● **FIGURE 20-27.** Large abdominal aortic aneurysm (*arrows*), only partially visualized on contrast angiogram. The rest of the sac is filled with thrombus.

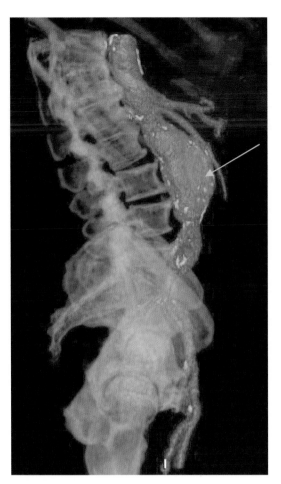

● **FIGURE 20-28.** CTA of an abdominal aortic aneurysm showing a large thrombus in the aneurysm not likely to be visible on a catheter angiogram.

Courtesy: Robert Falk MD, 3-DR Louisville, KY.

in conjunction prior to EVAR (Figures 20-27 and 20-28). Prior to open or endovascular repair the maximum transverse diameter of the aneurysm, its relationship to the renal arteries, presence of iliac artery or hypogastric artery aneurysm, stenosis of renal or iliac arteries, and presence of horse-shoe kidneys, etc., must be defined. The diagnostic modality must provide measurement of the neck and body of the AAA and of the iliac arteries. CTA is also excellent in defining the type of endoleak after EVAR before angiography to repair the endoleak (Figure 20-29).

Femoral approach is most common using 4- to 6-F pigtail or Omniflush catheter. Radial, brachial, or axillary approaches are also used. As a last resort, translumbar puncture can be done. For AAA, the pigtail or Omniflush catheter is positioned such that the tip is at T12-L1 level so that the side holes are at L1-L2 level. Contrast of 30 to 50 cc is injected. For abdominal or thoracic aortic stenosis, a translesional gradient can be measured as previously described. A gradient greater than 10 mm Hg is considered significant (Figure 20-17).

Visceral Artery Aneurysms

Open or endovascular repair has a class I indication for aneurysms greater than 2 cm in women of child-bearing age or in men or women undergoing liver transplant. They have Class IIa indication in men or in women who are beyond the child-bearing age. Splenic and hepatic artery aneurysms are not very common.[98,99] Most are found incidentally during imaging for other reasons. Most are asymptomatic but a rupture in pregnant women carries a very high mortality that may approach 70% for the mother and >90% for the

fetus.[100] In general population the rupture carries a mortality of 10% to 25%

SMA has 6% to 7% of all visceral aneurysms. Lower extremity aneurysms generally do not rupture but pose a danger of thromboembolism or vessel thrombosis. PA carries up to 70% of all LE aneurysms. CTA and MRA are the tests of choice.

Renal Artery

Renal artery stenosis (RAS) is a very common and progressive disease in patients with PAD. It is a relatively uncommon cause of hypertension.[101–103] A duplex US study of patients older than 65 years showed an incidence of 9.1% in men, 5.5% in women, 6.9% in white population, and 6.7% in black population.[102] In another series of 395 patients with abdominal aortic and ileofemoral disease, the incidence of RAS greater than 50% was 33% to 50%.[104] The incidence of significant RAS in patients who were undergoing coronary angiography who also underwent renal angiography was approximately 11% to 18%.[105–107] Conversely, the incidence of clinically significant CAD was 58% in patients with atherosclerotic RAS.[108] In 24% patients

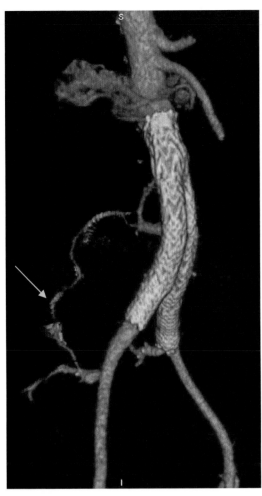

● **FIGURE 20-29.** CTA of an abdominal aortic endograft showing an endoleak via a collateral between Internal iliac and inferior mesenteric arteries (*arrow*).

Courtesy: Robert Falk MD, 3-DR Louisville, KY.

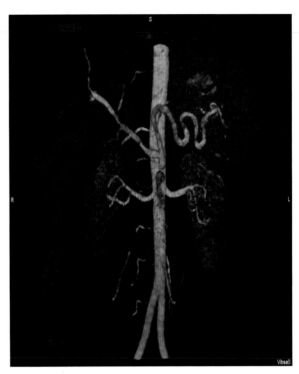

● **FIGURE 20-30.** (A and B) MRA of renal and mesenteric arteries showing normal vessels and abdominal aorta.

Courtesy: Robert Falk MD, 3-DR Louisville, KY.

Angiography

MRA has an ACC/AHA Class I indication as a screening tool for RAS (Figure 20-30). Similarly, CTA has Class I indication in patients with normal renal function. When the clinical suspicion is high and when the noninvasive tests are inconclusive, catheter angiography has Class 1 indication for the diagnosis of RAS (Figure 20-18).

MRA with gadolinium compared to catheter angiography has a sensitivity 90% to 100% and specificity of 76% to 94% in atherosclerotic RAS. For patients who have FMD, the accuracy of MRA is less.[117] MRA is the most expensive test diagnostic tool and other limitations are as discussed before. CTA has a sensitivity of 92% and specificity of 95% when compared to DSA.[118] Use of CTA is limited because of a risk of CIN. CTA with the old scanners had a sensitivity of 59% to 96% and specificity of 82% to 99% when compared to catheter angiography.[119–124] With the new scanners, they have improved to 91% to 92% and 99%, respectively.

Currently, catheter angiography is reserved for those patients whose diagnosis is not clear by noninvasive testing. It is also recommended in patients who are undergoing coronary or peripheral angiography in whom there is a high suspicion of RAS.

For contrast angiography, CFA approach is most common using 5- to 6-F short sheath. In severely tortuous ileofemoral vessels, a long 6 F sheath should be used. Brachial approach is used in patients with poor femoral approach or if the renal arteries are acutely downward angulated. Nonselective angiography is done first with a pigtail or

with end-stage renal disease (ESRD) and in need for dialysis, there was severe atherosclerotic RAS.[109] AS is by far the most common pathophysiological mechanism approaching 90% in patients with RAS. Fibromuscular dysplasia is found in approximately 10% of patients with RAS. There is also significant progression of RAS. In patients with less than 60% RAS, progression was 20% per year and in those with greater than 60% stenosis, there was complete occlusion in 5% cases at 1 year and 11% at 2 years.[110–112] Bilateral RAS is also common. In six different studies including 319 patients, it was found in 44% of cases.[113] renal atrophy and ESRD can develop in patients with RAS and RA occlusion.[114–116]

Renal arteries arise at L1–L2 level from the posterolateral aspect of the abdominal aorta. Right RA typically originates slightly higher than the left. Accessory renal arteries are also quite common and found in 25% to 35% of the general population. These usually supply the lower poles of the kidneys. They can arise anywhere from suprarenal aorta down to the iliac and are generally smaller in caliber. Main renal artery further branch into segmental, interlobar, arcuate, interlobular, and arterioles.

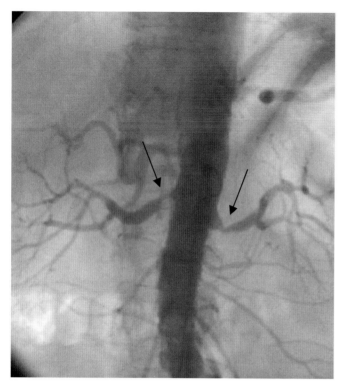

● **FIGURE 20-31.** Bilateral renal artery stenoses on flush angiography of abdominal aorta utilizing pigtail catheter.

Omniflush catheter positioned at L1-L2 level in AP view to look for ostia of the renal arteries and also to look for accessory renal arteries. DSA at 4 FPS with 30 mL non-ionic iso-osmolar contrast at the rate of 15 mL/s is usually injected (Figure 20-31). For selective renal angiography 4 to

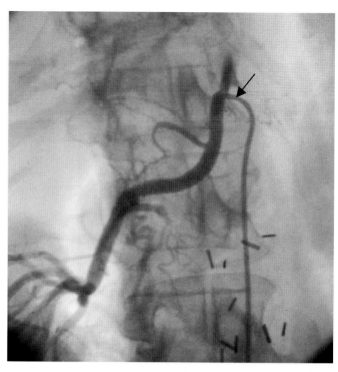

● **FIGURE 20-33.** Selective right renal artery angiography utilizing Cobra catheter.

5 F JR4, renal double curve, Cobra, IMA, SOS, or Hockey stick catheters can be used (Figures 20-32 to 20-34). For downward-angulated renals, reverse curve catheters, for example, Simmons or Omniselective can be utilized from the femoral approach or a straight MP catheter from the brachial approach. Contrast of 5 to 8 mL at 5 mL/s using DSA at 4 FPS will give excellent images. Usually an ipsilateral 15 to 30 degree oblique view will display the ostium and proximal renal artery. Another useful technique is to modify the LAO/RAO angulation under fluoroscopy while the catheter is engaged until the tip of the diagnostic

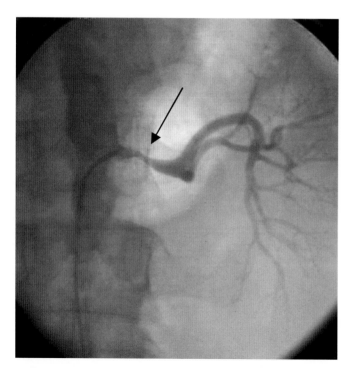

● **FIGURE 20-32.** Selective left renal artery angiography utilizing Judkin's right coronary catheter showing significant stenosis.

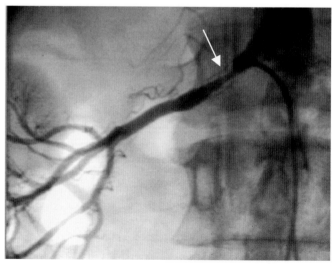

● **FIGURE 20-34.** Selective right renal artery angiography showing in-stent restenosis utilizing Judkin's right coronary catheter.

catheter is maximally opened. Cranial and caudal angulation can be used to open up the bifurcation lesions. Cineangiogram is prolonged until the nephrogram phase to assess the kidney size and regional perfusion of the kidney to optimize revascularization strategy.

No Touch Technique

Abdominal aorta frequently is severely atherosclerotic and there is risk of visceral or distal embolization of atheroma during manipulation of catheters. With this technique, a 0.14-inch wire is advanced through the catheter beyond the renal arteries. The catheter is manipulated toward the renal ostia without touching them, thus avoiding the scraping of the aortic intima.

In borderline lesions, a translesional gradient should be measured. A 0.014-inch pressure wire is most accurate. Alternatively, a 4 F diagnostic catheter is advanced beyond the lesion and gradient measured between the catheter and a 6 F sheath in the aorta. A systolic gradient greater than or equal to 20 mm Hg or a mean gradient of 10 mm Hg is considered significant. Vasodilators, for example, nitroglycerin 100 to 300 mg or Papaverine 20 to 30 mg intravenously can be used to augment the gradient. Intravascular ultrasound (IVUS) is also a very useful imaging modality in renal arteries to accurately assess the artery size and disease involvement of the ostia.

CIN is a significant risk and can be as high as 20% to 50% in patients with both chronic kidney disease and diabetes mellitus.[125,126] Iso-osmolar contrast agent Iodixinol showed less nephrotoxicity than low-osmolar agent Iohexol in one randomized trial.[127] In patients with creatinine clearance less than 60 mL/min and serum creatinine greater than 1.2 mg/dL, Mucomyst 600 mg twice a day decreased the incidence of CIN in patients undergoing coronary angiography.[128] In patients with renal insufficiency, CO_2 angiography can be done injecting 40 to 50 mL of CO_2 delivered by hand injection while the patient is holding breath using DSA. This will allow visualization of renal ostia to facilitate selective renal angiography. Gadolinium contrast or iodinated contrast in a 50:50 ratio with normal saline can also be used in patients with renal dysfunction.

Mesenteric Arteries

AS involvement of these arteries is common but mesenteric ischemia is uncommon. Mesenteric ischemia can also be caused by nonobstructive arterial disease in cases of low flow states. Two-thirds of the patients with intestinal ischemia are women with a mean age of 70 years and most have preexisting CAD.[129–131] Postprandial abdominal pain is almost always present as a symptom.

Celiac artery arises from the anterior surface of the aorta at T12 level. It travels inferiority for 1 to 3 cm before dividing into common hepatic, splenic, and left gastric arteries. SMA arises at the L1–L2 level and gives rise to middle colic and pancreatoduodenal arteries. IMA arises at L3–L4 level and gives rise to left colic and superior rectal arteries (Figure 20-35).

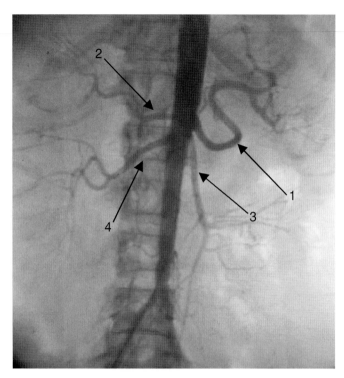

● **FIGURE 20-35.** Mesenteric vessel arteriogram showing (1) patent spenic, (2) common hepatic, (3) superior mesenteric, (4) and right renal arteries. Left renal artery is absent.

These vessels have rich collateral pathways. meandering mesenteric artery allows communication between SMA and IMA. Pancreatoduodenal artery communicates between celiac artery and SMA while IMA has collateral communications with the EIA. Occlusion of one of these arteries generally does not cause intestinal ischemia. Classical teaching was that severe stenosis or occlusion of two of the three of these arteries has to be present to cause this syndrome, but this is not considered entirely true now.[132,133] Single vessel disease, virtually always of the SMA, can cause intestinal ischemia (Figure 20-36). Patients in whom collateral circulation has been interrupted by prior surgery are especially prone to intestinal ischemia by single vessel involvement.

Duplex ultrasound, CTA, MRA with gadolinium enhancement, and catheter angiography with lateral abdominal aortography where noninvasive testing is not available or indeterminate, all have Class I indication in the diagnosis. In many cases, US is not very helpful because of the presence of bowel gas or patient body habitus. CTA and MRA are good for detecting proximal artery lesions. CTA, however, requires intravenous contrast. In case of acute intestinal ischemia, catheter angiography is the best test but it is limited by the time it may require in such emergencies. It can differentiate between occlusive versus nonocclusive disease. Sometimes the patient is not stable to undergo the procedure. Immediate laparotomy and surgical revascularization is the best approach in such cases.

Chronic intestinal ischemia is rare and almost always caused by AS.[134] Buerger's disease, FMD, and aortic dissection are very rare causes.

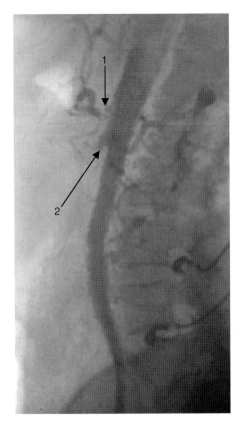

● **FIGURE 20-36.** Angiogram in a lateral projection showing critical stenosis of (1) celiac trunk and (2) 100% occlusion of SMA in a patient with severe mesenteric angina.

Courtesy: John Laird MD, Washington Hospital Center, Washington, DC.

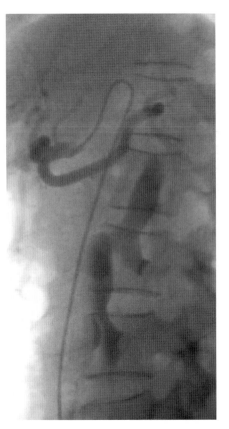

● **FIGURE 20-37.** Selective angiography of celiac trunk utilizing reverse curve Simmons catheter.

Catheter angiography has ACC/AHA Class I indication in patients with suspected nonocclusive intestinal ischemia whose condition does not improve rapidly with the treatment of the underlying disease, e.g., circulatory shock. It can also confirm vasospasm and vasodilator agents can be administered.[135–137]

CFA approach is most commonly used. Arm approach can be used if femoral approach is not feasible. A 4 to 5 F pigtail or Omniflush catheter is placed at T12-L1 level and 30–40 cc of contrast injected via power injector using DSA at 15 cc/s at 4 to 6 FPS. Lateral view will best visualize these vessels (Figures 20-37 and 20-38). An AP view should also be done to visualize the mesenteric circulation and the presence of any collateral vessels. "Arc of Riolan" (an enlarged collateral vessel connecting the left colic branch of the IMA with SMA) is an angiographic sign of proximal mesenteric arterial obstruction that is visible on the AP view.

Pelvis and Lower Extremity

Infra renal aorta and ileofemoral vessels are amongst the most commonly involved in atherosclerotic PAD. Ileofemoral involvement is more common in patents that have history of hypertension and smoking while below the knee, disease is commoner in diabetic population. Surgical

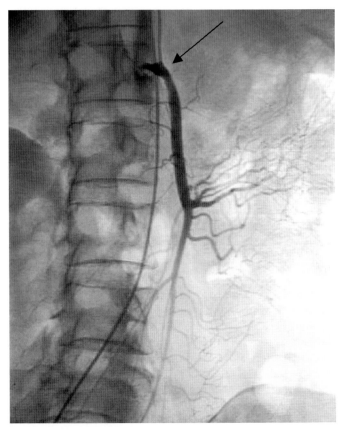

● **FIGURE 20-38.** Selective angiography of superior mesenteric artery utilizing reverse curve Simmons catheter.

revascularization in the ileofemoral region has a patency of >80%[138–140] but it is associated with significant mortality and morbidity. Endovascular revascularization is rapidly taking over as the first line of treatment in these cases.

AA bifurcates into common iliac arteries (CIA) at the L4-L5 level. CIA divides at L5-S1 junction into internal iliac artery (IIA) and external iliac artery (EIA). IIA courses posteromedially and EIA anterolaterally and exits the pelvis posterior to the inguinal ligament to become the CFA. The IMA takes off medially at the junction of EIA and CFA. The deep iliac circumflex artery takes off laterally and superiorly. CFA originates at the inguinal ligament and bifurcates at the lower part of the head of the femur into SFA anteromedially and DFA posterolaterally. DFA has two major branches, lateral and medial circumflex femoral arteries. These arteries along with the first perforating branch connect with the IIA via the superior and inferior gluteal and obturator arteries. Distally, its branches provide collaterals to the network around the knee, thus communicating with the popliteal and tibial vessels. Therefore, in cases of occlusion of SFA, the DFA becomes a very important source of collateral circulation.

The SFA becomes the popliteal artery (PA) as it enters the adductor canal (Hunters canal). PA runs posterior to the femur and gives sural and geniculate branches. Below the knee, the PA divides into anterior tibial artery (AT) that runs anterior and lateral to the tibia and continues into the dorsum of the foot as the dorsalis pedis artery (DP). After the takeoff of the AT, the PA continues as the tibioproneal trunk (TPT) that divides into posterior tibial and peroneal arteries. The peroneal artery runs between the AT and PT. It joins the PT above the ankle via its posterior division and the AT via its anterior division. PT runs behind the medial malleolus and gives medial and lateral plantar branches. The lateral plantar and distal DP joins to form the plantar arch.

Angiography

CTA and MRA are very good tools to delineate the anatomy (Figures 20-39 to 20-41). Compared to DSA, the MRA has shown a sensitivity of 97% and specificity of 99.2%.[141] Interest in this technology is growing as the sole diagnostic tool prior to surgical revascularization.[142] MRA in fact can be a better imaging modality than CTA and catheter angiography for below the knee vasculature (Figure 20-42). CTA is also excellent in the diagnosis but limited by CIN and radiation hazard.[143]

Contrast angiography is considered to be the gold standard (Figures 20-43 to 20-45). It should be reserved for the patients being considered for revascularization and should not be done for diagnostic purposes only if CTA or MRA facility is available. Initially a nonselective angiogram should be done. CFA, brachial, or radial approaches are used. Sheaths and catheters of 4 to 6 F are used. A PT or OF catheter is positioned at L4–L5 and 30 mL of contrast at 15 mL/s is injected with a power injector. DSA at 4 to 6 FPS should be utilized. In cases of known iliac artery obstruction, the catheter should be placed just below the renal

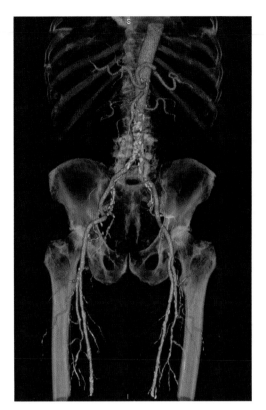

● **FIGURE 20-39.** CTA of abdominal aorta and pelvic arteries showing severe calcification of distal aorta, common and internal iliac arteries. Celiac trunk, superior mesenteric, and renal and inferior mesenteric arteries are patent.

Courtesy: Robert Falk MD, 3-DR Louisville, KY.

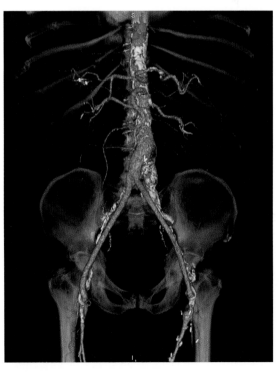

● **FIGURE 20-40.** CTA showing aortobifemoral and left femoral–distal bypass graft.

Courtesy: Robert Falk MD, 3-DR Louisville, KY.

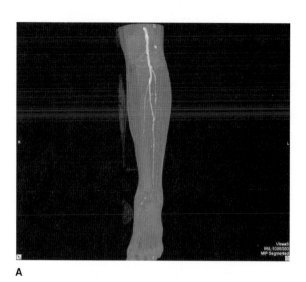

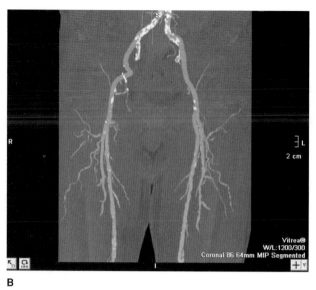

A   B

● **FIGURE 20-41.** "Thick maximal intensity projection" CTA of (A and B) left lower extremity arterial circulation and (C) bilateral ileo femoral arteries.

Courtesy: Robert Falk MD, 3-DR Louisville, KY.

arteries to look for collaterals from the lumbar branches. Selective iliac angiogram is typically done from the contralateral side using 4 to 5 F IMA or JR4 catheter. Other catheters, e.g., Simmons, Omniflush, or SOS, can be used as needed. An exchange length of 200 to 360 cm angled glide wire is advanced under flouro into the CFA or more distally and the catheter exchanged for a straight 4 to 5 F glide or MP catheter. A selective stepwise angiogram of the leg is performed. A 10 to 15 cc contrast is used at each step. For optimal below the knee angiogram, the catheter should be advanced to the distal SFA and vasodilators used. Interactive bolus chase technique as described before can also be used for nonselective angiography of both the legs.

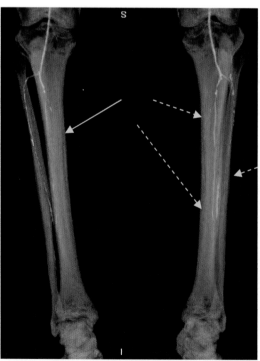

● **FIGURE 20-42.** MRA of below the knee arteries showing 100% occlusion of right posterior tibial artery (*solid arrow*) and 100% occlusion of all three arteries on the left (*dashed arrows*).

Courtesy: Robert Falk MD, 3-DR Louisville, KY.

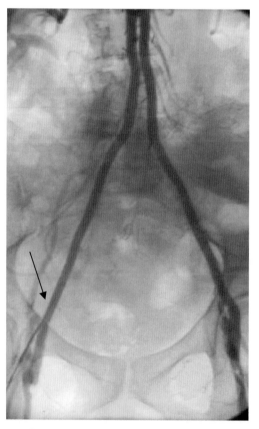

● **FIGURE 20-43.** Arteriogram of aorto bifemoral graft with the sheath inserted into the right limb of the graft (*arrow*).

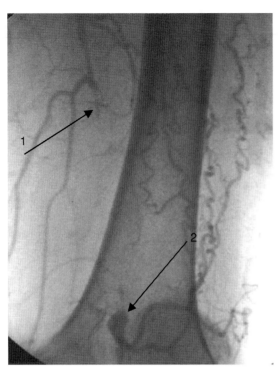

● **FIGURE 20-44.** (1) Hundred percent occlusion of left superficial femoral artery. (2) Collateral vessels reconstituting popliteal artery.

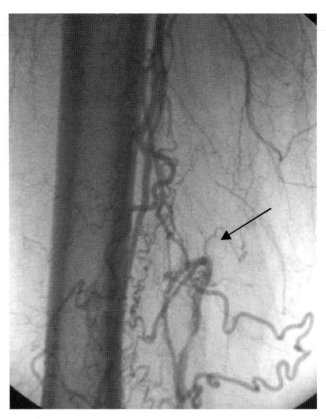

● **FIGURE 20-45.** Hundred percent occlusion of right SFA with extensive collateral vessels from deep femoral artery connecting with the popliteal artery in the same patient. This "mirror imaging" of AS frequently seen in the thigh vessels.

Another technique to engage the common iliac artery is to advance the angled glide wire in the catheter (usually pig tail) already in the abdominal aorta that was used for initial angiogram. The tip of the catheter is faced toward the contralateral iliac. The wire is advanced to "open up" the catheter and the catheter gently pulled down toward the aortic bifurcation. The glide wire will drop down into the common iliac artery as the catheter hooks the ostium of the common iliac. The catheter is then exchanged for the straight catheter as described above. This technique saves an extra step of engaging the contralateral iliac with another catheter first.

After the angiogram of the contra lateral leg is completed, the catheter is pulled just a few inches proximal to the tip of the insertion sheath in the ipsilateral leg and angiogram completed in a stepwise fashion. This can also be done with the sheath alone but a smaller catheter has less risk of causing dissection during angiography. Power injector, hand injection, or an "assist device" can be used. Contralateral angle of 30 to 40 degrees will open up the iliac artery bifurcation and 30 to 40 degrees ipsilateral angles will open up the vessels below the EIA. Lesions with greater the 50% diameter stenosis and translesional systolic gradient greater than 10 mm Hg are considered significant. If femoral approach is not feasible, then a brachial or radial approach utilizing straight catheters can also be used for selective angiography of each leg. Vasodilators, for example, NTG 100 to 300 mg, Papavarin 30 to 60 mg, or Tolazoline 12.5 to 25 mg can be used to optimize below the knee imaging and also to augment translesional radiant.[144]

High success rate with endovascular treatment has now encouraged most experienced operators to tackle below the knee PAD that was long thought to be only fit for surgical therapy. Patients with CLI who are being subjected to amputation should be given an option for peripheral vascular intervention even if it helps in the short-term healing of their infections and to prevent more proximal amputation.

● **VENOUS CIRCULATION**

With improvement in technology, enthusiasm is gaining momentum in the endovascular treatment of venous occlusive disease (VOD). The most common causes of VOD are coagulopathies, extrinsic compression from tumors, and thrombosis from iatrogenic catheters and wires. Venous enhanced subtracted peak arterial (VESPA) magnetic resonance venography is comparable to conventional venography in the diagnosis of femoral and iliac deep venous thrombosis.[145] CTA and MRA are both useful in the diagnosis of upper extremity and central VOD, stenoses, extrinsic masses, and pulmonary embolism.

Venous system parallels arterial system. The superficial veins in the infrainguinal region drain into the small saphenous vein, which drains into the popliteal vein, and into the greater saphenous vein that drains into the common femoral vein (CFV). The deep veins converge on the CFV that continues as the external iliac vein and combines with the internal iliac vein to form the common iliac veins which drain into the IVC that further drains into the right atrium of the heart.

Superficial upper extremity veins drain into the lateral cephalic and medial basilic veins that run along the arm. Cephalic vein empties into the axillary vein and basilic vein drain into the brachial vein. Deep veins drain into the brachial vein that continues as the axillary and subclavian veins. Each subclavian vein unites with the internal jugular vein to form the right and left innominate veins. They join together on the right side to form the superior vena cava (SVC) that empties into the right atrium.

Venous drainage from the pelvic area flows to internal iliac vein that joins with external iliac vein to form the common iliac vein. Venous drainage from abdominal viscera goes to IVC. The azygous and hemiazygous system of veins form an important link between IVC and SVC. The hemiazygous vein and accessory hemiazygous vein is located along the left side of thoracic vertebrae and receives blood from the left chest wall and lung and drain into the azygous vein. In two-thirds of cases, the hemiazygous vein communicates directly with the left renal vein. Azygous vein is located on the right side of the thoracic vertebrae and drains into the SVC at the level of T4. Distally, it connects to the IVC at the level of the renal vein.

Venogram

This is still considered the gold standard for VOD. Small amount of contrast through peripherally inserted catheters will provide visualization of the veins. Raising the arm improves central filling. For lower extremity angiography, venous access is obtained in the dorsum of the foot. DSA is used. For iliac veins 5 to 6 F sheath is inserted in the CFV and angiogram is obtained by hand injection of the contrast. For IVC, a pigtail or Omniflush catheter is inserted in CIV and 40 mL of contrast is injected. For pulmonary angiogram a 6 F angled pigtail or a Grollman catheter is advanced in the main pulmonary artery through a sheath in the CFV or IJ vein. Contrast at 30 mL at 15 mL/s is injected, and angiography acquired in AP and lateral views for each lung. If pulmonary artery pressure is high, then selective right and left pulmonary artery angiogram is obtained. Care should be taken in patients with preexisting LBBB because the catheter may cause RBBB, thus, causing complete heartblock.

● INTRAVASCULAR IMAGING

There are other intravascular imaging techniques that are less commonly used in routine catheter peripheral angiography. They can however be very useful in cases of ambiguous situations or where a decision to intervene is not clear cut.[146]

IVUS is the most widely available. IVUS catheter uses reflected sound waves to image vascular walls and structures in a two-dimensional tomographic format. Compared to cardiac echocardiogram, the catheters used in peripheral imaging have a much higher frequency, 20 to 40 MHz versus 2 to 5 MHz. Most new IVUS catheters are compatible with 6 F sheaths and guiding catheters. Over the wire and rapid exchange systems are available. In our center we use Boston Scientific Corp. system (Natwik, MA), unfractionated heparin at 70 units/kg is given intravenously during IVUS procedures. Intracoronary nitroglycerin is given prior to delivering the catheter at the area of interest. Automated pullback is done at 0.5 to 1 mm/s. Interpretation is based on recognition of blood–intima and media–adventitia interface. Lumina and adventitia are much brighter than the media creating a bright–dark–bright image. Angioscopy is not FDA-approved in the United States for clinical use. It is probably the best technique for imaging intravascular thrombus. It provides real-time color images of vascular surfaces and also gives information about atherosclerotic plaque and dissection flaps. Optical coherence tomography (OCT) generates real-time tomographic images from backscattered reflection of infrared light. It can be conceptualized as an optical analog of IVUS. It has 10 times higher resolution than conventional ultrasound. Imaging procedure is similar to IVUS; however, saline or contrast media must displace blood. There is only one system that is commercially available (Light bulb Imaging Inc., Westford. MA). A 0.014-inch imaging wire is inserted in the vessel distal to the occlusion balloon. The diagnostic accuracy of OCT for plaque characterization is confirmed by an ex vivo study of 3007 human AS specimens from aorta, carotid, and coronary arteries.[147] The complications of this procedure appear to be comparable to IVUS and angioscopy. However, data are lacking.

● ACKNOWLEDGMENT

We wish to thank and acknowledge all who have allowed us to reproduce their figures and tables.

REFERENCES

1. ACC/AHA Guidelines for the Management of Patients With Peripheral Arterial Disease (Lower Extremity, Renal, Mesenteric, and Abdominal Aortic). A Collaborative Report from the American Association for Vascular Surgery/Society for Vascular Surgery, Society for Cardiovascular Angiography and Interventions, Society for Vascular Medicine and Biology, Society of Interventional Radiology, and the ACC/AHA Task Force on Practice Guidelines (Writing Committee to Develop Guidelines for the Management of Patients With Peripheral Arterial Disease). *J Am Coll Cardiol.* 2006;47(6):1239–1312.

2. Criqui MH, Denenberg JO, Langer RD, et al. The epidemiology of peripheral arterial disease: importance of identifying the population at risk. *Vasc Med.* 1997;2:221–226.

3. Murabito JM, D'Agostino RB, Silbershatz H, et al. Intermittent claudication. A risk profile from The Framingham Heart Study. *Circulation.* 1997;96:44–49.

4. Isner JM, Rosenfield K. Redefining the treatment of peripheral artery disease. Role of percutaneous revascularization. *Circulation.* 1993;88:1534–1537.

5. Criqui MH. Peripheral arterial disease and subsequent cardiovascular mortality: a strong and consistent association. *Circulation.* 1990;82:2246–2247.

6. Hertzer NR. The natural history of peripheral vascular disease: Implications for its management. *Circulation.* 1991; 83(2 suppl):112–119.

7. Management of peripheral arterial disease (PAD). TASC Working Group. Trans Atlantic Inter-Society Consensus (TASC). *J Vasc Surg.* 2000;31:S1–S296.

8. Bellar GA, Bonow RO, Fuster V, et al. ACC Revised Recommendations for Training in Adult Cardiovascular Medicine Core Cardiology Training II (COCATS 2) (Revision of the 1995 COCATS Training Statement). American College of Cardiology, March 8, 2002.

9. White CJ, Ramee SR, Collins TJ, et al. Initial results of peripheral vascular angioplasty performed by experienced interventional cardiologists. *Am J Cardiol.* 1992;69:1249–1250.

10. Wexler L, Levin DC, Dorros G, et al. Training standards for physicians performing angioplasty: New developments. *Radiology.* 1991;178:19–21.

11. Guidelines for percutaneous transluminal angioplasty. Standards of Practice Committee of the Society of Cardiovascular and Interventional Radiology. *Radiology.* 1990;177:619.

12. Guidelines for performance of peripheral percutaneous transluminal angioplasty. The Society for Cardiac Angiography and Interventions Interventional Cardiology Committee Subcommittee on Peripheral Interventions. *Cathet Cardiovasc Diag.* 1988;21:128–129.

13. Pentecost MJ, Criqui MH, Dorros G, et al. Guidelines for peripheral percutaneous transluminal angioplasty of the abdominal aorta and lower extremity vessels. *Circulation.* 1994;84:511–531.

14. Spittell JA Jr, Nanda NC, Creager MA, et al. Recommendations for peripheral transluminal angioplasty: training and facilities. American College of Cardiology Peripheral Vascular Disease Committee. *J Am Coll Cardiol.* 1993;21:546–548.

15. Levin DC, Becker GJ, Dorros G, et al. Training standards for physicians performing peripheral angioplasty and other percutaneous peripheral vascular interventions. *J Vasc Intervent Radiol.* 2003;9(Pt2):S359–S361.

16. Babb JD, Collins TJ, Cowley MJ, et al. Revised guidelines for the performance of peripheral vascular interventions. *Cathet Cardiovasc Intervent.* 1999;46:21–23.

17. ACC/ACP/SCAI/SVMB/SVS Clinical Competence Statement on Vascular Medicine and Catheter-Based Peripheral Vascular Interventions. *J Am Coll Cardiol.* 2004;44(4):941–957.

18. Rofsky NM, Adelman MA. MR angiography in the evaluation of atherosclerotic peripheral vascular disease. *Radiology.* 2000;214:325–338.

19. Carpenter JP, Owen RS, Holland GA, et al. Magnetic resonance angiography of the aorta, iliac, and femoral arteries. *Surgery.* 1994;116:17–23.

20. Quinn SF, Sheley RC, Szumowski J, et al. Evaluation of the iliac arteries: comparison of two-dimensional time of flight magnetic resonance angiography with cardiac compensated fast gradient recalled echo and contrast-enhanced three-dimensional time of flight magnetic resonance angiography. *J Magn Reson Imaging.* 1997;7:197–203.

21. Ruehm SG, Hany TF, Pfammatter T, et al. Pelvic and lower extremity arterial imaging: diagnostic performance of three-dimensional contrast-enhanced MR angiography. *AJR Am J Roentgenol.* 2000;174:1127–1135.

22. Meaney JF, Ridgeway JP, Chakraverty S, et al. Stepping-table gadolinium-enhanced digital subtraction MR angiography of the aorta and lower extremity arteries: preliminary experience. *Radiology.* 1999;211:59–67.

23. Owen RS, Carpenter JP, Baum RA, et al. Magnetic resonance imaging of angiographically occult runoff vessels in peripheral arterial occlusive disease. *N Engl J Med.* 1992;326:1577–1581.

24. Rofsky NM, Johnson G, Adelman MA, et al. Peripheral vascular disease evaluated with reduced-dose gadolinium-enhanced MR angiography. *Radiology.* 1997;205:163–169.

25. Nelemans PJ, Leiner T, de Vet HC, et al. Peripheral arterial disease: meta-analysis of the diagnostic performance of MR angiography. *Radiology.* 2000;217:105–114.

26. Khilnani NM, Winchester PA, Prince MR, et al. Peripheral vascular disease: combined 3D bolus chase and dynamic 2D MR angiography compared with x-ray angiography for treatment planning. *Radiology.* 2002;224:63–74.

27. Maintz D, Tombach B, Juergens KU, et al. Revealing in-stent stenoses of the iliac arteries: comparison of multidetector CT with MR angiography and digital radiographic angiography in a phantom model. *AJR Am J Roentgenol.* 2002;179:1319–1322.

28. Lee VS, Martin DJ, Krinsky GA, et al. Gadolinium–enhanced MR angiography: artifacts and pitfalls. *AJR AM J Roentgenol.* 2000;175:197–205.

29. Sam AD 2nd, Morasch MD, Collins J, et al. Safety of gadolinium contrast angiography in patients with chronic renal insufficiency. *J Vasc Surg.* 2003;38:313–318.

30. Rubin GD, Shiau MC, Leung AN, et al. Aorta and iliac arteries: single versus multiple detector-row helical CT angiography. *Radiology.* 2000;215:670–676.

31. Martin ML, Tay KH, Flak B, et al. Multidetector CT angiography of the aortoiliac system and lower extremities: a prospective comparison with digital subtraction angiography. *AJR Am J Roentgenol.* 2003;180:1085–1091.

32. Willmann JK, Wildermuth S, Pfammatter T, et al. Aortoiliac and renal arteries: prospective intraindividual comparison of contrast-enhanced three-dimensional MR angiography and multi-detector row CT angiography. *Radiology.* 2003; 226:798–811.

33. Willmann JK, Mayer D, Banyai M, et al. Evaluation of peripheral arterial bypass grafts with multi-detector row CT angiography: comparison with duplex US and digital subtraction angiography. *Radiology.* 2003;229:465–474.

34. Ofer A, Nitecki SS, Linn S, et al. Multidetector CT angiography of peripheral vascular disease: a prospective comparison with intra-arterial digital subtraction angiography. *AJR Am J Roentgenol.* 2003;180:719–724.

35. Ota H, Takase K, Igarashi K, et al. MDCT compared with digital subtraction angiography for assessment of lower

extremity arterial occlusive disease: importance of reviewing cross-sectional images. *AJR Am J Roentgenol.* 2004;182:201–209.

36. Ricker O, Duber C, Schmiedt W, et al. Prospective comparison of CT angiography of the legs with intra-arterial digital subtraction angiography. *AJR Am J Roentgenol.* 1996; 166:269–276.

37. Napel S, Marks MP, Rubin GD, et al. CT angiography with spiral CT and maximum intensity projection. *Radiology.* 1992;185:607–610.

38. Lookstein RA. Impact of CT angiography on endovascular therapy. *Mt Sinai J Med.* 2003;70:367–374

39. Rubin GD, Schmidt AJ, Logan LJ, et al. Multi-detector row CT angiography of lower extremity arterial inflow and runoff: initial experience. *Radiology.* 2001;221:146–158.

40. Catalano C, Fraioli F, Laghi A, et al. Infrarenal aortic and lower extremity arterial disease: diagnostic performance of multi-detector row CT angiography. *Radiology.* 2004;231:555–563.

41. Beregi JP, Djabbari M, Desmoucelle F, et al. Popliteal vascular disease: evaluation with spiral CT angiography. *Radiology.* 1997;203:477–483.

42. Bluemke DA, Chambers TP. Spiral CT angiography: an alternative to conventional angiography. *Radiology.* 1995;195:317–319.

43. Huber PR, Leimbach ME, Lewis WL, et al. CO$_2$ angiography. *Catheter Cardiovasc Interv.* 2002;55:398–403.

44. Hawkins IF. Carbon dioxide digital subtraction arteriography. *AJR Am J Roentgenol.* 1982;139:19–24.

45. Weaver FA, Pentecost MJ, Yellin AE, Davis S, Finck E, Teitelbaum G. Clinical applications of carbon dioxide/digital subtraction arteriography. *J Vasc Surg.* 1991;13:266–272.

46. Kerns SR, Hawkins IF Jr, Sabatelli FW. Current status of carbon dioxide angiography. *Radiol Clin North Am.* 1995;33:15–29.

47. Kerns SR, Hawkins IF Jr. Carbon dioxide digital subtraction angiography: expanding applications and technical evolution. *AJR Am J Roentgenol.* 1995;164:735–741.

48. Caridi JG, Hawkins IF Jr. CO$_2$ digital subtraction angiography: potential complications and their prevention [see comment]. *J Vasc Intervent Radiol.* 1997;8:383–391.

49. Hawkins IF, Caridi JG. Carbon dioxide (CO$_2$) digital subtraction angiography: 26-year experience at the University of Florida. *Eur Radiol.* 1998;8:391–402.

50. Sullivan KL, Bonn J, Shaprio MJ, Gardiner GA. Venography with carbon dioxide as a contrast agent. *Cardiovasc Intervent Radiol.* 1995;18:141–145.

51. Forssmann W. Die Sondierung des rechten Herzens. *Klin Wochenschr.* 1929;8:2085.

52. Dos Santos R, Lama AC, Pereira-Caldas J. Arteriorgafa da aorta e dos vasos abdominalis. *Med Contempo.* 1929;47:93.

53. Bettmann MA, Heeren T, Greenfield A, et al. Adverse events with radiographic contrast agents: results of the SCVIR Contrast Agent Registry. *Radiology* 1997;203:611–620.

54. Waugh JR, Sacharias N. Arteriographic complications in the DSA era. *Radiology* 1992;182:243–246.

55. Baim DS. Proper use of cineangiographic equipment and contrast agents. In: Baim DS, Grossman W, eds. *Cardiac Catheterization, Angiography, and Intervention.* 6th ed. Philadelphia, PA: Lippincott, Williams, and Wilkins; 2000:15–34.

56. Balter S, Baim, DS. Cineangiographic imaging, radiation safety and contrast agents. In: Baim DS, Grossman W, eds. *Cardiac Catheterization, Angiography and Intervention.* 7th ed. Philadelphia: Lippincott, Williams, and Wilkins; 2006:31–33.

57. Sutton AG, Ashton VJ, Campbell PG, et al. A randomized prospective trial of ioxaglate 320 (Hexabrix) vs. iodixanol 320 (Visipaque) in patients undergoing percutaneous coronary intervention. *Catheter Cardiovasc Interv.* 2002;57:346–352.

58. Aspelin P, Aubry P, Fransson SG, et al. Nephrotoxic effects in high-risk patients undergoing angiography (iodixanol). *N Engl J Med.* 2003;348:491–499.

59. Schwab SJ, Hlatkey MA, Pieper KS, et al. Contrast nephrotoxicity—a randomized controlled trial of a nonionic and an ionic radiographic contrast agent. *N Engl J Med.* 1989; 320:149.

60. Steinberg EP, Moore RD, Powe NR, et al. Safety and cost effectiveness of high-osmolality as compared with low-osmolality contrast agents in patients undergoing cardiac angiography. *N Engl J Med.* 1992;326:425.

61. Bertrand ME, Esplugas E, Piessens J, et al. Influence of a non-ionic, iso-osmolar contrast medium (iodixanol) versus an ionic, low-osmolar contrast medium (ioxaglate) on major adverse cardiac events in patients undergoing percutaneous transluminal coronary angioplasty. *Circulation.* 2000;101:131–136.

62. Jaff MR, Macneill BD, Rosenfield K. Angiography of the aorta and peripheral arteries. In: Baim DS, Grossman W, eds. *Cardiac Catheterization, Angiography and Intervention.* 7th ed. Philadelphia: Lippincott, Williams, and Wilkins; 2006:257–258.

63. Millward SF, Burbridge BE, Luna G. Puncturing the pulseless femoral artery: a simple technique that uses palpation of anatomic landmarks. *J Vasc Intervent Radiol.* 1993;4:415–417.

64. Khangure MS, Chow KC, Christensen MA. Accurate and safe puncture of a pulse less femoral artery: an aid in performing iliac artery percutaneous transluminal angioplasty. *Radiology.* 1982;144:927–928.

65. Sacks D, Summers TA. Ante grade selective catheterization of femoral vessels with a 4- or 5-F catheter and safety wire. *J Vasc Intervent Radiol.* 1991;2:325–326.

66. Cohen DJ. Outpatient transradial coronary stenting: implications for cost-effectiveness. *J Invasive Cardiol.* 1996;8(suppl D):36D–39D.

67. Cooper CJ, El-Shiekh RA, Cohen DJ, et al. Effects of transradial access on quality of life and cost of cardiac catheterization: a randomized comparison. *Am Heart J.* 1999;138:430–436.

68. Mann T, Cowper PA, Peterson ED, et al. Transradial coronary stenting: comparison with femoral access closed with an arterial suture device. *Catheter Cardiovasc Interv.* 2000;49:150–156.

69. Campeau L. Entry sites for coronary angiography and therapeutic interventions: from the proximal to the distal radial artery. *Can J Cardiol.* 2001;17(3):319–325.

70. Campeau L. Percutaneous radial artery approach for coronary angiography. *Cathet Cardiovasc Diagn.* 1989;16:39.

71. Hovagim AR, Katz RI, Poppers PJ. Pulse oximetry for evaluation of radial and ulnar arterial blood flow. *J Cardiothorac Anesth.* 1989;3:27–30.

72. Barry WH, Levin DC, Green LH, et al. Left heart catheterization and angiography via the percutaneous femoral approach using an arterial sheath. *Cathet Cardiovasc Diagn.* 1979;5:401.

73. Nath PH, Soto B, Holt JH, Satler LF. Selective coronary angiography by translumbar aortic puncture. *Am J Cardiol.* 1983;52:425?

74. Hill BB, Zarins CK, Fogarty TJ. Endovascular repair of thoracic aortic aneurysms. In: White R, Fogarty T, eds. *Peripheral Endovascular Interventions.* New York, NY: Springer-Verlag; 1999:383–389.

75. Arko FR, Lee WA, Hill BB. Aneurysm-related death: primary endpoint analysis for comparison of open and endovascular repair. *J Vasc Surg.* 2002;36:297–304.

76. Crawford ES, Hess KR, Sati HJ. Ruptured aneurysm of the descending thoracic and thoracoabdominal aorta. *Ann of Surg.* 1991;213:417–426.

77. Ehrlich M, Grabenwoeger M, Cartes-Zumelzu F. Endovascular stent graft repair for aneurysms on the descending thoracic aorta. *Ann Thorac Surg.* 1998;66:19–24.

78. Endarterectomy for Asymptomatic Carotid Artery Stenosis-Executive Committee for the Asymptomatic Carotid Artery Stenosis Study. *JAMA.* 1995;273:1421–1428.

79. Carotid and Cerebral Angiography Performed by Cardiologists. Cerebrovascular Complications. *CCI.* 2002;55:277–280.

80. Beneficial effect of carotid endarterectomy in symptomatic patients with high-grade carotid stenosis. North American Symptomatic Carotid Endarterectomy Trial Collaborators. *N Engl J Med.* 1991;325:445–453.

81. MRC European Carotid Surgery Trial: interim results for symptomatic patients with severe (70%-99%) or with mild (0%-29%) carotid stenosis. European Carotid Surgery Trialists' Collaborative Group. *Lancet.* 1991;337:1235–1243.

82. Casserly IP, Yadav JS. Carotid intervention. In: Yadav JS, Casserly Ip, Sachar R, eds. *Manual of Peripheral Vascular Interventions.* Philadelphia, PA: Lippincott Williams, & Wilkins; 2005:84–86.

83. Mukherjee D, Rosenfield K. Vertebral artery disease. In: Yadav JS, Casserly Ip, Sachar R, eds. *Manual of Peripheral Vascular Interventions.* Philadelphia, PA: Lippincott Williams & Wilkins; 2005:110–111.

84. Phatouros CC, Higashida RT, Malek AM, et al. Endovascular treatment of noncarotid extra cranial cerebrovascular disease. *Neurosurg Clin N Am.* 2000;11(2):331–350.

85. Gabella G. Cardiovascular System. In: Williams PL, Bannister LH, Berry MM, eds. *Gray's Anatomy.* New York, NY: Churchill Livingstone; 1995:1505–1546.

86. Horejs D, Gilbert PM, Burstein S, Vogelzang RI. Normal aortoiliac diameters by CT. *J Comput Assist Tomogr.* 1988;12:602–603.

87. Ebaugh JL, Garcia ND, Matsumura JS. Screening and surveillance for abdominal aortic aneurysms: who needs it and when. *Semin Vasc Surg.* 2001;14:193–199.

88. Alcorn HG, Wolfson SK Jr, Sutton-Tyrrell K, et al. Risk factors for abdominal aortic aneurysms in older adults enrolled in The Cardiovascular Health Study. *Arterioscler Thromb Vasc Biol.* 1996;16:963–970.

89. Pedersen OM, Aslaksen A, Vik-Mo H. Ultrasound measurement of the luminal diameter of the abdominal aorta and iliac arteries in patients without vascular disease. *J Vasc Surg.* 1993;17:596–601.

90. Lanne T, Sandgren T, Sonesson B. A dynamic view on the diameter of abdominal aortic aneurysms. *Eur J Vasc Endovasc Surg.* 1998;15:308–312.

91. Johnston KW, Rutherford RB, Tilson MD, et al. Suggested standards for reporting on arterial aneurysms. Subcommittee on Reporting Standards for Arterial Aneurysms, Ad Hoc Committee on Reporting Standards, Society for Vascular Surgery and North American Chapter, International Society for Cardiovascular Surgery. *J Vasc Surg.* 1991;13:452–458.

92. Krupski WC, Selzman CH, Floridia R, et al. Contemporary management of isolated iliac aneurysms. *J Vasc Surg.* 1998;28:1–11; discussion 11–13.

93. Kasirajan V, Hertzer NR, Beven EG, et al. Management of isolated common iliac artery aneurysms. *Cardiovasc Surg.* 1998;6:171–177.

94. Rubin GD, Armerding MD, Dake MD, et al. Cost identification of abdominal aortic aneurysm imaging by using time and motion analysis. *Radiology.* 2000;215:63–70.

95. Turnipseed WD, Archer CW, Detmer DE, et al. Digital subtraction angiography and B-mode ultrasonography for abdominal and peripheral aneurysms. *Surgery.* 1982;92:619–626.

96. Bandyk DF. Preoperative imaging of aortic aneurysms: conventional and digital subtraction angiography, computed tomography scanning, and magnetic resonance imaging. *Surg Clin North Am.* 1989;69:721–735.

97. Galt SW, Pearce WH. Preoperative assessment of abdominal aortic aneurysms: noninvasive imaging versus routine arteriography. *Semin Vasc Surg.* 1995;8:103–107

98. Hallett JW Jr. Splenic artery aneurysms. *Semin Vasc Surg.* 1995;8:321–326.

99. Kasirajan K, Greenberg RK, Clair D, et al. Endovascular management of visceral artery aneurysm. *J Endovasc Ther.* 2001;8:150–155.

100. Angelakis EJ, Bair WE, Barone JE, et al. Splenic artery aneurysm ruptured during pregnancy. *Obstet Gynecol Surv.* 1993;48:145–148.

101. Holley KE, Hunt JC, Brown AL Jr, et al. Renal artery stenosis: a clinical–pathologic study in normotensive and hypertensive patients. *Lancet.* 1964;37:14–22.

102. Dustan HP, Humphries AW, Dewolfe VG, et al. Normal arterial pressure in patients with renal arterial stenosis. *JAMA.* 1964;187:1028–1029.

103. Scoble JE. The epidemiology and clinical manifestations of atherosclerotic renal disease. In: Novick AC, Scoble JE, Hamilton G, eds. *Renal Vascular Disease*. London, UK: WB Saunders; 1996:303–314.

104. Hansen KJ, Edwards MS, Craven TE, et al. Prevalence of renovascular disease in the elderly: a population based study. *J Vasc Surg*. 2002;36:443–451.

105. Olin JW, Melia M, Young JR, Graor RA, Risius B. Prevalence of atherosclerotic renal artery stenosis in patients with atherosclerosis elsewhere. *Am J Med*. 1990;88:46–51.

106. Harding MB, Smith LR, Himmelstein SI, et al. Renal artery stenosis: prevalence and associated risk factors in patients undergoing routine cardiac catheterization. *J Am Soc Nephrol*. 1992;2:1608–1616.

107. Weber-Mzell D, Kotanko P, Schumacher M, et al. Coronary anatomy predicts presence or absence of renal artery stenosis: a prospective study in patients undergoing cardiac catheterization for suspected coronary artery disease. *Eur Heart J*. 2002;23:1684–1691.

108. Jean WJ, al-Bitar I, Zwicke DL, et al. High incidence of renal artery stenosis in patients with coronary artery disease. *Cathet Cardiovasc Diag*. 1994;32:8–10.

109. Scoble JE, Maher ER, Hamilton G, Dick R, Sweny P, Moorhead JF. Atherosclerotic renovascular disease causing renal impairment—a case for treatment. *Clin Nephrol*. 1989; 31:119–122.

110. Zierler RE, Bergelin RO, Isaacson JA, Strandness DE. Natural history of atherosclerotic renal artery stenosis: A prospective study with duplex ultrasonography. *J Vasc Surg*. 1994;19:250–258.

111. Wright JR, Shurrab AE, Cheung C, et al. A prospective study of the determinants of renal functional outcome and mortality in atherosclerotic renovascular disease. *Am J Kidney Dis*. 2002;39(6):1153–1161.

112. Suresh M, Laboi P, Mamtora H, et al. Relationship of renal dysfunction to proximal arterial disease severity in atherosclerotic renovascular disease. *Nephrol Dial Transplant*. 2000;15(5):631–636.

113. Rimmer JM, Gennari FJ. Atherosclerotic renovascular disease and progressive renal failure. *Ann Intern Med*. 1993; 118:712–719.

114. Mailloux LU, Napolitano B, Bellucci AG, et al. Renal vascular disease causing end-stage renal disease, incidence, clinical correlates, and outcomes: a 20-year clinical experience. *Am J Kidney Dis*. 1994;24:622–629.

115. Guzman RP, Zierler RE, Isaacson JA, et al. Renal atrophy and arterial stenosis. A prospective study with duplex ultrasound. *Hypertension*. 1994;23:346–350.

116. Caps MT, Zierler RE, Polissar NL, et al. Risk of atrophy in kidneys with atherosclerotic renal artery stenosis. *Kidney Int*. 1998;53:735–742.

117. Mitsuzaki K, Yamashita Y, Sakaguchi T, et al. Abdomen, pelvis, and extremities: diagnostic accuracy of dynamic contrast-enhanced turbo MR angiography compared with conventional angiography-initial experience. *Radiology*. 2000;216:909–915.

118. Beregi JP, Elkohen M, Deklunder G, et al. Helical CT angiography compared with arteriography in the detection of renal artery stenosis. *AJR Am J Roenrtgenol*. 1996;167:495–501.

119. Halperin EJ, Rutter CM, Gardiner GA Jr, et al. Comparison of Doppler US and CT angiography for evaluation of renal artery stenosis. *Acad Radiol*. 1998;5:524–532.

120. Johnson PT, Halpern EJ, Kuszyk BS, et al. Renal artery stenosis: Ct angiography—comparison of real-time volume-rendering and maximum intensity projection algorithms. *Radiology*. 1999;211:337–343.

121. Kim TS, Chung JW, Park JH, et al. Renal artery evaluation: comparison of spiral CT angiography to intra-arterial DSA. *J Vasc Interv Radiol*. 1998;9:553–559.

122. Rubin GD, Duke MD, Napel S, et al. Spiral CT of renal artery stenosis: comparison of three-dimensional rendering techniques. *Radiology*. 1994;190:181–189.

123. Kawashima A, Sandler CM, Ernst Rd, et al. CT evaluation of renovascular disease. *Radiographics*. 2000;20:1321–1340.

124. Lufft V, Hoogestraat-Lufft L, Fels LM, et al. Contrast media nephropathy: intravenous CT angiography versus intra-arterial digital subtraction angiography in renal artery stenosis: a prospective randomized trial. *Am J Kidney Dis*. 2002;40:236–242.

125. Rihal CS, Textor SC, Grill DE, et al. Incidence and prognostic importance of acute renal failure after percutaneous coronary intervention. *Circulation*. 2002;105:2259–2264.

126. Parfrey PS, Griffiths SM, Barrett BJ, et al. Contrast material-induced renal failure in patients with diabetes mellitus, renal insufficiency or both. A prospective controlled study. *N Engl J Med*. 1989;320:143–149.

127. Aspelin P, Aubry P, Fransson SG, et al. Nephrotoxic effects in high-risk patients undergoing angiography. *N Engl J Med*. 2003;348:491–499.

128. Kay J, Chow WH, Chan TM, et al. Acetylcysteine for prevention of acute deterioration of renal function following elective coronary angiography and intervention: a randomized controlled trial. *JAMA*. 2003;289:553–558.

129. Ottinger LW, Austin WG. A study of 136 patients with mesenteric infarction. *Surg Gynecol Obstet*. 1967;124:251–261.

130. Hertzer NR, Beven EG, Humphries AW. Acute intestinal ischemia. *Ann Surg*. 1978;44:744–749.

131. Bergan JJ. Recognition and treatment of intestinal ischemia. *Surg Clin North Am*. 1967;47:109–126.

132. Mikkelsen WP. Intestinal angina: its surgical significance. *Surg Gynecol Obstet*. 1957;94:262–267; discussion, 267–269.

133. Buchardt Hansen HJ. Abdominal angina: results of arterial reconstruction in 12 patients. *Acta Chir Scand*. 1976;142: 319–325.

134. Fisher DF Jr, Fry WJ. Collateral mesenteric circulation. *Surg Gynecol Obstet*. 1987;164:487–492.

135. Kawauchi M, Tada Y, Asano K, et al. Angiographic demonstration of mesenteric arterial changes in postcoarctectomy syndrome. *Surgery*. 1985;98:602–604.

136. Siegelman SS, Sprayregen S, Boley SI. Angiographic diagnosis of mesenteric arterial vasoconstriction. *Radiology* 1974;112:533–542.

137. Nalbandian H, Sheth N, Dietrich R, et al. Intestinal ischemia caused by cocaine ingestion: report of two cases. *Surgery*. 1985;97:374–376.

138. Vitale GF, Inahara T. Extra peritoneal endarterectomy for iliofemoral occlusive disease. *J Vasc Surg.* 1990;12:409–413; discussion 414–415.

139. van den Dungen JJ, Boontje AH, Kropveld A. Unilateral iliofemoral occlusive disease: long-term results of the semiclosed endarterectomy with the ring-stripper. *J Vasc Surg.* 1991;14:673–677.

140. de Vries SO, Hunink MG. Results of aortic bifurcation grafts for aortoiliac occlusive disease: a meta-analysis. *J Vasc Surg.* 1997;26:558–569.

141. Cambria RP, Yucel EK, Brewster DC, et al. The potential for lower extremity revascularization without contrast arteriography: experience with magnetic resonance angiography. *J Vasc Surg.* 1993;17:1050–1056.

142. Sueyoshi E, Sakamoto I, Matsuoka Y, et al. Aortoiliac and lower extremity arteries: comparison of three-dimensional dynamic contrast-enhanced subtraction MR angiography and conventional angiography. *Radiology.* 1999;210:683–688.

143. Poletti PA, Rosset A, Didier D. Subtraction CT angiography of the lower limbs: a new technique for the evaluation of acute arterial occlusion. *AJR Am J Roentgenol.* 2004;183:1445–1448.

144. Legemate DA, Teeuwen C, Hoeneveld H, Eikelboom BC. Value of duplex scanning compared with angiography and pressure measurement in the assessment of aortoiliac arterial lesions. *Br J Surg.* 1991;78:1003–1008.

145. Fraser DG, Moody AR, Davidson IR, et al. Deep venous thrombosis: Diagnosis by using venous enhanced subtracted peak arterial MR venography versus conventional venography. *Radiology.* 2003;226(3):812–820.

146. Honda Y, Fitzgerald PJ, Yock PG. Intravascular Imaging techniques. In: Baim DS, Grossman W, eds. *Cardiac Catheterization, Angiography and Intervention.* 7th edition; Philadelphia, PA: Lippincott Williams & Wilkins; 2006:371–391.

147. Yabushita H, et al. Characterization of human atherosclerosis by optical coherence tomography. *Circulation.* 2002;106:1640–1645.

chapter 21

Intravascular Ultrasound in Peripheral Arterial Disease

Daniel H. Steinberg, MD / *Esteban Escolar, MD* / *Robert A. Gallino, MD* / *Neil J. Weissman, MD*

● INTRODUCTION

Intravascular ultrasound (IVUS) has become a standard imaging technique in high volume, experienced interventional laboratories, but most of its use is relegated to the coronary arteries. While conventional angiography provides a single-plane "shadow" of the vascular lumen, it has limited ability to accurately and reproducibly measure vessel stenosis and characterize plaque morphology. The high-definition, cross-sectional images of the arterial lumen and the arterial wall provided by IVUS allow a far more detailed analysis of the target vessel and peripheral interventional success. Nonetheless, IVUS has not enjoyed wide deployment in the peripheral interventional arena. This chapter will provide the information needed to utilize IVUS during peripheral interventions by reviewing the fundamentals of IVUS technology, image interpretation and standardized measurements, its general application during peripheral vascular interventions, and some specific considerations for each vascular territory.

● HISTORICAL PERSPECTIVE

One of the first IVUS catheters was designed in 1972s by Bom et al.[1] with the purpose of exploring the intracardiac chambers and cardiac structures. During the early and mid-1980s, new catheters were designed in order to evaluate and characterize the arterial structures. Because of their size and catheter stiffness, early clinical studies with IVUS in the late 1980s were done primarily in the periphery. In the early 1990s, rapid technical improvement in catheter design, transducer technology, and subsequently imaging quality produced clinically useful catheters. The standard IVUS catheter was reduced to 3.5 to 4.3 F catheter, which

led to marked growth of their use in coronary interventional cardiology research and practice. In the last 10 years, IVUS has moved from being solely a research tool to an established modality in clinical practice. While the use in the coronaries remains more common than in the peripheral arteries, the primary techniques, diagnostic utility, and therapeutic benefits remain similar.

IVUS serves three important clinical purposes—diagnosis, guiding the interventional strategy, and optimizing the interventional result. Starting with diagnosis, IVUS is the gold standard method to assess intermediate stenosis, ambiguous lesions, bifurcations, unusual lesion morphology (aneurysms, calcium, thrombi), in-stent restenosis, and any other unusual angiographic finding.[2] From an interventional perspective, IVUS has been utilized extensively as a guide to the procedure, aiding in selection of optimal strategy, adjuvant device utilization (rotational atherectomy, predilation, etc.) as well as selection of stent diameter and length.[3] Additionally, IVUS imaging enables optimization of stenting procedures, maximizing expansion and apposition, and identifying poststenting complications such as vessel rupture and dissection.

● TECHNOLOGY

Two different IVUS transducer technologies are currently available—solid state (or phase array) and mechanical (Figure 21-1).[4] Solid-state configuration has 64 transducer elements arranged as a collar around the catheter. The backscattered ultrasound information received from each transducer element is sent to a computer that performs real-time image reconstruction to formulate a cross-sectional image of the artery. The advantage of this catheter is that there are no mobile parts and therefore, no motion artifacts

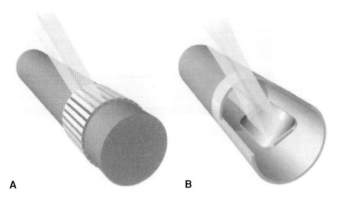

● **FIGURE 21-1.** IVUS transducers. (A) Phased array. (B) Mechanical.

Reproduced with permission from Yock PG, Fitzgerald PJ, Honda Y. Intravascular ultrasound. In: Topol EJ, ed. Interventional Cardiology. Philadelphia, PA: WB Saunders; 1999:801-818.

in the image. The principal disadvantage is a slightly lower spatial and temporal resolution than mechanical transducers and a "ring-down artifact," which is characterized by the appearance of bright halos around the IVUS catheter. This creates a small zone of uncertainty in the immediate area around the catheter and requires an additional corrective step in the calibration process[5] (Figure 21-2).

The second technology is a mechanical transducer, with a single rotating transducer mounted on a drive cable that allows a spinning transducer to build a tomography picture in real time. The resolution and dynamic ranges (gray scale) are superior with this method and clearer images can often be obtained. The disadvantage of a mobile drive shaft and transducers is the potential for an image artifact known as nonuniform rotational distortion (NURD). NURD (Figure 21-2) results from mechanical binding of the spinning transducer,[6] which can occur as a result of catheter kinking, excessive tightening of the hemostatic valve, or excessive vessel tortuosity.[5]

With coronary imaging, the transducers are typically between 30 and 40 MHz. This provides optimal resolution at a depth of penetration necessary for coronary arteries

and for small peripheral vessels such as the renal or infrapopliteal lower extremity arteries. The frequency of the catheters used in peripheral arteries range from 10 to 40 MHz transducers, depending on the size of the vessel being imaged and the necessary depth of penetration. There are currently two principal IVUS manufactures: Boston Scientific Corporation, Inc. (Maple Grove, MN) and Volcano Therapeutics (VT) (Rancho Cordova, CA). Both systems provide either a portable unit that can be wheeled from room to room of the catheterization laboratory or a permanent unit that is fully integrated into the catheterization laboratory (Figures 21-3A and 21-3B). Boston Scientific Corporation (BSC) has recently released Atlantis® PV Peripheral Imaging Catheter, mainly designed for aortic imaging (of aneurysms) with a wide field of view. It is an over-the-wire catheter requiring 8 F catheter introducer sheath and has a 15-MHz transducer capable of 25-cm pullback with 1 cm graduated markers for measurements. For other peripheral territories, BSC offers Sonicath® Ultra™ catheters ranging from 9 to 20 MHz as well as its coronary catheters, which are useful in renal and distal femoral arterial beds. VT has two catheters designed for peripheral vascular imaging. The detailed technical specifications of these catheters are summarized in Tables 21-1 and 21-2.

● IMPLEMENTATION, ACQUISITION, IMAGE INTERPRETATION, AND ANALYSIS

The important principles and steps necessary to integrate IVUS into the clinical setting are summarized in Table 12-3. Essentially, designation and training of appropriate IVUS technologists and interpreting physicians will allow for a seamless bridge between image acquisition, interpretation, and application. Once established, it can be expected that IVUS should add no more than a few minutes to the procedure time. A basic IVUS image acquisition protocol that can be used in a busy clinical lab is summarized in Table 12-4. The important point is that early identification for IVUS use allows the machine and catheter to be prepared so that imaging becomes a simple catheter exchange at the

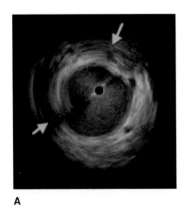
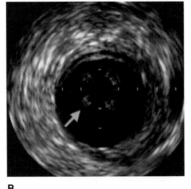
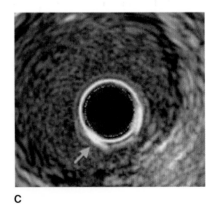

● **FIGURE 21-2.** IVUS artifacts. (A) NURD that is unique to mechanical systems. (B) Catheter defect producing artifact as bright straight lines around the catheter (arrow). (C) Ring-down artifact, seen as bright halos around the catheter (arrow).

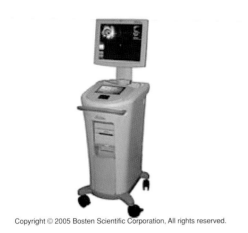

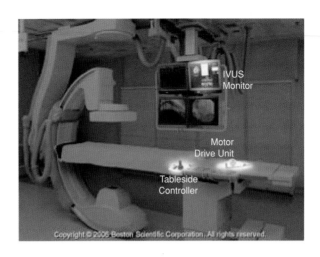

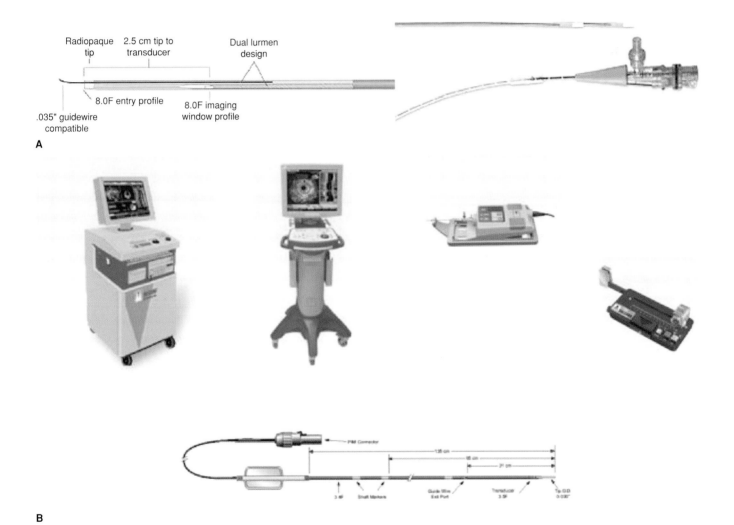

A

B

● **FIGURE 21-3.** IVUS Equipment. (A) Boston Scientific and (B) Volcano Therapeutics.

appropriate time. Motorized pullbacks are very useful in coronary arteries but can become time consuming in long peripheral lesions. If a long lesion is being imaged, a slow manual pullback often is sufficient as long as care is taken not to move "back and forth" and the rate of withdrawal is kept relatively slow and constant. If lesion length mea-

surements (or volume measurements) are needed, then a motorized pullback is required.

Successful IVUS image interpretation is dependent on understanding the fundamentals of the image formation and the anatomy of the arterial structure. IVUS image formation is based on the same principles as standard

TABLE 21-1. Boston Scientific Catheters for Peripheral Vascular Disease

	Sonicath® Ultra™ Catheters	Atlantis®
	3.2	Atlantis PV
Transducer frequency (MHz)	20	15
Maximal penetration (mm)	10	30
Usable length (mm)	135	95
Sheath compatibility (F)	6	8
Guide catheter compatibility (F)	7	NA
Typical use	Renal	Aorta/Iliac

NA, not applicable.

TABLE 21-2. VT Catheters for Peripheral Vascular Disease

	Visions PV 8.2	Visions PV .018 F/X
Transducer frequency (MHz)	10	20
Maximal penetration (mm)	60	24
Usable length (mm)	90	135
Sheath compatibility (F)	9	6
Guide catheter compatibility (F)	9	6
Typical use	Aorta/Iliac	Smaller arteries

TABLE 21-3. Starting an IVUS Program in the Catheterization Laboratory

1. Designate a specific IVUS technologist responsible for all practical aspects of IVUS imaging (equipment and catheter setup, image optimization, proper recording of IVUS imaging runs, patient, and procedure logs).

2. Designate a principle operator to be trained in IVUS image interpretation. With the time, this physician will pass the necessary knowledge to the rest of the operators allowing them to work independently with the help of the IVUS technologist.

3. Appropriate digital labeling: On screen labels should contain the timing of IVUS imaging (pre-, during-, or postprocedure), the procedure being performed, the target vessel, and location.

4. Modern equipment to the IVUS images in CD/DVD using the DICOM platform. Depending on the compression and quality use to save the data, up to eight patients with complete studies can be saved in a DVD.

TABLE 21-4. IVUS Image Acquisition

1. Verify that the catheter is compatible with the guide catheter and wide wire.

2. Flush the catheter free of air as air in the closed system produces black images that complicate image interpretation and continue flushing the catheter as it is introduced through the haemostatic valve.

3. Consider nitroglycerine 10–200 μg through the guide catheter in order to avoid vasospasm. (While this an essential step in coronary imaging, it may not be as important in larger peripheral vessels such as the aorta and iliac arteries).

4. Advance the catheter 3 or 5 cm distal to the segment to be interrogated. The catheter should advance smoothly without being forced. If the catheter is stuck in a lesion, it is generally due to an anatomic cause of interest. Turn the transducer on, as it will provide information useful for an interventional strategy (usually 360-degree calcification requiring plaque modification).

5. Connect catheter to automatic pullback device and initiate pullback. We recommend automatic pullback at rate of 1 mm/s in peripheral arteries as it provides improved image quality and increases accuracy of intended measurements. Upon completion the operator can readvance manually to further evaluate a particular area of interest.

6. Upon obtaining the image, the technologist can provide off-line information regarding lesion length, severity and morphology as well as reference diameters and landmarks.

7. Pull the catheter out, flush free of blood and store without bending to ensure catheter integrity for postprocedural use.

8. Repeat steps 1 to 7 with the same IVUS catheter for procedural and postprocedural guidance.

ultrasound imaging. An abrupt change in density (acoustic impedance) between adjacent tissue layers produces a strong reflection, resulting in an apparent boundary on the ultrasound image displayed on the screen. Applying this to vascular anatomy, the IVUS catheter is in the lumen where there is normal flowing blood, which reflects little to no sound and will appear black with a slight "speckle" from the blood cells. If blood cells are stagnant and have rouleaux formation, there will there be a substantial interface for the ultrasound to "bounce off." In this situation, blood appears bright on the screen. When ultrasound waves hit a very reflective object (such as a calcified plaque) most of the sound waves are reflected back toward the catheter, and the image obtained will be very bright (white) on the screen. Objects between these two extremes are displayed on a gray scale, with darker gray representing tissues with higher water or lipid content and lighter gray representing tissue that is more fibrous.

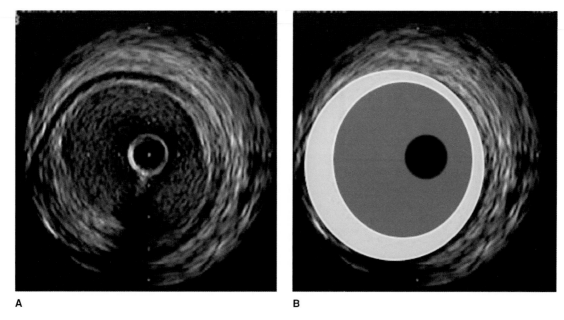

A   B

● **FIGURE 21-4.** Vessel layers. (A) IVUS image. (B) Corresponding color codes. Black denotes the IVUS catheter in the lumen. Red depicts the lumen with its outer border at the intimal border. Yellow depicts black and media with its outer border at the EEM. Outside the yellow circle is the adventitial layer.

Figure 21-4 depicts the normal three layers of the arterial wall depicted by IVUS. From the innermost to the outermost are the intima, media, and adventitia. The intima is composed of the endothelial cell layer and the underlying basal membrane with the internal elastic membrane representing external boundary of this layer. The media is composed of smooth muscle cells, elastin, and collagen and encircled by the external elastic membrane (EEM) representing the outer layer of the vessel. The adventitia is mainly composed of fibrous tissue. As can be seen in Figure 21-4, each of the arterial layers has different acoustic properties and each appears different (distinct) on the ultrasound screen. The intima reflects ultrasound and appears brighter than the blood in the lumen. The media, made mostly of homogenous smooth muscle cells, does not reflect a lot of ultrasound and is dark. The adventitia has "sheets" of collagen serving as several layers of interface for the ultrasound to be reflected off and is therefore very bright. While these layers are always present in muscular arteries, young people free of disease will have an intimal thickness below the resolution of IVUS and thus the three layers may be difficult to visualize (and it will appear as a "monolayer" with the blood apparently against the adventitia).

Standard IVUS measurements are shown in Figure 21-5. There are two primary interfaces: (1) the lumen-intima interface and (2) the media-adventitia interface. From these two "circles," virtually all required measurements can be obtained. The area enclosed by the lumen–intima interface is the luminal area. The area between the two interfaces is the plaque (or sometimes referred as the plaque and media or atheroma) area. The area enclosed by the media–adventitia interface is the vessel area (or media or EEM) area. Diameters are obtained by going through the center of the

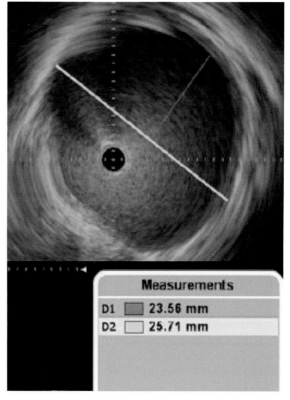

● **FIGURE 21-5.** IVUS measurements obtained in abdominal aorta. Red: minimum lumen diameter. Yellow: maximum lumen diameter.

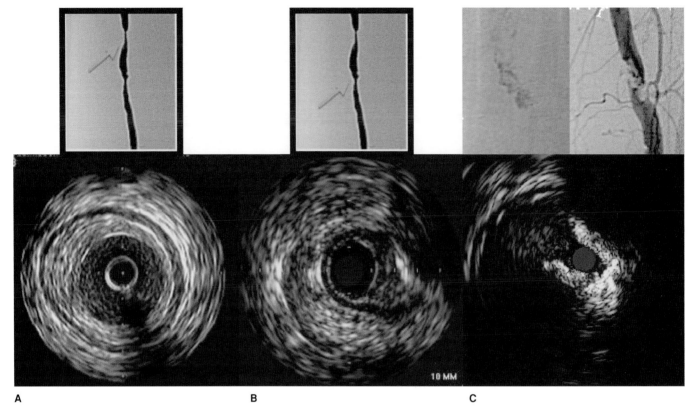

A   B   C

● **FIGURE 21-6.** Plaque morphology with angiographic appearance. (A) Fibrofatty. (B) Mixed. (C) Calcified.

image. These measurements are performed at the lesion and at the proximal and references. Furthermore, length measurements can be performed based on the amount of time it takes to get from one location to the next with a known pullback speed. Thus, the reported measures include reference lumen area and diameter, lesion area and minimal lumen diameter, and lesion length. These standard measurements can also be applied to stents (by adding another "circle" that follows the contour of the stent), enabling one to assess the stent deployment. In 2001, Mintz et al.[5] published the ACC consensus document on IVUS. Although this document refers primarily to coronary imaging, the principles outlined and the direct and derived measurements reviewed also pertain to peripheral imaging.

Plaque morphology can also be assessed by IVUS. Based on the degree of echogenicity, plaque can be characterized as soft (fatty), hard (fibrous), calcified, or mixed (Figure 21-6).[5,7–10] For instance, fatty plaque has a low echogenicity, where calcific plaque has high echogenicity and appears bright. Fibrous plaque has an intermediate echogenicity and mixed plaque contains more than one subtype.[5]

Intraluminal thrombus and dissection represent two additional tissue characteristics that can be seen by IVUS. Thrombus (Figure 21-7) is visualized as a mass in the lumen that often has a layered appearance. It is relatively echolucent and can occasionally be confused with atheroma or with stasis.[5,11] Dissection (Figure 21-8) is visualized as a discontinuity in the luminal wall with blood speckle be-

hind it. Five categories of dissection are intimal, medial or adventitial (depending on the depth to which a dissection penetrates), intramural hematoma, and intrastent.[5]

When IVUS is utilized to assess stents, standard luminal measurements apply. However, additional information should also be obtained including apposition, expansion, edge disease and, if present, intimal hyperplasia. Apposition (Figure 21-9) refers to whether the stent struts abut the vessel wall, with good stent apposition defined by stent struts in close-enough proximity to the vessel wall such that no flow between the stent strut and the wall occurs.[5,12] Expansion (Figure 21-10) refers to the stent minimum CSA compared to that of the reference segment[5] with adequate expansion (associated with a low risk of restenosis).[13] Stent edge issues include those of edge stenosis or dissection (both placing a particular vessel at higher risk for restenosis. Finally, neointimal hyperplasia (Figure 21-11) refers to the intimal growth within the stent.

● **CLINICAL APPLICATION**

IVUS is an imaging tool that is used for diagnosis, to guide intervention, and to assess for interventional success or complications. The following section provides an overview of the clinical applications of IVUS starting with a general clinical discussion and then addressing specific issues within each arterial bed. It is important to note that IVUS provides similar information regardless of the artery visualized. Specifically, IVUS gives the clinician information about

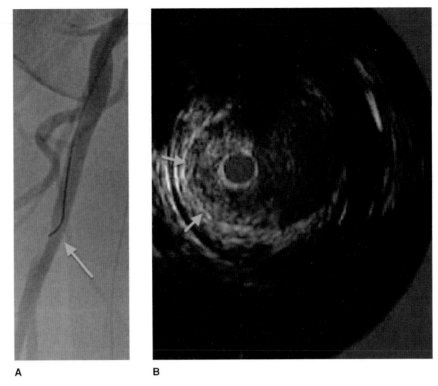

A   **B**

● **FIGURE 21-7.** Thrombus. (A) Angiography reveals minimal filling defect (arrow) corresponding to possible plaque or dissection. (B) IVUS confirms thrombus (arrowhead) from 6:00 to 11:00 around the catheter. Clearly visualized underneath thrombus are the intimal, medial, and adventitial layers.

vessel and lumen size, lesion composition, and lesion length, which helps guide the intervention. After the intervention, IVUS can be used to detect poststent complications such as stent underexpansion or malapposition, residual plaque, dissection, thrombus, hematoma, and rupture.

Diagnosis

As compared to angiography, IVUS provides high resolution, cross-sectional images of both the lumen and plaque. Thus, IVUS can more accurately determine the degree of luminal stenosis and the pattern/composition of the

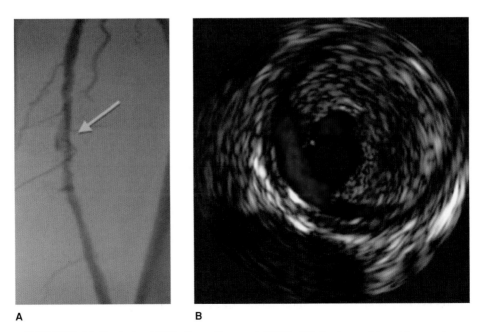

A   **B**

● **FIGURE 21-8.** Intimal SFA dissection post-PTCA. (A) Angiographic evidence of dissection (arrow). (B) IVUS confirms medial dissection (red color marks, blood flow within dissection plane).

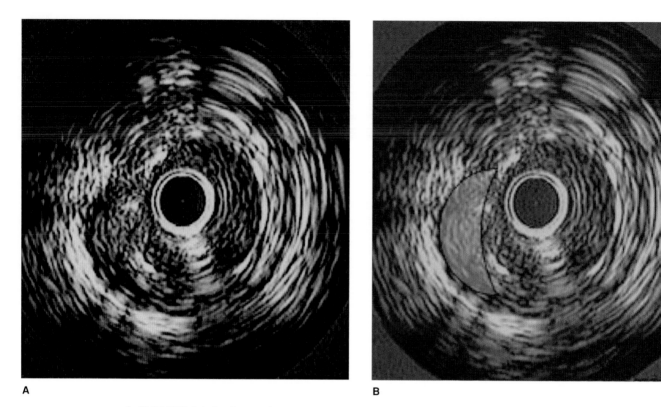

● **FIGURE 21-9.** Incomplete stent apposition. (A) IVUS image. (B) The yellow-shaded area denotes incomplete stent apposition to the vessel wall.

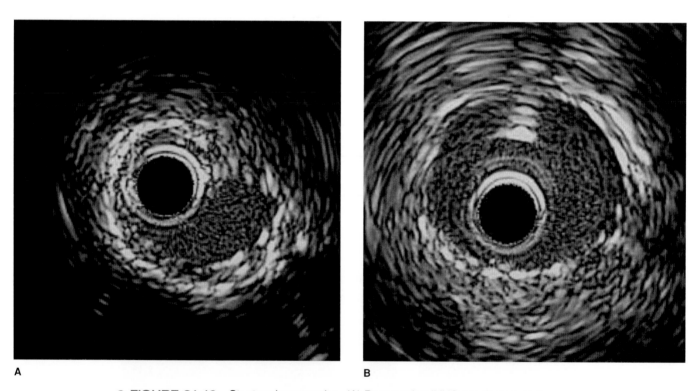

● **FIGURE 21-10.** Stent underexpansion. (A) Poststenting IVUS run demonstrating asymmetric underexpansion (arrows). (B) After high-pressure postdilation, symmetric/complete expansion is noted.

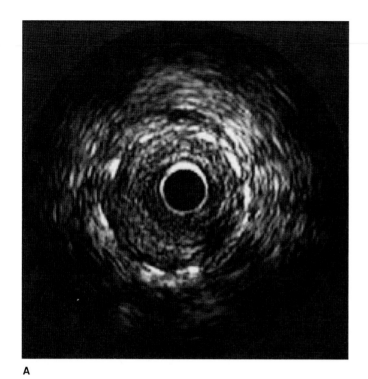

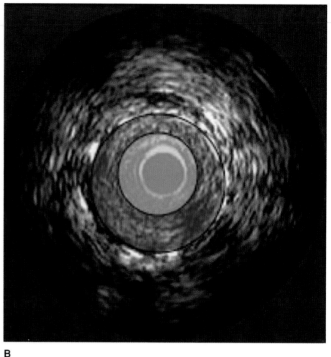

A

B

● **FIGURE 21-11.** Neointimal hyperplasia. (A) IVUS image. (B) The border of the green circle denotes the stent borders, the yellow circle denotes the lumen, and the green area represents neointimal hyperlasia.

stenotic lesion. For instance, a short and focal severe lesion is often readily apparent on angiography but diffuse disease may also be present; this could potentially alter the plan for treatment. Additionally, calcification and ulceration, two lesion characteristics that might require specific attention at the time of treatment, are readily visualized on IVUS imaging but not always apparent by angiography.

As an example of the importance of plaque morphology imaging, IVUS can easily determine whether a renal artery stenosis is caused by fibromuscular dysplasia or atherosclerotic disease. The echogenic characteristics of both the intima and the media with fibromuscular dysplasia and the absence of discrete plaque make it easily distinguishable from atherosclerotic disease. The stenosis from fibromuscular dysplasia can be treated with balloon dilation alone, without adjunctive stenting, whereby atherosclerosis may need stenting.

Guide to Intervention

When planning an interventional strategy, optimal results will more likely be obtained if there is a comprehensive understanding of lesion characteristics (including reference vessel diameter, lesion length, lesion composition, eccentricity, and calcification). Recognition of these characteristics enables the operator to deploy appropriately sized stents and use adjunctive equipment (such as atherectomy devices) when necessary.

While conventional angiography can provide clues to the above factors, IVUS imaging consistently provides this important information in a reliable fashion. With coronary interventions, preintervention IVUS can alter the strategy planned solely on the angiogram by as much as 40%.[3] Although not as robust, similar data in the peripheral literature exists for multiple arterial territories.[14,15] A representative case example is seen in Figure 21-12. In this case, fluoroscopy and angiography together demonstrate a complex, heavily calcified lesion in the SFA of this 61-year-old patient with known peripheral arterial disease and right lower extremity claudication at rest (Figure 21-12A). IVUS analysis revealed a heavy 270-degree concentric rim of calcium (Figure 21-12B). This lesion was debulked with a 2.5-mm Turbo Laser (Spectranetics, Colorado Springs, CO) revealing angiographic and IVUS results seen in Figure 21-12C. Specifically, the rim of calcium has been significantly fragmented thus allowing facilitated stent expansion. Finally, this lesion was stented at high pressure, yielding excellent angiographic and IVUS results as seen in Figure 21-12D.

With reference to stent sizing, IVUS can remove the guesswork implicit in choosing a stent based on luminal measurements. General consensus is to employ a stent diameter based on IVUS that corresponds to the larger of the proximal and distal reference lumens. This often leads to a significant upsizing of stents compared to conventional sizing with a goal of achieving a stent lumen of 80% to 90% of the average reference lumen.[16] Some experts, however,

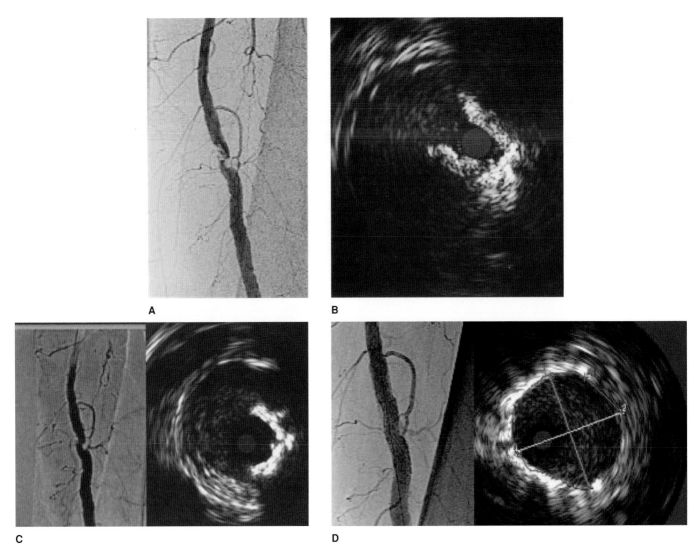

● **FIGURE 21-12.** Complex calcified lesion. (A) Angiography. (B) IVUS demonstrating a complex/severe lesion with a 270-degree rim of calcium. (C) Postlaser IVUS demonstrates that the calcification is more fragmented, permitting (D) full stent expansion.

base a stent size on "media-to-media" measurements, and therefore upsize even further.

Optimizing Final Results and Addressing Complications

Postintervention IVUS analysis provides an operator with the ability to evaluate procedural adequacy to a greater extent than angiography alone. For instance, thrombus (Figure 21-7) and vessel dissection (Figure 21-8) represent two complications often requiring further intervention that can be subtle on angiography but are obvious on IVUS. Additionally, stent malapposition (Figure 21-9) and underexpansion (Figure 21-10) are readily seen in vessels on which the corresponding angiogram reveals seemingly adequate results.

Regarding dissection, not only can IVUS imaging identify angiographically innapparent dissection but can aid in its treatment by allowing appropriate balloon sizing in order to tack down the dissection flap. An example of this is

shown in Figure 21-13. In this case, a 62-year-old man with right lower extremity claudication underwent diagnostic angiography revealing severe disease of the right SFA (Figure 21-13A). Post-PTCA, a large dissection flap was noted on IVUS imaging (Figure 21-13B). IVUS analysis of the proximal reference segment demonstrated a vessel diameter of 6 mm (Figure 21-13C) and with a 6-mm balloon the dissection was subjected to prolonged inflation with excellent angiographic and IVUS results depicted in Figure 21-13D. This case illustrates the utility of IVUS not only for detecting a significant procedural complication, but also its ability to guide appropriate resolution and optimize final results.

● CONSIDERATIONS IN SPECIFIC ARTERIAL TERRITORIES

Renal Artery (Table 21-5)

In 1991, Sheikh et al.[17] demonstrated the feasibility of IVUS imaging of the renal arteries, comparing it to contrast

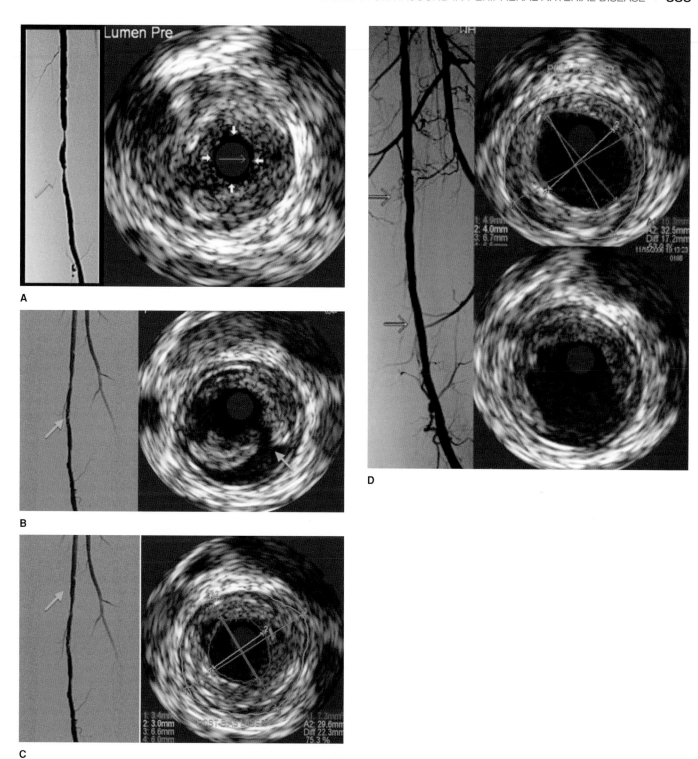

● **FIGURE 21-13.** Angioplasty complicated by dissection. (A) Pre-PTCA angiography on IVUS of a right SFA lesion in a 62-year-old man with right lower extremity claudication at rest. (B) Post-PTCA. A large dissection flap is noted on both angiography and IVUS (arrows). (C) In order to select a balloon with appropriate size to tack down the dissection, IVUS dimensions of the proximal reference vessel are obtained. In this case, the proximal reference diameter is 6 mm. (D) After a 6-mm balloon is inflated for 3 minutes, the proximal lumen cross-sectional area (top) has increased to 15.3 mm and the dissection flap (bottom) has been tacked down.

TABLE 21-5. Summary of Renal Artery IVUS Studies

Study	N	Purpose	Principal Findings
Shiekh et al.[17]	8	Diagnostic	Accurate angiographic and IVUS measurements. Postangioplasty dissection apparent on IVUS.
Leertouwer et al.[19]	22	Interventional	Additional treatment necessary in 6/18 patients with postangioplasty IVUS. Not seen on angiography.
Dangas et al.[15]	131	Interventional	Angiographic success in 100%. Post-IVUS led to additional dilation in 23.5%.

angiography. In this small series, IVUS measurements and digital angiography demonstrated high correlation with regard to lumen diameter ($r = 0.81$) and cross-sectional area ($r = 0.83$). Furthermore, by directly imaging all three layers of the arterial wall, IVUS could identify the mechanism of the renal arterial stenosis (RAS) as either fibromuscular dysplasia or atherosclerotic disease (an example of atherosclerosis and fibromuscular dysplasia is shown in Figure 21-14.[18]) Finally, IVUS imaging diagnosed postangioplasty dissection in three patients apparent by angiography in only one of the three.[17]

As a guide to intervention, Leertouwer et al.[19] reported on an initial experience of 22 patients with atherosclerotic RAS. After predilation, IVUS images were obtained in nine patients, resulting in selection of larger balloon sizes in five patients. In 18 patients, IVUS was performed poststenting, and led to additional interventional treatment in six patients (one for incomplete apposition, three for stent underexpansion, and two for distal lesions not seen on angiography). Additionally, vessel injury was noted in five patients (four dissection, one rupture) by IVUS, seen in only two patients by angiography.[19]

Investigators from the Washington Hospital Center evaluated IVUS-guided renal artery stenting in 131 patients with atherosclerotic RAS.[15] Interventions were performed on 153 renal artery segments. Angiography and IVUS demonstrated strong correlations between preintervention reference vessel ($r = 0.71$, $p < 0.0001$) and lesion minimal lumen diameter (MLD) ($r = 0.72$, $p < 0.0001$), lesion length ($r = 0.6$, $p < 0.0001$) and postintervention MLD ($r = 0.63$, $p < 0.0001$). However, while angiographic success was seen in all patients, IVUS analysis led to additional balloon dilatation in 36 (23.5%) cases. Factors leading to further intervention included incomplete stent apposition or expansion in 22 cases, dissection in 8 cases, and incomplete ostial stent coverage in 6 cases (incomplete ostial stent coverage is difficult to assess by angiography alone and carries a high risk of restenosis). In seven cases, findings on IVUS led to additional stenting.[15]

Additionally, case reports have demonstrated the utility of IVUS imaging as a guide to treatment of in-stent restenosis. In one case, IVUS evaluation revealed restenosis as a result of significant intimal hyperplasia and facilitated cutting balloon angioplasty of the segment with an excellent angiographic result confirmed by IVUS.[20] Another, more recent report, describes IVUS-guided deployment of 3.5 mm coronary paclitaxel-eluting stent to a proximal renal artery demonstrating severe in-stent restenosis with

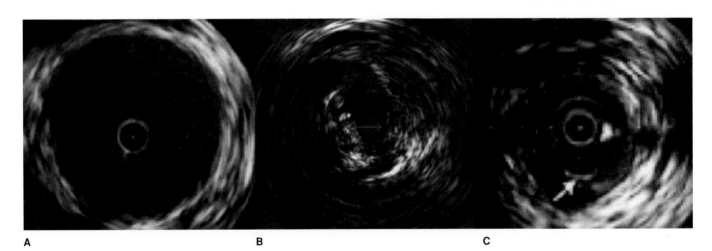

A   B   C

● **FIGURE 21-14.** Renal artery stenosis. Atherosclerosis and fibromuscular dysplasia. (A) Normal renal artery. (B) Atherosclerotic aorto-ostial renal artery stenosis characterized by a mildly calcific eccentric plaque. (C) Fibromuscular dysplasia characterized by a fixed, eccentric, and discrete membrane.

Reproduced with permission from Gowda MS, Loeb AL, Crouse LJ, Kramer PH. Complementary roles of color-flow duplex imaging and intravascular ultrasound in the diagnosis of renal artery fibromuscular dysplasia: should renal arteriography serve as the "gold standard"? J Am Coll Cardiol. 2003;41: 1305-1311.

excellent immediate and 6-month results confirmed by IVUS.[21]

Carotid Artery

Because of the risk of embolization, many operators have been somewhat hesitant to perform IVUS within the carotid vasculature. Safety, feasibility, and utility have since been demonstrated in more than 100 patients.[22–25]

The largest published experience with carotid IVUS imaging was in 98 consecutive patients,[26] No complications directly attributable to IVUS occurred in this series. While IVUS demonstrated excellent correlation with QCA of the reference vessels, a significantly smaller minimal lumen diameter was noted by IVUS as compared to angiography. Despite angiographic success in all patients, IVUS imaging identified the necessity for further intervention in 10% of patients. Furthermore, IVUS findings were found to be a predictor of complications; the IVUS-detected degree of superficial calcium was noted to be an independent and significant predictor of CVA at the time of the procedure.[26]

The same investigators recently reported on in-stent restenosis in carotid stents utilizing IVUS.[27] Of the patients included in the initial IVUS—carotid artery stent study,[26] 50 patients underwent 6-month IVUS follow-up. In those patients, a smaller minimum stent area and stent underexpansion was associated with increased intimal hyperplasia and restenosis. Again, no complications related to IVUS were noted.[27]

Aorta

When applied to aortic aneurysms and dissections, IVUS analysis is capable of providing real-time anatomic definition above that of computed tomography (CT) and angiography alone. In 1999, van Essen et al.[28] demonstrated consistent agreement between CT and IVUS with regards to both length ($r = 0.99$, $p < 0.001$) and diameter ($r = 0.93$, $p < 0.001$) measurements of the aneursym and proximal/distal neck ($r = 0.99$, $p < 0.001$) in a series of 16 patients with abdominal aortic aneurysms, although IVUS tended to slightly underestimate these dimensions compared to CT. In a series reported by Garret et al.,[14] IVUS altered the procedure in 28% of 78 cases by identifying, when compared to CT, differences in proximal neck diameter and lesion length. Additionally, IVUS analysis allowed endovascular repair in four patients who by CT were thought to have anatomy unsuitable for the procedure. In their series, although a causal relationship cannot be attributed to IVUS alone, there were no type I endovascular leaks at the conclusion of the procedure or at 20-month follow-up.[14] Other authors have reported on the usefulness of IVUS to accurately define aneurysm neck anatomy and optimally size aortic stent-grafts at the time of the procedure.[29–31]

For endovascular treatment of type B aortic dissections, IVUS was useful in identifying true versus false lumen as well as sites of entry and reentry within the dissection.[32] As illustrated by Koschyk et al.,[33] IVUS imaging can prove vital in excluding dissections that extend into the thorax

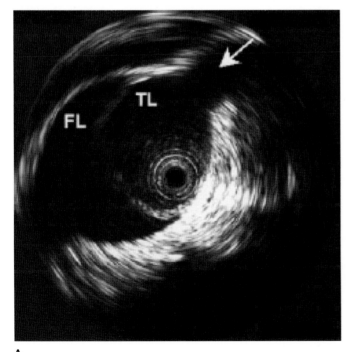 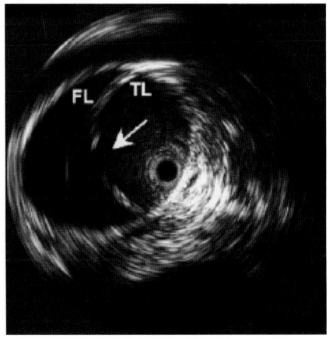

A   B

● **FIGURE 21-15.** Aortic dissection. (A) Side branch seen clearly in the true lumen—in this case, it is the right renal artery (arrow). (B) Entry point between the true and false lumen (arrow).

Reproduced with permission from Koschyk DH, Nienaber CA, Knap M, et al. How to guide stent-graft implantation in type B aortic dissection? Comparison of angiography, transesophageal echocardiography, and intravascular ultrasound. Circulation. 2005;112:I260-1264.

TABLE 21-6. Summary of Iliofemoral IVUS Studies

Study	N	Purpose	Findings
Navarro et al.[37]	44 (109 stents)	Interventional	Despite angiographic success, 28 lesions underwent further intervention (underexpansion, malapposition, dissection, thrombus, migration).
Buckley et al.[38]	52 (71 limbs)	Interventional	IVUS led to further intervention in 40% of limbs treated. In follow-up 100% of IVUS cases were free of repeat procedure vs. 77% of arteriography alone patients.
Gussenhoven et al.[40]	39	Interventional	After balloon angioplasty, decreased free lumen area and increased extent of dissection predicted restenosis.

from the abdomen and correctly identifying all entry sites between the true and false lumen. In this series, IVUS led to significant modification before the procedure in 5 of 25 dissections (4 with thoracic extension and 1 with a second angiographically unapparent entry site) and after the procedure (postdilation) in 7 patients.[33] The authors concluded that IVUS played an essential role in optimizing their results. An illustration of IVUS facilitated identification of entry site and side branches is provided in Figure 21-15.

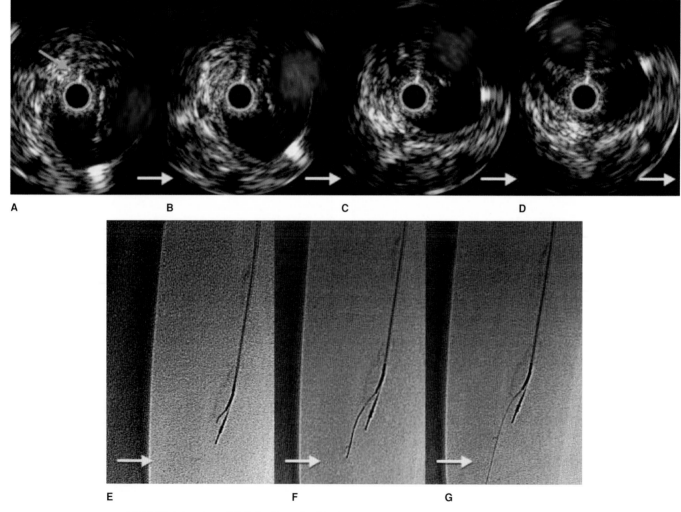

A   B   C   D

E   F   G

● FIGURE 21-16. IVUS facilitated subintimal reentry. (A) The IVUS probe is in the subintimal layer with the needle at 12-o'clock position (arrow) and the true lumen, represented in real-time by red color Doppler, from 3- to 8-o'clock position. (B, C, and D) With gradual rotation of the catheter, the true lumen is centered at the 12-o'clock position. (E) Needle puncture into the true lumen. (F and G) Guidewire advancement into the true lumen.

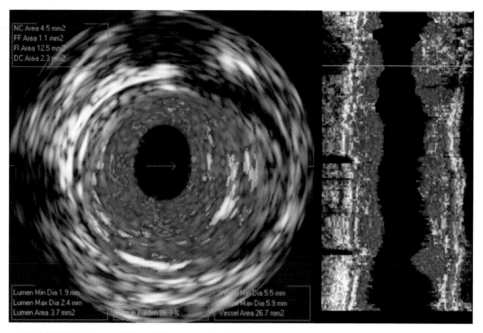

● **FIGURE 21-17.** Virtual histology. In this example from a superficial femoral artery, spectral analysis enables color-coding of the various components of plaque. Green: fibrous; white: calcified; red: necrotic; yellow: lipid.

Additionally, IVUS has been utilized to help treat post stent-graft intermittent claudication. In this situation, the false lumen essentially supplies a distal arterial bed, and once excluded by the stent graft, these arterial beds receive inadequate blood supply. Cases have been reported in which IVUS-guided fenestrations are placed within the graft to supply the false lumen and distal vessels with adequate blood flow and relief of claudication symptoms.[34]

Iliofemoral Arteries (Table 21-6)

In the mid-1990s, a few series on angioplasty with or without IVUS established the feasibility of IVUS in the iliac and infrailiac vessels. At the time of these studies, however, balloon angioplasty alone was standard. While angiographic vessel measurement correlate quite well with IVUS preintervention, it is well established from both the coronary and peripheral literature that the angiographic evaluation of postangioplasty vessels often overestimates lumen area and correlates poorly with IVUS measurements. Therefore, authors postulated that postangioplasty IVUS might influence one to use a stent in cases of residual stenosis.[35]

With the move toward routine stenting of iliac arteries, Arko et al.[36] demonstrated on prestenting IVUS that angiography alone underestimated vessel diameter in 25 of 40 aortoiliac occlusive lesions. Furthermore, poststenting IVUS revealed underexpansion in 40% of cases, necessitating postdilation.[36] Navarro et al.[37] reported on 44 patients undergoing IVUS-guided implantation of 109 stents. Despite angiographic success in all cases, 29 (27%) of these stents were found on postprocedural IVUS to be subop-

timally deployed (20 underexpanded stents, 3 malapposed stents, 4 arterial dissections, 1 thombosis, and 1 stent migration). Twenty-eight of these patients underwent modification with either further balloon dilation or repeat stenting. Successful angiographic and IVUS results were noted in 26 patients.[37]

In 2002, Buckley et al.[38] first reported a favorable effect on outcomes with IVUS in their study of 22 limbs treated with arteriography alone and 49 limbs treated with adjunctive IVUS. These investigators noted that despite angiographic success and a similar improvement in ankle-brachial indices, 40% of patients in the IVUS group underwent further balloon dilation because of stent malapposition. More importantly, in the angiography only group, early restenosis or occlusion occurred in four (18%) patients, all of whom at follow-up examination were documented by IVUS to have underexpanded stents. Secondary procedures were performed in none of the patients who underwent IVUS and 23% of those undergoing angiography alone ($p < 0.05$).[38]

In 1992, The et al.[39] investigated IVUS in SFA angioplasty, describing the mechanism of angioplasty (stretching) and commenting that overstretching was associated with dissection. Three years later, the EPISODE investigators reported on 39 patients undergoing IVUS-guided SFA angioplasty. They noted that while no characteristics on predilation IVUS appeared to influence 6-month outcomes, free lumen area and extent of dissection seen on IVUS significantly predicted 6-month failure.[40] In SFA and popliteal arteries, IVUS has the same utility to guide interventional procedures as it does in the carotid, renal, and iliac arteries.

A particularly interesting niche for IVUS in the iliac and femoral arteries pertains to the treatment of chronic total occlusion (CTO). Subintimal canalization is quite common while crossing a CTO, and when true-lumen reentry beyond the occlusion proves difficult, a number of reentry devices incorporating IVUS can aid in identification and reentry of the true lumen. In 2004, Casserly et al.[41] reported on two cases in which the CrossPoint TransAccess catheter (now called Pioneer, Medtronic Inc, Minneapolis, MN) was used to facilitate true lumen reentry and successfully revascularize the SFA. Investigators from St. Louis University recently reported on 87 chronic total occlusions and 24 in which the true lumen could not be re-entered with standard techniques (20 iliac, 4 femoral). In 21 of these cases, the Pioneer catheter was used to facilitate true-lumen reentry with technical success in all cases and continued patency at a mean of 5.8-month follow-up.[42] IVUS-guided true lumen reentry represents an important modality in treating iliac and femoral CTO. An example of this technique is depicted in Figure 21-16.

● SUMMARY

IVUS is a unique, real-time, cross-sectional imaging modality that provides a view of the artery unlike any other conventional imaging technique. Because of its ability to visualize the lumen, plaque, and arterial structures, it can assist peripheral artery diagnostic dilemmas and guide interventions to optimize results. Furthermore, IVUS can play an important role as a predictor, early identifier, and guide treatment for peripheral vascular interventional complications. In the future, enhanced software reconstruction including, for example, Virtual Histology (utilizing spectral analysis based on ultrasound to determine plaque composition, Figure 21-17)[43] may further enable tissue characterization and provide important guidance in both diagnostic and therapeutic arenas.

REFERENCES

1. Bom N, Lancee CT, Van Egmond FC. An ultrasound intracardiac scanner. *Ultrasonics.* 1972;10:72–76.

2. Di Mario C, Gorge G, Peters R, et al. Clinical application and image interpretation in intracoronary ultrasound. Study Group on Intracoronary Imaging of the Working Group of Coronary Circulation and of the Subgroup on Intravascular Ultrasound of the Working Group of Echocardiography of the European Society of Cardiology. *Eur Heart J.* 1998;19:207–229.

3. Mintz GS, Pichard AD, Kovach JA, et al. Impact of preintervention intravascular ultrasound imaging on transcatheter treatment strategies in coronary artery disease. *Am J Cardiol.* 1994;73:423–430.

4. Yock PG, Fitzgerald PJ, Honda Y. Intravascular ultrasound. In: Topol EJ, ed. *Interventional Cardiology.* Philadelphia, PA: WB Saunders; 1999:801–818.

5. Mintz GS, Nissen SE, Anderson WD, et al. American college of cardiology clinical expert consensus document on standards for acquisition, Measurement and Reporting of Intravascular Ultrasound Studies (IVUS). A report of the American College of Cardiology Task Force on Clinical Expert Consensus Documents. *J Am Coll Cardiol.* 2001;37:1478–1492.

6. ten Hoff H, Korbijn A, Smith TH, Klinkhamer JF, Bom N. Imaging artifacts in mechanically driven ultrasound catheters. *Int J Card Imaging.* 1989;4:195–199.

7. Hodgson JM, Reddy KG, Suneja R, Nair RN, Lesnefsky EJ, Sheehan HM. Intracoronary ultrasound imaging: correlation of plaque morphology with angiography, clinical syndrome and procedural results in patients undergoing coronary angioplasty. *J Am Coll Cardiol.* 1993;21:35–44.

8. Metz JA, Yock PG, Fitzgerald PJ. Intravascular ultrasound: basic interpretation. *Cardiol Clin.* 1997;15:1–15.

9. Mintz GS, Douek P, Pichard AD, et al. Target lesion calcification in coronary artery disease: an intravascular ultrasound study. *J Am Coll Cardiol.* 1992;20:1149–1155.

10. Nishimura RA, Edwards WD, Warnes CA, et al. Intravascular ultrasound imaging: in vitro validation and pathologic correlation. *J Am Coll Cardiol.* 1990;16:145–154.

11. Siegel RJ, Ariani M, Fishbein MC, et al. Histopathologic validation of angioscopy and intravascular ultrasound. *Circulation.* 1991;84:109–117.

12. Nakamura S, Colombo A, Gaglione A, et al. Intracoronary ultrasound observations during stent implantation. *Circulation.* 1994;89:2026–2034.

13. Moussa I, Moses J, Di Mario C, et al. Does the specific intravascular ultrasound criterion used to optimize stent expansion have an impact on the probability of stent restenosis? *Am J Cardiol.* 1999;83:1012–1017.

14. Garret HE Jr, Abdullah AH, Hodgkiss TD, Burgar SR. Intravascular ultrasound aids in the performance of endovascular repair of abdominal aortic aneurysm. *J Vasc Surg.* 2003;37:615–618.

15. Dangas G, Laird JR Jr, Mehran R, Lansky AJ, Mintz GS, Leon MB. Intravascular ultrasound-guided renal artery stenting. *J Endovasc Ther.* 2001;8:238–247.

16. Nissen SE, Yock P. Intravascular ultrasound: novel pathophysiological insights and current clinical applications. *Circulation.* 2001;103:604–616.

17. Sheikh KH, Davidson CJ, Newman GE, Kisslo KB, Schwab SJ. Intravascular ultrasound assessment of the renal artery. *Ann Intern Med.* 1991;115:22–25.

18. Gowda MS, Loeb AL, Crouse LJ, Kramer PH. Complementary roles of color-flow duplex imaging and intravascular ultrasound in the diagnosis of renal artery fibromuscular dysplasia: should renal arteriography serve as the "gold standard"? *J Am Coll Cardiol.* 2003;41:1305–1311.

19. Leertouwer TC, Gussenhoven EJ, van Overhagen H, Man in 't Veld AJ, van Jaarsveld BC. Stent placement for treatment of renal artery stenosis guided by intravascular ultrasound. *J Vasc Interv Radiol.* 1998;9:945–952.

20. Otah KE, Alhaddad IA. Intravascular ultrasound-guided cutting balloon angioplasty for renal artery stent restenosis. *Clin Cardiol.* 2004;27:581–583.

21. Kakkar AK, Fischi M, Narins CR. Drug-eluting stent implantation for treatment of recurrent renal artery in-stent restenosis. *Catheter Cardiovasc Interv.* 2006;68:118–122.

22. Reid DB, Diethrich EB, Marx P, Wrasper R. Intravascular ultrasound assessment in carotid interventions. *J Endovasc Surg.* 1996;3:203–210.

23. Wilson EP, White RA, Kopchok GE. Utility of intravascular ultrasound in carotid stenting. *J Endovasc Surg.* 1996;3:63–68.

24. Weissman NJ, Canos M, Mintz GS, et al. Carotid artery intravascular ultrasound: safety and morphologic observations during carotid stenting in 102 patients [abstract]. *J Am Coll Cardiol.* 2000;35(suppl A):10A.

25. Weissman NJ, Mintz GS, Dangas G, et al. Intravascular ultrasound lesion calcium predicts adverse clinical events after carotid artery stenting. *J Am Coll Cardiol.* 2000;35(suppl A):7A.

26. Clark DJ, Lessio S, O'Donoghue M, Schainfeld R, Rosenfield K. Safety and utility of intravascular ultrasound-guided carotid artery stenting. *Catheter Cardiovasc Interv.* 2004;63:355–362.

27. Clark DJ, Lessio S, O'Donoghue M, Tsalamandris C, Schainfeld R, Rosenfield K. Mechanisms and predictors of carotid artery stent restenosis: a serial intravascular ultrasound study. *J Am Coll Cardiol.* 2006;47:2390–2396.

28. van Essen JA, Gussenhoven EJ, van der Lugt A, et al. Accurate assessment of abdominal aortic aneurysm with intravascular ultrasound scanning: validation with computed tomographic angiography. *J Vasc Surg.* 1999;29:631–638.

29. van Essen JA, Gussenhoven EJ, Blankensteijn JD, et al. Three-dimensional intravascular ultrasound assessment of abdominal aortic aneurysm necks. *J Endovasc Ther.* 2000;7:380–388.

30. Tutein Noltenius RP, van den Berg JC, Moll FL. The value of intraoperative intravascular ultrasound for determining stent graft size (excluding abdominal aortic aneurysm) with a modular system. *Ann Vasc Surg.* 2000;14:311–317.

31. Slovut DP, Ofstein LC, Bacharach JM. Endoluminal AAA repair using intravascular ultrasound for graft planning and deployment: a 2-year community-based experience. *J Endovasc Ther.* 2003;10:463–475.

32. Koschyk DH, Nienaber CA, Knap M, et al. How to guide stent-graft implantation in type B aortic dissection? Comparison of angiography, transesophageal echocardiography, and intravascular ultrasound. *Circulation.* 2005;112:I260–1264.

33. Koschyk DH, Meinertz T, Hofmann T, et al. Value of intravascular ultrasound for endovascular stent-graft placement in aortic dissection and aneurysm. *J Card Surg.* 2003;18:471–477.

34. Husmann MJ, Kickuth R, Ludwig K, et al. Intravascular ultrasound-guided creation of re-entry sites to improve intermittent claudication in patients with aortic dissection. *J Endovasc Ther.* 2006;13:424–428.

35. Vogt KJ, Rasmussen JG, Just S, Schroeder TV. Effect and outcome of balloon angioplasty and stenting of the iliac arteries evaluated by intravascular ultrasound. *Eur J Vasc Endovasc Surg.* 1999;17:47–55.

36. Arko F, McCollough R, Manning L, Buckley C. Use of intravascular ultrasound in the endovascular management of atherosclerotic aortoiliac occlusive disease. *Am J Surg.* 1996;172:546–549.

37. Navarro F, Sullivan TM, Bacharach JM. Intravascular ultrasound assessment of iliac stent procedures. *J Endovasc Ther.* 2000;7:315–319.

38. Buckley CJ, Arko FR, Lee S, et al. Intravascular ultrasound scanning improves long-term patency of iliac lesions treated with balloon angioplasty and primary stenting. *J Vasc Surg.* 2002;35:316–323.

39. The SH, Gussenhoven EJ, Zhong Y, et al. Effect of balloon angioplasty on femoral artery evaluated with intravascular ultrasound imaging. *Circulation.* 1992;86:483–493.

40. Gussenhoven EJ, van der Lugt A, Pasterkamp G, et al. Intravascular ultrasound predictors of outcome after peripheral balloon angioplasty. *Eur J Vasc Endovasc Surg.* 1995;10:279–288.

41. Casserly IP, Sachar R, Bajzer C, Yadav JS. Utility of IVUS-guided transaccess catheter in the treatment of long chronic total occlusion of the superficial femoral artery. *Catheter Cardiovasc Interv.* 2004;62:237–243.

42. Jacobs DL, Motaganahalli RL, Cox DE, Wittgen CM, Peterson GJ. True lumen re-entry devices facilitate subintimal angioplasty and stenting of total chronic occlusions: initial report. *J Vasc Surg.* 2006;43:1291–1296.

43. Vince DG, Nair A, Klingensmith JD, Kuban BD, Margolis MP, Burgess V. Radiofrequency-tissue characterization and virtual histology. In: Waksman R, Serruys PW, eds. *Handbook of the Vulnerable Plaque.* London, UK: Taylor and Francis; 2004:327–342.

chapter 22

Arterial Diseases of the Eye

Robert J. Barnes, MD

The eye is proverbially the window to the soul, and literally a window into the vascular system. Evaluation of the retinal vasculature gives insight into multiple systemic diseases affecting the patient. Simply by evaluating the retina, one can determine diseases such as severe hypertension, diabetes mellitus, embolic disease, lupus, infection, and extended abdominal trauma.

● REVIEW OF OPHTHALMIC BLOOD SUPPLY

The eye is fed by the first branch of the internal carotid artery. This ophthalmic artery then branches off into the central retinal artery, the posterior ciliary arteries, and the muscular branches. The venous system is comprised of the posterior vortex veins, which drain into the superior and inferior orbital veins which then drain into the cavernous sinus; and the central retinal vein, which drains the retina and the optic nerve directly into the cavernous sinus.[1]

● HYPERTENSIVE RETINOPATHY

Systemic hypertension is diagnosed when the blood pressure is greater than 140 systolic and 90 diastolic measured on three separate occasions separated by at least 2 weeks. High blood pressure is extremely common to the industrialized countries. The ocular signs in hypertension are directly related to the rate and degree of systemic blood pressure. Atherosclerosis is a common finding in systemic hypertension. It can also occur in the normal aging population. The retinal changes seen in hypertension may overlap with those found in other retinal vascular diseases such as diabetes (Figure 22-1).[2]

Systemic hypertension is one of the most common diseases affecting patients throughout the world. The most common ocular manifestations include focal constriction and dilation of retinal arteries, narrowing and irregularity of the retinal arteries, AV nicking, blot retinal hemorrhages, microaneurysms, and cotton-wool spots. Several classification schemes have been used to stage hypertensive retinal changes. The most commonly accepted are the Keith-Wagener-Barker classification (Table 22-1) and the Scheie classification (Table 22-2). With these classification systems, one is able to evaluate the degree of hypertension systemically and begin therapy.

The treatment of hypertensive retinopathy consists of blood pressure control. No specific ocular therapy exists to reverse the changes. In case of accelerated hypertension or malignant hypertension, systemic diseases must be ruled out such as renal disease, polycystic kidney, renal stenosis, pheochromocytoma, and pregnancy.[4]

● RETINAL ARTERY OBSTRUCTION

Retinal artery obstructions are divided into two main types: central and branch, depending on the location of the obstruction. Central retinal artery occlusion is an acute stoppage of blood flow through the central retinal artery, leading to ischemia and nonperfusion of the retina. This is an abrupt, painless, severe loss of vision heralded by a cherry-red spot in the macula area. The peripheral retina becomes ischemic and white. The macula remains red secondary to choroidal blood flow. This is commonly referred to as an amaurosis fugax and is a term used to describe the situation with a painless loss of vision occurring. Emboli are seen only approximately 25% of the time. It is an indicator of carotid vascular disease approximately one-third of the time as opposed to giant cell arteritis, which is only found 5% of the time. Branch retinal artery occlusions have a similar presentation commonly associated with carotid vascular disease, cardiac valvular disease, or systemic clotting (Figure 22-3).[5]

Central retinal artery obstruction is rare. It is estimated to be seen in one patient out of 10 000 who visits to an ophthalmologist. Men are more common than women at a

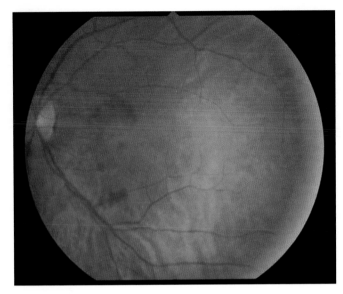

● **FIGURE 22-1.** Hypertensive retinopathy.

ratio of 2:1 with the onset being around 60 years of age. The majority of central retinal artery obstructions are caused by thrombus formation just proximal to the lamina cribrosa and are therefore not seen on ophthalmic examination. Atherosclerosis is the cause in most cases, although congenital anomalies of the central retinal artery, systemic coagulopathies, or low blood flow states may also be seen. In only 25% of the cases, an emboli is visible in the central retinal artery or one of its branches, suggesting that an embolic cause is not very common. Other diseases besides emboli that can lead to central retinal or branch retinal artery occlusion include shingles, optic neuritis, or mucormycosis. Systemic coagulopathies may be associated with both central and branch retinal artery obstructions. Other causes of obstructive retinopathy include radiation retinopathy, emboli associated with depot medication, injections such as steroids around the eye, and IV drug use.[6]

The hallmark of ocular manifestation of acute central retinal artery obstruction is an abrupt, painless loss of vision. Pain is unusual and if found is associated with ocular ischemic syndrome. Amaurosis fugax is seen in approximately 10% of the patients.

In rare situations, a patient may have a patent cilioretinal artery which perfuses the fovea and the patient may have normal central vision. The ophthalmic manifestation on clinical examination, the hallmark is a cherry-red spot of the macula, will not be seen in a patient with a ciliary retinal artery.

When a central retinal branch artery occlusion is found, systemic disease associated includes 60% of the time systemic hypertension, 25% of the time diabetes, and 50% of the cases have no definitive cause for the obstruction. Potential embolic sources are found less than 40% of the time in any type of arterial occlusion.

The most common association is significant ipsilateral carotid artery disease, which is present in approximately one-third of the patients. An embolic source from the heart is present in less than 10% of the cases. Other rare systemic diseases include blood-clotting abnormalities such as antiphospholipid antibodies, protein S deficiency, protein C deficiency, and antithrombin III deficiency.[7]

Common systemic conditions associated with central retinal artery obstruction include atherosclerotic cardiovascular disease such as carotid plaques or dissection, aortic plaques or dissection, cardiac disease such as valvular rheumatic fever, VSD (ventriculoseptal defects), cardiac myxoma, mural thrombus, and subacute bacterial endocarditis. Cancers including metastatic tumors, leukemia, and lymphoma have also been associated with vascular obstructive diseases.

TABLE 22-1. Keith-Wagener-Barker Classification	
Group 1	Moderate narrowing or sclerosis of the artery.
Group 2	Marked narrowing of the artery, exaggeration of the light reflex, and AV nicking.
Group 3	Arterial narrowing and focal constriction, retinal edema, cotton-wool spots, and hemorrhages.
Group 4	Same as group 3 plus papilledema.

TABLE 22-2. Scheie Classification	
Grade 0	No changes.
Grade 1	Barely detectable arterial narrowing.
Grade 2	Obvious arterial narrowing with focal irregularities.
Grade 3	Retinal hemorrhages exudates.
Grade 4	Same as group 3 plus papilledema[3] (Figure 22-2).

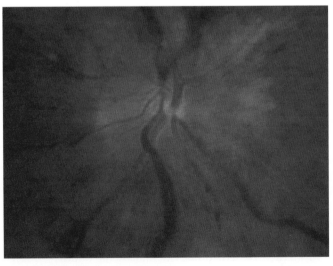

● **FIGURE 22-2.** Papilledema.

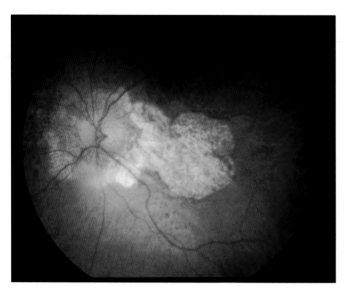

● FIGURE 22-3. Macular degeneration.

Medical procedures such as angiography, angioplasty, chiropractic neck manipulation, and cortical steroid injections around the eye have also been found to lead to vascular obstructive diseases. Systemic vasculitides such as temporal arteritis, Wegener's granulomatosis, inflammatory bowel disease, Kawasaki syndrome, systemic lupus, and polyarteritis nodosa have also been associated with retinal artery obstruction. Systemic infections such as syphilis—the great masquerader—have also been found associated with this syndrome.

Miscellaneous other diseases leading to vascular obstruction include amniotic fluid emboli, IV drug use, cocaine abuse, oral contraception, pregnancy, and migraines.

● **VENOUS OBSTRUCTION OF THE RETINA**

Venous obstruction of the retina is a relatively common finding second only to diabetes, more commonly affecting patients 50 years of age or older. Retinal vein obstructions are classified as whether they are central or branch. Although classified commonly together, they have significant differences leading to various outcomes for the eye. Specifically, ischemic venous obstructive diseases can lead to neovascular glaucoma of the eye and eventual blindness.[8]

Central retinal vein occlusion is 90% of the time in patients 50 years of age or older, more common in men than women. It is often associated with diabetes, hypertension, and atherosclerotic disease. Sedimentation rate elevation appears to be a risk factor in women only. Open-angle glaucoma is a relatively common finding in patients who have had a central retinal vein occlusion. Patients with a history of glaucoma are five times more likely to have a central retinal vein occlusion than those who do not. An acute angle-closure glaucoma may precipitate a central retinal vein occlusion.[9]

The exact pathogenesis of a central retinal vein occlusion seems to involve a thrombus at the central retinal vein near the lamina cribrosa, and why this occurs is unknown. Clini-cal findings include retinal hemorrhaging; dilated, tortuous veins in affected quadrants; disk edema; macular edema; and cotton-wool spots.

Central retinal vein occlusions can be broken down into nonischemic versus ischemic. Both involve hemorrhages throughout the retina in all four quadrants. However, with the ischemic version, approximately two-thirds of the patients go on to develop anterior segment neovascularization usually within 3 months, which then leads to neovascular glaucoma. Workup for venous occlusions would include a complete eye examination, blood pressure, complete blood count, partial thromboplastin time, antinuclear antibody, protein electrophoresis, and sedimentation rate.[10]

Patients with branch retinal vein occlusions have a similar prognostic fate and require a similar workup.

● **DIABETIC RETINOPATHY**

Diabetes mellitus is another very common disease affecting our patients today, and the best predictor of diabetic retinopathy is the duration of the disease. Patients who have had insulin-dependent diabetes for less than 5 years rarely show signs of diabetic retinopathy; however, of those who have had the disease from 5 to 10 years, approximately one-third will go on and develop retinopathy, and those of who have had diabetes for longer than 10 years, 70% to 90% will develop diabetic retinopathy. After 20 to 30 years, the incidence of diabetic retinopathy rises to 95%. Key features include microaneurysms, retinal hemorrhages, cotton-wool spots, lipid exudates, retinal edema, and retinal neovascularization. Diabetes mellitus is the leading cause of blindness in the western world and in the United States specifically.[11]

Diabetic retinopathy is divided into two main categories: nonproliferative phase and proliferative phase. The nonproliferative phase involves microaneurysm as the first detectable change. Macular edema and retinal thickening is commonly seen where capillaries leak fluid and blood, and lipid is deposited and is a leading cause of permanent blindness (Figure 22-4).

Proliferative diabetic retinopathy involves neovascularization of the retinal vessels which leads to increased leakage, lipid formation, and nonperfusion and eventual ischemia, which then leads to neovascularization. The ischemia associated with diabetic retinopathy leads to nonperfusion of the retina and eventual loss of function and blindness (Figure 22-5).

Cotton-wool spots often referred to as soft exudates of the nerve fiber layer are white, fluffy lesions of the nerve fiber layer caused by ischemia. Diagnosis of nonperfusion and diabetic retinopathy involve fluorescein angiography. Fluorescein angiography will demonstrate areas of nonperfusion and areas of neovascularization requiring laser photocoagulation. The Early Treatment Diabetic Retinopathy Study (ETDRS) found that intraretinal microvascular abnormalities, multiple retinal hemorrhages, venous beading, and loops seen on angiography are all significant risk factors for the development of proliferative retinopathy

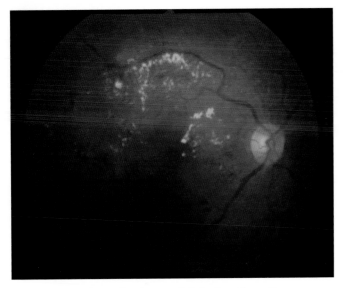

● **FIGURE 22-4.** Background diabetic retinopathy.

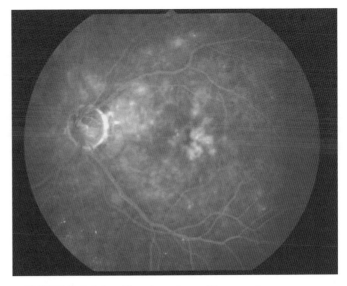

● **FIGURE 22-6.** Macular edema (fluorescein angiography).

(Figure 22-6). Treatment for severe diabetic retinopathy is panretinal photocoagulation (PRP). The Diabetic Retinopathy Study demonstrated that patients with high-risk eyes for developing diabetic retinopathy have a significant improvement with treatment with PRP. The exact mechanism by which PRP works remains unknown; however, the theory most advocate is that laser burns reduce the ischemic stimulation of the retina and release of vasoactive proteins. Focal laser also will seal off any leaky blood vessels, reducing lipid formation and hemorrhaging.[12]

The goal of panretinal photocoagulation is to cause regression of neovascularization in those patients having advanced proliferative phase (Figure 22-7). The ETDRS found that PRPs significantly retarded the development of neovascularization and reduce the amount of macular edema. Another therapy that has previously been used was peripheral retinal cryotherapy that, again, causes a focal scar

formation of the peripheral retina and therefore less oxygen demand and ischemic release of vasoproliferative substances. The final prognosis for most diabetic retinopathy is still poor despite the early treatment options that have been discovered by large studies. However, based on the Diabetic Retinopathy Study and the ETDRS, severe visual loss can be reduced by 95% by aggressive early intervention.[13]

● PROLIFERATIVE RETINOPATHIES

Proliferative retinopathies are a group of diseases associated with preretinal or optic nerve neovascularization. This group can be divided into two categories: one with associated systemic disease and the other associated with retinal or ocular disease. Those associated with systemic disease include diabetes, as previously discussed, hyperviscosity syndrome; aortic arch syndrome; carotid cavernous

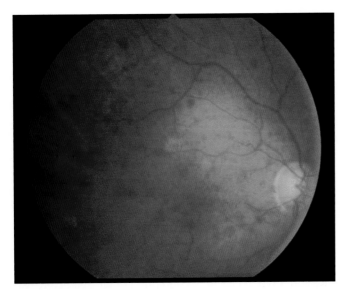

● **FIGURE 22-5.** Central retinal vein occlusion.

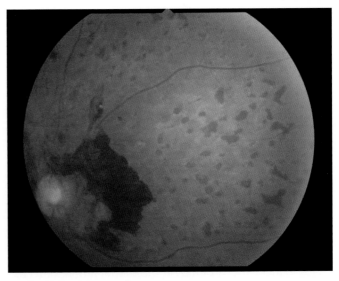

● **FIGURE 22-7.** Diabetic retinopathy.

fistula; multiple sclerosis; lupus; sickle cell disease; and sarcoidosis.

Diseases with proliferative retinopathy associated with strong hereditary components include sickling hemoglobinopathies such as SC disease, SS disease, and thalassemia. Those diseases associated purely with a retinal vascular or ocular inflammatory disease include Eales' disease, branch retinal vein occlusion, branch retinal artery occlusion, retinal emboli, retinopathy of prematurity (ROP), acute retinal necrosis, cocaine use, and choroidal melanoma. The number one cause of retinal neovascularization is diabetes mellitus, which has been discussed earlier. Hemoglobinopathies, SS disease, and SC disease are commonly associated with retinal neovascularization. Other diseases that are more uncommon include aortic arch syndrome. Patients with atherosclerosis involving the carotid artery or the aortic arch and patients with arteritis such as Takayasu's disease or syphilitic aortic involvement may go on and develop peripheral retinal neovascularization. Carotid cavernous fistulas where arterial blood enters the cavernous sinus venous system directly, bypassing the eye, and the consequential ischemia may stimulate retinal neovascularization. Multiple sclerosis has also been shown to develop peripheral venous sheathing and ischemia and may lead to neovascularization. Systemic lupus has also been associated with peripheral retinal neovascularization as well as sarcoidosis.[14]

Eales' disease is a bilateral disorder of young men, usually from India. They develop a peripheral retinal phlebitis and retinal nonperfusion. The etiology is unknown; however, frequently neovascularization of the retina is seen. The prognosis is good for this disease, but sometimes retinal photocoagulation is necessary.

● CHOROIDAL NEOVASCULAR DISEASES

Up to this point, most of the diseases that have been discussed involve retinal vasculature, but as stated earlier, the eye is fed by two branches of the ophthalmic artery, the central retinal artery and the choroidal vasculature. Most of the diseases that have been discussed so far involve the retinal vasculature. At this time, we will discuss abnormalities with the choroidal vasculature.

The choroid is a network of blood vessels underlying the retina that supply the outer half of the retinal architecture. The most common disease affecting the choroidal vasculature is macular degeneration or appropriately named age-related macular degeneration (ARMD).

ARMD is the most frequent cause of central vision loss among people aged 50 or older. The majority of the eyes that suffer vision loss are based on the damage from choroidal neovascularization. Choroidal neovascularization is the formation of new blood vessels in the choriocapillaris that erode into the retina, leading to hemorrhagic detachment of the retina, fibrosis, and vision loss. There are other diseases that affect the choriocapillaris and lead to choroidal neovascularizations, which will be discussed further on. ARMD affects severe vision loss on average aproximately

75 years of age. No significant difference is noted between sexes. Drusen or yellow deposits in the retina, which are focal excrescences of Bruch's membrane, are precursors to ARMD. ARMD is usually divided into non-neovascular or neovascular components. Non-neovascular macular degeneration is the most common form of this disease. It is often called the dry form of macular degeneration. The neovascular form is the growth of choroidal neovascular membranes with presentation of subretinal fluid, macular edema, and diskiform scar. This is frequently called the wet form of macular degeneration.[15]

Current treatment options for macular degeneration dry form involve vitamin therapy. The wet form at this point has had more significant new advances that are available. Previously, treatment has had more success with laser treatment. Currently, more successful treatment has been with antivascular endothelial growth factor (anti-VEGF) type drugs that are injected directly into the inside of the eye, which have shown vast improvements in the therapeutic options causing shrinkage of the neovascular membrane.

Other diseases causing choroidal neovascularization besides ARMD include angioid streaks, Best's disease, multifocal choroiditis, histoplasmosis, sarcoidosis, and toxoplasmosis (Figure 22-8).

Options for treatment for all of these forms of choroidal neovascularization have been improved with the injection of anti-VEGF drugs. Current treatment options for the wet form of macular degeneration involve multiple injections intraocularly of anti-VEGF drugs more than a 2-year period. This reduces the amount of damage from the choroidal neovascularization but does not stop the disease from progressing. Visual prognosis is poor for patients developing choroidal neovascularization.

Additional diseases leading to choroidal neovascularization include inflammatory infectious conditions such as histoplasmosis, toxoplasmosis, sarcoidosis, tuberculosis, syphilis, rubella, *Candida* endophthalmitis, toxocariasis,

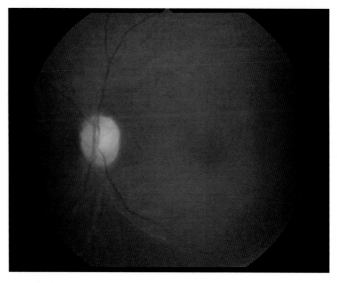

● **FIGURE 22-8.** Central retinal artery occlusion.

and pseudotumor cerebri. Tumors such as malignant melanoma, metastatic tumor, and choroidal hemangiomas can lead to choroidal neovascularizations. Trauma from choroidal rupture, laser photocoagulation, or surgical trauma can also lead to choroidal neovascularization.

RETINOPATHY OF PREMATURITY

Another vascular disease of the eye is seen in premature infants. ROP is a form of a proliferative retinopathy found in premature, low-birth-weight infants featuring abnormal proliferation of developing retinal blood vessels at the junction of vascularized and avascularized areas of the retina. First described in the 1940s was the association between retinopathy in prematurity and oxygen supplementation. ROP is a severe cause of visual loss in infants leading to severe visual impairment. ROP is a proliferative retinopathy that has a paradoxical relationship to oxygen levels. New vessel growth is induced initially by an ischemic avascular retina, but then as an infant of low birth weight receives supplemental oxygen therapy, there is a spurt of neovascularization that occurs, leading to extraretinal proliferation of blood vessels, macular dragging, tractional retinal detachment, retrolental fibroplasia, and glaucoma. The risk and severity of ROP are inversely proportional to birth weight, age, and oxygen use.[16]

The ocular manifestations of ROP include a classification system developed recently with stage I involving a thin, flat demarcation line between the vascular and avascular retina, stage II a ridge forming along the demarcation line that is elevated and thickened, stage III extraretinal fibrovascular proliferation along this ridge, and stage IV a fibrovascular mass formation and tractional retinal detachment.[17]

The differential diagnosis of ROP includes retinal blastoma, X-linked retinoschisis, Toxocara, toxocariasis, and Norrie's disease. Treatment for ROP involves cryotherapy, photocoagulation, and surgical repair of retinal detachments (Figure 22-9).

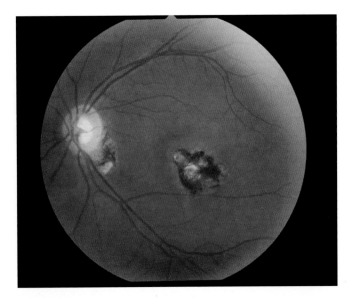

● **FIGURE 22-9.** Toxoplasmosis.

RETINAL ARTERIAL MACROANEURYSMS

These are unique aneurysms developing in the retinal blood vessels. They are usually localized saccular dilatations of the retinal arterial vessels within the first three branches of the central retinal artery, retinal hemorrhages, protein and lipid exudates, and macular edema. Retinal arterial macroaneurysms tend to occur in older patients, usually older than 60 years, and are commonly associated with hypertension. They may present as a hemorrhage in the vitreous or retina or as an exudative type picture.[18]

Retinal telangiectasias and a disease named Coats' disease are a unique group of diseases that are usually unilateral, more common in young men, and present with a white pupil. This is a congenital type anomaly that consists of abnormal telangiectatic segments of the arterial system of the eye. One would see lipid exudates and subretinal fluid. Coats' disease is a unique condition, and another subset of this is Leber's miliary aneurysm, which is a localized, less severe form of Coats' disease. This usually presents between the ages of 8 to 16 years. This is usually a diagnosis of exclusion after other vascular diseases are ruled out. The differential diagnosis would include retinoblastoma, ROP, retinal detachment, persistent hyperplasia of primary vitreous, cataract, toxocariasis, and Norrie's disease.

RADIATION RETINOPATHY AND VASCULAR DISORDERS

Radiation treatment to the eye for such diseases as ocular melanoma, retinoblastoma, or metastatic disease can lead to a progressive retinal vasculopathy. This would include retinal hemorrhaging, microaneurysms, exudates, cotton-wool spots, and optic nerve swelling. A general rule in patients who receive radiation doses of less than 2500 rads, or 25 Gy, in fractions of 200 rads or less at a time are likely to go on to develop significant retinopathy. Patients who are receiving radiation therapy and develop these retinal vascular disorders must also be ruled out for other diseases such as diabetic disease or vein occlusions.[19]

In summary, the eye affords us an opportunity to evaluate a patient's retinal vasculature and gives us great insight into its systemic system. A review of this chapter gives a brief description of a multitude of disease entities that affect a patient's systemic vascular system that can be easily evaluated and diagnosed by looking at the retinal vasculature.

ANTERIOR ISCHEMIC OPTIC NEUROPATHY

Anterior ischemic optic neuropathy is a presentation of a group of diseases with a rapid onset of painless unilateral vision loss. Frequently a visual field defect in an altitudinal picture is seen. The optic nerve can be swollen and then go on to develop pallor. In approximately 5% of the cases, an anterior ischemic optic neuropathy may be caused by temporal arteritis. Patients who have temporal arteritis usually have other symptoms associated with it including headache, jaw claudication, and temporal artery tenderness. Patients can also be seen with weight loss, fever, joint pain, and myalgia. Typically the patients, more commonly women, are older than 70 years. Measuring of the erythrocyte sedimentation rate is standard. Usually the sedimentation rate is more than 70 to 120 mm/h. Once an elevated sedimentation rate is discovered, prompt corticosteroid therapy and a confirmatory temporal artery biopsy are necessary. The unfortunate aspect to this disease is that one can have a normal sedimentation rate in an estimated 16% of biopsy-proven cases. One can also find elevated sedimentation rates with increasing age and other diseases such as malignancy or inflammatory disease and diabetes and not have temporal arteritis. Therefore, levels of plasma, fibrinogen, and C-reactive protein may aid in differentiation, as they tend to parallel the sedimentation rate only in vasculitis. Biopsies are frequently negative and therefore a minimum of 10 mm of artery must be analyzed, and sometimes, bilateral biopsies are recommended. Also, a negative biopsy does not necessarily rule out arteritis since there are frequently skipped lesions found and therefore an astute pathologist must be looking for these lesions through the complete submitted section.[20]

● TRAUMA AND THE EYE

Patients suffering trauma to the head with intracranial bleeding can develop frequently intraocular hemorrhaging. Vitreous hemorrhages can occur in approximately 3% to 5% of patients with intracranial bleeding. Subarachnoid bleeding from a cerebral aneurysm in particular is the most common underlying cause. Terson's syndrome is an intraocular hemorrhage associated with an acute intracranial bleed. It is bilateral with multiple posterior segment hemorrhages with retinal, intraretinal, and intravitreal locations. This is a term that was coined by Dr. Terson after seeing a patient with subarachnoid hemorrhage developing a vitreous hemorrhage (Figure 22-10).[2]

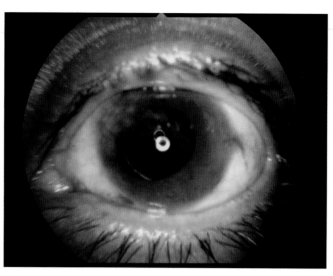

● **FIGURE 22-10.** Traumatic cataract/implant.

Purtscher's retinopathy is a retinal infarction with cotton-wool spot associated with severe trauma or other conditions. This is bilaterally seen and has associated retinal hemorrhaging and cotton-wool spots. It can be seen in head trauma, chest trauma, or long-bone injury. It can be seen as an amniotic fluid embolism or pancreatitis.[21]

● SHAKEN BABY SYNDROME

Unfortunately, we have seen a rise of child abuse in our society and throughout the world and therefore have been able to diagnose easily from an ocular examination cases of shaken baby syndrome. In this situation, one would see intraocular hemorrhages that can be bilateral or monocular with retinal or vitreous hemorrhage without any associated direct eye trauma. This occurs when a child has whiplash-like abuse. Frequently also associated is intracranial hemorrhaging, usually a subdural, cerebral edema, and other sites of trauma.[22]

REFERENCES

1. Harris A, Kagemann L. Assessment of human ocular hemodynamics. *Surv Ophthalmol.* 1998;42(6):509-533.

2. Flammer J, Pache M. Vasospasm in the role of pathogenesis to the eye. *Prog Retin Eye Res.* 2001;20(3):319-349.

3. Scheie HG. Evaluation of ophthalmic changes and hypertension. *Arch Ophthalmol.* 1953;49:117-138.

4. Hayreh SS. Prevalent misconceptions about acute retinal vascular occlusive disorders. *Prog Retin Eye Res.* 2005;24(4): 493-519.

5. Biousse V. Thrombolysis for central and artery occlusion. *J Neuroophthalmol.* 2007;27(3):215-230.

6. Beatty S. Acute occlusion of retinal arteries, current concepts and recent advances in diagnosis. *J Accid Emerg Med.* 2000;17(5):324-329.

7. Hayreh SS. Classification of central retinal vein occlusion. *Ophthalmology.* 1983;90:458-474.

8. Recchia FM. Systemic disorders associated with retinal vascular occlusion. *Curr Opin Ophthalmol.* 2000;11(6):462-467.

9. Sharma S. Systemic evaluation of acute retinal artery occlusion. *Curr Opin Ophthalmol.* 1998;9(3):1-5.

10. Celia C. Ocular ischemic syndrome. *Compr Ophthalmol.* 2000;8(1):17-28.

11. Kosmorsky GS. Sudden painless vision loss: optic nerve and circulatory disturbances. *Clin Geriatr Med.* 1999;15(1):1-13.

12. Yanko G. Prevalence of retinopathy in middle-aged and early diabetic men. *Br J Ophthalmol.* 1983;67:759-765.

13. Early Treatment of Diabetic Retinopathy Study Research Group. Fundus photographic risk factors for progression

of diabetic retinopathy. *Ophthalmology*. 1991;98:823-833.

14. Goldberg M. Sickle cell retinopathy. In: Duane TD, Tasman W, Jaeger EA, eds. *Duane's Clinical Ophthalmology*. Philadelphia: JP Lippincott; 1989:1-45.

15. Ciulla TA. Ocular perfusion and age-related macular degeneration. *Acta Ophthalmol Scand*. 2001;79(2):108-15.

16. Penn F. The influence of early PAO2 fluctuation on progression of retinopathy of prematurity. *Invest Ophthalmol*. 1995;1:36-67.

17. Pulido. Evaluation of eyes with advanced stages of retinopathy of prematurity using standardized echography. *Ophthalmology*. 1991;98:1099-1104.

18. Panton. Retinal arterial microaneurysms. *Br J Ophthalmol*. 1990;74:595-660.

19. Noble T. Central retinal artery occlusion: the presenting signs in radiation retinopathy. *Arch Ophthalmol*. 1994;112:1409-1410.

20. Hayreh SS. Anterior ischemic optic neuropathy. *Eye*. 1990;4:25-41.

21. Williams DF. Posterior segment manifestations of ocular trauma. *Retina*. 1990;10:S35-S44.

22. Levin AV. Ocular manifestations of child abuse. *Ophthalmology*. 1990;3:249-264.

23. Greven V. Retinal artery occlusions of the young. *Curr Opin Ophthalmol*. 1997;8(3):3-7.

24. Leishman R. The eye in general vascular disease: hypertension. *Br J Ophthalmol*. 1957;41:641-701.

25. Fineman H. Branch retinal artery occlusion as the initial sign of giant cell arteritis. *Am J Ophthalmol*. 1996;112:428-430.

chapter 23

Intracranial Arterial Disease

Ramachandra P. Tummala, MD / Babak S. Jahromi, MD, PhD / L. Nelson Hopkins, MD

● INTRODUCTION

All aspects of the management of intracranial arterial disease have undergone major transformations in the past two decades. Alternatives are now available for conditions previously treatable only with a single modality. Moreover, some conditions that would have been considered untreatable in the past now have safe and effective therapies. Although the credit for these advances is attributable to many factors, several fundamental achievements are recognized. First, the advances in noninvasive diagnostic neuroimaging, namely, computed tomographic (CT) and magnetic resonance (MR) imaging and their respective variants have resulted in the increased detection of asymptomatic vascular lesions and improved diagnostic sensitivity. As will be discussed later, this early detection presents a clinical dilemma in determining the appropriate management on the basis of the natural history of specific lesions. Second, the refinement of microneurosurgical techniques has resulted in improved surgical outcomes. This experience has also allowed us to recognize the limitations of cerebrovascular surgery. Third, the advances in neurological critical care have resulted in improved morbidity rates and shorter hospitalizations. Finally, the emergence of neuroendovascular therapy into a multidisciplinary field involving neurosurgeons, neurologists, and radiologists has changed practice patterns dramatically. The ongoing explosion in endovascular advances has allowed for catheter-based therapeutics in virtually every aspect of cerebrovascular disease.

In this chapter, the current concepts of the major categories of intracranial vascular disease are reviewed. Given the inherent limitations of covering such a broad subject in one chapter, some discussions are very cursory and superficial. The topics most likely to be encountered in clinical practice, namely, aneurysms, ischemic stroke, and arteriovenous malformations (AVMs), are treated more rigorously.

● STRUCTURE OF INTRACRANIAL ARTERIES

Histology

To gain insight into the numerous pathological conditions of the human intracranial arteries and to develop sound therapies for these disorders, a review of the gross and microscopic structure of normal arteries is necessary. The walls of the cerebral arteries are composed of three regions. From the lumen to the outer surface, these layers are the tunica intima, tunica media, and tunica adventitia. The intima is composed of an endothelial cell layer and the internal elastic lamina. The media is relatively thin and is composed of 4 to 20 smooth muscle layers that account for roughly half the thickness of the artery wall.[1] Collagen fibers and fibroblasts mostly comprise the adventitia. Innervation of the cerebral arteries is by myelinated and unmyelinated nerve fibers coursing in the adventitia or between the media and adventitia.[2]

There are notable differences between the structure of the intracranial and systemic arteries. The internal elastic lamina is extremely convoluted and well developed in the cerebral arteries.[3] The internal elastic lamina has long been thought to account for most of the mechanical strength of the artery.[4] Cerebral arteries have a smaller wall-to-lumen ratio than their systemic counterparts.[5] In contrast to peripheral arteries, intracranial arteries have few elastic fibers within the media. The external elastic lamina is absent, and the adventitia is poorly developed in the cerebral arteries. Unlike the well-developed fibrous layer seen in systemic arteries, the adventitia of intracranial arteries is sparse and composed of a loose network of connective tissue. Cerebral arteries generally do not have vasa vasorum. Instead, the cerebrospinal fluid (CSF) that surrounds these vessels in the subarachnoid space provides nutrients through the porous adventitia.[6] The adventitia also contains a distinct cell type that resembles the interstitial cells of Cajal; these cells may be responsible for rhythmic contraction of the arteries and may play a role in the regulation of cerebral blood flow (CBF).[2]

The conventional cerebral arterial structure described above becomes disorganized at bifurcation or branching points. Here, the internal elastic lamina is increasingly fenestrated, and the media is thin or absent. The smooth muscle cells are arranged in an organized, circumferential pattern around the lumen in straight segments of the arteries. However, the muscle cell orientation is random and multidirectional at branching points. In addition, asymmetric rings of connective tissue can be found encompassing the lumen at branching sites. Known as "intimal cushions," these structures are composed of connective tissue matrix and smooth muscle cells. These cushions are common in individuals older than 20 years of age, but their functional significance is unknown. It has been observed that the media layer is attenuated or absent under large intimal cushions.[7]

Angiographic Anatomy

Although cerebral angiography has been supplanted over the past two decades by noninvasive imaging for many diagnostic purposes, it has experienced a revival in recent years with the expansion of endovascular therapy. A thorough understanding of angiographic anatomy is mandatory before proceeding with any cerebrovascular intervention, either surgical or endovascular. In broad terms, the carotid artery and its intracranial branches are referred to as the anterior circulation, and the vertebrobasilar system is known as the posterior circulation.

Despite its invasiveness, cerebral angiography can be performed with low risk. More than 5500 diagnostic angiograms have been performed at the authors' institution during the past 8 years with a complication rate of 0.3% (Hopkins LN, personal communication, July 2007). Cerebral angiography is performed typically through a transfemoral route, although the radial or brachial arteries may be used to gain vascular access in cases of aortoiliac occlusive disease. For a thorough discussion on cerebral angiographic anatomy, refer the comprehensive works by Krayenbuhl and Yasargil,[8] Morris,[9] and Osborn.[10,11] A normal angiogram is shown in Figure 23-1 to serve as a guide for abnormal studies included later in this chapter.

● COLLATERAL CIRCULATION

In this section, we review briefly the main routes for collateral circulation that are important in the setting of intracranial or extracranial artery occlusion or that of therapeutic intervention. The collateral network of the brain includes anastomoses between the cerebral arteries themselves and between the cerebral arteries and the extracranial vessels. For a comprehensive discussion, refer the texts by Wojak[12] and by Marinkovic et al.[13] The anastomoses can be grouped into the following six categories based on location: Cervical, extracranial (in the head but outside the

cranium), extracranial–intracranial (EC–IC), intracranial–extracerebral, extracerebral–cerebral, and cerebral.

EC–IC Collaterals

EC–IC collaterals interconnect branches of the external carotid artery (ECA) and the internal carotid artery (ICA) or branches of the ECA and the vertebral artery (VA). These anastomoses are located primarily in the nasal cavity, orbit, and tympanic cavity. The therapeutic implications are realized when embolization through what seems to be a benign ECA branch leads to a profound neurological deficit. Furthermore, small branches from the ECA territory supply cervical nerve roots and cranial nerves.

Branches of the ophthalmic artery (off the ICA) form anastomoses with branches of the ECA, usually in the setting of ICA occlusion (Figure 23-2). Examples include connections between the angular branch of the facial artery and the dorsal nasal branch of the ophthalmic artery, between the frontal division of the superficial temporal artery (STA) (off the ECA) and the supratrochlear branch of the ophthalmic artery, and between the anterior deep temporal artery (off the internal maxillary artery) and the lacrimal branch of the ophthalmic artery.[13] The nasal and tympanic branches off the ECA also form anastomotic networks that may be important in chronic ICA occlusion. Persistent embryonic vessels, such as the persistent stapedial or hypoglossal arteries, also belong in the EC–IC category.

The ascending pharyngeal artery is a particularly dangerous vessel. The meningeal branch of the ascending pharyngeal artery forms anastomoses with the cavernous and petrous branches of the ICA. Other branches off this artery supply the trigeminal ganglion and lower cranial nerves. These branches have major implications during embolization of skull base tumors, especially those involving the jugular foramen. Rarely, the posterior inferior cerebellar artery may originate directly from the ascending pharyngeal artery rather than the VA.[12]

The occipital artery forms collaterals with the muscular branches of the VA and may reconstitute the distal VA in the setting of proximal occlusion. This artery may give rise to a stylomastoid branch that supplies the facial nerve as it exits the skull. We have had one case of a complete facial palsy developing after embolization of the occipital artery for a dural arteriovenous fistula (DAVF).

The internal maxillary artery forms several potentially dangerous anastomoses with branches of the ophthalmic artery and dural branches of the ICA. The middle meningeal artery, which arises proximally off the internal maxillary artery, is involved in many of these anastomoses. Additionally, the middle meningeal artery supplies the trigeminal ganglion and the first division of the trigeminal nerve.[12]

Cerebral Anastomoses

This group includes connections directly between the cerebral arteries. The circle of Willis is the best-known anastomotic structure in the brain. It provides connections

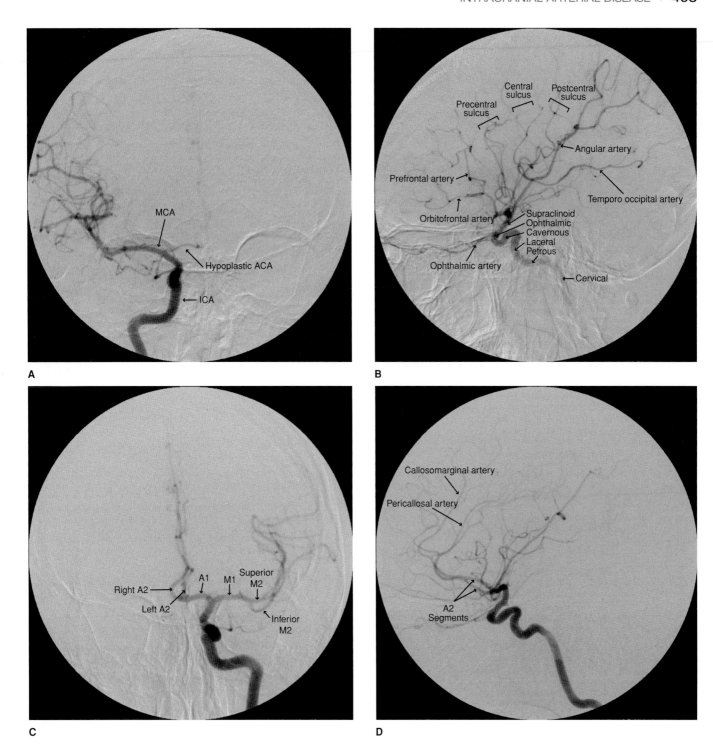

● **FIGURE 23-1.** Normal angiographic anatomy. Right ICA injection—(A) Anteroposterior and (B) lateral intracranial views. In this patient, the right ACA is hypoplastic (a hypoplastic A1 is a common anatomic variant); consequently, the MCA branches can be easily visualized on the lateral projection. MCA branches: orbitofrontal, prefrontal, precentral sulcus, central sulcus, postcentral sulcus, angular, temporo-occipital. ICA segments: supraclinoid, ophthalmic, cavernous, laceral, petrous, and cervical. Left ICA injection—(C) Anteroposterior and (D) lateral intracranial views. Reciprocally, the left A1 is dominant with filling across the anterior communicating artery to supply bilateral A2 segments. ACA segments: right A2, left A2, and A1. MCA segments: M1, superior M2, and inferior M2. (*continued*)

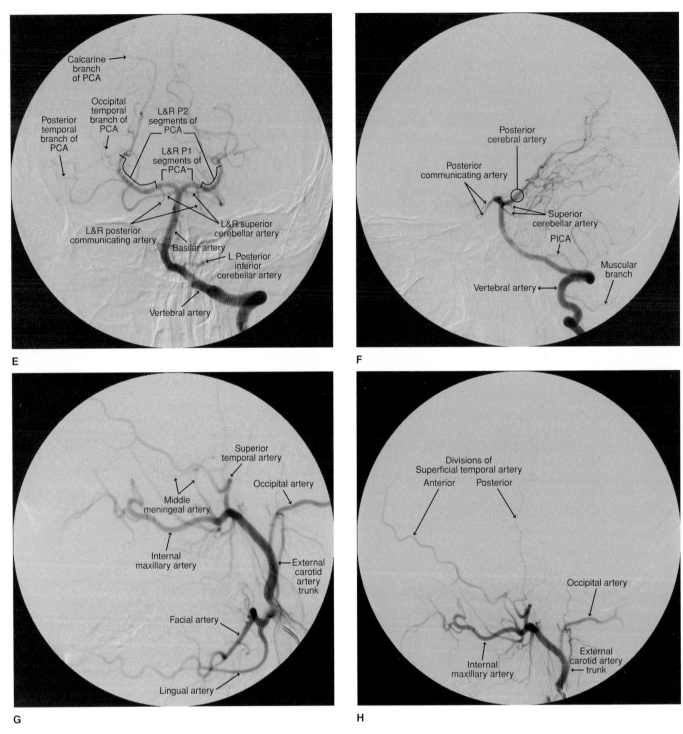

E

F

G

H

● **FIGURE 23-1.** (*Continued*) Left VA injection—(E) Anteroposterior and (F) lateral intracranial views. Right ECA injection lateral views—(G) Proximal and (H) distal views.

between the right and left ICA systems through the anterior communicating artery. In addition, the posterior communicating arteries (PCoA) connect the ICA system (anterior circulation) to the vertebrobasilar system (posterior circulation). It has the shape of an irregular polygon and is located mainly at the base of the frontal lobes. There are numerous anatomic variations of the circle of Willis, including agenesis or hypoplasia of certain components (see pp. 135-136 in Ref. 9). Under normal conditions, a hemodynamic balance

exists between the anterior and posterior circulation and between the right and left carotid circulation. A change in the balance, as seen with occlusive cerebrovascular disease, causes redistribution of blood through the circle of Willis. The complexity of these hemodynamic imbalances is responsible for the high frequency of aneurysm formation along branches of the circle of Willis.

There are numerous leptomeningeal anastomoses that form on the surface of the brain and that are important

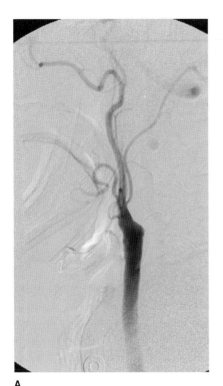
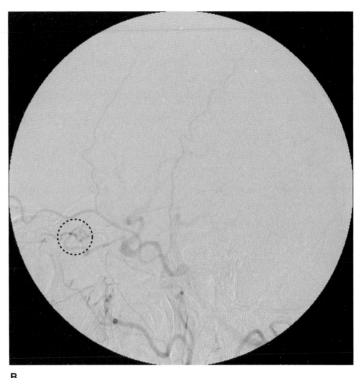

A   **B**

● FIGURE 23-2. External–internal carotid artery collaterals. This patient presented with a right hemispheric transient ischemic attack. A right common carotid artery injection demonstrated ICA occlusion at its origin. (A) Only the ECA branches are filling. (B) An intracranial view shows collaterals between the internal maxillary artery and ophthalmic artery (*dotted circle*) with resultant filling of the intracranial ICA proximally and distally.

in the setting of large artery occlusions. They occur in every major arterial territory. For example, a middle cerebral artery (MCA) occlusion may activate anastomoses between leptomeningeal branches of the MCA and the leptomeningeal branches of the anterior cerebral artery (ACA) or posterior cerebral artery (PCA). Another example is the anastomosis between the splenial artery (off the PCA) and the pericallosal artery (off the ACA) after occlusion of the ACA or PCA. These collaterals are seen on the lateral surface of the cerebral hemisphere. Connections between the anterior and posterior choroidal arteries occur in the choroid plexus of the lateral ventricle.

● INTRACRANIAL ANEURYSMS

Background

The main reason for concern about cerebral aneurysms is the consequences of their rupture and resultant subarachnoid hemorrhage (SAH). The most common cause of SAH is trauma; however, this discussion will focus on aneurysmal SAH. Cerebral aneurysms can be broadly classified by size, location, shape, and etiology. The causes of their formation and rupture are not well known. Unless noted otherwise, most of this discussion will focus on saccular lesions, which are the most common aneurysms by far. Once thought to be congenital, it is widely accepted that these lesions develop later in life.

Histological examination of saccular intracranial aneurysms reveals an absent or discontinuous internal elastic lamina, absence of the media at the aneurysm neck, deficient endothelium in the aneurysm lumen, and atherosclerotic changes in the parent vessel at the origin of the aneurysm. The walls of most small aneurysms are composed of discontinuous endothelium surrounded by fibrous adventitial tissue and no smooth muscle. Large (diameter between 1.0 and 2.5 cm) and giant aneurysms (≥2.5 cm diameter) may have more organized walls consisting of fibrous tissue, foam cells, and deposits of calcium.[14,15] It is believed that aneurysms form over a relatively short period of time, and either they rupture or they stabilize and remain unruptured.[16]

Pathogenesis

The reasons for aneurysm development and rupture are not known completely. It has been postulated that aneurysm formation may be related to the intimal cushions and defects of the media at the branching points described above,[17] but this has not been proven. Destruction of the internal elastic lamina seems to be the crucial event for aneurysm formation and is likely an early event that weakens the arterial wall.[4] Collagen also appears to play a role in aneurysm pathology. Part of the stabilization of the aneurysm is exuberant collagen formation, which leads to thickening of its wall. In fact, unruptured aneurysms have almost twice the collagen content of normal arteries. It is not known if this increased-collagen formation is a compensatory mechanism for the internal elastic lamina loss. In contrast, ruptured aneurysms have decreased and poorly organized collagen content.[18] Unlike normal arteries and unruptured aneurysms, ruptured lesions have a disrupted endothelial lining. Therefore, it has been proposed that endothelial injury may contribute to aneurysm formation and rupture.[19,20]

The ultimate source of the destruction of the internal elastic lamina and endothelium remains unknown, but an underlying inflammatory cause was proposed as early as the mid-19th century by Virchow.[19] T cells (natural killer cells) and macrophages have been found in both ruptured and unruptured aneurysms.[19] Additionally, lysosomal granule deposition and increased metalloproteinase activity has been observed within aneurysm walls.[21] These and other findings suggest at least a link between inflammation and aneurysm formation and, ultimately, rupture.[19] Because inflammatory changes are obligatory features of atherosclerosis,[22] aneurysm development may be part of an atherosclerotic spectrum in the parent vessel.

Debate continues regarding whether intracranial aneurysm pathogenesis has a genetic, acquired, or combined etiology. Support for a genetic mechanism comes from the association of aneurysms and several inheritable connective tissue disorders. These include autosomal dominant polycystic kidney disease, type IV Ehlers-Danlos syndrome (EDS) (see below), Marfan's syndrome, α_1-antitrypsin deficiency, neurofibromatosis type 1, and tuberous sclerosis—to list only a few.[23,24] The true incidence of aneurysms caused by these disorders is unknown because of their variable phenotypes. However, it seems these diseases are responsible only for a small percentage of aneurysms.

Familial intracranial aneurysms have been described for several decades. However, the pattern of inheritance is unknown. Some studies have shown up to a fivefold increase in aneurysm or SAH incidence in first-degree relatives of patients harboring intracranial aneurysms.[25,26] Regardless, the evidence has been sparse, and screening for asymptomatic intracranial aneurysms is not well defined. The yield of screening first-degree relatives and their lifetime risk of SAH are low when only one family member harbors an aneurysm.[27,28] The authors' strategy has been to evaluate first-degree relatives with CT angiography or MR angiography in families with two or more affected members. This is based on evidence that the yield from such screening is roughly 10%.[29,30] If the initial screening fails to reveal an aneurysm, we repeat a noninvasive study every 5 years in order to detect any de novo lesions.

Acquired risk factors are not well defined for SAH. Cigarette smoking is the one consistent factor identified in all studies to date. The estimated risk of SAH is up to 10 times higher in smokers than in nonsmokers. Smoking accelerates intracranial aneurysm growth, and continued smoking may increase the risk of de novo aneurysm development after an initial SAH.[31–34] Many reports have demonstrated the role of hypertension in increasing aneurysm development and rupture.[34,35] However, this risk does not seem to be as high as with smoking. While low-level alcohol consumption may lower SAH risk, high-level consumption and binge drinking seem to increase the risk.[33]

Epidemiology

Annual incidence rates of SAH are estimated between 9 and 15 cases per 100 000 persons.[36,37] This translates into roughly 30 000 cases of SAH in North America annually. However, there are considerable global variations in these figures. For example, a Finnish study reported an incidence as high as 30 per 100 000 person-years.[38] In contrast, a French study reported an incidence of 2.2 per 100 000.[39] In most studies, women have a 1.5 times greater incidence of SAH than men, with hormonal factors implicated for the gender inequity.[40] Unlike other types of stroke, SAH is unique with its female predilection. Studies from the United States have shown a more than two times greater risk for SAH in blacks than in whites.[41,42] The peak incidence of SAH is between 55 and 60 years of age. Indeed, our experience parallels the above figures in that the typical patient with SAH is a middle-aged female smoker.

The true prevalence of intracranial aneurysms remains unknown and is difficult to determine. It has been estimated at 5% on the basis of autopsy studies.[43] On the other hand, incidental aneurysms were detected in only 1% of cases during a random review of cerebral angiograms.[44] Not surprisingly, these studies are criticized for selection bias (e.g., what was defined as an aneurysm) and patient population. A prevalence of approximately 2% is generally assumed, as suggested by a contemporary meta-analysis.[45]

The outcome from aneurysmal SAH is dismal.[46] Approximately one-third of patients with a first SAH will die in the acute phase. One-third will remain with significant neurological disability. Only the remaining third will recover well from the hemorrhage and its sequelae.[37] Although there are some variations in these statistics from other studies, the above figures serve as easy reminders that the overall prognosis for SAH remains poor despite advances in initial resuscitation, aneurysm treatment, critical care, and treatment of cerebral vasospasm. Predictors of a good recovery from SAH include young age and good neurological function at presentation.[40]

Natural History

Given the gravity of SAH, knowledge of the natural history of cerebral aneurysms is important to understand the effects of treatment. In this section, the discussion has been limited to the known natural history of unruptured aneurysms. Knowing the natural history is particularly germane now that more aneurysms are being discovered with noninvasive imaging. The natural history of the aneurysm and the life expectancy of the patient must be matched against the risks of treatment.

Unfortunately, the natural history of intracranial aneurysms is not well established. Historically, the risk of rupture of an aneurysm was believed to be 1% to 2% per year. Of course, this risk can vary, depending on the patient and the aneurysm. Any contemporary discussion on the natural history must include the International Study of Unruptured Intracranial Aneurysms (ISUIA).[47,48] For this discussion, we focus on the ISUIA because of its influence on current practice patterns. The ISUIA was the largest systematic study undertaken to evaluate the natural history of unruptured aneurysms and to evaluate treatment risk. The study contained two parts. The first part, published in 1998, had both retrospective and prospective components.[47] In the retrospective cohort, 1937 aneurysms in 1449 patients from 53 centers were evaluated. These patients were subdivided into two groups:—those with previous SAH from another aneurysm and those without previous SAH. In the prospective arm, the surgical outcomes of unruptured aneurysms in 1172 patients were analyzed. For patients without previous SAH and with aneurysms <10 mm in size, the risk of rupture was 0.05% per year. Aneurysms <10 mm in patients with previous SAH had a rupture risk of 0.5% per year. Aneurysms >10 mm had a rupture risk of 1% per year in both groups. These rupture risks were much less than previously thought. The surgical morbidity of 15.7% was also much higher than reported in previous studies.[47] One major criticism of this study was that there was significant selection bias toward "low-risk" aneurysms because the "high-risk" lesions were selected out for treatment. In other words, the study did not represent *all* unruptured aneurysms, and therefore the unusually low rupture rates could not be applied to all lesions.[49,50]

The second part of the study[48] was published in 2003 and is ongoing. This part included 4060 patients, of whom 1692 patients harboring 2686 aneurysms were observed and 2368 atients were treated with surgery or coiling. Of the treated group, 1917 patients underwent surgery and 451 were treated with coiling. The risks associated with surgical and endovascular treatments were still higher than in previous reports at 12.6% and 9.8% at 1 year, respectively. Predictors of poor outcome from treatment included increased patient age, lesion diameter >12 mm, and aneurysm location in the posterior fossa. The rupture risk was 2.5% over 5 years for lesions involving the posterior circulation in patients with no previous SAH and 0% over 5 years for anterior circulation lesions. On the other hand, patients with previous SAH had 5-year rupture risks of 1.5% in the anterior circulation and 3.4% in the posterior circulation. The authors of the ISUIA proposed that there was no benefit in treating aneurysms <7 mm in size in patients with no previous SAH because of the low risk of rupture (0.1% per year) and the relatively high risk of treatment.[48] Once again, this part of the study has been criticized for selection bias because 534 of the 1692 patients selected for observation ultimately crossed over to treatment owing to concerns of rupture risk.[50]

One natural history study cited frequently to challenge the ISUIA is from Finland.[51] Most of the 142 patients in this study had previously suffered SAH and were followed without treatment for a mean of 19.7 years.[51] The annual incidence of rupture was approximately 1.3% in this cohort. Despite the criticisms of ISUIA and the debate over the exact aneurysm rupture risks, it seems the rupture risk is much less than previously thought. Furthermore, the clinical impact of the ISUIA cannot be disputed. Consequently, we have noted that a larger number of incidental aneurysms are being managed conservatively.

Clinical Characteristics and Diagnosis

It is widely recognized that a severe headache of sudden onset is a hallmark of aneurysmal SAH. The phrase "worst headache of my life" has become almost synonymous with aneurysm rupture. The headache is usually global and radiates to the neck and is often accompanied by nausea and vomiting. The patient typically has nuchal rigidity and photophobia. Transient loss of consciousness may be seen in one-third of patients. Seizures may be associated with SAH in 5% to 8% of patients. Focal neurological deficits may be seen from mass effect from large and giant aneurysms (see below). Cranial neuropathies may occur from compression by these aneurysms. For example, 30% of patients with ophthalmic artery aneurysms can have visual field deficits or monocular blindness.[52] Third cranial nerve palsies can occur with PCoA or basilar apex aneurysms. Posterior fossa aneurysms may cause tinnitus, trigeminal neuralgia, hemifacial spasm, facial weakness, or dysphagia from cranial nerve compression.

CT scanning usually confirms the diagnosis of SAH. Although the sensitivity of modern CT imaging exceeds 95% on the day of the ictus[53] and it decreases to 50% after 1 week and 30% by 2 weeks. CT is also important in the diagnosis of hydrocephalus, which occurs in 20% of patients with SAH or an associated intracerebral hemorrhage (ICH). The hydrocephalus may account for an initially poor grade on the neurological examination. If the clinical suspicion is high but CT fails to demonstrate SAH, a lumbar puncture is mandatory for diagnosis. Xanthochromia is the hallmark of SAH on lumbar puncture and occurs from lysis of erythrocytes in the CSF. Lumbar puncture is considered the gold standard for the diagnosis of SAH. However, at least 6 hours and preferably 12 hours should elapse after symptom onset to ensure the presence of xanthochromia and to reduce the chance of a false-negative result. Traumatic lumbar punctures can usually be differentiated from SAH. Bloody CSF that does not clear between the first and fourth tubes is highly suspicious of SAH. Furthermore, xanthochromia is absent in traumatic lumbar punctures, provided the sample is analyzed immediately.

In addition to neurological concerns, systemic manifestations of SAH are important. Cardiac abnormalities include arrhythmias, cardiac "stunning" with transient ventricular dysfunction, or myocardial infarction. Pulmonary disorders include aspiration pneumonia from decreased level of consciousness, neurogenic pulmonary edema, and bronchospasm.[54] Electrolyte disturbances are also seen, the most common being hyponatremia from cerebral salt wasting. The hypovolemia resulting from salt wasting may exacerbate cerebral vasospasm.

Once SAH is diagnosed, the aneurysm must be identified. This is classically done with cerebral angiography, which identifies the lesion in 85% of all SAH cases. If the first angiogram is unremarkable and the presence of an aneurysm is suspected, angiography is repeated in 1 week. CT angiography has been increasingly used to diagnose or exclude aneurysms, and its sensitivity has increased with improved multidetector, multislice technology that improves spatial and temporal resolution. The sensitivity of CT angiography is proportional to the size of the aneurysm. CT angiography sensitivities of 100% for aneurysms >4 mm, 94% for aneurysms 2 to 4 mm, and 50% for aneurysms <2 mm have been reported recently.[55] The accuracy of detecting aneurysms by CT angiography has been also been reported recently, with sensitivity of 98% and specificity of 100% in the setting of SAH.[56]

Aneurysm Location and Type

The most common locations for aneurysms in the anterior circulation are the anterior communicating artery, the ICA, and the MCA. Collectively, the ICA aneurysms, which include those at the ophthalmic artery, superior hypophyseal artery, PCoA, anterior choroidal artery, and at the ICA terminus, account for 40% of all aneurysms. Aneurysms of the PCoA alone account for half of the ICA aneurysms. Aneurysms of the MCA comprise 20% to 25% of all intracranial aneurysms.

In the posterior circulation, the basilar artery (BA) bifurcation is the most common location, accounting for 8% of all intracranial aneurysms. The posterior inferior cerebellar artery is the second most-frequent location, with 3% arising from this location. Less common are basilar trunk aneurysms and peripheral aneurysms off the major branches of the BA.

For completion, the authors mention intracavernous carotid artery aneurysms, i.e., aneurysms that arise from the ICA segment that lies within the cavernous sinus. These aneurysms are, by definition, extradural. Therefore, SAH from these lesions is rare unless part of the aneurysm protrudes into the subarachnoid space. Rupture of these aneurysms can cause a fistula between the ICA and the cavernous sinus. Life-threatening epistaxis may occur if the aneurysm ruptures directly into the adjacent sphenoid sinus. More commonly, unruptured aneurysms in this location become symptomatic by causing retroorbital pain, diplopia, or facial numbness. Diplopia and altered facial sensation result from cranial nerve (third, fourth, fifth, and sixth nerves) compression within the cavernous sinus.[57]

As mentioned, giant aneurysms are ≥2.5 cm in diameter **(Figure 23-3)**. These are fortunately rare lesions, and only 3% of intracranial aneurysms are in this category. The risk of rupture of these aneurysms is high, and one-third of patients harboring these lesions present with SAH. The remaining patients present with symptoms and signs from mass effect such as headache, seizures, altered mental status, or focal neurological deficits. Frequently, there is edema around these lesions, and their effects are similar to those of tumors. Many of these lesions contain thrombus as a result of turbulent blood flow, and the aneurysms may manifest with thromboembolism. Cerebral angiography may reveal only partial filling of the aneurysm because of thrombus, and MR imaging or CT scanning is necessary to delineate the true size of the lesion.

Pediatric aneurysms are rare and account for no more than 2% of all intracranial aneurysms.[58,59] Underlying disorders are present in more than one-half of these cases.[59] Infective causes such as endocarditis and sepsis were responsible for 25% of pediatric aneurysms in one series.[60] Although giant and fusiform aneurysms are rare in adults, a higher percentage of these complex lesions are found among infants and children.[58,61]

Infectious aneurysms, historically known as mycotic aneurysms, are uncommon and account for approximately 2% to 4% of all intracranial aneurysms.[62] They are usually found in association with infective endocarditis and subsequent septic embolization. Bacterial aneurysms tend to form distally in the cerebral circulation, most commonly in the distal MCA. They can form rapidly (within days) and develop from inflammatory necrosis of the vessel wall, starting in the adventitia and extending into the media. The weakened arterial wall then leads to aneurysm formation.[63] Consequently, these lesions do not have a well-defined neck. The incidence of clinically significant aneurysms within the setting of endocarditis can be as high as 5.4%.[64] These lesions can also develop from local spreading of an infection such as sinusitis, skull base osteomyelitis, or meningitis. In the setting of endocarditis, the infective organism is usually identified on blood culture. The most commonly identified bacteria are *Staphylococci* and *Streptococci*. Endocarditis must be included in the differential diagnosis of a febrile patient with neurological symptoms and signs. Infectious aneurysms are very friable and carry a high rupture rate. Either SAH or ICH occurs in 50% of patients.[62] The high morbidity and mortality from infectious aneurysms are caused by their high rupture rate and the severity of the underlying systemic illness. Fortunately, serial angiograms demonstrate that up to 50% of these aneurysms resolve or decrease in size with antibiotic therapy.[65] However, selected lesions require treatment, usually in the form of surgical or endovascular parent vessel sacrifice. Because these aneurysms are friable, direct clipping or coiling is not usually feasible. If parent vessel sacrifice is not possible, excision of the lesion and bypass may be necessary.

Traumatic aneurysms are even less common than infectious ones. They represent less than 1% of all aneurysms.[66,67] Most are associated with blunt head trauma and skull fractures, although 3.5% of patients with penetrating trauma have these lesions, particularly with low-velocity projectile injuries.[68] Traumatic aneurysms may also be iatrogenic lesions resulting from craniotomies or skull

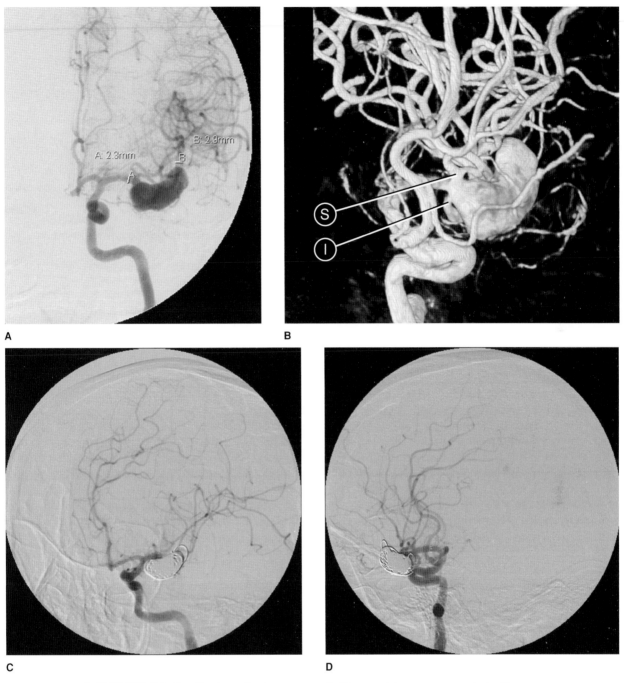

● **FIGURE 23-3.** Giant cerebral aneurysm. A 49-year-old woman presented with chronic headaches and was found to have (A) a giant left MCA aneurysm with a relatively wide neck. A three-dimensional view of the left ICA injection (AP projection) shows that the superior (S) and inferior (I) M2 divisions can be separated from the (B) aneurysm neck. Unlike the case with most MCA aneurysms, endovascular treatment of this lesion was undertaken. A Neuroform (Boston Scientific Target, Fremont, CA) stent was placed in the superior M2 division, followed by packing of the aneurysm with coils. (C and D) The final views showed minimal aneurysm neck residual with preservation of the M2 divisions.

base procedures. Their location may be divided into the peripheral cortical arteries or the large skull base arteries. The peripheral traumatic aneurysms typically involve the MCA distribution, while the basal traumatic lesions affect the cavernous, petrous, or supraclinoid ICA.[66] The distal ACA is also a fairly common location be-

cause of brain contusion against the falx cerebri. Damage to the internal elastic lamina may predispose to traumatic aneurysm formation. While the walls of saccular aneurysms are composed of intima and adventitia, those of traumatic aneurysms can be one of three types: true, false, or mixed.[69] True traumatic aneurysms result from partial arterial wall disruption caused by blunt injury. The trauma damages the intima and media while leaving the adventitia intact. In contrast, false aneurysms result from disruption of the full thickness of the artery wall, usually in the form of an arterial laceration. The false aneurysm does not contain any of the normal arterial elements; rather it is simply an organized thrombus formed after remodeling of the resultant hematoma from the laceration.[69] False aneurysms seem to be unstable lesions. Indeed, 50% of these aneurysms rupture within 2 weeks of the trauma. Mortality approaches 50% after rupture of these aneurysms.[70] The most common presentation of a traumatic aneurysm is a delayed deterioration following head trauma. Delayed, acute ICH should raise the suspicion of a traumatic aneurysm. Like infectious aneurysms, these lesions tend to arise from the distal cerebral arteries. Direct treatment with clipping or coiling is difficult, and parent vessel sacrifice is usually necessary. Endovascular placement of stents to span the injured region of the artery has emerged as an attractive option to reconstruct the vessel and avoid sacrifice of the parent artery.[71,72]

Treatment of Saccular Aneurysms

As mentioned above, the natural history for small intracranial aneurysms appears to be more benign than previously thought. The consequence is that many unruptured aneurysms are not treated and are followed radiographically. In this section, current therapeutic options for intracranial aneurysms are discussed. These are broad generalizations, and the nuances of surgical and endovascular treatment depend on the location, size, and morphology of the individual aneurysm and its relationship to other neurovascular structures. The goal of aneurysm therapy is to prevent rupture, or in the case of ruptured aneurysms, to prevent rehemorrhage. The traditional method has been open surgery and clipping of the aneurysm. The outcomes from aneurysm surgery have been optimized over the past four decades with the introduction of the operative microscope, development of microneurosurgical techniques, improvements in anesthesiology and intraoperative cerebral protection, and advanced neurocritical care. Over the past 15 years, endovascular therapy has emerged as a safe and effective method of treating certain aneurysms. The application of endovascular techniques has expanded significantly with the introduction of balloon- and stent-assisted coiling.

Surgical clipping provides essentially a permanent cure if complete obliteration is achieved. Even incompletely clipped aneurysms seem to have very low rupture rates. Long-term angiographic follow-up showed asymptomatic recurrence in only 2 of 135 lesions in one series of completely clipped aneurysms.[73] Additional benefits of surgery are the ability to reconstruct the parent vessel with clips, evacuation of any associated intracerebral hematoma from a ruptured aneurysm, and immediate collapsing of an aneurysm after clipping. The disadvantages of surgery include the potential need for brain retraction, prolonged general anesthesia during the procedure, potential injury to cranial nerves and arterial branches during dissection of the lesion, intraoperative aneurysm rupture, and prolonged convalescence after surgery. The 30-day morbidity and mortality rates associated with surgery for unruptured aneurysms range from 1% to 7% and from 4% to 15%, respectively.[74,75]

Coil embolization does not require craniotomy or brain retraction; aneurysm microdissection is also not necessary. Coiling involves microcatheterization of the aneurysm and packing the lesion with coils (Figure 23-4). The procedure is relatively safe with a mortality rate of less than 1% and a permanent morbidity rate of less than 10%.[76] However, incomplete aneurysm occlusion is more common with coiling than with surgery. Unlike clipping, endovascular treatment frequently results in aneurysm recanalization, especially in wide-necked and large aneurysms. These recanalization rates approach 30%,[77,78] although the impact of recanalization on hemorrhage rates is not clear (Figure 23-5). Even complete occlusion of the aneurysm may still result in recanalization from coil compaction. Therefore, one inherent disadvantage of coiling is the need for periodic follow-up evaluation and potential retreatment. Certain aneurysm morphologies, namely, wide-necked and large-sized lesions, present endovascular challenges as a result of the greater chance of coil herniation into the parent vessel. Some of these concerns have been addressed with balloon- and stent-assisted coiling and with three-dimensional coils that conform to the shape of the aneurysm. However, increased endovascular manipulation raises the chances of thromboembolic complications. The potential need for anticoagulants and antiplatelet agents during and after the endovascular procedures may confound adjunctive procedures, such as ventriculostomy, and other bedside procedures necessary in the setting of SAH.

Historically, poor-grade patients with ruptured aneurysms or inoperable lesions were selected for endovascular therapy. Posterior circulation aneurysms, particularly basilar tip aneurysms, are associated with higher surgical morbidity. The surgical mortality–morbidity rate approaches 15% to 20% for basilar tip aneurysms.[79] In contrast, MCA aneurysms are better suited for surgical clipping because of their relatively wide necks and close association of important branches that are at high risk for occlusion during endovascular therapy. As the experience with endovascular therapy has grown over the past decade, a selection bias has developed at many centers. Most patients in poor medical or neurological condition and many patients with posterior circulation aneurysms are treated with coiling, whereas patients with MCA aneurysms are referred for surgery. A fair appraisal of endovascular therapy must discriminate experience from the early 1990s to contemporary experience in this decade. This is a reflection of the rapid advancements in endovascular technology. For example, a comparison of these two eras showed procedure-related morbidity rates of 9.1% from 1990 to 1995 and 4.8% from 1996 to 2002.[80]

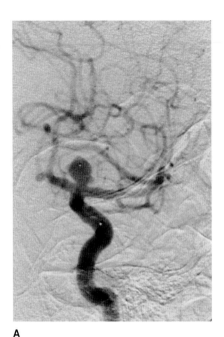
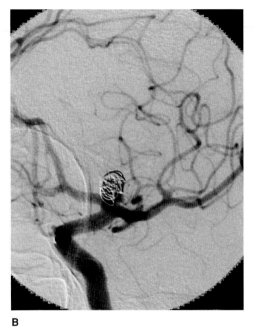
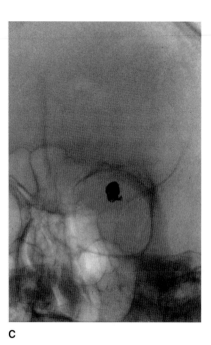

A   B   C

● **FIGURE 23-4.** Cerebral aneurysm. This 66-year-old man was found to have an incidental left ICA terminus aneurysm during a workup for minor head trauma. (A) An oblique view of the left ICA injection shows that the aneurysm has a slightly wide neck. The microcatheter is in a stable position within the aneurysm fundus. (B) Three-dimensional coils were used, and the coiling procedure was performed uneventfully. (C) A final anteroposterior fluoroscopic view shows good packing of the lesion without herniation of coils into the ACA or MCA.

To compare surgery against endovascular therapy, each treatment approach for ruptured and unruptured aneurysms has been considered here. The ISUIA and its impact on neurovascular practice have been discussed previously. The other major study that has shaped current aneurysm therapy is the International Subarachnoid Aneurysm Trial (ISAT).[81] ISAT was the first large-scale, randomized study comparing surgery and coiling for ruptured aneurysms. The study was designed to randomize patients with ruptured aneurysms thought to be suitable for either treatment. The trial was conducted mostly at European centers and demonstrated an absolute risk reduction of morbidity and mortality at 1 year of 6.9% in favor of endovascular therapy. The study was criticized for heavy selection bias because only 24% of patients enrolled were actually randomized.[82] The majority of randomized patients were in good clinical condition, and MCA and posterior circulation aneurysms were rare. The randomization obviously reflected inherent practice patterns described previously. Nonetheless, ISAT has provided level I evidence in support of endovascular therapy for certain ruptured aneurysms. It reiterates the notion that durability of treatment is not the immediate concern in SAH and that coiling offers improved short-term outcomes.

In contrast, the goal of treating an unruptured aneurysm is durable prevention of SAH. No prospective, randomized data is available for the treatment of unruptured aneurysms. In one review of 2500 patients, a morbidity rate of 18.5% was reported for surgical cases versus 10.6% for endovascular therapy.[83] Mortality rates in the same study were 2.3% versus 0.4% in favor of coiling. In the second part of ISUIA, 1-year surgical and endovascular morbidity rates of 12.6% and 9.8%, respectively, were reported.[48] However, this trial was not randomized, and many aneurysms were selected out for observation (see above).

● **CEREBRAL VASOSPASM**

Epidemiology

Cerebral vasospasm classically refers to a transient, self-limited constriction of cerebral arteries several days after exposure to subarachnoid blood, most frequently caused by rupture of a cerebral aneurysm. Cerebral vasospasm can refer to angiographic narrowing of cerebral blood vessels after SAH, neurological deficits caused by secondary ischemia from the resulting diminished blood flow, or both. Angiographic vasospasm is seen within 3 to 4 days of SAH, peaking in incidence and severity by day 6 to 8, and generally resolving by day 12.[84,85] Approximately 67% of patients demonstrate some degree of angiographic vasospasm in the second week after SAH,[86] with moderate-to-severe (vessel lumen narrowed by >25% of its original diameter) angiographic vasospasm seen in 30% of patients.[87,88] Those with more severe hemorrhage suffer from an increased incidence of severe vasospasm, with >50% narrowing seen in 55.9% of grade III to V patients.[89] Although vasospasm >50% is generally required before flow restriction results in clinical

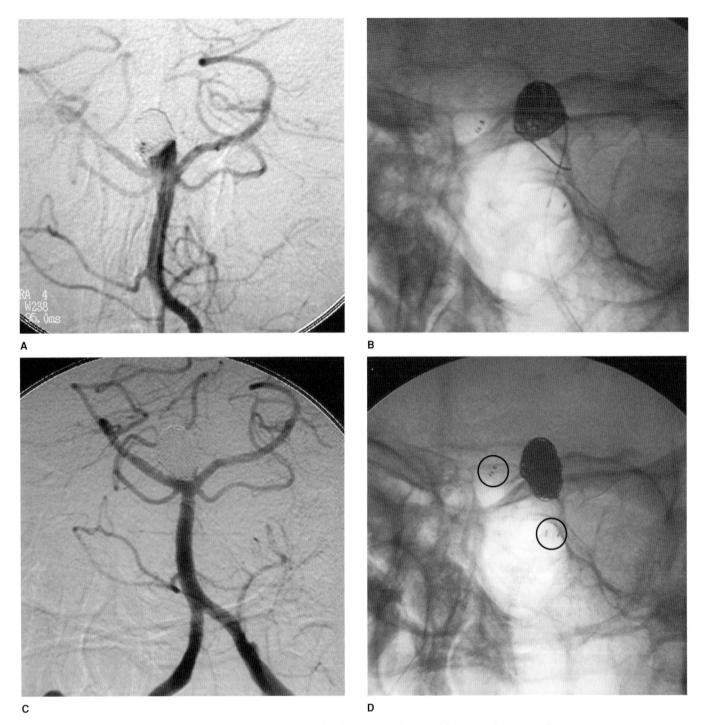

A

B

C

D

● **FIGURE 23-5.** Aneurysm recanalization. This 41-year-old man underwent coil embolization of a ruptured basilar tip aneurysm at an outside hospital and made a good recovery. He presented for follow-up evaluation and was found (by digital subtraction angiography [DSA]) to have significant recanalization of this (A) wide-necked aneurysm. (B) He underwent placement of a stent that spanned the distal BA and the right PCA (unsubtracted view). (C [DSA] and D [unsubtracted view]) The aneurysm was then coiled without herniation of the coils into either PCA (stent markers are *circled*).

ischemia,[90] other factors, such as location of spasm, collateral supply, and cerebral perfusion pressure, also influence whether ischemic symptoms become manifest. As a result, the incidence of clinical vasospasm is approximately half that of angiographic vasospasm and can be seen in up to one-third of patients.[86,89,91]

Pathogenesis

Extensive evidence points to the presence of subarachnoid blood clot as the chief etiology in cerebral vasospasm. The amount and location of subarachnoid blood predict the subsequent site and degree of cerebral vasospasm,[92,93] as does the rate of clearance of subarachnoid clot via endogenous means.[94] Hemoglobin within red blood cells is a key spasmogen,[95,96] although other components of the subarachnoid blood clot also contribute to vasospasm.[97] The underlying pathophysiology appears to be prolonged contraction of vascular smooth muscle cells rather than fibrosis or cellular proliferation,[98–100] as also evidenced by the ability of intra-arterial (IA) vasodilators such as papaverine and nicardipine to (at least transiently) ameliorate vasospasm.

Medical Management

Prophylaxis against cerebral vasospasm with oral nimodipine is considered standard of care in the treatment of SAH, because it significantly improves the odds of a good outcome and reduces death and disability owing to vasospasm.[101–104] However, once cerebral vasospasm becomes clinically apparent by causing neurological deficit(s), immediate/first-line therapy has traditionally involved the institution of so-called "triple-H" (hypertension, hemodilution, hypervolemia) therapy with use of increased fluids and/or pressors, particularly when access to endovascular treatment is limited or unavailable. Of the three components, induced *hypertension* is likely the most important,[105] with the common denominator of this approach being an increase in cerebral perfusion pressure, thereby enhancing both flow through a vasospastic segment and also collateral supply to the distal ischemic brain. Although never subjected to a randomized trial, outcomes with such treatment appear to be significantly better than the natural history of untreated vasospasm.[103,106]

Endovascular Management

Endovascular therapy for symptomatic cerebral vasospasm is generally undertaken after medical intervention has been deemed unsuccessful. It is important to rapidly maximize medical therapy to determine its efficacy or lack thereof and subsequent need for endovascular treatment because a delay in decision making can lead to fixed rather than reversible cerebral ischemic deficits. Endovascular options may be broadly categorized as IA infusion of vasodilators or balloon angioplasty. The first and most frequently used IA vasodilator drug is papaverine, initially described by Kaku et al.[107] and Kassell et al.[108] in 1992 for the treatment of vasospasm after aneurysmal SAH. Effects of papaverine are unfortunately short-lasting and include the potential side effects of raised intracranial pressure (ICP) and seizures, prompting renewed interest in IA calcium 2+ channel blockers, such as nicardipine[109] or verapamil,[110] or the treatment of vasospasm. Although side effects of IA calcium 2+ blockers (raised ICP in particular) are less frequent, their short-term effect has led to the adoption of balloon angioplasty, introduced in 1984 by Zubkov et al.[111] for symptomatic cerebral vasospasm. Current techniques with over-the-wire balloons provide a long-lasting, relatively safe treatment for vasospasm, although technical challenges diminish successful application in the ACA as a result of vessel angulation and tortuosity.[112,113] IA vasodilators still play a role in the treatment of distal vasospasm (inaccessible to balloon angioplasty) or in the pretreatment of very severe vasospasm in order to permit navigation by angioplasty balloons.

● ISCHEMIC STROKE

Epidemiology

The term "stroke" is all encompassing and includes ischemic stroke, ICH, and SAH. Annually, 15 million people worldwide suffer a stroke.[114] Of these, one-third die and one-third are permanently disabled.[114] Although the incidence of stroke is declining in industrial countries because of improved control of hypertension and smoking, the absolute numbers of strokes is increasing because of the aging population in these countries. Stroke is the third-leading cause of death in developed countries behind cardiovascular disease and cancer. In 2002, 10% of all deaths worldwide were attributed to stroke.[114] Ischemic strokes account for 87% of all strokes. Each year, approximately 700 000 people in the United States suffer a stroke.[115] Of these, 500 000 are first-time strokes. The estimated cost of stroke in the United States will exceed $62 billion in 2007.[115]

Etiology and Presentation

The hallmark feature of stroke is the sudden onset of neurological symptoms and signs. Focal neurological symptoms such as diplopia, weakness on one side, loss of sensation, dysarthria, aphasia, and visual field deficits are suggestive of ischemic stroke. In contrast, presentations of severe headache, seizures, alterations in level of consciousness, and vomiting are more likely to reflect hemorrhage.

Ischemic stroke can be classified by the type of vascular lesion or by the mechanism of ischemia. Numerous mechanisms may cause brain ischemia. Severe arterial stenosis or occlusion from atherosclerosis or thrombus may reduce perfusion in a purely hemodynamic fashion. Embolism may originate from a more proximal source and result in arterial occlusion. The small end-arteries in the deep gray matter may be affected by local atherosclerosis or lipohyalinosis. Miscellaneous causes of ischemic stroke include hypercoagulability, arterial dissection, arterial vasospasm, vasculitis, fibromuscular dysplasia, and moyamoya disease. Of all these causes, the four most frequent are large-vessel atherosclerosis, cardioembolism, small-vessel disease, and cryptogenic.[116] Extracranial large-arterial atherosclerosis, which is responsible for up to 40% of all ischemic strokes, is beyond the scope of this chapter. Intracranial atherosclerosis will be addressed later in this chapter.

Cardioembolism accounts for 15% to 30% of all ischemic strokes.[116] The most common cardiac sources of embolism include valvular disease such as mitral stenosis or regurgitation, endocarditis, mural thrombus following anterior myocardial infarction, left atrial appendage from atrial fibrillation, severe cardiomyopathies, and ventricular aneurysms. Less common is embolism from atrial myxoma or paradoxical right to left embolism from a patent foramen ovale.

A cardiac source is presumed when multiple infarcts involving more than one cerebral vascular territory are seen clinically or radiographically. Most embolic obstruction is cleared automatically within 48 hours through the homeostatic processes of recanalization and fibrinolysis.

Lacunar strokes also account for 15% to 30% of all ischemic strokes. These strokes involve the small vessels supplying the deep structures of the brain such as the basal ganglia and thalamus. These penetrating arteries can become stenotic or occluded by microatherosclerosis and lipohyalinosis. Uncontrolled hypertension and diabetes mellitus are often implicated with these strokes. Because these vessels are less than 400 μm in diameter, angiography is often unremarkable. Most lacunar strokes are diagnosed clinically with pure motor or sensory syndromes. MR imaging may demonstrate a small, deep infarct.

Characteristics of Specific Arterial Occlusions

In this section, the characteristics of specific large-vessel occlusions are outlined in the broadest terms. More specific descriptions can be found in standard neurology texts.

Occlusion of the main trunk of the MCA causes contralateral hemiparesis, contralateral anesthesia, ipsilateral gaze preference, and contralateral hemianopsia. If the dominant cerebral hemisphere is involved, the patient will also suffer from global aphasia. Involvement of the nondominant hemisphere leads to impaired spatial perception. Less severe combinations of these symptoms may occur, depending on occlusions of distal branches rather than the main trunk.

Infarction in the ACA territory typically results in paresis and anesthesia in the contralateral lower extremity. Motor neglect and disinclination to use the contralateral extremities may be observed. Bilateral ACA infarction is particularly devastating with resultant behavior and personality changes, severe apathy, incontinence, and muteness. These features are attributed to involvement of both the medial frontal lobes and the limbic structures.

Occlusion of the PCA usually causes a contralateral homonymous hemianopsia caused by injury to the occipital lobe. Proximal PCA occlusion may also injure the thalamus and midbrain because of the involvement of perforating branches. This typically results in contralateral loss of sensation, altered mental status, and impaired vertical gaze.

There are many brainstem infarction syndromes depending on the level (midbrain, pons, or medulla) and location in the brainstem. For interventional purposes, we have limited this discussion to vertebrobasilar occlusion. Rather than describing the dozens of brainstem syndromes, we will focus on what happens when the VA or BA itself are occluded. Occlusion of the BA or VA is more often the cause of brainstem infarction than occlusion of perforating branches.[117] The posterior circulation is easy to overlook as a source of stroke because of the wide spectrum of presentations, many of which are nonspecific. However, failure to recognize a VA or BA occlusion may have disastrous consequences. The posterior circulation should be considered in patients with bilateral or crossed (e.g., ipsilateral face and contralateral limb) motor and sensory signs, disconjugate eye movements or nystagmus, dysmetria and ataxia, involvement of cranial nerves, and altered levels of consciousness.

Malignant Cerebral Infarction

Classically, malignant infarction is described for large strokes involving the MCA. It is an emergency that carries a rate of mortality six to eight times higher than seen in other ischemic strokes. By definition, more than 50% of the MCA territory is involved with subsequent brain edema that may result in elevated ICP and eventual herniation and death.[118] Malignant MCA infarction may account for up to 10% of all ischemic strokes.[118] Besides the focal neurological deficit caused by the stroke itself, a progressive decline in the patient's level of consciousness is seen at approximately 48 hours after the onset of the stroke. In young patients with no baseline brain atrophy, clinical deterioration may begin as early as 12 hours from the onset.[119] Despite maximal medical management of intracranial hypertension, including osmodiuresis, hypothermia, and barbiturate coma, the mortality approaches 80%.[120]

Mechanical decompression of the edematous cerebral hemisphere through a hemicraniectomy has been performed for decades in numerous settings. Hemicraniectomy is very effective at reducing ICP and may be life-saving. Until recently, level I evidence supporting this procedure has been lacking. Controversial issues in the setting of stroke have been timing of hemicraniectomy and performance of this operation on left-sided lesions. The historical argument against left hemicraniectomy has been that survivors will remain globally aphasic and hemiplegic. In contrast, right-sided lesions may be more compatible with a functional outcome because of the absence of language involvement. One retrospective analysis concluded that hemicraniectomy reduced the mortality from malignant stroke to 24% and that patients with left-sided strokes had similar outcomes to those with right hemispheric strokes.[121] Additionally, patients younger than the age of 50 years seemed to have better outcomes. It has also been proposed that early (<24 hours from onset) hemicraniectomy improves outcomes.[122]

The effect of decompression on functional outcomes in these malignant strokes has been evaluated in three randomized controlled European trials.[123] These studies had similar design, and their data were pooled for analysis in a recent publication.[123] Two of the three trials were halted because the results showed a significant benefit of surgical decompression on mortality. The pooled analysis demonstrated a clear beneficial effect on survival and unfavorable outcome. However, these benefits were driven by an increase in patients with major disability. Therefore, the net benefit of surgical decompression must still be individualized.[124] The preliminary analysis did not show any significant difference in outcomes in patients decompressed within 23 hours versus 48 hours.[123]

The other classic surgical emergency occurs with large posterior fossa strokes. Although the stroke burden is small compared to that associated with a large MCA stroke, the posterior fossa is a much more confined space with little tolerance for brain edema. Mass effect in the posterior fossa can lead to compression of the fourth ventricle and hydrocephalus and eventual brain stem compression. These patients tend to improve with posterior fossa decompression in the form of suboccipital craniectomy.[125] These patients have survivable deficits (usually ataxia or dysmetria from cerebellar involvement), and their outcome is favorable if decompression is performed at the earliest signs of deterioration.

Medical Therapy

Medical management of ischemic stroke may be classified by its time course as emergent, thrombolytic, supportive, rehabilitative, and finally, preventative. Emergent and supportive measures are best reviewed in the recent guidelines from the AHA[126] and are summarized in Table 23-1 (rehabilitative and preventative treatments are outside the scope of this chapter). Medical thrombolytic treatment is primarily reviewed here, in contrast to interventional treatment, which is discussed in the subsequent section. The ischemic stroke imaging section follows both the medical and endovascular therapy sections because the reader will then know *why* we image and *what* we image for and will be aware of the *therapeutic implications of the imaging findings.*

On the basis of the first successful randomized controlled trial of intravenous (IV) thrombolysis for acute stroke, the National Institute of Neurological Disorders and Stroke (NINDS) trial,[127] administration of 0.9 mg/kg recombinant tissue plasminogen activator (rt-PA) within 3 hours of stroke onset is now recommended for suitable

---

TABLE 23-1. Medical Management of Acute Ischemic Stroke

1. Field management
   a. Secure airway, breathing, and circulation (ABCs), cardiac monitoring, IV access; administer supplemental oxygen (O_2) as needed; rule out hypoglycemia; keep nothing by mouth
   b. Transfer to closest designated stroke center or emergency department capable of handling acute stroke
2. Hospital management
   a. Maintain O_2 saturation >92%; intubate for airway protection as needed
   b. Normothermia (or hypothermia in context of neuroprotection trials)
   c. Continuous cardiac monitoring ≥24 hours; treatment of detected arrhythmias or ischemia
   d. Blood pressure:
      i. treat systolic blood pressure >220 mm Hg or diastolic blood pressure >120 mm Hg (185 and 110 mm Hg, respectively, if undergoing any thrombolytic intervention) with IV labetalol, nitropaste, or nicardipine infusion
      ii. determine underlying cause of and treat hypotension; optimize cardiac output
      iii. induce hypertension to improve cerebral blood flow in exceptional cases
   e. serum glucose: avoid hypoglycemia, treat glucose >140 mg/dL (goal 80–140 mg/dL)
3. Baseline diagnostics
   a. All patients: CT or MR imaging; serum glucose and electrolytes; renal function tests; cardiac enzyme levels; complete blood count; prothrombin time, partial thromboplastin time, international normalized ratio; electrocardiogram; O_2 saturation
   b. Select patients: liver function tests; toxicology screen; blood alcohol level; pregnancy test; arterial blood gas; chest X-ray; lumbar puncture (if SAH suspected); electroencephalogram (if seizure suspected)
4. Thrombolysis
   a. Rapid and accurate determination of onset, risk factors, and eligibility for treatment
   b. If eligible: IV and/or IA thrombolytic therapy (*see sections on ischemic stroke medical therapy and endovascular therapy*)
5. Supportive measures
   a. Setting: admission to comprehensive acute stroke unit is recommended
   b. Screening: lipid profile, dysphagia risk
   c. Prophylaxis: deep vein thrombosis; anticoagulation for atrial fibrillation; aspirin, 325 mg, within 24–48 hours of onset
   d. Treatment: medical or surgical treatment for brain edema or hemorrhage; antibiotics for urinary or pulmonary infections; avoid indwelling bladder catheters if possible; early mobilization
   e. Nutrition and hydration: nasogastric, nasoduodenal, or percutaneous endoscopic gastrotomy feedings if unable to swallow safely

---

Adapted from Adams HP Jr, del Zoppo G, Alberts MJ, et al. Guidelines for the early management of adults with ischemic stroke: a guideline from the American Heart Association/American Stroke Association Stroke Council, Clinical Cardiology Council, Cardiovascular Radiology and Intervention Council, and the Atherosclerotic Peripheral Vascular Disease and Quality of Care Outcomes in Research Interdisciplinary Working Groups: the American Academy of Neurology affirms the value of this guideline as an educational tool for neurologists. Stroke. 2007;38(5):1655-1711.

TABLE 23-2. Characteristics of Patients with Ischemic Stroke Who Could Be Treated with rt-PA

Diagnosis of ischemic stroke causing measurable neurological deficit

Neurological signs that are not clearing spontaneously or are not minor and isolated

Caution should be exercised in treating a patient with major deficits

Stroke symptoms that are not suggestive of SAH

Onset of symptoms <3 h before beginning treatment

No head trauma or prior stroke in the previous 3 months

No myocardial infarction in the previous 3 months

No gastrointestinal or urinary tract hemorrhage in the previous 21 days

No major surgery in the previous 14 days

No arterial puncture at a noncompressible site in the previous 7 days

No history of previous ICH

Blood pressure not elevated (systolic <185 mm Hg and diastolic <110 mm Hg)

No evidence of active bleeding or acute trauma (fracture) on examination

Not taking an oral anticoagulant or, if anticoagulant being taken, international normalized ratio ≤1.5

If receiving heparin in previous 48 h, activated partial thromboplastin time must be in normal range

Platelet count ≥100 000 mm³

Blood glucose concentration ≥50 mg/dL (2.7 mmol/L)

No seizures with postictal residual neurological impairments

CT does not show a multilobar infarction (hypodensity >1/3 cerebral hemisphere)

The patient or family members understand the potential risks and benefits from treatment

Reproduced with permission from Adams HP Jr, del Zoppo G, Alberts MJ, et al. Guidelines for the early management of adults with ischemic stroke: a guideline from the American Heart Association/American Stroke Association Stroke Council, Clinical Cardiology Council, Cardiovascular Radiology and Intervention Council, and the Atherosclerotic Peripheral Vascular Disease and Quality of Care Outcomes in Research Interdisciplinary Working Groups: the American Academy of Neurology affirms the value of this guideline as an educational tool for neurologists. Stroke. 2007;38(5):1655-1711.

candidates.[126] However, <1.25% of patients admitted to hospitals with strokes in the USA received rt-PA between 1999 and 2002.[128,129] This may be because of the strict eligibility requirements (Table 23-2[126]), lack of stroke centers or stroke experts, and a fear of ICH among front-line caregivers.

The original NINDS trial[127] demonstrated unequivocal benefit for rt-PA in acute stroke: infarct volumes were smaller on CT (15 vs. 24 mL),[130] inpatient stays were shorter with discharges to home occurring more frequently,[131] and patients were 32% more likely to have no or minimal disability at 3 months as measured on the Barthel index.[127] Efficacy of rt-PA was reflected by low

numbers needed to treat (NNT), with an NNT of 8 for no or minimal residual deficit (National Institutes of Health Stroke Scale [NIHSS] score of 0-1) and an NNT of 7 for achieving independence at 3 months (modified Rankin Scale [mRS] score of 0-2).[132] Subsequent criticism of baseline NIHSS score imbalance between treatment groups (more patients with NIHSS 0-5 were randomized to rt-PA, whereas more patients with NIHSS >20 were randomized to placebo) was addressed by a rigorous reanalysis that confirmed the benefit of rt-PA across all quintiles of the NIHSS.[133] Phase 4 clinical studies, such as the Standard Treatment with Alteplase to Reverse Stroke study, have also helped confirm the NINDS results, with a similar proportion (43%) of patients achieving independence (mRS 0-2) at 3 months following rt-PA treatment[134] as did those in the original NINDS trial. Meta-analysis of 15 postapproval publications found rates of symptomatic ICH (sICH), mortality, and excellent recovery (mRS 0-1) similar to those in the NINDS trial.[135] A more recent pooled analysis of all six rt-PA trials, Alteplase ThromboLysis for Acute Noninterventional Therapy in Ischemic Stroke, European and Australian Cooperative Acute Stroke Study, and NINDS, examined 2775 patients treated within 6 hours of onset (representing 99% of all patients treated with rt-PA within randomized trials) and found clear benefit of rt-PA despite a very strict definition of good outcome (mRS 0-1), with an odds ratio of 2.8 favoring treatment within the first 90 minutes and an odds ratio of 1.6 for the next 90 minutes after stroke onset.[136]

A key issue raised by the initial NINDS trial was increased sICH in patients receiving rt-PA (6.4%, vs. 0.6% in the placebo group). sICH was associated with higher NIHSS score, brain edema (acute hypodensity on CT scan) and mass effect on CT before treatment,[137] with benefit of rt-PA persisting despite hemorrhage. Risk of sICH may also increase with age.[138] Numerous authors have since demonstrated a similar safety profile for thrombolysis in both community and academic settings across the United States and Europe, with rates of sICH between 3.3% and 5.9%.[128,134–136,139]

IV thrombolysis is less efficacious (but likely still superior to placebo) in certain patient subgroups. Intuitively, patients with more severe strokes do worse.[133] Recanalization at 24 hours is much less frequent in diabetic patients possibly because of the higher endogenous levels of plasminogen activator inhibitor in these patients.[140] Patients older than 80 years benefit less than do those younger than 80 years: less independence at 3 months (mRS 0-2 achieved in 32%–36% vs. 62%–63%), higher mortality at 3 months (21%–40% vs. 5%–16%), and a questionably higher rate of sICH (2.6%–11.1% vs. 2.6%–6%).[141–143] Nevertheless, a subgroup analysis of NINDS data failed to show any age cutoff for benefit from rt-PA.[144] Patients receiving rt-PA within 3 hours with ICA-T occlusions (verified on CT angiography or MR angiography) fare worse than those with MCA occlusions,[145] but better than patients not receiving any thrombolysis at all.[146,147] Recent studies have discouraged subgroup analysis, pointing out that existing randomized trials of rt-PA are underpowered for such examinations.[148]

The most important factor for successful IV thrombolysis remains time from onset to treatment.[149] For example, Tomsick[132] calculates that delaying treatment in the first 90 minutes decreases the odds ratio of good outcome by approximately 1% per minute. Similarly, early recanalization strongly favors good outcome—half of patients with early (<2 hours) recanalization reach an mRS score of 0 to 1 at 3 months (vs. only 22% of patients without early recanalization),[150] and total infarct volumes rise with increasing time to recanalization.[151] Saver[152] estimates that the average patient with large vessel ischemic stroke looses, per hour, 120 million neurons, 830 billion synapses, and 714 km of myelinated fibers, effectively aging the brain 3.6 years per hour while untreated.

Given the importance of early recanalization for good outcome and the strict eligibility criteria for IV thrombolysis (Table 23-2[126]), attention has turned to more invasive IA treatment. The first randomized controlled trial of such therapy, the Prolyse in Acute Cerebral Thromboembolism (PROACT II) study, in which IA prourokinase was administered, demonstrated 66% recanalization (Thrombolysis in Myocardial Infarction [TIMI] grade 2–3 flow) of proximal M1 occlusions within 2 hours of treatment (vs. 18% in the placebo group).[153] By comparison, recanalization within 6 hours was seen only in 32% of patients receiving IV rt-PA,[151] and other investigators have shown even less recanalization rates at earlier time points (mean 2 hours): 12.5% for ICA or proximal MCA and 27.3% for distal MCA occlusions.[154] This contrasts with recanalization assessed at later time points, with recanalization rates documented by transcranial Doppler (TCD) imaging at 24 hours of 46.2%, 53.1%, and 68.4% for carotid-T, M1, and M2/distal occlusions, respectively.[140] These results have prompted a search for ways to enhance early thrombolysis with IV rt-PA, such as continuous transcranial ultrasound,[155] as well as various IA strategies alone or in combination with IV rt-PA.

Endovascular Therapy

Endovascular, IA, and interventional therapy for ischemic stroke all refer to transarterial procedures aimed at opening symptomatic occlusive lesions of the cerebral vasculature. These methods may be broadly grouped as (a) IA infusion of drugs, for example, thrombolytics or glycoprotein (GP) IIb/IIIa inhibitors; (b) mechanical disruption or maceration of IA clot, for example, with microwires, microcatheters, and/or snares; (c) clot retrieval, for example, with the Merci retrieval device (Concentric Medical, Mountainview, CA); (d) angioplasty; and (e) stenting.

The second PROACT II trial served as a landmark for endovascular therapy for stroke.[153] In PROACT II, IA recombinant prourokinase and placebo were compared in patients with acute M1 occlusions within 6 hours of onset (mean NIHSS score of 17, compared with 14 in the NINDS IV rt-PA trial[127]). Primary outcome (independence, defined as mRS 0–2 at 3 months) was

achieved in 40% of the treatment group and 18% of the placebo group (15% absolute benefit, 58% relative benefit, NNT = 7). TIMI 2 or 3 recanalization within 2 hours was seen in 66% of the prourokinase group versus 18% of the control group. There was a nonsignificant increase in sICH by day 10 (10% vs. 4%), and mortality was similar between the two groups (25% vs. 27% at 3 months). Even better results were later achieved with IA urokinase by Arnold et al.[156] in 78 patients presenting with M1 or M2 occlusions within 6 hours: 59% reached independence at 3 months and only 13% died, improving upon results obtained in the NINDS rt-PA trial.[127] Interestingly, even within the 3-hour window, results of IA thrombolytic therapy may equal or exceed those of IV treatment in the NINDS trial, with studies reporting 75% recanalization, 11% sICH (vs. 6.4% in NINDS), 22% mortality (vs. 17% in NINDS), and 50% excellent outcome (mRS 0-1) at 3 months (vs. 39% in NINDS).[157]

As expertise and familiarity with the potential benefits of endovascular therapy grew, investigators sought to incorporate it within the 3-hour IV rt-PA algorithm through a series of "bridging" trials that utilized a lesser dose of IV rt-PA (0.6 mg/kg). These included the Emergent Management of Stroke (EMS),[158] Interventional Management of Stroke (IMS-I),[159] IMS-II,[160] and IMS-III (currently recruiting). In comparison with the NINDS IV rt-PA trial, outcomes from IMS-II at 3 months suggest that combined IV-IA therapy is at least equivalent if not superior to IV rt-PA alone: 46% versus 39% independence (mRS ≥ 2), 53% versus 42% self-sufficiency in activities of daily living (Barthel Index 95-100), 16% versus 21% mortality, and 9.9% versus 6.6% sICH.[160] Remarkably, this was achieved with a higher proportion of patients with early ischemic changes on baseline CT (60% vs. 34%) and longer median delay to treatment (142 vs. 90 minutes) in IMS-II. IA thrombolysis may be feasible even after full (rather than bridging) doses of IV rt-PA, with studies reporting 72.5% recanalization, 40% independence (mRS 0-2) at 3 months, and 17% to 20% mortality with this approach in patients with a mean baseline NIHSS score of 18.[161,162] More recently, GP IIb/IIIa inhibitors have been added to the arsenal, with preliminary studies suggesting an acceptable safety profile in acute stroke without marked increase in the rates of sICH.[163–165]

Endovascular therapy also permits mechanical recanalization with clot-retrieval devices, thereby minimizing further use of thrombolytics or GP IIb/IIIa inhibitors. The most widely used such device remains the Merci clot retriever (Figure 23-6). Initial trials examined patients within 8-hour onset who were ineligible for IV thrombolysis and achieved 46% recanalization (≥TIMI 2) and mRS scores of 0 to 2 in 28%, with mortality in 4% at 3 months.[161,166] A subsequent trial that included the use of second-generation retriever devices showed improved results: 69% overall recanalization (54% with the device alone), 9% sICH, 34% mRS scores of 0 to 2, and 30% mortality at 3 months.[167] These results appear more promising when examined within the context of the patient population treated: stroke severity was significantly higher than

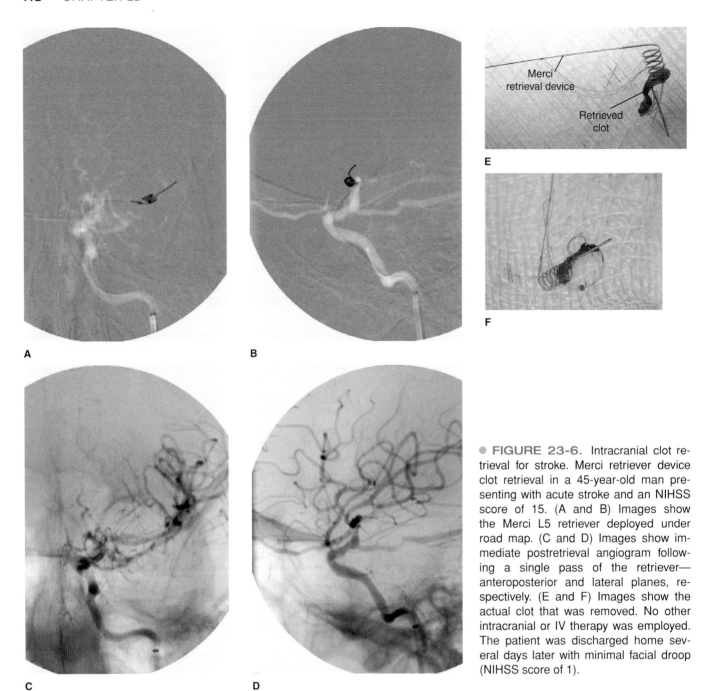

A

B

E

Merci retrieval device

Retrieved clot

F

C

D

● **FIGURE 23-6.** Intracranial clot retrieval for stroke. Merci retriever device clot retrieval in a 45-year-old man presenting with acute stroke and an NIHSS score of 15. (A and B) Images show the Merci L5 retriever deployed under road map. (C and D) Images show immediate postretrieval angiogram following a single pass of the retriever—anteroposterior and lateral planes, respectively. (E and F) Images show the actual clot that was removed. No other intracranial or IV therapy was employed. The patient was discharged home several days later with minimal facial droop (NIHSS score of 1).

in the NINDS IV rt-PA trial (mean NIHSS score of 19–20 vs. 14), time from onset was much longer (within 8 hours rather than 3 hours), and all were either ineligible for or had failed treatment with IV rt-PA.

Current endovascular intervention for stroke increasingly involves a "multimodality" approach, utilizing IA drugs, mechanical devices, angioplasty, and stenting in the hope that such an escalating strategy with potential synergy between the tools used will provide faster and better recanalization. Early results of such an approach show promise with a 63% recanalization rate and a 14% sICH rate, where combined use of thrombolytics and GP IIb/IIIa inhibitors and use of angioplasty or stenting favored increased recanalization.[165] In general, benefits of IA inter-

vention have resembled or exceeded those of IV rt-PA despite the fact that recipients have been mostly ineligible for the latter. These benefits appear to be long term, with Nedeltchev et al.[168] reporting 56% independence (mRS score, 0-2) and 23% mortality at 2 years following IA treatment of patients with acute stroke and mean baseline NIHSS score of 14 (equivalent to the NINDS trial). Rates of sICH after IA intervention tend to be comparable or slightly higher to those after IV rt-PA, which may be an acceptable tradeoff for better potential outcomes, especially in patients ineligible for IV rt-PA. Predictors of sICH after endovascular therapy for stroke include higher NIHSS score, longer time to recanalization, lower platelet counts, and higher glucose levels.[169,170]

Similar to the case with IV thrombolysis, less benefit is derived from IA therapy by certain patient groups, including diabetic patients and the elderly.[156] Those older than 80 years of age, in particular, fair worse: despite equivalent recanalization rates (79% vs. 68%), sICH (7% vs. 8%), and any ICH (39% vs. 37%), elderly patients show less excellent outcomes (mRS 0-1; 26% vs. 40%) and survival (57% vs. 80%) at 3 months' time.[171] However, these results remain superior to the generally dismal outcome of severe stroke in patients older than 80 years. Other subgroups may be defined by the site of the thrombus, with progressively worse outcomes with occlusion of the MCA, BA, and ICA.[172] Patients with vertebrobasilar thrombosis remain a special subgroup, where the grim prognosis associated with the natural history has spurred aggressive IA treatment up to 24 hours, and even 48 hours, after symptom onset. As reviewed by Ng et al.,[173] recanalization rates of up to 70% can be achieved with survival rates of 55% to 70%, whereas persistent vertebrobasilar occlusion heralds less than 10% chance of survival.

With ongoing rapid evolution of endovascular technique, further improvements in stroke care can be expected. Ultrasound-tipped microinfusion catheters (such as the EKOS catheter, EKOS Corporation, Bothell, WA) for IA thrombolysis[174]), upfront primary angioplasty for stroke,[175] and intracranial stenting in the setting of failed mechanical clot retrieval[176] are examples of recent advances in endovascular treatment of acute stroke. However, with increasing proliferation of devices and techniques, the need for randomized trials of stroke therapy has become clearer. One such trial, IMS-III, pits IV rt-PA against the EKOS catheter and the Merci retriever, with results expected in 2008 or 2009.

Imaging

Limited time availability during emergent management of acute ischemic stroke leads to imaging needs unlike those for hemorrhagic stroke, transient ischemic attack (TIA), or asymptomatic cerebrovascular disease, which will not be reviewed here. The following three broad categories of information should rapidly be sought, ideally by one or, at maximum, two imaging modalities, which in stroke remain CT, MR, and DSA in selected cases:

1. *Parenchymal*: Classically the first line of investigation to confirm diagnosis, distinguish between ischemic and hemorrhagic stroke, and determine stroke location and size. Noncontrast CT is generally used first because of superior speed and availability, whereas MRI provides better views of brain supplied by the posterior circulation.

2. *Vascular*: While initially not critical to decision-making in acute stroke, increasing availability of endovascular treatment options have made visualization of proximal or large-vessel occlusion more relevant in selected patients. Although modalities such as Doppler and TCD ultrasound imaging are operator-dependent and not universally available, CT angiography or MR angiography may simply be added to the initial modality chosen for parenchymal imaging. DSA is reserved for candidates for endovascular intervention.

3. *Perfusion*: New methods exist that provide clinicians with physiological data (rather than just anatomical data), permitting management of acute stroke based upon accurate visualization of infarcted core versus remaining penumbra at risk, rather than crude assessments of time from stroke onset. CT perfusion or MR perfusion imaging are now readily available (or can be added via simple software upgrades) at any center with CT or MR equipment. Xenon-CT, positron emission tomography (PET), and single photon emission computed tomography are less available options because of time or regulatory concerns.

Computed Tomography. CT remains the most readily available and rapid imaging modality in triage of acute ischemic versus hemorrhagic stroke. It is the only imaging criterion required in decisions regarding IV thrombolysis.[127] Although highly specific, it is less sensitive than MR imaging in detection of acute stroke, particularly for small or posterior fossa lesions. Plain CT imaging has specificity and positive predictive value (PPV) of 85% and 96%, respectively, whereas sensitivity and negative predictive value are 64% and 27%, respectively.[177] Sensitivity is increased to 71% with the use of variable gray-scale windowing,[178] 80% with multimodality CT (i.e., CT perfusion, contrast CT, CT angiography, and CT perfusion source images),[179] and approaches 100% for large territorial infarcts,[180] with only small lacunar or subcortical strokes being missed on multimodality CT imaging.

Attempts to increase the reliability and reproducibility of stroke diagnosis on noncontrast CT have lead to the development of the Alberta Stroke Programme Early CT Score (ASPECTS),[181] which provides a quantitative (10-point) assessment of MCA stroke burden on CT with high interobserver reliability in acute stroke. Lower ASPECT scores correlate well with more proximal occlusions[182] and have proven valuable for prognostication in acute stroke. When assessing dichotomized ASPECT scores, patients with low stroke burden (ASPECTS >7) on CT imaging incur less sICH after IV thrombolysis and have a higher chance of gaining independence (mRS $\geq$ 2).[181] Retrospective application of ASPECTS to IMS-I patients as compared with a matching cohort from the NINDS IV rt-PA trial suggested that patients with ASPECTS >7 do better with IV-IA therapy, whereas those with ASPECTS $\leq$ 7 do better with IV thrombolysis alone.[182] Similarly, PROACT II patients with ASPECTS > 7 experienced a 36.4% absolute benefit and a 3.2-fold decrease in risk of poor outcome after IA urokinase, compared with 6.4% absolute benefit and 1.2 risk ratio for those with ASPECTS $\leq$ 7. A similar dichotomous result for ASPECTS was not found in the NINDS IV rt-PA trial,[183] possibly

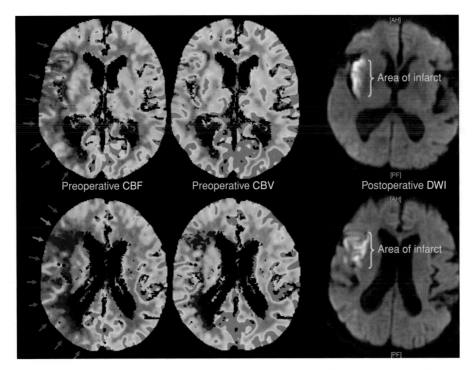

● **FIGURE 23-7.** CT Perfusion imaging in acute stroke. An 83-year-old man with paroxysmal atrial fibrillation presented with a right MCA stroke and an NIHSS score >10 at 14 hours after onset. CT perfusion imaging demonstrated large penumbra (decreased CBF but relatively preserved CBV, *blue arrows*) with a small area of established infarct (markedly decreased CBF as well as CBV, *red arrows*). Following combination therapy consisting of IA thrombolytic, GP IIb/IIIa inhibitor, mechanical retrieval, and intracranial angioplasty, complete (TIMI 3) revascularization was achieved. As a result, MR imaging several days later demonstrated only small stroke within the areas predicted by the CT perfusion findings; and the patient was discharged home without objective neurological deficit, with an mRS score of 0 at the 3-month follow-up evaluation.

because early CT changes (0–3 hours) may be reversible, whereas the later changes seen in PROACT II (3-6 hours) may represent fixed deficits. Indeed, more recent investigators have shown that early changes represented by focal swelling alone (rather than hypoattenuation) on CT images may represent the increased blood volume seen in salvageable penumbra rather than actual infarcted core.[184,185] Use of CT perfusion images rather than noncontrast CT increases prognostic accuracy of the ASPECT score, with final infarct mirroring cerebral blood volume (CBV) or CBF deficits when reperfusion is or is not achieved, respectively.[186]

Knowledge of regional blood flow in brain ischemia, although until recently not widely available, can be of great benefit to clinical decision making. In primates, reversible ischemia, cessation of electrical activity, and irreversible ischemia occur at 20 to 23, 18, and 10 to 12 mL/100 g per minute, respectively, matching human values for functional penumbra, flat EEG (during carotid artery clamping in endarterectomy studies), and cerebral infarction at thresholds of 14 to 22, 16 to 18, and 5 to 15 mL/100 g per minute, respectively (reviewed in Hoeffner et al.[187] and Heiss et al.[188]). With increasing availability of multidetector CT equipment and CT perfusion software packages,

clinicians can now rapidly assess CBF, CBV, and mean transit times (MTT) in ischemic brain. Although various algorithms exist from which to derive perfusion data, all such methods use CT equipment in cine mode to track the arrival and washout of IV contrast bolus and the associated parenchymal enhancement peak in real-time. CT perfusion is much more sensitive for stroke detection than plain CT,[179,180,189] and derived flow, volume, and transit time parameters have been well validated against Xenon-CT,[190] diffusion–perfusion MR imaging,[191] and PET.[192]

CT perfusion imaging permits differentiation of normal brain from ischemic penumbra (salvageable brain) and infarcted core (dead, unsalvageable brain). CBV appears critical in distinguishing penumbra from infarct: although both penumbra and infarcted core have decreased CBF, relative preservation or increase in CBV is what sets penumbra apart from infarcted core (Figure 23-7). At the simplest level, preserved or increased CBV may reflect the presence of dilated collaterals. Early investigators noted that CBV (rather than CBF or MTT) correlated better with final infarct volume, regardless of whether perfusion data was generated by CT[193] or MR[194] protocols. Importantly, it is preserved or increased CBV that determines what is salvageable penumbra *if* reperfusion happens:

Parsons et al.[195] found that *with* reperfusion of hypoperfused areas, 97%, 41%, and 3% of low, normal, and high CBV areas, respectively, progressed to infarct, whereas *without* reperfusion of hypoperfused areas, 94%, 63% and 94% of low, normal, and high CBV areas, respectively, went on to infarct. Other authors have suggested the use of relative ratios as more accurate, with CBF reduction beyond 66% (of the normal contralateral side) having 95% PPV for infarction regardless of recanalization.[196]

Combined analysis of CBF and CBV quantitative values may further increase CT perfusion accuracy. Murphy et al.[197] found that in stroke patients who experienced recanalization, CBF progressively decreased from normal to penumbral to infarcted gray matter (37.3 ± 5.0, 25.0 ± 3.82, and 13.3 ± 3.75 mL/100 g per minute, respectively) whereas CBV *increased* from normal to penumbral tissue but was markedly *decreased* in gray matter destined for infarction (1.78 ± 0.30 mL/100 g, 2.15 ± 0.43 mL/100 g, 1.12 ± 0.37 mL/100 g). Having noted divergent changes in CBF versus CBV in penumbral tissue, Murphy et al.[197] derived a multiplicative cutoff value of 31.3 (CBF × CBV) for $\geq 97\%$ sensitivity, specificity, and accuracy in distinguishing penumbra from infarcted core. Corresponding values for white matter are generally lower because of decreased metabolic needs.[196]

CT perfusion imaging is not without pitfalls. Current technology provides less cranial coverage than MR imaging (2–8 slices), although this will likely change with the advent of 256-detector CT. Small lacunar or subcortical strokes may be missed despite excellent accuracy with large territorial strokes.[180] Analysis and postprocessing are somewhat dependent on operator choice of arterial or venous region of interest.[198] CT perfusion also subjects patients to ionizing radiation. Although the radiation dose incurred by first-generation CT perfusion was roughly similar or less than that of a whole-head noncontrast CT,[199] this is not necessarily true with current multidetector CT; and investigators have examined ways of further reducing radiation dose by increasing scan intervals.[200]

Modern 64-slice CT scanners can provide near-DSA quality images of cervicocerebral vascular anatomy, with "arch-to-vertex" acquisition and analysis time of approximately 5 minutes for CT angiography. Combined CT, CT angiographic, and CT perfusion imaging is therefore now a routine part of a "CT Stroke Protocol" at the authors' institution, permitting treatment triage with knowledge of both the anatomy and physiology underlying acute cerebral ischemia within 15 minutes and <130 mL of iodinated contrast material. Other groups[179,180,201] have similarly noted benefits of combined CT angiography and CT perfusion imaging in rapid assessment of acute stroke, and Smith et al.[202] have demonstrated the safety of this approach without prior determination of a serum creatinine level.

Magnetic Resonace Imaging. MR imaging possesses two key advantages over CT in acute stroke: better soft-tissue resolution and increased sensitivity to water in tissue. The first attribute provides superior images of vasogenic edema associated with early (8–12 hours) stroke using conventional T2-weighted or fluid-attenuated inversion recovery sequences. Parenchymal edema is particularly well highlighted by fluid-attenuated inversion recovery sequences, which suppress confounding signal from free CSF. In particular, strokes that are small/lacunar or in brainstem/posterior fossa regions (otherwise poorly imaged by conventional CT owing to beam-hardening artifacts from the skull base) are better visualized on MR imaging. The second attribute forms the foundation of modern diffusion-weighted MR imaging (DWI) in ultra-early (<6 hours) stroke by using sequences that are sensitive to the diffusion of water molecules. DWI has a superior sensitivity (97%) and specificity (100%) to conventional MR imaging and noncontrast CT imaging in acute stroke.[203] At specialized centers, acute stroke MR imaging can be accomplished quickly, with some groups documenting 15 to 20 minutes door-to-door time.[204]

Similar to CT, MR imaging also provides clinicians with perfusion and angiographic images. Perfusion-weighted MR imaging (PWI) is based on tracking the arrival, peak, and washout of gadolinium and provides relative values for CBF, CBV, and MTT. Mismatch between MR DWI and PWI (DWI–PWI mismatch) is thought to represent ischemic penumbra at risk. Such MR perfusion data currently form the basis for several clinical trials attempting to extend the time window for IV thrombolysis. The addition of MR angiography provides clinicians with further information by visualizing the entire vascular tree, arch to vertex, in rotatable three-dimensional and multiplanar-reformatted projections.

MR imaging has several disadvantages. Concern for metal implants, increased susceptibility to motion artifact, difficulties with a relatively closed environment with respect to patients on mechanical ventilation or multiple intravenous drips, and recent FDA regulatory concerns regarding renal function in gadolinium-enhanced studies have all led to increased time screening for and then spent in the MR imaging suite, when compared to CT imaging. MR perfusion provides only relative estimates of CBF, CBV, and MTT, whereas CT perfusion provides absolute values that have been validated against Xenon-CT and PET.[205] Recent reports have dampened the enthusiasm for accuracy of MR perfusion in predicting true penumbra,[206,207] and DWI lesions may, at least in part, be reversible (reviewed in Schellinger et al.[208]). In some cases, MR imaging may even fail to show CT-documented hypoattenuation in lesions that are destined for infarction (the so called "reverse discrepancy").[209]

As discussed in the previous section, recent developments in CT perfusion have increased sensitivity for acute stroke; and at least one manufacturer currently markets equipment capable of near-complete (8 cm) cranial coverage. Furthermore, at least at the authors' institution, CT angiography has been found to be significantly better than MR angiography with respect to resolution, detail, and avoidance of common MR artifacts secondary to low or turbulent flow phenomena and vessel calcification. Because all stroke patients are usually first screened at our institution with emergent noncontrast CT (to determine hemorrhagic versus ischemic stroke and/or eligibility for IV or IA thrombolysis), we have found it relatively simple to proceed with the extra 10 minutes and <130 mL of contrast material necessary to provide CT perfusion and CT angiography information that has significantly influenced our decision making in stroke.

Digital Subtraction Angiography. DSA remains the "gold standard" for the assessment of cerebral vasculature in terms of resolution and flow information. DSA provides direct visualization of collateral cerebrovascular supply, and increased pial collaterals from the ACA territory in MCA stroke have been shown to correlate with lower final infarct volumes and better mRS scores at discharge.[210] However, catheter angiography takes time to organize and perform, whereas modern CT perfusion or CT angiographic imaging can provide preintervention cross-sectional maps of collateral supply, along with near-DSA quality images within 10 to 15 minutes. It must be kept in mind that DSA is not a prerequisite to and should not delay decisions regarding IV thrombolysis. As such, its use should be restricted to cases in which IA treatment is planned and should be performed at the institution capable of providing such treatment in order to avoid delays in therapy. Barr[211] has recommended the following when DSA is contemplated for the evaluation of acute stroke:

1. The study must be performed on a machine capable of true DSA and road-map imaging.
2. Efficient diagnostic technique is important to minimize contrast use because under emergent circumstances most patients are relatively dehydrated and may need subsequent intervention.
3. Primary ischemic territory should be imaged first, with relevant collateral supply visualized only as needed.
4. A "parenchygram" (high-contrast windowing of the capillary phase imaging) should be obtained to demonstrate areas of poor perfusion.
5. Proper sedation and blood-pressure management are critical: intubation may be necessary for patients with posterior fossa strokes in whom the level of consciousness or possibility of aspiration is a concern, those with left hemispheric strokes having language disability that may prevent them from being cooperative, or when a patient is restless or unable to cooperate or obtunded.

At the authors' institution, initial imaging of acute stroke is generally performed with noncontrast CT, proceeding immediately to CT angiographic or CT perfusion imaging if hemorrhage is not detected. IV thrombolysis is then rapidly administered if the patient is a suitable candidate and endovascular therapy is not contemplated. Should endovascular intervention be indicated—based on stroke severity (NIHSS score), proximal vessel occlusion, and large area of brain at risk—arrangements are rapidly made for cerebral angiography, with or without bridging IV rt-PA. MR imaging is generally performed acutely for small strokes not visualized on the initial CT scan or CT perfusion images or as part of a subsequent etiological workup to document final extent of stroke, evidence of previous strokes, hypertensive small vessel changes, and/or multiterritory infarcts suggestive of a cardioembolic rather than an arterioembolic cause.

• INTRACRANIAL ATHEROSCLEROSIS

Epidemiology

The true prevalence of intracranial stenosis is not well known, as no study has tested a large population-based cross-sectional sample for angiographically verifiable stenosis. Huang et al.[212] examined 1068 asymptomatic Chinese subjects with transcranial ultrasound and found 63 subjects (5.9%) had stenosis of the MCA. The overall prevalence of intracranial stenosis is higher in subjects who have suffered from any form of cerebrovascular ischemia: Wityk et al.[213] found that 22% to 24% of patients presenting with TIA or stroke had at least one intracranial lesion with ≥50% stenosis. Within this population, men had a higher prevalence of intracranial stenosis than women (29% vs. 14%, although both had a prevalence of 8% when symptomatic lesions alone were considered). Whites had more extracranial carotid artery disease (33% vs. 15%), but exhibited the same prevalence of intracranial stenosis.

Several studies of consecutive patients presenting with stroke or TIA estimate the incidence of symptomatic intracranial stenosis to be between 2.7 and 8% (Table 23-3).[213–215] When adjusted for age, education, diabetes, and cholesterol status, no significant racial differences were

TABLE 23-3. Incidence of Symptomatic Intracranial Stenosis in Large Consecutive Series of Patients Presenting with Stroke or TIA.*

Reference	No. of Patients	Angiography (%)	Symptomatic Intracranial Stenosis (%)
Sacco et al.[214] (1995)	438	45	8
Wityk et al.[213] (1996)	274	14	8
Thijs et al.[215] (2000)	1344	35	2.7

*Angiographic validation was not routinely obtained.

apparent.[214] Similarly, the risk of subsequent future stroke is not affected by race.[216] Younger age, insulin-dependent diabetes, and hypercholesterolemia favor intracranial rather than extracranial stenosis as a cause of the presenting stroke.[214]

Imaging

Given the challenges of accurately assessing vascular stenoses within the cranium, the gold standard remains cerebral angiography. In the Warfarin-Aspirin Symptomatic Intracranial Disease Study (WASID) study, which represents the best understanding of the natural history of intracranial stenosis to date, all patients were required to undergo angiography to accurately quantify the area of most severe stenosis.[217] This was then expressed as a percentage of the normal lumen proximally, distally, or on a feeding artery (in order of preference, should the first two segments also be diseased).[217] With current-generation 64-detector CT equipment, CT angiography represents the most accurate means of noninvasive imaging of the intracranial circulation. CT angiography has been shown to be vastly superior to MR angiography in sensitivity (98% vs. 70%) and PPV (93% vs. 65%), and equal or better than DSA (the latter particularly in slow-flow posterior circulation disease).[218] Most recently, the Stroke Outcomes and Neuroimaging of Intracranial Atherosclerosis trial (running concurrently with WASID as a sister trial) prospectively examined 407 patients from WASID across 46 centers in the United States, and found PPVs of only 36% and 59% for TCD and MR angiography, respectively, when compared against angiographically verified intracranial stenosis.[219] This may be explained by the absence of suitable cranial windows and operator dependence for TCD and flow or calcification artifacts that affect MR angiography. At the authors' institution, high-resolution three-dimensional DSA or CT angiography is primarily used as a screening test, with subsequent angiography usually performed with an intention to treat.

Natural History and Medical Management

Screening for asymptomatic intracranial stenosis is infrequently done and long-term follow up for this condition even less so. Consequently, few large series have specifically addressed the prognosis of asymptomatic intracranial stenosis. Komotar et al.[220] reviewed a large number of (small and mostly retrospective) series and concluded that the annual stroke rate for asymptomatic individuals was markedly less than for patients presenting with a stroke or TIA. Kremer et al.[221] examined 50 patients with incidental MCA stenosis and found a 0% annual risk of stroke or TIA, although only 12 of 50 patients had stenosis >50% by TCD criteria. Takahashi et al.[222] evaluated 2924 asymptomatic individuals who were not receiving any antiplatelet or anticoagulant therapy and identified those with intracranial stenosis (≥50% by MR angiography) and extracranial stenosis (ascertained by Doppler ultrasonography). Over a mean follow-up period of 63 months, the authors found the annual rate of ipsilateral ischemic events to be 1.1%, 0.6%, and 0.2% in patients with intracranial stenosis, in patients with intracranial but without extracranial stenosis, and in patients without any intracranial or extracranial stenosis, respectively. It may therefore be concluded that the excess stroke risk contributed by isolated asymptomatic intracranial stenosis alone is small.

Although the natural history of asymptomatic intracranial stenosis appears to be relatively benign, the natural history of symptomatic stenosis is believed to be much worse. Symptomatic patients are thus almost universally treated with various antiplatelet or anticoagulant agents. Consequently, series examining the "natural history" of intracranial stenosis actually reflect the outcome of medical management of symptomatic intracranial stenosis. Most literature on this topic has usually involved retrospective analysis of a relatively small number of patients. However, two recent prospective multicenter investigations stand out (Table 23-4), notably the WASID and Groupe d'Etude des Sténoses Intra-Crâniennes Athéromateuses symptomatiques (GESICA) studies. The investigators of the GESICA study performed follow-up in 102 patients with symptomatic intracranial stenosis ≥50% (63% of which were verified angiographically) for a mean of 23.4 months and examined the risk of recurrent stroke despite medical treatment.[223] The WASID investigators randomized 569 patients with angiographically verified symptomatic intracranial stenosis ≥50% to aspirin or warfarin and found no benefit for treatment with the latter.[224] WASID represents the largest series to date (prospective or otherwise) and with 100% angiographic verification and more than 4 years of follow-up, its conclusions represent the current gold standard for our understanding of the natural history of medically treated symptomatic intracranial stenosis. The population and overall results of WASID[216,224,225] and GESICA[223] were remarkably similar, with the key findings (also summarized in Table 23-4) being the following:

1. Risk of future stroke is markedly higher for intracranial stenosis of 70% to 99% versus 50% to 69% (Figure 23-8).
2. Risk of future stroke is markedly higher for patients presenting with stroke versus TIA.
3. Risk of future stroke is primarily early (median of 2 months from index event in GESICA, majority within 30 days in WASID (Figure 23-8).
4. Risk of future stroke is not affected by territory (anterior vs. posterior) of presenting event.
5. Risk of future stroke is not affected by whether patients were on antithrombotic medications at time of presenting event or not (WASID data[224]).

This data has important implications for interventional trials in symptomatic intracranial stenosis: one must determine which proportion of patients has ≥70% stenosis, how many present with stroke rather than TIA, and how early intervention should take place. For example, it may

TABLE 23-4. Summary of Studies Consisting of Patients with Stroke or Transient Ischemic Attack Attributable to Intracranial Stenosis ≥50%*

Study	Relevant Enrollment Criteria	No. Pts	Age (yrs)	Post. Circ.	Stroke as Qualifying Event (%)	Proportion of Stenosis ≥70%	Mean Stenosis (%)	Time to Tx (days)	30-Day TIA, Stroke, Death (%)	Ipsilateral TIA, Stroke, Death @ 1 yr (%)	@ 2 yr (%)	Other (mo)
Stenting												
ASSIST[237] (2007)	• Age 18–75, NIHSS <9 • ≥1 atherosclerosis risk factor	46	54	42	32.6	52%	NR	19.5	8.7	8.8	8.8	
Fiorella et al.[235] (2007)	• Consecutive patients • 95% failed antithrombotics • balloon-mounted coronary stents	44	64.8	100	NR	85%	82.5	NR	26.1	NR	NR	(43.5) 15%
Jiang et al.[233] (2007)	• ≥1 Vascular risk factors • >90% failed antithrombotics	121 92	52.4 53.2	41 31	38.1 36.2	All ≥70% All <70%	NR NR	49.9 53.1	4.8[†] 4.3[†]	7.2[†] 5.3[†]	8.2 8.3	
Jiang et al.[231] (2007)	• Consecutive patients,** 90/95% (BA/VA) failed antithrombotics	38 41	59 58	BA VA	34.2 36.6	71% 56%	76 70	34 41	5.1 1	9[‡] 1[‡]	NR	
Wingspan study[298] (2007)	• Age 18–80, mRS ≤3 • all failed antithrombotics	45	66	51	93.3	NR	74.9	NR	4.5	9.3	NR	(6) 7.1%
SSYLVIA[238] (2004)	• Age 18–80, mRS ≤3 • no ICH <30 d • no ipsilateral stroke >1/3 territory	61 43[†]	63.6	67 54[§]	60.7	NR	69.9	72.8	6.6 6.6[§]	13.1 14[§]	NR	
Angioplasty												
Marks et al.[239] (2006)	• Retrospective, across three institutions • 98% already on antiplatelet or anticoagulant therapy	120	62.3	49	55	92.5%	82.2	NR (~4–6 wk if stroke)	5.8	~9[¶]	~10[¶]	(60) ~11%[¶]
Marks et al.[299] (2005)	• Consecutive patients • failed antithrombotics	36	62.2	58	14	NR	84.2	NR	8.3	11.1	NR	(60) 15.3%

Study	Criteria										
WASID (2005–2006)[216][224,225]	• Age ≥40, mRS ≤3 • TIA/stroke within 90 d • all treated with ASA or warfarin • 100% angiographic verification	569	63.6	44	61 →Stroke only →Stroke only →TIA only →TIA only	37% →≥70% →<70% →≥70% →<70%	64	17	NA	11 →23 →8 →14 →3	14 →25 →11 →14 →8
GESICA[223] (2006)	• Age 18–80, mRS ≤2, NIHSS <15 • event within 6 mon • ≥2 vascular risk factors • all treated with antithrombotics • 63% angiographic verification	102	63.3	48	51.6	NR	NR	NA	NA	NR	13.7%
Qureshi et al.[300] (2003)	• Survivors of VBA TIA/stroke • retrospective, multicenter • 86% treated w/ antithrombotics • 65% angiographic verification	102	64	100	68.6	NR	NR	NA	NR	NR	7.8% (15)

*All studies included only patients with stroke or TIA attributable to intracranial stenosis ≥50%; All studies included 100% angiographic verification of degree of stenosis unless otherwise noted; Where treatment was used, results are only for elective patients (series including acute stroke are not included). Treatment with antithrombotics refers to any combination of antiplatelets and/or anticoagulants; Age/Time to treatment: Mean (or median, if mean is not reported); Wingspan: Wingspan self-expanding stent (Boston Scientific, Natick, MA); SSYLVIA: Neurolink balloon angioplasty, Neurolink balloon-mounted stent (Guidant Corporation, Menlo Park, CA); ASSIST: Apollo balloon-mounted stent (MicroPort Medical, Shanghai, China); GESICA: Data regarding medical treatment only.

† Perioperative and 1- and 2-year event rates do not include an additional 2.4% and 6.4% immediate perioperative event rate of asymptomatic SAH or ischemia requiring emergent intervention (for 70%–99% and 50%–69% stenoses, respectively).

‡ Authors report events per patient-years of cumulative follow up. Because stroke risk is higher closer to the index event, use of a fixed annual stroke rate represented by events per patient-years of cumulative follow up may underestimate the true early risk of stroke.

§ SSYLVIA results for intracranial stenting alone.

¶ Stroke rates are estimated from Figure 1 in the work of Marks et al.[239]

** Patients reported here form part of an overall group additionally reported by Jiang et al.[233] in their second publication in 2007. Both reports are subdivided by location or stenosis percentage to highlight specific differential risks and natural history. Stroke vs. TIA.

ASA, aspirin; ASSIST, Apollo Stent for Symptomatic atherosclerotic Intracranial Stenosis Treatment; BA, basilar artery; GESICA, Groupe d'Etude des Sténoses Intra-Crâniennes Athéromateuses symptomatiques; ICH, intracranial hemorrhage; mRS, modified Rankin scale; NIHSS, National Institutes of Health Stroke Scale; NA, not applicable; NR, not reported; SAH, subarachnoid hemorrhage; SSYLVIA, Stenting of Symptomatic Atherosclerotic Lesions in the Vertebral or Intracranial Arteries; TIA, transient ischemic attack; tx, treatment; VA, vertebral artery; VBA, vertebrobasilar artery; WASID, Warfarin-Aspirin Symptomatic Intracranial Disease Study.

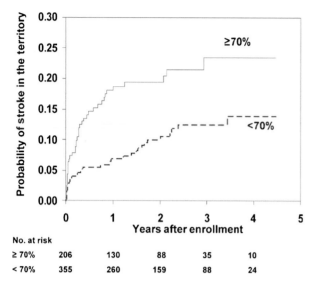

● FIGURE 23-8. Natural history of intracranial stenosis. Kaplan-Meier plot of probability of future stroke within territory of symptomatic stenosed artery showing significant difference (*p* < 0.001 log rank test) between intracranial stenoses ≥70% vs. <70%. Note the steep rise in the probability of a stroke within the first month.

Reproduced with permission from Kasner SE, Chimowitz MI, Lynn MJ, et al. Predictors of ischemic stroke in the territory of a symptomatic intracranial arterial stenosis. Circulation. 2006;113(4):555-563.

be difficult to improve upon the natural history of a patient presenting with a TIA and only 50% intracranial stenosis, particularly if months have passed from the initial event (Table 23-4). There are parallels between these findings from WASID and the conclusions from the North American Symptomatic Carotid Endarterectomy Trial[226,227] regarding symptomatic *extracranial* carotid disease: intracranial stenosis ≥70% carries a much higher risk than stenoses between 50% and 69%, presentation with stroke carries a grimmer prognosis than presentation with TIA, risk of recurrent stroke is early on, and stroke risk increases linearly with worsening intracranial stenosis from 50% to 89% but then decreases somewhat with critical stenosis of 90% to 99%, reminiscent of the near-occlusion category of extracranial carotid stenosis in the North American Symptomatic Carotid Endarterectomy Trial.

Endovascular Management

Intervention for symptomatic intracranial stenosis is now primarily accomplished by endovascular rather than open surgical means. The multicenter randomized EC–IC arterial bypass study conclusively demonstrated that surgical bypass worsened outcome in patients with MCA stenosis,[228] and surgical bypass of other cerebrovascular territories is considered even more technically difficult with concomitantly increased risk. As a result, bypass is now infrequently performed (usually within trials[229]) for chronic cerebral ischemia only when there is complete arterial occlusion and/or failure of endovascular management.

Endovascular treatment of intracranial atherosclerosis was advanced by the early pioneering work of Connors and Wojak,[230] who demonstrated good clinical results and increased safety using technical modifications including slow balloon inflation and balloon undersizing during intracranial angioplasty. Table 23-4 lists patient demographics and outcomes of modern large series examining intracranial angioplasty/stenting for symptomatic stenosis. Degree of stenosis (≥70% or <70%), presentation (TIA vs. stroke), and time to treatment are highlighted because of the critical importance of these factors in determining benefit over natural history where intervention was performed. Annual rates of ipsilateral stroke or TIA after endovascular treatment range between 5% and 14%, with most results clustering around 8% to 10% (with the exception of one report for vertebral stenting alone).[231] These results are in line with those from the most recent Cochrane metareview, which examined 1999 patients with angiographic stenosis ≥50% and found a perioperative stroke or death rate of 9.5%, with a further 5.6% at 1 year.[232]

A large proportion of ischemic events occur early after intervention, with risk factors including initial presentation with stroke rather than TIA,[233] presence of previous perforator stroke on MR imaging (8.2% vs. 0.8% risk of subsequent perforator stroke),[234] and use of balloon-mounted coronary stents in the posterior circulation (26.1% perioperative neurological mortality and morbidity).[235]

Restenosis >50% after intracranial stenting for symptomatic stenosis occurs in approximately one-third of patients across multiple studies and devices: 29.7% at a mean of 5.9 months for the Wingspan stent (Boston Scientific, Natick, MA),[236] 28% at a median of 7.4 months for the Apollo stent (MicroPort Medical, Shanghai, China),[237] and 32.4% at 6 months for the Neurolink stent (Guidant Corporation, Menlo Park, CA).[238] Results from angioplasty alone are not dissimilar: Marks et al.[239] noted 23.9% restenosis at a mean of 20 months after angioplasty (although only 58% of patients underwent angiographic follow up). This suggests that a significant proportion of intracranial plaques may show restenosis following intervention with current methods. A preliminary report suggests drugeluting stents may incur less restenosis (5% at a median of 4 months); however, 10% of stents could not be deployed and an overall perioperative complication rate of 12% was encountered.[240]

At present, conclusive evidence favoring intracranial stenting (± angioplasty) versus angioplasty alone for symptomatic intracranial atherosclerosis does not exist. Importantly, when comparing results from either technique to those with medical treatment alone (Table 23-4), the importance of rigorous patient selection becomes apparent: the patient presenting with nondisabling stroke caused by intracranial stenosis ≥70% is likely to derive significantly more benefit from early intervention than the patient presenting with TIA caused by stenosis of 50%. As techniques improve and intracranial-specific devices such as the Wingspan stent (Figure 23-9) undergo further

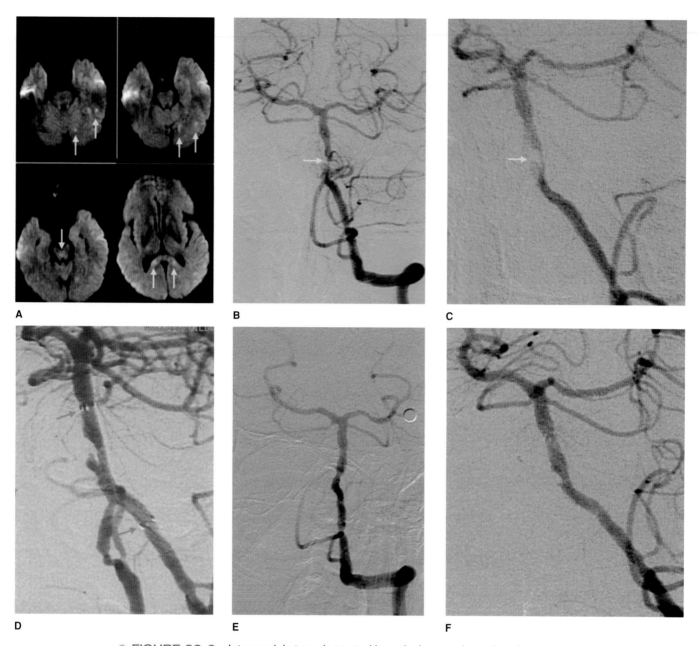

● **FIGURE 23-9.** Intracranial stenosis treat with angioplasty and stenting. A 63-year-old hypertensive diabetic male presented with (A) multiple BA strokes (*arrows*) while on warfarin. (B and C) Cerebral angiography demonstrated severe (>80%) stenosis of the mid-BA (*arrow* shown in both images). (D) He was treated with Gateway balloon angioplasty and Wingspan stenting (*arrows* show end of stent), (E and F) with excellent angiographic and clinical outcome at 6 months.

refinement, a trial of medical versus endovascular therapy may be justified. Future therapies will likely evolve beyond simple angioplasty ± stenting such as miniaturized atherectomy devices and/or eventually biological therapies alone.

● INTRACRANIAL ARTERIAL DISSECTION

Arterial dissection is known to occur in connective tissue disorders such as Marfan and EDS and fibromuscular dys-

plasia. There are six types of EDS; type IV is known as the vascular EDS caused by the high risk of arterial rupture or dissection in this subset. This disorder involves a structural defect in type III collagen.[241] Trauma tends to be the predisposing factor in the development of dissection in the extracranial arteries but not in the intracranial vessels. Most reported intracranial dissections have involved the posterior circulation. In extracranial dissection, pain may precede ischemic symptoms by several days. Intracranial dissection in adults usually presents with pain and neurological deficits simultaneously.[242] Cerebral hypoperfusion is thought to be the main mechanism for stroke in this setting, compared to thromboembolism in extracranial dissection.

The most common cause of childhood stroke is idiopathic.[243,244] However, with advanced noninvasive imaging, we may see that more cases of idiopathic stroke are actually caused by intracranial arterial dissection. Although pain is a frequent component of cerebral arterial dissection in adults, it is an inconsistent marker in children. Intracranial dissections in children tend to be spontaneous and occur mostly in males.[245,246] It is possible that some of the spontaneous dissections are because of an unknown defect of collagen.[247]

Intracranial dissections can lead to significant arterial stenosis or occlusion with subsequent ischemia or pseudoaneurysm formation. Pseudoaneurysm formation is likely because of the thin media layer in these arteries. The natural history of intracranial dissections is poorly understood; therefore, the most effective treatment has not been established. Intracranial dissecting aneurysms present most commonly with ischemic symptoms or SAH.[248] Dissecting aneurysms are most likely to involve the VA, and SAH is the presentation in the majority of these patients.[249] In contrast, most intracranial dissections in children occur in the anterior circulation.[245]

Historical data suggests a high stroke rate associated with intracranial dissections. Mortality from these strokes approaches 75% in some reports.[248,250,251] More favorable results have been reported in recent years with treatment.[242] Because the natural history is unknown and because of the high risk for ischemic sequelae, intracranial dissections are treated at our institution. Historical treatment options include medical management with antiplatelet agents or anticoagulants. Surgical treatment typically involves parent vessel sacrifice with or without bypass. Endovascular options have emerged recently including stenting of the dissected segment with coiling if there is an associated pseudoaneurysm. Although endovascular sacrifice of the vessel with coils is an option, the new reconstructive techniques with stents are attractive.[252,253]

● MISCELLANEOUS

Moyamoya Disease and Variants

Moyamoya disease is a chronic, occlusive cerebrovascular condition first reported in 1957. The term "moyamoya" refers to the "puffy" or "hazy" angiographic appearance of the collaterals that form in the setting of chronic ICA stenosis or occlusion.[254] Angiographic findings of moyamoya disease were first reported in 1963. To diagnose moyamoya disease, the following angiographic and clinical criteria must be fulfilled: (1) stenosis or occlusion of the ICA terminus bilaterally, (2) moyamoya vessels at the skull base, and (3) unknown etiology. It is important to stress that the cause of true moyamoya disease is unknown. However, moyamoya angiographic changes can occur in numerous other settings such as intracranial atherosclerosis, cranial irradiation, neurofibromatosis, tuberculosis, and sickle cell anemia.[255] Terms such as "moyamoya syndrome," "quasi-moyamoya disease," and "angiographic moyamoya" have been applied to these cases with known etiologies. Histological examination of moyamoya disease demonstrates fibrous thickening of the intima of the terminal ICA. Lipid deposits are seen occasionally within the proliferative intima.[256] Other prominent microscopic features are the tortuosity and duplication of the internal elastic lamina. Atherosclerotic plaque is not a feature of moyamoya disease.[257]

Patients with moyamoya disease typically present with TIAs or ischemic strokes. Intracranial hemorrhages occur less frequently. Although the disease can occur in all ages, the peak incidence is in children younger than the age of 10 years.[258] Although it has been described worldwide, there is a higher incidence of moyamoya disease in the Japanese and Koreans. A positive family history can be found in 10% of patients.[258] There is no known cure for moyamoya disease. Medical management involves antiplatelet or anticoagulation therapy. Surgical treatment of moyamoya disease, usually reserved for patients with recurrent symptoms while receiving medical therapy, involves direct or indirect bypass procedures. A bypass from the STA to a cortical branch of the MCA is the most commonly used direct procedure. In children, especially those younger than the age of 2 years, the STA is very small, and direct bypasses are difficult to perform. However, indirect bypasses have been effective in this population. Despite their formidable names, encephalo-duro-arterio-synangiosis and encephalo-myo-synangiosis are relatively straightforward procedures. In the encephalo-duro-arterio-synangiosis, the STA is dissected and placed directly on the pial surface of the brain. The encephalo-myo-synangiosis involves applying the temporalis muscle directly to the pial surface. The result of both indirect procedures is sprouting of collateral vessels in the ischemic brain territory.[259]

Hemorrhagic moyamoya disease is more common in adulthood. Increased hemodynamic stress within the fragile collaterals seen in moyamoya is thought to result in rupture of these vessels. Very small aneurysms occurring on these collateral vessels can also be a source of recurrent hemorrhage (Figure 23-10).[260] The prognosis is poorer for hemorrhagic moyamoya than for its ischemic counterpart. Mortality increases from 5% for the first hemorrhage to 25% for a second episode.[261] Management of these patients is focused on the prevention of rehemorrhage. Bypass surgery has been proposed to relieve the burden on these collaterals and thus reduce the risk of rehemorrhage.[260] Unfortunately, surgery does not appear to be as promising for hemorrhagic disease as it is for ischemia. In one retrospective survey of patients with hemorrhagic moyamoya disease, 28.3% of those treated conservatively developed recurrent hemorrhage, whereas 19.1% of patients who underwent surgery (direct or indirect bypass) suffered from recurrence.[262] Although surgery reduced recurrent hemorrhage in certain patients, the study failed to show statistical significance when compared to medical management.

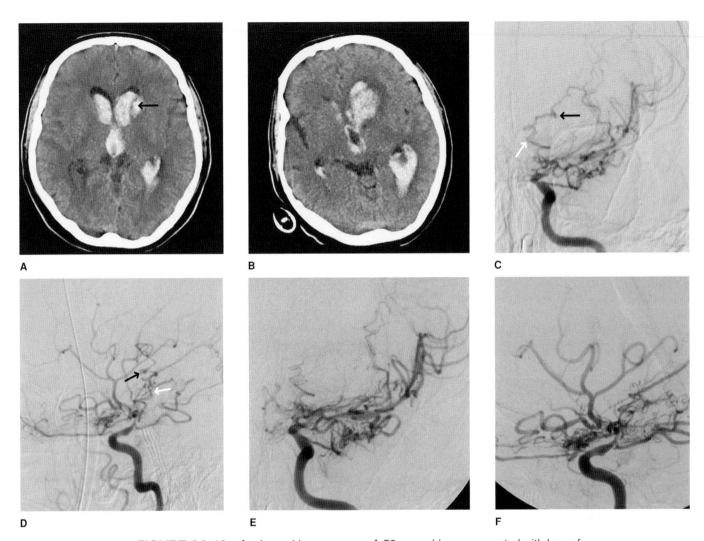

● **FIGURE 23-10.** Angiographic moyamoya. A 58-year-old man presented with loss of consciousness. Upon awakening, he had severe right hemiparesis and dysarthria. Noncontrast cranial (A) CT scan showed hemorrhage in the head of the left caudate nucleus (*arrow*) and diffuse intraventricular hemorrhage. The patient was managed with external ventricular drainage and recovered well. However, 2 weeks later, he developed sudden onset of coma and recurrent right hemiparesis. A follow-up (B) CT scan showed similar, recurrent hemorrhage. Cerebral angiography showed moyamoya changes bilaterally. (C) Anteroposterior and (D) lateral projections of the left common carotid artery injection demonstrated severe stenosis of the ICA terminus with the typical moyamoya appearance of collateral formation—a tiny aneurysm (*black arrow* shown in both images) is seen on a prominent medial lenticulostriate branch (*white arrow* shown in both images). This was likely the source of the recurrent hemorrhage. The patient was managed medically and recovered again. Angiography—(E) anteroposterior and (F) lateral—was repeated 1 week later, and there was no filling of the aneurysm or the distal medial lenticulostriate artery.

Vasculitis of the Central Nervous System (CNS)

Vasculitis is an inflammatory disorder of arteries and veins of all sizes. Structural vascular injuries can be seen histologically, and ischemia can occur in territories supplied by these vessels. CNS vasculitis may occur alone or may be associated with systemic vasculitic and connective tissue disorders. Primary angiitis (or vasculitis) of the CNS occurs without a known cause and is quite rare. In contrast, the more common secondary CNS vasculitis occurs in the setting of

known system diseases.[263] A basic diagnostic workup of all suspected CNS vasculitis includes analysis of CSF, thorough serology, and CT or MR imaging of the brain. Vasculitic lesions are nonspecific on MR imaging, but they are typically multifocal and bilateral and involve gray and white matter. In certain cases, catheter-based DSA and brain biopsy may be necessary for diagnosis. Angiographic features of vasculitis include segmental arterial stenosis, beading, occlusions, prolonged circulation time, and collateral formation in multiple territories (Figure 23-11).[264,265] Like noninvasive

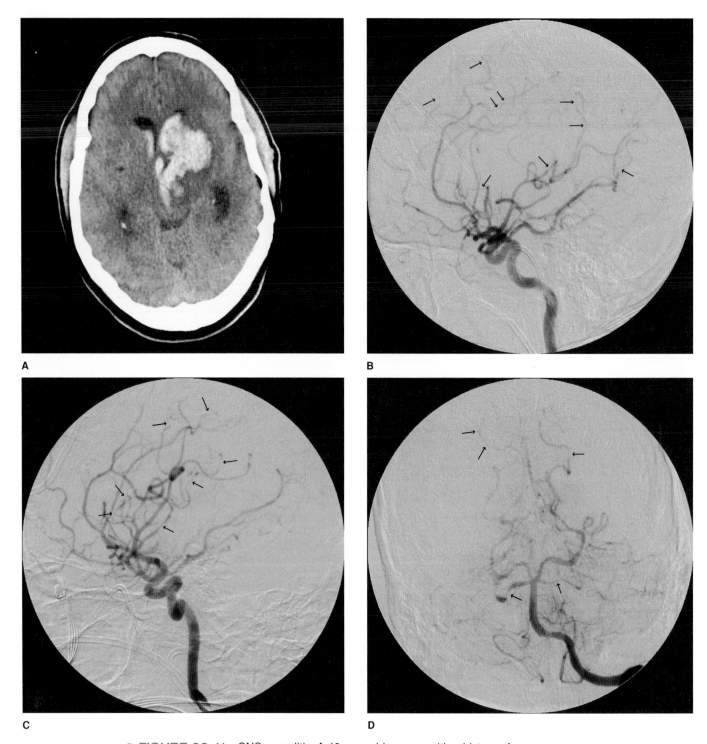

● **FIGURE 23-11.** CNS vasculitis. A 40-year-old woman with a history of myeloproliferative disorder presented with sudden onset of coma and right hemiparesis. Noncontrast cranial (A) CT scan demonstrated a large left basal ganglia hemorrhage with intraventricular extension. The patient did not have a history of hypertension, and an angiogram was performed to evaluate a source of the hemorrhage. (B) Lateral view of a right common carotid injection showed several focal areas of dilatation and stenosis in both the anterior and MCA territories (*arrows*). These findings were also noted on the (C) left carotid artery and (D) left VA injections (*arrows*). The angiographic findings were consistent with CNS vasculitis and the patient was started on high-dose intravenous steroid therapy. However, the patient's neurological examination never improved and she died within 10 days of admission.

studies, angiography is neither sensitive nor specific for vasculitis. A first angiogram may be diagnostic for vasculitis in less than 60% of cases.[264] However, serial cerebral angiography may be useful for monitoring the efficacy of therapy.[265]

Primary vasculitis of the CNS has been known by other names in the past, including isolated CNS vasculitis and granulomatous angiitis of the CNS. Primary CNS vasculitis (angiitis) is a more appropriate name as fewer than 50% of cases are truly granulomatous.[266] Although rare, this disease is important because of its often progressive and fatal outcome.[264] Cerebral ischemia with focal or multifocal infarction is the most common clinical presentation of primary CNS angiitis. However, ICH and SAH may result from focal angionecrosis.[264,267] Cerebral angiography is not a sensitive diagnostic test, and a normal angiogram does not necessarily exclude vasculitis.[268] Histological features of this disorder include segmental granulomatous lesions with a predominantly lymphocytic infiltrate. Up to 25% of cases have necrotizing vasculitic changes, similar to those seen in polyarteritis nodosa.[266]

Secondary CNS vasculitis is associated with systemic conditions including infections, malignancies, lymphoproliferative diseases, system connective tissue disorders, systemic vasculitides, drug hypersensitivity, or illicit drug use.[263] As a comprehensive review of these conditions is beyond the scope of this discussion, we will focus only on the salient features of secondary vasculitis. Vasculitis occurring with infection is usually caused by direct angioinvasion by the microorganism or because of the inflammatory host response to the infection. Infection-associated vasculitis is typically a small-vessel lymphocytic rather than necrotizing vasculitic response.[269] CNS vasculitis may complicate leukemias and other myeloproliferative disorders.

CNS manifestations in systemic lupus erythematosus is variable but may be as high as 75% of cases, although a noninflammatory vasculopathy is more common than true vasculitis.[270] CNS vasculitis is rarely associated with scleroderma, Sjögren's syndrome, and rheumatoid arthritis. Sarcoidosis affects the CNS in 5% of patients, but vasculitic changes are relatively uncommon. Behçet's syndrome is a systemic disease with well-documented CNS manifestations. Findings include venous thrombosis, demyelination, and a small cell lymphocytic vasculitis.[263]

Involvement of the CNS in systemic vasculitic diseases is variable. For example, CNS small-vessel necrotizing vasculitis is second only to renal complications as the cause of mortality in polyarteritis nodosa.[271] On the other hand, intracerebral involvement of the well-known and temporal (giant cell) arteritis is very uncommon.[263] Necrotizing vasculitis is also seen in illicit drug abuse. Widely recognized first in methamphetamine abusers, CNS vasculitis has been reported in cocaine, ephedrine, and heroin users as well.[272]

Amyloid Angiopathy

Cerebral amyloid angiopathy is caused by deposition of β-amyloid in the media and adventitia of the small arteries of the cerebral cortex. The classic histological appearance is congophilic with yellow-green birefringence under polarized light.[273] Although this pathological entity was recognized a century ago, its role in the lobar cerebral hemorrhages in elderly persons has been defined only in the past 30 years. Amyloid angiopathy often accompanies extracellular amyloid deposition in the form of plaques.[273] This histological substrate is also seen in Alzheimer's and other types of dementia. Amyloid angiopathy is responsible for asymptomatic cortical petechial hemorrhages, seen in most patients with amyloid-related lobar hemorrhages.[274] The incidence of cerebral amyloid angiopathy is age dependent and occurs rarely before the age of 55 years. As hypertension has become better controlled in the general population, the role of amyloid angiopathy in ICH has become more prominent. CT scans show classic lobar distribution of ICH (Figure 23-12). Gradient-echo sequences on MR imaging can identify petechial hemorrhages, allowing a presumptive diagnosis of amyloid angiopathy.[275]

● CEREBROVASCULAR MALFORMATIONS

Classification

Traditionally classified as AVMs, capillary telangiectasias, cavernous angiomas, and venous angiomas,[276] intracranial vascular malformations comprise a diverse and not entirely related group of diseases. A more systemic classification (adapted from Osborn, 1999[11]) divides cerebrovascular malformations by the location and type of nidus:

1. Dural
   a. DAVF
2. Cerebral
   a. with arteriovenous shunting
      i. AVM
         • plexiform nidus
         • mixed nidus (plexiform + fistulous)
      ii. AVF
         • single or multiple fistulae
         • mono- or multipedicular
   b. without arteriovenous shunting
      i. capillary malformation—also known as capillary telangiectasia
      ii. cavernous malformation—also known as cavernous angioma
      iii. venous malformation
         • developmental venous anomaly (DVA)
         • venous varix (but without associated AVM or AVF)

Dural Arteriovenous Fistulae

DAVF consist of an abnormal direct communication, located within the dura, between dural arterial vessels and dural veins. They are relatively rare, representing 10% to 15% of intracranial vascular malformations.[277] DAVF are believed to be acquired lesions, likely related to cerebral venous hypertension secondary to idiopathic or iatrogenic venous stenosis, occlusion, or thrombosis.[278] The nature

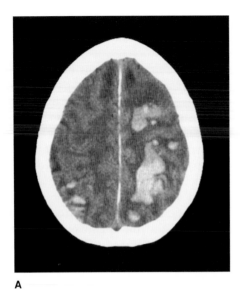 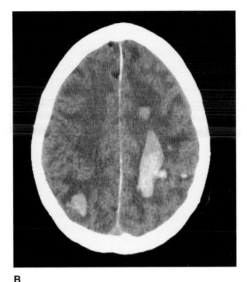

A   B

● **FIGURE 23-12.** Amyloid angiopathy. This 77-year-old woman presented with sudden onset on lethargy and right hemiplegia. Noncontrast (A and B) CT scans showed ICH bilaterally but mostly in the left frontal and parietal lobes. Cerebral angiography did not demonstrate any arteriovenous malformation or DAVF (not shown). This allowed for a presumptive diagnosis of amyloid angiopathy given the patient's age and lobar distribution of ICH. Consequently, brain biopsy was not done.

of the final venous outflow is key in the current Borden classification[279] of DAVF and our understanding of their presentation and natural history[280–282] (Table 23-5). Borden type I lesions are generally considered benign lesions, although a small risk (2%) exists that they may develop retrograde leptomeningeal venous drainage over time and thus progress to type II or III, mandating close observation of these patients.[281] Borden type II to III lesions have an ominous prognosis, requiring treatment to disconnect the retrograde leptomeningeal drainage by endovascular or surgical means.

Cerebral Arteriovenous Malformations and Fistulae

Cerebral AVMs consist of an entangled anastomosis of blood vessels with arteriovenous shunting within a central nidus with feeding arteries and draining veins. The nidus itself may be plexiform (AVM, most common), fistulous (AVF, i.e., a direct shunt without a true interposed "nidus," much more rare), or mixed. Classically, AVMs have a characteristic wedge shape with an apex at the ependymal surface of the lateral ventricle and the base of the wedge parallel to the overlying cerebral convexity. The prevalence of symptomatic cerebral AVMs is estimated to be 15 per 100 000 adults, whereas autopsy studies suggest an overall prevalence of 400 to 600 per 100 000, consistent with the low incidence of newly diagnosed AVMs at 1 to 2 per 100 000 per year.[283]

Approximately two-thirds of AVMs are diagnosed by presentation of the patient with ICH; another 18% to 27% of patients will present with seizure; and the rest are found in roughly equal proportions either incidentally or during workup for headaches or focal neurological deficits.[284] The subsequent natural history has proven contentious in the literature. Overall, unruptured AVMs have

TABLE 23-5. Venous Outflow of Dural Arteriovenous Fistulae Relative to Borden Classification, Presentation, and Natural History

Venous Outflow	Borden Type[279]	Relative Frequency[280] (%)	Presentation[280]		Natural History[281,282]		
			ICH (%)	NHND (%)	ICH	NHND	Mortality
RLVD	III	28	48	31	8.1% per year	6.9% per year	10.4% per year
DVS + RLVD	II	18	28	39	Similar to type III (above)		
DVS	I	54	0	2	ICH in only 1 of 68 patients followed conservatively for mean of 28 months[281]		

DVS, dural venous sinus; RLVD, retrograde leptomeningeal venous drainage; ICH, intracerebral hemorrhage; NHND, nonhemorrhagic neurological deficit.

TABLE 23-6. Spetzler-Martin[286] Grading for AVM*

Factor	Score
Size	
0–3 cm	+1
3–6 cm	+2
>6 cm	+3
Location in brain	
Noneloquent	+0
Eloquent	+1
Venous drainage	
Superficial alone	+0
Deep ± superficial	+1

Points are added for each anatomic feature, resulting in a grading score ranging from 1 to 5.

approximately 2% per year risk of hemorrhage, whereas ruptured AVMs have a higher risk of rehemorrhage (~6% per year), at least in the first year.[283–285] Factors that have been reported to be associated with increased risk of future AVM rupture include initial hemorrhagic presentation, older age, deep brain location, exclusive venous drainage, venous stenoses, and arterial aneurysms.[283–285]

Outcome following microsurgical resection of AVM can be predicted by the size, location, and venous drainage of the lesion as denoted by the Spetzler-Martin classification (Table 23-6),[286] with grades 4 to 5 incurring significant (>20%) permanent major morbidity.[287] As a result, patients harboring unruptured grade 4 or 5 AVMs undergo follow up expectantly at some centers.[288] With the addition of radiosurgical and endovascular tools, the proportion of AVMs amenable to successful and relatively safe obliteration has increased. Small (<3 cm) AVMs that are deep or within eloquent brain can be treated with radiosurgery, and preoperative endovascular embolization is now routinely used to facilitate subsequent surgery or radiotherapy by reducing the arterial supply and/or nidal volume.[289] Most AVMs are thereby now treated with multimodal therapy, with a combination of microsurgery, radiosurgery, and/or endovascular embolization being used (or at least considered).[290] Importantly, the initial decision to treat an AVM and the subsequent choice of method(s) require careful consideration of the specific procedural morbidities, the patient's age, and the institutional strengths at the treating facility.

Other

Cavernous malformations (also known as *cavernomas*) refer to abnormally enlarged collections of blood vessels without intervening brain parenchyma, characterized by endothelialized sinusoidal cavities without media or adventitia. Angiographically occult, these lesions are best seen on MR imaging. Cavernomas are rare (prevalence of approximately 0.5% to 0.7% on autopsy or MR imaging studies), are likely congenital but may be familial in up to 20% of patients (particularly Hispanics), and are often associated with a *DVA*, as described below.[291] Patients with cavernomas commonly present with seizures (36%), hemorrhage (25%), focal neurological deficits (20%), or headaches alone (6%).[292] Owing to their relative rarity, published annual hemorrhage rates vary, but most reports suggest an annual risk of ~0.5% to 1% for cavernomas without previous hemorrhage.[291] The hemorrhage rate is likely higher for those initially presenting with hemorrhage (4.5% in one study),[293] for deep-seated versus superficial lesions,[292] and for brainstem cavernomas.[294] Treatment generally consists of observation for patients with small, superficial, asymptomatic cavernomas and surgery for accessible lesions in patients with symptomatic hemorrhage or medically refractory seizures. Some have advocated radiotherapy for these lesions,[295] although this remains controversial.[291]

DVAs, also known as venous angiomas, are benign congenital anomalies of the cerebral venous drainage system. They are characterized by abnormally enlarged medullary venous channels centered on a draining venous trunk to resemble spokes around an umbrella stem. DVAs are the most common intracranial vascular malformation, with an overall incidence of 2% to 4%.[296] It is important to remember that a DVA drains normal brain and is a functional part of the individual's cerebral venous system. As such, isolated DVA are likely entirely benign,[296] with a very low symptomatic hemorrhage rate (0.34% per year) believed to be secondary to the known association of some DVAs with cavernomas.[297]

Capillary telangiectasia refers to collections of thin-walled, ectatic vascular channels resembling capillaries, with intervening brain parenchyma. Most frequently seen in the pons and basal ganglia, they are sporadic, angiographically occult benign lesions primarily found at autopsy or on MR imaging. Symptomatic capillary telangiectasia is rarely described, and no treatment is warranted.[291]

The orbit is primarily supplied by the ophthalmic artery. This artery is generally considered the first branch of the ICA as it exits the cavernous sinus. It enters the orbit through the optic foramen. Uncommonly, the ophthalmic artery may be a branch of the middle meningeal artery (branch of the ECA).

The central retinal artery is a branch of the ophthalmic artery. Both the central retinal artery and branch retinal arteries may become occluded. Central retinal artery occlusion manifests by painless and profound visual loss. It is virtually always unilateral, but may present at a later time in the contralateral eye.

Central retinal artery occlusion is most commonly caused by atherosclerotic plaque from carotid artery lesions. These may manifest as amaurosis fugax and funduscopically as Hollenhorst plaques. Other etiologies include a cardioembolic source, vasculitis, and small artery disease associated with hypertension and diabetes. Additional etiologies include hematological disorders, including sickle cell disease, hypercoagulable states, and hyperviscosity syndromes that are occasionally seen with leukemia and other hematologic malignancies.

Outcome for branch retinal artery occlusion may be better than central retinal artery occlusion. Central retinal artery occlusion is an ophthalmologic emergency and aggressive efforts should be made to reestablish the flow.

REFERENCES

1. Khurana VG, Smith LA, Weiler DA, et al. Adenovirus-mediated gene transfer to human cerebral arteries. *J Cereb Blood Flow Metab.* 2000;20(9):1360-1371.

2. Lee RM. Morphology of cerebral arteries. *Pharmacol Ther.* 1995;66(1):149-173.

3. Stephens RB, Stilwell DL. *Arteries and Veins of the Human Brain.* Springfield, IL: Charles C. Thomas; 1969.

4. Glynn LE. Medial defects in the circle of Willis and their relation to aneurysm formation. *J Pathol Bacteriol.* 1940;51:213-221.

5. Walmsley JG, Canham PB. Orientation of nuclei as indicators of smooth muscle cell alignment in the cerebral artery. *Blood Vessels.* 1979;16(1):43-51.

6. Zervas NT, Liszczak TM, Mayberg MR, Black PM. Cerebrospinal fluid may nourish cerebral vessels through pathways in the adventitia that may be analogous to systemic vasa vasorum. *J Neurosurg.* 1982;56(4):475-481.

7. Hassler O. Morphological studies on the large cerebral arteries, with reference to the aetiology of subarachnoid haemorrhage. *Acta Psychiatr Scand Suppl.* 1961;154:1-145.

8. Krayenbuhl H, Yasargil M. *Cerebral Angiography.* New York, NY: Thieme; 1982.

9. Morris PP. *Practical Neuroangiography.* 2nd ed. Philadelphia, PA: Lippincott Williams & Wilkins; 2007.

10. Osborn A. *Diagnostic Cerebral Angiography.* 1st ed. Philadelphia, PA: Lippincott Williams & Wilkins; 1998.

11. Osborn A. *Diagnostic Cerebral Angiography.* 2nd ed. Philadelphia, PA: Lippincott Williams & Wilkins; 1999.

12. Wojak JC. Fundamental neurovascular anatomy. In: Connors JJ, Wojak JC, eds. *Interventional Neuroradiology: Strategies and Practical Techniques.* Philadelphia, PA: Saunders; 1999:77-83.

13. Marinkovic S, Gibo H, Brigante L, Milisavljevic M, Donzelli R. *Arteries of the Brain and Spinal Cord: Anatomic Features and Clinical Significance.* Avellino, Italy: De Angelis Editore; 1997.

14. Stehbens WE. Histopathology of cerebral aneurysms. *Arch Neurol.* 1963;8:272-285.

15. Stehbens WE. *Pathology of Cerebral Blood Vessels.* St. Louis, MO: CV Mosby; 1972.

16. Wiebers DO, Whisnant JP, Sundt TM Jr, O'Fallon WM. The significance of unruptured intracranial saccular aneurysms. *J Neurosurg.* 1987;66(1):23-29.

17. Sekhar LN, Heros RC. Origin, growth, and rupture of saccular aneurysms: a review. *Neurosurgery.* 1981;8(2):248-260.

18. Canham PB, Finlay HM, Tong SY. Stereological analysis of the layered collagen of human intracranial aneurysms. *J Microsc.* 1996;183(pt 2):170-180.

19. Chyatte D. Pathology of intracranial aneurysms. In: LeRoux PD, Winn HR, Newell DW, eds. *Management of Cerebral Aneurysms.* Philadelphia, PA: Saunders; 2004:89-98.

20. Steiger HJ. Pathophysiology of development and rupture of cerebral aneurysms. *Acta Neurochir Suppl (Wien).* 1990;48:1-57.

21. Bruno G, Todor R, Lewis I, Chyatte D. Vascular extracellular matrix remodeling in cerebral aneurysms. *J Neurosurg.* 1998;89(3):431-440.

22. van der Wal AC, Becker AE, Das PK. Medial thinning and atherosclerosis—evidence for involvement of a local inflammatory effect. *Atherosclerosis.* 1993;103(1):55-64.

23. Schievink WI, Michels VV, Piepgras DG. Neurovascular manifestations of heritable connective tissue disorders. A review. *Stroke.* 1994;25(4):889-903.

24. Schievink WI. Genetics and aneurysm formation. *Neurosurg Clin N Am.* 1998;9(3):485-495.

25. De Braekeleer M, Perusse L, Cantin L, Bouchard JM, Mathieu J. A study of inbreeding and kinship in intracranial aneurysms in the Saguenay Lac-Saint-Jean region (Quebec, Canada). *Ann Hum Genet.* 1996;60(pt 2):99-104.

26. Gaist D, Vaeth M, Tsiropoulos I, et al. Risk of subarachnoid haemorrhage in first degree relatives of patients with subarachnoid haemorrhage: follow up study based on national registries in Denmark. *BMJ.* 2000;320(7228):141-145.

27. Ronkainen A, Miettinen H, Karkola K, et al. Risk of harboring an unruptured intracranial aneurysm. *Stroke.* 1998;29(2):359-362.

28. Schievink WI, Schaid DJ, Michels VV, Piepgras DG. Familial aneurysmal subarachnoid hemorrhage: a community-based study. *J Neurosurg.* 1995;83(3):426-429.

29. Raaymakers TW, Rinkel GJ, Ramos LM. Initial and follow-up screening for aneurysms in families with familial subarachnoid hemorrhage. *Neurology.* 1998;51(4):1125-1130.

30. Ronkainen A, Puranen MI, Hernesniemi JA, et al. Intracranial aneurysms: MR angiographic screening in 400 asymptomatic individuals with increased familial risk. *Radiology.* 1995;195(1):35-40.

31. Bonita R. Cigarette smoking, hypertension and the risk of subarachnoid hemorrhage: a population-based case-control study. *Stroke.* 1986;17(5):831-835.

32. Knekt P, Reunanen A, Aho K, et al. Risk factors for subarachnoid hemorrhage in a longitudinal population study. *J Clin Epidemiol.* 1991;44(9):933-939.

33. Longstreth WT Jr, Nelson LM, Koepsell TD, van Belle G. Cigarette smoking, alcohol use, and subarachnoid hemorrhage. *Stroke.* 1992;23(9):1242-1249.

34. Qureshi AI, Suri MF, Yahia AM, et al. Risk factors for subarachnoid hemorrhage. *Neurosurgery.* 2001;49(3):607-613.

35. Taylor CL, Yuan Z, Selman WR, Ratcheson RA, Rimm AA. Cerebral arterial aneurysm formation and rupture in 20767 elderly patients: hypertension and other risk factors. *J Neurosurg.* 1995;83(5):812-819.

36. Phillips LH II, Whisnant JP, O'Fallon WM, Sundt TM Jr. The unchanging pattern of subarachnoid hemorrhage in a community. *Neurology.* 1980;30(10):1034-1040.

37. Stapf C, Mast H, Sciacca RR, et al. The New York Islands AVM Study: design, study progress, and initial results. *Stroke.* 2003;34(5):e29-33.

38. Sarti C, Tuomilehto J, Salomaa V, et al. Epidemiology of subarachnoid hemorrhage in Finland from 1983 to 1985. *Stroke.* 1991;22(7):848-853.

39. Giroud M, Milan C, Beuriat P, et al. Incidence and survival rates during a two-year period of intracerebral and subarachnoid haemorrhages, cortical infarcts, lacunes and transient ischaemic attacks. The Stroke Registry of Dijon: 1985–1989. *Int J Epidemiol.* 1991;20(4):892-899.

40. Longstreth WT, Nelson LM, Koepsell TD, van Belle G. Subarachnoid hemorrhage and hormonal factors in women. A population-based case-control study. *Ann Intern Med.* 1994; 121(3):168-173.

41. Broderick JP, Brott T, Tomsick T, Huster G, Miller R. The risk of subarachnoid and intracerebral hemorrhages in blacks as compared with whites. *N Engl J Med.* 1992;326(11):733-736.

42. Labovitz DL, Halim AX, Brent B, Boden-Albala B, Hauser WA, Sacco RL. Subarachnoid hemorrhage incidence among Whites, Blacks and Caribbean Hispanics: the Northern Manhattan Study. *Neuroepidemiology.* 2006;26(3):147-150.

43. Housepian EM, Pool JL. A systematic analysis of intracranial aneurysms from the autopsy file of the Presbyterian Hospital, 1914 to 1956. *J Neuropathol Exp Neurol.* 1958;17(3):409-423.

44. Atkinson JL, Sundt TM Jr, Houser OW, Whisnant JP. Angiographic frequency of anterior circulation intracranial aneurysms. *J Neurosurg.* 1989;70(4):551-555.

45. Rinkel GJ, Djibuti M, Algra A, van Gijn J. Prevalence and risk of rupture of intracranial aneurysms: a systematic review. *Stroke.* 1998;29(1):251-256.

46. Johnston SC, Selvin S, Gress DR. The burden, trends, and demographics of mortality from subarachnoid hemorrhage. *Neurology.* 1998;50(5):1413-1418.

47. International Study of Unruptured Intracranial Aneurysms Investigators. Unruptured intracranial aneurysms—risk of rupture and risks of surgical intervention. *N Engl J Med.* 1998;339(24):1725-1733.

48. Wiebers DO, Whisnant JP, Huston J III, et al. Unruptured intracranial aneurysms: natural history, clinical outcome, and risks of surgical and endovascular treatment. *Lancet.* 2003; 362(9378):103-110.

49. Ecker RD, Hopkins LN. Natural history of unruptured intracranial aneurysms. *Neurosurg Focus.* 2004;17(5):E4.

50. Mocco J, Komotar RJ, Lavine SD, Meyers PM, Connolly ES, Solomon RA. The natural history of unruptured intracranial aneurysms. *Neurosurg Focus.* 2004;17(5):E3.

51. Juvela S, Porras M, Poussa K. Natural history of unruptured intracranial aneurysms: probability of and risk factors for aneurysm rupture. *J Neurosurg.* 2000;93(3):379-387.

52. Day AL. Aneurysms of the ophthalmic segment. A clinical and anatomical analysis. *J Neurosurg.* 1990;72(5):677-691.

53. van der Wee N, Rinkel GJ, Hasan D, van Gijn J. Detection of subarachnoid haemorrhage on early CT: is lumbar puncture still needed after a negative scan? *J Neurol Neurosurg Psychiatry.* 1995;58(3):357-359.

54. Vespa PM, Bleck TP. Neurogenic pulmonary edema and other mechanisms of impaired oxygenation after aneurysmal subarachnoid hemorrhage. *Neurocrit Care.* 2004;1(2):157-170.

55. Wintermark M, Uske A, Chalaron M, et al. Multislice computerized tomography angiography in the evaluation of intracranial aneurysms: a comparison with intraarterial digital subtraction angiography. *J Neurosurg.* 2003;98(4):828-836.

56. Agid R, Lee SK, Willinsky RA, Farb RI, Terbrugge KG. Acute subarachnoid hemorrhage: using 64-slice multidetector CT angiography to "triage" patients' treatment. *Neuroradiology.* 2006;48(11):787-794.

57. Linskey ME, Sekhar LN, Hirsch W Jr, Yonas H, Horton JA. Aneurysms of the intracavernous carotid artery: clinical presentation, radiographic features, and pathogenesis. *Neurosurgery.* 1990;26(1):71-79.

58. Ferrante L, Fortuna A, Celli P, Santoro A, Fraioli B. Intracranial arterial aneurysms in early childhood. *Surg Neurol.* 1988;29(1):39-56.

59. Norris JS, Wallace MC. Pediatric intracranial aneurysms. *Neurosurg Clin N Am.* 1998;9(3):557-563.

60. Allison JW, Davis PC, Sato Y, et al. Intracranial aneurysms in infants and children. *Pediatr Radiol.* 1998;28(4):223-229.

61. Sanai N, Quinones-Hinojosa A, Gupta NM, et al. Pediatric intracranial aneurysms: durability of treatment following microsurgical and endovascular management. *J Neurosurg.* 2006;104(2 suppl):82-89.

62. Ojemann RG. Infectious intracranial aneurysms. In: Ojemann RG, Ogilvy CS, Crowell RM, eds. *Surgical Management of Neurovascular Disease.* Baltimore, MD: Williams & Wilkins; 1995:368.

63. Molinari GF, Smith L, Goldstein MN, Satran R. Pathogenesis of cerebral mycotic aneurysms. *Neurology.* 1973;23(4):325-332.

64. Barrow DL, Prats AR. Infectious intracranial aneurysms: comparison of groups with and without endocarditis. *Neurosurgery.* 1990;27(4):562-573.

65. Morawetz RB, Karp RB. Evolution and resolution of intracranial bacterial (mycotic) aneurysms. *Neurosurgery.* 1984;15(1):43-49.

66. Benoit BG, Wortzman G. Traumatic cerebral aneurysms. Clinical features and natural history. *J Neurol Neurosurg Psychiatry.* 1973;36(1):127-138.

67. Soria ED, Paroski MW, Schamann ME. Traumatic aneurysms of cerebral vessels: a case study and review of the literature. *Angiology.* 1988;39(7, pt 1):609-615.

68. Aarabi B. Management of traumatic aneurysms caused by high-velocity missile head wounds. *Neurosurg Clin N Am.* 1995;6(4):775-797.

69. Parkinson D, West M. Traumatic intracranial aneurysms. *J Neurosurg.* 1980;52(1):11-20.

70. du Trevou M, Bullock R, Teasdale E, Quin RO. False aneurysms of the carotid tree due to unsuspected penetrating injury of the head and neck. *Injury.* 1991;22(3):237-239.

71. Hemphill JC III, Gress DR, Halbach VV. Endovascular therapy of traumatic injuries of the intracranial cerebral arteries. *Crit Care Clin.* 1999;15(4):811-829.

72. Lee CY, Yim MB, Kim IM, Son EI, Kim DW. Traumatic aneurysm of the supraclinoid internal carotid artery and an associated carotid-cavernous fistula: vascular reconstruction performed using intravascular implantation of stents and coils. Case report. *J Neurosurg.* 2004;100(1):115-119.

73. David CA, Vishteh AG, Spetzler RF, Lemole M, Lawton MT, Partovi S. Late angiographic follow-up review of surgically treated aneurysms. *J Neurosurg.* 1999;91(3):396-401.

74. Britz GW, Salem L, Newell DW, Eskridge J, Flum DR. Impact of surgical clipping on survival in unruptured and ruptured cerebral aneurysms: a population-based study. *Stroke.* 2004;35(6):1399-1403.

75. Raaymakers TW, Rinkel GJ, Limburg M, Algra A. Mortality and morbidity of surgery for unruptured intracranial aneurysms: a meta-analysis. *Stroke.* 1998;29(8):1531-1538.

76. Lanterna LA, Tredici G, Dimitrov BD, Biroli F. Treatment of unruptured cerebral aneurysms by embolization with guglielmi detachable coils: case-fatality, morbidity, and effectiveness in preventing bleeding—a systematic review of the literature. *Neurosurgery.* 2004;55(4):767-778.

77. Hayakawa M, Murayama Y, Duckwiler GR, Gobin YP, Guglielmi G, Vinuela F. Natural history of the neck remnant of a cerebral aneurysm treated with the Guglielmi detachable coil system. *J Neurosurg.* 2000;93(4):561-568.

78. Raymond J, Guilbert F, Weill A, et al. Long-term angiographic recurrences after selective endovascular treatment of aneurysms with detachable coils. *Stroke.* 2003;34(6):1398-1403.

79. Samson D, Batjer HH, Kopitnik TA Jr. Current results of the surgical management of aneurysms of the basilar apex. *Neurosurgery.* 1999;44(4):697-704.

80. Murayama Y, Nien YL, Duckwiler G, et al. Guglielmi detachable coil embolization of cerebral aneurysms: 11 years' experience. *J Neurosurg.* 2003;98(5):959-966.

81. Molyneux A, Kerr R, Stratton I, et al. International Subarachnoid Aneurysm Trial (ISAT) of neurosurgical clipping versus endovascular coiling in 2143 patients with ruptured intracranial aneurysms: a randomised trial. *Lancet.* 2002;360(9342):1267-1274.

82. Mueller-Kronast N, Jahromi BS. Endovascular treatment of ruptured aneurysms and vasospasm. *Curr Treat Options Neurol.* 2007;9(2):146-157.

83. Johnston SC, Wilson CB, Halbach VV, et al. Endovascular and surgical treatment of unruptured cerebral aneurysms: comparison of risks. *Ann Neurol.* 2000;48(1):11-19.

84. Bergvall U, Steiner L, Forster DM. Early pattern of cerebral circulatory disturbances following subarachnoid haemorrhage. *Neuroradiology.* 1973;5(1):24-32.

85. Weir B, Grace M, Hansen J, Rothberg C. Time course of vasospasm in man. *J Neurosurg.* 1978;48(2):173-178.

86. Dorsch NWC, King MT. A review of cerebral vasospasm in aneurysmal subarachnoid haemorrhage. Part I: incidence and effects. *J Clin Neurosci.* 1994;1:19-26.

87. Haley EC Jr, Kassell NF, Apperson-Hansen C, Maile MH, Alves WM. A randomized, double-blind, vehicle-controlled trial of tirilazad mesylate in patients with aneurysmal subarachnoid hemorrhage: a cooperative study in North America. *J Neurosurg.* 1997;86(3):467-474.

88. Kassell NF, Haley EC Jr, Apperson-Hansen C, Alves WM. Randomized, double-blind, vehicle-controlled trial of tirilazad mesylate in patients with aneurysmal subarachnoid hemorrhage: a cooperative study in Europe, Australia, and New Zealand. *J Neurosurg.* 1996;84(2):221-228.

89. Petruk KC, West M, Mohr G, et al. Nimodipine treatment in poor-grade aneurysm patients. Results of a multicenter double-blind placebo-controlled trial. *J Neurosurg.* 1988;68(4):505-517.

90. Saito I, Ueda Y, Sano K. Significance of vasospasm in the treatment of ruptured intracranial aneurysms. *J Neurosurg.* 1977;47(3):412-429.

91. Kassell NF, Torner JC, Haley EC Jr, Jane JA, Adams HP, Kongable GL. The International Cooperative Study on the Timing of Aneurysm Surgery. Part 1: overall management results. *J Neurosurg.* 1990;73(1):18-36.

92. Fisher CM, Kistler JP, Davis JM. Relation of cerebral vasospasm to subarachnoid hemorrhage visualized by computerized tomographic scanning. *Neurosurgery.* 1980;6(1):1-9.

93. Kistler JP, Crowell RM, Davis KR, et al. The relation of cerebral vasospasm to the extent and location of subarachnoid blood visualized by CT scan: a prospective study. *Neurology.* 1983;33(4):424-436.

94. Reilly C, Amidei C, Tolentino J, Jahromi BS, Macdonald RL. Clot volume and clearance rate as independent predictors of vasospasm after aneurysmal subarachnoid hemorrhage. *J Neurosurg.* 2004;101(2):255-261.

95. Macdonald RL, Weir BK. A review of hemoglobin and the pathogenesis of cerebral vasospasm. *Stroke.* 1991;22(8):971-982.

96. Mayberg MR, Okada T, Bark DH. The role of hemoglobin in arterial narrowing after subarachnoid hemorrhage. *J Neurosurg.* 1990;72(4):634-640.

97. Weir B, Macdonald RL, Stoodley M. Etiology of cerebral vasospasm. *Acta Neurochir Suppl.* 1999;72:27-46.

98. Findlay JM, Weir BK, Kanamaru K, Espinosa F. Arterial wall changes in cerebral vasospasm. *Neurosurgery.* 1989;25(5):736-746.

99. Macdonald RL, Weir BK, Grace MG, Martin TP, Doi M, Cook DA. Morphometric analysis of monkey cerebral arteries exposed in vivo to whole blood, oxyhemoglobin, methemoglobin, and bilirubin. *Blood Vessels.* 1991;28(6):498-510.

100. Mayberg MR, Okada T, Bark DH. The significance of morphological changes in cerebral arteries after subarachnoid hemorrhage. *J Neurosurg.* 1990;72(4):626-633.

101. Barker FGII, Ogilvy CS. Efficacy of prophylactic nimodipine for delayed ischemic deficit after subarachnoid hemorrhage: a metaanalysis. *J Neurosurg.* 1996;84(3):405-414.

102. Dorhout Mees SM, Rinkel GJ, Feigin VL, et al. Calcium antagonists for aneurysmal subarachnoid haemorrhage. *Cochrane Database Syst Rev.* 2007(3):CD000277.

103. Dorsch NWC. A review of cerebral vasospasm in aneurysmal subarachnoid haemorrhage: II. Management. *J Clin Neurosci.* 1994;1:78-92.

104. Tettenborn D, Dycka J. Prevention and treatment of delayed ischemic dysfunction in patients with aneurysmal subarachnoid hemorrhage. *Stroke*. 1990;21(12 suppl):IV85-89.

105. Jahromi BS, Macdonald RL. Vasospasm: diagnosis and medical management. In: Le Roux PD, Winn HR, Newell D, eds. *Management of Cerebral Aneurysms*. Philadelphia, PA: Saunders-Elsevier; 2004:455-487.

106. Macdonald RL. Cerebral vasospasm. *Neurosurg Q*. 1995;5:73-97.

107. Kaku Y, Yonekawa Y, Tsukahara T, Kazekawa K. Superselective intra-arterial infusion of papaverine for the treatment of cerebral vasospasm after subarachnoid hemorrhage. *J Neurosurg*. 1992;77(6):842-847.

108. Kassell NF, Helm G, Simmons N, Phillips CD, Cail WS. Treatment of cerebral vasospasm with intra-arterial papaverine. *J Neurosurg*. 1992;77(6):848-852.

109. Badjatia N, Topcuoglu MA, Pryor JC, et al. Preliminary experience with intra-arterial nicardipine as a treatment for cerebral vasospasm. *AJNR Am J Neuroradiol*. 2004;25(5):819-826.

110. Feng L, Fitzsimmons BF, Young WL, et al. Intraarterially administered verapamil as adjunct therapy for cerebral vasospasm: safety and 2-year experience. *AJNR Am J Neuroradiol*. 2002;23(8):1284-1290.

111. Zubkov YN, Nikiforov BM, Shustin VA. Balloon catheter technique for dilatation of constricted cerebral arteries after aneurysmal SAH. *Acta Neurochir (Wien)*. 1984;70(1-2):65-79.

112. Terry A, Zipfel G, Milner E, et al. Safety and technical efficacy of over-the-wire balloons for the treatment of subarachnoid hemorrhage-induced cerebral vasospasm. *Neurosurg Focus*. 2006;21(3):E14.

113. Zwienenberg-Lee M, Hartman J, Rudisill N, Muizelaar JP. Endovascular management of cerebral vasospasm. *Neurosurgery*. 2006;59(5, suppl 3):S139-S147.

114. Mackay J, Mensah G. *The Atlas of Heart Disease and Stroke*. Geneva, Switzerland: World Health Organization; 2004:50-53.

115. Rosamond W, Flegal K, Friday G, et al. Heart disease and stroke statistics—2007 update: a report from the American Heart Association Statistics Committee and Stroke Statistics Subcommittee. *Circulation*. 2007;115(5):e69-e171.

116. Sacco RL. Pathogenesis, classification, and epidemiology of cerebrovascular disease. In: Rowland LP, ed. *Merritt's Neurology*. 11th ed. Philadelpha, PA: Lippincott Williams & Wilkins; 2005:275-290.

117. Brust JCM. Cerebral infarction. In: Rowland LP, ed. *Merritt's Neurology*. 11th ed. Philadelpha, PA: Lippincott Williams & Wilkins; 2005:295-303.

118. Moulin DE, Lo R, Chiang J, Barnett HJ. Prognosis in middle cerebral artery occlusion. *Stroke*. 1985;16(2):282-284.

119. Qureshi AI, Suarez JI, Yahia AM, et al. Timing of neurologic deterioration in massive middle cerebral artery infarction: a multicenter review. *Crit Care Med*. 2003;31(1):272-277.

120. Hacke W, Kaste M, Bougousslavsky J, et al. for the European Stroke Initiative (EUSI) Executive Committee and the EUSI Writing Committee. European Stroke Initiative recommendations for stroke management – update 2003. *Cerebrovasc Dis*. 2003;16:311-337.

121. Gupta R, Connolly ES, Mayer S, Elkind MS. Hemicraniectomy for massive middle cerebral artery territory infarction: a systematic review. *Stroke*. 2004;35(2):539-543.

122. Schwab S, Steiner T, Aschoff A, et al. Early hemicraniectomy in patients with complete middle cerebral artery infarction. *Stroke*. 1998;29(9):1888-1893.

123. Vahedi K, Hofmeijer J, Juettler E, et al. Early decompressive surgery in malignant infarction of the middle cerebral artery: a pooled analysis of three randomised controlled trials. *Lancet Neurol*. 2007;6(3):215-222.

124. Berge E. Decompressive surgery for cerebral oedema after stroke: evidence at last. *Lancet Neurol*. 2007;6(3):200-201.

125. Hornig CR, Rust DS, Busse O, Jauss M, Laun A. Space-occupying cerebellar infarction. Clinical course and prognosis. *Stroke*. 1994;25(2):372-374.

126. Adams HP Jr, del Zoppo G, Alberts MJ, et al. Guidelines for the early management of adults with ischemic stroke: a guideline from the American Heart Association/American Stroke Association Stroke Council, Clinical Cardiology Council, Cardiovascular Radiology and Intervention Council, and the Atherosclerotic Peripheral Vascular Disease and Quality of Care Outcomes in Research Interdisciplinary Working Groups: the American Academy of Neurology affirms the value of this guideline as an educational tool for neurologists. *Stroke*. 2007;38(5):1655-1711.

127. The National Institute of Neurological Disorders and Stroke rt-PA Stroke Study Group. Tissue plasminogen activator for acute ischemic stroke. *N Engl J Med*. 1995;333(24):1581-1587.

128. Bateman BT, Schumacher HC, Boden-Albala B, et al. Factors associated with in-hospital mortality after administration of thrombolysis in acute ischemic stroke patients: an analysis of the nationwide inpatient sample 1999 to 2002. *Stroke*. 2006;37(2):440-446.

129. Dubinsky R, Lai SM. Mortality of stroke patients treated with thrombolysis: analysis of nationwide inpatient sample. *Neurology*. 2006;66(11):1742-1744.

130. The National Institute of Neurological Disorders and Stroke (NINDS) rt-PA Stroke Study Group. Effect of intravenous recombinant tissue plasminogen activator on ischemic stroke lesion size measured by computed tomography. *Stroke*. 2000;31(12):2912-2919.

131. Fagan SC, Morgenstern LB, Petitta A, et al. Cost-effectiveness of tissue plasminogen activator for acute ischemic stroke. NINDS rt-PA Stroke Study Group. *Neurology*. 1998;50(4):883-890.

132. Tomsick TA. Intravenous thrombolysis for acute ischemic stroke. *J Vasc Interv Radiol*. 2004;15(1, pt 2):S67-S76.

133. Ingall TJ, O'Fallon WM, Asplund K, et al. Findings from the reanalysis of the NINDS tissue plasminogen activator for acute ischemic stroke treatment trial. *Stroke*. 2004;35(10):2418-2424.

134. Albers GW, Bates VE, Clark WM, Bell R, Verro P, Hamilton SA. Intravenous tissue-type plasminogen activator for treatment of acute stroke: the Standard Treatment with Alteplase to Reverse Stroke (STARS) study. *JAMA*. 2000;283(9):1145-1150.

135. Graham GD. Tissue plasminogen activator for acute

ischemic stroke in clinical practice: a meta-analysis of safety data. *Stroke.* 2003;34(12):2847-2850.

136. Hacke W, Donnan G, Fieschi C, et al. Association of outcome with early stroke treatment: pooled analysis of ATLANTIS, ECASS, and NINDS rt-PA stroke trials. *Lancet.* 2004;363 (9411):768-774.

137. NINDS t-PA Stroke Study Group. Intracerebral hemorrhage after intravenous t-PA therapy for ischemic stroke. *Stroke.* 1997;28(11):2109-2118.

138. Larrue V, von Kummer RR, Muller A, Bluhmki E. Risk factors for severe hemorrhagic transformation in ischemic stroke patients treated with recombinant tissue plasminogen activator: a secondary analysis of the European-Australasian Acute Stroke Study (ECASS II). *Stroke.* 2001;32(2):438-441.

139. Wahlgren N, Ahmed N, Davalos A, et al. Thrombolysis with alteplase for acute ischaemic stroke in the Safe Implementation of Thrombolysis in Stroke-Monitoring Study (SITS-MOST): an observational study. *Lancet.* 2007;369 (9558):275-282.

140. Zangerle A, Kiechl S, Spiegel M, et al. Recanalization after thrombolysis in stroke patients: predictors and prognostic implications. *Neurology.* Jan 2, 2007;68(1):39-44.

141. Berrouschot J, Rother J, Glahn J, Kucinski T, Fiehler J, Thomalla G. Outcome and severe hemorrhagic complications of intravenous thrombolysis with tissue plasminogen activator in very old (> or = 80 years) stroke patients. *Stroke.* 2005;36(11):2421-2425.

142. Tanne D, Gorman MJ, Bates VE, et al. Intravenous tissue plasminogen activator for acute ischemic stroke in patients aged 80 years and older: the tPA stroke survey experience. *Stroke.* 2000;31(2):370-375.

143. van Oostenbrugge RJ, Hupperts RM, Lodder J. Thrombolysis for acute stroke with special emphasis on the very old: experience from a single Dutch centre. *J Neurol Neurosurg Psychiatry.* 2006;77(3):375-377.

144. Anon. Generalized efficacy of t-PA for acute stroke. Subgroup analysis of the NINDS t-PA Stroke Trial. *Stroke.* 1997; 28(11):2119-2125.

145. Linfante I, Llinas RH, Selim M, et al. Clinical and vascular outcome in internal carotid artery versus middle cerebral artery occlusions after intravenous tissue plasminogen activator. *Stroke.* 2002;33(8):2066-2071.

146. Georgiadis D, Oehler J, Schwarz S, Rousson V, Hartmann M, Schwab S. Does acute occlusion of the carotid T invariably have a poor outcome? *Neurology.* 2004;63(1):22-26.

147. Wunderlich MT, Stolz E, Seidel G, et al. Conservative medical treatment and intravenous thrombolysis in acute stroke from carotid T occlusion. *Cerebrovasc Dis.* 2005;20(5):355-361.

148. Lindley RI, Wardlaw JM, Sandercock PA. Alteplase and ischaemic stroke: have new reviews of old data helped? *Lancet Neurol.* 2005;4(4):249-253.

149. Marler JR, Tilley BC, Lu M, et al. Early stroke treatment associated with better outcome: the NINDS rt-PA stroke study. *Neurology.* 2000;55(11):1649-1655.

150. Labiche LA, Al-Senani F, Wojner AW, Grotta JC, Malkoff M, Alexandrov AV. Is the benefit of early recanalization

sustained at 3 months? A prospective cohort study. *Stroke.* 2003;34(3):695-698.

151. Molina CA, Montaner J, Abilleira S, et al. Time course of tissue plasminogen activator-induced recanalization in acute cardioembolic stroke: a case-control study. *Stroke.* 2001;32(12):2821-2827.

152. Saver JL. Time is brain—quantified. *Stroke.* 2006;37(1):263-266.

153. Furlan A, Higashida R, Wechsler L, et al. Intra-arterial prourokinase for acute ischemic stroke. The PROACT II study: a randomized controlled trial. Prolyse in Acute Cerebral Thromboembolism. *JAMA.* 1999;282(21):2003-2011.

154. Lee KY, Han SW, Kim SH, et al. Early recanalization after intravenous administration of recombinant tissue plasminogen activator as assessed by pre- and post-thrombolytic angiography in acute ischemic stroke patients. *Stroke.* 2007;38(1):192-193.

155. Alexandrov AV, Molina CA, Grotta JC, et al. Ultrasound-enhanced systemic thrombolysis for acute ischemic stroke. *N Engl J Med.* 2004;351(21):2170-2178.

156. Arnold M, Schroth G, Nedeltchev K, et al. Intra-arterial thrombolysis in 100 patients with acute stroke due to middle cerebral artery occlusion. *Stroke.* 2002;33(7):1828-1833.

157. Bourekas EC, Slivka AP, Shah R, Sunshine J, Suarez JI. Intraarterial thrombolytic therapy within 3 hours of the onset of stroke. *Neurosurgery.* 2004;54(1):39-46.

158. Lewandowski CA, Frankel M, Tomsick TA, et al. Combined intravenous and intra-arterial r-TPA versus intra-arterial therapy of acute ischemic stroke: Emergency Management of Stroke (EMS) Bridging Trial. *Stroke.* 1999;30(12):2598-2605.

159. Anon. Combined intravenous and intra-arterial recanalization for acute ischemic stroke: the Interventional Management of Stroke Study. *Stroke.* 2004;35(4):904-911.

160. IMS II Trial Investigators. The Interventional Management of Stroke (IMS) II Study. *Stroke.* 2007;38(7):2127-2135.

161. Kim DJ, Kim DI, Kim SH, Lee KY, Heo JH, Han SW. Rescue localized intra-arterial thrombolysis for hyperacute MCA ischemic stroke patients after early non-responsive intravenous tissue plasminogen activator therapy. *Neuroradiology.* 2005;47(8):616-621.

162. Shaltoni HM, Albright KC, Gonzales NR, et al. Is intra-arterial thrombolysis safe after full-dose intravenous recombinant tissue plasminogen activator for acute ischemic stroke? *Stroke.* 2007;38(1):80-84.

163. Abou-Chebl A, Bajzer CT, Krieger DW, Furlan AJ, Yadav JS. Multimodal therapy for the treatment of severe ischemic stroke combining GPIIb/IIIa antagonists and angioplasty after failure of thrombolysis. *Stroke.* 2005;36(10):2286-2288.

164. Deshmukh VR, Fiorella DJ, Albuquerque FC, et al. Intra-arterial thrombolysis for acute ischemic stroke: preliminary experience with platelet glycoprotein IIb/IIIa inhibitors as adjunctive therapy. *Neurosurgery.* 2005;56(1):46-55.

165. Gupta R, Vora NA, Horowitz MB, et al. Multimodal reperfusion therapy for acute ischemic stroke: factors predicting vessel recanalization. *Stroke.* 2006;37(4):986-990.

166. Smith WS, Sung G, Starkman S, et al. Safety and efficacy of mechanical embolectomy in acute ischemic stroke: results of the MERCI trial. *Stroke.* 2005;36(7):1432-1438.

167. Smith WS. Safety of mechanical thrombectomy and intravenous tissue plasminogen activator in acute ischemic stroke. Results of the multi Mechanical Embolus Removal in Cerebral Ischemia (MERCI) trial, part I. *AJNR Am J Neuroradiol.* 2006;27(6):1177-1182.

168. Nedeltchev K, Fischer U, Arnold M, et al. Long-term effect of intra-arterial thrombolysis in stroke. *Stroke.* 2006; 37(12):3002-3007.

169. Kase CS, Furlan AJ, Wechsler LR, et al. Cerebral hemorrhage after intra-arterial thrombolysis for ischemic stroke: the PROACT II trial. *Neurology.* 2001;57(9):1603-1610.

170. Kidwell CS, Saver JL, Carneado J, et al. Predictors of hemorrhagic transformation in patients receiving intra-arterial thrombolysis. *Stroke.* 2002;33(3):717-724.

171. Kim D, Ford GA, Kidwell CS, et al. Intra-arterial thrombolysis for acute stroke in patients 80 and older: a comparison of results in patients younger than 80 years. *AJNR Am J Neuroradiol.* 2007;28(1):159-163.

172. Gonner F, Remonda L, Mattle H, et al. Local intra-arterial thrombolysis in acute ischemic stroke. *Stroke.* 1998; 29(9):1894-1900.

173. Ng PP, Higashida RT, Cullen SP, Malek R, Dowd CF, Halbach VV. Intraarterial thrombolysis trials in acute ischemic stroke. *J Vasc Interv Radiol.* 2004;15(1, pt 2):S77-S85.

174. Mahon BR, Nesbit GM, Barnwell SL, et al. North American clinical experience with the EKOS MicroLysUS infusion catheter for the treatment of embolic stroke. *AJNR Am J Neuroradiol.* 2003;24(3):534-538.

175. Nakano S, Iseda T, Yoneyama T, Kawano H, Wakisaka S. Direct percutaneous transluminal angioplasty for acute middle cerebral artery trunk occlusion: an alternative option to intra-arterial thrombolysis. *Stroke.* 2002;33(12):2872-2876.

176. Sauvageau E, Samuelson RM, Levy EI, Jeziorski AM, Mehta RA, Hopkins LN. Middle cerebral artery stenting for acute ischemic stroke after unsuccessful Merci retrieval. *Neurosurgery.* 2007;60(4):701-706.

177. von Kummer R, Bourquain H, Bastianello S, et al. Early prediction of irreversible brain damage after ischemic stroke at CT. *Radiology.* 2001;219(1):95-100.

178. Lev MH, Farkas J, Gemmete JJ, et al. Acute stroke: improved nonenhanced CT detection—benefits of soft-copy interpretation by using variable window width and center level settings. *Radiology.* 1999;213(1):150-155.

179. Kloska SP, Nabavi DG, Gaus C, et al. Acute stroke assessment with CT: do we need multimodal evaluation? *Radiology.* 2004;233(1):79-86.

180. Maruya J, Yamamoto K, Ozawa T, et al. Simultaneous multi-section perfusion CT and CT angiography for the assessment of acute ischemic stroke. *Acta Neurochir (Wien).* 2005;147(4):383-392.

181. Barber PA, Demchuk AM, Zhang J, Buchan AM. Validity and reliability of a quantitative computed tomography score in predicting outcome of hyperacute stroke before thrombolytic therapy. ASPECTS Study Group. Alberta Stroke Programme Early CT Score. *Lancet.* 13 2000;355(9216):1670-1674.

182. Hill MD, Demchuk AM, Tomsick TA, Palesch YY, Broderick JP. Using the baseline CT scan to select acute stroke patients for IV-IA therapy. *AJNR Am J Neuroradiol.* 2006;27(8): 1612-1616.

183. Demchuk AM, Coutts SB. Alberta Stroke Program Early CT Score in acute stroke triage. *Neuroimaging Clin N Am.* 2005; 15(2):409-419.

184. Butcher KS, Lee SB, Parsons MW, et al. Differential prognosis of isolated cortical swelling and hypoattenuation on CT in acute stroke. *Stroke.* 2007;38(3):941-947.

185. Na DG, Kim EY, Ryoo JW, et al. CT sign of brain swelling without concomitant parenchymal hypoattenuation: comparison with diffusion- and perfusion-weighted MR imaging. *Radiology.* 2005;235(3):992-948.

186. Parsons MW, Pepper EM, Chan V, et al. Perfusion computed tomography: prediction of final infarct extent and stroke outcome. *Ann Neurol.* 2005;58(5):672-679.

187. Hoeffner EG, Case I, Jain R, et al. Cerebral perfusion CT: technique and clinical applications. *Radiology.* 2004;231(3): 632-644.

188. Heiss WD. Ischemic penumbra: evidence from functional imaging in man. *J Cereb Blood Flow Metab.* 2000;20(9):1276-1293.

189. Wintermark M, Fischbein NJ, Smith WS, Ko NU, Quist M, Dillon WP. Accuracy of dynamic perfusion CT with deconvolution in detecting acute hemispheric stroke. *AJNR Am J Neuroradiol.* 2005;26(1):104-112.

190. Wintermark M, Thiran JP, Maeder P, Schnyder P, Meuli R. Simultaneous measurement of regional cerebral blood flow by perfusion CT and stable xenon CT: a validation study. *AJNR Am J Neuroradiol.* 2001;22(5):905-914.

191. Wintermark M, Reichhart M, Cuisenaire O, et al. Comparison of admission perfusion computed tomography and qualitative diffusion- and perfusion-weighted magnetic resonance imaging in acute stroke patients. *Stroke.* 2002;33(8):2025-2031.

192. Kudo K, Terae S, Katoh C, et al. Quantitative cerebral blood flow measurement with dynamic perfusion CT using the vascular-pixel elimination method: comparison with H2(15)O positron emission tomography. *AJNR Am J Neuroradiol.* 2003;24(3):419-426.

193. Koenig M, Kraus M, Theek C, Klotz E, Gehlen W, Heuser L. Quantitative assessment of the ischemic brain by means of perfusion-related parameters derived from perfusion CT. *Stroke.* 2001;32(2):431-437.

194. Sorensen AG, Copen WA, Ostergaard L, et al. Hyperacute stroke: simultaneous measurement of relative cerebral blood volume, relative cerebral blood flow, and mean tissue transit time. *Radiology.* 1999;210(2):519-527.

195. Parsons MW, Pepper EM, Bateman GA, Wang Y, Levi CR. Identification of the penumbra and infarct core on hyperacute noncontrast and perfusion CT. *Neurology.* 2007;68(10): 730-736.

196. Schaefer PW, Roccatagliata L, Ledezma C, et al. First-pass quantitative CT perfusion identifies thresholds for salvageable penumbra in acute stroke patients treated with intra-arterial therapy. *AJNR Am J Neuroradiol.* 2006;27(1):20-25.

197. Murphy BD, Fox AJ, Lee DH, et al. Identification of penumbra and infarct in acute ischemic stroke using computed tomography perfusion-derived blood flow and blood volume measurements. *Stroke.* 2006;37(7):1771-1777.

198. Sanelli PC, Lev MH, Eastwood JD, Gonzalez RG, Lee TY. The effect of varying user-selected input parameters on quantitative values in CT perfusion maps. *Acad Radiol.* 2004;11 (10):1085-1092.

199. Wintermark M, Maeder P, Verdun FR, et al. Using 80 kVp versus 120 Vp in perfusion CT measurement of regional cerebral blood flow. *AJNR Am J Neuroradiol.* 2000;21 (10):1881-1884.

200. Wintermark M, Smith WS, Ko NU, Quist M, Schnyder P, Dillon WP. Dynamic perfusion CT: optimizing the temporal resolution and contrast volume for calculation of perfusion CT parameters in stroke patients. *AJNR Am J Neuroradiol.* 2004;25(5):720-729.

201. Esteban JM, Cervera V. Perfusion CT and angio CT in the assessment of acute stroke. *Neuroradiology.* 2004;46(9):705-715.

202. Smith WS, Roberts HC, Chuang NA, et al. Safety and feasibility of a CT protocol for acute stroke: combined CT, CT angiography, and CT perfusion imaging in 53 consecutive patients. *AJNR Am J Neuroradiol.* 2003;24(4):688-690.

203. Mullins ME, Schaefer PW, Sorensen AG, et al. CT and conventional and diffusion-weighted MR imaging in acute stroke: study in 691 patients at presentation to the emergency department. *Radiology.* 2002;224(2):353-360.

204. Sunshine JL, Tarr RW, Lanzieri CF, Landis DM, Selman WR, Lewin JS. Hyperacute stroke: ultrafast MR imaging to triage patients prior to therapy. *Radiology.* 1999;212(2):325-332.

205. Latchaw RE. Cerebral perfusion imaging in acute stroke. *J Vasc Interv Radiol.* 2004;15(1, pt 2):S29-S46.

206. Fiehler J, Foth M, Kucinski T, et al. Severe ADC decreases do not predict irreversible tissue damage in humans. *Stroke.* 2002;33(1):79-86.

207. Kucinski T, Naumann D, Knab R, et al. Tissue at risk is overestimated in perfusion-weighted imaging: MR imaging in acute stroke patients without vessel recanalization. *AJNR Am J Neuroradiol.* 2005;26(4):815-819.

208. Schellinger PD, Fiebach JB, Hacke W. Imaging-based decision making in thrombolytic therapy for ischemic stroke: present status. *Stroke.* 2003;34(2):575-583.

209. Kim EY, Ryoo JW, Roh HG, et al. Reversed discrepancy between CT and diffusion-weighted MR imaging in acute ischemic stroke. *AJNR Am J Neuroradiol.* 2006;27(9):1990-1995.

210. Christoforidis GA, Mohammad Y, Kehagias D, Avutu B, Slivka AP. Angiographic assessment of pial collaterals as a prognostic indicator following intra-arterial thrombolysis for acute ischemic stroke. *AJNR Am J Neuroradiol.* 2005;26(7):1789-1797.

211. Barr JD. Cerebral angiography in the assessment of acute cerebral ischemia: guidelines and recommendations. *J Vasc Interv Radiol.* 2004;15(1, pt 2):S57-S66.

212. Huang HW, Guo MH, Lin RJ, et al. Prevalence and risk factors of middle cerebral artery stenosis in asymptomatic residents in Rongqi County, Guangdong. *Cerebrovasc Dis.* 2007;24(1):111-115.

213. Wityk RJ, Lehman D, Klag M, Coresh J, Ahn H, Litt B. Race and sex differences in the distribution of cerebral atherosclerosis. *Stroke.* 1996;27(11):1974-1980.

214. Sacco RL, Kargman DE, Gu Q, Zamanillo MC. Race-ethnicity and determinants of intracranial atherosclerotic cerebral infarction. The Northern Manhattan Stroke Study. *Stroke.* 1995;26(1):14-20.

215. Thijs VN, Albers GW. Symptomatic intracranial atherosclerosis: outcome of patients who fail antithrombotic therapy. *Neurology.* 2000;55(4):490-497.

216. Kasner SE, Chimowitz MI, Lynn MJ, et al. Predictors of ischemic stroke in the territory of a symptomatic intracranial arterial stenosis. *Circulation.* 2006;113(4):555-563.

217. Samuels OB, Joseph GJ, Lynn MJ, Smith HA, Chimowitz MI. A standardized method for measuring intracranial arterial stenosis. *AJNR Am J Neuroradiol.* 2000;21(4):643-646.

218. Bash S, Villablanca JP, Jahan R, et al. Intracranial vascular stenosis and occlusive disease: evaluation with CT angiography, MR angiography, and digital subtraction angiography. *AJNR Am J Neuroradiol.* 2005;26(5):1012-1021.

219. Feldmann E, Wilterdink JL, Kosinski A, et al. The Stroke Outcomes and Neuroimaging of Intracranial Atherosclerosis (SONIA) trial. *Neurology.* 2007;68(24):2099-2106.

220. Komotar RJ, Wilson DA, Mocco J, et al. Natural history of intracranial atherosclerosis: a critical review. *Neurosurgery.* 2006;58(4):595-601.

221. Kremer C, Schaettin T, Georgiadis D, Baumgartner RW. Prognosis of asymptomatic stenosis of the middle cerebral artery. *J Neurol Neurosurg Psychiatry.* 2004;75(9):1300-1303.

222. Takahashi W, Ohnuki T, Ide M, Takagi S, Shinohara Y. Stroke risk of asymptomatic intra- and extracranial large-artery disease in apparently healthy adults. *Cerebrovasc Dis.* 2006;22(4):263-270.

223. Mazighi M, Tanasescu R, Ducrocq X, et al. Prospective study of symptomatic atherothrombotic intracranial stenoses: the GESICA study. *Neurology.* 2006;66(8):1187-1191.

224. Chimowitz MI, Lynn MJ, Howlett-Smith H, et al. Comparison of warfarin and aspirin for symptomatic intracranial arterial stenosis. *N Engl J Med.* 2005;352(13):1305-1316.

225. Kasner SE, Lynn MJ, Chimowitz MI, et al. Warfarin vs aspirin for symptomatic intracranial stenosis: subgroup analyses from WASID. *Neurology.* 2006;67(7):1275-1278.

226. North American Symptomatic Carotid Endarterectomy Trial Collaborators. Beneficial effect of carotid endarterectomy in symptomatic patients with high-grade carotid stenosis. *N Engl J Med.* 1991;325(7):445-453.

227. Barnett HJ, Taylor DW, Eliasziw M, et al. Benefit of carotid endarterectomy in patients with symptomatic moderate or severe stenosis. North American Symptomatic Carotid Endarterectomy Trial Collaborators. *N Engl J Med.* 1998;339 (20):1415-1425.

228. EC/IC Bypass Study Group. Failure of extracranial-intracranial arterial bypass to reduce the risk of ischemic stroke. Results of an international randomized trial. *N Engl J Med.* 1985;313(19):1191-1200.

229. Grubb RL Jr, Powers WJ, Derdeyn CP, Adams HP Jr, Clarke WR. The Carotid Occlusion Surgery Study. *Neurosurg Focus.* 2003;14(3):e9.

230. Connors JJ III, Wojak JC. Percutaneous transluminal angioplasty for intracranial atherosclerotic lesions: evolution of

technique and short-term results. *J Neurosurg.* 1999;91(3): 415-423.

231. Jiang WJ, Xu XT, Du B, et al. Long-term outcome of elective stenting for symptomatic intracranial vertebrobasilar stenosis. *Neurology.* 2007;68(11):856-858.

232. Cruz-Flores S, Diamond AL. Angioplasty for intracranial artery stenosis. *Cochrane Database Syst Rev.* 2006;3: CD004133.

233. Jiang WJ, Xu XT, Du B, et al. Comparison of elective stenting of severe vs moderate intracranial atherosclerotic stenosis. *Neurology.* 2007;68(6):420-426.

234. Jiang WJ, Srivastava T, Gao F, Du B, Dong KH, Xu XT. Perforator stroke after elective stenting of symptomatic intracranial stenosis. *Neurology.* 2006;66(12):1868-1872.

235. Fiorella D, Chow MM, Anderson M, Woo H, Rasmussen PA, Masaryk TJ. A 7-year experience with balloon-mounted coronary stents for the treatment of symptomatic vertebrobasilar intracranial atheromatous disease. *Neurosurgery.* 2007;61(2):236-243.

236. Levy EI, Turk AS, Albuquerque FC, et al. Wingspan in-stent restenosis and thrombosis: incidence, clinical presentation, and management. *Neurosurgery.* 2007;61(3):644-651.

237. Jiang WJ, Xu XT, Jin M, Du B, Dong KH, Dai JP. Apollo stent for symptomatic atherosclerotic intracranial stenosis: study results. *AJNR Am J Neuroradiol.* 2007;28(5):830-834.

238. SSYLVIA Study Investigators. Stenting of Symptomatic Atherosclerotic Lesions in the Vertebral or Intracranial Arteries (SSYLVIA): study results. *Stroke.* 2004;35(6):1388-1392.

239. Marks MP, Wojak JC, Al-Ali F, et al. Angioplasty for symptomatic intracranial stenosis: clinical outcome. *Stroke.* 2006;37(4):1016-1020.

240. Gupta R, Al-Ali F, Thomas AJ, et al. Safety, feasibility, and short-term follow-up of drug-eluting stent placement in the intracranial and extracranial circulation. *Stroke.* 2006; 37(10):2562-2566.

241. Germain DP. Clinical and genetic features of vascular Ehlers-Danlos syndrome. *Ann Vasc Surg.* 2002;16(3):391-397.

242. Chaves C, Estol C, Esnaola MM, et al. Spontaneous intracranial internal carotid artery dissection: report of 10 patients. *Arch Neurol.* 2002;59(6):977-981.

243. Dusser A, Goutieres F, Aicardi J. Ischemic strokes in children. *J Child Neurol.* 1986;1(2):131-136.

244. Williams LS, Garg BP, Cohen M, Fleck JD, Biller J. Subtypes of ischemic stroke in children and young adults. *Neurology.* 1997;49(6):1541-1545.

245. Fullerton HJ, Johnston SC, Smith WS. Arterial dissection and stroke in children. *Neurology.* 2001;57(7):1155-1160.

246. Schievink WI, Mokri B, Piepgras DG. Spontaneous dissections of cervicocephalic arteries in childhood and adolescence. *Neurology.* 1994;44(9):1607-1612.

247. Robertson WC Jr, Given CA II. Spontaneous intracranial arterial dissection in the young: diagnosis by CT angiography. *BMC Neurol.* 2006;6:16.

248. Farrell MA, Gilbert JJ, Kaufmann JC. Fatal intracranial arterial dissection: clinical pathological correlation. *J Neurol Neurosurg Psychiatry.* 1985;48(2):111-121.

249. Yamaura A, Ono J. Current diagnosis and treatment of intracranial dissecting aneurysms. *Neurosurg Q.* 1994:67-81.

250. Manz HJ, Vester J, Lavenstein B. Dissecting aneurysm of cerebral arteries in childhood and adolescence. Case report and literature review of 20 cases. *Virchows Arch A Pathol Anat Histol.* 1979;384(3):325-335.

251. Pessin MS, Adelman LS, Barbas NR. Spontaneous intracranial carotid artery dissection. *Stroke.* 1989;20(8):1100-1103.

252. Ahn JY, Chung SS, Lee BH, et al. Treatment of spontaneous arterial dissections with stent placement for preservation of the parent artery. *Acta Neurochir (Wien).* 2005;147(3):265-273.

253. Lylyk P, Cohen JE, Ceratto R, Ferrario A, Miranda C. Angioplasty and stent placement in intracranial atherosclerotic stenoses and dissections. *AJNR Am J Neuroradiol.* 2002; 23(3):430-436.

254. Suzuki J, Takaku A. Cerebrovascular "moyamoya" disease. Disease showing abnormal net-like vessels in base of brain. *Arch Neurol.* 1969;20(3):288-299.

255. Natori Y, Ikezaki K, Matsushima T, Fukui M. 'Angiographic moyamoya' its definition, classification, and therapy. *Clin Neurol Neurosurg.* 1997;99(suppl 2):S168-S172.

256. Yamashita M, Oka K, Tanaka K. Histopathology of the brain vascular network in moyamoya disease. *Stroke.* 1983;14(1): 50-58.

257. Fukui M, Kono S, Sueishi K, Ikezaki K. Moyamoya disease. *Neuropathology.* 2000;20(suppl):S61-S64.

258. Fukui M. Guidelines for the diagnosis and treatment of spontaneous occlusion of the circle of Willis ('moyamoya' disease). Research Committee on Spontaneous Occlusion of the Circle of Willis (Moyamoya Disease) of the Ministry of Health and Welfare, Japan. *Clin Neurol Neurosurg.* 1997; 99(suppl 2):S238-S240.

259. Hoffman HJ. Moyamoya disease and syndrome. *Clin Neurol Neurosurg.* 1997;99(suppl 2):S39-S44.

260. Iwama T, Morimoto M, Hashimoto N, Goto Y, Todaka T, Sawada M. Mechanism of intracranial rebleeding in moyamoya disease. *Clin Neurol Neurosurg.* 1997;99(suppl 2): S187-S190.

261. Saeki N, Nakazaki S, Kubota M, et al. Hemorrhagic type moyamoya disease. *Clin Neurol Neurosurg.* 1997;99(suppl 2):S196-S201.

262. Fujii K, Ikezaki K, Irikura K, Miyasaka Y, Fukui M. The efficacy of bypass surgery for the patients with hemorrhagic moyamoya disease. *Clin Neurol Neurosurg.* 1997;99(suppl 2):S194-S195.

263. Lie JT. Classification and histopathologic spectrum of central nervous system vasculitis. *Neurol Clin.* 1997;15(4):805-819.

264. Ozawa T, Sasaki O, Sorimachi T, Tanaka R. Primary angiitis of the central nervous system: report of two cases and review of the literature. *Neurosurgery.* 1995;36(1):173-179.

265. Wynne PJ, Younger DS, Khandji A, Silver AJ. Radiographic features of central nervous system vasculitis. *Neurol Clin.* 1997;15(4):779-804.

266. Lie JT. Angiitis of the central nervous system. *Curr Opin Rheumatol.* 1991;3(1):36-45.

267. Clifford-Jones RE, Love S, Gurusinghe N. Granulomatous angiitis of the central nervous system: a case with recurrent intracerebral haemorrhage. *J Neurol Neurosurg Psychiatry.* 1985;48(10):1054-1056.

268. Moore PM, Cupps TR. Neurological complications of vasculitis. *Ann Neurol.* 1983;14(2):155-167.

269. Lie JT. Vasculitis associated with infectious agents. *Curr Opin Rheumatol.* 1996;8(1):26-29.

270. Johnson RT, Richardson EP. The neurological manifestations of systemic lupus erythematosus. *Medicine (Baltimore).* 1968;47(4):337-369.

271. Travers RL, Allison DJ, Brettle RP, Hughes GR. Polyarteritis nodosa: a clinical and angiographic analysis of 17 cases. *Semin Arthritis Rheum.* 1979;8(3):184-199.

272. Kaye BR, Fainstat M. Cerebral vasculitis associated with cocaine abuse. *JAMA.* 1987;258(15):2104-2106.

273. Samandouras G, Teddy PJ, Cadoux-Hudson T, Ansorge O. Amyloid in neurosurgical and neurological practice. *J Clin Neurosci.* 2006;13(2):159-167.

274. Okazaki H, Reagan TJ, Campbell RJ. Clinicopathologic studies of primary cerebral amyloid angiopathy. *Mayo Clin Proc.* 1979;54(1):22-31.

275. Smith EE, Eichler F. Cerebral amyloid angiopathy and lobar intracerebral hemorrhage. *Arch Neurol.* 2006;63(1):148-151.

276. McCormick WF. The pathology of vascular ("arteriovenous") malformations. *J Neurosurg.* 1966;24(4):807-816.

277. Newton TH, Cronqvist S. Involvement of dural arteries in intracranial arteriovenous malformations. *Radiology.* 1969;93(5):1071-1078.

278. Szikora I. Dural arteriovenous malformations. In: Forsting M, ed. *Intracranial Vascular Malformations and Aneurysms.* Berlin, Germany: Springer-Verlag; 2004:101-141.

279. Borden JA, Wu JK, Shucart WA. A proposed classification for spinal and cranial dural arteriovenous fistulous malformations and implications for treatment. *J Neurosurg.* 1995;82(2):166-179.

280. Davies MA, TerBrugge K, Willinsky R, Coyne T, Saleh J, Wallace MC. The validity of classification for the clinical presentation of intracranial dural arteriovenous fistulas. *J Neurosurg.* 1996;85(5):830-837.

281. Satomi J, van Dijk JM, Terbrugge KG, Willinsky RA, Wallace MC. Benign cranial dural arteriovenous fistulas: outcome of conservative management based on the natural history of the lesion. *J Neurosurg.* 2002;97(4):767-770.

282. van Dijk JM, terBrugge KG, Willinsky RA, Wallace MC. Clinical course of cranial dural arteriovenous fistulas with long-term persistent cortical venous reflux. *Stroke.* 2002;33(5):1233-1236.

283. Cognard C, Spelle L, Pierot L. Pial arteriovenous malformations. In: Forsting M, ed. *Intracranial Vascular Malformations and Aneurysms.* Berlin, Germany: Springer-Verlag; 2004:39-100.

284. Al-Shahi R, Warlow C. A systematic review of the frequency and prognosis of arteriovenous malformations of the brain in adults. *Brain.* 2001;124(pt 10):1900-1926.

285. Stapf C, Mast H, Sciacca RR, et al. Predictors of hemorrhage in patients with untreated brain arteriovenous malformation. *Neurology.* 2006;66(9):1350-1355.

286. Spetzler RF, Martin NA. A proposed grading system for arteriovenous malformations. *J Neurosurg.* 1986;65(4):476-483.

287. Hamilton MG, Spetzler RF. The prospective application of a grading system for arteriovenous malformations. *Neurosurgery.* 1994;34(1):2-7.

288. Han PP, Ponce FA, Spetzler RF. Intention-to-treat analysis of Spetzler-Martin grades IV and V arteriovenous malformations: natural history and treatment paradigm. *J Neurosurg.* 2003;98(1):3-7.

289. Fiorella D, Albuquerque FC, Woo HH, McDougall CG, Rasmussen PA. The role of neuroendovascular therapy for the treatment of brain arteriovenous malformations. *Neurosurgery.* 2006;59(5, suppl 3):S163-S177.

290. Richling B, Killer M, Al-Schameri AR, Ritter L, Agic R, Krenn M. Therapy of brain arteriovenous malformations: multimodality treatment from a balanced standpoint. *Neurosurgery.* 2006;59(5, suppl 3):S148-S157.

291. Kuker W, Forsting M. Cavernomas and capillary telangiectasias. In: Forsting M, ed. *Intracranial Vascular Malformations and Aneurysms.* Berlin, Germany: Springer-Verlag; 2004:16-38.

292. Porter PJ, Willinsky RA, Harper W, Wallace MC. Cerebral cavernous malformations: natural history and prognosis after clinical deterioration with or without hemorrhage. *J Neurosurg.* 1997;87(2):190-197.

293. Kondziolka D, Lunsford LD, Kestle JR. The natural history of cerebral cavernous malformations. *J Neurosurg.* 1995;83(5):820-824.

294. Porter RW, Detwiler PW, Spetzler RF, et al. Cavernous malformations of the brainstem: experience with 100 patients. *J Neurosurg.* 1999;90(1):50-58.

295. Hasegawa T, McInerney J, Kondziolka D, Lee JY, Flickinger JC, Lunsford LD. Long-term results after stereotactic radiosurgery for patients with cavernous malformations. *Neurosurgery.* 2002;50(6):1190-1198.

296. Forsting M, Wanke I. Developmental venous anomalies. In: Forsting M, ed. *Intracranial Vascular Malformations and Aneurysms.* Berlin, Germany: Springer-Verlag; 2004:1-15.

297. McLaughlin MR, Kondziolka D, Flickinger JC, Lunsford S, Lunsford LD. The prospective natural history of cerebral venous malformations. *Neurosurgery.* 1998;43(2):195-201.

298. Bose A, Hartmann M, Henkes H, et al. A novel, self-expanding, nitinol stent in medically refractory intracranial atherosclerotic stenoses: the Wingspan study. *Stroke.* 2007;38(5):1531-1537.

299. Marks MP, Marcellus ML, Do HM, et al. Intracranial angioplasty without stenting for symptomatic atherosclerotic stenosis: long-term follow-up. *AJNR Am J Neuroradiol.* 2005;26(3):525-530.

300. Qureshi AI, Ziai WC, Yahia AM, et al. Stroke-free survival and its determinants in patients with symptomatic vertebrobasilar sten osis: a multicenter study. *Neurosurgery.* 2003;52(5):1033-1040.

chapter 24

Extracranial Carotid Disease

Timothy M. Sullivan, MD / Gustavo Oderich, MD

● ATHEROSCLEROTIC DISEASE OF THE CAROTID ARTERIES

Introduction

Cerebrovascular accident (CVA) is the third leading cause of death in the United States, surpassed only by heart disease and malignancy.[1] Stroke accounts for 10% to 12% of all deaths in industrialized countries. Almost one in four men and one in five women aged 45 years can expect to have a stroke if they live till 85 years of age. In a population of 1 million, 1600 people will have a stroke each year. Only 55% of these will survive 6 months, and a third of the survivors will have significant problems caring for themselves. As our population ages, the total number of people afflicted with stroke will continue to rise unless historic stroke rates decline in the future.[2]

The etiology of stroke is multifactorial. Ischemic stroke accounts for approximately 80% of all first-ever strokes, while intracerebral hemorrhage and subarachnoid hemorrhage are responsible for 10% and 5%, respectively. Of those strokes which are ischemic in nature, the majority are linked to complications of atheromatous plaques. The most frequent site of such an atheroma is the carotid bifurcation. Although the prevention of stroke in the general population has largely focused on the control of hypertension, a substantial number of strokes are preventable by the identification and treatment of carotid disease especially as the population ages.

Surgical endarterectomy of high-grade carotid lesions, both symptomatic and asymptomatic, has been identified as the treatment of choice for stroke prophylaxis in most patients when compared to "best medical therapy" (risk factor reduction and antiplatelet agents), as shown convincingly by the NASCET and ACAS studies.[3,4] More careful inspection of their respective results suggest that the risk of disabling stroke or death was 1.9% in NASCET, with a 3.9% risk of minor stroke. In ACAS, the risk of major stroke or death was 0.6% when one excludes the 1.2% risk of stroke caused by diagnostic arteriography (Table 24-1). Subsequently, carotid endarterectomy (CEA) has been performed in increasing numbers of patients, and now represents the most frequent surgical procedure performed by vascular surgeons. Despite the proven efficacy of CEA in the prevention of ischemic stroke, great interest has been generated in carotid angioplasty and stenting (CAS) as an alternative to surgical therapy. This chapter will examine the current role of CEA in the treatment of patients with stenosis of the cervical carotid arteries, will analyze the concept of "high-risk" CEA, and will discuss the evolving role of CAS.

Carotid Endarterectomy

The era of CEA was ushered in by the report of Eastcott, Pickering, and Robb in 1954. They treated a 66-year-old woman who had 33 episodes of transient cerebral ischemia (TIA); following operation, her symptoms resolved.[5] Despite publication of satisfactory surgical results, the efficacy of CEA came into question during the 1970s and 1980s. Among Medicare beneficiaries, the frequency of CEA declined from 1985 (61 273 per annum) to 1989 (46 571 per annum).[6] It was not until the 1990s that randomized trials of best medical therapy vs. CEA were undertaken. Following publication of the NASCET and ACAS trial results, the volume of CEA in the United States rose dramatically; again, among Medicare recipients, the incidence rose to 108 275 in 1996 following release of data from these trials. The Dartmouth Atlas of Vascular Health Care reported that the number of carotid endarterectomies performed between 1995 and 1997 nearly doubled, from 62 000 to 114 000 annually.[7]

The current indication for CEA include the following:

1. Asymptomatic high-grade stenosis (typically >70% by duplex ultrasound)

TABLE 24-1. Results of CEA for Symptomatic and Asymptomatic Carotid Stenosis

	Mortality (%)	Disabling Stroke (%)	Minor Stroke (%)
Symptomatic disease			
NASCET I[†] (>70% stenosis)	0.6	1.3	3.9
NASCET II[‡] (50%–69% stenosis)	1.2	1.6	4.0
Asymptomatic disease			
VA asymptomatic[§] (>50% stenosis)	1.9	1.0	1.4
ACAS[¶] (>60% stenosis)	0.4*	0.2*	0.5*

*Excludes 1.2% risk of stroke after angiography.
[†] Source: North American Symptomatic Carotid Endarterectomy Trial Collaborators. Beneficial effect of carotid endarterectomy in symptomatic patients with high-grade carotid stenosis. N Engl J Med 1991; 325:445-453.
[‡] Source: Benefit of carotid endarterectomy in patients with symptomatic moderate or severe stenosis. North American Symptomatic Carotid Endarterectomy Trial Collaborators. NEJM. 1998;339:1415-1425.
[§] Source: Hobson RW, Weiss DG, Fields WS, et al. Efficacy of carotid endarterectomy for asymptomatic carotid stenosis. The Veterans Affairs Cooperative Study Group. N Engl J Med 1993;328:221-227.
[¶] Source: Executive Committee for the Asymptomatic Carotid Atherosclerosis Study. Endarterectomy for asymptomatic carotid artery stenosis. JAMA 1995;273:1421-1428.

2. Symptomatic high-grade stenosis (typically >70% by duplex ultrasound)

3. Symptomatic patients with moderate (>50%) carotid stenosis. These lesions are typically associated with deep ulceration and failure of medical (antiplatelet) therapy.

With the advent of CAS, CEA has again come "under attack," despite its proven efficacy and durability in stroke prevention in patients with high-grade stenosis of the internal carotid artery (ICA).[8] Proponents of CAS have suggested that the results of NASCET and ACAS are not achievable in general practice outside selected centers of excellence. The question is a reasonable one; if the combined stroke and death rate of CEA in asymptomatic patients were more than 3%, there would be little benefit of operation in the asymptomatic population.[9] Both ACAS and NASCET included good-risk patients on the basis of reasonable life expectancy (so as to be available for follow-up) and exclusion of other potential causes of stroke (such as atrial fibrillation). Exclusion criteria included previous carotid surgery, prior myocardial infarction (MI), congestive heart failure (CHF), renal failure, unstable angina, and those requiring combined CEA and coronary bypass procedures. Tables 24-2 and 24-3 list inclusion and exclusion criteria for several important CEA and CAS trials. A review of 25 CEA studies reporting 30-day stroke and death rates by

Rothwell et al.[10] found a mortality rate of 1.3% in asymptomatic patients and 1.8% in symptomatic patients. The combined stroke and death rates were 3% in asymptomatic patients and 5.2% in those presenting with symptomatic carotid stenosis.

A number of studies have focused on NASCET and ACAS trial eligibility as they relate to the results of CEA in the general population. Lepore et al.[11] from the Ochsner Clinic reviewed 366 CEAs performed at their institution over a 2-year period. Surprisingly, 46% were found to be high risk based on NASCET and ACAS trial-ineligibility. Their cohort included 60% who presented with asymptomatic carotid stenosis; the remaining 40% had focal ipsilateral symptoms at presentation. The overall stroke and death rate (combined stroke and mortality, [CSM]) was 2.5%; trial-eligible "good risk" patients had a CSM of 1.5%, and the remainder (trial-ineligible) had a CSM of 3.6%. While there was a trend toward higher neurologic morbidity in trial-ineligible patients, this difference did not reach statistical significance ($p = 0.17$). These authors concluded that ineligibility for NASCET or ACAS should not be employed as a de novo indication for CAS. Illig et al.[12] examined the results of CEA at the University of Rochester in 857 patients. Stroke or death at 30 days occurred in 2.1%. Rates were similar in patients excluded from (2.7%) or included in (1.6%) NASCET and ACAS and in patients eligible (3.1%) or ineligible (2.1%) for ARCHeR, a CAS registry in high-risk patients. These rates did not differ according to whether exclusion or inclusion was based on anatomic risk, medical risk, or protocol exclusion; there was a trend, however, toward worse outcome in the high medical risk subgroup. Stroke and death rates were similar according to age, gender, repeat procedure, or the presence of contralateral occlusion.

Mozes et al.[13] examined the results of 776 consecutive CEAs from the Division of Vascular Surgery at the Mayo Clinic in Rochester, MN. Patients were categorized as "high risk" based on the inclusion and exclusion criteria for the SAPPHIRE trial of CAS with cerebral embolic protection. Of 776 CEAs, 323 (42%) were considered high risk based on the criteria listed in Table 24-4. Clinical presentation was similar in the high- and low-risk groups (Table 24-5). The overall postoperative stroke rate was 1.4% (symptomatic: 2.9%, asymptomatic: 0.9%). When comparing high- and low-risk CEAs, there was no statistical difference in stroke rate. Factors associated with significantly increased stroke risk were cervical radiation therapy, class III/IV angina, symptomatic presentation and age ≤60 years. Overall mortality was 0.3% (symptomatic: 0.5%; asymptomatic: 0.2%), not significantly different between the high- (0.6%) and low-risk groups (0.0%). Non-Q MI was more frequent in the high-risk group (3.1 vs. 0.9%; $p < 0.05$). Of note, the *only* MIs that occurred in the entire series were nontransmural (non-Q). A composite cluster of adverse clinical events (death, stroke, and MI) was more frequent in the symptomatic high-risk group (9.3% vs. 1.6%; $p < 0.005$), but not in the asymptomatic cohort. There was a trend for more major cranial nerve injuries in patients with local risk factors, such as high carotid

TABLE 24-2. Definition of High-Risk CEA: Major Exclusion Criteria of the NASCET/ACAS and Major Inclusion Criteria for Population-Based Studies on High-Risk CEA and for the SAPPHIRE Study

	Exclusion Criteria		Inclusion Criteria			
	NASCET	ACAS	Ouriel et al.[15] (2001)	Jordan et al.[21] (2002)	Gasparis et al.[20] (2003)	SAPPHIRE
Age	>79 y	>79 y			≥80y	>80 y
History	-Contralateral CEA <4 mo -Major surgical procedure <1 mo -Stroke in evolution	-Major surgical procedure <1 mo -Stroke in evolution		Major vascular procedure <1 mo		
Comorbidities						
Cardiac	-Unstable angina -Atrial fibrillation -Valvular heart disease -Symptomatic CHF -MI <6 mo	-Unstable angina -Atrial fibrillation -Valvular heart disease -Symptomatic CHF	-PTCA/CABG <6 mo -History of CHF	-Coronary procedure <1 mo -CABG <6 wk -Angina, NYHA 3/4 -EF <30% -MI <4 wk	-NYHA functional class III/IV -Canadian CVA heart failure functional class III/IV -CABG <6 mo -Steroid dependency -Oxygen dependency	-Open heart surgery <6 wk -MI <4 wk -Angina CCS class III/IV -CHF class III/IV -EF <30% -Abnormal cardiac stress test
Pulmonary	Lung failure	Lung failure with impact on 5-y survival	Severe COPD	-FEV₁ <1.0 liter -Home oxygen		-Chronic oxygen therapy -Resting pO₂ ≤60 mm Hg -Baseline hematocrit ≥50% -FEV₁ or DLCO ≤50% predicted
Renal	Kidney failure	Cr >3	Cr >3		Cr ≥3	
Other	-Uncontrolled HTN -Uncontrolled DM -Liver failure -Cancer, <50% 5-y survival	->180 systolic, 115 diastolic BP -Fasting glucose >400 -Liver failure -Cancer, <50% 5-y survival -Active ulcer disease -Coumadin				
Anatomic criteria	-Previous ipsilateral CEA -Tandem lesion >target stenosis	-Previous ipsilateral CEA -Tandem lesion >target stenosis -Cervical radiation treatment		-Previous ipsilateral CEA -Cervical radiation treatment -Contralateral carotid occlusion -High cervical lesion -Lesion below the clavicle	-Previous ipsilateral CEA -Cervical radiation treatment -Contralateral carotid occlusion -High cervical lesion	-Previous ipsilateral CEA -Severe tandem lesion -Cervical radiation treatment -Contralateral carotid occlusion -High cervical lesion (at least C₂) -Lesion below the clavicle -Contralateral laryngeal palsy

CHF, chronic heart failure; MI, myocardial infarction; HTN, hypertension; DM, diabetes mellitus; Cr, creatinine; BP, blood pressure; PTCA, percutaneous transluminal coronary angioplasty; CABG, coronary artery bypass graft; COPD, chronic obstructive pulmonary disease; NYHA, New York Heart Association; Canadian CVA, Canadian Cardiovascular Association; CCS, Canadian Cardiovascular Society; EF, ejection fraction; pO₂, partial oxygen pressure; FEV₁, forced expiratory volume in 1s; DLCO, diffusing capacity of the lung for carbon monoxide; C₂, second cervical vertebra.

TABLE 24-3. Exclusion Criteria, SAPPHIRE Trial

Acute stroke (≤48 h)
Staged elective procedure (within 30 d following the CEA)
    Elective percutaneous intervention
    Contralateral CEA
    Other elective operation
Synchronous operation
    CCA angioplasty/stenting or bypass
    Cardiac operation
    Noncardiac operation
Intracranial pathology
    Intracranial mass
    Aneurysm >9 mm
    Arteriovenous malformation
    Ventriculoperitoneal shunt

CEA, carotid endarterectomy; CCA, common carotid artery.

TABLE 24-5. Demographics and Frequency of Clinical Variables in Patients with High- and Low-Risk CEA

	High-Risk	Low-Risk	p
Number	323	453	
Presentation			
Asymptomatic	73%	73%	NS
TIA/amaurosis fugax	23%	22%	NS
Stroke	4%	5%	NS
Demographics			
Mean age	73 y	70 y	<0.0001
Male gender	67%	60%	<0.05
CV risk factors			
Smoking	71%	71%	NS
Arterial hypertension	88%	83%	NS
Dyslipidemia	76%	81%	NS
Diabetes mellitus	24%	24%	NS
Chronic CAD	55%	44%	0.01
Diagnostic studies			
Cardiac stress test	67%	47%	0.0001
Duplex US	97%	99%	NS
MRA	25%	22%	NS
Angiography	16%	11%	0.05
Operative technique			
Shunt	22%	13%	0.001
Patch	87%	89%	NS
Eversion CEA	2%	3%	NS

CEA, carotid endarterectomy; TIA, transient ischemic attack; CV, cardiovascular; CAD coronary artery disease; US, ultrasonography; MRA, magnetic resonance angiography; NS, not significant.

bifurcation, reoperation, and cervical radiation therapy (4.6% vs. 1.7%; $p < 0.13$). In 121 patients, excluded on the base of synchronous or immediate subsequent operations (who would have also been excluded from SAPPHIRE), the overall stroke (1.65%; $p = 0.69$), death (1.65%; $p = 0.09$), and MI (0.83%; $p = 0.71$) rates were not significantly different from the study population. The authors concluded that SAPPHIRE-eligible high-risk patients could undergo CEA with stroke and death rates well within accepted standards, and that patients with local risk factors were at higher risk for cranial nerve injuries, not necessarily stroke. These

TABLE 24-4. Number and Frequency of High-Risk Criteria in all Carotid Endarterectomies ($n = 776$); 84 Operations were Associated with More Than One High-Risk Criteria

High-Risk Criteria	Number (Frequency)
Positive cardiac stress test	109 (14%)
Age >80 y	85 (11%)
Contralateral carotid occlusion	66 (9%)
Pulmonary dysfunction	56 (7%)
High carotid bifurcation	36 (5%)
Carotid reoperation	27 (3%)
Left ventricular EF <30%	11 (1.4%)
NYHA class III/IV CHF	11 (1.4%)
NYHA class III/IV angina	8 (1%)
Cervical radiation therapy	6 (<1%)
Recent (<6 wk) cardiac operation	4 (<1%)
Contralateral laryngeal nerve palsy	2 (<1%)
Recent (<4 wk) MI	1 (<1%)

EF, ejection fraction; CHF, chronic heart failure; NYHA, New York Heart Association; MI, myocardial infarction.

data bring into question the application of CAS as an alternative to CEA, even in high-risk patients.

While the previously cited studies do not support the premise that operative risk is higher in patients excluded from NASCET and ACAS, or trials of CAS in high-risk patients, there may in fact be categories of patients in whom CEA may not be optimal therapy. Hertzer et al.[14] described the Cleveland Clinic experience for 2228 consecutive CEA procedures in 2046 patients from 1989 to 1995. The stroke and mortality rates for CEA as an isolated procedure were exemplary at 1.8% and 0.5%, respectively, for a combined rate of 2.3%. In addition, no statistical difference was found in stroke and mortality rates for asymptomatic patients, those presenting with hemispheric TIA, or those operated for stroke with minimal residua. Those patients having combined CEA and CABG had higher rates of perioperative stroke (4.3%) and death (5.3%) than those patients having isolated CEA. Carotid reoperations were also associated with higher stroke (4.6%) and death rates (2.0%). These data again lend credence to the idea that CEA can be performed safely in large groups of unselected patients, but may give some insight into categories of patients who are at increased risk for operative intervention.

A follow-up study from the Cleveland Clinic by Ouriel et al.[15] attempted to identify a subgroup of patients who, upon retrospective analysis, were at increased risk for CEA, and therefore might be better served by CAS. From a prospective database over 10-year period, 3061 carotid endarterectomies were examined. A high-risk cohort was identified, based on the presence of severe coronary artery disease (requiring angioplasty or bypass surgery within the 6 months prior to CEA), history of CHF, severe chronic obstructive pulmonary disease (COPD), or renal insufficiency (serum creatinine greater than 3 mg/dL). (Figures 24-1 and 24-2) The rate of the composite endpoint of stroke/death/MI was 3.8% for the entire group (stroke 2.1%; MI 1.2%; and death 1.1%). This composite end-

point occurred in 7.4% of those considered high risk ($n = 594$; 19.4%), significantly higher than in those in the low-risk ($n = 2467$; 80.6%) category (2.9%; $p = 0.008$). Patients in the high-risk group were further subdivided into those who had CEA alone and those in whom CEA was combined with CABG. Not surprisingly, the incidence of the composite endpoint was greater in those having combined CEA/CABG than those having CEA as an isolated procedure. In those having CEA alone, the risk of death was significantly greater in the high-risk group ($p < 0.001$). Importantly, however, while the risk of the combined endpoint stroke/death/MI was greater in the high-risk group, this

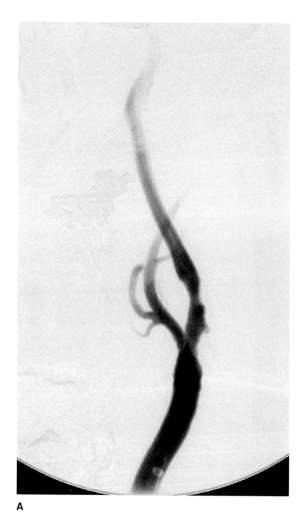

A

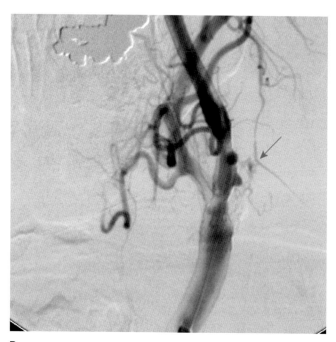

B

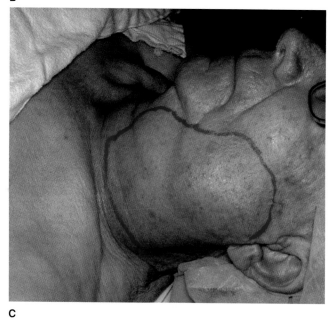

C

● **FIGURE 24-1.** (A and B) CAS in a symptomatic patient with an extremely calcified lesion. Note contrast extravasation on delayed angiographic image (*arrow*). (C) Cervical hematoma secondary to carotid artery rupture was managed nonoperatively.

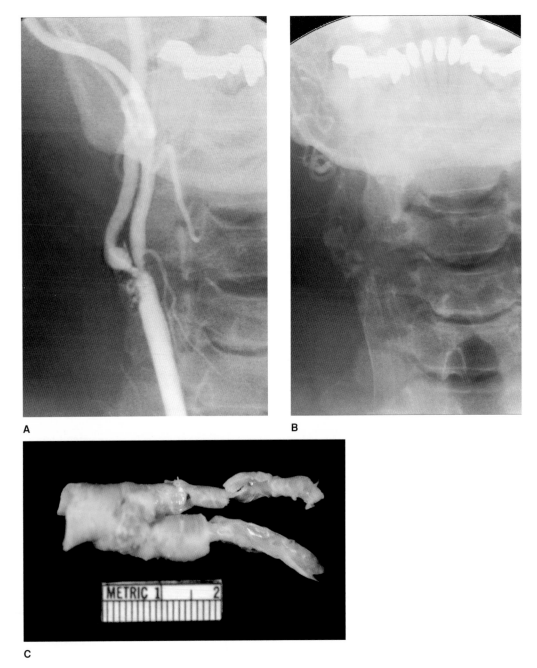

● FIGURE 24-2. (A) Angiography of a similarly calcified lesion of the right ICA. (B) Note calcification seen on plain radiograph. (C) Surgical specimen following CEA.

difference did not reach statistical significance ($p = 0.078$). In addition, the rates of the individual endpoints of MI and stroke did not differ statistically between the high- and low-risk groups. These data from the Cleveland Clinic vascular surgery registry seem to support the notion that patients enrolled in the multicenter trials of CEA (NASCET and ACAS) were likely similar to the low-risk group, while those in the high-risk group may not in fact have had such stellar outcomes if included in multicenter trials. Other authors have called into question the very idea of high-risk CEA; conflicting data exist as to factors such as high lesions, reoperations, cervical radiation, and contralateral carotid occlusion.[16–22] Subsequent trials have therefore focused

on medically compromised, high-risk patients as those who may benefit from an alternative procedure such as CAS.

High-Risk CEA

Significant disagreement exists regarding the definition of high-risk CEA. Based on data presented previously in this chapter, there is in fact a group of patients who are probably not best served by CEA—and should therefore be treated with CAS or with best medical therapy (especially asymptomatic patients felt to be at very high risk for any procedure). Tables 24-6 through 24-9 present data, principally from large single-center experiences, regarding the

TABLE 24-6. Risk of Perioperative Stroke and Death Following CEA in Large Series from Tertiary-Care Institutions

Institution	Time Period	Number of Patients	Symptomatic (%)	Stroke (%)	Death (%)
Cleveland Clinic	1989–1995	1924	39	1.8	0.5
University of Rochester	1993–2000	859	46	1.7	0.5
Ochsner Clinic	1996–1998	348	40	2.5	0.3
Stonybrook	1996–2001	788	39	0.8	0.4
University of Alabama	1998–2000	389	43	1.7	0.2
Mayo Clinic, Rochester	1998–2002	716	27	1.4	0.3
Total		5024			
Weighed average				1.6	0.4

performance of CEA in various subgroups typically deemed high risk. Several points deserve emphasis. In Table 24-6, more than 5000 carotid endarterectomies are compiled from six centers, with a composite risk of stroke and death of less than 2%; note that approximately 40% of patients in these series were symptomatic, the remaining 60% performed in asymptomatic patients. Nevertheless, the results are similar to those reported for the ACAS trial, which was an entirely asymptomatic cohort of patients. Elderly patients (>80 years) represent a particular challenge with both open surgery (CEA) and CAS; conflicting data exists in the peer-reviewed literature regarding which treatment is optimal. The data presented in Table 24-7 suggests that octogenarians are well treated with CEA, and that results compare favorably with those in younger patients. Those patients with contralateral internal carotid occlusion can also be safely treated with CEA compared to those with patent contralateral ICAs, as reflected in Table 24-8. Finally, patients having restenosis following prior CEA and those with radiation-induced carotid stenosis also have acceptable risks of stroke and death following operation; the major risk in this group of patients is that of cranial nerve injury, which can be debilitating (Table 24-9). These data suggest that the recommendation for CEA or CAS must be individualized, and that the traditional concept of "high-risk for CEA" may be challenged, especially in centers that excel in endarterectomy.

Finally, there are certain high-risk patients who are not well served by CAS who, if suitable for surgical intervention, may be well served by endarterectomy. Table 24-10 lists some *relative* contraindications and limitation to CAS for consideration. (Figures 24-1 to 24-3.)

Carotid Angioplasty/Stenting

The use of angioplasty and stenting techniques in the coronary and peripheral circulation stimulated an interest in the application of this technology to the carotid circulation, especially in those patients who are poor surgical candidates (Figure 24-4).

Indications: The basic indications for CAS do not differ from those of standard surgical carotid endarterectomy:

1. Asymptomatic lesions determined to be "high-grade," typically >70% by duplex ultrasound. Most clinical trials of CAS in asymptomatic patients require an *angiographic* stenosis of at least 80% for study inclusion.

2. Symptomatic patients (hemispheric TIA, amaurosis fugax, or stroke with minimal residua) with at least a 70% angiographic stenosis. While patients with symptomatic, ulcerated stenoses greater than 50% benefit from endarterectomy, this has not yet been extrapolated to carotid intervention.

A list of the possible indications for CAS in high-risk patients is listed in Table 24-11.

Results of CAS

Short-Term Results. The short-term results of CAS are largely dependent upon the presence or absence of cerebral embolization. With the relatively recent addition of cerebral protection to the procedure, associated stroke risk seems to have decreased. Admittedly, however, improvements in devices and technology have created a "moving target," making evaluation of results difficult at best.

Results from the SAPPHIRE[23] trial of CAS in high-risk patients have been published. This trial, which included a group randomized to CAS ($n = 159$) or CEA (151) is the only industry-sponsored FDA-approved trial to date which did in fact randomize patients. A separate registry was compiled of patients felt to be too high risk for surgery and underwent CAS ($n = 406$) or who were not suitable candidates for CAS and underwent CEA ($n = 7$). Importantly, the study sought to evaluate the combined endpoint of major adverse events (MAE) including stroke, death, and MI. Patients were independently evaluated by a certified neurologist before and after the procedure. Importantly, this trial was designed to support *noninferiority* of CAS compared with CEA. The majority of the randomized

TABLE 24-7. Risk of Perioperative Stroke and Death Following CEA in 80-Year-Old and Older Patients and in "Nonoctogenarians"

Authors/Institution/Year	Age Group (y)	Number of Patients	Symptomatic (%)	Stroke (%)	Death (%)	"Nonoctogenarians" Number/Stroke (%)/Death (%)
Plecha et al./Cleveland Vascular Society/1985	≥80	224	—	1.8	2.7	5778/1.8/1.5
Thomas et al./Melbourne, Australia/1996	>80	113	74	4.2	1.8	1705/2.7/1.9
O'Hara et al./Cleveland Clinic/1998	≥80	167	45	1.6	0.6	—/2.2/0.6
Perler et al./Maryland State/1998	≥80	1036	67	1.2	1.4	8882/1.0/1.9
Pruner et al./Milan, Italy/2003	>80	269	40	1.7	1.4	2474/1.2/0.3
Mozes et al./Mayo Clinic, Rochester/2004	≥80	109	39	0.9	0.0	667/1.5/0.3
Total		1918				19 506
Weighed average				1.5	1.5	1.4/1.5

TABLE 24-8. Risk of Perioperative Stroke and Death Following CEA in Patients with and Without Contralateral Carotid Occlusion

Authors/Institution/Year	Number of Patients	Symptomatic (%)	Stroke (%)	Death (%)	"No Contralateral Occlusion" Number/Stroke (%)/Death (%)
Sachs et al./Emory University/1984	54	59	5.6	0.0	410/2.0/0.8
Mackey et al./Tufts University/1990	63	57	4.8	0.0	535/2.6/1.1
Mattos et al./Southern Illinois University/1992	66	77	3.0	1.5	478/2.9/1.3
McCarthy et al./Northwestern University/1993	81	57	4.9	1.2	445/2.5/0.7
Coyle et al./Emory University/1995	116	48	1.7	2.6	956/2.5/1.5
Cao et al./University of Perugia, Italy/1995	55	75	0.0	0.0	110/2.7/1.0
Locati et al./Busto Arsizio, Cuggiono, Italy/2000	198	75	1.0	1.0	1068/0.9/0.3
Rockman et al./New York University/2002	338	62	3.0	0.6	2082/2.1/0.6
Mozes et al./Mayo Clinic/2004	67	25	3.0	1.5	709/1.3/0.1
Total	1038				6793
Weighed average			2.7	1.0	2.0/0.7

TABLE 24-9. Risk of Perioperative Stroke, Death and Cranial Nerve Injury Following CEA in Patients with Recurrent Carotid Artery Stenosis or Prior Cervical Radiation Therapy

Local "Risk Factor"	Author(s)/Institution/Year	Number of Patients	Symptomatic (%)	Stroke (%)	Death (%)	Cranial Nerve Injury All/Major (%)
Recurrent carotid stenosis	Das et al./Cleveland clinic/1985	61	51	1.5	3.1	9.2/1.5
	Bartlett/University of California, San Francisco/1987	94	70	4.3	2.0	19.8/—
	Meyer et al./Mayo Clinic/1994	82	92	6.5	4.3	—/—
	Mansour et al./Loyola University, Maywood/1997	69	66	4.8	0.0	7.3/1.2
	Hill et al./Stanford University/1999	40	50	0.0	0.0	7.2/0.0
	Hobson et al./New Jersey Medical School/1999	16	62	0.0	0.0	6.2/6.2
	O'Hara et al./Cleveland Clinic/2001	195	43	2.6	0.0	1.0/—
	Mozes et al./Mayo Clinic/2004	26	23	3.8	0.0	7.7/3.8
Total		583				
Weighed average				3.4	1.2	7.3/1.8
Prior cervical radiation	Francfort et al./Thomas Jefferson University Hospital, case report and review of literature/1989	20	73	4.0	0.0	—/—
	Rockman et al./New York University/1996	10	30	10.0	0.0	0.0/0.0
	Kashyap et al./University of California, Los Angeles/1999	24	73	0.0	0.0	23.0/0.0
	Friedell et al./Orlando Regional Medical Center/2000	10	50	0.0	0.0	0.0/0.0
	Leseche et al./Clichy, France/2003	27	60	3.3	3.3	0.0/0.0
Total		91				
Weighed average				3.0	1.0	7.8/0.0

TABLE 24-10. Limitations and Relative Contraindications to CAS

Unfavorable aortic arch anatomy
Severe tortuosity of the common or internal carotid
    arteries
Severely calcified/undilatable stenoses
Lesions containing fresh thrombus
Large amount of laminated thrombus at the site of
    patch angioplasty (prior CEA) on duplex ultrasound.
Extensive stenoses (longer than 2 cm)
Critical (99% and more) stenoses (string sign)
Lesions adjacent to carotid artery aneurysms
Contrast-related issues:
    Chronic renal insufficiency
    Previous life-threatening contrast reaction
Preload dependent states—severe aortic valvular
    stenosis
Age >>80 y

patients were asymptomatic; of the group randomized to CAS, 30.2% were symptomatic, and in the group randomized to CEA, 28.5% were symptomatic. At 30 days, the risk of stroke (CAS, 3.1%, CEA 3.3%, $p > 0.99$) in the two groups was almost identical. One patient in the CAS group (0.6%) and three patients in the CEA group (2.0%) died within 30 days; this difference did not reach statistical significance ($p = 0.36$). When periprocedural MI was examined, more patients in the CEA group suffered this complication (6.6%) than in the CAS group (4.4%), a difference that did reach significance ($p < 0.05$). Of note, the majority of the MI's were non-Q, identified on routine postprocedure laboratory studies, including 3 of 3 in the CAS group and 8 of 10 in the CEA cohort. The combined endpoint death/stroke/MI did not reach statistical significance (CAS 4.4%, CEA 9.9%, $p = 0.08$). At 1 year, those endpoints which reached statistical significance included major ipsilateral stroke (CAS 0%, CEA 3.3%, $p = 0.03$) and MI (CAS 2.5%, CEA 7.9%, $p = 0.04$). The reported results in the stent registry group included 20 strokes (4.9%), 9 deaths (2.2%), and 7 periprocedural MI's (1.7%) at 30 days.

The ARCHeR[24] trial represents another industry-sponsored study of a stent and protection device; it differs from SAPPHIRE in that it is a registry of high-risk patients rather than a randomized trial, and is a series of three multicenter, nonrandomized, prospective studies, which ultimately enrolled 581 high-risk patients from 48 centers. Angiographic stenosis of at least 50% for symptomatic patients and 80% for asymptomatic patients was required. The Accunet filter embolic protection device and the Acculink stent were utilized in this study; both devices were manufactured by Guidant, Inc. For the first portion of the study,

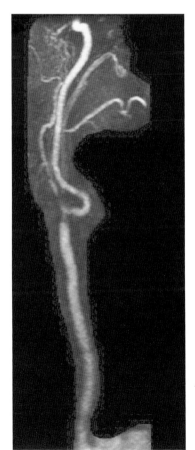

A

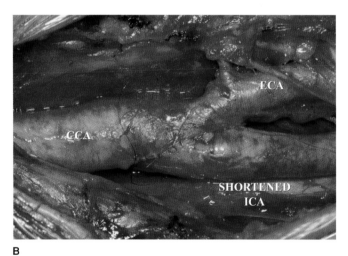

B

● **FIGURE 24-3.** (A) Magnetic resonance angiogram (MRA) shows tortuous ICA with high-grade stenosis. (B) Following eversion endarterectomy with ICA shortening and resolution of tortuosity.

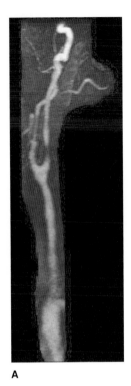
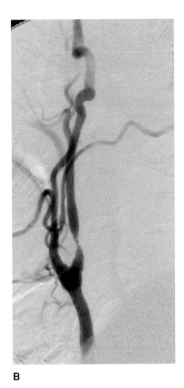
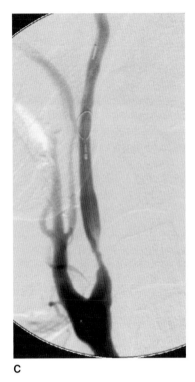
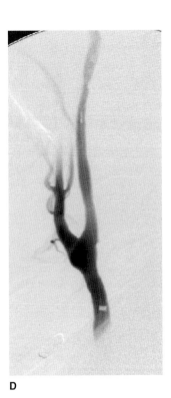

A   B   C   D

● **FIGURE 24-4.** (A) MRA identifies high-grade recurrent left internal carotid stenosis, 1.5 years following CEA. (B) Catheter angiography of the same lesion. (C) Filter has been deployed in the ICA. (D) Following angioplasty and stenting.

stents were placed without embolic protection, which was added in the latter two groups (422 patients). The primary endpoints were death, stroke, or MI at 30 days, and ipsilateral stroke from 31 to 365 days. The risk of the combined endpoint of stroke/death/MI at 30 days was 8.3%, and for stroke/death was 6.9% at 30 days; most strokes were minor. The risk of major/fatal stroke was 1.5%. The risk of ipsilat-

eral stroke at 1 year was 1.3%, yielding a primary composite endpoint of 9.6% at 1 year.

The EVA-3S study (Endarterectomy vs. Angioplasty in Patients with Severe Symptomatic Carotid Stenosis)[25] randomized symptomatic patients with > 60% carotid stenosis to + CAS or CEA. The trial, started in November 2000, was stopped in September 2005 at the recommendation of its Safety Committee. To participate, 20 academic and 10 nonacademic centers were required to have a neurologist (who was responsible for evaluating and following patients), a vascular surgeon who had performed at least 25 CEA (with no upper limit of stroke + death following CEA), and an interventional physician (who must have performed 12 CAS procedures or 35 interventions in the supra-aortic trunks, at least five of which were in the carotid artery); CAS operators had to have performed at least two procedures with a new device before it could be used in the trial. Patients with >60% de novo carotid artery stenoses, which were symptomatic, could be included in the study; exclusion criteria were similar to other trials. Patients were evaluated at 48 hours, 30 days, and 6 months posttreatment by a study neurologist. The primary endpoint was a composite of stroke and death at 30 days. Secondary endpoints included MI, TIA, cranial nerve injury, major local complications, and systemic complications within 30 days. In addition, ipsilateral stroke, any stroke, or any stroke or death from 31 days to last follow-up were evaluated.

Two-hundred and sixty-one patients underwent CAS, while 259 had CEA and were analyzed for primary outcome measures. Although the trial was designed to

TABLE 24-11. Indications for CAS in High-Risk Patients

1. Severe cardiac disease
   a. Requiring coronary PTA or CABG
   b. History of CHF
2. Severe COPD
   a. Requiring home oxygen
   b. FEV_1 <20% predicted
3. Severe chronic renal insufficiency
   a. Serum creatinine >3 mg/dL
   b. Currently on dialysis
4. Prior CEA (restenosis)
   a. Contralateral vocal cord paralysis
5. Surgically inaccessible lesions
   a. At or above the second cervical vertebra
   b. Inferior to the clavicle
6. Radiation-induced carotid stenosis
7. Prior ipsilateral radical neck dissection

demonstrate noninferiority, stenting was found to carry a greater risk than endarterectomy. The 30-day incidence of any stroke or death was 3.9% following CEA and 9.6% following CAS (with a relative risk of 2.5), a difference which was statistically significant. The 30-day incidence of disabling stroke or death was 1.5% following CEA and 3.4% following CAS, a relative risk of 2.2. Systemic complications were more frequent in the CEA group and major local complications were more common in the CAS group, but these differences did not reach statistical significance. Not surprisingly, cranial nerve injury was more common following CEA (7.7%). There was neither a difference in results from high-enrolling and low-enrolling centers, nor a difference when comparing experienced and less-experienced operators. The trial was stopped prematurely after enrollment of 527 patients because of "both safety and futility," as CAS carried significantly higher risk than CEA. The excess of primary outcome events after CAS was felt to be sufficient (one additional stroke with CAS for each 17 patients treated) for the Safety Committee to recommend stopping the trial. The authors note that the results of CEA were better than anticipated (based on previous pivotal trials), and conclude that the risks associated with endarterectomy have diminished significantly over time.

Thirty-day results from the SPACE[26] trial (Stent-protected angioplasty versus CEA in symptomatic patients) have been recently published. In this study, 1200 symptomatic patients (TIA or moderate stroke within 180 days) were randomized to CAS or CEA. The primary endpoints were ipsilateral ischemic stroke or death within 30 days of the procedure, analyzed on an intent-to-treat basis. The rate of death or stroke was 6.84% in the CAS group and 6.34% in the CEA group. The authors concluded that the study failed to prove the noninferiority of CAS compared with CEA (based on a p value of 0.09) and that the widespread use of CAS could not be justified.

These studies appear to have been well-designed and implemented, and their conclusions, given the data presented, seem valid. In addition, they are set against a backdrop of a systematic review[27] of five randomized trials comparing CAS with CEA which concluded that CEA is the current standard of care for patients with carotid stenosis. Given these results, it would seem that until data to the contrary are presented, endarterectomy is the treatment of choice for most patients with high-grade carotid artery stenosis; certain high-risk anatomic and physiologic subsets may be well treated with CAS, as suggested by the SAPPHIRE[23] study.

Stent Implantation, Restenosis, and Duplex Follow-up.

Restenosis has proven to be a substantial clinical problem following endovascular therapy in a number of vascular beds, including the coronary and renal arteries. Prior to the routine use of stents in conjunction with angioplasty (percutaneous transluminal angioplasty [PTA]), Crawley et al.[28] followed 12 patients with symptomatic carotid stenosis treated with PTA alone. The immediate angioplasty result decreased the mean percent stenosis from 82% to

51%. Six of the twelve showed further improvement in lumen diameter of >14% at 1 year, from a mean stenosis immediately post-PTA of 47% to 28% at follow-up angiography. Obviously, there is substantial arterial remodeling that occurs following carotid PTA. Schillinger et al.,[29] in a prospective study of 108 patients having CAS (with stenting), found restenosis of >50% in 6 patients (14%). Elevated levels of C-reactive protein (CRP) at 48 hours postintervention, indicative of a systemic inflammatory response, correlate strongly with restenosis at 6 months ($p = 0.01$). Both residual stenosis of 10% to 30% and restenosis following prior stent implantation were independent predictors of restenosis in this study. Khan et al.[30] identified, in a series of 222 patients having successful carotid artery stenting, a number of factors which were predictive of restenosis. By univariate analysis, female gender and age >75 years were statistically predictive of restenosis; by multivariate analysis, older age, female gender, implantation of multiple stents, and postprocedural percent stenosis were associated with an increased risk of restenosis. Christiaans et al.[31] also identified loss of proximal stent apposition as a risk factor for restenosis. In addition, in their series, most restenoses were found on routine follow-up and were asymptomatic, a finding confirmed by Lal et al.[32] These studies suggest that a number of patient-related and procedure-related factors are associated with restenosis following CAS. While the reported incidence of restenosis is quite variable, ranging from 1.8% to 75%, most studies report restenosis rates between 5% and 10% at 12 to 24 months.

Because of the nature of CAS—the plaque is not removed, simply displaced—the duplex criteria used to follow patients post-CEA may not apply. Robbin et al.,[33] reporting on patients treated at the University of Alabama at Birmingham by Yadav et al.,[23] prospectively studied 170 stented carotid arteries. Prospective duplex criteria for stenosis included peak systolic velocity greater than 125 cm/s, ICA:CCA ratio greater than 3, and intrastent doubling of velocity. Although very few stents showed significant restenosis, duplex was able to accurately identify restenosis, and correlated with angiographic findings at 1 year.

Clearly, based on this data, a baseline duplex following CAS, which can be correlated with the completion angiogram and followed over time, is imperative. This policy will lead to fewer false-positive duplex studies.

From the data presented, several recommendations regarding follow-up in patients having CAS can be made:

1. Duplex ultrasound follow-up of stented carotid arteries is an important tool to identify patients with restenosis. Early restenosis is typically secondary to myointimal hyperplasia.

2. As follow-up duplex ultrasound studies may be difficult to interpret based on traditional velocity criteria, a baseline study is imperative; this must be correlated with the degree of residual stenosis at the completion of the CAS procedure. Subsequent studies are

performed at 3, 6, and 12 months, and at 6- to 12-month intervals thereafter.

Current evidence suggests that a peak systolic velocity ≤150 cm/s in the ICA correlates with a normal vessel (0%–19% stenosis). Elevation of the peak systolic velocity and the ICA:CCA ratio (>80% increase) may be an even more important criterion in determining significant restenosis following CAS. Identification of high-grade restenosis typically warrants further evaluation with contrast angiography. Most patients having recurrent stenosis complicating CAS can be safely treated with repeat angioplasty.

Technical Aspects of CAS

Anatomy. The anatomy of the cerebral circulation, from the aortic arch to the capillary level, is important to the planning of CAS. Several anatomic considerations are particularly germaine to the procedure. The configuration of the aortic arch is perhaps the first anatomic challenge to consider. With advancing age, the apex of the arch tends to become displaced further distally. This change in arch configuration tends to make selective catheterization of the brachiocephalic vessels more challenging, and influences the choice of catheter to be used. The operator should become familiar with a variety of selective catheters; the author prefers the Simmons II catheter, as it provides for "deep" cannulation of the common carotid artery (CCA), facilitating ultimate passage of a guidewire for delivery of a sheath. As the level of the origin of the object vessel increases in distance from the dome of the arch, the degree of difficulty in obtaining guidewire and sheath access increases. Cannulation of a left CCA arising from a common brachiocephalic trunk (bovine arch) may be particularly difficult to access, and should be identified on preprocedural contrast- or MRA-aortography. Especially when starting to perform these interventions, a complete study, including the aortic arch and origins of the brachiocephalic trunks, is essential.

The presence of any tandem lesions along the course of the cerebral circulation is likewise important in treatment planning. Proximal CCA lesions may require intervention prior to ICA revascularization, in order to provide safe access to the ICA. Tortuosity of the ICA is also relevant; while most ICAs are relatively straight, extreme tortuosity may preclude safe passage of a guidewire or protection device, and may exclude patients from safe intervention. The anatomy and configuration of the external carotid artery (ECA) is typically not an important consideration in carotid intervention, even when this vessel is iatrogenically stenosed or covered with a bare stent.

Finally, collateral circulation (or lack thereof) through the circle of Willis is an important consideration which may profoundly influence procedural strategy. The status of the contralateral ICA, the vertebral-basilar system, and the intracranial collaterals may effect the type of embolic protection to be used. Anatomic variations in the circle of Willis are the rule rather than the exception. A "complete" circle is present in less than half of all cases.[34] Common variations include a hypoplastic (10%) or absent A1 segment, and plexiform(10%–33%) or duplicated (18%) anterior communicating artery. Anomalies of the posterior portion of the circle of Willis occur in half of all cases, including a hypoplastic (33%) or absent posterior communicating artery. Careful attention should be paid, on preprocedure angiography or intracranial MRA, to the anterior and posterior communicating arteries. Patients with limited collateral circulation may develop reversible neurologic symptoms with inflation of a protection balloon or during angioplasty of the target lesion. They may also be at higher risk for permanent neurologic deficts, as their limited collateral blood supply will be less likely to compensate for any iatrogenic arterial occlusions complicating the procedure.

Cerebral Protection During CAS. Stroke remains the most devastating complication of procedures, both surgical and interventional, directed at the extracranial carotid artery. Although a number of etiologies for stroke have been described, the majority are caused by cerebral embolization of atheromatous debris or thrombus. While CEA can be performed without mobilization and dissection of the carotid bulb, the same cannot be said for CAS, where the lesion must be crossed with a guidewire, balloon, and stent for treatment to occur. This has prompted the development of devices to prevent atheromatous embolization during critical portions of the procedure. Most would predict that unprotected angioplasty and stenting of high-grade, ulcerated carotid lesions would produce stroke rates of at least 25%. Nevertheless, even with relatively crude equipment and a lack of cerebral protection, early series of CAS produced stroke rates far below this level.

Even when cerebral emboli do not produce major stroke, they may in fact cause substantial cognitive impairment. Gaunt et al.,[35] in a prospective study of 100 patients monitored with TCD during CEA, found that microemboli were detected during 92% of procedures. While most emboli were characteristic of air (and not associated with adverse clinical events), more than 10 particulate emboli correlated with significant deterioration in postoperative cognitive function. Bickness et al.[36] studied the embolic potential of human carotid plaques during experimental angioplasty. An average of 133 emboli per angioplasty were measured; lesion severity correlated with increased maximum size of embolic particles ($p = 0.012$). Importantly, patients having been placed on statin therapy more than 4 weeks preoperatively had significantly fewer emboli of smaller size ($p = 0.022$). In the clinical arena, Tübler et al.,[37] using a distal balloon-occlusion system during CAS, found that the median number of particles, their maximum diameter, and their maximum area were significantly higher in patients who had periprocedural neurologic complications. Three phases of the procedure are associated with an increased risk of embolization: predilatation, stent deployment, and postdilatation.

Devices for Cerebral Embolic Protection. Three types of embolic protection are currently available for use in the carotid artery, either as part of FDA-approved clinical trials, or "off-label" use of devices approved for noncarotid use. These include distal balloon occlusion, distal filter protection, and reversal of internal carotid flow. Theron et al.[38] were the first to report on the use of an angioplasty technique involving temporary occlusion of the ICA during manipulation of ulcerated plaques. They subsequently reported on a triple-coaxial catheter system allowing angioplasty with cerebral protection in 13 patients. Cholesterol crystals, ranging in size from 600 to 1200 μm, were aspirated at the time of intervention. The PercuSurge Guardwire (Medtronic AVE, Santa Rosa, CA), which is approved for aortocoronary saphenous vein graft intervention, has been used in the MAVERIC trial of carotid intervention, and has been used extensively during off-label carotid intervention outside of FDA-approved clinical trials. Advantages of this device include its low profile and ease of crossing the target lesion, procedural simplicity, and its ability to aspirate large particulate debris following intervention. Disadvantages include potential incomplete occlusion of the ICA in patients with particularly large arteries (the device can be inflated from 3 mm to 6 mm diameter) and inability to aspirate exceptionally large particles into the suction catheter following intervention. In addition, as flow is diverted into the ECA, emboli may travel by this route and into the ipsilateral middle cerebral artery via periorbital and ophthalmic artery collaterals. Finally, a small percentage of patients with an incomplete circle of Willis and an "isolated" cerebral hemisphere may be intolerant of even temporary internal carotid occlusion. Whitlow et al.[39] evaluated the PercuSurge device in 75 CAS procedures. Four patients (5%) developed transient neurologic symptoms during balloon occlusion which resolved with deflation and restoration of internal carotid flow. Embolic material was aspirated from the internal carotid in all patients; none of the patients suffered major or minor stroke at 30 days.

A great deal of interest in filter protection devices has been generated, in an attempt to trap large particulate debris while maintaining flow in the internal carotid; this not only provides continued cerebral perfusion during intervention, but also allows angiography of the target vessel during various phases of the procedure. The pore size of all currently available filters is greater than 100 μm; as such they allow passage of smaller particles that may not cause clinically significant neurologic events, but which may cause silent neuronal injury. These filters may also be difficult to pass across particularly severe stenoses because of their larger profile when compared to balloon occlusion devices. Filters which are not completely apposed to the vessel wall may allow emboli to pass around the device and into the distal cerebral circulation.

Ohki et al.[40] reported on the use of a device which induces reversal of flow in the ICA by occluding the common and external carotid arteries via balloon occlusion of the external carotid and creation of a temporary AV shunt between the internal carotid and the femoral vein. This device, while potentially more cumbersome than other protection devices, may in fact produce "complete" protection by preventing *any* emboli from traveling to the intracranial circulation.

New et al.[41] reported their experience with 1202 CAS procedures from 1994 to 2002. During the study period, 33% of patients had a cerebral protection device used during their procedures. The overall stroke rate was 4.4%; the risk of stroke reached its maximum during the period from September 1996 to September 1997 (9.1%) and reached its nadir during the final year of the study (0.6%). The authors conclude that improvements in technique, equipment, pharmacotherapy and the use of neuroprotection have contributed significantly to improvements in results. Protection devices are not without potential problems and complications, including abrupt vessel closure secondary to iatrogenic dissection, inability to retrieve the device, transient loss of consciousness, and tremors and fasciculations secondary to device-induced cerebral ischemia. Nevertheless, it seems reasonable, based on the available evidence, to consider embolic cerebral protection devices in most cases of CAS.

Pharmacologic Adjuncts for the Prevention of Intraprocedural Stroke. The pharmacologic prevention of thromboembolic events during CAS is modeled after the literature regarding prevention of these events during percutaneous coronary interventions. Intravenous heparin should be administered to maintain an ACT of at least 250 to 300 seconds. Antiplatelet therapy consists of aspirin and clopidogrel orally prior to the procedure and for 1 month following the procedure. Antiplatelet therapy with glycoprotein IIB-IIIA antagonists has been shown to reduce thromboembolic complications during percutaneous coronary procedures. While there has been some interest in applying these agents to patients undergoing CAS, early data suggest that they offer no significant benefit[42] and may increase the risk of intracerebral hemorrhage.

Procedural Details. Regardless of the exact physical location of the procedure, access to high-quality imaging equipment is mandatory; portable C-arms are less adequate for this purpose. Patients are placed in a supine position; both groins are prepared routinely. The head is placed in a cradle and gently secured to decrease patient motion during critical portions of the procedure. The procedure is performed with the patient awake, although minimal sedation is acceptable particularly in anxious subjects.

The author's technique for CAS has evolved with time. The procedure, in its current iteration, is performed in the following steps, with few exceptions. Although one must, of course, be able to make adjustments to unanticipated situations, we encourage the operators to standardize the procedure as much as possible.

1. Retrograde femoral access with a 5-F sheath.
2. Full heparin anticoagulation (typically 100 mg/kg body mass) after arterial access is gained and prior to manipulation of catheters in the aortic arch and brachiocephalic vessels.

3. Following selective catheterization of the ipsilateral mid-distal CCA (typically with a Simmons II catheter), a selective arteriogram of the carotid bifurcation is performed, paying careful attention to choose a view which provides minimal overlap of the internal and external carotid arteries and provides maximum visualization of the target lesion. A complete cerebral arteriogram, if not performed previously, is performed as a baseline and to identify intracranial pathology such as aneurysms and AV communications.

4. We have utilized two techniques for advancing a sheath into the CCA: (1) The preferred technique is to place an exchange-length guidewire into the terminal branches of the ECA; our personal favorite is a stiff, angled glide wire (realizing that sheath exchange over this wire, given its lubricious nature, can be tricky). The diagnostic catheter and 5-F sheath are removed (while maintaining constant visualization of the guidewire in the ECA during this process) and a long (70 to 90 cm, depending on patient body habitus) 6-F sheath is advanced, with its dilator, into the CCA. If larger (>8 mm diameter) stents are to be utilized, a 7-F sheath may be required to allow for contrast injection around the stent delivery system. Care must be taken to identify the tip of the dilator, which is not radiopaque, as it may extend a significant distance from the end of the sheath, depending on the brand of sheath utilized. Obviously, inadvertently advancing the dilator into the carotid bulb may have disastrous consequences. In patients with short CCA's or low bifurcations, the sheath can be advanced over the dilator once the sheath edge (radiopaque marker) is past the origin of the CCA; (2) alternatively, the long sheath can be advanced into the transverse arch over a guidewire. The dilator is removed, and an appropriate selective diagnostic catheter is advanced into the CCA. This catheter must be substantially longer than the sheath, typically 100 cm or longer. A stiff guidewire is then advanced into the ECA. Using the wire *and* catheter for support (by pinning both at the groin), the sheath (without dilator) is advanced into the CCA. This technique may be advantageous in "hostile" arches, in that the catheter and wire provide more support than a wire alone, but risks "snowplowing" the edge of the sheath at the junction of the aortic arch and the innominate or left CCA (without the protection of the sheath dilator), causing dissection or distal embolization. One should not underestimate the importance of gaining and maintaining sheath access to the distal CCA: once the 0.035-inch guidewire is removed (and ultimately exchanged for a 0.014-inch wire), "support" for angioplasty and stent placement is provided solely by the sheath. If the sheath backs up into the aortic arch during the interventional procedure, it is virtually impossible to advance it into the CCA over a 0.014-inch guidewire or protection device. Patient selection and recognition of which arches to avoid are paramount to success. Particularly in difficult arches, deep inspiration or expiration may facilitate sheath advancement by subtly changing the configuration of the brachiocephalic origins once guidewire access has been obtained. Alternatively, in patients in whom a sheath *cannot* be advanced into the CCA, a preshaped guiding sheath or catheter can be seated in the proximal CCA; while potentially facilitating an otherwise impossible intervention, guiding catheters provide a less stable position, and should be used only if no other reasonable alternative exists.

5. For patients with an occluded ECA, sheath access to the common carotid may be difficult. We have utilized two techniques to overcome this challenge: (1) A stiff 0.035-inch wire with a preshaped "J" can be placed into the distal CCA, taking care to avoid the bulb and bifurcation. The "J" configuration prevents guidewire traversal of the lesion. A stiff wire with a shapeable tip can be used to the same end; (2) Alternatively, a wire with variable diameter (0.018-inch tip, enlarging to 0.035-inch more proximally) can be used to cross the internal carotid lesion, giving additional guidewire support to facilitate sheath advancement. While a reasonable option, this technique ultimately necessitates crossing the target lesion twice.

6. Once the sheath is in place, the guidewire and dilator are removed. We prefer to attach the sheath sidearm to a slow, continuous infusion of heparin–saline solution to avoid stagnation of blood in the sheath. A selective angiogram of the carotid bifurcation is then performed through the sheath, again demonstrating the area of maximal stenosis, the extent of the lesion, and normal ICA and CCA above and below the lesion. Road mapping, if available, is helpful in crossing the lesion with an embolic protection device or guidewire. The majority of procedures are now performed with the aid of an embolic protection device.

7. It is wise to have determined an activated clotting time (ACT) prior to crossing the lesion and performing CAS. For patients in whom balloon occlusion of the ICA is being utilized for embolic protection, an ACT maintained at >300 seconds is desired. If a filter-type device or standard guidewire is employed, an ACT >250 seconds is likely sufficient. The interventional team should discuss, in detail, the steps that will subsequently be performed, so that all members are "on the same page." Balloons should be flushed and prepped (with special care to remove all air from the system in the unlikely event of balloon rupture), the stent opened and on the table, and the crossing guidewire/embolic protection device prepped. For de novo lesions, we typically administer atropine (0.5 to 1.0 mg intravenously) as prophylaxis against bradycardia during balloon inflation in the carotid

bulb; for restenoses following CEA, this may not be necessary. The monitoring nurse/CRNA should be alerted that balloon inflation may cause significant hemodynamic instability (bradycardia, hyptension).

8. The guidewire/embolic protection device (0.014 inch) is advanced across the lesion, with the aid of road mapping. Care should be taken when inserting the device through the sheath valve, as the tip can be damaged at this juncture. If a protection device is utilized, it should be deployed into the distal extracranial ICA, just prior to the horizontal petrous segment. For balloon-occlusion devices, *absence* of flow in the ICA must be demonstrated; for filter devices, apposition of the device to the ICA must be documented, along with flow in the ICA through the device (and should be documented after each step during the intervention, to detect a filter occluded with debris) (Figures 24-5 and 24-6).

9. The lesion is predilated with a 5.0-mm angioplasty balloon, typically with a monorail or "rapid exchange" platform. The balloon can be advanced into the distal CCA prior to crossing the lesion with the guidewire/protection device to save time. Typically, relatively low inflation pressures (4–6 mm Hg) are required to achieve balloon profile. After the predilation balloon is removed, another bifurcation angiogram is performed through the sheath (unless distal balloon occlusion is utilized, in which case the ICA will not be visualized; in these circumstances, the distal stent must be placed based on predetermined bony landmarks and the location of the CCA bifurcation).

10. The stent is then deployed after confirmation of accurate position. Our current preference is to utilize nitinol stents, most commonly extending an 8 to 10 mm (diameter) × 30 mm (length) stent from the ICA into the CCA, covering the ECA origin. Nitinol stents may have a tendency to "jump" distally when deployed rapidly (despite manufacturers' claims to the contrary), which may cause one to miss the target lesion. As such, we typically expose/deploy two or three stent rings and wait for 5 to 7 seconds, allowing the distal stent to become fully expanded, well-opposed and attached to the ICA above the lesion. Subsequently, the remainder of the stent can be deployed more rapidly with little worry that it will migrate. The diameter of the stent must be sized to the largest portion of the vessel, typically the distal CCA (and not the ICA); it is important to avoid unopposed stent in the CCA, which may become a nidus for thrombus formation. Unconstrained stent diameter should be at least 10% (approximately 1–2 mm) larger than the maximum CCA diameter. On occasion, the lesion will be limited to the ICA well above the carotid bifurcation, allowing for a shorter stent isolated to the ICA.

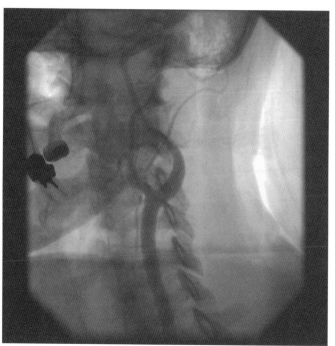

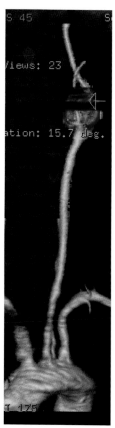

● **FIGURE 24-5.** (A) Catheter angiogram of carotid body tumor. Note splaying of internal and external carotid arteries at the bifurcation. (B) CT angiogram in the same patient highlights the tumor (*arrow*).

A

B

● **FIGURE 24-6.** (A) MRA. Symptomatic aneurysm of the right carotid bifurcation associated with a stenosis of the proximal ICA. (B) Surgical repair with interposition greater saphenous vein graft.

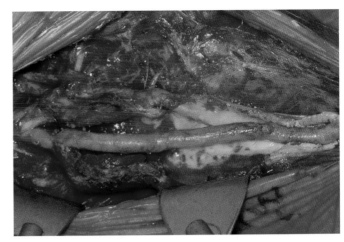

B

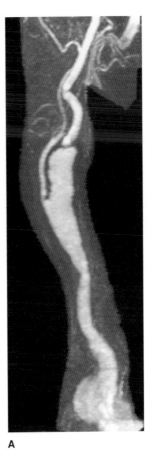

A

11. If necessary, the lesion is postdilated with a 5-mm balloon; larger balloons are rarely necessary. Our tendency has been to predilate with a larger balloon (5 mm diameter), avoiding postdilation if possible. A residual stenosis of 10% or so is completely acceptable; the goal is protection from embolic stroke, not necessarily a perfect angiographic result.

12. A completion angiogram of the carotid bulb/bifurcation and distal extracranial ICA is performed *prior to* removing the guidewire/device wire to assure that a dissection or occlusion has not occurred. Severe vasospasm can sometimes be encountered (and can mimic dissection). Watchful waiting and, on occasion, administration of vasodilators through the sheath (nitroglycerine in 100 μg aliquots) will usually resolve this problem. On occasion, the wire must be removed before spasm will resolve completely, but this should be undertaken only after dissection is excluded. After the wire is removed, a completion angiogram of the carotid and intracranial circulation is performed in two views.

13. We typically do not reverse the heparin anticoagulation, and obtain access-site hemostasis with a percutaneous closure device.

Following the procedure, the patient is monitored in the recovery area for approximately 30 minutes and is then transferred to a monitored floor. Admission to an intensive care unit is typically not necessary. Patients are allowed to ambulate in 2 to 3 hours if a closure device is utilized, and allowed to resume a regular diet. An occasional patient will suffer prolonged hypotension from carotid sinus stimulation; this can be managed with judicious fluid administration, pharmacologic treatment of bradycardia, and occasionally with intravenous pressors such as dopamine. A rare patient will experience prolonged hypotension which must be treated with oral agents; phenylephrine and midodrine are both acceptable for this purpose.

Regardless of the exact technique utilized for CSSA, like surgical CEA, proper patient selection, procedural standardization, and meticulous attention to detail are mandatory for success.

Complications Following CAS. Embolic stroke is the most common serious complication reported for CAS; its incidence may be affected by the use of cerebral protection devices. Advanced age and the presence of long or multiple lesions have been implicated as independent predictors of stroke. As with most procedures, there is a significant learning curve that must be overcome. Other complications have also been cited, including prolonged bradycardia and hypotension, deformation of balloon-expandable stents, stent thrombosis, and Horner's syndrome. Cerebral hyperperfusion with associated seizures and intracranial hemorrhage have also been reported.

Future Directions. Based on the preliminary results of clinical trials of CAS in high-risk patients, it appears that the results of this procedure are equivalent to CEA in this subgroup. The addition of cerebral protection, along with improvements in stents and better patient selection will likely add to its safety. The next logical question to be asked is "Can good-risk patients be safely treated with CAS?" The Carotid Revascularization Endarterectomy versus Stent Trial[43] will attempt to provide a definitive answer. This important study contrasts the relative efficacy of CEA and CAS in preventing primary outcomes of stroke, MI or death at 30 days, and ipsilateral stroke at 4-year follow-up. The primary criteria for eligibility are carotid stenosis of at least 50% and hemispheric TIA or nondisabling stroke. It is anticipated that 2500 patients will be randomized. The outcome is not anticipated for a number of years, but randomization is the only way to definitively answer the question at hand.

External Carotid Disease and Carotid Stump Syndrome

In cases of internal carotid occlusion, the ECA may provide significant perfusion to the intracranial circulation via a rich collateral network. These collaterals include communications via the superficial temporal artery to the ophthalmic artery, the occipital artery to the vertebral artery, and leptomeningeal collaterals which connect the middle meningeal artery to the anterior cerebral branch of the ICA. In patients with ICA occlusion and atherosclerotic disease of the ECA, emboli may travel to the retinal or intracranial circulatory beds. Patients will most commonly present with ocular symptoms (amaurosis fugax), but will occasionally develop focal hemispheric symptoms. Indications for treatment include symptomatic patients with ipsilateral ICA occlusion who have failed medical (antiplatelet) therapy and in whom other potential causes of cerebral ischemia have been excluded.[44] Treatment of asymptomatic patients is not warranted. Surgical therapy includes endarterectomy of the ECA, patch angioplasty, and exclusion of an ICA cul-de-sac if present.

The ECA may be patched with a "flap" of ICA, obviating the need for a prosthesis.

Carotid stump syndrome results from occlusion of the ICA and persistence of a "stump" or cul-de-sac of ICA at its origin. Thrombotic debris can embolize through a patent, nondiseased ECA into the retinal or cerebral beds. Treatment has typically been surgical, as described above. Recent reports suggest that endovascular therapy may have a role in this relatively infrequent condition.[45,46]

⬤ NONATHEROSCLEROTIC CAROTID DISEASE

Carotid Fibromuscular Dysplasia

Fibromuscular dysplasia (FMD) is a noninflammatory, nonatherosclerotic vasculopathy that affects medium-sized muscular arteries, including the ICA. A number of mech-

anisms have been postulated, including ischemia of the arterial media in long, nonbranching segments that result in web-like dysplastic lesions. The majority of cases are seen in females in their fourth or fifth decades of life, and with the more frequent use of noninvasive imaging, increasing numbers of cases are identified, many of which are asymptomatic. Approximately 65% of patients will have bilateral disease. Previous reports suggested a 20% to 50% incidence of associated aneurysms of the ipsilateral carotid siphon or middle cerebral artery, although a meta-analysis by Cloft et al.[47] suggests that the incidence may be closer to 7%. Twenty percent of patients with carotid FMD will also have fibromuscular disease of the vertebral arteries.

The diagnosis of carotid FMD is typically made on angiography or MRA. Duplex ultrasound may occasionally, but not consistently, make the diagnosis. The classis "string of beads" appearance (Figure 24-7) is typical of medial fibrodysplasia. Intimal fibroplasia appears as a smooth, tapered narrowing on contrast angiography. The differential diagnosis includes atypical atherosclerotic lesions, inflammatory vasculitis such as Takayasu's, neurofibromatosis, vascular spasm, and connective tissue diseases such as Ehlers-Danlos.

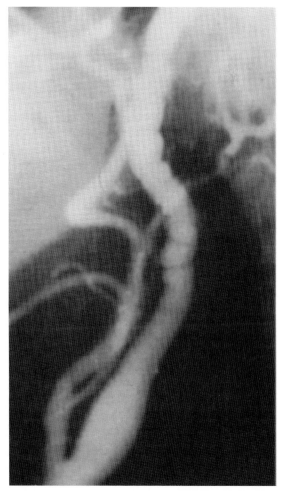

⬤ **FIGURE 24-7.** Catheter angiogram. FMD of the ICA.

Stewart et al.[48] followed 49 patients with carotid FMD; over a 7.5-year period of time, 35 asymptomatic patients initially followed expectantly had no strokes. In addition, of 14 patients who presented with TIA, only one had another event during the follow-up period, highlighting the often-benign course of this condition. Corrin et al.[49] followed 79 patients for 5 years; only three had focal cerebral ischemic events. As suggested by Curry and Messina[50] in their review, the incidence of asymptomatic disease is unknown; lesions become symptomatic by producing cerebral embolization. Treatment is reserved for symptomatic lesions.

Symptomatic patients with carotid FMD may be treated by surgical or endovascular means. Those with associated kinks and coils may be best served with a surgical approach, wherein the redundant artery can be straightened and at the same time, the associated webs can be dilated. Graduated internal dilatation of the ICA was first introduced by Morris et al.[51] in 1967; the technique involves mobilization of the ICA, opening the vessel under heparin anticoagulation, and passage of olive-tipped metal dilators of increasing diameter. The ICA is allowed to backbleed following each dilatation to prevent distal embolization. In a series of 118 dilatation procedures in 79 patients, Effney et al.[52] reported three strokes and eight TIAs. More recently, PTA has been advocated for the treatment of symptomatic patients.

Carotid Dissection. Arterial dissection occurs when hemorrhage into the arterial wall produces separation of the layers of the artery. It may develop in the subintimal space or in the subadventitial space; the former are associated with an increased risk of thrombus formation, while the latter are associated with aneurysm formation. The dissection typically originates in the proximal ICA and progresses variable distances distally, often terminating at the carotid canal within the petrous segment of the temporal bone. Carotid artery dissections may be spontaneous or traumatic in nature. Patients with carotid FMD and connective tissue diseases (Ehlers-Danlos type IV, Marfan's syndrome) are at increased risk of spontaneous dissection; in most patients, however, an underlying etiology cannot be determined. Traumatic dissection may be caused by a wide variety of seemingly innocuous events, including neck hyperextension and vigorous coughing. In addition, direct blunt trauma, penetrating injuries, and iatrogenic catheter-induced trauma may be associated.

Carotid artery dissection may be found incidentally, but the hallmark clinical picture includes neck pain, headache, Horner's syndrome (from injury to the cervical sympathetic fibers adjacent to the internal carotid within its bony canal), pulsatile tinnitus, and focal neurologic defect.[53] Neurologic symptoms, ranging in severity from TIA to frank stroke, result from carotid occlusion (in the absence of adequate collateralization from the remaining cerebral arteries) or from distal embolization. Symptom onset may be delayed, but typically occurs within hours to days.

The diagnosis of carotid dissection has typically been made by catheter-based angiography. Increasingly, however,

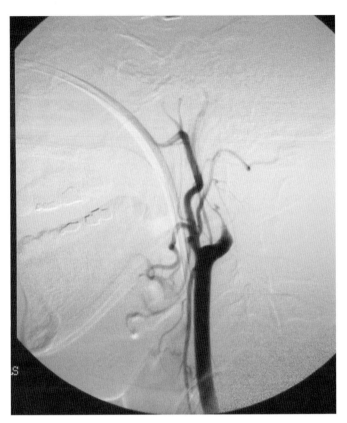

● **FIGURE 24-8.** Spontaneous dissection of the ICA.

other modalities such as ultrasound, MRA, and CT angiography have been utilized.[54–56] Classic angiographic features include tapered narrowing or occlusion of the proximal ICA, which begins a few centimeters from the ICA origin, sometimes associated with an aneurysm at the base of the skull, and are diagnostic (Figure 24-8).

The treatment of carotid artery dissections is evolving, and includes a broad spectrum ranging from antiplatelet therapy to surgical revascularization. Typically, patients with spontaneous carotid artery dissection who are asymptomatic or have a small, stable neurologic defect are treated with heparin anticoagulation, and then converted to coumadin for 3 to 6 months. For patients with severe neurologic defects, anticoagulation with heparin is often contraindicated because of the risk of converting a bland (ischemic) infarction into a hemorrhagic one. Chandra et al.[57] reviewed a 10-year experience with spontaneous dissection of the carotid and vertebral arteries in 20 patients (21 arteries). The majority were diagnosed with magnetic resonance angiography (MRA). Twenty of twenty-one cases were treated with heparin anticoagulation; one patient with persistent symptoms despite anticoagulation was treated with stent placement; this patient subsequently suffered an intracranial hemorrhage. Most reports suggest that the prognosis following carotid artery dissection is quite good. In a series by Treiman et al.[58] in 24 patients, of those who presented without neurologic defect and were treated with anticoagulation, only one developed a stroke in follow-up. In a study from Mokri et al.,[59] of 36 patients with spontaneous dissection, 85% had excellent or complete recovery. In contrast, Biousse et al.[60] reported that more than half of 80 patients who presented with dissection developed stroke. Endovascular therapy with angioplasty and stent placement has some appeal in the treatment of patients who fail medical therapy. Edgell et al.[61] reported on seven patients (12 arteries) with spontaneous dissection treated for the following indications: enlarging pseudoaneurysm, contraindication to or failure of anticoagulation, and compromised cerebral blood flow. Five of the seven patients had FMD as an underlying cause. One patient had hemorrhagic conversion of a preexisting ischemic stroke; the remainder had no neurologic complications following their procedure. Others have reported on the use of covered stents for similar pathology.[62]

Surgical therapy may be indicated for patients who fail medical therapy. Muller et al.[63] reported on 48 patients (50 arteries) treated surgically for chronic dissections that had failed medical therapy. The mean period of anticoagulation prior to operation was 9 months. Indication for operative repair included aneurysmal dilatation or persistent high-grade stenosis. The majority of dissections (70%) were spontaneous; the remainder were posttraumatic. Operative intervention included resection and vein graft interposition in 40, thromboendarterectomy with patch closure in three, graduated dilation in two, and carotid ligation (for dissections that extended to the skull base) in five. Ten percent of patients developed minor stroke, and 58% developed cranial nerve palsy, the majority of which were temporary. In follow-up, only one patient developed a recurrent neurologic defect.

Treatment of patients with posttraumatic dissection must be individualized. Dissections secondary to penetrating trauma are typically treated surgically with arterial repair. In dissections secondary to blunt trauma, patients who are asymptomatic or have minimal neurologic defects are typically treated medically with heparin; if full anticoagulation is contraindicated, antiplatelet therapy may suffice. In general, these patients are managed in a similar manner to those who present with spontaneous dissection. For patients with more severe degrees of neurologic impairment and a large stroke on CT or MR, heparin is typically avoided and antiplatelet therapy instituted, in an attempt to prevent conversion to a hemorrhagic infarction.[64]

Carotid Body Tumors. Carotid body tumors are neoplasms of the paraganglion cells, known by a variety of names including carotid body tumor, cervical paraganglioma, and chemodectoma. They are felt to arise from the afferent ganglion of the glossopharyngeal nerve, are typically located at the cervical carotid bifurcation, and are adherent to the adventitia of the ECA and ICA. Their primary blood supply is from the ECA, which is important in the operative approach to these difficult tumors, and is typically benign in nature. Most carotid body tumors present as an asymptomatic neck mass; a minority will experience pain, hoarseness, or symptoms related to neuroendocrine secretions. Diagnosis can be made by duplex ultrasound,

which may identify a "splaying" of the carotid bifurcation; definitive diagnosis is made by CT angiography, MRA, or catheter-based angiography (Figure 24-5).

All carotid body tumors should be considered for resection in good-risk patients, as their natural history is one of continued expansion. Smaller tumors are typically easier to resect, and carry a smaller risk of injury to adjacent neurologic structures. Radiation therapy may provide some palliation in patients who cannot withstand operation.[65]

Preoperative embolization of the tumor, to decrease intraoperative blood loss, may be indicated in those lesions greater than 5 cm in diameter.[66] While the risk of stroke with surgical resection has decreased over time, the principal risk of surgery remains that of cranial nerve injury, which occurs in 20% to 30% of patients. The risk of cranial nerve injury and stroke are directly related to tumor size.[67,68] The technique of surgical excision includes dissection of the tumor from the periadventitial arterial plane and careful identification of adherent cranial nerves. As noted, approximately 20% of patients will experience permanent cranial nerve injury, and another 20% will have temporary defects, typically involving the hypoglossal and marginal mandibular nerves. On occasion, the tumor arises from the vagus nerve, which must be sacrificed in order to accomplish complete tumor excision. Long-term results are excellent; more than 90% of patients will have no evidence of recurrence, and survival is similar to age- and sex-matched controls.

Aneurysms of the Extracranial Carotid Artery. True aneurysms represent approximately half of all reported carotid artery aneurysms; the remainder are secondary to infection, prior carotid surgery, dissection, and trauma. True aneurysms of the carotid, like most peripheral aneurysms, are more common in men. Most occur at the carotid bulb, and approximately 10% of patients will have bilateral disease.[69] The majority of aneurysms are asymptomatic, although of those presenting to a vascular surgical service, more than half may have symptoms of TIA or stroke. Rupture is an infrequent event. Surgical repair is indicated for all symptomatic aneurysms, and in asymptomatic aneurysms greater than 2 cm in diameter in good-risk patients. Most often, the aneurysm is resected and arterial replacement performed with saphenous vein or a synthetic conduit (Figure 24-6).

Vasculitis Involving the Carotid Arteries. Takayasu's arteritis is an inflammatory disease affecting the aorta and its primary branches, including the brachiocephalic trunks. It is thought to be an autoimmune disease, and likely represents a spectrum that includes giant cell arteritis. The diagnosis is often one of exclusion, as patients may present with a variety of vague symptoms including fever and malaise, upper extremity "claudication," visual changes, TIA, and stroke. The diagnosis is typically made by radiographic studies, especially MRA, which identifies aortic thickening.[70] Corticosteroids are the mainstay of treatment; a minority of patients will require surgical repair. Fields et al.[71]

reported on operative results in 42 patients treated at the Mayo Clinic from a Takayasu's registry of 251 patients. The majority (38/42) of patients having operation were female, with a median age of 29 years. Mean duration of symptoms prior to operation was 5.6 months, although 13 patients underwent surgery for acute presentation or failure of medical management. In the majority, operation was indicated for occlusive symptoms, and in 52%, involvement of the arch and abdominal vessels was identified. There were no operative deaths, MIs, or strokes. Three patients had early graft thrombosis, and 11 patients required graft revision at a mean follow-up of 6.7 years; five of these had active disease at presentation. The authors conclude that a minority of patients with Takayasu's require operation, that revision is more frequently required in those with active disease, and that when necessary, surgical repair is safe. Long-term survival was excellent; mortality was 4% at 5 and 10 years.

Giant cell (temporal) arteritis is an inflammatory condition that affects medium-sized and large arteries, most commonly affecting the aortic arch and its branches, the ICA, and the ECA. In contrast to Takayasu's arteritis, age at presentation is typically in the sixth or seventh decade. The classic presentation is of an elderly female who develops constitutional symptoms (such as fever, malaise, weight loss), subsequent jaw ischemia (from involvement of the ECA), and tenderness overlying the superficial temporal artery. Ocular symptoms (amaurosis fugax, ischemic optic neuritis) may also occur, and may proceed to blindness if not treated aggressively. Diagnosis is made by identification of elevated serologic markers (ESR and CRP), and by temporal artery biopsy. The mainstay of treatment is corticosteroids. Surgical therapy is infrequently necessary, but may be indicated in patients with progressive upper or lower extremity symptoms.[72,73]

• CONCLUSION

At the present time, CEA remains the treatment of choice for the majority of patients, both symptomatic and asymptomatic, with carotid occlusive disease. The results of CEA, although variable from center to center and among individual operators, are exemplary. Certain patients at increased risk for CEA (a definition that is undergoing continued refinement) are well served by CAS. The challenge of each individual vascular physician is to identify which therapy (medical, surgical, or endovascular) best suits the individual patient.

REFERENCES

1. U.S. Bureau of the Census. *Statistical Abstract of the United States*. 112th ed. Washington, DC; 1992.

2. Bonita R. Epidemiology of stroke. *Lancet*. 1992;339:342-344.

3. North American Symptomatic Carotid Endarterectomy Trial Collaborators. Beneficial effect of carotid endarterectomy in symptomatic patients with high-grade carotid stenosis. *N Eng J Med*. 1991;325:445-453.

4. Executive Committee for the Asymptomatic Carotid Atherosclerosis Study. Endarterectomy for asymptomatic carotid artery stenosis. *JAMA*. 1995;273:1421-1428.

5. Eastcott HHG, Pickering GW, Robb CG. Reconstruction of the internal carotid artery in a patient with intermittent attacks of hemiplegia. *Lancet*. 1954;2:994-996.

6. Hsia DC, Krushat WM, Moscoe LM. Epidemiology of carotid endarterectomies among Medicare beneficiaries. *J Vasc Surg*. 1992;16:201-208.

7. Huber TS, Seeger JM. Dartmouth atlas of vascular health care review: impact of hospital volume, surgeon volume, and training on outcome. *Vasc Surg*. 2001;34:751-756.

8. Menzoian JO. Presidential address: carotid endarterectomy, under attack again! *J Vasc Surg*. 2003;37:1137-1141.

9. Chaturvedi S, Aggarwal R, Murugappan A. Results of carotid endarterectomy with prospective neurologist follow-up. *Neurology*. 2000;55:769-772.

10. Rothwell PM, Slattery J, Warlow CP. A systematic comparison of the risks of stroke and death due to carotid endarterectomy for symptomatic and asymptomatic stenosis. *Stroke*. 1996;27:266-269.

11. Lepore MR, Sternbergh C, Salartash K, Tonnessen B, Money SR. Influence of NASCET/ACAS trial eligibility on outcome after carotid endarterectomy. *J Vasc Surg*. 2001;34:581-586.

12. Illig KA, Zhang R, Tanski W, Benesch C, Sternbach Y, Green RM. Is the rationale for carotid angioplasty and stenting in patients excluded from NASCET/ACAS or eligible for ARCHeR justified? *J Vasc Surg*. 2003;37:575-581.

13. Mozes G, Sullivan T, Torres-Russotto D, et al. Carotid endarterectomy in SAPPHIRE-eligible 'high-risk' patients: implications for selecting patients for carotid angioplasty and stenting. *J Vasc Surg*. 2004;39:958-965.

14. Hertzer NR, O'Hara PJ, Mascha EJ, Krajewski LP, Sullivan TM, Beven EG. Early outcome assessment for 2228 consecutive carotid endarterectomy procedures: the Cleveland Clinic experience from 1989 to 1995. *J Vasc Surg*. 1997;26:1-10.

15. Ouriel K, Hertzer NR, Beven EG, et al. Preprocedural risk stratification: identifying an appropriate population for carotid stenting. *J Vasc Surg*. 2001;33:728-732.

16. Rockman CB, Riles TS, Landis R, et al. Redo carotid surgery: an analysis of materials and configurations used in carotid reoperations and their influence on perioperative stroke and subsequent recurrent stenosis. *J Vasc Surg*. 1999;29:72-80.

17. Kashyap VS, Moore WS, Quinones-Baldrich WJ. Carotid artery repair for radiation-associated atherosclerosis is a safe and durable procedure. *J Vasc Surg*. 1999;29:90-96.

18. Sundt TM Jr, Houser OW, Sharbrough FW, Messick JM Jr. Carotid endarterectomy: results, complications, and monitoring techniques. *Adv Neurol*. 1977;16:97-119.

19. Rothwell PM, Slattery J, Warlow CP. Clinical and angiographic predictors of stroke and death from carotid endarterectomy: systematic review. *BMJ*. 1997;315:1571-1577.

20. Gasparis AP, Ricotta L, Cuadra SA, et al. High-risk carotid endarterectomy: act or fiction. *J Vasc Surg.* 2003;37:40-46.

21. Jordan WD, Alcocer F, Wirthlin DJ, et al. High-risk carotid endarterectomy: challenges for carotid stent protocols. *J Vasc Surg.* 2002;35:16-22.

22. Reed AB, Gaccione P, Belkin M, et al. Preoperative risk factors for carotid endarterectomy: defining the patient at high risk. *J Vasc Surg.* 2003;37;1191-1199.

23. Yadav JS, Wholey MH, Kuntz RE, et al. Protected carotid artery stenting versus endarterectomy in high-risk patients. *N Engl J Med.* 2004;351:1493-1501.

24. Gray WA, Hopkins LN, Yadav S, et al. Protected carotid stenting in high surgical risk patients: the ARCHeR results. *J Vasc Surg.* 2006;44:258-269.

25. Mas JL, Chatellier G, Beyssen B, et al. Endarterectomy versus stenting in patients with severe, symptomatic carotid stenosis. *N Engl J Med.* 2006;355:1660-1671.

26. SPACE collaborative group. 30 day results from the SPACE trial of stent-protected angioplasty versus carotid endarterectomy in symptomatic patients: a randomized non-inferiority trial. *Lancet.* 2006;368:1239-1247.

27. Coward LJ, Featherstone RL, Brown MM. Safety and efficacy of endovascular treatment of carotid artery stenosis compared with carotid endarterectomy: a Cochrane systematic review of the randomized evidence. *Stroke.* 2005;36:905-911.

28. Crawley F, Clifton A, Markus H, Brown MM. Delayed improvement in carotid artery diameter after carotid angioplasty. *Stroke.* 1997;28:574-579.

29. Schillinger M, Exner M, Mlekusch W, et al. Acute-phase response after stent implantation in the carotid artery: association with 6-month in-stent restenosis. *Radiology.* 2003;227:516-521.

30. Khan MA, Liu MW, Chio FL, et al. Predictors of restenosis after successful carotid artery stenting. *Am J Cardiol.* 2003;92(7):895-897.

31. Christiaans MH, Ernst JMPG, Suttorp MJ, van den Berg JC, et al. Restenosis after carotid angioplasty and stenting: a follow-up study with duplex ultrasonography. *Eur J Vasc Endovasc Surg.* 2003;26(2):141-144.

32. Lal BK, Hobson RW, Goldstein J, et al. In-stent recurrent stenosis after carotid artery stenting: life table analysis and clinical relevance. *J Vasc Surg.* 2003;38(6):1162-1169.

33. Robbin ML, Lockhart ME, Weber TM, et al. Carotid artery stents: early and intermediate follow-up with Doppler US. *Radiology.* 1997;205:749-756.

34. Osborn A. *Diagnostic Cerebral Angiography.* 2nd ed. Philadelphia, PA: Lippincott Williams & Wilkins; 1999:111.

35. Gaunt ME, Martin PJ, Smith JL, et al. Clinical relevance of intraoperative embolization detected by transcranial Doppler ultrasonography during carotid endarterectomy: a prospective study of 100 patients. *Br J Surg.* 1994;81:1435-1439.

36. Bickness CD, Cowling MG, Clark MW, et al. Carotid angioplasty in a pulsatile flow model: factors affecting embolic potential. *Eur J Vasc Endovasc Surg.* 2003;26:22-31.

37. Tübler T, Schlüter M, Dirsch O, et al. Balloon-protected carotid artery stenting: relationship of periprocedural neurological complications with the size of particulate debris. *Circulation.* 2001;104:2791-2796.

38. Theron J, Courtheoux P, Alachkar F, et al. New triple coaxial catheter system for carotid angioplasty with cerebral protection. *Am J Neuroradiol.* 1990;11:869-874.

39. Whitlow PL, Lylyk P, Londero H, et al. Carotid artery stenting protected with an emboli containment system. *Stroke.* 2002;22:1308-1314.

40. Ohki T, Parodi J, Veith FJ, et al. Efficacy of a proximal occlusion catheter with reversal of flow in the prevention of embolic events during carotid artery stenting: an experimental analysis. *J Vasc Surg.* 2001;33(3):504-509.

41. New G, Roubin GS, Iyer SS, et al. Outcomes from carotid artery stenting in over 1000 cases from a single group of operators. *J Am Coll Cardiol.* 2003;41(suppl A):868.

42. Hofmann R, Kerschner K, Steinwender C, Kypta A, Bibl D, Leisch F. Abciximab bolus injection does not reduce cerebral ischemic complications of elective carotid artery stenting: a randomized study. *Stroke.* 2002;33(3):725-727.

43. Hobson RW. CREST: background, design, and current status. *J Vasc Surg.* 2000;13:139-143.

44. Gertler JP, Cambria RP. The role of external carotid endarterectomy in the treatment of ipsilateral internal carotid occlusion: a collective review. *J Vasc Surg.* 1987;6:158-167.

45. Naylor AR, Bell PR, Bolia A. Endovascular treatment of carotid stump syndrome. *J Vasc Surg.* 2003;38:593-595.

46. Nano G, Dalainas I, Casana R, et al. Endovascular treatment of carotid stump syndrome. *Cardiovasc Intervent Radiol.* 2006;29:140-142.

47. Cloft HJ, Kallmes DF, Kallmes MH, et al. Prevalence of cerebral aneurysms in patients with fibromuscular dysplasia: a reassessment. *J Neurosurg.* 1998;88:436-440.

48. Stewart MT, Moritz MW, Smith RB, et al. The natural history of carotid fibromuscular dysplasia. *J Vasc Surg.* 1986;3:305-310.

49. Corrin LS, Sandok BA, Houser OW. Cerebral ischemic events in patients with carotid artery fibromuscular dysplasia. *Arch Neurol.* 1981;38:616-618.

50. Curry TK, Messina LM. Fibromuscular dysplasia: when is intervention warranted? *Semin Vasc Surg.* 2003;16:190-199.

51. Morris GC Jr, Lechter A, DeBakey ME. Surgical treatment of fibromuscular disease of the carotid arteries. *Arch Surg.* 1968;96:636-643.

52. Effney DJ, Ehrenfeld WK, Stoney RJ, et al. Why operate on carotid fibromuscular dysplasia? *Arch Surg.* 1980;115:1261-1265.

53. Baumgartner RW, Bogousslavsky J. Clinical manifestations of carotid dissection. *Front Neurol Neurosci.* 2005;20:70-76.

54. Benninger DH, Caso V, Baumgartner RW. Ultrasound assessment of cervical artery dissection. *Front Neurol Neurosci.* 2005;20:87-101.

55. Paciaroni M, Caso V, Agnelli G. Magnetic resonance imaging, magnetic resonance and catheter angiography for diagnosis of cervical artery dissection. *Front Neurol Neurosci.* 2005;20:102-118.

56. Taschner CA, Leclerc X, Lucas C, Pruvo JP. Computed tomography angiography for the evaluation of carotid artery dissections. *Front Neurol Neurosci.* 2005;20:119-128.

57. Chandra A, Suliman A, Angle N. Spontaneous dissection of

the carotid and vertebral arteries: the 10-year UCSD experience. *Ann Vasc Surg.* 2007;21:178-185.

58. Treiman GS, Treiman RL, Foran RF, et al. Spontaneous dissection of the internal carotid artery: a nineteen year clinical experience. *J Vasc Surg.* 1996;24:597-607.

59. Mokri B, Sundt TM Jr, Houser OW, et al. Spontaneous dissection of cervical internal carotid artery. *Ann Neurol.* 1986;19:126-138.

60. Bogousslavsky J, Despland PA, Regli F. Spontaneous carotid dissection with acute stroke. *Arch Neurol.* 1987;44:137-140.

61. Edgell RC, Abou-CheblA, Yadav JS. Endovascular management of spontaneous carotid artery dissection. *J Vasc Surg.* 2005;42:854-860.

62. Assadian A, Senekowitsch C, Assadian O, et al. Combined open and endovascular stent grafting of internal carotid artery fibromuscular dysplasia: long term results. *Eur J Vasc Endovasc Surg.* 2005;29:345-349.

63. Muller BT, Luther B, Hort W, et al. Surgical treatment of 50 carotid dissections: indications and results. *J Vasc Surg.* 2000;31:980-988.

64. Mokri B, Piepgras DG, Houser OW. Traumatic dissections of the extracranial internal carotid artery. *J Neurosurg.* 1988; 68:189-197.

65. Schild SE, Foote RL, Buskirk SJ, et al. Results of radiotherapy for chemodectomas. *Mayo Clin Proc.* 1992;67:537-540.

66. Kasper GC, Welling RE, Wladis AR, et al. A multidisciplinary approach to carotid paragangliomas. *Vasc Endovasc Surg.* 2006;40:467-474.

67. Shamblin WR, ReMine WH, Sheps SG, et al. Carotid body tumor: clinicopathological analysis of 90 cases. *Am J Surg.* 1971;122:732-739.

68. Hallett JW, Nora JD, Hollier LH, et al. Trends in the neurovascular complications of surgical management for carotid body and cervical paragangliomas: a 50-year experience with 153 tumors. *J Vasc Surg.* 1988;7:284-291.

69. Painter TA, Hertzer NR, Beven EG, et al. Extracranial carotid aneuryms: report of six cases and a review of the literature. *J Vasc Surg.* 1985;2:312-318.

70. Kissin EY, Merkel PA. Diagnostic imaging in Takayasu's arteritis. *Curr Opin Rheumatol.* 2004;16:31-37.

71. Fields CE, Bower TC, Cooper LT, et al. Takayasu's arteritis: operative results and influence of disease activity. *J Vasc Surg.* 2006;43:64-71.

72. Weyand CM, Bartley GB. Giant cell arteritis: new concepts in pathogenesis and implications for management. *Am J Ophthamol.* 1997;123:392-395.

73. Hunder GG, Bloch DA, Michel BA, et al. The American College of Rheumatology 1990 criteria for the classification of giant cell arteritis. *Arth Rheum.* 1990;33:1122-1128.

chapter 25

Vertebrobasilar Disease

Monica Simionescu, MD / *Michael Schneck, MD*

● INTRODUCTION

Vertebrobasilar arterial disease has a heterogeneous, clinical presentation that depends on the underlying pathophysiology of the lesion. Regardless of etiology, however, vertebrobasilar arterial strokes can be devastating and have, until recently, been associated with a high rate of death and disability. With technical advances in neuroimaging and endovascular procedures, as well as data from randomized, clinical trials on stroke prevention and management of acute stroke, we have gained a better understanding of the pathophysiology and treatment options for vertebrobasilar disease. Although currently there is not always definitive data to guide the treatment of choice, immediate expert evaluation by a stroke neurologist may help in selecting the appropriate imaging modality and treatment plan that can often be lifesaving.

● ANATOMY

Vertebral Artery

The anatomic course of the vertebral artery (VA) is divided into four segments. The first segment (V1) lies between the origin of VA from the subclavian artery (SA) and the transverse foramen of C5 or C6. The second segment (V2) is located within the transverse foramina from C5 or C6 to C2. The third segment (V3), also known as the vertebral siphon, courses posteriorly and laterally between the atlas and occiput. The fourth segment (V4) is the intracranial portion of the VA; the vessel pierces the dura mater and enters the cranium through the foramen magnum, then courses medially and superiorly to merge with the opposite VA at the level of pontomedullary junction giving rise to the basilar artery (BA).

The left VA originates directly from the aortic arch in approximately 8% of cases. Asymmetry between the vertebral arteries is found in 66% of cases with the left VA being dominant in 45% cases.[1] The VA has three major intracranial branches: anterior spinal artery, posterior spinal artery, and posterior inferior cerebellar artery (PICA).

The anterior spinal artery is a midline unpaired vessel formed by anastamosis of two branches from each VA. It originates at the level of the olivary nucleus to the conus medullaris and descends caudally to supply to the ventral surface of the medulla and the anterior two-thirds of the spinal cord.

The posterior spinal artery is a branch of either the VA or PICA and supplies the posterior third of the spinal cord.

The PICA is usually the largest branch of the distal intracranial portion of the VA, branching in close proximity to the BA origin. Fifteen percent of individuals lack one PICA and 5% have a hypoplastic PICA. Additionally, a PICA originating from the proximal BA directly or from a common trunk with AICA can be occasionally seen.[1] The lateral medulla, inferior cerebellar vermis, and inferior surface of the cerebellum are supplied by the PICA.

Basilar Artery

The BA lies ventral to the pons and extends from the pontomedullary junction to the pontomesencephalic junction where it bifurcates into its terminal branches, the posterior cerebral arteries (PCAs). It is responsible for the vascular supply of the pons, midbrain, cerebellum, labyrinth, cochlea, thalamus, subthalamus, and temporooccipital lobes. The branches of BA can be divided into three groups: paramedian, long circumferential, and short circumferential branches.

Paramedian arteries branch perpendicular to the BA and penetrate the pons feeding a paramedian wedge of the pontine parenchyma. In the distal part of the BA, close to the bifurcation, there are paramedian vessels, also known as interpeduncular vessels that supply the midbrain and the subthalamus.

Short circumferential arteries enter the brachium pontis and are responsible for the vascular supply of ventrolateral part of the pons. Long circumferential arteries ensure the blood supply to the pontine tegmentum and to the cerebellum. Anterior inferior cerebellar artery (AICA) and superior cerebellar artery (SCA) are also considered long circumferential vessels in addition to unnamed smaller branch vessels.

The AICA is a branch of the proximal BA and supplies the lateral, caudal pons (facial, trigeminal, vestibular and cochlear nuclei, spinothalamic tract, root of seven and eighth cranial nerves), brachium pontis, floculonodular lobe, and the ventral part of cerebellar hemispheres. The internal auditory artery typically branches off of AICA and only occasionally derives directly from the BA. Its vascular territory includes the auditory, vestibular, and facial nerve.

The SCA is a branch of the distal BA, just below the bifurcation into the PCAs. It has a close anatomic relation with the oculomotor nerve in the subarachnoid space, which passes superior to the SCA and inferior to the PCA. The vascular territory of the SCA includes the rostral pontine tegmentum, brachium conjunctivum, superior vermis, and cerebellar hemispheres.

The PCAs are "terminal branches" of the BA. The course of each PCA can be divided in four segments: P1 to P4. More than 25% of humans have a persistent, primitive, and vascular pattern in which the PCA arises from the ICA and where the connection between BA and PCA remains vestigial.

P1, also known as the interpeduncular segment, extends from the bifurcation to the junction of posterior communicating artery. It provides paramedian branches to the midbrain and thalamoperforating branches to the medial thalamus. Percheron's artery is an anatomic variant in which the two thalamoperforating pedicles arise from a common trunk from one PCA. P2, the ambient segment of the PCA, extends from the posterior communicating artery, in the ambient cistern, to the quadrigeminal cistern. The main branches of P2 are the medial and lateral posterior choroidal arteries that supply the choroid plexus of lateral ventricle. These branches also supply the pretectal region, pulvinar and posterolateral thalamus, as well as the thalamo-geniculate pedicle for the posterolateral thalamus. P3, the quadrigeminal segment, courses in the quadrigeminal cistern to the anterior part of the calcarine fissure. P4 is the part of PCA above the tentorial edge, entering the anterior part of the calcarine fissure. Cortical branches of the PCA, which usually arise from P3 or P4, include anterior temporal, posterior temporal, parieto-occipital, and calcarine arteries. The dorsal callosal artery is a branch of the parieto-occipital artery and supplies the splenium of corpus callosum.

● ETIOPATHOLOGY

Common causes of posterior circulation ischemic stroke can be divided into large-vessel disease, small-vessel disease, and cardioembolism.

Large-Vessel Disease

Atherosclerosis is the leading cause of vertebrobasilar disease and its distribution varies, depending on race and sex. White men have predominantly extracranial large artery atherosclerosis; blacks, Asians, and women have predominantly intracranial large-vessel disease.[2] The origin of the VA is a frequent site of atherosclerotic lesions. These lesions are commonly associated with atherosclerotic plaques at the level of carotid and coronary arteries, as well as peripheral vascular disease, hypertension, hypercholesterolemia, and smoking.[1] Common intracranial locations of plaques are at the level where the VA pierces the dura and the proximal and middle BA. Pathology of the plaques consists of fatty streaks and fibrous tissue with often superimposed calcifications. Macroscopically the vessel will appear stenosed or occluded. As in coronary arterial disease, a complicated plaque, with hemorrhage, ulceration, or in situ thrombosis, is often responsible for the stroke mechanism either from in situ thrombosis with secondary vessel occlusion or artery-to-artery thrombembolic material propagated to downstream branches. Aortic arch atheroma that is also associated with artery-to-artery embolism may also sometimes be a cause of posterior circulation cerebral ischemia.[1] BA atherosclerotic plaque, located in the proximal or middle portion of the BA, often can occlude the origin of paramedian perforators producing a particular pattern of paramedian pontine or midbrain infarction.[3] BA atherothrombosis can be either isolated or occur in the context of widespread posterior circulation atherosclerosis, with intracranial VA stenosis or occlusion being most common. In the context of multiple vessel stenosis or occlusion, an infarct in the territory of the affected posterior circulation vessels more likely is a result of hypoperfusion as opposed to in situ thrombosis.[4]

Dissection of the VA, spontaneous or traumatic, usually occurs in the extracranial segments, with V1 and V3 being predominantly affected because of increased mobility of the vessels within the vertebral canals of the cervical spine.[5] Intimal tear and accumulation of blood between the layers of arterial wall can result in stenosis caused by subintimal dissection, or aneurismal dilatation of the vessel wall, with possible superimposed thrombosis, caused by subadventitial dissection. Subsequently, strokes may be related to hemodynamic mechanisms associated with stenosis or thromboembolic mechanism in the context of a thrombosed aneurysm.[5] Dissections may be posttraumatic or may occur in relation with precipitating factors such as neck hyperextension or rotation. Attribubeted causes of cervicocerebral dissection have included minor sports or motor vehicle trauma chiropractic manipulations, and even simply coughing, sneezing, or vomiting. An underlying structural defect of the arterial wall, causing an arteriopathy, can sometimes be identified in association with cervicocephalic dissections. Among such conditions are fibromuscular dysplasia, cystic medial necrosis, Ehlers-Danlos syndrome type IV, Marfan's syndrome, autosomal dominant polycystic kidney disease,

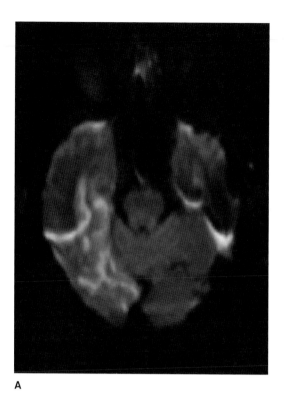
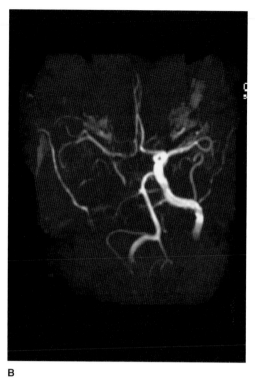

A   B

● **FIGURE 25-1.** (A) MRI/DWI showing a right PCA territory acute infarct in a 71-year-old man with left-sided dysmetria and homonymous hemianopsia. (B) MRA showing an absent right PCA as well as nonvisualization of the right ICA.

osteogenesis imperfecta type I, and α_1-antitrypsin deficiency.

Dolichoectatic VA or BA is reported as a rare cause of posterior circulation stroke in the absence of atherosclerosis or vascular risk factors.[3] Posterior circulation aneurysms can sometimes be associated with ischemic strokes resulting from several mechanisms. These include artery-artery embolism, in situ thrombosis, ischemia caused by compression and traction of posterior fossa structures, or vasospasm secondary to aneurismal leak[1] (Figure 25-1).

Small-Vessel Disease

Lipohyalinosis is the most common pathologic lesion associated with small-vessel disease. Small penetrating arteries are occluded with hyaline material, subsequently resulting in lacunar infarcts. These lesions are usually seen in the context of hypertension.

Cardioembolism

Fifteen to twenty percent of all ischemic strokes occur as a result of cardiac emboli to the brain. Cardioembolism in the posterior circulation is often associated with distal BA occlusion or distal PCA branch occlusions. Common cardiac sources with a high embolic potential include atrial fibrillation, acute myocardial infarction, infective endocarditis, rheumatic mitral stenosis, mechanical prosthetic heart valves, and dilated cardiomyopathy. Interatrial septal aneurysm, patent foramen ovale (PFO), bioprosthetic

valves, and atrial flutter are associated with a lower risk of cardioembolic stroke. Congenital heart disease a common cause of cardioembolic stroke in children is being seen more frequently in young adults as children with congenital heart disease survive longer.[3]

Rare Causes

There are rare causes responsible for strokes in both the anterior and posterior circulation such as hypercoagulable states, septic arteritis, aspergillosis, sickle-cell disease, systemic lupus erythematous, and granulomatous angiitis. Among rare conditions causing strokes with a predilection for the posterior circulation are Behcet syndrome, Fabry disease, syphilitic arteritis, and neurofibromatosis.[1]

● PATHOPHYSIOLOGY

The mechanisms responsible for ischemia are in situ thrombosis, embolic occlusion, hemodynamic hypoperfusion, and vasospasm. Normal cerebral blood flow (CBF) at rest is 50 to 55 mL/100 g/min. When CBF is less than 18 mL/100 g/min, neuronal electrical activity is disturbed; when CBF is less than 8 mL/100 g/min, membrane failure and cell death ensues. The brain region surrounding the infarct, also known as the ischemic penumbra, has reduced blood flow though above the threshold for absolute cell death and that tissue is therefore potentially salvageable. Ischemia triggers endothelial activation at the level of microvessels, with secondary accumulation of inflammatory mediators. Hypoxia in the precapillary arteries stimulates expression of vascular endothelial growth factors (VEGF) that is involved in angiogenesis and neovascularization.

At the level of the posterior circulation, there are multiple collaterals that can maintain blood flow via both extracranial and intracranial vessels. Intracranially, the long circumferential arteries AICA, PICA, and SCA establish an important collateral network that can compensate for cerebellar or brainstem ischemia. The brainstem tegmentum, caused by multiple collaterals, is usually resistant to ischemia whereas the lateral medullary region, caused by poor collaterals, is usually vulnerable to ischemia.[1] Development of collateral vessels and recanalization of the occluded vessels are important factors that influence the prognosis of vertebrobasilar disease.

● CLINICAL MANIFESTATIONS

Posterior circulation stroke has a variety of clinical presentations depending on the affected region and the underlying pathology.[6] The most common symptoms and signs suggestive of vertebrobasilar disease are listed in Table 25-1. Patients may have transitory symptoms completely resolving in less then 24 hours, clinically defined as transient ischemic attacks (TIAs) or may have permanent deficits reflecting infarction of the brain parenchyma, clinically defined as ischemic strokes. TIAs usually last 15 to 60 minutes and present with at least two symptoms or signs. Isolated recurrent dizziness or vertigo has traditionally been thought to be a sign of peripheral vestibular dysfunction rather than a manifestation of vertebrobasilar ischemia.[6] The true frequency of isolated dizziness associated with vertebrobasilar ischemia may be found to be more common in the future with increased frequency of MR imaging of patients with these symptoms, however.

Posterior circulation ischemic strokes can present with different syndromes depending on the occluded vessel that are discussed in the etiopathologic context.

Extracranial VA Disease

Atherosclerotic stenosis or occlusion of the extracranial VA can be asymptomatic or can present with TIAs or strokes secondary to embolic occlusion of distal branches. Lesions limited to the extracranial VA often develop slowly, so extensive collaterals from the external carotid artery, occipital branches, the subclavian artery, or thyrocervical trunk, may develop. Vertebrobasilar TIAs are seen in approximately 50% of patients with extracranial VA atherosclerotic disease, and the most common symptoms associated with this clinical scenario include dizziness, blurred vision, and gait ataxia.[7] Strokes are usually embolic to the distal branches of posterior circulation but these strokes are rare, however, compared with the otherwise high incidence of cardiac embolic lesions.[1]

VA dissection presents with neck pain or occipital headache followed in approximately 90% cases by ischemic manifestations in the brainstem, cerebellum, thalamus, or cerebral hemispheric regions supplied by the posterior circulation. Cervical spinal cord ischemia is a rare complication associated with VA dissection.[5]

Intracranial VA Disease

Intracranial VA occlusion may be asymptomatic, or may present with TIAs or infarcts in the medulla or cerebellum. These syndromes have well known clinical characteristics and will be discussed separately.

Lateral Medullary Syndrome (Wallenberg). The characteristic clinical presentation is nausea, vomiting, vertigo, gait ataxia, ipsilateral cerebellar signs and symptoms, dysarthria, dysphagia, crossed sensory pattern with decreased sensation in the ipsilateral face and contralateral body, ipsilateral Horner syndrome, and occasionally hiccups (singultus). Clinicoanatomic correlations of Wallenberg syndrome are detailed in Table 25-2. Because of destruction of vestibular nuclei and their connections with the cerebellum as well as with the labyrinth, abnormalities

TABLE 25-1. Common Symptoms and Signs of Vertebrobasilar Ischemia

Symptoms	Signs
Dizziness	Ataxia
Vertigo	Nystagmus
Nausea	Vomiting
Coordination and balance difficulties	Cerebellar signs
Double vision or bilateral loss of vision	Oculomotor palsies
Unilateral, bilateral, or alternating motor or sensory symptoms	Unilateral, bilateral, or alternating weakness or sensory loss
Slurred speech	Dysarthria
Swallowing difficulties	Dysphagia
Headache	

TABLE 25-2. Clinicoanatomic Correlations of Wallenberg Syndrome

Signs & Symptoms	Lesions
Nausea, vomiting, vertigo Ocular motor abnormalities	Vestibular nuclei & their connections
Dysphagia, dysarthia Vocal cord paralysis	Nucleus ambiguus
Ipsilateral face sensory loss	Spinal trigeminal nucleus and tract
Contralateral body pain and temperature sensory loss	Spinothalamic tract
Ipsilateral cerebellar signs	Restiform body (inferior cerebellar peduncle)
Ipsilateral Horner syndrome	Descending sympathetic fibers

of eye movements such as skew deviation, nystagmus, smooth pursuit, or saccades difficulties may occur. Mild ipsilateral facial paresis is reported with this syndrome, and is probably related to either rostral extension of the infarct or destruction of cortico-bulbar fibers after decussation that loop inferiorly and then ascend to the facial nucleus. Caudal extension of the infarct may affect the corticospinal tract after the pyramidal decussation and may produce an ipsilateral motor deficit. This latter syndrome is known as the submedullary syndrome of Opalski.[8]

Medial Medullary Syndrome (Dejerine's Anterior Bulbar Syndrome).

This syndrome results from destruction of medially medullary structures: the hypoglossal nucleus and nerve, medial lemniscus, and medullary pyramid. Clinically, it presents with ipsilateral tongue paresis, atrophy and fasciculations, contralateral loss of position and vibration, and contralateral motor deficit with face spring, respectively (Figure 25-2).

Hemimedullary Syndrome (Babinski-Nageote).

This syndrome is the result of a combination of the medial and lateral medullary syndromes.

PICA Infarcts.

The PICA vascular distribution can be divided into medial PICA (mPICA) supplying the lateral medulla and the dorsomedial caudal cerebellum, and lateral PICA (l-PICA) supplying the lateral caudal cerebellum. Isolated complete PICA territory infarcts are rarely reported.

These infarcts are usually associated with AICA or SCA ischemia, and clinically present with a high tendency for edema, brainstem compression, and tonsillar herniation.[9] The medial PICA syndrome presents with a complete or incomplete Wallenberg syndrome. Lateral PICA infarcts presents with either isolated vertigo or vertigo associated with ipsilateral cerebellar syndrome.

BA Disease

BA occlusions can be thrombotic or embolic. Thrombotic BA occlusion usually affects the proximal or midportion of the BA and is clinically characterized by the gradual progression of symptoms over variable intervals of time reported from a few hours to more than 2 weeks.[1] Signs and symptoms of pontine ischemia with gradual progression without improvement is a poor, prognostic sign. Alternating transient hemiparesis or inappropriate laugh ("fou rire prodromique") is classically described as heralding BA occlusion. Coma or a "locked-in syndrome" follows. BA embolism that usually presents with sudden onset is clinically related to "top of the basilar syndrome," because of anatomic narrowing of the distal BA and lodging of embolic material at this level.

Coma is secondary to destruction of the ascending activating reticular formation in the pontine tegmentum. Apneustic breathing pattern, pinpoint but reactive pupils, and decerebrate postures are often present and may suggest the pontine localization of coma.

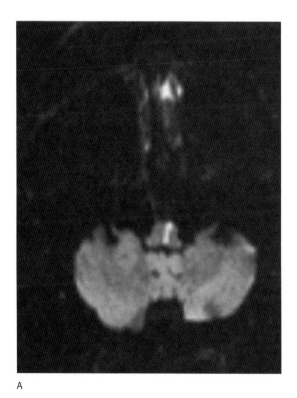
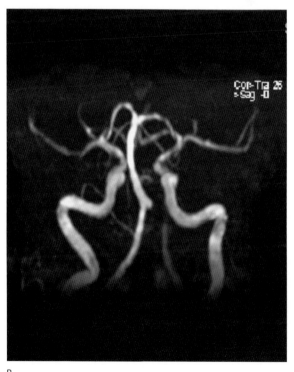

A

B

● **FIGURE 25-2.** (A) MRI/DWI showing a left medial medullary acute infarct in a 70-year-old patient with right hemiplegia and left tongue deviation. (B) MRA illustrating lack of flow in the distal left VA.

TABLE 25-3. Neuro-Ophthalmologic Signs in BA Occlusion

Ocular bobbing—sudden and brief conjugate downward movements of the eyes	Accentuated vertical eye roving when the horizontal gaze is lost
Skew deviation	Asymmetric lesions of vestibular nuclei and their connections
Conjugate horizontal gaze palsy	Paramedian pontine reticular formation (PPRF)
Internuclear ophthalmoplegia (INO)—limited adduction in one eye with nystagmus in abducting eye	Medial longitudinal fasciculus (MLF) ipsilateral to limited adduction
One-and-a-half syndrome—INO plus horizontal gaze palsy	MLF and PPRF
Ptosis	Descending sympathetic fibers
Pinpoint pupils	Descending sympathetic fibers
Vertical nystagmus	Vestibular connections

Locked-in syndrome is anatomically correlated with bilateral, ventral, and pontine lesions. Clinically, it presents with quadriplegia caused by bilateral corticospinal tract involvement, mutism, bilateral facial paresis, and horizontal eye movements caused byinvolvement of bilateral corticobulbar fibers. Consciousness is preserved because the dorsal pontine tegmentum is spared. Vertical eye movements are also preserved because of sparing of the ri-MLF which is located in the midbrain.

Neuro-ophthalmologic signs described in association with BA occlusion and their anatomic correlation are presented in Table 25-3.

Top of the BA Syndrome presents with a constellation of signs and symptoms related to midbrain, thalamus, and temporo-occipital lobes infarcts (Figure 25-3). Eye movement abnormalities include vertical gaze paresis, convergence defects, nystagmus, skew deviation, and retraction of upper eyelids (Collier's sign). Pupils are either small and reactive, or fixed in midposition. Visual defects such as homonymous hemianopia, cortical blindness, or simultanagnosia often occur. Sleep disturbances, behavioral abnormalities, motor or sensory deficits are also described.[8]

AICA infarcts. The AICA vascular supply includes the lateral caudal pons, middle cerebellar peduncle (brachium pontis), and flocculus. Clinically, these infarcts can present with isolated cerebellar signs, isolated vertigo, or with

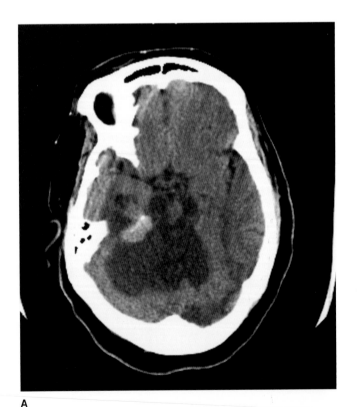

A

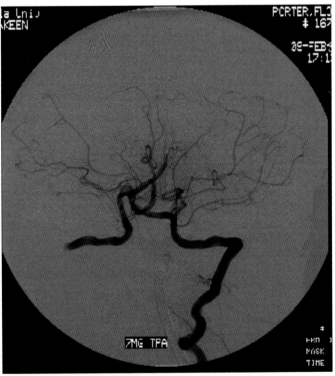

B

● **FIGURE 25-3.** (A) Unenhanced CT scan showing hypodensities in both cerebellar hemispheres, vermis, and midbrain as well as compression of the fourth ventricle in a 68-year-old woman presenting with top of the basilar syndrome. (B) Catheter cerebral angiogram showing distal basilar occlusion.

a lateral pontine syndrome associated with a ventral cerebellar syndrome. Complete AICA infarcts characteristically present with vertigo, nausea, vomiting, nystagmus, ipsilateral deafness and facial paresis, ipsilateral ataxia, crossed sensory symptoms with ipsilateral face sensory loss for all modalities, contralateral body sensory loss to pain and temperature, ipsilateral Horner syndrome, and an ipsilateral conjugate lateral gaze palsy (floccular lesion). AICA infarcts are considered to be rare. However, their clinical significance is important because of case reports in which they heralded subsequent BA occlusion.[8,9]

SCA infarcts present with signs and symptoms of lateral, rostral brainstem involvement in association with dorsal, rostral, and cerebellar involvement. Classically described syndromes of SCA include nausea, vomiting, nystagmus, ipsilateral intention tremor, ipsilateral ataxia (superior cerebellar peduncle or brachium conjunctivum), contralateral body sensory loss, hearing impairment (lateral lemniscus), and ipsilateral Horner syndrome (descending oculosympathetic fibers).[8,9]

PCA infarct presentation varies depending on the site of occlusion. P1 occlusions may produce midbrain, thalamic, and temporo-occipital infarcts. Occlusion of P2 segments proximal to the thalamogeniculate pedicle are associated with a posterolateral thalamic infarct and posterior cortical ischemia. Occlusions distal to the thalamogeniculate pedicle usually produce infarcts in the distal hemispheric branches of PCA. Common signs and symptoms include visual field deficits, visual and color agnosia, visual hallucinations, prosopagnosia caused by occipital branches occlusion or amnesia, and/or memory problems or agitated delirium caused by mesial temporal branches ischemia. Occlusion of a dorsal callosal artery in the dominant hemisphere is clinically associated with a characteristic syndrome of alexia without agraphia caused by destruction of crossing association fibers from the contralateral angular gyrus. The same lesion in the nondominant hemisphere produces contralateral visual neglect.[8]

Thalamic infarcts are classically described as four different characteristic syndromes of which three are related to posterior circulation branches: paramedian thalamic infarct, posterolateral thalamic infarct, and dorsal thalamic infarct. Paramedian thalamic infarction is related to occlusion of thalamoperforate vessels branching from P1 segment and clinically presents with somnolence, memory difficulties, mood changes, and vertical gaze palsy. In the presence of Percheron's artery, caused by bilateral thalamic paramedian ischemia, coma is the usual clinical presentation. Posterolateral thalamic infarcts, caused by ischemia in the thalamogeniculate pedicle from P2 segment, present usually with contralateral sensory loss to all modalities, dysesthesias, and involuntary movements with choreoathetoid appearance. The anatomic correlation is with a lesion of the ventral posterolateral thalamic nucleus (VPL) referred by the eponym of the "syndrome Dejerine-Roussy." Dorsal thalamic infarcts, secondary to occlusion of posterior choroidal arteries, present clinically

TABLE 25-4. Classical Lacunar Syndromes with the Posterior Circulation Localization	
Syndromes	*Localization*
Pure motor stroke	Basis pontis
Pure sensory stroke	VPL thalamus
Sensory-motor stroke	Basis pontis
Ataxic hemiparesis	Basis pontis
Dysarthria-clumsy hand syndrome	Basis pontis

with visual field defects caused by involvement of the lateral geniculate body, sensory symptoms caused by partial involvement of VPL, and language difficulties especially in the dominant hemisphere, caused by pulvinar involvement.[8,9]

Lacunar syndromes are small, ischemic infarcts resulting from occlusion of perforating vessels. There are at least 20 lacunar syndromes described in the literature. Five of them are well recognized and frequently described: pure motor, pure sensory, sensory-motor, ataxic hemiparesis, and dysarthria-clumsy hand syndrome. Occlusions of the perforating vessels of BA, SCA, or PCA are responsible for different lacunar infarcts that are described. Summaries of the classical lacunar syndromes as well as the specific pontine and mesencephalic syndromes in the posterior circulation, with their clinical manifestation, are presented in Tables 25-4 to 25-6.

Bilateral VA Disease

Bilateral VA stenosis or occlusion at the origin is usually associated with good collateral flow and subsequently these patients are either asymptomatic or present with TIAs that are precipitated by low blood pressure, suggesting a hemodynamic mechanism[1] (Figure 25-4). The symptoms tend to develop gradually, with recurrent TIAs presenting before permanent deficits occur. Bilateral intracranial VA occlusion presentation depends on the collateral flow, site of occlusion and associated BA lesions. Patients with bilateral VA occlusion below PICA are often symptomatic, presenting with ischemia in the cerebellum, pontine, and midbrain tegmentum. Associated BA occlusive disease carries a particularly poor prognosis.[10]

Widespread Posterior Circulation Atherosclerosis

Patients with multiple, vascular risk factors often have BA occlusion associated with intracranial or extracranial VA stenosis or occlusion. Clinically they present with recurrent TIAs that progress to stroke in multiple cerebellar artery territories. Bilateral paramedian pontine infarctions often coexist. Case series in the literature suggest that despite the severity of the lesions, prognosis is better when compared with BA embolic strokes.[5]

TABLE 25-5. Pontine Syndromes

Millard-Gubler syndrome—ventrocaudal pons	Contralateral hemiplegia Ipsilateral fascicular CN VI, VII—ipsilateral lateral rectus paresis; ipsilateral peripheral facial paresis
Raymond syndrome—ventral medial pons	Contralateral hemiplegia Ipsilateral fascicular VI—paresis of ipsilateral lateral rectus
Foville syndrome—dorsal pons	Contralateral hemiplegia Ipsilateral VI nucleus, PPRF, or both—ipsilateral horizontal gaze palsy Ipsilateral VII—ipsilateral peripheral facial paresis
Marie-Foix syndrome—lateral pons	Contralateral hemiparesis Ipsilateral cerebellar signs Variable contralateral pain and temperature loss (spinothalamic tract)
Paramedian pontine syndromes	Sensory-motor syndrome Pure motor stroke Ataxic hemiparesis Dysarthria-clumsy hand syndrome Pseudobulbar palsy (bilateral lesions)

Border-zone Ischemia in the Posterior Circulation

There are few case reports in the literature of border-zone ischemia in the posterior circulation. Cerebellum border-zone ischemia occurs mainly in the anastomotic zones between PICA and SCA or between right and left SCA at the level of the cerebellar cortex. Reported infarcts are small.

TABLE 25-6. Mesencephalic Syndromes

Weber's syndrome—ventral midbrain	Contralateral hemiplegia Ipsilateral fascicular III nerve palsy (with involvement of pupillary fibers)
Benedikt's syndrome— ventral midbrain tegmentum	Contralateral involuntary movements, intention tremor, hemichorea, or hemiathetosis (red nucleus) Ipsilateral fascicular III nerve palsy (with involvement of pupillary fibers)
Claude's syndrome—dorsal midbrain tegmentum	Contralateral cerebellar signs (brachium conjunctivum) Ipsilateral fascicular III nerve palsy (with involvement of pupillary fibers)
Parinaud syndrome— dorsal midbrain	Upward gaze palsy Convergence retraction nystagmus Lid retraction (Collier's sign) Lid lag Pseudoabducens palsy Pupillary light-near dissociation

The mechanism of these strokes is not clear and hypotension vulnerability is only hypothesized.[1]

DIAGNOSTIC APPROACH

In the emergency department setting, nonenhanced head CT scan is a good and rapid method to rule out intracranial hemorrhages. However, it has limitations in visualizing posterior fossa structures which are mainly the target in vertebrobasilar disease, and has no value in visualizing the vessels. MRI and MRA offer a better way to assess the location and the size of the infarct and the integrity and anatomic variations of the arteries. Diffusion-weighted images combined with ADC maps are especially helpful in determining the acuteness of the lesion. Combined CT scan perfusion and CT scan angiography is an alternative option that has recently been utilized to a greater extent particularly for those patients who cannot undergo MR studies. MRI/MRA, however, offers an accurate and quick assessment of the size of the infarct and the surrounding ischemic penumbra as well as the extracranial and intracranial vessels. Diagnostic catheter angiography has limited but certain indications in defining cervicocephalic dissections, nonatherosclerotic vasculopathies, or cerebral vasculitis. Catheter angiography as a method of localizing the occluded vessel is otherwise used only when intra-arterial pharmacologic thrombolytic or mechanical thrombectomy is contemplated. When evaluating stroke patients, in addition to imaging of the brain and extracranial and intracranial vessels, evaluation of the aortic arch and the heart are mandatory in order to better define the underlying pathology.

Transthoracic echocardiogram should be routinely performed in all stroke patients but whenever a cardiac source of embolism or a right to left shunt are clinically suspected, transesophageal echocardiography (TEE) may be

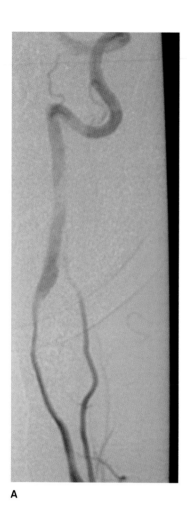

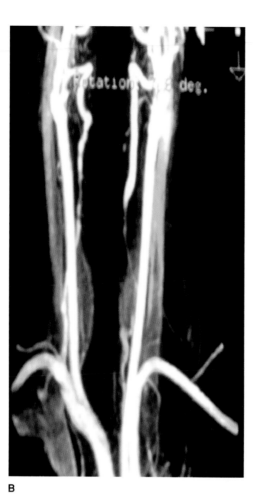

● **FIGURE 25-4.** (A) Catheter cerebral angiogram showing bilateral VA dissection in a 34-year-old presenting with delayed neck pain and vertigo. (B) MRA 3 months later, with similar findings. The initial and subsequent MRIs of the brain were normal (not shown).

A

B

appropriate. Telemetry monitoring is also routinely recommended in order to identify paroxysmal arrhythmias.

● TREATMENT

Acute Treatment

Thrombolytic Therapy. Acute therapeutic options for posterior circulation ischemic stroke are very similar with the ones available for anterior circulation. The only FDA approved therapy that a showed better outcome at 3 months was intravenous recombinant tissue plasminogen activator (rt-PA) administered within 3 hours of symptoms onset. The approval was based on the National Institute of Neurological Disorders and Stroke (NINDS) trial published in 1995.[11] At 6 months and 1 year follow-up, the same investigators were able to prove a sustained benefit of rt-PA treated patients.[12] Early treatment within 90 minutes is associated with the highest benefit.[13] However, the risk of intracranial hemorrhage is 10 times higher in treated patients (6.4% compared with 0.6% in the placebo group). The risk of hemorrhage following iv-TPA is increased in association with larger infarcts, early CT scan changes, age, cardiac disease, diabetes mellitus, and borderline low platelets.[14] Inclusion and exclusion criteria should be closely followed, as protocol violations are associated with a higher risk of symptomatic intracranial hemorrhage.[15] The seminal paper that led to FDA approval of rt-PA for acute ischemic

stroke is the first step toward more aggressive therapeutic options in order to improve recovery, but it lacks information regarding monitoring of vessel recanalization or about the comparative benefits of thrombolysis for anterior versus posterior circulation stroke. A few case series suggest that intravenous rt-PA for vertebrobasilar infarcts, especially for BA occlusion, even beyond 3 hours, may be safe and associated with better outcomes.[16,17] Recanalization and good long-term recovery were reported in up to 52% cases with BA occlusion treated with intravenous rt-PA within 12 hours for acute onset and 48 hours for gradual onset.[16]

BA occlusion, however, is a catastrophic disease, with a reported mortality between 85% and 95% if recanalization is not achieved.[18] Hence, experimental intra-arterial rt-PA which is associated with reported rates of recanalization between 44% and 80% has been increasingly considered for patients with suspected BA occlusions.[19] Clinicians should be aware that the reported risk of intracranial hemorrhage and fatalities are approximately 8% and 53%, respectively, whenever considering this experimental therapy.[18,19] Moreover, a recent meta-analysis comparing intravenous with intra-arterial thrombolysis for BA occlusion suggested that there was no significant difference in death, dependency, or survival between the two approaches, with only slightly higher chances of recanalization after intra-arterial therapy.[20]

Factors that appear to influence recanalization in BA occlusion include age, BA segment, mechanism of occlusion, and clinical presentation. Advanced age, longer segment occlusions thrombotic occlusions, and coma with tetraplegia are considered poor prognostic factors. Based on current evidence, it is not clear which dose, thrombolytic agent, or time window is best for posterior circulation strokes. However, there is a general consensus that the time window is longer for vertebrobasilar circulation when compared to the carotid circulation. Combined intravenous and intra-arterial protocols are also under investigation for ischemic stroke but, to date, the pilot trials could only demonstrate that clinical outcomes and intracranial hemorrhage rates were similar to the NINDS intravenous rt-PA trial, and the numbers of posterior circulation strokes were too few to make any conclusions about specific benefits in this circulation.[21]

Mechanical embolectomy with the MERCI catheter alone (or other similar devices) or in combination with intra-arterial rt-PA is FDA approved for acute clot removal within 8 hours of symptoms onset. The MERCI -II trial is a prospective, single-arm, nonrandomized, multicenter study in which treated patients showed no improved outcome compared with historic controls and the reported procedural complications was 13%. Its clinical efficacy for acute stroke remains, as yet, unproven.[22]

New Approaches. Combined rt-PA with glycoprotein (GP) IIb/IIIa receptor blockers such as tirofiban or eptifibatide in small studies reported promising results, but their role in the therapy of acute stroke needs further validation with prospective, randomized controlled trials. Newer thrombolytic agents such as tenectoplase and desmoteplase are under current investigation. Defibrinogenating agents (Anacrod) administered within 3 hours or direct thrombin inhibitors (Argatroban) administered within 12 hours of stroke symptoms onset also showed promise, but more studies are needed to establish their efficacy.

Other Therapies

Unfractionated heparin and low-molecular-weight (LMW) heparin in the setting of acute stroke was systematically reviewed in the Cochrane database in 2004 and failed to show benefits in mortality, morbidity, stroke recurrence, or stroke progression.[23] This conclusion should however be judged cautiously considering that the trials reviewed had several limitations and did not appropriately evaluate adjusted intravenous anticoagulation in selected stroke subtypes, especially large-vessel atherosclerotic disease. Recent evidence suggests that intravenous heparin within a 3-hour window for nonlacunar stroke is associated with better outcomes and decrease mortality, with a rate of symptomatic intracranial hemorrhage of 6.2% (compared to 1.4% in the control group) and a rate of asymptomatic intracranial hemorrhage of 11% (compared to 10% in the control group).[24] Based on anecdotal evidence, there is a general consensus that adjusted intravenous unfractionated heparin might help in

selected clinical situations including cerebral venous thrombosis, extracranial cervicocephalic arterial dissections, intracardiac thrombus associated with severe valvular disease, low-ejection fraction, or mechanical heart valves, and intraluminal arterial thrombus. Progressing stroke is a controversial, yet unproved indication that requires further investigation. A noncontrast head CT scan is mandatory before initiation of anticoagulation. Large infarcts, uncontrolled hypertension, and bleeding diathesis are contraindications for early intravenous anticoagulation. In general, indiscriminate use of intravenous unfractionated heparin or LMW heparins, even in the posterior circulation, should be discouraged.

Antiplatelet agents are considered for acute treatment in patients who are not candidates for thrombolytic therapy. Based on a Cochrane database review, aspirin 160 to 325 mg daily given within 48 hours of symptoms onset is associated with decreased risk of early recurrent ischemic stroke and better long-term outcome, without a major risk of hemorrhagic complications for both anterior and posterior circulation ischemic stroke.[25] Acceptable alternatives to aspirin for intolerant patients are clopidogrel and ticlopidine, although there are no trials to evaluate the role of these agents in the setting of acute stroke.

Secondary Stroke Prevention

Oral anticoagulation with warfarin is indicated for both primary and secondary stroke prophylaxis in the presence of a cardioembolic source. In the context of atrial fibrillation, warfarin is associated with a relative risk reduction of 68% and 67% for primary and secondary prevention, respectively, compared with only 21% relative risk reduction with the use of aspirin.[26] Patients with mechanical heart valves should be anticoagulated with warfarin with a target INR of 3.5, unless contraindicated. For bioprosthetic valves warfarin with a target INR of 2.0 to 3.0 for 3 months is the accepted recommendation followed by antiplatelet therapy thereafter. Following acute large anterior wall myocardial infarction (MI), MI with apical hypokinesia, left ventricular thrombus, or low-ejection fraction, a 3 to 6-month course of anticoagulation in conjunction with low-dose aspirin is recommended.[27] Based on current data, there is not sufficient evidence to support anticoagulation with warfarin for stroke prevention in the context of aortic arch atheroma or patent foramen ovale related strokes.[28] However, there are selected situations, including cerebral venous thrombosis and extracranial cervicocephalic arterial dissections in which, after initiation of intravenous heparin, oral warfarin is continued for 3 to 6 months. In the case of cerebral venous thrombosis, anecdotal evidence, and small, randomized trials suggest there is benefit for anticoagulation even in the face of hemorrhagic conversion of the stroke. Case series suggest that patients with hypercoagulable states, such as antiphospholipid antibody syndrome (APAS) should also be treated with oral anticoagulation for secondary stroke prevention but the role of anticoagulation in primary prevention of stroke in patients with APAS is less clear and the lack of randomized data hampers our understanding of the absolute benefit of anticoagulation versus antiplatelet therapy in APAS.[29] Oral anticoagulation with warfarin failed to prove benefit over aspirin in the setting of noncardioembolic stroke or stroke caused by intracranial atherosclerosis.[30,31]

Antiplatelet agents are the mainstay of medical therapy for secondary stroke prevention in both the anterior and posterior circulation. Aspirin in doses ranging from 50 to 1300 mg daily reduces the combined risk of stroke, MI and vascular death by approximately 25%.[32] The major side effect is gastrointestinal hemorrhage, in up to 5% cases. Ticlopidine proved to be superior to aspirin in prevention of nonfatal stroke or death. However, because of thrombocytopenia (occurring in 1/5000 cases) and, severe reversible neutropenia (occurring in 0.85% cases) ticlopidine is rarely used.[33,34] Clopidogrel is a newer thienopyridine that has supplanted ticlopidine in the management of atherosclerotic vascular disease. The CAPRIE trial showed that Clopidogrel 75 mg daily compared to aspirin 325 mg daily is better in reducing the combined risk of stroke, MI, or vascular death (8.7% relative risk reduction).[35] Two studies evaluated the advantage of combining aspirin with clopidogrel compared to clopidogrel alone (MATCH) or aspirin alone (CHARISMA).[36,37] The MATCH trial looked at patients with stroke or TIA who were at particular high risk for recurrent events. Both trials failed to prove a statistically significant superiority of combination therapy for secondary stroke prevention and showed higher risk of hemorrhagic complication. However, clinicians should be aware that combination therapy of clopidogrel 75 mg daily and aspirin 75 to 325 mg daily proved to reduce the relative risk of stroke, MI, or vascular death in patients with acute coronary syndromes (CURE trial).[38] As such, the current approach for ischemic stroke is to use clopidogrel monotherapy in the absence of a cardiac indication for combination therapy.

The combination of 25 mg aspirin twice daily and 200 mg extended release (ER) dipyridamole for secondary stroke prevention was assessed in two studies: European Stroke Prevention Study-2 (ESPS-2) and European and Australian Stroke Prevention Reversible Ischemia Trial (ESPRIT).[39,40] Both studies showed an additive effect of the combination compared to each component and to placebo. ESPS-2 reported a 37% relative risk reduction in fatal and nonfatal stroke at 2 years, but for fatal stroke and MI the benefit was modest. ESPRIT reported a 20% relative risk reduction per year for a combined end point of stroke, MI or vascular death, but included only patients with minor strokes or TIA. The, PRoFESS trial was designed to compare clopidogrel 75 mg daily with the combination of low-dose aspirin and ER dipyridamole and results of that trial are anticipated within the next 1 to 2 years.[41]

Risk factor control should be a routine measure, in conjunction with antithrombotic drugs, for secondary stroke prevention. Blood pressure (BP) control is the most powerful way to prevent stroke, as lowering the diastolic BP above 90 mm Hg by 5 to 6 mm will reduce stroke mortality with 42%[42] and control of systolic hypertension is equally effective. Recent evidence suggests that high-dose atorvastatin in patients with recent stroke or TIA also decreased the overall incidence of stroke.[43]

Interventional Procedures for Secondary Stroke Prevention

Angioplasty and stenting for vertebrobasilar disease are an available but unproven therapeutic option for symptomatic large-vessel intracranial atherosclerotic stenoses. In the SSylvia trial, a small prospective nonrandomized, multicenter case series using the Neurolink® device, the rate of complications was relatively high and extracranial VA stenting appeared to be associated with a higher rate of restenosis compared to carotid artery stenting.[44] Angioplasty for intracranial symptomatic vertebrobasilar ischemia decreased the degree of stenosis by more then 40% with an overall risk of stroke or death of 28% in a case series of 25 patients.[45] Elective stenting of symptomatic BA stenosis was reported to be safe in a case series of 12 patients; however, urgent revascularization for symptomatic intracranial atherosclerotic stenosis was associated with a 50% rate of periprocedural complications including intracranial hemorrhage, disabling stroke, major extracranial hemorrhage, or death.[46,47] Balloon angioplasty followed by deployment of a self-expanded microstent had been used in 15 patients with symptomatic intracranial stenosis refractory to medical treatment, without mortality or morbidity associated with the procedure. The case series included nine patients with posterior circulation disease (48*—Wingspan article). That nonrandomized case registry, using the Wingspan stent device, was recently updated with 45 patients described. The 30-day-mortality was of 4.4% and a stroke recurrence at 6 months of 7.1% for the 45 patients. In this series, 22 patients had posterior circulation disease (13 VA and 9 BA trunks).

Various extracranial-intracranial (EC-IC) bypasses for posterior circulation ischemia are reported, proving that these procedures are feasible but they are currently associated with a higher risk (mortality up to 20%) and a lower patency rate (78%–100%) compared to anterior circulation bypass.[48] Surgical reconstruction for extracranial VA in a large retrospective case series showed a patency rate of 80% and a survival rate of 70% at 5 years with an overall risk of stroke and death of 5.1%.[49]

In general, the evidence for these interventional approaches is mainly anecdotal. Therefore, these techniques should be considered only for patients with recurrent symptoms despite aggressive medical treatment and only in the context of a team with extensive experience in the field.

● SPECIAL TOPICS

Vasculitis

The posterior circulation can be affected in the context of either primary central nervous system (CNS) vasculitis or a systemic vasculitis.

Isolated CNS angiitis also known as granulomatous angiitis of the CNS is a rare condition characterized by inflammation restricted to small cerebral and leptomeningeal arteries. Clinical manifestations are in general nonspecific, reflecting a diffuse CNS involvement with possible superimposed focal findings. There is no specific noninvasive test to support the diagnosis. CSF analysis usually shows increased protein and lymphocytic pleocytosis because of leptomeningeal involvement. Brain MRI usually suggests a diffused white and gray matter disease. MRA has a low-diagnostic yield because of its limitation in visualizing small vessels. Cerebral angiogram may be normal or may show a "beading" pattern, but this is only a marker of vasculitis and does not give any information about the etiology of the disease. The diagnosis is made only in the absence of systemic necrotizing vasculitis, after excluding other inflammatory, autoimmune, toxic, or infectious etiologies. In selected cases, in which there is a strong clinical suspicion, a combined brain and leptomeningeal biopsy can confirm the diagnosis. The biopsy is indicated mainly when it is not possible to differentiate between vasculitis, lymphoma, or infection after extensive laboratory and imaging tests.

Giant cell arteritis is an inflammatory condition affecting medium and large vessels with a predilection for the head and neck, hence explaining the usual clinical presentation with headache and vision loss. Intracranial vessels are rarely affected and strokes are an uncommon but potential serious complication of the disease. There is a predilection for posterior circulation strokes in this clinical scenario and the mechanisms include artery to artery embolism, subclavian steel, or local stenosis or occlusion secondary to inflammation.

Takayasu's arteritis is a large-vessel granulomatous arteritis that can affect extracranial carotid or vertebral arteries thus leading ischemic strokes.

Herpes zoster associated angiitis is a recognized late complication of herpes zoster ophthalmicus because of cerebral vessel vasculitis mainly in the territory of middle cerebral artery branches and only rare extending to ipsilateral posterior cerebral arteries. Contralateral hemiparesis occurs weeks to months after the varicella-zoster infection and there are anecdotal reports of resolving of the symptoms without any treatment. A hypothesized mechanism is viral spreading from the eye to the surrounding vessels.

Systemic vasculitidies that affect the CNS include systemic lupus erythematosis (SLE), polyarteritis nodosa, rheumatoid arthritis, Wegener granulomatosis, Sjogren syndrome, scleroderma, cryoglobulinemia, lymphomatoid granulomatosis, malignant atrophic papulosis (Degos' disease), and Behcet disease. Generally the mechanism of CNS involvement is because of small-vessel vasculitis in these syndromes. In SLE, cerebral infarction can also be secondary to local thrombosis because of a hypercoagulable condition associated to antiphospholipid antibody syndrome or to thrombotic thrombocytopenic purpura, cardioembolism caused by nonbacterial thrombotic endocarditis (Libmann-Sacks), or cerebral venous thrombosis. Hemorrhages, including subarachnoid hemorrhage (SAH)

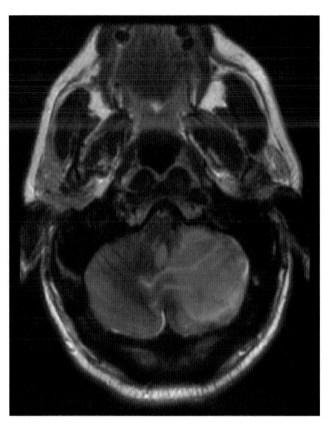

● **FIGURE 25-5.** MRI/FLAIR showing a left cerebellar infarct with compression of the fourth ventricle in a 48-year-old hypertensive man presenting with nausea, vomiting, and left side dysmetria; MRA was normal (not shown).

are also described in association with SLE, but are less common than ischemic strokes. Posterior circulation infarcts secondary to compression of VA are also seen in rheumatoid arthritis in association with a compressive cervical myelopathy as a complication of C1–C2 subluxation (Figure 25-5). Both arterial and venous thrombosis is described in Behcet disease and Degos' disease.

Other CNS vasculopathies of unknown etiology that affect specific vessels include Susac's syndrome, Cogan syndrome, and Eales disease. Susac's syndrome is a retinocohleocerebral vasculopathy presenting with blindness, deafness, and encephalopathy, affecting mainly young females, and should be considered in the differential diagnosis of multiple sclerosis. Cogan syndrome presents with anterior chamber inflammation (keratitis, scleritis, or episcleritis) and vestibulocohlear dysfunction. Eales disease is an isolated primary retinal vasculopathy affecting mainly young males.

CNS vasculitis is treated with different combinations of corticosteroids and cytotoxic agents. However, the response to therapy is typically poor and the condition is associated with a grim prognosis.[1,50]

Aneurysms

The overall prevalence of unruptured cerebral aneurysms in the anterior and posterior circulation is estimated at 5%

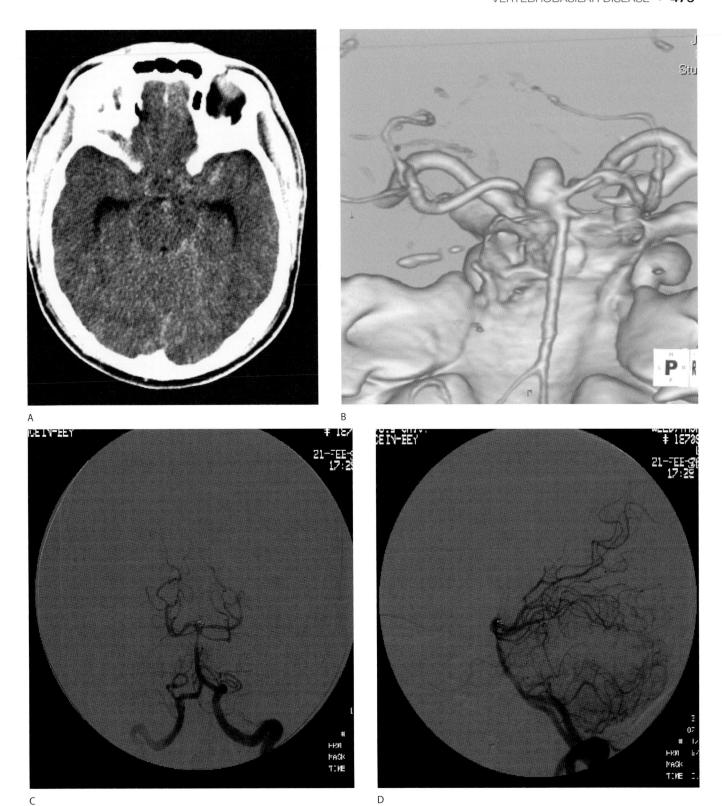

● **FIGURE 25-6.** (A) Unenhanced CT scan showing subarachnoid hemorrhage in a 38-year-old man presenting with severe headache and mild alteration in level of consciousness (Glasgow Coma Scale = 13). (B) CTA of the same patient showing a basilar tip aneurysm that was subsequently coiled. (C) Cerebral angiogram anteroposterior view. (D) lateral view showing the coiled tip of the basilar aneurysm.

based on radiologic and autopsy series. Only 15% of unruptured aneurysms are located in the posterior circulation, with the BA tip being the most common aneurysmal location, followed by the VA-PICA junction[51] (Figure 25-6). Etiopathologically, aneurysms can be classified as saccular, fusiform, infectious or mycotic, and traumatic. Saccular aneurysms, also known as berry aneurysms, are the most common type, are described as thin-walled protrusions of the vessels, and are usually considered acquired lesions related with hemodynamic stress. Fusiform aneurysms involve the entire vessel circumference and their preferential location is in the BA. Mycotic and traumatic aneurysms are found in selected patients and are usually located in the peripheral branches. Multiple aneurysms are found in up to 20% to 30% of patients. Inherited conditions associated with a high incidence of intracranial aneurysms include adult autosomal dominant polycystic kidney disease, Ehlers-Danlos type IV, familial aldosteronism type I, and moya-moya disease. The prevalence of intracranial aneurysms in first-degree relatives of patients with aneurysms is double compared to general population regardless of the presence of a hereditary syndrome. Cigarette smoking, hypertension, and estrogen deficiency are predisposing factors for aneurysm formation.[52]

Clinically unruptured aneurysms are usually asymptomatic, and are discovered incidentally. Rarely, local compression or ischemia secondary to thromboembolism occur leading to nonspecific symptoms such as headache, visual acuity loss, facial pain, or TIA-like episodes. Ruptured intracranial aneurysms present with subarachnoid hemorrhage (SAH) and the gold standard for diagnosis in this clinical scenario remains catheter cerebral angiogram.

The natural history of an unruptured intracranial aneurysm depends on the size, location, and prior history of SAH. The subsequent prevalence of aneurysmal rupture has been variously estimated at more than 0.5% when an unruptured cerebral aneurysm is first identified. Posterior circulation aneurysm seems to have a higher rate of rupture compared to anterior circulation aneurysms. The International Study of Unruptured Intracranial Aneurysms (ISUIA) showed that the 5-year cumulative rupture rates in patients without a prior history of SAH were 2.5%, 14.5%, 18.4%, and 50% for 7 mm, 7 to 12 mm, 13 to 24 mm, and greater than 25 mm aneurysms, respectively. Aneurysms less then 7 mm have an annual rate of rupture of 0.1%.[53] Treatment decisions in the light of these data should be individualized. Risks and benefits should be clearly presented to the patient, who ultimately will be able to make an educated choice.

Treatment of a ruptured aneurysm can be achieved by either surgical clipping or endovascular coiling, depending on multiple factors including aneurysm size, location, geometry, associated morbidity, patient preferences, and physician experience. The International Subarachnoid Aneurysmal Trial (ISAT) showed that for aneurysms that are amenable to both procedures, endovascular coiling is associated with significant higher rates of survival free of disability at 1 year, and this result was persistent at 7 years in a follow-up study. Because of the greater risk of surgical intervention in the posterior circulation, coiling of aneurysms has become the preferred approach to treating these lesions. Rebleeding risk is low but higher with endovascular coiling as compared with surgery.[54,55] As in the case of unruptured aneurysms, optimal treatment of ruptured intracranial aneurysms remains controversial and should be individualized and approached within a team of interventionalists and neurosurgeons, at specialized centers which have both surgical and interventional capabilities.

REFERENCES

1. Mohr JP, Choi DW, Grotta JC, Weir B, Wolf PA. *Stroke Pathophysiology, Diagnosis, and Management.* Philadelphia, PA: Churchill Livingstone; 2004:207-274, 575-602, 775-784.

2. Caplan LR, Gorelick PB, Hier DB. Race, sex, and occlusive cerebrovascular disease: a review. *Stroke.* 1986;17:648-655.

3. Bogousslavsky J, Regli F, Maeder P, Meuli R, Nader J. The etiology of posterior circulation infarcts: a prospective study using magnetic resonance imaging and magnetic resonance angiography. *Neurology.* 1993;43:1528-1533.

4. Voetsch B, Dewitt LD, Pessin MS, Caplan LR. Basilar artery occlusive disease in the New England medical center posterior circulation registry. *Arch Neurol.* 2004;61:496-504.

5. Schievink WI. Spontaneous dissection of the carotid and vertebral arteries. *N Engl J Med.* 2001;344:898-906.

6. Savitz SI, Caplan LR. Vertebrobasilar disease. *N Engl J Med.* 2005;325(25):2618-2626.

7. Bogousslavsky J, Moncayo-Gaete J. Vertebrobasilar transient ischemic attacks. *Medlink Neurol.* 2006. http://www.medlink.com.

8. Biller J, Brazis PW, Masdeu JC. *Localization in Clinical Neurology.* 5th ed. Philadelphia, PA: Lippincott Williams & Wilkins; 2007:349-381, 521-555.

9. Amarenco P. Cerebellar stroke syndromes. In: Bogousslavsky J, Caplan L, eds. *Strokes Syndromes.* 2nd ed. Cambridge, UK: Cambridge University Press, 2001:Chap 42 540-556.

10. Shin H-K, Yoo K-M, Chang H-M, Caplan LR. Bilateral intracranial vertebral artery disease in the New England medical center posterior circulation registry. *Arch Neurol.* 1999; 56:1353-1358.

11. The National Institute of Neurological Disorders and Stroke rt-PA Stroke Study Group. Tissue plasminogen activator for acute ischemic stroke. *N Engl J Med.* 1995;333:1581.

12. Kwiatkowski, TG, Libman, RB, Frankel, M, et al. Effects of tissue plasminogen activator for acute ischemic stroke at one year. *N Engl J Med.* 1999;340:1781.

13. Marler JR, Tilley BC, Lu M, et al. Early stroke treatment associated with better outcome: the NINDS rt-PA stroke study. *Neurology.* 2000;55:1649.

14. Tanne D, Kasner SE, Demchuk AM, et al. Markers of increased risk of intracerebral hemorrhage after intravenous recombinant tissue plasminogen activator therapy for acute ischemic stroke in clinical practice: the Multicenter rt-PA Stroke Survey. *Circulation.* 2002;105:1679.

15. Katzan IL, Furlan AJ, Lloyd LE, et al. Use of tissue-type plasminogen activator for acute ischemic stroke: the Cleveland area experience. *JAMA.* 2000;283:1151.

16. Lindsberg PJ, Soinne L, Tatlisumak T, et al. Long-term outcome after intravenous thrombolysis of basilar artery occlusion. *JAMA.* 2004;292:1862.

17. Montavont A, Nighoghossian N, Derex L, et al. Intravenous r-tPA in vertebrobasilar acute infarcts. *Neurology.* 2004;62:1854-1856.

18. Lindsberg P, Soinne L, Roine RO, Tatlisumak T. Options for recanalization therapy in basilar artery occlusion. *Stroke.* 2005;36(2):203-204.

19. Arnold M, Nedeltchev K, Schroth G, et al. Clinical and radiological predictors of recanalization and outcome of 40 patients with acute basilar artery occlusion treated with intra-arterial thrombolysis. *J Neurol Neurosurg Psychiatry.* 2004;75(6):857-862.

20. Lindsberg PJ, Mattle HP. Therapy of basilar artery occlusion: a systematic analysis comparing intra-arterial and intravenous thrombolysis. *Stroke.* 2006;37:922.

21. The IMS Study Investigators. Combined intravenous and intra-arterial recanalization for acute ischemic stroke: the Interventional Management of Stroke Study. *Stroke.* 2004;35:904.

22. Smith WS, Sung G, Starkman S, et al. Safety and efficacy of mechanical embolectomy in acute ischemic stroke: results of the MERCI trial. *Stroke.* 2005;36:1432.

23. Gubitz G, Sandercock P, Counsell C. Anticoagulants for acute ischaemic stroke. *Cochrane Database Syst Rev.* 2004:CD000024.

24. Carmelingo M, Salvi P, Belloni G, Gamba T, Cesana BM, Mamoli A. Intravenous heparin started within the first 3 hours after onset of symptoms as a treatment for acute nonlacunar hemispheric cerebral infarctions. *Stroke.* 2005;36(11):2415-2420.

25. Sandercock P, Gubitz G, Foley P, Counsell C. Antiplatelet therapy for acute ischaemic stroke. *Cochrane Database Syst Rev.* 2003:CD000029.

26. Atrial Fibrillation Investigators. Risk factors for stroke and efficacy of antithrombotic therapy in atrial fibrillation: analysis of pooled data from five randomized controlled trials. *Arch Intern Med.* 1994;154:1449-1457.

27. Harrington R, Becker R, Ezekowitz M, et al. Antithrombotic therapy for coronary artery disease. *Chest.* 2004;126:513S-548S.

28. Alberts G, Amarenco P, Easton J, et al. Antithrombotic and thrombolytic therapy for ischemic stroke. *Chest.* 2004;126:483S-512S.

29. Khamashta MA, Cuadrado MJ, Mujic F, Taub NA, Hunt BJ, Hughes GVR. The management of thrombosis in the antiphospholipid antibody syndrome. *N Engl J Med.* 1995;332:993-997.

30. Mohr J, Thomson J, Lazar R, et al. A comparison of warfarin and aspirin for the prevention of recurrent ischemic stroke. *N Engl J Med.* 2001;345:1444-1451.

31. Chimowitz MI, Lynn MJ, Howlett-Smith H, et al. Comparison of warfarin and aspirin for symptomatic intracranial arterial stenosis. *N Engl J Med.* 2005;352:1305-1316.

32. Antithrombotic Trialist's Collaboration (ATC). Collaborative meta-analysis of randomised trials of antiplatelet therapy for prevention of death, myocardial infarction, and stroke in high risk patients. *BMJ.* 2002;324:71-86.

33. Hass WK, Easton JD, Adams HP, et al. A randomized trial comparing ticlopidine hydrochloride with aspirin for the prevention of stroke in high-risk patients. *N Engl J Med.* 1989;321:501.

34. Gorelick PB, Richardson D, Kelly M, et al. Aspirin and ticlopidine for prevention of recurrent stroke in black patients: a randomized trial. *JAMA.* 2003;289:2947.

35. CAPRIE Steering Committee. A randomised, blinded, trial of clopidogrel versus aspirin in patients at risk of ischaemic events (CAPRIE). *Lancet.* 1996;348:1329.

36. Diener HC, Bogousslavsky J, Brass LM, et al. Aspirin and clopidogrel compared with clopidogrel alone after recent ischaemic stroke or transient ischaemic attack in high-risk patients (MATCH): randomised, double-blind, placebo-controlled trial. *Lancet.* 2004;364:331.

37. Bhatt DL, Fox KA, Hacke W, et al. Clopidogrel and aspirin versus aspirin alone for the prevention of atherothrombotic events. *N Engl J Med.* 2006;354:1706.

38. Yusuf S, Zhao F, Mehta SR, et al. Effects of clopidogrel in addition to aspirin in patients with acute coronary syndromes without ST-segment elevation. *N Engl J Med.* 2001;345:494.

39. Diener HC, Cunha L, Forbes C, et al. European Stroke Prevention Study 2. Dipyridamole and acetylsalicylic acid in the secondary prevention of stroke. *J Neurol Sci.* 1996;143:1.

40. Halkes PH, van Gijn J, Kappelle LJ, et al. Aspirin plus dipyridamole versus aspirin alone after cerebral ischaemia of arterial origin (ESPRIT): randomised controlled trial. *Lancet.* 2006;367:1665.

41. Sacco RL, Diener H-C, Yusuf S; PRoFESS Steering Committee and Study Group. Prevention regimen for effectively avoiding second strokes (PRoFESS) [Abstract]. Presented at the 30th International Stroke Conference, American Stroke Association. New Orleans, LA; 2005.

42. Collins R, Peto R, MacMahon S, et al. Blood pressure, stroke, and coronary heart disease. part 2, short-term reductions in blood pressure: overview of randomized drug trials in their epidemiological context. *Lancet.* 1990;335:827.

43. Amarenco P, Bogousslavsky J, Callahan A III, et al. High-dose atorvastatin after stroke or transient ischemic attack. *N Engl J Med.* 2006;355(6):549-559.

44. Lutsep HL, Barnwell SL, Mawad M, et al. Stenting of Symptomatic Atherosclerotic Lesions in the Vertebral or Intracranial Arteries (SSYLVIA): study results. [abstract]. *Stroke.* 2003;34:253-253.

45. Gress DR, Smith WS, Dowd CF, Van HV, Finley RJ, Higashida RT. Angioplasty for intracranial symptomatic vertebrobasilar ischemia. *Neurosurgery.* 2002;51:23-27.

46. Gomez CR, Misra VK, Liu MW, et al. Elective stenting of symptomatic basilar artery stenosis. *Stroke.* 2000;31:95-99.

47. Gupta R, Schumacher HC, Mangla S, et al. Urgent endovascular revascularization for symptomatic intracranial atherosclerotic stenosis. *Neurology*. 2003;61:1729-1735.

48. Henkes H, Miloslavski E, Lowens S, et al. treatment of intracranial atherosclerotic stenosis with balloon dilatation and self-expanding stent deployment (WingSpan). *Neuroradiology*. 2005;47:222-228.

49. Bose A, Hartmann M, Henkes H, et al. A novel, self-expanding, nitinol stent in medically refractory intracranial atherosclerotic stenosis: the Wingspan study. *Stroke*. 2007; 38(5):1531-1537.

50. Amin-Hanjani S, Charbel FT. Is extracranial-intracranial bypass surgery effective in certain patients? *Neurol Clinics*. 2006; 24(4):729-743.

51. Berguer R, Flynn LM, Kline RA, Caplan L. Surgical reconstruction of the extracranial vertebral artery: management and outcome. *J Vasc Surg*. 2000;31:9-18.

52. Younger DS. Vasculitis of the nervous system. *Curr Opin Neurol*. 2004;17:317.

53. Stehbens WE. Aneurysms and anatomic variation of cerebral arteries. *Arch Pathol*. 1963;75:45.

54. Schievink WI. Intracranial aneurysms. *N Engl J Med*. 1997; 336:28.

55. Wiebers DO, Whisnant JP, Huston J, et al. Unruptured intracranial aneurysms: natural history, clinical outcome, and risks of surgical and endovascular treatment. *Lancet*. 2003; 362:103-110.

56. Molyneax A, Kerr R, Stratton I, et al. International Subarachnoid Aneurysm Trial (ISAT) of neurosurgical clipping versus endovascular coiling in 2143 patients with ruptured intracranial aneurysms: a randomized trial. *Lancet*. 2002;360:1267-1274.

57. Molyneax A, Kerr R, Yu LM. International Subarachnoid Aneurysm Trial (ISAT) of neurosurgical clipping versus endovascular coiling in 2143 patients with ruptured intracranial aneurysms: a randomized comparison of effects on survival, dependency, seizures, rebleeding, subgroups, and aneurysm occlusion. *Lancet*. 2005;366:809-817.

chapter 26

Ascending Thoracic Aorta

Jose D. Amortegui, MD / *Thomas E. Gaines, MD*

This chapter is intended to provide a clinically oriented discussion of proximal aortic disease emphasizing not only the more common problems seen in clinical practice such as ascending aneurysms and dissection but also to serve as an initial reference for many less common conditions that are generally encountered only occasionally or in specialized circumstances. A discussion of congenital aortic disease is included since an ever-increasing number of patients are now surviving into adulthood and will be encountered by vascular specialists.

● EMBRYOLOGY

The primordial heart and the vascular system appear in the middle of the third week of embryonic development. As the pharyngeal arches form during the fourth and fifth weeks of development, they are supplied by arteries—the aortic arches—that arise from the aortic sac and terminate in the dorsal aortae. Initially, the paired dorsal aortae run through the entire length of the embryo, but they soon fuse to form a single dorsal aorta, just caudal to the pharyngeal arches (Figure 26-1). When the primordial ventricle contracts, blood is pumped through the bulbus cordis and truncus arteriosus into the aortic sac, from which it is distributed to the aortic arches in the pharyngeal arches. The blood then passes into the dorsal aortae for distribution to the embryo.

During the fifth week of development, active proliferation of mesenchymal cells in the walls of the bulbus cordis results in the formation of bulbar ridges, similar ridges form in the truncus arteriosus. The bulbar and truncal ridges undergo a 180-degree spiraling. The spiral orientation of the bulbar and truncal ridges results in the formation of a spiral aorticopulmonary septum when the ridges fuse. This septum divides the bulbus cordis and truncus arteriosus into two arterial channels, the aorta and pulmonary trunk (Figure 26-2). The final transformation of the truncus arterio-

sus, aortic sac, aortic arches, and dorsal aorta into the adult arterial pattern are shown in Figure 26-3.[1]

● CONGENITAL LESIONS

Congenital heart disease (CHD) occurs in 0.4% to 0.8% of live births. Excluding bicuspid aortic valve (BAV) and aortic valve stenosis, conotruncal abnormalities represent only 10% to 15% of congenital heart lesions. The incidence of CHD does not seem to vary by race.[2]

Some environmental exposures, maternal illnesses, or exposure to drugs can increase the likelihood of developing CHD; infants of diabetic mothers are at increased risk of developing CHD in general and conotruncal defects such as truncus arteriosus in particular. Exposure to retinoic acids is also associated with conotruncal defects. Although CHD is often considered a sporadic event, some cases result from inherited genetic traits. There is an increased recurrence risk of CHD when either a parent or a sibling is affected.[2,3]

Truncus Arteriosus

Truncus arteriosus (TA) or persistent TA is a rare anomaly, comprising between 1% and 4% of all cases of congenital heart disease. TA results from failure of truncal ridges and aorticopulmonary septum to develop normally and to divide the truncus arteriosus into the aorta and pulmonary trunk. The exact cause of this condition is unknown, but up to 40% of the patients have microdeletions in the chromosome band 22q11. In this anomaly, a single arterial trunk, the TA, arises from the heart by way of a semilunar valve and supplies the systemic, pulmonary, and coronary circulations. A large perimembranous, infundibular ventricular septal defect (VSD) is present below the TA anomaly. The number of truncal valve cusps varies from two to as many as six.[1,4–6] Other associated abnormalities include right aortic arch in 30% of patients, interrupted aortic arch (IAA) in

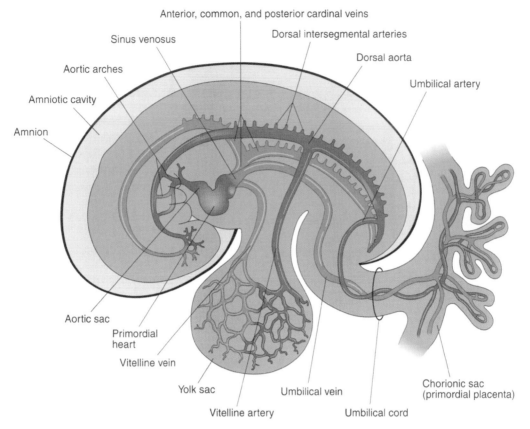

● **FIGURE 26-1.** Embryonic cardiovascular system (at approximately 26 days).

Reproduced with permission from Moore K, Persaud TVN. The cardiovascular system. In: Before We Are Born. Essentials of Embryology and Birth Defects, 6th ed. Philadelphia, PA: WB Saunders; 2003:264.

10% of the patients, which almost always occurs between the left common carotid and the left subclavian artery, and evidence of DiGeorge syndrome with hypocalcemia in 33% of the patients.[5]

This anomaly is divided in four types according to the Collett and Edwards' classification, which is based on the origin of the pulmonary artery. Type I, a short pulmonary trunk emerges from the left lateral wall of the common arterial trunk and divides into right and left pulmonary branches. In type II, the pulmonary arteries arise either independently or via a common orifice from the posterior wall of the common arterial trunk, this is the most common type of persistent TA, type I and II constitute 85% of cases. In type III, the pulmonary arteries arise from the lateral aspects of the truncus. In type IV, no true pulmonary arteries are present, and the lungs are supplied by arteries arising from either the aortic arch or the descending aorta.[5,7] In 1965, Van Praaghs proposed the other commonly cited classification that also includes four types. Type A1 is identical to the type I of Collett and Edwards. Type A2 includes Collett and Edwards type II and most cases of type III, namely, those with separate origin of the branch pulmonary arteries from the left and right lateral aspects of the common trunk. In type A3, only one pulmonary artery (right or left) is present, and one lung is supplied by either a bronchial artery or an aberrant pulmonary artery arising from the aor-

tic arch. Type A4 is defined by the coexistence of an IAA (Figure 26-4).[4–6]

Pathophysiology. The main pathophysiologic consequences of truncus arteriosus are the mandatory mixing of systemic and pulmonary venous blood at the level of the VSD and truncal valve, which leads to arterial saturations near 85%, and the presence of a nonrestrictive left-to-right shunt. Additionally, truncal valve stenosis or regurgitation, left ventricular outflow tract obstruction, and stenosis of the pulmonary artery branches can further contribute to both pressure and volume loading of the ventricles. These factors lead to severe heart failure early in life. Increased pulmonary vascular resistance may develop as early as 6 months of age, leading to poor results with surgical repair. Pulmonary blood flow increases in type I, remains normal in types II and III, and decreases in type IV.[4,5]

Clinical Manifestations and Diagnosis. The clinical signs of truncus arteriosus vary with age and depend on the level of pulmonary vascular resistance. Patients usually present in the neonatal period with signs and symptoms of congestive heart failure (CHF) secondary to increased pulmonary blood flow and mild to moderate cyanosis, which may be seen immediately after birth. A history of dyspnea with feeding, failure to thrive, and frequent respiratory

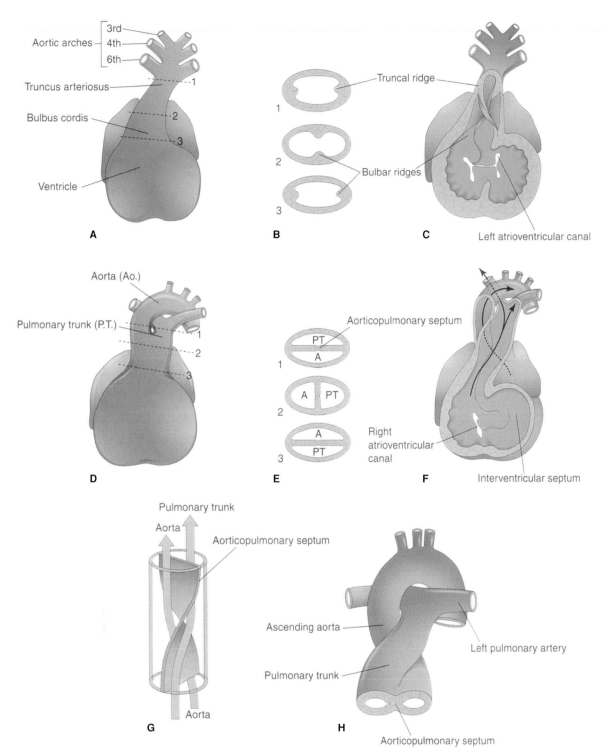

● FIGURE 26-2. Partitioning of the bulbus cordis and truncus arteriosus. (A) Ventral aspect of the heart at 5 weeks. (B) Transverse sections of the truncus arteriosus and bulbus cordis, illustrating the truncal and bulbar ridges. (C) The ventral wall of the heart and truncus arteriosus have been removed to demonstrate these ridges. (D) Ventral aspect of the heart after partitioning of the truncus arteriosus. (E) Sections through the newly formed aorta (A) and pulmonary trunk (PT) show the aorticopulmonary septum. (F) Six weeks. The ventral wall of the heart and pulmonary trunk have been removed to show the aorticopulmonary septum. (G) Diagram illustrating the spiral form of the aorticopulmonary septum. (H) Drawing showing the great arteries twisting around each other as the leave the heart.

Reproduced with permission from Moore K, Persaud TVN. The cardiovascular system. In: Before We Are Born. Essentials of Embryology and Birth Defects, 6th ed. Philadelphia, PA: WB Saunders; 2003:264.

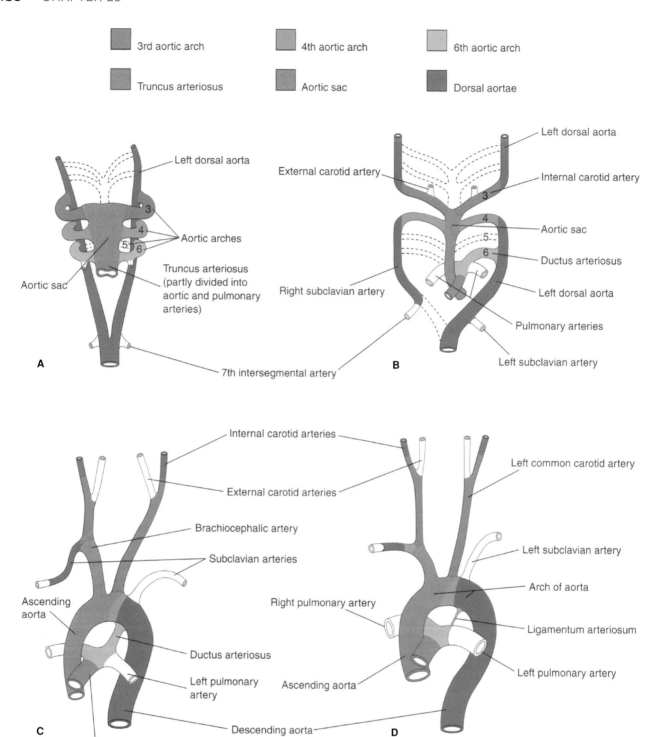

Legend:
- 3rd aortic arch
- 4th aortic arch
- 6th aortic arch
- Truncus arteriosus
- Aortic sac
- Dorsal aortae

A
- Left dorsal aorta
- Aortic arches
- Truncus arteriosus (partly divided into aortic and pulmonary arteries)
- Aortic sac
- 7th intersegmental artery

B
- External carotid artery
- Left dorsal aorta
- Internal carotid artery
- Aortic sac
- Ductus arteriosus
- Left dorsal aorta
- Pulmonary arteries
- Right subclavian artery
- Left subclavian artery

C
- Internal carotid arteries
- External carotid arteries
- Brachiocephalic artery
- Subclavian arteries
- Ascending aorta
- Ductus arteriosus
- Left pulmonary artery
- Descending aorta
- Pulmonary trunk

D
- Left common carotid artery
- Left subclavian artery
- Arch of aorta
- Right pulmonary artery
- Ligamentum arteriosum
- Ascending aorta
- Left pulmonary artery

● FIGURE 26-3. Arterial changes that result during transformation of the truncus arteriosus, aortic sac, aortic arches, and dorsal aortae into the adult pattern. The vessels that are not colored are not derived from these structures. (A) Aortic arches at 6 weeks. By this stage, the first two aortic arches have disappeared. (B) Aortic arches at 7 weeks. The parts of the dorsal aortae and aortic arches that normally disappear are indicated in with broken lines. (C) Arterial arrangement at 8 weeks. (D) Arterial vessels of a 6-month-old infant.

Reproduced with permission from Moore K, Persaud TVN. The cardiovascular system. In: Before We Are Born. Essentials of Embryology and Birth Defects, 6th ed. Philadelphia, PA: WB Saunders; 2003:264.

Collett & Edwards

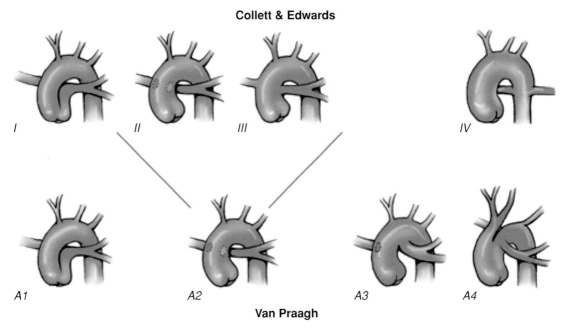

Van Praagh

● **FIGURE 26-4.** Anatomic subtypes of truncus arteriosus (TA), according to the classification systems of both Collett and Edwards (I, II, III) and the Van Praaghs (A1, A2, A3, A4).

Reproduced with permission from Karamlou TB, Shen I, Ungerleider RM. Congenital heart disease. In: Brunicardi FC, ed. Schwartz's Principles of Surgery. 8th ed. New York, NY: McGraw-Hill; 2005:611.

infections is usually present in infants. The peripheral pulses are bounding with a wide pulse pressure. The second heart sound is loud and single. A harsh pan-systolic murmur may be noted at the left sternal border and suggest VSD, and occasionally a diastolic murmur may be heard in the presence of truncal regurgitation.[4,5]

Chest radiography shows increased pulmonary flow and cardiomegaly. As mentioned above a right aortic arch may be seen in 30% of cases. The ECG shows normal sinus rhythm with biventricular hypertrophy. Echocardiography is sufficient to confirm the diagnosis and fully characterize the various anatomic features in most patients. Echocardiography shows three diagnostic findings: A large VSD directly under the truncal valve, a large single great artery that arises from the heart and nonvisualization of the pulmonary valve, and only one semilunar (truncal) valve is seen. Cardiac catheterization can be helpful in cases where pulmonary hypertension is suspected or to further delineate coronary artery abnormalities, which can be present in up to 50% of the subjects. Coronary abnormalities include stenotic ostia, a high or low takeoff, and abnormal branching or course.[4,5]

Treatment. Without surgery most infants die of CHF within 6 to 12 months. If pulmonary blood flow is restricted by the development of pulmonary vascular disease, the patient may survive into early adulthood. The cause of death in unrepaired patients usually is cardiac arrest or multiple organ failure in the face of systemic perfusion that is inadequate to meet the body's metabolic demands with progressive metabolic acidosis and myocardial dysfunction.[5,8]

Truncus arteriosus is an indication for surgery and repair should be done in the neonatal period before the development of pulmonary hypertension and Eisenmenger's physiology. Surgical repair is done with cardiopulmonary bypass (CPB). Repair is based on modifications of the Rastelli procedure and consists of separation of the pulmonary arteries from the aorta, closure of the aortic defect, and VSD closure. For type I a valved or valveless conduit, preferentially aortic homograft, is placed between the right ventricle and the pulmonary artery in order to reconstruct the right ventricular outflow tract. For types II and III, a circumferential band of the truncus, which contains both pulmonary artery orifices, is removed. This cuff is connected to the right ventricle by a valved or valveless Dacron tube. Aortic continuity is restored with a tubular Dacron graft. Severe truncal valve insufficiency occasionally requires truncal valve replacement, which can be done with a cryopreserved allograft. Severe truncal regurgitation, IAA, and coexistent coronary anomalies are risk factors for perioperative death and poor outcome. Pulmonary artery banding is reserved for patients who have increased pulmonary blood flow and are not deemed suitable candidates for definitive repair.[4,5,9,10] Surgical mortality rate is 10% to 30%. For those surviving the initial postoperative period, the survival rate at 10 to 20 years is in excess of 60%, with most deaths resulting from sequelae of delayed repair (pulmonary vascular obstructive disease), reinterventions, or residual/recurrent physiologic abnormalities.[9,11–13]

Follow-up every 4 to 12 months is required to detect late complications. Progressive truncal valve insufficiency may develop, and truncal valve replacement may be needed. A small conduit needs to be changed to a larger size, usually by 2 to 3 years of age. Calcification of the valve in the conduit may occur within 1 to 5 years, which requires re-operation. Ventricular arrhythmias may develop because of right ventriculotomy.[5,9,11,13]

Aortopulmonary Window Defect

Aortopulmonary window defect (APW) is a rare congenital lesion that accounts for less than 1% of all congenital heart lesions. APW results from failure of the spiral septum to completely divide the embryonic truncus arteriosus; this is a consequence of failure of the conotruncal ridges to fuse. The spiral septum normally divides the truncus into the aorta and the pulmonary artery. No genetic associations or environmental risk factors are known. The APW consists of a large communication between the ascending aorta and the main pulmonary artery that usually occurs as a single defect that begins above the sinuses of valsalva on the left lateral wall of the aorta (Figure 26-5). The presence of a pulmonary and an aortic valve and an intact ventricular septum distinguishes this anomaly from truncus arteriosus. More than half of the patients have some other associated lesions that include but are not limited to coronary artery anomalies, patent ductus arteriosus (PDA), atrial septal defect (ASD), VSD, IAA, and tetralogy of Fallot.[4,8,14,15]

Pathophysiology. The main pathophysiologic event in APW is that of a large left-to-right shunt with increased pulmonary blood flow. Volume overload and increased pulmonary blood flow lead to progressive left ventricular dysfunction and early development of CHF, these patients are particularly susceptible to Eisenmenger syndrome at an early age because of combined systolic and diastolic runoff into the pulmonary circulation. Aortic arch obstruction and IAA are usually associated with APW, and they act as an obstruction to systemic flow and further increase the left-to-right shunt. Perfusion to the lower body is therefore dependent on flow through the ductus arteriosus. Closure of the ductus results in severe hypoperfusion of the lower body, increased pulmonary blood flow, and CHF.

Clinical Manifestations and Diagnosis. Infants usually present with symptoms of heart failure during early infancy, occasionally minimal cyanosis, frequently respiratory tract infections, tachypnea with feedings, and failure to thrive. Peripheral pulses are bounding. There is usually a systolic murmur with a mid-diastolic component as a result of the increased blood flow across the mitral valve. The second heart sound is loud and does not split.[8]

The ECG shows left or biventricular hypertrophy, chest radiography demonstrates cardiomegaly, prominence of the pulmonary artery, and increased pulmonary blood flow. Echocardiogram shows enlargement of the left-sided heart chambers and the window defect. Cardiac catheterization reveals a left-to-right shunt at the level of the pulmonary artery, and manipulation of the catheter from the main pulmonary artery directly into the ascending aorta is diagnostic.[8] Cardiac catheterization is usually reserved for those patients who present after 6 months of age or to any patient at risk of pulmonary hypertension. If pulmonary resistance is elevated, testing for reversibility with vasodilators should be performed since the presence of irreversible pulmonary hypertension is a contraindication for surgery.

Treatment. The APW should be surgically corrected during infancy or as soon as it is diagnosed to avoid the development of pulmonary hypertension. Spontaneous closure is not known to occur. Surgery is performed with CPB. The defect is exposed from the anterior aspect of the aorta, the main pulmonary artery, or the APW itself, and the defect in the aorta and pulmonary artery are corrected with a patch; and any other associated anomalies should be repaired at the same time.[14,15]

The patient will require lifelong echocardiographic follow-up to monitor for the development of aortic or pulmonary artery stenosis. The mortality rate reflects the changes that have occurred in pediatric cardiac surgery over time, with a mortality of 37% in the early series when simple ligation or transection of the defect was performed, to 0% in later years with the approach described above. The risk of mortality depends upon the presence or absence of associated anomalies, being less than 10% and 0% respectively.[14,15]

● FIGURE 26-5. Classification of aortopulmonary window. (A) Type I proximal defect. (B) Type II distal defect. (C) Type III total defect.

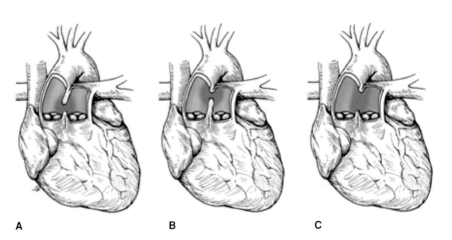

A   B   C

Hypoplastic Left Heart Syndrome

The hypoplastic left heart syndrome (HLHS) is defined as a spectrum of cardiac malformations with normally aligned great arteries without a common atrioventricular (AV) junction, characterized by underdevelopment of the left heart with significant hypoplasia of the left ventricle including atresia, stenosis, or hypoplasia of the aortic or mitral valve, or both, and hypoplasia of the ascending aorta and aortic arch.[16]

HLHS, therefore, is made up of several pathologic cardiac phenotypes. At the severe end of the spectrum are found those patients with aortic and mitral atresia with a virtually nonexistent left ventricle. At the mild end of the spectrum are those patients with hypoplasia of the aortic and mitral valves, but without intrinsic valvar stenosis or atresia, and milder degrees of left ventricular hypoplasia.[16]

The etiology of the HLHS is unknown. The reported prevalence of HLHS is 0.2 per live births and is more common in males (3:2 to 2:1). Several other associated congenital anomalies have been reported, including anomalous venous return, transposition or malposition of the great arteries, VSD, and AV canal defect.[17]

Multiple classifications and definitions have been used in the past, creating confusion and a lack of consistency in previous reports. In 2005 an International Pediatric and Congenital Cardiac Code was accepted based on work from the Society of Thoracic Surgeons and the European Association for Cardio-Thoracic Surgery. This is a very extensive and detailed classification that goes beyond the scope of this chapter, and readers are referred to it for further details.[16]

At birth, the right ventricle provides output to the pulmonary circulation via the ductus arteriosus to the systemic circulation. The pulmonary and aortic pressures are equal in both systole and diastole. Blood returning from the pulmonary veins into the left atrium cannot flow into the left ventricle, and patency of the foramen ovale is imperative. There is mixing of pulmonary and systemic venous return, but the relative contribution of each varies depending on the underlying anatomy. The restrictive nature of the ASD can produce postcapillary pulmonary hypertension, leading not only to pulmonary edema and increased cyanosis, but also a decrease in flow of blood to the lungs, with less volume overload on the right ventricle.[18,19]

Clinical Manifestations and Diagnosis. A grayish blue color of the skin is soon apparent after birth and denotes a combination of cyanosis and hypoperfusion. The diagnosis is usually made in the first day of life. Signs of heart failure are usually apparent in the first days of life. The peripheral pulses are weak or absent. Cardiac examination reveals a dominant right ventricular impulse, a single second heart sound, and a nonspecific systolic murmur at the left lateral border. Chest radiography shows cardiomegaly and increase pulmonary blood flow. ECG shows right atrial enlargement and right ventricular hypertrophy. Echocardiography is diagnostic. Cardiac catheterization is not usually necessary.[8]

Treatment. If left untreated, the vast majority of children with HLHS will die within 7 to 10 days of birth. Survival for patients with HLHS became a possibility in 1980 when Norwood et al. described a staged palliative surgical approach including aortic arch reconstruction. Shortly thereafter, heart transplantation for infants and small children also became feasible.[20] In the preoperative management it is mandatory to maintain ductal patency to avoid systemic and coronary hypoperfusion and to prevent excessive pulmonary blood flow. A relative hypoxemia should be maintained (70%–80%), in order to prevent pulmonary vasodilatation since this would increase pulmonary blood flow and would decrease systemic perfusion.[18]

Three surgical approaches have evolved over the years: A multistage reconstructive surgery based on a single ventricle physiology popularized by Norwood, cardiac replacement proposed by Bailey, and a biventricular repair as used in patients at the mild end of the spectrum of hypoplastic heart syndrome, as well as for those patients with aortic atresia with a VSD and well-developed left ventricle. The first two approaches can be used in any patient with HLHS, the biventricular approach can be used in very few patients.[16]

The Norwood operation is defined as an aorticopulmonary connection and neoaortic arch construction resulting in univentricular physiology and pulmonary blood flow controlled with a calibrated systemic-to-pulmonary artery shunt, or a right ventricle to pulmonary artery conduit, or rarely a cavopulmonary connection.[16]

The principles of the Norwood operation are as follows: First, establishment of a permanent communication between the right ventricle and aorta by transection of the pulmonary trunk and creation of an anastomosis between the pulmonary trunk and the ascending aorta and aortic arch. Second, limitation of blood flow to the lungs to attenuate the development of pulmonary hypertension. This is accomplished by a calibrated systemic-to-pulmonary artery shunt, or a right ventricle to pulmonary artery conduit, or rarely a cavopulmonary connection. Third, creation of a satisfactory interatrial communication by an atrial septotomy in order to ensure unobstructed pulmonary venous return to the tricuspid valve. Fourth, the PDA is ligated. Finally, the adequacy of the coronary arterial perfusions assured. This first stage is performed in the first 2 weeks of life.[16,21]

In a second surgery performed at 4 to 6 months of age, a form of the hemi-Fontan operation or construction of a bidirectional superior cavopulmonary shunt is done and the systemic-to-pulmonary artery shunt is removed. Finally, in a third operation performed at 12 to 18 months after the second surgery, physiologic correction is achieved by separating the systemic and pulmonary circulations using a Fontan-type procedure. Multiple variations in this technique have been reported, trying to fulfill more reliably the surgical criteria for the first stage of palliation and to prepare the patient to become an optimal candidate for the Fontan operation.[16,21]

Factors associated with poor outcome include prematurity, low birth weight, chromosomal and other extracardiac abnormalities, additional intracardiac lesions, older age, small aorta, poor preoperative right ventricular function, and obstructed pulmonary venous return.[20,22,23]

Cardiac transplantation offers the advantage of replacement of an abnormal circulation with a normal 4-chamber heart in a single operation. Disadvantages of this approach are the limited availability of donors and the need for life-long immunosuppression and risk of rejection.

As mentioned before, the biventricular repair is applicable only in patients at the milder end of the spectrum of the HLHS. These include three groups of patients: Those with hypoplasia of the structures of the left ventricle and aorta without intrinsic valvar stenosis or atresia (the so-called hypoplastic left heart complex), those with critical aortic stenosis with left ventricular hypoplasia, and finally those with aortic atresia with VSD and a well-developed left ventricle. The surgery consists of an extensive enlargement of the aortic arch and ascending aorta with a pulmonary homograft and closure of the atrial and VSDs.[16]

Chang et al.[17] analyzed data of 1986 infants (younger than 30 days) with HLHS in the United States. The overall inhospital mortality was 40.9% (812/1986). Only 407 patients (20.5%) underwent surgery, 346 (17.4%) had the Norwood procedure, and 61 (3.1%) had a heart transplantation. A trend was seen in the increasing percentage of patients treated with the Norwood procedure, from <8% in 1988 to 34% in 1997. The percentage of patients who were treated with heart transplantation remained stable. The overall inhospital mortality for patients who underwent the Norwood procedure was 46%. The inhospital mortality rate for patients with the Norwood procedure decreased from 64% in 1988 to close to 30% in 1997. The overall inhospital mortality rate was significantly lower in the heart transplantation group than in the Norwood procedure group (26.2% vs. 46%). From this data one can appreciate the fact that comfort care is still the most common strategy. Comfort care is the predominant option offered to families of infants with HLHS in other countries such as Japan and the United Kingdom.

Bove et al.[22] reported a hospital survival of 93% for 85 patients with standard risks and 53% for 15 patients considered to be at high risk in patients who underwent the Norwood procedure. Similar results have been reported by others.[23–26] The mortality for the second and third stage of the correction is lower, with survival for both procedures greater than 95%.[25,27,28] The 5-year survival is approximately 70%.[24,25]

Transposition of the Great Arteries

Transposition of the great arteries (TGA) is the most common cause of cyanotic heart disease in newborn infants; it accounts for approximately 5% of all congenital heart defects and is more common in males than in females as well as in infants of diabetic mothers. There is no race predilection. The hallmark of the TGA is ventriculoarterial discordance. In typical cases, the aorta is located anteriorly and to the right of the pulmonary artery and arises from right ventricle carrying desaturated blood to the body, while the pulmonary trunk arises posteriorly from the left ventricle carrying oxygenated blood to the lungs. This configuration is known as D-transposition of the great arteries (D-TGA). Survival in these neonates is provided by an ASD, the ductus arteriosus, and/or a VSD, which permits some mixture of oxygenated and deoxygenated blood. The exact etiology of this anomaly is unknown and is presumed to be multifactorial. This defect is thought to result from the failure of the conus arteriosus to develop normally during incorporation of the bulbus cordis into the ventricles. Defective neural crest cell migration may also be involved.[1,5]

Other associated anomalies include VSD, coarctation of the aorta (COA), IAA, pulmonary atresia, subaortic or valvular aortic stenosis, coronary anomalies, and overriding of the AV valves.[29,30]

D-TGA results in parallel pulmonary and systemic circulations, with patient survival depending on intracardiac mixing. There is increased pulmonary blood flow, which causes left atrial enlargement and a left-to-right shunt through the foramen ovale.

Clinical Manifestations and Diagnosis. Infants with D-TGA and intact ventricular septum are cyanotic at birth. The clinical course and manifestations depend on the extent of intercirculatory mixing and the presence of associated anatomic lesions. Those with a VSD may take longer time to become cyanotic. Signs of congestive heart failure develop during the newborn period. Physical findings depend on the presence of associated lesions and include a single and loud second heart sound. No murmur is heard if the ventricular septum is intact and, if there is a VSD, a systolic murmur is present. ECG shows right ventricular hypertrophy. Biventricular hypertrophy may be present in infants with a large VSD, PDA, or pulmonary vascular obstructive disease. Chest radiography reveals the classic egg-shaped configuration with a narrow superior mediastinum. Echocardiography is diagnostic and usually provides the anatomic and functional information necessary for management of these infants. Cardiac catheterization is rarely required, except in those infants requiring surgery in the neonatal period to assess the suitability of the left ventricle to support the systemic circulation.[4,5]

The natural progression consists of progressive hypoxia and acidosis resulting in death unless mixing of blood improves. CHF develops in the first week of life. Without surgical repair, death occurs in 30% by the first week, 50% by the end of the first month, and 90% by the end of the first year. Those patients with an intact ventricular septum are the sickest group and develop pulmonary vascular obstructive disease early in life. Patients with a VSD or a large PDA are the least cyanotic group but the most likely ones to develop CHF and pulmonary vascular disease. The presence of VSD and pulmonary stenosis protects from pulmonary vascular disease and allows a longer survival without surgery.[5]

Treatment. Before surgical repair certain measures are required. The ductus arteriosus should be kept open or reopened with the infusion of prostaglandin in order to improve arterial oxygenation. Balloon atrial septotomy should be performed in order to improve intracardiac mixing. If an adequate interatrial communication exists, this procedure is not required. In older infants or those for whom the balloon septotomy was only temporarily successful, blade atrial septotomy may be performed.[5]

Several procedures have been described for the repair of TGA. The procedures can be grouped into those that redistribute right- and left-sided flow at the level of the atrium, the ventricle, and the great arteries.

The Mustard and the Senning operations are performed at the atrial level. In the Mustard operation, the pulmonary and systemic blood return is redirected at the atrial level through a pericardial or prosthetic baffle. In the Senning operation, the blood return from the pulmonary veins is redirected through the tricuspid valve to the systemic right ventricle by means of an atrial flap fashioned from the free wall of the right atrium plus redirection of systemic venous flow from both the superior and inferior vena cava, through the mitral valve to the pulmonary left ventricle by using the intra-atrial septum. These atrial switch procedures result in a physiologic correction, but not an anatomic one, as the systemic circulation is still based on the right ventricle. Long-term complications include atrial conduction disturbances, sick sinus syndrome, supraventricular arrhythmias, right ventricular failure, tricuspid valve insufficiency, sudden death, superior or inferior vena cava syndrome, and pulmonary vascular obstructive disease.[4,5,31,32]

The Rastelli operation is used in patients with VSD and severe pulmonary stenosis. The redirection of flow is accomplished at the ventricular level. The left ventricle output is directed to the aorta by creating an interventricular tunnel between the VSD and the aortic valve. The pulmonary artery is disconnected from the left ventricle and a conduit is placed between the right ventricle and the pulmonary artery.[5]

In the arterial switch or Jatene procedure, the great arteries are divided proximally, the coronary arteries are reimplanted in the pulmonary trunk, and the distal great arteries are connected to the proximal end of the other great artery (distal aorta to pulmonary trunk and distal pulmonary artery to proximal aorta). The Damus-Kaye-Stansel operation is used in patients with VSD and subaortic stenosis. In this procedure the pulmonary artery is divided proximal to the bifurcation and anastomosed end to side to the ascending aorta by using a Dacron or Gore-Tex tube, the aortic valve is closed, the VSD is closed, and a conduit is placed between the right ventricle and the distal pulmonary artery. The most common complications is pulmonary artery stenosis at the site of the anastomosis. Other complications include complete heart block and aortic regurgitation or stenosis. Arrhythmias are rare.[5,7,33]

The surgical approach depends on the age of the patient at presentation and the presence of associated congenital cardiac lesions. The arterial switch is considered the procedure of choice in the majority of the cases, since it is associated with fewer complications and restores the normal physiologic relationships of systemic and pulmonary arterial flow. The Senning operation is reserved for those patients with unfavorable coronary anatomy, for late referral, or for patients with TGA and pulmonary vascular obstructive disease. The timing of surgery depends on the presence and size of a PFO, ASD, VSD, PDA, pulmonary stenosis, and aortic stenosis. The arterial switch is performed in the first 2 weeks of life before the left ventricular mass decreases to the point at which it would not be able to generate adequate pressure to perfuse the systemic circulation.

The inhospital mortality for the arterial switch is less than 8%, with a 5-year and 15-year survival greater than 80%.[29,30,32–35] Factors associated with increased mortality include unfavorable coronary anatomy, the presence of a VSD, arch pathology, and delayed sternal closure.[29,30,35] The inhospital mortality for the Senning procedure is usually less than 15%.[31]

L-TGA or Congenitally Corrected Transposition of the Great Arteries. L-TGA or congenitally corrected TGA occurs in less than 1% of all patients with congenital heart disease. In this case, the right atrium is to the right of the left atrium. The right atrium empties into the anatomic left ventricle through the mitral valve, and the left atrium empties in the anatomic right ventricle through the tricuspid valve. There is an inversion of the ventricular chambers with their corresponding AV valves. The aorta is located to the left of the pulmonary artery. Oxygenated blood returns into the left atrium, passes to the anatomic right ventricle, and is then ejected into the aorta.[5]

Theoretically, no functional abnormality exists, but in most cases there are associated intracardiac defects, AV conduction disturbances, and arrhythmias. VSD is present in 80% of the cases. Pulmonary stenosis is present in 50% of patients and is usually associated with VSD. Dextrocardia is present in nearly 50% of subjects and there is usually inversion of the coronary arteries. Patients are usually asymptomatic when there are no associated defects. Most patients with associated defects become symptomatic in the first months of life. Medical and surgical management is dictated by the associated anomalies.[5]

Interrupted Aortic Arch

IAA is an uncommon anomaly, accounting for less than 1% of all congenital heart lesions. There is no gender or race predilection. IAA is defined as an absence of luminal continuity between the ascending and descending aorta, representing an extreme form of COA in which the aortic arch is atretic or a segment of the aortic arch is absent.

In the majority of cases there is a concomitant VSD or PDA. Other associated anomalies include ASD, truncus arteriosus, APW, TGA, HLHS, double-outlet right ventricle, AV canal defect, BAV, mitral valve anomalies, and subaortic stenosis. Up to 50% of patients have associated DiGeorge syndrome.[36–39]

Approximately half of patients with IAA have a deletion in the chromosome band 22q11. The T-box gene *TBX1* appears to be responsible for most aspects of the DiGeorge

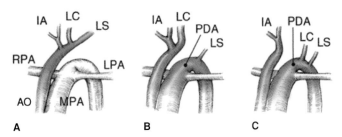

● **FIGURE 26-6.** Anatomic types of interrupted aortic arch. (A) Interruption distal to the left subclavian artery. (B) Interruption between the left subclavian and left carotid arteries. (C) Interruption between the left carotid and innominate arteries. AO = aorta; IA = innominate artery; LC = left carotid artery; LPA = left pulmonary artery; LS = left subclavian artery; MPA = main pulmonary artery; PDA = patent ductus arteriosus; RPA = right pulmonary artery.

phenotype. IAA type A seems to have a different etiology from IAA type B. Three-fourths of patients with IAA type B have the deletion, while few patients with IAA type A have the deletion.[40,41]

IAA is classified into three types based on the location of the interruption (Figure 26-6). In type A, the interruption occurs distal to the left subclavian artery (20%–30% of the cases). In type B, the interruption occurs between the left subclavian artery and the left carotid artery (70%–80% of the cases); an aberrant right subclavian artery is commonly associated with this type. In type C, the interruption is between the innominate artery and the left carotid artery (1%–5%).[36,38,39]

Clinical Manifestations and Diagnosis. Signs usually appear in the first days of life and include dyspnea, cyanosis, decreased peripheral pulses, and signs of CHF; findings become more accentuated when the ductus begins to close. Chest radiography shows cardiomegaly with increased pulmonary blood flow. In patients with DiGeorge syndrome, the upper mediastinum is narrow because of the absence of a thymus. ECG may show right ventricular hypertrophy. Echocardiography is usually diagnostic.[5]

Treatment. If the IAA is left untreated, most patients die in 4 to 10 days, usually following closure of the ductus arteriosus. These subjects are ductus dependent; therefore, the ductus should be kept open with the use of prostaglandin E1 in order to avoid systemic hypoperfusion and to prevent an excessive pulmonary flow. Relative hypoxia should be maintained in order to prevent pulmonary vasodilatation since this would increase the pulmonary blood flow and decrease systemic perfusion.

The preferred surgical approach is aortic repair followed by closure of the VSD. The correction can be performed in one or two stages. In the single stage procedure, the repair consists of direct end-to-end anastomosis between the ascending and descending aorta. In some cases a graft is required for the repair. In the same operation, other associated anomalies are corrected. In the staged procedure,

reconstruction of the aortic arch is performed by anastomosing the divided end of the left carotid artery to the descending aorta, ligation of the PDA, and pulmonary artery banding. The second stage of the procedure consists of closure of the VSD, debanding of the pulmonary artery, and pulmonary arterial reconstruction. Other procedures might be needed depending on the presence of associated anomalies. Initial inhospital mortality is usually less than 15% in most series, with long-term survival of 70% to 80% at 5 to 15 years. The most important factor associated with worse outcome is the presence of complex anomalies; other risk factors are increased age at the time of surgery, low weight, type B IAA, and the presence of the DiGeorge syndrome.[36–39]

Vascular Rings

Vascular rings comprise less than 1% of congenital heart lesions. Vascular rings can produce tracheal and esophageal compression. Respiratory symptoms are more common in younger patients and dysphagia is more common in older children. Although these anomalies are mainly identified in childhood, there are reports of these occurring in adults as well.[42] Vascular rings have been generally divided into four classes: double aortic arch, right aortic arch, innominate compression, and pulmonary sling. Double aortic arch and right aortic arch are the two most common forms.[43]

Double Aortic Arch. Double aortic arch is a rare anomaly that is characterized by a complete vascular ring encircling the trachea and esophagus. A double aortic arch is responsible for 50% of all vascular ring anomalies. There is no gender or race predilection. The vascular ring results from persistence of the fourth arches and failure of the distal part of the right dorsal aorta to disappear. In more than 70% of the patients the right aortic arch is dominant and passes posterior to the trachea and esophagus. Associated anomalies include VSD, ASD, PDA, COA, and tetralogy of Fallot. Less frequently associated anomalies include truncus arteriosus, TGA, pulmonary atresia, and HLHS.[1,44,45] Chromosome 22q11 deletions are present in 20% of patients with double aortic arch.[46]

Symptoms result from compression of the esophagus and trachea by the vascular ring. The severity of symptoms depends on the degree of compression by the vascular ring. The onset of symptoms is usually at birth but can be as late as 3 years of age. Respiratory symptoms are more common than gastrointestinal and cardiac symptoms. The most common respiratory symptoms are stridor and wheezing. Other respiratory symptoms include coughing, choking, upper and lower respiratory infection, dyspnea, increased oral secretions and, aspiration. The most common gastrointestinal symptom is choking with feeds. Other symptoms include dysphagia, failure to thrive, emesis, and cyanosis with feedings. Lastly, cardiac features include murmurs, cyanosis, chest pain, and CHF. Chest radiography sometimes shows narrowing of the trachea. An esophagogram will demonstrate an indentation in the esophageal wall. Echocardiography, MRI, or CT are diagnostic. Arch predominance is best determined by echocardiography or MRI. Aortic angiography is rarely needed.[44,45,47]

The treatment of a double aortic arch is surgical. Alsenaidi et al.[44] in their series of 81 patients, approached the repair through a left lateral thoracotomy in 72 patients and median sternotomy in 5 patients. Surgery consists of resection of the atretic arch, ligation of the PDA or ligamentum arteriosus, and complete and thorough mobilization of the trachea and esophagus. Right side dominance was present in 56 patients (71%), left dominance in 16 (20%), and equal dominance in 7 patients (9%). Inhospital mortality was 3% and 5-year survival was 96%. Long-term outcome is excellent. Similar results were reported by Bonnard et al. and Backer et al.[45,47] in a more heterogeneous group of patients that included other vascular ring abnormalities. Video-assisted thoracoscopic surgery has been reported in this population with good results.[48]

Right Aortic Arch. When the entire right dorsal aorta persists and the distal part of the left dorsal aorta involutes, a right arch results. When there is a right aortic arch, the arrangement of the three branches is reversed.[1] Several types of vascular rings exist in which the aortic arch is right sided and they share the defining feature of all vascular rings, namely, encirclement of the trachea and esophagus by connected segments of the aortic arch and its branches. A right aortic arch may occur without forming a vascular ring. The presence or absence of a vascular ring in the setting of a right aortic arch depends on the branching of the brachiocephalic vessels and the location of the ductus arteriosus.[49]

Two primary forms of vascular ring with a right aortic arch exist. In the most frequent form, an aberrant origin of the left subclavian artery from a retroesophageal diverticulum (diverticulum of Kommerell) is present, which originates as the last branch of the aortic arch. The ring is completed by a left-sided ductus arteriosus (or its remnant ligamentum arteriosum) passing from the aberrant left subclavian artery to the proximal left pulmonary artery. In this type, the brachiocephalic vessels originate from the arch in mirror-image fashion with a left innominate artery as the first branch followed by the right common carotid and subclavian arteries. A left-sided ductus arteriosus or ligamentum arteriosum passes between the descending aorta and the proximal left pulmonary artery.[49]

As with double aortic arch, anomalies associated with right aortic arch include VSD, ASD, PDA, COA, and tetralogy of Fallot. Less frequently associated anomalies are truncus arteriosus, TGA, pulmonary atresia, and HLHS.[1,44,45] Chromosome 22q11 deletions are frequently present in patients with right aortic arch.[41,46]

Clinical manifestations are similar to those for double aortic arch, although patients with a right aortic arch tend to present later than those with a double aortic arch. The most common symptoms are stridor, wheezing, and choking with feeds. Chest radiography sometimes shows narrowing of the trachea. An esophagogram shows an indentation in the esophageal wall. Echocardiography, MRI, or CT are diagnostic. Aortic angiogram is rarely needed.[45,47]

Surgical division of the vascular ring is indicated in any patient with symptoms of airway or esophageal compression and in patients undergoing surgery for repair of associated cardiovascular or thoracic anomalies. The procedure is performed through a left thoracotomy, the ductus arteriosus, or the ligamentum arteriosum is divided, and complete and thorough mobilization of the trachea and esophagus are performed. Results are similar to those for double aortic arch.[45,47,48]

Tracheal compression is caused by a more distal and posterior origin of the innominate artery. Patients present with stridor. Life-threatening symptoms may present as the innominate artery compresses the trachea anteriorly by more than 75% of the original tracheal lumen as it courses from the left of the mediastinum to the right arm.[43] Bronchoscopy is essential at the time of surgery to confirm the diagnosis and results of repair. Suspension of the aorta and innominate artery to the sternum is the treatment of choice, with excellent results and minimal morbidity and mortality.[50]

Pulmonary artery slings are not true rings. The left pulmonary artery originates from the right pulmonary artery and encircles the distal trachea and right mainstem.[43] Approximately 30% to 50% are associated with complete tracheal rings ranging from short segments to the entire length. Patients are usually younger than 2 years and present with stridor, wheezing, or respiratory distress. The procedure of choice to establish the diagnosis is echocardiography while a bronchoscopy is key to the assessment of tracheal stenosis. An esophagogram may show a distinctive anterior pulsatile indentation of the esophagus that is pathognomonic. Correction is accomplished by dividing and reanastomosing the left pulmonary artery anterior to the trachea to the main pulmonary artery, simultaneous resection, or tracheoplasty is also performed. Median sternotomy is the preferred approach.[51]

Sinus of Valsalva Aneurysm

Sinus of valsalva aneurysm (SVA) develops as gradual bulging of a sinus of valsalva into the right atrium or the right ventricle. It is more common in Orientals and the male-to-female ratio is approximately 2 to 4:1. SVA is an uncommon defect responsible for 0.1% to 3.5% of all congenital heart lesions. In the United States and Western countries it is present in less than 0.3% of the congenital lesions. The right coronary sinus is more frequently involved (70%–90%), followed by the noncoronary sinus (10%–30%) and the left coronary sinus (<1%–6%). The aneurysm may rupture into the right ventricle (60%–90%), right atrium (10%–40%), or left atrium (<5%).[52–55]

The most commonly associated cardiac defects is VSD, which is present in more than 40% of patients; other associated anomalies include ASD, pulmonary valvular stenosis, subaortic stenosis, BAV, and COA.[52–55]

The essential lesion in the vast majority of cases is progressive separation of the aortic media of the sinus from the aortic valve cusp. The congenital weakness in this region gradually gives away under aortic pressure to form an aneurysm. A deficiency of normal elastic tissue and abnormal development of the bulbus cordis have been associated with the development of SVA. Acquired SVA are even less common than congenital aneurysms. Acquired aneurysm are caused by conditions that cause degeneration of the media including infections (syphilis, bacterial or fungal endocarditis or tuberculosis), atherosclerosis, cystic medial necrosis, connective tissue disorders, inflammatory diseases (Takayasu's arteritis, Behcet's disease), direct trauma, or surgical complications during the repair of a VSD or removal of a calcified aortic or mitral valve.[52,55,56]

Clinical Manifestations and Diagnosis. Unruptured aneurysms are asymptomatic and produce no signs, but occasionally can cause compression and distortion of surrounding structures. Aneurysm rupture usually occurs in the third or fourth decade of life and is accompanied by chest pain, dyspnea, palpitations, syncope, myocardial ischemia, arrhythmias, a machinery-like murmur, and bounding peripheral pulses with the development of CHF. In more than 50% of cases there is a sudden onset of symptoms with life-threatening hemodynamic deterioration as a consequence of acute aortic regurgitation, coronary steal, or massive left-to-right shunt. In a small subset of patients with small perforations that remain limited or increase in size gradually, patients may remain asymptomatic for a prolonged period until symptoms of CHF develop. Sudden cardiac death may result from tamponade, myocardial ischemia, conduction disturbances, or arrhythmias.[53–55,57] Chest radiography shows cardiomegaly with increased pulmonary blood flow. Sometimes it is possible to visualize the bulging caused by the aneurysm. Echocardiography is diagnostic in most cases. CT has not been widely used to diagnose SVA. MRI has proven very useful in the diagnosis of SVA. MRI and cine MRI may define the anatomy precisely, demonstrate wall thickness, the presence of thrombus, and small perforations better than aortography. Diagnostic cardiac catheterization is rarely necessary although can be useful in evaluating the hemodynamic significance of the rupture, associated cardiac defects, and coronary anatomy.[53,55]

Treatment. Small- to moderate-sized asymptomatic unruptured aneurysms are usually followed. Surgical repair is indicated for symptomatic unruptured aneurysms and aneurysms that cause hemodynamic alterations, including significant aortic regurgitation and ventricular outflow tract obstruction. Other indications include infection, malignant arrhythmias, acute ostial coronary artery obstruction, associated congenital defects, and rupture. In the latter case, surgery should be done as soon as possible to avoid the development of CHF.[52,53,55]

Surgical repair with patch closure is preferred over simple closure. In some cases it is also necessary to perform aortic root and/or aortic valve replacement (AVR) or reconstruction. When other congenital lesions are present, repair is performed during the same procedure. Mortality is usually less than 2% with good long-term results.[52–54] More recently, encouraging results have been described with endovascular techniques including the deployment of occluders (Amplatzer device).[56,58,59] Factors associated with a poor outcome include the presence of simultaneous VSD and aortic regurgitation.[60]

Bicuspid Aortic Valve

The BAV is a common congenital cardiac anomaly with a prevalence that varies from 0.5% to 2% in the general population. It is more common in men with a male-to-female ratio of 2:1. There is a familial predisposition with up to 10% of first-degree relatives having the diagnosis of BAV as well. Inheritance is likely autosomal dominant with variable expressivity and incomplete penetrance. Thus, echocardiographic family screening is recommended for all first-degree relatives of patients with BAV, this would be important not only to search for a dilated aorta but also to prevent endocarditis.[61,62]

More than 50% of patients with BAV have other congenital cardiovascular malformations including PDA, VSD, supravalvular aortic stenosis (Williams's syndrome), left heart obstructing lesions (Shone's syndrome), coronary artery anatomic variants, and abnormalities of the aortic wall such as COA, aortic dissection (AD), and aortic root dilatation. Valvular complications include aortic stenosis, aortic regurgitation, and infective endocarditis. While COA is relatively uncommon, approximately 50% of patients with COA have a BAV. The presence of BAV in patients with COA confers a markedly increased risk of AD. After surgical correction of COA, BAV is the strongest clinical predictor of aortic wall complications in these patients, regardless of the type of repair or the presence of hypertension.[61] AD may complicate BAV in the absence of COA or hypertension. BAV is reported in up to 30% of patients with ascending AD, and the prevalence is significantly higher in younger patients. AD occurs earlier in life in patients with BAV. When AD complicates BAV, the average age of the patient is 54 years compared to 62 for the patient with a tricuspid aortic valve (TAV). AD occurs 5 to 10 times more frequently in patients with a BAV compared with patients with a normal aortic valve.[61]

Aortic dilatation is the most common vascular complication in patients with BAV. Up to 50% to 70% of adults with BAV have echocardiographic evidence of aortic dilatation; therefore, all patients with a diagnosed BAV should be screened for the development of thoracic aorta aneurysm. Aortic dilatation typically involves the aortic root and ascending aorta whereas it is not present in the descending and abdominal aorta. Dilatation can also involve the aortic arch, especially in those patients older than the age of 40 years. Up to 20% of patients with dilated aortic root have a BAV. Aortic dilatation can occur in the absence of valve dysfunction. Aortic size is significantly larger in BAV patients compared to patients with TAV and the same degree of valve dysfunction.[61-63]

Clinical Manifestations and Diagnosis. The great majority of patients with BAV are asymptomatic and physical examination is normal. If symptoms are present, they relate to the development of aortic stenosis or regurgitation or both. The initial diagnosis is usually suspected when a systolic ejection murmur is noted on routine physical examination. Chest radiography may show aortic valve calcification. Other nonspecific findings such as cardiomegaly occur when there is chronic regurgitation. Radiographic features of associated anomalies such as aortic dilatation or rib notching in the case of COA may appear. Transthoracic echocardiography is usually diagnostic. Transesophageal echocardiography (TEE) is useful in those cases in which the transthoracic echocardiogram cannot provide a full assessment of the valve and is better for evaluation of the aortic root and for AD. MRI and CT have a very high sensitivity and specificity with the advantage of providing information about the other associated anomalies and the extent of aortic involvement.[61,62]

Treatment. Patients should be educated about the potential for valve lesion progression, the risk of infective endocarditis, and the possibility of aortic aneurysm and AD. Good dental hygiene and antibiotic prophylaxis are important. Even after AVR, patients with BAV remain at risk for aortic root dilatation and AD. Long-term follow-up, not only of valve function, but also for aortic enlargement is recommended. As mentioned, first-degree relatives should also be monitored. Patients may respond favorably to risk-factor modifications including following a heart-healthy diet, avoidance of cigarette smoking, and treatment of hyperlipidemia. Patients with valvular insufficiency and/or aortic dilatation should avoid strenuous isometric exercise and contact sports. Hypertension must be controlled. Beta-blockers reduce shear stress and may limit matrix remodeling, but whether this prevents aortic dilatation and decreases the risk of AD in patients with BAV has not been proven. As with any other thoracic aneurysm, beta-blockers are recommended when aortic dilatation is already present.[61,62]

The indications for replacement of a BAV with stenosis or regurgitation are well established and are identical to those for replacement of a diseased TAV. However, patients undergoing AVR for BAV are younger than those with TAV, making the decision to implant a mechanical versus bioprosthetic valve more complex.[61]

The indications for resection of an aneurysm involving the ascending aorta in patients with BAV are shown in Table 26-1. For those with a diameter of 3.5 to 4.5 cm in whom aortic replacement is not indicated, reduction aortoplasty has been suggested with or without external synthetic wrapping to prevent further dilatation. This measure is still controversial and not widely accepted.[61,62]

Options for aortic replacement in patients with BAV include replacement of the supracoronary ascending aorta

---

TABLE 26-1. Indications for Resection of Aneurysm Involving the Ascending Aorta in Patients with BAV[61,62]

Aortic diameter greater than 5.0–5.5 cm
Aortic ratio >1.5 or 1.4 in women who wish to become pregnant
Growth rate greater than 3–5 mm/y
Symptomatic aneurysm
Large sinus of valsalva aneurysm associated with BAV
Patients with BAV undergoing valve replacement for valve dysfunction who have an aortic diameter greater than 4–5 cm or a ratio >1.4

BAV = bicuspid aortic valve.

---

with a tube graft, replacement of the aortic root and ascending aorta with reimplantation of the coronary arteries (Bentall procedure), and valve-sparing aortic replacement. The Bentall procedure is the technique of choice according to most authors since it addresses both problems at the same time (the BAV and the aorta), and because it is the best surgical option to avoid future reoperation and aortic complications in the BAV cohort who are usually relatively young and have a long life expectancy at the time of surgery. The Ross procedure (replacement of the aortic valve with pulmonary autograft) should be used cautiously, if at all, in most patients with BAV, because it has been noted that these patients have progressive dilatation of the pulmonary autograft and higher reoperation rates than with other techniques of aortic valve and/or ascending aorta replacement.[61,62]

● MARFAN'S SYNDROME

Marfan's syndrome (MFS) is a systemic disorder of connective tissue caused by mutations in the *FBN1* gene that encodes the extracellular matrix protein fibrillin 1. The condition is inherited in an autosomal dominant manner with complete penetrance but demonstrates variable expression with significant intra- and interfamilial variation. Approximately 25% of cases are sporadic.

Epidemiology

The incidence of classic MFS is approximately 2 to 3 per 10 000 individuals with worldwide occurrence and no sex predilection. Before the era of open-heart surgery, the majority of patients with MFS died prematurely of rupture of the aorta, with an average life expectancy of 45 years. More recently, life expectancy approaches that of unaffected individuals.[64,65]

Clinical Manifestations

MFS is a multisystem disorder with manifestations typically involving the cardiovascular, skeletal, and ocular systems.

The most striking manifestation is the overgrowth of the long bones with a reduced upper to lower body segment ratio (0.85 vs. 0.93 in normal subjects) and arm span exceeding height (ratio >1.05); other skeletal abnormalities include pectus excavatum or pectus carinatum, long fingers (arachnodactyly), mild to moderate joint laxity, scoliosis, flat feet, and some craniofacial alterations. Lens dislocation, severe myopia, flat cornea, hypoplastic iris, and increased axial length of the globe are among the ocular manifestations. Other manifestations of the MFS are restrictive lung disease, spontaneous pneumothorax, skin striae, inguinal hernia and increased risk of surgical and recurrent hernias, and ectasia of the dura that could be manifested as back pain.[64,65]

Cardiovascular manifestations include thickening of the AV valves and often associated with prolapse and regurgitation that can lead to heart failure and death. AV valvular insufficiency is the leading cause of morbidity and mortality in young children. Mitral valve prolapse is the most prevalent valvular abnormality, affecting 35% to 100% of patients. Aortic valve dysfunction presents later in life in 15% to 44% of patients and is secondary to stretching of the aortic annulus by an expanding root aneurysm. In some cases there are supraventricular or ventricular arrhythmias as well as QT interval prolongation. Aortic aneurysm and dissection remain the most life-threatening manifestation of MFS. This finding is age dependent, necessitating life-long monitoring. Dilation of the aorta is found in 50% of children and progresses with time. The dilatation is generally greatest and often restricted to the aortic root (Figure 26-7). The most important determinants of dissection are diameter and a family history of dissection. The severity of the aortic disease is related to the degree of aortic dilatation and to the length of the dilated segment. Patients with acute dissection often present with severe chest pain, frequently radiating along the path of the dissection. This path almost always begins at the aortic root (type A in the Stanford scheme or type I in the DeBakey classification)

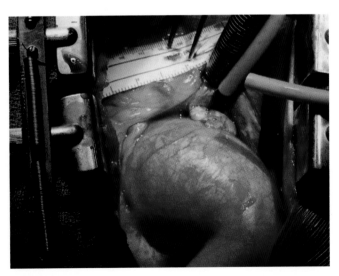

● **FIGURE 26-7.** Aortic root aneurysm in a patient with MFS.

and dissection can remain isolated (type II) or propagate to the descending aorta (type III). Death is usually caused by pericardial tamponade secondary to rupture into the pericardium.[64,65]

Management

Routine monitoring of aortic growth is essential to decrease the risk of AD. Yearly assessment by transthoracic echocardiography allows serial measurements of the proximal aorta. CT and MRI can provide accurate images. More frequent imaging is indicated if the aortic size is approaching the threshold for surgery or if there is rapid growth. Beta-blockers to delay aneurysm progression and dissection are considered the standard of care. The rationale for this treatment is to decrease proximal aortic shear stress. Patients receiving beta-blockers demonstrate slower aortic root growth, fewer cardiovascular complications (aortic regurgitation, dissection, congestive heart failure), and improved survival. Primarily because of the risk of acute AD, patients should be advised against contact sports, competitive athletics, and isometric exercise.[64,65] The management of noncardiovascular manifestations of MFS is beyond the scope of this chapter and the reader may review references.

Surgical repair of the aorta is recommended when the diameter reaches 5 cm in adults. Earlier surgery is recommended when the rate of growth is greater than 1 cm per year or when there is significant aortic regurgitation. The value of elective repair was illustrated in a series of 675 patients from Johns Hopkins in which the 30-day mortality for elective repair, urgent repair (within 7 days after surgical consultation), or emergency repair (within 24 hours of consultation) was 1.5%, 2.6%, and 11.7%, respectively.[66]

Composite surgical replacement of the aortic root and valve was pioneered by Bentall. Modifications of this technique have evolved with various methods of coronary reimplantation. More recent approaches spare the native aortic valve (Figure 26-8). The valve sparing procedure obviates the risk of thromboembolism and warfarin-associated morbidity associated with a mechanical prosthetic valve. In the majority of patients with aortic root aneurysm the pathologic abnormality involves dilatation of the aortic root rather than an abnormality of the valve leaflets.[64,65] In a retrospective analysis of 220 consecutive patients undergoing aortic valve sparing aortic root replacement, including 40% with MFS, David et al.[67] reported low rates of valve related complications with a freedom from moderate or severe aortic insufficiency at 10 years of 85% ± 5% for all patients, and 84% ± 6% for patients with MFS. The freedom from valve replacement at 10 years was 95% ± 3%. The operative mortality was low at 1.3%. The overall survival was just slightly less than that of the general population, and the rates of thromboembolism, bleeding, and endocarditis were lower than what has been reported for mechanical valves. Karck et al.[68] in a series of 119 patients with MFS, compared composite graft (CG) replacement

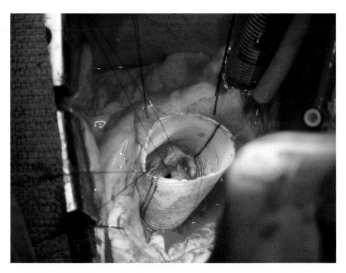

● **FIGURE 26-8.** Aortic valve sparing replacement of aortic root aneurysm.

with mechanical valved conduits ($n = 74$) and valve sparing aortic root replacement ($n = 45$). Early postoperative mortality was 6.8% among patients with CG replacement and 0% in patients with valve-sparing surgery. Freedom from reoperation and death after 5 years was 92% and 89% in patients with CG and 84% and 96% in patients with valve-sparing procedure. Thromboembolic complications or late postoperative bleeding were significantly higher in patients undergoing CG replacement.

In general, stent grafts should not be used in patients with MFS. An exception is in patients with previous aortic replacement operations complicated by a late localized false aneurysm or dissection of more distal aortic segments, the mortality for a second surgery in this population has been reported as high as 33%.[69] Stent grafting in this situation has been reported to be feasible, successful, and a safer alternative than a repeat thoracotomy.[65,70-72]

After repair of the ascending aorta, the arch and the descending aorta are sites at risk for subsequent aneurysm and dissections, prompting the need for routine imaging of the entire aorta. An MRA or a CTA is recommended at 6 to 12 months intervals. Beta-blockers should be continued indefinitely after surgery to reduce the risk of distal aortic complications.[65]

Women with MFS are at increased risk for dissection during pregnancy. The risk for dissection is low if the aortic root diameter is <4.0 cm. Beta-blockers and serial echocardiography should be continued throughout the pregnancy. Cardiovascular complications are more likely if the aorta is >4 cm or if the aortic root diameter increases rapidly, which occurs primarily in the third trimester. If possible, surgical repair of an enlarged aortic root should be done prepartum. The decision about the method of delivery depends on individual circumstances, but a vaginal delivery can be considered if the patient has no aortic dilatation or dissection. The stress of labor should be reduced by means of epidural anesthesia and efforts should be made to shorten the second stage of labor.[65]

● EHLERS-DANLOS

Ehlers-Danlos syndrome (EDS) is a heterogeneous group of hereditable disorders of connective tissue, characterized by skin extensibility, joint hypermobility, and tissue fragility. Prevalence ranges from 1 per 10 000 to 1 per 20 000 births and there is no gender or race predilection. To date, 11 variants of EDS have been identified but more than one-third of persons with EDS do not fit into a single type; overlap is common. The syndrome formerly known as type IV EDS or Sack-Barabas syndrome is now called vascular EDS according to the currently most widely accepted classification, the Villefranche classification.[73] Vascular EDS is the focus of this review. Type III collagen is encoded by a single gene, *COL3A1*, and is an essential structural component of blood vessels, intestine, uterus, and other structural elements. Type III collagen is decreased or absent in patients with vascular EDS and this accounts for the characteristic features of this population. The disease is inherited in an autosomal dominant fashion and accounts for less than 4% of all cases of EDS.[74-76]

Clinical Features of Vascular Ehlers-Danlos Syndrome

Clinical diagnosis of vascular EDS is made on the basis of four major diagnostic criteria: distinctive facial features, thin and translucent skin, easy bruising, and arterial, intestinal, or uterine fragility or rupture. Minor diagnostic criteria include hypermotility of small joints, tendon and muscle rupture, clubfoot, early-onset of varicose veins, arteriovenous or carotid-cavernous sinus fistula, pneumothorax, gingival recession, and family history. The presence of any two or more of the major criteria is highly indicative of the diagnosis.[73] Unlike other types of EDS, vascular EDS is associated with little skin hyperextensibility. The diagnosis is confirmed by the demonstration that cultured fibroblasts synthesize abnormal type III procollagen or by the identification of a mutation in the *COL3A1* gene.

Patients have a shortened lifespan with a median life expectancy of 45 to 50 years. Vascular complications are the leading cause of death in patients with vascular EDS. Sudden death can occur after visceral perforation or after rupture of a large vessel. Arterial rupture is unpredictable and surgical repair is difficult because of tissue fragility. Involvement of arteries in the thorax and abdomen account for 50% of the vascular complications; however, any anatomical location can be involved, with a predilection for medium-sized arteries. Approximately 25% of subjects have complications by the age of 20 years and more than 80% by the age of 40 years.[74-77] Although subjects with vascular EDS have a higher risk for arterial dissection and rupture, subjects with the classic type (types I and II) and those with the hypermobility type (type III) show a propensity for aortic root dilation with a reported incidence of 28%.[78] Pepin et al.[76] reported on 419 subjects with vascular EDS, a total of 131 subjects died, of 103 deaths caused by arterial rupture, 78 involved thoracic or abdominal vessels. Oderich et al.[79]

reported 132 vascular complications in 24/31 patients with vascular EDS, including 6 subjects with aortic arch complications and 10 involving the thoracic aorta; most vascular complications were arterial dissections, or arterial tears resulting in contained hematomas, false aneurysm, or intracavitary bleeding. As discussed in the following chapter, most aneurysms associated with vascular EDS are false aneurysms.

There are currently no specific treatments, and medical interventions are limited to symptomatic treatments, precautionary measures, and genetic counseling. Strenuous exercise and contact sports should be avoided. Medications interfering with platelet or coagulation function are contraindicated.[74,75]

Surgery can pose a life-threatening risk to these patients. Management is challenging because of extreme tissue fragility, risk of massive bleeding, anastomotic disruption, poor healing, and easy dehiscence. Oderich et al. and Freeman et al.[79,80] reported a 23% incidence of complications in patients with vascular EDS who underwent arteriography; therefore, noninvasive diagnostic studies should be preferred unless embolization of bleeding is considered. In the Oderich et al. series,[79] major morbidity occurred after 14 vascular procedures (46%) and late graft-related complications occurred in 40% of the arterial reconstructions. The traditional recommendation when dealing with vascular complications of vascular EDS has been a conservative approach, with operative treatment reserved for patients presenting with imminent life-threatening bleeding. Patients treated conservatively for aneurysm (or pseudoaneurysm) need close follow-up (3–6 months) to assess expansion rate.[74,75,79,80] When surgical management is the best option, special considerations should be kept in mind and extreme caution is mandatory with any maneuver. Precautionary measures include gentle and atraumatic handling of tissues. Even the usual ways of handling arteries can cause more arterial tears. Use of soft, protected arterial clamps or balloon occlusion is preferable to standard arterial clamps. Anastomosis should be tensionless and sheer tension must be avoided using interrupted horizontal mattress sutures reinforced with pledgets. The anastomosis should be covered with a cuff made of Dacron or Teflon to buttress the repair.[77,79–81]

Osteogenesis imperfecta (OI) results from a defect in type I collagen fibers. It is inherited in an autosomal dominant fashion and there are several clinical subtypes described. Vascular complications of OI include aneurysms of nearly any territory including cerebral, aorta, and peripheral. ADs as well as valvular heart disease have been reported in patients with OI. Vascular repair can be complicated by the friability of the tissue including bleeding complications and the theoretical potential for late pseudoaneurysm development. Figure 26-9 is an example of an ascending thoracic aortic aneurysm in a patient with OI. This was discovered in an OI patient who underwent 64 slice coronary CT angiography to investigate chest pain. This imaging modality was specifically used in order to avoid an invasive diagnostic procedure as well as to de-

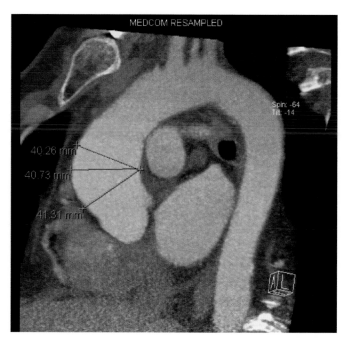

● **FIGURE 26-9.** Ascending aortic aneurysm in a patient with osteogenesis imperfecta.

tect any incidental vascular findings, such as the aneurysm which was found.

● ANEURYSM

An aneurysm is defined as a localized dilatation of an arterial segment greater than 50% above its normal size. In the case of the adult ascending aorta, this means a diameter greater than 3.5 to 4.0 cm. The combination of dilatation of the ascending aorta and aortic annulus is termed annuloaortic ectasia.[82]

The estimated incidence of thoracic aortic aneurysmal disease with an associated elevated risk for dissection (TAAD) is 6 cases per 100 000 person-years. It is more common in male than female subjects (2–4:1) and the mean age at diagnosis is 60 to 70 years. Sixty percent of TAAD involve the aortic root and/or ascending aorta, 40% involve the descending aorta, 10% involve the aortic arch, and 10% involve the thoracoabdominal aorta, with some involving more than one segment.[63]

Etiology and Pathogenesis

Aneurysms of the ascending aorta result from an intrinsic microstructural abnormality of the aortic media. The reader is referred to the following chapter for a detailed discussion of the pathogenesis. Frequent etiologies of ascending aorta aneurysm are those associated with heritable disorders of the aortic media including familial TAAD, BAV, MFS, and Turner's syndrome. Ascending aneurysms are rarely associated with atherosclerosis, and many are idiopathic. Some aneurysms are caused by inflammatory arteritides such as syphilis and giant cell arteritis (GCA).

Familial Thoracic Aortic Aneurysm Syndrome. An inherited pattern for TAAD has been reported in up to 22% of patients who do not have MFS. The predominant inheritance pattern is autosomal dominant with varying degrees of penetrance. Patients with familial TAAD are younger than those with sporadic TAAD (mean age of 58 years vs. 65 years) but older than those with MFS (mean age of 27 years). The growth rate of ascending aneurysms in familial TAAD patients is higher than in sporadic cases suggesting a more virulent pattern of disease. First-order relatives of patients with familial TAAD should be screened for thoracic aneurysms as well.[63,83,84]

Atherosclerosis is an infrequent cause of ascending thoracic aneurysm, and patients with ascending thoracic aneurysm usually have decreased systemic atherosclerotic disease. Conversely, atherosclerosis is the most common cause of descending aorta aneurysm.[63,85]

Turner's syndrome is caused by the absence of one set of genes of the X chromosome—the karyotype representation if 45X. This anomaly is present in 1 of every 2000 live birth females in the United States. Turner's syndrome is associated with a number of cardiovascular anomalies, including COA and BAV. This population is at increased risk for AD and rupture; therefore, it is recommended that all women with Turner's syndrome undergo a complete cardiac evaluation and echocardiographic or MRI examination at least every 5 years and before attempting assisted reproduction in order to detect thoracic aneurysms.[63,86]

Natural History

The most devastating complication of TAAD is dissection, which may lead to arterial occlusion, end-organ ischemia, and rupture. The growth rate for thoracic aneurysm varies from 0.07 to 0.15 cm/y with a mean of approximately 0.10 cm/y. Patients with pulmonary disease, MFS or familial thoracic aortic aneurysm have a higher growth rate. Aneurysm size is the most important determinant for complications including dissection, rupture, and death. The risk of rupture or dissection and death are shown in Table 26-2. At a size greater than 6 cm, the risk of rupture increases 27-fold. The 5-year survival for patients with aneurysm less than 5 cm is 80%, for those with aneurysm 5 to 5.9 cm is 78%, and for those with aneurysm ≥6 cm is 56%. There is variation in individual aneurysm growth rates; therefore, all aneurysms should be followed up with regular surveillance imaging to monitor growth.[63,84,87]

Clinical Manifestation and Diagnosis. Most patients are asymptomatic at the time of the diagnosis since most findings are incidental on imaging studies for other indications, but when symptomatic, the most common complaint is chest pain. Aneurysms of the aortic root may cause secondary aortic regurgitation, which may be manifested as a diastotic murmur or heart failure. When the aneurysm is large, patients may have signs of local mass effect, including compression of the trachea or mainstem bronchus causing cough, dyspnea, wheezing, or recurrent pneumonia. Compression of the esophagus is manifested by dysphagia, compression of the recurrent laryngeal nerve causes hoarseness, and compression of the superior vena cava causes distended neck veins. Erosion into surrounding structures may result in hemoptysis, hematemesis, or gastrointestinal bleeding. Rupture of thoracic aneurysm into the pericardium results in acute tamponade, rupture into the pleura usually results in massive hemothorax with rapid exanguination and death. Clinical manifestations of aneurysm complicated with acute dissection will be discussed in another part of this chapter.[63,88]

Chest radiography may show mediastinal widening, enlargement of the aortic knob, tracheal deviation, and/or loss of the retrosternal space in the lateral view. CT or MRI are very accurate in the diagnosis of thoracic aneurysm with sensitivities and specificities very close to 100%. The location and extent of the aneurysm and the relationship to major branch vessels and surrounding sturtures are readily demonstrated. The size of the aneurysm, the presence of dissection, intimal flaps, mural thrombus, intramural hematoma (IMH), and rupture may also be elucidated. The usefulness of transthoracic echocardiography is limited to the aortic root since visualization of other parts of the ascending aorta is difficult. TEE can potentially evaluate much of the ascending aorta and demonstrate intimal flaps associated with dissection. Cardiac catheterization should be performed in patients with history of coronary artery disease or those older than 40 years of age. Catheterization may also be helpful for the evaluation of the left ventricular function and the degree of aortic valve insufficiency, although this information can be readily obtained by echocardiography.[63,88]

Treatment. All aneurysms must be treated with risk-factor reduction including smoking cessation. Hypertension should be controlled regardless of the aneurysm size. Patients should be placed on beta-blockers to control the blood pressure and reduce the shear stress in the aortic wall. Patients should avoid strenuous isometric exercise since it is associated with the development of AD. Aerobic exercise is generally safe. If the patient is going to engage in vigorous aerobic exercise, it is prudent to obtain an exercise treadmill test on beta-blockers and/or other antihypertensives in order to assess the response to exercise and ensure that the

---

TABLE 26-2. Risk of Rupture, Dissection, or Death in Patients with Ascending Aorta Aneurysm[63,84,87]

Aneurysm Size	Risk of Rupture or Dissection/Y	Risk of Death/y	Combined Risk of Rupture, Dissection or Death/y
<5 cm	2%	4%	5.5%
5–5.9 cm	3%	5%	7%
≥6 cm	6.9%	11.8%	15.6%

TABLE 26-3. Indications for Surgical Repair of Ascending Aorta Aneurysm[62,63,84]

Diameter of ≥5.5 cm
Diameter ≥5 cm in patients with high risk of aortic rupture (Marfan's, Ehlers-Danlos, familial thoracic aortic aneurysm, and bicuspid aortic valve)
Growth rate ≥0.5 cm/y
Symptomatic aneurysm

systolic blood pressure does not rise above 180 mm Hg. Patients with thoracic aneurysm should be screened for the presence of concomitant aneurysms in the descending and abdominal aorta. Once the diagnosis of thoracic aneurysm is made and there is no surgical indication, patients should be followed with serial imaging examination every 6 months initially and then annually if the aneurysm remains stable.[62,63]

Indications for repair of ascending aorta aneurysm are showed in Table 26-3. The mortality of an elective ascending thoracic aneurysm repair is 2.5% to 5%. Complications include stroke in approximately 1% to 8% of the patients and myocardial infarction in approximately 5%.[84,89] Thoracic aortic repair requires CPB. The aneurysm is resected and replaced with a tube of Dacron. When there is compromise of the aortic root with associated aortic regurgitation or stenosis, a Bentall procedure is indicated. This consists in the use of a composite tube graft and a prosthetic valve, and reimplantation of the coronary arteries. An alternative to the Bentall procedure in those patients with dilation of the aortic root and normal aortic valve leaflets is a valve-sparing procedure, a root replacement technique developed by Yacoub, David and others.[67,90,91] The valve-sparing procedure has increased in popularity in recent years because it obviates the long-term complications of a prosthetic aortic valve and lifelong anticoagulation. The technique consists of excising the sinuses of valsalva while sparing the aortic leaflets, sewing a Dacron graft to the aortic annulus, and reimplanting the aortic valve leaflets within the graft to restore their normal anatomic configuration.

In a series with 220 patients who had a valve sparing root replacement, David et al.[67] had a operative mortality of 1.3%, freedom from moderate or severe aortic insufficiency at 10 years of 85%, freedom from AVR at 10 years was 95% and 88% survival at 10 years. 88% of the patients were in functional class I and 10% in class II.

For arch aneurysm repair, the brachiocephalic arteries are reimplantated into the tube graft as an en-bloc patch or can be anastomosed individually to branched prosthetic arch grafts. The latter allows for a selective antegrade cerebral perfusion, which may reduce the chances for neurologic dysfunction.[63,92]

Serial evaluations (CT or MRI) should be performed every 3 to 6 months during the first postoperative year and every 6 months thereafter.

● AORTIC DISSECTION

Aortic dissection is defined as a separation of the layers of the aortic wall resulting from a partial thickness tear, which allows pulsatile blood to create a false passage. The true lumen is usually smaller and is lined by intima; the false lumen is lined by the media. Typically, flow in the false lumen is slower than in the true lumen, and the false lumen often dilates and becomes aneurysmal. AD has a prevalence of 0.5 to 3.5/100 000/y with a mortality rate of 3.2 to 3.6/100 000/y. The most common cause of death in this population is aortic rupture. AD is more common in men (men-to-women ratio 1.5–3:1) and usually presents in the seventh decade of life.[93–97] Up to 65% to 85% of the intimal tears occur in the ascending aorta (type A) and 15% to 20% in the descending aorta (type B).[93,96,97]

Mechanisms that weaken the aortic wall and lead to higher wall stress can induce aortic dilatation and aneurysm formation, eventually resulting in AD or rupture.

Multiple conditions are associated with an increased risk of AD, and include inherited diseases such as MFS, Ehler-Danlos syndrome, familial thoracic aortic aneurysm, BAV, COA, atherosclerosis, syphilis and other infections, Turner's syndrome, arteritis, cocaine use, previous cardiac and/or ascending aortic surgery, and trauma. Iatrogenic causes include catheter-based interventional procedures, CPB, aortic cross-clamping, and intra-aortic balloon pumping. Tobacco use, hypertension, and hypercholesterolemia all contribute to wall stiffness and to an increased vulnerability to shear stress with subsequent aneurysm formation and dissection. Overall, more than 70% of patients presenting with acute dissection have associated hypertension.[93,94,98,99]

Aortic Dissection Classification

The classification of AD is based upon the site of the intimal tear and the extent of the dissection. There are two commonly used classifications for AD. The Stanford classification and the DeBakey classification (Figure 26-10). In the Stanford classification, dissection is divided into types A and B. Type A dissection involves the ascending aorta and the entry site may be located anywhere along the aorta. Type B dissection is confined to the descending aorta. In the DeBakey classification there are four categories. In types I and II the intimal tear is located in the ascending aorta. In DeBakey type I dissection, the hematoma extends for a variable distance beyond the ascending aorta, in type II, the dissection is limited to the ascending aorta. In type III the dissection originates in the descending aorta. In type IIIA the dissection is limited to the descending aorta and in type IIIB extends to the abdominal aorta.

Clinical Manifestation and Diagnosis

AD is classified as acute or chronic based upon the duration of symptoms at presentation. Dissections are considered acute when symptoms are present for less than 2 weeks. Rapid diagnosis of AD is important since it is associated

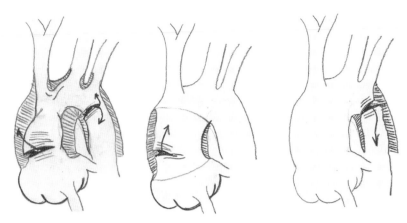

● **FIGURE 26-10.** Aortic dissection classification.

DeBakey type I   DeBakey type II   DeBakey type III

Stanford type A   Stanford type B

with a high early mortality rate. The mortality for acute AD is 1% to 2% per hour for the first 24 to 48 hours. The most common causes of death are aortic rupture, stroke, visceral ischemia, and cardiac tamponade. Chronic presentation is unusual since up to 85% of the patients who do not have surgery for an acute ascending dissection will die in the first 2 weeks.[93–95,98,100]

AD should be considered in the differential diagnosis of patients presenting with myocardial ischemia, syncope, chest pain, back pain, stroke, and acute heart failure. Symptoms and presentation vary according to the anatomic disruption caused by the dissection. The typical patient with acute AD is a male in his sixties with a history of hypertension who suffers an abrupt onset of chest pain. The pain is described as sharp, the location could change as the dissection extends. In type A (type I and II) dissections, the pain is usually located retrosternally, whereas in type B (type III) dissections it is interscapular in the back. Up to 20% of patients may present with syncope or stroke. Syncope could indicate the presence of pericardial tamponade, obstruction of cerebral vessels, or activation of baroreceptors. When there is aortic regurgitation, the patient may present with symptoms of heart failure. Other symptoms may arise as branches of the aorta are compromised by the dissection, including myocardial ischemia caused by coronary occlusion, paraplegia caused by the compromise of the intercostal arteries, acute renal failure because of the involvement of the renal arteries, and mesenteric ischemia. Physical findings may include loss of pulses, neurologic deficits, signs associated with the mass effect of the aorta as described previously in the aortic aneurysm section. A diastolic murmur of aortic regurgitation is present in 50% of the patients with proximal AD. Shock may be a presenting sign, resulting from tamponade, coronary compression, acute aortic valve incompetence, or loss of blood and exsanguination.[93–95,98]

Laboratory testing plays a minor role in the assesment of acute AD, but is useful to exclude other diseases. An assay of circulating smooth-muscle myosin heavy-chain protein, a protein specific to smooth muscle that is released from damaged aortic medial smooth muscle has been shown to have a sensitivity of 90% and specificity of 97% to diagnose acute dissection when measured in the initial 3 hours after the onset of the symptoms. Limitations include the availability of the test and the fact that it is only effective in the first 24 hours after the onset of the symptoms. ECG helps to differentiate from myocardial ischemia; although in cases of dissection with involvement of the coronary ostia, patients will have both conditions. Twenty percent of patients with ascending AD will have evidence of acute ischemia.[94,98,100]

The goals of the imaging studies are to confirm the diagnosis, classify the dissection, delineate the extent of the dissection, differentiate the true and false lumen, distinguish between communicating and noncommunicating dissection, localize internal flaps, assess branch involvement, detect aortic regurgitation, and detect extravasation. The classic radiologic sign characteristic of AD is a wide mediastinum. Other radiographic signs include a double shadow of the aortic wall or a disparity in the size of the ascending and descending aorta. A chest radiograph is abnormal in 60% to 90% of cases of AD but a normal test is not sufficient to rule out AD. The overall sensitivity is 64% and the specificity is 86% but is lower (sensitivity 47%) for involvement of the proximal aorta. Transthoracic echocardiography is usually limited by its inability to evaluate the ascending aorta and the aortic arch. The overall sensitivity is 70% to 80% with a specificity of 93% to 96%. TEE is the preferred ultrasound modality. TEE is usually diagnostic with a sensitivity of 90% to 98% and specificity of 89% to 95%. Disadvantages include its invasive nature, the anatomic blind spot in the distal ascending aorta and aortic arch associated with the air-filled trachea and left main stem bronchus, and it is operator dependant. CT is fast, accurate, and noninvasive; it has an average sensitivity better than 95% and specificity of 90% to 100%. Limitations are related to the diagnosis of aortic regurgitation, and occasionally to tear localization and detection of subtle dissections. MRI has a sensitivity and specificity close to 100%. It allows visualization of the vascular compartment, the vessel wall, and its surrounding tissue and provides functional information of the imaged vasculature, and may be useful for the evaluation of aortic insufficiency. Limitations are related to the time of acquisition of the images and the availability in the ER setting. The specificity of aortography is better than 95% but its sensitivity may be lower than other techniques, as low as 88%. Limitations include its inability to identify the false lumen when it is totally thrombosed or when it has slow flow, inability to evaluate wall thickness or the presence of IMHs, its invasive nature, and potential for trauma caused by wires and catheters. The role of aortography today is as a component of endovascular therapy and not so much as a diagnostic tool. Intravascular ultrasound (IVUS) has close to 100% sensitivity and specificity. It is especially useful when the aortography is not diagnostic. Limitations include the evaluation of aortic regurgitation, pericardial effusion, and its invasive nature. A high level of clinical suspicion followed by prompt imaging is the most important diagnostic tool. A patient with a high probability of disease should undergo a second investigation if the findings of the first are negative.[94,98,101]

Treatment. Initial management of an acute AD includes pain control and control of the associated hypertension. The goal of the initial medical treatment is to decrease the blood pressure and the shearing force of myocardial contractility in order to decrease the propagation of the dissection. The systolic blood pressure should be kept between 100 and 120 mm Hg. Beta-blockers are the drug of choice for blood pressure control. Beta-blockers reduce the force of left ventricular ejection and shear stress on the aortic wall. If beta-blockers are not enough to control the blood pressure, vasodilators are the second-line of treatment, but they should always be used in combination with the beta-blockers.[94,98]

Acute type A (type I and II) dissection is a surgical emergency. The aim of surgical intervention in type A aortic dissection is the prevention of aortic rupture or the development of pericardial tamponade. It is also important to correct aortic regurgitation and limitations to coronary blood flow. The principles of the surgical repair are excision of the intimal tear, obliteration of the entry into the false lumen, and reconstruction of the aorta. If the aortic root diameter is normal without aortic valve insufficiency, a tubular graft is an adequate option for repair (supracomissural replacement). If the aortic valve is involved, a valve-sparing procedure may be attempted but if this is not possible, a composite tube graft is the indicated repair (Bentall procedure). The distal connection of the tube graft is made to the uninvolved ascending aorta in type A (type II) dissection. In all other patients, replacement is carried to the junction of the ascending aorta and arch or beyond that level. For almost all dissections, an open distal anastomosis of the graft and the conjoined aortic wall layers in the arch portions is made using a period of circulatory arrest. Rarely a very limited dissection in the ascending aorta may be repaired with a cross-clamp on the distal ascending aorta. If an entry tear is located in the arch, the distal graft to aortic anastomosis is usually made in such a manner to replace the arch beyond the entry-bearing portion. In some cases total replacement of the aortic arch may be indicated. In the case of an arch aneurysm extending into the descending aorta, an "elephant trunk" extension of the arch graft is left extending into the descending aneurysm for possible later anastomosis to a descending aortic graft. The hospital mortality for acute type A (type I and II) dissection after surgical repair is 15% to 30%, well below the 50% to 85% mortality with only medical treatment. For repair of chronic dissection the mortality is 10% to 20%. This improved mortality is explained by the fact that the repair is performed on a more elective basis, and the aortic tissues are usually more mature, stronger, and more manageable. Neurologic complications occur in 6% to 15% of patients with ascending or arch involvement. The 5-year survival after surgical repair varies from 80% to 95%, and 10-year survival from 30% to 60%.[93–95,97,99,100,102,103] The risk of death is increased in patients who present with or develop pericardial tamponade, involvement of the coronary arteries, or malperfusion of the brain. Other factors associated with a high inhospital mortality are age older than 70 years, hypotension, renal failure, and pulse deficits. Iatrogenic AD carries a mortality that is slightly higher than noniatrogenic dissections.[100]

Kallenbach et al.[102] compared three procedures (supracommissural repair, Bentall, and valve-sparing technique) in 295 patients with type A dissection. The perioperative mortality and incidence of neurologic complications was similar between groups. The 5-year survival was similar as well, 80%, 85%, and 89%, respectively. Patients with supracommissural repair had a higher rate of reoperation for aortic valve problems and dilatation of the aortic root. The use of endovascular techniques is limited to type B dissection where good results with low morbidity and mortality has been reported. Disease of the aortic arch is sometimes amendable to endovascular repair as well. The experience with endovascular techniques in type I and II dissection is limited to a few reports; therefore, its use is not yet well supported, although this is a field in constant development.[100,101,104,105]

Nearly one-third of patients surviving the initial treatment for an acute dissection will experience dissection extension or aortic rupture or will require surgery for aortic aneurysm formation within 5 years. The risk is substantial in the first few months after initial therapy.[105] The majority of late deaths following primary repair are caused by rupture of the aorta. The two main indications for reoperation are aneurysm formation remote from the initial repair and dissections that were improperly repaired. The rate of reoperation for type I and type II dissection is approximately 10% at 5 years and up to 40% at 10 years.[94,102]

MRI and CT are the techniques of choice for follow-up. The goals of follow-up are to detect signs of aortic expansion, aneurysm formation, signs of leakage at anastomoses or stent graft sites and malperfusion. Regular assessment of the aorta should be performed 1, 3, 6, and 12 months after the acute event, followed by evaluations every 6 to 12 months thereafter. The single most important medical issue in these patients is to maintain a blood pressure less than 120/80 mm Hg. All dissection patients should receive lifelong treatment with beta-blockers.[94,98,100]

INTRAMURAL HEMATOMA AND PENETRATING ULCER

Aortic IMH is one form of a collection of aortic pathology termed acute aortic syndromes, also included are AD and aortic penetrating ulcer. IMH is considered a precursor of dissection. Two different pathophysiologic processes have been suggested for IMH. In the case of IMH without intimal disruption, the hematoma may originate from the spontaneous rupture of a vasa vasorum in the media resulting in an aortic wall infarct and hematoma formation. A second explanation for the development of IMH is that it may be caused by small intimal tears that are not visualized with conventional imaging studies. Another type of IMH is associated with an atherosclerotic ulcer that penetrates into the internal elastic lamina and allows hematoma formation within the media. The causes for IMH are similar to those for AD.[100,106,107]

Patients with IMH tend to be older than those with AD. They are usually in their late sixties compared to the late fifties and early sixties in the case of the classic AD. The gender distribution is the same as in aortic dissection, with 60% to 70% being men.[108–110] The prevalence of IMH in patients with suspected AD varies between 5% and 30%. In the natural progression of the disease, progression occurs in 60% to 70% of the patients, acute AD develops in 28% to 47% of the patients, aortic rupture in 21% to 47% and regression is observed only in 10% to 30% of patients.[94,98,111]

Most IMH, 50% to 80%, are located in the descending aorta. There are two types of IMH. Type I shows a smooth inner aortic lumen, the diameter is usually less than 3.5 cm, and the wall thickness greater than 0.5 cm; echo-free spaces are found in less than one-third of the patients. Type II IMH occurs with aortic atherosclerosis. A rough inner aortic surface with severe aortic sclerosis is characteristic. The aorta is usually larger than 3.5 cm and calcium deposits are usually found. The mean wall thickness is 1.3 cm with a range of 0.5 to 4 cm. Echo-free spaces are found in 70% of the subjects.[94,108]

Clinical manifestations are similar to those of acute AD. Abrupt onset of chest or back pain is the most common symptom. IMH tends to be a more segmental process. Aortic insufficiency, and vascular complications, such as myocardial ischemia, stroke, visceral ischemia, and pulse deficits are less common than in acute AD.[100,108,109]

For diagnosis, CT, MRI and TEE have an accuracy greater than 90%, and a sensitivity close to 100%. The normal aortic wall thickness is less than 3 mm by any imaging modality; therefore, aortic wall thickness greater than 5 mm is sufficient for diagnosis of IMH in patients with symptoms suggesting an acute aortic syndrome. A hematoma thickness ≥11 mm and an aortic diameter ≥48 mm are associated with a worse outcome.[106,110,112]

Initial management of IMH includes pain control and control of the associated hypertension. Involvement of the ascending aorta is sometimes considered an indication for urgent surgery because of the inherent risk of rupture, tamponade, or compression of the coronary ostia. Surgery may be indicated in type A IMH and initial medical therapy in patients with type B IMH. The hospital mortality for type A IMH with surgical treatment is 8% to 14% and with medical therapy it is 36% to 55% in the first 30 days. Hospital mortality is associated with the proximity of the IMH to the aortic valve. The closer the hematoma to the aortic valve, the higher the mortality.[100,108,110,111]

As with those patients with AD, regular assessment of the aorta should be performed 1, 3, 6, and 12 months after the acute event, followed by evaluations every 6 to 12 months thereafter. The use of beta-blockers have shown to improve long-term outcome.[108,111]

Penetrating Ulcer

In a penetrating aortic ulcer, an atheromatous plaque ulcerates and disrupts the internal elastic lamina, burrowing deeply through the intima into the media. When an atherosclerotic ulcer penetrates into the media, the media is exposed to pulsatile arterial flow, which causes hemorrhage into the wall that may lead to IMH. Ulceration of atherosclerotic aortic plaques that can lead to AD or perforation often complicates IMH and appears as an ulcer-like projection into the hematoma. The presence of an ulcer in an IMH is associated with a higher rate of progressive disease in patients with IMH. Aortic ulcers are present most often in the descending and abdominal aorta. Symptomatic ulcers with signs of deep erosion are more prone to rupture than others.[94,100,107,113,114] Those in the descending and more distal aorta may be readily treated by endovascular techniques.

TUMORS OF THE AORTA

Primary tumors of the aorta are extremely rare. In a review article by Seelig et al.,[115] they found 86 cases reported in the literature since the first description in 1873. The vast majority of the cases were diagnosed at the time of autopsy or at histologic examination of thromboembolic material that suggested the presence of an upstream intra-aortic tumor. In this review, there were 59 male patients (67.8%) and the mean age at diagnosis was 60 years with a range of 3 months to 82 years. Tumor was diagnosed at the following locations: abdominal aorta 39 (44.8%), thoracic aorta 39 (44.8%), and thoracoabdominal aorta 9 (10.4%). The vast majority of these tumors have been of mesenchymal origin. The prognosis of primary malignant aortic tumors is poor. Of the 86 cases described, 72% had metastases. Metastases were located in bone (28.8%), kidneys (27.1%), liver (23.7%), adrenals (20.3%), and lungs (15.3%). The mean survival rate of patients in whom the diagnosis could be established was 14 months.

In another review by Chiche et al.,[116] 132 patients were analyzed. In this report, similar to that of Seeling et al., 63.7% were male and the mean age at the time of diagnosis was again 60 years. The locations of primary tumors were in the descending thoracic aorta (34.9%), abdominal aorta (27.3%), thoracoabdominal aorta (26.5%), and ascending aorta and aortic arch (11.3%). Pain was the presenting symptom in 25.9% of the cases. More specific presentations involved occlusive manifestations that varied depending on the location of the tumor and the acute or chronic nature of the obstruction. Occlusive symptoms result from acute embolic ischemia (20%), intermittent claudication of the lower extremities (15.5%), severe renovascular hypertension (19.2%), intestinal infarction (11.1%), and abdominal angina (2.9%). Rare complications included stroke, ischemia of the upper extremities, rupture, fistula to the bronchus, fistula to the vena cava, fistula to the esophagus, secondary gastrointestinal bleeding caused by metastasis, or ischemic ulceration of the intestinal wall. Some patients may present with findings similar to those reported in patients with vasculitis—general fatigue, weight loss, and increased sedimentation rate. Patients with signs of arteritis not responding to steroid therapy should undergo further examination for vascular malignancy.[117]

Of the 132 cases analyzed by Chice et al.,[116] angiosarcoma was diagnosed in 34 cases (25.8%), intimal sarcoma in 27 (20.5%), malignant fibrous histiocytoma in 20 (15.2%), leiomyosarcoma in 19 (14.3%), and undifferentiated sarcoma in 12 (9%). The remaining cases included miscellaneous tumors such as fibromyxosarcoma, fibrosarcoma, hemangiopericytoma, chondrosarcoma, and myoma. Tumors were located in the intimal layer in 62.9% of the cases, intramural in 18.2%, in all three layers in 10.6%, and unmentioned in 8.3%. The tumors usually progress through the aortic lumen or wall to the supra-aortic trunks or visceral arteries. Metastases were documented in 82.2% of the cases with a distribution similar to that reported by Seelig et al. Isolated metastases were present in 50% of the cases, isolated tumor emboli in 26.6%, and combined metastases and tumor emboli in 23.6%. Mean survival was 16 months with a median of 7 months. Cumulative overall survival rates at 3 and 5 years were 11.2% and 8%, respectively. In surgically treated patients, the survival at 3 and 5 years were 16.5% and 11.8%, respectively.

Salm[118] described three morphologic types of primary aortic tumors. The first two, intraluminal and intimal tumors, are usually polypoid and extend intraluminally. The third group includes tumors arising in the media and adventitia and exhibiting mainly mural growth. Wright et al.[119] proposed a classification that combined the intraluminal and intimal tumors in one group (and differentiates them as obstructing or nonobstructing) and mural tumors in the second group.

Retrograde arteriography should be avoided because of the potential of embolization. In most cases arteriography shows a nonspecific pattern mimicking simple mural thrombus or aneurysm.[115,116] MRI is considered the most reliable imaging study for diagnosis and is more precise at differentiating normal aortic wall from tumor, and tumor from thrombus. MRI also provides excellent contrast between the aortic lumen and surrounding structures. Transesophageal ultrasound may be useful in patients with tumor involving the ascending aorta, aortic arch, and descending thoracic aorta. Ultrasound can delineate the extent of the intra-aortic mass and mobile intra-aortic components.[115,116]

In the majority of cases, surgery has been performed before the lesion was identified as a tumor, and subsequent procedures were therefore required. Chiche et al.[116] suggest resection with prosthetic replacement as the best option not only because it can be curative if there are no undetectable metastases but also because it reduces the risk of recurrence if there are metastases. If the patient is not a surgical candidate, and a large intra-aortic mass is identified, therapeutic anticoagulation should be recommended.[115]

The operative mortality rate is high (17%). The most frequent causes of early postoperative death were embolism resulting in mesenteric or renal infarction, strokes and aortic occlusion. Surgical treatment seems more likely to be effective than radiation therapy and/or chemotherapy. Factors associated with worse survival are intimal lesions, tumors involving the ascending aorta, aortic arch, or upper thoracoabdominal aorta.[116]

● VASCULITIS

Vasculitis is defined by the presence of leukocytes in the vessel wall with reactive damage to mural structures. Loss of integrity leads to bleeding and compromise of the lumen leading to tissue ischemia and necrosis. Vasculitis may occur as a primary process or may be secondary to other underlying diseases. Inflammation of the aorta and its major branches occurs in a number of disorders, including more commonly GCA, Takayasu's arteritis, and isolated ascending aortitis. Other diseases that cause aortitis, although rarely, include syphilis, tuberculosis, rheumatoid arthritis, spondyloarthropathies, Behcet's disease, Kawasaki disease, COA, lupus, ergotism, and neurofibromatosis.[120–122]

Isolated Ascending Aortitis

In their retrospective study of 45 patients with noninfectious ascending aortitis, Miller et al.[122] found that 21 cases (47%) were classified as isolated aortitis, 14 (31%) as GCA, 6 (14%) as Takayasu's arteritis, 2 (4%) as rheumatoid, and 2 (4%) were unclassified. Patients with isolated aortitis were older than 50 years and 76% were female. The most common symptoms were back or chest pain, fever, and fatigue. Ascending aortic aneurysm was present in 95% of cases (19/21). Pathologic analysis showed that medial necrosis may represent the primary abnormality and that the inflammatory response may be secondary. No evidence of systemic disease or extra-aortic vasculitis was present in any of these patients. These authors state that the two features that are most helpful for distinguishing isolated aortitis from the other form of ascending aortitis are clinical rather than microscopic. They include the absence of systemic disease and the favorable outcome in the absence of anti-inflammatory treatment. In this series, only 2/21 patients received steroids, 14 patients were alive without disease at the time of follow-up, one had recurrent disease, and 4 died of causes unrelated to aortic disease. Similar findings have been described by Rojo-Leyva and Kerr.[123,124]

Takayasu's Arteritis

Takayasu's arteritis, also known as pulseless disease, occlusive thromboaortopathy, or Martorell syndrome, is an idiopathic, inflammatory, nonautoimmune, granulomatous vasculopathy that affects all the layers of large vessels, mainly the aorta and its main branches. Vessel inflammation leads to wall thickening, fibrosis, stenosis or occlusive lesions, and to a hypercoagulable state that predisposes to thrombus formation. If disease progression is rapid, fibrosis can be inadequate leading to aneurysm formation. Takayasu's arteritis is more common in Asian countries, India, and Mexico. The incidence in the United States is approximately 2.6 cases per million per year. Takayasu's arteritis is more common in females than in males with a ratio of 8 to 9:1.[120,125,126]

Clinical Manifestation and Diagnosis. A two stage process has been suggested with a prepulseless phase characterized by nonspecific inflammatory features, followed by a chronic phase with the development of vascular insufficiency, in some cases with intermittent flares. The disease usually presents in the second or third decade of life. Nonspecific symptoms include low-grade fever, night sweats, malaise, weight loss, arthralgia, myalgia, and mild anemia. The most typical symptoms are the result of ischemia in organs supplied by stenotic vessels. Characteristic features include decreased or absent pulses associated with limb claudication, asymmetric pulses, vascular bruits, blood pressure discrepancy between limbs, and hypertension. Subclavian artery involvement is common and a stenotic lesion proximal to the origin of the vertebral artery can lead to subclavian steal syndrome. Angina can result from compromise of the coronary arteries, and mesenteric angina from visceral arterial compromise. Other symptoms and findings include headaches, carotidynia, jaw claudication, chest wall pain, Takayasu's retinopathy, aortic regurgitation secondary to dilatation of the ascending aorta, CHF, neurologic features secondary to hypertension or ischemia as postural dizziness, seizures, TIA, stroke, amaurosis, dermatologic manifestations such as erythema nodosum, ulcerated nodular lesions, and erythema multiforme. The pulmonary arteries may be involved in up to 50% of the patients; however, symptoms related to pulmonary arteritis are uncommon and include chest pain, dyspnea, and hemoptysis. Pulmonary hypertension may occur.[120,125,126] Diagnostic criteria for Takayasu's arteritis are shown in Table 26-4. The four most important complications are Takayasu retinopathy, secondary hypertension, aortic regurgitation, and aneurysm formation. Takayasu's arteritis is associated with significant morbidity and mortality. Twenty percent of patients have a self-limited, monophasic inflammatory episode. The remaining subjects have a progressive or relapsing course. The overall 15-year survival rate is 90% to 95%.[120,125,126]

Laboratory findings reflect the inflammatory process but are mostly nonspecific. Anemia of chronic disease is common. Acute phase reactants such as elevated erythrocyte sedimentation rate (ESR), elevated CRP, and hypoalbu-

TABLE 26-4. Criteria for the Diagnosis of Takayasu's Arteritis*

Age at disease onset $\leq$40 y
Claudication of extremities
Decreased brachial artery pulse
Difference of >10 mm Hg in systolic blood pressure between arms
Bruit over subclavian arteries or aorta
Arteriographic narrowing or occlusion of the aorta, its primary branches or large arteries in the proximal upper or lower extremities.

Diagnosis requires at least three of the six criteria.
Data from Johnston SL, Lock RJ, Gompels MM. Journal of clinical pathology; Takayasu arteritis: a review [review]. Br Med Assoc. 2002; 55:481(6). http://find.galegroup.com.proxy.lib.utk.edu:90/itx/infomark. do?&contentSet = IAC-Documents&type = retrieve&tabID = T002& prodId=ITOF&docId = A89923777&source = gale&srcprod = ITOF &userGroupName = tel_a_utl&version = 1.0. Accessed November 20, 2006.

minemia are frequent. Tissue biopsy has almost no role in the diagnosis of Takayasu's arteritis since histologic examination of the great vessels is usually possible only at the time of surgery or postmortem. Arteriography remains the gold standard for diagnosis. MRI/MRA is steadily replacing angiography as the gold standard, having the advantages of a noninvasive procedure. In addition to the evaluation of luminal stenosis, MRI provides information about vessel wall thickness, edema, and contrast enhancement. These findings may indicate early vascular inflammation and are useful to monitor patients and to differentiate between active and inactive disease. Disadvantages of the MRA are the poor image quality of distal vessels and the inability to evaluate for calcified plaques, making discrimination between vasculitic and atherosclerotic disease difficult. High-resolution ultrasound is very useful in carotid disease but the aorta cannot currently be imaged with it. Similar to MRI/MRA, CTA also has a high sensitivity and specificity but requires contrast administration and is also poor for the evaluation of distal vessels. PET scanning has been shown to be useful in monitoring disease activity and response to treatment but is limited by the lack of information on arterial wall morphology or luminal blood flow.[126,127]

Treatment. The goals of treatment are to arrest the progression of existing lesions and prevention of new lesions. Steroids constitute the first line of treatment. Steroids decrease inflammatory symptoms and the ESR and improve pulses in approximately 60% of the patients. However, symptom relapse occurs in 50% when the steroids are weaned. Other medications that have been used with some success include cyclophosphamide, azathioprine, methotrexate, and mycophenolate mofetil. These agents are used in cases of steroid resistance or in combination with steroids to reduce side effects.[120,125] A new strategy that has been used with some success but has no long-term follow-up is antitumor necrosis factor agents (etanercept and infliximab).[128–130]

The diagnosis of Takayasu's arteritis is usually made when stenotic or occlusive lesions have already occurred. These lesions are usually not reversible with medical treatment and may require surgical repair. Indications for surgery include hypertension with critical renal artery stenosis, claudication limiting activities of daily living, cerebrovascular ischemia or critical stenosis of three or more cerebral vessels, moderate aortic regurgitation, and cardiac ischemia with confirmed coronary artery disease. Stenosis of the aortic arch is a surgical indication in order to prevent strokes. Thoracic aneurysm should also be repaired in an early stage, usually when larger than 5 cm. Surgery is preferred when the disease is quiescent in order to avoid complications, which include restenosis, anastomotic failure, thrombosis, bleeding, and infection. Overall, good results are achieved with bypass grafts; the restenosis rate is 20% to 30%, with a survival at 20 years of approximately 75%. Patch angioplasty, endarterectomy, and endovascular procedures have a greater risk of restenosis and occlusion although angioplasty could be useful in short-segment stenosis. A 13% rate of anastomotic aneurysm at 20-year follow-up has been reported. Based on this, CT, MRI, or ultrasound are recommended to screen for this complication.[120,125,126,131,132] Matsuura et al.[133] reported long-term outcomes in 90 patients with AVR for aortic regurgitation secondary to Takayasu's arteritis. Sixty-three patients had AVR and 27 CG. The hospital mortality was 5.6%. Five-year survival was 88% and 15-year survival was 76%. Detachment of the prosthetic valve occurred in 11.1% of patients with AVR and in 3.7% of patients with CG. Late dilatation of the residual ascending aorta occurred in 11.1% of those with AVR and in 3.7% of those with CG. The same group reported a series of 21 patients with Takayasu's arteritis and aortic arch replacement, 14 patients had associated aortic regurgitation and 12 had main branches lesions.[134] Total arch replacement was performed in 14 patients and hemi arch replacement in 7. Hospital mortality was 4.8% (1/21), 5-year survival was 85% and 82.7% at 10 years. Five patients required aortic replacement for dilatation of the remaining aorta and 2 patients required AVR for recurrent aortic regurgitation after a valve-sparing aortic root replacement.

Giant Cell Arteritis

GCA, also known as temporal arteritis or cranial arteritis is a systemic, chronic, idiopathic vascular disease. It is the most common vasculitis of large- and medium-sized vessels. The disease involves the arteries originating from the aortic arch and most characteristically the temporal arteries. The female-to-male ratios is 3:2 and it affects almost exclusively subjects older than 50 years.[122,135,136]

In a population-based cohort study,[137] some large vessel complication (aneurysm or dissection) was found in 27% of the cohort (46/168), of these, 11% (18/168) were present in the thoracic aorta; although the exact location in the thoracic aorta was not reported, 17/18 patients had some degree of aortic insufficiency. Stenosis of aortic arch branches was present in 13% of patients (21/168) but no patient had stenosis of the thoracic aorta. Margos et al.[138] in a comparative study between patients with GCA and healthy volunteers, found that compared with healthy subjects, aortic distensibility and aortic strain are decreased in patients with GCA; patients with GCA also have an increased incidence of aortic regurgitation and increased aortic root and ascending aortic diameter. These changes may be caused by the granulomatous inflammatory process in the inner portion of the media, and the resulting fragmentation of elastic fibers in the aortic wall.

Clinical Manifestations and Diagnosis. Typical symptoms of GCA include headache, scalp tenderness, abnormal temporal arteries, jaw claudication, polymyalgia rheumatica, visual alterations including blindness, and nonspecific constitutional symptoms as weight loss, anorexia, malaise, fatigue, and fever. Patients with large artery complications including stenosis and aneurysm often have few of the typical symptoms of GCA, and as a result early disease may be unrecognized. Patients with large-vessel arteritis may present with claudication, and occasionally with subclavian steal syndrome. On clinical examination, as in those with other large-vessel arteritides, patients may have vascular bruits, asymmetry in blood pressure and pulses and signs of tissue hypoperfusion. The aortitis usually becomes evident when signs of acute AD appear. These include chest pain, dyspnea, pulselessness, and hypotension caused by rupture or aortic valve regurgitation. Patients can also present with signs of CHF caused by aortic valve regurgitation secondary to annuloaortic ectasia. Factors associated with aortic aneurysm or dissection include an aortic insufficiency murmur, hyperlipidemia, coronary artery disease, and elevated ESR with symptoms of polymyalgia. Renal involvement is not common.[135–137,139]

Acute phase reactants, and more frequently ESR and CRP, are usually elevated. Chronic disease anemia is present in more than 50% of patients. Temporal artery biopsy should be obtained, although it is not always diagnostic in those patients with large-vessel arteritis. MRI/MRA or CTA are required for diagnosis of large-vessel GCA, and are also useful to evaluate the extent and degree of activity of the disease. PET scanning is not useful in the evaluation of medium-size vessels but has value in the case of large-vessel involvement.[135,140]

Treatment. GCA is usually a self-limited disease with an average duration of 2 years. Steroids are the mainstay of treatment and most of the patients have good response. Surgery is rarely required. Contrary to Takayasu's arteritis, no other medications have proven to be useful. Low-dose aspirin reduces the risk of cranial ischemic complications. If symptoms of large-vessel stenosis persist despite adequate anti-inflammatory therapy, balloon angioplasty is a good option. Surgical intervention is indicated in ascending aorta aneurysm greater than 5 cm or if the aneurysm is symptomatic. In those cases in which surgical repair is indicated because of ascending aneurysm, it has been suggested that both, the aortic root and the ascending aorta should be replaced even when the root is macroscopically normal, since patients in whom the aortic root is preserved present later with SVAs that requires surgical repair.[135,139]

Patients with GCA appear to have a survival similar to the general population. Those patients with large-vessel GCA have the same survival as those patients with GCA without large-vessel involvement, but those with thoracic AD have a significant increased mortality.[141]

Other Aortic Vasculitis

Syphilis is a venereal disease caused by the spirochete *Treponema Pallidum*. Syphilis was once the most common cause of ascending thoracic aorta aneurysm, but in the era of antibiotics is a rare cause. Untreated syphilis progresses through 4 stages: primary, secondary, latent, and tertiary. Tertiary syphilis affects the cardiovascular system in 80% to 85% of the cases and the CNS in 5% to 10%. Latency may last from a few years to as many as 25 years before the destructive lesions of tertiary syphilis become manifest. Cardiovascular syphilis affects mainly the ascending aorta and results from endarteritis obliterans with subse-

quent medial necrosis, aortitis, and aneurysm formation. This may cause incompetence of the aortic valve and narrowing of the coronary ostia. Syphilitic aortitis should be suspected whenever linear calcifications are noted on chest radiographs of the ascending aorta, a finding seldom seen in arteriosclerotic disease. Syphilitic aneurysms rarely dissect. Surgical treatment is indicated in the case of a syphilitic aneurysm.[142,143]

Behcet's disease is a rare multisystem vasculitic disorder of unknown etiology. Small vessels are the predominant site of inflammation, and it can affect both arteries and veins. Large vessel involvement is seen in up to a third of the patients. The inflammatory process at arterial sites is acute and destructive, resulting in rapid formation of true and/or false aneurysms with an increased incidence of rupture and bleeding. There is also a thrombotic and occlusive component. The aorta is the most common place of aneurysm formation and can be associated with aortic valve regurgitation. Surgical repair is generally indicated for the treatment of aneurysms because of the risk of rupture and for the treatment of severe or symptomatic aortic valve regurgitation. Adjunctive treatment with steroids and immunosuppressive agents and possibly with anticoagulants and anti-aggregants antiplatelets agents may also be indicated.[144,145]

REFERENCES

1. Moore K, Persaud TVN. The cardiovascular system. In: *Before We Are Born. Essentials of Embryology and Birth Defects.* 6th ed. Philadelphia, PA: Saunders; 2003:264.

2. Goldmuntz E. The epidemiology and genetics of congenital heart disease. *Clin Perinatol.* 2001;28:1-10.

3. Wren C, Birrell G, Hawthorne G. Cardiovascular malformations in infants of diabetic mothers. *Heart.* 2003;89:1217-1220.

4. Karamlou TB, Shen I, Ungerleider RM. Congenital heart disease. In: Brunicardi FC, ed. *Schwartz's Principles of Surgery.* 8th ed. New York, NY: McGraw-Hill; 2005:611-644.

5. Park MK. Specific congenital heart defects. In: *Pediatric Cardiology for Practitioners.* 4th ed. Philadelphia, PA: Mosby; 2002.

6. Chiu I, Wu S, Chen M, Chen S, Wang J. Anatomic relationship of the coronary orifice and truncal valve in truncus arteriosus and their surgical implication. *J Thorac Cardiovasc Surg.* 2002;123:350-352.

7. Restivo A, Piacentini G, Placidi S, Saffirio C, Marino B. Cardiac outflow tract: a review of some embryogenetic aspects of the conotruncal region of the heart. *Anat Rec A Discov Mol Cell Evol Biol.* 2006;288:936-943.

8. Behrman RE, Kliegman RM, Jenson HB. Congenital heart disease. In: Behrman RE, Kliegman RM, Jenson HB, eds. *Nelson Textbook of Pediatrics.* 17th ed. Philadelphia, PA: Saunders; 2004.

9. Brown JW, Ruzmetov M, Okada Y, Vijay P, Turrentine MW. Truncus arteriosus repair: outcomes, risk factors, reoperation and management. *Eur J Cardiothorac Surg.* 2001;20:221-227.

10. Miyamoto T, Sinzobahamvya N, Kumpikaite D, et al. Repair

of truncus arteriosus and aortic arch interruption: outcome analysis. *Ann Thoracic Surg.* 2005;79:2077-2082.

11. Alexiou C, Keeton BR, Salmon AP, Monro JL. Repair of truncus arteriosus in early infancy with antibiotic sterilized aortic homografts. *Ann Thorac Surg.* 2001;71:S371-S374.

12. Thompson LD, McElhinney DB, Reddy VM, Petrossian E, Silverman NH, Hanley FL. Neonatal repair of truncus arteriosus: continuing improvement in outcomes. *Ann Thorac Surg.* 2001;72:391-395.

13. Tlaskal T, Hucin B, Kucera V, et al. Repair of persistent truncus arteriosus with interrupted aortic arch. *Eur J Cardio Thorac Surg.* 2005;28:736-741.

14. Backer CL, Mavroudis C. Surgical management of aortopulmonary window: a 40-year experience. *Eur J Cardiothorac Surg.* 2002;21:773-779.

15. Erez E, Dagan O, Georghiou GP, Gelber O, Vidne BA, Birk E. Surgical management of aortopulmonary window and associated lesions. *Ann Thorac Surg.* 2004;77:484-487.

16. Tchervenkov CI, Jacobs JP, Weinberg PM, et al. The nomenclature, definition and classification of hypoplastic left heart syndrome. *Cardiol Young.* 2006;16:339-368.

17. Chang RK, Chen AY, Klitzner TS. Clinical management of infants with hypoplastic left heart syndrome in the United States, 1988–1997. *Pediatrics.* 2002;110:292-298.

18. Sidi D. Hypoplasia of the left ventricle and the physiology of the norwood circulation. *Cardiol Young.* 2004;14(suppl 3):77-80.

19. Nelson DP, Schwartz SM, Chang AC. Neonatal physiology of the functionally univentricular heart. *Cardiol Young.* 2004;14(suppl 1):52-60.

20. Goldberg CS, Gomez CA. Hypoplastic left heart syndrome: new developments and current controversies. *Semin Neonatol.* 2003;8:461-468.

21. Jacobs ML. The norwood procedure for hypoplastic left heart syndrome. *Cardiol Young.* 2004;14(suppl 1):34-40.

22. Bove EL. Results of the norwood operation for hypoplastic left heart syndrome. *Cardiol Young.* 2004;14(suppl 3):85-89.

23. McGuirk SP, Stickley J, Griselli M, et al. Risk assessment and early outcome following the norwood procedure for hypoplastic left heart syndrome. *Eur J Cardiothorac Surg.* 2006;29:675-681.

24. Tweddell JS, Hoffman GM, Mussatto KA, et al. Improved survival of patients undergoing palliation of hypoplastic left heart syndrome: lessons learned from 115 consecutive patients. *Circulation.* 2002;106:I82-I89.

25. Jaquiss RDB, Siehr SL, Ghanayem NS, et al. Early cavopulmonary anastomosis after norwood procedure results in excellent fontan outcome. *Ann Thorac Surg.* 2006;82:1260-1266.

26. Pizarro C, Malec E, Maher KO, et al. Right ventricle to pulmonary artery conduit improves outcome after stage I norwood for hypoplastic left heart syndrome. *Circulation.* 2003;108(suppl 1):II155-II160.

27. Mosca RS, Kulik TJ, Goldberg CS, et al. Early results of the fontan procedure in one hundred consecutive patients with hypoplastic left heart syndrome. *J Thorac Cardiovasc Surg.* 2000;119:1110-1118.

28. Douglas WI, Goldberg CS, Mosca RS, Law IH, Bove EL. Hemi-fontan procedure for hypoplastic left heart syndrome: outcome and suitability for fontan. *Ann Thorac Surg.* 1999;68:1361-1367; discussion 1368.

29. Dodge-Khatami A, Kadner A, Berger F, Dave H, Turina MI, Pretre R. In the footsteps of senning: lessons learned from atrial repair of transposition of the great arteries. *Ann Thorac Surg.* 2005;79:1433-1444.

30. Williams WG, McCrindle BW, Ashburn DA, Jonas RA, Mavroudis C, Blackstone EH. Outcomes of 829 neonates with complete transposition of the great arteries 12–17 years after repair. *Eur J Cardiothorac Surg.* 2003;24:1-10.

31. Hutter PA, Kreb DL, Mantel SF, Hitchcock JF, Meijboom EJ, Bennink GBWE. Twenty-five years' experience with the arterial switch operation. *J Thorac Cardiovasc Surg.* 2002;124:790-797.

32. Kang N, de Leval MR, Elliott M, et al. Extending the boundaries of the primary arterial switch operation in patients with transposition of the great arteries and intact ventricular septum. *Circulation.* 2004;110:II123-II127.

33. Sarris GE, Chatzis AC, Giannopoulos NM, et al. The arterial switch operation in europe for transposition of the great arteries: a multi-institutional study from the european congenital heart surgeons association. *J Thorac Cardiovasc Surg.* 2006;132:633-639.

34. Legendre A, Losay J, Touchot-Kone A, et al. Coronary events after arterial switch operation for transposition of the great arteries. *Circulation.* 2003;108(suppl 1):II186-II190.

35. Prifti E, Crucean A, Bonacchi M, et al. Early and long term outcome of the arterial switch operation for transposition of the great arteries: predictors and functional evaluation. *Eur J Cardiothorac Surg.* 2002;22:864-873.

36. Brown JW, Ruzmetov M, Okada Y, Vijay P, Rodefeld MD, Turrentine MW. Outcomes in patients with interrupted aortic arch and associated anomalies: a 20-year experience. *Eur J Cardiothorac Surg.* 2006;29:666-673; discussion 673-674.

37. Schreiber C, Eicken A, Vogt M, et al. Repair of interrupted aortic arch: results after more than 20 years. *Ann Thorac Surg.* 2000;70:1896-1900.

38. Morales DLS, Scully PT, Braud BE, et al. Interrupted aortic arch repair: aortic arch advancement without a patch minimizes arch reinterventions. *Ann Thorac Surg.* 2006;82:1577-1584.

39. McCrindle BW, Tchervenkov CI, Konstantinov IE, et al. Risk factors associated with mortality and interventions in 472 neonates with interrupted aortic arch: a congenital heart surgeons society study. *J Thorac Cardiovasc Surg.* 2005;129:343-350.

40. Marino B, Digilio MC, Persiani M, et al. Deletion 22q11 in patients with interrupted aortic arch. *Am J Cardiol.* 1999;84:360-361.

41. Yagi H, Furutani Y, Hamada H, et al. Role of TBX1 in human del22q11.2 syndrome. *Lancet.* 2003;362:1366-1373.

42. Grathwohl KW, Afifi AY, Dillard TA, Olson JP, Heric BR. Vascular rings of the thoracic aorta in adults. *Am Surg.* 1999;65:1077-1083.

43. Backer CL, Mavroudis C. Congenital heart surgery nomenclature and database project: vascular rings, tracheal stenosis, pectus excavatum. *Ann Thorac Surg.* 2000;69:S308-S318.

44. Alsenaidi K, Gurofsky R, Karamlou T, Williams WG, McCrindle BW. Management and outcomes of double aortic arch in 81 patients. *Pediatrics.* 2006;118:e1336-e1341.

45. Backer CL, Mavroudis C, Rigsby CK, Holinger LD. Trends in vascular ring surgery. *J Thorac Cardiovasc Surg.* 2005;129:1338-1346.

46. McElhinney DB, Clark I, Bernard J, et al. Association of chromosome 22q11 deletion with isolated anomalies of aortic arch laterality and branching. *J Am Coll Cardiol.* 2001;37:2114-2119.

47. Bonnard A, Auber F, Fourcade L, Marchac V, Emond S, Revillon Y. Vascular ring abnormalities: a retrospective study of 62 cases. *J Pediatr Surg.* 2003;38:539-543.

48. Koontz CS, Bhatia A, Forbess J, Wulkan ML. Video-assisted thoracoscopic division of vascular rings in pediatric patients. *Am Surg.* 2005;71:289-291.

49. McElhinney DB, Wernovsky G. Vascular rings, right aortic arch. www.imedicine.com. Accessed May 15, 2006.

50. Adler SC, Isaacson G, Balsara RK. Innominate artery compression of the trachea: diagnosis and treatment by anterior suspension. A 25-year experience. *Ann Otol Rhinol Laryngol.* 1995;104:924-927.

51. Fiore AC, Brown JW, Weber TR, Turrentine MW. Surgical treatment of pulmonary artery sling and tracheal stenosis. *Ann Thorac Surg.* 2005;79:38-46.

52. Li F, Chen S, Wang J, Zhou Y. Treatment and outcome of sinus of valsalva aneurysm. *Heart Lung Circulation.* 2002;11:107-111.

53. Vural KM, Sener E, Tasdemir O, Bayazit K. Approach to sinus of valsalva aneurysms: a review of 53 cases. *Eur J Cardiothorac Surg.* 2001;20:71-76.

54. Harkness JR, Fitton TP, Barreiro CJ, et al. A 32-year experience with surgical repair of sinus of valsalva aneurysms. *J Card Surg.* 2005;20:198-204.

55. Feldman DN, Roman MJ. Aneurysms of the sinuses of valsalva. *Cardiology.* 2006;106:73-81.

56. Chang CW, Chiu SN, Wu ET, Tsai SK, Wu MH, Wang JK. Transcatheter closure of a ruptured sinus of valsalva aneurysm. *Circ J.* 2006;70:1043-1047.

57. Gaio G, Santoro G, Iacono C, et al. Non-surgical treatment of ruptured sinus of valsalva aneurysm. *Int J Cardiol.* 2006;113:e44-e45.

58. Arora R, Trehan V, Thakur AK, Mehta V, Sengupta PP, Nigam M. Transcatheter closure of congenital muscular ventricular septal defect. *J Interv Cardiol.* 2004;17:109-115.

59. Abidin N, Clarke B, Khattar RS. Percutaneous closure of ruptured sinus of valsalva aneurysm using an amplatzer occluder device. *Heart.* 2005;91:244.

60. Naka Y, Kadoba K, Ohtake S, et al. The long-term outcome of a surgical repair of sinus of valsalva aneurysm. *Ann Thorac Surg.* 2000;70:727-729.

61. Braverman AC, Guven H, Beardslee MA, Makan M, Kates AM, Moon MR. The bicuspid aortic valve. *Curr Probl Cardiol.* 2005;30:470-522.

62. Cecconi M, Nistri S, Quarti A, et al. Aortic dilatation in patients with bicuspid aortic valve. *J Cardiovasc Med (Hagerstown).* 2006;7:11-20.

63. Isselbacher EM. Thoracic and abdominal aortic aneurysms. *Circulation.* 2005;111:816-828.

64. Judge DP, Dietz HC. Marfan's syndrome. *Lancet.* 2005;366: 1965-1976.

65. Milewicz DM, Dietz HC, Miller DC. Treatment of aortic disease in patients with Marfan syndrome. *Circulation.* 2005; 111:e150-e157.

66. Gott VL, Greene PS, Alejo DE, et al. Replacement of the aortic root in patients with Marfan's syndrome. *N Engl J Med.* 1999;340:1307-1313.

67. David TE, Feindel CM, Webb GD, Colman JM, Armstrong S, Maganti M. Long-term results of aortic valve-sparing operations for aortic root aneurysm. *J Thorac Cardiovasc Surg.* 2006;132:347-354.

68. Karck M, Kallenbach K, Hagl C, Rhein C, Leyh R, Haverich A. Aortic root surgery in Marfan syndrome: comparison of aortic valve-sparing reimplantation versus composite grafting. *J Thorac Cardiovasc Surg.* 2004;127:391-398.

69. Alexiou C, Langley SM, Charlesworth P, Haw MP, Livesey SA, Monro JL. Aortic root replacement in patients with Marfan's syndrome: the southampton experience. *Ann Thorac Surg.* 2001;72:1502-1507.

70. Ince H, Rehders TC, Petzsch M, Kische S, Nienaber CA. Stent-grafts in patients with Marfan syndrome. *J Endovasc Ther.* 2005;12:82-88.

71. Fleck TM, Hutschala D, Tschernich H, et al. Stent graft placement of the thoracoabdominal aorta in a patient with Marfan syndrome. *J Thorac Cardiovasc Surg.* 2003;125: 1541-1543.

72. Baril DT, Carroccio A, Palchik E, et al. Endovascular treatment of complicated aortic aneurysms in patients with underlying arteriopathies. *Ann Vasc Surg.* 2006;20:464-471.

73. Beighton P, De Paepe A, Steinmann B, Tsipouras P, Wenstrup RJ. Ehlers-Danlos syndromes: revised nosology, Villefranche, 1997. Ehlers-Danlos National Foundation (USA) and Ehlers-Danlos Support Group (UK). *Am J Med Genet.* 1998;77:31-37.

74. Germain DP. Clinical and genetic features of vascular Ehlers-Danlos syndrome. *Ann Vasc Surg.* 2002;16:391-397.

75. Germain DP, Herrera-Guzman Y. Vascular Ehlers-Danlos syndrome. *Ann Genet.* 2004;47:1-9.

76. Pepin M, Schwarze U, Superti-Furga A, Byers PH. Clinical and genetic features of Ehlers-Danlos syndrome type IV, the vascular type. *N Engl J Med.* 2000;342:673-680.

77. Bergqvist D. Ehlers-Danlos type IV syndrome. A review from a vascular surgical point of view. *Eur J Surg.* 1996;162:163-170.

78. Wenstrup RJ, Meyer RA, Lyle JS, et al. Prevalence of aortic root dilation in the Ehlers-Danlos syndrome. *Genet Med.* 2002;4:112-117.

79. Oderich GS, Panneton JM, Bower TC, et al. The spectrum, management and clinical outcome of Ehlers-Danlos syndrome type IV: a 30-year experience. *J Vasc Surg.* 2005; 42:98-106.

80. Freeman RK, Swegle J, Sise MJ. The surgical complications of Ehlers-Danlos syndrome. *Am Surg.* 1996;62:869-873.

81. Maltz SB, Fantus RJ, Mellett MM, Kirby JP. Surgical complications of Ehlers-Danlos syndrome type IV: case report and review of the literature. *J Trauma.* 2001;51:387-390.

82. Yun KL. Ascending aortic aneurysm and aortic root disease. *Coron Artery Dis.* 2002;13:79-84.

83. Albornoz G, Coady MA, Roberts M, et al. Familial thoracic aortic aneurysms and dissections-incidence, modes of inheritance, and phenotypic patterns. *Ann Thorac Surg.* 2006;82:1400-1405.

84. Elefteriades JA. Natural history of thoracic aortic aneurysms: indications for surgery, and surgical versus nonsurgical risks. *Ann Thorac Surg.* 2002;74:S1877-S1880; discussion S1892-S1898.

85. Achneck H, Modi B, Shaw C, et al. Ascending thoracic aneurysms are associated with decreased systemic atherosclerosis. *Chest.* 2005;128:1580-1586.

86. Postellon D. Turner syndrome. www.imedicine.com. Accessed August 25, 2006.

87. Davies RR, Goldstein LJ, Coady MA, et al. Yearly rupture or dissection rates for thoracic aortic aneurysms: simple prediction based on size. *Ann Thorac Surg.* 2002;73:17-27; discussion 27-28.

88. Tseng E, Camacho M. Thoracic aortic aneurysm. www. imedicine.com. Accessed December 6, 2005.

89. Zehr KJ, Orszulak TA, Mullany CJ, et al. Surgery for aneurysms of the aortic root: a 30-year experience. *Circulation.* 2004;110:1364-1371.

90. Yacoub MH, Gehle P, Chandrasekaran V, Birks EJ, Child A, Radley-Smith R. Late results of a valve-preserving operation in patients with aneurysms of the ascending aorta and root. *J Thorac Cardiovasc Surg.* 1998;115:1080-1090.

91. David TE, Ivanov J, Armstrong S, Feindel CM, Webb GD. Aortic valve-sparing operations in patients with aneurysms

of the aortic root or ascending aorta. *Ann Thorac Surg.* 2002; 74:S1758-S1761.

92. Strauch JT, Spielvogel D, Lauten A, et al. Technical advances in total aortic arch replacement. *Ann Thorac Surg.* 2004;77:581-590.

93. Hagan PG, Nienaber CA, Isselbacher EM, et al. The international registry of acute aortic dissection (IRAD): new insights into an old disease. *JAMA.* 2000;283:897-903.

94. Erbel R, Alfonso F, Boileau C, et al. Diagnosis and management of aortic dissection. *Eur Heart J.* 2001;22:1642-1681.

95. Meszaros I, Morocz J, Szlavi J, et al. Epidemiology and clinicopathology of aortic dissection. *Chest.* 2000;117:1271-1278.

96. Clouse WD, Hallett JW Jr, Schaff HV, et al. Acute aortic dissection: population-based incidence compared with degenerative aortic aneurysm rupture. *Mayo Clin Proc.* 2004;79:176-180.

97. Chiappini B, Schepens M, Tan E, et al. Early and late outcomes of acute type A aortic dissection: analysis of risk factors in 487 consecutive patients. *Eur Heart J.* 2005;26:180-186.

98. Mukherjee D, Eagle KA. Aortic dissection–an update. *Curr Probl Cardiol.* 2005;30:287-325.

99. Tsai TT, Evangelista A, Nienaber CA, et al. Long-term survival in patients presenting with type A acute aortic dissection: insights from the international registry of acute aortic dissection (IRAD). *Circulation.* 2006;114:I350-I356.

100. Tsai TT, Nienaber CA, Eagle KA. Acute aortic syndromes. *Circulation.* 2005;112:3802-3813.

101. Atkins MD Jr, Black JHIII, Cambria RP. Aortic dissection: perspectives in the era of stent-graft repair. *J Vasc Surg.* 2006;43(suppl A):30A-43A.

102. Kallenbach K, Oelze T, Salcher R, et al. Evolving strategies for treatment of acute aortic dissection type A. *Circulation.* 2004;110:II243-II249.

103. Jault F, Rama A, Lievre L, et al. Chronic dissection of the ascending orta: surgical results during a 20-year period (previous surgery excluded). *Eur J Cardiothorac Surg.* 2006;29:1041-1045.

104. Leurs LJ, Bell R, Degrieck Y, Thomas S, Hobo R, Lundbom J. Endovascular treatment of thoracic aortic diseases: combined experience from the EUROSTAR and United Kingdom Thoracic Endograft registries. *J Vasc Surg.* 2004;40:670-679.

105. Nienaber CA, Eagle KA. Aortic dissection: new frontiers in diagnosis and management: part II: therapeutic management and follow-up. *Circulation.* 2003;108:772-778.

106. Song JK. Diagnosis of aortic intramural haematoma. *Heart.* 2004;90:368-371.

107. Ganaha F, Miller DC, Sugimoto K, et al. Prognosis of aortic intramural hematoma with and without penetrating atherosclerotic ulcer: a clinical and radiological analysis. *Circulation.* 2002;106:342-348.

108. Evangelista A, Mukherjee D, Mehta RH, et al. Acute intramural hematoma of the aorta: a mystery in evolution. *Circulation.* 2005;111:1063-1070.

109. Motoyoshi N, Moizumi Y, Komatsu T, Tabayashi K. Intramural hematoma and dissection involving ascending aorta:

the clinical features and prognosis. *Eur J Cardiothoracic Surg.* 2003;24:237-242.

110. Maraj R, Rerkpattanapipat P, Jacobs LE, Makornwattana P, Kotler MN. Meta-analysis of 143 reported cases of aortic intramural hematoma. *Am J Cardiol.* 2000;86:664-668.

111. von Kodolitsch Y, Csosz SK, Koschyk DH, et al. Intramural hematoma of the aorta: predictors of progression to dissection and rupture. *Circulation.* 2003;107:1158-1163.

112. Song JM, Kim HS, Song JK, et al. Usefulness of the initial noninvasive imaging study to predict the adverse outcomes in the medical treatment of acute type A aortic intramural hematoma. *Circulation.* 2003;108(suppl 1):II324-II328.

113. Macura KJ, Corl FM, Fishman EK, Bluemke DA. Pathogenesis in acute aortic syndromes: aortic dissection, intramural hematoma, and penetrating atherosclerotic aortic ulcer. *AJR Am J Roentgenol.* 2003;181:309-316.

114. Cho KR, Stanson AW, Potter DD, et al. Penetrating atherosclerotic ulcer of the descending thoracic aorta and arch. *J Thorac Cardiovasc Surg.* 2004;127:1393-1401.

115. Seelig MH, Klingler PJ, Oldenburg WA, Blackshear JL. Angiosarcoma of the aorta: report of a case and review of the literature. *J Vasc Surg.* 1998;28:732-737.

116. Chiche L, Mongredien B, Brocheriou I, Kieffer E. Primary tumors of the thoracoabdominal aorta: surgical treatment of 5 patients and review of the literature. *Ann Vasc Surg.* 2003;17:354-364.

117. Bohner H, Luther B, Braunstein S, Beer S, Sandmann W. Primary malignant tumors of the aorta: clinical presentation, treatment, and course of different entities. *J Vasc Surg.* 2003;38:1430-1433.

118. Salm R. Primary fibrosarcoma of aorta. *Cancer.* 1972;29:73-83.

119. Wright EP, Glick AD, Virmani R, Page DL. Aortic intimal sarcoma with embolic metastases. *Am J Surg Pathol.* 1985; 9:890-897.

120. Johnston SL, Lock RJ, Gompels MM. Journal of clinical pathology; Takayasu arteritis: a review [review]. *Br Med Assoc.* 2002;55:481-486. http://find.galegroup.com.proxy. lib.utk.edu:90/itx/infomark. do?&contentSet = IAC-Documents&type = retrieve&tabID = T002&prodId = ITOF&docId = A89923777&source = gale&srcprod = ITOF&userGroupName = tel_a_utl&version = 1.0. Accessed November 20, 2006.

121. Weyand CM, Goronzy JJ. Medium- and large-vessel vasculitis. *N Engl J Med.* 2003;349:160-169.

122. Miller DV, Isotalo PA, Weyand CM, Edwards WD, Aubry MC, Tazelaar HD. Surgical pathology of noninfectious ascending aortitis: a study of 45 cases with emphasis on an isolated variant. *Am J Surg Pathol.* 2006;30:1150-1158.

123. Rojo-Leyva F, Ratliff NB, Cosgrove DM III, Hoffman GS. Study of 52 patients with idiopathic aortitis from a cohort of 1204 surgical cases. *Arthritis Rheum.* 2000;43:901-907.

124. Kerr LD, Chang YJ, Spiera H, Fallon JT. Occult active giant cell aortitis necessitating surgical repair. *J Thorac Cardiovasc Surg.* 2000;120:813-815.

125. Liang P, Hoffman GS. Advances in the medical and surgical treatment of Takayasu arteritis. *Curr Opin Rheumatol.* 2005;17:16-24.

126. Kerr GS, Hallahan CW, Giordano J, et al. Takayasu arteritis. *Ann Intern Med.* 1994;120:919-929.

127. Kissin EY, Merkel PA. Diagnostic imaging in Takayasu arteritis. *Curr Opin Rheumatol.* 2004;16:31-37.

128. Hoffman GS, Merkel PA, Brasington RD, Lenschow DJ, Liang P. Anti-tumor necrosis factor therapy in patients with difficult to treat Takayasu arteritis. *Arthritis Rheum.* 2004;50:2296-2304.

129. Della Rossa A, Tavoni A, Merlini G, et al. Two Takayasu arteritis patients successfully treated with infliximab: a potential disease-modifying agent? *Rheumatology (Oxford).* 2005;44:1074-1075.

130. Tanaka F, Kawakami A, Iwanaga N, et al. Infliximab is effective for Takayasu arteritis refractory to glucocorticoid and methotrexate. *Intern Med.* 2006;45:313-316.

131. Liang P, Tan-Ong M, Hoffman GS. Takayasu's arteritis: vascular interventions and outcomes. *J Rheumatol.* 2004;31: 102-106.

132. Miyata T, Sato O, Koyama H, Shigematsu H, Tada Y. Long-term survival after surgical treatment of patients with Takayasu's arteritis. *Circulation.* 2003;108:1474-1480.

133. Matsuura K, Ogino H, Kobayashi J, et al. Surgical treatment of aortic regurgitation due to Takayasu arteritis: long-term morbidity and mortality. *Circulation.* 2005;112:3707-3712.

134. Matsuura K, Ogino H, Matsuda H, et al. Surgical outcome of aortic arch repair for patients with Takayasu arteritis. *Ann Thorac Surg.* 2006;81:178-182.

135. Bongartz T, Matteson EL. Large-vessel involvement in giant cell arteritis. *Curr Opin Rheumatol.* 2006;18:10-17.

136. Gonzalez-Gay MA, Barros S, Lopez-Diaz MJ, Garcia-Porrua C, Sanchez-Andrade A, Llorca J. Giant cell arteritis: disease patterns of clinical presentation in a series of 240 patients. *Medicine (Baltimore).* 2005;84:269-276.

137. Nuenninghoff DM, Hunder GG, Christianson TJ, McClelland RL, Matteson EL. Incidence and predictors of large-artery complication (aortic aneurysm, aortic dissection, and/or large-artery stenosis) in patients with giant cell arteritis: a population-based study over 50 years. *Arthritis Rheum.* 2003;48:3522-3531.

138. Margos PN, Moyssakis IE, Tzioufas AG, Zintzaras E, Moutsopoulos HM. Impaired elastic properties of ascending aorta in patients with giant cell arteritis. *Ann Rheum Dis.* 2005;64:253-256.

139. Gelsomino S, Romagnoli S, Gori F, et al. Annuloaortic ectasia and giant cell arteritis. *Ann Thorac Surg.* 2005;80:101-105.

140. Gonzalez-Gay MA, Lopez-Diaz MJ, Barros S, et al. Giant cell arteritis: laboratory tests at the time of diagnosis in a series of 240 patients. *Medicine (Baltimore).* 2005;84:277-290.

141. Nuenninghoff DM, Hunder GG, Christianson TJ, McClelland RL, Matteson EL. Mortality of large-artery complication (aortic aneurysm, aortic dissection, and/or large-artery stenosis) in patients with giant cell arteritis: a population-based study over 50 years. *Arthritis Rheum.* 2003;48:3532-3537.

142. Liu P. Syphilis. www.imedicine.com. Accessed August 1, 2006.

143. Tramont EC. Treponema pallidum (syphilis). In: Medell G, Bennet J, Dolin R, eds. *Principles and Practice of Infectious Diseases.* 6th ed. Philadelphia, PA: Churchill Linvingstone; 2005:2768-2784.

144. Calamia KT, Schirmer M, Melikoglu M. Major vessel involvement in Behcet disease. *Curr Opin Rheumatol.* 2005;17:1-8.

145. Tsui KL, Lee KW, Chan WK, et al. Behcet's aortitis and aortic regurgitation: a report of two cases. *J Am Soc Echocardiogr.* 2004;17:83-86.

chapter 27

Ascending Thoracic Aorta and Aortic Arch

Thomas E. Gaines, MD

The diagnosis and management of disorders of the ascending aorta and aortic arch remain as formidable challenges in cardiovascular medicine and surgery. Until the advent of the modern era of cardiac surgery with cardiopulmonary bypass, this region of the aorta was all but inaccessible to any surgical intervention and even now definitive medical therapies remain elusive. Accurate diagnosis requires the sophisticated, yet now readily available, imaging techniques developed over the past few decades and rarely can be made on clinical grounds alone. While not as prevalent as atherosclerotic peripheral and coronary arterial occlusive disease, diseases of the proximal aorta are common enough that cardiovascular specialists are inevitably confronted with them in many different clinical settings. The sometimes enigmatic but dramatic and lethal presentation of ascending aortic dissection (AD) has attracted considerable public attention in recent years (See, for example, the 2004 Pulitzer Prize winning series by Kevin Helliker and Thomas Burton of *The Wall Street Journal*). Dissection and rupture, often occurring in otherwise vigorous individuals, are catastrophic biomechanical failures, and the end result of many different aortic pathologies. Aneurysmal degeneration is a common manifestation of proximal aortic disease and precedes many, but not all, instances of dissection. Congenital disease often involves obstructive lesions while atherosclerosis in this region does not. Yet even in the absence of luminal narrowing or aneurysm, the changes in aortic compliance or stiffness that accompany disease and aging have important pathophysiologic effects not only downstream in other organ systems but upstream in the heart.

In this chapter the focus is on the anatomy, microstructure, functional mechanics, and pathophysiology of the proximal aorta. This field encompasses a broad range of disciplines from multiple areas of clinical medicine, genetics, cell biology, and biomedical engineering and an attempt has been made to integrate information derived from all these areas to provide a basic level of understanding of the function, structure, and pathologies and their systemic ramifications of this unique segment of the arterial system. The preceding chapter is designed to provide a more immediately clinical discussion.

PROXIMAL AORTIC STRUCTURE AND MECHANICS

Macrostructure

The ascending aorta includes the aorta from the level of the aortic valve to the origin of the brachiocephalic artery. It is further divided into the sinus portion containing the three sinuses of valsalva and the tubular portion. The aortic valve, aortic sinuses, and coronary ostia are integral elements of the sinus portion of the aorta. The proximal aorta from the ventricular outlet to the tubular part of the ascending aorta including the sinotubular junction (STJ) is called the aortic root. The precise anatomy of the aortic root[1] is of considerable clinical importance in the surgical treatment of both aneurysmal disease and aortic valvular disease. The aortic arch, which gives rise to the brachiocephalic, left common carotid, and left subclavian arteries, extends transversely from the ascending aorta to the descending thoracic aorta distal to the subclavian origin. The region where the aortic arch joins the descending thoracic aorta is termed the aortic isthmus and is an area of important aortic pathology including coarctation and the intimal tear initiating

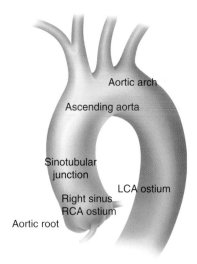

● **FIGURE 27-1.** Anatomic diagram of the proximal aorta showing the three divisions, aortic root, ascending aorta, and aortic arch. There are three sinuses of valsalva, the right, left, and noncoronary sinuses, each of which has an associated aortic valve cusp. The two coronary ostia arise from the right and left sinuses.

dissection and a likely site of traumatic rupture associated with deceleration injuries (Figure 27-1).

With the exception of the trilobed sinus portion, the proximal aorta is generally round in cross-section when distended at physiologic pressures. Therefore, its size and related mechanical properties can be associated with its diameter. While in childhood the dimensions of the normal aorta bear a relationship to body size,[2] in adults, aortic luminal diameters are independent of weight, height, and body surface area. In a study involving 70 adults aged 17 to 89 and free of signs of cardiovascular disease, helical CT scanning was used to measure luminal diameters of the thoracic aorta at defined points from the sinuses to the diaphragm. The diameters tapered from a maximum of 3.2 ($\pm$0.42 SD) cm in men and 2.9 $\pm$ 0.38 cm in women in the ascending aorta to 2.51 $\pm$ 0.34 cm in men and 2.27 $\pm$ 0.31 cm in women at the diaphragm. Other than the small (within 1 SD) association with sex, the only important correlate was age, confirming a roughly one millimeter per decade increase in aortic diameters found in an earlier study.[3]

The aortic wall is composed of three layers: The intima, the media, and the adventitia. The normal intima consists of a single layer of highly biochemically active endothelial cells, a subendothelial connective tissue layer, and the internal elastic lamina. The media is composed of vascular smooth muscle cells (VSMCs), which are also biochemically active, and an extracellular matrix. The extracellular matrix contains elastin, collagen, and glycoproteins including fibrillin microfibrils and imparts unique elastomeric properties to the aortic wall.[4] The outer limit of the media is bounded by the external elastic lamina. The adventitia is composed of collagen containing connective tissue and includes nerve fibers and the vaso vasora that

supply the outer layers of the media. The inner layers of the media receive nutrient supply from the aortic lumen. Anatomic variation in aortic wall thickness in the absence of disease, is determined by the number of concentric fibromuscular layers in the media, and is linearly related to aortic diameter, not only in man but also remarkably across multiple mammalian species of markedly different size.[5]

Microstructure

The unique, mechanical distensibility and elastic recoil of the aorta and its pathophysiologic features are dependent upon the structural architecture and complicated developmental and homeostatic processes of the media. The basic structure involves the lamellar unit which consists of two fenestrated elastic lamellae encasing smooth muscle cells and extracellular matrix components.[6] A simplified schematic representation has been presented by Dingemans et al.[7] (Figure 27-2) who found 53 to 78 concentric, lamellar layers in their study of human ascending aortas.

Elastic lamellae and their interconnections are made up of elastic fibers that demonstrate "a bewildering jigsaw of molecular interactions involving fibrillin, elastin, and various microfibril-associated molecules...".[8] Microfibrils are structural elements found in most tissues and most abundantly associated with basement membranes and elastic fibers. An important milestone in the understanding of microfibril biology has been the discovery of fibrillin as a major glycoprotein in microfibrils.[9] Fibrillins exist in at least three isoforms whose primary structures are dominated by calcium binding epidermal growth factor (cbEGF) domains that adopt a rodlike structure in the presence of calcium.[8] Fibrillin molecules also have compact, globular regions that

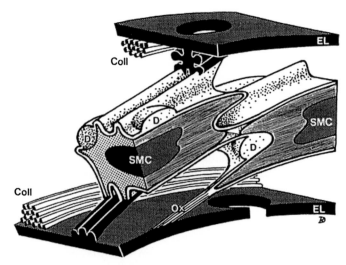

● **FIGURE 27-2.** Schematic representation of the relationships of smooth muscle cells and extracellular matrix.

Reproduced, with permission, Dingemans KP, Teeling P, Lagendijk JH, Becker AE. Extracellular matrix of the human aortic media: an ultrastructural histochemical and immunohistochemical study of the adult aortic media. Anat Rec. 2000;258:1–14.

appear to be related to their capacity for extensibility.[10] Elastic fiber development involves the deposition of tropoelastin, the soluble precursor of elastin, on a preformed matrix of fibrillin-rich microfibrils and, under appropriate conditions, elastin undergoes a process of ordered self-aggregation called coacervation and becomes cross-linked by lysyl oxidase.[8] Elastic fibers are thus a composite material composed of cross-linked elastin and fibrillin-rich microfibrils and arranged in fenestrated elastic lamellae with irregular protrusions that reach toward smooth muscle cells. Fibulin-5 is an extracellular matrix protein abundantly expressed in great vessels, cardiac valves, and other elastic tissues during embryogenesis as well as in adult life and appears to have a critical function as a scaffold protein organizing links between elastic fibers and cells.[11] Based on studies of comparative anatomy, the incorporation of elastin with the system of microfibrils appears to be necessary to support the high pressure closed circulatory systems of higher vertebrates.[12] Recognizing the critical roles of tropoelastin, fibrillin-1, and fibulin-5 in the formation and maintenance of elastic fibers and their attachments and interactions with vascular cells, brings the promise of bioengineered vascular grafts with the mechanical characteristics of normal arteries.[13]

Elastic fiber biology is associated with more than 30 reported molecules (Table 27-1).[4]

Immunoelectron microscopy of specimens of adult human ascending aorta have revealed important observations on the relationships of collagen, fibrillin, fibronectin, elastin, and VSMCs in the aortic media.[7] Thick collagen fibers containing types I, III, and V collagen are closely associated with elastic lamellae. Collagen fibers are most numerous close to elastic lamellae and are oriented circumferentially, roughly parallel to the main axis of the VSMCs, and to the irregular protrusions of the elastic lamellae extending into the interlamellar space. Collagen fibers more centrally in the interlamelar space are thin and more randomly oriented. Elastic lamellae are nearly straight in distended aortas but wavy in those prepared in a collapsed state. Collagen fibrils in the adventitia are on an average very thick compared with most collagen fibrils in the media, but those in the intima are thinner. Within the media, fibril diameters are strikingly variable. The shapes of the collagen fibrils on cross-section are also highly variable with most being rounded but others irregular and angular especially near the adventitia. Some of these collagen fibrils, irregularly shaped on cross section, appeared to be loose and spiraled when seen longitudinally and may be degenerated forms. Type VI collagen as well as fibrillin was found in the oxytalen fibers that connect smooth muscle cells to the elastic elements with the actual cell attachments involving fibronectin. Type IV collagen, which generally seems to be a major basement membrane component, was found in aggregates located further from cell surfaces than fibronectin.[7]

The proteoglycans dermatan sulfate, heparan sulfate, and chondroitin sulfate were also demonstrated in the work cited above in the matrix material of aortic elastic lamellae. Of the extracellular structures described only the cell-associated fibronectin positive layers, the elastin-associated material, and the oxytalan fibers were devoid of proteoglycans. Dermatan (decorin) was associated with collagen fibers and is thought to be related to the control of collagen fibrillogenesis, heparan (perlecan) was found within basal laminalike material, where it is thought to be a binding site for growth factors and cytokines, and the large interstitial chondroitin proteoglycans (versican) seem to function in maintaining shape and sustaining the compression generated by pulsatile forces.[7]

The embryologic development and homeostatic processes of the aortic media are clearly more complicated than a static view of its microstructure. VSMCs possess receptor mechanisms that allow the detection and a corresponding response to shear stress and tension as well as other cell-signaling events.[14] This response involves matrix modifications such as the deposition of collagen fibers, tropoelastin, or microfibrils resulting from the activation of transcription factors and subsequent gene expression. The aortic wall is best viewed as an intricate biochemical mechanism having its origin in the developing embryo and subject to a continuum of development, growth, maintenance, and senescence. While the aorta develops as a component of the embryonic circulatory system, most of its functional life is spent under very different conditions of vessel geometry, blood pressure and, therefore, wall tension since the aorta grows and blood pressure increases steadily from the embryonic state to adulthood with further changes occurring with senescence. The corresponding microstructure changes as well since aortic mesodermal cells respond to these factors in a more or less continuous way as can be seen from bioengineering studies designed to produce substitute autologous arteries.[15–17] There is an active and on going cell-mediated maintenance program for structural proteins, but as with most tissues, repair functions are not unlimited especially with the loss of cellular elements.

One class of molecules known to be important in matrix development and homeostasis are the matrix metalloproteinases (MMPs) and their antagonist tissue inhibitors of MMPs (TIMPs). Remodeling is an important element of tissue growth and morphogenesis and this requires matrix degradation, which seems to be one component of MMP function. However, MMPs have a more expansive regulatory role in several extracellular matrix processes including cell migration, proliferation, and apoptosis as well as angiogenesis and wound healing.[18]

Mechanical Properties of the Proximal Aorta

Blood is delivered to the proximal aorta in boluses depending upon the stroke volume and pressure generated by left ventricular systole, by the intrinsic impedance of the ventricular outflow tract and aortic root, peripheral vascular resistance, and by the viscosity of the blood. This event causes a pulse wave of flow and pressure that is repeated with every heartbeat. However, when blood reaches the arterioles and capillaries; pressure is nearly constant and

TABLE 27-1. Elastic Fiber Associated Molecules

Molecule	Site	Clinical Association
Amyloid	Some microfibrils	Amyloidosis
BigH3 (keratoepithelin)	Elastic fiber/collagen interface	
Biglycan	Elastic fiber core	
Collagen III	External structural support for elastic fibers	Vascular Ehlers-Danlos syndrome
Collagen VIII	Some elastic fibers	
Collagen XVI	Dermal microfibrils	
Collagen VI	Some microfibrils	
Decorin	Microfibrils	
Elastin	Elastic fiber core	Supravalvular aortic stenosis, William's syndrome, cutis laxa
Elastin-binding protein	Newly secreted tropoelastin	
Emilin-1	Elastin-microfibril interface	
Emilin-2	Elastin-microfibril interface	
Endostatin α_1-XVIII	Vascular elastic fibers	
Fibrillin-1	Microfibrils	Marfan's syndrome
Fibrillin-2	Microfibrils	
Fibrillin-3	Microfibrils	
Fibulin-1	Elastic fiber core	
Fibulin-2	Elastin-microfibril interface	
Fibulin-5	Elastic fiber—cell interface	Cutis laxa
LOXL		Lysyl-oxidase like protein
LOXL2		
Elastic Fiber Associated Molecules		
LTBP-1	Some microfibrils	Latent TGFbeta binding protein
LTBP-2	Microfibrils/elastic fibers	
LTBP-3		
LTBP-4		
Lysyl oxidase (LOX)	Microfibrils/tropoelastin	
MAGP-1	Microfibrils	Microfibril associated glycoprotein
MAGP-2	Some microfibrils	
MFAP-1	Some microfibrils	Microfibril associated protien
MFAP-3	Some microfibrils	
MFAP-4 (MAGP-36)	Some microfibrils	
TGFBR1		Transforming growth factor beta receptor, familial thoracic aneurysm, Loeys-Dietz syndrome
TGFBR2		
Tropoelastin	Elastic fibre core	
Versican	Some microfibrils	
Vitronectin	Some microfibrils	

flow continuous. Much of the attenuation of the amplitude of flow and pressure waves occurs in the aorta. The ratio of flow pulse amplitude to mean flow decreases by more than threefold from the aortic arch to the femoral artery.[19] This phenomenon is a result of the unique elastic properties of the aortic wall which allow a calibrated level of distension and elastic recoil with each ventricular systole and thereby produce a diastolic counterpulsation qualitatively similar to that produced by the intra-aortic balloon pump used to augment the hemodynamics of a failing heart (Figure 27-3). Shadwick[20] points out that this

pulse amplitude attenuation may serve to minimize the hydraulic power requirements of the heart by lowering the energy cost of accelerating and decelerating the blood mass in each cycle and to minimize the drag force imposed by flow on the endothelial cells lining the small vessels. There is, however, some energy lost in this process of elastic recoil. When an artery is subjected to inflation-deflation cycles, viscoelasticity, in distinction to pure elasticity, will cause the pressure-volume curve for deflation to fall below that for inflation, forming a hysteresis loop. The area enclosed in this loop represents the 15% to 20% of total strain energy

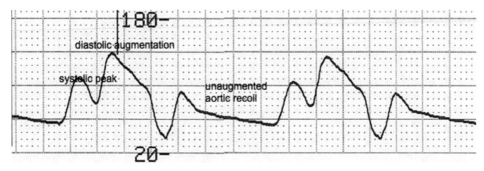

● **FIGURE 27-3.** Aortic pressure tracing from a patient with an intra-aortic balloon pump demonstrating marked diastolic augmentation resulting from diastolic balloon inflation distal to the site of the pressure measurement. The unaugmented subsequent beat shows a lower peak pressure but higher end diastolic pressure resulting from intrinsic aortic recoil. In this older patient with some degree of aortic stiffening the dicrotic notch is somewhat atypical with no secondary upstroke at the onset of the native aorta's unaugmented diastolic recoil.

input lost with each systole. Together with blood viscosity the viscoelasticity of the artery wall prevents reflected pressure waves from resonating in the arterial system.[20]

A conceptual model of the relationships of arterial pressure and flow, termed the *Windkessel* ("air chamber") was developed by Otto Frank.[21] The model considers the circulatory system as a closed hydraulic circuit consisting of a pump connected to a chamber partially filled with incompressible water but containing a pocket of compressible air to simulate aortic compliance and elastic recoil. Thus these properties of the aorta are sometimes called Windkessel properties. The model has undergone many modifications to allow it to accurately predict measurable circulatory parameters. A four element Windkessel has been presented with elements corresponding to physiologic concepts that produces waveforms with excellent fidelity to those observed in vivo[22] (Figure 27-4).

Elastic behavior is an intrinsic property of materials under conditions of loading. In the least complicated situation, that of a simple spring, the deformation (strain), or change in length of the spring relative to its original length, is directly proportional to the load placed upon it (stress). This simple relationship is linear, (E = stress/strain, where E is a constant) and the deformation is purely elastic with the material returning to its exact original state only under ideal (theoretical) conditions. Deformations that result in a permanent change in the material are termed plastic while those that result in hysteresis or the loss of energy with return toward the original configuration are termed viscoelastic. Nevertheless, materials are characterized by the modulus of elasticity (E) calculated from the stress-strain relationship, which is not a simple linear one in the case of viscoelastic, multicomponent materials. The higher this value, the stiffer the material and conversely the lower the number, the more compliant the material is. Materials demonstrating elastic behavior also have a yield point where excess strain results in plastic deformation and a point, the tensile strength, which defines the limits of structural integrity. Figure 27-5 demonstrates stress-strain curves for descending thoracic aortic strips. At low stress levels elas-

tic behavior is dominated by the mechanical properties of elastin and at high levels near the yield point by the properties of collagen.

The aortic wall can be considered as a cylinder composed of microscopic springs that are oriented longitudinally, circumferentially, and radially within the thickness of its wall. When the aorta is pressurized, the circumferential and longitudinal springs are stretched and the radial springs are compressed. The aorta tends to dilate and/or elongate, and its wall thins. The moduli of elasticity for these different sets of "springs" are not necessarily the same. If they were, the material would be termed isotropic. If the material displays different degrees of stiffness depending on the orientation of loading it is termed anisotropic. Since the aorta has a complex composite structure when its properties are viewed as a whole it is anisotropic. To simplify analysis, the volume of tissue comprising the aortic wall is often considered to be constant, that is, the wall is incompressible and there are proportionate changes in thickness, length, and diameter. The precise form of these proportionate changes in strain, occurring in a given two dimensions, is an intrinsic material property known as Poisson's ratio. For anisotropic materials this ratio will differ, as does the modulus of elasticity depending upon the direction of loading. Further, the stress (tension) on the innermost layers of "springs" may not necessarily be the same as on those in the outer layers and this appears to be the case in arteries.[23] It has been shown that there exists residual strain with different levels of tension in the inner and outer layers of the aortic wall when no pressure load distends the aorta, as in a beam of prestressed concrete.[24] This phenomenon serves to equalize wall tension across the thickness of the aortic wall during pressure loading and has been quantified by calculating the "opening angle." That is, the angle created between the two end points and the midpoint of the circumference of a cylindrical segment of aortic tissue cut open longitudinally (which may actually be greater than 180 degrees with the aorta turning itself inside out)[25] (Figure 27-6).

Using a two-dimensional analysis considering average longitudinal (axial) and circumferential stress and strain,[26]

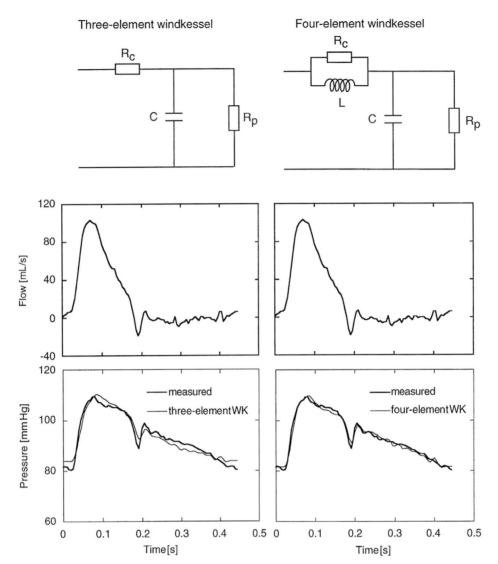

● FIGURE 27-4. Three and four element Windkessel models, displayed by analogy to circuit diagrams, designed to create high fidelity predictions of arterial pressure and flow based on measurable circulatory parameters. R_p represents peripheral resistance or mean pressure divided by mean flow. C represents total arterial compliance or the sum of volume changes in all arterial segments divided by pressure changes and is mainly determined by the elastic properties of large arteries, primarily the proximal aorta. R_c represents the characteristic resistance which is determined by the local inertia and local compliance of the very proximal aorta based on wave transmission theory. L is an inertial term (total arterial inertance) included in the four element model and is dependent upon blood density, arterial segment lengths and cross-sectional areas summed over all arterial segments. The middle panels are measured flow curves in an animal model and the lower panels represent corresponding model-derived and measured pressure curves for the same animal.

Reproduced, with permission, from Stergiopulos N, Westerhof BE, Westerhof N. Total arterial inertance as the fourth element of the windkessel model. Am J Physiol. 1999;276:H81–H88.

the average circumferential Kirchhoff wall stress (τ_c) can be given by the relation:

$$\tau_c = P(r_i)/h(\lambda_c)^2,$$

where P is the luminal pressure, r_i the inner luminal radius, h the vessel thickness, and λ_c the circumferential stretch ratio (the ratio of the circumference at load to that at no load which is different for the outer and inner layers and this

difference becomes larger the thicker the cylinder wall). Similarly, the average Kirchhoff longitudinal stress (τ_z) can be given by

$$\tau_z = P(r_i)/h[(r_i) + (r_o)](\lambda_z)^2,$$

where r_o is the outer luminal radius and λ_z is the longitudinal stretch ratio.

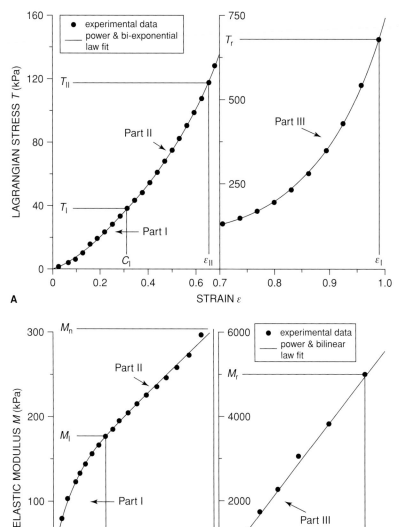

A

● **FIGURE 27-5.** (A) Typical stress–strain curve of a longitudinal strip from the descending thoracic aorta. (B) The data in (A) are presented in the form of an elastic modulus-stress curve that consists of a nonlinear (part I) and two linear parts (II and III). The transition points are shown, which constitute the limits of the three parts. TI, epsilon I, and MI designate stress, strain, and elastic modulus at the transition point from part I to II of the curves, while TII, epsilon II, MII denote the respective quantities at the transition point from part II to III.

Reproduced, with permission, from Sokolis DP, Kefaloyannis EM, Kouloukoussa M, Marinos E, Boudoulas H, Karayannacos PE. A structural basis for the aortic stress-stress relation in uniaxial tension. J Biomech. 2006;39:1651–1662.

B

It can be seen, therefore, that the average circumferential or longitudinal wall stress is directly proportional to the pressure in the vessel and its radius and is inversely proportional to the thickness of the vessel wall. For infinitesimal deformations the stretch ratio terms become insignificant, approaching one. This analysis expands the familiar "law of Laplace" which states that wall tension is proportional to the product of pressure and radius and underscores the relentless rise in wall tension that accompanies the growth of aneurysms. The wall thickness component is also important since one can see the purely geometric component in aortic weakening that is associated with wall thinning from destructive processes. Additionally, it can be seen how small vessels can be pressurized to the same extent as the aorta and yet be thin-walled. At physiologic pressures, in normal arteries, it has been empirically determined that the ratio of internal radius to wall thickness is between 7:1 and 10:1[27]

so that circumferential wall tension is approximately 10 times the blood pressure. If an aneurysm doubles the aortic radius, the corresponding wall tension is 20 times the blood pressure if the wall thickness is maintained and even higher if the aneurysm is thin walled.

Cardiac dynamics have been shown to increase longitudinal (axial) ascending aortic stress independent of aortic distending pressure. It is known from a careful analysis of cine aortograms that there exists axial downward displacement of the aortic root during systole and an associated twisting deformation as well.[28] The degree of axial displacement significantly increases local stress in the region above the STJ. Subjects with aortic insufficiency demonstrate significantly greater axial displacement and those with poor contractile function significantly less than the norm.[28] In addition to the effect of vigorous cardiac contraction on the strain induced in the proximal aorta, it has been shown,

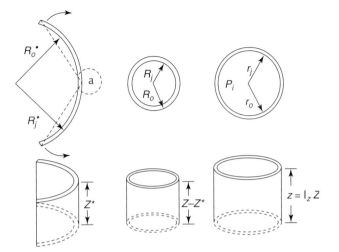

● **FIGURE 27-6.** The cylinder model for evaluating aortic mechanical properties including a depiction of the opening angle alpha.

Reproduced, with permission, from Okamoto RJ, Xu H, Kouchoukos NT, Moon MR, Sundt TM III. The influence of mechanical properties on wall stress and distensibility of the dilated ascending aorta. J Thorac Cardiovasc Surg. 2003;126:842–850.

based on a finite element analysis, that blood flow asymmetry through the aortic root results in 21% and 10% greater wall stress in the right and noncoronary sinuses, respectively, as compared to the left.[29] Therefore, the convexity or greater curvature side of the proximal aorta is subject to higher regional stresses no doubt affecting the propensity for stress-induced damage.

The third dimension of aortic wall mechanics is also important. While longitudinal and axial stresses are tensile during loading and unloading of the aorta during each cardiac cycle, radial stresses may actually change from compressive during systole to tensile during diastole depending upon the residual strain in the outer layers of the media. That is, as the aorta is depressurized, the differential strain energies resident in different layers of the aorta will tend to pull the layers apart, especially if the magnitude of this differential stress exceeds the blood pressure at that point. This has important implications for the development of intramural hematoma and AD. Further, in vivo, there are additional stress and strain components related to the shear forces exerted on intimal surfaces by flowing blood and at curves and branch points. These shearing forces are of no consequence when considering the mechanical properties of isolated aortic segments in a physiology laboratory but may be of considerable importance in the local, microscopic analysis of aortic function and pathophysiology.

Creep is a materials property that is relevant to most mechanical systems. Materials with persistent or repeated loading to levels below the yield point exhibit small but cumulative plastic deformation over time. Collagen,[30] elastin, and other structural elements of the aortic wall are subject to this process. Therefore, the aorta dilates over time as is clearly seen by the one millimeter per decade increase in aortic size that accompanies aging.[3] Fatigue is yet another

relevant material process by which catastrophic failure under conditions of repeated loading can occur at loads well below the yield point. Considering that, at an average heart rate of only 60, the aorta will be subjected to 31 536 000 loading cycles per year, fatigue characteristics of its constituent elements are obviously of major importance.

Micromechanical Model of the Aortic Wall

The aorta functions to provide a predefined degree of distension when pressurized, with a limit at peak systole, and then elastic recoil as has been described. It has been difficult to purify and test elastin without contaminating microfibrils; however, recent studies reveal a linear stress-strain response with equal stiffness in circumferential and axial directions. Isolated elastin appears to have an elastic modulus of approximately 80 kPa,[31] whereas the elastic modulus of fibrillin-rich microfibrils is approximately 80 MPa or three orders of magnitude greater.[32] Collagen fibers are even stiffer with an elastic modulus between 300 and 2500 MPa and maximum strains of only 3% to 4%[27] and provide the outer limit of vessel wall distension.

Since stress-strain curves (see Figure 27-5) demonstrate a smooth transition between the elastic compliance of elastin and the stiffness of collagen, there must exist a mechanism to dampen this transition. In the classic Maxwell model of viscoelasticity, the elastic component is represented by a spring and the transition damper by a dashpot (analogous to the device attached to a spring-loaded door to keep it from slamming shut). The precise microstructural mechanism for this coupling remains to be defined but a model can be proposed from available research. A modified Maxwell model[33] has been described using the disconnecting hook element of Wiederhielm[34] to describe the relationship of smooth muscle cells, elastin, and collagen in human brachial arteries. This model has been criticized on the basis of additional engineering measurements made on collagenase digested specimens by Van Bavel et al. in rat mesenteric arteries and a serial element model proposed[35] (Figure 27-7 and Figure 27-8). This serial element model may better explain the collagen data since excessive strains exceeding the 3% to 4% observed for collagen fibers may be required for the hook model. In electron micrographs, collagen exists in substantial circumferential bundles and pericellular interlacing fibrils.[36] Sokolis and collegues have described a three part constitutive mathematical expression for the nonlinear stress-strain relationship of the aortic wall represented graphically in Figure 27-5,[37] the first part corresponding to low stresses up to a uniaxial load of 40 kPa (which would roughly correspond to an intraluminal pressure of 30 torr), the second part up to 120 kPa (intraluminal pressure roughly 90 torr), and the third part for higher stresses. Attempting to correlate the three part stress-strain observation with aortic microstructure, micrographs of rabbit descending aorta were fixed at various stress levels from each of the three parts and demonstrated progressive straightening of wavy elastic lamellae through part I, then extension and compaction in parts II and III. Collagen remained

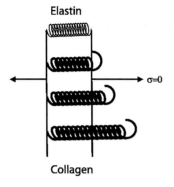

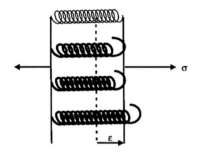

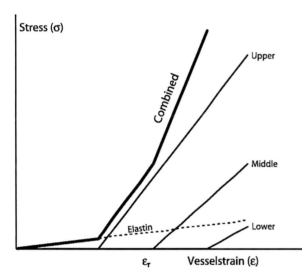

● **FIGURE 27-7.** The hook-on model of the elastin-collagen interaction with predicted stress-strain curves. Note the significant strains required of the initial collagen fibers to be engaged before longer fibers "hook on."

Reproduced, with permission, from VanBavel E, Siersma P, Spaan JA. Elasticity of passive blood vessels: a new concept. Am J Physiol Heart Circ Physiol. 2003;285:H1986–H2000.

corrugated through part I but tended to reorient toward the direction of stress. During stressing into part II, the collagen fibers continued to reorient and some began to uncoil. Well into part III the collagen fibers were almost straight and densely packed (Figure 27-9). In this study of uniaxial, longitudinal loading, circumferentially oriented elastic fibers, and collagen bundles did not change from their unstressed wavy, or tangled appearance suggesting that these circumferential elements are not tensioned with orthogonal uniaxial loading and are not firmly attached to the longitu-

dinal elements. This feature allows for differential biaxial distensibility since orthogonal elements must slide over one another, yet also facilitates separation of layers under radial tension (as in dissection or intramural hematoma). Silver et al.[38] have proposed that at least some of the collagen fibrils in the media are in series with smooth muscle cells and this collagen-smooth muscle cell network is in parallel with parallel networks of collagen and elastic tissue, as in the model of VanBavel et al.

Smooth muscle cells in the aortic media have been termed *spannmuskeln* and those in muscular distributing arteries *ringmuskeln* by Benninghof (Figure 27-10)[27] with the latter arrangement functioning to regulate arterial caliber and the former configuration, unique to the aorta, and large elastic arteries, providing for the maintenance of aortic distensibility. As described above, proximal aortic *spannmuskeln* are suspended in the interlamellar space (see Figure 27-2), likely under tension, given that their long axis of orientation is circumferential, parallel to the orientation of the major collagen fibers. It appears that oxytalen fibers containing fibrillin microfibrils as well as type VI collagen are responsible for suspending smooth muscle cells under tension along with elastic lamellar extensions. That these VSMC-elastic lamellar connections are likely of considerable mechanical strength has been demonstrated by Dingemans et al. in an ultrastructural study of severely pathologic areas of aorta where these connections often remained intact.[39] Since elastic lamellae are wavy in the unstressed state and the waviness resolves under tension, it appears that the fibrillin-rich microfibrils within elastic fiber extensions and oxytalen fibers become tensioned along with VSMCs, which shift from a radial-tilt along waves of elastic lamellae to a more nearly straight circumferential orientation. Fibrillin-rich microfibrils are much stiffer than elastin, approaching the lower limit of collagen stiffness but are, to some degree, extensible.[10] Further, microfibrils are incorporated into elastic fiber structure perhaps in a parallel configuration with elastin within microelements and creating a serial microelement arrangement as proposed by van Bavel et al. and Silver et al. with the elastin-fibrillin-smooth muscle cell interaction acting as the "dashpot" at strains below those at which collagen fibers are engaged. Once elastic lamellar deformation has occurred, smooth muscle cells and microfibrils are tensioned, and, after some small additional strain, given the high elastic modulus of microfibrils, the much tougher, stiff collagen fibers are tensioned preventing further strain on all elastic elements and acting like a door stop. This arrangement would allow for smooth muscle cell signaling in response to tension and strain both for elastic and nonextensible components as well as explaining the three part wall tension-radius curves. Since fibrillin with its EGF domains is intimately involved in this mechanical cell signaling mechanism, interference with the fibrillin-smooth muscle cell relationship could have important pathophysiologic implications for the maintenance not only of microfibrils but for collagen and elastic fibers as well.

It is noteworthy that oxytalen fibers, collagen fibers, and smooth muscle cells are oriented in a circumferential or

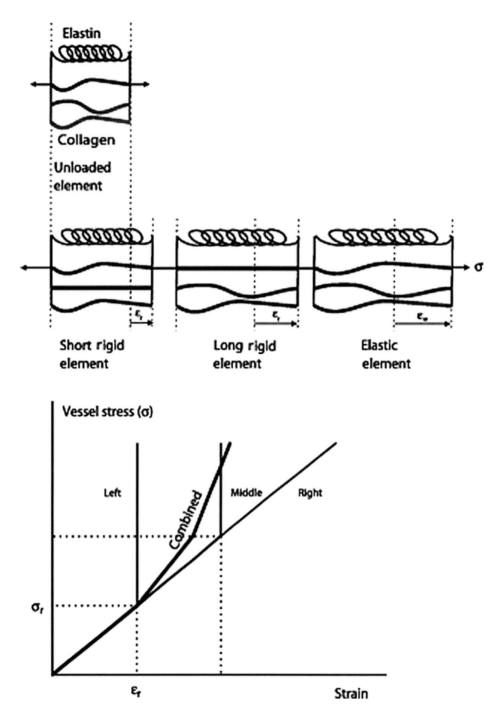

● FIGURE 27-8. Serial element model of the elastin-collagen interaction with predicted stress-strain curves.

Reproduced, with permission, from VanBavel E, Siersma P, Spaan JA. Elasticity of passive blood vessels: a new concept. Am J Physiol Heart Circ Physiol. 2003;285:H1986–H2000.

tangential direction with fewer fibers providing radial inter-lamellar connections. This allows the sliding of orthogonally oriented elements and adjacent lamellae as outlined above. Additionally, this arrangement provides plains of dissection allowing the surgical technique of endarterectomy that involves removal of the intima and most severely damaged inner layers of the media. Not surprisingly, in a study of pig aortas, the radial tensile properties were considerably different from longitudinal or circumferential ones demonstrating a much lower elastic modulus, calculated immediately prior to tissue failure, with failure occurring at lower levels of stress than would be required for disruption in other directions.[40] As has been described, radial forces are generally compressive rather than tensile with pressurization of the aorta; however, radial tension is to be expected in the propagation of AD.

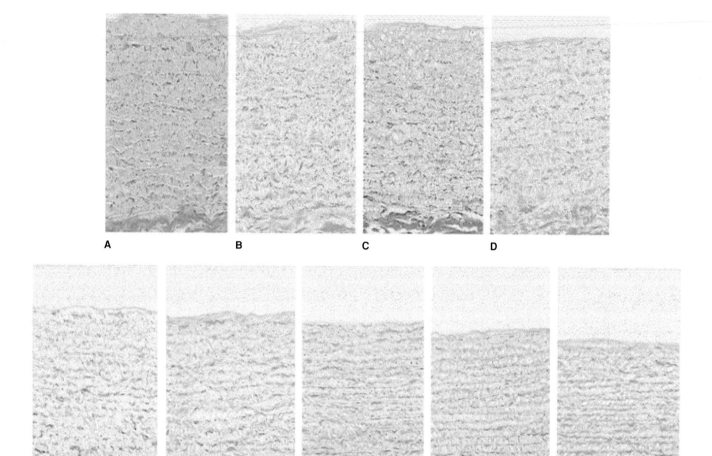

● **FIGURE 27-9.** Longitudinal sections of the aortic wall fixed while subjected to progressive levels of stress. Collagen fibers are stained red and smooth muscle cell nuclei black. The tortuosity of collagen fibers is highest (A) and (B), and remains unchanged in (C) and (E), yet, in these figures, collagen fibers are progressively reoriented with increasing stress toward the longitudinal direction. In (G), a large number of reoriented fibers are straightened in the region of the tunica media close to the adventitia, and finally in (I), only straightened fibers are observed through the entire media (Sirus red, × 20).

Reproduced, with permission, from Sokolis DP, Kefaloyannis EM, Kouloukoussa M, Marinos E, Boudoulas H, Karayannacos PE. A structural basis for the aortic stress-strain relation in uniaxial tension. J Biomech. 2006;39:1651–1662.

● PATHOPHYSIOLOGY OF PROXIMAL AORTIC DISEASE

Animal Models of Aortic Disease

In a remarkable experiment in aortic pathophysiology, Opitz et al. created a bioengineered aortic graft by seeding autologous VSMCs on a bioresorbable scaffold. After dynamically culturing the cells an endothelial layer was added and an additional intestinal submucosal wrap was applied and the grafts implanted in the descending aorta of juvenile sheep, creating a three layered neoaorta. All was well at 3 months with a confluent endothelial layer and no sign of dilation or occlusion. However by 6 months, there was severe degeneration of the graft with significant dilation and thrombus formation. Although histology showed layered tissue formation with alternating layers of VSMCs and matrix elements resembling native aorta, the elastin content of the grafts was significantly reduced compared to native aorta. Elastin and elastic fibers are therefore absolutely essential to prevent aneurysmal degeneration of collagen-bounded vascular structures.[17]

Genetically engineered mice have been created with several different deficits in elastic fiber components and have added greatly to the understanding of ascending aortic homeostasis and pathophysiology. A mutant mouse line was created with an internally deleted fibrillin-1 gene (the

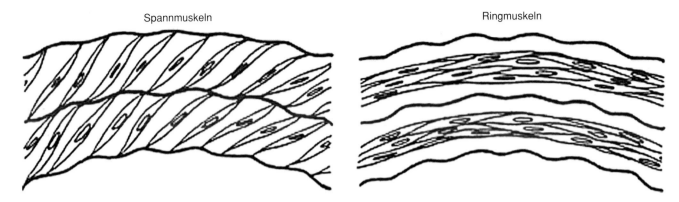

Spannmuskeln

Ringmuskeln

● **FIGURE 27-10.** Diagram illustrating *spannmuskeln* and *ringmuskeln*. Spannmuskeln are found in the aorta and large elastic arteries. Ringmuskeln are found in muscular distributing arteries. Arterioles are largely ringmuskeln with small amounts of connective tissue. This arrangement facilitates the function of elastic recoil in the aorta and pressure wave dampening in the large distributing arteries, while in muscular distributing arteries and arterioles it facilitates regulation of vessel caliber and flow distribution.

Reproduced, with permission, from Dobrin PB. Mechanical properties of arteries. Physiol Rev. 1978;58:397–460.

mutant allele mgΔ) reducing fibrillin-1 expression more than 10-fold. Homozygous mgΔ mice die soon after birth of vascular complications but exhibit normal elastic fibers between focal lesions and heterozygous mgΔ mice survive into adulthood appearing phenotypically normal, thus demonstrating the predominant role of fibrillin-1 in homeostasis rather than embryogenesis of elastic fibers.[41] Another mutant allele of fibrillin-1, the mgR allele, creates a hypomorphic mutation with homozygous animals demonstrating a fivefold reduction in fibrillin-1 gene expression. These mice have become a model for the study of Marfan's syndrome (MFS) demonstrating many of its phenotypic manifestations including vascular lesions, kyphosis and skeletal abnormalities, diaphragmatic hernias, and pulmonary insufficiency with early death at 3 to 6 months of age. Vascular lesions were characterized by intimal hyperplasia, medial calcification, and smooth muscle invasion of the intima with ectopic collagen and elastin deposition. Monocytic infiltration of the media occurred with fragmentation of elastic lamellae, loss of elastin content, and aneurysm formation[41] Elastin null mice die of obstructive arterial disease related to subendothelial cell proliferation and smooth muscle cell reorganization. Phenotypically, the hemizygous counterparts of elastin-null mice resemble patients with supravalvular aortic stenosis (SVAS). Fibulin-1 null mice die shortly after birth of blood vessel rupture and fibulin-5 null mice demonstrate a generalized deficit of elastic tissue with stiff tortuous aortas, emphysema, and loose skin.[8]

Pathophysiology of Clinical Proximal Aortic Defects

The pathophysiology of proximal aortic disease clearly involves a complex interaction of genetic abnormalities, developmental miscues, environmental factors, and injury. The results include several clinical outcomes. Traumatic penetration or rupture of the aortic wall may lead to exsanguinating hemorrhage, pseudoaneurysm formation, or pericardial tamponade since the ascending aorta is an intrapericardial structure. There are macrostructural developmental abnormalities of aortic alignment, patency, conotruncal septation, aortic arch branching, and sidedness. Aortic wall microstructural disorders, many congenital in origin, lead to the formation of aneurysms, intramural hematoma, and dissection. Atherosclerosis and inflammatory disease lead to degeneration of the aortic wall with the development of penetrating ulcers, distal embolization of atheromatous material, calcification, aneurysms, and rupture. Loss of normal, physiologic aortic compliance from aortic wall disease is associated with hypertension and has important consequences both for cardiac function and for downstream vascular and end-organ function.

Pathophysiology of Morphologic Macrostructural Defects

The precise, pathogenetic mechanisms for congenital malformations affecting the proximal aorta remain largely undetermined; however, an outline can be constructed. Embryogenesis involves genes and gene products with specific signaling functions. Interference with the genes themselves or with the signals or their reception increases the likelihood of aberrant structure.

The chromosomal defect, 22q11.2 deletion (DiGeorge syndrome), is characterized by aortic and cardiac anomalies, T-cell deficits, facial and palatal defects, and thyroid and parathyroid defects. More than 30 genes are deleted in the syndrome, but the resulting haploinsufficiency of the TBX1 gene appears to be the major determinant of the phenotype since isolated TBX1 mutations cause a very similar clinical picture.[42] Significant aortic defects associated with 22q11 deletion are right-sided aortic arch, an abnormal aortic arch branching pattern, both abnormal sidedness and branching abnormalities, and truncus arteriosus.[43] The TBX1 gene is a member of the T-box gene family found to be essential for normal heart development.[44]

The CFC1 gene, a member of the EGF-CFC (epidermal growth factor-Cripto/FRL-1/Cryptic) family which encodes extracellular proteins participating in early embryogenesis, is associated with heterotaxy (abnormal sidedness) and mutations have been implicated in some cases of isolated transposition of the great arteries and double outlet right ventricle.[45] Low expression VEGF haplotypes are associated with an increased risk of tetralogy of Fallot.[46] Thus alterations in the amplitude and precision of cell-signaling by the products of haploinsufficient genes, underexpressed gene products, or abnormal proteins result in diverse but stereotypical anomalies.

Since the expression of a normal phenotype or an aberrant one may depend upon slight differences in the configuration of a protein signal or of a mutated transcriptional regulator, such as Nkx2.5,[47] complex patterns, and incomplete penetrance result with few families demonstrating classic mendelian inheritance. Evidence from fetal screening of subsequent first-degree relatives of probands with congenital heart disease supports this interpretation.[48]

It is apparent that fetal environmental factors may be important in some cases with maternal diabetes known to be a significant risk factor for transposition of the great arteries as well as ventricular septal defect and other forms of congenital heart disease.[49] In a case control study in Finland, maternal first trimester upper respiratory infection was found to be a significant risk factor for hypoplastic left heart syndrome.[50] Eghtesady has suggested that hypoplastic left heart syndrome may be analogous to rheumatic heart disease with maternal antibodies to group A beta-hemolytic streptococci crossing the placenta leading to an immune mediated injury to the developing left ventricle or left-sided valves through a mechanism of molecular mimicry.[51] A recent report of monochorionic twins where one twin had hypoplastic left heart syndrome and the other a bicuspid aortic valve (BAV)[52] supports the interpretation that some factors such as antigenic mimicry in developing valvular tissue and maternal antibody interference in the embryonic response to flow patterns and developing mesenchymal cell signaling cause a perturbation with multiple related but not precisely predictable outcomes.

Pathophysiology of Wall Defects Leading to Aneurysm and Dissection in the Thoracic Aorta

The development of thoracic aneurysms and dissection (TAAD) results from a defect in aortic wall microstructure that renders the aorta incapable of resisting plastic deformation or material failure under physiologic loading conditions. Defects involving elastic fibers are likely responsible for most proximal aortic aneurysms, while dissection and rupture represent a failure of collagen fibers or their connections. Aneurysm and dissection of the ascending aorta are often not associated with atherosclerosis in contrast to these processes occurring in the more distal aorta, and in fact, patients manifesting these conditions have a lower incidence of atherosclerosis, as determined by a lesser degree of vascular calcification, not only involving the aorta itself but coronary arteries as well.[53]

Elastic Fiber Defects. Elastic fiber defects frequently result from mutations of genes encoding for microfibril proteins or matrix proteins involved in the maintenance and cellular interactions of elastic fibers. While some defects may be acquired later in life, heritable defects observed in families allow for the identification and characterization of the genes and gene products involved.

MFS (OMIM154700) is caused by a defect in the activity of the fibrillin I gene (FBN1), mapped to 15q21.1. The syndrome is characterized by cardiovascular defects including proximal aortic aneurysm, skeletal abnormalities with overgrowth of long bones, ocular abnormalities including ectopia lentis, restrictive lung disease related to thoracic bony deformities, spontaneous pneumothorax and bleb disease, striae atrophica of the skin, and dural ectasia. More than 500 mutations have been identified with more than 90% representing private mutations unique to an individual or family.[54] Dominance in MFS is felt to be caused by a dominant-negative effect resulting from adverse activity of the mutant protein on the deposition, stability, or function of the normal protein encoded by the normal copy of FBN1. Haploinsufficiency of the normal protein, however, also seems critical for the development of the Marfan's phenotype.[54]

Mutations in the genes encoding for transforming growth factor beta (TGFbeta) receptors 1 and 2 (TGFBR1 and 2) are an important cause of proximal aortic aneurysm and dissection. Affected kindreds with TGFBR2 mutations have been seen not only with proximal aortic involvement but with descending and abdominal aortic, pulmonary artery, carotid, cerebral, renal, and popliteal aneurysms.[55] A phenotype very similar to MFS but lacking ocular findings has been termed MFS type II (MFS2) and documented to have TGFBR2 mutations.[56] TGFBR2 has been mapped to 3p24-25. Wide phenotypic variability is seen in TGFBR2 mutations. An important phenotype is the Loeys-Dietz syndrome.[57] This syndrome consists of severe aortic and branch vessel aneurysmal disease and arterial tortuosity, craniofacial involvement consisting of crainiosynostosis, cleft palate, hypertelorism, bifid uvula, structural brain abnormalities, and may include mental retardation. Skeletal abnormalities, translucent skin, patent ductus, and atrial septal defects were also seen. This has been termed Loeys-Dietz syndrome type I (LDS I). Loeys-Dietz syndrome type II is defined as a phenotype with similar vascular findings but resembling vascular Ehlers-Danlos syndrome (EDS) in other respects such as joint laxity, translucent skin, bowel or splenic rupture, or rupture of the gravid uterus. LDS patients have a characteristically more virulent propensity for aortic rupture than patients with MFS or other familial aneurysm syndromes but, unlike vascular EDS patients, aortic surgery can generally be successfully accomplished.[57]

TGFBR1 mutations are also associated with LDS phenotypes and map to 9q 33-34.

Cutis laxa syndromes form a heterogeneous group of connective tissue disorders characterized by loose, sagging skin, sometimes caused by mutations in the elastin (ELN) gene but also caused by mutations in fibulin genes.[58] An autosomal resessive form of fibulin-4 deficiency results in cutis laxa and ascending aortic aneurysms as well as vascular tortuosity, developmental emphysema, hernias, joint laxity, and pectus excavatum.[59] The fibulin-4 (FBLN4) or EGF-containing fibulinlike extracellular matrix protein 2 (EFEMP2) gene maps to 11q13 (OMIM 604633). Pseudoxanthoma elasticum (PXE) is an elastic tissue disorder caused by mutations in the gene encoding for the transmembrane transporter protein adenosine triphosphate binding cassette (ABC)-C6 and results in calcification of elastic fibers in the skin eyes, and cardiovascular system.[60] An association of a PXE phenotype associated with beta-thalassemia and ascending aneurysm has been described.[61]

ELN gene disorders affecting the aorta observed clinically do not primarily involve elastic fiber degredation and aneurysm formation but rather haploinsufficiency states associated with hyperplastic intimal lesions resulting in SVAS and segmental arterial occlusion. Homozygous ELN mutations are likely not compatible with life. Two forms of the disorder have been characterized. The first involves isolated ELN mutations mapped to 7q11.2 (OMIM 185500) and the second a multiple gene deletion most often involving the hemizygous deletion of a 1.5-mB interval at 7q11.23 (OMIM 194050). The latter defect is associated with the Williams-Beuren syndrome phenotype which consists of SVAS, elfin facies, hypercalcemia, growth deficiency, and developmental delay. The mechanism of smooth muscle cell proliferation is unclear, but it has been suggested that insoluble elastin may either initiate an antimitogenic signal or block mitogenic signals[62] transduced by EGF-type molecules. Thus, the homeostatic response to local tension and flow is distorted and rather than a normal smooth muscle cell response resulting in elastic fiber and collagen development and homeostasis an inappropriate cellular proliferation results.

Isolated familial ascending aortic aneurysm and dissection (TAAD) defects have been mapped to 5q and 16p in addition to 3p, 9q, 11q, and 15q as mentioned above (OMIM 607086). Mutations in MYH11, mapped to 16p12.2-p13.13, represent a defect primarily of a VSMC protein rather than elastic fiber proteins per se. The mutation affects the smooth muscle myosin heavy chain resulting in marked aortic stiffness and large areas of medial degeneration with very low smooth muscle cell content. Affected kindreds demonstrate autosomal dominant inheritance with TAAD and patent ductus.[63]

Bicuspid Aortic Valve and Proximal Aortic Aneurysm. BAV is a heritable defect[64] with a significant likelihood of associated ascending aortic aneurysm. While it has been debated as to whether the aneurysm is related primarily to the hemodynamic properties of the bicuspid valve,[65] sub-stantial evidence supports the notion that there exists a concomitant aortic wall defect.[66–69] Subjects with BAVs represent a heterogenous group; some with two symmetric leaflets, some with fusion of two fairly normal-sized leaflets and a correspondingly smaller second leaflet, and others with varying degrees of asymmetry. Some bicuspid valves are regurgitant and others stenotic and some with varying degrees of both hemodynamic conditions. The resulting flow dynamics are obviously variable as are the configurations of aneurysmal disease. The most common configuration, often associated with aortic stenosis involves primarily the ascending aorta above the STJ while a phenotype observed in younger males involves the aortic root.[70] Ascending aneurysms often show characteristic asymmetry with bulging and elongation toward the convexity.[71] Nevertheless, studies on tissue samples in BAV subjects compared to control subjects add to our understanding of the pathophysiology of aortic dilation. Fedak et al. found that the proximal aorta of BAV subjects had a lower fibrillin-1 content, albeit with a pattern of significant overlap with controls, in ascending aortic samples (in the anterior aorta one cm above the STJ) as well as in pulmonary artery samples. Additionally, an increase in proMMP-2 was discovered in both locations but only in the aortic specimens was there an increase in MMP-2 itself. Elastin, collagen, and MMP-9 were not different than in controls.[67] Cotrufo et al. compared tissue samples obtained from the convexity (greater curvature) and the concavity (lesser curvature) of the ascending aorta 2 cm above the STJ in BAV subjects and in controls. BAV subjects had decreased types I and III collagen in both the convexity and concavity but the magnitude of the reduction was significantly greater in the convexity. Type IV collagen levels were increased in the dilated BAV aortas and more so in subjects with stenotic as opposed to regurgitant lesions. Levels of mRNA for type I collagen were noted to be diminished from normal in BAV aortas with regurgitant valves but similar to controls in those with stenotic valves. Tenascin, a protein with crucial roles in embryonic development and tissue remodeling involving collagen, was virtually absent in controls but present in dilated BAV aortas and to a greater degree in the convexity of regurgitant valve cases.[65] It therefore appears that hemodynamic factors play a significant role in modulating the effects of an intrinsic defect in aortic structural maintenance that favors degredation of smooth muscle cells, elastic components, and collagen despite a local stress environment that should favor conservation or reinforcement of these elements. This suggests a role for gene regulation defects; however no such genetic locus has been mapped or specific genes identified at this point.

Primary Collagen Defect: Vascular EDS. Vascular EDS IV is caused by structural defects in the pro α_1-III chain of collagen III encoded by COL3A1.[72] Patients with this defect have a median survival of 48 years with death resulting most frequently from arterial rupture.[73] Obstetric complications and spontaneous bowel rupture are also commonly associated with morbidity and mortality in vascular

EDS.[73,74] Since there may be significant phenotypic overlap with other defects such as type II Loeys-Dietz syndrome which results from TGFBR1 or 2 mutations, descriptions of patients without a molecular diagnosis may be misleading. Vascular EDS patients do not have aneurysmal disease but present with arterial rupture or dissection of normal-sized arteries. Surgical treatment of ascending AD is often unsuccessful.[75,76] In the series of vascular EDS patients reported from the Mayo clinic,[75] three cases of ascending AD were described with two operative deaths and the third dying a few years later of rupture of an anastomotic pseudoaneurysm from the aortic repair. When aneurysms do occur they are likely pseudoaneurysms.[77,78] This defect demonstrates the role of type III collagen reinforcement in the integrity of the aortic wall, with collagen fibers preventing catastrophic deformation of the elastin-microfibril-smooth muscle cell complex.

While vascular EDS is not primarily associated with true aneurysms, other forms of EDS are associated with a significant incidence of aortic root dilation.[79] Thus, some forms of collagen likely play a role in the connections among fibrillin microfibers and VSMCs.

Matrix Degredation and TAAD. The role of MMPs has been investigated in the pathogenesis of ascending aortic aneurysm and dissection. MMP-1 and MMP-9 expression have been found to be significantly increased over controls in human TAAD specimens obtained at surgery.[80] The highest levels of MMP-9 expression were found in dissection specimens and MMP-2 expression was also higher for dissection than aneurysm. TIMP-1 was not different from controls and TIMP-2 was actually increased in the patient group suggesting at least some degree of modulation of the increased elastase and collagenase activity. Nevertheless, the ratio of MMP-9 to TIMP-1 was significantly elevated in both aneurysm and dissection groups suggesting an imbalance favoring structural degradation. In experimental models of abdominal aortic and descending aortic aneurysms in mice induced by bathing the external surface of the aorta in a $CaCl_2$ solution both MMP-2 and MMP-9 are apparently required to produce aneurysms[81,82] since mice deficient in MMP-2 or MMP-9 failed to develop aneurysms despite $CaCL_2$ induction. While these studies did not involve the ascending aorta, the $CaCl_2$ induction mechanism may be relevant to the ascending aorta since the elastic fiber defects known to produce ascending aneurysms involve molecules such as fibrillin with Ca-binding EGF domains and these molecules are likely significantly affected by excess calcium. It may be that cell-signalling properties are more significantly altered than mechanical properties and that inappropriate activation of cellular activities involving MMP secretion and apoptosis underlie the pathogenesis of these aneurysms. This would be consistent with the dominant negative effect of a single mutant FBN1 allele as proposed for MFS. In a study of aortic specimens obtained from the anterior proximal aorta adjacent to the STJ, Boyum et al. discovered that aneurysms associated with a BAV demonstrated higher levels of MMP-2 and MMP-9 activity than those associated with tricuspid valves in a group that did not include MFS patients or dissection patients. TIMP-1 and -2 activities were not significantly different.[83] This finding would also support the notion of inappropriate signaling related to some intrinsic defect in BAV patients. Despite the association of emphysema and ascending aneurysm in some MFS and other TAAD phenotypes, it is interesting that no association has been made between TAAD and α_1-antitrypsin deficiency. Further, no definitely characterized TIMP deficit has been found in association with TAAD although one would expect such a heritable deficit to exist.

Medial Degeneration and Apoptosis. VSMCs are the metabolic factories responsible for the production and maintenance of collagen, elastic fiber elements, and other extracellular matrix proteins in the aortic media. Cystic medial degeneration (CMD) is a noninflammatory process involving the proximal aorta and characterized by loss of VSMCs with associated elastin fragmentation, focal fibrosis, and accumulation of acid mucopolysaccharides (glycoprotiens) and collagen in a patchy distribution.[84] In a study of AD specimens, Ihling et al. demonstrated clear evidence of apoptosis or progammed cell death as the cause for VSMC loss. The tumor suppressor gene p53 was found more prominently in the VSMCs of dissected aortas in association with Bcl2 associated protein X (Bax) a proapoptotic protein of the Bcl2 family which consists of both pro- and antiapoptotic peptides.[84] Complementary techniques including TUNEL labeling, biochemical DNA fragmentation analysis, electron microscopy, and ASP/c-jun staining further support an apoptosis mechanism rather than some other source of direct cellular injury. Schmid and colleagues have also demonstrated strong evidence for apoptosis of VSMCs in material from aneurysmal ascending aortas in patients with both tricuspid and BAV. The process appeared worse in BAV aortas.[85,86] Increased deposition of types I and III collagen as a result of elevated connective tissue growth factor expression was found in AD specimens removed at surgery by Wang and colleagues[87] suggesting a remodeling process that replaces elastic tissue with nondistensible collagen.

Morphology of TAAD Affecting the Proximal Aorta

McKusick described the classic form of aortic root aneurysm associated with MFS as "... predominant involvement of the base of the aorta or most of the ascending aorta (in progressively lesser degree as one passes away from the heart, usually with rather sharp stopping of the alterations at the mouth of the innominate artery)...".[88] This pattern has been termed annuloaortic ectasia and characteristically stops proximal to the innominate artery origin (Figures 27-11 and 27-12). The coronary ostia are displaced superiorly and the aortic sinuses are aneurysmal. Aneurysms associated with BAV are usually asymmetric

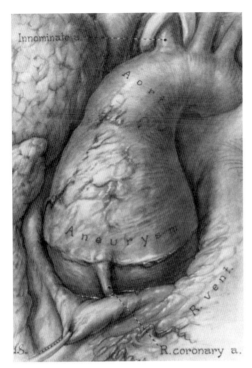

● **FIGURE 27-11.** Annuloaortic ectasia. An aneurysm of the ascending aorta in a patient with Marfan's syndrome is depicted from this early surgical paper of Bahnson and Nelson. The sinuses of valsalva the sinotubular junction and the proximal ascending aorta are most prominently involved.

Reproduced, with permission, from Bahnson HT, Nelson AR. Cystic medial necrosis as a cause of localized aortic aneurysms amenable to surgical treatment. Ann Surg. 1956;144:519–529.

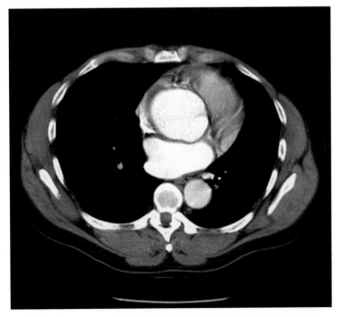

● **FIGURE 27-12.** Computed tomographic scan of a patient with an ascending aortic aneurysm involving the aortic root. Note the line of lucency in the opacified aortic root caused by the left coronary cusp of the aortic valve.

bulging, toward the convexity[71] and a smaller group, phenotypically similar to MFS annuloaortic ectasia as has been discussed above. Surprisingly, aortic wall thickness is not generally diminished or may be slightly increased in aneurysmal ascending aortas[25,88,89] (at least until the aneurysm reaches larger diameters greater than 6 cm—see below). Aneurysms may extend into the aortic arch and descending aorta; however, it is likely that aneurysms originating distal to the innominate artery origin are more likely to arise from atherosclerotic degeneration than those in the ascending aorta.

AD represents the final mode of failure for a large proportion of proximal aortic aneurysms. Larson and Edwards, in an extensive autopsy study of AD in 161 cases,[90] were able to identify an intimal tear in each case. Those cases where the tear originated in the ascending aorta, comprising 75% of the total group, had grade 3 or 4 atherosclerosis at the site of the intimal tear in only 9%, as opposed to this finding in 80% of cases where the tear originated in the descending aorta. Lansman et al. in a surgical series of 168 patients with acute dissection reported 139 cases of Stanford type A (type A involves the ascending aorta whereas type B only the descending aorta) with 60% having solitary ascending aortic tears and 30% having arch tears.[91] Eight type A cases had descending tears, 11 multiple tears, and in four cases an intramural hematoma but no tear was found. In the author's experience most ascending tears are transverse and linear, similar in appearance to those seen in patients with traumatic tears at the aortic isthmus associated with deceleration injuries, although in the latter instance the tears are more often completely circumferential and involve the full thickness of the aorta with the hematoma contained by the mediastinal pleura, while ascending tears and those descending tears associated with dissection are often less than circumferential and extend only into the outer layers of the media. A final breech of the aortic adventitia containing the false channel results in intrapericardial hemorrhage, tamponade, and death. Loss of support for the aortic valve, with resultant acute aortic insufficiency, and myocardial ischemia from coronary ostial dissection are additional potentially fatal consequences of Stanford type A AD.

Microstructural Pathology in Proximal Aortic TAAD

Cystic medial necrosis (or Erdheim's cystic medionecrosis) was once thought to be a more or less homogenous pathologic entity explaining the development of ascending aortic disease[92]; however it was also recognized that patients had typical pathologic findings with or without other elements of MFS[88] calling this concept into question. In a recent surgical series, 513 patients having resection of ascending aortic tissue, of whom 479 had TAAD as the primary indication for surgery, were reviewed.[93] Histologic findings included CMD in 209 cases defined as fragmentation and/or loss of elastic fibers associated with or without pools of glycoproteins. Laminar medial necrosis defined as coagulative necrosis of medial smooth muscle cells with collapse of elastic lamellae was found in 100 patients and coexisted with CMD, AD, aortitis, and other lesions in all but two. Of 109 patients with AD only 56 had CMD. Ninety patients were found to have normal media, 57% of whom had BAV. Thus significant aortic pathology can exist with some aortic tissue samples from involved aortas showing little or no histologic abnormality by light microscopy.

It has been discovered that histopathologic changes associated with ascending aneurysms vary with location within the aneurysm, the asymmetric collagen distribution in BAV aortas mentioned above providing one example. In ascending aneurysms associated with tricuspid aortic valves, the area of maximal dilation (MDA) demonstrates more advanced changes, with evidence of ineffective healing, while in the transition area (TA) immediately adjacent to normal aorta an active stage of the disease. In their study of these patients, Kirsch et al.[89] noted that overall aortic thickness was similar in the two areas but with an increase in adventitial thickness and a loss of media in the MDA. An increase in microvessels and macrophage infiltration was seen in the TA more than in the MDA. VSMCs were more abundant in the MDA but had lost their typical lamellar organization, whereas lamellar organization was preserved in the TA.

Dingemans and colleagues have made important ultrastructural observations from surgical and autopsy specimens obtained from dissected aortas. Comparisons were made with MFS and non-MFS patients and with normal aortic controls. There was a "striking similarity" between MFS and non-MFS aortas and every patient aorta studied contained large, relatively normal areas. Large dissections were always found in the outer third of the media, often only a few lamellar units from the adventitia or actually on the medial-adventitial border. Most patient aortas had fibrotic areas from which nearly all VSMCs had disappeared but some elastic lamellae remained. Normal aortas in subjects over 35 sometimes had transverse mural tears with sharp margins but in patient aortas an average of 20 transverse tears were identified and 30% of the tears were within 20 microns of large dissections. Tears were found in thick and compact elastic lamellae rather than in degenerated areas. While many areas maintained numerous elastic extensions and microfibrils (connections to VSMCs), a smaller number of adjacent areas contained smooth lamellae lacking elastic extensions and associated with isolated rounded elastin deposits likely representing detached extensions. The only clear microfibrillar abnormality was the focal loss of microfibrils associated with elastic extensions leading to detachment of VSMCs from elastic lamellae. Inflammatory cells were scarce in the media providing little support for the notion that inflammatory release of proteolytic enzymes plays any role in the pathogenesis of AD.[39]

Mechanisms of TAAD

Aneurysm Formation. Based upon this data some generalizations about the mechanisms of TAAD can be formulated. Ascending aneurysms are likely initiated by the degradation of the fibrillin-rich microfiber components of the elastic lamellar—VSMC complex (Figure 27-13). As outlined above, these microfiber elements contribute to the midrange stiffness of the aortic wall in the transition from highly compliant elastin to essentially noncompliant collagen, and are involved in the attachments of VSMCs to elastic lamellae. Therefore, degradation of fibrillin microfibers would not only increase the compliance of the aortic wall microelement effected and increase its length at any given pressure (more than 30 torr where there is a normal compliance transition and below which the compliance of elastin alone is operative) but also result in the detachment of VSMCs. If enough microelements of the aortic wall are affected the aorta will dilate and elongate. The aorta would also become measurably more compliant which is indeed the case for smaller-sized aneuryms (see below).

Maintenance of elastic lamellae is likely a major function of VSMCs and controlled by mechanical signals transduced through microfiber attachments. If the VSMC loses the attachments, the signal response would be one for "no stress" and degradation and probably even apoptosis of the cell. This would initiate a second phase of aneurysm formation whereby elastic and cellular components are lost. The affected microelement would eventually become nothing but collagen fibers. Since this defective microelement is connected in a linear series with other microelements resisting a circumferential or axial deformation and has no ability to recoil, that series of microelements will become longer, especially if several of its constituent microelements are similarly affected. The whole string of microelements will therefore not participate in subsequent loading cycles to the same extent as adjacent strings of microelements. This may result in additional nonmaintenance and apoptotic signals with the appearance of MMPs, tenascin, and other remodeling proteins and degradation of the collagen support of that string of microelements. While this process may result in a subsequent stress-induced signal to bolster the local collagen support from adventitial fibroblasts, the defective strings of medial microelements lacking VSMCs are incapable of restoring lost elastic components.

This process would then create a patch of more dilated, stiffer aortic wall that may provoke local supraphysiologic stress in the more normal adjacent strings of microelements and make aortas so affected weaker and more prone to AD and rupture.

To compound the degenerative process further, microelements dependent only upon the integrity of inextensible collagen fibers would continue to gradually lengthen since creep and fatigue are unmitigated by the viscoelastic absorption of energy by the "dashpot" mechanism. This would result in progressive plastic deformation of collagen even in the face of remaining cell signals promoting collagen reinforcement, since, responding to strain, the signal would be incrementally behind the elongation process.

Expression of MMPs, tenascin, and matrix degradation is to be expected in the remodeling process and not directly the result of inflammatory cell infiltration, a feature supported by the lack of inflammatory cells seen in

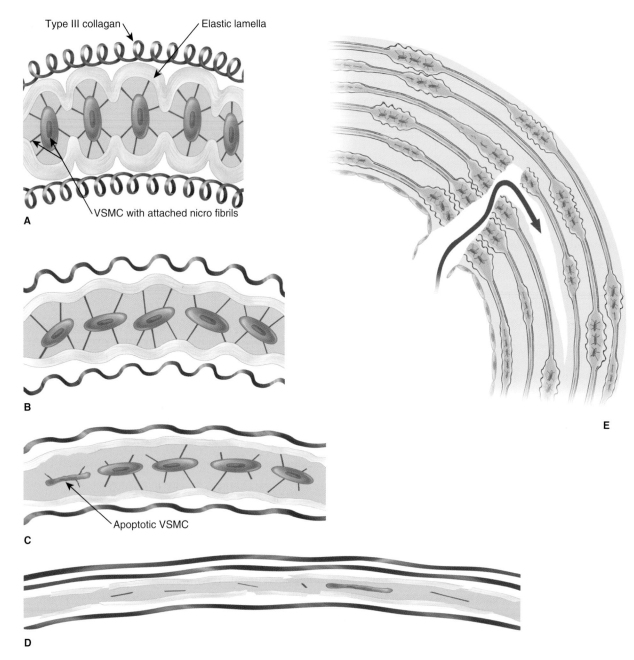

● FIGURE 27-13. Schematic representation of the stages of ascending aneurysm development. In (A), the aorta is not distended. Collagen fibers are coiled, the elastin is wavy, and VSMCs are suspended in the intercellular matrix by microfibers and type IV collagen. In (B), the aorta is pressurized. The thick type III collagen fibers begin to uncoil but at physiologic pressures the load is borne by elastin–fibrillin microfibril/type IV collagen-VSMC complexes and collagen fibers in most microelements remain slack until the extreme limit of distension. Microelements likely exist in a series arrangement within lamellae as described and may be of differing lengths. In (C), microfibers degenerate and there is associated apoptosis of VSMCs. The microelement becomes more compliant because its distensibility depends only upon that of elastin unmodified by the properties of attached microfibril-VSMC components. In (D), the VSMCs and microfibers have disappeared and the elastin components that depend upon fibrillin microfibers and VSMCs for their maintenance degenerate and no longer are load-bearing. The involved microelement assumes the dimension of its constituent type III collagen fibers with no capacity for elastic recoil and the microelement contributes to the permanent lengthening of the series of microelements in which it lies, contributing to permanent dilation and thinning of the aorta. In(E), a medial tear extends through the inner, more normal lamellae. In cases of aortic dissection this tear extends to the outer lamellae.

histologic samples of most proximal aortic aneurysms and is in contrast to the findings associated with atherosclerotic aneurysms involving more distal aortic segments. The fact that histologic sections taken from fragments of aneurysmal tissue show patchy areas of CMD, LMD, or even no pathologic change is compatible with this mechanism. The missing elastic lamellae-VSMC connections require electron microscopy to detect, the process is patchy, and affected lamellae and VSMCs may look normal in the unloaded, fixed state. Precisely how the initial loss of elastic extensions occurs is less clear and there seem to be multiple abnormalities that can be responsible, including abnormal fibrillin-1, TGFbeta receptor defects, and intrinsic VSMC defects as discussed earlier. In the case of mutated fibrillin-1 it would appear that mistaken EGF signaling results in a nonmaintenance signal for elastin-microfibril-cellular connections.

Dissection and Intramural Hematoma. Ascending AD (Figures 27-14 to 27-16) develops in the same milieu as do aneurysms. A mural tear occurs (a process seen in multiple areas in dissected aortas and occasionally in "normal" aortas), extends through the intima into the outer lamellae of the media and, as a result of shear stress on the edge of the tear coupled with longitudinal stress pulling the edges of the tear apart, pressurized blood gains entry into the interlamellar plain. Since there is very little interlamellar, radial, tensile strength as has been discussed and since the interlamellar plane may extend the entire length of the aorta and out into its branches, the dissection may involve all these areas. With the process set in motion by the loss of elastic extensions to VSMCs, apoptosis, and matrix degredation discussed above, not only is there elongation and dilation of the aorta but there are corresponding focal areas of aortic stiff-

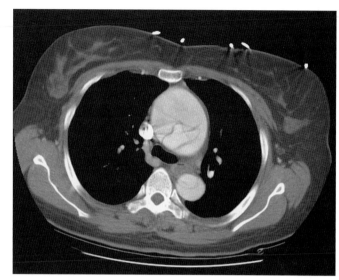

● **FIGURE 27-14.** Image from a computed tomographic scan of a patient with a bicuspid aortic valve and ascending aneurysm who developed acute type A aortic dissection. She required an emergency aortic root and hemiarch replacement utilizing not only cardiopulmonary bypass but a period of profound hypothermia and total circulatory arrest. Postoperatively she remains at risk for dilation and potential rupture of the remaining thoracic aorta since in the majority of cases blood flow into the false lumen persists. Further, the noncompliant ascending and arch prosthesis results in higher wall tension in the remaining aorta.

ening and loss of the energy absorbing "dashpot" function of the elastin-microfibril-VSMC-collagen coupling interaction described earlier. The mural tear does not involve these abnormal areas that have been remodeled from the compliant tissue responsible for aortic *Windkessel* properties to

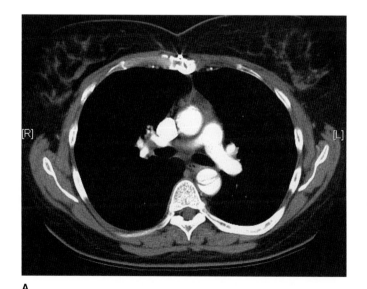

A

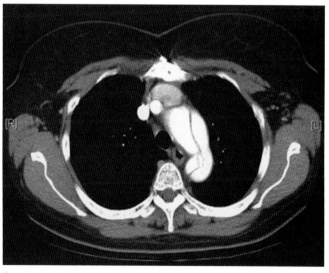

B

● **FIGURE 27-15.** (A and B). Images from a computed tomographic scan of the patient from Figure 15 made postoperatively showing the graft in the ascending aorta but residual flow in the false channel and overall dilation of the aorta involving the distal arch and descending aorta. The remaining aorta remains at risk for progressive dilation of the false lumen.

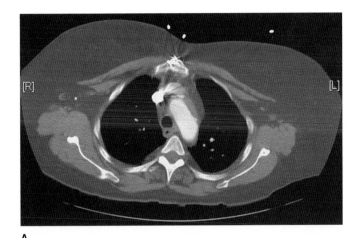

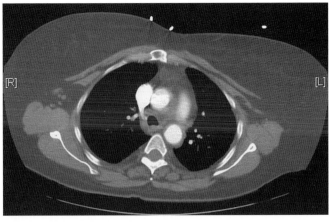

A

B

● FIGURE 27-16. (A and B). Images from a postoperative computed tomographic scan of another patient showing obliteration of the false channel leaving only wall thickening to mark the extent of the dissection. In both cases, Bioglu (tradename) surgical adhesive was used in an attempt to relaminate the dissected layers in the arch; however in the patient in Figures 15 and 16 there were very likely additional medial tears in the descending aorta that permitted continued entry into the false channel despite sealing the accessible areas in the arch.

tough, nonextensible material with the properties of a bag made of layers of collagen, through which the dissection can nevertheless propagate. The mural tear involves adjacent more normal elastic lamellae that are forced to absorb supraphysiologic strain energy. The combination of shear forces and longitudinal loading which creates the transverse defect are magnified by the downward displacement of the aortic root, particularly with aortic insufficiency and higher levels of inotropy, creating an area of high stress just above the STJ.[28] Although circumferential stress underlies the growth of aneurysms, mural tears are almost never longitudinal and circumferential stresses do not cause dissection. Further, while there are thick bundles of collagen oriented circumferentially that do not resist axial loading there are relatively thinner intralamellar collagen fibers oriented axially. Since the remodeling process creates medial thinning and adventitial thickening, associated with collagen deposition in the adventitia,[89] the inner, longitudinal collagen fibers are most vulnerable to rupture.

Dissection results from catastrophic collagen failure. In the case of vascular EDS, there is little evidence for true aneurysm formation or elastic fiber deficits and dissection occurs because of a defect of type III collagen by a similar mechanism but at lower levels of wall stress. TGFBR1 and 2 mutations may cause defects that have a greater affect on collagen homeostasis than FBN1 or other TAAD mutations since some TGFBR mutations are associated with LDS which has phenotypic overlap with vascular EDS.

In some cases atherosclerotic ulceration may be the site of mural entry for an ascending dissection as was suggested by the 9% of cases in the series of Larson and Edwards who had high-grade atherosclerosis at the tear site in the ascending aorta. Atherosclerotic ulceration is a much more common mechanism for entry into the interlamellar dissection plane for dissections originating in the arch or descending aorta.[90] Such ulceration (Figure 27-17) may re-

sult in rupture, intramural hematoma, and dissection and are a source of acute aortic syndromes, a group that includes penetrating ulcer, intramural hematoma, and acute dissection. Intramural hematomas (IMH) may occur from rupture of vaso vasora or in association with small mural tears that allow bleeding into the interlamellar space of an aorta with high levels of residual strain. Most commonly this occurs in older patients with stiffer aortas. Significant atherosclerotic disease with extensive medial involvement is protective toward the development of dissection or the

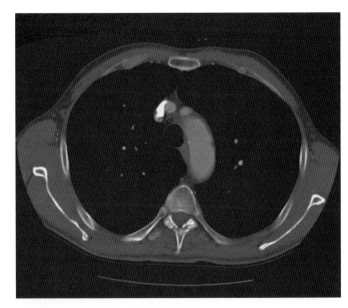

● FIGURE 27-17. Aortic arch image from a computed tomographic scan of a patient with an atherosclerotic ulcer arising in an area of wall thickening. The patient had otherwise unexplained chest pain at the time of presentation when the lesion was discovered and has been subsequently followed with medical treatment for blood pressure control and statin therapy.

enlargement of IMH since the interlamellar planes may be destroyed.

Mechanics of Proximal Aortic Aneurysm and Dissection

Despite extensive, mechanical, and physiologic research, a practical, in vivo means of assessing mechanical properties that allows the accurate prediction of aortic catastrophe across the range of patients seen in clinical practice remains a work in progress. Advances have been made in recent years by the study of aneurysmal aortic tissue obtained at surgery[25,94] and by the analysis of operative measurements and imaging data. Koullias et al.[95] studied ascending aortic aneurysms in vivo at the time of surgery for aneurysm repair and calculated distensibility, wall stress, and an incremental (tangential) elastic modulus (Einc) at a defined blood pressure, using an analysis based on circumferential stress and strain. A cylindrical model for the aneurysm shape is assumed as well. Since these parameters reflect an analysis only of circumferential loading and rupture and dissection result from axial loading, as has been described, there are inherent limitations in the model's ability to precisely predict rupture. Further, aneurysm shapes are variable, often not cylindrical but more spherical at the point of maximum dilation or eccentric as in the case of BAV. While a spherical shape may actually diminish circumferential wall stress (WS) (Pr/2h instead of Pr/h), there may be increased longitudinal wall stress at the transition zone from the cylindrical to the spherically shaped area especially if there is a loss of compliance in the spherical region. A more precise prediction of stress patterns based on aneurym shape can be made with a finite element analysis applied to high resolution three-dimensional images.[96] Such an analysis, however, is limited by its restriction to a static mode of loading and necessary assumptions of homogeneity in the aortic wall. Nevertheless, the analysis of Koullias et al. in conjunction with laboratory studies of the tensile properties of aneurysmal aortic tissue specimens provides important insights into the mechanical behavior of aneurysms in situ. In their study of 33 aneuryms and 20 normal aortas,[95] it was found that aortic distensibility is actually supernormal for small aneurysms less than 4 cm and does not fall below normal levels until the aneurysm exceeds 5 cm in diameter but falls to a very low level above 6 cm. Aneurysms greater than 4 cm showed a progressive rise in Einc until those over 6 cm had a value 5 times normal. These data demonstrate the virtual disappearance of functioning elastic elements by the time the aneurysm reaches 6 cm. Further, calculated WS was 857 ± 290.8 kPa for aneurysms greater than 6 cm at a systolic blood pressure of 220 torr. Interestingly, wall thickness was fairly constant until aneurysms exceeded 6 cm when it was 35% thinner, perhaps demonstrating the final compaction of elastic fiber-deficient lamellae. In the study of Vorp et al., tensile strength of longitudinally oriented ascending aortic aneurysm strips was 1180 ± 240 kPa whereas that for circumferentially oriented strips was 1210 ± 90 kPa. The corresponding values for normal aortas were 1800 kPa and 1710 kPa, respectively. This demonstrates a signif-

icant weakening in the aneurysm patients and shows the narrow margin between a blood pressure spike and catastrophe with the confidence range for tensile strength and WS overlapping. AD has been observed to occur in association with extreme physical exertion, especially weight lifting. In a cohort of 31 patients collected by Hatzaras et al.[97] AD occurred under such circumstances at a mean aortic diameter of 4.63 cm. To achieve a WS exceeding 1800 kPa in an otherwise healthy aorta would require a blood pressure spike in excess of 1000 torr, which seems unlikely. Therefore some form of aortic wall pathology must coexist in these patients and indeed this may be the case since muscular strength training has been shown to increase proximal aortic stiffness.[98]

This analysis of the mechanical properties of aneurysms supports the policy of elective operation for ascending aneurysms at 5.5 cm diameter given the marked deterioration of strength and mechanical properties at diameters above 6 cm. This has been the empirically generated recommendation for some time. Nevertheless there are some patients whose aortic wall pathology provokes a greater risk of rupture at smaller sizes, apparently related to a more virulent deterioration of collagen support. The standard recommendation for MFS patients is for elective surgery at 5 cm, a growth rate exceeding 1 cm/y, or for small aneurysms with a family history of dissection at a size less than 5 cm.[54] For patients with LDS it has been advised that elective surgical repair occur at 4 cm in adolescents and adults or when the aortic annulus exceeds 1.8 cm and the maximal ascending aortic dimension exceeds the 99th percentile for children. In this group, AD often occurs in childhood at aortic diameters well below 5 cm.[57] Patients with BAV also require special consideration since late AD and sudden death after aortic valve replacement (AVR) are significantly more likely than in AVR patients with tricuspid valves.[99,100] A policy of ascending aortic replacement at the time of AVR when the ascending aorta exceeds 4.5 cm is advocated by Borger et al.[100]

Proximal Aortic Stiffening

Loss of aortic compliance commonly accompanies aging and provides an important measure of biologic age.[101] In an MRI study, regional aortic compliance was greatest in the ascending aorta, lower in the arch, and lowest in the descending aorta and decreased with age. Athletes had significantly higher compliance than age-matched controls.[102] Isolated systolic hypertension (ISH) is associated with aortic stiffening and aging. However, in an analysis of data from the ENIGMA study,[103] there also exists a younger population with ISH, most of whom had an elevated stroke volume in conjunction with an increased pulse wave velocity (PWV). An increased PWV suggests aortic stiffening in the absence of an elevated stroke volume. A subset of these subjects had an elevated PWV but normal stroke volume suggesting that premature aortic stiffening may be responsible for their ISH. Graft replacement of the ascending aorta, an iatrogenic form of aortic stiffening since no currently available conduit material can duplicate the *Windkessel* properties of the native aorta, results in increased blood pressure, wall tension, and rate of pressure rise in the residual aorta.[104] The end result of progressive stiffening of the native aorta is a rigid, calcified tube with essentially no compliance, termed a porcelain aorta by surgeons. Aside from the difficulty encountered in attempts to suture material with the properties of alternating layers of egg shell and butter, aortic stiffening has important pathophysiologic implications. Increased aortic stiffness as measured by PWV results in an increase in all-cause and cardiovascular mortality and it has been estimated that the mortality risk associated with a 5 m/sec elevation of PWV is equivalent to aging 10 years.[105] Aortic stiffness is correlated with atherosclerosis, a likely major contributing cause, based on a monkey study of induced and regressed atherosclerosis.[106] Endothelial dysfunction is significantly associated with a loss of proximal aortic compliance as well.[107] Left ventricular hypertrophy (LVH) is associated with loss of arterial distensibility[108] and among patients with heart failure, a loss of aortic distensibility is associated with diminished exercise capacity independent of ejection fraction.[109] Direct catheter measurements of aortic distensibility in humans demonstrate a significant relationship between coronary artery disease and deterioration of aortic elastic properties.[110] It is thought that cerebral and renal microvascular disease develop as a consequence of a loss of elastic compliance in the central arterial system resulting in systolic hypertension, increased pulse pressure, and increased pulse wave velocity, with transmission of unmodulated pulsations to the microvessels of the brain and kidneys, since perfusion of these organs is unique in that the carotid and renal arteries provide little resistance to flow.[111]

While it is felt that drugs offer little direct benefit on the degenerated aorta, the angiotensin antagonists, calcium channel blockers, and nitrates are thought to reduce wave reflections associated with a loss of arterial compliance and central pulse pressure thereby mitigating the effects of systolic hypertension associated with aortic stiffening.[111] Exercise training is also beneficial, possibly as a result enhanced endothelial function and vascular remodeling although there is some controversy about the effects of excercise on arterial compliance.[112] While aerobic exercise has beneficial effects on measures of arterial compliance and systolic blood pressure, muscular strength training may have deleterious effects and has been shown to reduce proximal aortic compliance and raise pulse pressure.[98] Cigarette smoking results in impaired peripheral vascular endothelial function associated with decreased central arterial distensibility, most marked in the carotid arteries, and involving all segments of the aorta with an associated increase in PWV.[113] Aortic elastic properties show an acute deterio-ration on either active cigarette smoking or passive inhalation of tobacco smoke as demonstrated in a catheterization-based human subjects study.[114] It may be that VSMC contraction underlies this acute change since other apparently etiologic factors such as atherosclerosis appear to result in chronic, degenerative changes. In a study of pigs, bilateral vagotomy distal to the origin of the recurrent laryngeal nerves was associated with an increase in both collagen and elastin density and decreased VSMC density which resulted in aortic stiffening and increased tensile strength.[115] This may also implicate cholinergic VSMC stimulation as a mechanism for nicotinic effects in the aorta, possibly acutely resulting in activation of contractile proteins and subsequent chronic remodeling.

Proximal Aortic Atherosclerosis and Cerebrovascular Events

The presence of severe atherosclerosis of the ascending aorta in the absence of dissection or aneurysm with which it is rarely associated became a major concern with the recognition that surgical manipulation of an affected aorta was associated with a high risk of intraoperative stroke.[116] Further, patients presenting with ischemic stroke and no obvious embolic source have a much higher likelihood of echocardiographically evident, >4 mm aortic arch plaques than those with another possible cause.[117] In a study of 1957 coronary bypass patients assessed for the presence and severity of ascending aortic atherosclerosis by intraoperative epiaortic ultrasound, Davila-Roman et al. concluded that ascending atherosclerosis is a marker for severe atherosclerotic disease, is a direct cause of cerebral atheroembolism, and is an independent predictor of long-term neurologic events and mortality following coronary bypass surgery.[118] Ascending aortic wall thickness of >4 mm detected by intraoperative ultrasonography was prevalent in 26% of 387 patients selected for follow-up by Schachner et al. after coronary bypass surgery and was associated with an increased risk of late stroke.[119] In this same patient population the risk for an ascending aortic wall thickness >4 mm was correlated with age (mean age of patients with atheromas was 70 years), an elevated creatinine, higher EuroSCORE (European system for cardiac operative risk evaluation), and descending aortic wall thickness.[120] In the experience of the author, ongoing cigarette smoking is also a significant correlate. Epiaortic ultrasound scanning is therefore recommended to direct modifications in cardiac surgical techniques to prevent atheroembolic strokes in elderly smokers and in those with other atherosclerosis risk factors since it has been shown that inspection and palpation of the ascending aorta is not adequately sensitive in such patients.[120]

REFERENCES

1. Anderson RH. Clinical anatomy of the aortic root. *Heart.* 2000;84:670-673.

2. Hager A, Kaemmerer H, Rapp-Bernhardt U, et al. Diameters of the thoracic aorta throughout life as measured with helical computed tomography. *J Thorac Cardiovasc Surg.* 2002;123: 1060-1066.

3. Rammos S, Apostolopoulou SC, Kramer HH, et al. Normative angiographic data relating to the dimensions of the aorta

and pulmonary trunk in children and adolescents. *Cardiol Young.* 2005;15:119-124.

4. Kielty CM, Baldock C, Lee D, Rock MJ, Ashworth JL, Shuttleworth CA. Fibrillin: from microfibril assembly to biomechanical function. *Philos Trans R Soc Lond B Biol Sci.* 2002;357:207-217.

5. Wolinsky H, Glagov S. Comparison of abdominal and thoracic aortic medial structure in mammals. Deviation of man from the usual pattern. *Circ Res.* 1969;25:677-686.

6. Wolinsky H, Glagov S. A lamellar unit of aortic medial structure and function in mammals. *Circ Res.* 1967;20:99-111.

7. Dingemans KP, Teeling P, Lagendijk JH, Becker AE. Extracellular matrix of the human aortic media: an ultrastructural histochemical and immunohistochemical study of the adult aortic media. *Anat Rec.* 2000;258:1-14.

8. Kielty CM, Sherratt MJ, Shuttleworth CA. Elastic fibres. *J Cell Sci.* 2002;115:2817-2828.

9. Sakai LY, Keene DR, Engvall E. Fibrillin, a new 350-kD glycoprotein, is a component of extracellular microfibrils. *J Cell Biol.* 1986;103:2499-2509.

10. Baldock C, Siegler V, Bax DV, et al. Nanostructure of fibrillin-1 reveals compact conformation of EGF arrays and mechanism for extensibility. *Proc Natl Acad Sci U S A.* 2006;103:11922-11927.

11. Yanagisawa H, Davis EC, Starcher BC, et al. Fibulin-5 is an elastin-binding protein essential for elastic fibre development in vivo. *Nature.* 2002;415:168-171.

12. Faury G. Function-structure relationship of elastic arteries in evolution: from microfibrils to elastin and elastic fibres. *Pathol Biol (Paris).* 2001;49:310-325.

13. Stephan S, Ball SG, Williamson M, et al. Cell-matrix biology in vascular tissue engineering. *J Anat.* 2006;209:495-502.

14. Lehoux S, Tedgui A. Cellular mechanics and gene expression in blood vessels. *J Biomech.* 2003;36:631-643.

15. Isenberg BC, Tranquillo RT. Long-term cyclic distention enhances the mechanical properties of collagen-based media-equivalents. *Ann Biomed Eng.* 2003;31:937-949.

16. Kanda K, Matsuda T. Mechanical stress-induced orientation and ultrastructural change of smooth muscle cells cultured in three-dimensional collagen lattices. *Cell Transplant.* 1994;3:481-492.

17. Opitz F, Schenke-Layland K, Cohnert TU, et al. Tissue engineering of aortic tissue: dire consequence of suboptimal elastic fiber synthesis in vivo. *Cardiovasc Res.* 2004;63:719-730.

18. Vu TH, Werb Z. Matrix metalloproteinases: effectors of development and normal physiology. *Genes Dev.* 2000;14:2123-2133.

19. Milnor WR. *Hemodynamics.* Philadelphia, PA: Williams & Wilkins; 1982.

20. Shadwick RE. Mechanical design in arteries. *J Exp Biol.* 1999;202:3305-3313.

21. Frank O. Die Grundform des arteriellen pulses. *Zeitung fur Biologie.* 1899;37:483-526.

22. Stergiopulos N, Westerhof BE, Westerhof N. Total arterial inertance as the fourth element of the windkessel model. *Am J Physiol.* 1999;276:H81-H88.

23. Chuong CJ, Fung YC. Three-dimensional stress distribution in arteries. *J Biomech Eng.* 1983;105:268-274.

24. Sundt TM III. Residual strain in the aorta. *J Thorac Cardiovasc Surg.* [author reply]. 2006;131:1420,1;1421-1422.

25. Okamoto RJ, Xu H, Kouchoukos NT, Moon MR, Sundt TM III. The influence of mechanical properties on wall stress and distensibility of the dilated ascending aorta. *J Thorac Cardiovasc Surg.* 2003;126:842-850.

26. Guo X, Kassab GS. Variation of mechanical properties along the length of the aorta in C57bl/6 mice. *Am J Physiol Heart Circ Physiol.* 2003;285:H2614-H2622.

27. Dobrin PB. Mechanical properties of arterises. *Physiol Rev.* 1978;58:397-460.

28. Beller CJ, Labrosse MR, Thubrikar MJ, Robicsek F. Role of aortic root motion in the pathogenesis of aortic dissection. *Circulation.* 2004;109:763-769.

29. Grande KJ, Cochran RP, Reinhall PG, Kunzelman KS. Stress variations in the human aortic root and valve: the role of anatomic asymmetry. *Ann Biomed Eng.* 1998;26:534-545.

30. Jager IL. A model for the stability and creep of organic materials. *J Biomech.* 2005;38:1459-1467.

31. Gundiah N, B Ratcliffe M, A Pruitt L. Determination of strain energy function for arterial elastin: experiments using histology and mechanical tests. *J Biomech.* 2006;40:586-594.

32. Sherratt MJ, Baldock C, Haston JL, et al. Fibrillin microfibrils are stiff reinforcing fibres in compliant tissues. *J Mol Biol.* 2003;332:183-193.

33. Bank AJ, Wang H, Holte JE, Mullen K, Shammas R, Kubo SH. Contribution of collagen, elastin, and smooth muscle to in vivo human brachial artery wall stress and elastic modulus. *Circulation.* 1996;94:3263-3270.

34. Wiederhielm CA. Distensibility characteristics of small blood vessels. *Fed Proc.* 1965;24:1075-1084.

35. VanBavel E, Siersma P, Spaan JA. Elasticity of passive blood vessels: a new concept. *Am J Physiol Heart Circ Physiol.* 2003;285:H1986-H2000.

36. Clark JM, Glagov S. Transmural organization of the arterial media. The lamellar unit revisited. *Arteriosclerosis.* 1985;5:19-34.

37. Sokolis DP, Kefaloyannis EM, Kouloukoussa M, Marinos E, Boudoulas H, Karayannacos PE. A structural basis for the aortic stress-strain relation in uniaxial tension. *J Biomech.* 2006;39:1651-1662.

38. Silver FH, Snowhill PB, Foran DJ. Mechanical behavior of vessel wall: a comparative study of aorta, vena cava, and carotid artery. *Ann Biomed Eng.* 2003;31:793-803.

39. Dingemans KP, Teeling P, van der Wal AC, Becker AE. Ultrastructural pathology of aortic dissections in patients with Marfan syndrome: comparison with dissections in patients without Marfan syndrome. *Cardiovasc Pathol.* 2006;15:203-212.

40. MacLean NF, Dudek NL, Roach MR. The role of radial elastic properties in the development of aortic dissections. *J Vasc Surg.* 1999;29:703-710.

41. Pereira L, Lee SY, Gayraud B, et al. Pathogenetic sequence for aneurysm revealed in mice underexpressing fibrillin-1. *Proc Natl Acad Sci U S A.* 1999;96:3819-3823.

42. Baldini A. The 22q11.2 deletion syndrome: a gene dosage perspective. *SciWorld Journal.* 2006;6:1881-1887.

43. McElhinney DB, Driscoll DA, Emanuel BS, Goldmuntz E. Chromosome 22q11 deletion in patients with truncus arteriosus. *Pediatr Cardiol.* 2003;24:569-573.

44. Plageman TF Jr, Yutzey KE. T-box genes and heart development: putting the "T" in heart. *Dev Dyn.* 2005;232:11-20.

45. Goldmuntz E, Bamford R, Karkera JD, dela Cruz J, Roessler E, Muenke M. CFC1 mutations in patients with transposition of the great arteries and double-outlet right ventricle. *Am J Hum Genet.* 2002;70:776-780.

46. Lambrechts D, Devriendt K, Driscoll DA, et al. Low expression VEGF haplotype increases the risk for tetralogy of Fallot: a family based association study. *J Med Genet.* 2005;42:519-522.

47. Schott JJ, Benson DW, Basson CT, et al. Congenital heart disease caused by mutations in the transcription factor NKX2-5. *Science.* 1998;281:108-111.

48. Gill HK, Splitt M, Sharland GK, Simpson JM. Patterns of recurrence of congenital heart disease: an analysis of 6,640 consecutive pregnancies evaluated by detailed fetal echocardiography. *J Am Coll Cardiol.* 2003;42:923-929.

49. Wren C, Birrell G, Hawthorne G. Cardiovascular malformations in infants of diabetic mothers. *Heart.* 2003;89:1217-1220.

50. Tikkanen J, Heinonen OP. Risk factors for hypoplastic left heart syndrome. *Teratology.* 1994;50:112-117.

51. Eghtesady P. Hypoplastic left heart syndrome: rheumatic heart disease of the fetus? *Med Hypotheses.* 2006;66:554-565.

52. Mu TS, McAdams RM, Bush DM. A case of hypoplastic left heart syndrome and bicuspid aortic valve in monochorionic twins. *Pediatr Cardiol.* 2005;26:884-885.

53. Achneck H, Modi B, Shaw C, et al. Ascending thoracic aneurysms are associated with decreased systemic atherosclerosis. *Chest.* 2005;128:1580-1586.

54. Judge DP, Dietz HC. Marfan's syndrome. *Lancet.* 2005;366:1965-1976.

55. Pannu H, Fadulu VT, Chang J, et al. Mutations in transforming growth factor-beta receptor type II cause familial thoracic aortic aneurysms and dissections. *Circulation.* 2005;112:513-520.

56. Disabella E, Grasso M, Marziliano N, et al. Two novel and one known mutation of the TGFBR2 gene in Marfan syndrome not associated with FBN1 gene defects. *Eur J Hum Genet.* 2006;14:34-38.

57. Loeys BL, Schwarze U, Holm T, et al. Aneurysm syndromes caused by mutations in the TGF-beta receptor. *N Engl J Med.* 2006;355:788-798.

58. Loeys B, Van Maldergem L, Mortier G, et al. Homozygosity for a missense mutation in fibulin-5 (FBLN5) results in a severe form of cutis laxa. *Hum Mol Genet.* 2002;11:2113-2118.

59. Hucthagowder V, Sausgruber N, Kim KH, Angle B, Marmorstein LY, Urban Z. Fibulin-4: a novel gene for an autosomal recessive cutis laxa syndrome. *Am J Hum Genet.* 2006;78:1075-1080.

60. Christen-Zach S, Huber M, Struk B, et al. Pseudoxanthoma elasticum: evaluation of diagnostic criteria based on molecular data. *Br J Dermatol.* 2006;155:89-93.

61. Farmakis D, Vesleme V, Papadogianni A, Tsaftaridis P, Kapralos P, Aessopos A. Aneurysmatic dilatation of ascending aorta in a patient with beta-thalassemia and a pseudoxanthoma elasticum-like syndrome. *Ann Hematol.* 2004;83:596-599.

62. Urban Z, Riazi S, Seidl TL, et al. Connection between elastin haploinsufficiency and increased cell proliferation in patients with supravalvular aortic stenosis and Williams-Beuren syndrome. *Am J Hum Genet.* 2002;71:30-44.

63. Zhu L, Vranckx R, Khau Van Kien P, et al. Mutations in myosin heavy chain 11 cause a syndrome associating thoracic aortic aneurysm/aortic dissection and patent ductus arteriosus. *Nat Genet.* 2006;38:343-349.

64. Cripe L, Andelfinger G, Martin LJ, Shooner K, Benson DW. Bicuspid aortic valve is heritable. *J Am Coll Cardiol.* 2004;44:138-143.

65. Cotrufo M, Della Corte A, De Santo LS, et al. Different patterns of extracellular matrix protein expression in the convexity and the concavity of the dilated aorta with bicuspid aortic valve: preliminary results. *J Thorac Cardiovasc Surg.* 2005;130:504-511.

66. Hahn RT, Roman MJ, Mogtader AH, Devereux RB. Association of aortic dilation with regurgitant, stenotic and functionally normal bicuspid aortic valves. *J Am Coll Cardiol.* 1992;19:283-288.

67. Fedak PW, de Sa MP, Verma S, et al. Vascular matrix remodeling in patients with bicuspid aortic valve malformations: implications for aortic dilatation. *J Thorac Cardiovasc Surg.* 2003;126:797-806.

68. Nistri S, Sorbo MD, Marin M, Palisi M, Scognamiglio R, Thiene G. Aortic root dilatation in young men with normally functioning bicuspid aortic valves. *Heart.* 1999;82:19-22.

69. Nistri S, Sorbo MD, Basso C, Thiene G. Bicuspid aortic valve: abnormal aortic elastic properties. *J Heart Valve Dis.* 2002;11:369,73; discussion 373-374.

70. Della Corte A, Bancone C, Quarto C, et al. Predictors of ascending aortic dilatation with bicuspid aortic valve: a wide spectrum of disease expression. *Eur J Cardiothorac Surg.* 2007;31:397-405.

71. Bauer M, Gliech V, Siniawski H, Hetzer R. Configuration of the ascending aorta in patients with bicuspid and tricuspid aortic valve disease undergoing aortic valve replacement with or without reduction aortoplasty. *J Heart Valve Dis.* 2006;15:594-600.

72. Beighton P, De Paepe A, Steinmann B, Tsipouras P, Wenstrup RJ. Ehlers-Danlos syndromes: revised nosology, Villefranche, 1997. Ehlers-Danlos National Foundation (USA) and Ehlers-Danlos Support Group (UK). *Am J Med Genet.* 1998;77:31-37.

73. Pepin M, Schwarze U, Superti-Furga A, Byers PH. Clinical and genetic features of Ehlers-Danlos syndrome type IV, the vascular type. *N Engl J Med.* 2000;342:673-680.

74. Perdu J, Boutouyrie P, Lahlou-Laforet K, et al. Vascular Ehlers-Danlos syndrome. *Presse Med.* 2006;35:1864-1875.

75. Oderich GS, Panneton JM, Bower TC, et al. The spectrum, management and clinical outcome of Ehlers-Danlos syndrome type IV: a 30-year experience. *J Vasc Surg.* 2005;42: 98-106.

76. Laporte-Turpin E, Marcoux MO, Machado G, et al. Lethal aortic dissection in a 13-year-old boy with a vascular Ehlers-Danlos syndrome. *Arch Pediatr.* 2005;12:1112-1115.

77. Barabas AP. Ehlers-Danlos syndrome type IV. *N Engl J Med.* [author reply]. 2000;343:366;368.

78. Pyeritz RE. Ehlers-Danlos syndrome. *N Engl J Med.* 2000; 342:730-732.

79. Wenstrup RJ, Meyer RA, Lyle JS, et al. Prevalence of aortic root dilation in the Ehlers-Danlos syndrome. *Genet Med.* 2002;4:112-117.

80. Koullias GJ, Ravichandran P, Korkolis DP, Rimm DL, Elefteriades JA. Increased tissue microarray matrix metalloproteinase expression favors proteolysis in thoracic aortic aneurysms and dissections. *Ann Thorac Surg.* 2004;78:2106, 2110; discussion 2110-2111.

81. Longo GM, Xiong W, Greiner TC, Zhao Y, Fiotti N, Baxter BT. Matrix metalloproteinases 2 and 9 work in concert to produce aortic aneurysms. *J Clin Invest.* 2002;110:625-632.

82. Ikonomidis JS, Barbour JR, Amani Z, et al. Effects of deletion of the matrix metalloproteinase 9 gene on development of murine thoracic aortic aneurysms. *Circulation.* 2005;112: I242-1248.

83. Boyum J, Fellinger EK, Schmoker JD, et al. Matrix metalloproteinase activity in thoracic aortic aneurysms associated with bicuspid and tricuspid aortic valves. *J Thorac Cardiovasc Surg.* 2004;127:686-691.

84. Ihling C, Szombathy T, Nampoothiri K, et al. Cystic medial degeneration of the aorta is associated with p53 accumulation, Bax upregulation, apoptotic cell death, and cell proliferation. *Heart.* 1999;82:286-293.

85. Schmid FX, Bielenberg K, Schneider A, Haussler A, Keyser A, Birnbaum D. Ascending aortic aneurysm associated with bicuspid and tricuspid aortic valve: involvement and clinical relevance of smooth muscle cell apoptosis and expression of cell death-initiating proteins. *Eur J Cardiothorac Surg.* 2003; 23:537-543.

86. Schmid FX, Bielenberg K, Holmer S, et al. Structural and biomolecular changes in aorta and pulmonary trunk of patients with aortic aneurysm and valve disease: implications for the Ross procedure. *Eur J Cardiothorac Surg.* 2004;25: 748-753.

87. Wang X, LeMaire SA, Chen L, et al. Increased collagen deposition and elevated expression of connective tissue growth factor in human thoracic aortic dissection. *Circulation.* 2006;114:I200-1205.

88. Mckusick VA. The cardiovascular aspects of Marfan's syndrome: a heritable disorder of connective tissue. *Circulation.* 1955;11:321-342.

89. Kirsch EW, Radu NC, Gervais M, Allaire E, Loisance DY. Heterogeneity in the remodeling of aneurysms of the ascending aorta with tricuspid aortic valves. *J Thorac Cardiovasc Surg.* 2006;132:1010-1016.

90. Larson EW, Edwards WD. Risk factors for aortic dissection: a necropsy study of 161 cases. *Am J Cardiol.* 1984;53:849-855.

91. Lansman SL, McCullough JN, Nguyen KH, et al. Subtypes of acute aortic dissection. *Ann Thorac Surg.* 1999;67: 1975,1978; discussion 1979-1980.

92. Bahnson HT, Nelson AR. Cystic medial necrosis as a cause of localized aortic aneurysms amenable to surgical treatment. *Ann Surg.* 1956;144:519-529.

93. Homme JL, Aubry MC, Edwards WD, et al. Surgical pathology of the ascending aorta: a clinicopathologic study of 513 cases. *Am J Surg Pathol.* 2006;30:1159-1168.

94. Vorp DA, Schiro BJ, Ehrlich MP, Juvonen TS, Ergin MA, Griffith BP. Effect of aneurysm on the tensile strength and biomechanical behavior of the ascending thoracic aorta. *Ann Thorac Surg.* 2003;75:1210-1214.

95. Koullias G, Modak R, Tranquilli M, Korkolis DP, Barash P, Elefteriades JA. Mechanical deterioration underlies malignant behavior of aneurysmal human ascending aorta. *J Thorac Cardiovasc Surg.* 2005;130:677-683.

96. Borghi A, Wood NB, Mohiaddin RH, Xu XY. 3D geometric reconstruction of thoracic aortic aneurysms. *Biomed Eng Online.* 2006;5:59.

97. Hatzaras I, Tranquilli M, Coady M, Barrett PM, Bible J, Elefteriades JA. Weight lifting and aortic dissection: more evidence for a connection. *Cardiology.* 2007;107:103-106.

98. Bertovic DA, Waddell TK, Gatzka CD, Cameron JD, Dart AM, Kingwell BA. Muscular strength training is associated with low arterial compliance and high pulse pressure. *Hypertension.* 1999;33:1385-1391.

99. Russo CF, Mazzetti S, Garatti A, et al. Aortic complications after bicuspid aortic valve replacement: long-term results. *Ann Thorac Surg.* 2002;74:S1773,S1776; discussion S1792-S1799.

100. Borger MA, Preston M, Ivanov J, et al. Should the ascending aorta be replaced more frequently in patients with bicuspid aortic valve disease? *J Thorac Cardiovasc Surg.* 2004; 128:677-683.

101. Bulpitt CJ, Cameron JD, Rajkumar C, et al. The effect of age on vascular compliance in man: which are the appropriate measures? *J Hum Hypertens.* 1999;13:753-758.

102. Mohiaddin RH, Underwood SR, Bogren HG, et al. Regional aortic compliance studied by magnetic resonance imaging: the effects of age, training, and coronary artery disease. *Br Heart J.* 1989;62:90-96.

103. McEniery CM, Yasmin, Wallace S, et al. Increased stroke volume and aortic stiffness contribute to isolated systolic hypertension in young adults. *Hypertension.* 2005;46:221-226.

104. Scharfschwerdt M, Sievers HH, Greggersen J, Hanke T, Misfeld M. Prosthetic replacement of the ascending aorta increases wall tension in the residual aorta. *Ann Thorac Surg.* 2007;83:954-957.

105. Laurent S, Boutouyrie P, Asmar R, et al. Aortic stiffness is an independent predictor of all-cause and cardiovascular mortality in hypertensive patients. *Hypertension.* 2001;37:1236-1241.

106. Farrar DJ, Bond MG, Riley WA, Sawyer JK. Anatomic correlates of aortic pulse wave velocity and carotid artery elasticity during atherosclerosis progression and regression in monkeys. *Circulation.* 1991;83:1754-1763.

107. Nigam A, Mitchell GF, Lambert J, Tardif JC. Relation between conduit vessel stiffness (assessed by tonometry) and endothelial function (assessed by flow-mediated dilatation) in patients with and without coronary heart disease. *Am J Cardiol.* 2003;92:395-399.

108. Girerd X, Laurent S, Pannier B, Asmar R, Safar M. Arterial distensibility and left ventricular hypertrophy in patients with sustained essential hypertension. *Am Heart J.* 1991;122:1210-1214.

109. Rerkpattanapipat P, Hundley WG, Link KM, et al. Relation of aortic distensibility determined by magnetic resonance imaging in patients > or = 60 years of age to systolic heart failure and exercise capacity. *Am J Cardiol.* 2002;90:1221-1225.

110. Stefanadis C, Stratos C, Vlachopoulos C, et al. Pressure-diameter relation of the human aorta. A new method of determination by the application of a special ultrasonic dimension catheter. *Circulation.* 1995;92:2210-2219.

111. O'Rourke MF, Safar ME. Relationship between aortic stiffening and microvascular disease in brain and kidney: cause and logic of therapy. *Hypertension.* 2005;46:200-204.

112. Petersen SE, Wiesmann F, Hudsmith LE, et al. Functional and structural vascular remodeling in elite rowers assessed by cardiovascular magnetic resonance. *J Am Coll Cardiol.* 2006;48:790-797.

113. Wiesmann F, Petersen SE, Leeson PM, et al. Global impairment of brachial, carotid, and aortic vascular function in young smokers: direct quantification by high-resolution magnetic resonance imaging. *J Am Coll Cardiol.* 2004;44:2056-2064.

114. Stefanadis C, Vlachopoulos C, Tsiamis E, et al. Unfavorable effects of passive smoking on aortic function in men. *Ann Intern Med.* 1998;128:426-434.

115. Sokolis DP, Zarbis N, Dosios T, et al. Post-vagotomy mechanical characteristics and structure of the thoracic aortic wall. *Ann Biomed Eng.* 2005;33:1504-1516.

116. Mills NL, Everson CT. Atherosclerosis of the ascending aorta and coronary artery bypass. Pathology, clinical correlates, and operative management. *J Thorac Cardiovasc Surg.* 1991;102:546-553.

117. Amarenco P, Cohen A, Tzourio C, et al. Atherosclerotic disease of the aortic arch and the risk of ischemic stroke. *N Engl J Med.* 1994;331:1474-1479.

118. Davila-Roman VG, Murphy SF, Nickerson NJ, Kouchoukos NT, Schechtman KB, Barzilai B. Atherosclerosis of the ascending aorta is an independent predictor of long-term neurologic events and mortality. *J Am Coll Cardiol.* 1999;33:1308-1316.

119. Schachner T, Zimmer A, Nagele G, Laufer G, Bonatti J. Risk factors for late stroke after coronary artery bypass grafting. *J Thorac Cardiovasc Surg.* 2005;130:485-490.

120. Schachner T, Nagele G, Kacani A, Laufer G, Bonatti J. Factors associated with presence of ascending aortic atherosclerosis in CABG patients. *Ann Thorac Surg.* 2004;78:2028-2032; discussion 2032.

chapter 28

Aortic Arch Vessels and Upper Extremity Arteries

David C. Cassada, MD / Trent L. Prault, MD

Loss of arm and hand function arguably carries higher morbidity than that of the leg, as there seems to be an unspoken stigma associated with arm or hand loss. Upper extremity function is critical to human interaction within the environment. Hand strength, sensation, and other complex functions protect and provide for human survival and socialization.

Vascular disorders of the upper extremities result in symptoms ranging in severity from nuisance to limb-threatening. Patients with arm-related vascular pathology are encountered by physicians with lesser frequency than lower extremity vascular disease, making diagnosis and treatment unfamiliar to many clinicians who are otherwise skilled in the care of vascular disease. It is paramount that the clinician be able to recognize many of the upper extremity arterial disorders to prevent both overly aggressive treatment, as well as treatment omissions that could lead to tissue loss. This chapter serves to provide an overview of the diagnosis and treatment of frequently encountered vascular disease patterns of the arm.

The arm's arterial supply consists of the brachiocephalic vessels of the aortic arch, as well as the run-off arterial anatomy of the upper extremities. The disease processes are broken down into three major groups: arterial occlusive/embolic disease, arterial inflammatory disease, and aneurysmal disease of the branch vessels and upper extremities.

In approximately 92% of the population, the aortic anatomy includes, from right to left, the innominate artery, the right common carotid artery, (succeeded across the arch by the origin of the left common carotid artery), and the left subclavian artery. Depending on congenital formation and obliteration of primordial arches allowing for tortuous changes. Over time, the origins of the great vessels can vary in their initiation across the curve of the aortic arch. In general, the more proximal the take-off of the great vessels from the ascending aortic arch, the more difficult catheter-based access becomes when endovascular surgery is performed for subclavian and carotid arterial disease (Figure 28-1).[1,2]

In 2% to 6% of patients, the left common carotid artery takes its origin from the innominate artery. This arrangement termed *bovine arch*, can increase the complexity of intervention for innominate arterial disease, as the majority of cerebral inflow is dependent upon the innominate artery. In general, the innominate artery is the largest branch arising from the arch of the aorta. Its origin occurs at the upper border of the second right costal cartilage and because of the angulation of the aortic arch, it is found anterior to the left carotid in the anterior–posterior plane. The innominate artery typically gives off no branches but in 1% of patients a thyroidea IMA takes origin and supplies blood to the lower part of the thyroid body.[1]

The right common carotid artery arises from the innominate artery behind the right sternoclavicular articulation. The left common carotid artery takes its origin from the highest point in the aortic arch. The left common carotid is typically longer than the right carotid, and takes its origin deeper within the thorax. The left subclavian artery occupies the position posteriorly and slightly left and lateral to this.[3,4]

Anomalies in aortic arch anatomy can occur during developmental obliteration of the six primordial aortic arches. One observed anomaly includes the origin of the right subclavian artery from the lower aortic arch at the level of the aortic isthmus, crossing posterior to the aerodigestive tract as a result of the partial persistence of a right aortic arch.

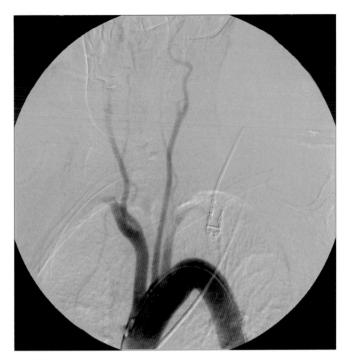

● **FIGURE 28-1.** Great vessels arising far right within the aortic arch present challenges in the endovascular treatment of both occlusive and aneurysmal disease of Axillo-subclavian arterial segments.

Chronic compression by aerodigestive structures can result in subclavian arterial aneurysmal degeneration, manifesting as dysphagia or airway-obstructive symptoms.

The number of arch vessels can also be increased from three to four where the right carotid and subclavian arteries arise directly from the aortic arch with the innominate being absent. Based on primordial arch anatomy, this arrangement can be highly variable, and the number of trunks from the arch may be increased to five or six. In such cases, the external and internal carotid arteries can rise separately from the main aortic arch. In rare cases, where six branches are encountered, there are also separate origins of the vertebral arteries directly from the aortic arch. Because of the rare potential variety of arch anatomic configurations, there can be any combination of these anomalies with new challenges presented during the management of aortic arch disease.

● **GIANT CELL ARTERITIS**

Giant cell arteritis (GCA) is termed *temporal arteritis* or *cranial arteritis*. This is a systemic vasculitis affecting segmental portions of the aortic arch and great vessel anatomy.[5–7] Early signs of this disease process can include headache and partial or complete vision loss as a result of dissection or end-arterial obliteration.[8,9] Further catastrophic consequences of GCA can include aortic aneurysmal rupture and cerebral or coronary hypoperfusion syndrome. Additionally, the axillary and brachial arteries can be affected resulting in rapid onset of forearm and hand claudication symptoms. The aortic arch and its branches, particularly the medium diameter branches, are the blood vessels most

affected. Rarely, lower abdominal branch vessels including renal, mesenteric, and iliofemoral arteries as well as the coronary arteries can be affected.[7]

GCA can cause an array of changes to include stenosis, frank occlusion or aneurysmal dilatation. Microscopically the vascular wall is infiltrated with inflammatory cells, particularly monocytes and CD-4 positive T cells, as macrophages are found to penetrate throughout the arterial wall. Multinuclear giant cells are observed and found closely related to the disrupted internal elastic membrane, likely because of the activity of proteolytic enzymes.[7,10] Loss of this membrane and medial necrosis can cause formation aneurysms or thickening of the wall acute bouts of arteritis resulting in stenosis or occlusion.

Early signs of GCA include headache, poor appetite, muscle pain, loss of weight and febrile status. Within weeks, severe headaches and jaw claudication can occur.[5,6,11] If these symptoms are in fact caused by GCA, 40% of untreated patients may proceed to permanent vision impairment to include blindness, ipsilateral to the affected arteries.

Many patients with GCA demonstrate underlying polymyalgia rheumatica (PMR). PMR can present as pain in the shoulder and hip girdles with weakness and muscle pain during motion.[12] Classic symptoms and presentation are rare, therefore, unilateral headaches, particularly those with visual changes, should prompt consideration of GCA and result in the appropriate testing to include measurement of Westergren sedimentation rate (WSR or ESR) and C-reactive proteins (CRP). A WSR greater than 50 mm/h is of concern for GCA but often can exceed 100 mm/h in patients with severe GCA. CRP is noted to be increased in 92% of patients and although this is a nonspecific test, it can be sensitive in detecting GCA. Elevated white blood cell count, platelet count and liver enzymes occur in roughly 30% of patients with GCA. Occasionally, GCA can also be associated with increased anticardiolipin antibodies, compounding the obliterative process because of the associated thrombophilia.[5,7,8,10]

Treatment of GCA requires confirmation of diagnosis with arterial biopsy done at a low threshold based upon clinical presentation. In patients in their sixth or seventh decade of life, new onset of severe headaches, jaw claudication, or bilateral arm claudication, with or without systemic signs of inflammation, could indicate GCA. Evaluation should include noninvasive arterial waveform testing, arterial biopsy and occasionally arteriography.[6] Duplex evaluation of the temporal artery demonstrates the "halo sign." Waveform plethysmography of the upper extremities may suggest bilateral proximal axillo-subclavian or brachial artery occlusive disease. Brisk onset of such disease is consistent with acute GCA and may present as arm and hand claudication during performance of tasks (Figure 28-2).[7]

Unilateral headaches, with or without visual changes and positive ESR and CRP, should prompt vessel biopsy to confirm the diagnosis. Biopsy of the temporal artery should include a minimum 2-cm segment with a longer segment obtained if possible, thereby improving the pathologic

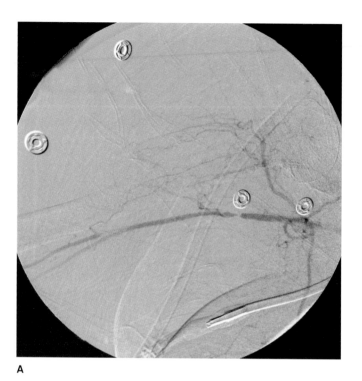

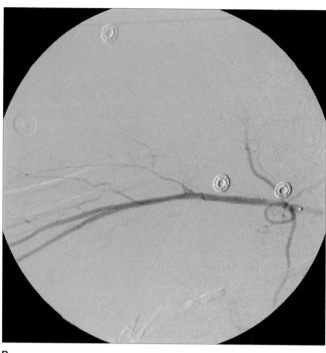

A

B

● **FIGURE 28-2.** (A) GCA can involve segment of the axillary and brachial segments of the upper extremity arterial anatomy. (B) Although the treatment of GCA generally requires the use of steroids to resolve arterial inflammation, occasionally endovascular therapy or surgical bypass can be performed for tissue-threatening occlusive lesions. Here a self-expanding stent is deployed to improve arm arterial runoff in a patient with hand tissue loss.

sampling of the vessel, as well as the sensitivity and specificity of this clinical test to confirm GCA.[10]

The acute treatment of GCA includes the administration of corticosteroids. Prednisone can be initiated at a dose of 1 mg/kg per day. However, in those with impending vision loss, prednisone should be administered in a dose of at least 20-mg three times daily. Once the active phase of the disease is controlled, the dose is consolidated to a single daily dose until the vasculitis resolves completely, after which steroid taper is possible. Corticosteroid treatment can be guided by normalization of ESR and CRP. Other medications have included various forms of immunosuppressive drugs, with variable proven clinical efficacy.[5]*

Surgical bypass for the complications of GCA is typically not performed in the inflammatory setting of acute vasculitis. Where tissue threat is present, principles of surgery include bypass from normal inflow vessels to relatively healthy target vessels while trying to avoid the inclusion of acutely diseased segments in the anastomotic zones of the revascularization. There seems to be little role for endovascular therapy beyond diagnostic imaging of diseased arteries in planning for medical and/or surgical therapy. However, in those patients with severe comorbidities, angioplasty is a reasonable treatment strategy to avoid tissue loss.

● **RADIATION-INDUCED ARTERITIS**

Radiation-induced arteritis is seen increasingly in patients who have undergone radiation in the treatment of malig-

nancies earlier in life. Ionizing radiation tends to injure rapidly dividing cells and is therefore effective in cancer cells. However, adjacent tissue radiation can result in damage to normal mitotic cells and can result in chronic radiation damage of the vascular tree.[13]

Endothelial cells are exquisitely radiosensitive. Initially there can be swelling and exfoliation of endothelial cells, which can lead to obstruction of small blood vessels by thrombosis as subintimal collagen is exposed to blood cell constituents. Therefore, the acute damage of small diameter cells results in characteristic "sausage segment" with irregular stenotic occlusion of these vessels. In larger diameter vessels, there can also be damage to the vaso vasora with chronic medial fibrosis producing a narrowed arterial lumen which may require revascularization, depending upon its location within the great vessel anatomy.[13]

● **SMALLER ARTERIAL DISEASES OF THE UPPER EXTREMITY**

In the majority of patients with ischemic changes of the hand, there is a relationship to small vessel obstructive disease. The small vessel arterial disease results in symptoms related to vasospasm or obstruction of the small digital arteries of the hand. The vasospastic processes can result in a waxing and waning of ischemic changes, coolness, pain, and numbness. Color changes are often initially observed which may make the patient particularly aware that there is an arterial problem with their digits. Vasospasm can ultimately lead to loss of portions of the digits if the disease goes un-checked.

RAYNAUD'S SYNDROME

Raynaud's Syndrome (RS) is the most commonly encoun-tered upper extremity arterial disease process. RS manifests as intermittent digital ischemia in response to environmen-tal cooling of the hand. This can be exacerbated by high cat cholinergic states such as during periods of emotional or physical stress. RS has a classic presentation of tri-colored changes proceeding from white to blue to red, although one or more phases of this color progression may be absent. RS is seen in the cooler and damper climates typical to the United States, Great Britain, and Scandinavia.[14,15]

RS is subdivided into vasospastic and thrombo-obstruc-tive subgroups. Those with vasospastic RS can be observed as having normal plethysmographic waveforms when symp-toms are not present. Vasospasms result in a marked in-crease in the obstructive characteristics of peaked plethys-mographic waveforms ("nipple sign") in the fingertips, cor-relating with symptoms. A large portion of the patients (approaching 50%) can proceed to obstructive RS as the va-sospasm results in intraluminal small vessel obliteration suf-ficient to overcome systemic pressure distending forces.[15]

Treatment of RS initially includes major lifestyle modi-fications including the liberal use of gloves for thermal pro-tection from environmental cold stress. Patients are encour-aged to avoid handling cold objects, and to refrain from submerging their hands in cold water. They are also coun-seled regarding rapid changes in environmental tempera-tures such as proceeding into an air-conditioned indoor set-ting from an otherwise warm day. Underlying life stressors are identified and addressed as is appropriate. Initial phar-macological therapy includes the use of calcium channel blocking medications, and antiplatelet medications.[14–16] Some physicians recommend medications to alter the rhe-ology of red blood cells to decrease small vessel blood viscosity. Long-acting vasodilators, such as nifedipine (avail-able in a 30-mg slow-release formulation) as well as an an-tiplatelet medication, can be effective.

Patients refractory to these measures can be treated with either needle directed pharmacological sympathec-tomy or surgical sympathectomy focusing efforts on the second thoracic segment of the sympathetic ganglia. There are also multiple treatment regimens dependent upon phar-macological sympatholytic agents (primarily alpha adreno-ceptor blockade) to affect vasodilatation during severe vasospasm.[15,17]

Connective tissue diseases can be associated with RS al-though literature review shows a wide variation in associa-tion. Most commonly, these diseases include scleroderma, lupus, polymyositis, and rheumatoid arthritis. Many pa-tients with some connective tissue disease will manifest RS during fulminant courses of their disease process; however, an aggressive search for connective tissue diseases will of-ten be nondiagnostic in those patients presenting with RS alone.[14]

There are other causes for RS as a secondary process related to primary disease or traumatic insult. Ergot derived drug toxicity and β-adrenoceptor blocking medications can initiate RS as well as acquired arterial occlusive conditions. Arterial thoracic outlet syndrome can also be complicated by secondary RS and the surgical treatment may include T2 sympathectomy to improve vasodilation after thoracic outlet decompression and revascularization.

BUERGER'S DISEASE

Thromboangiitis obliterans or *Buerger's Disease* (BD) is char-acterized by thrombosis of small and medium-sized arteries in the extremities with associated arterial wall leukocyte infiltrate.[18,19] A large number of patients suffering from BD will have only upper extremity manifestations; how-ever, 40% of these may also demonstrate lower extremity disease. Patients with BD are predominately men in their fourth decade who often abuse tobacco. The age of onset is especially important in suspicion of this disease, as it al-most always occurs before 45 years of age. This is further suggested by noninvasive evidence of the absence disease proximal to the elbow in the upper extremity, and proxi-mal to the knee in the lower extremity. Although strongly suspected, tobacco abuse alone does not constitute a sole risk factor for BD.

Arteriographic findings with BD include normal appear-ing inflow vessels with the presence of "cork screw" changes in the small and medium vessels of the distal extremity and digits. The corkscrew changes result in obliteration of nor-mal arterial lumens as a result of the inflammatory changes within the vessel. Collaterals are formed as the adventitial vaso vasora form large channels to perfuse the distal extrem-ity. As the collaterals form, they are ectatic and irregular, resulting in the "cork screw" appearance.

Treatment includes extensive counseling regarding to-bacco use, as well as psychological counseling, and the pos-sible use of pharmacologic agents to break habitual smok-ing. It is still important to refrain from pharmacological nicotine substitutes, as these medications tend to exacer-bate peripheral vasospasm, which may worsen the BD.[18] There are clinical reports of the use of pharmacologic sym-pathectomy to treat acute bouts of digital ischemia, and rarely the use of surgical sympathectomy of both the lower and upper extremities to abate the disease process. Up to 40% of patients will proceed to digit loss and/or major por-tions of extremities. This is likely because of the high recidi-vism rate of those who attempt tobacco abstinence. There is limited relief after the use of long-acting calcium channel blockers and/or sympathectomy.[20]

OCCUPATIONAL UPPER EXTREMITY VASCULAR DISEASE

Exposure to traumatic or regular use of vibrating instru-ments such as jackhammers and mortar screws can result in chronic small vessel arterial disease. The initiating factors are thought to be vasospasm especially where cold exposure is involved, followed by arterial obliteration.

Other traumatic injuries to hand arterial vessels can occur in certain lines of work where the hand is used as a blunt force to move or align objects. As such, pounding of the hypothenar imminence of the hand results in "hyperthenar hammer syndrome" where the distal most segment of the ulnar artery is traumatized at the wrist. This can result in aneurysmal changes with ischemia secondary to thrombosis or distal embolization. Arteriography is often diagnostic and can help plan small vessel repair where incomplete palmar arch anatomy precludes resection and ligation of the diseased arterial segment.

● AORTIC ARCH RECONSTRUCTION

Management of aortic arch arterial disease requires many considerations. For occlusive disease, the clinician must consider the fact that there is redundancy of cerebral inflow to both the anterior and posterior circulation making even short segment occlusive lesions tolerable by the patient. Therefore, not every occlusion requires treatment. Left subclavian arterial occlusive disease is the most common complete occlusion found in patients with extracranial cerebrovascular disease. This is followed by left common carotid artery disease, and brachiocephalic occlusive lesions. Left subclavian arterial occlusive disease is usually well-tolerated by patients, absent most of which are neurologic symptoms (i.e., although patients may have subclavian steal, they do *not* have subclvavian steal *syndrome*). Often there is no reason to treat great vessel disease at this level.

Symptoms can include neurologic deficits resulting from arterial embolic phenomenon to include transient ischemic attacks and strokes of the anterior and posterior circulation. Additionally, hemodynamic factors must be considered such as subclavian steal syndrome of posterior circulation, whereby there is observed reversal of vertebral blood flow to supply the upper extremity runoff basin when the resistance of the arm capillary bed is lower than that of the posterior fossa run off. Interestingly, symptoms can sometimes be provoked after deflating a blood pressure cuff on the affected arm. The resultant low resistance to the arm "steals" more blood from posterior circulation—thus, causing symptoms.

Radiographic subclavian steal anatomy can be observed absent the symptoms associated with subclavian steal syndrome. Typically, a patient with true subclavian steal syndrome will complain of vertebral-basilar related symptoms such as effort-induced dizziness, dizziness at rest, blurred vision, and even nausea and vomiting. In patients presenting with these symptoms, a pressure gradient between the arms of 20 mm Hg systolic blood pressure can indicate that the anatomy producing subclavian steal syndrome could be present. The "Dieter test" can be useful to provoke symptoms in a patient with borderline symptoms. In this test, a blood pressure cuff is applied to the affected extremity and inflated above the systolic pressure. The cuff is then rapidly deflated. This results in hyperemic flow to the arm and exacerbation of any vertebral artery flow reversal and steal—potentially evoking neurological symptoms. Diagno-

sis can be made with noninvasive imaging such as MRA and CTA with image reconstruction to determine the extent of subclavian artery occlusive disease, as well as proximity to the origin of the ipsilateral vertebral artery. Dyanamic kinking of the proximal subclavian artery during respirations (the "Dieter sign") has been described; since it represents a pseudostenosis, invasive treatment should be avoided (Figure 28-3).

Other considerations for subclavian steal syndrome include the presence of common and internal carotid artery disease, as well as intracranial vascular anatomy, which may play an important role in the presence of subclavian steal syndrome. Despite the subclavian steal syndrome that is observed clinically in select patients, chronic occlusion of the proximal left subclavian artery is surprisingly well-tolerated by a significant number of patients where there is a robust collateral arterial network supplying both the intracranial runoff and the axillo-subclavian segment. It is likely that fewer than 30% of these lesions will ever come to clinical significance and are therefore rarely treated.

In symptomatic patients with demonstrated subclavian steal syndrome related to proximal subclavian artery occlusive, it is reasonable to consider catheter-based therapy. The appeal of such therapy includes avoiding the cardiovascular stress of general anesthesia and operative exposure, as well as reducing arterial occlusive times related to cross-clamping of the subclavian artery and the ipsilateral common carotid artery. Important to consider is prior coronary revascularization, where the ipsilateral internal mammary artery may provide inflow to the myocardial vessels pending on patent graft function. In this subset of patients, there can be observed subclavian steal with associated anginal symptoms ("coronary subclavian steal syndrome"). Careful consideration is made prior to treating these patients either by endovascular or open technique given the potential for worsened complicating myocardial ischemia and myocardial infarction.

Both subclavian and axillary arterial lesions can be approached either antegrade by a femoral artery access or retrograde by brachial or radial artery access.[21,22] The best candidates are those patients who have lesions that are not involving the origin of the vertebral or internal mammary artery (Figure 28-4). Whether the antegrade or retrograde approach is planned, aortic arch arteriography is important and is generally performed through a femoral approach, using a pigtail catheter. Imaging of the arch and great vessel origins is important to define the exact location of the vessel ostium, so that ballooning and stenting of these lesions can be done with great precision. Often a guide wire is left positioned against the outer curve of the aortic arch to help determine where the great vessel origin takes place during the variability of the cardiac cycle.[23]

The best lesions indicated for angioplasty and/or stenting are those which are remote from the subclavian region, both well proximal and isolated from the vertebral artery. A lesion juxtaposed to the vertebral artery may be best treated with open surgery since intervention may result in vertebral artery dissection and compromise vertebral artery

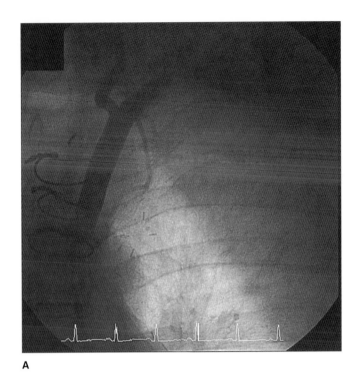

A

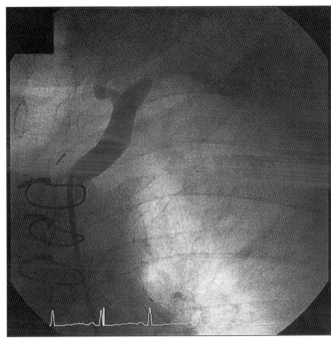

B

● **FIGURE 28-3.** The Dieter sign represents dynamic subclavian artery obstruction with respiration. (A) With inspiration the artery is straightened. (B) With expiration there is apparent stenosis.

Reproduced, with permission, from Dieter RS, et al. Description of a new angiographic sign: dynamic left subclavian artery obstruction. Vasc Dis Manage. 2006;3:298–299.

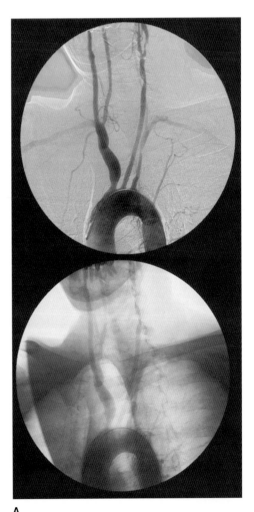

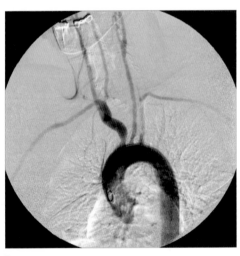

B

● **FIGURE 28-4.** These images show upper extremity (A) with and (B) without evocative maneuvers that reveal extrinsic compression of the sublcavian and/or axillary artery. Without such maneuvers, these periodic compressive forces would not be evident, and potentially not seen during the evaluation of the patient with arterial thoracic outlet syndrome. Areas of extrinsic compression can represent damage to the arterial wall intima, and are potentially sources for thromboembolic disease of the hand.

A

blood flow. Such a complication can have catastrophic consequences, which may not be addressed quickly enough to avoid neurological morbidity using a less invasive procedure. Some have utilized protection strategies for complex lesions involving the vertebral artery. Balloon diameter within the subclavian artery is typically chosen between 6 and 8 mm. The subclavian artery is quite soft and rupture of this vessel can result in acute intrathoracic bleeding which can be fatal. Therefore, computer-assisted measuring of the vessel prior to intervention is critical to treatment planning; others have used IVUS or a marker catheter during angiography for sizing. Once angioplasty is performed, completion angiography is reviewed to look for evidence of recurrent stenosis greater than 20% of the normal luminal diameter of the vessel, or the presence of a subclavian artery dissection. Thereafter, a balloon expandable or self-expanding stent can be placed to assure wide patency of the treated vessel and also to reapproximate any intimal flaps to prevent ongoing dissection or acute occlusion during the perioperative period.[23]

There is little long-term data regarding the use of stents in the proximal subclavian arteries. In one study by Peterson et al; there is a report of 20 consecutive brachiocephalic interventions using catheter-based technology for stenosis ranging from 85% to 95% diameter narrowing.[22] A technical success rate of 100% is reported as well as a nonincidence of any periprocedural untoward events. Long-term outcomes and restenosis data is incomplete in this series, and cannot be compared to open surgical data. In a separate study, proximal subclavian artery angioplasty and stenting was performed in the treatment of coronary steal syndrome after coronary revascularization using internal mammary artery in 14 patients. Again, this study did not reveal any significant periprocedural morbidity or mortality and a 29-month patency was cited at 100%. From this data, it seems that there is clearly a role for angioplasty and/or stenting in the proximal subclavian artery in select patients with symptoms of subclavian steal syndrome or arm claudicating symptoms.[21]

Other considerations during treatment for axillo-subclavian artery occlusive disease include the morphology of the vascular lesion. If there is associated aneurysmal disease or ulceration within the plaque, strong consideration should be made favoring open surgery to provide a more durable repair, potentially avoiding the complication of upper extremity or posterior circulation embolic phenomenon (thoracic outlet syndrome must be ruled out for distal lesions prior to undertaking an endovascular treatment since these lesions are best treated initially with surgical decompression). More recently, there has been clinical experience with the use of embolic protection devices to include occlusive balloons and filter wires to control embolic disease. Given these advances in technology, some authors favor the use of endovascular treatment for proximal subclavian lesions over open surgical technique.[22]

Open surgical management of proximal arterial occlusive lesions consists of two basic techniques, subclavian to carotid arterial transposition and carotid to subclavian by-

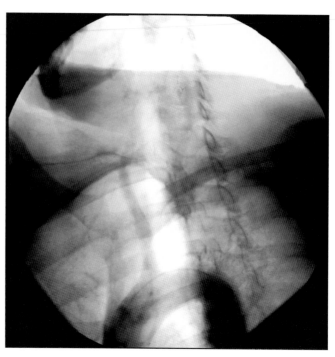

● **FIGURE 28-5.** The complete absence of great vessel origins on vascular imaging generally precludes safe endovascular intervention, and surgical bypass become the treatment of choice in those patients with cerebrovascular symptoms or arm ischemic symptoms.

pass, both providing inflow to the upper extremity as well as vertebral or internal mammary arteries (Figure 28-5). Subclavian artery transposition has the adherent advantage of avoiding the use of bypass graft conduit.[24,25] In the neck, nonautogenous materials such as polytetrafluoroethylene and modified Dacron polyester seem to have an advantage where dynamic movement in the neck and shoulder girdle can lead to graft kinking. The ridged nature of such manmade materials tends to resist kinking during routine range of motion use of the neck and upper extremity.

Subclavian to carotid transposition requires general anesthesia and involves proximal mobilization and transection of the subclavian artery with end-to-side transposition of this vessel to the common carotid artery. Such an operation has challenging technical aspect as the subclavian artery needs to be dissected deep within the thoracic outlet and loss of control of the proximal subclavian artery can lead to intrathoracic and mediastinal hemorrhage which may be difficult to control acutely. The remaining subclavian artery stump needs to be oversewn in a secure fashion using permanent monofilament suture to prevent postoperative bleeding or pseudoaneurysm formation in the remaining stump.[26]

During the course of subclavian artery transposition, there is occlusion of both the subclavian artery and the common carotid artery so it is important to have knowledge of the intracranial arterial anatomy optimally including a patent and complete circle of Willis. If there is uncertainty as to the extent of collateral circulation, distal common carotid artery stump pressures can be measured while intraoperative systolic blood pressure is maintained at 150 mm Hg or greater. A pressure of at least 30 mm Hg within the distal stump would indicate adequate collateral blood flow to tolerate the relative ischemic time during the reconstruction. The reconstruction should be brisk, yet meticulous, with excellent communication between the surgeon and anesthesiologist to maintain cerebral perfusion pressures by manipulating the intraoperative blood pressure and maintaining a systolic 150 mm Hg or greater.[24]

If coronary revascularization exists, based on internal mammary artery bypass, this technique may be unsuitable as proximal subclavian occlusion could precipitate myocardial infarction during the obligate ischemic period of subclavian artery cross-clamping. Carotid subclavian transposition, when done correctly, can demonstrate long-term patency rates exceeding 80%. Perioperative mortality should be less than or equal to 1% with a brief hospital stay. These assumptions are made based on the experience of the surgeon with prior operations and the ability to complete a well-orchestrated operation.[24]

Carotid to subclavian bypass may be a better option when there is extensive proximal subclavian artery occlusive disease or there is compromised intracranial blood flow, such that two vessel cross clamping cannot be tolerated without unacceptable cerebral ischemia. It can also be a treatment of choice where coronary blood flow is dependent on an IMA bypass graft, as proximal subclavian arterial clamping may not be necessary.[24]

Access is made to both the common carotid artery and the subclavian artery with close proximal dissection within the thoracic outlet. A short-segment 6- or 8-mm polytetrafluoroethylene or Dacron graft is selected, and placed in such a position as not to compromise the phrenic nerve and also to be resistant to kinking during range of motion.[26] Manipulation of the arm should be carried out after conclusion of the operation to assure no graft kinking occurs.

More distal extremity revascularizations to the axillary and brachial artery are best done with autogenous material such as reversed or nonreversed greater saphenous vein. The saphenous vein provides a healthy conduit which is relatively resistant to intimal hyperplasia. There is better size matching on the distal vessel and crossing of the shoulder girdle and even the elbow joint can be successfully achieved with reasonable patency rates over time. Primary patency rate of the carotid-subclavian artery bypasses should be in excess of 90%, but major complications can include thoracic duct injury on the left, resulting in limb fistula or chylothorax, Horner's syndrome, cranial nerve injury, graft infection, or possible phrenic injury. The morbidity of such an operation should be similar to that of carotid-subclavian transposition and is again dependent on the experience of the surgeon performing the operation.[24]

● ARTERIAL THORACIC OUTLET SYNDROME

It is important that the clinician pay special attention to arm and hand complaints by sorting out the different vascular

related diseases to prevent morbidity related to arterial disease of the arm.

Thoracic outlet syndrome (TOS) is defined by symptoms and clinical findings that can vary in description from one authoritative source to the next. TOS contains references to multiple anatomic sites of neurovascular compression, all generally located around the scalene musculature, and the first thoracic rib and the clavicle, resulting in end-organ dysfunction. Morbidity includes ischemic and embolic arterial disease, venous-occlusive disease, and neuropathic disease.[27–29] The vascular components of TOS can have objective measures to specify the diagnosis and describe the pathophysiology, while neurogenic TOS carries the challenge of trying to interpret a location of neurocompression based upon history, symptoms, and often-subjective clinical findings.[30] These complicating factors can lead to significant time delay in diagnosing TOS. When arterial compromise results from TOS, delay in treatment can severely compromise functional outcome because of the ongoing arterial damage and thromboembolic events, potentially leading to permanent neurologic damage.[31–35]

In a review of our own experience with TOS at the University of Tennessee Knoxville, we found the clinical course of arterial TOS is largely determined by correct early identification of those patients at risk for arterial compression (Table 28-1). Unfortunately, because of the confusing nature of symptoms many patients have had prior diagnoses ascribed to explain pain and numbness, and a large subset have even had non-TOS operations that preceded vascular examination.[30] As time progresses, further arterial damage occurs with aneurysmal degeneration of the artery, thromboembolism, and permanent loss of runoff vessels to the arm and hand.[36] Although technical success is possible in the revascularization after longstanding disease, there can be a loss in function and pain likely related to chronic ischemia. Clinical awareness of TOS is therefore paramount to recognizing and appropriately treating patients early, before permanent arm impairment occurs.

The bony boundaries of the thoracic outlet include the transverse processes of the lower cervical vertebrae, the first

TABLE 28-1. Examples of Potential Risk Factors for the Development or Exacerbation of Extrinsic Arterial Compression in TOS, as Seen in the Described Series Review

• Shelf stocking	3
• MVC	3
• Repetitive labor	5
• Healthcare	2
• COPD/coughing	2
• Baseball pitcher	1
• Cheerleader	1
• Computer	2
• No identified risk	3

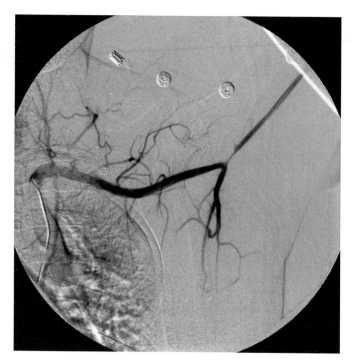

● **FIGURE 28-6.** Sub-humeral brachial artery compression is seen particularly in athletes where damage to segments under traction can result in aneurysm formation and/or digital thromboembolization.

thoracic rib and clavicle.[37] This bony framework provides the platform for the musculature that completes the "fixed" points of the thoracic outlet. The transverse processes of C4 through C7 are invested with the tendinous origin of the anterior and middle scalene, which inserts onto the anterior and lateral superior surfaces of the first rib. These muscles have a teleological role in ventilation, and are rarely recruited in the healthy adult during periods of ventilatory exertion as a portion of the "accessory" muscles of breathing.

Cervical ribs can exist with variation in size and "completeness," ranging from complete C7 ribs that insert 3/4 of the length along the first rib to small rudimentary ribs with fibrous bands that connect to the first rib.[38] These bony and fibrous elements are well described and raise the floor of the scalene triangle, leading to an increased fulcrum of the artery and lower trunk of the brachial plexus where it exits the interscalene space.[37] Where a cervical rib exists with symptoms, there is no opportunity for relief by physical therapy alone, and surgery is needed to eliminate the possibility of ongoing subclavian artery damage.

Diagnosis of arm ischemic changes from TOS can be made based upon history and physical examination. Digital plethysmography with the arms placed in positional, evocative maneuvers can help confirm the diagnosis. Compression of the subclavian artery most often occurs at the insertion of the anterior scalene muscle upon the anterior first thoracic rib, and elevation with abduction of the arm

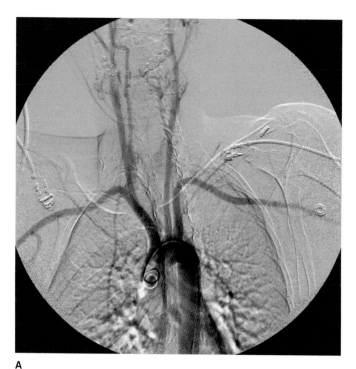

A

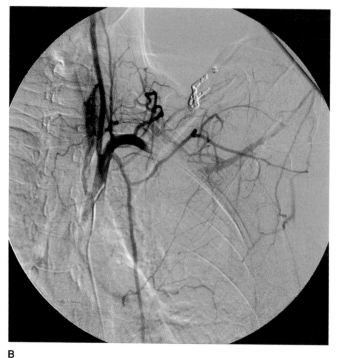

B

● **FIGURE 28-7.** (A and B) Evocative maneuvers performed during the course of arteriography may be required to reveal sites of extrinsic arterial compression. This series was obtained during the evaluation of a patient with digital ulceration caused by thromboembolism developed during the course of manual labor requiring overhead arm tasks.

accentuates the extrinsic compression with subsequent pulse waveform dampening. Those patients with a fixed diminution in the pulse or with frank ischemic changes caused by embolism should proceed to arteriography both to confirm the diagnosis and to plan therapy consisting of thrombus clearance with revascularization of the damaged arterial segments.[39] This author prefers to avoid percutaneous thrombolytics as morcellation of the thrombus can lead to distal embolization and loss of precious digital runoff vessels. Controlled open thrombectomy of the major burden of thrombus can be performed safely, followed by the administration of urokinase or tissue plasminogen activator to dissolve small residual thrombus debris.

In our series of patients, we have observed three separate sites of arterial compression as a cause for arm ischemia either because of the ongoing embolization or arterial occlusion. These include the anterior scalene insertion point on the first rib, (just posterior to the insertion of pectoralis minor on the first rib), and under the humeral head because of traction on the circumflex humeral branch vessels (Figure 28-6). To elucidate the exact location of arterial injury during arteriography, evocative maneuvers should be performed to include Adson's maneuver and the "military

tuck" position (Figure 28-7). If thrombus is seen, residing in the vessel at any of these shoulder girdle locations, the evocative maneuvers are avoided, and adequate data will include only a runoff sequence to determine the degree of distal embolic disease.

In our review of 23 patients undergoing treatment for arterial TOS, 95% had complete resolution of hand emboli, with no further events after surgery. There was 80% technical success for patients undergoing revascularization. A single failure accounts for further loss of runoff and failure of graft patency after surgery in a patient with thrombophilia. This unfortunate patient underwent hand amputation after three failed attempts at thrombectomy and graft revision.

Postoperative morbidity was common and included temporary or chronic neuropathic pain, ischemic nerve injury with contracture, temporary phrenic nerve dysfunction, and pneumothorax. The greatest number of complications was encountered in the group undergoing revascularization; however, decompression alone accounted for a significant number of untoward events (Figure 28-8).

Patients undergoing revascularization failed to return to gainful employment during the study interval and 63% undergoing decompression alone were able to return to work with physician-guided modifications to their manual responsibilities. In all cases, the surgeon played an active role as patient advocate in obtaining disability leave, interacting with employment safety officers, and providing depositions in the event of worker's compensation determination. All patients treated by physical therapy alone were eventually able to return to the workforce with specific restrictions imposed, while 60% of those undergoing decompression

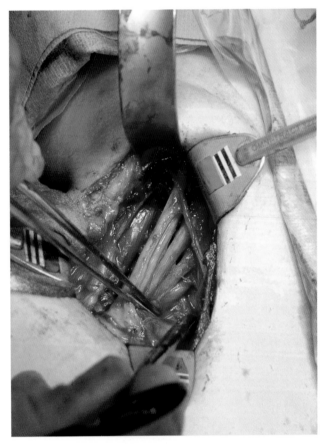

● **FIGURE 28-8.** Intraoperative exposure of the interscalene space during thoracic outlet decompression for dynamic arterial compression. Although relatively rarely performed, this intervention can help salvage extremities threatened by ongoing arterial injury during the course of every day tasks.

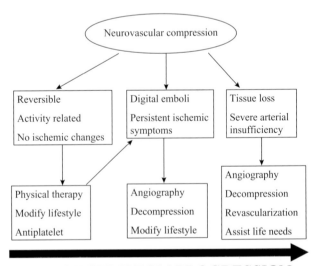

TIME OF SYMPTOM PROGRESSION

● **FIGURE 28-9.** Proposed algorithm for the treatment of arterial TOS. Symptoms and arterial injury can progress in a time-based fashion, requiring more aggressive treatment ranging from physical therapy with antiplatelet pharmacology to complex surgery with the goals of arterial decompression and vessel reconstruction. Although arm salvage is generally the rule, longstanding embolic and ischemic damage can lead to functional destruction of the arm and hand.

were eventually able to perform an occupation (Figure 28-9). All patients undergoing decompression and revascularization were rendered disabled for the study period. Time to diagnosis seemed to correlate closely with the degree of arterial damage and need for aggressive intervention. The best method of improving outcome in these difficult cases is to generate a wider clinical understanding and awareness of arterial TOS with primary care providers who have the important role of directing patients to the appropriate vascular specialist for treatment.

REFERENCES

1. Gray H. *Anatomy, Descriptive and Surgical*. 15th ed. New York, NY: Bounty Books; 1977:480-482.

2. Feldtman RW, Buckley CJ, Bohannon WT. How I do it: cervical access for carotid artery stenting. *Am J Surg*. 2006; 192(6):779-781.

3. Loftus CM, Kreswik TF. *Carotid Artery Surgery*. New York, NY: Stuttgart, Thieme; 2000:343-353.

4. Heitzman RE. *The Mediastinum*. St. Louis, MO: CV Mosby; 1977:124-157.

5. Soubrier M, Dubost JJ, Ristori JM. Polymyalgia rheumatica: diagnosis and treatment. *Joint Bone Spine*. 2006;73(6):599-605.

6. Schwedt TJ, Dodick DW, Caselli RJ. Giant cell arteritis. *Curr Pain Headache Rep*. 2006;10(6):415-420.

7. Jennette JC, Falk RJ. Small-vessel vasculitis. *N Engl J Med*. 1997;337:1512-1523.

8. Paraskevas KI, Boumpas DT, Vrentzos GE, Mikailidis DP. Oral and ocular/orbital manifestations of temporal arteritis: a disease with deceptive clinical symptoms and devastating consequences. *Clin Rheumatol*. 2007;26(7):1044-1048. Epub December 16, 2006.

9. Durkin SR, Athanasiov PA, Compton JL. Polymyalgia rheumatica and giant cell arteritis—an ophthalmic emergency. *Aust Fam Physician*. 2006;35(11):889-891.

10. Imrich R, Bosak V, Rovensky J. Polymyalgia rheumatica and temporal arteritis: the endocrine relations and the pathogenesis. *Endocr Regul*. 2006;40(3):83-89.

11. Evans RW. Diagnostic testing for chronic daily headache. *Curr Pain Headache Rep*. 2007;11(1):47-52.

12. Sourbrier M, Dubost JJ, Ristori JM. Polymyalgia rheumatica: diagnosis and treatment. *Joint Bone Spine*. 2006;73(6):599-605.

13. Modrall JG, Sadjadi J. Early and late presentations of radiation arteritis. *Semin Vasc Surg*. 2003;16(3):209-214.

14. Carpentier PH, Satger B, Poensin D, Maricq HR. Incidence and natural history of raynaud phenomenon: a long-term follow-up (14 years) of a random sample from the general population. *J Vasc Surg*. 2006;44(5):1023-1028.

15. Bart PA, Waeber B. Understanding Raynaud's phenomenon: towards a better treatment. *Rev Med Suisse*. 2006;2(48):93-96.

16. Cooke JP, Marshall JM. Mechanisms of raynaud's disease. *Vasc Med*. 2005;10(4):293-307.

17. Thune TH, Ladegaard L, Licht PB. Thorascopic sympathectomy for Raynaud's phenomenon—a long term follow-up study. *Eur J Vasc Endovasc Surg*. 2006;32(2):198-202.

18. Puechal X, Fiessinger JN. Thromboangiitis obliterans or Buerger's disease: challenges for the rheumatologist. *Rheumatology (Oxford)*. 2007;46(2):192-199.

19. Subhashree AR, Gopalan R, Krishnan KB, Shekar N. Buerger's disease: clinical and histomorphological study. *Indian J Pathol Microbiol*. 2006;49(4);540-542.

20. Ozaki, CK Seegar JM. *"Buerger's Disease"* Current therapy in Vascular Surgery. 4th ed. St. Louis, MO: Mosby; 2001:151-154.

21. Westerband A, Rodriguez J, Venkatesh R, Dietchrich E. Endovascular therapy in prevention and management of coronary-subclavian steal. *J Vasc Surg*. 2003;38(4):699-703.

22. Peterson BG, Resnich SA, Morasch MD, Hassouon HT, Eskandari MK. Aortic arch vessel stenting: a single-center experience using cerebral protection. *Arch Surg*. 2006;141(6):560-563.

23. Edwards WH Jr, Edwards WH Sr. Subclavian to carotid arterial transposition. In: Ernst C, Stanley J, eds. *Current Therapy in Vascular Surgery*. 4th ed. St. Louis, MO: Mosby; 2001: 90-97.

24. Loftus CM, Kresowik TF. Extrathoracic revascularization of innominate artery lesions. In: *Carotid Artery Surgery*. New York, NY: Stuttgart, Thieme; 2000:348-351.

25. Rutherford RB. Vascular exposures. In: *Atlas of Vascular Surgery*. Philadelphia, PA: WB Saunders; 1993:241-251.

26. Cleveland TJ. Subclavian and axillary artery angioplasty and stenting. In: *Vascular and Endovascular Surgical Techniques*. 4th ed. London, UK: WB Saunders; 2001:295-303.

27. Thomas GI. Perspectives in vascular surgery: diagnosis and treatment of thoracic outlet syndrome. *Vasc Surg*. 1995;8(2):1-27.

28. Patton GM. Arterial thoracic outlet syndrome. *Hand Clin*. 2004;20(10):107-111.

29. Degeorges R, Reynaud C, Becquemin JP. Thoracic outlet syndrome surgery: long-term functional results. *Ann Vasc Surg*. 2004;18(5):558-565.

30. Edgelow PI. Neurovascular consequences of cumulative trauma disorders affecting the thoracic outlet: a patient centered treatment approach. In: Donatelli R, ed. *Physical Therapy of the Shoulder*. 4th ed. Edinburgh, UK: Churchill Livingston; 2004.

31. Cornier JM, Amrane M, Ward A, et al. Arterial complications of the thoracic outlet syndrome: fifty-five operative cases. *J Vasc Surg*. 1989;9(6):778-787.

32. Sanders RJ. *Thoracic Outlet Syndrome: A Common Sequela of Neck Injuries*. Vail. CO: Maple-Vail Book Manufacturing Group; 1991.

33. Liu JE, Tahmoush AJ, Roos DB, et al. Shoulder-arm pain from cervical bands and scalene muscle abnormalities. *J Neurol Sci*. 1995;128;175-180.

34. Hagberg M, Wegman DH. Prevalence Rates and Odds Ratios of Shoulder-Neck Diseases in Different Occupational Groups. *Br J Ind Med*. 1987;44(9):602-610.

35. Davidovic LB, Kostic DM, Jakovljevic NS, et al. Vascular thoracic outlet syndrome. *World J Surg*. 2003;27(5):545-550.

36. Pascarelli EF, Hsu YP. Understanding work-related upper extremity disorders: clinical findings in 485 computer users, musicians, and others. *J Occup Rehabil*. 2001;11(1):1-21.

37. Ritter A, Sensat ML, Harn SD. Thoracic outlet syndrome: a review of the literature. *J Dent Hyg*. 1999;73(4):205-207.

38. Guidotta TL. Occupational repetitive strain injury. *Am Fam Physician*. 1992;45(2):585-592.

39. Durham JR, Yao JS, Pearce WH, et al. Arterial injuries in the thoracic outlet syndrome. *J Vasc Surg*. 1995;21(1):57-70.

chapter 29

Descending Thoracic Aorta

Daniel Alterman, MD / *Raymond A. Dieter III, MD*

INTRODUCTION

Acute aortic syndrome presents challenging diagnostic and therapeutic disease. Intramural hematoma (IMH), penetrating aortic ulcer, aortic dissection (AD), and aneurysm can all have a similar clinical presentation with advanced disease. Many of these syndromes have undergone significant revision in terms of classification and therapeutic strategy in the last 30 years. The increasing sophistication and speed of computed tomographic (CT) scan has raised it to a prominent role in the evaluation of this disease. The exact role endovascular intervention will play in the treatment algorithms remains to be determined. Despite the benefit of modern imaging and this collective experience, it remains a highly morbid malady.

EMBRYOLOGY

The embryonic vascular system begins formation in the third week of gestation. From the primitive aortic sac arise six ventral paired aortic arches. These pass laterally around the primitive gut to terminate in the paired dorsal aortae. Eventually, there is fusion of the paired dorsal aortae. The first pair of aortic arches contributes to formation of maxillary and external carotid arteries. The second pair contributes to formation of the stapedial arteries. The third pair contributes to formation of the common and internal carotid arteries. The left fourth aortic arches contribute to form the aortic arch and the right fourth arch contributes to formation of the right subclavian artery. The fifth pair of aortic arches usually has no anatomic contribution. An association between persistent fifth aortic arch and chromosome 22q11.2 deletion has been described.[1] The left sixth aortic arch contributes to formation of the left pulmonary artery and the ductus arteriosus. The right sixth aortic arch contributes to formation of the right pulmonary artery.

ANATOMY

The descending thoracic aorta arises from the aortic arch just after the origin of the left subclavian artery, at the inferior border of the fourth thoracic vertebrae. This point of transition is termed the aortic isthmus. In adults, the average diameter of the descending thoracic aorta is 2.8 cm in men and 2.6 cm in women.[2] This narrows as it descends into the abdomen. It terminates as it enters the abdomen via the diaphragmatic aortic hiatus, at the 12th intercostal space. The thoracic aorta descends in the posterior mediastinum to the left of the vertebral column and gradually shifts to the midline at the aortic hiatus. It is surrounded by the thoracic aortic plexus. Anteriorly, the left pulmonary hilum crosses with the left main bronchus and left pulmonary artery being closely associated. Continuing inferiorly, the esophagus, pericardium, and diaphragm are also situated at the anterior border of the thoracic aorta. As the thoracic aorta descends, the esophagus crosses anteriorly and then laterally at the diaphragm. Posteriorly, the hemiazygous vein and anterior vertebral column are associated. Laterally, it is closely applied to the inferior lobe of the left lung. Medially, the esophagus, thoracic duct, and azygous vein are closely associated. There are bronchial, esophageal, intercostal, mediastinal, pericardial, subcostal, and superior phrenic branches of the descending thoracic aorta. The main artery supplying the lower spinal cord (artery of Adamkiewicz) typically arises from a left-sided intercostal artery between the 9th and 12th intercostal spaces. The wall of the aorta is composed of thin inner intima, a thicker middle media, and a thinner outer adventitia containing vasa vasorum. During systole, the elastic laminae of the robust media distend and create potential energy, which is transmitted during the diastolic phase.

● THORACIC AORTIC ANEURYSM

Epidemiology

The estimated incidence of thoracic aortic aneurysm (TAA) was 0.37/100 000 person-years.[3] The incidence has been reported to be rising dramatically in the past 40 years, with a recent estimate of 10.4/100 000 person-years.[4] The median age of diagnosis ranges from 64.5 to 68.5 years and the mean 58 to 70.5 years. Men tend to have a higher incidence than women with an average ratio of 1.9:1, but the reported range varies from 0.9:1 to 17:1.[5] Several risk factors have a strong association with TAA formation. Of those having TAA, greater than 70% have hypertension and at least 80% are smokers.[5] Other associated risks are coronary artery disease, chronic renal failure, cerebrovascular disease, peripheral vascular disease, visceral occlusive disease, chronic obstructive pulmonary disease (COPD), and diabetes mellitus.[5] A recent study of TAAs, dissections and pedigrees revealed that 21.5% of non-Marfan syndrome patients had an inherited pattern. Seventy-six percent were transmitted autosomally dominant with a varying penitiance.[6]

Pathophysiology

An aneurysm has been defined as a permanent localized dilation of an artery having at least a 50% increase in diameter compared to the expected normal diameter of the artery. The average diameter of the descending thoracic aorta is 2.8 cm in men and 2.6 cm in women.[2] It is more accurate to define the size of aneurysm based on expected size of age, gender, and body surface area (BSA) matched controls. This data is available in the Pearce et al. paper[2] (see Figure 29-1). An imbalance of enzymatic degradation as well

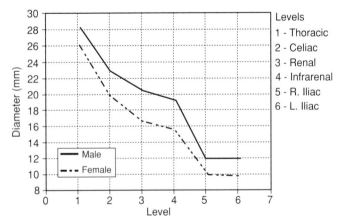

● **FIGURE 29-1.** Normal diameter of aorta, tapering from thoracic to iliac levels; male and female.

Reproduced, with permission, from Pearce WH, Slaughter MS, LeMaire S, Salyapongse AN, Feinglass J, McCarthy WJ, Yao JS. Aortic diameter as a function of age, gender, and body surface area. Surgery. 1993;114: 691–697.

as genetically defective structural elements has been implicated in aneurysm formation. Deficiency of other proteins, as occurs with Marfan's syndrome with deficient fibrillin, is associated with aortic aneurysm also. There is also an association between bicuspid aortic valve and TAA.

Turner syndrome is associated with aortic dilation in approximately 6.3% of those affected according to one survey.[7] The most common congenital anomaly of the heart is bicuspid aortic valve. Aortic root dimensions were found to be significantly larger in a group of young men with biscup aortic valve.[8] Up to 15% to 20% of TAA or AD maybe familial.[9] Several specific loci have been identified to be associated with familial syndrome, specifically 16p12.2–p13.3, 5q13–q14, 3p24–p25, and 11q23.2–q24.[9] Collagen and elastin contribute significant structural support to the aorta. Elastin allows mobility throughout the cardiac cycle. A paucity of elastin is found in the wall of an aneurysm and can be experimentally depleted by elastase, resulting in dilation of the aortic wall.[10] Dilation of the aorta leads to increased wall tension according to La Place's law $T = (P \times r)/2t$, where T is wall tension, P is distending pressure, r is the radius, and t is the wall thickness. This principle may also explain the well-documented logarithmic growth of TAA. Collagen types I and III are abundant in the wall of the aorta. A deficiency or increased destruction of collagen via collagenase has been implicated in formation of aneurysm.[4] Cystic medial degeneration is commonly found in TAA.[11] Atherosclerosis is typically found in descending TAA.[12] Of TAAs, about 40% involve the descending aorta.[11] TAAs are often part of a multifocal aneurysmal disease. In a review of 217 patients operated for TAA by Crawford, 68% of these had multiple aneurysms with the most common association being with infrarenal abdominal aortic aneurysm (AAA). Additionally, of 1076 patients treated for AAA, 12% were found to have additional aneurysms.[13] Of patients with thoracoabdominal aortic aneurysm (TAAA), aneurysms of the renal artery occurred an average 2.7% and in peripheral arteries (such as iliac, femoral, or popliteal) an average of 4.2%.[5] These data emphasize both the systemic nature of this disease as well as the importance of adequate screening for associated aneurysmal disease upon discovery of one site.

Natural History

The natural history of descending TAA is one of progressive enlargement with risk of rupture. Both the size of the aneurysm and the rate of expansion have significant impact on development of complications. The natural history of AAAs is more clearly defined than TAA. Part of the reason for this is the heterogeneity in the literature, often included in these series are a mixture of aneurysm extents as well as different acute aortic syndromes. There is a faster expansion of AAA compared with TAA. Masuda found an average expansion of TAA to be 1.3 mm/year compared with 3.9 mm/year of AAA.[14] The rate of expansion is influenced by initial aneurysm size, with aneurysms >5 cm having a higher rate of expansion.[15] The most common cause of death in patients with untreated TAA is aortic rupture.[16] A series by Dapunt et al. estimated change in TAA diameter to be 0.43 cm at 1 year with largest rate of expansion in smokers and aneurysm size >5 cm at presentation.[15] Coady reported annual aneurysm growth rate of 0.12 cm/year of descending TAA to be greater than ascending TAA of 0.09 cm/year, with a mean size of 5.2 cm at initial presentation.[17] While a larger aneurysm carries a higher risk of rupture, smaller TAA (those between 4 and 5 cm) also have a significant risk of rupture and death.

Classification

The extent of involvement of TAAA is defined according to the Crawford classification[18] (see Figure 29-2). Type I extends from above the sixth intercostal space, near the left subclavian artery, to the root of mesenteric vessels but not to the infrarenal aorta. Type II extends from above the sixth intercostal space to the infrarenal aorta and usually to the bifurcation as well. Type III arise below the sixth intercostal space of the thoracic aorta and extend to the infrarenal aorta as type II does. Type IV runs the length of the abdominal aorta from diaphragm to the bifurcation.[18]

Risk Stratification

Predicting the risk of rupture has been evaluated by several authors by proposed formula. As a result of review of 67 patients by Dapunt, a formula was proposed to predict the rate of change of maximal diameter.[15]

$$Y = aX^b,$$

where Y is the change in diameter, $a = 0.0167$, X is the initial diameter, and $b = 2.1$.

Juovonen reviewed a series of 114 patients and reported the following factors to be associated with the risk in rupture in descending TAA; maximal aneurysm diameter, older

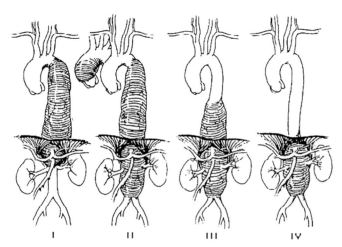

● **FIGURE 29-2.** Crawford classification of thoracoabdominal aortic aneurysm.

Reproduced, with permission, from LeMaire SA, Miller CC 3rd, Conklin LD, Schmittling ZC, Köksoy C, Coselli JS. A new predictive model for adverse outcomes after elective thoracoabdominal aortic aneurysm repair. Ann Thorac Surg. 2001;71:1233–1238.

age, uncharacteristic pain and history of COPD.[19] Based on multivariate risk factor analysis, the following formula was proposed to predict 1-year risk of rupture.

$$\ln \lambda = -21.055 + 0.093 \, (\text{age}) + 0.841 \, (\text{pain})$$
$$+ 18.22 \, (\text{COPD}) + 0.643$$
$$(\text{descending diameter in cm}),$$

where pain and COPD = 1 if present and 0 if absent. Probability of rupture within 1 year = $1 - e^{1\lambda(365)}$.

Descending TAA tend to rupture at a larger size (median diameter 7.2 cm) compared with ascending or arch aneurysms (median diameter 5.9 cm).[17] A review of 165 patients with TAA led to proposal of a similar formula to predict risk of rupture. Risk factors identified included aneurysm size, COPD, age, and uncharacteristic pain. A more rapid growth rate was seen with smokers.

$$\ln \lambda = -21.055 + 0.0093 \, (\text{age}) + 0.841 \, (\text{pain})$$
$$+ 1.282 \, (\text{COPD}) + 0.643$$
$$(\text{descending diameter in cm}),$$

where pain and COPD = 1 if present and 0 if absent. Probability of rupture within 1 year = $1 - e1^{\lambda(365)}$.

An attempt was made to validate the above formulae by Schimada et al.[16] This review of 88 patients with TAA again demonstrate exponential enlargement over time. When this data was compared with the above formulas, the Coady formula underestimated growth by 0.8 mm while the Dapunt formula overestimated growth by 1.5 mm. The decision to operate will be more straightforward in some patients and will obviate the need for calculation as above. Current indications include presence of symptoms, evidence of dissection, accelerated growth rate (>10 mm/year), or diameter 6 to 7 cm.[18,20] Some patients will not be adequately evaluated by the above formula because there are other possible risks such as development of serious cough with associated recurrent laryngeal nerve irritation with rapid aneurysmal expansion. Additionally, comorbidities may dictate the urgency of repair as well. New onset or increasing severity of pain will also lead to earlier repair. Based on recent review of 721 patients with TAA, the mean rate of rupture or dissection of TAA is 2% for aneurysm <5 cm, 3% for 5 to 5.9 cm, and 6.9% for aneurysms 6 cm or larger.[21] The biggest dilemma about decision to operate arises in a patient who has a relatively asymptomatic TAA. The above formula maybe useful in these patients to help estimate risk of rupture. The decision to operate on TAA should be based on expected morbidity of the proposed intervention compared with the expected morbidity of no operation. A review of 1509 surgical repairs of TAAAs by Crawford reported predictors of complication and complication rates. Neurologic complication such as paraplegia or paraparesis occurred in 16%, neurogenic bladder in 0.5%, renal failure requiring dialysis in 9%, postoperative stroke in 3%, pulmonary embolus in 1%, pulmonary complication in 33%, cardiac complication in 12%, bleeding requiring reoperation in 7%, sepsis in 8%, gastrointestinal complication in

7%, and coagulopathy in 4%.[22] The major cause of post-operative morbidity is occurrence of paraplegia or paraparesis. Several protective strategies have been adopted to minimize this occurrence. Heparinization, mild hypothermia, aggressive reattachment of critical intercostal arteries (T8 to L1), and cerebrospinal fluid drainage have been advocated.[23]

A recent meta-analysis reports a benefit for cerebrospinal fluid drainage to prevent paraplegia.[24] Risk factors for post-operative complication after elective repair of TAA were identified as preoperative renal insufficiency, older age, a symptomatic aneurysm, and type II aneurysm. A formula was created based on review of this series to predict adverse outcome.[23] An adverse outcome was defined as operative death, paraplegia or paraparesis, stroke, or acute renal failure requiring dialysis.

$$\text{Risk} = \text{odds}/(1 + \text{odds}),$$
$$\text{odds} = \exp\,[(\text{age} \times 0.272) + (C_2 \times 0.8945)$$
$$+ (\text{symptoms} \times 0.5504) + (\text{renal} \times 1.2612)$$
$$- 4.6597],$$

where age is given in years, $C_2 = 1$ for type 2 aneurysm and 0 for types I, III or IV, symptoms = 1 or 0, renal = 1 or 0 for preoperative renal insufficiency.

This model has not been validated prospectively. It does emphasize known risk factors for complicated disease. The authors say they use this risk calculation and balance it against calculated risk of rupture, and recommend surgery when risk of rupture exceeds risk of adverse outcome.

Evaluation

Diagnostic imaging includes chest radiograph, contrast aortogram, contrast-enhanced computed tomography (CT) scan, magnetic resonance angiography (MRA), and transthoracic and transesophageal echocardiography.[11] On supine chest radiograph, widening of the mediastinum (>8 cm at aortic arch) is about 80% sensitive and 50% specific. Widening of the left paraspinal stripe and deviation of the trachea or esophagus to the right are greater than 80% specific but sensitivity is low.[25] Thoracic aortography yields sensitivity almost 100% and specificity of 98% for traumatic aortic injury.[25] CT scan is 99.3% specific and about 90% sensitive for detecting aneurysm (Figure 29-3). MRA is almost 100% sensitive and specific for detecting aneurysm.(Figure 29-4).[25] An important potential pitfall to be aware of when evaluating cross-sectional imaging is transverse slice through torturous area where the aorta is angulated or curving. This is common in the elderly. This can result in a false-positive read for aneurysm.

Plain film chest radiograph is often used as an initial study with chest complaint. Several criteria have been associated with aortic disease on chest radiograph. Widening of the aortic contour, widening of the mediastinal shadow, tracheal shift to the right or distortion of the left main bronchus, displacement of intimal calcification greater than 6 mm into the aortic shadow, kinking or tortuosity of the

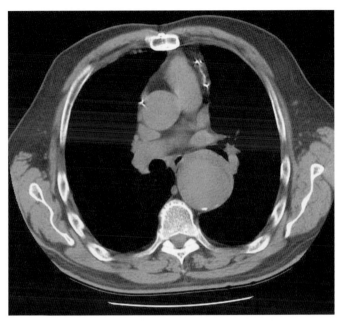

● **FIGURE 29-3.** CT scan of descending thoracic aorta aneurysm with compression, left bronchus.

aorta, opacification of the pulmonary window, and blurring of the aortic contour. A ratio of mediastinal width to chest width exceeding 0.25 has been used although some sources say up to 0.45 is acceptable.[26] Chest radiography has a sensitivity of 64% and specificity of 86% for detecting aortic disease, with the percentage being lower for ascending aortic disease.[26] Magnetic resonance imaging (MRI) is an accurate method to image patients with suspected aortic aneurysm or dissection. There is high soft tissue contrast and the ability to finely evaluate the aortic lumen and wall. An advantage when compared with the potentially nephrotoxic and allergenic CT contrast media is that MRI gadolinium-based contrast media are safer and have less renal toxicity.[27] Specific considerations apply when evaluating aneurysm disease with MRI/MRA. Accurate measurements of the outer aortic diameter are best obtained without angiographic enhancement. Also, the adventitia is not well visualized on MRA. MRI is also highly accurate for the detection of AD. Because of the length of the study, MRI has limitations in the emergent setting and is restrictive in terms of monitoring equipment.

Transesophageal echocardiography (TEE) offers high-resolution images as a result of the proximity of the esophagus and thoracic aorta. The ascending aorta and aortic root are directly anterior to the esophagus. From the level of the aortic arch to the diaphragm, the aorta and esophagus are close in their course. The newer biplane probes allow better imaging of the aorta compared with the monoplane transducer. In the evaluation of AD, reported sensitivity ranges from 97% to 99% and specificity from 77% to 100%.[28] The sensitivity is higher for dissections of the ascending aorta, however.[29] The finding of an undulating intimal flap in the aorta is the most definitive finding for AD.[29] This modality also allows assessment of aortic valve function, cardiac

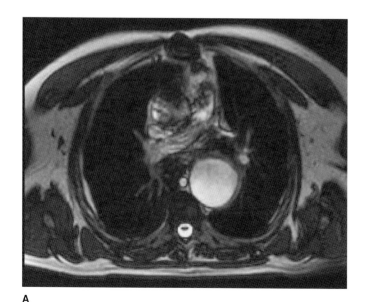

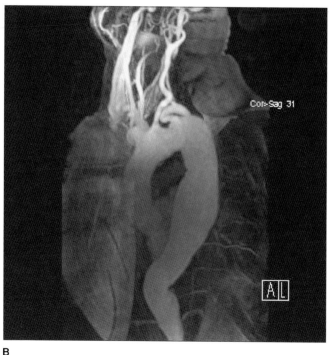

A

B

● **FIGURE 29-4.** MRI images demonstrating descending thoracic aortic aneurism.

function, blood flow in false and true lumens and thrombus, and frequently visualization of coronary ostia. It is advantageous to be able to evaluate the coronary ostia for operative planning in the case of a proximal dissection. Typically, this has been done with preoperative coronary angiography. Compared with MRI or CT, it is not as good at detecting thrombus in the false lumen as well as evaluating the entire length of the aorta.[28] The ascending aorta and proximal arch are incompletely evaluated by TEE.[30] TEE is a good adjunct to follow TAA, however, as some areas are incompletely visualized. It is very useful for aortic valve assessment with known TAA, which is an important consideration in surgical decision. TEE avoids the potential risks of aortography, which may include embolus with possible stroke, possible retrograde extension of the dissection, and site complications. There are certain patients who will not tolerate a TEE. It is not suitable for those with known esophageal varices, stricture, or tumors. It may produce vasovagal reaction and there is the risk of perforation.[29]

Medical Treatment

Medical management consists of minimizing risk factors for aneurysm growth. Beta blockade is the standard recommendation titrated to a systolic blood pressure of 100 to 120 mm Hg. Long-term beta-blockade therapy has been demonstrated to be effective in slowing the rate of aortic dilatation in patients with Marfan's syndrome.[31] The foundation of this treatment is derived from experimental data of turkeys prone to spontaneous aortic rupture having improved survival when propranolol was added to the

feed.[32] In addition to blood pressure control and heart rate control, this also reduces $\Delta P/\Delta t$, the so-called antiimpulse therapy.[25]

Surgical Treatment

It is unclear exactly which TAA should be repaired and which should be observed. Distinguishing between the risk of nonoperative and operative treatment is key but often difficult in the absence of clear guidelines for each patient. Careful risk assessment and knowledge of the natural history of TAA will guide this decision. For elective repair, a TAA of 7 cm or larger should be repaired.[14] Crawford recommends repairing TAA and TAAA greater than 5 cm in a good-risk patient and in symptomatic patients.[33] Lobato and colleagues gathered prospective data on 31 patients with TAA of less than 60 mm and deemed high risk for surgery or who had refused surgical therapy.[20] They recommend elective repair when the initial anterior–posterior diameter is 5 cm or greater with an annual growth rate of at least 10 mm. However, during their 47-month follow-up, nine patients with initial aneurysm size of 4 to 4.9 cm had rupture.[20] An unanswered question remains what is the best treatment for aneurysms 4 to 5 cm, especially those with a smaller growth rate than 10 mm annually. Operative mortality for type I Crawford TAAA is reported to range between 5% and 8%.[5]

Endovascular Treatment

Endovascular repair (EVAR) of the thoracic aorta has seen increasing utilization. The position of the proximal point

TABLE 29-1. Anatomic Endograft Zones of Thoracic Aorta

Zone 0: Ascending aorta to distal innominate artery origin
Zone 1: Arch distal innominate artery origin to distal left carotid origin
Zone 2: Arch–distal left carotid to distal left subclavian
Zone 3: Descending thoracic aorta–distal left subclavian to mid-descending thoracic aorta
Zone 4: Distal descending thoracic aorta

of the endograft is defined according to four anatomic divisions of the proximal aorta proposed by Ishimaru.[34] These zones (Table 29-1) are based anatomically on a line drawn tangent to the distal side of each of the arch branches (see Figure 29-5).

A recent review by Iyer examined their 6-year experience with 70 cases of EVAR of the thoracic aorta. EVAR was used for TAA in 63% and 30-day mortality was 1/70. Other lesions included one aortoesophageal fistula, seven traumatic rupture, and eight type B dissections. Postoperative endoleak occurred in 23% and endovascular failure in 11%. The majority of these repairs were done with the Tal-

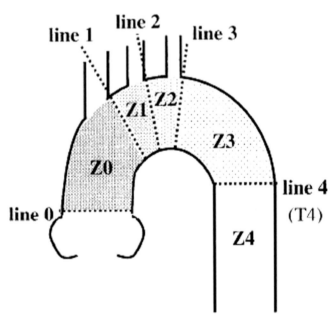

● **FIGURE 29-5.** An anatomical map of each landing zone bordered by lines delineating the distal sides of the branch arteries of the aortic arch. The position of the proximal end of the endograft is classified according to this system. Z, zone; T, thoracic vertebral level.

Reproduced, with permission, from Mitchell RS, Ishimaru S, et al. First International Summit on Thoracic Aortic Endografting: Roundtable on Thoracic Aortic Dissection as an Indication for Endografting. J Endovasc Ther 2002;9:II-98-II-105.)

ent self-expanding endograft system and five with Zenith system. Graft access was via common femoral artery, iliac artery via retroperitoneal exposure, or directly to the aorta via laparotomy. Systemic heparin was only used in one case and pharmacologic hypotension was used with graft deployment. For arch lesions, extra-anatomic bypass is used to enlarge the proximal landing zone (as with zone 1 or some zone 2 repairs). When more than one graft component is used, a 4 to 5 cm overlap is utilized. Cerebrospinal fluid drain was placed in 70% of patients and there was only one case of peripheral neuropraxia documented at 30 days with no paraplegia. Acute renal failure and conversion to open occurred in 4%. At 5 years, about 70% of the total treated patients were free from secondary endovascular intervention.[35] A similar report by Criado examined their 4-year experience of 47 thoracic lesions with 31 TAA and 16 type B dissections. The mean size of TAA treated was 6.8 cm (4.8 to 10.7 cm). A 4% 60-day mortality was reported. There was no paraplegia or stroke. These report as well as several older reports are adding to the growing body of evidence that may make EVAR of thoracic lesions the procedure of choice in the future. It should be recalled however that the reported 30-year experience of Crawford demonstrated a 30-day survival rate of 92% (1386/1509).[22] Long-term results of EVAR have yet to be determined but initial reports are promising. What remains to be answered are what lesions will provide the best long-term outcomes with endovascular approach and which should be treated with open repair.

A phenomenon known as postimplantation syndrome has been described after aortic endograft placement.[34] This consists of leukocytosis, mild thrombocytopenia, and postoperative fever. This may represent inflammation of the aortic wall to the graft. Conservative treatment with aspirin is recommended and typically resolves spontaneously.

● **THORACIC AORTIC DISSECTION**

Epidemiology

Incidence of AD has been estimated to be 2.9/100 000/year incidence. Other estimates have ranged from 0.5 to 4.04/100 000/year. Average age at dissection is about 63.4 years with a male-to-female ratio 1.55: 1.[36,37]

Natural History

The physician of King George II, Dr Nicholls, first described AD on autopsy in 1760.[38] Despite the significant advances in technology, the mortality of AD remains high. Type A dissection carries a higher rate of complication and mortality. After the acute onset of symptoms of AD, the mortality maybe as high as 1% per hour.[39] Predictors of in-hospital death include age >69 years, hypotension or cardiac tamponade, renal failure, and pulse deficits.[38] A trend toward improved survival with AD has been seen in recent years.[40] Erbel and colleagues reported survival rates of 52% for type I dissection, 69% for type II dissection, and 70% for type III dissection.[41] The IRAD data reports mortality of type A dissection to be 26% with surgical treatment and 58% without it. Mortality of type B dissection was 10.7% with medical treatment and 31.4% with surgical treatment[37] hence, the difference in treatment of ascending versus descending thoracic ADs.

Classifcation

AD is typically classified based on anatomical location and time from onset. Those involving the ascending aorta are Stanford type A dissection and those not involving the ascending aorta and distal to the left subclavian artery are Stanford type B. DeBakey type I AD involves the entire aorta, type II just the ascending portion, and type III the descending portion (see Figure 29.6). Within 14 days of the initial dissection is designated the acute phase. Presentation after 14 days of the acute phase is designated a chronic dissection (see Figure 29.6).

Svensson and colleagues have defined five types of AD, which includes the classically described type and its variants.[42] Type 1 involves an intimal tear creating a flap between true and false aneurysm, allowing flow of blood through a false channel. Type 2 is described as an IMH (see following section). Type 3 is an intimal tear without creation of false lumen. Type 4 is a penetrating ulcer to the adventitia. Type 5 is related to iatrogenic cause or trauma, such as injury with endovascular catheter. Mortality of iatrogenic AD is higher than noniatrogenic (35% vs. 24%).[8]

Etiology for type A iatrogenic AD includes cardiac surgery (69%), coronary angiography or intervention (27%), and renal angioplasty (4%). For iatrogenic aortic type B dissection, coronary angiography or intervention is primarily implicated (87%) and cardiac surgery secondarily (12%).[43] Sequelae of iatrogenic AD include myocardial ischemia or infarction (36% and 15%), limb ischemia (14%), and 30-day mortality of 35%.[43] In addition to endovascular injury, another iatrogenic etiology is the association with cardiac surgery. Type A AD is rare after heart surgery with an incidence of about 0.12%.[44] This is frequently attributed to surgical trauma of the aorta and the patients underlying diseased vessels. Off-pump aortocoronary bypass surgery is associated with a higher risk of AD compared with on-pump and maybe resulting from a risk of injury associated with aortic sideclamp and the subsequent pulsatile pressure at that site.[44]

Pathophysiology

Mechanisms that weaken the aortic wall can induce aortic dilation, eventually leading to dissection or rupture. The most commonly implicated mechanism for this weakening is hypertension. Risk factors were analyzed in data from the International Registry of Acute Aortic Dissection (IRAD).[37] Of 464 patients registered, 72% had history of hypertension, 5% had history of diabetes or Marfan syndrome. Risk factors associated with AD are long-standing

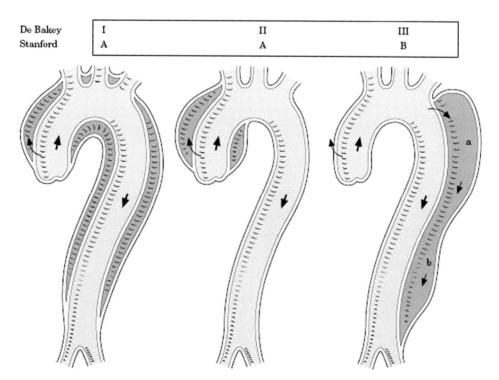

● **FIGURE 29-6.** Classification of aortic dissection: DeBakey and Stanford types.

Reproduced, with permission, from Erbel R, Alfonso F, Boileau C, et al. Diagnosis and management of aortic dissection: recommendations of the Task Force on Aortic Dissection, European Society of Cardiology. Eur Heart J 2001;22:1642.

hypertension, connective tissue disorders, bicuspid aortic valve, coarctation, vasculitis, dyslipidemia, cocaine, blunt trauma, genetics, and introgenic injuries.[43] The role of various entities such as cystic medial necrosis and atherosclerosis have been discussed as playing a central role in AD but these are found to play a role in only a minority of cases.[36]

Evaluation

Up to 55% of patients will die without a correct antemortem diagnosis of aortic dissection.[39] A high index of suspicion is necessary as well as rapidly implemented therapeutic plan. The sudden onset of severe chest pain is a cardinal symptom; however up to 20% of patients may not manifest this condition.[39] Differential diagnosis of AD includes acute coronary syndromes (ACS), aortic regurgitation, aortic aneurysm, musculoskeletal pain, pericarditis, mediastinal tumor, pleuritis, pulmonary embolus, cholecystitis, and atherosclerotic or cholesterol embolism.[41] Common presenting signs and symptoms are intense paroxysmal thoracic pain, syncope, hypotension, congestive heart failure, pulse loss, and evidence of branch obstruction such as cerebrovascular accident or paraplegia. A new onset diastolic aortic insufficiency murmur may also be a key finding. From the IRAD data, only 31.6% had aortic regurgitation and 15.1% had pulse deficit.[37] Of presenting symptoms reported, 95% reported abrupt onset of pain to chest and back, severe in nature and typically sharp or tearing in quality. This is contrasted to the pressure or tight sensation of angina. On imaging with chest X-ray, 61.6% had widened mediastinum and 50% had abnormal aortic contour.[37]

See "Evaluation of TAA" for a discussion of the imaging modalities. Initial diagnostic steps should include an EKG, chest radiograph, and a definitive imaging study, most commonly CT (Figure 29.7). The role and sensitivity of TEE, CT scan, MRI, and aortography are discussed in the previous sections. The role for coronary angiography is useful preoperatively to define the coronary anatomy. However, angiography is not without risk and is difficult in this setting and therefore is often not done. Only 25% of patients with acute dissection have significant coronary artery disease.[39]

Treatment

The main goal of medical therapy is to decrease the force of left ventricular contraction. The primary treatment of type B AD is medical therapy. Early mortality with medical therapy ranges from 8% to 12%.[45] Treatment focuses on halting progression of dissection by decreasing "impulse-force" ($\Delta P/\Delta t$). This is accomplished with using beta-blocker, calcium-channel blocker, nitroglycerin, and sodium nitroprusside (in this ascending order) to obtain target systolic blood pressure <120 mm Hg, mean arterial pressure <80 mm Hg, and heart rate <65 beats/min. When these goals are achieved, a transition to oral equivalent is pursued until target parameters are stable. General supportive therapy also includes aggressive pain control, deep venous thrombosis prophylaxis, nutritional support, and pulmonary therapy.[45] Risk factors for early mortality are rupture, renal failure, peripheral ischemia, and need for laparotomy. Endovascular treatment of AD is a recent addition to the treatment armamentarium. Stent graft closure of the proximal entry tear was introduced in 1999.[46,47] The standard of care for type B AD has been medical therapy, focusing on blood pressure and heart rate control. Surgical treatment in the acute setting has been reserved for complicated course such as a type A, worsening pain, enlarging diameter of false lumen, rupture, or end-organ ischemia. Paraplegia is not usually considered an indication as it is rarely reversible. Chronically, aneurysm formation is the main indication.

Mortality with surgical treatment has been reported up to 27% with elective surgery and greater than 50% with emergent surgery. Survival rates at 5 years have been reported between 32% and 60% with optimal medical and surgical treatment.[48] Stroke and paraplegia are the most concerning complications of surgical treatment and occur up to 21% of the time. Recently, short- and mid-term data have begun to accrue on the endovascular treatment of AD. However, these studies are nonrandomized and observational, making direct comparison with medical and surgical treatment complex. A meta-analysis of mostly (96%) type B AD treated with endovascular stent-grafting reported on 609 cases.[49] Thirty-day mortality for acute AD was 9.8% vs. 3.2% with chronic AD. Technical success rate is quite high in skilled hands (>98%). Perioperative stroke occurred in 1.9% and paraplegia in 0.8%. At 19 months follow-up, about 75% had thrombosed the false lumen. Continued perfusion of the false lumen has been identified as the main predictor of adverse outcome over the long term.[49,50] Successful endovascular stent-graft treatments of acute type A AD have been reported.[51] Requisite for this treatment is

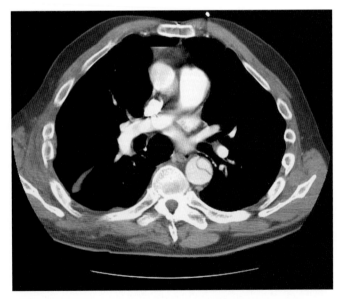

● **FIGURE 29-7.** CT scan of chest with dissection of descending thoracic aorta. The intimal flap is well visualized.

a functional aortic valve (no high-grade insufficiency) and an adequate landing zone above the coronary ostia. A key issue in endovascular treatment of AD is the timing of the repair. Late rupture has been reported in 2% to 9% of the patients.[49,50] This emphasizes the need for life-long follow-up with patients treated with stent-graft. A randomized trial comparing medical, surgical, and endovascular treatments is not currently available.

● TRAUMA/LACERATION

Blunt aortic rupture is the second leading cause of death after head injury, in motor vehicle accidents.[52] Deceleration injury is the leading mechanism of rupture of the thoracic aorta, and this kind of aortic tear maybe full in thickness or partial in thickness. A shearing force is generated between the mobile aorta and points of fixation, the majority of these being at the ligamentum arteriosum. Other less common sites of blunt injury do include the ascending arch, distal descending, or abdominal aorta. Incidence of blunt aortic injury is estimated to be about 8000 per year with about 85% dying on the scene.[52] Recent data outlining contemporary treatment and outcomes report a morality of 31% of those reaching the hospital alive, with 63% of these deaths attributable to aortic rupture.[53] The timing of diagnosis varied with both immediate finding on imaging as well as postmortem diagnosis in some of these patients. Associated injuries are common and maybe extensive and often involve neurologic, orthopedic, pulmonary, cardiac, gastrointestinal, or solid organ systems. The mean injury severity score (ISS) was 42.1. Widening of the mediastinum is the most characteristic radiographic feature. Chest radiograph findings on admission may also include apical cap, left pleural effusion, first or second rib fracture, tracheal deviation, depression of the left mainstream bronchus, or deviation of the nasogastric tube. Chest x-rays may also be "normal or negative." Symptoms may consist of back pain and blood pressure difference between limbs or dyspnea. Because of the frequency of associated injuries, evaluation and diagnosis requires a high index of suspicion and appropriate imaging. Nonoperative management (e.g., beta blockade therapy) of these injuries have been used, with modest success, as a temporizing measure while other severe injuries are addressed such as major head injury, extensive burns, sepsis, or large contaminated wounds.[54] Imaging options are aortography, CT scan, and TEE. Aortogram is the gold standard and in most series is superior to CT scan and TEE.[55] Thoracic aortography has a high sensitivity of almost 100% with a specificity of 98% for traumatic aortic injury.[25] This imaging is not as portable as a TEE and not readily available in the trauma-receiving area, making it less accessible. CT scan (Figure 29.8) has been reported as having sensitivity and specificity close to 93% and 100%, and TEE close to 75% and 100%.[56]

Operative repair is indicated and generally involves a "clamp-and-sew" technique or utilizing a bypass mechanism such as left heart bypass. The primary concern with clamp and sew is rising risk of paraplegia; however, distal perfusion does not negate this complication. Because of the high incidence of associated injuries and morbidity, immediate surgery is not always optimal. Patients with active extravasation or hemodynamic instability secondary to the aortic injury who are surgical candidates should be immediately repaired. Otherwise, aggressive blood pressure control initially with beta-blockers and intensive monitoring allows intervention on a recovered patient with heparinization for distal perfusion. Open repair via a left thoracotomy and clamping proximal to the left subclavian usually requires an interposition graft. Distal perfusion and use of heparin is often contraindicated at presentation secondary to associated injuries (i.e., intracranial hemorrhage, pulmonary contusion, solid organ lacerations, or orthopedic injuries).

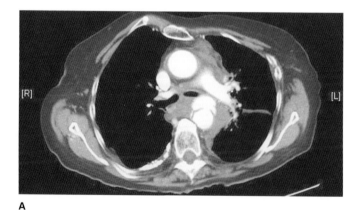

A

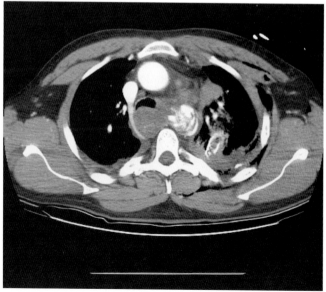

B

● **FIGURE 29-8.** Blunt descending thoracic aortic injury. (A) Contrast extravasation (B) Compression of the aorta by extensive hematoma is demonstrated.

EVAR may now be the procedure of choice in the acute setting because of the lower incidence of complications and mortality.[57]

MARFAN SYNDROME

Marfan syndrome is associated with mutations in the fibrillin-1 protein and occurs in approximately 1/3000 to 5000 individuals.[58,59] The identified mutation of *FBN1* gene has been linked to chromosome 15q15-21.3.[60]

There is significant mutational heterogeneity among patients who fulfill the Ghent criteria for diagnosis of Marfan's syndrome.[61] The life expectancy has increased in recent years and this maybe attributable to improvements in surgical therapy.[62] The introduction of composite valve graft technique for replacement of the aortic valve and root by Bentall in 1968 has led to more durable techniques and better long-term survival.[63,64] Surgical therapy of associated aortic aneurysm prolongs life expectancy by about 30 years.[65] Finkbohner et al. reviewed 192 patients undergoing surgical treatment of aortic aneurysm secondary to Marfan syndrome. Of the affected relatives who did not have surgical therapy, 50% died by age 30 years compared with age 60 years of the surgical-treated cohort.[65] Median survival in 1972 was 48 years compared with 72 years in 1993.[62] The mechanism of death usually includes rupture of the aorta into the pericardial sac with subsequent pericardial tamponade. Frequent monitoring of the aortic size and valve function is indicated. Activity restrictions involve prevention of contact sports and limitations of isometric exercise. Medical treatment to delay progression of aneurysm involves β-blocker and calcium channel antagonist therapy. These have been demonstrated to slow aortic growth in adult and pediatric patients with Marfan syndrome.[31,64] Recommendations for elective replacement of the ascending aorta are when the diameter of the aorta exceeds 5 to 5.5 cm.[66] In general, the occurrence of dissection and regurgitation is directly related to the size of the aortic root. However, acute dissections may occur when the aortic diameter is <5 cm and careful risk assessment is needed.[31] Dilation limited to the sinuses of valsalva has a better prognosis than if the aortic dilation is generalized and involves the proximal ascending aorta.[67] Rapid growth (>1 cm/year), aortic regurgitation, and family history of early dissection may lead to repair when the aortic diameter is <5 cm.[59] Elective repair is safe and has had a 30-day mortality of 1.5%, rising to 12% with emergent surgery.[68] Previously, composite valve graft with reimplantation of the coronary ostia was the standard treatment for Marfan syndrome patients who had aneurysm or dissection of the ascending aorta. Valve-sparing techniques were introduced by Yacoub and David.[69,70] While the valve-sparing aortic root replacement is safe and reliable, patients must understand the possibility of a second surgery if the native valve fails. The Yacoub technique involves remodeling with two aortic suture lines and the David technique involves reimplantation with three aortic suture lines.[71] Long-term data comparing valve-sparing procedure versus composite valve graft in patients with Marfan syndrome is lacking.

EHLERS-DANLOS SYNDROME

Ehlers-Danlos syndrome is a heterogeneous heritable connective tissue disease. At least six types have been characterized. Joint laxity and tissue fragility are the main findings. The vessels are prone to aneurysm. Incidence is estimated to be about 1/5000. Aortic disease is seen in type IV Ehlers-Danlos.[43] Surgical therapy is complicated by tissue fragility.

ARTERITIS—TAKAYASU'S

Aortic vasculitis may lead to dilation by weakening with intramural inflammation and may eventually to aortic rupture, regurgitation, or dissection. There is destruction of the medial elastic fibers that maintain the strength of the aortic wall. Takayasu's arteritis is a chronic giant-cell vasculitis that affects the aorta and main branches.[72] Incidence is estimated to be between 0.12 and 0.26 cases/100 000/year.[73] Multiple vascular sites and organ systems are involved and diagnostic criteria proposed by Ishikawa emphasizes this.[74] Glucocorticoids constitute the main medical therapy, with refractory disease using combination therapy involving methotrexate or azathioprine.[75] There is a risk of valve detachment or anastomotic aneurysm after aortic root or valve replacement. A review of 90 patients who underwent surgery for aortic valve regurgitation had a 15-year survival rate of 76%.[76]

PENETRATING ATHEROSCLEROTIC ULCER/INTRAMURAL HEMATOMA

Advanced atherosclerosis creates plaque that may ulcerate. Progression of this ulceration in the aorta can be catastrophic. Clinical presentation of patients with acute aortic syndromes (i.e., dissection, aneurysm rupture, penetrating ulcer, or IMH) is similar but the pathophysiology and radiographic findings differ. Penetrating ulcer of the thoracic aorta was first described in 1934 by Shennan.[77] This principally affects elderly hypertensive men. Multiple ulcers may occur and the most common site is the mid and distal descending thoracic aorta. These ulcerations may occur in normal caliber or aneurysmal aortas, but is more frequent in enlarged portions.[77] Penetrating ulcer occurs in frequent association with IMH in the descending thoracic aorta, while IMH without penetrating ulcer is more frequent in the ascending portion.[78,79] IMH is a variant of AD and represents intramedial thickening areas of noncommunicating blood. Aortic IMH was first described by Krukenberg in 1920 as "dissection without intimal tear."[79] The etiology of IMH is unclear but it maybe related to spontaneous rupture of the vasa vasorum, leading to hematoma formation or caused by atherosclerotic ulcer penetration through the internal elastic lamina, allowing hematoma to form in the media. There is potential of these lesions to regress or to progress to aneurysm, dissection, or rupture. The presence of penetrating ulcer with IMH places the patient at high risk for complications.

Of 1010 patients with acute aortic syndrome, 5.7% of these had IMH.[80] In this series, mortality was similar to those with classic AD. In-hospital mortality for IMH based upon site of origin includes 60% in aortic root, 30% to 50% in ascending aorta, 7% in proximal descending aorta, and 13% in the distal descending aorta.[80]

Diagnosis of penetrating ulcer is made by CT findings of contrast material-filling ulcer of the aorta without false lumen or dissection flap/tear.[79,81] MRI, TEE, and aortography also have a role in diagnosis. MRI may overestimate ulcer size because of blood flow adjacent to the ulcer. Extensive aortic calcifications are often seen with these lesions also.[81] Chest radiographs commonly show pleural effusion (left greater than right) and widened mediastinum.[82] A distinction has been made between the behavior of IMH with and without penetrating ulcer. Patients with IMH-associated penetrating ulcer who present with symptoms typically have a progressive course and require aggressive therapy. Those with IMH without penetrating ulcer, particularly those isolated to the descending thoracic aorta, tend to be stable.[79] Factors associated with disease progression in IMH patients with penetrating ulcer are severe pain, worsening pleural effusion, proximal aortic lesions, a maximal ulcer depth of 13.7 mm, and width of 21.1 mm.[79]

Typically, patients with IMH of the ascending aorta have surgical graft replacement and those involving the descending aorta are treated with antihypertensive therapy initially.[79] This recommendation was supported by the experience of Muluk and colleagues.[83] Patients with descending thoracic aorta IMH have a better long-term prognosis than those with type B AD.[84] Predictors for progression of descending IMH include age older than 70 years and new ulcer-like projection. The natural history of this disease is not fully defined and identification of subsets, beyond the above-mentioned groups, that benefit from early surgical repair is needed. It is agreed that a patient with acute, refractory pain and having IMH associated with penetrating ulcer should be surgically treated. EVAR of ruptured penetrating ulcer of the descending thoracic aorta has been described.[85] Recent midterm results are promising for the endovascular treatment of descending thoracic aorta penetrating ulcer disease. Brinster and colleagues treated 21 patients with such disease and reported 30-day mortality of 0% and overall mortality of 4.8%.[86] The requirement of a short segment of endoluminal stent graft maybe an advantage in terms of less potential for spinal ischemia and risk of paralysis. This was confirmed with an earlier experience by Demers.[87] Prospective and randomized data are lacking however.

● TUMORS

Less than 100 cases of primary aortic tumor have been reported. A premortem diagnosis maybe possible by symptomatology such as the case of a young woman with embolic phenomenon to her lower extremity.[88] The rest are typically found either at operation or postmortem. Most of these are found to be malignant and a type of sarcoma. Reported survival with malignant primary tumor of the aorta is very poor.[88]

● FISTULA—BRONCHIAL/ESOPHAGEAL

Aortoesophageal fistula arises from a variety of conditions and is fatal unless rapidly corrected. Esophageal cancer, TAA, penetrating ulcer of the aorta, trauma, and previous thoracic surgery have all been implicated.[89] Given the circumstances of diagnosis, operation carries significant morbidity. Recurrence of fistula maybe frequent.[90] EVAR have been attempted for both bronchial and esophageal fistula.[91] Successful reports are available; however, the risk of graft infection is a consideration. This maybe a palliative maneuver in a patient deemed high risk and with a likely poor mortality irrespective of the type of treatment. Aortobronchial fistula typically presents with hemoptysis and is fatal unless accurately diagnosed. After aortic surgery, it may present between 3 weeks and 25 years later.[92] Endovascular treatment has been effective for this condition and may require pulmonary resection as well or repair of bronchus with a pericardial patch.

● SURGERY-DESCENDING THORACIC AORTA

The descending thoracic aorta is usually approached via left thoracotomy. Median sternotomy or the "clam shell" with thoracotomy and transverse sternotomy can be utilized if the ascending aorta or aortic arch is involved but have limited role. If an aneurysm extends below the diaphragm, a thoracoabdominal incision can provide exposure down to the iliac arteries. The level at which the aneurysm begins will affect the interspace of optimal incision. If the proximal descending thoracic aorta is involved, the fourth intercostal space with a "hinged" rib or resection of the fifth rib allows access to this area. Most surgical repair of aneurysm and transections will require graft placement. However, occasionally a simple tear maybe treated primarily.

One of the concerning complications after aortic surgery is paralysis or paraplegia. The best method to protect the spinal cord has been extensively researched and improvements have been made. However, none of the methods have removed the risk and some are still debated. For example, papers supporting the use of distal perfusion with left heart bypass or full cardiopulmonary bypass even with deep hypothermic circulatory arrest have been published with paraplegia rates of approximately 2.3%.[93,94] However, Coselli reports equally impressive results with the clamp-and-sew technique.[95] Cerebral spinal fluid drainage has been shown to decrease the incidence of paraplegia in thoracoabdominal aneurysm repair[96] as has cooling.[97] Svensson also recommends reattaching intercostal arteries below T-8 for descending thoracic aneurysms and T-6 to L-2 for thoracoabdominal repairs along with keeping the patients hypertensive.[98] Increased cross-clamp times, extent of aneurysm, dissection, and acute presentation of the patient also play a role in outcome.

Compared to historic reports of paralysis being 41%, recent adjuncts have decreased the incidence to approximately 3% to 7% in elective procedures. Thirty-day mortality rates for open cases ranges from 4.4% to 19% in the reviewed articles with surgery before 1990, coronary artery disease, renal dysfunction, and acute presentation being other predictors of outcome.

Endovascular stenting of the descending thoracic aorta is becoming an attractive alternative to open repair. It can be done through smaller incisions or in conjunction with open repair. However, despite the "minimally invasive" approach, it also is not free of complications. In a recent review of 145 selected patients including 92 patients with descending aortic pathology, there was a primary success rate of 94.5%. Short-term mortality rate was 6.2% with three strokes, two patients with acute renal failure, one acute respiratory failure, and seven type 1 endoleaks.[99] Spinal cord ischemia is also a complication reported in approximately 6% of the patients.[100] As with open repair, this may occur in a delayed fashion and respond to cerebral spinal fluid drainage and/or arterial pressure augmentation.

● COARCTATION OF THE AORTA

Coarctation of the aorta (CoA) is a narrowing that obstructs blood flow. It represents 5% to 8% of all congenital heart defects.[101] The most common form is a localized narrowing of the descending thoracic aorta just distal to the left subclavian artery, justaductal. However, it may occur anywhere in the aorta or maybe diffuse hypoplasia often involving the aortic arch. The exact etiology is not known. Different theories include extension of ductal tissue into the aortic wall or hemodynamic factors that decrease flow through the aortic arch secondary to left ventricular outflow obstruction (i.e., aortic stenosis, mitral disorders, ventricular septal defects). Genetics also play a role as coarctation is one of the most common cardiac defects associated with Turner's syndrome[102] and can be transmitted with incomplete penetrance autosomally dominant.[103] Pseudocoarctation of the aorta results from an elongated or tortuous aorta with kinking but no obstruction to flow.

Patients with coarctation of the aorta usually present during infancy, however a second group presents later in life. Infants often have severe narrowing with blood flow to the lower body dependant on a patent ductus arteriosus (PDA) and may have other associated cardiac defects. In patients with poor collaterals, ductal closure can result in lower body end-organ ischemia and heart failure secondary to left ventricular overload. Symptoms may occur acutely resulting in shock. Prostaglandin E can be used to open the ductus in such settings.[104] Prostaglandin E has also been reported to relieve aortic obstruction without opening the ductus, supporting the theory of ductal tissue in growth and contracture.[105]

The second group of patients will present later in life with upper body hypertension. Aneurismal dilation of the aorta or intercostals arteries, dissection, rupture, endocarditis, intracranial hemorrhage, heart failure, and lower extremity claudication may also be the presenting symptom. Chest radiograph may reveal rib notching or the "3" sign. Physical examination should reveal decreased femoral pulses with upper body hypertension. Echocardiogram is usually diagnostic, noninvasive, and can identify associated cardiac anomalies. CT and magnetic resonance imaging are other noninvasive studies that are diagnostic (Images A and B). Cardiac catheterization is usually not warranted unless there are other associated anomalies.

Both endovascular and surgical repair are options. Balloon angioplasty offers a less invasive route but has a high recurrence rate, 41% in one series of infants and neonates.[106]

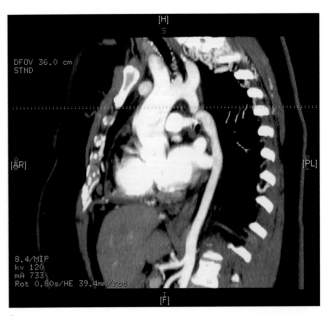

A

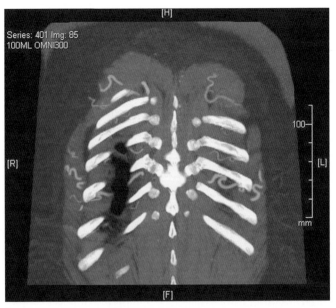

B

● **FIGURE 29-9.** (A) CT scan demonstrating aortic coarctation in a 48 year old. (B) Intercostal collateral as a result of the coarctation.

Stenting has been reported in a neonate in an emergency setting with the stented segment later resected at surgery.[107] EVAR has also been utilized in children and young adults with good short-term results.[108]

There are multiple surgical options available depending on the complexity of the coarctation. Subclavian flap aortoplasty, resection with end-to-end anastomosis, patch aortoplasty with other materials, and graft placement have all been utilized. The two most common are subclavian flap and resection with primary anastomosis often in an extended end-to-end fashion. A left thoracotomy is the normal surgical approach with a sternotomy utilized when there are other associated cardiac anomalies. In older patients, large intercostal arterial collaterals can be problematic at surgery. Extra anatomic grafts are also of value in adults. The may originate on the ascending aorta, arch, subclavian, or axillary artery and terminate at the descending thoracic aorta, abdominal aorta, or femoral arteries. Recent studies suggest that operative mortality is less than 3% and recoarctation up to 15% for isolated lesions.[104,108] Mortality and recoarctation is higher in patients with complex lesions involving the aortic arch. Use of partial bypass should be considered for those patients with inadequate collaterals to help decrease the incidence of postoperative paraplegia.[109] Patients should be followed long-term for hypertension and restenosis.

● PATENT DUCTUS ARTERIOSUS

The ductus arteriosus is derived from the sixth aortic arch. It usually connects the main or left pulmonary artery to the descending thoracic aorta. In utero, it serves to bypass the nonfunctioning lungs and usually closes shortly after birth. Closure is initiated by an increase in oxygen tension and a decrease in prostacyclin and prostaglandin E2. The smooth muscle in the media, arranged more longitudinally and spirally as opposed to circumferentially in the aorta, contracts. Over the next couple of weeks, the ductus becomes fibrosed, resulting in the ligamentum arteriosus.

PDA represents 5% to 10% of congenital heart defects occurring in up to 0.7% of the population and approaching 50% in premature infants weighing less than 1500 g.[110] The patency of the ductus is intentionally maintained in some forms of congenital heart disease (i.e., coarctation of the aorta) with postaglandin E1 or stenting.[111]

The degree of symptoms is dependent on the resistance of flow through the ductus and resultant left to right shunt. Size, length, internal diameter, and configuration all relate to the resistance. A large PDA may cause heart failure early in life manifested by tachypnea, tachycardia, and poor feeding. Smaller, less symptomatic ones may not be identified until later in life when a murmur is heard on examination. Infective arteritis and aneurysm formation are other complications. Adult PDAs have been found and are sometimes calcified, making closure more difficult. A continuous "machinery" type murmur maybe heard at the left sternal boarder; however physical findings can be absent. Signs of heart failure or Eisenmenger's syndrome usually only occur in patients with long standing shunts. Chest X-rays may be normal or may demonstrate cardiomegaly and increased pulmonary vascular volumes. Echocardiogram is usually diagnostic and other studies such as magnetic resonance imaging or CT are not needed. Arteriography is utilized if pulmonary hypertension is suspected to determine if it is fixed or reversible.

Gross reported the first successful surgical closure of a PDA in 1939, which included the use of medicines, catheters, and surgery. Indomethacin has been reported to result in closure of 40% to 75%. Larger PDA, low birth weight, low platelet counts, early surfactant use, and severity of illness have been identified as predictors of failure of medical treatment.[112,113] Transcatether closures utilizing coils and Amplatzer duct occluder depend on the size of the PDA. These are also limited in smaller neonates. Residual shunts have been reported in 3% to 30% including adults.[114] Other complications include migration or embolization of the device, hemolysis, partial pulmonary artery obstruction, arteriovenous fistulas, and vocal cord paralysis.

Surgical treatment of the PDA ranges from posterolateral, limited, or axillary thoracotomy, video-assisted thorascopic surgery or thoracoscopy, transpleural or extrapleural approaches. Potts clamps for division and oversewing, suture ligature, and clips are used for occlusion. In adults with calcified PDAs, median sternotomy with patch closure on pump via the pulmonary artery maybe advisable. Recannulation although rare, recurrent laryngeal nerve injury, chylothorax and bleeding are the main complications.[110,115,116]

In one prospective study of neonates undergoing PDA ligation, 7 of 61 patients evaluated using a flexible laryngoscopy had vocal cord paralysis. Only 2 of the 7 patients had strider or feeding problems. It was felt that compensation occurred early and there were generally no long-term problems with the airway or feeding.[117] Mortality from surgery is usually low and related to other comorbid conditions.

REFERENCES

1. Lee ML, Chen HN, Chen M, et al. Persistent fifth aortic arch associated with 22q11.2 deletion syndrome. *J Formos Med Assoc.* 2006;105:284-289.

2. Pearce WH, Slaughter MS, LeMaire S, et al. Aortic diameter as a function of age, gender, and body surface area. *Surgery.* 1993;114:691-697.

3. Bickerstaff LK, Pairolero PC, Hollier LH, et al. Thoracic aortic aneurysms: a population-based study. *Surgery.* 1982; 92:1103-1108.

4. Clouse WD, Hallett JW Jr, Schaff HV, Gayari MM, Ilstrup DM, Melton LJ 3rd. Improved prognosis of thoracic aortic aneurysms: a population-based study. *JAMA.* 1998; 280:1926-1929.

5. Panneton JM, Hollier LH. Nondissecting thoracoabdominal aortic aneurysms: Part I. *Ann Vasc Surg.* 1995;9:503-514.

6. Albornoz G, Coady MA, Roberts M, et al. Familial thoracic aortic aneurysms and dissections—incidence, modes of

inheritance, and phenotypic patterns. *Ann Thorac Surg.* 2006;82:1400-1405.

7. Lin AE, Lippe B, Rosenfeld RG. Further delineation of aortic dilation, dissection, and rupture in patients with turner syndrome. *Pediatrics.* 1998;102:e12.

8. Nistri S, Sorbo MD, Marin M, Palisi M, Scognamiglio R, Thiene G. Aortic root dilatation in young men with normally functioning bicuspid aortic valves. *Heart.* 1999;82:19-22.

9. Khau Van Kien P, Mathieu F, Zhu L, et al. Mapping of familial thoracic aortic aneurysm/dissection with patent ductus arteriosus to 16p12.2-p13.13. *Circulation.* 2005;112:200-206.

10. Crawford ES, Cohen ES. Aortic aneurysm: a multifocal disease. Presidential address. *Arch Surg.* 1982;117:1393-1400.

11. Isselbacher EM. Thoracic and abdominal aortic aneurysms. *Circulation.* 2005;111:816-828.

12. Alexander JJ, Miguel R, Graham D. Low density lipoprotein uptake by an endothelial-smooth muscle cell bilayer. *J Vasc Surg.* 1991;13:444-451.

13. MacSweeney ST, Powell JT, Greenhalgh RM. Pathogenesis of abdominal aortic aneurysm. *Br J Surg.* 1994;81:935-941.

14. Masuda Y, Takanashi K, Takasu J, Morooka N, Inagaki Y. Expansion rate of thoracic aortic aneurysms and influencing factors. *Chest.* 1992;102:461-466.

15. Dapunt OE, Galla JD, Sadeghi AM, et al. The natural history of thoracic aortic aneurysms. *J Thorac Cardiovasc Surg.* 1994;107:1323-1332; discussion 1332-1333.

16. Shimada I, Rooney SJ, Pagano D, et al. Prediction of thoracic aortic aneurysm expansion: validation of formulae describing growth. *Ann Thorac Surg.* 1999;67:1968-1970; discussion 1979-1980.

17. Coady MA, Rizzo JA, Hammond GL, Kopf GS, Elefteriades JA. Surgical intervention criteria for thoracic aortic aneurysms: a study of growth rates and complications. *Ann Thorac Surg.* 1999;67:1922-1926; discussion 1953-1958.

18. Crawford ES, Crawford JL, Safi HJ, et al. Thoracoabdominal aortic aneurysms: preoperative and intraoperative factors determining immediate and long-term results of operations in 605 patients. *J Vasc Surg.* 1986;3:389-404.

19. Juvonen T, Ergin MA, Galla JD, et al. Prospective study of the natural history of thoracic aortic aneurysms. *Ann Thorac Surg.* 1997;63:1533-1545.

20. Lobato AC, Puech-Leao P. Predictive factors for rupture of thoracoabdominal aortic aneurysm. *J Vasc Surg.* 1998;27:446-453.

21. Davies RR, Goldstein LJ, Coady MA, et al. Yearly rupture or dissection rates for thoracic aortic aneurysms: simple prediction based on size. *Ann Thorac Surg.* 2002;73:17-27; discussion 27-28.

22. Svensson LG, Crawford ES, Hess KR, Coselli JS, Safi HJ. Experience with 1509 patients undergoing thoracoabdominal aortic operations. *J Vasc Surg.* 1993;17:357-368; discussion 368-370.

23. LeMaire SA, Miller CC 3rd, Conklin LD, Schmittling ZC, Koksoy C, Coselli JS. A new predictive model for adverse outcomes after elective thoracoabdominal aortic aneurysm repair. *Ann Thorac Surg.* 2001;71:1233-1238.

24. Cina CS, Abouzahr L, Arena GO, Lagana A, Devereaux PJ, Farrokhyar F. Cerebrospinal fluid drainage to prevent paraplegia during thoracic and thoracoabdominal aortic aneurysm surgery: a systematic review and meta-analysis. *J Vasc Surg.* 2004;40:36-44.

25. Fishman JE. Imaging of blunt aortic and great vessel trauma. *J Thorac Imaging.* 2000;15:97-103.

26. von Kodolitsch Y, Nienaber CA, Dieckmann C, et al. Chest radiography for the diagnosis of acute aortic syndrome. *Am J Med.* 2004;116:73-77.

27. Roberts DA. Magnetic resonance imaging of thoracic aortic aneurysm and dissection. *Semin Roentgenol.* 2001;36:295-308.

28. Wiet SP, Pearce WH, McCarthy WJ, Joob AW, Yao JS, McPherson DD. Utility of transesophageal echocardiography in the diagnosis of disease of the thoracic aorta. *J Vasc Surg.* 1994;20:613-620.

29. Cigarroa JE, Isselbacher EM, DeSanctis RW, Eagle KA. Diagnostic imaging in the evaluation of suspected aortic dissection. Old standards and new directions. *N Engl J Med.* 1993;328:35-43.

30. Blanchard DG, Kimura BJ, Dittrich HC, DeMaria AN. Transesophageal echocardiography of the aorta. *JAMA.* 1994;272:546-551.

31. Shores J, Berger KR, Murphy EA, Pyeritz RE. Progression of aortic dilatation and the benefit of long-term beta-adrenergic blockade in marfan's syndrome. *N Engl J Med.* 1994;330:1335-1341.

32. Simpson CF, Kling JM, Palmer RF. Beta-aminopropionitrile-induced dissecting aneurysms of turkeys: Treatment with propranolol. *Toxicol Appl Pharmacol.* 1970;16:143-153.

33. Crawford ES, Hess KR, Cohen ES, Coselli JS, Safi HJ. Ruptured aneurysm of the descending thoracic and thoracoabdominal aorta. analysis according to size and treatment. *Ann Surg.* 1991;213:417-425; discussion 425-426.

34. Mitchell RS, Ishimaru S, Ehrlich MP, et al. First international summit on thoracic aortic endografting: roundtable on thoracic aortic dissection as an indication for endografting. *J Endovasc Ther.* 2002;9 Suppl 2:II98-II105.

35. Iyer VS, Mackenzie KS, Tse LW, et al. Early outcomes after elective and emergent endovascular repair of the thoracic aorta. *J Vasc Surg.* 2006;43:677-683.

36. Meszaros I, Morocz J, Szlavi J, et al. Epidemiology and clinicopathology of aortic dissection. *Chest.* 2000;117:1271-1278.

37. Hagan PG, Nienaber CA, Isselbacher EM, et al. The international registry of acute aortic dissection (IRAD): new insights into an old disease. *JAMA.* 2000;283:897-903.

38. Tsai TT, Nienaber CA, Eagle KA. Acute aortic syndromes. *Circulation.* 2005;112:3802-3813.

39. Spittell PC, Spittell JA, Jr, Joyce JW, et al. Clinical features and differential diagnosis of aortic dissection: experience with 236 cases (1980 through 1990). *Mayo Clin Proc.* 1993;68:642-651.

40. Clouse WD, Hallett JW Jr, Schaff HV, et al. Acute aortic dissection: population-based incidence compared with degenerative aortic aneurysm rupture. *Mayo Clin Proc.* 2004;79:176-180.

41. Erbel R, Oelert H, Meyer J, et al. Effect of medical and surgical therapy on aortic dissection evaluated by transesophageal

echocardiography. Implications for prognosis and therapy. The European Cooperative Study Group on Echocardiography. *Circulation*. 1993;87:1604-1615.

42. Svensson LG, Labib SB, Eisenhauer AC, Butterly JR. Intimal tear without hematoma: an important variant of aortic dissection that can elude current imaging techniques. *Circulation*. 1999;99:1331-1336.

43. Nienaber CA, Eagle KA. Aortic dissection: new frontiers in diagnosis and management: Part I: from etiology to diagnostic strategies. *Circulation*. 2003;108:628-635.

44. Chavanon O, Carrier M, Cartier R, et al. Increased incidence of acute ascending aortic dissection with off-pump aortocoronary bypass surgery? *Ann Thorac Surg*. 2001;71:117-121.

45. Estrera AL, Miller CC 3rd, Safi HJ, et al. Outcomes of medical management of acute type B aortic dissection. *Circulation*. 2006;114:I384-I389.

46. Dake MD, Kato N, Mitchell RS, et al. Endovascular stent-graft placement for the treatment of acute aortic dissection. *N Engl J Med*. 1999;340:1546-1552.

47. Nienaber CA, Fattori R, Lund G, et al. Nonsurgical reconstruction of thoracic aortic dissection by stent-graft placement. *N Engl J Med*. 1999;340:1539-1545.

48. Eggebrecht H, Herold U, Kuhnt O, et al. Endovascular stent-graft treatment of aortic dissection: determinants of post-interventional outcome. *Eur Heart J*. 2005;26:489-497.

49. Eggebrecht H, Nienaber CA, Neuhauser M, et al. Endovascular stent-graft placement in aortic dissection: a meta-analysis. *Eur Heart J*. 2006;27:489-498.

50. Bernard Y, Zimmermann H, Chocron S, et al. False lumen patency as a predictor of late outcome in aortic dissection. *Am J Cardiol*. 2001;87:1378-1382.

51. Zimpfer D, Czerny M, Kettenbach J, et al. Treatment of acute type a dissection by percutaneous endovascular stent-graft placement. *Ann Thorac Surg*. 2006;82:747-749.

52. Smith RS, Chang FC. Traumatic rupture of the aorta: still a lethal injury. *Am J Surg*. 1986;152:660-663.

53. Fabian TC, Richardson JD, Croce MA, et al. Prospective study of blunt aortic injury: multicenter trial of the american association for the surgery of trauma. *J Trauma*. 1997;42:374-380; discussion 380-383.

54. Fisher RG, Oria RA, Mattox KL, Whigham CJ, Pickard LR. Conservative management of aortic lacerations due to blunt trauma. *J Trauma*. 1990;30:1562-1566.

55. Sturm JT, Hankins DG, Young G. Thoracic aortography following blunt chest trauma. *Am J Emerg Med*. 1990;8:92-96.

56. Vignon P, Boncoeur MP, Francois B, Rambaud G, Maubon A, Gastinne H. Comparison of multiplane transesophageal echocardiography and contrast-enhanced helical CT in the diagnosis of blunt traumatic cardiovascular injuries. *Anesthesiology*. 2001;94:615-622; discussion 5A.

57. Tehrani HY, Peterson BG, Katariya K, et al. Endovascular repair of thoracic aortic tears. *Ann Thorac Surg*. 2006;82:873-877; discussion 877-878.

58. Judge DP, Dietz HC. Marfan's syndrome. *Lancet*. 2005;366:1965-1976.

59. Milewicz DM, Dietz HC, Miller DC. Treatment of aortic disease in patients with marfan syndrome. *Circulation*. 2005;111:e150-e157.

60. Dietz HC, Cutting GR, Pyeritz RE, et al. Marfan syndrome caused by a recurrent de novo missense mutation in the fibrillin gene. *Nature*. 1991;352:337-339.

61. Loeys B, Nuytinck L, Delvaux I, De Bie S, De Paepe A. Genotype and phenotype analysis of 171 patients referred for molecular study of the fibrillin-1 gene FBN1 because of suspected Marfan syndrome. *Arch Intern Med*. 2001;161:2447-2454.

62. Silverman DI, Burton KJ, Gray J, et al. Life expectancy in the marfan syndrome. *Am J Cardiol*. 1995;75:157-160.

63. Bentall H, De Bono A. A technique for complete replacement of the ascending aorta. *Thorax*. 1968;23:338-339.

64. Rossi-Foulkes R, Roman MJ, Rosen SE, et al. Phenotypic features and impact of beta blocker or calcium antagonist therapy on aortic lumen size in the Marfan syndrome. *Am J Cardiol*. 1999;83:1364-1368.

65. Finkbohner R, Johnston D, Crawford ES, Coselli J, Milewicz DM. Marfan syndrome. Long-term survival and complications after aortic aneurysm repair. *Circulation*. 1995;91:728-733.

66. Kouchoukos NT, Dougenis D. Surgery of the thoracic aorta. *N Engl J Med*. 1997;336:1876-1888.

67. Roman MJ, Rosen SE, Kramer-Fox R, Devereux RB. Prognostic significance of the pattern of aortic root dilation in the Marfan syndrome. *J Am Coll Cardiol*. 1993;22:1470-1476.

68. Gott VL, Greene PS, Alejo DE, et al. Replacement of the aortic root in patients with Marfan's syndrome. *N Engl J Med*. 1999;340:1307-1313.

69. de Oliveira NC, David TE, Ivanov J, et al. Results of surgery for aortic root aneurysm in patients with marfan syndrome. *J Thorac Cardiovasc Surg*. 2003;125:789-796.

70. Birks EJ, Webb C, Child A, Radley-Smith R, Yacoub MH. Early and long-term results of a valve-sparing operation for marfan syndrome. *Circulation*. 1999;100:II29-II35.

71. Miller DC. Valve-sparing aortic root replacement in patients with the Marfan syndrome. *J Thorac Cardiovasc Surg*. 2003;125:773-778.

72. Hata A, Noda M, Moriwaki R, Numano F. Angiographic findings of Takayasu arteritis: new classification. *Int J Cardiol*. 1996;54 Suppl:S155-S163.

73. Vanoli M, Bacchiani G, Origg L, Scorza R. Takayasu's arteritis: a changing disease. *J Nephrol*. 2001;14:497-505.

74. Ishikawa K. Diagnostic approach and proposed criteria for the clinical diagnosis of Takayasu's arteriopathy. *J Am Coll Cardiol*. 1988;12:964-972.

75. Hoffman GS, Leavitt RY, Kerr GS, Rottem M, Sneller MC, Fauci AS. Treatment of glucocorticoid-resistant or relapsing takayasu arteritis with methotrexate. *Arthritis Rheum*. 1994;37:578-582.

76. Matsuura K, Ogino H, Kobayashi J, et al. Surgical treatment of aortic regurgitation due to Takayasu arteritis: long-term morbidity and mortality. *Circulation*. 2005;112:3707-3712.

77. Troxler M, Mavor AI, Homer-Vanniasinkam S. Penetrating atherosclerotic ulcers of the aorta. *Br J Surg*. 2001;88:1169-1177.

78. Nienaber CA, Richartz BM, Rehders T, Ince H, Petzsch M. Aortic intramural haematoma: natural history and predictive factors for complications. *Heart*. 2004;90:372-374.

79. Ganaha F, Miller DC, Sugimoto K, et al. Prognosis of aortic intramural hematoma with and without penetrating atherosclerotic ulcer: a clinical and radiological analysis. *Circulation*. 2002;106:342-348.

80. Evangelista A, Mukherjee D, Mehta RH, et al. Acute intramural hematoma of the aorta: a mystery in evolution. *Circulation*. 2005;111:1063-1070.

81. Coady MA, Rizzo JA, Hammond GL, Pierce JG, Kopf GS, Elefteriades JA. Penetrating ulcer of the thoracic aorta: what is it? how do we recognize it? how do we manage it? *J Vasc Surg*. 1998;27:1006-1015; discussion 1015-1016.

82. Kazerooni EA, Bree RL, Williams DM. Penetrating atherosclerotic ulcers of the descending thoracic aorta: evaluation with CT and distinction from aortic dissection. *Radiology*. 1992;183:759-765.

83. Muluk SC, Kaufman JA, Torchiana DF, Gertler JP, Cambria RP. Diagnosis and treatment of thoracic aortic intramural hematoma. *J Vasc Surg*. 1996;24:1022-1029.

84. Kaji S, Akasaka T, Katayama M, et al. Long-term prognosis of patients with type B aortic intramural hematoma. *Circulation*. 2003;108 Suppl 1:II307-II311.

85. Brittenden J, McBride K, McInnes G, Gillespie IN, Bradbury AW. The use of endovascular stents in the treatment of penetrating ulcers of the thoracic aorta. *J Vasc Surg*. 1999;30:946-949.

86. Brinster DR, Wheatley GH 3rd, Williams J, Ramaiah VG, Diethrich EB, Rodriguez-Lopez JA. Are penetrating aortic ulcers best treated using an endovascular approach? *Ann Thorac Surg*. 2006;82:1688-1691.

87. Demers P, Miller DC, Mitchell RS, Kee ST, Chagonjian L, Dake MD. Stent-graft repair of penetrating atherosclerotic ulcers in the descending thoracic aorta: mid-term results. *Ann Thorac Surg*. 2004;77:81-86.

88. Das AK, Reddy KS, Suwanjindar P, et al. Primary tumors of the aorta. *Ann Thorac Surg*. 1996;62:1526-1528.

89. Reardon MJ, Brewer RJ, LeMaire SA, Baldwin JC, Safi HJ. Surgical management of primary aortoesophageal fistula secondary to thoracic aneurysm. *Ann Thorac Surg*. 2000;69:967-970.

90. da Silva ES, Tozzi FL, Otochi JP, de Tolosa EM, Neves CR, Fortes F. Aortoesophageal fistula caused by aneurysm of the thoracic aorta: successful surgical treatment, case report, and literature review. *J Vasc Surg*. 1999;30:1150-1157.

91. Leobon B, Roux D, Mugniot A, et al. Endovascular treatment of thoracic aortic fistulas. *Ann Thorac Surg*. 2002;74:247-249.

92. Algaba Calderon A, Jara Chinarro B, Abad Fernandez A, Isidoro Navarrete O, Ramos Martos A, Juretschke Moragues MA. Recurrent hemoptysis secondary to an aortobronchial fistula. *Arch Bronconeumol*. 2005;41:352-354.

93. Estrera AL, Miller CC 3rd, Chen EP, et al. Descending thoracic aortic aneurysm repair: 12-year experience using distal aortic perfusion and cerebrospinal fluid drainage. *Ann Thorac Surg*. 2005;80:1290-1296; discussion 1296.

94. Patel HJ, Shillingford MS, Mihalik S, Proctor MC, Deeb GM. Resection of the descending thoracic aorta: outcomes after use of hypothermic circulatory arrest. *Ann Thorac Surg*. 2006;82:90-95; discussion 95-96.

95. Coselli JS, LeMaire SA, Conklin LD, Adams GJ. Left heart bypass during descending thoracic aortic aneurysm repair does not reduce the incidence of paraplegia. *Ann Thorac Surg*. 2004;77:1298-1303; discussion 1303.

96. Coselli JS, Lemaire SA, Koksoy C, Schmittling ZC, Curling PE. Cerebrospinal fluid drainage reduces paraplegia after thoracoabdominal aortic aneurysm repair: results of a randomized clinical trial. *J Vasc Surg*. 2002;35:631-639.

97. von Segesser LK, Marty B, Mueller X, et al. Active cooling during open repair of thoraco-abdominal aortic aneurysms improves outcome. *Eur J Cardiothorac Surg*. 2001;19:411-415; discussion 415-416.

98. Svensson LG. Paralysis after aortic surgery: in search of lost cord function. *Surgeon*. 2005;3:396-405.

99. Civilini E, Melissano G, Chiesa R. Endovascular treatment of thoracic aortic pathology: lessons learned. *Acta Chir Belg*. 2006;106:323-331.

100. Cheung AT, Pochettino A, McGarvey ML, et al. Strategies to manage paraplegia risk after endovascular stent repair of descending thoracic aortic aneurysms. *Ann Thorac Surg*. 2005;80:1280-1288; discussion 1288-1289.

101. Rao PS. Coarctation of the aorta. *Curr Cardiol Rep*. 2005;7:425-434.

102. Papp C, Beke A, Mezei G, Szigeti Z, Ban Z, Papp Z. Prenatal diagnosis of turner syndrome: report on 69 cases. *J Ultrasound Med*. 2006;25:711-717; quiz 718-720.

103. Towbin JA, Belmont J. Molecular determinants of left and right outflow tract obstruction. *Am J Med Genet*. 2000;97:297-303.

104. Korbmacher B, Krogmann ON, Rammos S, et al. Repair of critical aortic coarctation in neonatal age. *J Cardiovasc Surg (Torino)*. 2002;43:1-6.

105. Liberman L, Gersony WM, Flynn PA, Lamberti JJ, Cooper RS, Stare TJ. Effectiveness of prostaglandin E1 in relieving obstruction in coarctation of the aorta without opening the ductus arteriosus. *Pediatr Cardiol*. 2004;25:49-52.

106. Patel HT, Madani A, Paris YM, Warner KG, Hijazi ZM. Balloon angioplasty of native coarctation of the aorta in infants and neonates: Is it worth the hassle? *Pediatr Cardiol*. 2001;22:53-57.

107. Fink C, Peuster M, Hausdorf G. Endovascular stenting as an emergency treatment for neonatal coarctation. *Cardiol Young*. 2000;10:644-646.

108. Marshall AC, Perry SB, Keane JF, Lock JE. Early results and medium-term follow-up of stent implantation for mild residual or recurrent aortic coarctation. *Am Heart J*. 2000;139:1054-1060.

109. Backer CL, Stewart RD, Kelle AM, Mavroudis C. Use of partial cardiopulmonary bypass for coarctation repair through a left thoracotomy in children without collaterals. *Ann Thorac Surg*. 2006;82:964-972.

110. Leon-Wyss J, Vida VL, Veras O, et al. Modified extrapleural ligation of patent ductus arteriosus: a convenient surgical approach in a developing country. *Ann Thorac Surg*. 2005;79:632-635.

111. Sivakumar K, Francis E, Krishnan P, Shahani J. Ductal stenting retrains the left ventricle in transposition of great arteries with intact ventricular septum. *J Thorac Cardiovasc Surg*. 2006;132:1081-1086.

112. Godambe S, Newby B, Shah V, Shah PS. Effect of indomethacin on closure of ductus arteriosus in very-low-birthweight neonates. *Acta Paediatr*. 2006;95:1389-1393.

113. Boo NY, Mohd-Amin I, Bilkis AA, Yong-Junina F. Predictors of failed closure of patent ductus arteriosus with indomethacin. *Singapore Med J*. 2006;47:763-768.

114. Chaowu Y, Shihua Z, Shiliang J, et al. Transcatheter closure of patent ductus arteriosus with severe pulmonary arterial hypertension in adults. *Cardiol Young*. 2000;6:644-666.

115. Mandhan PL, Samarakkody U, Brown S, et al. Comparison of suture ligation and clip application for the treatment of patent ductus arteriosus in preterm neonates. *J Thorac Cardiovasc Surg*. 2006;132:672-674.

116. Vanamo K, Berg E, Kokki H, Tikanoja T. Video-assisted thoracoscopic versus open surgery for persistent ductus arteriosus. *J Pediatr Surg*. 2006;41:1226-1229.

117. Pereira KD, Webb BD, Blakely ML, Cox CS Jr, Lally KP. Sequelae of recurrent laryngeal nerve injury after patent ductus arteriosus ligation. *Int J Pediatr Otorhinolaryngol*. 2006;70:1609-1612.

chapter 30

Abdominal Aorta

J. William Mix, MD / Sridevi R. Pitta, MD / Jeffrey P. Schwartz, MD / J. Michael Tuchek, DO / Robert S. Dieter, MD, RVT / Michael B. Freeman, MD

● INTRODUCTION

The abdominal aorta is frequently affected by both degenerative and occlusive disease. Since these diseases of the aorta frequently afflict the elderly, and with an aging U.S. population, surgical and endovascular treatment of aortic disease is common in a vascular specialist's practice. Approximately 42 000 operations for the treatment of abdominal aortic aneurysms (AAA) were performed in the United States in 2003.[1,2] Though in the past open surgical therapy for aortic diseases was the primary therapy, endovascular therapy of aortic diseases has emerged as an acceptable alternative to open aortic reconstruction and expanded the treatment options for those who treat aortic lesions. Advances in graft materials, surgical technique, and perioperative care have led to a marked reduction in perioperative morbidity and mortality with improvements in long-term results. With proper patient selection and appropriate procedure choice, the management of aortic diseases is one of the most rewarding areas of a modern vascular specialist's practice.

● ANATOMY

The abdominal aorta is the final segment of the aorta and the continuation of the thoracic aorta beginning at the median aortic hiatus and terminating at the level of fourth lumbar vertebra by dividing into two common iliac arteries. The average diameter of the abdominal aorta is 2 cm (range of 1.4–3 cm). The abdominal aorta is frequently classified as suprarenal or infrarenal segments (Figure 30.1). The branches of the abdominal aorta are subdivided as either ventral, lateral, or dorsal. The ventral branches are unpaired visceral branches consisting of the celiac artery, the superior mesenteric artery, and the inferior mesenteric artery. The lateral branches are primarily paired visceral branches including the suprarenal artery, renal artery, and ovarian or testicular arteries. The inferior phrenic artery is also a lateral branch but is a paired parietal branch. The lumbar and sacral arteries are the dorsal branches of the abdominal aorta.

● ABDOMINAL AORTIC ANEURYSMS

Though obstructive, atherosclerotic changes of the abdominal aorta are a frequent finding in the aging population, AAA is the most common disease of the abdominal aorta that requires treatment. First described by Vesalius, a 16th century anatomist, AAAs are defined by a diameter 50% greater than the expected diameter. This is frequently accepted to be a size of 3 cm or greater. When less than 50% diameter enlargement is encountered, it is defined as arteriomegaly or ectasia.

Pathogenesis

More than 90% of all AAAs are caused by degenerative changes of the aortic wall. However, atherosclerosis cannot be the sole factor leading to AAA development. Since the atherosclerosis theory does not completely explain the development of either occlusive or aneurysmal changes in the aorta of similar patients, aneurysmal changes of the abdominal aorta must be caused by a more complex degenerative mechanism than just atherosclerosis.

The most important matrix proteins in the aortic wall, which can be affected by aneurysmal changes and lead to AAA, are elastin and collagen. These proteins are arranged in such a manner to withstand intense arterial pressures, with the principal load-bearing element in the aorta being elastin. In the normal aorta, there is a gradual but marked reduction in the number of medial elastin layers from the

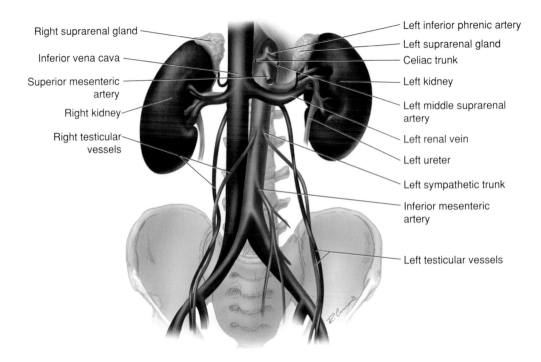

Right suprarenal gland

Inferior vena cava

Superior mesenteric artery

Right kidney

Right testicular vessels

Left inferior phrenic artery

Left suprarenal gland

Celiac trunk

Left kidney

Left middle suprarenal artery

Left renal vein

Left ureter

Left sympathetic trunk

Inferior mesenteric artery

Left testicular vessels

● **FIGURE 30-1.** Abdominal aorta and its relation to its surrounding structures.

proximal thoracic aorta (60–80 layers) to the infrarenal aorta (28–32 layers), accompanied by medial thinning and intimal thickening in the more distal aorta.[3,4] Halloran and colleagues described a marked 58% decrease in elastin content between the suprarenal and infrarenal aorta and noted that this was the only location within the aorta where the proportion of elastin decreases relative to collagen.[3] Because elastin fragmentation and degeneration is observed histologically in aneurysm walls, these observations may help explain the predilection for aneurysm formation in the infrarenal aorta.

Proteolytic degradation of medial elastin fibers and collagen degradation leading to the weakening and dilatation of the aortic wall is the most predominant pathophysiologic concept of aneurysm development.[5] The medial layer destruction in aortic aneurysms is associated with an inflammatory response of the media and adventitia with infiltration of T and B lymphocytes, mast cells, and macrophages in response to oxidized lipids within the intima. Degradation and thinning of aortic media in response to these changes implies that these cells maybe responsible for the noted increase in proteolytic enzymes relative to their inhibitors. Numerous reports have documented increased expression and activity of matrix metalloproteinases (MMPs) in the wall of aortic aneurysms.[6–9] MMPs are the zinc- and calcium-dependent proteolytic enzymes that are produced by macrophages. Smooth muscle cells and inflammatory cytokines are known to upregulate MMP production. There is an abundant wealth of data in the literature to suggest alterations in MMPs, including MMP-1 (collagenase-1), MMP-3 (Stromelysin-1), MMP-2 and MMP-9 (gelati-

nases), and MMP-12 (macrophage elastase), leading to AAA development.[10,11] MMP-9 is of particular interest because it is the most abundant elastolytic proteinase having activity against insoluble elastin fibers. Abundantly expressed in aneurysm infiltrating macrophages at the site of tissue damage, MMP-9 as well as its synthesis is directly correlated with aneurysm size.[12] Further evidence that MMP-9 may play a role in AAA pathogenesis was shown when an experimental murine model for aortic aneurysm targeting the deletion of the MMP-9 gene prevented aneurysmal degradation. Two potent elastolytic cysteine proteases, cathepsins S and K, may also play a role in AAA pathogenesis. These proteases are overexpressed in atherosclerotic plaques by macrophages and smooth muscle cells in the presence of proinflammatory cytokines found in aneurysm atheroma. Inhibition of proteases is also thought to play a part in AAA development. Cystatin C is the most abundant extracellular inhibitor of cysteine proteases and is severely reduced in aneurysmal lesions. The imbalance between cysteine proteases and cystatin C maybe responsible for the arterial wall remodeling in aneurysmal diseases.[12–15]

Histologic studies of AAAs have shown elastin fragmentation and chronic medial and adventitial inflammation. This differs from aortic occlusive disease, which shows inflammation of the intimal plaque. This transmural inflammatory infiltrate seems to be the key process for development of AAA, but its cause is not understood. Some studies have found *Chlamydia pneumoniae* in the wall of AAAs, which suggested that infection could be a possible causative agent for transmural inflammation. In rabbit models, *Chlamydia* can induce AAA. Other authors suggest an autoimmune source of chronic, transmural inflammation. An autoimmune component was hypothesized since the inflammatory cellular infiltrate of AAAs have shown the presence of B lymphocytes, plasma cells, and large amounts of immunoglobulin. Tilson and coworkers have identified a 40-kDa matrix protein, which may mediate an autoimmune response leading to aneurysm formation.[16] Termed *aortic aneurysm antigenic protein* (AAAP-40), it is immunoreactive with IgG isolated from the aneurysm wall.[17]

In addition to reduced elastin content in the infrarenal aorta, hemodynamic and structural factors unique to this location predispose the infrarenal aorta to aneurysm formation. Reflected waves from the aortic bifurcation increase pulsatility and wall tension in the distal, less compliant atherosclerotic aorta. Absence of vasa vasorum in the infrarenal aorta has been suggested to reduce nutrient supply and potentiate degeneration. More recently, Xia and coworkers proposed an autoimmune mechanism for aneurysm formation and found that immunoreactive protein is more conspicuously expressed in the abdominal aorta compared with the thoracic aorta.[17,18] This may explain the increased frequency of aneurysms in this location.

AAA development also has a genetic component reflected by an increased prevalence of AAA seen in siblings and first-degree family members. The defects in genes of connective tissue lines, especially the collagen III gene responsible for Ehlers-Danlos syndrome type IV, play a mechanistic role in the formation of some aneurysms. Any connective tissue disease, which negatively affects microfibrillar integrity, may lead to AAA development. Patients with Marfan's syndrome, a disease of defective fibrillin, are particularly prone to aneurysmal disease.

Evidence also suggests that there maybe other independent, nonatherosclerotic AAA-forming pathways similar to chronic obstructive pulmonary disease (COPD). Lederle et al. conducted a systematic review of the relative risk of smoking on aortic aneurysms compared to other smoking-related diseases. The mechanism is still unclear, but smoking can lead to decreased aortic elasticity and induce MMP production by macrophages leading to degeneration of collagen and elastin of the arterial media and ultimately the development of an aortic aneurysm.

Less common causes of AAA include infection, cystic medial necrosis, vasculitis, trauma, and anastomotic pseudoaneurysms. Aortic aneurysms are rare in children and are most commonly associated with infection from umbilical artery catheters.

Epidemiology

Rupture of AAA is the 13th leading cause of death in men older than 55 years of age.[19] It is therefore important to know the epidemiology and etiology to help identify and reduce the mortality from AAA. The exact prevalence of AAA varies according to the criteria and methodology used.[20] The first epidemiologic information was obtained from necropsy studies with an increased prevalence after the age of 55 years. An incidence of 4.7% in men 65 to 74 years old with a peak incidence of 5.9% by the age of 80 years was found. The prevalence among women was 1.2% between 65 and 74 years of age increasing to 4.5% above 90 years of age.[21] Various estimates from screening studies have shown that the prevalence of AAA varies depending on age group screened, diagnostic method, criteria used to define AAA, and associated risk factors. AAA prevalence in the Wanhainen study ranged from 3.6% to 16.9% in men and 0.8% to 9.4% in women, depending on the different definition and diagnostic techniques used. The Aneurysm Detection and Management (ADAM) study identified AAAs in 4.6% of patients screened (infrarenal aorta 3 cm or larger) and 1.4% had an infrarenal aneurysm 4 cm or larger.[22] Age, male gender, smoking, and family history had the most significant positive associations with AAA. Female gender, diabetes mellitus, and black race had negative associations with AAA. A family history of AAA has been documented in the literature with 15% to 25% of patients with AAA having a first-degree relative with an AAA. In a systematic review of the literature, it has been found that smoking and aortic aneurysm are closely linked. The relative risk associated with aortic aneurysm related events was 3 to 6 compared to 1 to 2 for coronary artery disease and 5 to 12 for COPD.[23] The Veteran's Administration cooperative study demonstrated that smoking was also an associated risk factor for 4 cm or greater AAA in 75% of AAA cases, with the association between smoking and AAA increasing with the number of years of tobacco use. High cholesterol levels, coronary artery disease, peripheral arterial disease, COPD, and hypertension have also been positively associated with AAA.

Clinical Features

The majority of patients with AAA are asymptomatic with the AAA detected on routine physical examination or seen incidentally by noninvasive imaging. Occasionally the patient may note the ability to feel their heartbeat in their stomach, which leads to the diagnosis of an AAA. Symptoms of AAA are secondary to acute aneurysm sac expansion or rupture. The pathognomic features of a symptomatic or ruptured AAA are abdominal or back pain and pulsatile abdominal mass. Most ruptured AAAs are tender on palpation and associated with hypotension.

The presence of a pulsatile mass between the xiphoid and umbilicus when palpating the abdomen in a nonobese patient is the best way to detect an AAA on physical examination (Figure 30.2). Unfortunately, abdominal palpation has limited sensitivity for detecting AAA. The sensitivity of this technique depends on the AAA size, the obesity of the patient, the skill of the examiner, and the focus of the examination. The abdominal examination may detect large, easily palpable AAAs, but by itself cannot exclude

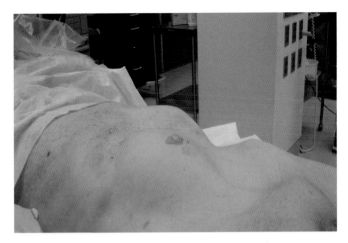

● **FIGURE 30-2.** Abdominal aortic aneurysm is seen as a midline pulsatile swelling below the xiphoid region on physical examination of the abdomen.

the presence of an aneurysm. Small aneurysms may not be detectable by physical examination and obesity can hide even large AAAs. Moreover, physical examination cannot reliably distinguish between a clinically relevant AAA and an ectatic/tortuous aorta. Patients with hypertension and widened pulse pressure as well as patients with abdominal masses overlying the aorta may also lead to the incorrect diagnosis of an AAA.

Diagnosis

Various diagnostic modalities are available to detect, measure, and monitor AAA. Plain abdominal x-ray or lumbosacral spine x-ray may demonstrate aortic wall calcifications. Measurements of the aneurysm may overestimate the size of the AAA because of the 20% magnification of the AAA by these types of x-ray. Ultrasonography (US) has been widely used in many published studies for AAA screening and has a sensitivity of 95% with near 100% specificity when used with adequate quality assurance.[17] It is a useful tool to distinguish aneurysms from other conditions and there is a high degree of correlation between aneurysm size measured by US and operative size in both transverse and longitudinal diameter. Reported advantages for ultrasound include its simplicity and relatively low cost. It can be used to perform serial measurements of aneurysm growth, rapidly identify rupture, and to distinguish aneurysms from other conditions. The major limitation of US is that the abdominal aorta might not be well visualized as a result of obesity, excessive bowel gas, periaortic disease, or scarring from previous abdominal surgery. Moreover, the US measurements of the suprarenal aorta are not as reliable because of difficulty in visualization. Also noted was modest interobserver variability in US measuring of AP and transverse aneurysm diameters.[23-26] Many physicians will generally follow patients with US surveillance until they reach the size of approximately 4 to 4.5 cm in diameter at which time more accurate monitoring with computed tomography (CT) imaging maybe utilized. Although

it can be helpful for postoperative evaluation of endografts, it provides insufficient data for preoperative endograft planning.

Unlike US, contrast-enhanced spiral CT scanning provides more accurate information about the size, shape, and three-dimensional configuration of the AAA, independent of body habitus. CT scan can also provide more accurate anatomic information and better visualization of the suprarenal aorta and the iliac arteries. Compared to US, the major disadvantages of CT include its expense, use of iodinated contrast, and the radiation dose received.

Magnetic resonance imaging (MRI) in combination with magnetic resonance angiography (MRA) is another modality, which is as accurate as CT but more expensive and less available. Furthermore, it is not tolerated in claustrophobic patients and those with certain metallic implants. There is less familiarity with its use and image manipulation for endograft planning is less user-friendly. Unlike CT, bony landmarks are less well visualized. Gadolinium-based MR contrast agents, once thought to be safe in patients with chronic kidney disease, has now been associated with nephrogenic fibrosing dermopathy. This limits its use in this patient subpopulation.

Aortography, particularly digital subtraction angiography (DSA), is an excellent tool in defining perianeurysmal anatomy, particularly visceral and renal arteries (Figure 30.3). It can underestimate the size of aneurysms in the presence of nonspecified mural thrombus. Therefore, it is not useful in determining the size of AAA. Angiography is expensive and associated with the use of contrast and ionizing radiation. It is the most invasive imaging modality available in imaging AAA.

Natural History

The natural history of an AAA is expansion and rupture, with rupture being the most dreaded complication of AAA. The risk of rupture increases with the diameter of the aneurysm, as predicted by LaPlace's law. According to Laplace's law, the wall tension of the AAA is directly proportional to the radius and blood pressure and inversely proportional to the wall thickness. Rupture risk also increases with an increased rate of expansion and certain comorbid conditions, particularly COPD. According to the UK Small Aneurysm Trial, 25% of patients with a ruptured AAA died without ever reaching the hospital, 51% died in the hospital without undergoing surgery, 13% died within 30 days of surgery (46% operative mortality rate), and only 11% survived beyond 30 days.[27,28] The short-term mortality (30 days) associated with elective surgical repair is 2.7% to 5.8%, based on ADAM and UK Small Aneurysm Trial[28,29]. Aneurysm rupture is associated with a mortality rate of 60% to 90%.[30] The risk of rupture is independently associated with female gender, larger initial aneurysm diameter, current smoking, and higher mean blood pressure. Although aneurysms are less frequently observed in women, AAA in women has a threefold increased risk of rupture

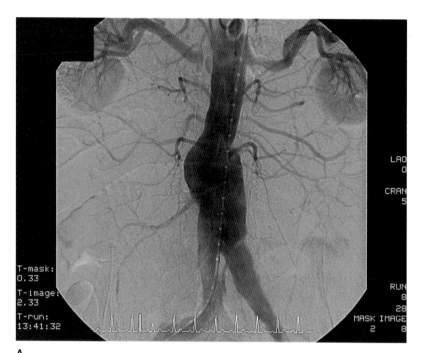

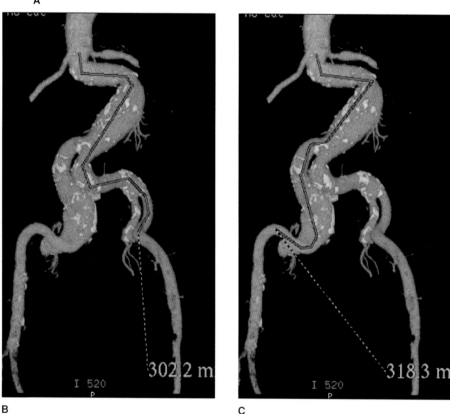

● FIGURE 30-3. Examples of angiography (A) and CT reconstructions (B, C) to define aneurysm morphology and guide endograft selection.

A

B   C

compared to men with similar sized aneurysms. According to the UK Small Aneurysm Trial, women with a 4 to 5.5 cm AAA are at four times higher risk of rupture compared to men. The reason most often cited for this phenomenon relates to the smaller aortic diameter and the classical recommendations for repairing aneurysms when they reach 5 to 5.5 cm.

The annual risk of rupture of an AAA with a diameter of 5.5 to 5.9 cm is 9.4%, 10.2% for an AAA between 6 and 6.9 cm, 19.1% for an AAA between 6.5 and 6.9 cm, and 32.5% for an AAA of 7 cm or larger.[27,28,31] The rate of expansion is also an important determinant of rupture. The mean rate of expansion in ruptured aneurysms is 0.82 cm/year compared to 0.42 cm/year in nonruptured aneurysms. Effective control of blood pressure and cessation of smoking are likely to diminish the risk of rupture.

The routine screening of asymptomatic patients has not been shown to be cost-effective for patients younger than 65 years of age because of the low prevalence of AAA. Patients with a family history of AAA or men older than 65 years of age with history of smoking or hypertension may benefit from aneurysm screening. This has been addressed by major trials like the Multicenter Aneurysm Screening Study (MASS). A single normal ultrasonographic scan at age 65 years in men virtually rules out significant aneurysm disease for life. Presently, Medicare has approved US screening for high-risk individuals when they enter the program at the age of 65 years.

Management

All patients with AAA should have aggressive cardiovascular risk factor modification. Arguably, blood pressure should be controlled with ACE inhibitors and possibly beta-blockers. Patients should undergo routing surveillance of AAAs to determine aneurysm morphology, growth rate, and absolute sizes. After the initial diagnosis, a follow-up imaging study at 6 months is often indicated to determine the growth curve for the aneurysm. If there is no rapid expansion and the aneurysm is under 4 cm in diameter, then annual surveillance is reasonable. Beyond 4 to 4.5 cm, the AAA should be followed every 6 months. Surgical intervention is recommended when the size of the aneurysm is above 5 to 5.5 cm in diameter, when it is expanding rapidly at a rate of more than 0.5 cm in 6 months, or when symptomatic. Options for surgical repair include the traditional transperitoneal route or a retroperitoneal approach. The transperitoneal approach is the most widely used approach for infrarenal aortic disease. The advantages being faster opening and closing of the incision, the ability to explore the concomitant abdominal organs, and better access to the right iliac and right renal arteries, which facilitates repair of these vessels. The retroperitoneal approach is preferred in patients with scarring from intraabdominal inflammation or previous surgery. It can also be used to access the aorta through the contralateral retroperitoneum in patients with colostomy or ileostomy. The operative steps are detailed in Figure 30.4(A–C).

The mortality associated with elective surgery is 2.7% to 5.8% and increases to 19% for urgent aortic repair and at least 50% for repair of a ruptured aortic aneurysm.[28,29] According to the ACC/AHA guidelines, open surgical repair is recommended for patients with low or average risk of operative complications. High-risk patients need to be evaluated closely to determine their fitness for repair.

Endovascular Repair

Although endovascular aneurysm repair (EVAR) is recommended for patients with high risk of complications with open repair, it is gaining popularity because of its lower morbidity, quicker recovery times, and lower early mortality. The EVAR-1 trial is a randomized controlled trial of 1082 patients enrolled between 1999 to 2003 comparing 30-day mortality between elective endovascular repair or open AAA repair. The study results demonstrated a 30-day mortality in the EVAR group of 1.7% vs. 4.7% in the open repair group ($p = 0.009$), but more secondary interventions were required with endovascular repair (9.8% vs. 5.8%). The EVAR group also had a significantly shorter hospital stay (7 vs. 12 days), compared to open repair.[32]

Further benefits for EVAR over open AAA repair were demonstrated in the Dutch Randomized Endovascular Aneurysm Management (DREAM) trial. The DREAM trial was a multicenter, randomized trial comparing open repair with endovascular repair in 345 patients with at least 5 cm aneurysms. The study outcomes were operative (30-day) mortality and severe complications. The operative mortality rate in the endovascular repair group was 1.2% vs. 4.6% in the open-repair group. The combined rate of operative mortality and severe complications in endovascular group was 4.7% vs. 9.8% in the open-repair group. The study concluded that the endovascular repair is preferable to open repair in patients with AAA of at least 5 cm in diameter.[33]

Despite the benefit shown for EVAR, its use in those unfit for open repair was brought into question by the EVAR-2 trial. EVAR-2 was a randomized controlled trial of EVAR outcomes in patients unfit for open repair of AAA. The study randomized 338 patients aged 60 years or older with at least 5.5 cm AAAs to receive either EVAR or no intervention. The primary endpoint of the study was all-cause mortality. Secondary endpoints were aneurysm-related mortality, health-related quality of life (HRQL), postoperative complications, and hospital costs. The 30-day operative mortality in the EVAR group was 9% (13 of 150, 95% CI 5–15) and the no intervention group had a rupture rate of 9 per 100 person years (95% CI 6.0–13.5). There was no significant difference between the EVAR group and the no intervention group for all-cause mortality (hazard ratio 1.21, 95% CI 0.87–1.69, $p = 0.25$). Moreover, there was no difference in aneurysm-related mortality or HRQL scores. The mean hospital costs per patient over 4 years in the no intervention group were £8649 less than in the EVAR group. The study concluded that EVAR repair or observation has no difference in all-cause or aneurysm-related mortality after 4 years in this high-risk surgical group.[34]

The major advantages of EVAR include reductions in major morbidity, intubation time, hospital stay, blood loss, and a faster return to normal activity after the repair. Despite the apparent early advantages to EVAR, long-term outcomes are equivalent to open surgery in both observational studies and randomized trials. The survival advantage associated with endovascular repair has been shown to be lost after 1 year. As shown in the DREAM trial, the cumulative survival at 2 years was not different with EVAR or open repair yet EVAR was associated with increased repeat interventions.[35] The EVAR-2 trial also did not show survival difference between EVAR or no intervention at 4 years in those patients unfit for open repair.[34,36] These observations have led many vascular specialists to temper their initial enthusiasm for endovascular treatment of AAA.

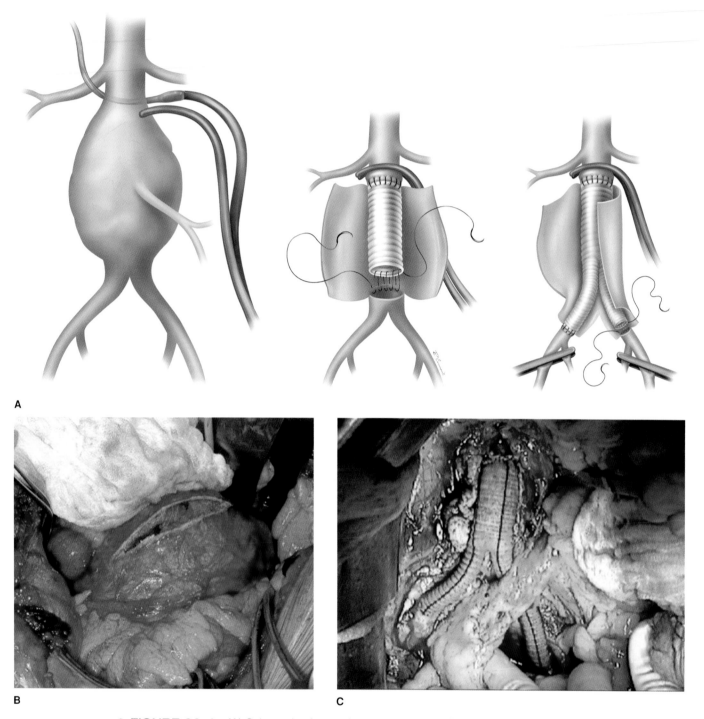

● **FIGURE 30-4.** (A) Schematic of steps for open repair. (B&C) Photos of open repair.

Endovascular repair involves femoral artery access, placement of an endoluminal stent-graft via the iliac arteries, and deployment of an aortobiiliac stent graft, excluding the aneurysmal lumen from pressurized blood flow and thus minimizing the risk of rupture. A variety of endografts are commercially available (Figure 30.5). Prior to EVAR, thin cut (≤3 mm) contrast-enhanced spiral CT is the only imaging modality necessary to plan the placement of a stent graft. Intraoperative angiography, and in selected cases intravascular ultrasound (IVUS), are essen-

tial to determine the appropriate size and length of endograft needed. Anatomic considerations for preoperative EVAR planning include proximal neck length/diameter, distal neck length/diameter, total length, neck angulation, femoral/iliac artery diameters, mesenteric and accessory renal artery locations, as well as occasionally an aberrant artery of Adamkowicz. (Figures 30.6 and 30.7). Follow-up of patients after endovascular repair is typically done at 1 and 6 months, and annually thereafter with CT angiography though US maybe used in selected

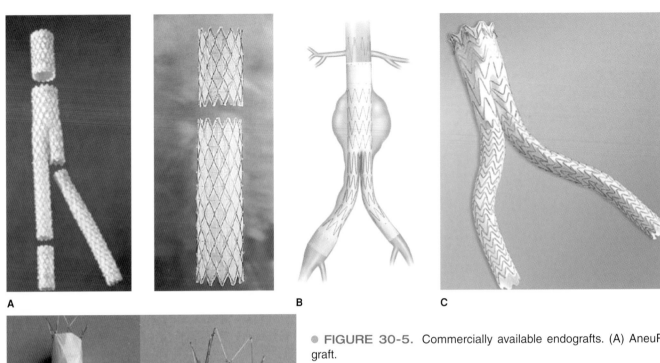

A

B

C

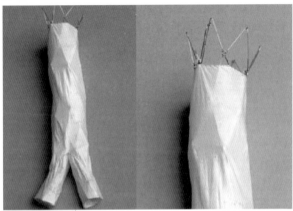

● **FIGURE 30-5.** Commercially available endografts. (A) AneuRx graft.

Courtesy of Medtronic, Inc, Minneapolis, MN.
(B) Zenith flex AAA endovascular graft.

Courtesy of Cook Medical, Bloomington, IN.
(C) Gore excluder bifurcated endoprosthesis—assembled bifurcated graft.

Reproduced, with permission, from Kinney TB, Rivera-Sanfeliz GM, Ferrara S. Stent grafts for abdominal and thoracic disease. Appl Radiol. 2005;34:9-19.
(D) Endologix graft.

Courtesy of Endologix, Irvine, CA.

D

cases. Abdominal plain films can be utilized to look for graft migration. Post-EVAR evaluation includes aneurysm diameter, presence of an endoleak, or graft migration/integrity.

Post-EVAR complications include endoleak, endotension, endograft limb occlusion, endograft migration, and postimplantation syndrome. An endoleak is defined as a persistent flow of blood into the aneurysm sac after EVAR and is classified into types I to IV. Endoleak can lead to pressurization of the aneurysm sac with aneurysmal expansion and rupture. About 20% to 40% of patients develop endoleaks after EVAR.

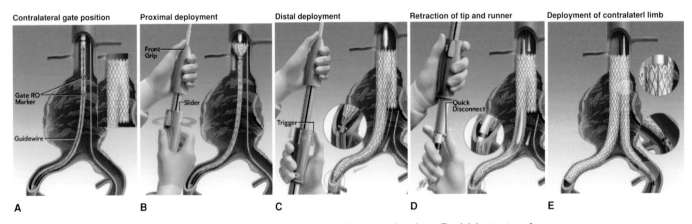

A B C D E

● **FIGURE 30-6.** (A–E) Images representing stepwise AneuRx AAA stent graft deployment.

Courtesy of Medtronic, Inc, Minneapolis, MN.

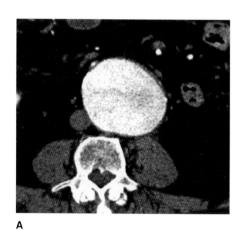
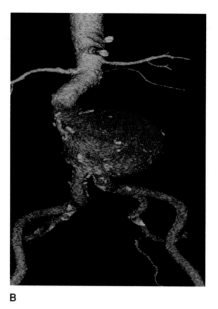
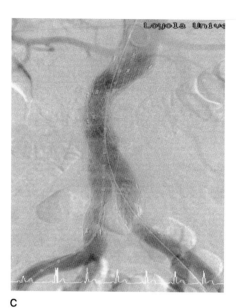

A B C

● **FIGURE 30-7.** (A) CT scan showing abdominal aortic aneurysm of size 8 cm. (B) CT-angiography image of the AAA Pre-AneuRx. (C) Post implant angiogram image of AneuRx reveals successful exclusion of the aneurysm.

A type I endoleak is caused by inadequate seal at either the proximal (Ia) or distal (Ib) attachment site, and has an incidence up to 10%. Appropriate oversizing of the proximal portion of the endograft by at least 10% to 20%, as recommended by the graft manufacturers, should reduce the rate of type I endoleaks. Risk factors for type I leaks include over- or undersizing of the proximal/distal attachment sites, short seal zones, and significant angulation at the fixation zones. The classic dogma is that during implantation, if a type I (or type III) endoleak is encountered, the procedure is not complete until this is corrected.

Type II endoleaks are secondary to retrograde flow of blood into the aneurysm sac from aortic branch vessels (the inferior mesenteric artery or lumbar arteries). Type II endoleaks are the most common, occurring after 10% to 25% of all EVARs. It is rare for type II leaks to lead to significant pressurization or expansion of an aneurysm sac. Most patients with type II endoleaks can be followed closely with serial imaging studies. If aneurysm sac expansion occurs on surveillance imaging, several treatment options are available to eliminate retrograde flow into the sac. Embolization of branch arteries, thrombogenic packing of the aneurysmal sac, laparoscopic branch ligation, or conversion to open repair are methods to treat type II leaks. The timing of the occurrence of type II endoleak (early vs. late) as well as sac enlargement (either in diameter or volume) is a predictor for subsequent intervention.

Type III endoleaks are caused by graft tear or a leak from attachment sites of modular components ("modular disconnect"). Like type I endoleaks, type III leaks result in systemic pressurization of the aneurysm sac and should be repaired. The repair is often accomplished by sealing of the leak with the placement of another endograft component, such as a cuff proximally or extension limb distally.

Type IV endoleaks are caused by graft porosity. The incidence of type IV endoleak is diminishing as a result of modifications in graft materials. Angiographically, this appears as a diffuse blush from the endograft into the aneurysm sac. Most type IV endoleaks, when identified at the time of surgery, can be followed and will show resolution on follow-up CT imaging.

Classically, endotension is defined as the persistent pressurization of the aneurysm sac in the absence of an endoleak. It likely results from aortic pulsatility against thrombus or undetectable endoleaks.[31] Endotension can lead to sac rupture and enlargement. The clinical significance of endotension needs further study. There are ongoing newer modalities including multidimensional CT angiography measurements or implantable pressure transducers, which are being examined to measure endotension, identify endoleaks, and aneurysm sac expansion.[37]

Postimplantation syndrome is an acute inflammatory response developing within the first few weeks following endovascular stent placement. Its etiology is unknown but is thought to be related to AAA thrombus formation and is associated with the development of fever, leukocytosis, and elevated C-reactive protein (CRP). Most symptoms related to postimplantation syndrome will resolve within 6 weeks.

Medical Management

Medical therapy is beneficial in patients with aneurysms of all sizes, though no significant single therapy has been clearly shown to inhibit the progression of aneurysm growth. The risk of aneurysm formation increases by 20% to 25% with continued smoking and is a major risk factor for aneurysm growth and rupture. Hence smoking cessation should be strongly emphasized. The current ACC/AHA guidelines recommend the control of lipids and blood pressure similar to patients with atherosclerotic disease (coronary heart disease equivalent). All patients with AAA should be on statin therapy for secondary prevention of cardiovascular events. There is experimental and limited retrospective data suggesting statin therapy might suppress aneurysm growth possibly via an anti-inflammatory effect, but more human studies will be needed to prove this observation. ACE inhibitors have also been suggested to reduce the likelihood of aneurysm growth/rupture, however there is no level I evidence to support its use.[38]

Inflammatory Abdominal Aortic Aneurysms

Inflammatory AAAs are a subset of AAAs representing less than 5% of all aneurysms. They are a distinct clinical entity marked by thickening of the aneurysm wall anteriorly and laterally, perianeurysmal and retroperitoneal fibrosis. This extensive inflammatory reaction frequently involves the vena cava, renal vein, duodenum, and ureters. Inflammatory aneurysms are thought to have an inheritance of specific HLA alleles with a higher incidence of HLA-DRB1. Traditionally, they present with a triad of abdominal/flank pain, fever, and constitutional symptoms. On CT scan, a "halo" sign is often seen with an anterior predominance of inflammatory tissue, which will enhance with intravenous contrast administration. The operative risk associated with inflammatory aneurysms is higher with an operative mortality of 7.9 versus 2.4% for traditional AAAs. Preoperative recognition of an inflammatory aneurysm may facilitate the selection of a left retroperitoneal approach to avoid the most inflamed portion of the aneurysm. Although not extensively studied, an endovascular approach maybe used for this subset of aneurysms. Meta-analysis of EVAR in inflammatory aortic aneurysms of the abdominal aorta showed a primary technical success rate of 95.6% with regression of the aneurysm sac median diameter by 11 mm over a mean follow-up of 18 months after endovascular repair. Of 43 patients with periaortic fibrosis prior to the stent graft, 22 (51.2%) patients showed complete regression, 18 (41.8%) remained unchanged, and 3 (7.0%) showed inflammatory progression after EVAR. Renal impairment resolved in 11 (45.8%) of 24 patients. Reinterventions were required in 8 patients. The procedure-related and follow-up (18 months) mortality rates were 0% and 13.0%, respectively. The study concluded that EVAR of inflammatory aortic aneurysm is feasible and excludes the aneurysm effectively, reduces periaortic fibrosis, and improves renal impairment in most patients with very low periprocedural and midterm mortality (18 months).[6]

● INTRAMURAL HEMATOMA

Intramural hematoma (IMH) is a variant of aortic dissection and categorized as an acute aortic syndrome. The exact cause for IMH is debatable but is thought to be produced by a rupture of the vasa vasorum into the aortic media without a demonstrable intimal tear or intraluminal flow. However, it is also thought that IMH can result from a microtear too small to visualize on imaging studies, causing luminal blood flow, which later occludes.[7]

Epidemiology and Diagnosis

Since IMH of the abdominal aorta is considered a variant of aortic dissection, they share similar predisposing risk factors and symptoms. Historically, IMH has been underdiagnosed but because of recent advances in imaging techniques there has been an increased prevalence of IMH.

IMH can be classified as either traumatic or nontraumatic. The International Registry of Aortic Disease (IRAD) registry found the prevalence of nontraumatic IMH among acute aortic syndromes at the rate of 5.7% while it ranged from 10% to 30% in other reports. Distal aortic IMH accounts for 60% of cases, while 40% IMH are proximal.[39]

Generally, IMH cannot be distinguished clinically from a localized aortic dissection and imaging studies are necessary for accurate diagnosis. The aortography criteria used to detect classic intimal flap and double luminal flow in aortic dissection cannot be used to diagnose IMH. Aortography has a low detection rate for IMH because of the absence of an intimal tear and failure to opacify the thrombosed false lumen. Hence, newer, less noninvasive imaging like CT/CTA and MRI/MRA are used to detect and monitor abdominal aortic IMH. The use of MRI in IMH is limited but can provide high-quality images noninvasively without the need for iodinated intravascular contrast. With T1-weighted images, IMH has an isodense intensity, whereas T2-weighted images show a high-intensity signal by formation of methemoglobin. MRI can estimate the age of thrombus through fat-suppressed technique and by assessing methemoglobin versus oxyhemoglobin signals.

IMH on CT is defined by the presence of a circular- or crescent-shaped area of high attenuation along the aortic wall (without an intimal flap), which fails to enhance after injection of contrast medium. An aortic wall thickness ≥ 5 mm is used to diagnose IMH as the normal thickness of the aorta is usually less than 3 mm by any imaging modality. This should be distinguished from a AAA with intraluminal thrombus/atheroma (Figure 30.8).

Treatment

The natural history, prognosis, and treatment of abdominal aortic IMH is not well understood.[40] Abdominal aortic IMH can have a variable clinical course in that it may remain as a limited hemorrhage, progress to an aortic dissection or aneurysm, or regress on medical therapy. The presence of a maximum aortic diameter of ≥ 40 mm or maximal aortic wall thickness of ≥ 10 mm are independent predictors for rupture of IMH.[41] IMH have a high rate of resorption compared to aortic dissection regardless of the affected site. IMH without penetrating ulcer or other high-risk features (diameter, wall thickness) usually has a stable course. Acute IMH involving the descending aorta has an in-hospital mortality of 10%, which is similar to a descending type B aortic dissection. However, patients with abdominal IMH had no in-hospital mortality in the IRAD registry.[39]

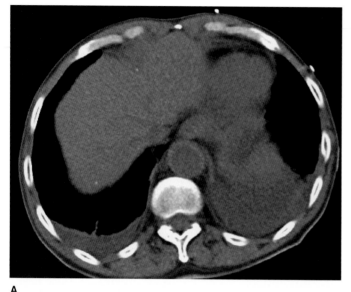

A

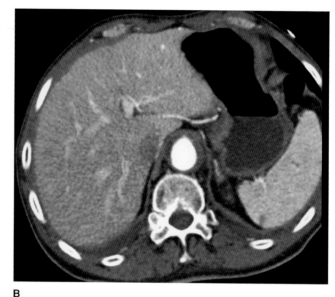

B

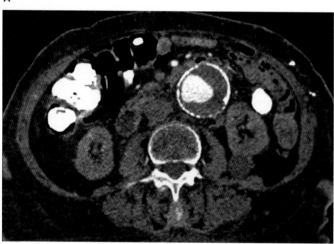

C

● **FIGURE 30-8.** (A to C) Computed tomographic images of the abdominal aorta revealing a significant abdominal aortic aneurysm with intraluminal thrombus and atheroma.

The treatment of IMH is uncertain owing to the absence of randomized trials. General recommendations include empirical medical management for IMH and serial aortic imaging surveillance similar to classic type B aortic dissections. A retrospective study of 53 patients with acute IMH showed a 0% in-hospital mortality rate. All patients were initially treated medically. Eleven patients (20%) with IMH showed progression with the development of aortic dissection or aortic enlargement in follow-up imaging (mean follow up periods of 53 ± 43 months) and two patients (2%) ultimately underwent surgery. The survival rates at 1, 2, and 5 years were 100%, 97%, and 97%, respectively. In another study, Song et al. evaluated the outcomes on medically treated IMH with an in-hospital mortality of 1% and a 3-year survival rate of 87% for distal IMH. This study also demonstrated that 78% of cases resulted in resorption and localized dissection occurred in 16% on follow-up imaging.[8]

Complications develop less often in patients with IMH than in those with acute aortic dissection. Patients with uncomplicated IMH not associated with rupture, organ ischemia, or severe pain can be treated with blood pressure control during the acute phase. The optimal medical treatment for uncomplicated descending aortic IMH includes beta-blockers and calcium channel blockers.

The mortality associated with surgical therapy for IMH is 15%.[9,39] Surgical intervention for IMH is recommended for intractable pain, inability to control the blood pressure, branch vessel compromise, maximum diameter of the affected aorta ≥50 to 60 mm, rapid enlargement of the affected aortic segment, development and rapid enlargement of an ulcer like lesion, and rupture of the affected aorta. Surgery involves the resection of the affected areas and the placement of a Dacron interposition graft. The role of endovascular stenting in IMH is not well defined but is gaining acceptance. Long-term follow-up is similar to aortic dissection and includes imaging at 1, 6, and 12 months after discharge and annually thereafter.

● PENETRATING AORTIC ULCER

Penetrating aortic ulcer (PAU) is a potentially lethal condition and is thought to occur when an ulcerated atheromatous plaque erodes through the intimal layer of the

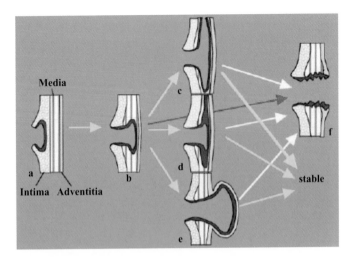

● **FIGURE 30-9.** The image features the concept of penetrating atherosclerotic ulcer of the aorta and disease process.

Reproduced, with permission, from Hayashi H, Matsuoka Y, Sakamoto I, et al. Penetrating atherosclerotic ulcer of the aorta: imaging features and disease concept. Radiographics. 2000;20:995-1005.

aorta lamina into the media/adventitial layers (Figure 30.9). The PAU can progress along the media extending the hematoma and stretching the adventitia, leading to IMH, pseudoaneurysm, or life-threatening sequelae such as aortic aneurysms, dissection (Figure 30.10) (though less frequently than IMH), and rupture[42] (Figure 30.11). It is classified as an acute aortic syndrome and shares some clinical features with aortic dissection and IMH though it may have a higher risk of rupture. The incidence of abdominal aortic penetrating ulcers is approximately 3.7%, with a mean age of 73 years. The majority of patients have hypertension and usually present with abdominal or back/flank pain.[43] PAU usually occurs in the most atherosclerotic areas of the aorta, predominantly involving the descending thoracic aorta and less commonly, the infrarenal aorta.

PAU needs to be distinguished from aortic dissection or IMH as it has a different prognosis and management. Diagnosis of PAU maybe confirmed by CT/CTA, MRI/MRA, or aortography and, less commonly duplex ultrasound (Figure 30.12).[44] Aortography often demonstrates the presence of an aortic ulcer but is limited because of the invasive nature and high incidence of false-negative results if the image intensifier is not in the proper projection angle. Duplex imaging, CT, and MRI demonstrate an irregular crater-like outpouching with jagged edges and associated atheromatous plaque. Extensive aortic calcifications are frequently seen on contrast-enhanced CT imaging and can distinguish PAU from IMH, pseudoaneurysm, and contained rupture. MRI has the advantage of multiplanar imaging without contrast. MRI is also superior to CT in helping to distinguish periaortic tumors involving the aortic wall from extra-aortic hematoma caused by a ruptured PAU.[45]

PAU requires close follow-up to monitor the potential progression of the disease in order to initiate therapy before serious complications occur. The natural history and

management of PAU is not well-defined compared to aortic dissection or IMH. PAU generally have a benign course, however complications including transmural aortic rupture, dissection, embolization, pseudoaneurysm formation, or progressive aneurysmal dilatation occur in up to 40% of patients.[46] The management of PAU depends on the presence or absence of symptoms and associated morphological features. Symptomatic patients are at a higher risk of developing complications. The symptoms might resolve after the initial treatment and remain stable for years. However, for those that develop worsening symptoms, the initial treatment parallels that of type B aortic dissection involving intravenous analgesics to reduce pain and antihypertensives to reduce blood pressure and thus the risk of rupture. Medical therapy should be continued if the symptoms abate and no progression of PAU is noted on follow-up imaging. If the patient develops persistent or recurrent pain, hemodynamic instability, or radiological progression (hematoma expansion, pseudoaneurysm formation, rupture, or dissection), surgical therapy is recommended. Open surgical repair is the gold standard for PAU. It involves local excision of the affected aortic segment and Dacron graft interposition. As it frequently affects the elderly with advanced atherosclerosis, surgery is associated with a high morbidity and mortality. Because of the risks of surgical repair, endovascular treatment is a new alternative in selected patients. Endovascular repair involves sealing of a penetrating ulcer by the stent-graft and reducing wall stress, thus providing stabilization to the diseased aortic segment. The effectiveness of endovascular repair in PAU of the infrarenal aorta was retrospectively studied by Tsuji et al. in four patients with Gianturco Z-stent covered with a thin-walled Dacron graft. Their postoperative course was uneventful after stent-grafting with no endoleak or aneurysm expansion seen during the mean follow-up of 14 months.[47] A prospective observational study of 348 patients undergoing abdominal aortic procedures by endovascular treatment showed a total of 13 patients with abdominal PAUs. All 13 patients underwent endovascular treatment and were followed with CT at 1, 4, and 12 months after the intervention, and yearly thereafter. Their primary technical success was 100% with no postoperative deaths and only one major complication (transient ischemic attack). There were no endoleaks, aneurysm formation, or stent graft failure during a mean follow-up period of 26 months.[43] Hence, endovascular grafting appears feasible, safe, and a less invasive alternative to open surgical repair.

● **AORTIC PSEUDOANEURYSM**

A pseudoaneurysm of the aorta is the disruption of the aortic wall, which results in a contained rupture (Figure 30.13). This is in contrast to true aneurysms of the aorta in which all three layers are intact. Pseudoaneurysms of the abdominal aorta are a rare finding and account for 5% of all pseudoaneurysms and less than 1% of all abdominal aneurysms. The etiology of pseudoaneurysms include infection, surgical puncture, vascular graft degeneration, and

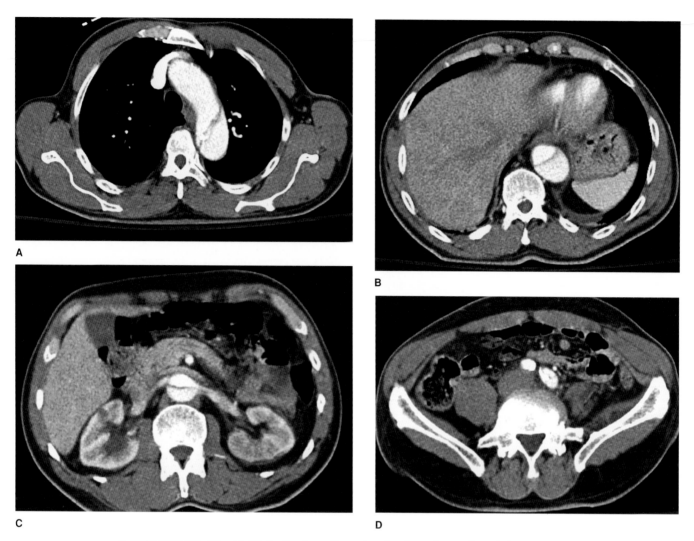

FIGURE 30-10. (A–D) Aortic dissection extending from the aortic arch in the region of the left subclavian artery with involvement of the entire thoracoabdominal aorta, extending into the left renal artery and left common iliac artery. No evidence of active contrast extravasation.

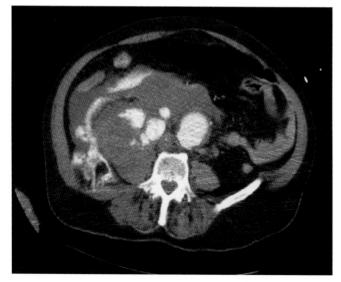

FIGURE 30-11. Ruptured abdominal aortic aneurysm.

trauma. Pseudoaneurysms of the abdominal aorta are often diagnosed late or after catastrophic complications. Abdominal or back pain caused by compression of retroperitoneal structures, renovascular hypertension, embolization to the distal extremities, acute abdominal or retroperitoneal hemorrhage, or palpable abdominal mass are frequently observed signs and symptoms at presentation. The diagnosis requires a high level of suspicion for pseudoaneurysm especially in patients with a history of previous aortic surgery or trauma. Duplex US, MRI, and CT scanning aid in the diagnosis, and in selected cases, arteriography can provide additional diagnostic and anatomic information. Although small asymptomatic pseudoaneurysms maybe followed with serial imaging studies, larger ones require repair because of the high mortality associated with rupture. Depending on the site and proximity to other abdominal aortic side branches, either open or endovascular surgery maybe performed to prevent leak or hemorrhage. Stent graft placement for infected aortic pseudoaneurysms

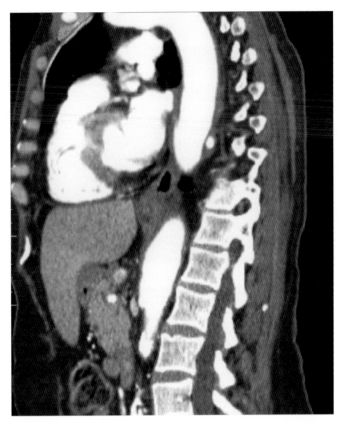

● **FIGURE 30-12.** Ulcerated plaque of the abdominal aorta.

can be used as a temporizing measure before surgical repair in high risk cases.[48,49]

● **TRAUMA TO THE ABDOMINAL AORTA**

Traumatic injuries to the abdominal aorta are unusual but a potentially lethal event. They can be classified as penetrating, nonpenetrating (blunt), or iatrogenic. In a study of blunt trauma with an incidence of 0.3% aortic injuries, 20% involved the abdominal aorta.[50] Blunt traumatic aortic injuries commonly involve the descending aorta near the origin of the left subclavian artery (at the ligamentum arteriosum where the aorta is relatively fixed) because of rapid deceleration accidents. While blunt trauma accounts for a higher percentage of thoracic aortic injuries, abdominal aortic injuries are most likely caused by penetrating trauma. Most are caused by penetrating trauma secondary to assault while only 15% of the injuries are caused by blunt trauma. The lower incidence of blunt aortic trauma is thought to be due to the aorta's relatively protected position.[50,51] Penetrating injuries from gun shots, knives, or shrapnel can lead to intimal injury, pseudoaneurysm, or perforation. Almost all the abdominal aortic injuries secondary to penetrating trauma will also involve surrounding visceral structures.

Blunt abdominal injuries usually include crushing or direct blows, high-speed motor vehicle accidents, and seat belt injuries. These injuries are caused by both direct and indirect forces. In the rapid deceleration of a high-speed collision, seat belts act as a fulcrum of rotation. Subsequently,

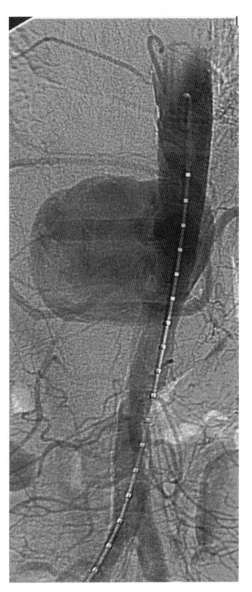

● **FIGURE 30-13.** Aortic pseudoaneurysm.

the viscera and aorta are subjected to direct compression between the spine and lap seat belt, which can lead to intimal injury. The indirect forces are created by shearing forces from the acute flexing of the abdominal aorta subjecting it to higher deceleration forces than the mesenteric arteries. The presence of atherosclerosis increases the susceptibility of the aorta to blunt abdominal trauma and the disruption of weakened intima. Abdominal aortic lesions in traumatic injuries include a spectrum ranging from simple contusion and IMH to intimal disruption, dissection, pseudoaneurysm formation, or rupture.

Abdominal aortic injuries can also be secondary to iatrogenic trauma. Iatrogenic dissections can be sustained at any site from aortic clamping during aortic surgery or from aortic cannulation during cardiac surgery or as a result of guidewires and catheters used during angiographic procedures. Full thickness aortic perforations or pseudoaneurysms have been reported following spinal surgery and retroperitoneal periaortic lymph node sampling. Injuries to the abdominal aorta have also occurred during placement of laparoscopic trocars.

The clinical presentation of an aortic injury is acute in 70% of the cases, with the patient presenting with either acute arterial insufficiency or an acute abdomen with exsanguinating hemorrhage or visceral ischemia. The most common presenting symptoms include abdominal pain, tachycardia, and ecchymosis of the flank area. Intimal disruption is the most common anatomic lesion. CT angiography provides the best diagnostic study to help with decisions regarding management.

According to a population-based study of aortic trauma in Scotland, of the patients who survived to the emergency department, 55% of patients died in the emergency department and 32% underwent operative repair, with an operative mortality of 59%. Overall mortality was reported to be 86%.[50] Outcomes after vascular trauma are poor and the physician should have a high index of suspicion in patients with a seat-belt injury, lumbar spine injury, or a crushing force to the abdomen. An abnormal distal vascular examination should also arouse suspicion. Prompt recognition and surgical treatment are essential in the management of traumatic aortic injuries and key to a patient's survival and good long-term outcome. Knowledge of anatomic relationships between the viscera and affected vessels forms the basis for directed surgical dissection, optimal exposure, and lasting repair of vessels. Urgent surgical repair of an abdominal aortic injury is necessary for the unstable patient or those with threatened extremities. The presence of an expanding hematoma, shock, or threatened extremities mandates emergency operative exploration and repair. Operative treatment is performed by direct aortic repair, Dacron graft replacement, or exclusion with extra-anatomic bypass. Because of the sheaering force involved in the injury, there is often an associated bowel injury with varying degrees of gastrointestinal contamination. The risk of infection after placement of prosthetic material in a potentially infected field is 2.5% where the aorta is concerned. The use of extra-anatomic bypasses has been recommended by some for both blunt and penetrating injuries because of the high incidence of associated bowel injuries. In the stable patient with viable limbs, treatment with placement of endovascular stent-grafts may provide a less invasive option in the face of intra-abdominal contamination.[52]

• PRIMARY AORTIC TUMORS

Primary aortic tumors of the aorta are extremely rare lesions and are almost always malignant. Only 111 cases have been reported in literature. They are classified into two categories according to the site of occurrence in the aortic wall. Intimal tumors comprise the first category originating from the mesenchymal cells of the intima. They are polypoid tumors, which grow along the endothelial surface into the aortic lumen. These tumors include intimal sarcoma, undifferentiated sarcoma, malignant fibrous histiocytoma, angiosarcoma of endothelial origin, and leiomyosarcoma. The second category is the adventitial or mural aortic tu-

mor, which arises within the media or adventitia and exhibits mural growth. In a study of 29 patients with aortic tumors, those involving the intima accounted for 62.9% of cases, mural in 18.2%, all three layers in 10.6%, and unmentioned in 8.3%.[53] Review of the literature on primary tumors of the thoracoabdominal aorta by Chiche et al. showed a male-to-female ratio of 1.7:1 with a mean age of 59.7 ± 1.13 years at the time of diagnosis. Primary aortic tumors are most common in the thoracic aorta; however 26.5% of aortic tumors are found in the abdominal aorta.[54] Clinical manifestations are nonspecific and subtle, mimicking atherosclerotic or atheroembolic disease. Since the majority of primary tumors are intimal tumors, they can acutely embolize or cause occlusive symptoms such as blue toe syndrome, acute onset ischemia, intermittent claudication of the lower extremity, severe renovascular hypertension, intestinal infarction, or abdominal angina.[55] Less than 5% of tumors are identified preoperatively. They are often misdiagnosed as thrombus, atherosclerotic plaque, pseudoaneurysm, aneurysm, or aortic dissection. Angiography shows nonspecific findings, mimicking simple mural thrombus or aneurysm. Because of the potential risk for detachment of a polypoid tumor and embolization, aortography should be avoided if possible. MRI is the most reliable imaging technique for diagnosis of primary aortic tumors. With gadolinium, MRI provides excellent contrast between the aortic lumen, aortic wall, and surrounding structures and is more precise than CT in differentiating aortic wall tumor from thrombus. Duplex imaging of the abdominal aorta can also help identify intraluminal defects.

As a result of delayed diagnosis, treatment of primary aortic tumors is usually initiated at an advanced stage and is generally associated with a poor prognosis. Distant metastatic disease located primarily in the bone, kidneys, liver, adrenal glands, and the lungs was identified in 82.2% of cases around the time of diagnosis. Median survival is 7 months and cumulative overall survival rates at 3 and 5 years were 11.2% and 8%, respectively. Owing to the lack of data, the best way to manage aortic tumors remains controversial. Surgical resection remains the best option because it offers the best chance for cure if there are no detectable metastases and reduces the risk of local recurrence if there are metastases. For those treated surgically, the median duration of survival is 10 months, with the cumulative survival rates at 3 and 5 years being 16.5% and 11.8%.[54,56] Curative resection cannot be achieved in up to 50% surgically treated patients because of failure to make accurate preoperative or intraoperative diagnosis and technical difficulties preventing complete resection. Since many of the tumors were mistaken for thrombus, surgical techniques leaving the aortic wall in place (endarterectomy) resulted in residual tumor left behind. The efficacy of external beam radiation therapy and/or systemic chemotherapy for residual disease has not been well-defined. In patients with high operative risk or metastases, endovascular treatment could be used as a palliative procedure for the treatment of an occlusive or embolic aortic lesion. Unfortunately, treatment is mostly nonsurgical, supportive, and palliative in patients with diffuse primary aortic tumor.

AORTIC OCCLUSIVE DISEASE

Acute Aortic Occlusion

Acute aortic occlusion of the abdominal aorta is a vascular catastrophe most commonly because of in situ thrombosis of a severely diseased atherosclerotic aorta or less frequently saddle embolus. Acute thrombosis is related to underlying atherosclerotic disease, hypercoagulable states, and low flow states secondary to cardiac dysfunction or severe volume depletion. Acute aortic occlusion is defined as symptom onset of less than 2 weeks. A retrospective review of patients with acute abdominal aortic obstruction identified common comorbid risk factors such as smoking, diabetes mellitus, and preexisting peripheral vascular disease. The most common presenting symptom is the acute onset of bilateral lower extremity ischemia or exacerbation of existing chronic ischemia. Other clinical presentations can vary from neurologic symptoms of the lower extremities (paresthesia, paralysis), abdominal symptoms with pain because of the involvement of associated vascular structures, or acute hypertensive crisis because of the extension of thrombus into the renal arteries. The absence of bilateral femoral pulses associated with ischemic signs/symptoms of both lower extremities is a key finding in acute aortic occlusion. Early recognition of acute aortic occlusion is important as prognosis is time-dependent. In a reported series of acute aortic occlusion, coronary atherosclerotic heart disease, recent myocardial infarction, and peripheral vascular disease were more frequently associated with the thrombotic versus embolic group. The thrombotic group was also associated with an overall lower mortality compared to the embolic group (12% vs. 31%).[57,58]

Imaging studies for the diagnosis of an acute aortic occlusion include CTA, MRA, or invasive angiography. Angiography is useful in both confirming the diagnosis and planning therapy; however because of the nature of the disease, vascular access is limited to an upper extremity or translumbar approach. CT or MR angiography can provide the key information without the need for direct access to the arterial system. The early preoperative management of acute aortic occlusion includes systemic anticoagulation, volume resuscitation, and optimizing cardiac function. Surgical treatment for acute aortic occlusion includes bilateral transfemoral embolectomy for saddle emboli, aortoiliac bypass, or axillobifemoral bypass. Alternatively, in selected high-risk patients, thrombolytic therapy and mechanical rheolytic thrombectomy followed by stent placement of severely diseased arterial segments can be associated with a lower mortality than surgical therapy.[59]

Chronic Abdominal Aortic Occlusion

Chronic atherosclerotic infrarenal occlusion is uncommon and is caused by chronic progression of atherosclerotic disease. Mostly noted in heavy smokers (98%), the mean age of patients with chronic infrarenal abdominal aortic occlusion is 57 years. The most common symptoms noted in patients with infrarenal, chronic aortic occlusion are claudication (81%), rest pain (25%), tissue loss (15%), and impotence in 81% of men. It is commonly associated with other arterial diseases including mesenteric artery stenosis and renal artery stenosis. Management includes aortic reconstruction and bypass, transaortic endarterectomy, proximal thrombectomy, or extra-anatomic remote bypass. Recently, endovascular treatment has also been utilized for revascularization. Lifelong antiplatelet therapy is suggested to prevent future thromboembolic events.[60]

Hypoplastic (Small) Aortic Syndrome

Hypoplastic (small) aortic syndrome occurs mostly in women and exhibits a characteristic clinical picture. The classic example is a younger female about 50 years of age with a history of heavy smoking, who has localized aortoiliac disease. These women also have a predilection for visceral (renal and mesenteric) occlusive disease. Common angiographic findings of hypoplastic aortic syndrome include small aorta, iliac, and femoral vessels; a high aortic bifurcation; and occlusive disease often strikingly localized to the distal aorta or aortic bifurcation. The major clinical features at presentation are hypertension and arterial insufficiency of the lower extremities. The surgical intervention involves prosthetic reconstruction or aortoiliac endarterectomy with patch angioplasty.[61] Vascular reconstruction in patients with hypoplastic aortic syndrome are associated with lower patency rates than those reported when the aorta is normal in size.

Middle Aortic Syndrome

Middle aortic syndrome (MAS) is an uncommon condition characterized by segmental narrowing (coarctation) of the proximal abdominal aorta and ostial stenosis of its visceral and renal branches. MAS primarily affects children and young adults. The classic presentation of MAS is a young adult patient with renovascular hypertension, weak femoral pulses, and a systolic bruit in the abdomen. The tissues from these aortic lesions exhibit marked subendothelial fibroplasias, but no inflammation. Other etiologies of this syndrome include secondary granulomatous vasculitis from Takayasu's arteritis and neurofibromatosis secondary to von Reckinghausens disease. MAS is usually diagnosed using CT/CTA, MRI/MRA, or conventional aortography. Surgical revascularization with aortoaortic bypass or aortic resection with interposition grafting is usually recommended for symptomatic patients.[62]

INFECTIOUS AORTITIS

Introduction

Aortitis is the inflammatory process involving one or more layers of the aortic wall (intima, media, adventitia) and caused by various mechanisms. Infectious aortitis can be caused by tuberculosis, syphilis, bacteria, or fungus. It results from either septic embolization, bacteremia, or extension from a contiguous site of infection. Infectious aortitis can result from a diverse array of organisms such as *Streptococcus pneumonia, group A Streptococcus,* or *Haemophilus influenzae* in the preantibiotic era, while *Staphylococcus aureus* and *Salmonella* (frequently associated with sickle cell anemia) are currently the most prevalent infecting organisms of the abdominal aorta,[63] Infectious aortitis, if untreated, can lead to mycotic aneurysm formation but is a rare (0.7%) cause of all aneurysms.[64] Risk factors for aortic infection include endocarditis (older series), elderly population, chronic immunosuppression, and diabetes mellitus. Infected aneurysms have a poor outcome because of their sometimes aggressive presentation, high rupture risk, and complex aneurysm location requiring revascularization of branch vessels. Since they often occur in patients who are immunocompromised, aortic infections are associated with high perioperative morbidity and mortality.

Mycotic Aneurysm

Mycotic aneurysms of the aorta are rare, accounting for 0.7% to 1.3% of all aneurysms. They maybe termed primary or secondary, depending on whether the aneurysm originated from infectious degeneration of the aortic wall or from secondary infection of an existing AAA. Despite being termed mycotic aneurysms, the majority of infected aneurysms are caused by bacterial infection. The term mycotic aneurysm is currently used to describe any type of infected aneurysm regardless of its pathogenesis.

Primary mycotic aneurysm is the dilatation of an artery caused by destruction of the vessel wall by an infection in a previously normal arterial wall or through secondary infection of a preexisting aneurysm. A number of routes account for infection of an arterial wall including septic embolization to the vasa vasorum or contiguous infective focus extending to the arterial wall (e.g., from penetrating trauma, bacterial seeding of an atherosclerotic plaque, or extension of an abdominal infection). Other predisposing factors are age and impaired immunity, including alcoholism and chronic immunosuppression. The organisms usually involved include *Staphylococcus aureus, Streptococcus* spp, *Salmonella* (in some series, 35%–40% of infected aneurysms), *Treponema pallidum,* and fungi (e.g., Candida and Cryptococcus). The classic clinical presentation is a painful, pulsatile, enlarging mass with associated fevers. The diagnosis maybe suspected based on imaging studies but confirmed by positive blood cultures or ultimately by the isolation of an organism in the aneurysmal tissue. Ultrasound, CT/CTA, and MRI/MRA are useful imaging modalities that can identify mycotic aneurysms. Infected aortic aneurysms have an aggressive presentation and are associated with significant mortality. Predictors of death in patients with an infected aortic aneurysm are extensive peri-aortic infection, female gender, *Staphylococcus aureus* infection, aneurysm rupture, and suprarenal location. Since *Salmonella* bacteria can invade the normal intima and

causes early aneurysm rupture, it is also associated with a virulent course and poor survival.[65,66]

A combined timely surgical intervention along with prolonged medical therapy provides reasonable outcomes. Isolated medical therapy is associated with a high mortality because of the significant risk of rupture. Early surgical debridement and revascularization prevents the rupture of the aneurysm, controls hemorrhage in cases of rupture, confirms the diagnosis, and may help control the associated sepsis. Open surgical procedures are the standard of care for infected aortic aneurysms and, however, are associated with a mortality in the range of 20% to 40% in previously published reports. Most deaths are attributed to sepsis. Infrarenal abdominal aortic mycotic aneurysms have a better survival compared to suprarenal aneurysms.[67,68] Surgical options include in situ graft placement or extra-anatomic bypass. Extra-anatomic bypass should be considered to avoid placing prosthetic graft material in an infected field (e.g., axillary bifemoral) but is associated with 20% rate of stump disruption, 20% to 29% rate of amputation, and 20% rate of reinfection. In situ reconstruction has been utilized in suprarenal mycotic aneurysms and in infrarenal aneurysms to avoid aortic stump disruption. This procedure requires diligent debridement of infected tissue and prolonged periods of antibiotic therapy. In situ reconstruction with cryopreserved arterial allografts can also be used as alternative treatment in mycotic aneurysm or infected aortic prosthetic grafts as standard surgical management.[69] Antimicrobial therapy should be continued for at least 6 weeks or longer, as it helps in eradication of the pathogen and prevents recurrent infection.

● SYPHILITIC AORTITIS

Syphilitic aortitis has declined in incidence since the advent of antibiotics, particularly penicillin. Clinical manifestations are insidious in onset, taking up to 15 to 30 years from primary infection to aneurysm formation. The aneurysms can occur anywhere in the aorta but mostly involve the ascending aorta, aortic arch, and descending thoracic aorta (thought to be caused by the rich lymphatic network) and rarely the abdominal aorta. The infection initially localizes to the adventitia of the aortic wall in the primary infection stage. The infection eventually invades the media via lymphatics around the vasa vasorum and results in endarteritis obliterans of the vasa vasorum of the aorta, leading to medial necrosis with destruction of elastic tissue, resulting in aneurysm formation; these rarely dissect. Treatment of the early syphilitic stage (uncomplicated aortitis) with antimicrobial therapy frequently prevents late complications. The treatment at later symptomatic stages is more involved, often requiring surgical reconstruction.

● TUBERCULOUS AORTITIS

Infection of the abdominal aorta with *Mycobacterium tuberculosis* is a rare sequelae of latent tuberculosis. There was a decline in tuberculosis prior to 1980 but there has been a resurgence owing to an increased number of immunosuppressed patients, particularly those with HIV/AIDS. The mechanism for tuberculous aortitis involves the direct spread from adjacent tuberculous tissue (e.g., retroperitoneal lymph nodes to the abdominal aorta), hematogenous spread to intimal lesions (such as atherosclerotic plaque), septic embolization to the vessels, or lymphatic spread to the arterial wall. Tuberculous aortitis has various consequences including aneurysm formation, which can lead to rupture, dissection, or fistulous connections to adjacent structures (particularly, the duodenum or colon). Furthermore, complete degeneration, stenosis, or constriction and perivascular fibrosis have been observed. Patients can present with nonspecific symptoms of fever and pulmonary problems. Testing includes skin testing with PPD, plain chest radiographs, tissue cultures, and imaging with ultrasound, computer tomography, and magnetic resonance imaging. These may demonstrate the granulomatous nature of disseminated tuberculosis. The overall mortality from rupture of tuberculous aortitis is high. The treatment is surgical resection, aortic reconstruction with in situ graft placement or extra-anatomic bypass and long-term antituberculous therapy.

● VASCULITIS

Takayasu arteritis (TA) and giant cell arteritis affect large arteries, with the potential of abdominal aorta involvement. TA, also known as "pulseless disease," has its highest prevalence in Asians, affecting predominantly women (80% to 90%) with the age of onset between 10 to 40 years. According to the American Association of Rheumatology, in order to make the diagnosis, at least three of the six criteria need to be met: (1) age of onset ≤40 years; (2) claudication of extremities; (3) decreased pulse of one or both brachial arteries; (4) difference of at least 10 mm Hg in systolic blood pressure between the arms; (5) bruit over one or both subclavian arteries or the abdominal aorta; and (6) arteriographic narrowing or occlusion of the entire aorta, its primary branches or large arteries of the proximal upper or lower extremities, not caused by arteriosclerosis, fibromuscular dysplasia, or other causes. It has a close association with HLA B5 or B52 and B39 haplotype. According to the international conference on TA, there are five types (I to V) based upon angiography. Type IV involves only the abdominal aorta and has increased predilection to Asian Indians presenting as hypertension because of the involvement of the renal arteries or suprarenal aortic stenosis. The histological features in TA are of a destructive immune response in the aortic wall with invasion of T-lymphocytes, fibrous thickening of the adventitia, increased production of cytokines and adhesion molecules resulting in stenosis, and occlusion and aneurysm formation of the involved segment of the aortic wall. TA is a progressive disease with 80% to 90% 5-year survival on follow-up studies. The outcome is predicted by the course of the disease as well as complications which arise (such as hypertension or aneurysm formation). The diagnosis is made by clinical features and imaging of the vascular tree by CT, MRI, and aortography,

demonstrating smoothly tapered luminal narrowing or occlusion with thickening of the arterial wall. MRI in the early stages of TA can visualize concentric wall thickening, edema of the inflamed vessel; contrast can enhance the wall in chronic stage and helps to noninvasively assess the vascular tree. Treatment of TA includes corticosteroids, percutaneous transluminal angioplasty/stent, or bypass grafts when there is irreversible arterial stenosis causing significant ischemic symptoms. Angioplasty is preferable as it is a cost-effective, simple procedure compared to surgical revascularization. However, it is less successful in long stenoses or occlusions and when the artery is heavily scarred.

Giant cell arteritis (GCA, temporal arteritis) is a chronic vasculitis of large- and medium-sized arteries. The age group affected is usually above 50 years again with a predisposition to women. It most frequently involves the cranial branches originating from the aortic arch. A study from Olmsted county showed GCA patients are 2.4 times more likely to develop isolated AAAs compared to other persons of the same age and sex in the county. Aortic aneurysms are a late and potentially serious complication of GCA and aortic dissection can occur in the absence of aneurysm. It is difficult to distinguish it from TA as it involves large arteries, granulomatous changes on histology, and respond to steroids. But the age of onset, presence of shoulder stiffness (association with polymyalgia rheumatica), tender scalp with upper extremity vascular involvement distinguishes it from TA. Magnetic resonance imaging/angiography are preferred imaging studies. Corticosteroids are the mainstay of treatment and, when initiated early, can prevent the late complications of aneurysm formation. Surgical or endovascular treatment is required for dissections/aneurysms.

● AORTOENTERIC FISTULA

Aortoenteric fistula (AEF) represents one of the most challenging conditions faced by vascular surgeons. AEFs are classified as to their location and etiology (Figure 30.14). Primary AEF is a communication between the aorta and the bowel lumen. The communication most commonly occurs between an infrarenal aortic aneurysm and the third or fourth portion of the duodenum. Primary AEF occurs spontaneously and is associated with aortic or gastrointestinal diseases. Usually, the aortic aneurysm results from a degenerative process and is sterile. The remainder of cases is associated with aortitis or mycotic aneurysm commonly caused by low-grade *Staphylococcus* infection. Other rare causes of primary AEF are associated with peptic ulcer disease, neoplasms, pancreatic pseudocyst, ingested foreign body, diverticulitis, appendicitis, and radiation injury.

Secondary AEFs occur in the setting of a prior aortic reconstruction with prosthetic material. There are two forms of secondary AEF. The first type is a communication between the aortic lumen and the bowel lumen at the aortic-to-graft suture line. Massive GI bleeding is frequently associated with this form of AEF. The second type, termed graft-enteric erosion (GEE), is a result of mechanical erosion of the bowel and resultant infection of the graft.

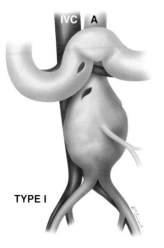

TYPE I

Primary (aortic aneurysm)

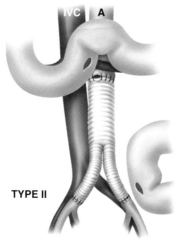

TYPE II

Secondary (aneurysm graft)

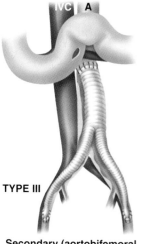

TYPE III

Secondary (aortobifemoral graft)

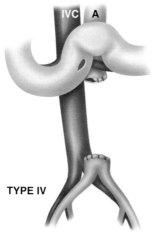

TYPE IV

Secondary (infrarenal stump)

● **FIGURE 30-14.** Types of aortoenteric fistulas. Type I: primary aortoenteric fistula caused by spontaneous erosion of gut. Types II to IV: secondary aortoenteric fistulas occur following surgical interventions. Type II: following prosthetic replacement of abdominal aorta. Type III: following aortobifemoral prosthetic graft. Type IV: communication between infrarenal aortic stump and gut following removal of infected infrarenal aneurysm.

The GEE occurs in the middle of the graft away from the suture line. This form of AEF often lends itself to intermittent low-grade GI hemorrhage.

The diagnosis of AEF requires a high level of clinical suspicion in patients presenting with gastrointestinal bleeding and a history of aortic surgery. These patients often have a "herald bleed," which maybe manifested as melena or hematemesis. The clinical diagnosis is difficult to make and is usually done intraoperatively, but should be suspected in any patient who presents with abdominal pain, pulsatile abdominal mass, and gastrointestinal hemorrhage. Survival is dependent upon prompt diagnosis and surgical intervention. Computed tomography may confirm the diagnosis, but does not always rule out the possibility of AEF. Upper endoscopy is a useful tool to rule out other gastroduodenal sources of bleeding. Aortography may help in the diagnostic algorithm, but if the diagnosis cannot be ruled out, exploratory laparotomy is mandatory. The ultimate goal is prevention of AEFs before they occur. The available data suggest that the following technical points should be followed at the time of the initial aortic reconstruction including careful attention to sterile technique, careful retraction of the bowel to avoid tension and ischemia, and closure of

the aneurysm wall and retroperitoneum after aortic reconstruction to allow total exclusion of the aortic graft from the bowel.[70]

Once the diagnosis of AEF is made, expeditious surgical treatment is the only treatment associated with success. The goals of treatment are to stop the hemorrhage, repair the defect in the GI tract, debridement of infected tissue, and restoration of limb perfusion. The classic management of AEF includes graft resection, debridement of the retroperitoneum, repair of the enteric defect, and extra-anatomic bypass to restore lower extremity perfusion. Though endografts for treatment of AEF have been reported in selected high-risk patients, the concern for graft infection in long-term follow-up limits their usefulness in most patients.

● **AORTOCAVAL FISTULA**

Aortocaval fistula is a communication between the high flow of the aorta and the low-pressure system of the vena cava. The fistula can be spontaneous (primary aortocaval fistula) or maybe secondary to trauma. Most spontaneous aortocaval fistulas are caused by an erosion of an infrarenal AAA into the inferior vena cava. The sudden erosion of an AAA into the vena cava can result in symptoms of ruptured AAA and retroperitoneal hemorrhage. Alternatively, the fistula may form a stable, chronic arteriovenous fistula.

Aortocaval fistula is an uncommon complication of AAA and has an incidence of less than 1% to 2% in elective AAA surgical series, while it is noted in 6.3% of patients in one ruptured AAA study with a 14-year follow up. Traumatic fistulae between the aorta and vena cava may also occur after spine surgery. The surgeon operating through the disk space may notice massive bleeding or unexplained hypotension during the case.

Aortocaval fistulae result in a marked decrease in peripheral vascular resistance. This decrease in peripheral resistance is responsible for all the systemic effects. The mean arterial pressure decreases and central venous pressure increases. The resultant compensatory mechanisms are increased in cardiac output owing to increases in heart rate, ejection fraction, and venous return. In addition, the renin-angiotensin-aldosterone axis is activated. These compensatory mechanisms can result in high output congestive heart failure.

The diagnosis of aortocaval fistula is made intraoperatively in 30% to 50% of cases. Clinical manifestations are variable and include abdominal and back pain caused by local compression of adjacent structures. They also manifest neurologic signs of paresis caused by venous hypertension of vertebral veins. Edema from venous hypertension, arterial insufficiency from decreased distal arterial flow, and high output congestive heart failure (CHF) are other manifestations of aortocaval fistula. Duplex imaging and CT scan are utilized to assist with the diagnosis of aortocaval fistulas. Arteriography can be used to confirm the fistula in the absence of thrombosis. The diagnosis maybe difficult in cases of contained rupture and should be suspected by the surgeon if there is the presence of unexplained venous hypertension.

The treatment of aortocaval fistula is mandatory because they continue to grow and may cause systemic symptoms if observed. The safest approach is to close the fistula from within the arterial lumen after opening the artery because dissection around the vena cava and iliac veins can be hazardous. Recently endografts have also been reported to successfully treat aortocaval fistula.

• AORTOURETERIC FISTULA

Aortoureteric fistula or ureteroarterial fistula results from the constant pulsation from an aneurysm on the ureter or from erosion from the ureter (e.g., from ureteral stents) into the aorta. The predisposing conditions are previous genitourinary or pelvic surgery, ureteral stent placement, radiation therapy, previous abdominal aorta surgery, and underlying vascular pathology. Aortoureteral fistulas are rare and generally present with intermittent hematuria or frank major urinary bleeding. The diagnosis is made by ureterography and selective arteriography. The management approach is surgical intervention with ligation or removal of the involved artery and ureter. In cases of massive bleeding from a aortoureteral fistula, endovascular treatment maybe at-tempted. Endovascular treatment helps in achieving immediate hemostasis while minimizing surgical exposure.

• CONGENITAL LESIONS OF ABDOMINAL AORTA

The abdominal aorta is the least common site for congenital abnormalities, and mostly present as stenosis. Congenital abdominal aortic coarctation (Figure 30.15) is because of underdeveloped aortic segment and occurs in isolation or in conjunction with lesions of the renal artery (stenosis). The aortic tissues exhibit marked subendothelial fibroplasias but no inflammation. MAS or mid-aortic dysplastic syndrome is the aortic coarctation of the distal thoracic aorta, abdominal aorta, or both, and is congenital in origin. Other etiologies of this syndrome include secondary granulomatous vasculitis from TA and others from Von Reckinghausens disease. The patients may have symptomatic renovascular hypertension or claudication. Surgical revascularization with aortoaortic bypass or aortic resection with interposition grafting is usually recommended for symptomatic patients.

• VON RECKLINGHAUSEN'S (NEUROFIBROMATOSIS TYPE I)

Von Recklinghausen's (neurofibromatosis type I) disease is an autosomal dominant disorder and is often accompanied by vascular anomalies of the aorta and its branches. The exact incidence of vascular manifestations are unknown but are attributed to proliferation of Schwann cells within the arterial walls followed by secondary degenerative changes and fibrosis. Vascular abnormalities include aneurysm, stenosis, arteriovenous malformations, invasion, or arterial compression by tumor. It frequently involves aortic, renal, or mesenteric vessels. Symptoms might manifest in childhood or early adulthood and renovascular hypertension is the most frequent presentation as the renal artery is the most frequently involved artery. There are reported cases of abdominal aortic coarctation of the aorta by neurofibromatous disease. Treatment depends on the age of the patient and type of lesion. Surgical intervention is recommended for patients with renal artery hypertension unresponsive to medical therapy, abdominal aortic coarctation with chronic mesenteric ischemia, or disabling claudication. Endovascular repair of aneurysms in this disease is not widely reported but maybe utilized in selected patients.

• PSEUDOXANTHOMAELASTICUM (GRONBLAD-STRANDBERG SYNDROME)

Pseudoxanthomaelasticum (Gronblad-Strandberg syndrome) is an autosomal recessively inherited disorder and is associated with the accumulation of mineralized and fragmented elastic fibers in the skin, Bruch's membrane in the retina, and vessel walls. The genetic abnormality is in ATP-binding cassette, subfamily C (CFTR/MRP), member 6 (ABCC6). There is disruption of arterial elastic tissue which may contribute to atherogenesis in PXE. Although

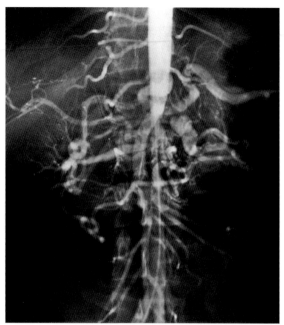

A

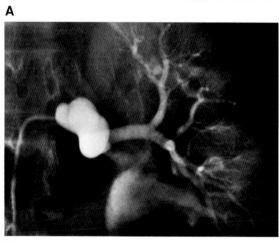

B

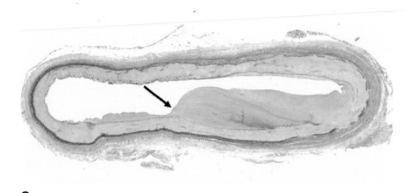

C

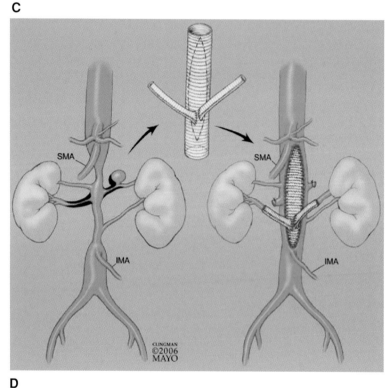

D

● **FIGURE 30-15.** (A) Abdominal aortic coarctation revealed on abdominal aortogram. (B) Bilateral renal artery stenoses and a large left renal artery aneurysm. (C) Renal artery specimen shows fibromuscular dysplasia with predominance of neointimal thickening. (D) Illustration summarizes preoperative angiographic findings and the operative treatment with a longitudinal abdominal aortoplasty and bilateral renal artery.

Reproduced, with permission, from Oderich GS, Sullivan TM, Bower TC, et al. Vascular abnormalities in patients with neurofibromatosis syndrome type I: clinical spectrum, management, and results. J Vasc Surg. 2007;46:475-484.

generally a disease of medium and small vessels, abdominal aortic occlusion has been reported. It should be suspected in young patients presenting with intermittent claudication without risk factors. Fluorescein angiography reveals angioid streaks of PXE. The management is difficult as the vascular disease is diffuse, often involving distal vessels.

REFERENCES

1. Cowan JA Jr, Dimick JB, Henke PK, Rectenwald J, Stanley JC, Upchurch GR Jr. Epidemiology of aortic aneurysm repair in the United States from 1993 to 2003. *Ann N Y Acad Sci.* 2006;1085:1-10.

2. Isselbacher EM. Diseases of the Aorta. In: Braunwald E, Zipes DP, Libby P, Bonow R, eds. Braunwald's Heart Disease: A Textbook of Cardiovascular Medicine. 7th ed. New York, NY: Saunders, 2004:1403-1435.

3. Halloran BG, Davis VA, McManus BM, Lynch TG, Baxter BT. Localization of aortic disease is associated with intrinsic differences in aortic structure. *J Surg Res.* 1995;59(1):17-22.

4. Wolinsky H, Glagov S. Comparison of abdominal and thoracic aortic medial structure in mammals. Deviation of man from the usual pattern. *Circ Res.* 1969;25(6):677-686.

5. Davies MJ. Aortic aneurysm formation: lessons from human studies and experimental models. *Circulation.* 21 1998; 98(3):193-195.

6. Puchner S, Bucek RA, Rand T, et al. Endovascular therapy of inflammatory aortic aneurysms: a meta-analysis. *J Endovasc Ther.* 2005;12(5):560-567.

7. Isselbacher EM. Intramural hematoma of the aorta: should we let down our guard? *Am J Med.* 2002;113(3):244-246.

8. Song JK, Kim HS, Song JM, et al. Outcomes of medically treated patients with aortic intramural hematoma. *Am J Med.* 2002;113(3):181-187.

9. Sawhney NS, DeMaria AN, Blanchard DG. Aortic intramural hematoma: an increasingly recognized and potentially fatal entity. *Chest.* 2001;120(4):1340-1346.

10. Saito S, Zempo N, Yamashita A, Takenaka H, Fujioka K, Esato K. Matrix metalloproteinase expressions in arteriosclerotic aneurysmal disease. *Vasc Endovascular Surg.* Jan-Feb 2002;36(1):1-7.

11. Xiong W, Knispel R, Mactaggart J, Baxter BT. Effects of tissue inhibitor of metalloproteinase 2 deficiency on aneurysm formation. *J Vasc Surg.* 2006;44(5):1061-1066.

12. Longo GM, Buda SJ, Fiotta N, et al. MMP-12 has a role in abdominal aortic aneurysms in mice. *Surgery.* 2005;137(4): 457-462.

13. Shi GP, Sukhova GK, Grubb A, et al. Cystatin C deficiency in human atherosclerosis and aortic aneurysms. *J Clin Invest.* 1999;104(9):1191-1197.

14. McMillan WD, Tamarina NA, Cipollone M, Johnson DA, Parker MA, Pearce WH. Size matters: the relationship between MMP-9 expression and aortic diameter. *Circulation.* 1997;96(7):2228-2232.

15. Goodall S, Crowther M, Hemingway DM, Bell PR, Thompson MM. Ubiquitous elevation of matrix metalloproteinase-2 expression in the vasculature of patients with abdominal aneurysms. *Circulation.* 2001;104(3):304-309.

16. Tilson MD, Ozsvath KJ, Hirose H, Xia S. A genetic basis for autoimmune manifestations in the abdominal aortic aneurysm resides in the MHC class II locus DR-beta-1. *Ann N Y Acad Sci.* 1996;800:208-215.

17. Xia S, Ozsvath K, Hirose H, Tilson MD. Partial amino acid sequence of a novel 40-kDa human aortic protein, with vitronectin-like, fibrinogen-like, and calcium binding domains: aortic aneurysm-associated protein-40 (AAAP-40) [human MAGP-3, proposed]. *Biochem Biophys Res Commun.* 1996;219(1):36-39.

18. U.S. Preventive Services Task Force. Screening for abdominal aortic aneurysm: recommendation statement. *Ann Intern Med.* 2005;142(3):198-202.

19. Silverberg E, Boring CC, Squires TS. Cancer statistics, 1990. *CA Cancer J Clin.* 1990;40(1):9-26.

20. Wanhainen A, Bjorck M, Boman K, Rutegard J, Bergqvist D. Influence of diagnostic criteria on the prevalence of abdominal aortic aneurysm. *J Vasc Surg.* 2001;34(2):229-235.

21. Bengtsson H, Bergqvist D, Sternby NH. Increasing prevalence of abdominal aortic aneurysms. A necropsy study. *Eur J Surg.* 1992;158(1):19-23.

22. Lederle FA, Johnson GR, Wilson SE, et al. Yield of repeated screening for abdominal aortic aneurysm after a 4-year interval. Aneurysm Detection and Management Veterans Affairs Cooperative Study Investigators. *Arch Intern Med.* 2000;160(8):1117-1121.

23. Lederle FA, Nelson DB, Joseph AM. Smokers' relative risk for aortic aneurysm compared with other smoking-related diseases: a systematic review. *J Vasc Surg.* 2003;38(2):329-334.

24. Lederle FA, Walker JM, Reinke DB. Selective screening for abdominal aortic aneurysms with physical examination and ultrasound. *Arch Intern Med.* 1988;148(8):1753-1756.

25. McGregor JC, Pollock JG, Anton HC. The diagnosis and assessment of abdominal aortic aneurysms by ultrasonography. *Ann R Coll Surg Engl.* 1976;58(5):388-392.

26. Lederle FA. Ultrasonographic screening for abdominal aortic aneurysms. *Ann Intern Med.* 2003;139(6):516-522.

27. Brown LC, Powell JT. Risk factors for aneurysm rupture in patients kept under ultrasound surveillance. UK Small Aneurysm Trial Participants. *Ann Surg.* 1999;230(3):289-296; discussion 296-297.

28. Lederle FA, Johnson GR, Wilson SE, et al. Rupture rate of large abdominal aortic aneurysms in patients refusing or unfit for elective repair. *JAMA.* 2002;287(22):2968-2972.

29. The United Kingdom Small Aneurysm Trial Participants. Long-term outcomes of immediate repair compared with surveillance of small abdominal aortic aneurysms. *N Engl J Med.* 2002;346(19):1445-1452.

30. Singh K, Bonaa KH, Jacobsen BK, Bjork L, Solberg S. Prevalence of and risk factors for abdominal aortic aneurysms in a population-based study: The Tromso Study. *Am J Epidemiol.* Aug 1 2001;154(3):236-244.

31. Powell JT, Brown LC. The natural history of abdominal aortic aneurysms and their risk of rupture. *Adv Surg.* 2001;35:173-185.

32. Greenhalgh RM, Brown LC, Kwong GP, Powell JT, Thompson SG. Comparison of endovascular aneurysm repair with open repair in patients with abdominal aortic aneurysm (EVAR trial 1), 30-day operative mortality results: randomised controlled trial. *Lancet.* 2004;364(9437):843-848.

33. Prinssen M, Verhoeven EL, Buth J, et al. A randomized trial comparing conventional and endovascular repair of abdominal aortic aneurysms. *N Engl J Med.* 2004;351(16):1607-1618.

34. EVAR Trial participants. Endovascular aneurysm repair and outcome in patients unfit for open repair of abdominal aortic aneurysm (EVAR trial 2): randomised controlled trial. *Lancet.* 2005;365(9478):2187-2192.

35. Blankensteijn JD, de Jong SE, Prinssen M, et al. Two-year outcomes after conventional or endovascular repair of abdominal aortic aneurysms. *N Engl J Med.* 2005;352(23): 2398-2405.

36. Dieter R, Laird JR. Endovascular abdominal aortic aneurysm repair. In: King SB, Yeung AC, eds. Interventional Cardiology. New York: McGraw-Hill, 2006:561-575.

37. Pacanowski JP, Stevens SL, Freeman MB, et al. Endotension distribution and the role of thrombus following endovascular AAA exclusion. *J Endovasc Ther.* 2002;9(5):639-651.

38. Huang W, Alhenc Gelas F, Osborne-Pellegrin MJ. Protection of the arterial internal elastic lamina by inhibition of the

renin-angiotensin system in the rat. *Circ Res.* 1998;82(8): 879-890.

39. Evangelista A, Mukherjee D, Mehta RH, et al. Acute intramural hematoma of the aorta: a mystery in evolution. *Circulation.* 2005;111(8):1063-1070.

40. Vilacosta I, San Roman JA, Ferreiros J, et al. Natural history and serial morphology of aortic intramural hematoma: a novel variant of aortic dissection. *Am Heart J.* 1997; 134(3):495-507.

41. Sueyoshi E, Imada T, Sakamoto I, Matsuoka Y, Hayashi K. Analysis of predictive factors for progression of type B aortic intramural hematoma with computed tomography. *J Vasc Surg.* 2002;35(6):1179-1183.

42. Harris JA, Bis KG, Glover JL, Bendick PJ, Shetty A, Brown OW. Penetrating atherosclerotic ulcers of the aorta. *J Vasc Surg.* 1994;19(1):90-98; discussion 98-99.

43. Piffaretti G, Tozzi M, Lomazzi C, Rivolta N, Caronno R, Castelli P. Endovascular repair of abdominal infrarenal penetrating aortic ulcers: a prospective observational study. *Int J Surg.* 2007;5(3):172-175.

44. Hayashi H, Matsuoka Y, Sakamoto I, et al. Penetrating atherosclerotic ulcer of the aorta: imaging features and disease concept. *Radiographics.* 2000;20(4):995-1005.

45. Yucel EK, Steinberg FL, Egglin TK, Geller SC, Waltman AC, Athanasoulis CA. Penetrating aortic ulcers: diagnosis with MR imaging. *Radiology.* 1990;177(3):779-781.

46. Eggebrecht H, Baumgart D, Schmermund A, et al. Penetrating atherosclerotic ulcer of the aorta: treatment by endovascular stent-graft placement. *Curr Opin Cardiol.* 2003;18(6):431-435.

47. Tsuji Y, Tanaka Y, Kitagawa A, et al. Endovascular stent-graft repair for penetrating atherosclerotic ulcer in the infrarenal abdominal aorta. *J Vasc Surg.* 2003;38(2):383-388.

48. Borioni R, Garofalo M, Seddio F, Colagrande L, Marino B, Albano P. Posttraumatic infrarenal abdominal aortic pseudoaneurysm. *Tex Heart Inst J.* 1999;26(4):312-314.

49. Takach TJ, Cervera RD, Gregoric ID. Aortic pseudoaneurysm. *Tex Heart Inst J.* 2005;32(2):235-237.

50. Tambyraja AL, Scollay JM, Beard D, et al. Aortic trauma in Scotland—a population based study. *Eur J Vasc Endovasc Surg.* 2006;32(6):686-689.

51. Lassonde J, Laurendeau F. Blunt injury of the abdominal aorta. *Ann Surg.* 1981;194(6):745-748.

52. Gunn M, Campbell M, Hoffer EK. Traumatic abdominal aortic injury treated by endovascular stent placement. *Emerg Radiol.* 2007;13(6):329-331.

53. Thalheimer A, Fein M, Geissinger E, Franke S. Intimal angiosarcoma of the aorta: report of a case and review of the literature. *J Vasc Surg.* 2004;40(3):548-553.

54. Chiche L, Mongredien B, Brocheriou I, Kieffer E. Primary tumors of the thoracoabdominal aorta: surgical treatment of 5 patients and review of the literature. *Ann Vasc Surg.* 2003; 17(4):354-364.

55. Khan A, Jilani F, Kaye S, Greenberg BR. Aortic wall sarcoma with tumor emboli and peripheral ischemia: case report with review of literature. *Am J Clin Oncol.* 1997;20(1):73-77.

56. Seelig MH, Klingler PJ, Oldenburg WA, Blackshear JL. Angiosarcoma of the aorta: report of a case and review of the literature. *J Vasc Surg.* 1998;28(4):732-737.

57. Babu SC, Shah PM, Nitahara J. Acute aortic occlusion—factors that influence outcome. *J Vasc Surg.* 1995;21(4):567-572; discussion 573-565.

58. Surowiec SM, Isiklar H, Sreeram S, Weiss VJ, Lumsden AB. Acute occlusion of the abdominal aorta. *Am J Surg.* Aug 1998;176(2):193-197.

59. Buth J, Cuypers P. The diagnosis and treatment of acute aortic occlusions. *J Mal Vasc.* 1996;21(3):133-135.

60. Ligush J Jr, Criado E, Burnham SJ, Johnson G Jr, Keagy BA. Management and outcome of chronic atherosclerotic infrarenal aortic occlusion. *J Vasc Surg.* 1996;24(3):394-404; discussion 404-405.

61. Magnoni F, Pisano E, Cirelli M, Tarantini S, Pedrini L. Abdominal aortic hypoplasia: clinical and technical considerations. *Cardiovasc Surg.* 1994;2(6):760-762.

62. Connolly JE, Wilson SE, Lawrence PL, Fujitani RM. Middle aortic syndrome: distal thoracic and abdominal coarctation, a disorder with multiple etiologies. *J Am Coll Surg.* 2002; 194(6):774-781.

63. Miller DV, Oderich GS, Aubry MC, Panneton JM, Edwards WD. Surgical pathology of infected aneurysms of the descending thoracic and abdominal aorta: clinicopathologic correlations in 29 cases (1976 to 1999). *Hum Pathol.* 2004; 35(9):1112-1120.

64. Oderich GS, Panneton JM, Bower TC, et al. Infected aortic aneurysms: aggressive presentation, complicated early outcome, but durable results. *J Vasc Surg.* 2001;34(5):900-908.

65. Ting AC, Cheng SW. Repair of Salmonella mycotic aneurysm of the paravisceral abdominal aorta using in situ prosthetic graft. *J Cardiovasc Surg (Torino).* 1997;38(6):665-668.

66. Hsu RB, Lin FY, Chen RJ, Hsueh PR, Wang SS. Antimicrobial drug resistance in salmonella-infected aortic aneurysms. *Ann Thorac Surg.* 2005;80(2):530-536.

67. Fillmore AJ, Valentine RJ. Surgical mortality in patients with infected aortic aneurysms. *J Am Coll Surg.* 2003;196(3):435-441.

68. Hsu RB, Chen RJ, Wang SS, Chu SH. Infected aortic aneurysms: clinical outcome and risk factor analysis. *J Vasc Surg.* 2004;40(1):30-35.

69. Zhou W, Lin PH, Bush RL, et al. In situ reconstruction with cryopreserved arterial allografts for management of mycotic aneurysms or aortic prosthetic graft infections: a multi-institutional experience. *Tex Heart Inst J.* 2006;33(1): 14-18.

70. Dieter RA, Jr., Blum AS, Pozen TJ, Kuzycz G. Endovascular repair of aortojejunal fistula. *Int Surg.* 2002;87(2):83-86.

chapter 31

Mesenteric Artery Disease

Pranab Das, MD / Aravinda Nanjundappa, MD, RVT / John P. Pacanowski Jr., MD / M. Habeeb Ahmed, MD, RVT / Michael L. Eng, MD / Raymond A. Dieter Jr., MD, MS

● INTRODUCTION

The mesenteric arterial bed receives 10% to 35% of total cardiac output. Diseases of this extensive arterial bed can be a cause of significant mortality and morbidity. Ischemia of the mesenteric vasculature is caused by a reduction in the blood flow either from a systemic low flow state or from local impairment of the flow. Sudden onset of intestinal hypoperfusion from occlusive or nonocclusive obstruction of arterial or venous blood flow causes acute mesenteric ischemia. Chronic mesenteric ischemia is the result of episodic or constant intestinal hypoperfusion usually among patients with systemic atherosclerosis.

● ANATOMY

Mesenteric circulation has numerous variations in its blood supply to the visceral organs. Delineation and understanding of these various patterns of mesenteric circulation is important. Fortunately, with the advent of current imaging technology and digital angiography, it is now quite possible to accurately study the major vessels, pathologies, and aberrations of these vessels as well their branches, and the collaterals in every patient.

Embryology

The mesenteric vessels arise from the primitive ventral segmental arteries. All but three of these segmental arteries regress as development proceeds.[1] The 10th, 13th, and 21st or 22nd artery give rise to the celiac, superior mesenteric, and inferior mesenteric artery (IMA) to supply the foregut, midgut, and the hindgut, respectively. Figure 31.1 shows the embryologic origin of mesenteric arteries.

Arterial Supply of the Intestines

Arterial supply of the mesenteric bed is characterized by a unique, well-developed network of collateral circulation. Presence of this collateral network is protective to a great extent against transient perturbation in the vascular supply of the intestines. Ischemia can develop even in the background of this rich collateral network if the insult persists for a prolonged period or if the insult affects a large area of vasculature.[2,3]

The blood supply predominantly occurs through three major branches of the abdominal aorta. Figure 31.2 shows the splanchnic arteries and the collateral circulation.

Celiac Axis. Celiac axis (CA) is the largest of the three arteries, and originates anteriorly from the aorta. After origin, it trifurcates into common hepatic, splenic, and left gastric arteries. The common hepatic artery may provide significant collateral flow to the intestine through its first branch, the gastroduodenal artery as well as the anterior and posterior pancreaticoduodenal arcades.

Superior Mesenteric Artery. The superior mesenteric artery (SMA) arises anteriorly, 1 to 3 cm distal to the celiac artery, and forms a more acute angle. It courses almost parallel to the aorta proximally before curving toward the right lower quadrant terminating as the ileocolic artery. It also gives rise to the inferior pancreaticoduodenal artery, several ileal and jejunal branches, the middle colic artery, and the right colic artery. The middle colic artery supplies the proximal to midtransverse colon, and the right colic artery supplies mid to distal ascending colon. The ileocolic artery supplies the distal ileum, cecum, and the proximal ascending colon.

Inferior Mesenteric Artery. The IMA artery is smaller in caliber, originates from the infrarenal aorta 5 to 8 cm distal

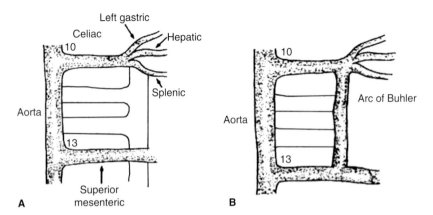

● **FIGURE 31-1.** Embryologic origin of the visceral arteries. (A) The celiac trunk and the superior mesenteric artery arise from the 10th and 13th segmental arteries, respectively. (B) The arc of Buhler residual communications between the 10th and 13th segmental arteries.

Reproduced, with permission, from Rosenblum GD, Boyle CM, Schwartz LB. The mesenteric circulation. Anatomy and physiology. Surg Clin North Am. 1997;77:289-307.

to the SMA. It gives rise to left colic artery, the sigmoid arteries, and the hemorrhoidal arteries. It provides perfusion to the distal transverse colon, descending colon, and the rectum. The superior hemorrhoidal artery, the continuation of the IMA descends into the pelvis between the layers of the mesentery of the sigmoid colon, form a series of loops around the lower end of the rectum, and communi-cate with the middle hemorrhoidal branches of the internal iliac artery, and with the inferior hemorrhoidal branches of the internal pudendal artery.

Collateral Circulation: Three major collateral networks in the mesenteric arterial circulation are responsible for rendering splanchnic bed relatively resistant to ischemic insult unless two of the three mesenteric arteries are

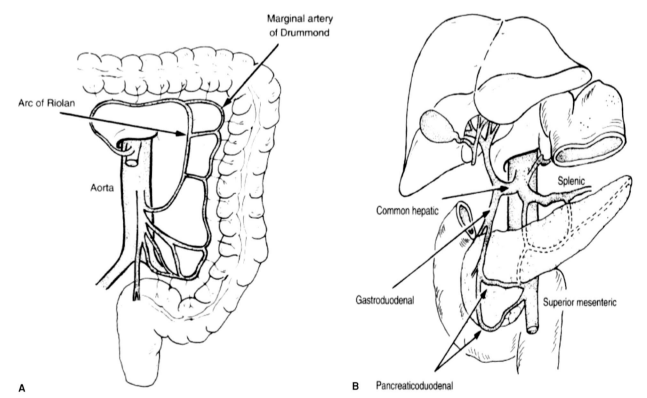

● **FIGURE 31-2.** Collateral circulation of the splanchnic circulation. (A) The marginal artery of Drummond and the arc of Riolan, which form anastomotic communications between the SMA and IMA. (B) Collaterals between the celiac and superior mesenteric artery via pancreaticoduodenal arteries.

Reproduced, with permission, from Rosenblum GD, Boyle CM, Schwartz LB. The mesenteric circulation: Anatomy and physiology. Surg Clin North Am 1997;77:289-307.

simultaneously diseased. The CA and the SMA via superior and inferior pancreaticoduodenal arteries, the SMA and IMA via middle colic and left colic arteries (primarily anastomose through the marginal artery of Drummond and the Arc of Riolan), and the IMA and internal iliac artery via superior hemorrhoidal artery and middle rectal arteries comprise these collateral networks. Symptomatic manifestations of intestinal ischemia depend on the site of stenoses in relation to these collateral networks. If stenosis is mainly before the collateral network, patient may not develop symptoms at all. However, if stenoses occur either after the collateral network or both before and after the collateral network, symptoms develop readily.

● PATHOPHYSIOLOGY

Regulation of mesenteric vascular tone can be either by intrinsic autoregulation or by extrinsic control. Following sudden fall in intestinal hypoperfusion, direct arterial smooth muscle relaxation ensues. Metabolic response to adenosine and other metabolites of ischemia are the proposed mechanism of this arteriolar relaxation.[4,5] Autoregulation continues to maintain intestinal perfusion across the range of mean arterial pressure of 50 to 75 mm Hg. A broad array of neurohumoral factors such as gastrin, glucagon, and secretin as well as other vasoactive petides such as bradykinin, serotonin, histamine, and prostaglandins are thought to contribute to the regulation of the mesenteric blood supply. Autonomic nervous system, renin angiotensin system, and vasopressin all play important roles in the control of splanchnic blood supply. Sudden reduction in blood supply to the intestine initiates the changes associated with organ ischemia, and compromises the mucosal barrier function. Because of extensive collateral network, and efficient oxygen extraction, intestine can sustain substantial ischemic injury for several hours. Following restoration of blood supply, reperfusion injury can cause further deleterious effects catalyzed by oxygen-free radicals and other toxins. Following brief period of ischemia, reperfusion injury causes most of the damage, whereas after prolonged ischemia, hypoxic damage predominates. Both reperfusion injury and prolonged ischemia result in loss of cellular integrity, and eventual cell necrosis.

● ETIOLOGY

Mesenteric ischemia can be acute or chronic.

Acute Mesenteric Ischemia: Table 31.1 enlists various risk factors of mesenteric ischemia. Acute mesenteric ischemia accounts for 60% to 70% of mesenteric ischemia. The diagnosis of acute mesenteric ischemia maybe present in up to 1 in every 1000 patients admitted to acute care hospitals and is bound to increase as our aging population is on the rise. Advanced age, low cardiac output state, atherosclerotic cardiovascular disease, recent myocardial infarction, cardiac arrhythmias, valvular heart disease, and intra-abdominal neoplasms are specific risk factors for acute mesenteric ischemia.[2] Formation of oxygen-free radicals during ischemia causes injury to the bowel wall, and allows

TABLE 31-1. Risk Factors for Mesenteric Ischemia

a. Mesenteric thrombosis
  i. Atherosclerosis
b. Mesenteric embolism
  i. Cardiac arrhythmia with left atrial appendage thrombus
  ii. Left ventricular apical thrombus following myocardial infarction
  iii. Prosthetic valve
  iv. Rheumatic valve disease
  v. Vegetations from infective endocarditis
c. Nonobstructive mesenteric ischemia
  i. Low output state
    1. Congestive heart failure
    2. Cardiac arrhythmia
    3. Postcardiac surgery
    4. Cardiomyopathy
  ii. Mesenteric vasoconstriction
    1. Medications: digitalis, vasopressors
    2. Hypovolemia
    3. Septic shock
    4. Hemoconcentration
    5. Postabdominal surgery
d. Mesenteric venous thrombosis
  i. Prothombotic state
    1. Antithrombin III deficiency
    2. Protein C deficiency
    3. Protein S deficiency
    4. Factor V Leiden mutation
    5. Antiphospholipid antibody syndrome
    6. Oral contraceptives
    7. Pregnancy
    8. Neoplasms
  ii. Hematologic
    1. Polycythemia vera
    2. Essential thrombocytosis
    3. Paroxysmal nocturnal hemoglobinuria
  iii. Intra-abdominal inflammatory state
    1. Pancreatitis
    2. Peritonitis
    3. Inflammatory bowel disease
    4. Diverticulitis
  iv. Post operative state
    1. Postlaparotomy
    2. Splenectomy
    3. Sclerotherapy
  v. Parasitic infection
    1. Ascaris lumbricoides
  vi. Other causes
    1. Cirrhosis
    2. Portal hypertension
    3. Blunt abdominal trauma
    4. Decompression sickness

systemic release of endotoxins from the infarcted bowels. The endotoxemia thus ensued following restoration of flow can lead to DIC, shock, adult respiratory distress syndrome (ARDS), and even multiorgan system failure. Acute mesenteric ischemia carries a mortality rate up to 60% among hospitalized patients.[2]

Arterial Embolism

Embolization to the SMA is the most frequent cause of acute mesenteric ischemia. In response to acute occlusion, concomitant vasoconstriction may further compromise arterial perfusion, thus exacerbating the ischemic insult. Because of larger caliber and narrow angle at the take-off at its origin, SMA is more susceptible to embolization unlike IMA, which is of smaller caliber and thus is very rarely affected by arterial emboli.[6–9] Typically, the emboli originate in the heart in an akinetic or aneurysmal left ventricular apex following an infarction, in the left atrial appendage in atrial fibrillation, and in valve cusps with vegetations in infective endocarditis. Rarely, a paradoxical embolism from the venous thrombus may cross an unrecognized right to left shunt (generally, a patent foramen ovale). Occasionally, atheromatous aortic arch with mobile plaques either spontaneously or with catheter manipulation in the aorta during an endovascular procedure may contribute to SMA embolism. Emboli usually become lodged at major branch points within the SMA where the distal vessel tends to taper. This is typically just beyond the origin of the middle colic artery, although emboli at more distal branch points have been identified. Proximal SMA perfusion maybe maintained, ensuring viability of the jejunum and resulting in a clear demarcation of the affected intestinal segment at the time of laparotomy. In about 15% of patients, emboli may occlude the SMA at its origin, and in 20%, emboli may affect multiple vascular beds.[2,6] Fig-

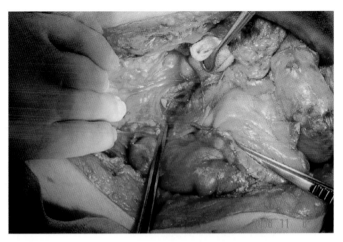

● **FIGURE 31-4.** Surgery for mesenteric ischemia.
Courtesy of Raymond A. Dieter Jr., MD.

ure 31.3 shows appearance of small intestine during acute mesenteric ischemia. Figures 31.4 and 31.5 depict surgical procedures for acute mesenteric ischemia. Figure 31.6 shows an angiogram showing acute SMA occlusion from an embolus.

Arterial Thrombosis

Thrombosis of the mesenteric arteries occurs at the ostia (aorto-ostial), or very proximal segments of the mesenteric arteries. Thrombosis of the residual lumen of the diseased mesenteric artery may occur during a period of relative hypotension, or reduced flow.[10] Dehydration may also precipitate thrombosis in elderly patients.[11] Sometimes, intramural hemorrhage into an atheromatous plaque may lead to complete occlusion of the vessel lumen. Although atherosclerosis is the commonest cause of mesenteric arterial thrombosis, arterial dissection either as a result of extension of an aortic dissection or localized dissection (spontaneous or iatrogenic) may also cause thrombosis. Fibromuscular dysplasia (FMD) and Takayasu's arteritis may

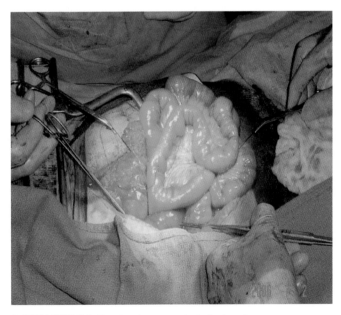

● **FIGURE 31-3.** Acute mesenteric ischemia.
Courtesy of Dr. Raymond A. Dieter Jr, MD.

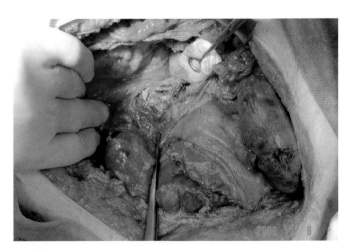

● **FIGURE 31-5.** Resection of small bowel for mesenteric ischemia.
Courtesy of Raymond A. Dieter Jr, MD.

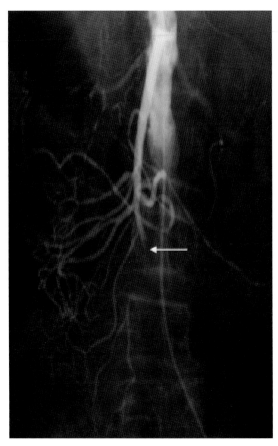

● **FIGURE 31-6.** Selective angiography of SMA shows an abrupt cutoff of the SMA caused by embolus.

Reproduced, with permission, from Martinez JP, Hogan GJ. Mesenteric ischemia. Emerg Med Clin N Am. 2004;22:900-928.

also cause thrombosis of the mesenteric arteries. Rarely, arterial thrombosis may occur with underlying hypercoagulable state.[12]

Mesenteric Venous Thrombosis

Although this chapter focuses on arterial diseases, mesenteric venous thrombosis (MVT) is an important cause of mesenteric ischemia, and will be briefly discussed here. The development of thrombus in the portal and superior mesenteric venous system may induce intestinal ischemia. Hypercoagulable state, traumatic injury, smoking, portal hypertension, splenectomy, malignancies of the portal region, obstruction of the venous flow, and intra-abdominal infection are risk factors commonly associated with mesenteric vein thrombosis.[13,14] In contrast to other etiologies of acute mesenteric ischemia, patients with MVT are typically younger, between the ages of 30 and 60 years, and predominantly women. Inherited hypercoagulable states account for the majority of cases of venous thrombosis. Activated protein C resistance, prothrombin 20210 A gene mutation, deficiencies of protein C & S, antithrombin III deficiency, and antiphospholipid antibody syndrome (APS) are present in that order. Among the acquired hypercoagulable state,

paroxysmal nocturnal hemoglobinuria and myeloproliferative syndromes are commonly associated with MVT.[14] The primary pathophysiologic process associated with venous thrombosis is an increase in portal and mesenteric venous pressure. This increased hydrostatic pressure leads to luminal fluid sequestration and bowel wall edema. The resultant relative hypovolemia and hemoconcentration lead to vasoconstriction and ultimately infarction. The arterial response to venous thrombosis may persist well after the venous obstruction has been corrected. Figure 31.7 shows normal mesenteric venous circulation and Figure 31.8 shows a computed tomography (CT) of abdomen with MVT.

Nonocclusive Mesenteric Ischemia

Hypoperfusion of the mesenteric vascular bed and resultant reactive vasoconstriction among patients with advanced atherosclerotic vascular disease leads to nonocclusive mesenteric ischemia (NOMI). Low output cardiac state following a large myocardial infarction or an episode of congestive heart failure, hypovolemia following blood loss or diuretic use, cardiac arrhythmias, sepsis, aortic insufficiency, drugs such as digoxin and alpha adrenergic agonists (pseudoephedrine, amphetamines), cocaine use, postcardiac surgery, especially those requiring long aortic cross-clamp time or inotropic support, and postdialysis are associated with NOMI.[15–18] NOMI can also occur as a result of mesenteric arterial spasm following repair of aortic coarctation and revascularization procedures for chronic mesenteric ischemia.

Chronic Mesenteric Ischemia. Chronic mesenteric ischemia refers to episodic or constant intestinal hypoperfusion that usually develops among patients with mesenteric atherosclerotic disease.[19] Patients typically develop abdominal pain (intestinal angina) within 1 hour of eating that lasts typically 1 to 2 hours. Larger and fatty meals tend to worsen symptoms readily.[20] Typically, patients will have marked weight loss as they develop fear of food, and want to eat frequent small meals to avoid worsening of their pain. Disease of other vascular trees such as coronary and peripheral arteries often coexist, and risk factors of systemic atherosclerosis including diabetes, hypertension, and smoking are often present.[21,22] Figure 31.9 shows mesenteric stenosis causing chronic mesenteric ischemia. Figure 31.10 depicts development of collaterals in splanchnic artery occlusions.

Unusual Causes of Chronic Mesenteric Ischemia

MECHANICAL CAUSES

> *Mesenteric Arterial Dissection*: The causes of spontaneous arterial dissection of the splanchnic arteries are uncertain. Atherosclerosis, cystic medial necrosis, and primary muscular dysplasia are thought to be contributory. Dissection can present either as intra-abdominal hemorrhage (abdominal apoplexy) or mesenteric ischemia.[23]

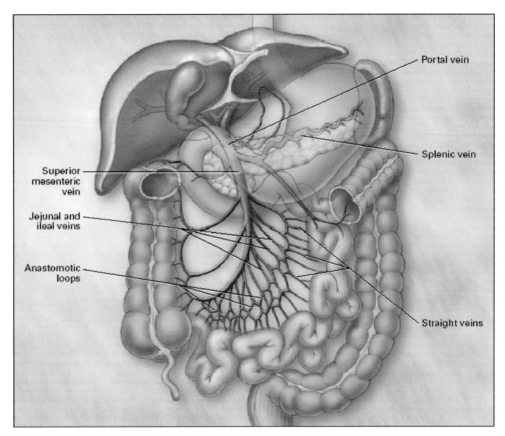

● **FIGURE 31-7.** Normal mesenteric venous circulation.

Reproduced, with permission, from Kumar S, Sarr MG, Kamath PS. Mesenteric venous thrombosis. N Engl J Med. 2001;345:1683-1688.

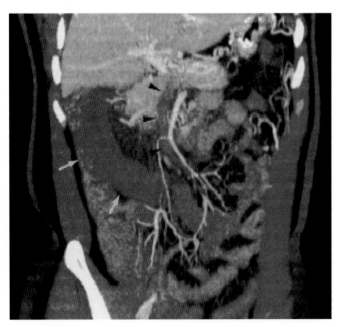

● **FIGURE 31-8.** Acute mesenteric venous thrombosis. Multidetector CT of intestinal infarction showing no bowel wall enhancement of affected bowel loop (arrows) and extensive superior mesenteric vein thrombosis (arrowheads).

Reproduced, with permission, from: Kim AY, Ha HK. Evaluation of suspected mesenteric ischemia: efficacy of radiologic studies. Radiol Clin North Am. 2003;41:327-342.

Median Arcuate Ligament Syndrome: Median arcuate ligament syndrome is caused by compression of the celiac or SMA by the median arcuate ligament of the diaphragm. Two anatomic variants have been described.[23] In one, CA alone is compressed; in the other, both CA and SMA are compressed. It occurs in young individuals, mostly women. The pain produced by celiac compression could be ischemic or neural in origin caused by fibrosis of celiac ganglion.[23,24] In many patients, this syndrome progresses to thrombosis of celiac artery. Median arcuate ligament syndrome is unusual in that only one mesenteric artery needs to be involved to produce symptoms. The classical presentations are upper abdominal pain on eating, with associated weight loss, and a loud epigastric systolic bruit. The bruit occurs throughout systole, and the initial part of diastole. During inspiration, the bruit is loudest owing to caudal displacement of aorta and CA with the celiac band moving in cranial direction. Angiography, especially lateral aortography, shows compression of CA by the median arcuate ligament during deep expiration and is diagnostic. Compression of CA by the arcuate ligament produces a concave defect in the superior aspect of the celiac trunk just beyond its origin. This defect often increases with expiration,

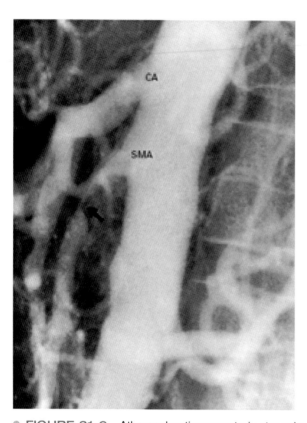

● **FIGURE 31-9.** Atherosclerotic mesenteric stenosis causing chronic mesenteric ischemia as shown by small arrow.

Reproduced, with permission, from Ansari A, Decesare R, Images in clinical medicine: mesenteric ischemia. N Eng J Med. 2000; 343(13):937.

and decreases or disappears with inspiration. Duplex ultrasonography can measure blood flow in the SMA and CA. Contrast-induced CT scan and MR angiogram may also be used to demonstrate a compression. Surgery is the treatment of choice for median arcuate ligament syndrome. Division of the obstructing diaphragmatic fibers and denervation of the celiac ganglion is the most commonly performed operative procedure. Endovascular treatment maybe used in conjunction with surgical procedure. Balloon dilation of the CA or SMA or arterial reconstruction following surgical division may offer more symptomatic relief compared to surgical division alone.[23,25] Figures 31.11 to 31.14 show relation of median arcuate ligament to the celiac and SMA.

Retroperitoneal Fibrosis: Retroperitoneal fibrosis is a rare disorder characterized by inflammatory and fibrotic changes of the retroperitoneal space. It has been associated with the use of methysergide, an antimigraine agent.[26] Rarely, this can occur with inflammatory aneurysms. Ureteral obstruction is a common finding in this disorder. Although arterial obstruction is rare, obstruction of the abdominal aorta or its branches (celiac or mesenteric arteries) can occur and cause chronic intestinal ischemia.[27] Surgical resection of the fibrotic tissue to relieve

the arterial obstruction maybe attempted in symptomatic patients, though maybe technically difficult.

Neurofibromatosis: Neurofibromatosis (Von Recklinghausen's disease) is an autosomal dominant, neurocutaneous disorder and characterized by café-au-lait spots, mental retardation, seizure disorder, and multiple neurofibromas. Intimal and adventitial layers of the vascular system are distorted by presence of neurofibromas within these layers. This may eventually lead to vascular compromise, and thereby intestinal ischemia.[28]

Radiation: Exposure to radiation therapy leads to chronic fibrosis and cicatrisation (formation of scar tissue) of the mural and extramural tissue, and thereby can cause obstruction of one of the splanchnic vessels leading to mesenteric ischemia.[23]

DRUGS

Digitalis: Digitalis, a cardiac glycoside, produces contraction of vascular smooth muscles in vitro and in vivo. Thus, among patients with preexisting mesenteric atherosclerosis, digitalis-induced vasoconstriction may lead to mesenteric ischemia, particularly NOMI.[29,30]

Cocaine: It is a sympathomimetic and local anesthetic alkaloid. A very popular recreational drug, and at present widely abused, it can cause numerous cardiovascular and cerebrovascular complications such as myocardial infarction, stroke, and arrhythmia by causing arterial vasoconstriction.[31] By similar mechanism, cocaine causes intestinal vasoconstriction and ischemia regardless of its mode of administration.[32]

Ergotamines: The ergot alkaloids, especially ergotamine are potent arterial vasoconstrictors. Chronic and repetitive use of ergot alkaloids may thus lead to intense intestinal vasoconstriction and subsequent mesenteric ischemia.[33]

Vasopressors: Alpha adrenergic agonists such as ephedrine, pseudoephedrine, amphetamines, and vasopressin can cause vasoconstriction and intestinal ischemia.[34,35]

CLINICAL FEATURES. Accurate diagnosis of acute mesenteric ischemia remains a clinical challenge while early and prompt diagnosis is the key to improving patient survival. Table 31.2 describes clinical features of four major causes of acute mesenteric ischemia. Heightened awareness and adequate knowledge of the varied clinical presentations while maintaining a high index of suspicion play vital roles in making an expedient diagnosis of acute mesenteric ischemia.

Rapid onset of severe periumbilical abdominal pain, often out of proportion to physical findings, is the commonest presentation of acute mesenteric ischemia. This apparent inconsistency between the presenting symptoms and

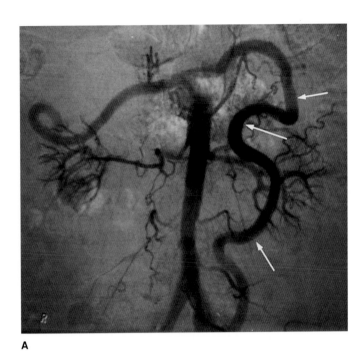

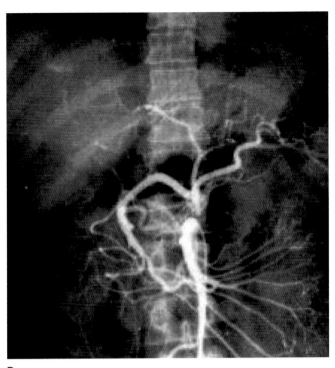

A   **B**

● **FIGURE 31-10.** Collateral network in chronic mesenteric ischemia. (A) Angiogram showing marginal artery of Drummond (*arrows*) in chronic SMA occlusion.

Reproduced, with permission, from Martinez JP, Hogan GJ. Mesenteric ischemia. Emerg Med Clin N Am. 2004;22:900-928.
(B) Angiogram of SMA in celiac occlusion showing collateral filling of celiac branches through the gastroduodenal artery. Also noted are replaced right hepatic artery and replaced left hepatic artery from the SMA and left gastric artery.

Reproduced, with permission, from Rosenblum GD, Boyle CM, Schwartz LB. The mesenteric circulation: Anatomy and physiology. Surg Clin North Am 1997;77:289-307.

paucity of physical findings, which has been a major hurdle in making an accurate diagnosis, is unfortunately the sine qua non of acute mesenteric ischemia.[2,9] Unlike most of the atherosclerotic vascular disease, mesenteric ischemia does not predominate in men. Among patients with arterial embolism and thrombosis causing mesenteric ischemia, the symptom onset is drastic. However, among patients with MVT, symptoms are more insidious in onset. Several clues to the etiology of ischemia maybe present. Acute abdominal pain followed by rapid and forceful bowel evacuation strongly suggests SMA emboli. Acute abdominal pain that develops after percutaneous arterial interventions in which catheters traverse the visceral aorta or abdominal pain among patients with risk factors of systemic emboli such as atrial fibrillation or recent myocardial infarction should suggest mesenteric emboli as the cause of acute intestinal ischemia.[21] A history of abdominal pain for several months followed by acute worsening suggests mesenteric artery thrombosis. Patients with NOMI may not present with abdominal pain in up to 25% of cases, and may present as unexplained abdominal distension and gastrointestinal bleeding. Nausea and vomiting, and less commonly diarrhea maybe seen. In patients with NOMI, the clinical picture maybe overshadowed by the precipitating disorders

such as hypotension, congestive heart failure, arrhythmia, and hypovolemia.[8,15] The stool may contain occult blood in up to 75% of the patients, and bloody diarrhea is not uncommon. Feculent breath may herald intestinal necrosis. Unexplained abdominal distention may herald intestinal infarction and maybe present early in the course. Mental confusion maybe present in the elderly.[36]

When physical findings suggestive of an acute intra-abdominal catastrophe are present, bowel infarction may have already ensued, and the chances of survival for these elderly patients are already compromised. Abdominal examination maybe normal initially or reveal only abdominal distension. But as the disease progresses, abdomen becomes grossly distended, bowel sounds become absent, and peritoneal signs develop.

● **DIAGNOSIS**

Laboratory Testing

A complete blood count with differential, electrolyte panel, coagulation studies, liver function tests, and an amylase level should be drawn in any patient suspected of having an acute abdominal pain. The findings of leucocytosis, metabolic acidosis, and elevated amylase level are

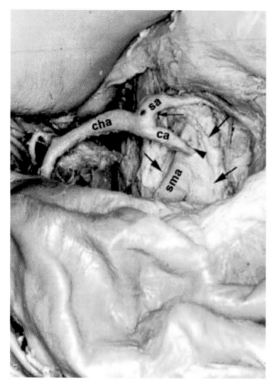

● **FIGURE 31-11.** Relation of median arcuate ligament to the celiac artery (CA) and superior mesenteric artery (SMA). The median arcuate ligament (big arrows) was moved aside, showing CA with a notch (*arrowhead*) caused by median arcuate ligament. SA, splenic artery; CHA, common hepatic artery.

Reproduced, with permission, from Petrella S, Rodrigues CFS, Sgrott EA, Fernandez GJM, Marques SR, Prates JC. Relationship of the celiac trunk with median arcuate ligament of the diaphragm. Int J Morphol. 2006;24:263-274.

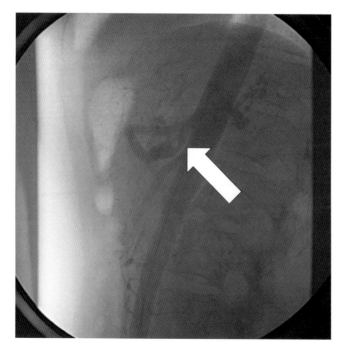

● **FIGURE 31-12.** Median arcuate ligament syndrome involving celiac artery, as shown by the arrow.

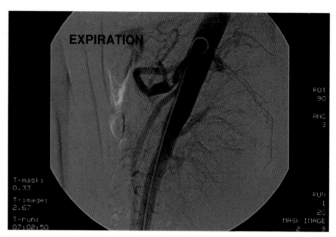

● **FIGURE 31-13.** Median arcuate ligament syndrome, shown on expiration.

associated with more advanced ischemia and most likely, nonviable bowel. Significant base deficit can occur early in patients with SMA occlusion and intestinal infarction without hypotension. This can occur within 8 to 16 hours of symptom onset, and may precede the physical findings, laboratory data, and radiologic studies suggestive of intestinal infarction. Conditions other than SMA occlusion causing abdominal pain do not cause the base deficit unless associated with cardiogenic shock.[37] Serum lactate level is also very helpful in diagnosis in case of intestinal ischemia. Elevated serum lactate level is found in one study to be 100% sensitive, and 42% specific for intestinal ischemia/infarction.[38] Serum D-dimer levels maybe elevated in patients with acute ischemia and maybe a useful marker, although nonspecific.[39] Alpha-glutathione S-transferase (alpha-GST) and intestinal fatty acid-binding protein (I-FABP) are found to be elevated inpatients with ischemia, and may prove to be useful in diagnosing mesenteric ischemia and infarction.[40,41]

Plain Radiography

Plain abdominal x-rays may be normal in early ischemia. Later in the course of ischemia, x-rays may show formless

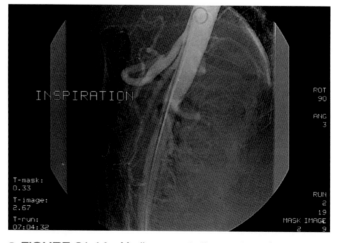

● **FIGURE 31-14.** Median arcuate ligament syndrome, shown on inspiration.

TABLE 31-2. Differential Clinical Features of Major Causes of Acute Mesenteric Ischemia

	Arterial Thrombosis	Arterial Embolism	Nonocclusive Mesenteric Ischemia	Mesenteric Venous Thrombosis
Incidence (%)	50	25	20	5
Age	Elderly	Elderly	Elderly	Younger
Gender predominance	Female	Male	Male	Female
Clinical presentations	Gradual and progressive postprandial pain	Sudden onset abdominal pain	Progressive vague abdominal pain and distension	More insidious abdominal pain with distension, and ascites
Mortality	Very high	High	Highest	Lowest
Prior symptoms	Intestinal angina	No	No	No

loops of bowel, ileus, or thickening of the bowel wall with "thumbprinting," suggestive of submucosal edema. Any radiological findings are late signs of ischemia, and portend an ominous outcome.[42] Figure 31.15 shows radiographic pictures of acute mesenteric ischemia.

Duplex Ultrasonography. Duplex ultrasound can assess flow in the SMA and the portal vein. Although duplex ultrasonography is not the first line imaging study for suspected acute mesenteric ischemia, this can be useful in detecting thrombus and occlusion of these vessels. But, duplex can only assess the proximal part of the major vessels, good windows are not possible in presence of fluid filled loops of bowels, and in NOMI, duplex can be normal. Duplex ultrasound has an overall accuracy of approximately 90% for detection of >70% diameter stenoses or occlusions of the celiac and superior mesenteric arteries when performed in highly experienced laboratories.[21,42,43]

Computed Tomography Scanning

CT scanning is helpful in diagnosing mesenteric ischemia. Early signs include bowel wall thickening and luminal dilation, and are nonspecific. Late signs such as gas in the bowel wall (pneumatosis) and mesenteric or portal venous gas are suggestive of necrotic bowel and are very specific for intestinal necrosis. Contrast-enhanced CT scanning is the procedure of choice in diagnosing acute MVT. Lack of opacification of the mesenteric veins after contrast injection is diagnostic of MVT. CT angiography (CTA) now allows three-dimensional (3D) reconstruction of vessels and enables the physician to visualize the vessel in a way almost similar to conventional angiography and holds the potential to replace conventional angiography as a noninvasive means of diagnosing acute mesenteric ischemia.[43–45]

Magnetic Resonance Angiography

Magnetic resonance angiography (MRA) with gadolinium greatly enhances vascular visualization. Like duplex ultrasound, it is useful in evaluating CA and SMA, but limited in evaluation of IMA and peripheral branches. Moreover, it

is expensive, cumbersome, and not available readily. MRA may be falsely negative in NOMI.[43–45]

Basic Electrical Rhythm

Basic electrical rhythm (BER) (Figure 31.16) is the underlying slow wave electrical activity of the gastrointestinal tract and is detectable by measuring magnetic fields generated by transabdominal superconducting quantum interference devices (SQUIDs). Preliminary animal studies have shown alterations in BER detectable by SQUIDs within 30 minutes of induced ischemia.[46]

Angiography. Angiography remains the gold standard for diagnosing acute and chronic mesenteric ischemia. It has a sensitivity of over 90% in detecting both occlusive and nonocclusive forms of intestinal ischemia. Both anteroposterior and lateral aortography should be obtained. Lateral aortography delineates the typical ostial lesions, whereas frontal view may show the presence of an enlarged "Arc of Riolan," an angiographic sign of proximal mesenteric artery obstruction (an enlarged collateral vessel connecting left colic branch of IMA with the SMA). Abrupt cutoff of a vessel without evidence of any collateral flow is diagnostic of acute mesenteric ischemia. In the SMA embolus, this cutoff develops 3 to 10 cm distal to the origin of the SMA. In SMA thrombosis, the entire SMA often is not visualized, the so-called "naked aorta"; this reflects occlusion of the SMA at the site of atherosclerosis usually at its origin. A prominent "meandering artery" denotes enlargement of the marginal artery of Drummond in response to the chronic atherosclerotic disease. In addition to this diagnostic utility, therapeutic intervention if warranted at the time of diagnostic angiogram such as administration of vasodilators (e.g., papaverine) or thrombolytics have shown to improve outcome in patients with acute mesenteric ischemia. Prompt and accurate diagnosis made in an expedient manner by angiography has shown to improve mortality in these highly morbid patients. In spite of these advantages, there are certain negative aspects of angiography and these are to be considered as well during the planning of management of these sick patients. It is invasive, time-consuming, and

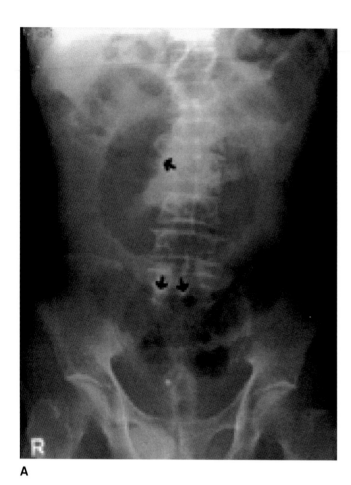

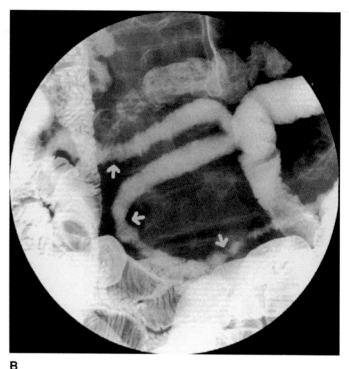

B

A

● **FIGURE 31-15.** Radiographic appearance of acute mesenteric ischemia. (A) Plain radiograph showing multiple loops of distended bowels in AMI.

Reproduced, with permission, from Martinez JP, Hogan GJ. Mesenteric ischemia. Emerg Med Clin N Am. 2004;22:900-928.

(B) Barium study of intestinal ischemia showing diffuse luminal narrowing of distal small intestine with prominent thickening of valvulae conniventes and shallow thumbprinting in a patient with superior mesenteric vein thrombosis.

Reproduced, with permission, from Kim AY, Ha HK. Evaluation of suspected mesenteric ischemia: efficacy of radiologic studies. Radiol Clin North Am 2003;41:327-342.

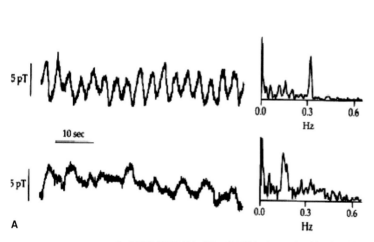

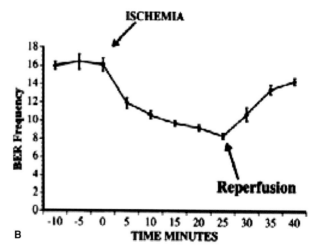

● **FIGURE 31-16.** BER in intestinal ischemia.

Reproduced, with permission, from Richards WO, Garrard CL, Allos SH, Bradshaw LA, Staton DJ, Wikswo JP. Noninvasive diagnosis of mesenteric ischemia using a SQUID magnetometer. Ann Surg. 1995;221:696-704.

can cause bleeding from the access site, and may lead to nephrotoxicity from the dye.[44]

● TREATMENT

The mainstay of therapy in acute mesenteric ischemia is to restore blood flow at the earliest possible before irreversible ischemia has ensued. Early diagnosis is the only way of achieving this goal. Despite this, there is still a 60% mortality rate.[18,21] Figures 31.17 to 31.20 describe the management algorithm for mesenteric ischemia.

General Therapeutic Measures

Aggressive hemodynamic monitoring and support, correction of metabolic acidosis, and placement of nasogastric tube for gastric decompression are very important in early management. Patient should be kept nothing by mouth; and a Foley catheter for monitoring of urine output is recommended.

Broad Spectrum Antibiotics

Broad-spectrum antibiotics should be started immediately as mesenteric ischemia is suspected. Antibiotic therapy

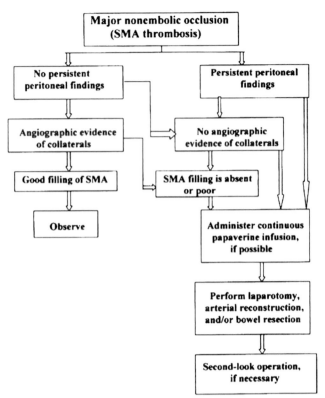

● **FIGURE 31-18.** Algorithm for SMA thrombosis.

Reproduced, with permission, from Brandt LJ, Boley SJ. AGA technical review on intestinal ischemia. Gastroenterology 2001;118:954.

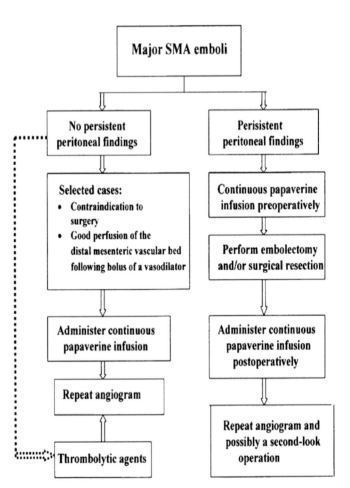

● **FIGURE 31-17.** Algorithm for management of SMA emboli.

Reproduced, with permission, from Brandt LJ, Boley SJ. AGA technical review on intestinal ischemia. Gastroenterology. 2001;118:954-968.

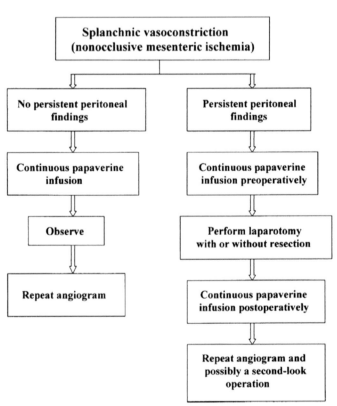

● **FIGURE 31-19.** Algorithm for NOMI.

Reproduced, with permission, from Brandt LJ, Boley SJ. AGA technical review on intestinal ischemia. Gastroenterology. 2001;118:954-968.

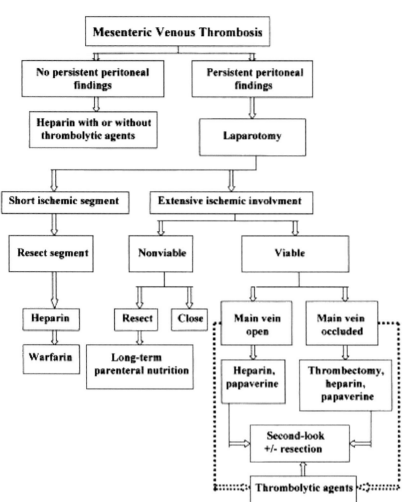

● **FIGURE 31-20.** Management algorithm for acute MVT.

Reproduced, with permission, from Brandt LJ, Boley SJ. AGA technical review on intestinal ischemia. Gastroenterology. 2001;118:954.

could protect against bacterial translocation in the ischemic segment.

Anticoagulation

Institution of heparin for anticoagulation is important in management of ischemia. Immediate heparin if no signs of bowel infarction and deferred heparin for 48 hours if infarction has already occurred are the preferred strategies.

Vasoconstrictors

Dopamine and norepinephrine are to be avoided. Digitalis should also be avoided. If treatment for hypotension is required, dobutamine, low-dose dopamine, or milrinone are to be preferred as initial agents.

Surgery

Surgery should not be delayed in patients suspected or diagnosed of having intestinal perforation or gangrene. If diagnosis is in doubt, following initial stabilization of the patients, an expedient mesenteric angiography will be imperative in making an accurate diagnosis as this improves survival up to 67% if done within 12 hours of presentation as compared to earlier reported survival of only 30%.[3,10]

Table 31.3 details various surgical procedures for mesenteric revascularization.[22]

Superior Mesenteric Artery Embolus

Once diagnosed, early surgical embolectomy has been the mainstay of treatment.[47,48] This is achieved by an arteriotomy distal to the emboli, and then advancement of a balloon-tipped embolectomy catheter for retrieval of the embolus. Palpation of the SMA pulses allow surgeon to resect any nonviable segment. Resection should be limited to frankly necrotic bowel, and any bowel of questionable viability should be reexamined at a second look laparotomy in 24 to 48 hours. Intraoperative Doppler ultrasound[49] and intravenous fluorescein injection followed by examination of the bowel under Wood's Lamp are indirect ways of confirming tissue viability.[50]

Percutaneous interventions including transcatheter lytic therapy, balloon angioplasty, and stenting are recommended as class IIb (level of evidence C) therapy in the treatment of acute mesenteric ischemia.[21] Given the high operative mortality of these patients, percutaneous revascularization is an option. Alternative therapy for SMAE is local, intraarterial infusion of thrombolytic therapy during angiography especially if done within 8 hours of

TABLE 31-3. Surgical Procedures for Mesenteric Revascularization

Reconstructive

Grafts: Synthetic or autologous
    Bypass
    Patch
    Interposed segment
    Y grafts
    Multiple

Endarterectomy
    Trapdoor

Angioplasty
    Operative

Anastomosis
    End to side
    End to end
    To branch vessel

Transplantation of origin

Resectional
    Small or large bowel resection
    Enterostomy

Adhesions or bands:
    Lysis
    Resection

Open angioplasty/vascular dilation
    Through aorta
    Through side
    Through primary vessel

presentation in absence of bowel infarction and contraindications to thrombolysis.[51] Concomitant intraarterial papaverine administration maybe beneficial in alleviating vasoconstriction.[2] If patient develops progressive ischemia following thrombolysis, surgical exploration is mandatory. Long-term management of SMAE involves administration of warfarin to prevent future emboli. However, even after successful percutaneous revascularization, most of these patients may still require laparotomy with surgical exploration and maybe at risk of endotoxemia, leading to disseminated intravascular coagulation or respiratory distress syndrome as release of toxins from infracted bowel into the circulation takes place following restoration of flow. This potential ischemia-reperfusion injury maybe better contained by surgical revascularization rather than endovascular revascularization.

Mesenteric Artery Thrombosis

As mesenteric artery thrombus usually occurs in the setting of atherosclerosis, thrombectomy alone may not confer a durable outcome. So, thrombectomy in conjunction with surgical revascularization followed by arterial reconstruction and resection of the nonviable intestine is the preferred strategy especially if peritoneal signs are present.[2,52] In absence of peritoneal signs and with angiographic evidence of good collateral flow, heparin anticoagulation is justified for short term. In presence of peritoneal signs, poor collateral flow, and decreased SMA filling, continuous papaverine injection, and laparotomy is indicated.[47] Long-term aspirin may reduce the risk of recurrence of mesenteric ischemia in the future.

Mesenteric Venous Thrombosis. In patients with MVT with signs of peritonitis, emergent laparotomy with resection of the necrotic bowel is recommended. Papaverine maybe infused to relieve associated arterial spasm. A second look operation should then be performed 12 to 24 hours after the first operation.[54,56] Immediate heparinization for 7 to 10 days after surgery, and warfarin for 3 to 6 months should then be administered. Duration of warfarin should be longer if a hypercoagulable state is present.[55] However, these patients need close observation, and if signs of peritonitis develop, immediate laparotomy is indicated in these patients. Successful venous thrombolysis with fibrinolytic agents (streptokinase, urokinase, and TPA) while administered antergrade via the SMA, retrograde via the internal jugular vein, and transhepatically via the hepatic vein is also reported to be effective in acute MVT, although not widely recommended at this time.

Nonocclusive Mesenteric Ischemia

Since NOMI does not result from thrombosis or embolization, surgery in NOMI is reserved for patients with bowel infarction requiring resection. Alpha-agonists, digitalis, and vasopressors are avoided. In addition to making attempts to reverse the underlying condition, administration of papaverine via angiographic catheter during SMA angiography remains the mainstay of therapy in NOMI. Papaverine is administered at 30 to 60 mg/hr and the infusion is generally continued for 24 hours with close monitoring of the hemodynamic status. In patients without any peritoneal signs, repeat angiography in 24 hours allows assessment of bowel viability. If peritoneal signs develop in stable patients, papaverine may even be attempted. For persistent peritoneal signs, laparotomy is indicated. Papaverine in those cases should be continued intraoperatively and postoperatively. Concomitant heparin therapy (intravenous) may prevent thrombosis in the cannulated vessel.[57–59] Iloprost, a prostacycline analogue with vasodilating and fibrinolytic activity, has been shown to increase SMA flow in porcine model without significantly decreasing mean arterial blood pressure, yet improving mucosal hypercarbia and intramucosal PH.[60] If proven in clinical trials, this maybe a useful agent in the treatment of NOMI without the need of direct SMA infusion.

Chronic Mesenteric Ischemia

When indicated, chronic mesenteric ischemia can be treated by either surgical revascularization or percutaneous transluminal angioplasty (PTA) with or without stent.

Surgical Revascularization. Surgical procedures in the treatment of chronic mesenteric ischemia are retrograde bypass grafting, antegrade bypass grafting, transaortic endarterectomy, local arterial endarterectomy with patch angioplasty, thrombectomy, and SMA reimplantation. Bypass grafting (from supraceliac or infrarenal aorta) endarterectomy and reimplantations are usually preferred reconstructive techniques, and the choice mostly depends on the individual operator choice and experience.[61] Mateo and colleagues[62] reported early and late outcomes of a series of 85 patients who underwent elective surgery for symptomatic mesenteric arterial disease. There were 8% early postoperative deaths (<35 days), but 5-year survival rate was 64%, and 3-year symptom-free survival was 81%. Advanced age at operation, cardiac disease, hypertension, and additional occlusive disease were predictors of mortality. Concomitant aortic replacement, renal failure, advanced age, and complete revascularization were associated with postoperative morbidity and mortality. Results from several other studies evaluating long-term results of surgical revascularization have shown that primary graft patency at 5 years ranged from 57% to 69%, and 5-year survival ranged from 63% to 77%. Mortality from surgical procedures varies widely from 0% to 11%, but up to 50% among patients with acute on chronic disease.[61,63] Revascularization of asymptomatic intestinal arterial stenoses except in patients undergoing aortic/renal surgery for other indications is not indicated.[21]

Percutaneous Revascularization. PTA of mesenteric arteries is ideally done in conjunction with a vascular surgeon. PTA can be done via brachial or femoral access as determined by the angle of origin of the vessels from the aorta. Femoral access is usually ergonomically easier, whereas brachial access is preferred when SMA has a downsloping course after its origin. Ostial lesions are approached with a "no touch technique" or "telescoping technique." Cannulation of the mesenteric artery is usually done with a 0.014″ wire and the lesion is preferentially treated with predilation with a low-profile, semicompliant balloon.[64,65] Suboptimal result after balloon angioplasty is defined as residual stenosis of >50% or a flow-limiting dissection. In these situations, a balloon expandable stent can be used for ostial and proximal lesions, whereas self-expanding stents can be used for mid to distal lesions. As aggressive balloon sizing can be detrimental with its attendant risks, balloon/stent to artery ratio should ideally be 1:1. PTA of intestinal arterial stenoses is indicated in patients with chronic intestinal ischemia as Class I indication (level of evidence B).[21] Kasirajan et al., in their case series of 28 patients undergoing PTA of mesenteric arteries, have reported long-term outcomes as compared to a historical cohort of surgically revascularized patients for CMI.[66] During their 3.5 years of follow-up, although there was no difference in early in-hospital complications or mortality between two groups, percutaneously revascularized patients had higher incidence of symptom recurrence. A retrospective, single center study by Silva et al.[67] has demonstrated 96% procedural success

and 88% clinical success with relief of symptoms among patients with chronic mesenteric ischemia. Even on longer follow-up at mean duration of 38 ± 15 months, 79% of these patients remained alive, only 17% had recurrence of symptoms, and 29% had restenosis. In another retrospective study of 60 patients undergoing endovascular versus open mesenteric revascularization, Sivamurthy et al.[68] have shown that 30-day mortality and 3-year survival between these two methods were similar, but surgical group had better symptom relief. Brown et al.,[68] in a small series of 14 patients with mesenteric stenting for CMI, have reported higher risk of restenosis, symptom recurrence, and the need for reintervention with stenting compared to a historical cohort of surgical patients. Angioplasty and stenting thus have low inherent mortality and morbidity, yet a very high procedural and clinic success rate. This option of percutaneous intervention of mesenteric arterial stenoses thus seems very attractive and viable. Atkins et al.[70] reported 20% symptom recurrence requiring reintervention both after surgical and percutaneous revascularization. Although in-hospital outcomes were similar between these two methods of revascularization, primary patency was lower in stenting group needing earlier reintervention.

Thus, in the early stages of chronic mesenteric ischemia, medical and endovascular techniques remain the most effective. CMI caused by stenotic arteriosclerotic lesions are better treated by PTA, whereas chronic arterial occlusions are better managed by surgical revascularization.[71]

● VASCULITIS OF MESENTERIC ARTERIES

The mesenteric arteries are generally affected by medium to small vessel vasculitides. Vasculitides affecting the mesenteric vessels are part of generalized systemic process, and can present as systemic, intestinal, or extraintestinal symptoms.[72]

Clinical Features

The clinical manifestations maybe acute and severe or chronic. Abdominal pain, gastrointestinal bleeding, nausea and vomiting, and diarrhea are some of the common intestinal symptoms. Postprandial abdominal pain and weight loss are symptoms of chronic mesenteric ischemia. Bowel infarction, perforation, and peritonitis are rare complications of vasculitis.

Systemic Lupus Erythematosus. This is a vasculitis of small- and medium-sized vessels with gastrointestinal manifestations in up to 50% of cases. Abdominal pain, usually intermittent and insidious spanning over several months, is characteristic of systemic lupus erythematosus (SLE). Patients with SLE presenting with chronic abdominal pain should alert the physician of mesenteric vasculitis. Mesenteric vasculitis may lead to potentially life-threatening complications such as bowel infarction, septic shock, and bowel perforation. Risk factors that are known to predispose a patient with SLE to mesenteric vasculitis are peripheral vasculitis and central nervous system lupus.[72]

Pathology demonstrates occlusion of several mesenteric and intramural vessels with organized thrombi associated with inflammation. Treatment of SLE with gastrointestinal involvement needs aggressive, pulse doses of systemic methylprednisolone and cyclophosphamide therapy.

Antiphospholipid Antibody Syndrome. APS can present with SLE or as an isolated disorder. As APS is a hypercoagulable state, its manifestations affecting the gastrointestinal tract are mostly from mesenteric arterial and venous thrombosis. APS is diagnosed if at least one of the clinical criteria (recurrent venous or arterial thrombosis, recurrent fetal loss, persistent thrombocytopenia, livedo reticularis) and at least one of the laboratory criteria (IgG or IgM anticardiolipin antibody, anti-B2 glycoprotein 1 antibody, lupus anticoagulant) are positive on at least two occasions more than 3 months apart.[73] Treatment of APS should therefore involve long-term, and maybe life-term anticoagulation.

Polyarteritis Nodosa. This systemic necrotizing arteritis of small- and medium-sized arteries can affect virtually any organ with the exception of the lungs. Unlike other systemic vasculitides (microscopic polyarteritis, Wegener's granulomatosis, and Churg-Strauss syndrome), polyarteritis nodosa (PAN) is not associated with antineutrophil cytoplasmic antibodies (ANCA). Granulomatous inflammation does not occur in PAN, but disruption in the internal and external elastic lamina contributes to aneurysmal dilation of the affected vessels. Skin, kidney, musculoskeletal, and gastrointestinal systems are typically involved. When mesenteric vessels are affected, gastrointestinal bleeding, infarction, hemorrhage, and perforation may occur with a mortality of 75% to 100%. Mesenteric angiography shows multiple aneurysms and irregular constrictions in the large vessels with occlusion of smaller penetrating arteries.[74,75] Diagnostic criteria of PAN are enlisted in Table 31.4.[76] Treatment with cyclophosphamide and corticosteroids has been successful in improvement in survival and relief of symptoms. PAN related to hepatitis B infection or hairy cell leukemia responds to treatment of these underlying diseases.

Buerger Disease. This is a nonatherosclerotic segmental inflammatory vasculopathy that most commonly affects the small- and medium-sized arteries, veins, and nerves of the extremities (arms and legs). Typically seen among young male smokers before the age of 40 to 45 years, there are reports of increasing prevalence among women ranging from 11% to 23%. The prevalence of the disease among all patients varies from as low as 0.5% to 5.6% in Western Europe to as high as 45% to 63% in India, 16% to 66% in Japan, and Korea, and 80% in Israel among Jews of Ashkenazi ancestry.[77,78] Pathologically, there is a highly cellular and inflammatory thrombus with relative sparing of the vessel wall. The acute phase reactants (ESR and CRP) and immunological markers (circulating immune complexes, cryoglobulins, and complement levels) are typically normal in this disease. Angiograms of the affected vessels

---

TABLE 31-4. Diagnostic criteria for PAN*

1. Otherwise unexplained weight loss >4 kg
2. Livedo reticularis
3. Testicular pain or tenderness
4. Myalgia (excluding that of the shoulder and hip girdle), weakness of muscles, tenderness of muscles, or polyneuropathy
5. Mononeuropathy or polyneuropathy
6. New onset diastolic blood pressure >90 mm Hg
7. Elevated levels of serum blood urea nitrogen (>40 mg/dL) or Creatinine (>1.5 mg/dL)
8. Evidence of hepatitis B virus infection via serum antibody or antigen serology
9. Characteristic angiographic abnormalities not resulting from noninflammatory disease process
10. A biopsy of small or medium sized artery containing polynuclear cells

Presence of at least 3 of the criteria has a sensitivity and specificity of 82% and 87% for diagnosis of PAN.

---

are likely to show multiple occlusions with collateralization ("corkscrew collaterals") around the areas of occlusion. Mesenteric arteries can also be involved in this vasculopathy, leading to mesenteric ischemia. The only proven strategy to prevent disease progression is immediate cessation of smoking in any form. Figure 31.21 illustrates Buerger disease.

Churg-Strauss Syndrome. Churg-Strauss syndrome also affects small- and medium-sized vessels, and present as characteristic triad of allergic rhinitis, asthma, and peripheral eosinophilia.[79] Most patients with this disease respond to high-dose steroid therapy. Diagnostic criteria for Churg-Strauss syndrome is enlisted in Table 31.5.

Henoch-Schonlein Purpura. Mostly a disease of children, Henoch-Schonlein purpura (HSP) is a small vessel vasculopathy with gastrointestinal involvement in up to 50% of cases. Patients with gastrointestinal involvement may present with colicky abdominal pain, nausea, vomiting, diarrhea, and gastrointestinal bleeding. It is self-limiting, resolving spontaneously in majority of cases, and rarely needs systemic steroids or immunosuppressive agents in recalcitrant cases.[80] Diagnosis is confirmed by demonstration of immunoglobulin A (IgA) deposition on skin or kidney biopsy.

Takayasu's Disease. A medium/large vessel vasculopathy of the aorta and its major branch vessels, it typically involves aortic arch branches, although can extend into the mesenteric and renal arteries. Often, because of chronic progression of the disease, collaterals develop in patients with visceral artery involvement, and they remain

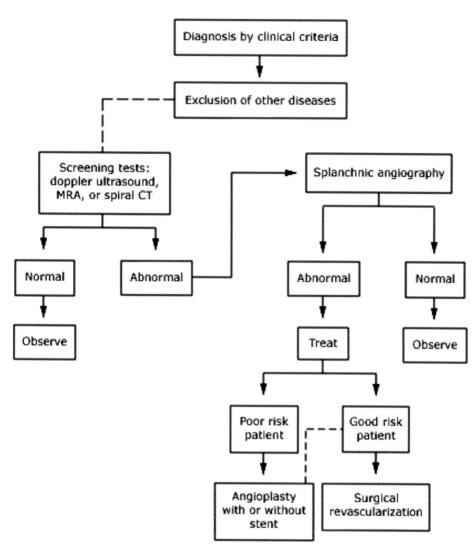

● **FIGURE 31-21.** Management of CMI. Solid lines indicate accepted management plan. Dashed lines indicate alternate management plan. MRA, magnetic resonance angiography; CT, computed tomography.

Reproduced, with permission, from Brandt LJ, Boley SJ. AGA technical review on intestinal ischemia. Gastroenterology 2001;118:954.

asymptomatic for a long time. Intestinal ischemia maybe brought on by thrombosis of main visceral arteries that propagate into the collateral vessels. Women are predominantly affected mostly in their early ages between 10 and 40 years. The prevalence is very high among the Asians. Gastrointestinal involvement with mesenteric ischemia can occur and manifest as abdominal pain, diarrhea, and bleeding. Diagnostic criteria for Takayasu's arteritis is listed in Table 31.6.[81]

Behcet's Syndrome. A necrotizing vasculitis predominantly affecting young males, it is characterized by uveitis, aphthous stomatitis, and genital ulcers. Meseneteric vessels are rarely involved and cause mesenteric ischemia mostly by occlusion of arteries with organized thrombi. New international criteria[82] for diagnosis of Behcet's disease require the presence of recurrent oral aphthous ulcers (at least three times a year) plus two of the following four criteria: (1) recurrent genital ulcers; (2) uveitis; (3) skin lesions (erythema nodosum, pseudovasculitis, papulopustular lesions, and acneiform nodules); and (4) a positive pathergy test (a papule of 2 mm or more in size developing 24 to 48 hours after oblique insertion of a 20 to 25 gauge needle

---

TABLE 31-5. Diagnostic Criteria for Churg-Strauss Syndrome*

1. Asthma (a history of wheezing or the finding of wheezing on expiration)
2. Eosinophilia of >10% on differential white blood cell count
3. Mononeuropathy (including multiplex) or polyneuropathy
4. Migratory or transient pulmonary opacities detected radiographically
5. Paranasal sinus abnormality
6. Biopsy containing a blood vessel showing the accumulation of eosinophils in extravascular areas

Presence of 4 or more of the criteria yields a sensitivity of 85% and specificity of 99.7%.

TABLE 31-6. Diagnostic Criteria for Takayasu's Arteritis

1. Age at onset ≤40 years
2. Claudication of the extremities
3. Decreased pulsation of one or both brachial arteries
4. Difference of at least 10 mm Hg in systolic blood pressure between the arms
5. Bruit over one or both subclavian arteries or the abdominal aorta
6. Arteriographic narrowing or occlusion of the entire aorta, its primary branches, or large arteries in the proximal upper or lower extremities, not caused by atherosclerosis, fibromuscular dysplasia, or other causes

Presence of 3 or more criteria yields a sensitivity and specificity of 90.5% and 97.8%, respectively, for Takayasu's arteritis.

into the skin). Although the symptoms can wax and wane, systemic disease is typically treated with steroids and immunosuppressive agents such as azathioprine, cyclosporine, or cyclophosphamide.

Diagnosis

Most patients will have systemic manifestations and will have already been diagnosed before the onset of mesenteric symptoms.

Laboratory Testing. Erythrocyte sedimentation rate (ESR) is almost always elevated. Specific serological markers are also helpful in making specific diagnosis such as antinuclear antibody (ANA) and antidouble-stranded DNA antibody for SLE, antinuclear cytoplasmic antibodies (ANCA) for PAN, and antiphospholipid antibody for APS. Tissue biopsies are confirmatory in most of these vasculitides.

Imaging Studies. CT scan and barium studies are nonspecific in diagnosing early cases of mesenteric vasculitis. Angiography is useful in diagnosing PAN, Buerger disease, and Takayasu's arteritis.

Endoscopy. Endoscopy at times maybe used for tissue biopsies if other accessible biopsy sites are not readily available. Endoscopy should be done with extreme caution as there is an increased risk of perforation from this instrumentation.

Treatment. Treatment of vasculitides is aimed at treating the underlying systemic disease with aggressive immunosuppressive therapy and corticosteroids. Surgical intervention is indicated in patients with mesenteric infarction or intestinal perforation.

● FIBROMUSCULAR DYSPLASIA

FMD is nonatheroclerotic, noninflammatory angiopathy primarily of medium-sized arteries, leading to arterial stenoses and symptoms of ischemia. It is seen in mostly in young women with an incidence of 1%. Although this disease predominantly involves renal and cerebral arteries, mesenteric arteries are involved in about 9% of the total cases.[83,84] Table 31.7 enlists the arterial distribution of FMD. Unless severe, FMD may go undiagnosed and less likely to be considered in the differential diagnosis as it maybe mistaken for more commoner pathology such as atherosclerosis, thrombosis, or even vasculitis. Genetics may play a role in the development of FMD, and is most likely to be inherited as an autosomal dominant pattern with variable penetrance. Mechanical factors such as cyclic stretching of arterial smooth muscle cells and trauma to the blood vessel wall may also contribute to the development of FMD. Ischemia of the arterial wall by occlusion of the vasa vasorum may potentially lead to increased accumulation of connective tissue and myofibroblasts as a reparative process leading to FMD. Smoking may also predispose to FMD in a dose–response relationship. FMD can have three different pathological morphologies. Medial fibroplasia is the commonest and has classic "strings of beads" appearance. The beading is larger than the caliber of the normal artery and is confined to the middle to distal portion of the artery. Media is typically involved, whereas the intima, internal elastic lamina, and adventitia are spared. Medial fibroplasia causes thickened fibromuscular ridges alternating with mural thinning and aneurysms. Intimal fibroplasia occurs in less than 10% of patients. Angiographically, it may appear as a focal, concentric stenosis or a long tubular stenosis.

TABLE 31-7. Arterial Involvement in Fibromuscular Dysplasia

Arteries Involved	Frequency of Involvement (%)
Renal arteries	60–75
Bilateral	35
Extracranial cerebrovascular circulation (carotid or vertebral arteries)	25–30
Associated intracranial aneurysm	7–50
Multiple vascular beds	28
Other arterial beds (iliac, popliteal, splanchnic, hepatic, coronary, subclavian, brachial, aorta, superficial femoral, tibial, or peroneal)	Uncommon, exact frequency unknown

Fibromuscular dysplasia may be a generalized process; in rare case, it has also been identified in the venous system.
Reproduced, with permission, from Olin JW. Thromboangitis obliterans. N Engl J Med. 2000;343: 864-869.

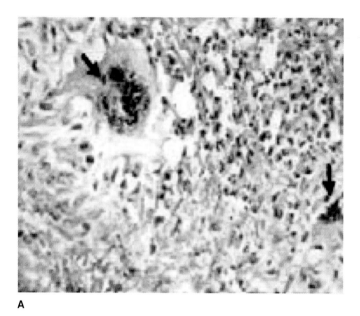

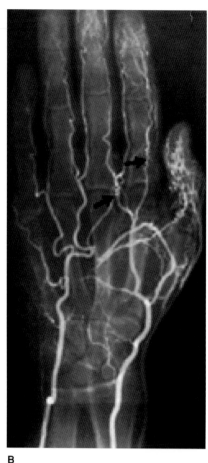

● **FIGURE 31-22.** (A) Pathology and (B) angiograms of Buerger disease.

Reproduced, with permission, from Olin JW. Thromboangitis obliterans. N Engl J Med. 2000;343:864-869.

B

Adventitial (periarterial) fibroplasia is the rarest of all varieties of FMD. Angiographically, it may appear as sharply localized, tubular stenosis.

Symptoms of mesenteric FMD include nausea, vomiting, abdominal pain, anorexia, and weight loss. Although symptomatic FMD is rare, and because of collateral network, ischemia is uncommon unless two major arteries are severely involved. At times, presence of an abdominal bruit gives clue to the diagnosis.

Diagnosis of FMD is challenging. Duplex ultrasonography, CTA, and even MRA are useful imaging modalities in the initial work-up and characteristic appearance on the angiography are further suggestive of the diagnosis. A histopathological diagnosis is needed for confirmation.

Symptomatic mesenteric FMD may require revascularization. Focal FMD can be treated by PTA. But FMD is diffuse, majority of patients eventually require surgical revascularization treatment. Data on the outcomes of surgical revascularization are mixed. In one study,[85] following revascularization of mesenteric stenosis, patients had resolution of symptoms with minimal postoperative mortality or morbidity. On the contrary, a study by Howard et al.[86] had shown poor outcome of surgery of mesenteric arteries for FMD and was complicated by multiorgan failure and death. Patients with diffuse mesenteric FMD become symptomatic at a very advanced stage of the disease

and surgery is then poorly tolerated. Figure 31.22 illustrates FMD in renal arteries.

● **MESENTERIC ARTERY ANEURYSMS**

Aneurysms of mesenteric arteries are not so uncommon. Based on autopsy reports, the prevalence of mesenteric artery aneurysms is estimated to be up to 10%. About 25% of these aneurysms are complicated by ruptures that carry a mortality rate ranging 25% to 70%.[87] Most of the splanchnic aneurysms will require surgical intervention. The use of endovascular coils and stent grafts have been reported and may gain popularity as experience and follow-up develops. Figures 31.23 through 31.26 illustrate the distribution and types of various splanchnic aneurysms.

Etiology

The causes of mesenteric artery aneurysm are listed in Table 31.8.

Splenic Artery Aneurysm. Splenic artery aneurysms are more prevalent among multiparous women, in patients with splenomegaly such as portal hypertension, and following orthotopic liver transplantation. Increased splenic blood flow is likely to be the contributing factor in the development of splenic artery aneurysms among these patients. Most of the aneurysms occur at the distal third of

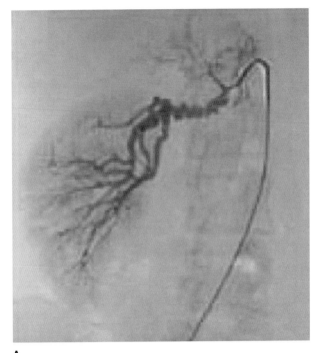

A

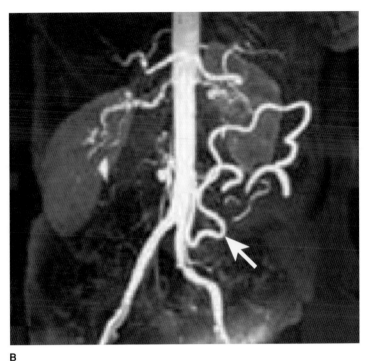

B

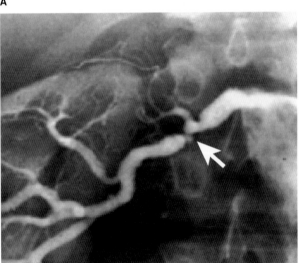

C

● FIGURE 31-23. (A–C) Imaging of fibromuscular dysplasia.
Reproduced, with permission, from Slovut DP, Olin JW. Fibromuscular dysplasia: current concepts. N Engl J Med. 2004;350:1862-1871.

the splenic artery, are saccular, and involve the bifurcation. Risk of rupture is markedly increased among pregnant patients, and with aneurysms larger than 2 cm in diameter. If symptomatic, these aneurysms mostly present as left upper quadrant pain. When ruptured, complications such as hypovolemic shock or gastrointestinal bleeding causes increased mortality, especially among pregnant patients with a 75% maternal and 95% fetal mortality. Elective surgery for splenic artery aneurysm is indicated for symptomatic aneurysms, aneurysms larger than 2 cm, and aneurysms of any size present in pregnant women or in women of childbearing age. Ruptured aneurysms are treated with splenectomy. Percutaneous coil embolization maybe performed for all splenic aneurysms except for those present in the hilum, which are best treated by splenectomy. Proximal artery aneurysms are treated by sim-

ple surgical ligation and midartery aneurysms are treated by aneurysmectomy followed by end to side anastomosis. While elective surgery has minimal surgical mortality, emergency surgery has a mortality rate as high as 40%. Close follow-up of the splenic aneurysms measuring 1 to 2 cm is therefore recommended with an imaging study every 6 months. Splenic aneurysms associated with portal hypertension are treated by transcatheter coil embolization as increased vascularity may make the surgical treatment difficult. Splenic artery pseudoaneurysms are better treated by surgery.

Celiac Artery Aneurysm. Celiac artery aneurysm occurs mostly among middle-aged individuals, and has equal occurrence among both sexes. Upper abdominal pain, dysphagia, and gastrointestinal bleeding are common presenting

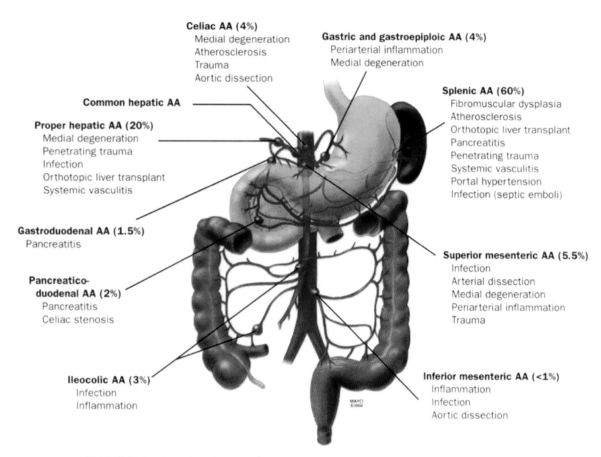

Celiac AA (4%)
Medial degeneration
Atherosclerosis
Trauma
Aortic dissection

Gastric and gastroepiploic AA (4%)
Periarterial inflammation
Medial degeneration

Common hepatic AA

Proper hepatic AA (20%)
Medial degeneration
Penetrating trauma
Infection
Orthotopic liver transplant
Systemic vasculitis

Splenic AA (60%)
Fibromuscular dysplasia
Atherosclerosis
Orthotopic liver transplant
Pancreatitis
Penetrating trauma
Systemic vasculitis
Portal hypertension
Infection (septic emboli)

Gastroduodenal AA (1.5%)
Pancreatitis

Pancreatico-
duodenal AA (2%)
Pancreatitis
Celiac stenosis

Superior mesenteric AA (5.5%)
Infection
Arterial dissection
Medial degeneration
Periarterial inflammation
Trauma

Ileocolic AA (3%)
Infection
Inflammation

Inferior mesenteric AA (<1%)
Inflammation
Infection
Aortic dissection

● **FIGURE 31-24.** Distribution of splanchnic artery aneurysms (AA). Prevalence of percentage of all splanchnic artery aneurysms and sites of splanchnic artery aneurysms are indicated.

Reproduced, with permission, from Pasha SF, Gloviczki P, Stanson AW, Kamath PS. Splanchnic artery aneurysms. Mayo Clin Proc. 2007;82:472-479.

symptoms. Celiac aneurysms are usually treated by surgical ligation followed by aortohepatic bypass or direct aortic reimplantation. Ruptured aneurysms are managed by either surgical ligation or percutaneous coil embolization.

Hepatic Artery Aneurysm. Hepatic artery aneurysm accounts for 20% of mesenteric aneurysms. Most of the hepatic aneurysms are pseudoaneurysms, and may follow interventional procedures. Most of the symptomatic hepatic artery aneurysms present as right upper quadrant pain.

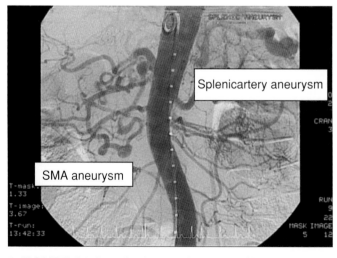

Splenicartery aneurysm

SMA aneurysm

● **FIGURE 31-25.** Angiogram showing an SMA and splenic artery aneurysm.

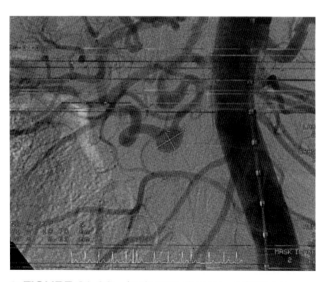

● **FIGURE 31-26.** Angiogram showing an SMA aneurysm.

TABLE 31-8. Etiology of Splanchnic Artery Aneurysms

True aneurysms

Common causes
    Arteriosclerosis
    Fibromuscular dysplasia
    Cystic medial necrosis
    Portal hypertension

Uncommon causes

Autoimmune /collagen vascular diseases
    Polyaretritis nodosa
    Systemic lupus erythematosus
    Takayasu's arteritis
    Ehlers-Danlos syndrome
    Marfan syndrome
    Neurofibromatosis

Hypertension

Congenital

Alpha-antitrypsin deficiency

Pseudoaneurysms

Common causes
    Inflammatory conditions
        Pancreatitis
    Blunt or penetrating abdominal trauma
    Anastomotic pseudoaneurysms (after orthotopic liver
        transplantation)
    Percutaneous intervention of biliary tract
    Arterial dissection

Uncommon causes

Infectious diseases
    Mycotic aneurysms
    Syphilis
    Infective endocarditis
    Tuberculosis

Adapted from Pasha SF, Gloviczki P, Stanson AW, Kamath PS. Splanchnic artery aneurysms. Mayo Clin Proc. 2007;82:472-479.

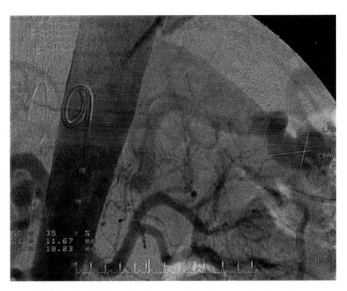

● **FIGURE 31-27.** Angiogram showing a splenic artery aneurysm.

Obstructive jaundice from compression by the aneurysm of the bile duct, erosion into the biliary tract, or gastrointestinal bleeding following rupture are more serious presentations of hepatic artery aneurysms. Most aneurysms are extrahepatic and occur mostly in men older than 60 years of age. Multiple aneurysms and nonatherosclerotic aneurysms are associated with increased risk of rupture and thus warrant intervention. Surgical ligation with or without vascular reconstruction are the preferred mode of management for these aneurysms although transcatheter coil embolization or endograft stenting are reserved for patients with high surgical risks.

Superior Mesenteric Artery Aneurysm. Superior mesenteric artery aneursym occurs both in men and women equally. Infective endocarditis, especially with nonhemolytic streptococci, staphylococci, or gram-negative bac-

teria account for most of the SMA aneurysms. These aneurysms occur among young men younger than 50 years of age with a history of intravenous drug use. Nearly 50% of patients present with rupture with a mortality rate of up to 30%. SMA aneurysms are usually symptomatic, and may present with abdominal pain with or without mesenteric ischemia, or gastrointestinal bleeding. Surgical ligation is advised for patients with low surgical risks. Transcatheter coil embolization or endograft stenting are reserved for high surgical risk patients or for patients not willing to have surgery. Beta-blockers may protect against rupture and should be used when these aneurysms are medically managed. Figures 31.21 and 31.27 show SMA and splenic artery aneurysm.

Pancreaticoduodenal and Gastroduodenal Artery Aneurysms. Pancreaticoduodenal and gastroduodenal artery aneurysms are usually the sequelae of pancreatitis or of pancreatoduodenectomy. Epigastric pain is the commonest presentation of these aneurysms. Erosion into the pancreatic duct may cause hemosuccus pancreaticus (bleeding into the pancreatic duct). Erosion into a pancreatic pseudocyst may cause a pulsatile pseudocyst. Either surgical ligation with or without vascular reconstruction or endovascular exclusion with transcatheter coil embolization or stent-grafting is recommended for treatment of these aneurysms.

Diagnosis

Abdominal plain radiograph may reveal calcification, and often provides early clues to a diagnosis of visceral artery aneurysm. Diagnosis of a splanchnic artery aneurysm is usually made with one of the imaging modalities. Ultrasonography has a very low sensitivity and is compromised by bowel gas and obesity. Computed tomography (CT) helps to even detect small aneurysms with excellent delineation of anatomical details. Magnetic resonance imaging (MRI) can also provide a great clarity of the splanchnic vessel aneurysms, but is often cumbersome and not readily available. Angiography is the diagnostic study of choice as it provides the elaborative details of the aneurysms, and at the same time offers the scope of catheter interventions if warranted.

INTESTINAL ARTERIOVENOUS MALFORMATIONS

Arteriovenous malformations (AVMs) of the gastrointestinal tract are rare sources of gastrointestinal bleeding, and are categorized into three clinical groups depending on lesion location and age at presentation. Angiodysplasia is the commonest form of intestinal AVMs, which are solitary and localized lesions usually found in the right colon, and manifest later in life usually after the age of 50 years. Angiodysplasias are common among the elderly, and also among patients with aortic stenosis. Less common are the AVMs of small intestine, usually occurring in younger patients and present as massive bleeding with negative diagnostic workups. Most often, these patients would end up undergoing several blind intestinal resections. Rarest variety of AVMs constitutes hereditary hemorrhagic telengiectasia (HHT) also called Osler-Weber-Rendu syndrome.

HHT is an autosomal dominant disorder with varying penetrance. Presence of at least three of the four criteria confirm the diagnosis of HHT: (1) spontaneous and recurrent epistaxis; (2) multiple mucocutaneous telangiectasia; (3) visceral involvement, most commonly of gastrointestinal, pulmonary, cerebral, and hepatic AVMs; and (4) a first-degree relative with HHT. The exact etiology of HHT is not entirely known. However, presence of mutation involving endoglin, a membrane glycoprotein needed for maintaining endothelial integrity on chromosome 9, and mutation of activin-receptor like kinase, ALK-1, a transdermal growth factor β (TGF-β) receptor on chromosome 12 are implicated in the causation of AVMs seen in HHT. HHT is not present at birth. Epistaxis, the earliest sign, occurs in childhood. Pulmonary AVMs occur at puberty, and gastrointestinal and mucocutaneous signs occur with increasing age. Nearly 30% of HHT will have pulmonary AVMs, 30% with hepatic AVMs, and 10% to 20% with cerebral AVMs. Dyspnea, hemoptysis, and playpnea-orthodeoxia are common symptoms of pulmonary AVMs. Cerebral abscesses, cerebrovascular accidents, or transient ischemic attacks are common neuroembolic manifestations of HHT and occur exclusively in patients with pulmonary AVMs with right to left shunts. Cerebral AVMs may present with headache, seizures, or cerebral hemorrhage. Hepatic AVMs mostly present with high-output cardiac failure (left to right shunt), portal hypertension, biliary disease, and hepatic encephalopathy. Screening of the family members with HHT should be carried out with history, focused physical examination, chest X-ray, contrast echocardiogram, and cerebral MRI.

TABLE 31-9. Complications of Splanchnic Artery Aneurysms

1. Intraperitoneal rupture
   a. Hemoperitoneum
   b. Hypovolemic shock
2. Intrahepatic subcapsular rupture
3. Retroperitoneal hemorrhage
4. Gastrointestinal hemorrhage
   a. Hemobilia
   b. Hemosuccus pancreaticus
   c. Herald bleed
5. Arteriovenous fistula formation
   a. Portal hypertension
   b. Ascites
   c. Variceal bleeding
6. Obstructive jaundice
7. Acute mesenteric ischemia

Reproduced, with permission, from Pasha SF, Gloviczki P, Stanson AW, Kamath PS. Spalnachnic artery aneurysms. Mayo Clin Proc. 2007;82:472-479.

Treatment

In some studies, splanchnic artery aneurysms have been found to be more common than the abdominal aortic aneurysms in the autopsy studies. Advancement in imaging technology with the CT, MRI, and digital angiography has led to easier detection of asymptomatic aneurysms as an incidental finding when these tests are ordered for other reasons. Multiple aneurysms maybe detected in one third of these patients. Although mostly asymptomatic, mortality from rupture of a visceral aneurysm is very high (50%–75%) even with an emergency surgery whereas elective repair has a low mortality rate (less than 15%). Close follow-up of the splanchnic aneurysms is therefore required to minimize the rate of rupture and thus to reduce mortality. Although presentations of these aneurysms vary, symptoms of abdominal pain, abdominal bruits, or a pulsatile mass should raise the suspicion of a splanchnic artery aneurysm. Table 31.9 describes the complications of splanchnic artery aneurysms. Surgical repair (aneurysmectomy with or without arterial reconstruction) or percutaneous exclusion (coil embolization or endograft stenting) of the aneurysms are the modalities commonly used to treat these aneurysms. While surgery is commonly preferred, percutaneous treatment is reserved for high surgical risk patients. Symptomatic aneurysms, enlarging aneurysms, or large aneurysms (>2 cm) require prompt interventions.[85]

SEGMENTAL ARTERIAL MEDIOLYSIS

Segmental arterial mediolysis (SAM) is an acute; self-limiting; noninflammatory visceral arteriopathy of unclear etiology that is very rare but affects mainly the mesenteric vasculature.[90] Vacuolization and subsequent lysis of the smooth muscle cells of the mesenteric arterial walls leading to aneurysmal dilation of the arteries are characteristics of this disease. Vacuolization initially starts in the outer media with sparing of the internal elastic lamina and the intima but in the advanced stage, it progresses to be transmural. SAM most commonly presents with painful abdominal distension, intra-abdominal hemorrhage, and hypotension or shock from aneurysmal ruptures of the mesenteric arteries. Pathology remains to be the gold standard for making a diagnosis of SAM; however, digital subtraction angiography or CT angiography demonstrating characteristic arterial involvement while maintaining a high degree of clinical suspicion is probably enough in most cases to clinch a diagnosis of SAM. An estimated mortality of up to 50% may be seen in the acute phase of this disease. Surgical interventions including segmental resection of the diseased segment and end-to-end anastomosis are the mainstay of management. However, transcatheter arterial embolization of the involved artery may be useful and feasible in treatment of SAM, although very close monitoring following coil embolization is imperative for these patients as morphological evolution can ensue very rapidly among these patients.[91]

SMA SYNDROME (OR WILKIE SYNDROME)

SMA syndrome or Wilkie syndrome is characterized by constellation of symptoms resulting from the compression of the transverse part of the duodenum against the aorta by the SMA. Abdominal pain, abdominal distension, nausea, or vomiting may be the manifest presentations of this syndrome as a result of chronic, intermittent, or acute complete or acute partial duodenal obstruction. As the transverse part of duodenum course between the aorta and SMA, any condition that alters this aortomesenteric angle (such as thin body habitus, skeletal deformities, surgical interventions of the spine, etc.) can predispose to this syndrome. Most patients may only need conservative treatment while surgery may be reserved for the nonresponders. Barium X-rays or CT of abdomen is usually helpful in clinching the diagnosis.

NUTCRACKER SYNDROME

Nutcracker syndrome, also known renal vein entrapment syndrome, results from the compression of the left renal vein between the abdominal aorta and SMA. This is associated with hematuria, left flank pain, nausea, and/or vomiting. This is diagnosed with left renal venography (the gold standard test), or with CT. Treatment may include endovascular stenting, renal vein reimplantation, or gonadal vein embolization.

CONCLUSION

Mesenteric vascular disease is quite a common, yet highly lethal disease. Treatment of this disease should be immediate, aggressive, and accurate. Adequate knowledge of the disease with a high degree of suspicion is a must for prompt and effective treatment of these patients. The decision to perform a mesenteric angiogram in patients with high-risk features of mesenteric arterial disease should not be delayed, and a multidisciplinary approach should be followed in treating these patients.

REFERENCES

1. Rosenblum GD, Boyle CM, Schwartz LB. The mesenteric circulation. Anatomy and physiology. *Surg Clin North Am.* 1997;77:289-307.

2. McKinsey JF, Gewertz BL. Acute mesenteric ischemia. *Surg Clin North Am.* 1997;77:307-318.

3. Boley SJ, Brandt LJ, Sammartano RJ. History of mesenteric ischemia. The evolution of a diagnosis and management. *Surg Clin North Am.* 1997;77:275-288.

4. Boley SJ, Frieber W, Winslow PR, et al. Circulatory responses to acute reduction of superior mesenteric arterial flow. *Physiologist.* 1969;12:180.

5. Zimmerman BJ, Granger DN. Reperfusion injury. *Surg Clin North Am.* 1992;72:65-83.

6. Cappell, MS. Intestinal (mesenteric) vasculopathy. I. Acute superior mesenteric arteriopathy and venopathy. *Gastroenterol Clin North Am.* 1998;27:783-825.

7. Burns BJ, Brandt LJ. Intestinal ischemia. *Gastroenterol Clin N Am.* 2003;32:1127-1143.

8. Tendler DA, LaMont JT. Acute mesenteric ischemia. Up to date 2007 edition.

9. Martinez JP, Hogan GJ. Mesenteric ischemia. *Emerg Med Clin N Am.* 2004;22:900-928.

10. Stoney RJ, Cunningham CG. Acute mesenteric ischemia. *Surgery.* 1993;114:489-490.

11. Wilson DB, Mostafvi K, Craven TE, Ayerdi J, Edwards MS, Hansen KJ. Clinical course of mesenteric artery stenosis in elderly Americans. *Arch Intern Med.* 2006;166:2095-2100.

12. Thomas DP, Roberts HR. Hypercoagulability in venous and arterial thrombosis. *Ann Intern Med.* 1997;126:638-644.

13. Rhee RY, Gloviczki P. Mesenteric venous thrombosis. *Surg Clin North Am.* 1997;77:327-338.

14. Kumar S, Sarr MG, Kamath PS. Mesenteric venous thrombosis. *N Engl J Med.* 2001;345:1683-1688.

15. Bassiouny HS. Nonocclusive mesenteric ischemia. *Surg Clin North Am.* 1997;77:319-326.

16. Garofalo M, Borioni R, Nardi P, et al. Early diagnosis of acute mesenteric ischemia after cardiopulmonary bypass. *J Cardiovasc Surg (Torino).* 2002;43:455-459.

17. Diamond S, Emmett M, Henrich WL. Bowel infarction as a cause of death in dialysis patients. *JAMA.* 1986;256:2545-2547.

18. Brandt LJ, Boley SJ. AGA technical review on intestinal ischemia. *Gastroenterology.* 2000;118:954-968.

19. Moawad J, Gewertz BL. Chronic meseneteric ischemia. Clinical presentation and diagnosis. *Surg Clinic North Am.* 1997; 77:357-369.

20. Poole JW, Sammartano RJ, Boley SJ. Hemodynamic basis of pain of chronic mesenteric ischemia. *Am J Surg.* 1987; 153:171-176.

21. Hirsch AT, Haskal ZJ, Hertzer NR, et al. ACC/AHA 2005 Guidelines for the management of patients with peripheral arterial disease. *J Am Coll Cardiol.* 2006;47:1239-1312.

22. Dieter RA, Kuzycz G, Dieter RA III, Dieter RS. Visceral arterial obstructive disease. In: Chang JB, ed. *Textbook of Angiology.* Berlin: Springer; 2000;545-558 [chap. 45].

23. Krupski WC, Selzman CH, Whitehill TA. Unusual causes of mesenteric ischemia. *Surg Clinic North Am.* 1997;77:472-503.

24. Dunbar JD, Molnar W, Berman FF, Marable SA. Compression of the celiac trunk in abdominal angina: preliminary report of 15 cases. *Am J Roentgenol.* 1956;95:731-744.

25. Reilly LM, Ammar AD, Stoney RJ, Ehrenfeld WK. Late results following operative repair for celiac compression syndrome. *J Vasc Surg.* 1985;2:79-91.

26. Graham JR, Suby HI, LeCompte PR, et al. Fibrotic disorders associated with methysergide therapy for headache. *N Engl J Med.* 1966;274:359-368.

27. Ketz J, Vogel R. Abdominal angina as a complication of methysergide maleate therapy. *JAMA.* 1967;199:124-126.

28. Brunner H, Stacher G, Banki H, Grabner G. Chronic mesenteric arterial insufficiency caused by vascular neurofibromatosis. *Am J Gastroenterol.* 1974;62:442-447.

29. Levinsky RA, Lewis RM, Bynum TE, Hanley HG. Digoxin induced intestinal vasoconstriction. *Circulation.* 1975;52:130-136.

30. Shanbour LL, Jacobson ED. Digitalis and the mesenteric circulation. *Dig Dis.* 1993;17:826-827.

31. Lange RA, Cigarrola RG, Yancy CW Jr, et al. Cocaine-induced coronary artery vasoconstriction. *N Engl J Med.* 1989; 321:1557-1562.

32. Brown DN, Rosenholtz MJ, Marshall JB. Ischemic colitis related to cocaine abuse. *Am J Gastroenterol.* 1994;89:1558-1561.

33. Holmes G, Marten E, Tabua S. Mesenteric vascular occlusion in pregnancy: suspected ergot poisoning. Med J Aust 1969;2:1009-1111.

34. Bernadi RS. Vascular complications of superior mesenteric artery infusion with pitressin in treatment of bleeding esophageal varices. *Am J Surg.* 1974;127:757-761.

35. Schneider RP. Ischemic colitis caused by decongestants? *J Clin Gastroenterol.* 1995;21:335-336.

36. Ruotolo RA, Evans SRT. Mesenteric ischemia in the elderly. *Clin Geriatr Med.* 1999;15:527-557.

37. Brooks DH, Carey LC. Base deficit in superior mesenteric artery occlusion, an aid to early diagnosis. *Ann Surg.* 1973;352-356.

38. Lange H, Jackel R. Usefulness of plasma lactate concentration in the diagnosis of acute abdominal disease. *Eur J Surg.* 1994;160:381-384.

39. Acosta S, Nilsson TK, Bjorck M. Preliminary study of D-dimer as a possible marker of acute bowel ischemia. *Br J Surg.* 2001;88:385-388.

40. Gearhart SL, Delaney CP, Senagore AJ, et al. Prospective assessment of the predictive value of alpha-glutathione S-transferase for intestinal ischemia. *Am Surg.* 2003;69:324-329.

41. Kanda T, Fujii H, Tani T, et al. Intestinal fatty acid-binding protein is a useful diagnostic marker for mesenteric infarction in humans. *Gastroenetrology.* 1996;110:339-343.

42. Klein HM, Lensing R, Klosterhalfen B, et al. Diagnostic imaging of mesenteric infarction. *Radiology.* 1995;197:79-82.

43. Jamieson WG, Marchuk S, Rowsom J, Durand D. The early diagnosis of massive acute intestinal ischaemia. *Br J Surg.* 1982;69 Suppl:S52-S53.

44. Bakal CW, Sprayregen S, Wolf EL. Radiology in intestinal ischemia. Angiographic diagnosis and management. *Surg Clin North Am.* 1992;72:125-141.

45. Kim AY, Ha HK. Evaluation of suspected mesenteric ischemia: efficacy of radiologic studies. *Radiol Clin North Am.* 2003;41:327-342.

46. Seidel SA, Bradshaw LA, Ladipo JK, Wikswo JR Jr, Richards WO. Noninvasive detection of ischemic bowel. *J Vasc Surg.* 1999;30:309-319.

47. Boley SJ, Sprayregen S, Siegelman SJ, Veith FJ. An aggressive roentgenologic and surgical approach to acute mesenteric ischemia. *Surg Ann.* 1973;5:355-378.

48. Boley J, Feinstein FR, Sammartano R, Brandt LJ. New concepts in the management of emboli of the superior mesenteric artery. *Surg Gynecol Obstet.* 1981;153:561-569.

49. Reinus JF, Brandt LJ, Boley SJ. Ischemic diseases of the bowel. *Gastroenterol Clin North Am.* 1990;19:319-343.

50. Carter MS, Fantini GA, Sammartano RJ, Mitsudo S, Silverman DG, Boley SJ. Qualitative and quantitative fluorescein fluorescence in determining intestinal viability. *Am J Surg.* 1984;147:117-123.

51. McBride KD, Gaines PA. Thrombolysis of a partially occluding superior mesenteric artery thromboembolus by infusion of streptokinase. *Cardiovasc Intervent Radiol.* 1994;17: 164-166.

52. Cho JS, Carr JA, Jacobsen G, et al. Long-term outcome after mesenteric artery reconstruction: a 37-year experience. *J Vasc Surg.* 2002;35:453-460.

53. Klempnauer J, Grothues F, Bektas H, Pichlmayr R. Long-term results after surgery for acute mesenteric ischemia. Surgery 1997;121:239-243.

54. Levy P, Krausz MM, Manny J. The role of second-look procedure in improving survival time for patients with mesenteric venous thrombosis. *Surg Gynecol Obstet.* 1990;170:287-291.

55. Petitti DB, Strom BL, Melmon KL. Duration of warfarin anticoagulant therapy and the probabilities of recurrent thromboembolism and hemorrhage. *Am J Med.* 1986;81:255-259.

56. Grieshop RJ, Dalsing MC, Cikrit DF, et al. Acute mesenteric venous thrombosis: revisited in a time of diagnostic clarity. *Am Surg.* 1991;57:573-577.

57. Trompeter M, Brazda T, Remy CT, et al. Non-occlusive mesenteric ischemia: etiology, diagnosis, and interventional therapy. *Eu Radiol.* 2002;12:1179-1187.

58. Anatharaju A, Van Thiel DH. Non-occlusive mesenteric ischemia: reality. *J Gastroenetrol.* 2002;37:876.

59. Ward D, Vernava AM, Kaminski DL, et al. Improved outcome by identification of high-risk nonocclusive mesenteric ischemia, aggressive re-exploration, and delayed anastomosis. *Am J Surg.* 1995;170:557-580.

60. Kang H, Manasia A, Rajamani S, et al. Intravenous iloprost increases mesenteric blood flow in experimental acute nonocclusive mesenteric ischemia. *Crit Care Med.* 2002;30:2528-2534.

61. Shanley CJ, Ozaki CK, Zelenock GB. Bypass grafting for chronic mesenteric ischemia. *Surg Clin North Am.* 1997;77: 381-395.

62. Mateo RB, O'Hara PJ, Hertzer NR, Mascha EJ, Beven EG, Krajewski LP. Elective surgical treatment of symptomatic chronic mesenteric occlusive disease: early results and late outcomes. *J Vasc Surg.* 1999;29:821-831.

63. Park WM, Cherry KJ Jr, Chua HK, et al. Current results of open revascularization for chronic mesenteric ischemia: a standard for comparison. *J Vasc Surg.* 2002;35:853-859.

64. Raza JA, Miller M, Dieter RS, Clavijo LC, Stoner MC, Nanjundappa A. Diagnosis and non-surgical management of mesenteric ischemia. Vascular disease management. ISSN: 1553-8036. 2006;3(2):223-228.

65. Matsumoto AH, Tegtmeyer CJ, Fitzcharles EK, et al. Percutaneous transluminal angioplasty of visceral arterial stenoses: results and long-term clinical follow-up. *J Vasc Interv Radiol.* 1995;6:165-174.

66. Kasirajan K, O'Hara PJ, Gray BH, et al. Chronic mesenteric ischemia: open surgery versus percutaneous angioplasty and stenting. *J Vasc Surg.* 2001;33:63-71.

67. Silva JA, White CJ, Collins TJ, et al. Endovascular therapy for chronic mesenteric ischemia. *J Am Coll Cardiol.* 2006;47:944-950.

68. Sivamurthy N, Rhodes JM, Waldman DL, Green RM, Davies MG. Endovascular versus open mesenteric revascularization: immediate benefits do not equate with short-term functional outcomes. *J Am Coll Surg.* 2006;202:859-867.

69. Brown DJ, Schermerhorn ML, Powell RJ, et al. Mesenteric stenting for chronic mesenteric ischemia. *J Vasc Surg.* 2005;42:268-274.

70. Atkins MD, Kwolek CJ, Lamuraglia GM, Brewster DC, Chung TK, Cambria RP. Surgical revascularization versus endovascular therapy for chronic mesenteric ischemia. *J Vasc Surg.* 2007;45:1162-1171.

71. Gray BH, Sullivan TM. Mesenteric vascular disease. *Curr Treat Opt Cardiovasc Med.* 2001;3:195-206.

72. Apstein MD. Gastrointestinal manifestations of vasculitis. www.uptodate.com. Accessed March 24, 2008.

73. Lockshin MD. Antiphopholipid antibody. Babies, blood clots, biology. *JAMA.* 1997;277:1549-1551.

74. Guillevin L, Le Thi Huong D, Godeau P, Jais P, Wechsler B. Clinical findings and prognosis of polyarteritis nodosa and Churg-Strauss angiitis: a study of 165 patients. *Br J Theumatol.* 1988;27:258-264.

75. Zizic TM, Classen JN, Stevens MB, et al. Acute abdominal complications of systemic lupus erythematosus and polyarteritis nodosa. *Am J Med.* 1982;73:525-531.

76. Lightfoot RW, Michet BA, Bloch DA, et al. The American College of Rheumatology 1990 criteria for the classification of polyarteritis nodosa. *Arthritis Rheum.* 1990;33:1088-1093.

77. Kobayashi M, Kurose K, Kobata T, Hida K, Sakamoto S, Matsubara J. Ischemic intestinal involvement in a patient with Buerger disease: case report and literature review. *J Vasc Surg.* 2003;38:170-174.

78. Olin JW. Thromboangitis obliterans. *N Engl J Med.* 2000; 343:864-869.

79. Masi AT, Hunder GG, Lie JT, et al. American College of Rheumatology 1990 criteria for the classification of Churg-Strauss syndrome. *Arthritis Rheum.* 1990;33:1094-1100.

80. Blanco R, Martinez-Taboada VM, Rodriguez-Valverde V, et al. Henoch- Schonlein purpura in adulthood and childhood: two different expressions of the same syndrome. *Arthritis Rheum.* 1997;40:859-864.

81. Arend WP, Michel BA, Block DA, et al. The American College of Rheumatology 1990 criteria for the classification of Takayasu arteritis. *Arthritis Rheum.* 1990;33:1129-1134.

82. Criteria for diagnosis of Behcet's disease. International study group for Behcet's disease. *Lancet.* 1990;335:1078-1080.

83. Slovut DP, Olin JW. Fibromusular dysplasia: current concepts. *N Engl J Med.* 2004;350:1862-1871.

84. Guill CK, Benavides DC, Rees C, Fenves AZ, Burton EC. Fatal mesenteric fibromuscular dysplasia: a case report and review of the literature. *Arch Intern Med.* 2004;164:1148-1153.

85. Babu SC, Shah PM. Celiac territory ischemic syndrome in visceral artery occlusion. *Am J Surg.* 1993;166:227-230.

86. Howard TR, Brooks DL, Flynn TC, Seeger JM. Multiple organ dysfunction after mesenteric artery revascularization. *J Vasc Surg.* 1993;18:459-460.

87. Pasha SF, Gloviczki P, Stanson AW, Kamath PS. Spalnachnic artery aneurysms. *Mayo Clin Proc.* 2007;82:472-479.

88. Petrella S, Rodrigues CFS, Sgrott EA, Fernandez GJM, Marques SR, Prates JC. Relationship of the celiac trunk with median arcuate ligament of the diaphragm. *Int J Morphol.* 2006;24:263-274.

89. Richards WO, Garrard CL, Allos SH, Bradshaw LA, Staton DJ, Wikswo JP. Noninvasive diagnosis of mesenteric ischemia using a SQUID magnetometer. *Ann Surg.* 1995;221:696-704.

90. Slavin RE, Saeki K, Bhagavan B, et al. Segmental arterial mediolysis: a precursor of fibromuscular dysplasia? *Mod pathol.* 1995;8:287-294.

91. Shimohira M, Ogino H, Sasaki S, et al. Transcatheter arterial embolization for segmental arterial mediolysis. *J endovasc Ther.* 2008;15:493-497.

chapter 32

Renal Artery Disease

Brian Guttormsen, MD / *Giorgio Gimelli, MD*

Major advancements in vascular imaging techniques have facilitated the diagnosis of renovascular disease, and modern medical therapies as well as surgical and percutaneous interventional techniques offer the clinician a wide array of therapeutic tools in the management of renovascular disease. Despite these developments however, the indications for medical therapy versus surgical or percutaneous revascularization are controversial, and the clinician's ability to predict the effect of revascularization on clinical outcomes remains limited.

Vascular lesions affecting the renal artery can be caused by atherosclerosis, fibromuscular dysplasia (FMD), aneurysms, congenital or traumatic arteriovenous fistula (AVF), extrinsic compression, trauma, and embolization. The overwhelming majority of arterial artery lesions, however, are secondary to either atherosclerosis or FMD, which will be discussed below. A separate section will be dedicated to renal artery aneurysms, arteriovenous malformations (AVMs), and spontaneous renal artery dissections.

● PREVALENCE AND NATURAL HISTORY

Fibromuscular Dysplasia

Often clinically silent and discovered incidentally, FMD accounts for less than 10% of cases of renal artery stenosis (RAS), and although it can affect the intima, in the majority of cases it involves the media, resulting in the typical "string of beads" appearance (Figure 32-1).[1] The cause remains largely unknown; however it may have a genetic component and it is more frequent in hypertensive patients and smokers.[2] FMD usually affects women between 15 and 50 years of age, but it can be also observed in males and older patients as well.[1] It occurs most frequently in the renal artery, but can also involve the carotid and vertebral arteries, sometimes in association with intracranial aneurysms, as well as other visceral vessels.[1,3,4]

In a series of angiogram of potential renal donors, incidental renal FMD was found in 3.8% patients, 75% of whom were females; in another study of patients with resistant hypertension screened with angiography, 16% had FMD.[5,6] Because it is a disease of young patients with few cardiovascular risk factors, FMD is easily distinguishable from atherosclerotic RAS. FMD, unlike atherosclerotic RAS, tends to affect the mid and distal portion of the renal artery, and not the ostium. Its appearance can sometimes resemble vasculitis, but FMD is not an inflammatory process and it lacks the systemic manifestations and abnormal markers typical of vasculitis.

The severity of stenosis can be difficult to accurately measure with both noninvasive testing as well as with catheter-based angiography, but progression of disease has been documented in up to 37% of patients.[7,8]

Atherosclerotic Renal Artery Stenosis

Atherosclerosis accounts for approximately 90% of all renovascular lesions, and it usually involves the ostium and the proximal portion of the artery, although occasionally it can extend more distally.[9]

Atherosclerosis of the renal artery is more prevalent in the elderly, in patients with diabetes, and in patients with evidence of coronary or peripheral vascular disease elsewhere. In elderly white and black patients participating in the Cardiovascular Health Study (CHS), the prevalence of significant (≥60%) RAS detected by renal duplex sonography was 6.8%.[10] Renovascular disease was not correlated to ethnicity, but was independently associated with age, hyperlipidemia, and hypertension. In a series of hypertensive patients undergoing coronary angiography, 19% had ≥50% stenosis and 7% had ≥70% stenosis by quantitative angiographic analysis. In a larger series of 3987 patients undergoing coronary angiography, aortography demonstrated ≥75% RAS in 4.8% patients.[11] In 3.7% patients, the renal

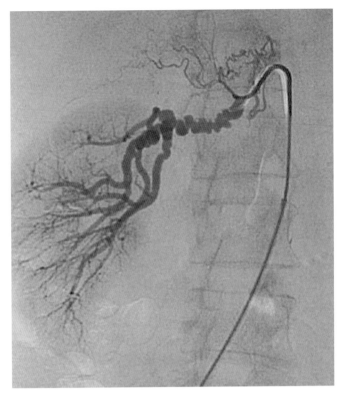

● **FIGURE 32-1.** Fibromuscular dysplasia with "string of beads" appearance involving the mid and distal portions of the renal artery. Differently from atherosclerotic renovascular disease, FMD typically spares the ostium of the renal artery.

Reprinted with permission from Slovut DP, Olin JW. Fibromuscular dysplasia. N Engl J Med. 2004;350(18):1862–1871.

arteries were affected bilaterally.[12] In patients with aortic aneurysms, aorto-occlusive or lower-extremity occlusive disease greater than 50% stenosis was present in more than 30% of patients.[13]

The increased prevalence of RAS in patients with coronary or peripheral arterial disease reflects the systemic nature of atherosclerosis and the overlapping existence of the disease in multiple vascular beds.

Atherosclerotic RAS is a progressive disease. In a series of 295 kidneys followed by renal artery duplex scans, the 3-year cumulative incidence of renal artery disease progression stratified by initial degree of stenosis was 18%, 29%, and 49% for renal artery classified as normal, with <60% stenosis and with ≥60% stenosis, respectively.[14] In this study, there were nine occlusions which occurred in patients who had ≥60% stenosis at the time of initial evaluation. Schreiber et al., however, have reported progression to total occlusion in 39% of patients with ≥75% stenosis at renal arteriography.[15] In the Dutch Renal Artery Stenosis Intervention Cooperative study, a randomized trial of medical therapy versus balloon angioplasty for the treatment of hypertension in RAS patients, progression to complete occlusion occurred in 16% of patients treated medically.[16]

Besides the initial degree of stenosis, other factors related to disease progression include diabetes mellitus and hypertension; interestingly, progression of RAS is also found in patients in whom optimal blood pressure control has been achieved with medical therapy.[17]

RAS can result in decreased renal size. In a series of 204 kidneys in 122 subjects, Caps et al. reported a 2-year cumulative incidence of renal atrophy of 5.5%, 11.7%, and 20.8% in kidneys with normal renal arteries, with <60% stenosis and with ≥60% stenosis.[18] Furthermore, RAS is the documented cause of end-stage renal artery disease (ESRD) in up to 15% of patients initiating dialysis each year, and in these patients, the overall prognosis is worse than in ESRD secondary to other etiologies.[19,20] Even in patients who have not reached ESRD, the presence of RAS is related to increased mortality, with 2-year survival rates of 96% in patients with unilateral RAS, 74% with bilateral RAS and 47% in RAS affecting a solitary functioning kidney.[21,22]

● PATHOPHYSIOLOGY

Renovascular Hypertension

Experimental studies of renovascular hypertension pioneered by Goldblatt et al. demonstrated that renal artery obstruction is followed by an increase in arterial blood pressure, and identified important differences in the pathophysiology of hypertension in unilateral and bilateral RAS.[23]

In unilateral RAS, the normal kidney counterbalances the pressor mechanisms triggered by the stenotic kidney. Reduction in perfusion of the affected kidney causes renin release, leading to the formation of angiotensin II and, in turn, to increased plasma aldosterone levels, sodium retention in the underperfused kidney, and peripheral vascular resistance. The contralateral kidney counterregulates by responding to increased pressure with urinary sodium excretion ("sodium natriuresis") and suppression of renin release, which tend to lower blood pressure and decrease perfusion pressure in the stenotic kidney. This, in turn, leads to increased renin and angiotensin production in a self-perpetuating cycle. In this situation, systemic hypertension is secondary to the pressor effect of angiotensin II. In fact, blockade of angiotensin action in the "two-kidney, one clip" rat model can completely prevent the increase in systolic blood pressure, at least in the early phases.[24]

Angiotensin II, however, can also increase blood pressure by modulating autonomic nervous system activity, resulting in neurogenic vasoconstriction, and has complex effects on the formation of reactive oxygen species with vasoconstrictive properties, as demonstrated by the detection of increased levels of isoprostanes in experimental models.[25,26] Recent work has demonstrated impaired endothelial function, as assessed by response of forearm blood flow to acetylcholine, in patients with renovascular hypertension, with improvement after renal angioplasty, thus suggesting that excessive oxidative stress may indeed be involved in impaired endothelium-dependent vasodilatation.[27]

Vasoconstriction can also be mediated by endothelin and thromboxane A2, both upregulated in renovascular hypertension.[28,29] The complex interplay of these diverse mechanisms varies individually and over time, partially explaining the difficulties in predicting reversal of hypertension after renal artery revascularization procedures. During the early phases of renovascular hypertension, treatment of RAS may indeed result in the resolution of the blood pressure abnormalities, but in later stages, when angiotensin II levels maybe lower or normal and hypertension may have transitioned to a less reversible state, it may become ineffectual.

In bilateral RAS, or in RAS affecting a solitary kidney, the "one-kidney, one clip" (1K1C) rat experimental model exposes a different mechanism in the pathophysiology of hypertension, one in which the entire renal mass is underperfused. In this case, activation of the renin-angiotensin-aldosterone system is not counterbalanced by a normal contralateral kidney, and pressure natriuresis cannot occur. Hence volume expansion ensues, resulting in hypertension and circulatory congestion. Finally, the positive volume status can result in normalization of renal perfusion, resulting in decreased plasma renin and angiotensin II. In this situation, volume expansion is critical. However, if volume status is reduced by sodium restriction and/or diuresis, hypertension will return to its renin-mediated form; hence sodium and volume expansion can suppress the renin-angiotensin system even in renovascular disease.[30,31]

Differences in function and hormonal status in unilateral and bilateral RAS portend diagnostic and clinical implications. Side-to-side differences between the kidneys have in fact been employed in a variety of diagnostic tests and preinterventional functional studies, which have been largely supplanted by the advent of modern diagnostic imaging studies.

Patients with bilateral RAS are more prone to vascular congestion and pulmonary edema, tend to have more severe hypertension, can experience deterioration in renal function with angiotensin-converting enzyme (ACE) inhibitors and angiotensin II receptor blockers (ARB), and have a higher mortality.[32,33]

Ischemic Nephropathy

The term "ischemic nephropathy" refers to the deterioration of renal function occurring in renovascular disease, and which can lead to ESRD in 14% to 20% of affected patients.[19,34]

The nature of ischemic nephropathy is complex and multifactorial. Since the main function of the kidney is filtration, renal blood flow is among the highest of all organs, and only 10% is necessary for this organ's metabolic needs.[35] Furthermore, the kidney is capable of autoregulating blood flow in the presence of RAS of up to 75% diameter reduction and, in conditions of impaired perfusion, oxygen delivery can be maintained by the development of collaterals from the adrenal and lumbar arteries.[36] Given the oversupply of oxygenated blood, some authors have therefore suggested the alternative term of "azotemic renovascular disease" or "hypoperfusion injury" to describe the parenchymal changes resulting from chronic renal hypoperfusion, ultimately leading to fibrosis and ESRD.

In acute ischemic renal injury, rapid changes in perfusion can damage the outer medulla, which is less efficiently autoregulated than the cortex, thus resulting in acute tubular necrosis (ATN). In chronic hypoperfusion, however, the medulla is protected at the expenses of cortical blood flow, and the gradual reduction in renal perfusion results in the interplay of protective mechanisms, which result in morphologic and functional changes different from the ones observed in acute ischemic injury, and which remain incompletely elucidated.[37]

Proposed pathways activated in chronic renal hypoperfusion, and which can lead to parenchymal injury and interstitial fibrosis, are depicted in Figure 32-2, and involve the complex and interrelated effects of angiotensin II, nitric oxide (NO), endothelin, vasodilating and vasoconstrictive prostaglandins, and a variety of cytokines.

Angiotensin II maintains glomerular filtration pressure and glomerular filtration rate (GFR) by constricting the efferent arterioles, but its effects in the kidney also include local inflammatory responses, cell hypertrophy, and hyperplasia, which are mostly mediated by AT1 receptors.[38] In fact, when angiotensin I is infused in rat experimental models, it results in focal and segmental glomerulosclerosis, which can be prevented by the AT1 blocker losartan.[39] Other angiotensin II effects also include vascular smooth muscle proliferation, mesangial cell growth, platelet aggregation, activation of adhesion molecules and macrophages, induction of gene transcription for proto-oncogenes, and oxidation of low-density lipoproteins.[37,40]

Angiotensin II-mediated vasoconstriction is modulated by endogenous vasodilator prostaglandins and by NO, limiting the potentially ischemic effects of this hormone.[41] NO downregulates gene expression of angiotensin II-type 1 receptor, a mechanism possibly implicated in the antiatherogenic effects of NO.[42] NO also inhibits the growth of vascular smooth muscle cells, mesangial cell hypertrophy and hyperplasia, as well as synthesis of extracellular matrix.[37,43] In RAS, diminished "shear stress" distal to the stenotic segment results in the production of NO, while decreased renal perfusion causes release of renin and generation of angiotensin II, thus shifting the balance in favor of vasoconstriction mediated by angiotensin II and by vasoconstrictive prostaglandins such as thromboxane. In fact, as RAS progresses, regulation of blood flow becomes less dependent on NO and more dependent on prostaglandins.[44]

While the synthesis of prostaglandins such as prostacycline and prostaglandin E2 protect the kidney from ischemia, thromboxane A2 mediates some of the deleterious effects of angiotensin II, and its synthesis increases in renovascular hypertension.[29] Many of the vascular effects of angiotensin II are mediated by endothelin, a very powerful vasoconstrictive peptide, which is released from the renal epithelial cells in renal ischemia after stimulation by thrombin and cytokines like transforming growth factor-beta (TGF-β), interleukin-1, and tumor necrosis factor (TNF).[45,46] These and other mechanisms, such as the generation of free oxygen radicals, interact with each other,

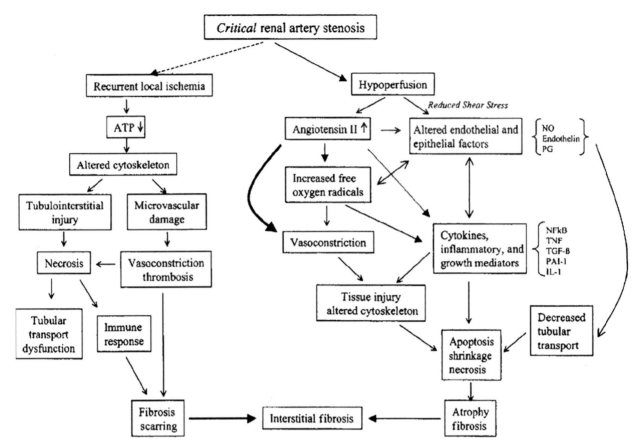

● **FIGURE 32-2.** Proposed mechanisms of parenchymal injury and interstitial fibrosis secondary to renal hypoperfusion. The figure outlines the complex and interrelated effects of angiotensin II, nitric oxide (NO), endothelin, vasodilating and vasoconstrictive prostaglandins, and of a variety of other cytokines. Some of these alterations develops in the absence of true ischemia.

Reprinted with permission from Lerman L, Textor SC. Pathophysiology of ischemic nephropathy. Urol Clin North Am. 2001;28(4):793–803, ix.

eventually resulting in renal scarring even in the absence of "true" renal ischemia.[26]

The complexity and variability of these interactions in different individuals is another factor that makes predictions on the recovery of kidney function after revascularization difficult, and explains why patients with impaired renal function before revascularization may have no significant increase in their GFR after percutaneous or surgical interventions.[31,47]

● **CLINICAL MANIFESTATIONS OF RENOVASCULAR DISEASE (TABLE 32-1)**

RAS can be often asymptomatic and found incidentally and, as reviewed above, it is usually secondary to either FMD or atherosclerosis.[6,13] Although incidentally discovered RAS is common, renovascular hypertension occurs only in 1% to 5% of all patients with hypertension.[13,48]

The predominant manifestation of FMD is hypertension, most commonly in patients younger than 30 years and predominantly in women. Atherosclerotic RAS typically occurs in patients older than 50 years, and can be accompanied by other clinical manifestations of atherosclerosis, renal insufficiency, or by recurrent episodes of congestive heart failure and pulmonary edema.[9,49] Accelerated and malignant hypertension are both suggestive of RAS, but renovascular hypertension can also present less

TABLE 32-1. Clinical Manifestations of Renovascular Disease

Asymptomatic	Incidental
Renovascular hypertension	Accelerated hypertension Malignant hypertension Resistant hypertension
Ischemic nephropathy	Renal insufficiency Kidney atrophy
Cardiovascular manifestations	Recurrent pulmonary edema Angina pectoris Stroke

dramatically, and can sometimes be difficult to differentiate from essential hypertension.[50] Characteristics such as the absence of a family history of essential hypertension, duration of hypertension of less than 1 year, and the presence of an abdominal bruit and hypokalemia are more suggestive of the diagnosis of renovascular hypertension.[9,51] RAS can be associated with both systolic and diastolic hypertension, but the diagnosis should be more strongly suspected in the presence of new-onset diastolic hypertension in patients older than 55 years.

Another common presentation of renovascular hypertension is the development of resistant hypertension in patients with previously well-controlled blood pressure, as defined by failure to reduce blood pressure to less than 140/90 mm Hg with a regimen of three drugs, which include a diuretic.[52]

A discrepancy in renal size can also be a clue to the presence of renovascular hypertension, and should prompt further diagnostic investigations.[13,53]

Azotemia in the setting of therapy with an ACE inhibitor maybe an indication of bilateral RAS or of RAS of a solitary functioning kidney, underscoring the vasoconstrictive role of angiotensin II on the efferent arterioles to preserve GFR in these situations.[54]

Patients with recurrent "flash" pulmonary edema, or with angina pectoris in the absence of any other causes, should also be evaluated for RAS. In the first case, symptoms maybe secondary to bilateral RAS, when pressure natriuresis cannot occur and vascular congestion ensues, while in the latter increased left ventricular afterload may play a role.[32,55,56] In these cases, renal artery revascularization can result in a marked symptomatic improvement, possibly also as a result of improved blood pressure control.[55,57]

A summary of clinical clues suggestive of RAS is reported in Table 32-2. It is important to understand, however, that the differences between the clinical manifestation of RAS and those of essential hypertension can be small, and that none of the clinical characteristics mentioned above has, in itself, a high predictive value for RAS. Nevertheless, a recent study, which combined the presence of vascular disease in other vascular districts with abdominal bruits, body weight, smoking, and other factors into a clinical score, found it to be of good predictive value for RAS in patients referred for resistant hypertension.[5]

● DIAGNOSTIC EVALUATION

Although a perfect test to diagnose RAS does not exist, modern imaging tests such as renal duplex ultrasonography, magnetic resonance angiography (MRA), and computed tomographic angiography (CTA) have become quite accurate and sophisticated in detecting the presence of RAS, as well as in assessing the anatomy of the kidney and adjacent structures. Importantly, none of these tests requires discontinuation of patients' antihypertensive treatment, a major advantage in comparison to older diagnostic modalities such as captopril renography and peripheral plasma renin activity. The choice of which one of the major imaging modalities

---

TABLE 32-2. Clinical Predictors of Renal Artery Stenosis

Hypertension
Onset of hypertension before age of 30 years or after after age 55 years
Accelerated or malignant hypertension in any age group
Hypertension resistant to three or more antihypertensive drugs including a diuretic
Acute onset or worsening of previously well controlled hypertension in any age group
Renal Functional or Anatomic Abnormalities
Impairment of renal function or acute renal failure associated with ACE inhibitors
Hypertension with unexplained renal dysfunction
Unilateral reduction in kidney size
ESRD without a known cause
Unexplained hypokalemia in a hypertensive patient

Cardiac Symptoms
Recurrent pulmonary edema
Recurrent CHF without apparent cause
Angina pectoris in the absence of critical coronary artery disease

Atherosclerosis Elsewhere
Epigastric abdominal or flank bruit
Peripheral arterial disease affecting the lower extremities or the carotid arteries
Aorto-iliac disease
Abdominal aortic aneurysm
Severe coronary artery disease

ESRD, end-stage renal disease; CHF, congestive heart failure.

---

should be used depends on a variety of factors, including local availability and expertise, as well as cost. Potential advantages and disadvantages of each technique will be described below.

Renal Duplex Ultrasonography

Renal artery duplex combines B-mode imaging with Doppler velocity measurements of blood flow. It provides information on location and degree of RAS, measurement of kidney size, and visualization of possible adjacent processes such as obstruction, masses, or abdominal aortic aneurysms. In addition, an assessment of intrinsic small vessel renovascular disease can be obtained, and a prediction on blood pressure response to revascularization can be made.[58] Duplex ultrasonography is the least expensive of the imaging modalities, does not require the use of intravenous contrast, and with improvement in modern hardware and software, can provide visualization of the entire renal artery, including its distal portion. The overall sensitivity and specificity of duplex ultrasonography compared with arteriography are 98% and 98%, respectively.[59] Potential disadvantages include prolonged examination time (up to 45–60 minutes), as well as its dependence on operator

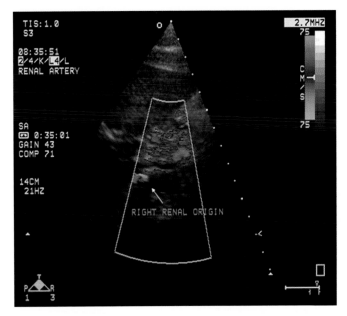

● **FIGURE 32-3.** Renal duplex ultrasonography. Transverse view of the right renal artery origin shows flow turbulence at the site of the stenosis.

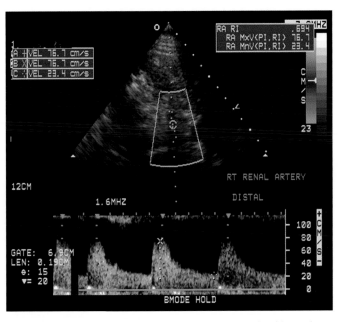

● **FIGURE 32-4.** Renal duplex ultrasonography. Normal Doppler spectrum from the right renal artery. Note the typical "low resistance" flow pattern, with rapid systolic upstroke and gradual diastolic decay with persistent forward flow in diastole.

skills as well as on patient's body habitus. Duplex ultrasonography can be technically quite challenging, especially in obese patients or in the presence of abdominal gas, hence this diagnostic test is preferentially conducted by experienced technicians in the morning and on fasting patients.

Usually the examination begins in the longitudinal plane, with the patient supine, acquiring velocity data from the celiac trunk and superior mesenteric arteries. The peak systolic velocity in the aorta is obtained just distally to the superior mesenteric artery; this will be used to calculate the renal artery-to-aorta velocity ratio. Using a transverse approach, the examination continues with location of the origin of the renal arteries from the aorta.[60] The right renal artery is usually easier to find than the left (Figure 32-3). Since the left renal artery is difficult to follow all the way to the kidney from the anterior approach, the patient can be positioned in the right lateral decubitus, scanning from the left posterolateral approach.[61] For the right, the patient can be positioned in the left lateral decubitus.

Kidney size and morphology are evaluated. The peak systolic and end diastolic velocities are then obtained from the proximal, mid and distal renal artery, bilaterally, and from the segmental arteries in the upper and lower poles of the kidneys. Attention should be paid to the possible presence of accessory renal arteries.

Renal arteries as well as segmental and interlobar arteries are characterized by low resistance (Figure 32-4). The renal-to-aortic ratio (RAR) is calculated by dividing the peak systolic velocity of the renal artery by the peak systolic velocity of the aorta. A normal ratio is <3.5. A renal-to-aorta peak systolic velocity ratio ≥3.5 combined with a peak systolic velocity at the lesion of >180 to 200 cm/s is consistent with ≥60% RAS (Figure 32-5). If the end-diastolic velocity is ≥150 cm/s, the stenosis is likely to

be ≥80%.[59,62] A significant stenosis should be accompanied by poststenotic turbulence and spectral broadening in the abnormal waveforms. Damping of the arterial signal distal to the stenotic lesion, defined numerically by acceleration index or acceleration time, and usually described visually as "pulsus parvus and tardus," is also consistent with severe RAS (Figure 32-6). When no flow can be detected in the

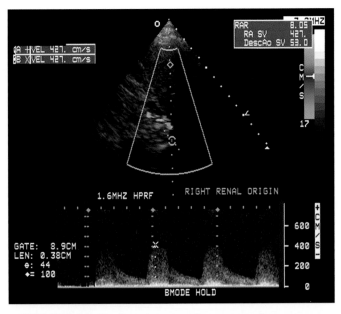

● **FIGURE 32-5.** Renal duplex ultrasonography. Hemodynamically significant stenosis at the origin of the right renal artery, with a peak systolic velocity of 427 cm/s, and a renal artery/aortic ratio of 8.05, both well above the cutoffs of 200 cm/s and 3.5.

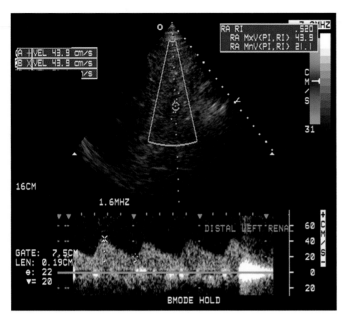

● **FIGURE 32-6.** Renal duplex ultrasonography. Intrarenal vessel imaging in a patient with severe left renal artery stenosis, demonstrating low-amplitude signals with prolonged systolic acceleration time ("tardus and parvus" pattern).

renal artery, low parenchymal Doppler velocities support the diagnosis of an occluded renal artery. In these cases the kidney is usually small (<9 cm in length).[59]

Since treatment of a stenotic renal artery does not guarantee a positive clinical response, several investigators have sought to identify other duplex criteria to predict a positive outcome after revascularization. The "resistance index" (RI), calculated as RI = (1 − [end-diastolic velocity/peak systolic velocity]) × 100, is being used to evaluate renal parenchymal disease, and has been studied by Radermacher and others in 138 patients undergoing angioplasty or surgery.[58] An RI >80 found to identify patients in whom angioplasty or surgery will not improve renal function, blood pressure, or kidney survival. Although this is a potentially useful tool, it can be falsely elevated in patients with decreased cardiac output.

In conclusion, duplex imaging plays an important role in the diagnosis of RAS, but it can be technically demanding and time-consuming, especially in obese individuals or when excessive bowel gas is present. In our practice, we have found this tool very valuable in the follow-up of patients who have undergone renal artery stenting, in whom MRA accuracy maybe hindered by stent artifacts and the administration of intravenous contrast might be undesirable. In these patients, Duplex ultrasound has been in fact shown to be an excellent technique, with high sensitivity and specificity for the diagnosis of in-stent restenosis when a threshold peak systolic velocity ≥226 cm/s and a RAR ≥2.7 are used.[63]

Computed Tomographic Angiography

Recent technologic advancements leading to the development of multidetector computed tomography (MDCT)

have resulted in increased speed of image acquisition and high spatial resolution, making CTA a reliable and accurate modality to evaluate renovascular disease.[64–66]

The initial image output is in sets of sequential or overlapping axial images, and postprocessing of volumetric data is required to create three-dimensional angiographic representations.[67] Sensitivity and specificity of CTA in the diagnosis of RAS have both been reported to be in excess of 90%,[66,68] but it is important that the area of acquisition is extensive enough to detect the presence of accessory renal arteries.[67] Furthermore, a study designed to visualize the renal arteries should include imaging of the iliac and femoral arteries in case any revascularization intervention should be needed. Advantages of CTA over catheter-based angiography include the fact that it is not invasive, and that adjacent anatomic structures can also be examined. Compared to MRA, CTA has higher spatial resolution and is less affected by artifacts caused by the presence of calcium or previously implanted metallic stents. CTA is also much less operator-dependent than duplex ultrasonography.

The most obvious disadvantage of CTA, however, is that it requires the administration of nephrotoxic iodinated contrast. Although the rapid acquisition of images allows reduction in contrast use, the typical amount of dye necessary for a CTA of the renal arteries can in fact exceed 100 mL.[69,70] Additional limitations include exposure of patients to ionizing radiation, potential difficulties in estimating the degree of stenosis when arterial wall calcification is present, and lengthy postprocedure processing time. Furthermore, CTA, as well as duplex ultrasonography and MRA, is not as accurate as catheter-based angiography in the assessment of RAS secondary to FMD.[1]

Magnetic Resonance Arteriography (Figure 32-7)

Magnetic resonance arteriography (MRA) of the peripheral arterial circulation was initially performed without the use of contrast, using the so-called 2D time-of-flight technique. With this approach, acquisition times were prolonged and motion artifacts resulted in image degradation. The use of the gadolinium-enhanced gradient echo technique has significantly decreased acquisition times (now down to 20–40 seconds) and improved the accuracy of MRA, which, in contrast to CTA, does not require ionizing radiation and can be performed in patients with renal insufficiency, congestive heart failure, and dye allergy. Differently from renal duplex ultrasonography, MRA is less operator-dependent and allows visualization of surrounding anatomical structures as well as of accessory renal arteries.[71] Furthermore, MRA may play a role in the physiologic assessment of renovascular disease by determining glomerular filtration rate (gadolinium clearance) and assessing renal perfusion.[72–74]

Contrast-enhanced MRA of the abdominal aorta and its branches has become the screening imaging test of choice for RAS in many institutions, and has reached a sensitivity

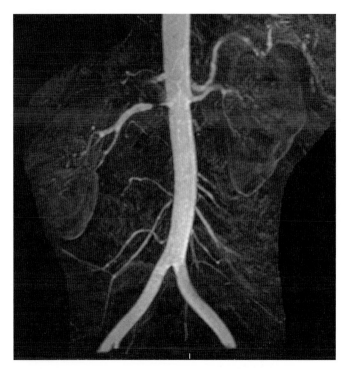

● **FIGURE 32-7.** Gadolinium-enhanced magnetic resonance angiogram demonstrating a right renal artery stenosis and a normal left renal artery. This technique allows visualization and measurement of kidney size.

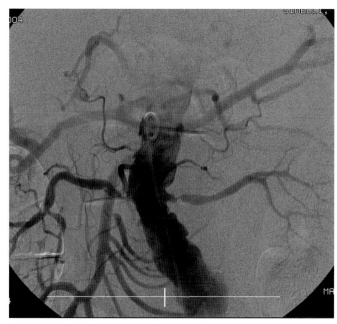

● **FIGURE 32-8.** Digital subtraction angiogram demonstrating diffuse atherosclerosis of the abdominal aorta and bilateral renal artery stenosis. The angiogram was obtained injecting 20 mL of iodinated contrast at 20 mL/s via power injector.

and specificity in excess of 90%.[75–77] MRA's spatial resolution of approximately 1 mm, however, remains inferior to digital subtraction angiography (DSA), and this maybe an issue in imaging the distal renal artery. While the aorta and the proximal portion of the renal artery do not significantly move with respiration, there is persistent craniocaudal motion of the distal portion of the artery, even during fast, breathhold contrast-enhanced MRA.[78] For this reason, MRA is ideally suited to screen for atherosclerotic renal artery disease but not FMD, where DSA remains the most accurate diagnostic method.[1] Other limitations of MRA include the presence of pacemakers and other non-MRA-compatible metallic objects, as well as its inability, at least for the time being, to reliably identify in-stent restenosis in patients followed after percutaneous renal artery revascularization. For these patients, renal duplex ultrasonography remains the preferred technique, although MRI-compatible stents are being developed and may become available in the near future.[79]

Catheter-Based Angiography

Contrast angiography remains the gold standard for diagnosis and the assessment of the severity of both atherosclerotic and fibrodysplastic RAS. It allows evaluation of the abdominal aorta, renal arteries, and branch vessels, the presence of accessory renal arteries, as well as cortical blood flow and renal dimensions. Furthermore, pressure gradients across a RAS can be obtained to evaluate its hemodynamic signifi-

cance. DSA has become available in many institutions and, although its resolution is inferior to film, it permits the use of lower concentrations of iodinated contrast, as well as of alternative contrast agents such as CO_2 and gadolinium.[67]

Typically, an abdominal aortogram is performed prior to selective catheterization of the renal artery, usually positioning a pigtail catheter at the lower edge of the first lumbar vertebra and power-injecting 15 to 20 mL of dye at 20 mL/s (Figure 32-8).

The abdominal aortogram will provide information regarding the aorta itself, the position of the renal arteries, and the presence of accessory arteries as well as of aortic or renal artery calcification. In most instances, the aortogram provides adequate visualization of the renal arteries, but if optimal imaging or pressure gradient measurement are needed, selective catheterization becomes necessary. This can be achieved with a variety of different 4-F to 6-F diagnostic catheters. Whatever catheter shape is used, the goal is to achieve selective cannulation of the renal artery without excessive catheter manipulation, especially when evaluating atherosclerotic RAS, since aortic atheromas are often adjacent or contiguous to the renal artery lesion and distal embolization can occur. In visualizing the renal arteries, it is important to recognize that they originate posteriorly from the aorta; therefore, it maybe necessary to obtain ipsilateral oblique projections (15°–30°) to optimally outline the ostium and the proximal segments of the vessels. Furthermore, angiography should be performed long enough to image the renal cortex and assess renal size and perfusion.[80]

The obvious disadvantages of catheter-based angiography are its invasiveness, the exposure of patients to ionizing radiation, and the use of nephrotoxic contrast. In patients with renal insufficiency, however, alternative contrasts such as CO_2 and gadolinium can be used. When compared to conventional angiography in the identification of RAS of more than 60%, CO_2 angiography with DSA has a sensitivity and a specificity of 83% and 99%, respectively.[81,82] Gadolinium, either alone or with CO_2, can also provide good images in patients with renal insufficiency.[83–85] In these patients, proper hydration, minimization of contrast load, along with the use of either CO_2 or gadolinium and prophylaxis with sodium bicarbonate and/or acetylcysteine, are strategies that maybe adopted to minimize the incidence of nephrotoxicity.

Captopril Renography

Captopril renography, also known as captopril scintigraphy, consists of two sequential isotope renograms before and after the administration of an ACE inhibitor. In unilateral RAS, the GFR of the stenotic kidney will fall after captopril administration, whereas it will increase in the normal kidney, resulting in asymmetric renal uptake of the filtered radioactive isotope.[86] Captopril renography is of limited value in patients with renal insufficiency of with bilateral RAS and, although it was widely used in the past, it has become a secondary screening modality after duplex ultrasonography, MRA, and CTA.

● TREATMENT MODALITIES

Medical Therapy

Medical therapy in patients with renal artery disease related to atherosclerotic vascular disease is critical to minimize cardiovascular morbidity and mortality, and to slow disease progression in other vascular districts. Medical therapy includes antihypertensive drugs, antiplatelet agents, and lipid reduction as outlined in the recent National Cholesterol Education Program Executive Summary, as well as smoking cessation and therapeutic lifestyle changes.[87] Hypertension control in patients with renovascular hypertension can be particularly difficult, and frequently the combination of multiple agents becomes necessary. All classes of antihypertensive medications maybe used safely.[88] In particular, agents that block the renin-angiotensin system such as ACE inhibitors and angiotensin receptor blockers can be effective in up to 75% to 80% of patients with renovascular disease.[89] Cholesterol-lowering drugs, particularly hMG coA reductase inhibitors or "statins," are of critical importance in achieving low-density lipoprotein levels of ≤100 mg/dL in most patients and of ≤70 mg/dL in higher-risk subsets of patients with diabetes or established coronary artery disease.[87]

Antiplatelet drugs, particularly aspirin, should be recommended to all patients with evidence of atherosclerotic vascular disease, and smoking cessation should be pursued aggressively.

Surgical Therapy

Before the advent of more aggressive medical therapy for atherosclerosis and of new percutaneous modalities, surgery was frequently used in the treatment of renovascular disease. Several operative techniques have been described including aortorenal bypass, extra-anatomic renal bypass (with the graft originating from a vessel other than the aorta), renal artery reimplantation, and renal endarterectomy. Technique selection varies, as no single procedure offers optimal results for all types of renovascular disease. Several factors influence this decision including severity and location of disease, concomitant aortic disease, redundancy of the renal artery, and operator experience. Aortorenal bypass utilizes various conduits including saphenous veins grafts, the hypogastric artery, or synthetic conduits such as Dacron or polytetrafluoroethylene (PTFE). Figure 32-9 illustrates both the end-to-side and end-to-end anastamosis techniques.[90] The choice of graft depends on a number of factors; however, most utilize saphenous vein conduits unless the available vein is particularly small (<4 mm in diameter). Patients can also undergo concomitant aortic endarterectomy if necessary. Perioperative mortality ranges from 2.1% to 6%.[91–95] Early graft failure is typically related to technical problems with rates ranging from 1.4% to 10%.[9,93–95] Early graft failure is the strongest predictor of perioperative mortality with other being coronary artery disease, poorly controlled arterial hypertension (HTN), and the need for combined aortic procedures.[91] Surgical morbidity rates depend on the population studied, ranging from 11% to 16%, with potential complications including myocardial infarction, stroke, bleeding, infection, congestive heart failure, respiratory failure, and arrhythmias.[93,94,96–98] Long-term patency rates range from 82% to 95.5%.[91,92,95,99]

The long-term efficacy of these grafts to improve hypertension control or renal insufficiency has not been studied in a statistically rigorous fashion. Available series are plagued by nonrandomized design and multiple differing definitions for improvement of HTN control, HTN cure, and improvement or stabilization of renal function. Despite these differences and lack of statistical rigor, multiple studies have documented hypertension cure or improvement in 50% to 91% of patients.[94–96,98,99] Improvement of renal function has been demonstrated in 12.5% to 49% of patients.[94,96–100] Surgical revascularization of fibromuscular disease is safer and equally efficacious as compared to those patients with atherosclerosis.[94,95]

In recent years, aging population and increasing frequency of cardiovascular comorbidities have changed the profile of the renovascular disease patient.[97] Today's patients are older and have more advanced atherosclerosis with multiple comorbid conditions, and this has fostered the application of techniques that are less traumatic to a frequently severely diseased aorta. Bypass operations, which

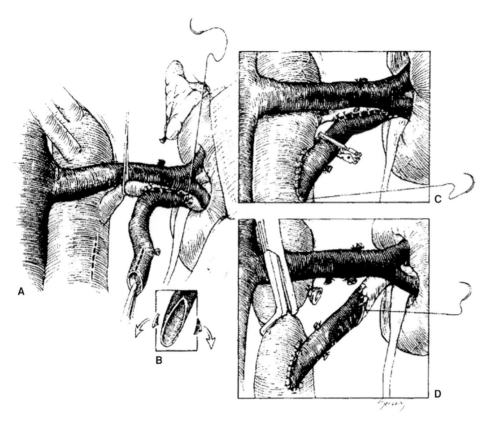

● **FIGURE 32-9.** Technique for end-to-side (A, B, and C) and end-to-end aortorenal bypass grafting (D).

Reprinted with permission from Benjamin ME, Dean RH. Techniques in renal artery reconstruction: Part I. Ann Vasc Surg. 1996; 10(3):306–314.

use extra-anatomic sites from vessels other than the aorta such as the splenic, mesenteric, hepatic, and iliac arteries, are performed more frequently, and this trend is illustrated in a series from the Cleveland Clinic where the use of aorto-renal bypass has decreased from 72% of all surgical renal revascularization procedures between 1975 and 1980 to 27% of surgeries performed between 1981 and 1984.[95] The durability and patency rates of these extra-anatomic bypass sites as well as the surgical complication rates, effects on blood pressure control, and stabilization of renal function compare favorably to the more traditional aortorenal approaches.[91,98]

Another surgical approach to renal artery revascularization is thromboendarterectomy, most suitable for those patients with ostial atheroscleriosis particularly of multiple renal arteries.[101] Transaortic endarterectomy can be performed simultaneously if necessary. This procedure is however contraindicated in the presence of preaneurysmal degeneration of the aorta and transmural aortic calcification.[101] The outcomes compare favorably to bypass techniques.[102] Renal artery reimplantation is utilized when the stenosis is ostial and the vessel is of sufficient length to allow the vessel to be reimplanted into the aorta in a slightly more caudal position.[101] This is the least frequently used technique among those described.

Percutaneous Therapy

Percutaneous therapy for renovascular disease has largely supplanted surgery; it is associated with a lower incidence of adverse events, equivalent outcome in terms of hyper-tension control, and lower cost compared to surgery.[103–105] The first description of balloon angioplasty for renovascular disease was provided by Gruntzig and coauthors in 1978,[106] and balloon angioplasty remains the treatment of choice in patients with uncontrolled hypertension and renovascular disease secondary to FMD.[107,108]

To date, there are three randomized controlled trials of balloon angioplasty compared to medical therapy in patients with atherosclerotic renovascular disease.[16,109,110] These trials are limited by small number of patients enrolled and frequent crossover from the medical to the percutaneous group. Probably the most widely cited publication is the DRASTIC trial, which randomized 106 patients with >50% stenosis and diastolic hypertension despite treatment with two antihypertensive medications to either balloon angioplasty or medical therapy.[16] Primary endpoints were systolic and diastolic blood pressures at 3 and 12 months. At 3 months, there was a statistically significant improvement in blood pressure control in the balloon angioplasty arm; 1-year analysis, however, showed no difference in blood pressure control between the two groups. Importantly, 22 of the 50 patients in the medical therapy group had crossed over to the angioplasty arm for persistently difficult to control blood pressure, and patients in the angioplasty group required significantly fewer antihypertensive medications. The absence of any blood pressure difference at 12 months led the authors to conclude that angioplasty was of little benefit over medical therapy in treating hypertension and RAS. Opponents of percutaneous therapy for renovascular disease have argued that this trial demonstrates the ineffec-tiveness of catheter-based therapy in these patients. With the high degree of crossover reported, however, a definite conclusion based upon its results is very difficult to draw.

Stenting has largely supplanted balloon angioplasty in the catheter-based treatment of renovascular disease. A randomized trial of stenting versus balloon angioplasty in 84 patients with ostial renovascular disease demonstrated improved procedural success and patency rates with stenting; however, there were no significant differences in HTN control or improvement in renal function.[111] Two meta-analyses have analyzed the success and durability of renal artery stenting.[112,113] Initial angiographic success rates were significantly improved compared to balloon angioplasty at 96% to 100% with no significant difference in complication rates. The ability of renal artery stenting to improve blood pressure control and renal function has been studied in multiple series. A meta-analysis demonstrated an overall HTN cure rate of 20% and improved HTN control in 49%, and improvement in renal function in 30% with stabilization of renal function in 38% of patients,[112] With similar complication rates and improved initial and long-term angiographic success, it is safe to say that renal artery stenting is the percutaneous treatment of choice in patients with RAS.

Although not necessarily true in the past, nowadays procedural techniques for percutaneous renal intervention utilize much the same equipment as coronary interventions.

The choice of guide catheter is determined by the angle with which the renal artery arises off the aorta. Most commonly, retrograde access via the femoral artery is used. A very sharp caudal angle of origin of the renal artery may however require an antegrade approach using the radial or brachial arteries to achieve optimal guide-catheter engagement. Interventions are usually performed using a 6 or 7 French system with commonly used guide-catheters with shapes such as the Judkins-Right series, the "renal standard curve," "renal double curve," and "hockey stick." Engagement of the guide catheter can be performed directly or using a telescoping technique.

High-grade ostial lesions with concomitant aortic plaque can increase the risk for atheroembolism. The recently proposed "no-touch" technique attempts to minimize trauma to the vessel ostium, at least theoretically lessening the risk of atheroembolism to the renal parenchyma. With this technique, a 0.035-inch "J-tip" guidewire is advanced just past the guide-catheter tip, to lean against the abdominal aorta above the renal artery, thus keeping the catheter away from the aortic wall (Figure 32-10). Once the guide-catheter is directed toward the ostium of the renal artery and visualization of the renal artery is obtained by subselective injection of contrast, a 0.014″ guidewire is navigated past the target lesion into the distal renal vessel. The 0.035″ guidewire is then withdrawn from the catheter, allowing it

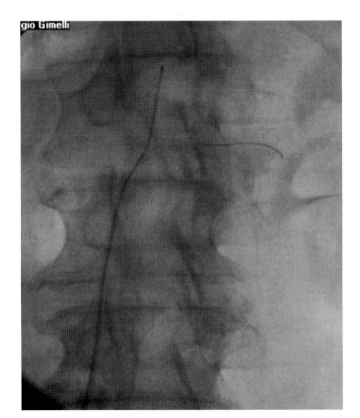

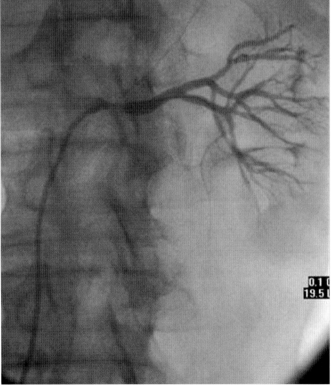

● **FIGURE 32-10.** The "no-touch" technique is used to selectively engage the left renal artery. A 0.035″ soft wire protrudes from the tip of the guide-catheter, leaning against the abdominal aorta above the renal artery and keeping the catheter from scraping the aortic wall. Using nonselective injections of diluted contrast, a 0.014″ wire is used to cross the target lesion. Once the 0.014″ is in position, the 0.035″ is removed.

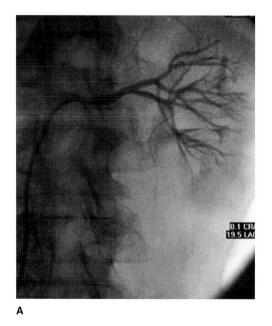 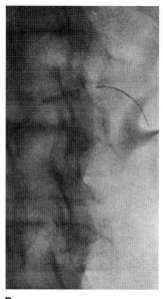 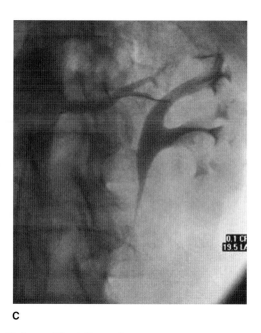

A   B   C

● FIGURE 32-11. Guide-catheter selectively engaged in the Ostium of the left renal artery (A). Balloon predilatation (B) followed by stenting of the left renal artery. The final result is demonstrated in (C).

to gently slide into or adjacent to the ostium of the renal artery over the 0.014″ wire (Figure 32-11). Predilatation of the target lesion is especially recommended in aorto-ostial atherosclerotic lesions and is typically performed with a balloon approximately 1 mm less than the measured diameter of the vessel.

The two balloon-expandable stents specifically approved by the FDA for use in failed renal angioplasty are the Palmaz stent (Cordis Corporation) and the Double Strut stent (Medtronic Corporation), but the most frequently used stents have been approved for biliary tree interventions. In ostial lesions, after the stent is deployed, its proximal portion can be "flared" with a slightly oversized balloon protruding into the aorta. Stent placement should be confirmed in two views. Careful attention to contrast dye load is required, especially in patients at high risk for contrast nephropathy. As mentioned above, gadolinium and CO_2 can be used as alternative contrast agents at least during some parts of the intervention.

Adjuvant pharmacology before and after renal artery percutaneous intervention has not been systematically studied. Heparin to maintain an activated clotting time of 250 to 300 seconds is frequently used as the anticoagulant of choice during interventional procedures; most interventionalists are quite familiar with its use and it can be easily reversed with protamine. Patients are usually pretreated with aspirin, which is continued indefinitely. The use of clopidogrel seems theoretically necessary following percutaneous intervention; however, there are no controlled studies exploring its use in the renal artery. Other possible intraprocedural anticoagulants such as glycoprotein 2B3A receptor antagonists and direct thrombin inhibitors such as bilvalrudin have not been formally studied in renal interventions.

Complications related to percutaneous intervention can be related to vascular access, guide catheter engagement, wiring of the artery, balloon and stent deployment or contrast administration.

As with all percutaneous procedures, complications related to vascular access are the most frequent and include groin and retroperitoneal hematomas and bleeding, psuedoaneurysm, AVF, and infection. Atheroembolism to the kidney parenchyma, bowel, or lower extremities can occur and result in renal failure, bowel ischemia, or digital ischemia. Renal artery dissection is typically treated with stenting. Distal wire perforation should be treated with reversal of anticoagulation and coiling if necessary. Perforation should be treated with prolonged balloon inflation, reversal of anticoagulation, or possibly the deployment of a covered stent graft. In cases not responding to percutaneous treatment, surgery maybe necessary. Rocha-Singh and others reported in-hospital adverse events in 4.5% of patients and 2-year adverse events in 19.7% with 14.4% of these being target lesion revascularization.[114]

Like coronary artery stenting, restenosis remains the Achille's heel of renal artery stenting. Reported rates of restenosis range from 11% to 23% with two meta-analyses reporting rates of 16% and 17%.[9,112,113] Multiple studies have examined clinical and angiographic predictors of restenosis.[115–117] These studies have demonstrated that a larger minimum luminal diameter is the only factor consistently associated with a lower incidence of restenosis. In one series of 748 patients, a stent diameter ≤5 mm was associated with an odds ratio of 2.31 for target vessel revascularization as compared to those with a diameter >5 mm.[117] The type of stent can also have an impact on restenosis. Gold-coated stents are associated with a significantly increased rate of restenosis compared to stainless steel stents.[118] The treatment of restenosis remains somewhat controversial with very limited data. Described modalities for the treatment of restenosis include repeat balloon angioplasty, stenting, cutting balloon angioplasty, and vascular brachytherapy.[119–122] More recently, the use of drug-eluting stents for the treatment of in-stent restenosis has been described.[123,124]

Another possible complication of percutaneous renal intervention is distal embolization into the kidney parenchyma; this, along with the use of nephrotoxic contrast, could potentially be the cause for the deterioration in renal function sometimes observed after these interventions. One small series demonstrated that embolization after surgical revascularization of the renal arteries was associated with worse survival.[125] Atheroemblosim related to aortic angiography has been reported and could have similar deleterious effects.[126] The true incidence, risk factors, and consequences of renal atheroemboli following renal angiography remain, however, unknown. Several studies have examined the utilization of distal protection devices in renal artery stenting in an attempt to prevent atheroembolism.[127,128] These series have examined the effects of distal balloon occlusion devices and filter wires and have reported retrieval of debris in 65% to 100% of patients. The Cardiovascular Outcomes in Renal Atherosclerotic Lesions (CORAL) trial in patients with HTN and RAS is currently enrolling and using embolic protection devices in all patients randomized to stenting, although the study will not have a control arm where distal protection is not used. There are potential complications and limitations associated with deployment of the currently available distal protection devices. For their use, a 2-cm landing zone is ideally required distal to the lesion, and although this is usually the case in the saphenous vein grafts for which the devices were developed, it may not be in short or bifurcating renal arteries.

Filters and occlusive balloons can also potentially cause distal vessel trauma, resulting in perforation or dissection; wire kinking and filter entrapment are also potential concerns in tortuous renal with unfavorable take-off from the aorta. Whether distal protection will become an integral part of percutaneous renal intervention remains a topic of active investigation; meanwhile, however, their use should be considered in patients with severe atherosclerosis of the abdominal aorta, baseline renal insufficiency, single functional kidney, and when the anatomy is suitable.

Patient selection remains a very challenging part of renal revascularization, given the variable response in blood pressure control or kidney function. Several series have attempted to find clinical, laboratory, or angiographic predictors of improved blood pressure or renal outcomes.[129–131] Factors independently associated with improvement in renal function include higher baseline serum creatinine and left ventricular function.[129] Predictors of improvement in blood pressure include bilateral RAS, higher baseline blood pressure, female gender, and pelvis/parenchymal ratio of >1. Dieter et al. have recently demonstrated that pulse pressure inversely correlates to the outcome of renal artery interventions. Patients with a high pulse pressure tend not to respond to treatment while those with a more normal pulse pressure have improvements in blood pressure and renal function after intervention on renal artery stenosis (personal communication from the author). Recently, investigators have looked for a possible association between brain type natruretic peptide (BNP) and improvement in HTN control following renal intervention.[132] These authors examined a series of 27 patients with RAS and measured BNP before, during, and after intervention. They were able to show that a higher initial BNP and a more significant drop in BNP after intervention were independently associated with improved blood pressure control after intervention. Certainly, this study will need to be performed in a larger group; however it highlights the ongoing quest for a test to identify patients who will benefit from renal revascularization.

In summary, the majority of renal revascularizations are performed today using stenting and this technique has been shown to be durable and effective in achieving improvement in renal arterial diameter. Further studies will be required to improve patient selection, choose the most appropriate adjuvant pharmacology, define the role of distal embolic protection devices, and to prevent and optimally treat in-stent restenosis.

● OTHER CAUSES OF RENOVASCULAR DISEASE

Arteriovenous Malformations and Arteriovenous Fistulas

Renal AVMs are anomalous congenital communications between the arterial and venous systems of the kidney, with no intermediate capillary vessels (Figure 32-12).[133] Renal AVMs are rare, with an incidence of 1 per 30 000 in a large series of autopsies.[133] They can be divided into two types, cirsoid and cavernomatous.[134,135] Cirsoid AVMs are the most common type and are formed of multiple spiral-shaped arteriovenous communications in the form of a renal mass near the collecting system. Cavernomatous AVMs are instead composed of a cystic cavity with a single artery entering it and draining vein.[133,134] AVMs are usually unilateral, but bilateral AVMs have been reported.[136,137]

Acquired lesions are referred to as AVFs and are much more common than AVMs, representing 75% to 80% of all anomalous renal arteriovenous communications.[133,134] AVFs can be caused by trauma, malignant disease, or nephrectomy, but the most common cause is percutaneous renal artery biopsy.[133,138] Renal AVMs can be asymptomatic, but usually present with gross hematuria, which is the most common symptom and has been reported in 72% to 80% of cases.[139–141] Gross hematuria is more frequent in AVMs than in acquired fistulas.[141] Renin-mediated arterial hypertension can be present in both AVMs and AVFs, but more often in AVFs (50% vs. 25%, respectively). Other less common clinical findings include flank pain or tenderness, cardiomegaly with or without congestive

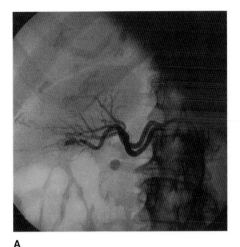
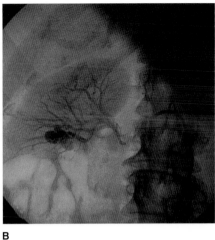
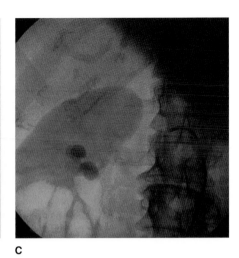

A   B   C

● **FIGURE 32-12.** (A, B, and C) Arteriovenous malformation in the left renal artery.

Courtesy of Robert Dieter, MD, RVT.

heart failure, and abdominal bruits.[133,139,141] When patients present with gross hematuria, the initial evaluation is usually performed with intravenous pyelography (IVP) and CT scan. IVP can be normal but may show filling defects of the dilated vessels as well as blood clots. Ultrasonography is usually the first diagnostic technique employed when the diagnosis of AVM is suspected.[142] Color Doppler ultrasonography can demonstrate the vascular nature of the lesion showing high-velocity turbulent flow. Spiral CT scan with contrast administration may demonstrate a vascular mass and renal vein dilatation, but cannot differentiate AVMs from hypervascular solid lesions.[143] MRI and MRA reveal the vascular nature of the lesion, but may fail to differentiate AVMs from aneurysms.[141] Angiography remains the standard for the diagnosis of renal AVMs, and demonstrates single or multiple arteriovenous communications and early visualization of the draining renal veins and inferior vena cava, possibly with a decreased nephrogram distal to the AVM, and is necessary to guide therapeutic percutanous interventions.[135,141,144]

Treatment of AVMs should be tailored to the individual. Asymptomatic patients require no treatment, while more aggressive management is reserved for patients with severe hematuria, intraparenchymal hemorrhage, severe and resistant hypertension, recurrent renal or urethral colics, as well for those with heart failure.[135] When treatment is necessary, transarterial embolization should be tried first, while surgery should be reserved when this approach fails or in very large AVMs.[135,144,145]

Embolization agents used include platinum coils, glue, plastic polymers, gelatin sponges as well as absolute alcohol.[145–148] Surgical approaches include nephrectomy and ligation of the feeding vessels; surgical procedures that spare renal parenchyma are preferred and can be performed in conjuction with endovascular techniques.[135,144]

Spontaneous Dissection of the Renal Artery

Spontaneous dissection of the renal artery (SDRA) is a rare disease, and its clinical presentation may vary.[149–151]

The causes are not known, and changes in the media and vasa-vasorum are among the possible etiologic factors. Although FMD can coexist with dissecting aneurysms in 9.1% of FMDs, SDRA is probably a separate entity.[152] Renal artery dissection can be an incidental finding, and can be found bilaterally in 20% to 25% of the cases.[150,153] Patients, however, often present more dramatically with new or accelerated hypertension and impaired renal function, flank pain, and hematuria, as well as with neurological symptoms.[150,154–156] The natural history is not known, but severe hypertension can result in target organ damage, encephalopathy, and severe cardiovascular complications including sudden death.[153,157]

The diagnosis of renal artery dissection is primarily made by angiography, usually performed to rule out renovascular causes of elevated blood pressure. Whereas standard aortography maybe sufficient to outline dissections of the renal artery's ostium and proximal segment, selective angiography is usually necessary when the dissection extends to the terminal branches of the artery.[154]

Treatment of SDRA is controversial.[151] Medical therapy can be an acceptable first approach when SDRA is accompanied by hypertension, but endovascular or surgical treatment maybe necessary for refractory cases or in severely damaged kidneys.

The role of endovascular treatment of SDRA has not been well established, but this approach seems reasonable in ostial and proximal renal artery dissections. For more distal disease, arterial artery reconstruction either in situ or ex situ followed by autotransplantation can achieve restoration of normal arterial anatomy and renal perfusion.[154,156] The only indications for nephrectomy are severely damaged kidneys with dissections affecting inaccessible intrarenal branches and severe parenchymal alterations.[154]

Renal Artery Aneurysm (Figure 32-13)

Renal artery aneurysm represents a rare diagnosis with the prevalence in the general population reported at between 0.01% and 1%.[158] Renal artery aneurysms represent 22%

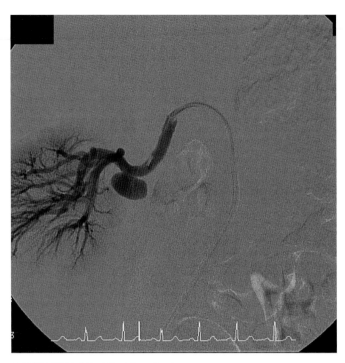

● **FIGURE 32-13.** Renal artery aneurysm.
Courtesy of Robert Dieter, MD, RVT.

of all visceral artery aneurysms.[159] Clinicians will typically encounter this diagnosis as an incidental finding on an imaging study such as CT scan or MRI; however patients can present with hypertension, renal dysfunction, hematuria, flank pain, and rarely rupture. The most common etiologic agents are atherosclerosis and FMD. The natural history of renal artery aneurysms is unknown, but the incidence of rupture is thought to increase with size. Mortality rates following rupture are reported at 10%.[160]

Indications for treatment of renal artery aneurysm in symptomatic patients include hypertension, hematuria, flank pain, and pregnancy. The reported incidence of rupture with pregnancy is as high as 80% mandating treatment in pregnant patients.[158] The size at which to intervene in an asymptomatic patient is unknown. Some authors have advocated for intervention in aneurysms as small as 1.5 cm if they are increasing in size while others have suggested intervening in those aneurysms >2 cm.[160,161] This question will likely remain unanswered given the infrequency with which this diagnosis is encountered.

Treatment options include both surgical and percutaneous techniques. Historically, these lesions have been treated with open surgical anuerysmectomy with good operative outcomes. In a series from Michigan, 121 patients were treated operatively for renal artery aneurysms.[162] There were no perioperative deaths and all but two grafts remained patent during a mean follow-up of 91 months. Percutaneous treatment is limited to case reports with reported techniques including placement of stent grafts, coiling and exclusion with covered stents.[160,163–165] The long-term durability of these techniques with regard to patency and prevention of rupture remains unknown.

REFERENCES

1. Slovut DP, Olin JW. Fibromuscular dysplasia. *N Engl J Med.* 2004;350(18):1862-1871.

2. Pannier-Moreau I, Grimbert P, Fiquet-Kempf B, et al. Possible familial origin of multifocal renal artery fibromuscular dysplasia. *J Hypertens.* 1997;15(12 Pt 2):1797-1801.

3. Pollock M, Jackson BM. Fibromuscular dysplasia of the carotid arteries. *Neurology.* 1971;21(12):1226-1230.

4. Dayes LA, Gardiner N. The neurological implications of fibromuscular dysplasia. *Mt Sinai J Med.* 2005;72(6):418-420.

5. Krijnen P, van Jaarsveld BC, Steyerberg EW, Man in 't Veld AJ, Schalekamp MA, Habbema JD. A clinical prediction rule for renal artery stenosis. *Ann Intern Med.* 1998;129(9):705-711.

6. Cragg AH, Smith TP, Thompson BH, et al. Incidental fibromuscular dysplasia in potential renal donors: long-term clinical follow-up. *Radiology.* 1989;172(1):145-147.

7. Kincaid OW, Davis GD, Hallermann FJ, Hunt JC. Fibromuscular dysplasia of the renal arteries. Arteriographic features, classification, and observations on natural history of the disease. *Am J Roentgenol Radium Ther Nucl Med.* 1968;104(2):271-282.

8. Goncharenko V, Gerlock AJ Jr, Shaff MI, Hollifield JW. Progression of renal artery fibromuscular dysplasia in 42 patients as seen on angiography. *Radiology.* 1981;139(1):45-51.

9. Safian RD, Textor SC. Renal-artery stenosis. *N Engl J Med.* 2001;344(6):431-442.

10. Hansen KJ, Edwards MS, Craven TE, et al. Prevalence of renovascular disease in the elderly: a population-based study. *J Vasc Surg.* 2002;36(3):443-451.

11. Conlon PJ, Little MA, Pieper K, Mark DB. Severity of renal vascular disease predicts mortality in patients undergoing coronary angiography. *Kidney Int.* 2001;60(4):1490-1497.

12. Rihal CS, Textor SC, Breen JF, et al. Incidental renal artery stenosis among a prospective cohort of hypertensive patients undergoing coronary angiography. *Mayo Clin Proc.* Apr 2002;77(4):309-316.

13. Olin JW, Melia M, Young JR, Graor RA, Risius B. Prevalence of atherosclerotic renal artery stenosis in patients with atherosclerosis elsewhere. *Am J Med.* 1990;88(1N):46N-51N.

14. Caps MT, Perissinotto C, Zierler RE, et al. Prospective study of atherosclerotic disease progression in the renal artery. *Circulation.* 1998;98(25):2866-2872.

15. Schreiber MJ, Pohl MA, Novick AC. The natural history of atherosclerotic and fibrous renal artery disease. *Urol Clin North Am.* 1984;11(3):383-392.

16. van Jaarsveld BC, Krijnen P, Pieterman H, et al. The effect of balloon angioplasty on hypertension in atherosclerotic renal-artery stenosis. Dutch Renal Artery Stenosis

Intervention Cooperative Study Group. *N Engl J Med.* 2000; 342(14):1007-1014.

17. Dean RH, Kieffer RW, Smith BM, et al. Renovascular hypertension: anatomic and renal function changes during drug therapy. *Arch Surg.* 1981;116(11):1408-1415.

18. Caps MT, Zierler RE, Polissar NL, et al. Risk of atrophy in kidneys with atherosclerotic renal artery stenosis. *Kidney Int.* 1998;53(3):735-742.

19. Scoble JE, Maher ER, Hamilton G, Dick R, Sweny P, Moorhead JF. Atherosclerotic renovascular disease causing renal impairment—a case for treatment. *Clin Nephrol.* 1989; 31(3):119-122.

20. Mailloux LU, Napolitano B, Bellucci AG, Vernace M, Wilkes BM, Mossey RT. Renal vascular disease causing end-stage renal disease, incidence, clinical correlates, and outcomes: a 20-year clinical experience. *Am J Kidney Dis.* 1994;24(4): 622-629.

21. Olin JW. Renal artery disease: diagnosis and management. *Mt Sinai J Med.* 2004;71(2):73-85.

22. Conlon PJ, O'Riordan E, Kalra PA. New insights into the epidemiologic and clinical manifestations of atherosclerotic renovascular disease. *Am J Kidney Dis.* 2000;35(4):573-587.

23. Goldblatt H. Experimental renal hypertension; mechanism of production and maintenance. *Circulation.* 1958;17(4, part 2):642-647.

24. DeForrest JM, Knappenberger RC, Antonaccio MJ, Ferrone RA, Creekmore JS. Angiotensin II is a necessary component for the development of hypertension in the two kidney, one clip rat. *Am J Cardiol.* 1982;49(6):1515-1517.

25. Fink GD. Long-term sympatho-excitatory effect of angiotensin II: a mechanism of spontaneous and renovascular hypertension. *Clin Exp Pharmacol Physiol.* 1997;24(1):91-95.

26. Lerman LO, Nath KA, Rodriguez-Porcel M, et al. Increased oxidative stress in experimental renovascular hypertension. *Hypertension.* 2001;37(2 part 2):541-546.

27. Higashi Y, Sasaki S, Nakagawa K, Matsuura H, Oshima T, Chayama K. Endothelial function and oxidative stress in renovascular hypertension. *N Engl J Med.* 2002;346(25):1954-1962.

28. Firth JD, Ratcliffe PJ. Organ distribution of the three rat endothelin messenger RNAs and the effects of ischemia on renal gene expression. *J Clin Invest.* 1992;90(3):1023-1031.

29. Anderson CB, Tannenbaum JS, Sicard GA, Etheredge EE. Renal thromboxane synthesis in excised kidney distal to renovascular lesions. *JAMA.* 1984;251(23):3118-3120.

30. Gavras H, Brunner HR, Thurston H, Laragh JH. Reciprocation of renin dependency with sodium volume dependency in renal hypertension. *Science.* 1975;188(4195):1316-1317.

31. Garovic VD, Textor SC. Renovascular hypertension and ischemic nephropathy. *Circulation.* 2005;112(9):1362-1374.

32. Messina LM, Zelenock GB, Yao KA, Stanley JC. Renal revascularization for recurrent pulmonary edema in patients with poorly controlled hypertension and renal insufficiency: a distinct subgroup of patients with arteriosclerotic renal artery occlusive disease. *J Vasc Surg.* 1992;15(1):73-80; discussion 80-72.

33. Missouris CG, Belli AM, MacGregor GA. "Apparent" heart failure: a syndrome caused by renal artery stenoses. *Heart.* 2000;83(2):152-155.

34. Simon P, Benarbia S, Charasse C, et al. [Ischemic renal diseases have become the most frequent causes of end stage renal disease in the elderly]. *Arch Mal Coeur Vaiss.* 1998;91(8): 1065-1068.

35. Epstein FH. Oxygen and renal metabolism. *Kidney Int.* 1997;51(2):381-385.

36. Yune HY, Klatte EC. Collateral circulation to an ischemic kidney. *Radiology.* 1976;119(3):539-546.

37. Lerman L, Textor SC. Pathophysiology of ischemic nephropathy. *Urol Clin North Am.* 2001;28(4):793-803, ix.

38. Kontogiannis J, Burns KD. Role of AT1 angiotensin II receptors in renal ischemic injury. *Am J Physiol.* 1998;274(1 Pt 2): F79-F90.

39. Zou LX, Imig JD, von Thun AM, Hymel A, Ono H, Navar LG. Receptor-mediated intrarenal angiotensin II augmentation in angiotensin II-infused rats. *Hypertension.* 1996;28(4):669-677.

40. Matsusaka T, Hymes J, Ichikawa I. Angiotensin in progressive renal diseases: theory and practice. *J Am Soc Nephrol.* 1996;7(10):2025-2043.

41. Stebbins CL, Symons JD, Hageman KS, Musch TI. Endogenous prostaglandins limit angiotensin-II induced regional vasoconstriction in conscious rats. *J Cardiovasc Pharmacol.* 2003;42(1):10-16.

42. Ichiki T, Usui M, Kato M, et al. Downregulation of angiotensin II type 1 receptor gene transcription by nitric oxide. *Hypertension.* 1998;31(1 Pt 2):342-348.

43. Bachmann S, Mundel P. Nitric oxide in the kidney: synthesis, localization, and function. *Am J Kidney Dis.* 1994; 24(1):112-129.

44. Tokuyama H, Hayashi K, Matsuda H, et al. Stenosis-dependent role of nitric oxide and prostaglandins in chronic renal ischemia. *Am J Physiol Renal Physiol.* 2002;282(5): F859-865.

45. Dohi Y, Hahn AW, Boulanger CM, Buhler FR, Luscher TF. Endothelin stimulated by angiotensin II augments contractility of spontaneously hypertensive rat resistance arteries. *Hypertension.* 1992;19(2):131-137.

46. Ritthaler T, Gopfert T, Firth JD, Ratcliffe PJ, Kramer BK, Kurtz A. Influence of hypoxia on hepatic and renal endothelin gene expression. *Pflugers Arch.* 1996;431(4):587-593.

47. Textor SC, Wilcox CS. Renal artery stenosis: a common, treatable cause of renal failure? *Annu Rev Med.* 2001;52: 421-442.

48. Harding MB, Smith LR, Himmelstein SI, et al. Renal artery stenosis: prevalence and associated risk factors in patients undergoing routine cardiac catheterization. *J Am Soc Nephrol.* 1992;2(11):1608-1616.

49. Olin JW. Atherosclerotic renal artery disease. *Cardiol Clin.* 2002;20(4):547-562, vi.

50. Davis BA, Crook JE, Vestal RE, Oates JA. Prevalence of renovascular hypertension in patients with grade III or IV hypertensive retinopathy. *N Engl J Med.* 1979;301(23):1273-1276.

51. Simon N, Franklin SS, Bleifer KH, Maxwell MH. Clinical

characteristics of renovascular hypertension. *JAMA*. 1972; 220(9):1209-1218.

52. Chobanian AV, Bakris GL, Black HR, et al. The Seventh Report of the Joint National Committee on Prevention, Detection, Evaluation, and Treatment of High Blood Pressure: the JNC 7 report. *JAMA*. 2003;289(19):2560-2572.

53. Gifford RW, Jr., McCormack LJ, Poutasse EF. The atrophic kidney: its role in hypertension. *Mayo Clin Proc*. 1965; 40(11):834-852.

54. Textor SC, Tarazi RC, Novick AC, Bravo EL, Fouad FM. Regulation of renal hemodynamics and glomerular filtration in patients with renovascular hypertension during converting enzyme inhibition with captopril. *Am J Med*. 1984;76(5B):29-37.

55. Gray BH, Olin JW, Childs MB, Sullivan TM, Bacharach JM. Clinical benefit of renal artery angioplasty with stenting for the control of recurrent and refractory congestive heart failure. *Vasc Med*. 2002;7(4):275-279.

56. Diamond JR. Flash pulmonary edema and the diagnostic suspicion of occult renal artery stenosis. *Am J Kidney Dis*. 1993;21(3):328-330.

57. Khosla S, Kunjummen B, Manda R, et al. Prevalence of renal artery stenosis requiring revascularization in patients initially referred for coronary angiography. *Catheter Cardiovasc Interv*. 2003;58(3):400-403.

58. Radermacher J, Chavan A, Bleck J, et al. Use of Doppler ultrasonography to predict the outcome of therapy for renal-artery stenosis. *N Engl J Med*. 2001;344(6):410-417.

59. Olin JW, Piedmonte MR, Young JR, DeAnna S, Grubb M, Childs MB. The utility of duplex ultrasound scanning of the renal arteries for diagnosing significant renal artery stenosis. *Ann Intern Med*. 1995;122(11):833-838.

60. Strandness DE, Jr. Duplex scanning in diagnosis of renovascular hypertension. *Surg Clin North Am*. 1990;70(1):109-117.

61. Isikoff MB, Hill MC. Sonography of the renal arteries: left lateral decubitus position. *AJR Am J Roentgenol*. Jun 1980; 134(6):1177-1179.

62. Hoffmann U, Edwards JM, Carter S, et al. Role of duplex scanning for the detection of atherosclerotic renal artery disease. *Kidney Int*. 1991;39(6):1232-1239.

63. Bakker J, Beutler JJ, Elgersma OE, de Lange EE, de Kort GA, Beek FJ. Duplex ultrasonography in assessing restenosis of renal artery stents. *Cardiovasc Intervent Radiol*. 1999;22(6): 475-480.

64. Lookstein RA. Impact of CT angiography on endovascular therapy. *Mt Sinai J Med*. 2003;70(6):367-374.

65. Elkohen M, Beregi JP, Deklunder G, Artaud D, Mounier-Vehier C, Carre AG. A prospective study of helical computed tomography angiography versus angiography for the detection of renal artery stenoses in hypertensive patients. *J Hypertens*. 1996;14(4):525-528.

66. Kim TS, Chung JW, Park JH, Kim SH, Yeon KM, Han MC. Renal artery evaluation: comparison of spiral CT angiography to intra-arterial DSA. *J Vasc Interv Radiol*. 1998;9(4):553-559.

67. Fisher JEO, Jeffrey W. Renal artery stenosis. Clinical evaluation. In: Saunders E, ed. *Vascular Medicine*. Philadelphia, PA; 2006:343.

68. Willmann JK, Wildermuth S, Pfammatter T, et al. Aortoiliac and renal arteries: prospective intraindividual comparison of contrast-enhanced three-dimensional MR angiography and multi-detector row CT angiography. *Radiology*. 2003;226(3):798-811.

69. Sandstede JJ, Kaupert C, Roth A, Jenett M, Harz C, Hahn D. Comparison of different iodine concentrations for multidetector row computed tomography angiography of segmental renal arteries. *Eur Radiol*. 2005;15(6):1211-1214.

70. Lufft V, Hoogestraat-Lufft L, Fels LM, et al. Contrast media nephropathy: intravenous CT angiography versus intraarterial digital subtraction angiography in renal artery stenosis: a prospective randomized trial. *Am J Kidney Dis*. 2002;40(2): 236-242.

71. De Cobelli F, Venturini M, Vanzulli A, et al. Renal arterial stenosis: prospective comparison of color Doppler US and breath-hold, three-dimensional, dynamic, gadolinium-enhanced MR angiography. *Radiology*. 2000;214(2):373-380.

72. Soulez G, Oliva VL, Turpin S, Lambert R, Nicolet V, Therasse E. Imaging of renovascular hypertension: respective values of renal scintigraphy, renal Doppler US, and MR angiography. *Radiographics*. 2000;20(5):1355-1368; discussion 1368-1372.

73. Grist TM. Magnetic resonance angiography of renal artery stenosis. *Am J Kidney Dis*. 1994;24(4):700-712.

74. Niendorf ER, Grist TM, Lee FT, Jr., Brazy PC, Santyr GE. Rapid in vivo measurement of single-kidney extraction fraction and glomerular filtration rate with MR imaging. *Radiology*. 1998;206(3):791-798.

75. Snidow JJ, Johnson MS, Harris VJ, et al. Three-dimensional gadolinium-enhanced MR angiography for aortoiliac inflow assessment plus renal artery screening in a single breath hold. *Radiology*. 1996;198(3):725-732.

76. Rieumont MJ, Kaufman JA, Geller SC, et al. Evaluation of renal artery stenosis with dynamic gadolinium-enhanced MR angiography. *AJR Am J Roentgenol*. 1997;169(1):39-44.

77. Fain SB, King BF, Breen JF, Kruger DG, Riederer SJ. High-spatial-resolution contrast-enhanced MR angiography of the renal arteries: a prospective comparison with digital subtraction angiography. *Radiology*. 2001;218(2):481-490.

78. Vasbinder GB, Maki JH, Nijenhuis RJ, et al. Motion of the distal renal artery during three-dimensional contrast-enhanced breath-hold MRA. *J Magn Reson Imaging*. 2002;16(6):685-696.

79. Buecker A, Spuentrup E, Ruebben A, et al. New metallic MR stents for artifact-free coronary MR angiography: feasibility study in a swine model. *Invest Radiol*. 2004;39(5):250-253.

80. Reginelli JPCCJ. Renal artery intervention. In: Wilkins LW, ed. *Peripheral Vascular Interventions*. Philadelphia, PA; 2005:175.

81. Schreier DZ, Weaver FA, Frankhouse J, et al. A prospective study of carbon dioxide-digital subtraction vs standard contrast arteriography in the evaluation of the renal arteries. *Arch Surg*. 1996;131(5):503-507; discussion 507-508.

82. Hawkins IF, Jr., Wilcox CS, Kerns SR, Sabatelli FW. CO_2 digital angiography: a safer contrast agent for renal vascular imaging? *Am J Kidney Dis*. 1994;24(4):685-694.

83. Spinosa DJ, Hagspiel KD, Angle JF, Matsumoto AH, Hartwell GD. Gadolinium-based contrast agents in angiography and interventional radiology: uses and techniques. *J Vasc Interv Radiol.* 2000;11(8):985-990.

84. Spinosa DJ, Matsumoto AH, Angle JF, et al. Safety of CO(2)- and gadodiamide-enhanced angiography for the evaluation and percutaneous treatment of renal artery stenosis in patients with chronic renal insufficiency. *AJR Am J Roentgenol.* 2001;176(5):1305-1311.

85. Spinosa DJ, Matsumoto AH, Hagspiel KD, Angle JF, Hartwell GD. Gadolinium-based contrast agents in angiography and interventional radiology. *AJR Am J Roentgenol.* 1999;173(5):1403-1409.

86. Nally JV, Barton DP. Contemporary approach to diagnosis and evaluation of renovascular hypertension. *Urol Clin North Am.* 2001;28(4):781-791.

87. Executive Summary of The Third Report of The National Cholesterol Education Program (NCEP) Expert Panel on Detection, Evaluation, And Treatment of High Blood Cholesterol In Adults (Adult Treatment Panel III). *JAMA.* 2001; 285(19):2486-2497.

88. Hirsch AT, Haskal ZJ, Hertzer NR, et al. ACC/AHA 2005 guidelines for the management of patients with peripheral arterial disease (lower extremity, renal, mesenteric, and abdominal aortic): executive summary a collaborative report from the American Association for Vascular Surgery/Society for Vascular Surgery, Society for Cardiovascular Angiography and Interventions, Society for Vascular Medicine and Biology, Society of Interventional Radiology, and the ACC/AHA Task Force on Practice Guidelines (Writing Committee to Develop Guidelines for the Management of Patients With Peripheral Arterial Disease) endorsed by the American Association of Cardiovascular and Pulmonary Rehabilitation; National Heart, Lung, and Blood Institute; Society for Vascular Nursing; TransAtlantic Inter-Society Consensus; and Vascular Disease Foundation. *J Am Coll Cardiol.* 2006;47(6):1239-1312.

89. Textor SC. ACE inhibitors in renovascular hypertension. *Cardiovasc Drugs Ther.* 1990;4(1):229-235.

90. Benjamin ME, Dean RH. Techniques in renal artery reconstruction: Part I. *Ann Vasc Surg.* 1996;10(3):306-314.

91. Cambria RP, Brewster DC, L'Italien GJ, et al. The durability of different reconstructive techniques for atherosclerotic renal artery disease. *J Vasc Surg.* 1994;20(1):76-85; discussion 86-77.

92. Lawrie GM, Morris GC, Jr., Glaeser DH, DeBakey ME. Renovascular reconstruction: factors affecting long-term prognosis in 919 patients followed up to 31 years. *Am J Cardiol.* 1989;63(15):1085-1092.

93. Libertino JA, Bosco PJ, Ying CY, et al. Renal revascularization to preserve and restore renal function. *J Urol.* 1992; 147(6):1485-1487.

94. Hansen KJ, Starr SM, Sands RE, Burkart JM, Plonk GW, Jr., Dean RH. Contemporary surgical management of renovascular disease. *J Vasc Surg.* 1992;16(3):319-330; discussion 330-333.

95. Novick AC, Ziegelbaum M, Vidt DG, Gifford RW, Jr., Pohl MA, Goormastic M. Trends in surgical revascularization for renal artery disease. Ten years' experience. *JAMA.* 1987;257(4):498-501.

96. Cherr GS, Hansen KJ, Craven TE, et al. Surgical management of atherosclerotic renovascular disease. *J Vasc Surg.* 2002; 35(2):236-245.

97. Bredenberg CE, Sampson LN, Ray FS, Cormier RA, Heintz S, Eldrup-Jorgensen J. Changing patterns in surgery for chronic renal artery occlusive diseases. *J Vasc Surg.* 1992;15(6):1018-1023; discussion 1023-1014.

98. Reilly JM, Rubin BG, Thompson RW, Allen BT, Anderson CB, Sicard GA. Long-term effectiveness of extraanatomic renal artery revascularization. *Surgery.* 1994;116(4):784-790; discussion 790-791.

99. Steinbach F, Novick AC, Campbell S, Dykstra D. Long-term survival after surgical revascularization for atherosclerotic renal artery disease. *J Urol.* 1997;158(1):38-41.

100. Chaikof EL, Smith RB, 3rd, Salam AA, et al. Ischemic nephropathy and concomitant aortic disease: a ten-year experience. *J Vasc Surg.* 1994;19(1):135-146; discussion 146-148.

101. Hansen KJ, Wilson DB, Edwards MS. Surgical revascularization of atherosclerotic renovascular disease: state of the art. *Perspec Vasc Surg Endovasc Ther.* 2004;16(4):281-295.

102. Clair DG, Belkin M, Whittemore AD, Mannick JA, Donaldson MC. Safety and efficacy of transaortic renal endarterectomy as an adjunct to aortic surgery. *J Vasc Surg.* 1995;21(6): 926-933; discussion 934.

103. Weibull H, Bergqvist D, Bergentz SE, Jonsson K, Hulthen L, Manhem P. Percutaneous transluminal renal angioplasty versus surgical reconstruction of atherosclerotic renal artery stenosis: a prospective randomized study. *J Vasc Surg.* 1993; 18(5):841-850; discussion 850-852.

104. Xue F, Bettmann MA, Langdon DR, Wivell WA. Outcome and cost comparison of percutaneous transluminal renal angioplasty, renal arterial stent placement, and renal arterial bypass grafting. *Radiology.* 1999;212(2):378-384.

105. Bettmann MA, Dake MD, Hopkins LN, et al. Atherosclerotic Vascular Disease Conference: Writing Group VI: revascularization. *Circulation.* 2004;109(21):2643-2650.

106. Gruntzig A, Kuhlmann U, Vetter W, Lutolf U, Meier B, Siegenthaler W. Treatment of renovascular hypertension with percutaneous transluminal dilatation of a renal-artery stenosis. *Lancet.* 1978;1(8068):801-802.

107. Tegtmeyer CJ, Elson J, Glass TA, et al. Percutaneous transluminal angioplasty: the treatment of choice for renovascular hypertension due to fibromuscular dysplasia. *Radiology.* 1982;143(3):631-637.

108. Sos TA, Pickering TG, Saddekni S, et al. The current role of renal angioplasty in the treatment of renovascular hypertension. *Urol Clin North Am.* 1984;11(3):503-513.

109. Webster J, Marshall F, Abdalla M, et al. Randomised comparison of percutaneous angioplasty vs continued medical therapy for hypertensive patients with atheromatous renal artery stenosis. Scottish and Newcastle Renal Artery Stenosis Collaborative Group. *J Hum Hypertens.* 1998;12(5):329-335.

110. Plouin PF, Chatellier G, Darne B, Raynaud A. Blood pressure outcome of angioplasty in atherosclerotic renal artery stenosis: a randomized trial. Essai Multicentrique Medicaments vs Angioplastie (EMMA) Study Group. *Hypertension.* 1998;31(3):823-829.

111. van de Ven PJ, Kaatee R, Beutler JJ, et al. Arterial stenting and balloon angioplasty in ostial atherosclerotic renovascular disease: a randomised trial. *Lancet.* 1999;353(9149):282-286.

112. Leertouwer TC, Gussenhoven EJ, Bosch JL, et al. Stent placement for renal arterial stenosis: where do we stand? A meta-analysis. *Radiology.* 2000;216(1):78-85.

113. Isles CG, Robertson S, Hill D. Management of renovascular disease: a review of renal artery stenting in ten studies. *QJM.* 1999;92(3):159-167.

114. Rocha-Singh K, Jaff MR, Rosenfield K. Evaluation of the safety and effectiveness of renal artery stenting after unsuccessful balloon angioplasty: the ASPIRE-2 study. *J Am Coll Cardiol.* 2005;46(5):776-783.

115. Vignali C, Bargellini I, Lazzereschi M, et al. Predictive factors of in-stent restenosis in renal artery stenting: a retrospective analysis. *Cardiovasc Intervent Radiol.* 2005;28(3):296-302.

116. Lederman RJ, Mendelsohn FO, Santos R, Phillips HR, Stack RS, Crowley JJ. Primary renal artery stenting: characteristics and outcomes after 363 procedures. *Am Heart J.* 2001;142(2):314-323.

117. Bates MC, Rashid M, Campbell JE, Stone PA, Broce M, Lavigne PS. Factors influencing the need for target vessel revascularization after renal artery stenting. *J Endovasc Ther.* 2006;13(5):569-577.

118. Nolan BW, Schermerhorn ML, Powell RJ, et al. Restenosis in gold-coated renal artery stents. *J Vasc Surg.* Jul 2005; 42(1):40-46.

119. Stoeteknuel-Friedli S, Do DD, von Briel C, Triller J, Mahler F, Baumgartner I. Endovascular brachytherapy for prevention of recurrent renal in-stent restenosis. *J Endovasc Ther.* 2002;9(3):350-353.

120. Reilly JP, Ramee SR. Vascular brachytherapy in renal artery restenosis. *Curr Opin Cardiol.* 2004;19(4):332-335.

121. Munneke GJ, Engelke C, Morgan RA, Belli AM. Cutting balloon angioplasty for resistant renal artery in-stent restenosis. *J Vasc Interv Radiol.* 2002;13(3):327-331.

122. Bax L, Mali WP, Van De Ven PJ, Beek FJ, Vos JA, Beutler JJ. Repeated intervention for in-stent restenosis of the renal arteries. *J Vasc Interv Radiol.* 2002;13(12):1219-1224.

123. Zeller T, Rastan A, Rothenpieler U, Muller C. Restenosis after stenting of atherosclerotic renal artery stenosis: is there a rationale for the use of drug-eluting stents? *Catheter Cardiovasc Interv.* 2006;68(1):125-130.

124. Kakkar AK, Fischi M, Narins CR. Drug-eluting stent implantation for treatment of recurrent renal artery in-stent restenosis. *Catheter Cardiovasc Interv.* 2006;68(1):118-122; discussion 123-124.

125. Krishnamurthi V, Novick AC, Myles JL. Atheroembolic renal disease: effect on morbidity and survival after revascularization for atherosclerotic renal artery stenosis. *J Urol.* 1999;161(4):1093-1096.

126. Scolari F, Tardanico R, Zani R, et al. Cholesterol crystal embolism: a recognizable cause of renal disease. *Am J Kidney Dis.* 2000;36(6):1089-1109.

127. Holden A, Hill A. Renal angioplasty and stenting with distal protection of the main renal artery in ischemic nephropathy: early experience. *J Vasc Surg.* 2003;38(5):962-968.

128. Henry M, Henry I, Klonaris C, et al. Renal angioplasty and stenting under protection: the way for the future? *Catheter Cardiovasc Interv.* 2003;60(3):299-312.

129. Zeller T, Frank U, Muller C, et al. Predictors of improved renal function after percutaneous stent-supported angioplasty of severe atherosclerotic ostial renal artery stenosis. *Circulation.* 2003;108(18):2244-2249.

130. Rocha-Singh KJ, Mishkel GJ, Katholi RE, et al. Clinical predictors of improved long-term blood pressure control after successful stenting of hypertensive patients with obstructive renal artery atherosclerosis. *Catheter Cardiovasc Interv.* 1999;47(2):167-172.

131. Burket MW, Cooper CJ, Kennedy DJ, et al. Renal artery angioplasty and stent placement: predictors of a favorable outcome. *Am Heart J.* 2000;139(1 Pt 1):64-71.

132. Silva JA, Chan AW, White CJ, et al. Elevated brain natriuretic peptide predicts blood pressure response after stent revascularization in patients with renal artery stenosis. *Circulation.* 2005;111(3):328-333.

133. Munoz IA, Bustos GA, Pardal AG, et al. Heart failure and severe pulmonary hypertension secondary to a giant renal arteriovenous malformation. *J Ultrasound Med.* 2006; 25(7):933-937.

134. Kawashima A, Sandler CM, Ernst RD, Tamm EP, Goldman SM, Fishman EK. CT evaluation of renovascular disease. *Radiographics.* 2000;20(5):1321-1340.

135. Crotty KL, Orihuela E, Warren MM. Recent advances in the diagnosis and treatment of renal arteriovenous malformations and fistulas. *J Urol.* 1993;150(5 Pt 1):1355-1359.

136. Minetti E, Montoli A. Images in clinical medicine. Bilateral renal arteriovenous malformation. *N Engl J Med.* 2004; 351(10):e9.

137. Ullian ME, Molitoris BA. Bilateral congenital renal arteriovenous fistulas. *Clin Nephrol.* 1987;27(6):293-297.

138. Cho KJ, Stanley JC. Non-neoplastic congenital and acquired renal arteriovenous malformations and fistulas. *Radiology.* 1978;129(2):333-343.

139. Yazaki T, Tomita M, Akimoto M, Konjiki T, Kawai H, Kumazaki T. Congenital renal arteriovenous fistula: case report, review of Japanese literature and description of non-radical treatment. *J Urol.* 1976;116(4):415-418.

140. Takaha M, Matsumoto A, Ochi K, Takeuchi M, Takemoto M, Sonoda T. Intrarenal arteriovenous malformation. *J Urol.* 1980;124(3):315-318.

141. Chatziioannou A, Mourikis D, Kalaboukas K, et al. Endovascular treatment of renal arteriovenous malformations. *Urol Int.* 2005;74(1):89-91.

142. Cisternino SJ, Malave SR, Neiman HL. Congenital renal arteriovenous malformation: ultrasonic appearance. *J Urol.* 1981;126(2):238-239.

143. Honda H, Onitsuka H, Naitou S, et al. Renal arteriovenous malformations: CT features. *J Comput Assist Tomogr.* 1991; 15(2):261-264.

144. Kopchick JH, Bourne NK, Fine SW, Jacobsohn HA, Jacobs SC, Lawson RK. Congenital renal arteriovenous malformations. *Urology.* 1981;17(1):13-17.

145. Takebayashi S, Hosaka M, Kubota Y, Ishizuka E, Iwasaki A, Matsubara S. Transarterial embolization and ablation of renal arteriovenous malformations: efficacy and damages in

30 patients with long-term followup. *J Urol.*1998;159(3): 696-701.

146. Bischoff W, Pohle W, Goerttler U. Treatment of arteriovenous angiomas of the kidney: surgical intervention and intraarterial embolization. *J Urol.* 1979;122(6):825-828.

147. Beaujeux R, Saussine C, al-Fakir A, et al. Superselective endo-vascular treatment of renal vascular lesions. *J Urol.* 1995;153(1):14-17.

148. Takebayashi S, Hosaka M, Ishizuka E, Hirokawa M, Matsui K. Arteriovenous malformations of the kidneys: ablation with alcohol. *AJR Am J Roentgenol.* 1988;150(3):587-590.

149. Beroniade V, Roy P, Froment D, Pison C. Primary renal artery dissection. Presentation of two cases and brief review of the literature. *Am J Nephrol.* 1987;7(5):382-389.

150. Smith BM, Holcomb GW, Richie RE III, Dean RH. Renal artery dissection. *Ann Surg.* 1984;200(2):134-146.

151. Edwards BS, Stanson AW, Holley KE, Sheps SG. Isolated renal artery dissection, presentation, evaluation, management, and pathology. *Mayo Clin Proc.* 1982;57(9):564-571.

152. Harrison EG, Jr., Hunt JC, Bernatz PE. Morphology of fibromuscular dysplasia of the renal artery in renovascular hypertension. *Am J Med.* 1967;43(1):97-112.

153. Mathieu D, Abbou C, Meunier S, Larde D, Vasile N. Primary dissecting aneurysm of the renal artery. *Urol Radiol.* 1983;5(1):17-21.

154. Lacombe M. Isolated spontaneous dissection of the renal artery. *J Vasc Surg.* 2001;33(2):385-391.

155. Gewertz BL, Stanley JC, Fry WJ. Renal artery dissections. *Arch Surg.* 1977;112(4):409-414.

156. van Rooden CJ, van Baalen JM, van Bockel JH. Spontaneous dissection of renal artery: long-term results of extracorporeal reconstruction and autotransplantation1. *J Vasc Surg.* 2003;38(1):116-122.

157. Esayag-Tendler B, Yamase H, Ramsby G, White WB. Accelerated hypertension with encephalopathy due to an isolated dissection of a renal artery branch vessel. *Am J Kidney Dis.* 1994;23(6):869-873.

158. Bulbul MA, Farrow GA. Renal artery aneurysms. *Urology.* 1992;40(2):124-126.

159. Deterling RA, Jr. Aneurysm of the visceral arteries. *J Cardiovasc Surg (Torino).* 1971;12(4):309-322.

160. Pershad A, Heuser R. Renal artery aneurysm: successful exclusion with a stent graft. *Catheter Cardiovasc Interv.* 2004; 61(3):314-316.

161. Hageman JH, Smith RF, Szilagyi E, Elliott JP. Aneurysms of the renal artery: problems of prognosis and surgical management. *Surgery.* 1978;84(4):563-572.

162. Henke PK, Cardneau JD, Welling TH, III, et al. Renal artery aneurysms: a 35-year clinical experience with 252 aneurysms in 168 patients. *Ann Surg.* 2001;234(4):454-462; discussion 462-463.

163. Bui BT, Oliva VL, Leclerc G, et al. Renal artery aneurysm: treatment with percutaneous placement of a stent-graft. *Radiology.* 1995;195(1):181-182.

164. Centenera LV, Hirsch JA, Choi IS, Beckmann CF, Gillard CS, Libertino J. Wide-necked saccular renal artery aneurysm: endovascular embolization with the Guglielmi detachable coil and temporary balloon occlusion of the aneurysm neck. *J Vasc Interv Radiol.* 1998;9(3):513-516.

165. Tan WA, Chough S, Saito J, Wholey MH, Eles G. Covered stent for renal artery aneurysm. *Catheter Cardiovasc Interv.* 2001;52(1):106-109.

chapter 33

Lower Extremity Peripheral Arterial Disease

Ravi K. Ramana, DO / Bruce E. Lewis, MD / Robert S. Dieter, MD, RVT

● INTRODUCTION

Lower extremity peripheral arterial disease (LEPAD) is a major cause of poor quality of life, disability, and significant morbidity and mortality in the United States.[1-17] In this chapter, LEPAD is used to refer to any arterial disease affecting the lower extremity, including occlusive, aneursymal, and vasculitic disease states. Even when asymptomatic, LEPAD has been shown to decrease mobility and bone mineral density[8,9,12,18]; leads to foot ulcers and amputations[8,19]; and be a strong predictor of subsequent cardiovascular (CV) disease, nonfatal CV events (e.g., myocardial infarction and stroke), and mortality.[6,10,20] Standard therapy for LEPAD should include antiplatelet therapy and be directed at control of risk factors including smoking cessation, lipid management, strict diabetic therapy, and control of blood pressure[21] in attempts to stop progression of the systemic atherosclerotic process. Current therapy on symptomatic disease includes exercise therapy, antiplatelet medications, and a variety of percutaneous interventional and surgical procedures. Therefore, early diagnosis and appropriate therapy for LEPAD can significant improve quality of life and decrease significant morbidity and CV mortality.

This chapter will attempt to concisely

- review the epidemiology and determined risk factors of LEPAD,
- discuss the embryologic development and subsequent normal and variant anatomic features of LE vasculature,
- summarize the classification and grading schemata for LEPAD,
- discuss the pathophysiology underlying LEPAD and limb ischemia,

- review the common and uncommon etiologies of LEPAD,
- discuss the typical clinical presentation, physical examination findings, and natural history of LEPAD,
- summarize the various diagnostic modalities for LEPAD,
- review the medical and nonpharmacologic therapies for LEPAD,
- discuss the percutaneous and surgical revascularization procedures for LEPAD and outline the appropriate clinical indications for use of each therapy,
- discuss more specific therapy for critical limb ischemia (CLI), and
- summarize the current investigations and future directions in the treatment of LEPAD.

● EPIDEMIOLOGY

Prevalence

It is without question that LEPAD is a common disease process affecting a significant portion of the adult population. There are a reported 413 000 discharges per year with chronic peripheral arterial disease (PAD), 88 000 inpatient lower extremity arteriographies, and nearly 30 000 discharges involving patients who had undergone embolectomy or thrombectomy of the lower limb arterial vasculature.[22] Numerous epidemiologic studies have been performed in attempts to accurately quantify the prevalence of LEPAD in the adult population and although these studies have reported a variety of rates, most experts and consensus statements agree that up to 12 million individuals in the United States are affected by PAD. The variability found in these numerous studies evaluating

LEPAD is widely attributable to the differing clinical presentations (namely asymptomatic individuals), clinical definitions, diagnostic modalities, or specific patient subpopulations used in each study.

The Framingham Heart Study was the first to address the prevalence of LEPAD in a large population sample in 1948. The initial and long-term follow-up data, which based the diagnosis of LEPAD exclusively on intermittent claudication symptoms, reported the prevalence of LEPAD to be 7.3%. In addition, this study was the first to report the incidence of LEPAD was higher in the elderly, a finding which has been consistently reproduced. However, their data suggesting a higher incidence in males has not been as well validated.[16,23,24] However, the overall prevalence rates reported in this cohort study is a gross underestimate, since LEPAD often may present in asymptomatic forms that can only be detected via noninvasive or invasive imaging. Therefore, more recent studies have used other modalities to diagnosis LEPAD in further attempt investigate the prevalence of LEPAD in the general and specific patient populations. These studies have revealed a number of epidemiologic characteristics and disease comorbid risk factors that result in a higher prevalence in certain patient populations.

One such study attempted to elucidate the prevalence of large-vessel and small-vessel LEPAD in a small population. Their assessment involved traditional questionnaires, physical examination, and noninvasive testing (segmental blood pressure, flow velocity, postocclusive reactive hyperemia, and pulse reappearance half-time). Results revealed a nearly 12% and 16% prevalence of large- and small-vessel lower extremity disease, respectively. Interestingly, the prevalence of large-vessel disease, but not isolated small-vessel disease, was significantly correlated with patients who were male and older than 60 years of age. These results demonstrate a significant fivefold underestimate of LEPAD when compared to symptoms of claudication, but a twofold overestimate of LEPAD when compared to pulse abnormalities on physical examination.[14]

A national, community-based PAD detection program (PARTNERS) used 350 local primary care sites to identify patients who were deemed higher risk for PAD: Age more than 70 years, or age more than 50 years with a history of diabetes and/or tobacco abuse. Findings revealed a 29% incidence of PAD, defined as an ankle–brachial index (ABI) less than 0.9.[13] Similarly, a European population study evaluating more than 7000 patients, found nearly a 20% frequency of LEPAD in patients 55 years and older, with nearly 60% frequency in men elder than 85 years of age.[13,16]

Interestingly, in nearly all of the patients diagnosed by abnormal ABIs or other noninvasive imaging in these studies, only 1% to 22% of the patients had self-reported claudication or symptoms by Rose questionnaire.[13,16,25–29] This strongly supports the notion that most patients with LEPAD remain either asymptomatic, have limited their activities to avoid claudication symptoms, are limited by other comorbid conditions, or simply attritibute their symptoms to their increasing age. Yet, it is important to note that

nearly 10% of these "asymptomatic" patients have advanced PAD with severe obstruction to blood flow,[17] and all carry an increased risk of future CV events.[14,16,17,30,31]

Risk Factors

Numerous risk factors for the development of LEPAD have been identified (Figure 33-1). And since the vast majority of LEPAD is caused by occlusive atherosclerotic disease, risk factors for the development and/or progression of LEPAD are nearly identical to those which can lead to cardiac and cerebrovascular atherosclerotic disease.[21] The strongest correlations exist with elderly age and variably male gender (as discussed above). Other comorbidities including tobacco abuse, diabetes mellitus, hypertension, and hyperlipidemia and the relative risk—each of these relays onto the development of LEPAD are discussed below (Figure 33-1). Also, the coexistence of these risk factors relates synergistic effects on the development of LEPAD—one study reported a relative risk increase of 2.3 to 3.3 to 6.3 in patients with one, two, or three risk factors (tobacco abuse, hypertension, and diabetes) present, respectively.[32]

Tobacco Abuse. The association between smoking and PAD and subsequent claudication symptoms was first

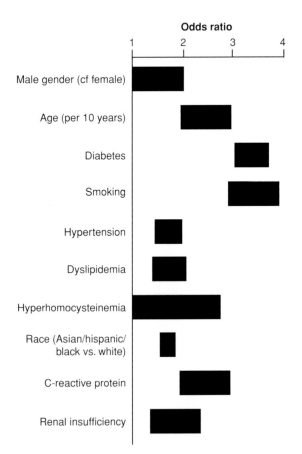

● **FIGURE 33-1.** Odd ratios for risk factors developing PAD.

Source: Reprinted with permission from Elsevier in Norgren L, Hiatt WR, Dormandy JA, et al. Inter-Society Consensus for the Management of Peripheral Arterial Disease (TASC II). J Vasc Surg 2007;45(1): S5-S67.

described in 1911.[33] Tobacco abuse is a strong predictor of the development and progression of LEPAD[15] as studies have reported a two- to sixfold risk of development of LEPAD compared to nonsmokers.[5,16,34–36] In fact, tobacco abuse has been demonstrated to have a significantly higher relative risk for the development of PAD compared with the traditional atherosclerotic risk factors.[34] Also, there is a strong, dose-dependent (i.e., number of packs per day and number of pack-years smoked) predictor of the development of LEPAD, risk of amputation, peripheral graft occlusion, and mortality.[33,37–39]

Diabetes. Numerous epidemiologic studies have reported a strong association between diabetes and an increased prevalence of PAD.[40,41] Specifically, studies have reported that for every 1% increase in hemoglobin A1C levels, there is an associated 26% increased risk of PAD.[42] Even patients with insulin resistance (and not diabetes) carry an increased risk of PAD.[43] Moreover, other studies have demonstrated a two- to fourfold higher prevalence of LEPAD (defined as ABI <0.9) in patients with diagnosed diabetes.[7,15,16,44–46] A large cohort study reported that 30.3% of patients with diabetes also had previously known or newly diagnosed PAD.[13] PAD in diabetic patients is more aggressive, with early large vessel involvement in addition to standard microangiopathy.[33] Also, patients with longstanding diabetes are more likely to have more severe LEPAD[47,48] and suffer from claudication symptoms.[33] In addition, moderate-to-severe PAD in diabetic patients may be asymptomatic because of diabetic peripheral neuropathy.[12] Thus, the risk of a diabetic patient to develop LEPAD and possibly chronic CLI is correlated to the severity and duration of the diabetes.[46,49] Diabetic patients who develop LEPAD have a nearly 10-fold increased risk for need to undergo a major amputation as compared to nondiabetic patients with LEPAD.[47,50–54]

Hypertension. Chronically elevated blood pressure results in increased shear stress against the vessel wall and causes subsequent endothelial damage. This disrupted endothelium acts as a nidus for inflammation, platelet adhesion, and cholesterol deposition (i.e., the atherosclerotic process). Therefore, it is not surprising that the majority of epidemiologic studies evaluating LEPAD have reported a strong, independent association between the presence of systolic hypertension and LEPAD.[36,55–59] Specifically, patients with a diagnosis of hypertension carry a 1.50 to 2.20 odds ratio of having or developing LEPAD compared to nonhypertensives. In addition, the presence of hypertension increased the risk of the development of claudication symptoms claudication up to fourfold, and the risk was proportional to the severity of hypertensive disease.[35]

Hyperlipidemia. Since the underlying cause of the vast majority of LEPAD is atherosclerosis, it is logic that hyperlipidemia predisposes a patient to the development and/or progression of LEPAD. However, extensive epidemiologic research in this area has proved inconsistent results. The majority of initial trials provided evidence that elevated total cholesterol levels was associated with an increased risk

of developing LEPAD.[34,58,59,60] Specifically, the incidence of LEPAD increases by 5% to 10% for each 10 mg/dL rise in total cholesterol.[23,60] Other trials have reported that high-density lipoprotein (HDL) cholesterol is protective against the development of LEPAD.[61–63] Therefore, a measure to combine these values (e.g., non-HDL cholesterol and a total to HDL cholesterol ratio) have reported patients in this highest quartile having nearly four times the claudication risk than those patients in the lowest quartile.[36,64] In addition, further studies have confirmed elevated low-density lipoprotein (LDL) levels to be associated with LEPAD and the development of claudication symptoms.[16,23,34,45,65] In addition, one study reported patients with PAD had significantly higher levels of VLDL cholesterol, IDL cholesterol, triglycerides, VLDL triglycerides, and IDL triglycerides.[63] However, evidence to support isolated hypertriglyceridemia as a risk factor for LEPAD is conflicting,[66–70] as most studies report a nonsignificant relationship following multivariate analysis.[34,71]

Homocysteinemia. Homocysteine (Hcy), an amino acid, is determined by both genetic and dietary factors and has been proven to have thrombotic and arteriosclerotic properties[72] via direct toxicity to the endothelium, increasing DNA synthesis in vascular smooth muscles, and causing oxidation of LDL.[72–74] In addition, previous studies have shown that elevated levels of serum Hcy appear to act as an independent predictor for PAD. Another study compared peak serum Hcy levels following a standard methionine loading test in normal subjects and in patients with known early PAD (diagnosed prior to 55 years of age). In this study, hyperhomocystenemia was detected in 28% of patients with known early PAD and in none of the normal subjects.[75] More specifically, a case–control study which defined hyperhomocysteinemia as a fasting Hcy level greater than 12 μmol/L or greater than 38 μmol/L 6 hours postmethionine load (dose of 100 mg/kg). The relative risk for a patient with only an elevated fasting Hcy, only elevated postload Hcy level, or both was 1.6, 1.5, and 2.5, respectively.[76,77] This risk factor has been shown to be more significant in patients with noninsulin dependent diabetes.[78] Additionally, a thorough meta-analysis reported that hyperhomocysteinemia's effect on the development of PAD was independent of serum cholesterol, diabetes mellitus, smoking, or hypertension.[72,76]

A prospective study following 351 patients with symptomatic LEPAD or cerebrovascular disease who were followed more than a 3-year period reported an increased risk of all-cause mortality, death from CV causes, and progression of coronary heart disease.[79] Although a more recent study suggested that elevated levels of serum Hcy did not predict progression of large- or small-vessel LEPAD.[80] In addition, patients with elevated serum Hcy levels who undergo lower extremity revasclurazation procedures are more likely to have failure of their vascular intervention.[81]

C-reactive Protein. Previous research[82,83] have shown that low-grade inflammation and therefore elevated inflammatory markers (e.g., C-reactive protein [CRP]) are present in patients with atherosclerotic disease is coronary and cerebral vascular beds. But more recently, a prospective study evaluated apparently healthy males with baseline serum CRP levels who subsequently developed symptoms of intermittent claudication or necessitated revascularization during a 60-month follow-up period. The findings support that patients who developed symptomatic LEPAD had significantly higher baseline CRP levels (1.4 vs. 0.99 mg/L), and the risk of developing symptomatic LEPAD increased with each increasing quartile of baseline serum CRP level (e.g., highest quartile had relative risk of 4.1 vs. patients who remained asymptomatic). The predictive value of CRP levels was independent of presence of hyperlipidemia, hypertension, and/or diabetes.[83] A more recent study suggested that an elevated level of serum hsCRP is predictive of progression of large-vessel (as evidenced by a decline in ABI measurements), but not small-vessel LEPAD.[80]

Ethnicity. Until recently, it has been difficult to assess any correlation with ethnicity and the risk of development of LEPAD since most previous large trials and registries involved non-Hispanic white patients. However, in more recent trials that have had larger percentages of minority patients, it is apparent that non-Hispanic blacks have an increased rate of LEPAD when compared to non-Hispanic whites.[7,84] Specifically, studies have reported that black race is associated with a greater than twofold risk of developing PAD.[44,85–87] This relationship persisted after multivariable analysis was made for traditional atherosclerotic risk factors, such as hypertension and diabetes.[88] In addition, there appears to be an increased risk of developing PAD in Mexican Americans when compared to non-Hispanic whites.[7,84]

On the other hand, other studies have reported other ethnic groups (e.g., Hispanics, Asians, Native Americans) as having a lower prevalence of PAD when compared to non-Hispanic white patients.[88–91] Therefore, studies to assess the relationship between ethnicity and nontraditional atherosclerotic risk factors (e.g., various markers of inflammation) with the development of LEPAD.

Specific High Risk Groups. In addition to disease comorbidities, specific patient populations have been found to have extremely high rates of LEPAD. These subpopulations include patients who are hospitalized with known CAD (40%)[91]; or have known abdominal aortic aneurysms[92] (46%), chronic renal insufficiency (27%),[93] or previous renal or cardiac transplantation.[94,95]

Genetic Influence and Protective Risk Factors. Although previous studies, including the Framingham Heart Study, have clearly shown a genetic component to the development of coronary artery disease, there has been no objective evidence correlating a positive family history of LEPAD as a risk factor for the development of LEPAD.[33] On the other hand, few patient characteristics have been elucidated that appear to incur a protective effect on the development of LEPAD and/or symptoms of claudication. The positive protective factors include regular physical activity[96] and moderate alcohol intake.[97]

Coexistence with Coronary Artery, Carotid Artery, and Renal Artery Disease. Since atherosclerosis is the major underlying disease process of LEPAD, CAD, carotid artery disease, and renal artery disease, it is intuitive that patients diagnosed with one of these disease processes have a significantly higher risk for coexistence of another of these conditions. In general, patients with LEPAD are two- to four-times more likely to have underlying CAD or carotid artery disease than those patients that do not have LEPAD[98] (Figure 33-2). A prospective study, completed in a long-term health care facility, revealed a 33% to 58% prevalence of

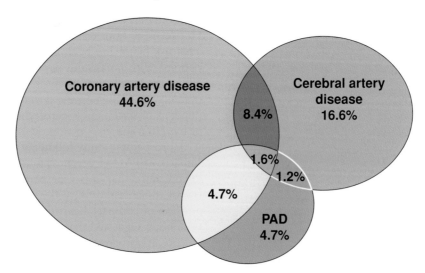

● **FIGURE 33-2.** Coexistent prevalence of peripheral, coronary, and cerebrovascular arterial disease.

Source: Reprinted with permission from Elsevier in Norgren L, Hiatt WR, Dormandy JA, et al. Inter-Society Consensus for the Management of Peripheral Arterial Disease (TASC II). J Vasc Surg 2007;45(1):S5-S67.

TABLE 33-1. Coexistent Prevalence of Carotid and Renal Arterial Disease in an Aortoiliac Artery Disease Population

	n	% (95% CI)
CAS > 50%	47	28.0 (21.2–34.8)
RAS > 60%	67	39.9 (32.5–47.3)
CAS > 50% or RAS > 60%	64	38.1 (30.8–45.4)
CAS > 50% and RAS > 60%	25	14.9 (9.5–20.3)

CAS, carotid artery stenosis; RAS, renal artery stenosis; CI, confidence interval.
Source: Miralles M, Corominas A, Cotillas J, Castro F, Clara A, Vidal-Barraquer F. Screening for carotid and renal artery stenoses in patients with aortoiliac disease. Ann Vasc Surg. 1998;12(1):17-22.

coexistence of symptomatic coronary artery disease, PAD, and/or atherothrombotic brain infarctions in their patient population.[84] Another study suggest that in patients with known LEPAD, angiographically proven coronary heart disease can be seen in up to 90%.[99,100] Similar studies have reported more than one-fourth of patients undergoing coronary angiography prior to elective LEPAD revascularization surgery have severe triple-vessel coronary artery disease.[101] Furthermore, an autopsy study which evaluated the coronary arteries in elderly patients (mean age 63 years) who had undergone amputation of at least one lower extremity because of severe LEPAD revealed that 92% of subjects had severe atherosclerotic narrowing (>75% of CSA) of at least one major epicardial vessels.[102] Although the association is less dramatic, it appears that in patients with known LEPAD, carotid artery disease is seen in up to 25% of patients.[33,102] However, these patients rarely have any history of clinically significant cerebrovascular events (less than 5%).[33]

In addition, a smaller study of patients undergoing elective aortoiliac surgery revealed nearly 40% of patients showed >60% stenosis in one or both renal arteries as assessed by renal duplex scanning. These patients were more likely to have significant renal artery stenosis if the planned aortoiliac surgery was secondary to obstructive arterial disease rather than abdominal aortic aneurysm (43% vs. 29%), or had an ABI less than 0.5 (73% coprevalence rate).[103] Although not yet supported by clinical data, some suggest that in patients with PAD, the presence of significant renal artery stenosis portends a higher mortality rate[33] (Table 33-1).

● ANATOMICAL AREAS OF INTEREST

Embryology. Early in development, the embryologic dorsal aorta develops three sets of branches, including the (dorsal and ventral) intersegmental arteries which give rise to vasculature of the head, neck, body wall, vertebral column, and limbs. The median sacral artery is the small continuation of the dorsal aorta beyond the bifurcation at the iliac arteries. The fifth intersegmental artery which becomes the lumbar and lateral sacral arteries, together with an axial artery that develops along the central axis of the limb, supply blood to each leg limb bud. This original axial artery, which develops as a continuation of the internal iliac artery, terminates into a plexus where it joins the femoral artery. The axial artery, then progressively degenerates and is represented in the adult only as a small sciatic (ischiatic), inferior gluteal, popliteal, and distal section of the peroneal artery. Thereafter, the majority of the limb blood supply is derived from the external iliac artery. For instance, the obturator artery, tibial arteries, and proximal part of the popliteal artery develop much later in utero[104] (Figure 33-3).

In vast majority of patients with normal arterial anatomy, the abdominal aorta bifurcates into the common iliac arteries at the level of the fourth and fifth lumbar vertebrae (Figure 33-4). Each common iliac artery travels laterally and caudally and gives rise to small branches to the peritoneum, lumbar musculature, ureters, and occasionally iliolumbar or accessory renal arteries. The common iliac artery terminates by dividing into the hypogastric and external iliac artery, the latter supplying blood to the lower extremity. The hypogastric artery provides blood to the pelvis, buttocks, genitalia, and medial thigh. In addition, the common iliac gives rise to small branches to the peritoneum, lumbar musculature, ureters, and occasionally iliolumbar or accessory renal arteries (Figures 33-5 and 33-6). In addition, there is an extensive collateral circulation present involving the iliac and pelvic vasculature (Figure 33-7).

The external iliac artery courses to the inguinal ligament and becomes the common femoral artery (CFA) just distal to the lateral circumflex and inferior epigastric arteries. The first portion of the CFA, which is enclosed in a fibrous sheath (i.e., the femoral sheath), subsequently divides into the deep profunda femoral artery (PFA) and the superficial femoral artery (SFA) (Figures 33-8 to 33-10). From its posterolateral origin at the CFA, the PFA travels deep behind the adductor longus and adductor magnus, feeding blood to the posterior thigh musculature and acts as an important source of collateral flow to the distal vessels. More specifically, the PFA gives off the lateral and medial femoral circumflex, perforating and muscular arteries.

As the SFA courses along the upper third and middle part of the thigh, it is contained in the femoral triangle (Scarpa's triangle) and adductor canal (Hunter's canal), respectively. Major branches of the SFA include the superficial epigastric, superficial iliac circumflex, superficial and deep external pudendal, and various muscular branches. The SFA ends as it passes into the adductor canal and becomes the popliteal artery. In turn, the popliteal artery gives off blood supply to numerous cutaneous, muscular (to the posterior thigh and lower leg musculature), and genicular arterial branches (Figure 33-11). At the lower border of the popliteus muscle, the popliteal artery divides into the anterior tibial artery and tibioperoneal, which further divides into the peroneal and posterior tibial (PT) arteries. Also, surrounding the knee is a complex network of vessels that constitutes a superficial and deep plexus (Figure 33-12).

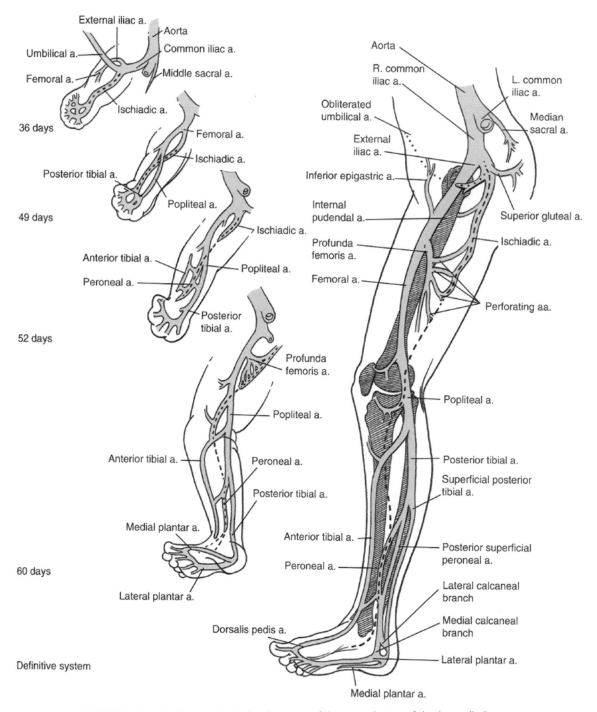

● **FIGURE 33-3.** Embryologic development of the vasculature of the lower limb.

Source: Reprinted with permission from Elsevier in Larsen WJ, Sherman LS, Potter SS, and Scott WJ.
Human Embryology. 3rd ed. Philadelphia, PA: Churchill Livingstone; 1993.

For the majority of its course, the anterior tibial artery travels along the interosseous membrane supplying the front of the leg via the tibial recurrent, fibular, maelle-olar, and more muscular artery branches (Figure 33-13). At the lower part of the leg, the anterior tibial artery lies along the tibia and becomes the dorsalis pedis artery. In contrast, the majority of the blood supply to posterior lower leg musculature arises from the PT artery. As the PT artery travels on the tibial side of the leg to the posterior aspect of

the ankle, it gives rise to several branches including malleo-lar, medial calcaneal, muscular, and the peroneal artery. The peroneal artery travels down the medial side of the fibula and terminates into lateral calcaneal branches.

The majority of the blood supply to the foot is from the dorsalis pedis artery, peroneal artery, and the distal branches of the PT artery (Figure 33-14). Initially, the anterior tibial artery gives rise to the anterior (medial and lateral) malle-olar arteries that arise above the ankle and travel through

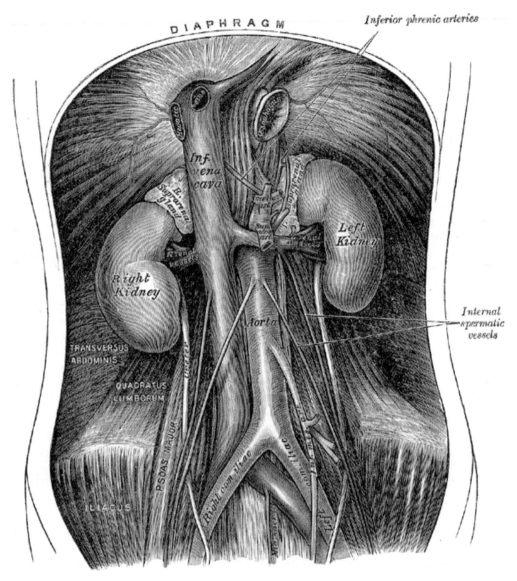

● **FIGURE 33-4.** Branches of the abdominal aorta.

Source: Reprinted with permission from Elsevier in Standring S, ed. Gray's Anatomy. The Anatomical Basis of Clinical Practice. 39th ed. Philadelphia, PA: Churchill Livingstone; 2005.

the sides of the ankle, and anastomose distally with the (medial and lateral) plantar arteries (Figure 33-15). Also, the dorsalis pedis artery branches include the tarsal (medial and lateral), arcuate, and deep plantar arteries. The tarsal arteries provide blood supply to the medial and lateral borders of the foot, and anastomose distally with the branches of the malleolar and lateral plantar arteries. The arcuate artery gives off the second, third, and fourth dorsal metatarsal arteries and subsequent digital branches. The dorsalis pedis terminates into the bifurcation of the first dorsal metatarsal and deep plantar artery (Figure 33-16). These arteries mainly supply the halux and sole of the foot, respectively. Lastly, the PT artery gives rise to the calcaneal arteries (supplying the heel) and nutrient artery (supplying the navicular bone). The PT ends at the takeoff of the medial and lateral plantar arteries. The smaller medial plantar artery courses toward the base of the halux and supplies

blood flow to the halux and musculature on the medial portion of the foot. On the other hand, the lateral plantar artery tranverses laterally to join with the deep plantar branch of the dorsalis pedis artery (the plantar arch). This artery acts as the major blood supply of the lateral foot musculature; second, third, and fourth metatarsals; and digits.[105]

Variant Anatomy. Minor alterations in the above described anatomy; considered merely normal variants, occur in the general population. For example, the level of aortic bifurcation varies and may be seen below the level of the iliac crest. Levels of bifurcation and relative lengths of the each of the described arteries can vary. Cases have been reported of patients with absence of the CFA, SFA, and/or PFA[106]; duplication of the SFA and/or PFA[107]; SFA bifurcation again after the origin of the PFA; or the popliteal artery trifurcating directly into the anterior tibial, PT, and

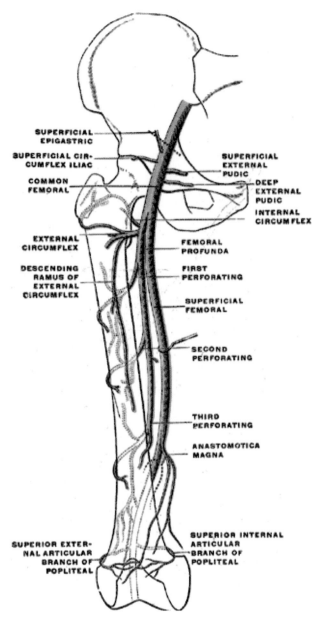

● **FIGURE 33-5.** Collateral circulation around the hip and thigh.

Source: Reprinted with permission from Elsevier in Standring S, ed. Gray's Anatomy. The Anatomical Basis of Clinical Practice. 39th ed. Philadelphia, PA: Churchill Livingstone; 2005.

peroneal artery[106] (Figure 33-17). Also, there appears to be a clear association with some chromosomal abnormality syndromes (e.g., disorganization-like syndrome, campomelic syndrome, congenital abnormalities of the lower limb) and abnormalities in lower leg vasculature.[108–110] Other rare causes of LEPAD include gelatinous dystrophy, Leriche-Fontaine aneursymal dystrophy, and anterior tibial hypoplasia.[111]

Persistence of Sciatic (Ischiatic) Artery. The sciatic artery is an embryologic continuation of the internal iliac artery into the popliteal–tibial arteries. In early embryologic

development, it serves as the major source of blood supply to the lower limb bud. In normal embryologic development, the sciatic artery involutes once the femoral arteries form and provide the majority of blood to the lower extremity.[112] Normal adult remnants of the proximal sciatic artery are the proximal portions of the anterior and superior gluteal arteries, the artery to the sciatic nerve, and the popliteal and peroneal arteries[112,113] (Figure 33-18). However, in less than 0.5% of adults, the embryologic sciatic artery persists. In most cases, this occurs when the femoral arterial vasculature (specifically, the SFA) fails to develop properly.[112] In these patients, the persistent sciatic artery (PSA) may continue to be the major blood supply to the lower extremity as a continuation from the internal iliac artery to the popliteal artery.[114–116] Five types of PSA anomalies have been described in attempt to better compare outcomes from different centers: Type I—complete PSA with continuity from the internal iliac to the popliteal artery with the femoral system ending as the saphenous artery; Type II—complete PSA associated with aplastic external iliac and femoral arteries and normal superficial femoral and popliteal arteries; Type III—incomplete PSA with the femoral system ending as the saphenous and sural arteries; Type IV—incomplete PSA with hypoplasia of the sciatic artery in the thigh with the femoral system as the dominant supply to the lower extremity; and Type V—incomplete PSA with hypoplasia of both the femoral and the sciatic arteries with limb atrophy.[117] Of more clinical importance, there is an estimated 44% incidence of aneurysmal dilatation in these persistent sciatic arteries.[115] Other vascular findings that can be seen in conjunction with persistent sciatic arteries include abnormal iliac and hypogastric arteries,[118–120] and various venous anomalies.[119–122]

Most commonly, a PSA is an incidental finding. However, patients with this disorder may present with abnormal lower extremity pulses, claudication, sciatic pain (via compression of the adjacent sciatic nerve), a pulsatile mass in the buttocks, or rupture.[115,118,122–124] Diagnosis can be readily made by ultrasound, computed tomography (CT), magnetic resonance imaging, or angiography. Treatment is not necessary for asymptomatic patients with persistent sciatic arteries. However, aneursymal sciatic arteries should be occluded by surgical ligation or transcatheter embolization in attempts to prevent distal embolization or rupture.[112] In select patients, bypass revascularization from an adequate proximal (femoral) artery to the distal limb vasculature may be necessary.[116,125,126]

● **CLASSIFICATION**

There are two major schemes to characterize PAD: The Fontaine and Rutherford Classifications. The severity of a patient's disease process is based on symptoms, evidence of tissue damage, and/or tissue loss. The Fontaine classification includes four stages (Table 33-2). Fontaine I represents asymptomatic individuals; Stages IIa and IIb describe individuals with mild and moderate claudication, respectively; Stage III includes patients with ischemic rest pain;

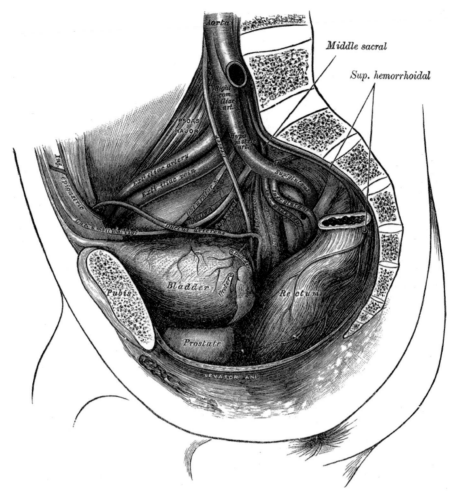

● **FIGURE 33-6.** Arterial system of the pelvis.

Source: Reprinted with permission from Elsevier in Standring S, ed. Gray's Anatomy. The Anatomical Basis of Clinical Practice. 39th ed. Philadelphia, PA: Churchill Livingstone; 2005.

and patients with ischemic ulcerations or gangrene are classified as Fontaine Stage IV. Similarly, the newer Rutherford classification divides PAD into five grades (0-IV), which include six categories: Rutherford Grade 0 represents asymptomatic individuals; Grade I signifies claudication symptoms of varying severity; Grade II describes patients with ischemic rest pain; and Grades III and IV include patients with tissue loss, ulceration, or gangrene.[33,127]

● ETIOLOGY

The most common cause of LEPAD is systemic, atherosclerotic disease. However, LEPAD may also be caused by degenerative disorders that affect arterial wall structure and subsequent dilation[99] including Marfan syndrome, Ehlers-Danlos syndrome (EDS), and cystic medical necrosis. The disorders that lead to thromboembolic phenomenon or inflammatory changes, in the vessel wall, may also lead LEPAD (Table 33-3).

Atherosclerosis

The most common cause of asymptomatic and symptomatic LEPAD is atherosclerosis. Studies have shown that this disease is a complex, chronic, active immunoinflammatory and fibroproliferative process. The atherosclerotic plaques begin with macrophages and cholesterol deposition into intact, but leaky endothelium. These complexes become oxidized and, in turn, become proinflammatory, prothrombotic, and chemotaxic via the MMP, tissue factor and further macrophage recruitment. This inflammatory process promotes further cholesterol deposition and plaque formation. The process continues as smooth muscle cell proliferation occurs in attempt to heal and repair arterial injury. This fibroproliferative process may thicken the plaque's cap, but also may become voluminous and result in symptomatic stenosis.[127,128] These plaques may continue to remain stable or become unstable, the latter often referred to as "vulnerable" plaques. These vulnerable plaques have been defined to have a (1) thin fibrous cap, (2) necrotic; lipid rich core, and (3) dense macrophage infiltration.[129] Once a vulnerable plaque ruptures, circulating platelets adhere to the necrotic core and monocytes secrete tissue factor promoting thrombosis or embolization.[1]

Patients with (and without) underlying atherosclerosis may present with an embolic phenomenon that leads to symptoms of LEPAD. Patients with known atherosclerosis

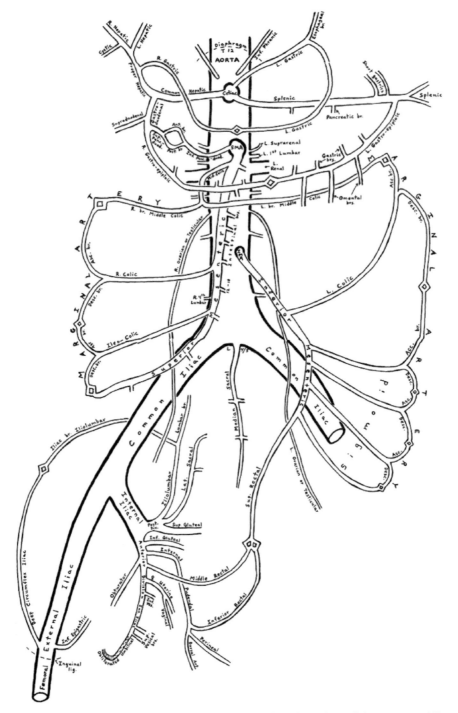

● **FIGURE 33-7.** Extensive collateral circulation of the branches of the aorta and iliac vessels.

Source: Adapted from Agur, Grant's Atlas of Anatomy, 9th ed. and S. Meltzer, Medical Class of 1991.

are prone to cholesterol plaque rupture and subsequent thrombosis or distal atheroembolization resulting in thrombosis. Other conditions (e.g., primary prothrombotic diseases, atrial fibrillation, prosthetic valves, aneurysmal disease, ventricular thrombus, or endocarditis) predispose patients to an embolic event that may affect large or medium-sized arterial vessels.[99] Embolic events may classically appear on angiography with multiple filling defects, filling defects at bifurcations, meniscus sign, and/or lack of collateral or notable atherosclerotic disease.[33]

Abdominal Coarctation of the Aorta

Claudication secondary to abdominal (infrarenal) coarctation of the aorta with/without severe hypoplasia of the aortoiliac femoral arterial system has been reported.[130–134]

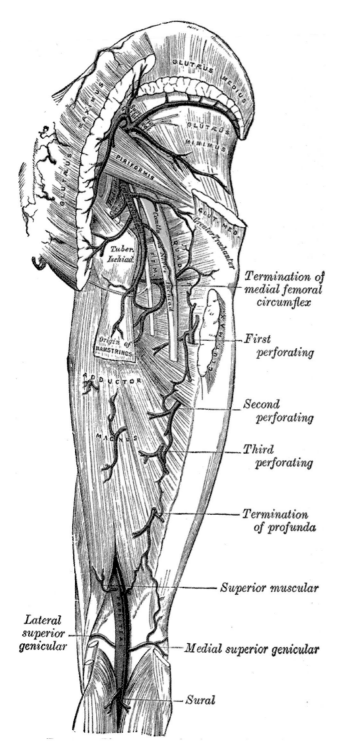

● **FIGURE 33-8.** Arterial system of the gluteal and posterior femoral regions.

Source: Reprinted with permission from Elsevier in Standring S, ed. Gray's Anatomy. The Anatomical Basis of Clinical Practice. 39th ed. Philadelphia, PA: Churchill Livingstone; 2005.

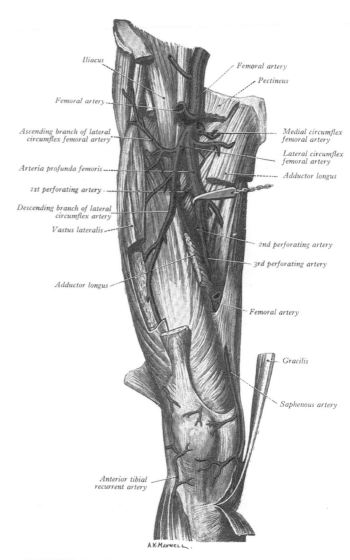

● **FIGURE 33-9.** Arterial system of the profunda femoral artery.

Source: Reprinted with permission from Elsevier in Standring S, ed. Gray's Anatomy. The Anatomical Basis of Clinical Practice. 39th ed. Philadelphia, PA: Churchill Livingstone; 2005.

Aneurysmal Disease and Acute Dissection

Diseases of the arterial wall (e.g., atherosclerosis, connective tissue disorders, trauma, nonspecific inflammatory changes, etc.) can lead to local weakening and subsequent aneurysm formation. In the case of atherosclerosis, the exact mechanism of aneurysm formation is unknown. Although it is likely because of a combination of compromise of oxygen and nutrients to the media and aortic wall shear stress from hypertension. This scenario leads to ischemic injury to the media producing local weakening and damage (to the media and elastic membrane) to the vessel wall. Subsequently, this weakening allows dilatation of the aorta that (based on Laplace's law) results in further wall tension stress and further dilatation of the vessel lumen. This process may be accentuated by an active inflammatory and proteolytic process. Also, these aneursymal lesions are

Typically, these patients present with hypertension, cardiac failure, claudication, or decreased lower extremity pulses.[130,131,133–135] Diagnosis can be confirmed with contrast aortography and standard treatment is surgical bypass revascularization.

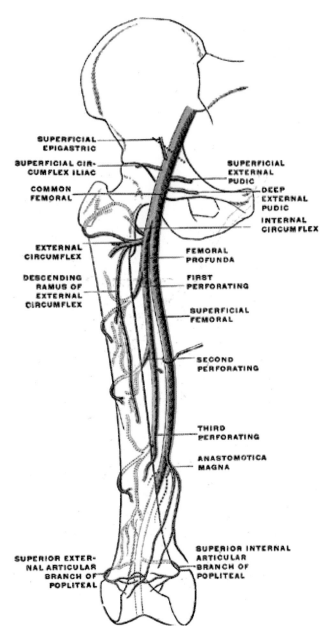

● FIGURE 33-10. Arterial system of the superficial femoral region.

Source: Reprinted with permission from Elsevier in Standring S, ed. Gray's Anatomy. The Anatomical Basis of Clinical Practice. 39th ed. Philadelphia, PA: Churchill Livingstone; 2005.

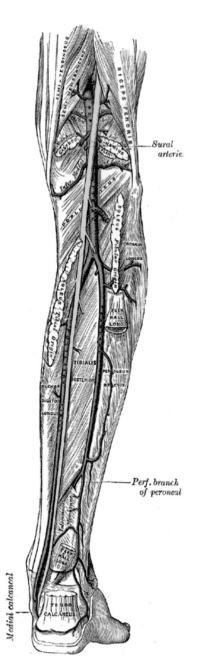

● FIGURE 33-11. Arterial system of the popliteal, PT, and peroneal region.

Source: Reprinted with permission from Elsevier in Standring S, ed. Gray's Anatomy. The Anatomical Basis of Clinical Practice. 39th ed. Philadelphia, PA: Churchill Livingstone; 2005.

predisposed to dissection that may cause distal ischemia via rupture or lumen occlusion.

In addition, as a result of nonlaminar flow through the aneursymal segment, blood stasis may occur predisposing the patient to lumen thrombus formation. This thrombus material may embolize distally and produce ischemic symptoms.

Aneurysmal disease can be seen in any arterial vascular bed. Most commonly, it affects the aorta with and without combination with more distal peripheral arterial beds. The most commonly occurring peripheral arterial aneurysms are popliteal artery aneurysms (PAAs), which account for up to

85% of all peripheral arterial aneurysms, and are most often because of underlying atherosclerosis.[135] These aneurysms, defined when the artery is greater than 1.5 cm, are often bilateral and associated with abdominal aortic aneurysms.[136] These aneurysms may be asymptomatic if small, but also may present as symptomatic disease (e.g., claudication/rest pain or leg pain/numbness as a result of mass effect and compression). PAAs may present with acute limb ischemia caused by acute vessel thrombosis (Figure 33-19), distal embolization or rupture—all historically carrying a high rate of limb loss.[137]

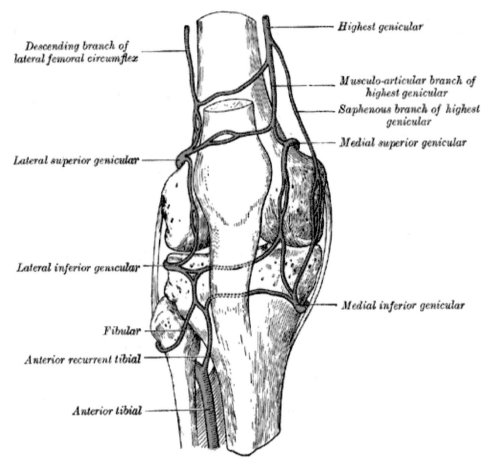

Descending branch of lateral femoral circumflex

Lateral superior genicular

Lateral inferior genicular

Fibular

Anterior recurrent tibial

Anterior tibial

Highest genicular

Musculo-articular branch of highest genicular

Saphenous branch of highest genicular

Medial superior genicular

Medial inferior genicular

● **FIGURE 33-12.** Arterial anastomoses of the knee joint.

Source: Reprinted with permission from Elsevier in Standring S, ed. Gray's Anatomy. The Anatomical Basis of Clinical Practice. 39th ed. Philadelphia, PA: Churchill Livingstone; 2005.

In contrast, aneurysms involving the CFA are rare but also are a marker of possibly aneurismal disease elsewhere (Figure 33-20). Common femoral artery aneurysms (CFAA) can be classified anatomically as Type I, in which the aneurysm ends before the bifurcation of the CFA into the superficial femoral and profunda femoris arteries, and Type II, in which the aneurysm involves the orifice of the profunda femoris artery.

However, aneursymal disease isolated to the iliac system (IIAA) can be seen in 2% to 7% of patients affected with intra-abdominal aneurysms. Of note, these isolated iliac aneurysms are mostly asymptomatic but do carry a high rate of rupture, embolization, thrombosis, compression of adjacent structures, and significant operative mortality.[138,139]

Connective Tissue Disorders

Ehlers-Danlos Syndrome. EDS is a disorder consisting of nine distinct subtypes, all of which are characterized by abnormal collagen and subsequent hyperelasticity of the skin and hypermobile joints. The diagnosis of EDS is based on the clinical presentation: Patients typically present in the third decade with hyperplastic and fragile skin, hypermobile joints, or spontaneous rupture of arteries in the legs

with ensuing ecchymosis.[140–143] Currently, there is no specific therapy for patients with EDS. Since patients with Type IV and IX (Menkes' Syndrome) have been found to have an increased risk of arterial aneurysm formation and possible arterial (e.g., popliteal, femoral, iliac, and aorta) dissection or rupture, it would be prudent for these patients to undergo serial ultrasound evaluations for early detection of aneurysm formation. However, surgical repair of detected aneurysms may be complicated by the increased friability of tissues and pseudoaneursym formation.[144–146]

Pseudoxanthoma Elasticum. Pseudoxanthoma elasticum is a rare, inherited connective tissue disorder that results in abnormal elastic fibers. Pseudoxanthoma elasticum most commonly presents in the second to fourth decade of life[147] with symptoms related to elastic degeneration of the skin, eyes, gastrointestinal system, or arteries (18% present with intermittent claudication).[148–150] All arterial beds may be affected and is manifested as progressive luminal narrowing with severe arterial calcification that may lead to complete occlusion.[148–150] Treatment consists of avoidance of dietary calcium and standard (albeit often extensive) revascularization interventions for only symptomatic stenosis.[151]

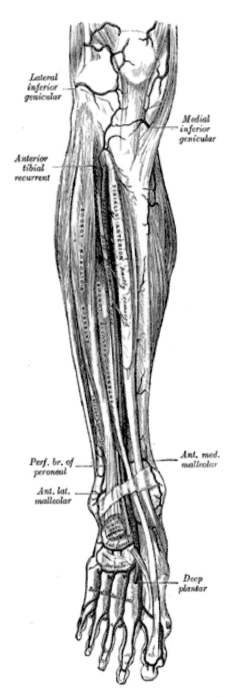

● **FIGURE 33-13.** Arterial system of the tibial and dorsal pedis regions.

Source: Reprinted with permission from Elsevier in Standring S, ed. Gray's Anatomy. The Anatomical Basis of Clinical Practice. 39th ed. Philadelphia, PA: Churchill Livingstone; 2005.

Fibromuscular Dysplasia. Fibromuscular dysplasia (FMD) is a disease affecting medium- and small-sized arteries. It is most commonly seen affecting the renal or carotid arterial vasculature, although there have been reports of isolated abnormalities of the iliac and lower limb vasculature.[152] Histologic examination most often reveals medial dysplasia with or without fibrosis of the elastic membrane in the diseased vessel wall. Specifically in isolated cases of lower limb vasculature, the abnormality

has been theorized to be attributable to arteritis, previous thigh injury, or thromboembolic events with recanalization of the artery.[152] Diagnosis can be made by angiography revealing a classic "string of beads" appearance reflecting diseased, thickened fibromuscular ridges adjacent to thin, less involved arterial wall segments. Treatment consists of PTA or surgical revascularization for symptomatic patients. In addition, these patients presenting with FMD of the lower extremity should be routinely screened for similar disease in the carotid and renal vasculature.

Adventitial Cystic Disease. Cystic adventitial disease, whereas intramural mucin-containing cysts occur between the media and adventitial layers of the vessel wall, has been reported to cause claudication. This condition more commonly affects the popliteal and femoral artery, and presents as sudden calf claudication aggravated by knee flexion.[153,154] However, this condition was first described affecting the external iliac artery.[155] Diagnosis can be made using Doppler ultrasound, CT, or MR. Also, contrast angiography may depict a smooth, curvilinear stenosis (scimitar sign) or hour-glass narrowing. Treatment may include cyst evacuation or aspiration, patch angioplasty, or surgical resection with vein bypass.[154,156,157]

Vasculitis

Vasculitides consist of a large, variable group of chronic inflammatory disorders that result in damage to the blood vessel structure. These conditions result in a reduced peripheral blood flow caused by endothelial dysfunction and/or vascular obstructions.[158] A broad range of vasculitic disease states exists, since any vessel type, vessel size, and vascular bed can be affected. (Of note, limb ischemia may develop acutely with inflammatory processes such as HIV arteriopathy).[33]

Thromboangiitis Obliterans. Thromboangiitis obliterans (TO or Buerger disease) is an inflammatory disorder resulting in stenosis and obstruction of medium- and small-sized vessels in the distal arms and legs. The disease typically affects young Asian males (although women and the elderly have been reported) with heavy tobacco use. Although the underlying pathophysiology of TO is unclear, it is suggested that it may be an autoimmune reaction against a component of tobacco. Histologic examination reveals leukocyte and fibroblast infiltration leading to perivascular fibrosis and recanalization. Also, endothelin-1, a potent vasoconstrictor, may be elevated in patients with TO.[159–161] Patients with TO often present with claudication or ischemic rest pain in the hand or foot. In more severe cases, ulcerations and gangrene of the fingers and toes may occur.

Diagnosis is supported by angiography depicting smooth, tapering segmental lesions in the distal vasculature and/or classic "corkscrew" appearance of arteries resulting from vascular damage at sites of occlusions (Figure 33-21). In contrast to other vasculitidis, TO does not affect arteries outside the limb vasculature (e.g., visceral, pulmonary,

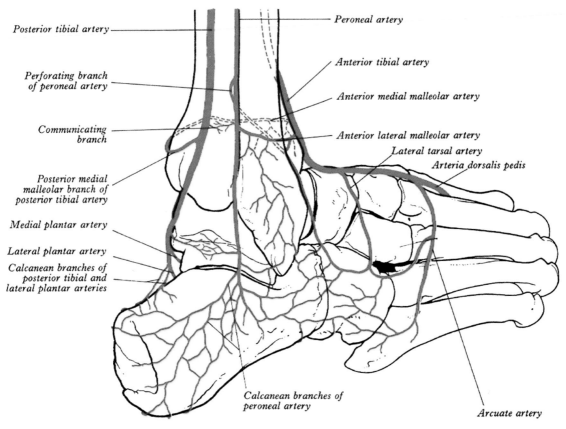

● **FIGURE 33-14.** Arterial anastomoses of the ankle joint.

Source: Reprinted with permission from Elsevier in Standring S, ed. Gray's Anatomy. The Anatomical Basis of Clinical Practice. 39th ed. Philadelphia, PA: Churchill Livingstone; 2005.

renal, cerebral vasculature). To date, there has been no data to support the benefit for use of antiplatelet, anticoagulant, or anti-inflammatory medications in these patients. The only effective treatment for Buerger disease is immediate and complete cessation of tobacco use. Results with sympathectomy to control the vasospastic component of the disorder has been have been suboptimal. In end-stage patients, attempts with omentopexy (pedicled omental transplantation) to the affected limb to avoid amputation have been promising with nearly 85% limb-salvage rates.[162,163]

Takayasu Arteritis. Most commonly, Takayasu's arteritis (TA) affects the aortic arch and its branches (large- and medium-sized vessels) of young women. The underlying pathophysiology of TA is unclear, but immunopathogenic mechanisms have been suggested. Histologic examination suggests a panarteritis with inflammatory infiltrates, occasional giant cells, marked intimal proliferation and fibrosis, scarring of the media, and degeneration of the elastic lamina.[164] Affected patients may complain of fever, fatigue or be noted to have new-onset hypertension, aortic insufficiency, or suffer a cerebrovascular event. In severe cases, patients may present with arm and/or leg claudication. Often, these patients will have evidence of arterial occlusive disease on physical examination with appreciable bruits and significantly dimished (or absent) peripheral pulses. Diag-

nosis can be confirmed by ultrasound and MR (evidenced by thickening of the aortic wall) or contrast angiography (revealing stenosis, poststenotic dilatation, aneurysm formation and occlusion of the aorta with possible involvement of its major branches). Most patients respond to prednisone therapy, but methotrexate may be useful. Additional revascularization via endovascular or surgical bypass revascularization also may be needed for significant stenosis.

Giant Cell Arteritis. Giant cell arteritis (GCA or temporal arteritis) is the most common adult type of vasculitis that occurs almost exclusively in the elderly population. This disorder typically affects the carotid artery and its branches, but may affect any large- or medium-sized artery, including, but rarely, the lower extremities. Nearly half of GCA patients are found to have polymyalgia rheumatica. Classic presenting symptoms include headache or scalp tenderness, jaw claudication, proximal muscle pain, fever or blurred vision. If severe and left untreated, it may progress to blindness. The underlying mechanism of this disease is unknown, but likely related to an autoimmune reaction or elevated levels of endothelin-1, a potent vasoconstrictor.[159–161] Histologic examination reveals a panarteritis with leukocyte infiltrates in the vessel wall with frequent giant cell formation. Diagnosis is made the clinical scenario, elevated sedimentation rate, and confirmed by biopsy of the temporal

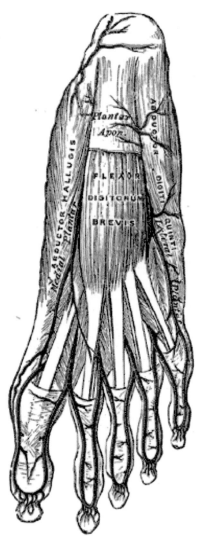

● FIGURE 33-15. Plantar arteries of the foot—superficial dissection.

Source: Reprinted with permission from Elsevier in Standring S, ed. Gray's Anatomy. The Anatomical Basis of Clinical Practice. 39th ed. Philadelphia, PA: Churchill Livingstone; 2005.

(affected) artery. The current treatment for TA is prednisone therapy. Smaller studies have reported response to therapy with methotrexate and tumor necrosis factor blockers.

Behcet Disease. Behcet disease, presumed to be immune mediated, presents typically as a triad of mouth ulcers, genital ulcers, and eye inflammation. But, in less common instances, it may include a panarteritis affecting even the limb arteries. Vascular symptoms include claudication or a lower extremity mass that can be as a result of aneursymal formation or occlusion of an affected arterial bed. The underlying histopathology reveals fragmentation of the vessel wall's elastic fibers, degeneration of vasa vasorum with perivascular round cell infiltrate.[165,166] Diagnosis can be made with CT or angiography. Treatment usually includes immune-mediated medications and possible surgical resection and/or bypass revascularization. However, surgical re-

pair is complicated by the diseased delicate vessel walls, which predispose the patient to pseudoaneurysm at the site of anastomosis or thrombosis of the bypass grafts.[166–169]

Other Etiologies

Vasospastic (Raynaud) Disease. Abnormal peripheral vasospasm, first described by Maurice Raynaud in 1862,[170] is often caused by increased vascular tone in response to cold or emotional stimuli. Classic presentation occurs in three phases: First, the digits main arterial branches constrict resulting in paleness, numbness, pain or parasthesias; second, the digits become cyanotic and become purple or black in appearance; and third, the blood flow is reestablished with postischemic hyperemia and the digits appear purple. The pathophysiology of this condition is unclear, although many believe it is a result of endothelial dysfunction. The abnormal vascular tone may be a primary (Raynaud disease) or secondary phenomenon (usually because of an underlying collagen vascular disease). The diagnosis of Raynaud disease is entirely based on clinical presentation and there are no laboratory or imaging tests needed for confirmation (although some may be done to rule out other etiologies). Treatment for Raynaud disease includes avoidance of sudden cold exposure, cessation of tobacco use, and avoidance of sympathomimetic medications (e.g., decongestatnts, amphetamies, etc.). Cases that are more resistant may be treated with calcium channel blockers, other vasodilators, sympatholytic agents, and prostaglandins.

Pernio (Chilbain's Disease). Similar in clinical presentation to Raynaud disease, pernio is an inflammatory condition characterized by raised red and blue, pruritic lesions located on the pretibial area and toes. In severe cases, these lesions may blister or ulcerate. Typically, these lesions last less than 3 weeks. Pernio is caused by an abnormal vasomotor tone response to cold exposure, and therefore most likely to present in the spring and autumn (during cold, damp conditions). Pernio may be idiopathic or secondary to an underlying disorder (e.g., chronic myelomonocytic leukemia, macroglobulinemia, cyroglobulinemia, antiphospholipid antibody syndrome, or anorexia nervosa). A variant of pernio is chilblain lupus erythematosus that manifests as similar lesions over the dorsal interphalangeal joints. These patients often have abnormal serology (antinuclear antibody and/or rheumatoid factor) and a small proportion progress to develop systemic lupus. Diagnosis can be confirmed by lesion biopsy revealing dermal edema, perivascular lymphocytic infiltrate ("fluffy edema" of vessel walls) and epidermal spongiosis or necrosis. Treatment consists of keeping affected areas warm and dry. Several other studies have suggested that vasodilator medications, such as calcium channel blockers, or ultraviolet light therapy may have clinical benefit in treating and preventing episodes.

Ergot Toxicity. Rare cases of claudication and digital ischemia may be secondary to ergot toxicity (e.g., St. Anthony's fire), most commonly seen in younger females being

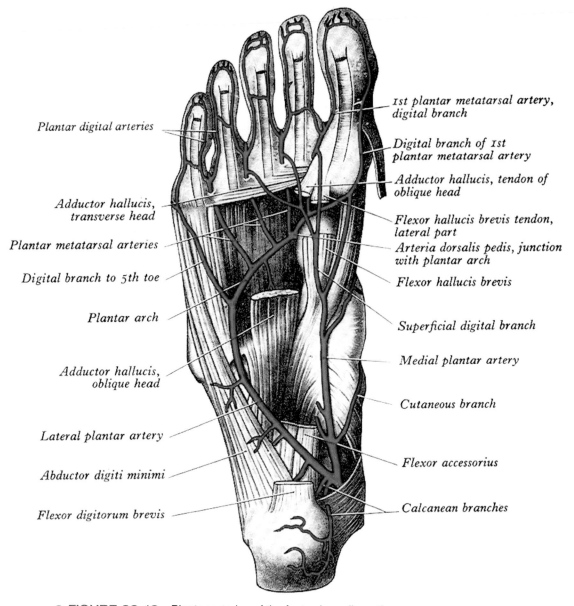

● **FIGURE 33-16.** Plantar arteries of the foot—deep dissection.

Source: Reprinted with permission from Elsevier in Standring S, ed. Gray's Anatomy. The Anatomical Basis of Clinical Practice. 39th ed. Philadelphia, PA: Churchill Livingstone; 2005.

treated with ergot derivatives for migraines. Typical symptoms are a result of an acute vasospastic episode initially occurring in the SFA and progressing distally.[171-173] Diagnosis can be made with contrast angiography which classically reveals diffuse and segmental vasospasm seen as a smooth narrowing of the vessels.[174] Treatment includes discontinuation of smoking, caffeine intake or any other offending ergot product. Additional vasodilator therapy (nitroprusside or nifedipine) may be necessary in severe or refractory cases.

Popliteal Artery Entrapment Syndrome. First described in 1879, the popliteal artery entrapment syndrome is a rare anatomic abnormality (0.2%–3% of adults) consisting of an anomalous popliteal artery, which courses around the gas-

trocnemius muscle, resulting in intermittent vascular compression (i.e., entrapment) between the muscle and medial femoral condyle.[175-177] The compression can lead to vessel wall fibrosis, stenosis, thrombosis, aneurismal dilatation, and distal microembolization.[175] This abnormality is caused by abnormal embryologic development of the gastrocnemius and popliteal artery (although cases have been reported following femoropopliteal bypass surgery because of the similar misplacement of the venous graft.[175] Based on Insua's classification, there are four variants of this entrapment syndrome, but most cases are secondary to an abnormal course of the popliteal artery or abnormal insertion site of the medial head of the gastrocnemius.[178] In rare cases, acquired entrapment syndrome may occur following surgical procedures.[175,177-180]

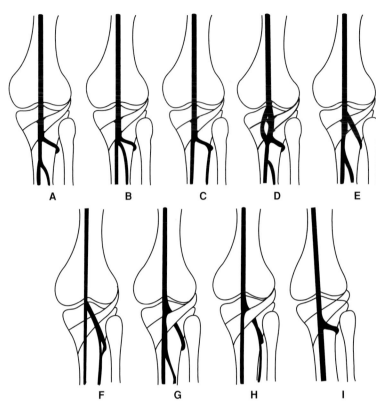

A, Normal.
B, Trifurcating popliteal artery.
C, Peroneal artery arising from low anterior tibial artery.
D, "Island" popliteal artery (very rare); this pattern was not identified in our series.
E, High anterior tibial origin passing superficial to popliteus muscle.
F, Same as E with peroneal artery arising from anterior tibial artery.
G, Same as E with anterior tibial artery passing deep to popliteus muscle.
H, Same as F except anterior tibial artery passes deep to popliteus muscle.
I, Absent posterior tibial artery.

● **FIGURE 33-17.** Anatomic variants of the popliteal artery.

Source: Mauro MA, Jaques PF, Moore M. The popliteal artery and its branches: embryologic basis of normal and variant anatomy. AJR Am J Roentgenol. 1988;150(2):435-437.

Although a rare entity, history of sudden, unilateral calf claudication with parathesia and numbness while walking—but not running—in a young, athletic male should raise the clinician's suspicion of this disorder. Diagnosis should be confirmed by angiography (performed with leg straight and in flexion), or more recently, by CT of the popliteal fossa.[175] The treatment of choice is surgical release of the gastrocnemius muscle, grafting of the damaged artery with a vein graft resulting in normal blood flow to the lower limb.[175,181]

In addition, there are several case reports of other muscular or surrounding (e.g., Baker's cyst, bony prominence, or venous aneurysm) structures constricting or compressing large arteries. For example, adductor canal compression syndrome occurs in cases where an abnormal band of tissue, originating from the adductor magnus muscle, courses across the SFA. Patients with this abnormality often are asymptomatic, but may have claudication with exercise as a result of the compression of the artery within the adductor canal. This condition may result in arterial damage and thrombotic events and can be treated with surgical ligation of the compressing tissue bands.[182] Other case reports have described the passage of the femoral artery through the sartorius muscle.[183]

Iliac Artery Entrapment Syndrome. Similarly, patients with external iliac endofibrosis (iliac artery compression)

may complain of leg pain with exercise—most commonly with high-performance cycling. Initial reports suggested the leg pain was as a result of the compression of the iliac artery at the inguinal ligament (because of the position of a cyclist).[184,185] Others suggest the symptoms that occur with exercise are secondary to marked intimal thickening and subsequent significant stenosis. Treatment of symptomatic patients may be PTA/stent, surgical endarterectomy, or surgical bypass revascularization.[185]

Pseudoocclusion. Some patients who present with symptoms of lifestyle limiting claudication or ischemic pain and undergo angiography are not found to have severely stenotic or occlusive lesions. Instead, these patients are found to have symptoms as a result of the external compression of arteries. For example, intermittent popliteal occlusion can occur with marked extension of the knee with or without plantar flexion.[186,187] In more rare instances, popliteal artery compression can occur with the knee in neutral position. Pseudoocclusion of the popliteal artery must be differentiated from popliteal entrapment syndrome that also often occurs with only extreme dorsal flexion of the ankle. Evidence that might suggest pseudoocclusion as a cause of the symptoms includes normal angiographic appearance with change in position (e.g., knee flexed) (Figure 33-22), angiographic appearance out of proportion to an ABI measurement, lack of contralateral

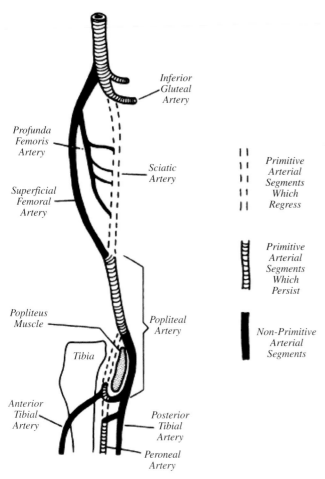

● **FIGURE 33-18.** Diagram showing embryologic development of PSA.

Source: Mauro MA, Jaques PF, Moore M. The popliteal artery and its branches: embryologic basis of normal and variant anatomy. AJR Am J Roentgenol. 1988;150(2):435-437.

disease or collateral circulation. Patients with pseudoocclusion, and therefore proven normal arterial anatomy, should not undergo mechanical intervention.[188]

Miscellaneous. Other causes of LEPAD include trauma (including iatrogenic), pseudoanueryms (PSA), and arteriovenous fistulas (AVF). A pseudoaneursym is a contained disruption of the intimal and medial layers of a vessel wall. A PA may result from blunt trauma,[189] an iatrogenic cause (e.g., arterial puncture), or dehiscence of a surgical anastomosis. Patients with PA located in the lower limb vasculature may remain asymptomatic or complain of swelling, a pulsatile mass, parasthesias, localized pain, or claudication. Symptomatic PA may be successfully treated with ultrasound-guided compression, thrombin injection, endovascular ligation or stent implantation, or via open surgical repair. In addition, these PA may become complicated by infection, most commonly by *Staphlyococcus*. Patients with infected PA most often present following a percutaneous arterial access or synthetic graft bypass revascularization procedure and require surgical excision and bypass revascularization with (commonly) the superficial femoropopliteal vein.[190]

Arteriovenous fistulas (AVF) are abnormal communications between an artery and vein, which bypasses the capillary bed. These defects may be congenital or acquired (as a complication to cardiac catheterization, etc.). Other reports have presented patients presenting with claudication because of the spontaneous arteriovenous fistulas of the lower extremities.[191] AVFs may be asymptomatic, but can present as a pulsatile mass that may result in chronic venous insufficiency and/or distal ischemia. Duplex ultrasound or angiography can confirm the diagnosis. Treatment of large/symptomatic AVFs include surgical excision.

Other modes of trauma injury include penetrating injuries, gunshot wounds or blunt trauma. Patients with traumatic vascular injury may present either hemodynamically stable or unstable. Diagnosis can be made on physical examination (e.g., evidence of distal ischemia, absent or diminished peripheral pulses, or expanding hematoma) or by

TABLE 33-2. The Two Major Schemes to Characterize PAD: The Fontaine and Rutherford Classifications

Fontaine		Rutherford		
Stage	Clinical	Grade	Category	Clinical
I	Asymptomatic	0	0	Asymptomatic
IIa	Mild claudication	I	1	Mild claudication
IIb	Moderate-to-severe claudication	I	2	Moderate claudication
		I	3	Severe claudication
III	Ischemic rest pain	II	4	Ischemic rest pain
IV	Ulceration or gangrene	III	5	Minor tissue loss
		III	6	Major tissue loss

Source: Reprinted with permission form Elsevier in Norgren L, Hiatt WR, Dormandy JA, et al. Inter-Society Consensus for the Management of Peripheral Arterial Disease (TASC II). J Vasc Surg 2007. 45(I):S5-S67.

TABLE 33-3. Differential Diagnosis in the Etiology of LEPAD and Claudication Symptoms

Anuerysmal disease
Arthritis
Atherosclerosis
Baker's cyst
Coarctation of the abdominal aorta
Chronic compartment syndrome
Cystic adventitial disease
Ischemic intermittent claudication
Emboli
Endofibrosis of the external iliac artery
FMD
Lymphangitis
Musculoskeletal
Myositis
Nerve root compression
Neuropathy
Phlebetis
Popliteal entrapment
Reflex sympathetic dystrophy
Spinal stenosis
Trauma
Vasculitis
Vascular tumors
Venous claudication

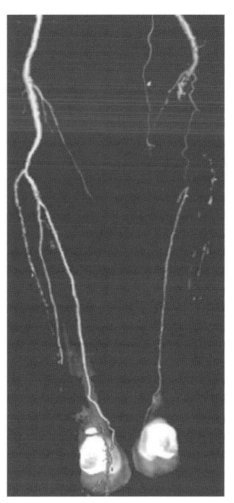

● **FIGURE 33-19.** CT images of thrombosis of the left popliteal artery with proximal aneurysal dilatation.

preoperative angiography. These patients should be treated with surgical bypass revascularization (utilizing saphenous vein or PTFE grafts) or arteriorrhaphy.[192]

● **CLINICAL PRESENTATION**

Asymptomatic

The overwhelming percentage of patients with LEPAD are asymptomatic. On the basis of previous data, nearly 90% of all PAD patients would be missed if ABI testing was reserved only for patients with classic claudication symptoms.[193] Therefore, further objective evaluation of high-risk asymptomatic patients is necessary.

Claudication

The most common presenting symptom in patients with LEPAD are atypical symptoms. However, intermittent claudication, defined as pain in the leg musculature with ambulation which is relieved by a short rest, is the earliest and most common classic presenting symptom in patients with LEPAD affecting 2% to 5% of the Unites States population older than 55 years,[21,33] with prevalence of claudication symptoms increasing with age.[33] However, the rates of reported intermittent claudication by patients greatly underestimates the prevalence of LEPAD in the general population (Figure 33-23). This is likely a result of many elderly patients who are unable to walk far enough to experience

claudication symptoms caused by other comorbidities including congestive heart failure, chronic obstructive pulmonary disease, and/or osteoarthritis. Yet, less than 25% of patients with claudication will have significant progression of their disease.[194] This stabilization of the disease process may be as a result of the development of collateral vessels, metabolic adaptation of ischemic muscle, or change in the patient's behavioral or activity patterns.[33] It is important to realize that not all subjective complaints of leg pain is claudication. Therefore, it is imperative for the clinician to have a thorough understanding of the various causes of leg discomfort (Table 33-3).

Critical Limb Ischemia

CLI, defined as pain that occurs at rest in the affected limb or impending limb loss, is secondary to a severe reduction of blood flow in the affected tissue bed.[99] These patients have tissue perfusion that is inadequate to maintain the *resting* metabolic needs of the affected limb. In a patient presenting with limb ischemia, it is mandatory that the clinician quickly determine if the disease process is acute or chronic CLI because the diagnostic methodology, therapeutic

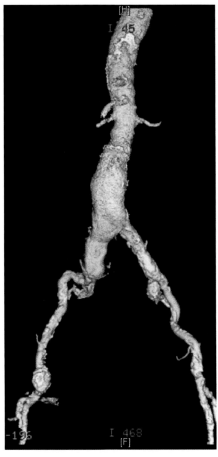

● **FIGURE 33-20.** CT image of right common femoral aneurysm.

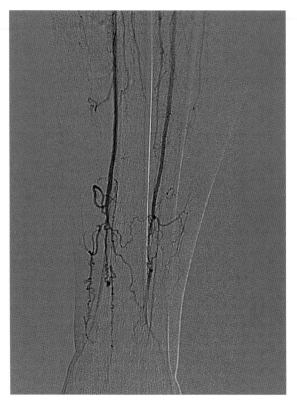

● **FIGURE 33-21.** Contrast angiography depicting smooth, tapering segmental lesions in the distal vasculature and/or classic "corkscrew" appearance in a patient with TO.

regimen, and prognosis for each is strikingly different. In general, chronic ischemic disease is defined as the presence of symptoms for more than 2 weeks.[33]

Chronic CLI

The most common symptoms of chronic CLI are rest pain, ischemic ulcers and gangrene. Rest pain as a result of severe, chronic tissue ischemia is most often located in the forefoot or toes and is not easily attenuated by standard analgesics. Since the discomfort is often worsened when the patient is supine or when the limb is elevated, it is very common for the patient to complain of the symptoms at night or while sleeping. On the other hand, ischemic ulcers often originate in patients with an ABI <0.3, T_cPO_2 <40%, ankle pressures <50 mm Hg, and/or toe pressures <30 mm Hg. These ulcers are most commonly seen at the site of non-healing minor trauma sites and may lead to osteomyelitis. These ulcers are most often dry, painful, and are located at sites of local pressure (e.g., lateral malleolus, metatarsal heads, and distal aspects of toes). Lastly, gangrene occurs when the arterial blood supply is unable to meet the metabolic needs of resting tissue.[195] It is typified by cyanotic, anesthetic tissue and can either characterized as "dry" or "wet." Dry gangrene appears hard and most often occurs in the distal toes, with clear demarcation between healthy

and necrotic tissue. In contrast, wet gangrene appears moist, swollen and may blister and carries a more severe prognosis.

Most CLI is secondary due severe atherosclerotic disease, but may be due to by a variety of diverse etiologies. But, when caused by atherosclerotic disease, CLI is a sign of severe, diffuse, or multisegmental disease.[99] Additional factors that contribute to the development and progression of CLI include diabetes, heart failure, infection, skin breakdown, or skin/tissue injury.[99] Therefore, the clinician must understand the likelihood of concomitant severe coronary and cerebrovascular disease and the subsequent greater risk of CV ischemic events[6,13,196–198] when determining the appropriate treatment strategy for a patient with CLI.

Acute CLI

Acute ischemia of the lower extremity can result from thrombosis of a preexisting atherosclerotic lesion or more commonly from an acute embolic event (Figure 33-24). It may present as either a focal event because of embolic disease or a diffuse ischemic event secondary to an abrupt occlusion of a previously stenotic area.[199] The size and consequently the level of obstruction of the embolus generally dictate the patients' symptoms, clinical signs, and the anatomic territory at risk. A more proximal obstruction by the embolus leads to a larger territory at risk, but usually a less severe presentation of ischemia because of

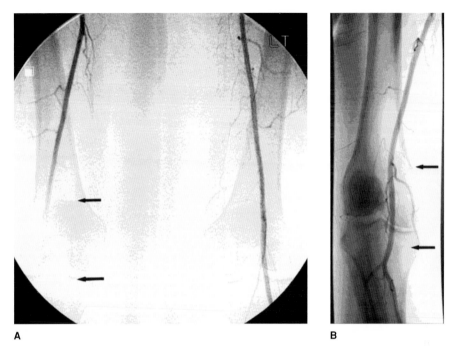

A   B

● **FIGURE 33-22.** Contrast angiography depicting pseudoocclusion of the left popliteal artery. The knee is in (A) normal supine position and (B) slightly flexed.

Source: Reprinted with permission from Wiley-Liss, Inc., a subsidiary of John Wiley & Sons, Inc. Jones WT III, Gray BH. Arteriographic evidence of pseudoocclusion of the popliteal artery: don't be fooled. Catheter Cardiovasc Interv. 2006;68(4):522-525.

collaterals. Patients who have embolization to the small digital end arterioles, quite often present with ischemic ("blue") toes that are extremely painful.

When acute limb ischemia presents as a diffuse process, the patient may experience an abrupt onset of pain, coolness, numbness and paralysis of the affected limb. In the majority of cases, acute limb ischemia is secondary to thrombo-

sis of a ruptured atherosclerotic (e.g., "vulnerable") plaque, thrombosis of a previously placed bypass graft, or embolization to the lower extremity from a cardiac or proximal aneursymal source[99,200] (although less commonly from a paradoxical or tumor embolus). When acute limb ischemia is a result of thrombosis of an existing plaque, the thrombosis tends to propogate proximally in the artery, up to the

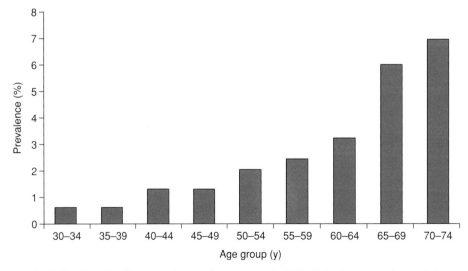

● **FIGURE 33-23.** The prevalence of symptomatic LEPAD in the general population.

Source: Reprinted with permission from Elsevier in Norgren L, Hiatt WR, Dormandy JA, et al. Inter-Society Consensus for the Management of Peripheral Arterial Disease (TASC II). J Vasc Surg 2007;45(1):S5-S67.

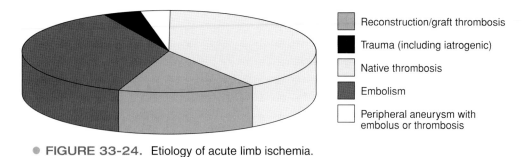

Reconstruction/graft thrombosis

Trauma (including iatrogenic)

Native thrombosis

Embolism

Peripheral aneurysm with embolus or thrombosis

● **FIGURE 33-24.** Etiology of acute limb ischemia.

Source: Reprinted with permission from Elsevier in Norgren L, Hiatt WR, Dormandy JA, et al. Inter-Society Consensus for the Management of Peripheral Arterial Disease (TASC II). J Vasc Surg 2007;45(1):S5-S67.

previous major side branch. In addition, there may be distal propogation of the thrombosis as a result of the resultant low flow state. During an embolic event, the subsequent occlusion often occurs at a branch point in the arterial tree.[99]

Acute limb ischemia caused by embolization is most likely to present as sudden, severe, pain in the affected limb. In comparison, acute limb ischemia caused by thrombosis may present more gradually. In either case, the pain often is less dependant on position and localized than that of CLI. Associated signs and symptoms of acute limb ischemia are the six P's: Pain, paralysis, paresthesias, pulselessness, pallor, and polar (cold). Typically, the line of transition in temperature or color is one limb segment below the level of occlusion. Common findings of early ischemia include loss of light touch sensation, 2-point discrimination, proprioception, and vibratory perception. Findings of motor dysfunction or pain on passive movement is indicative of advanced ischemia and impending limb loss.[99] However, it is important to note that in patients with previous neurosensory defects (such as diabetic neuropathy), pain may not be present. Also, pedal pulses may be normal in cases of microembolization.

Blue Toe Syndrome

Focal acute limb ischemic events are characterized by a sudden appearance of a cold, painful forefoot/toe in the presence or absence of strong pedal pulses. In addition, there may be evidence of petechaie or cyanosis on the soles of the ischemic foot. The "blue toe syndrome (BTS)" often suggests embolic showering from a proximal atherosclerotic lesion.

Classically, patients with BTS have dusky or bluish demarcated lesions on one or multiple toes (occasionally bilaterally) in the presence of pedal pulses. In addition, there may be evidence of petechaie or cyanosis on the soles of the ischemic foot. Cholesterol emboli incite an intense inflammatory reaction and when coupled with embolization to the renal parenchyma can lead to acute renal failure, elevated sedimentation rate with hypocomplementemia, plasma and urinary eosinophilia, a urine sediment with modest proteinuria, and livedo reticularis.

BTS can develop either spontaneously or secondary to plaque disruption during trauma, angiography/

catheterization, intra-aortic balloon pump counterpulsation, or (cardio) vascular surgery. The source of embolization is often a proximal atherosclerotic plaque, but may include proximal aneurysms (e.g., abdominal aortic aneurysm (AAA) or popliteal artery aneurysms). Since it appears that the underlying lesions that result in BTS may be multiple and can be found at various levels in the arterial tree, it can be difficult to determine the exact source of embolization. Avoiding further manipulation of the aorta is advised and hence, noninvasive diagnostic tests (e.g., Magnetic resonance angiography [MRA], CT-A, duplex) are advocated as first line.

Although, it is not possible to consistently determine the severity or extent of acute limb ischemia, a classification scheme has been constructed in attempts to further detail this disease process (Table 33-4).

● NATURAL HISTORY AND RISKS

Natural History

The natural history of patients with LEPAD has been well documented in previous studies. Patients with asymptomatic LEPAD or claudication symptoms may clinically improve, stabilize or deteriorate with possible ensuing revascularization and/or amputation (Figure 33-25). Initial studies which investigated the natural history of LEPAD reported that only 25% of these patients will *significantly* deteriorate, but only 7% and 12% patients requiring a major amputation at 5 and 10 years, respectively.[194] More recent studies confirm that the majority of patients with asymptomatic, but objectively defined LEPAD (per abnormal ABI or angiography), will not have any limiting claudication symptoms at 5 years.[33] In addition, these studies report an improved rate of major amputation of 2% at 5 years,[33,194] which likely is attributable to the current availability of more limb-salvage techniques. This small subset of patients, most often deteriorate within the first year of diagnosis compared to the years thereafter. Also, it appears that patients with an ABI <0.5 or ankle pressure <60 mm Hg have an increased risk for amputation than those patients that do not. Interestingly, studies suggest that the presence of symptoms do not indicate a higher risk of disease progression.[33] Also, patients with diabetes mellitus,

TABLE 33-4. Separation of Threatened Versus Viable Extremities

		Findings		Doppler Signals	
Category	Description/Prognosis	Sensory Loss	Muscle Weakness	Arterial	Venous
I. Viable	Not immediately threatened	None	None	Audible	Audible
II. Threatened					
a. Marginal	Salvageable if promptly treated	Minimal (toes) or none	None	Inaudible (often)	Audible
b. Immediate	Salvageable with immediate revascularization	More than toes, associated with rest pain	Mild, moderate	Inaudible (usually)	Audible
III. Irreversible	Major tissue loss or permanent nerve damage inevitable	Profound, anesthetic	Profound, paralysis (rigor)	Inaudible	Inaudible

Source: Reprinted with permission form Elsevier in Norgren L, Hiatt WR, Dormandy JA, et al. Inter-Society Consensus for the Management of Peripheral Arterial Disease (TASC II). J Vasc Surg 2007. 45(I):S5-S67.

tobacco abuse, or severely abnormal ABI (less than 0.5) were more likely to have progressive LEPAD.[50,51,201,202]

In patients with critical leg ischemia, it is difficult to accurately define the *natural* history of the disease process since most patients will undergo a revascularization procedure. However, the overall prognosis is grim. In patients who develop chronic limb ischemia, the risk of major amputation is greater than 10% in a 3-month follow-up period[203] and approximately 40% will lose their limb within 6 months.[204–206] One large cohort study involving patients suffering from CLI (defined as rest ischemic pain, ulceration and/or gangrene), 1 and 2 years mortality rates neared 22% and 33%, respectively, and was not altered by surgical revascularization procedures.[203]

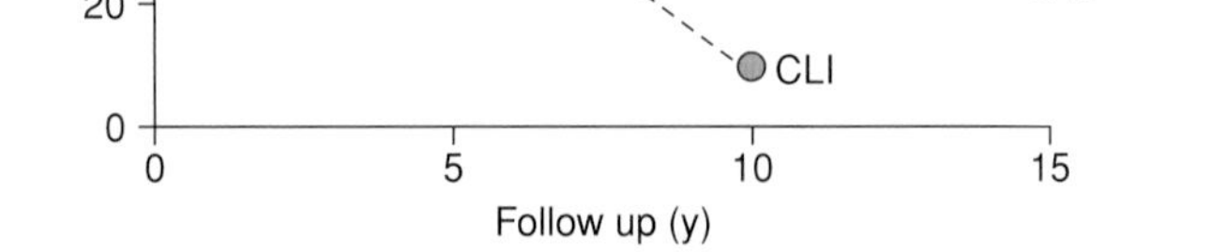

● **FIGURE 33-25.** Survival rates in patients with LEPAD dependent on symptomology.
IC, intermittent claudication; CLI, critical limb ischemia.

Source: Reprinted with permission from Elsevier in Norgren L, Hiatt WR, Dormandy JA, et al. Inter-Society Consensus for the Management of Peripheral Arterial Disease (TASC II). J Vasc Surg 2007;45(1):S5-S67.

Additional research has suggested that more than 80% of patients who present with CLI will be dead within 10 years.[204–206]

Risks

Several short and long-term cohort studies have shown significant risk of CV morbidity and increased mortality rates in patients with LEPAD. However, these patients are more commonly afflicted by the consequences of the underlying systemic atherosclerotic process (e.g., myocardial infarction, stroke, incident congestive heart failure) than by progression of the LEPAD. CAD is the most common cause of death among these patients, accounting for approximately 50% of their mortality. In addition, patients with known PAD have an increased risk of anginal symptoms and a 2% to 3% annual incidence of nonfatal myocardial infarction Other catastrophic vascular events, namely stroke or ruptured abdominal aneurysms, account for 20% to 30% of the remaining deaths.[33]

Interestingly, the severity of the LEPAD infers a greater risk of CV morbidity and mortality: Analysis of studies report a statistically significant increase in mortality with each 0.1 decrement in the ABI[44] (Figure 33-26). In so much, that an ABI less than 0.5 confers more than a fivefold increase in nonfatal CV events,[207] and an ABI less than 0.4 predicts a nearly 70% mortality at 10 years.[208]

Patients with large-vessel LEPAD (as defined in various studies by ABI < 0.9, abnormal segmental blood pressures, abnormal image findings or flow velocity by Doppler ultrasound) have a relative risk of approximately 3.0 for all-cause mortality, 6.0 for CV death, and nearly 7.0 for death related to coronary heart disease compared to patients without LEPAD more than a 10-year period.[6] Several other studies confirmed this data in various patient subgroups including patients with advanced age[44] and hypertension.[20] More specifically, patients with *symptomatic* large-vessel LEPAD

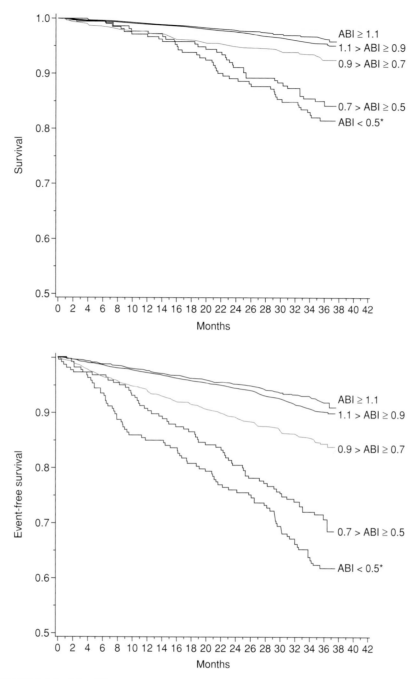

● FIGURE 33-26. Three-year survival and event-free survival rates according to ABI.

Source: Reprinted with permission from Diehm C, Lange S, Darius H, et al. Association of low ankle brachial index with high mortality in primary care. Eur Heart J. 2006;27(14):1743-1749.

are at a 15-fold increase in CV and coronary heart disease-related deaths.[6]

Similar studies have reported that LEPAD patients have been shown to have an increased risk of angina, coronary artery bypass graft surgery, congestive heart failure, and nonfatal or fatal myocardial infarction.[196,20,209–217] In addition, LEPAD predicts increased mortality in these patients with acute myocardial infarction[218–220] or undergoing percutaneous coronary intervention,[221] or coronary artery bypass graft surgery.[222] Also, patients with LEPAD are at

increased risk for TIA,[196] nonfatal stroke,[223] and worse outcomes once a cerebrovascular event occurs.[224]

● **DIAGNOSTIC MODALITIES**

The clinician can initiate an appropriate, focused work-up only after a thorough understanding of the patient's subjective complaints, medical history, and physical examination. However, the history and standard physical examination alone have a very low accuracy in the diagnosis of LEPAD.

TABLE 33-5. Summary Table of Diagnostic Modalities

Angioscopy
ABI
Bedside Doppler ultrasound
CTA
Contrast angiography
Digital subtraction angiography
Doppler velocity waveform analysis
Duplex arterial ultrasound
Exercise ABI and TBI
History and physical examination
Intravascular ultrasound
Magnetic resonance angiography
Optical coherence tomography
Pressure gradient wire measurements
Pulse volume recording
Segmental limb pressure and continuous wave
  Doppler

Therefore, many patients require more objective measures of LEPAD be used (Table 33-5).

Clinical History and Standard Questionnairres

The vast majority of patients with LEPAD are asymptomatic. The lack of symptoms is most likely because of either mild, nonflow limiting obstructive disease, or a sedentary lifestyle which does not induce ischemic symptoms. The most common presenting symptom of LEPAD is intermittent claudication. Other clinical presentations include atypical leg pain, ischemic ulcers, or chronic and acute limb ischemia (see above). Important aspects of any reported symptoms include the timing, symmetry (i.e., symptoms in the contralateral limb), use of potentially vasospastic medications, abuse of nonprescription drugs (especially tobacco), and occupational exposures.

Also, one must closely review the comorbid medical conditions that the patient has been, and maybe even has not been, diagnosed with previously. Specifically, one must ascertain if the patient has a known history of atherosclerosis in another vascular bed (e.g., coronary, carotid, or renal). Additionally, a prior history of atrial fibrillation or flutter, severe left ventricular dysfunction, aortic plaqueing, aneurysmal disease, or intracardiac shunts (e.g., patent foramen ovale or atrial septal defect)[99] raises the probability that thromboembolic disease may be a culprit of any lower extremity symptoms. Other constitutional symptoms, such as fever, weight loss, night sweats, malaise, arthralgias, and myalgias may be indicative of an inflammatory vasculitic process. Any previously diagnosed hematologic, rheumatologic, or malignant diseases raises the suspicion for vasospasm, vasculitis, or hypercoaguable conditions.

In addition to obtaining a standard medical history, the clinician may find a standardized questionnaire to help elucidate symptoms of claudication or LEPAD. Presently, three standardized forms originally created to assess and standardize patients' symptoms in previous trials regarding LEPAD can be effectively used in clinical practice: The Rose and Edinburgh questionnaires. The Rose questionnaire, developed in 1962, has been shown only to correctly identify 10% patients with an abnormal ABI.[20] In addition, numerous epidemiologic studies have shown only moderately sensitivity (~65%) but high specificity (90%–100%) in detecting intermittent claudication.[196] Therefore, in efforts to improve upon the questionnaire's diagnostic accuracy, the Edinburgh claudication questionnaire (ECQ) was created as a modification of the Rose questionnaire in 1962. In an initial small study of 300 patients, the ECQ had a reported sensitivity of 91% and sensitivity of 99% in the diagnosis of intermittent claudication.[225] Thirdly, the San Diego Claudication Questionnaire was developed in order to further evaluate leg-specific symptoms and evaluate thigh, buttock and calf pain.[55]

Physical Examination

In general, a complete physical examination should also focus on evidence of underlying systemic disorders that are risk factors for the development of LEPAD. For example, close attention must be given to determine signs of end-organ damage caused by underlying hypertension (retinopathy, fourth heart sound, abdominal bruits), hyperlipidemia or hyperlipoproteinemia (arcus, hollenhorst plaque, xanthomas, etc.), or diabetes (signs of peripheral neuropathy, diabetic ulcers). Patients with systemic inflammatory, rheumatologic, or vasculitic disease may appear chronically ill or cachetic. These patients also present with synovitis, nail pitting, prominent nailbed capillary loops, and skin lesions (e.g., erythema nodosum, pyoderma gangrenosum, petechial rash, or palpable purpura). However, the constellation of fever, rash, petechiae, and nail findings also warrants the consideration of infective endocarditis with embolization to the lower extremities. Other additional findings of embolization (atheroembolic or endocarditis) underlying the process include hemorrhages near the optic discs with white spots in the center (Roth spots), Osler nodes, Janeway lesions, and splinter hemorrhages under the nail beds.

Because of the high prevalence of asymptomatic LEPAD in patients with risk factors for atherosclerosis, it is reasonable to perform an office-based screening for LEPAD in all patients referred to a vascular specialist by assessing pulses, auscultating for bruits, palpating for abdominal aortic aneurysms, and measuring blood pressures in both arms. All central and peripheral pulses should be palpable and symmetric throughout their course. When palpating for arterial pulsations, it is important to assess the volume of the pulse and the apparent condition of the vessel wall. Pulse volume is most commonly reported on a scale of 0 to 2 (0, absent; 1, decreased; 2, normal).[226] Pulses that should be appreciable in healthy patients include the femoral, popliteal, dorsalis pedis, and PT arteries. Significant narrowing of the vasculature may manifest as reduced/absent pulses and/or bruits.[227] However, patients with isolated occlusion of the internal iliac artery or stenosis of the common or external iliac artery pay have normal femoral and pedal pulses at rest and after exercise, but buttocks claudication and/or impotence in males.[33]

The femoral artery should be palpated just caudal to the inguinal ligament, halfway between the anterosuperior iliac spine and the pubic symphysis.[227] The popliteal artery can be best appreciated with the patient's hip and knee slightly flexed and the clinician's fingers tucked into the popliteal fossa.[228] The PT artery can be palpated below and behind the medial malleolus.[229] Lastly, the dorsal pedis pulse is most often detected with the patient's foot in slight dorsiflexion and the clinician palpating nearly halfway down the dorsum of the foot, just lateral to the extensor tendon of the first toe.[227,219] However, absent pedal pulses can be an indicator of LEPAD with only moderate sensitivity and specificity.[230] In less than 10% of patients, pulses may not be present because of congenital absence of the artery—most commonly the dorsalis pedis artery.[226] At the same time, auscultation to appreciate bruits should be performed over the iliac (2 cm lateral from the umbilicus halfway toward the inguinal ligament), common femoral, superficial femoral, and popliteal artery areas.[228] The presence of a bruit may indicate the presence of a stenosis, extrinsic compression of the vessel, or other abnormality.

Other helpful clues on physical examination include capillary refill time and the Buerger test. Capillary refill can be determined by applying firm pressure for 5 seconds on the plantar aspect of the halux. After releasing pressure in a patient without LEPAD, normal skin color should return in 5 seconds.[231] In patients with severe LEPAD, it may take up to 20 seconds for the pallor to dissipate.[226] Also, pallor can sometimes be induced on the soles of the feet by elevation of the foot above the level of the heart and repeated dorsiflexion and plantar flexion of the ankle. Then, the leg may be slowly lowered until the reddish hue returns (known as the "angle of circulatory insufficiency"). The test is considered abnormal if the angle of circulatory insufficiency is less than 0 degrees (i.e., patient's leg needs to hang off the table for baseline color to return).[231,232] This maneuver assesses the rate of blood flow, which in turn reflects the severity of stenosis and adequacy of collateral vessels.[232]

To perform the Buerger test, the patient is placed supine and his leg is raised to 90 degrees or until the clinician notes the development of pallor (known as the "vascular angle"). In cases of CLI, this angle is often less than 30 degrees.[226] Then, the leg may be slowly lowered until the reddish hue returns (known as the "angle of circulatory insufficiency"). The test is considered abnormal if the angle of circulatory insufficiency is less than 0 degrees (i.e., patient's leg needs to hang off the table for baseline color to return).[231] Venous refill time may be determined by raising the leg for 30 to 60 seconds and then returned to the horizontal position. An abnormal test, indicative of severe arterial ischemia,

is suggested if the veins take greater than 5 seconds to refill.[226]

Patients with distal limb segments with chronic ischemia may have distal limb segments that appear purple (dependent rubor), which is attributable to skin capillaries becoming dilated with deoxygenated blood.[226] Additonally, the examiner may appreciate noticeable skin color changes, especially when closely compared to the contralateral limb. The most common signs of acute arterial insufficiency are pulselessness, pallor, poikilothermia, pain, parasthesia, and/or polar (coldness). Additional signs of chronic arterial insufficiency include cool skin, noticeable petechiae, persistent cyanosis or pallor, pedal edema resulting from prolonged dependency, smooth and "bronzing" skin, focal hair loss, muscle atrophy, thickened and brittle toenails, and subcutaneous fat atrophy of the digital pads.[226,228,232]

The development of skin fissures and nonhealing ulcers at areas of minor trauma and digital gangrene may also indicate chronic arterial insufficiency (although they may be seen in acute arterial insufficiency).[233] Arterial ulcers typically have a pale base, sharply demarcated borders, a typical "punched out" appearance and usually involve the tips of the toes or the heel of the foot, develop at sites of pressure, and vary in size (3 mm and greater).[232] These ulcers, which most commonly occur at the lateral malleolus, tips of the toes, and/or metatarsal heads, can often be differentiated from venous ulcers which occur on the medial malleolus and are usually painless.[228] Although the presence of skin ulceration strongly suggests atherosclerotic disease, the clinician still must consider embolic disease, Buerger disease, or vasculitis.[99] In cases of atheroembolism, livedo reticularis, a mottled, "fishnet" reticular pattern can be seen on the lower extremities. The discoloration is typically pink or purplish in color that worsens with cold exposure. This finding also is seen in Raynaud syndrome, collagen vascular diseases, and hyperviscosity syndromes.[226]

Bedside Doppler Ultrasound

Following a thorough physical examination, the use of a rapid, bedside Doppler examination of the lower extremity may be helpful in patients in whom the clinician is considering the diagnosis of LEPAD. In a study evaluating more than 200 patients, a "PAD score" was calculated based on the number of ausculatated arterial components, grade of peripheral pulse, and history of myocardial infarction which included the number of ausculted components and grade of palpated pulses of both PT arteries and the history of myocardial infarction. Patients with a score of less than 6 (or less than 4 when only one limb was assessed), made the diagnosis of LEPAD highly more likely (LR 7.80). These investigators suggested using this simple Doppler examination to determine which patients should be referred for ABI testing.[234]

Ankle–Brachial Index

The most commonly used objective measurement for the assessment of LEPAD are ABIs because of its ease of use, noninvasive nature, high sensitivity and specificity (95% and nearly 100% respectively, when compared to angiography),[235,236] and lack of expense. An ABI can be readily calculated by dividing the highest ankle systolic pressure (dorsalis pedis or PT artery measured blood pressure at the level of the malleolus) by the highest brachial systolic pressure.[21] Although methods to quantitate systolic pressures vary (including auscultation with a stethoscope, oscillometric, or Doppler ultrasound), no study has shown one method to be more superior. Traditionally, this technique is done using Doppler ultrasound: A suggested method of obtaining ABI includes placing the patient in a supine position, inflating the sphygmomanometer cuff 2 to 3 cm above the point of pulse measurement, and slowly releasing cuff pressure. Then a Doppler ultrasound probe, placed at the point of pulse measurement, is used to determine systolic pressure defined as the systolic pressure during which the Doppler signal returns.[235] But, a small study which evaluated the use of automated oscillometry (i.e., "automated ABIs") compared to standard Doppler ultrasound determined that an automated ABI is a reliable and easier method in diagnosing LEPAD (correlation coefficient 0.78).[237] However, it is important that the methodology guiding patients' serial examinations be consistent over time.

An ABI of <0.9 indicates an abnormal result.[228] An ABI of 0.71 to 0.90, 0.41 to 0.70, and 0.40 and less represents mild, moderate, and severe LEPAD, respectively.[238] However, these measurements do not necessarily reflect the current clinical status of the patient. But, in general, ischemic rest pain most often occurs when ABIs are less than 0.50, while clinical ischemic or gangrene occur when ABIs are less than 0.20.[235] In asymptomatic patients older than the 65 years and without prior diagnosis of CAD or PAD, 10% have an ABI <0.9.[98] Thus, this easily obtainable objective measurement can provide important data about subclinical atherosclerosis. However, the association between clinical and subclinical disease with angiographic assessment of LEPAD suggest that patients with an abnormal ABI already have significantly advanced atherosclerosis.[6,16,35,58,60]

More specifically, studies have shown that ABIs measurements correlate with severity of disease[44] and act as an independent predictor for future vascular events such as myocardial infarction, congestive heart failure, or CV-related death.[44,239] A large prospective observational study, which followed nearly 7000 consecutive patients more than a 3-year period, reported an overall 2.5-fold increased risk for CV event or death in patients with a baseline ABI less than 0.9. In addition, patients with an ABI less than 0.5 were at a nearly fivefold increased risk for CV event or death.[207]

This data has been supported by other large observational, cohort studies.[223,240]

A similar large observational study reported the rate of new clinical LEPAD events was significantly associated with the presence of an abnormal ABI at baseline examination. However, the absolute risk of developing *symptomatic* LEPAD was less than that of developing other CV disease events (e.g., angina or stroke), or the risk for all-cause mortality.[33,44] Even in those patients with previous CV events, an abnormal ABI predicts a higher risk of recurrent events and mortality.[98] These patients remain at higher risk even after coronary revascularization.

On the other hand, ABIs may be falsely normal (in cases of moderate stenosis of the infrarenal abdominal aorta, common iliac arteries, or bilateral subclavian stenosis) or elevated. ABI values greater than 1.3 are most often because of heavily calcified, noncompliant arteries (e.g., medial calcification of the tibial vessels).[226] However, in these patients with noncompressible vessels, measurement of an absolute systolic blood pressure of less than 30 mm Hg at the toe will often imply that amputation may be required if revascularization is not performed.[33] Also, since abnormally elevated ABIs also have been associated with increased mortality, further investigation in attempts to diagnose LEPAD or other underlying disease processes still is necessary.[228,235,241,242]

Exercise ABI and Toe–Brachial Index

In patients with classic claudication symptoms but a normal or borderline ABI measurement at rest, it is reasonable to repeat ABI measurements following an exercise challenge. With intermediate lesions, there may be no pressure decrease across the stenosis at rest, but with increased flow velocity with exercise (or other forms of induced hyperemia), these lesions may become hemodynamically significant. A typical exercise regimen consists of a constant-speed; constant-grade treadmill test at 2 mile/h at a 12% incline for up to 5 minutes or until maximal (not initial) claudication discomfort occurs.[99,226] Once the exercise is complete, an ABI is measured every minute until preexercise baseline measurement is reached.[99] A normal response to exercise is peripheral vasodilatation and therefore a slight increase or no change in ankle systolic pressures when compared to resting blood pressures. However, in patients with LEPAD, this vasodilatation results in a significant blood pressure gradient at the level and distal to the stenosis. Therefore, the arterial limb pressure decreases, the ABI decreases, and a fall of 15 mm Hg in ankle systolic pressure in response to exercise is considered diagnostic of significant LEPAD.[226]

For those patients who are unable to perform on a treadmill, they can be asked to stand and perform repeated pedal plantar-flexions with their knees fully extended (e.g., "toe raises"). Once the patient reaches maximal discomfort or has performed 50 repetitions, an "exercise" ABI measurement may be obtained.[243] The decrease in ankle pressure 30 seconds after cuff deflation is analogous to that observed 1 minute after initial claudication symptoms begin on an treadmill.[33] In addition, exercise ABIs may also be useful in assessing clinical response to a revascularization procedure or in long-term monitoring in patients with LEPAD.[226] Also, the clinician can perform an ABI after simulating "maximal hyperemic response" by inflating a blood pressure cuff to suprasystolic levels for a short period of time then released.

Also, if LEPAD is suspected but the ABI is normal or elevated, a toe–brachial index (TBI) measurement may be performed. Since medial calcification does not typically affect digital vasculature, these distal vessels do not become noncompressible. Therefore, a more accurate assessment of LEPAD may be obtained by use of a small, occlusion cuff on the first or second toe. The toe pressure is approximately 30 mm Hg less than the ankle pressure, and a TBI less than 0.7 is considered abnormal.[33,226]

Segmental Limb Pressure with Continuous Wave Doppler

When a patient is found to have abnormal ABIs, it is reasonable to attempt to detect the level of arterial obstruction using segmental limb pressures (SLP) with continuous wave Doppler (CWD) measurements. This test is readily available in the majority of vascular laboratories. A series of limb pressure cuffs are placed on the upper and lower thigh, calf, ankle, transmetatarsal region, and halux. Systolic blood pressure at each respective limb segment is determined by inflating the pneumatic cuff to 20 to 30 mm Hg above the known systolic pressure and then detecting the pressure at which blood flow occurs during cuff deflation by CWD. Most commonly, the Doppler probe is placed over the PT artery as it courses inferior and posterior to the medial malleolus or over the dorsalis pedis artery on the dorsum of the forefoot (whichever artery provides the highest ABI). The cuffs are slowly deflated, and the pressure at each level is measured. In the iliac and femoral arteries, a 70% to 90% obstruction will result in a significant pressure gradient. Specifically, a systolic pressure decrease of 20 to 30 mm Hg or more between any two consecutive limb segment levels strongly suggests a stenosis in the arterial segment proximal to the most caudal cuff. Also, differences in systolic pressure measurements between limbs infers a significant arterial obstruction proximal to the cuffs.[226,232] Even though the accuracy of segmental limb pressures is limited by calcified, noncompressible arterial vessels, when obtained with pulse volume recordings, the diagnostic accuracy to detect significant LEPAD is more than 95% (discussed below).[244] Further limitations of SLP include missing intermediate lesions that do not produce a resting pressure gradient and the inability to differentiate between a severe stenosis and complete occlusion.[33]

Pulse Volume Recording

Pulse volume recordings (PVR) are a qualitative study to assess the extent of LEPAD. The waveforms are acquired with a cuff system (including a pneumoplethysmograph) to detect changes in volume, pulse contour, and pulse amplitude throughout the cardiac cycle.[243] The cuff system is inflated to approximately 60 mm Hg and a plethysmographic tracing is obtained at various levels including the thigh, calf, ankle, metatarsal region, and toe. The pulse volume curves are dependent on local arterial blood pressure and vessel wall distensibility.[231] A normal volume curve has a steep

upstroke, a sharp systolic peak, a narrow pulse width, a dicrotic notch, and a downslope bowing to the baseline (similar to an arterial waveform).[245] In patients with significant LEPAD, the slope of the upstroke flattens, the peak becomes rounded and has as a wider pulse width, the dicrotic notch disappears, and the downslope bows away from the baseline[243] (Figure 33-27). In severely diseased limbs, the waveforms become significantly attenuated, and may even appear as flat and nonpulsatile ("dampened") waveforms in cases of CLI.[226,232]

When arterial waveforms exhibit these attenuated changes at the transmetatarsal or toe level relative to the ankle level, small vessel disease must be strongly considered.[243] And, unlike ABIs and segmental limb pressures, PVR may provide accurate information regarding arterial blood flow in the setting of noncompressible vessels. In addition, detailed analysis of the pulse waves may help determine the location of the arterial stenosis; the culprit lesion is located between the normal and abnormal PVR.[232] When used alone, PVR measurements are 85% accurate in detecting significant occlusive lesions compared with angiography. This accuracy improves to nearly 95% if PVR measurements are used in conjunction with SLP.[244]

Duplex Arterial Ultrasound

Duplex arterial ultrasound imaging is an accurate, easy, inexpensive, noninvasive study to assess anatomic and functional properties of the lower extremity vasculature. In comparison to contrast angiography, the overall sensitivity and specificity of duplex arterial ultrasound imaging to detect stenosis or occlusions is 92% and 97%, respectively.[226] More specifically, the sensitivity and specificity of detecting stenosis in the aortoiliac arteries (86% and 97%) was greater than detecting stenosis in the femoropoplitieal (80% and 96%), and tibial and peroneal vessels (83% and 84%).[246] A thorough ultrasound examination includes gray scale B-mode ultrasound imaging, pulsed Doppler velocity measurements, and color coding of Doppler-shift information. Although the major limitation of the test is its operator dependency, optimal measurements are more likely when using a standard probe (with a 7.5 to 10 MHz transducer), the vessel is studied in the sagittal plane, and the probe is angled no more than 60 degrees from the longitudinal axis of the studied.[225,231] Other noted limitations include the inability to accurately assess the aortoiliac arterial segments in patients with large body habitus, signal "drop out" in calcified vessels, and decreased sensitivity for severe stenosis in the presence of multiple, "tandem" lesions.[243]

Any characteristics regarding the vasculature or stenotic lesions are made from the Doppler waveform and increases in peak systolic velocity. For example, intimal medial thickening or atherosclerotic plaque may be evident on gray scale B-mode ultrasound imaging. Intimal medial thickening of the popliteal artery has been shown to be predictive of the presence of LEPAD. Specifically, one study evaluated the incidence of increased carotid and popliteal artery intimal medial thickness (IMT) by noninvasive ultrasound in

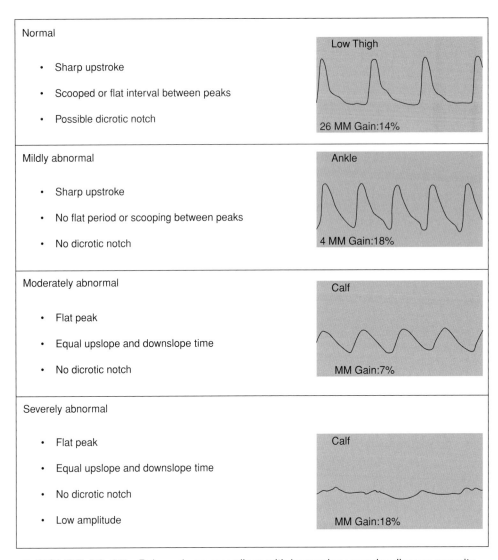

● **FIGURE 33-27.** Pulse volume recordings with increasing vascular disease severity.

Source: Guidelines for noninvasive vascular laboratory testing: a report from the American Society of Echocardiography and the Society of Vascular Medicine and Biology. Vascular Med. 2006;19:955-972 and is reproduced with the permission of the copyright holder, the American Society of Echocardiography; www.asecho.org.

patients with and without documented CAD and/or LEPAD. This study reported that the prevalence of PAD increased across the IMT quartiles, with the lowest disease in participants with the smallest IMT and the highest disease prevalence in participants with the largest IMT.[247]

During a Doppler ultrasound study, pulsed wave signals allow determination of the blood flow velocity within the arterial lumen. More specifically, a doubling in peak systolic velocity at the site of an atherosclerotic plaque indicates at least a 50% diameter stenosis, a threefold increase in velocity suggests at least a 75% stenosis, while a complete arterial occlusion generates no Doppler signal.[226,232] Therefore, from a clinical standpoint, most often vessels are characterized into five categories: Normal; 1% to 19% stenosis (change in Doppler waveform but not peak systolic velocity); 20% to 49% stenosis (increases of 30%–100% in peak systolic velocity compared to a normal vessel segment); 50% to 99% stenosis (increases of greater than 100% peak

systolic velocity with loss of early diastolic flow reversal); and complete occlusion.[226,243]

In addition, color Doppler ultrasound imaging provides more information on the location of obstructive lesions. For example, in normal arteries, blood flow is laminar with the highest velocities at the center of the lumen. Therefore, a normal color Doppler image is mostly homogeneous in color and intensity. But, in the presence of an arterial stenosis, blood flow velocity increases through the narrowed lumen that results in turbulent flow distal to the stenosis. This turbulent flow leads to changes in color imaging, which may then be superimposed onto the gray scale ultrasound images creating a real-time display of intraluminal blood flow velocity. In addition, pulsed Doppler velocity measurements often are then made at these areas of turbulent flow for further assessment of blood flow velocity.[232]

Also, duplex ultrasound imaging may be helpful in detecting steal phenomena, pseudoaneurysms, arterial

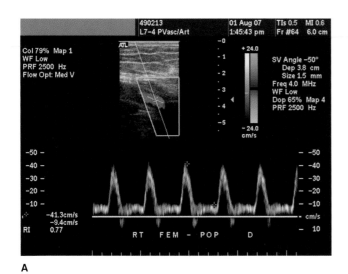

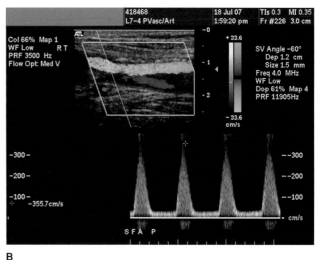

A   **B**

● **FIGURE 33-28.** Doppler velocity waveform analysis. (A) Normal waveform and (B) an abnormal waveform in a patient with significant peripheral arterial disease.

dissections, and is often used to assess whether a lesion is amenable to angioplasty and then for surveillance of patients after therapy. However, when used in this clinical setting, the clinician must appreciate that the duplex arterial ultrasound may overestimate residual stenosis.[226] Also, duplex ultrasound is now widely used to guide *therapy* for pseudoaneurysms via compression or thrombin injection.

Doppler Velocity Waveform Analysis

Doppler velocity waveforms, which provide further information regarding extent and location of LEPAD, are commonly used in conjunction with segmental limb pressure measurements and can be used in place of PVR.[226] Analysis can be recorded using CWD over the major lower extremity arterial vessels. In normal vasculature, the waveform is triphasic—systolic forward flow, brief reversal of flow in early diastole, and subsequent forward flow in late diastole (Figure 33-28). In mild arteriosclerotic disease, the reverse component is lost and the waveforms may appear biphasic.[243] As the disease process progresses, the forward flow becomes continuous and the waveform appears monophasic. In severe disease, the waveform amplitude is attenuated. Acceleration time (AT) can be used to assess for in-flow (e.g., iliac) stenosis with an AT in the CFA greater than 133 ms suggestive of proximal stenosis.

Computed Tomographic Angiography

Computed tomographic angiography (CTA), using intravenous administration of radiocontrast dye, is used to opacify and therefore clearly visualizes the lower extremity vasculature. These rapid sequence acquisition allows for detailed images from the suprarenal abdominal aorta to the ankles (Figure 33-29).[243]

Recent advancements in CT scanners can acquire raw images that can be constructed into 3-dimensional images

and manipulated to allow for detailed inspection of significant arterial lesions. Therefore, CTA allows for excellent visualization of normal, diseased, or previously revascularized lower extremity arteries and adjacent extravascular structures in multiple anatomic planes.[248]

Compared to standard contrast angiography, the sensitivity and specificity for detecting occlusions by CTA using

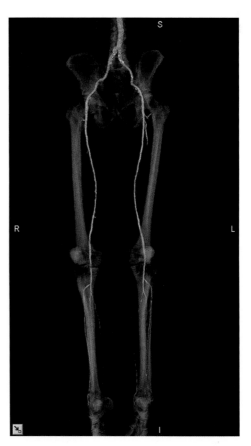

● **FIGURE 33-29.** CT of the lower extremities.

single detector technology are 85% to 100% and 98% to 100%, respectively. For nonobstructive lesions (stenosis less than 50%), the sensitivity and specificity is near 85% and specificity lesions greater than 75%; for stenosis of 50% to 99%, the sensitivity and specificity is near 80% to 93% and 95% to 97%.[243] The use of newer generation multidetector scanners improves this accuracy. And further studies have shown that evaluation of peripheral arterial stents and evaluation of peripheral arterial bypass grafts is at least comparable to duplex ultrasound.[249,250] In fact, some studies suggest that the accuracy of CTA is good enough to be used in patients with known LEPAD that are being considered for a revascularization procedure.[251]

Advantages to CTA (over MRA) include the ability to use in patients with previously placed stents, metal surgical clips, or pacemakers. Also, CTA may allow for visualization of vessel calcification (vs. MRA), which allows the clinician to construct more appropriate revascularization strategies. Disadvantages to the use of CTA include moderate doses of ionizing radiation, suboptimal visualization of tibeal anatomy,[252] and possible complications from contrast dye (e.g., nephropathy or allergic reaction).[127]

Magnetic Resonance Angiography

MRA refers to a set of pulse sequences in magnetic resonance imaging that allow for exquisite imaging of vascular structures and their lumen (Figure 33-30A and 33-30B).[226] The principle role of MRA in patients with LEPAD is to provide a detailed reconstruction of the peripheral vessels when planning revasularization therapy. It may also be used for detection of LEPAD in patients at high risk for LEPAD,

with aneurysmal, inflammatory, or embolic disease, or with previous graft revascularization.[226] Commonly, a single bolus of contrast is injected and followed down through the popliteal and tibioperoneal arteries (i.e., "bolus chase" technique).

Specifically, gadolinium contrast-enhanced (CE) MRA is the standard imaging technique for LEPAD. In comparison to contrast angiography, its sensitivity and specificity to detect LEPAD is greater than 93% and 96%, respectively.[253] Studies have suggested so much that the diagnostic accuracy of MR is acceptable to be used in patients with known LEPAD that are being considered for a revascularization procedure.[246] However, in some studies, MRA is inferior to DSA in the evaluation of iliac inflow disease and tibial vessel anatomy.[253]

Phase-contrast sequences are not routinely used, but may be helpful when information regarding anatomic and functional physiologic data is necessary (e.g., quantify flow across a stenosis). Suggested MRA protocols for the evaluation of LEPAD include 2-dimensional MR-DSA, coronal 3-dimensional CE-MRA bolus chase, or axial 2-dimansional TOF for tibioperoneal vessels.[225] However, technical specifics regarding these protocols are beyond the scope of this discussion.

Advantages of MR to CTA or angiography include the lack of need for nephrotoxic contrast dye. Disadvantages to MRA include artifacts (motion, susceptibility, coverage, timing, and resolution). In addition, MR with gadolinium rarely may result in nephrogenic fibrosing dermopathy/nephrogenic systemic fibrosis (NFD/NSF).[254] Also, it is highly operator dependent and is time consuming. The presence of permanent pacemakers, defibrillators, or other

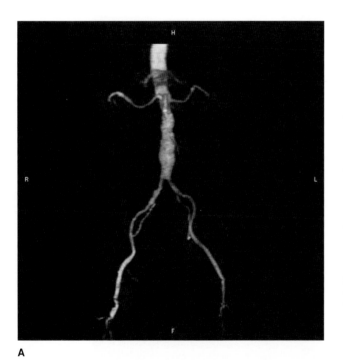
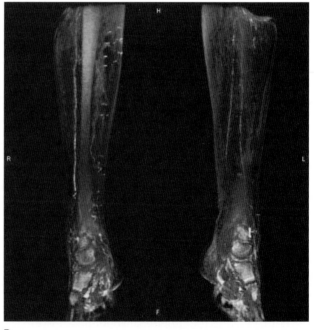

A   **B**

● **FIGURE 33-30.** MRA revealing significant (A) aortoiliac and (B) infrapopliteal vascular disease.

metallic implants is a contraindication to undergoing MRA. However, most patients with endovascular stents and non-metallic prosthetic cardiac valves can safely undergo MRA testing.

Catheter-Based Contrast Angiography and Digital Subtraction Angiography

Catheter-based contrast angiography (i.e., conventional or contrast angiography) remains the gold standard for the definitive diagnosis of LEPAD. In addition, it allows for the direct measurement of intra-arterial blood pressures, arterial waveforms, and lesion gradients. However, rarely is it used simply for the diagnosis of LEPAD. Instead, it is reserved for patients with known LEPAD that are being considered for or undergoing a revascularization procedure. Conventional angiography allows for the use of pressure-sensing wire or IVUS to further evaluate a stenotic lesion. And although there is no firm consensus on the definition of a "significant gradient," it is common practice to assume any resting peak systolic gradient of 5 mm Hg or an increase greater than 10 mm Hg following vasodilator challenge is indicative of a hemodynamically significant lesion.[255] Also, if a lesion is determined significant and amenable to revascularization, it is immediately accessible at the time of the diagnostic catheterization.

Contrast angiography, using radioiodinated contrast material to opacify the lower extremity vasculature, is most commonly done via a retrograde transfemoral catheterization. However, in cases of aortic occlusion when transfemoral catheterization is not feasible, the aorta may be visualized via an upper extremity approach (brachial, axillary, or radial) or translumbar approach. In addition, many catheterization laboratories now routinely use digital subtraction techniques (DSA) after the administration of intra-arterial injections of contrast material. More specifically, an injection of contrast into the aorta allows visualization of the aorta and iliac arteries, and an injection of contrast into the iliofemoral segment permits imaging of the femoral, popliteal, tibial, and peroneal arteries (photo). Some laboratories use bolus chase acquisition to visualize the entire lower extremity in one subtracted pass.

It is appropriate to begin each angiographic study with an abdominal aortogram performed with a catheter (pig-tailed, racket, or SOS types) at the level of L1-L2. This allows the clinician to quickly visualize the distal aorta and origin of the iliac and femoral vessels, along with the renal arteries. DSA images are commonly performed with approximately 20 mL of iso-osmolar contrast injected at a rate of 10 mL/s. Other textbooks suggest a slightly modified approach using a multi-hole catheter (pigtail or Omni Flush) that is placed at the L4-L5 level. An automatic power injection in the AP projection at 15 mL/s for 2 seconds then will adequately opacify the aortoiliac bifurcation and common iliac arteries. If an iliac artery occlusion is known or suspected, the catheter instead should be repositioned just caudal to the renal arteries to enhance visualization of possible collateral flow from the lumbar arteries. When DSA is

used, an image rate of 4 frames/s and 2 frames/s is sufficient for visualization of the suprapopliteal and infrapopliteal arteries, respectively. For further evaluation of the distal aorta including runoff vessels, the pigtail catheter may be lowered to the L2-L3 level and contrast should be injected at 8 mL/s for 10 seconds (or 4 mL/s for 10 seconds if each leg is injected separately) (bolus chase technique). Contralateral and ipsilateral (usually 30–45 degrees angulation) may be necessary to clearly visualize the iliac and femoral bifurcations. However, conventional angiography of the iliac arteries also may be done from an ipsilateral femoral artery access site by retrograde injections through the sheath or through a catheter placed retrograde in the common iliac artery. Angiography can also be performed through a contralateral femoral artery approach after selective engagement of the target common iliac vessel with an Omni Flush, glide catheter, Cobra, SOS-OMNI, hook, or internal mammary catheter. The standard views for iliac angiography are the contralateral 30- to 40-degree oblique angle, which allows better visualization of the common iliac bifurcation into the internal and external iliac arteries. Usually, hand injections of 10 mL of contrast is adequate.

Similarly, the lower leg segments can be studied via an ipsilateral or contralateral access site (involving engagement of the aortoiliac bifurcation and contralateral iliac system as described above). The standard set-up for assessing the common femoral bifurcation is 30 to 45 degrees of ipsilateral oblique angulation, which allows better visualization of the CFA bifurcation into the superficial femoral and profunda femoris arteries. A Hand injection of 6- to 8-mL contrast with DSA is acceptable practice. Best angulation to view the SFA is an AP view with minor angulation if a stenosis is suspected. The popliteal, tibeoperoneal trunk and trifurcation are best visualized in an ipsilateral 30-degree angle. Lastly, infrapopliteal vasculature is best imaged with an AP or ipsilateral oblique angulation. And although the distal runoff vessels can be assessed with these several, segmental injections, many catheterization laboratories institute one "moving table" run to assess the distal lower extremity vasculature. These distal arteries may be optimally viewed after the administration of vasodilating agents.[255]

Disadvantages to conventional angiography include exposure to modest doses of radiation, complications for contrast (e.g., nephropathy or allergic reaction), and complications from arterial puncture (e.g., bleeding, vessel wall trauma, infection, etc.).

Other Diagnostic Modalities

As stated above, angiography with or without digital subtraction is the gold standard accepted methed for guiding endovascular procedures in the treatment of LEPAD. However, other modalities to assess the morphology and/or hemodynamic significance of intermediate lesions may be useful in select cases. The adjunctive techniques include pressure gradient and duplex velocity measurements, intravascular ultrasound, angioscopy, and optical coherence tomography.[99] Also, these imaging modalities may be used as an adjunct to balloon angioplasty to detect dissection, stent underdeployment, stent thrombosis, and to predict restenosis risk.

● RECOMMENDATIONS FOR SCREENING OF THE ASYMPTOMATIC PATIENT

As stated above, there is considerable morbidity and mortality related to symptomatic, and even asymptomatic, LEPAD. Recently, there have been several medical communities and professional organizations have attempted to describe appropriate screening practices for asymptomatic individuals. In so much, this subject has been met with differing opinions.

The United States Preventitive Services Force (USPSF), an independent private sector panel of experts in prevention and primary care, has issued a recommendation statement recommending against routine screening for PAD in all asymptomatic individuals (Class D recommendation: Evidence is ineffective or that harm outweighs benefits). Their recommendations are based on the belief that: (1) the prevalence of LEPAD is low in the asymptomatic population, (2) the treatment of asymptomatic LEPAD has not been shown to improve health outcomes, and (3) screening of asymptomatic individuals could lead to harm, including false-positive results, subsequent workups, and adverse effects of these work-ups (e.g., complications from an angiographic procedure, medical, or surgical therapy).[256]

However, this recommendation seems contrary to the results of the PARTNERS Trial and similar studies and perpetuates misconceptions regarding LEPAD. Many argue that the detection and subsequent aggressive therapy of LEPAD does indeed lead to improved health outcomes. Numerous studies support that the asymptomatic patient is not necessarily a "no-risk" patient.[257–260] Indeed, LEPAD is considered a coronary equivalent and all such patients should have aggressive secondary risk factor modification. Therefore, the American College of Cardiology/American Heart Association (ACC/AHA) Guidelines for LEPAD conclude that the diagnosis of LEPAD should be evaluated via a resting ABI measurement in only asymptomatic patients who are deemed at higher risk: Patients with exertional leg symptoms, patients aged 5 to 69 years who have CV risk factors, patients elder than 70 years of age, and patients with a 10-year CV risk between 10% and 20%. Results from a detailed history (including or not including a standard questionnaire) and an ABI then should guide possible additional diagnostic testing and/or the initiation of behavioral, medical, endovascular, and/or surgical therapy (Figure 33-31).[99] Other recommendations have included mandatory screening with an ABI every 5 years in high-risk patient subgroups such as diabetes.[12]

● GENERAL PRINCIPLES OF NONINVASIVE TREATMENT

As previously stated, most patients with LEPAD are asymptomatic. And rarely, patients with claudication symptoms

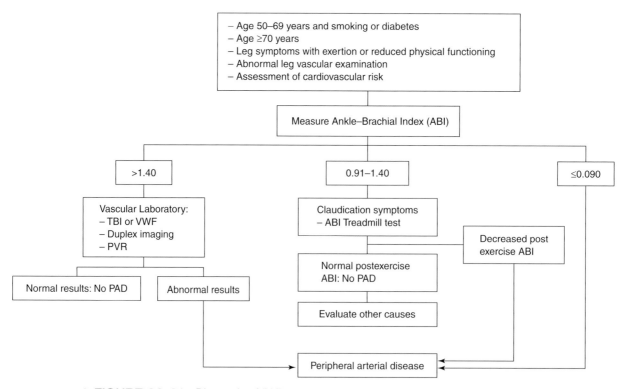

● **FIGURE 33-31.** Diagnosis of PAD.

Source: Reprinted with permission from Elsevier in Norgren L, Hiatt WR, Dormandy JA, et al. Inter-Society Consensus for the Management of Peripheral Arterial Disease (TASC II). J Vasc Surg 2007;45(1):S5-S67.

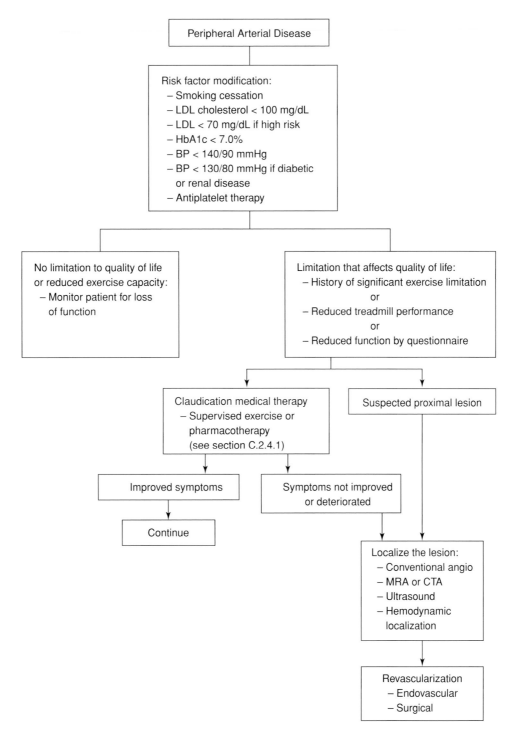

● **FIGURE 33-32.** Treatment of asymptomatic and symptomatic LEPAD.

Source: Reprinted with permission from Elsevier in Norgren L, Hiatt WR, Dormandy JA, et al. Inter-Society Consensus for the Management of Peripheral Arterial Disease (TASC II). J Vasc Surg 2007;45(1):S5-S67.

do progress to CLI and/or amputation. However, all claudicants are at a greater risk of death from cardiac and cerebrovascular events. Therefore, aggressive treatment with structured exercise, medical therapy, and treatment of underlying related comorbidities is of critical importance in patients with LEPAD (Figure 33-32). Unfortunately, despite these significantly greater risks and rates of morbidity and mortality, patients with LEPAD are less likely to re-

ceive appropriate treatment for atherosclerotic risk factors in clinical practice.[13,261,262] For example, epidemiologic studies evaluating the prevalence of antiplatelet therapy in outpatient clinical practice suggest that only 54% of newly diagnosed LEPAD and 71% of known PAD and CAD patients were prescribed antiplatelet medications; and 44% of newly diagnosed LEPAD and 56% of known PAD and CAD patients were prescribed lipid-lowering medications.[13]

Behavioral Modication Therapy

Exercise Therapy. The mechanisms behind exercise providing clinical benefit in patients with claudication is still under investigation. Ernst and Matrai et al.[263] support the hemorheologic hypothesis which states that exercise induces improved blood supply via decreased blood viscosity and the ability of autologous red cells to be filtered. Other research suggests that exercise-induced improved blood flow occurs as a result of an increase in the oxidative capacity of skeletal muscle which leads to greater oxygen extraction.[264] These beneficial effects do not appear to be a result from an improvement in ABI measurements or promotion of vascular collateral growth.[265] In addition, previous concern regarding the risk of exercise-induced long-term attenuation of the inflammatory response (via production of muscle ischemia and local oxidant stress response, free-radical formation, neutrophil activation, and subsequent endothelial damage) appears to be offset by the improvement in claudication symptoms.

A large meta-analysis reported that a structured, supervised exercise program for LEPAD patients with claudication symptoms improved maximum walking time by 150%. These improvements were seen after 4 weeks of exercise therapy and were sustained in patients participating in long-term exercise programs.[264] This clinical improvement was a larger improvement compared to those taking pentoxifylline (20%) or cilostazol (50%),[264] and in similar studies more effective than antiplatelet therapy or angioplasty, but was equal to the effects found from surgical revascularization.[265]

Therefore, it is appropriate for a clinician to prescribe a supervised clinic or hospital-based program consisting of short periods of treadmill walking alternating with periods of rest throughout a 1-hour exercise session, occurring at least three times weekly.[264] Patients should stop walking when claudication symptoms become moderate; rest until symptoms resolve; then continue exercising. Clinical benefits have been greatest with patients training on a treadmill, achieving a high level of claudication pain during exercise, and exercise programs lasting at least 6 months.[33,266] Clinicians prescribing a home-based, patient-constructed exercise session may not have as significant improvements in claudication symptoms.

Weight Loss. Based on the available literature, it does not appear that obesity maintains a constant independent positive relationship with PAD. Instead, the data report conflicting findings. Specifically, there are have been several studies that failed to report a significant relationship between obesity and PAD after multivariable adjustment.[60,71,267-269] It is possible that maybe more accurate predictors of PAD, as it is for CAD and myocardial risk, are central obesity, intra-abdominal adipose tissue, and/or increased waist-to-hip ratios and not just an elevated BMI.[57,270] On the other hand, there is data that suggests that an elevated BMI or weight is protective against the development of PAD.[34,35,44] Nonetheless, since obesity has been strongly implicated in the development of other PAD risk factors (e.g., diabetes, hypertension, and hyperlipidemia), it may be prudent to encourage and support a weight-loss plan in patients presenting with asymptomatic or symptomatic PAD.

Smoking Cessation. Smoking cessation among patients with claudication often significantly reduces the frequency and severity of their symptoms.[59,60,271-273] In fact, these observational studies have demonstrated an improvement in physiologic and functional assessments of the patients' lower extremity vasculature. However, some patients do not experience symptom improvement. But, more importantly, convincing data has reported a reduction in CV events, amputation rates and overall mortality in patients with LEPAD who successfully cease smoking.[271-273] In one study of patients with intermittent claudication, the 10-year survival rate in former smokers compared to continued smokers was 82% and 46%, respectively.[272]

Therefore, in efforts to possibly improve quality of life and increase survival, it is mandatory that any patient with LEPAD discontinue use of all tobacco products. Success of patients' attempts to stop smoking may be improved by physician advice/support, nicotine replacement and buprioprion. Other newer medications, such as varenicline, also have been shown to significantly aid in smoking cessation regimen. The clinician must be aware that there have been reports of behavioral changes while on varenicline—particularly depression and suicide.

Pharmacologic Therapy

Antiplatelet Medications. A large meta-analysis reviewed the randomized controlled trials assessing the effect of antiplatelet therapy (vs. placebo) in over 135 000 patients at high risk for a CV ischemic event.[274] Overall, patients with PAD ($n = 9706$) randomized to antiplatelet therapy had a significant 23% relative risk reduction (5.8% vs. 7.1% event rates with antiplatelet and placebo therapy, respectively) in subsequent nonfatal myocardial infarction, stroke, and vascular death. The majority of these reductions occurred in patients who were prescribed aspirin therapy, with further analysis revealing no additional clinical benefit in aspirin regiments of greater than 150 mg daily. Furthermore, other studies have shown that daily aspirin therapy was found to reduce the risk of LEPAD necessitating revascularization by 46%.[275] In addition, dipyridamole added to standard aspirin therapy resulted in no further reduction of measured CV endpoints. However, the use of clopidogrel and ticlopidine resulted in a trend to further reduce the risk of combined vascular endpoints by 10% to 12% when compared to aspirin therapy.[274]

In the CAPRIE study, patients defined as high risk for subsequent CV events were randomized to daily aspirin (325 mg) versus clopidogrel (75 mg) therapy. Three-year follow-up revealed a relative risk reduction of 8.7% in myocardial infarction, ischemic stroke or death in patients assigned to clopidogrel (Figure 33-33A). More specifically, in the subset of patients with known arterial obstructive

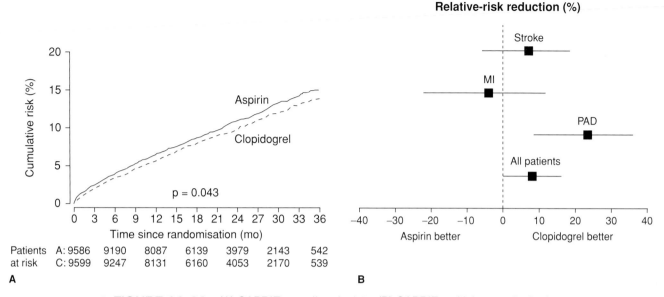

● **FIGURE 33-33.** (A) CAPRIE overall endpoints. (B) CAPRIE multiple vascular bed endpoints.

Source: Reprinted with permission from Investigators C. A randomised, blinded, trial of clopidogrel versus aspirin in patients at risk of ischaemic events (CAPRIE). CAPRIE Steering Committee. Lancet 1996;348(9038):1329-1339.

disease in multiple vascular beds, there was a 24% relative risk reduction (3% absolute risk reduction) in CV endpoints (Figure 33-33B). Therefore, the CAPRIE data suggested that patients with significant arteriosclerosis in multiple vascular beds may benefit from clopidogrel therapy versus aspirin therapy in prevention of ischemic CV endpoints.[276]

More recently, the results of the CHARISMA trial have been reported.[277] This trial, which randomized patients at high risk of heart attack, stroke, or CV death, was designed to assess whether adding clopidogrel to aspirin therapy provided any benefit over aspirin monotherapy in preventing the occurrence of CV events. In the subgroup of patients with established, *symptomatic* atherothrombotic disease were evaluated, data analysis suggested a 12% relative risk reduction (6.9% vs. 7.9% combined event rates) in myocardial infarction, stroke, or CV. However, this same study suggested that use of clopidogrel in addition to aspirin in patients with only multiple vascular risk factors (i.e., asymptomatic individuals) did not result in a reduction in CV endpoints and may result in increased harm—including bleeding rates.

Ticlopidine, another antiplatelet medication, has been shown to significantly increase pain-free walking distance.[278] But use of this medicine has been limited because of the reports of neutropenia, TTP, aplastic anemia. Other antiplatelet medications, such as picotamide, trifusal, and ketanserin, have not been shown to be more effective than aspirin for preventing CV events in patients with LEPAD.[274] A smaller study suggested that picotamide, a platelet thromboxane A2 synthase inhibitor and thromboxane receptor antagonist, reduced the risk of death by nearly 45% in patients with documented PAD

and diabetes mellitus when compared to standard aspirin therapy.[279] However, further data is needed before the use of this medication can be recommended.

Therefore, based on the current data, it is appropriate to place all *asymptomatic* patients with LEPAD on daily aspirin therapy (75–325 mg daily) and consider those patients with *symptomatic* LEPAD for dual-antiplatelet therapy of clopidogrel (75 mg daily) and aspirin (75–162 mg daily) or clopidogrel (75 mg daily) alone in effort to reduce the risk of subsequent CV events. Of course, these recommendations are made with assumption that the patient has no contraindications to antiplatelet therapy and/or does not have a high risk of bleeding complications.

Cilostazol, a phophodiesterase Type 3 inhibitor, induces vasodilatation and inhibits platelet aggregation. A meta-analysis of randomized controlled trials reported that cilostazol significantly improved pain-free walking distance and maximum walking distance versus placebo.[280,281] However, there was no significant difference in rates of CV or all-cause mortaliy. In addition, this medication remains contraindicated in patients with concomitant congestive heart failure, as this class of medications have been suggested to increase cardiac mortality.[264,280,282]

In addition, it seems reasonable that intra-arterial or intravenous infusion of vasodilators may help decrease ischemic pain and/or improve ulcer healing in patients with CLI. There have been only a few studies to support the use of pentoxifylline, PGE-1 or intravenous iloprost to reduce ischemic pain and improve ulcer healing.[283–286] However, these medications seem to have no effect on rates of amputation or mortality. In addition, currently there is no evidence to support the use of cilostazol or oral iloprost in this patient population.[99,287]

Antithrombotic Medications. In addition to platelet activation, thrombin generation plays a central role in the development of occlusive LEPAD. In addition, previous trials have shown in patients with coronary artery disease, that high-intensity oral anticoagulation (INR greater than 2.8) or moderate-intensity (INR 2–3) oral anticoagulation with aspirin therapy significantly reduced rates of myocardial infarction, stroke, and CV death. However, these clinical event benefits came with a risk of increased bleeding.[288,289]

More specifically, there have been numerous, smaller trials[290–294] evaluating the safety and efficacy of oral anticoagulation in patients with LEPAD (albeit the majority of patients in these trials had a recent surgical revascularization procedure). Studies have not consistently shown any significant reduction in adverse clinical outcomes, but rather an increased risk of bleeding with the use of these medications.[295] Therefore, there has been no established proven role for heparin or warfarin in the standard treatment of patients with stable LEPAD. A recent multinational, multicenter RCT evaluated the use of moderate intensity oral anticoagulation (target INR 1.8–3.5) plus antiplatelet (aspirin, ticlopidine, or clopidogrel) therapy versus antiplatelet therapy alone in patients with symptomatic or severe (defined as ischemic rest pain, nonhealing ulcers, previous limb amputation, or revascularization).[296] This trial reported that combining oral anticoagulation therapy with antiplatelet therapy does not provide a statistically significant benefit over antiplatelet therapy alone in reducing rates CV death, myocardial infarction, or stroke at nearly 4 years (combined event rates of 12.2% vs. 13.3%). In fact, patients on combined oral anticoagulation and antiplatelet therapy more frequently experienced life-threatening bleeds (4% vs. 1.2%, RR 3.41). Therefore, the use of warfarin should be reserved for patients deemed high risk for bypass graft restenosis or occlusion (e.g., prosthetic grafts, infrageniculate grafts, etc.) may benefit from chronic warfarin therapy.[297,298] In summary, there is no current recommendation to treat LEPAD with combined oral anticoagulation and antiplatelet therapy.[299] Studies investigating newer anticoagulation agents, such as Factor Xa inhibitors, are ongoing.

Angiogenic Growth Factors. Angiogenic growth factors have been shown in animal models to improve the development of collateral blood vessel formation (angiogenesis) and increase the caliber of preexisting arteriolar collateral connections (arteriogenesis),[300] and therefore have positive effects on symptoms and clinical outcomes in atherosclerotic disease.[301–303] The majority of the current research has focused on the use and efficacy of recombinant bFGF and gene transfer of VEGF. Several, nonrandomized trials evaluating intra-arterial and intramuscular administration of gene transfer therapy with a VEGF plasmid DNA resulted in minor improvements in angiographic blood flow, histologic evidence of new blood vessel formation, an increase in ABI, and healing of ischemic ulcers.[304–307] However, larger randomized trials have shown a similar improvement of angiographic blood flow but conflicting data on its effects on ABIs, rates of restenosis after PTA, amputation rates, ulcer healing, or ischemic pain.[308–311]

Miscellaneous. Previous research has show that L-arginine may inhibit the development of atherosclerosis, improve flow-mediate vasodilatation, and reduce monocyte adhesiveness and reduce platelet aggregability.[312] A small series of patients with CLI were treated with L-arginine, a precursor to nitric oxide (vasodilator). All treated patients had improvement in ischemic pain symptoms and improvement in ulcer healing.[312] Also, studies have suggested that the use of gingko biloba may significantly increase pain-free walking distance.[313,314] Other randomized trials have evaluated the efficacy of naftidrofuryl, pentoxifylline, garlic, testosterone, ketanserin, buflomedil, defibrotide, levocarnitine, propionyl-L-carnitine, isovolemic hemodilution, and chelation therapy.[33] Several trials have shown an improvement in maximal walking distances (with naftidrofuryl, levocarnitine, and propionyl-L-carnitine),[315–320] the majority have not shown a consistent significant benefit to support their medical use.[282,319,321–323]

Modification of Other Comorbidities

As discussed above, comorbid conditions such as diabetes, hypertension and hyperlipidemia are risk factors in the development and progression of LEPAD. Therefore, it is imperative that patients with LEPAD receive aggressive medical management of these disease processes. Unfortunately, in comparison to patients with known CAD or PAD, previous studies have suggested that patients with newly diagnosed PAD were less intensely treated for hyperlipidemia and hypertension.[13]

Diabetes Mellitus. Current guidelines recommend a target glycosylated hemoglobin level of less than 7.0%,[324] but also recommends an A1C as "close to normal" (<6%) without significant hypoglycemia.[33] However, clinical trial evidence to support aggressive glycemic control to reduce CV event rates in patients with diabetes and PAD is sparse. Data from the UK Prospective Diabetes Study (UKPDS) suggests that intensive glycemic control with a suphonlyurea or insulin resulted in a nonsignificant 16% risk reduction for myocardial infarction or sudden death when compared to diet control.[325] This same database reported no significant difference in all-cause mortality between the treatment and control groups. In addition, it appears that the most clinical benefit in aggressive glycemic control is in reduction of microvascular (retinopathy, renal failure), and not macrovascular (myocardial infarction, stroke, amputation, or death caused by PAD) endpoints.[326]

Hypertension. Hypertension is a significant risk factor for the development of PAD and contributes to the pathogenesis of atherosclerosis.[327,328] Therefore, in patients with hypertension, aggressive treatment is necessary to reduce the risk of stroke, myocardial infarction, heart failure, and death (i.e., goal of less than 130 mm Hg systolic over 80 mm Hg diastolic).[329,330] However, in patients with LEPAD, treatment of elevated blood pressure may result in decreased limb perfusion, worsened claudication, or CLI.[99] Yet, most patients are able to tolerate antihypertensive medications without significant.

In the past, there was concern that beta-blocker medications might lead to peripheral vasoconstriction and subsequent worsened ischemia in patients with LEPAD. However, there is very little data to support this concern.[331,332] In fact, several beta-blocker medications possess "intrinsic sympathomimetic activity (ISA)" which theoretically cause peripheral vasodilatation. And since, a considerable subset of patients with PAD have symptomatic CAD, the use of beta-blocker medications to reduce the risk of reinfarction and overall survival, is merited (Class I Indication).[99] Currently, there is no absolute contraindication for the use of beta-blocker medications in patients with LEPAD, but should be used with caution in patients with severe disease.

In addition, the Heart Outcomes Prevention Evaluation (HOPE) study demonstrated that therapy with an ACE-inhibitor, ramipril, significantly reduced the risk of CV death, myocardial infarction, and stroke in patients with known PAD by nearly 25%.[333] Other trials investigating ACE-inhibitor therapy in patients with PAD have reported improvements in maximal walking distance without a significant change in ABI measurements.[334] Therefore, ACE-inhibitors are indicated for the use in symptomatic or asymptomatic patients with LEPAD and hypertension.[335]

Also, one small study has suggested that the use of a calcium channel antagonist, verapamil, in patients who had recently undergone PTA for symptomatic LEPAD resulted in a trend toward reduced restenosis rates.[336]

Hyperlipidemia. Although there have been numerous trials investigating the effects of lipid-lowering therapy in patients with known coronary atherosclerotic disease, there are fewer trials evaluating the same regimen for patients with documented PAD. However, a review of seven randomized control trials suggest that therapy was associated with a nonsignificant trend in reduction of mortality and a significant improvement in angiographic appearance on follow-up. Depending on each trial, there were conflicting results regarding improvement in nonfatal CV events, ABI measurements, maximum walking distance, or symptomatic improvement. The disparity of these studies may be a result of some trial therapy protocols not resulting in significant reduction in lipid levels compared to controls.[337] However, several larger trials have reported a significant reduction in CV events in patients with PAD and coexisting CAD when treated with statin medications.[338–340] Nonetheless, it is prudent to aggressively treat patients with documented LEPAD with lipid-lowering agents in attempts to prevent progression and some regression (by QCA) of atherosclerotic disease, restenosis of previously treated symptomatic lesions, or other systemic CV endpoints.[341] Current recommendations suggest a target LDL cholesterol level <70 mg/dL or non-HDL cholesterol level <130

mg/dL. In addition, treatment to increase HDL levels with niacin has been associated with regression of femoral and reduction of progression of coronary atherosclerosis.[342,343] Therefore, in patients with PAD current recommendations suggest a target HDL cholesterol level greater than 40 mg/dL in males and greater than 50 mg/dL in females.[99]

Homocysteinemia. Patients with known hyperhomocysteinemia who have taken low- or high-dose folic acid supplementation have shown a modest decrease in serum Hcy levels (200 μg/d of folic acid resulting in an average 4 μmol/L reduction in Hcy levels). However, similar studies have suggested that there is a plateau response with no additional lowering of serum Hcy levels after 6 weeks of intensive therapy (including 1000 μg folic acid, 0.4 mg cobalamin, and 12.2 mg pyridoxine).[72] Although this data supports the efficacy of medical therapy to lower serum Hcy levels, there is no current clinical data to suggest folate therapy improves CV endpoints.[344]

Summary of Behavioral and Medical Therapy

Therefore, based on the current medical literature, all patients with diagnosed LEPAD should be strongly encouraged and supported to stop smoking. All these patients should be encouraged to remain physically active, and be enrolled in a supervised exercise program if claudication symptoms occur. Patients with LEPAD should be treated at least with antiplatelet medications (aspirin for asymptomatic and possibly aspirin and clopidogrel for symptomatic patients), a statin medication, and an antihypertensive irrespective of their baseline cholesterol and blood pressure measurements. Patients with underlying diabetes, hyperlipidemia or hypertension should be aggressively treated. Lastly, obese patients with LEPAD should be encouraged to lose weight. Failure of these measures to improve symptoms or progression of LEPAD should lead to consideration of more invasive therapy.

● GENERAL PRINCIPLES OF INVASIVE REVASCULARIZATION TREATMENT

Indications

Regardless of the clinical presentation, the main therapeutic goals of any revascularization therapy are limb preservation, improvement on quality of life, and reduction of CV complications from the underlying systemic atherosclerotic process. Currently, there are three major indications to consider revascularization in patients with LEPAD: Refractory claudication, chronic CLI, and acute CLI. These entities will be discussed below.

Claudication. It is uncommon for patients with claudication symptoms to require revascularization therapy. However, a patient with claudication symptoms can be considered for a percutaneous or surgical revascularization procedure if he has an inadequate response to exercise and pharmacologic therapies, continues to have a severe disability or decreased quality of life because of these symptoms, has a lack of significant comorbid conditions, and has a occlusive lesion that appears to have a low risk and high probability of initial and long-term success following intervention.[33] Patients fulfilling this criteria should undergo further imaging studies (CTA, MR, and/or angiography) to elucidate their arterial anatomy and help the clinician determine the most appropriate mode of revascularization (surgical vs. percutaneous). Patients who undergo some form of revascularization for claudication, almost universally have significant improvement or elimination of the symptoms.

However, there is additional data to suggest that younger patients who fulfill this criteria have a more aggressive form of atherosclerosis. Trials evaluating the efficacy of surgical bypass revascularization in these younger patients have consistently revealed higher rates of graft failure, need for graft revision, amputation, and mortality.[345–347] Therefore, in patients younger than 50 years with refractory claudication, surgery should be avoided if possible.[99]

Chronic CLI. The treatment goal of CLI is relief of ischemic pain (often necessitating narcotic medications), promote ulcer healing, prevent amputation, improve quality of life, and prolong survival. The risk of limb loss is unacceptably high in the presence of ischemic rest pain, ischemic ulceration, or gangrene.[21] Previous literature has proven balloon angioplasty with and without adjunctive stenting and surgical revascularization to helpful in these clinical scenarios. The revascularization procedure of choice is dependent on anatomy of the lesion.[348]

Acute CLI. Acute limb ischemia requires immediate diagnosis and treatment. Patients presenting with acute limb ischemia have an approximate 30% and 20% rate of limb loss or hospital mortality, respectively.[349] Patients presenting with acute limb ischemia and a salvageable extremity should undergo immediate evaluation to determine the level of arterial obstruction and subsequent revascularization (Class I indication, level of evidence B).[99] However, patients with acute limb ischemia and a nonviable extremity should not undergo a revascularization procedure (Class III indication, level of evidence B).[99]

Determining the Appropriate Revascularization Strategy

Currently, patients with LEPAD causing refractory claudication or CLI may benefit from endovascular or surgical modes of revascularization. In determining the most likely beneficial type of revascularization, the treating clinician(s) can be guided by recommendations made based on the available clinical data. The cornerstone in determining the appropriate therapeutic pathway is understanding the standardized TransAtlantic Inter-Society Consensus (TASC) morphologic classification of iliac and femoropopliteal lesions (Figures 33-34 and 33-35).[33] The consensus recommendations for patients with clinically significant aortoiliac or femoropopliteal disease is that endovascular procedures are the treatment of choice in TASC Type A and B lesions, and surgical revascularization remain the treatment of choice in TASC Type C and D lesions. However, in 2007, the most effective initial revascularization strategy in patients with TASC Type C lesions and severe comorbidities which may complicate an open surgical revascularization procedure, may be endovascular therapy.[33]

However, in the last decade, there have been tremendous advancements in the technology and experience in treating LEPAD via endovascular techniques. Although surgical bypass revascularization remains an effective treatment for patients presenting with refractory claudication or CLI, endovascular therapy is considered by many to be the initial treatment of choice. Nonetheless, in all these complex cases, it is even more important to consider patients' preference, comorbid conditions and suitability (or unsuitability) for a specific type of revascularization strategy. For example, in patients with severe comorbidities that may predict greater risk of perioperative adverse events (e.g., cardiac ischemia, cardiomyopathy, or severe lung disease), it is appropriate to initially attempt endovascular therapy regardless the lesion type.

Percutaneous Intervention Treatment Modalities

As stated above, the clinical efficacy of endovascular interventions treating LEPAD is based on the lesion morphology (TASC lesion type) and clinical presentation. In addition, prior to performing an endovascular intervention, it is recommended that the clinician assess the hemodynamic significance of a lesion by obtaining translesional pressure gradients with and without vasodilator challenges. Endovascular therapy should only be done in cases where a significant pressure gradient exists (defined as a mean gradient of 10 mm Hg or 15% peak systolic pressure gradient at rest or after administration of a vasodilator).[99,350–353]

Arterial Access. Appropriate arterial puncture and access is imperative to a successful peripheral intervention. In the vast majority of patients, the CFA lies atop the femoral head and is the ideal entry for arterial access. Depending on the level of interest of a peripheral angiography and/or endovascular interventions, arterial access may be initiated with a contralateral, ipsilateral, or tibial/pedal approach. A contralateral approach may be most appropriate when there is iliac (other than a proximal common iliac stenosis) and significant SFA disease. In contrast, an antegrade approach has been described[354] and may be most useful when evaluating infrapopliteal disease. Furthermore, use of intra-arterial vasodilators are recommended for intrapopliteal interventions, as these arteries can be quite sensitive to manipulation.[355]

Percutaneous Balloon Angioplasty. Percutaneous Balloon Angioplasty (PTA) has been shown to be a relatively simple endovascular technique with high procedural success rates in Type A and B lesions. Restenosis in the

Type A lesions

- Unilateral or bilateral stenoses of CIA
- Unilateral or bilateral single short (≤3 cm) stenosis of EIA

Type B lesions

- Short (≤3 cm) stenosis of infrarenal aorta
- Unilateral CIA occlusion
- Single or multiple stenosis totaling 3–10 cm involving the EIA not extending into the CFA
- Unilateral EIA occlusion not involving the origins of internal iliac or CFA

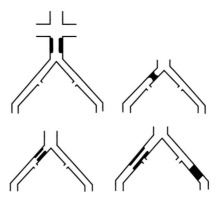

Type C lesions

- Bilateral CIA occlusions
- Bilateral EIA stenoses 3–10 cm long not extending into the CFA
- Unilateral EIA stenosis extending into the CFA
- Unilateral EIA occlusion that involves the origins of internal iliac and/or CFA
- Heavily calcified unilateral EIA occlusion with or without involvement of origins of internal iliac and/or CFA

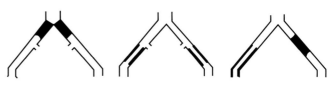

Type D lesions

- Infrarenal aortoiliac occlusion
- Diffuse disease involving the aorta and both iliac arteries requiring treatment
- Diffuse multiple stenoses involving the unilateral CIA, EIA, and CFA
- Unilateral occlusions of both CIA and EIA
- Bilateral occlusions of EIA
- Iliac stenoses in patients with AAA requiring treament and not amenable to endograft placement or other lesions requiring open aortic or iliac surgery

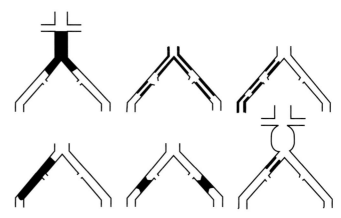

● **FIGURE 33-34.** Morphologic classification of iliac lesions.

Source: Reprinted with permission from Elsevier in Norgren L, Hiatt WR, Dormandy JA, et al. Inter-Society Consensus for the Management of Peripheral Arterial Disease (TASC II). J Vasc Surg 2007;45(1):S5-S67.

infrainguinal vasculature is likely because of the low blood flow rates, high resistance, and long lesions. Specific factors which have been shown to lead to more favorable clinical outcomes with PTA include short lesion length, good peripheral runoff, symptoms of claudication versus CLI, the absence of diabetes, and nontotal occlusive lesions.[356–366] Further trials comparing endovascular to surgical revascularization therapy in patients with LEPAD amenable to PTA have reported no significant difference in resolution of claudication symptoms, improvement in ABI measurements, patency rates, or mortality.[367–369] These trials have shown that long-term patency rates following endovascular intervention is greatest in common iliac artery lesions and then progressively decrease down the lower extremity arterial vasculature.[99] Trials have reported 1-year patency rates of iliac PTA alone and iliac stenting of approximately 78% and 90%, respectively.[33,370] Numerous trials evaluating these same treatment modalities in the femoropopliteal arteries have reported patency rates more than 60% and 50% at 1 and 3 years, respectively.[33] Other predictors of restenosis

Type A lesions

- Single stenosis ≤10 cm in length
- Single occlusion ≤5 cim in length

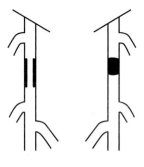

Type B lesions

- Multiple lesions (stenoses or occlusions), each ≤ 5 cm
- Single stenosis or occlusion ≤15 cm not involving the infrageniculate popliteal artery
- Single or multiple lesions in the absence of continuous tibial vessels to improve inflow for a distal bypass
- Heavily calcified occlusion ≤5 cm in length
- Single popliteal stenosis

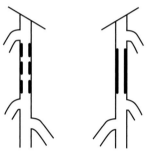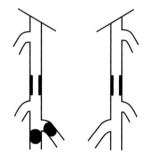

Type C lesions

- Multiple stenoses or occlusions totaling >15 cm with or without heavy calcification
- Recurrent stenoses or occlusions that need treatment after two endovascular interventions

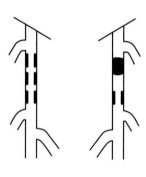

Type D lesions

- Chronic total occlusions of CFA or SFA (>20 cm, involving the popliteal artery)
- Chronic total occlusion of popliteal artery and proximal trifurcation vessels

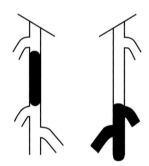

● FIGURE 33-35. Morphologic classification of femoropopliteal lesions.

Source: Reprinted with permission from Elsevier in Norgren L, Hiatt WR, Dormandy JA, et al. Inter-Society Consensus for the Management of Peripheral Arterial Disease (TASC II). J Vasc Surg 2007;45(1):S5-S67.

or reocclusion include longer lesion length, muscular (distributing) arteries, multiple or diffuse lesions, small residual vessel diameter, poor peripheral runoff, diabetes, female gender, renal failure, smoking, and presentating symptomatology of CLI (vs. claudication).[350,356–366,370]

In the setting of severe infrapopliteal disease, there is increasing data is supportive for the use of endovascular treatment. Specifically, studies investigating infrapopliteal PTA with provisional stenting have demonstrated nearly 90%

procedural success rates and improved ABI measurements and maximum walking distance.[355,371] Also, it is important to note that clinical success of PTA in the setting of CLI may be superior to angiographic success since after wound healing is attained, recurrent restenosis is unlikely to lead to recurrent ulcer formation.[372]

Stents. The efficacy of stenting is mostly seen in long, eccentric, or heavily calcified lesions where by elastic recoil, residual stenosis and flow-limiting dissections is seen after PTA. These complications are theoretically avoided with the use of endovascular stenting via refixation of the intimal flaps to the arterial wall or resisting elastic recoil of the treated vessel wall.[373,374] Therefore, as with technologic advancements and clinical improvements in percutaneous coronary interventions, the introduction of stent implantation in patients with LEPAD have led to improved clinical outcomes and have allowed for more complex lesions to be treated via endovascular methods. In the 1980s, first-generation bare-metal stents, namely the Palmaz (Cordis, Miami, FL) and the Wallstent (Boston Scientific, Natick, MA), were introduced to LEPAD endovascular interventions. Several trials have investigated the efficacy of primary versus provisional stenting in the endovascular treatment of certain patient subgroups with LEPAD.[375–380] One prospective trial reported that patients with iliac artery stenosis that were treated with PTA with selective stent placement (in cases in which the residual mean pressure gradient was greater than 10 mm Hg) had better symptomatic improvement compared with patients treated with primary stent placement.[381] Based on this data, primary or provisional stenting is an acceptable therapeutic modality in the treatment of common and external iliac artery disease.[99]

However, in one review of the efficacy of bare-metal stents (excluding nitinol stents, as discussed below) in femoropopliteal interventions reported patency rates of 67% at 1- and 58% at 3-year follow-up.[33] These late failures were a result from restenosis and mechanical compression of the deployed stents.[382] Since the use of balloon-expandable stainless steel stents in femoropopliteal disease was associated with favorable initial results without significant improvement in longer-term patency rates when compared to PTA (and in some studies worse results), there was no recommendation made for primary stenting as an initial treatment modality for femoropopliteal LEPAD interventions with balloon-expandable stents (especially because of the concerns of stent compression).[33]

In 1996, the Wallstent (Boston Scientific, Natick, MA) was approved as the first self-expanding stent for clinical use following suboptimal iliac artery PTA. Since then, several similar devices have been introduced. Trials comparing traditional PTA to self-expanding stents, and comparing self-expanding stent designs to one another[383] for the endovascular treatment of iliac or femoropopliteal lesions have reported similar immediate procedural success, MACE rates, freedom from target lesion revascularization, and 1-year patency rates (87%–91%). Also, these trials have consistently shown a significant improvement in ABI measurements, claudication symptoms, and ulcer healing. Potential adverse effects of self-expanding stents include release wire breakage and stent deployment failure.[383–386]

Nitinol (a unique material combining nickel and titanium) stents are constructed in a simple coil or mesh design, and are more likely to resist external deformation.[387] Multiple trials that have investigated the patency rates following nitinol stent deployment for femoropopliteal disease (and using historical comparison patency rates of PTA alone) reported significantly greater short- and long-term patency rates (76%–90% and 76% at 1- and 3-year, respectively).[387–390] In fact, some trials suggest the 1 year patency rates are comparable to surgical bypass revascularization, even in patients with complex atherosclerotic disease.[391]

Yet, the enthusiasm behind the use of nitinol stents in endovascular treatment of infrainguinal LEPAD has been slowed by unexpected reported rates of stent–fracture. Studies attempting to elucidate the factors leading to stent fracture have implicated th superficial course of the artery with crossing of flexion points (common femoral or popliteal artery)[392] or compression, torsion, and elongation from the surrounding musculature.[393] However, another study has shown that a significant amount of the mechanical stress onto the stent may be is not restricted to these flexion or compression sites, but rather be transmitted to the stent material as a result of the pulsatile blood flow.[394]

Although many of these stent–fractures initially were thought to be clinically insignificant, other trials suggest a strong correlation with higher restenosis rates.[382] But, a randomized trial comparing primary nitinol stent implantation to PTA with provisional stenting in the treatment of SFA disease revealed significantly lower restenosis rates at 6- and 12-months (24% vs. 43% and 37% vs. 63%, respectively) in the patients undergoing primary stent therapy. Also, patients who underwent primary stent implantation reported improved maximal walking capacity during follow-up.[395] Long-term follow-up and results from additional randomized trials (e.g., RESILIENT and Zilver PTX Trial) are needed to clarify the optimal role for stenting in femoropopliteal endovascular interventions.

Currently, there is limited data to strongly support the use of stents in infrapopliteal interventions. A small study comparing the use of sirolimus-eluting stents to bare-metal stents in an infrapopliteal artery reported significantly improved short-term patency rates (92% vs. 68%, respectively) and less target vessel revascularization.[396] But, the most common indications for use of stents in the peroneal/tibial arteries remain flow-limiting dissections and vascular recoil.[355]

Therefore, many suggest that self-expanding stents are most beneficial in the treatment of tortuous arteries or femoropopliteal lesions that are located at bifurcation points or areas that might be prone to external compression (via external trauma or adjacent muscle activity).[397]

Aneursymal Disease. More specifically, studies have addressed the feasibility and efficacy of the use of endovascular stented grafts for the use of specific isolated peripheral aneursymal disease. For example, although some controversy exists about the appropriate time to treat asymptomatic PAAs, the vast majority of literature supports repair of PAAs that are symptomatic or greater than 2 cm in size.[135,137,398] Until recently, surgery (including surgical bypass of the aneurysmal segment with ligation of the popliteal artery proximal and distal to the area of disease

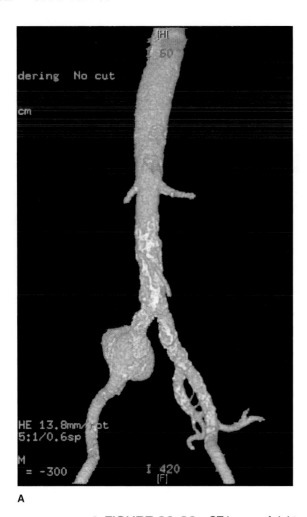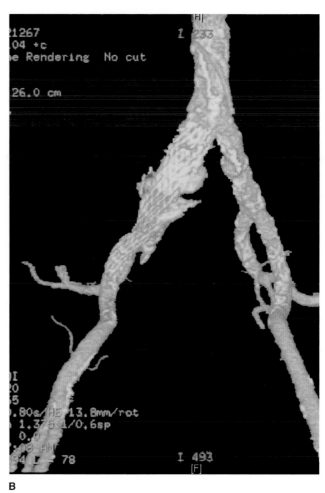

A **B**

● **FIGURE 33-36.** CT image of right common iliac aneurysm (A) before and (B) after endovascular repair.

and additional use of embolectomy or thrombolysis with acute thrombosis cases) was considered the only standard form of treatment. However, more recent experience has supported the use of endovascular repair via deployment of a stent graft (at least in surgical high-risk patients). In prospective studies which used stent grafts for the treatment of PAAs that excluded patients with poor distal runoff, 2-year patency rates were up to 90%.[399,400]

Although, no prospective natural history data exists, isolated iliac aneursyms >3 to 4 cm are recommended to undergo repair because of an unacceptable risk of rupture.[401] The iliac artery aneurysm can be approached surgically or endovascularly. Currently, endovascular approaches for treatment of CFAAs are limited because the femoral artery crosses the inguinal canal/crease and is therefore prone to repeated flexion and extension stress. Therefore, stents are less effective at this location because of theoretic kinking, fracture, migration, or metal fatigue. In addition, the standard surgical repair, suggested for aneurysms that are symptomatic or greater than 2.5 cm in size, is not extensive and is usually well tolerated.

Several studies have shown that the use of endovascular stents for the treatment of isolated iliac aneursymal disease is safe and efficacious with excellent rates of imme-diate technical success (∼100%), follow-up graft patency (95%–100%) and complications (including endoleak, embolization, graft thrombosis, ischemia, etc.).[138,139,402–404] (Figure 33-36).

Drug-Eluting Stents. Presently, there is little data to support the use of drug-eluting stents in endovascular therapy of LEPAD. Two randomized trials evaluating the efficacy of sirolimus-eluting nitinol stents versus uncoated nitinol stents in patients with SFA stenoses or occlusions revealed only a small, nonsignificant reduction in restenosis rates beyond 12 months of treatment. In addition, patients who received multiple or longer sirolimus-eluting stents appeared to have an increased risk of stent fracture.[394,405] Further investigation needs to be completed to assess the clinical severity of these stent fractures. Therefore, there is no current indication for the primary use of drug-eluting stents in the endovascular treatment of LEPAD. Although efficacy with drug-eluting stents has been show in the infrapopliteal vasculature, proper randomized trials are still needed.

Biodegradable Stents. There is immense amount of research in the field of intravascular stent technology. Biodegradable stents represent a possible technologic advancement to limit foreign-body (deployed stent) reaction leading to intimal hyperplasia. Further recommendations regarding the use and efficacy of biodegradable stents in endovascular therapy for LEPAD only can be made following completion of ongoing and future clinical trials.

Other Percutaneous Techniques. A number of complex interventional techniques have been explored in attempts to reduce restenosis rates following catheter-based endovascular intervention of LEPAD. These modalities, when compared to PTA or stenting, have not consistently been proven to be superior.[394,406-420] However, these techniques may prove useful in the treatment of certain patient and/or lesion types.

Subintimal Angioplasty. Initially described in 1989,[421] subintimal angioplasty (also referred to as the Percutaneous Intentional Extraluminal Revascularization [PIER] technique) entails intentionally passing a guidewire into the subintimal space prior to and extending beyond the occlusion (i.e., an iatrogenic subintimal dissection). The wire then is redirected back within the true lumen distal to the lesion and subintimal angioplasty is performed. This results in the creation of a new pathway for blood to pass to the distal circulation. This technique is most often used with lesions that are not amenable to standard guidewire and PTA techniques (e.g., highly calcified occlusions, long lesions, flush SFA occlusions, and diffuse tandem lesions).[382] Patency rates for subintimal angioplasty range from 53% to 92%.[422,423] However, technical failure rates are as high as 26% and are most often attributable to the inability to recannulate the true vessel lumen distal to the lesion.[424] Also, it is important that in the absence of adequate distal runoff, this procedure is contraindicated because a procedural failure could lead to ischemia without a surgical alternative. Furthermore, distal reentry should be as proximal as possible in the true lumen to avoid unnecessary propogation of the dissection.

Excisional (Direct) Atherectomy. An excisional atherectomy device approved in 2003, the SilverHawk (FoxHollow Technologies, Redwood City, CA), is available for use in infrainguinal vessel interventions. The device uses a rotating blade to shave plaque away from the vessel wall. As it is excised, the atherosclerotic debris is collected at the tip of the device and then removed from the patient. This technique may prove to be most useful in CFA,[425] ostial disease and popliteal artery lesions.[382]

Excisional Laser Therapy. Another form of excisional technique involves the use of a catheter-based laser light that delivers short bursts of ultraviolet energy. This energy (wavelength of 308 nm) removes plaque, thrombus or calcium deposits by photoacoustic (i.e., not thermal) ablation without disrupting the vessel endothelium. By performing excimer laser angioplasty, the treating clinician may debulk the plaque/thrombus and liquefy the occluding lesion without significant distal embolization.[426] One prospective reg-

istry evaluated patients with CLI (deemed not be suitable for bypass surgery) who underwent excimer laser angioplasty followed by PTA with optional stenting. Although the majority of these patients had long femoropopliteal or tibial artery lesions (TASC Type D lesions), the study reported only a 45% adjunctive stent use, an 86% immediate procedural success rate, and a 92% limb-salvage rate at 6 months.[426] The PELA trial randomized patients presenting with claudication with long, total SFA occlusions to excimer laser-assisted PTA versus PTA alone. Procedural success was 85% in the laser group (with a 28% reduction in stent use) compared to 91% in the PTA group. After 12 months, patency rates and functional status improvement were similar in both groups.[427] Therefore, it has been suggested that excimer laser-assisted angioplasty for CLI offers procedural success and limb-salvage rates with decreased need for adjunctive stenting in patients deemed unsuitable for surgical bypass revascularization. In addition, some studies have suggested that laser excimer therapy is helpful in crossing chronic occlusions via a "step-by-step" technique in which the laser is used to create a wire channel.[426,428-430]

Cutting Balloon Angioplasty. Cutting balloon angioplasty (CBA) attempts to reduce vascular injury, elastic recoil and distal dissection during endovascular treatment of an occluded vessel. The device, using three or four fixed blades, cut into and scores the stenotic plaque as the balloon is inflated. This allows for lower balloon inflation pressures and subsequently less vessel wall distention and trauma (theoretically leading to more controlled dissections) compared to PTA. Initial studies of CBA in femoropopliteal disease have reported more than 90% procedural success rates and nearly 90% patency and limb-salvage rates at 1 year.[431,432] However, one study reported an increased risk of vessel perforation (20%); these perforations were all treated successfully with stenting.[431]

Rotational Atherectomy. High-speed rotational atherectomy (RA), first described in 1989,[433] is performed using a rotating abrasive burr that is designed to debulk atherosclerotic plaque by producing small particles (~7–15 μm in diameter) that are washed away across the capillary bed and filtered by the reticuloendothelial system.[434] Further studies have suggested that RA diminishes plaque volume with abrasion, as opposed to fracturing plaque, and therefore has potential to minimize acute vessel injury and avoid disruption of soft elastic tissue.[435] On the other hand, RA may cause severe distal embolization of atherosclerotic debris, which may further compromise the distal runoff in these patients.[436]

Early studies evaluating the efficacy of RA revealed very high procedural success rates with more than 80% shorter-term patency rates.[437] More recent trials have confirmed the high procedural success rate, but have been unable to duplicate these impressive short- and long-term success rates.[416,438]

Cryoplasty. Another catheter-based modality is cryoplasty, a technique in which an angioplasty balloon is inflated with liquid nitrous oxide at a targeted, stenotic lesion. The endovascular device (PolarCath, Boston Scientific Corporation, Natick, MA) cools the lesion to less than 10 degrees Celsius which results in reduced vessel elasticity, a more homogenous dilation and therefore less medial injury and/or flow-limiting dissections. To date, this device has been studied most often with SFA interventions, although literature to support its use in popliteal and tibial artery lesions exists. A small, prospective study reported a high immediate procedural success (82%) with good clinical results: Eighty percent of patients had improved ABI measurements, 89% of patients reported improvement in claudication symptoms, and 75% of patients were free of target-vessel repeat revascularization at 3 years.[439] Only 9% of these patients required adjunctive stenting at the time of the cryoplasty procedure. Several other nonrandomized studies have confirmed these procedural and clinical results.[440,441]

Endovascular Radiation. Previous research has shown that catheter based; endovascular radiation therapy (i.e., intravascular brachytherapy [IB]) inhibits neointimal hyperplasia and therefore possibly reduces significant restenosis following PTA.[442,443] IB requires transient placement of gamma- or beta-emitting radiation seeds or wires (delivered within an indwelling arterial catheter) into the diseased vasculature. Theoretically, this "localized" radiation therapy penetrates the arterial wall endothelium and breaks the bonds of single-stranded DNA in rapidly dividing cells. Therefore, proliferation of smooth muscle cells and fibroblasts is slowed, collagen synthesis is decreased, which leads to reduced target lesion restenosis.[444,445]

Initially, a small number of randomized studies reported IB to be beneficial in reducing short-term restenosis rates when used after PTA in femoropopliteal disease.[412,414,446–448] The highest benefit was seen in patients with lesions that were longer, previously treated with PTA or completely occluded lesions.[446] However, a large randomized trial investigating the efficacy of gamma radiation for the prevention of restenosis after PTA of SFA disease failed to show any significant benefit in clinical or angiographic endpoints at 1 year.[449] In addition, as seen in intracoronary brachytherapy, the use of IB in the treatment of LEPAD can be complicated by injury to normal adjacent vessels, edge stenosis, delayed healing of dissections, artery spasm, thrombosis, and/or late thrombotic occlusions.[447,450] Therefore, there is no current specific indication for the use of intravascular brachytherapy in the treatment of LEPAD.

Surgical Intervention Treatment Modalities

Numerous studies have compared the patency rates of bypass grafts constructed constructed with autogenous vein grafts (from the ipsilateral or contralateral leg or arm) have been compared to synthetic grafts. Although there is some variation in patency rates between these studies, it is apparent that superior clinical results are obtained with use of an autogenous vein graft when compared to synthetic grafts (5-year patency rates of 73% vs. 39%, respectively).[451] However, in patients when a sufficient vein graft is not available, the use of a synthetic (most often PTFE) is acceptable. Of note, patients in need of more distal anastomosis (e.g., femoral–tibial bypass) have a much higher rate of graft failure, need for graft revision, or amputation; These patients should not receive synthetic bypass grafts constructed as a result of unacceptably high rates of graft failure and subsequent amputation.[452,453] Often, when a surgical bypass fails (as opposed to following an endovascular therapy), the limb is acutely ischemic and threatened.

The most effective surgical therapy for patients with hemodynamically significant; occlusive LEPAD involving the aortoiliac arterial system (i.e., inflow disease or aortoiliac) who are deemed most appropriate for surgical revascularization, is aortobifemoral bypass. Numerous studies and registries have reported with 5- and 10-year patency rates of 85% and 80%, respectively.[454] In this procedure, a bifurcating synthetic graft is attached proximally end to end with the distal abdominal aorta (most often distal to the origin of the renal arteries) and distally to the common or deep femoral arteries. Specifically, in cases with severe occlusive disease that involves only the distal aortic bifurcation, localized aortoiliac endarterectomy may be effective. Other types of effective surgical revascularization procedures for inflow disease include aortoiliac bypass, femorofemoral bypass, axillofemoral bypass, axillofemoral–femoral bypass, and iliac endarterectomy.[99]

In patients with significant LEPAD involving the arterial vasculature beyond the iliac artery (i.e., outflow disease, the CFA and distal), the most common surgical revascularization procedure is a femoral–popliteal bypass. This surgical method carries nearly 70% patency rates at 5 years,[455–457] with patency rates near 80% when bypass is done to an above the knee anastomosis.[455] Other surgical revascularization procedures used for the treatment of outflow disease include femoral–tibial bypass and profundaplasty.

Thrombolytic Therapy

A systematic review of previous literature regarding thrombolytic therapy concluded that intra-arterial (vs. intravenous) infusion resulted in improved clinical efficacy and reduced bleeding complications. The infusion catheter should be placed within the thrombus under fluoroscopic guidance for the best clinical results. Also, high-dose infusions may result in faster lysis, but at the cost of increased bleeding rates and no improved overall clinical outcomes.[458] Power-pulse spray technique may allow for equivalent lysis with less exposure to thrombolytics.

Limb Salvage and Amputation

For the greatest chance of clinical success, it is necessary for the treating endovascular clinician to obtain "restoration of straight-line flow" to the pedal arch in one or more of the pedal arteries. This can be predicted by a postprocedure ABI greater than 0.7 or an ankle systolic pressure greater than 50 mm Hg. Also, it is imperative that the patency of the pedal arch is confirmed.[459] For example, a significant improvement in inflow may reduce or eliminate ischemic rest pain, but pulsatile flow to the foot is needed for optimal healing of ischemic ulcers and/or gangrene. Therefore, following correction of inflow disease, if the ABI is less than 0.7, correction of the outflow disease must be strongly considered.[460]

Clinical success of an endovascular procedure can be measured by relief of ischemic rest pain, improvement in healing of ulcers, and, most importantly, preservation of the diseased limb (e.g., avoidance of major amputation).[459] Several studies have reported high rates of clinical success in patients presenting with CLI and treated with PTA (procedural success rates more than 90% and 5-year limb-salvage rates of 77%–91%).[460]

Following an attempted limb-salvage revascularization procedure, it is important to address local wound care. After defining the level of adequate circulation following the revascularization, the patient may require local (digit, ray, midfoot, or symes) amputation or aggressive (including bone excision) debridement of any wounds.[33]

Although many patients presenting with limb ischemia can be successfully treated with surgical or percutaneous revascularization, in patients with occlusive disease nonamenable to revascularization (up to 60% cases), nonviable extremities, or extensive tissue necrosis amputation can be lifesaving. Therefore, patients with nonviable extremities should undergo amputation. The amputation surgery should attempt to salvage as many joint as possible (in attempt to facilitate rehabilitation efforts) and the level of viable tissue/amputation can most often be made at the time of surgery. If amputation is significantly delayed, the patient becomes dangerously susceptible to gangrene, infection, sepsis, rhabdomyolysis, myocardial infarction, and/or death.

Specific Treatment of Acute CLI

The majority of cases of acute CLI is secondary to a sudden embolic, traumatic injury, or reconstruction occlusions (Figure 33-24).[33] As a result of the severity of acute CLI, these patients require prompt and aggressive medical therapy initiated at the time of diagnosis, and emergent revascularization therapy immediately considered. Initial evaluation of these patients must determine the severity of acute limb ischemia (ALI) and if the limb viable, is its viability threatened, and/or are there irreversible changes that preclude limb salvage.[33] Viability in these limbs is suggested by minimal sensory and motor loss with audible Doppler signals (Table 33-4). Appropriate therapeutic intervention is then guided by the severity of ALI (Figure 33-37).

It is imperative that patients with acute limb ischemia receive intravenous heparin (except in cases of heparin antibodies) followed by a continuous infusion as soon as the diagnosis is made.[461] The goal of heparinization is to prevent progression of the occluding embolus or thrombus. Following the initiation of heparin therapy, it is necessary to carefully evaluate the patient and determine the duration of ischemia and viability of the affected extremity. Based on this information, the clinician can more easily determine the appropriate ensuing therapy. Currently, there is no evidence to suggest the antiplatelet medications in the setting of ALI improves clinical outcomes of the affected limb(s) (although these patients should be these medications to reduce the risk of systemic vascular events and long-term progression of their underlying atherosclerotic disease).

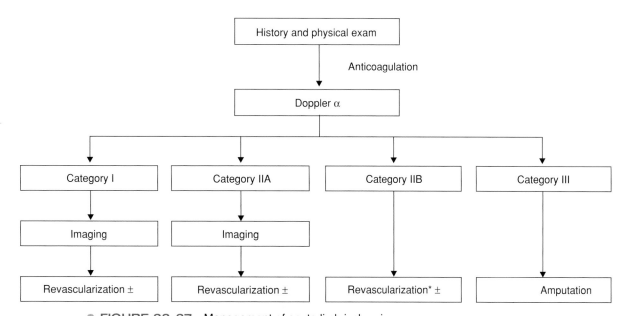

● FIGURE 33-37. Management of acute limb ischemia.

Source: Reprinted with permission from Elsevier in Norgren L, et al. Inter-Society Consensus for the Management of Peripheral Arterial Disease (TASC II). J Vasc Surg 2007;45(1):S5-S67.

Patients with ischemic extremities deemed viable, may undergo surgical revascularization, percutaneous revascularization, or undergo thrombolytic therapy. The appropriate therapy can be best guided after determining the duration of ischemia and following urgent lower extremity angiography to define the patient's arterial anatomy and disease process. Specifically, it is important to note if the ischemic lesion appears to be due to an embolus or thrombus, and the location and length of the lesion. In patients with occlusive suprainguinal lesions or trauma injury, open surgical revascularization may be the preferred initial therapeutic modality. On the other hand, many cases of infrainguinal occlusions resulting in ALI are often successfully treated with endovascular techniques. A general rule of thumb is that embolisms should be treated with embolectomies and thrombosis considered for thrombolytic therapy. If it is determined that surgery is the best and definitive procedure, delaying an operation to perform angiography or other imaging studies may not be necessary and proceeding directly to surgery may be best for the patient.

Surgical Revascularization Therapy. Patients who present with ischemia caused by an embolic event should undergo emergent surgical revascularization as irreversible damage to tissue and nerves can occur after only 4 hours of ischemia. In most cases, an embolectomy is curative of the occlusion and ischemic event. However, intraoperative thrombolytic therapy may be used if there is concern for or evidence of small emboli in the distal arterial circulation. In addition, a fasciotomy may be necessary to prevent the compartment syndrome.

Percutaneous Revascularization Therapy. Over the past decade, technologic advancements in catheters, guidewires, stents and other adjunctive therapies have made percutaneous transluminal angioplasty (PTA) an effective and beneficial therapy in many patients with acute limb ischemia. A large trial randomized 450 patients with severe limb ischemia caused by outflow disease (i.e., infrainguinal disease) to PTA or surgical bypass revascularization. Clinical endpoints following revascularization revealed no difference in mortality at 30 days or amputation-free survival up to 3 years. However, there were significantly higher rates of immediate technical failure (20% vs. 15%), morbidity (57% vs. 41%), and need for reintervention (26% vs. 18%) in patients who initially underwent PTA (57% vs. 41%).[348] Therefore, these findings support the notion that in patients presenting with CLI and severe comorbidities or shorter life expectancies (less than 2 years) that initial therapy with PTA is an acceptable therapeutic modality; However, surgery should be considered as a primary treatment modality for other patients.

Several randomized trials comparing catheter-directed thrombolytic therapy to surgical bypass revascularization for patients presenting with acute occlusion of native arteries or bypass grafts. Many of these trials suggested thrombolytic therapy to be a superior therapy with higher amputation-free survival (75% vs. 52%) and overall survival (84% vs. 58%) at 1 year.[462] More recent trials have shown that the benefit of thrombolytic therapy is limited to those patients with symptoms less than 2 weeks. Also, in patients with symptoms greater than 2 weeks who had received thrombolytic therapy there were higher rates of recurrent ischemia and major amputation than those with who initially had undergone surgical bypass revascularization.[463,464]

Large randomized trials compared thrombolytic therapy versus surgical therapy in patients with acute lower extremity limb ischemia.[464–466] These studies concluded that in patients with ischemic symptoms of less than 2 weeks, that there were no differences in amputation-free survival (72% vs. 75%, respectively) or overall mortality (65% vs. 70%, respectively) at 1 year in patients who had received thrombolytic therapy versus surgical revascularization.[465,466] However, there was an increased risk of bleeding in those patients receiving thrombolytic therapy (12.5% vs. 5.5%).[465] In addition, many studies have shown that up to 60% patients who are initially treated with thrombolytic therapy may still require surgical revascularization procedures within 6 months.[465,467] However, these surgical procedures are often less complex than those surgeries of patients who initially underwent surgical revascularization.[463,465]

Therefore, two major organizations concluded that catheter-based thrombolytic therapy is effective and beneficial in patients presenting with acute limb ischemia of less than 2 weeks duration.[99,461] However, patients with overwhelming limb ischemia may not tolerate the time necessary to perform thrombolysis; these patients should promptly be directed to surgical revascularization.

In addition, there have been smaller trials evaluating the use of percutaneous thrombectomy devices (e.g., aspiration thrombectomy and mechanical thrombectomy) in patients with acute limb ischemia of less than 2 weeks duration. Combined analysis suggests high procedural success rates (greater than 90%) and limb-salvage rates (89%). Therefore, in patients with contraindications to thrombolytics and surgical bypass revascularization, the use of these devices should be considered.

Blue Toe Syndrome. There is a high rate of mortality in patients with BTS. Initial attempts at aggressive medical therapy including statins and antiplatelet agents are indicated. All patients should have aggressive wound care, hydration, and attention to renal function. There has been no consistent data with the use of vasodilators of any type. Early literature suggested that anticoagulation with heparin/coumadin may further provoke embolization although this has not been well tested. If the proximal source is an aneurysm, then exclusion of the aneurysm is indicated, even if the aneurysm is not at a size that would traditionally warrant repair. For patients with severely atherosclerotic aortas ("shaggy" aortas), surgical bypass or exclusion with a stent graft (although, with a known risk to further dislodge emboli), have been advocated by some. Rarely, axillary–bifemoral bypass with CFA ligation has been performed.

Surveillance Following Revascularization. Based on the ACC/AHA Guidelines, patients who have undergone surgical bypass revascularization should undergo "periodic" evaluations for 2 years that include: assessment of continuation or progression of claudication; physical examination including pulse examination; duplex imaging of the entire length of the graft with peak systolic velocity measurements; and rest and exercise ABIs.[99] Prophylactic intervention for restenosis increases the graft survival rate.

REFERENCES

1. Garcia LA. Epidemiology and pathophysiology of lower extremity peripheral arterial disease. *J Endovasc Ther.* 2006;13 (suppl 2):II3-II9.

2. Dormandy JA. Management of peripheral arterial disease. TASC Working Group. TransAtlantic Inter-Society Consensus (TASC). *J Vasc Surg.* 2000;31:S5-S74.

3. Pentecost MJ, Criqui MH, Dorros G, et al. Guidelines for peripheral percutaneous transluminal angioplasty of the abdominal aorta and lower extremity vessels. *Circulation.* 1994;89:511-531.

4. Weitz JI, Byrne J, Clagett GP, et al. Diagnosis and treatment of chronic arterial insufficiency of the lower extremities: a critical review. *Circulation.* 1996;94:3026-3049.

5. Smith GD, Shipley MJ, Rose G. Intermittent claudication, heart disease risk factors, and mortality: the Whitehall study. *Circulation.* 1990;82:1925-1931.

6. Criqui MH, Langer RD, Fronek A, et al. Mortality over a period of 10 years in patients with peripheral arterial disease. *N Engl J Med.* 1992;326(6):381-386.

7. Gregg EW, Sorlie P, Paulose-Ram R, et al. Prevalence of lower-extremity disease in the U.S. adult population ≥40 years of age with and without diabetes. *Diabetes Care.* 2004; 27(7):1591-1597.

8. Mayfield JA, Reiber GE, Sanders LJ, et al. Preventative foot care in people with diabetes. *Diabetes Care.* 1998;21:2161-2177.

9. McDermott MM, Greenland P, Liu K, et al. Leg symptoms in peripheral arterial disease: associated clinical characteristics and functional impairment. *JAMA.* 2001;286:1599-1606.

10. Mohler E. Peripheral arterial disease: identification and implications. *Arch Intern Med.* 2003;163:2306-2314.

11. Harrington C, Zagari MJ, Corea J, Klitenic J. A cost analysis of diabetic lower-extremity ulcers. *Diabetes Care.* 2000; 23(9):1333-1338.

12. American Diabetes Association Consensus Panel. Peripheral arterial disease in people with diabetes. *Diabetes Care.* 2003; 26(12):3333-3341.

13. Hirsch AT, Criqui MH, Treat-Jacobson D, et al. Peripheral arterial disease detection, awareness, and treatment in primary care [see comment]. *JAMA.* 2001;286(11):1317-1324.

14. Criqui MH, Fronek A, Barrett-Connor E, Klauber MR, Gabriel S, Goodman D. The prevalence of peripheral arterial disease in a defined population. *Circulation.* 1985;71(3):510-515.

15. Criqui MH, Denenberg JO, Langer RD, Fronek A. The epidemiology of peripheral arterial disease: importance of identifying the population at risk. *Vasc Med.* 1997;2(3):221-226.

16. Meijer WT, Hoes AW, Rutgers D, Bots ML, Hofman A, Grobbee DE. Peripheral arterial disease in the elderly: the Rotterdam Study. *Arterioscler Thromb Vasc Biol.* 1998;18(2): 185-192.

17. Fowkes FHE, Cawood EH, et al. Edinburgh Artery Study. *Int J Epidemiol* 1991;20:384-392.

18. Vogt MT, Cauley JA, Kuller LH, Nevitt MC. Bone mineral density and blood flow to the lower extremities: the study of osteoporotic fractures. *J Bone Miner Res.* 1997;12(2):283-289.

19. Sumpio BE. Foot ulcers. *N Engl J Med.* 2000;343(11):787-793.

20. Newman AB, Sutton-Tyrrell K, Vogt MT, Kuller LH. Morbidity and mortality in hypertensive adults with a low ankle/arm blood pressure index. *JAMA.* 1993;270(4):487-489.

21. Ouriel K. Peripheral arterial disease [see comment]. *Lancet.* 2001;358(9289):1257-1264.

22. Gillum RF. Peripheral arterial occlusive disease of the extremities in the United States: hospitalization and mortality. *Am Heart J.* 1990;120(6, pt 1):1414-1418.

23. Murabito JM, D'Agostino RB, Silbershatz H, Wilson WF. Intermittent claudication. A risk profile from The Framingham Heart Study. *Circulation.* 1997;96(1):44-49.

24. Kannel WB, Skinner JJ Jr, Schwartz MJ, Shurtleff D. Intermittent claudication. Incidence in the Framingham Study. *Circulation.* 1970;41(5):875-883.

25. Al Zahrani HA, Al Bar HM, Bahnassi A, Abdulaal AA. The distribution of peripheral arterial disease in a defined population of elderly high-risk Saudi patients. *Int Angiol.* 1997;16(2):123-128.

26. Binaghi F, Fronteddu PF, Cannas F, et al. Prevalence of peripheral arterial occlusive disease and associated risk factors in a sample of southern Sardinian population. *Int Angiol.* 1994;13(3):233-245.

27. Cheng SW, Ting AC, Lau H, Wong J. Epidemiology of atherosclerotic peripheral arterial occlusive disease in Hong Kong. *World J Surg* 1999;23(2):202-206.

28. Coni N, Tennison B, Troup M. Prevalence of lower extremity arterial disease among elderly people in the community. *Br J Gen Pract.* 1992;42(357):149-152.

29. Gallotta G, Iazzetta N, Milan G, Ruocco A, Napoli C, Postiglione A. Prevalence of peripheral arterial disease in an elderly rural population of southern Italy. *Gerontology.* 1997; 43(5):289-295.

30. McKenna M, Wolfson S, Kuller L. The ratio of ankle and arm arterial pressure as an independent predictor of mortality. *Atherosclerosis.* 1991;87(2-3):119-128.

31. Vogt MT, Wolfson SK, Kuller LH. Lower extremity arterial disease and the aging process: a review. *J Clin Epidemiol* 1992; 45(5):529-542.

32. Da Silva A, Widmer LK, Ziegler HW, Nissen C, Schweizer W. The Basle longitudinal study: report on the relation of initial glucose level to baseline ECG abnormalities, peripheral artery disease, and subsequent mortality. *J Chronic Dis.* 1979; 32(11-12):797-803.

33. Inter-Society Consensus for the Management of Peripheral Arterial Disease. TransAtlantic Inter-Society Consensus (TASC II). *Eur J Vasc Endovasc Surg* 2007;33(suppl A):S5-S75.

34. Fowkes FG, Housley E, Riemersma RA, et al. Smoking, lipids, glucose intolerance, and blood pressure as risk factors for peripheral atherosclerosis compared with ischemic heart disease in the Edinburgh Artery Study. *Am J Epidemiol.* 1992; 135(4):331-340.

35. Kannel WB, McGee DL. Update on some epidemiologic features of intermittent claudication: the Framingham Study. *J Am Geriatr Soc.* 1985;33(1):13-18.

36. Bowlin SJ, Medalie JH, Flocke SA, Zyzanski SJ, Goldbourt U. Epidemiology of intermittent claudication in middle-aged men. *Am J Epidemiol.* 1994;140(5):418-430.

37. Price JF, Mowbray PI, Lee AJ, Rumley A, Lowe GD, Fowkes FG. Relationship between smoking and cardiovascular risk factors in the development of peripheral arterial disease and coronary artery disease: Edinburgh Artery Study. *Eur Heart J.* 1999;20(5):344-353.

38. Powell JT, Edwards RJ, Worrell PC, Franks PJ, Greenhalgh RM, Poulter NR. Risk factors associated with the development of peripheral arterial disease in smokers: a case–control study. *Atherosclerosis.* 1997;129(1):41-48.

39. Kannel WB, Shurtleff D. The Framingham Study. Cigarettes and the development of intermittent claudication. *Geriatrics.* 1973;28(2):61-68.

40. Pyorala K, Laakso M, Uusitupa M. Diabetes and atherosclerosis: an epidemiologic view. *Diabetes Metab Rev* 1987;3(2): 463-524.

41. Donahue RP, Orchard TJ. Diabetes mellitus and macrovascular complications. An epidemiological perspective. *Diabetes Care.* 1992;15(9):1141-1155.

42. Selvin E, Marinopoulos S, Berkenblit G, et al. Meta-analysis: glycosylated hemoglobin and cardiovascular disease in diabetes mellitus. *Ann Intern Med.* 2004;141(6):421-431.

43. Muntner P, Wildman RP, Reynolds K, Desalvo KB, Chen J, Fonseca V. Relationship between HbA1 c level and peripheral arterial disease. *Diabetes Care.* 2005;28(8):1981-1987.

44. Newman AB, Siscovick DS, Manolio TA, et al. Ankle–arm index as a marker of atherosclerosis in the Cardiovascular Health Study. Cardiovascular Heart Study (CHS) Collaborative Research Group. *Circulation.* 1993;88(3):837-845.

45. Hiatt WR, Hoag S, Hamman RF. Effect of diagnostic criteria on the prevalence of peripheral arterial disease. The San Luis Valley Diabetes Study. *Circulation.* 1995;91(5):1472-1479.

46. Beks PJ, Mackaay AJ, de Neeling JN, de Vries H, Bouter LM, Heine RJ. Peripheral arterial disease in relation to glycaemic level in an elderly Caucasian population: the Hoorn study. *Diabetologia.* 1995;38(1):86-96.

47. Jude EB, Oyibo SO, Chalmers N, Boulton AJ. Peripheral arterial disease in diabetic and nondiabetic patients: a comparison of severity and outcome. *Diabetes Care.* 2001;24(8): 1433-1437.

48. Al-Delaimy WK, Merchant AT, Rimm EB, Willett WC, Stampfer MJ, Hu FB. Effect of type 2 diabetes and its duration on the risk of peripheral arterial disease among men. *Am J Med.* 2004;116(4):236-240.

49. Katsilambros NL, Tsapogas PC, Arvanitis MP, Tritos NA, Alexiou ZP, Rigas KL. Risk factors for lower extremity arterial disease in non-insulin-dependent diabetic persons. *Diabet Med.* 1996;13(3):243-246.

50. McDaniel MD, Cronenwett JL. Basic data related to the natural history of intermittent claudication. *Ann Vasc Surg.* 1989;3(3):273-277.

51. Dormandy JA, Murray GD. The fate of the claudicant-a prospective study of 1969 claudicants. *Eur J Vasc Surg.* 1991; 5(2):131-133.

52. Most RS, Sinnock P. The epidemiology of lower extremity amputations in diabetic individuals. *Diabetes Care.* 1983; 6(1):87-91.

53. Silbert S, Zazeela H. Prognosis in arteriosclerotic peripheral vascular disease. *J Am Med Assoc.* 1958;166(15):1816-1821.

54. Schadt DC, Hines EA Jr, Juergens JL, Barker NW. Chronic atherosclerotic occlusion of the femoral artery. *JAMA.* 1961;175:937-940.

55. Criqui MH, Denenberg JO, Bird CE, Fronek A, Klauber MR, Langer RD. The correlation between symptoms and noninvasive test results in patients referred for peripheral arterial disease testing. *Vasc Med.* 1996;1(1):65-71.

56. Rose GA. The diagnosis of ischaemic heart pain and intermittent claudication in field surveys. *Bull World Health Organ.* 1962;27:645-658.

57. Vogt MT, Cauley JA, Kuller LH, Hulley SB. Prevalence and correlates of lower extremity arterial disease in elderly women. *Am J Epidemiol.* 1993;137(5):559-568.

58. Bainton D, Sweetnam P, Baker I, Elwood P. Peripheral vascular disease: consequence for survival and association with risk factors in the Speedwell prospective heart disease study. *Br Heart J.* 1994;72(2):128-132.

59. Dagenais GR, Maurice S, Robitaille NM, Gingras S, Lupien PJ. Intermittent claudication in Quebec men from 1974-1986: the Quebec Cardiovascular Study. *Clin Invest Med.* 1991;14(2):93-100.

60. Ingolfsson IO, Sigurdsson G, Sigvaldason H, Thorgeirsson G, Sigfusson N. A marked decline in the prevalence and incidence of intermittent claudication in Icelandic men 1968–1986: a strong relationship to smoking and serum cholesterol—the Reykjavik Study. *J Clin Epidemiol.* 1994;47 (11):1237-1243.

61. Horby J, Grande P, Vestergaard A, Grauholt AM. High density lipoprotein cholesterol and arteriography in intermittent claudication. *Eur J Vasc Surg.* 1989;3(4):333-337.

62. Bradby GV, Valente AJ, Walton KW. Serum high-density lipoproteins in peripheral vascular disease. *Lancet.* 1978;2 (8103):1271-1274.

63. Senti M, Nogues X, Pedro-Botet J, Rubies-Prat J, Vidal-Barraquer F. Lipoprotein profile in men with peripheral

vascular disease. Role of intermediate density lipoproteins and apoprotein E phenotypes. *Circulation*. 1992;85(1):30-36.

64. Ridker PM, Stampfer MJ, Rifai N. Novel risk factors for systemic atherosclerosis: a comparison of C-reactive protein, fibrinogen, homocysteine, lipoprotein(a), and standard cholesterol screening as predictors of peripheral arterial disease. *JAMA*. 2001;285(19):2481-2485.

65. Sanderson KJ, van Rij AM, Wade CR, Sutherland WH. Lipid peroxidation of circulating low density lipoproteins with age, smoking and in peripheral vascular disease. *Atherosclerosis*. 1995;118(1):45-51.

66. Novo S, Avellone G, Di Garbo V, et al. Prevalence of risk factors in patients with peripheral arterial disease. A clinical and epidemiological evaluation. *Int Angiol*. 1992;11(3):218-229.

67. Mowat BF, Skinner ER, Wilson HM, Leng GC, Fowkes FG, Horrobin D. Alterations in plasma lipids, lipoproteins and high density lipoprotein subfractions in peripheral arterial disease. *Atherosclerosis*. 1997;131(2):161-166.

68. Mendelson G, Aronow WS, Ahn C. Prevalence of coronary artery disease, atherothrombotic brain infarction, and peripheral arterial disease: associated risk factors in older Hispanics in an academic hospital-based geriatrics practice. *J Am Geriatr Soc*. 1998;46(4):481-483.

69. Harris LM, Armstrong D, Browne R, et al. Premature peripheral vascular disease: clinical profile and abnormal lipid peroxidation. *Cardiovasc Surg*. 1998;6(2):188-193.

70. Greenhalgh RM, Rosengarten DS, Mervart I, Lewis B, Calnan JS, Martin P. Serum lipids and lipoproteins in peripheral vascular disease. *Lancet*. 1971;2(7731):947-950.

71. Murabito JM, Evans JC, Nieto K, Larson MG, Levy D, Wilson PW. Prevalence and clinical correlates of peripheral arterial disease in the Framingham Offspring Study. *Am Heart J*. 2002;143(6):961-965.

72. Boushey CJ, Beresford SA, Omenn GS, Motulsky AG. A quantitative assessment of plasma homocysteine as a risk factor for vascular disease. Probable benefits of increasing folic acid intakes. *JAMA*. 1995;274(13):1049-1057.

73. Tsai JC, Perrella MA, Yoshizumi M, et al. Promotion of vascular smooth muscle cell growth by homocysteine: a link to atherosclerosis. *Proc Natl Acad Sci U S A*. 1994;91(14):6369-6373.

74. Heinecke JW, Rosen H, Chait A. Iron and copper promote modification of low density lipoprotein by human arterial smooth muscle cells in culture. *J Clin Invest*. 1984;74:1890-1894.

75. Clarke R, Daly L, Robinson K, et al. Hyperhomocysteinemia: an independent risk factor for vascular disease. *N Engl J Med*. 1991;324(17):1149-1155.

76. Robinson K, Arheart K, Refsum H, et al. Low circulating folate and vitamin B6 concentrations: risk factors for stroke, peripheral vascular disease, and coronary artery disease. European COMAC Group. *Circulation*. 1998;97(5):437-443.

77. Graham IM, Daly LE, Refsum HM, et al. Plasma homocysteine as a risk factor for vascular disease. The European Concerted Action Project. *JAMA*. 1997;277(22):1775-1781.

78. Hoogeveen EK, Kostense PJ, Beks PJ, et al. Hyperhomocysteinemia is associated with an increased risk of cardiovascular disease, especially in non-insulin-dependent diabetes mellitus: a population-based study. *Arterioscler Thromb Vasc Biol*. 1998;18(1):133-138.

79. Taylor LM Jr, Moneta GL, Sexton GJ, Schuff RA, Porter JM. Prospective blinded study of the relationship between plasma homocysteine and progression of symptomatic peripheral arterial disease. *J Vasc Surg*. 1999;29(1):8-19; discussion 21.

80. Aboyans V, Criqui MH, Denenberg JO, Knoke JD, Ridker PM, Fronek A. Risk factors for progression of peripheral arterial disease in large and small vessels. *Circulation*. 2006;113(22):2623-2629.

81. Currie IC, Wilson YG, Scott J, et al. Homocysteine: an independent risk factor for the failure of vascular intervention. *Br J Surg*. 1996;83(9):1238-1241.

82. Ridker PM, Cushman M, Stampfer MJ, Tracy RP, Hennekens CH. Inflammation, aspirin, and the risk of cardiovascular disease in apparently healthy men. *N Engl J Med*. 1997;336(14):973-979.

83. Ridker PM, Cushman M, Stampfer MJ, Tracy RP, Hennekens CH. Plasma concentration of C-reactive protein and risk of developing peripheral vascular disease. *Circulation*. 1998;97(5):425-428.

84. Aronow WS, Ahn C. Prevalence of coexistence of coronary artery disease, peripheral arterial disease, and atherothrombotic brain infarction in men and women > or = 62 years of age. *Am J Cardiol*. 1994;74(1):64-65.

85. McDermott MM, Fried L, Simonsick E, Ling S, Guralnik JM. Asymptomatic peripheral arterial disease is independently associated with impaired lower extremity functioning: the women's health and aging study. *Circulation*. 2000;101(9):1007-1012.

86. Zheng ZJ, Sharrett AR, Chambless LE, et al. Associations of ankle–brachial index with clinical coronary heart disease, stroke and preclinical carotid and popliteal atherosclerosis: the Atherosclerosis Risk in Communities (ARIC) Study. *Atherosclerosis*. 1997;131(1):115-125.

87. Kullo IJ, Bailey KR, Kardia SL, Mosley TH Jr, Boerwinkle E, Turner ST. Ethnic differences in peripheral arterial disease in the NHLBI Genetic Epidemiology Network of Arteriopathy (GENOA) study. *Vasc Med*. 2003;8(4):237-242.

88. Criqui MH, V Vargas, Hoe E, et al. Ethnicity and peripheral arterial disease. *Circulation*. 2002;105:e113.

89. Curb JD, Masaki K, Rodriguez BL, et al. Peripheral artery disease and cardiovascular risk factors in the elderly. The Honolulu Heart Program. *Arterioscler Thromb Vasc Biol* 1996;16(12):1495-1500.

90. Fabsitz RR, Sidawy AN, Go O, et al. Prevalence of peripheral arterial disease and associated risk factors in American Indians: the Strong Heart Study. *Am J Epidemiol*. 1999;149(4):330-338.

91. Dieter RS, Tomasson J, Gudjonsson T, et al. Lower extremity peripheral arterial disease in hospitalized patients with coronary artery disease. *Vasc Med*. 2003;8(4):233-236.

92. Sukhija R, Aronow WS, Yalamanchili K, Sinha N, Babu S. Prevalence of coronary artery disease, lower extremity peripheral arterial disease, and cerebrovascular disease in 110

men with an abdominal aortic aneurysm. *Am J Cardiol.* 2004;94(10):1358-1359.

93. O'Hare AM, Glidden DV, Fox CS, Hsu CY. High prevalence of peripheral arterial disease in persons with renal insufficiency: results from the National Health and Nutrition Examination Survey 1999-2000. *Circulation.* 2004;109(3): 320-323.

94. Erdoes LS, Hunter GC, Venerus BJ, et al. Prospective evaluation of peripheral vascular disease in heart transplant recipients. *J Vasc Surg.* 1995;22(4):434-440; discussion 40-42.

95. Cofan F, Nunez I, Gilabert R, et al. Increased prevalence of carotid and femoral atherosclerosis in renal transplant recipients. *Transplant Proc.* 2001;33(1-2):1254-1256.

96. Housley E, Leng GC, Donnan PT, Fowkes FG. Physical activity and risk of peripheral arterial disease in the general population: Edinburgh Artery Study. *J Epidemiol Community Health.* 1993;47(6):475-480.

97. Camargo CA Jr, Stampfer MJ, Glynn RJ, et al. Prospective study of moderate alcohol consumption and risk of peripheral arterial disease in U.S. male physicians. *Circulation.* 1997; 95(3):577-580.

98. Stoffers HE, Rinkens PE, Kester AD, Kaiser V, Knottnerus JA. The prevalence of asymptomatic and unrecognized peripheral arterial occlusive disease. *Int J Epidemiol.* 1996; 25(2):282-290.

99. Hirsch AT, Haskal ZJ, Hertzer NR, et al. ACC/AHA 2005 guidelines for the management of patients with peripheral arterial disease (lower extremity, renal, mesenteric, and abdominal aortic): executive summary a collaborative report from the American Association for Vascular Surgery/Society for Vascular Surgery, Society for Cardiovascular Angiography and Interventions, Society for Vascular Medicine and Biology, Society of Interventional Radiology, and the ACC/AHA Task Force on Practice Guidelines (Writing Committee to Develop Guidelines for the Management of Patients With Peripheral Arterial Disease) endorsed by the American Association of Cardiovascular and Pulmonary Rehabilitation; National Heart, Lung, and Blood Institute; Society for Vascular Nursing; TransAtlantic Inter-Society Consensus; and Vascular Disease Foundation. *J Am Coll Cardiol.* 2006;47(6): 1239-1312.

100. Golomb BA, Dang TT, Criqui MH. Peripheral arterial disease: morbidity and mortality implications. *Circulation.* 2006;114(7):688-699.

101. Hertzer NR, Beven EG, Young JR, et al. Coronary artery disease in peripheral vascular patients. A classification of 1000 coronary angiograms and results of surgical management. *Ann Surg.* 1984;199(2):223-233.

102. Mautner GC, Mautner SL, Roberts WC. Amounts of coronary arterial narrowing by atherosclerotic plaque at necropsy in patients with lower extremity amputation. *Am J Cardiol.* 1992;70(13):1147-1151.

103. Miralles M, Corominas A, Cotillas J, Castro F, Clara A, Vidal-Barraquer F. Screening for carotid and renal artery stenoses in patients with aortoiliac disease. *Ann Vasc Surg.* 1998;12(1): 17-22.

104. Larsen WJ, Sherman LS, Potter SS, et al. *Human Embryology.* 3rd ed. Philadelphia, PA: Churchill Livingstone; 1993.

105. Standring S, ed. *Gray's Anatomy. The Anatomical Basis of Clinical Practice.* 39th ed. Philadelphia, PA: Churchill Livingstone; 2005.

106. Schmidt J, Paetz B, Allenberg JR. Bilateral congenital aplasia of the deep femoral arteries. *Ann Vasc Surg.* 1990;4(5):498-501.

107. Kantarci F, Mihmanli I, Aksoy H, Barutca H, Gurses B, Kaynak K. Duplication of the superficial femoral artery diagnosed primarily on the basis of color Doppler ultrasonography. *J Ultrasound Med.* 2003;22(6):641-643.

108. Woods CG, Treleaven S, Betheras FR, Sheffield LJ. 'Disorganization-like syndrome' with 47, XXY and unilateral narrowing of the common iliac artery. *Clin Dysmorphol.* 1995;4(1):82-86.

109. Rodriguez JI. Vascular anomalies in campomelic syndrome. *Am J Med Genet.* 1993;46(2):185-192.

110. Levinsohn EM, Hootnick DR, Packard DS Jr. Consistent arterial abnormalities associated with a variety of congenital malformations of the human lower limb. *Invest Radiol.* 1991; 26(4):364-373.

111. Kim M, Dupuy JP, Dany F. Embryology, anomalies, dystrophy and pathology of the lower limbs arteries (author's transl). *J Mal Vasc.* 1981;6(3):187-192.

112. Brantley SK, Rigdon EE, Raju S. Persistent sciatic artery: embryology, pathology, and treatment. *J Vasc Surg.* 1993;18(2): 242-248.

113. Mauro MA, Jaques PF, Moore M. The popliteal artery and its branches: embryologic basis of normal and variant anatomy. *AJR Am J Roentgenol.*1988;150(2):435-437.

114. Martin KW, Hyde GL, McCready RA, Hull DA. Sciatic artery aneurysms: report of three cases and review of the literature. *J Vasc Surg.* 1986;4(4):365-371.

115. Williams LR, Flanigan DP, O'Connor RJ, Schuler JJ. Persistent sciatic artery. Clinical aspects and operative management. *Am J Surg.* 1983;145(5):687-693.

116. McLellan GL, Morettin LB. Persistent sciatic artery: clinical, surgical, and angiographic aspects. *Arch Surg.* 1982;117 (6):817-822.

117. Sultan SA, Pacainowski JP, Madhavan P, et al. Endovascular management of rare sciatic artery aneurysm. *J Endovasc Ther.* 2000;7(5):415-422.

118. Cowie TN, Mc KN, Mc LN, Smith G. Unilateral congenital absence of the external iliac and femoral arteries. *Br J Radiol.* 1960;33:520-522.

119. Greebe J. Congenital anomalies of the iliofemoral artery. *J Cardiovasc Surg (Torino).* 1977;18(3):317-323.

120. Nicholson RL, Pastershank SP, Bharadwaj BB. Persistent primitive sciatic artery. *Radiology.* 1977;122(3):687-689.

121. Wright FW. Persistent axial or sciatic artery of the lower limb in association with hemihypertrophy. *Clin Radiol.* 1964; 15:291-292.

122. Youngson GG, Taylor B, Rankin R, Heimbecker RO. Persistent sciatic artery: a case report. *Can J Surg.* 1980;23(5):466-467.

123. Clark FA Jr, Beazley RM. Sciatic artery aneurysm: a case report including operative approach and review of the literature. *Am Surg.* 1976;42(1):13-16.

124. Thomas ML, Blakeney CG, Browse NL. Arteriomegaly of persistent sciatic arteries. *Radiology.* 1978;128(1):55-56.

125. Mayschak DT, Flye MW. Treatment of the persistent sciatic artery. *Ann Surg.* 1984;199(1):69-74.

126. Sottiurai VS, Omlie W. Femoral artery hypoplasia and persistent sciatic artery with blue toe syndrome: a case report, histologic analysis and review of the literature. *Int Angiol.* 1994;13(2):154-159.

127. Dieter RS, Chu WW, Pacanowski JP Jr, McBride PE, Tanke TE. The significance of lower extremity peripheral arterial disease. *Clin Cardiol.* 2002;25(1):3-10.

128. Ross R. Atherosclerosis—an inflammatory disease. *N Engl J Med.* 1999;340(2):115-126.

129. Schaar JA, Muller JE, Falk E, et al. Terminology for high-risk and vulnerable coronary artery plaques. Report of a meeting on the vulnerable plaque, June 17 and 18, 2003, Santorini, Greece. *Eur Heart J.* 2004;25(12):1077-1082.

130. Park TC, Hamre DW, Porter JM. Nonatherosclerotic causes of lower extremity claudication. *Ann Vasc Surg.* 1992; 6(6):541-549.

131. Roques X, Bourdeaud'hui A, Choussat A, et al. Coarctation of the abdominal aorta. *Ann Vasc Surg.* 1988;2(2):138-144.

132. Cohen JR, Birnbaum E. Coarctation of the abdominal aorta. *J Vasc Surg* 1988;8(2):160-164.

133. Graham LM, Zelenock GB, Erlandson EE, Coran AG, Lindenauer SM, Stanley JC. Abdominal aortic coarctation and segmental hypoplasia. *Surgery.* 1979;86(4):519-529.

134. Rossi MA. Infrarenal aortic coarctation and diffuse hypoplasia of the aortoiliac–femoral system. *Acta Cardiol.* 1997;52(4):373-379.

135. Wain RA, Hines G. A contemporary review of popliteal artery aneurysms. *Cardiol Rev.* 2007;15(2):102-107.

136. Wychulis AR, Spittell JA Jr, Wallace RB. Popliteal aneurysms. *Surgery.* 1970;68(6):942-952.

137. Mousa AY, Beauford RB, Henderson P, et al. Update on the diagnosis and management of popliteal aneurysm and literature review. *Vascular.* 2006;14(2):103-108.

138. Parsons RE, Marin ML, Veith FJ, Parsons RB, Hollier LH. Midterm results of endovascular stented grafts for the treatment of isolated iliac artery aneurysms. *J Vasc Surg.* 1999; 30(5):915-921.

139. Boules TN, Selzer F, Stanziale SF, et al. Endovascular management of isolated iliac artery aneurysms. *J Vasc Surg.* 2006; 44(1):29-37.

140. Serry C, Agomuoh OS, Goldin MD. Review of Ehlers-Danlos syndrome. Successful repair of rupture and dissection of abdominal aorta. *J Cardiovasc Surg (Torino).* 1988;29(5):530-534.

141. Pope FM, Narcisi P, Nicholls AC, Liberman M, Oorthuys JW. Clinical presentations of Ehlers Danlos syndrome type IV. *Arch Dis Child.* 1988;63(9):1016-1025.

142. Imahori S, Bannerman RM, Graf CJ, Brennan JC. Ehlers-Danlos syndrome with multiple arterial lesions. *Am J Med.* 1969;47(6):967-977.

143. Barabas AP. Vascular complications in the Ehlers-Danlos syndrome, with special reference to the "arterial type" or Sack's syndrome. *J Cardiovasc Surg (Torino)* 1972;13(2):160-167.

144. Wright CB, Lamberth WC, Ponseti IV, Hanson J. Successful management of popliteal arterial disruption in Ehlers-Danlos syndrome. *Surgery.* 1979;85(6):708-712.

145. Valverde A, Tricot JF, de Crepy B, Bakdach H, Djabbari K. Innominate artery involvement in type IV Ehlers-Danlos syndrome. *Ann Vasc Surg.* 1991;5(1):41-45.

146. Hunter GC, Malone JM, Moore WS, Misiorowski RL, Chvapil M. Vascular manifestations in patients with Ehlers-Danlos syndrome. *Arch Surg.* 1982;117(4):495-498.

147. Slade AK, John RM, Swanton RH. Pseudoxanthoma elasticum presenting with myocardial infarction. *Br Heart J.* 1990;63(6):372-373.

148. Wolff HH, Stokes JF, Schlesinger BE. Vascular abnormalities associated with pseudoxanthoma elasticum. *Arch Dis Child.* 1952;27(131):82-88.

149. Wahlqvist ML, Fox RM, Beech AM, Favilla I. Peripheral vascular disease as a mode of presentation of pseudoxanthoma elasticum. *Aust N Z J Med.* 1977;7(5):523-525.

150. Viljoen D. Pseudoxanthoma elasticum (Gronblad-Strandberg syndrome). *J Med Genet.* 1988;25(7):488-490.

151. Carter DJ, Woodward DA, Vince FP. Arterial surgery in pseudoxanthoma elasticum. *Postgrad Med J.* 1976;52(607):291-292.

152. Raso AM, Conforti M, Cassatella R, et al. Acute lower limb thrombosis caused by a congenital fibrous ring of the superficial femoral artery. *Minerva Cardioangiol.* 2001;49(2):147-151.

153. Owen ER, Speechly-Dick EM, Kour NW, Wilkins RA, Lewis JD. Cystic adventitial disease of the popliteal artery—a case of spontaneous resolution. *Eur J Vasc Surg.* 1990;4(3):319-321.

154. Flanigan DP, Burnham SJ, Goodreau JJ, Bergan JJ. Summary of cases of adventitial cystic disease of the popliteal artery. *Ann Surg.* 1979;189(2):165-175.

155. Ishikawa K. Cystic adventitial disease of the popliteal artery and of other stem vessels in the extremities. *Jpn J Surg.* 1987; 17(4):221-229.

156. Fox RL, Kahn M, Adler J, et al. Adventitial cystic disease of the popliteal artery: failure of percutaneous transluminal angioplasty as a therapeutic modality. *J Vasc Surg.* 1985;2(3):464-467.

157. di Marzo L, Peetz DJ Jr, Bewtra C, Schultz RD, Feldhaus RJ, Anthone G. Cystic adventitial degeneration of the femoral artery: is evacuation and cyst excision worthwhile as a definitive therapy? *Surgery.* 1987;101(5):587-593.

158. Kavanaugh A, O-MN, ed. *The Role of the Vascular Endothelium in the Pathogenesis of Vasculitis.* New York, NY: Marcel Dekker; 1992.

159. von Bierbrauer A, Ehlenz K, Herzog P, Cassel W, von Wichert P. Plasma endothelin concentration during cold provocation in primary Raynaud's syndrome. *Dtsch Med Wochenschr.* 1995;120(25-26):902-906.

160. Schiffrin EL, Intengan HD, Thibault G, Touyz RM. Clinical significance of endothelin in cardiovascular disease. *Curr Opin Cardiol.* 1997;12(4):354-367.

161. Kadono T, Kikuchi K, Kubo M, Fujimoto M, Tamaki K. Serum concentrations of basic fibroblast growth factor in collagen diseases. *J Am Acad Dermatol.* 1996;35(3, pt 1):392-397.

162. Hoshino S, Hamada O, Iwaya F, Takahira H, Honda K. Omental transplantation for chronic occlusive arterial diseases. *Int Surg.* 1979;64(5):21-29.

163. Agarwal VK. Long-term results of omental transplantation in chronic occlusive arterial disease (Buerger's disease). *Int Surg.* 2005;90(3):167-174.

164. Braunwald E, Fauci AS, Kasper DL, et al. *Harrison's Principles of Internal Medicine.* Colombus, OH: McGraw-Hill; 2001.

165. Park JH, Han MC, Bettmann MA. Arterial manifestations of Behcet disease. *AJR Am J Roentgenol.* 1984;143(4):821-825.

166. Hamza M. Large artery involvement in Behcet's disease. *J Rheumatol.* 1987;14(3):554-559.

167. Yazici H, Pazarli H, Barnes CG, et al. A controlled trial of azathioprine in Behcet's syndrome [see comment]. *N Engl J Med.* 1990;322(5):281-285.

168. Little AG, Zarins CK. Abdominal aortic aneurysm and Behcet's disease. *Surgery.* 1982;91(3):359-362.

169. Jenkins AM, Macpherson AI, Nolan B, Housley E. Peripheral aneurysms in Behet's disease. *Br J Surg.* 1976;63(3):199-202.

170. Raynaud M. *On Local Asphyxia and Symmetrical Changes to the Extremities.* London, UK: New Sydenham Society; 1888.

171. Tanner JR. St. Anthony's fire, then and now: a case report and historical review. *Can J Surg.* 1987;30(4):291-293.

172. Wells KE, Steed DL, Zajko AB, Webster MW. Recognition and treatment of arterial insufficiency from cafergot. *J Vasc Surg.* 1986;4(1):8-15.

173. Baader W, Herman C, Johansen K. St. Anthony's fire: successful reversal of ergotamine-induced peripheral vasospasm by hydrostatic dilatation. *Ann Vasc Surg.* 1990;4(6):597-599.

174. McKiernan TL, Bock K, Leya F, et al. Ergot induced peripheral vascular insufficiency, non-interventional treatment. *Cathet Cardiovasc Diagn.* 1994;31(3):211-214.

175. Van Damme H, Ballaux JM, Dereume JP. Femoro-popliteal venous graft entrapment. *J Cardiovasc Surg.* 1988;29(1):50-55.

176. Mentha C. Malposition and extrinsic stenosis of the popliteal artery caused by the musculotendinous compression of the internal gemellus muscle. *J Chir (Paris).* 1966;91(4):489-500.

177. Haimovici H, Sprayregen S, Johnson F. Popliteal artery entrapment by fibrous band. *Surgery.* 1972;72(5):789-792.

178. Insua JA, Young JR, Humphries AW. Popliteal artery entrapment syndrome. *Arch Surg.* 1970;101(6):771-775.

179. Gibson MH, Mills JG, Johnson GE, Downs AR. Popliteal entrapment syndrome. *Ann Surg.* 1977;185(3):341-348.

180. Baker WH, Stoney RJ. Acquired popliteal entrapment syndrome. *Arch Surg.* 1972;105(5):780-781.

181. Rich NM, Collins GJ Jr, McDonald PT, Kozloff L, Clagett GP, Collins JT. Popliteal vascular entrapment. Its increasing interest. *Arch Surg.* 1979;114(12):1377-1384.

182. Verta MJ Jr, Vitello J, Fuller J. Adductor canal compression syndrome. *Arch Surg.* 1984;119(3):345-346.

183. Banjo AO. Anomaly of the femoral artery passage through the substance of sartorius muscle. Clinical consequences. *Afr J Med Med Sci.* 1995;24(4):343-346.

184. Abraham P, Chevalier JM, Loire R. External iliac artery end-ofibrosis in a young cyclist. *Circulation.* 1999;100:38.

185. Rousselet MC, Saint-Andre JP, L'Hoste P, Enon B, Megret A, Chevalier JM. Stenotic intimal thickening of the external iliac artery in competition cyclists. *Hum pathol.* 1990; 21(5):524-529.

186. Erdoes LS, Devine JJ, Bernhard VM, Baker MR, Berman SS, Hunter GC. Popliteal vascular compression in a normal population. *J Vasc Surg.* 1994;20(6):978-986.

187. Hoffmann U, Vetter J, Rainoni L, Leu AJ, Bollinger A. Popliteal artery compression and force of active plantar flexion in young healthy volunteers. *J Vasc Surg.* 1997;26(2):281-287.

188. Jones WT III, Gray BH. Arteriographic evidence of pseudoocclusion of the popliteal artery: don't be fooled [see comment]. *Catheter Cardiovasc Interv.* 2006;68(4):522-525.

189. Schena S, Owens CA, Hassoun HT, Kibbe MR. Delayed presentation of a posttraumatic superficial femoral artery pseudoaneurysm. *J Am Coll Surg.* 2006;203(2):250-251.

190. Bell CL, Ali AT, Brawley JG, et al. Arterial reconstruction of infected femoral artery pseudoaneurysms using superficial femoral–popliteal vein. *J Am Coll Surg.* 2005;200(6):831-836.

191. Straton CS, Tisnado J. Spontaneous arteriovenous fistulas of the lower extremities: angiographic demonstration in five patients with peripheral vascular disease. *Cardiovasc Interv Radiol.* 2000;23(4):318-321.

192. Asensio JA, Kuncir EJ, Garcia-Nunez LM, Petrone P. Femoral vessel injuries: analysis of factors predictive of outcomes. *J Am Coll Surg.* 2006;203(4):512-520.

193. Beckman JA, Jaff MR, Creager MA. The United States preventive services task force recommendation statement on screening for peripheral arterial disease: more harm than benefit? *Circulation.* 2006;114(8):861-866.

194. Bloor K. Natural history of arteriosclerosis of the lower extremities. *Ann R Coll Surg Engl.* 1961;28:36.

195. DeWeese JA, Leather R, Porter J. Practice guidelines: lower extremity revascularization. *J Vasc Surg.* 1993;18(2):280-294.

196. Leng GC, Lee AJ, Fowkes FG, et al. Incidence, natural history and cardiovascular events in symptomatic and asymptomatic peripheral arterial disease in the general population. *Int J Epidemiol.* 1996;25(6):1172-1181.

197. Mukherjee D, Lingam P, Chetcuti S, et al. Missed opportunities to treat atherosclerosis in patients undergoing peripheral vascular interventions: insights from the University of Michigan Peripheral Vascular Disease Quality Improvement Initiative (PVD-QI2). *Circulation.* 2002;106(15):1909-1912.

198. Grundy SM, Pasternak R, Greenland P, Smith S Jr, Fuster V. AHA/ACC scientific statement: assessment of cardiovascular risk by use of multiple-risk-factor assessment equations: a statement for healthcare professionals from the American Heart Association and the American College of Cardiology. *J Am Coll Cardiol.* 1999;34(4):1348-1359.

199. Karmody AM, Powers SR, Monaco VJ, Leather RP. "Blue toe" syndrome. An indication for limb salvage surgery. *Arch Surg.* 1976;111(11):1263-1268.

200. Nasser TK, Mohler ER III, Wilensky RL, Hathaway DR. Peripheral vascular complications following coronary interventional procedures. *Clin Cardiol.* 1995;18(11):609-614.

201. Juergens JL, Barker NW, Hines EA Jr. Arteriosclerosis obliterans: review of 520 cases with special reference to pathogenic and prognostic factors. *Circulation.* 1960;21:188-195.

202. Cronenwett JL, Warner KG, Zelenock GB, et al. Intermittent claudication. Current results of nonoperative management. *Arch Surg.* 1984;119(4):430-436.

203. The ICAI Group. Long-term mortality and its predictors in patients wtih critical limb ischemia. *Eur J Vasc Endovasc Surg.* 1997;14:91-95.

204. Norgren L, Alwmark A, Angqvist KA, et al. A stable prostacyclin analogue (iloprost) in the treatment of ischaemic ulcers of the lower limb. A Scandinavian-Polish placebo controlled, randomised multicenter study. *Eur J Vasc Surg.* 1990; 4(5):463-467.

205. Lowe GD, Dunlop DJ, Lawson DH, et al. Double-blind controlled clinical trial of ancrod for ischemic rest pain of the leg. *Angiology.* 1982;33(1):46-50.

206. Belch JJ, McKay A, McArdle B, et al. Epoprostenol (prostacyclin) and severe arterial disease. A double-blind trial. *Lancet.* 1983;1(8320):315-317.

207. Diehm C, Lange S, Darius H, et al. Association of low ankle brachial index with high mortality in primary care. *Eur Heart J.* 2006;27(14):1743-1749.

208. Jelnes R, Gaardsting O, Hougaard Jensen K, Baekgaard N, Tonnesen KH, Schroeder T. Fate in intermittent claudication: outcome and risk factors. *Br Med J (Clin Res Ed).* 1986;293(6555):1137-1140.

209. Sadanandan S, Cannon CP, Gibson CM, Murphy SA, DiBattiste PM, Braunwald E. A risk score to estimate the likelihood of coronary artery bypass surgery during the index hospitalization among patients with unstable angina and non-ST-segment elevation myocardial infarction. *J Am Coll Cardiol.* 2004;44(4):799-803.

210. Ostergren J, Sleight P, Dagenais G, et al. Impact of ramipril in patients with evidence of clinical or subclinical peripheral arterial disease. *Eur Heart J.* 2004;25(1):17-24.

211. Ogren M, Hedblad B, Engstrom G, Janzon L. Prevalence and prognostic significance of asymptomatic peripheral arterial disease in 68-year-old men with diabetes. Results from the population study 'Men born in 1914' from Malmo, Sweden. *Eur J Vasc Endovasc Surg.* 2005;29(2):182-189.

212. Newman AB, Shemanski L, Manolio TA, et al. Ankle–arm index as a predictor of cardiovascular disease and mortality in the Cardiovascular Health Study. The Cardiovascular Health Study Group. *Arterioscler Thromb Vasc Biol.* 1999;19(3):538-545.

213. Narins CR, Zareba W, Moss AJ, et al. Relationship between intermittent claudication, inflammation, thrombosis, and recurrent cardiac events among survivors of myocardial infarction. *Arch Intern Med.* 2004;164(4):440-446.

214. Minakata K, Konishi Y, Matsumoto M, et al. Influence of peripheral vascular occlusive disease on the morbidity and mortality of coronary artery bypass grafting. *Jpn Circ J.* 2000;64(12):905-908.

215. Kornitzer M, Dramaix M, Sobolski J, Degre S, De Backer G. Ankle/arm pressure index in asymptomatic middle-aged males: an independent predictor of ten-year coronary heart disease mortality. *Angiology.* 1995;46(3):211-219.

216. Kallero KS. Mortality and morbidity in patients with intermittent claudication as defined by venous occlusion plethysmography. A ten-year follow-up study. *J Chronic Dis.* 1981;34(9-10):455-462.

217. SHEP Cooperative Research Group. Prevention of stroke by antihypertensive drug treatment in older persons with isolated systolic hypertension. Final results of the Systolic Hypertension in the Elderly Program (SHEP). *JAMA.* 1991; 265(24):3255-3264.

218. Pardaens J, Lesaffre E, Willems JL, De Geest H. Multivariate survival analysis for the assessment of prognostic factors and risk categories after recovery from acute myocardial infarction: the Belgian situation. *Am J Epidemiol.* 1985; 122(5):805-819.

219. Eagle KA, Rihal CS, Foster ED, Mickel MC, Gersh BJ. Long-term survival in patients with coronary artery disease: importance of peripheral vascular disease. The Coronary Artery Surgery Study (CASS) Investigators. *J Am Coll Cardiol.* 1994;23(5):1091-1095.

220. Behar S, Zion M, Reicher-Reiss H, Kaplinsky E, Goldbourt U. Short- and long-term prognosis of patients with a first acute myocardial infarction with concomitant peripheral vascular disease. SPRINT Study Group. *Am J Med.* 1994;96(1):15-19.

221. Saw J, Bhatt DL, Moliterno DJ, et al. The influence of peripheral arterial disease on outcomes: a pooled analysis of mortality in eight large randomized percutaneous coronary intervention trials. *J Am Coll Cardiol.* 2006;48(8):1567-1572.

222. Pokorski RJ. Effect of peripheral vascular disease on long-term mortality after coronary artery bypass graft surgery. *J Insur Med.* 1997;29(3):192-194.

223. Leng GC, Fowkes FG, Lee AJ, Dunbar J, Housley E, Ruckley CV. Use of ankle brachial pressure index to predict cardiovascular events and death: a cohort study. *BMJ.* 1996; 313(7070):1440-1444.

224. Tonelli C, Finzi G, Catamo A, et al. Prevalence and prognostic value of peripheral arterial disease in stroke patients. *Int Angiol.* 1993;12(4):342-343.

225. Leng GC, Fowkes FG. The Edinburgh Claudication Questionnaire: an improved version of the WHO/Rose Questionnaire for use in epidemiological surveys. *J Clin Epidemiol.* 1992;45(10):1101-1109.

226. Rajagopalan S, Mukkerjee D, Mohler R. *Manual of Vascular Diseases.* Philadelphia, PA: Lippincott Williams & Wilkins; 2005.

227. Woods BO. Clinical evaluation of the peripheral vasculature. *Cardiol Clin.* 1991;9(3):413-427.

228. Khan NA, Rahim SA, Anand SS, Simel DL, Panju A. Does the clinical examination predict lower extremity peripheral arterial disease? *JAMA.* 2006;295(5):536-546.

229. Orient J. *Sapira's Art of Science of Bedside Diagnosis.* 2nd ed. Philadelphia, PA: Lippincott Williams & Wilkins; 2000.

230. Criqui MH, Fronek A, Klauber MR, Barrett-Connor E, Gabriel S. The sensitivity, specificity, and predictive value of traditional clinical evaluation of peripheral arterial disease: results from noninvasive testing in a defined population. *Circulation.* 1985;71(3):516-522.

231. Insall RL, Davies RJ, Prout WG. Significance of Buerger's

test in the assessment of lower limb ischaemia. *J R Soc Med.* 1989;82(12):729-731.

232. Braunwald E, ed. *Braunwald's Heart Disease: A Textbook of Cardiovascular Medicine.* 7th ed. Saunders; 2004.

233. DeGowan R, ed. *DeGowan & DeGowan's Bedside Diagnostic Examination.* 5th ed. New York, NY: MacMillan; 1987.

234. Farkouh ME, Oddone EZ, Simel DL. Improving the clinical examination for a low ankle–brachial index. *Int J Angiol.* 2002;11:41-45.

235. Sacks D, Bakal CW, Beatty PT, et al. Position statement on the use of the ankle–brachial index in the evaluation of patients with peripheral vascular disease: a consensus statement developed by the standards division of the society of cardiovascular and interventional radiology. *J Vasc Interv Radiol.* 2002;13(4):353.

236. Ouriel K, McDonnell AE, Metz CE, Zarins CK. Critical evaluation of stress testing in the diagnosis of peripheral vascular disease. *Surgery.* 1982;91(6):686-693.

237. Beckman JA, Higgins CO, Gerhard-Herman M. Automated oscillometric determination of the ankle–brachial index provides accuracy necessary for office practice. *Hypertension.* 2006;47(1):35-38.

238. Sumner DS, Strandness DE Jr. The relationship between calf blood flow and ankle blood pressure in patients with intermittent claudication. *Surgery* 1969;65(5):763-771.

239. Doobay AV, Anand SS. Sensitivity and specificity of the ankle–brachial index to predict future cardiovascular outcomes: a systematic review. *Arterioscler Thromb Vasc Biol.* 2005;25(7):1463-1469.

240. Hooi JD, Kester AD, Stoffers HE, Rinkens PE, Knottnerus JA, van Ree JW. Asymptomatic peripheral arterial occlusive disease predicted cardiovascular morbidity and mortality in a 7-year follow-up study. *J Clin Epidemiol* 2004;57(3):294-300.

241. O'Hare AM, Katz R, Shlipak MG, Cushman M, Newman AB. Mortality and cardiovascular risk across the ankle–arm index spectrum: results from the Cardiovascular Health Study. *Circulation.* 2006;113(3):388-393.

242. Resnick HE, Lindsay RS, McDermott MM, et al. Relationship of high and low ankle brachial index to all-cause and cardiovascular disease mortality: the Strong Heart Study. *Circulation.* 2004;109(6):733-739.

243. Begelman S, Jaff MR. Noninvasive diagnostic strategies for peripheral arterial disease. *Cleve Clin J Med.* 2006;73(S4): S22-S29.

244. Rutherford RB, Lowenstein DH, Klein MF. Combining segmental systolic pressures and plethysmography to diagnose arterial occlusive disease of the legs. *Am J Surg.* 1979;138(2): 211-218.

245. Darling RC, Raines JK, Brener BJ, Austen WG. Quantitative segmental pulse volume recorder: a clinical tool. *Surgery.* 1972;72(6):873-877.

246. Koelemay MJ, den Hartog D, Prins MH, Kromhout JG, Legemate DA, Jacobs MJ. Diagnosis of arterial disease of the lower extremities with duplex ultrasonography. *Br J Surg.* 1996;83(3):404-409.

247. Burke GL, Evans GW, Riley WA, et al. Arterial wall thickness is associated with prevalent cardiovascular disease in middle-aged adults. The Atherosclerosis Risk in Communities (ARIC) Study. *Stroke.* 1995;26(3):386-391.

248. Muhs BE, Gagne P, Sheehan P. Peripheral arterial disease: clinical assessment and indications for revascularization in the patient with diabetes. *Curr Diab Rep.* 2005;5(1):24-29.

249. Willmann JK, Mayer D, Banyai M, et al. Evaluation of peripheral arterial bypass grafts with multi-detector row CT angiography: comparison with duplex US and digital subtraction angiography. *Radiology.* 2003;229(2):465-474.

250. Goldman CK, Morshedi-Meibodi A, White CJ, Jaff MR. Surveillance imaging for carotid in-stent restenosis. *Catheter Cardiovasc Interv.* 2006;67(2):302-308.

251. Kock MC, Adriaensen ME, Pattynama PM, et al. DSA versus multi-detector row CT angiography in peripheral arterial disease: randomized controlled trial. *Radiology.* 2005;237(2):727-737.

252. Abul-Koudoud O. Diagnosis and risk assessment of lower extremity peripheral arterial disease. *J Endovasc Ther.* 2006; 13(SII):10-18.

253. Cambria RP, Kaufman JA, L'Italien GJ, et al. Magnetic resonance angiography in the management of lower extremity arterial occlusive disease: a prospective study. *J Vasc Surg* 1997;25(2):380-389.

254. Boyd AS, Zic JA, Abraham JL. Gadolinium deposition in nephrogenic fibrosing dermopathy. *J Am Acad Dermatol.* 2007;56(1):27-30.

255. Baim D, ed. *Grossman's Cardiac Catheterization, Angiography, and Intervention.* 7th ed. Lippincott Willams & Wilkins; 2005.

256. USPSTF. *Recommendation Statement: Screening for Peripheral Arterial Disease.* Washington, DC; 2005.

257. Gonzalez-Gay MA, Garcia-Porrua C. Epidemiology of the vasculitidies. Rheumatic Diseases Clinics of North America 2001;27:729-749.

258. Johnston SL, Lock RJ, Gompels MM. Takayasu arteritis: a review. *J Clin Pathol.* 2002;55(7):481-486.

259. Cid MC, Font C, Coll-Vinent B, Grau JM. Large vessel vasculitides. *Curr Opin Rheumatol.* 1998;10(1):18-28.

260. Langford CA, Sneller MC. New developments in the treatment of Wegener's granulomatosis, polyarteritis nodosa, microscopic polyangiitis, and Churg-Strauss syndrome. *Curr Opin Rheumatol.* 1997;9(1):26-30.

261. McDermott MM, Mehta S, Ahn H, Greenland P. Atherosclerotic risk factors are less intensively treated in patients with peripheral arterial disease than in patients with coronary artery disease. *J Gen Intern Med.* 1997;12(4):209-215.

262. Rehring TF, Sandhoff BG, Stolcpart RS, Merenich JA, Hollis HW Jr. Atherosclerotic risk factor control in patients with peripheral arterial disease. *J Vasc Surg.* 2005;41(5):816-822.

263. Ernst EE, Matrai A. Intermittent claudication, exercise, and blood rheology. *Circulation.* 1987;76(5):1110-1114.

264. Lumsden AB, Rice TW. Medical management of peripheral arterial disease: a therapeutic algorithm. *J Endovasc Ther.* 2006;13(suppl 2):II19-II29.

265. Stewart KJ, Hiatt WR, Regensteiner JG, Hirsch AT. Exercise training for claudication. *N Engl J Med.* 2002;347(24):1941-1951.

266. Gardner AW, Poehlman ET. Exercise rehabilitation programs for the treatment of claudication pain. A meta-analysis. *JAMA*. 1995;274(12):975-980.

267. Meijer WT, Grobbee DE, Hunink MG, Hofman A, Hoes AW. Determinants of peripheral arterial disease in the elderly: the Rotterdam study. *Arch Intern Med*. 2000;160(19):2934-2938.

268. Hooi JD, Kester AD, Stoffers HE, Overdijk MM, van Ree JW, Knottnerus JA. Incidence of and risk factors for asymptomatic peripheral arterial occlusive disease: a longitudinal study. *Am J Epidemiol*. 2001;153(7):666-672.

269. Ness J, Aronow WS, Ahn C. Risk factors for symptomatic peripheral arterial disease in older persons in an academic hospital-based geriatrics practice. *J Am Geriatr Soc*. 2000;48(3):312-314.

270. Thorne A, Lonnqvist F, Apelman J, Hellers G, Arner P. A pilot study of long-term effects of a novel obesity treatment: omentectomy in connection with adjustable gastric banding. *Int J Obes Relat Metab Disord*. 2002;26(2):193-199.

271. Quick CR, Cotton LT. The measured effect of stopping smoking on intermittent claudication. *Br J Surg*. 1982;69(suppl):S24-S26.

272. Jonason T, Bergstrom R. Cessation of smoking in patients with intermittent claudication. Effects on the risk of peripheral vascular complications, myocardial infarction and mortality. *Acta Med Scand*. 1987;221(3):253-260.

273. Faulkner KW, House AK, Castleden WM. The effect of cessation of smoking on the accumulative survival rates of patients with symptomatic peripheral vascular disease. *Med J Aust*. 1983;1(5):217-219.

274. Antithrombotic Trialists' Collaboration. Collaborative meta-analysis of randomised trials of antiplatelet therapy for prevention of death, myocardial infarction, and stroke in high risk patients. *BMJ*. 2002;324(7329):71-86.

275. Goldhaber SZ, Manson JE, Stampfer MJ, et al. Low-dose aspirin and subsequent peripheral arterial surgery in the Physicians' Health Study. *Lancet*. 1992;340(8812):143-145.

276. Investigators C. A randomised, blinded, trial of clopidogrel versus aspirin in patients at risk of ischaemic events (CAPRIE). CAPRIE Steering Committee. *Lancet*. 1996;348(9038):1329-1339.

277. Bhatt DL, Fox KA, Hacke W, et al. Clopidogrel and aspirin versus aspirin alone for the prevention of atherothrombotic events. *N Engl J Med*. 2006;354(16):1706-1717.

278. Balsano F, Coccheri S, Libretti A, et al. Ticlopidine in the treatment of intermittent claudication: a 21-month double-blind trial. *J Lab Clin Med*. 1989;114(1):84-91.

279. Neri Serneri GG, Coccheri S, Marubini E, Violi F. Picotamide, a combined inhibitor of thromboxane A2 synthase and receptor, reduces 2-year mortality in diabetics with peripheral arterial disease: the DAVID study. *Eur Heart J*. 2004;25(20):1845-1852.

280. Thompson PD, Zimet R, Forbes WP, Zhang P. Meta-analysis of results from eight randomized, placebo-controlled trials on the effect of cilostazol on patients with intermittent claudication. *Am J Cardiol*. 2002;90(12):1314-1319.

281. Dawson DL, Cutler BS, Hiatt WR, et al. A comparison of cilostazol and pentoxifylline for treating intermittent claudication. *Am J Med*. 2000;109(7):523-530.

282. Hankey GJ, Norman PE, Eikelboom JW. Medical treatment of peripheral arterial disease. *JAMA*. 2006;295(5):547-553.

283. The European Study Group. Intravenous pentoxifylline for the treatment of chronic critical limb ischaemia. *Eur J Vasc Endovasc Surg*. 1995;9(4):426-436.

284. Trubestein G, Diehm C, Gruss JD, Horsch S. Prostaglandin E1 in chronic arterial disease—a multicenter study. *Vasa Suppl*. 1987;17:39-43.

285. The ICAI Study Group. Prostanoids for chronic critical leg ischemia. A randomized, controlled, open-label trial with prostaglandin E1. Ischemia Cronica degli Arti Inferiori. *Ann Intern Med* 1999;130(5):412-421.

286. The Ciprostene Study Group. The effect of ciprostene in patients with peripheral vascular disease (PVD) characterized by ischemic ulcers. *J Clin Pharmacol*. 1991;31(1):81-87.

287. The Oral Iloprost in severe Leg Ischaemia Study Group. Two randomised and placebo-controlled studies of an oral prostacyclin analogue (Iloprost) in severe leg ischaemia. *Eur J Vasc Endovasc Surg*. 2000;20(4):358-362.

288. Anand SS, Yusuf S. Oral anticoagulants in patients with coronary artery disease. *J Am Coll Cardiol*. 2003;41(4 suppl S):62S-69S.

289. Anand SS, Yusuf S. Oral anticoagulant therapy in patients with coronary artery disease: a meta-analysis. *JAMA*. 1999;282(21):2058-2067.

290. Sarac TP, Huber TS, Back MR, et al. Warfarin improves the outcome of infrainguinal vein bypass grafting at high risk for failure. *J Vasc Surg*. 1998;28(3):446-457.

291. Kretschmer G, Herbst F, Prager M, et al. A decade of oral anticoagulant treatment to maintain autologous vein grafts for femoropopliteal atherosclerosis. *Arch Surg*. 1992;127(9):1112-1115.

292. Arfvidsson B, Lundgren F, Drott C, Schersten T, Lundholm K. Influence of coumarin treatment on patency and limb salvage after peripheral arterial reconstructive surgery. *Am J Surg*. 1990;159(6):556-560.

293. Johnson WC, Williford WO. Benefits, morbidity, and mortality associated with long-term administration of oral anticoagulant therapy to patients with peripheral arterial bypass procedures: a prospective randomized study. *J Vasc Surg*. 2002;35(3):413-421.

294. Chesney CM, Elam MB, Herd JA, et al. Effect of niacin, warfarin, and antioxidant therapy on coagulation parameters in patients with peripheral arterial disease in the Arterial Disease Multiple Intervention Trial (ADMIT). *Am Heart J*. 2000;140(4):631-636.

295. Cosmi B, Conti E, Coccheri S. Anticoagulants (heparin, low molecular weight heparin and oral anticoagulants) for intermittent claudication. *Cochrane Database Syst Rev*. 2001;(3):CD001999.

296. The WAVE Investigators. The effects of oral anticoagulants in patients with peripheral arterial disease: rationale, design, and baseline characteristics of the Warfarin and Antiplatelet Vascular Evaluation (WAVE) trial, including a meta-analysis of trials. *Am Heart J*. 2006;151(1):1-9.

297. LeCroy CJ, Patterson MA, Taylor SM, Westfall AO, Jordan WD Jr. Effect of warfarin anticoagulation on below-knee polytetrafluoroethylene graft patency. *Ann Vasc Surg*. 2005;19(2):192-198.

298. Dagher NN, Modrall JG. Pharmacotherapy before and after revascularization: anticoagulation, antiplatelet agents, and statins. *Semin Vasc Surg.* 2007;20(1):10-14.

299. Anand S, Yusuf S, Xie C, et al. Oral anticoagulant and antiplatelet therapy and peripheral arterial disease. *N Engl J Med.* 2007;357(3):217-227.

300. Ito WD, Arras M, Scholz D, Winkler B, Htun P, Schaper W. Angiogenesis but not collateral growth is associated with ischemia after femoral artery occlusion. *Am J Physiol.* 1997;273(3, pt 2):H1255-H1265.

301. Collinson DJ, Donnelly R. Therapeutic angiogenesis in peripheral arterial disease: can biotechnology produce an effective collateral circulation? *Eur J Vasc Endovasc Surg.* 2004; 28(1):9-23.

302. Yang HT, Deschenes MR, Ogilvie RW, Terjung RL. Basic fibroblast growth factor increases collateral blood flow in rats with femoral arterial ligation. *Circ Res.* 1996;79(1):62-69.

303. Takeshita S, Zheng LP, Brogi E, et al. Therapeutic angiogenesis. A single intraarterial bolus of vascular endothelial growth factor augments revascularization in a rabbit ischemic hind limb model. *J Clin Invest.* 1994;93(2):662-670.

304. Isner JM, Walsh K, Symes J, et al. Arterial gene therapy for therapeutic angiogenesis in patients with peripheral artery disease. *Circulation* 1995;91(11):2687-2692.

305. Isner JM, Pieczek A, Schainfeld R, et al. Clinical evidence of angiogenesis after arterial gene transfer of phVEGF165 in patient with ischaemic limb. *Lancet.* 1996;348(9024):370-374.

306. Isner JM. Arterial gene transfer of naked DNA for therapeutic angiogenesis: early clinical results. *Adv Drug Deliv Rev.* 1998;30(1-3):185-197.

307. Baumgartner I, Pieczek A, Manor O, et al. Constitutive expression of phVEGF165 after intramuscular gene transfer promotes collateral vessel development in patients with critical limb ischemia. *Circulation.* 1998;97(12):1114-1123.

308. Tateishi-Yuyama E, Matsubara H, Murohara T, et al. Therapeutic angiogenesis for patients with limb ischaemia by autologous transplantation of bone-marrow cells: a pilot study and a randomised controlled trial. *Lancet.* 2002;360 (9331):427-435.

309. Shyu KG, Chang H, Wang BW, Kuan P. Intramuscular vascular endothelial growth factor gene therapy in patients with chronic critical leg ischemia. *Am J Med.* 2003;114(2):85-92.

310. Makinen K, Manninen H, Hedman M, et al. Increased vascularity detected by digital subtraction angiography after VEGF gene transfer to human lower limb artery: a randomized, placebo-controlled, double-blinded phase II study. *Mol Ther.* 2002;6(1):127-133.

311. Lederman RJ, Mendelsohn FO, Anderson RD, et al. Therapeutic angiogenesis with recombinant fibroblast growth factor-2 for intermittent claudication (the TRAFFIC study): a randomised trial. *Lancet.* 2002;359(9323):2053-2058.

312. Weiland D. The effects of L-arginine on Symptomatic Patients with Nonreconstructable Vascular Disease. *Wounds.* 2006;18(8):238-244.

313. Horsch W, Kogel J, Schiefer M. Effect of experimental temperature on the in vitro liberation of salicylic acid-suspension ointments. *Pharmazie.* 1974;29(1):63-64.

314. Pittler MH, Ernst E. Ginkgo biloba extract for the treatment of intermittent claudication: a meta-analysis of randomized trials. *Am J Med.* 2000;108(4):276-281.

315. Lehert P, Comte S, Gamand S, Brown TM. Naftidrofuryl in intermittent claudication: a retrospective analysis. *J Cardiovasc Pharmacol.* 1994;23(suppl 3):S48-S52.

316. Spengel F, Clement D, Boccalon H, Liard F, Brown T, Lehert P. Findings of the Naftidrofuryl in Quality of Life (NIQOL) European study program. *Int Angiol.* 2002;21(1):20-27.

317. Kieffer E, Bahnini A, Mouren X, Gamand S. A new study demonstrates the efficacy of naftidrofuryl in the treatment of intermittent claudication. Findings of the Naftidrofuryl Clinical Ischemia Study (NCIS). *Int Angiol.* 2001;20(1):58-65.

318. Hiatt WR, Regensteiner JG, Creager MA, et al. Propionyl-L-carnitine improves exercise performance and functional status in patients with claudication. *Am J Med.* 2001; 110(8):616-622.

319. Brevetti G, Diehm C, Lambert D. European multicenter study on propionyl-L-carnitine in intermittent claudication. *J Am Coll Cardiol.* 1999;34(5):1618-1624.

320. Boccalon H, Lehert P, Mosnier M. Effect of naftidrofuryl on physiological walking distance in patients with intermittent claudication. *Ann Cardiol Angeiol (Paris).* 2001;50(3):175-182.

321. Jepson RG, Kleijnen J, Leng GC. Garlic for peripheral arterial occlusive disease. *Cochrane Database Syst Rev.* 2000;(2): CD000095.

322. Price JF, Leng GC. Steroid sex hormones for lower limb atherosclerosis. *Cochrane Database Syst Rev.* 2002;(1): CD000188.

323. Villarruz MV, Dans A, Tan F. Chelation therapy for atherosclerotic cardiovascular disease. *Cochrane Database Syst Rev.* 2002;(4):CD002785.

324. American Diabetes Association. Standards of medical care for patients with diabetes mellitus. *Diabetes Care.* 2001; 24(suppl 1):S33-S43.

325. Intensive blood-glucose control with sulphonylureas or insulin compared with conventional treatment and risk of complications in patients with type 2 diabetes (UKPDS 33). UK Prospective Diabetes Study (UKPDS) Group. *Lancet.* 1998;352(9131):837-853.

326. Marso SP, Hiatt WR. Peripheral arterial disease in patients with diabetes. *J Am Coll Cardiol.* 2006;47(5):921-929.

327. Simon AC, Levenson J, Maarek B, Bouthier J, Safar ME. Evidence of early changes of the brachial artery circulation in borderline hypertension. *J Cardiovasc Pharmacol.* 1986; 8(suppl 5):S36-S38.

328. McGill HC Jr, McMahan CA, Tracy RE, et al. Relation of a postmortem renal index of hypertension to atherosclerosis and coronary artery size in young men and women. Pathobiological Determinants of Atherosclerosis in Youth (PDAY) Research Group. *Arterioscler Thromb Vasc Biol.* 1998; 18(7):1108-1118.

329. Mehler PS, Coll JR, Estacio R, Esler A, Schrier RW, Hiatt WR. Intensive blood pressure control reduces the risk of cardiovascular events in patients with peripheral arterial disease and type 2 diabetes. *Circulation* 2003;107(5):753-756.

330. Psaty BM, Smith NL, Siscovick DS, et al. Health outcomes associated with antihypertensive therapies used as first-line agents. A systematic review and meta-analysis. *JAMA*. 1997; 277(9):739-745.

331. Solomon SA, Ramsay LE, Yeo WW, Parnell L, Morris-Jones W. Beta blockade and intermittent claudication: placebo controlled trial of atenolol and nifedipine and their combination. *BMJ*. 1991;303(6810):1100-1104.

332. Radack K, Deck C. Beta-adrenergic blocker therapy does not worsen intermittent claudication in subjects with peripheral arterial disease. A meta-analysis of randomized controlled trials. *Arch Intern Med*. 1991;151(9):1769-1776.

333. Yusuf S, Sleight P, Pogue J, Bosch J, Davies R, Dagenais G. Effects of an angiotensin-converting-enzyme inhibitor, ramipril, on cardiovascular events in high-risk patients. The Heart Outcomes Prevention Evaluation Study Investigators. *N Engl J Med*. 2000;342(3):145-153.

334. Overlack A, Adamczak M, Bachmann W, et al. ACE-inhibition with perindopril in essential hypertensive patients with concomitant diseases. The Perindopril Therapeutic Safety Collaborative Research Group. *Am J Med*. 1994; 97(2):126-134.

335. Ahimastos AA, Lawler A, Reid CM, Blombery PA, Kingwell BA. Brief communication: ramipril markedly improves walking ability in patients with peripheral arterial disease: a randomized trial. *Ann Intern Med*. 2006;144(9):660-664.

336. Schweizer J, Kirch W, Koch R, Hellner G, Uhlmann K. Effect of high dose verapamil on restenosis after peripheral angioplasty. *J Am Coll Cardiol*. 1998;31(6):1299-1305.

337. Leng GC, Price JF, Jepson RG. Lipid lowering therapy in the treatment of lower limb atherosclerosis. *Eur J Vasc Endovasc Surg*. 1998;16(1):5-6.

338. Cannon CP, Braunwald E, McCabe CH, et al. Intensive versus moderate lipid lowering with statins after acute coronary syndromes. *N Engl J Med*. 2004;350(15):1495-1504.

339. Pedersen TR, Kjekshus J, Pyorala K, et al. Effect of simvastatin on ischemic signs and symptoms in the Scandinavian simvastatin survival study (4S). *Am J Cardiol*. 1998; 81(3):333-335.

340. MRC/BHF Heart Protection Study of cholesterol lowering with simvastatin in 20536 high-risk individuals: a randomised placebo-controlled trial. *Lancet*. 2002;360(9326): 7-22.

341. Grundy SM, Cleeman JI, Merz CN, et al. Implications of recent clinical trials for the National Cholesterol Education Program Adult Treatment Panel III Guidelines. *J Am Coll Cardiol*. 2004;44(3):720-732.

342. Blankenhorn DH, Azen SP, Crawford DW, et al. Effects of colestipol-niacin therapy on human femoral atherosclerosis. *Circulation*. 1991;83(2):438-447.

343. Taylor AJ, Sullenberger LE, Lee HJ, Lee JK, Grace KA. Arterial Biology for the Investigation of the Treatment Effects of Reducing Cholesterol (ARBITER) 2: a double-blind, placebo-controlled study of extended-release niacin on atherosclerosis progression in secondary prevention patients treated with statins. *Circulation*. 2004;110(23):3512-3517.

344. Liem A, Reynierse-Buitenwerf GH, Zwinderman AH, Jukema JW, van Veldhuisen DJ. Secondary prevention with folic acid: effects on clinical outcomes. *J Am Coll Cardiol*. 2003;41(12):2105-2113.

345. Green RM, Abbott WM, Matsumoto T, et al. Prosthetic above-knee femoropopliteal bypass grafting: five-year results of a randomized trial. *J Vasc Surg*. 2000;31(3):417-425.

346. Olsen PS, Gustafsen J, Rasmussen L, Lorentzen JE. Long-term results after arterial surgery for arteriosclerosis of the lower limbs in young adults. *Eur J Vasc Surg*. 1988;2(1):15-18.

347. Reed AB, Conte MS, Donaldson MC, Mannick JA, Whittemore AD, Belkin M. The impact of patient age and aortic size on the results of aortobifemoral bypass grafting. *J Vasc Surg*. 2003;37(6):1219-1225.

348. Adam DJ, Beard JD, Cleveland T, et al. Bypass versus angioplasty in severe ischaemia of the leg (BASIL): multicentre, randomised controlled trial. *Lancet*. 2005;366(9501):1925-1934.

349. Yeager RA, Moneta GL, Taylor LM Jr, Hamre DW, McConnell DB, Porter JM. Surgical management of severe acute lower extremity ischemia. *J Vasc Surg*. 1992;15(2):385-391; discussion 92-93.

350. Palmaz JC, Laborde JC, Rivera FJ, Encarnacion CE, Lutz JD, Moss JG. Stenting of the iliac arteries with the Palmaz stent: experience from a multicenter trial. *Cardiovasc Intervent Radiol*. 1992;15(5):291-297.

351. Udoff EJ, Barth KH, Harrington DP, Kaufman SL, White RI. Hemodynamic significance of iliac artery stenosis: pressure measurements during angiography. *Radiology*. 1979; 132(2):289-293.

352. Tetteroo E, van Engelen AD, Spithoven JH, Tielbeek AV, van der Graaf Y, Mali WP. Stent placement after iliac angioplasty: comparison of hemodynamic and angiographic criteria. Dutch Iliac Stent Trial Study Group. *Radiology*. 1996; 201(1):155-159.

353. Kinney TB, Rose SC. Intraarterial pressure measurements during angiographic evaluation of peripheral vascular disease: techniques, interpretation, applications, and limitations. *AJR Am J Roentgenol*. 1996;166(2):277-284.

354. Botti CF Jr, Ansel GM, Silver MJ, Barker BJ, South S. Percutaneous retrograde tibial access in limb salvage. *J Endovasc Ther*. 2003;10(3):614-618.

355. Morshedi-Meibodi AD, Dieter RS. Endovascular treatment of infrapopliteal lesions. *Endovascular Today*. July 2006:43-46.

356. Stokes KR, Strunk HM, Campbell DR, Gibbons GW, Wheeler HG, Clouse ME. Five-year results of iliac and femoropopliteal angioplasty in diabetic patients. *Radiology*. 1990;174(3, pt 2):977-982.

357. Soder HK, Manninen HI, Jaakkola P, et al. Prospective trial of infrapopliteal artery balloon angioplasty for critical limb ischemia: angiographic and clinical results. *J Vasc Interv Radiol*. 2000;11(8):1021-1031.

358. Sapoval MR, Chatellier G, Long AL, et al. Self-expandable stents for the treatment of iliac artery obstructive lesions: long-term success and prognostic factors. *AJR Am J Roentgenol*. 1996;166(5):1173-1179.

359. Lofberg AM, Karacagil S, Ljungman C, et al. Percutaneous transluminal angioplasty of the femoropopliteal arteries in

limbs with chronic critical lower limb ischemia. *J Vasc Surg.* 2001;34(1):114-121.

360. Laborde JC, Palmaz JC, Rivera FJ, Encarnacion CE, Picot MC, Dougherty SP. Influence of anatomic distribution of atherosclerosis on the outcome of revascularization with iliac stent placement. *J Vasc Interv Radiol.* 1995;6(4):513-521.

361. Johnston KW, Rae M, Hogg-Johnston SA, et al. 5-year results of a prospective study of percutaneous transluminal angioplasty. *Ann Surg.* 1987;206(4):403-413.

362. Johnston KW. Iliac arteries: reanalysis of results of balloon angioplasty. *Radiology.* 1993;186(1):207-212.

363. Jamsen T, Manninen H, Tulla H, Matsi P. The final outcome of primary infrainguinal percutaneous transluminal angioplasty in 100 consecutive patients with chronic critical limb ischemia. *J Vasc Interv Radiol.* 2002;13(5):455-463.

364. Bull PG, Mendel H, Hold M, Schlegl A, Denck H. Distal popliteal and tibioperoneal transluminal angioplasty: long-term follow-up. *J Vasc Interv Radiol.* 1992;3(1):45-53.

365. Brown KT, Moore ED, Getrajdman GI, Saddekni S. Infrapopliteal angioplasty: long-term follow-up. *J Vasc Interv Radiol.* 1993;4(1):139-144.

366. Bakal CW, Sprayregen S, Scheinbaum K, Cynamon J, Veith FJ. Percutaneous transluminal angioplasty of the infrapopliteal arteries: results in 53 patients. *AJR Am J Roentgenol.* 1990;154(1):171-174.

367. Holm J, Arfvidsson B, Jivegard L, et al. Chronic lower limb ischaemia. A prospective randomised controlled study comparing the 1-year results of vascular surgery and percutaneous transluminal angioplasty (PTA). *Eur J Vasc Surg.* 1991;5(5):517-522.

368. Wolf GL, Wilson SE, Cross AP, Deupree RH, Stason WB. Surgery or balloon angioplasty for peripheral vascular disease: a randomized clinical trial. Principal investigators and their Associates of Veterans Administration Cooperative Study Number 199. *J Vasc Interv Radiol.* 1993;4(5):639-648.

369. Wilson SE, Wolf GL, Cross AP. Percutaneous transluminal angioplasty versus operation for peripheral arteriosclerosis. Report of a prospective randomized trial in a selected group of patients. *J Vasc Surg.* 1989;9(1):1-9.

370. Dieter RS, Laird JR. Overview of restenosis in peripheral arterial interventions. *Endovascular Today.* October 2004:36-38.

371. Krankenberg H, Sorge I, Zeller T, Tubler T. Percutaneous transluminal angioplasty of infrapopliteal arteries in patients with intermittent claudication: acute and one-year results. *Catheter Cardiovasc Interv.* 2005;64(1):12-17.

372. Tsetis D, Belli AM. The role of infrapopliteal angioplasty. *Br J Radiol.* 2004;77(924):1007-1015.

373. Zorger N, Manke C, Lenhart M, et al. Peripheral arterial balloon angioplasty: effect of short versus long balloon inflation times on the morphologic results. *J Vasc Interv Radiol.* 2002;13(4):355-359.

374. Gray BH, Sullivan TM, Childs MB, Young JR, Olin JW. High incidence of restenosis/reocclusion of stents in the percutaneous treatment of long-segment superficial femoral artery disease after suboptimal angioplasty. *J Vasc Surg.* 1997;25(1):74-83.

375. Zdanowski Z, Albrechtsson U, Lundin A, et al. Percutaneous transluminal angioplasty with or without stenting for femoropopliteal occlusions? A randomized controlled study. *Int Angiol.* 1999;18(4):251-255.

376. Vroegindeweij D, Vos LD, Tielbeek AV, Buth J, vd Bosch HC. Balloon angioplasty combined with primary stenting versus balloon angioplasty alone in femoropopliteal obstructions: A comparative randomized study. *Cardiovasc Intervent Radiol.* 1997;20(6):420-425.

377. Schillinger M, Mlekusch W, Haumer M, Sabeti S, Ahmadi R, Minar E. Angioplasty and elective stenting of de novo versus recurrent femoropopliteal lesions: 1-year follow-up. *J Endovasc Ther.* 2003;10(2):288-297.

378. Muradin GS, Bosch JL, Stijnen T, Hunink MG. Balloon dilation and stent implantation for treatment of femoropopliteal arterial disease: meta-analysis. *Radiology.* 2001;221(1):137-145.

379. Grimm J, Muller-Hulsbeck S, Jahnke T, Hilbert C, Brossmann J, Heller M. Randomized study to compare PTA alone versus PTA with Palmaz stent placement for femoropopliteal lesions. *J Vasc Interv Radiol.* 2001;12(8):935-942.

380. Cejna M, Thurnher S, Illiasch H, et al. PTA versus Palmaz stent placement in femoropopliteal artery obstructions: a multicenter prospective randomized study. *J Vasc Interv Radiol.* 2001;12(1):23-31.

381. Klein WM, van der Graaf Y, Seegers J, et al. Dutch iliac stent trial: long-term results in patients randomized for primary or selective stent placement. *Radiology.* 2006;238(2):734-744.

382. Lyden SP, Shimshak TM. Contemporary endovascular treatment for disease of the superficial femoral and popliteal arteries: an integrated device-based strategy. *J Endovasc Ther.* 2006;13(suppl 2):II41-II51.

383. Ponec D, Jaff MR, Swischuk J, et al. The Nitinol SMART stent vs Wallstent for suboptimal iliac artery angioplasty: CRISP-US trial results. *J Vasc Interv Radiol.* 2004;15(9):911-918.

384. Vorwerk D, Gunther RW, Schurmann K, Wendt G. Aortic and iliac stenoses: follow-up results of stent placement after insufficient balloon angioplasty in 118 cases. *Radiology.* 1996;198(1):45-48.

385. Martin EC, Katzen BT, Benenati JF, et al. Multicenter trial of the wallstent in the iliac and femoral arteries. *J Vasc Interv Radiol.* 1995;6(6):843-849.

386. Zollikofer CL, Antonucci F, Pfyffer M, et al. Arterial stent placement with use of the Wallstent: midterm results of clinical experience. *Radiology.* 1991;179(2):449-456.

387. Laird JR. Limitations of percutaneous transluminal angioplasty and stenting for the treatment of disease of the superficial femoral and popliteal arteries. *J Endovasc Ther.* 2006;13(suppl 2):II30-II40.

388. Sabeti S, Schillinger M, Amighi J, et al. Primary patency of femoropopliteal arteries treated with nitinol versus stainless steel self-expanding stents: propensity score-adjusted analysis. *Radiology.* 2004;232(2):516-521.

389. Mewissen MW. Self-expanding nitinol stents in the femoropopliteal segment: technique and mid-term results. *Tech Vasc Interv Radiol.* 2004;7(1):2-5.

390. Lugmayr HF, Holzer H, Kastner M, Riedelsberger H, Auterith A. Treatment of complex arteriosclerotic lesions with nitinol stents in the superficial femoral and popliteal arteries: a midterm follow-up. *Radiology.* 2002;222(1):37-43.

391. Dorrucci V. Treatment of superficial femoral artery occlusive disease. *J Cardiovasc Surg (Torino)*. 2004;45(3):193-201.

392. Babalik E, Gulbaran M, Gurmen T, Ozturk S. Fracture of popliteal artery stents. *Circ J*. 2003;67(7):643-645.

393. Rosenfield K, Schainfeld R, Pieczek A, Haley L, Isner JM. Restenosis of endovascular stents from stent compression. *J Am Coll Cardiol*. 1997;29(2):328-338.

394. Duda SH, Pusich B, Richter G, et al. Sirolimus-eluting stents for the treatment of obstructive superficial femoral artery disease: six-month results. *Circulation*. 2002;106(12):1505-1509.

395. Schillinger M, Sabeti S, Loewe C, et al. Balloon angioplasty versus implantation of nitinol stents in the superficial femoral artery. *N Engl J Med*. 2006;354(18):1879-1888.

396. Siablis D, Kraniotis P, Karnabatidis D, Kagadis GC, Katsanos K, Tsolakis J. Sirolimus-eluting versus bare stents for bailout after suboptimal infrapopliteal angioplasty for critical limb ischemia: 6-month angiographic results from a nonrandomized prospective single-center study. *J Endovasc Ther*. 2005;12(6):685-695.

397. Jahnke T, Voshage G, Muller-Hulsbeck S, Grimm J, Heller M, Brossmann J. Endovascular placement of self-expanding nitinol coil stents for the treatment of femoropopliteal obstructive disease. *J Vasc Interv Radiol*. 2002;13(3):257-266.

398. Nelson PR, Anthony Lee W. Endovascular treatment of popliteal artery aneurysms. *Vascular*. 2006;14(5):297-304.

399. Antonello M, Frigatti P, Battocchio P, et al. Open repair versus endovascular treatment for asymptomatic popliteal artery aneurysm: results of a prospective randomized study. *J Vasc Surg*. 2005;42(2):185-193.

400. Tielliu IF, Verhoeven EL, Zeebregts CJ, Prins TR, Span MM, van den Dungen JJ. Endovascular treatment of popliteal artery aneurysms: results of a prospective cohort study. *J Vasc Surg*. 2005;41(4):561-567.

401. Kasirajan V, Hertzer NR, Beven EG, O'Hara PJ, Krajewski LP, Sullivan TM. Management of isolated common iliac artery aneurysms. *Cardiovasc Surg*. 1998;6(2):171-177.

402. Sanchez LA, Patel AV, Ohki T, et al. Midterm experience with the endovascular treatment of isolated iliac aneurysms. *J Vasc Surg*. 1999;30(5):907-913.

403. Matsumoto K, Matsubara K, Watada S, et al. Surgical and endovascular procedures for treating isolated iliac artery aneurysms: ten-year experience. *World J Surg*. 2004;28(8):797-800.

404. Caronno R, Piffaretti G, Tozzi M, et al. Endovascular treatment of isolated iliac artery aneurysms. *Ann Vasc Surg*. 2006;20(4):496-501.

405. Duda SH, Bosiers M, Lammer J, et al. Sirolimus-eluting versus bare nitinol stent for obstructive superficial femoral artery disease: the SIROCCO II Trial. *J Vasc Interv Radiol*. 2005;16(3):331-338.

406. Zehnder T, von Briel C, Baumgartner I, et al. Endovascular brachytherapy after percutaneous transluminal angioplasty of recurrent femoropopliteal obstructions. *J Endovasc Ther*. 2003;10(2):304-311.

407. Waksman R, Laird JR, Jurkovitz CT, et al. Intravascular radiation therapy after balloon angioplasty of narrowed femoropopliteal arteries to prevent restenosis: results of the PARIS feasibility clinical trial. *J Vasc Interv Radiol*. 2001; 12(8):915-921.

408. Vroegindeweij D, Tielbeek AV, Buth J, Schol FP, Hop WC, Landman GH. Directional atherectomy versus balloon angioplasty in segmental femoropopliteal artery disease: two-year follow-up with color-flow duplex scanning. *J Vasc Surg*. 1995;21(2):255-268; discussion 68-69.

409. Sidawy AN, Weiswasser JM, Waksman R. Peripheral vascular brachytherapy. *J Vasc Surg*. 2002;35(5):1041-1047.

410. Saxon RR, Coffman JM, Gooding JM, Natuzzi E, Ponec DJ. Long-term results of ePTFE stent–graft versus angioplasty in the femoropopliteal artery: single center experience from a prospective, randomized trial. *J Vasc Interv Radiol*. 2003;14(3):303-311.

411. Nakamura S, Conroy RM, Gordon IL, et al. A randomized trial of transcutaneous extraction atherectomy in femoral arteries: intravascular ultrasound observations. *J Clin Ultrasound*. 1995;23(8):461-471.

412. Minar E, Pokrajac B, Maca T, et al. Endovascular brachytherapy for prophylaxis of restenosis after femoropopliteal angioplasty : results of a prospective randomized study. *Circulation*. 2000;102(22):2694-2699.

413. Lammer J, Pilger E, Decrinis M, Quehenberger F, Klein GE, Stark G. Pulsed excimer laser versus continuous-wave Nd:YAG laser versus conventional angioplasty of peripheral arterial occlusions: prospective, controlled, randomised trial. *Lancet*. 1992;340(8829):1183-1188.

414. Krueger K, Landwehr P, Bendel M, et al. Endovascular gamma irradiation of femoropopliteal de novo stenoses immediately after PTA: interim results of prospective randomized controlled trial. *Radiology* 2002;224(2):519-528.

415. Jeans WD, Murphy P, Hughes AO, Horrocks M, Baird RN. Randomized trial of laser-assisted passage through occluded femoro-popliteal arteries. *Br J Radiol*. 1990;63(745):19-21.

416. Jahnke T, Link J, Muller-Hulsbeck S, Grimm J, Heller M, Brossman J. Treatment of infrapopliteal occlusive disease by high-speed rotational atherectomy: initial and mid-term results. *J Vasc Interv Radiol*. 2001;12(2):221-226.

417. Jahnke T, Andresen R, Muller-Hulsbeck S, et al. Hemobahn stent–grafts for treatment of femoropopliteal arterial obstructions: midterm results of a prospective trial. *J Vasc Interv Radiol*. 2003;14(1):41-51.

418. Fisher CM, Fletcher JP, May J, et al. No additional benefit from laser in balloon angioplasty of the superficial femoral artery. *Eur J Vasc Endovasc Surg*. 1996;11(3):349-352.

419. Duda SH, Poerner TC, Wiesinger B, et al. Drug-eluting stents: potential applications for peripheral arterial occlusive disease. *J Vasc Interv Radiol*. 2003;14(3):291-301.

420. Belli AM, Cumberland DC, Procter AE, Welsh CL. Follow-up of conventional angioplasty versus laser thermal angioplasty for total femoropopliteal artery occlusions: results of a randomized trial. *J Vasc Interv Radiol*. 1991;2(4):485-488.

421. Bolia A, Brennan J, Bell PR. Recanalisation of femoro-popliteal occlusions: improving success rate by subintimal recanalisation. *Clin Radiol*. 1989;40(3):325.

422. Treiman GS, Whiting JH, Treiman RL, McNamara RM, Ashrafi A. Treatment of limb-threatening ischemia with percutaneous intentional extraluminal recanalization: a preliminary evaluation. *J Vasc Surg*. 2003;38(1):29-35.

423. Nydahl S, Hartshorne T, Bell PR, Bolia A, London NJ. Subintimal angioplasty of infrapopliteal occlusions in critically ischaemic limbs. *Eur J Vasc Endovasc Surg.* 1997;14(3):212-216.

424. McCarthy RJ, Neary W, Roobottom C, Tottle A, Ashley S. Short-term results of femoropopliteal subintimal angioplasty. *Br J Surg.* 2000;87(10):1361-1365.

425. Dieter RS, Pacanowski JR Jr, Ahmed MH, Mannebach P, Nanjundappa A. FoxHollow atherectomy as a treatment modality for common femoral artery occlusion. *WMJ.* 2007; 106(2):90-91.

426. Laird JR, Zeller T, Gray BH, et al. Limb salvage following laser-assisted angioplasty for critical limb ischemia: results of the LACI multicenter trial. *J Endovasc Ther.* 2006;13(1):1-11.

427. Laird J. Peripheral Excimer Laser Angioplasty (PELA) Trial Results. In: TCT Annual Meeting; 2002; Washington, DC.

428. Dieter RS, Laird JR. Nonstent endovascular treatment of SFA Occlusions. *Endovascular Today.* March 2006:59-64.

429. Boccalandro F, Muench A, Sdringola S, Rosales OR. Wireless laser-assisted angioplasty of the superficial femoral artery in patients with critical limb ischemia who have failed conventional percutaneous revascularization. *Catheter Cardiovasc Interv.* 2004;63(1):7-12.

430. Konig CW, Pusich B, Tepe G, et al. Frequent embolization in peripheral angioplasty: detection with an embolism protection device (AngioGuard) and electron microscopy. *Cardiovasc Intervent Radiol.* 2003;26(4):334-339.

431. Ansel GM, Sample NS, Botti IC Jr, et al. Cutting balloon angioplasty of the popliteal and infrapopliteal vessels for symptomatic limb ischemia. *Catheter Cardiovasc Interv.* 2004;61(1):1-4.

432. Rabbi JF, Kiran RP, Gersten G, Dudrick SJ, Dardik A. Early results with infrainguinal cutting balloon angioplasty limits distal dissection. *Ann Vasc Surg.* 2004;18(6):640-643.

433. Fourrier JL, Bertrand ME, Auth DC, Lablanche JM, Gommeaux A, Brunetaud JM. Percutaneous coronary rotational angioplasty in humans: preliminary report. *J Am Coll Cardiol.* 1989;14(5):1278-1282.

434. Rubartelli P, Niccoli L, Alberti A, et al. Coronary rotational atherectomy in current practice: acute and mid-term results in high- and low-volume centers. *Catheter Cardiovasc Interv.* 2004;61(4):463-471.

435. Hoffmann R, Mintz GS, Kent KM, et al. Comparative early and nine-month results of rotational atherectomy, stents, and the combination of both for calcified lesions in large coronary arteries. *Am J Cardiol.* 1998;81(5):552-557.

436. Simpson JB, Selmon MR, Robertson GC, et al. Transluminal atherectomy for occlusive peripheral vascular disease. *Am J Cardiol.* 1988;61(14):96G-101G.

437. Henry M, Amor M, Ethevenot G, Henry I, Allaoui M. Percutaneous peripheral atherectomy using the rotablator: a single-center experience. *J Endovasc Surg.* 1995;2(1):51-66.

438. Zacca NM, Raizner AE, Noon GP, et al. Treatment of symptomatic peripheral atherosclerotic disease with a rotational atherectomy device. *Am J Cardiol* 1989;63(1):77-80.

439. Lyden SP. Polarcath cryoplasty: 9 month IDE Trial update. In: 31st Global Vascular and Endovascular Issues, Techinques and Horizon; 2004; Cleveland, OH.

440. Weichmann BaK, SE. Cryoplasty for treating femoropopliteal occlusive disease. *Endovascular Today* June 2005:76-79.

441. Laird J, Jaff MR, Biamino G, et al. Cryoplasty for the treatment of femoropopliteal arterial disease: results of a prospective, multicenter registry. *J Vasc Interv Radiol.* 2005; 16(8):1067-1073.

442. Wiedermann JG, Marboe C, Amols H, Schwartz A, Weinberger J. Intracoronary irradiation markedly reduces restenosis after balloon angioplasty in a porcine model. *J Am Coll Cardiol.* 1994;23(6):1491-1498.

443. Waksman R, Rodriguez JC, Robinson KA, et al. Effect of intravascular irradiation on cell proliferation, apoptosis, and vascular remodeling after balloon overstretch injury of porcine coronary arteries. *Circulation.* 1997;96(6):1944-1952.

444. Fischer-Dzoga K, Dimitrievich GS, Schaffner T. Effect of hyperlipidemic serum and irradiation on wound healing in primary quiescent cultures of vascular cells. *Exp Mol Pathol.* 1990;52(1):1-12.

445. Mukherjee D, Moliterno DJ. Brachytherapy for in-stent restenosis: a distant second choice to drug-eluting stent placement. *JAMA.* 2006;295(11):1307-1309.

446. Pokrajac B, Potter R, Maca T, et al. Intraarterial (192) Ir high-dose-rate brachytherapy for prophylaxis of restenosis after femoropopliteal percutaneous transluminal angioplasty: the prospective randomized Vienna-2-trial radiotherapy parameters and risk factors analysis. *Int J Radiat Oncol Biol Phys.* 2000;48(4):923-931.

447. Bonvini R, Baumgartner I, Do DD, et al. Late acute thrombotic occlusion after endovascular brachytherapy and stenting of femoropopliteal arteries. *J Am Coll Cardiol.* 2003; 41(3):409-412.

448. Krueger K, Zaehringer M, Bendel M, et al. De novo femoropopliteal stenoses: endovascular gamma irradiation following angioplasty—angiographic and clinical follow-up in a prospective randomized controlled trial. *Radiology* 2004; 231(2):546-554.

449. Waksman R. Results of the PARIS Trial. In: TCT Annual Meeting; 2003; Washington, DC.

450. Kipshidze N, Serruys PW, Moses J, Fareed J, ed. *Textbook of Interventional Cardiovascular Pharmacology.* 1st ed. London, UK: Informa Healthcare; 2007.

451. Johnson WC, Lee KK. A comparative evaluation of polytetrafluoroethylene, umbilical vein, and saphenous vein bypass grafts for femoral–popliteal above-knee revascularization: a prospective randomized Department of Veterans Affairs cooperative study. *J Vasc Surg.* 2000;32(2):268-277.

452. Veith FJ, Gupta SK, Ascer E, et al. Six-year prospective multicenter randomized comparison of autologous saphenous vein and expanded polytetrafluoroethylene grafts in infrainguinal arterial reconstructions. *J Vasc Surg* 1986;3(1):104-114.

453. Baldwin ZK, Pearce BJ, Curi MA, et al. Limb salvage after infrainguinal bypass graft failure. *J Vasc Surg.* 2004;39(5):951-957.

454. de Vries SO, Hunink MG. Results of aortic bifurcation grafts for aortoiliac occlusive disease: a meta-analysis. *J Vasc Surg.* 1997;26(4):558-569.

455. Hunink MG, Wong JB, Donaldson MC, Meyerovitz MF, Harrington DP. Patency results of percutaneous and surgical revascularization for femoropopliteal arterial disease. *Med Decis Making*. 1994;14(1):71-81.

456. Oskam J, van den Dungen JJ, Boontje AH. Thromboendarterectomy for obstructive disease of the common iliac artery. *Cardiovasc Surg*. 1996;4(3):356-359.

457. Nicoloff AD, Taylor LM Jr, McLafferty RB, Moneta GL, Porter JM. Patient recovery after infrainguinal bypass grafting for limb salvage. *J Vasc Surg*. 1998;27(2):256-263; discussion 64-66.

458. Kessel DO, Berridge DC, Robertson I. Infusion techniques for peripheral arterial thrombolysis. *Cochrane Database Syst Rev*. 2004;(1):CD000985.

459. Nanjundappa A LJ. Critical limb ischemia. *Endovascular Today*. 2006:36-40.

460. Bernstein EF, Rhodes GA, Stuart SH, Coel MN, Fronek A. Toe pulse reappearance time in prediction of aortofemoral bypass success. *Ann Surg*. 1981;193(2):201-205.

461. Clagett GP, Sobel M, Jackson MR, Lip GY, Tangelder M, Verhaeghe R. Antithrombotic therapy in peripheral arterial occlusive disease: the Seventh ACCP Conference on Antithrombotic and Thrombolytic Therapy. *Chest*. 2004;126(3 suppl):609S-626S.

462. Ouriel K, Shortell CK, DeWeese JA, et al. A comparison of thrombolytic therapy with operative revascularization in the initial treatment of acute peripheral arterial ischemia. *J Vasc Surg*. 1994;19(6):1021-1030.

463. Weaver FA, Comerota AJ, Youngblood M, Froehlich J, Hosking JD, Papanicolaou G. Surgical revascularization versus thrombolysis for nonembolic lower extremity native artery occlusions: results of a prospective randomized trial. The STILE Investigators. Surgery versus Thrombolysis for Ischemia of the Lower Extremity. *J Vasc Surg*. 1996;24(4):513-521; discussion 21-23.

464. Results of a prospective randomized trial evaluating surgery versus thrombolysis for ischemia of the lower extremity. The STILE trial. *Ann Surg*. 1994;220(3):251-266; discussion 66-68.

465. Ouriel K, Veith FJ, Sasahara AA. A comparison of recombinant urokinase with vascular surgery as initial treatment for acute arterial occlusion of the legs. Thrombolysis or Peripheral Arterial Surgery (TOPAS) Investigators. *N Engl J Med*. 1998;338(16):1105-1111.

466. Ouriel K, Veith FJ, Sasahara AA. Thrombolysis or peripheral arterial surgery: phase I results. TOPAS Investigators. *J Vasc Surg*. 1996;23(1):64-73; discussion 4-5.

467. Diffin DC, Kandarpa K. Assessment of peripheral intraarterial thrombolysis versus surgical revascularization in acute lower-limb ischemia: a review of limb-salvage and mortality statistics. *J Vasc Interv Radiol*. 1996;7(1):57-63.

chapter 34

Medical Therapy of Intermittent Claudication

Manu Rajachandran, MD / Robert M. Schainfeld, DO

The medical therapy of intermittent claudication is founded on two fundamental precepts (Table 34-1). The most compelling of these is that peripheral arterial disease is evidence for systemic atherosclerosis. Affected patients most likely have concomitant coronary artery and cerebrovascular diseases. As a result, they are at increased risk for adverse clinical outcomes including myocardial infarction, stroke, and death. These patients also frequently manifest symptoms of intermittent claudication, resulting in impaired functional status, or symptoms of critical limb ischemia—rest pain, ulcers, or gangrene, which ultimately threaten the viability of the limb. Therefore, management of these patients must employ therapeutic strategies that decrease their risk of cardiovascular events, reduce mortality, improve functional capacity and quality of life, and preserve limb integrity. In contrast to the relative intangibility of vascular risk reduction, symptomatic improvement in peripheral arterial disease after the institution of appropriate medical therapy can often become apparent to the patient within a matter of weeks or a few months and can significantly enhance a patient's quality of life.

● PENTOXIFYLLINE

Pentoxifylline was the first drug approved by the U.S. Food and Drug Administration (FDA) in 1984 for the treatment of claudication. It is a methylxanthine derivative that increases intracellular levels of cyclic adenosine monophosphate (cAMP). The drug improves red cell and white cell deformability, lowers plasma fibrogen concentrations, and possesses antiplatelet effects.[1] The drug's clinical effects have however been somewhat lackluster. Although pentoxifylline increased maximal treadmill walking distance by 12% as compared with placebo in one randomized clinical

US trial, there was no difference between the two groups in the increase in maximal treadmill walking distance when compared to baseline.[2] Another study found only a 21% (nonsignificant) increase in maximal treadmill walking distance in patients treated with pentoxifylline as compared to placebo.[3] Most recently, a trial that compared pentoxifylline, cilostazol, and placebo found that cilostazol was the sole agent that improved pain-free and maximal walking distances compared with placebo.[4] Patients randomized to pentoxifylline in this study fared as well as those randomized to the placebo arm in terms of symptom relief. A meta-analysis found a net benefit of only an additional 44 m in the maximal distance walked on a treadmill (95% CI, 14–74 m) in patients treated with pentoxifylline.[5]

In addition to the marginal clinical benefit afforded by pentoxifylline in improving exercise capacity, use of the drug is hobbled by a paucity of information with regard to its impact on function status and quality of life. Importantly, with the recent and now routine inclusion of quality of life questionnaires into clinical drug trial designs for claudication, pentoxifylline failed to demonstrate improvement in daily functional status as assessed by the Walking Impairment Questionnaire (WIQ) or Medical Outcomes Scale Health Survey (MOS SF-36), when compared to cilostazol.[4]

It has been recently postulated that pentoxifylline may possess the potential to alter the natural history of peripheral arterial disease (PAD). The facts supporting this hypothesis, however, deserve close scrutiny. Although the use of pentoxifylline was associated with a reduction in hospital expenditures without a greater overall cost of PAD-related care, the drug did not alter the risk of PAD-related hospitalization.[6] Compliance with taking pentoxifylline

TABLE 34-1. Pharmacological Treatment for Intermittent Claudication

Drug/study	No. of Subjects	Dosage	Duration (months)	Change in MWD (%)*	p Value	ACC/AHA[8] Guidelines (Class/Level of Evidence)
Pentoxifylline						
Porter et al.[2]	128	1.2 g	6	12	0.19	
Lindgarde et al.[3]	150	1.2 g	6	21	0.09	
Hood et al.[5]	511	Varied	Varied	30	<0.05	
Dawson et al.[4]	698	1.2 g	6	0	0.82	II_b/A
Cilostazol						
Dawson et al.[11]	81	200 mg	3	73	<0.01	
Money et al.[12]	239	200 mg	4	32	<0.001	
Beebe et al.[13]	516	200 mg	6	82	<0.001	
Dawson et al.[14]	698	200 mg	6	33	<0.001	I/A
Propionyl levocarnitine						
Brevetti et al.[25]	114	2 g	12	41	<0.01	
Brevetti et al.[24]	245	1–3 g	6	27	0.049	II_b/B
Naftidrofuryl						
Adhoute et al.[27]	94	600 mg	6	32	<0.001	
Trübestein et al.[29]	104	600 mg	3	16	0.02	
Moody et al.[30]	108	600 mg	6	11	0.27	NC
Buflomedil						
Trübestein et al.[31]	113	600 mg	3	55	<0.01	NC
Prostaglandins						
Lievre et al.[35]	424	Beraprost 120 μg (oral)	6	25	0.004	
Mohler et al.[36]	897	Beraprost 120 μg (oral)	6	17	NS	III/A
L-Arginine						
Maxwell et al.[38]	41	8 g	2 wks	23	NS	II_b/B
Defibrotide						
Strano et al.[48]	227	400–800 mg	6	50	<0.01	NC

NC, not classified; NS, not significant.
*% Change in MWD = Net Improvement in maximal walking distance compared to placebo.

reduced the frequency of invasive vascular procedures during the first year in a small group of claudicators.[7]

Pentoxifylline is administered in a dose of 400 mg 3 times daily with meals, but maybe reduced to 400 mg twice daily if gastrointestinal or central nervous system side effects occur. Because of its nearly complete absorption with some first-pass metabolism and renal excretion route, precaution needs be taken in patients with renal impairment, as metabolites may accumulate. It is relatively well tolerated with rare reported side effects, which include dyspepsia, nausea, vomiting, headache, and dizziness.

The results of clinical trials demonstrating the efficacy of pentoxifylline in improving treadmill walking distance have been equivocal and there are insufficient data to presently justify its generalized use in PAD (Table 34-1). The current ACC/AHA guidelines for the management of PAD advise that pentoxifylline maybe considered as second-line, alternative therapy to cilostazol to improve walking distance in patients with intermittent claudication (Class IIb, level of

evidence: A). Furthermore, the guidelines clearly state that the clinical effectiveness of pentoxifylline as therapy for intermittent claudication is marginal and not well established (level of evidence: C).[8]

● CILOSTAZOL

Cilostazol was the second agent approved by the FDA in 1999 for the symptomatic treatment of claudication. It functions as a phosphodiesterase type III inhibitor, thereby increasing the intracellular levels of cyclic AMP through its inhibition of proteolysis. This drug has a plethora of therapeutic mechanisms including the inhibition of platelet aggregation and arterial thrombogenesis, and the inhibition of smooth-muscle cell proliferation. Cilostazol amplifies the effects of prostacyclin and promotes direct smooth-muscle cell relaxation, leading to arterial vasodilatation.[9,10] The precise mechanism of this drug's dramatic effects on reducing claudication symptoms and improving ambulatory capacity remains elusive and maybe multifactorial.

Cilostazol has undergone intensive clinical scrutiny, with no less than eight randomized controlled clinical trials examining its efficacy. Of these, four trials are large enough to warrant review; these were randomized, placebo-controlled enrolling a total of 1534 claudicants.[4,11–13] In all four trials, cilostazol improved pain-free and maximal walking distance by 35% to 50% as compared to placebo. In three of the trials, cilostazol demonstrated a significant improvement in functional status and walking performance compared to placebo using both the MOS SF-36 and walking impairment questionnaire criteria. The WIQ data from these trials indisputably established the superiority of this drug over placebo in improving both walking distance and speed over placebo.[12,13] In these trials, a significantly greater number of patients treated with cilostazol noted a dramatic subjective improvement in exercise capacity and quality of life, which ultimately is the most compelling indication for its "first line" use in claudication.

Cilostazol (50 mg twice daily) also has been shown to increase maximal walking distance on treadmill exercise testing. Cilostazol demonstrated a greater improvement in walking distance when compared to pentoxifylline and placebo in a large randomized clinical trial. The increase in the absolute claudication distance of 107 m (54%) with cilostazol eclipsed that observed with pentoxifylline of 64 m (30%) or placebo of 65 m (34%), after 6 months of treatment. Drug withdrawal in this study resulted in a rapid decline of the walking distance within 6 weeks, providing further evidence that the initial improvement in walking distance was solely the effect of cilostazol itself. In comparison, withdrawal of pentoxifylline therapy, like that of placebo drug in this study, resulted in no change in claudication symptoms or in exercise capacity from baseline.[14]

Ancillary benefits associated with cilostazol therapy in clinical trials include an increase in ankle-brachial indicies (ABI),[12] significant increases in high-density lipoprotein (HDL) cholesterol by 10%, and lowering of triglycerides by 15% with greater effects demonstrated in patients with higher baseline triglycerides.[15] Patients with diabetes treated with cilostazol showed a significant reduction in carotid intimal-medial thickening on duplex ultrasound analysis.[16] Once again in this study, as in many others, the modest increase noted in the ABI (9%) was not consonant with the dramatic and reproducible improvement in claudication symptoms in those patients randomized to the drug.

The standard cilostazol dosage of 100 mg twice daily provides the optimal efficacy, but patients who experience side effects may benefit from reducing the initial dosage to 50 mg twice daily.[13]

The pharmacokinetics of cilostazol are notable for its extensive hepatic metabolism by the 3A4 isoform of cytochrome P450 (CYP3A4) and by the 2C19 and 1A2 isoforms with the formation of active metabolites and predominant renal excretion.[10] Although no recommendations have been put forward regarding the issue of dose ad-

justment in patients with renal or hepatic impairment, caution is advised in the use of this drug in the context of moderate or severe liver dysfunction.[17,18] Adjustment to dosage should be instituted during coadministration of agents that inhibit CYP3A4 or CYP2C19 such as ketoconazole, itraconazole, erythromycin, diltiazem, omeprazole, and consumption of large quantities of grapefruit juice, in excess of one quart daily.

The most frequent side effects are headache, which affects approximately 34% of patients as compared to 14% of patients taking placebo, followed by diarrhea, palpitations and dizziness.[10] Despite the reported side effects, cilostazol has been well tolerated, as exemplified by the similar rates of discontinuation of the drug amongst patients receiving placebo or pentoxifylline in clinical trials.[13] Although cilostazol is safe to be taken in conjunction with aspirin, there exists only limited safety data on combinations with clopidogrel.[19]

Cilostazol is contraindicated in patients with congestive heart failure, although it has not been shown in any clinical trial to precipitate or exacerbate this complication. The contraindication is based upon the fact that other phosphodiesterase 3 inhibitors such as milrinone, which was developed as an inotropic agent for the treatment of heart failure, have been associated with excess cardiac mortality in patients with New York Heart Association Class III–IV heart failure.[20] Cilostazol labeling is now accompanied by a "black-box" warning that it is contraindicated in patients with heart failure of any magnitude. In clinical trials involving more than 2000 patients treated with cilostazol followed for up to 6 months, no appreciable increase in cardiovascular death (0.6%) in cilostazol-treated vs. 0.5% in placebo-treated patients was observed. Myocardial infarction was also rare, occurring in 1.5% and 1.1% of cilostazol-treated and placebo-treated patients, respectively.[9]

The current ACC/AHA guidelines recommend cilostazol 100 mg twice daily as an effective therapy to improve symptoms and walking distance in patients with lower extremity PAD and intermittent claudication (in the absence of heart failure). The recommendations also state that a therapeutic trial of cilostazol should be considered in all patients with lifestyle-limiting claudication. Both these recommendations are class I, level of evidence: A.[8]

Given the theoretical concern regarding the risk of the drug in patients with heart failure, each individual physician needs to tailor his experience and comfort level as to the role of routine screening for evidence of congestive heart failure (CHF), interim assessment of risk–benefit ratio on subsequent ischemic events and monitoring of cardiac rate, and rhythm during commencement of therapy.[21]

● LEVOCARNITINE AND PROPIONYL LEVOCARNITINE

Metabolic derangements in the exercising lower extremity skeletal muscles of PAD patients have been well documented. As a result of these abnormalities in carnitine metabolism, there is a deficiency of carnitine and concomitant accumulation of acylcarnitine in PAD, which correlate with the degree of impairment in exercise performance.[22]

Levocarnitine and propionyl levocarnitine (PLC) has been shown to improve metabolism and exercise capacity of ischemic muscles. A trial conducted with levocarnitine, 2 g twice daily, improved maximal treadmill walking distance, but the acylated form of carnitine, PLC, was even more effective in improving maximal walking distance when administered in an equimolar dose.[23] In two double-blind, placebo-controlled, multicenter trials enrolling 730 patients, both the pain-free and maximal walking distance improved more in patients receiving PLC than in those receiving placebo. The mean walking distance (MWD) increased between 62% and 73% in subjects receiving PLC as compared to 46% with placebo by intention-to-treat analysis.[24,25] In a subgroup analysis of 114 patients with a MWD of less than 250 m, there was an improvement in walking distances with PLC, with an increase in MWD of 98% (155 m) compared with a 54% (95 m) increase in the placebo arm ($p < 0.05$).[25] This study may identify a target population of patients that would benefit from carnitine therapy.

Mirroring this objective improvement in exercise performance, a recent trial noted a similar improvement in perceived functional status when employing the Walk Impairment Questionnaire and the Medical Outcome Scale Health Survey (MOS SF-36), in patients randomized to PLC versus placebo.[10]

The optimal dose, although not clearly established, appears to be 2 g daily, which seems to achieve the greatest benefit. The agent is well tolerated, with minimal side effects including occasional headaches and gastrointestinal symptoms.

The ACC/AHA guidelines state that the effectiveness of PLC as a therapy to improve walking distance in patients with claudication is not well established (Class IIb, level of evidence: B).[8] As a result, this agent has not been approved in the United States for the treatment of claudication.

● NAFTIDROFURYL

Naftidrofuryl is one of two available agents approved for use in Europe for the symptomatic treatment of claudication. The drug appears to exert its effect through its antagonism of 5-hydroxytryptamineserotonine receptors; this results in the reduction of platelet and erythrocyte aggregation and enhancement of aerobic metabolism in ischemic tissue. Although a number of randomized, controlled trials have been conducted, a review of five of the largest of these concluded that naftidrofuryl solely improved pain-free treadmill walking distance (PFWD) without affecting the maximal walking distance.[26–29] Furthermore, a randomized trial of 188 patients enrolled with severe claudication (Fontaine classification IIb) failed to confirm an improvement in either PFWD or MWD.[30]

The dose recommended for clinical use is 600 to 800 mg daily (divided into two or three doses). Naftidro-furyl is well tolerated with associated only mild gastrointestinal symptoms. It is not available in the United States.

● BUFLOMEDIL

Buflomedil has been used in select countries around the world, although not available in the United States. It functions as a vasodilator, through its adrenolytic and weak calcium antagonistic effects. It is believed to exert its benefits by improved blood rheology, facilitating platelet disaggregation and enhancing RBC deformability. Data supporting its clinical efficacy has been conflicting in the few small trials that have been conducted.

In a randomized trial comprising 93 claudicators, the buflomedil-treated group showed an improvement in PFWD by 100% and MWD by 97%, compared with placebo (38% and 42%, respectively).[31] A small study comparing buflomedil to pentoxifylline or nifedipine failed to show an improvement in PFWD with buflomedil or nifedipine as compared to pentoxifylline.[32] Buflomedil is taken at a dose of 600 mg daily with observed side effects of dyspepsia, headache, dizziness, erythema, and pruritis.

● PROSTAGLANDINS

Prostaglandins, such as prostaglandin I_2 (PGI_2), prostaglandin E_1, (PGE_1), and their analogs, have shown promise in the treatment of patients with critical limb ischemia and when administered intravenously in patients with intermittent claudication. These agents are potent vasodilators and possess antiplatelet properties, which make them attractive for potential use in the treatment of PAD.

Although there are only a few studies examining this drug in patients with claudication, one such open label study demonstrated a benefit of PGE_1 infusion when added to an exercise program. An increase in MWD of 371% was seen when a 4-week infusion of PGE_1 was added to exercise; not surprisingly, exercise in and of itself, in this study, conveyed a 99% increase in MWD.[33] One randomized clinical trial of a novel lipid-based moiety of PGE_1 enrolled 90 patients, randomized to the drug and to placebo. Patients randomized to prostaglandin therapy enjoyed a significant improvement in MWD and quality of life. After 8 weeks of therapy with three different dosage regimens administered 5 d/wk, there was a dose-related improvement in the above measured parameters.[34]

Recent trials of oral analogs of prostaglandins using PGI_2 (beraprost) failed to show a statistically significant improvement in walking distance compared with placebo. Furthermore, the drug was poorly tolerated at higher doses secondary to its side effects. Subsequently, a randomized controlled trial of beraprost in patients with claudication found a statistically significant improvement in PFWD and MWD as well as a reduction in cardiovascular events in those patients randomized to the drug.[35] A similar study conducted in the United States however did not substantiate these results and failed to show any benefit with beraprost compared to placebo in exercise capacity.[36]

The reported constellation of side effects of these agents include headache, flushing, and gastrointestinal intolerance. These agents are not FDA approved in the United States for the treatment of claudication or critical limb ischemia. ACC/AHA guidelines presently state that oral vasodilator prostaglandins such as beraprost and iloprost are not effective medications to improve walking distance in patients with claudication (class III, level of evidence: A).[8]

L-ARGININE

L-Arginine has been shown to induce nitric oxide formation and improve endothelial-dependent vasodilatation in patients with atherosclerosis. Nitric oxide maybe useful in the treatment of chronic limb ischemia through its vasodilatory, antiplatelet, and antiproliferative effects. Small studies have shown improvement in PFWD and MWD following treatment of claudication patients with this compound. These effects were quite prolonged, lasting 6 weeks after discontinuation of drug, and were associated with an improvement in endothelium-dependent vasodilatation.[37] Comparable benefits were observed when an L-arginine-enriched food bar was recommended as a nutritional supplement for patients with PAD. This resulted in an improvement in PFWD of 66% and MWD of 23% in the group receiving the supplement twice daily, as compared to the group that received placebo and once daily supplementation.[38]

The current ACC/AHA guidelines state that the effectiveness of L-arginine for patients with intermittent claudication is not well established (class IIb, level of evidence: B).[8]

ANGIOGENIC GROWTH FACTORS

Angiogenic growth factors, such as vascular endothelial growth factor (VEGF) and basic fibroblast growth factor (bFGF), are mitogenic agents that promote the development of new collateral channels in models of peripheral limb ischemia.[39] Regional intramuscular gene transfer using angiogenic growth factors, such as fibroblast growth factor 1 (FGF-1),[40] $VEGF_{121}$,[41] $VEGF_{165}$,[42,43] VEFG-C,[44] or hypoxia-inducible factor 1 (HIF-1), appears to be pharmacokinetically more practical and efficient. Although the bulk of experience with the use of growth factors has revolved around patients with critical limb ischemia, a renewed interest has arisen surrounding their application in the management of patients with intermittent claudication. In a small (19 patient) phase I trial, subjects were randomized to one of three doses of bFGF or placebo. An improvement of calf blood flow as measured by plethysmography was observed in the higher dose of FGF at 1 month by 66% and by 153% at 6 months.[45] The Therapeutic Angiogenesis with FGF-2 For Intermittent Claudication (TRAFFIC) study was a larger phase II trial employing recombinant FGF-2 infusion in patients with claudication. The preliminary findings of this trial included an improvement in the MWD at 90 days after a single infusion of recombinant FGF-2 compared to placebo.[46] However, the salutary effects of the drug were not sustained in the long-term; there was no substantial benefit seen at 6-month follow-up, and there was no added benefit after repeat infusions of the medication.

The concept that neovascularization could be augmented by administering bone marrow or circulating endothelial progenitor cells (EPCs) have previously been shown to contribute to vascular endothelium. The demonstrated role of EPCs and the physiologic response to ischemia has led to the exploration of strategies employing them for neovascularization in ischemic disease. As a result, preliminary trials are underway utilizing the injection of autologous CD 34-positive cells for symptomatic relief in patients with severe intermittent claudication.

DEFIBROTIDE

Defibrotide is a polydeoxyribonucleotide that modulates endothelial function, decreases the levels of tissue plasminogen activator inhibitor, and increases levels of tissue plasminogen activator. The compound also stimulates prostacyclin release and inhibits platelet aggregation. A meta-analysis of 10 placebo-controlled trials enrolling 743 patients, found a 73-m improvement in MWD in patients treated with the defibrotide versus placebo.[47,48] The usual dose regimen is 200 to 400 mg twice daily. The drug is, however, not available for use at present.

ANTIPLATELET AGENTS

This class of agents includes aspirin, dipyridamole, cilostazol, ticlopidine, and clopidogrel. To date, there is no evidence to support the use of aspirin as solo therapy or in combination with other antiplatelet agents for the symptomatic treatment of claudication.[49,50] However, these agents are useful in reducing cardiovascular events in this patient population. The single drug that has comparatively more data available on its use is ticlopidine, an adenosine diphosphate antagonist. An extremely potent antiplatelet agent, ticlopidine, has been shown in several small randomized trials to demonstrate a modest improvement in claudication symptoms. In one study of 151 claudication patients, both the PFWD and MWD were increased as compared to a group of patients subjected to placebo.[51] However, another placebo-controlled, randomized trial examined the effects of the drug in 169 patients failed to demonstrate a similar benefit on treadmill walking distance in the ticlopidine-treated cohort.[52]

As of yet, there is no compelling, supporting data for the routine use of antiplatelet agents in the symptomatic treatment of claudication. However, given the proven cardioprotective benefit of these drugs, demonstrated in multiple trials, they should be a vital part of the medical regimen in patients with peripheral arterial disease.[53]

KETANSERIN

Ketanserin is a selective S_2-serotonin receptor blocker that acts as a vasodilator. It decreases blood viscosity and is also postulated to dilate collateral vessels. The clinical data studying this drug is conflicting, with a small placebo-controlled study showing an improvement in walking distance.[54] However, a multicenter trial of 179 patients did not demonstrate an improvement in treadmill walking distance when compared to placebo.[55] Ketanserin is not available in the United States.

α-TOCOPHEROL

An active form of vitamin E, α-tocopherol, is a lipid-soluble antioxidant free-radical scavenger. Despite several small studies demonstrating a modest improvement in claudication with use of the drug, α-tocopherol's role in the treatment of claudication should be viewed with skepticism.[56,57] Not only is there limited data supporting its use, but the results of the Heart Outcome Prevention Evaluation (HOPE) trial were negative with regard to the impact of vitamin E on cardiovascular events in a high-risk population of patients, many of whom had peripheral arterial disease.[58]

CHELATION THERAPY

Chelation therapy involves the administration of ethylenediamine tetraacetic acid (EDTA) that is theorized to function as a mobilizer of calcium in atherosclerotic plaques and thus resulting in regression of these lesions. A randomized, double-blind, placebo-controlled trial involving 153 claudication patients found that chelation therapy did not positively improve any objective or subjective parameters, such as walking distance, oxygen tension, ABIs, angiographic appearance, or subjective complaints of symptoms.[59] The potential side effects of this therapy are hypoglycemia and renal failure.

OTHER DRUGS

Studies examining the effects of other available agents for the symptomatic improvement of claudication have generated at best, negative, and at worst, adverse results. These included testosterone,[60] cinnarizine,[61] inositol niacinate,[62] verapamil,[63] anticoagulants, low-molecular weight heparin,[64] aminophylline,[65] and NM-702,[66] a novel phosphodiesterase inhibitor.

Although preliminary results of studies with ginko biloba in treating claudication have seemed promising, the routine use of this compound remains controversial. A recent meta-analysis of eight randomized trials showed an improvement of a mere 33 m in PFWD as compared to placebo.[67] Owing to the fact that none of these agents have been evaluated in large clinical trials, their routine use should not be advocated, pending further future investigation as to their safety and efficacy.

ANTIBIOTICS

The role of infection in the genesis of atherosclerosis and the concept of treating infection to prevent cardiovascular events remain among the more controversial topics in vascular medicine, and therefore the current management guidelines for peripheral arterial disease do not address this particular subject. Nevertheless, pharmacological research is currently investigating the potential role of antibiotics in the treatment of patients with PAD and notably their ability to augment exercise capacity. There are a number of putative mechanisms by which antibiotic therapy can impact the clinical course of atherosclerosis and the natural history of intermittent claudication. Antibiotics may mitigate the inflammatory vascular effects resulting from chronic vascular infection. These drugs may also blunt the detrimental inflammatory effects of chronic ischemia on muscle metabolism, a process that has been demonstrated in in vitro models of vascular disease.[68]

Chlamydia pneumoniae is the infectious agent most convincingly associated with development and progression of atherosclerosis. Several epidemiological studies have demonstrated an association between chlamydia pneumoniae seropositivity and atherosclerosis of the lower limb vasculature.[69] However, substantial controversy on this subject still exists and the precise beneficial effect of antibiotic treatment on the course of atherosclerosis in chlamydia pneumoniae seropositive patients remains to be elucidated.

In a small placebo-controlled trial, including 40 patients who were seropositive for chlamydia pneumoniae, 20 patients received roxithromycin 300 mg daily for 30 days and the other 20 were given placebo. The primary end-points included the number of revascularization procedures and the walking distance between the groups at 2.7 years of follow-up. The results showed a limitation of walking distance to 200 m or less observed in four patients (20%) in the roxithromycin group compared with 13 patients (65%) in the placebo group. The effect of macrolide treatment was significant on preinterventional walking distance ($p = 0.025$) as well as on the walking distance assessed at the end of the study ($p = 0.04$). Furthermore, the secondary endpoint of need for future revascularization procedures showed a clear-cut difference between the two study groups: five vascular interventions requiring percutaneous transluminal angioplasty (PTA) were observed in four patients (20%) in the roxithromycin group and 29 events requiring PTA or bypass surgery in nine patients (45%) in the placebo group.[70]

The PROVIDENCE trial is an ongoing prospective, randomized, double-blind study of rifamycin, an antichlamydia drug in the treatment of seropositive PAD patients. The primary objectives are to evaluate the progression of peripheral arterial occlusive disease in patients randomized to either rifamycin or placebo following a 3-month course of drug. The primary end-point of PROVIDENCE-I is to demonstrate improvement in maximum walking distance at 6 months in treated PAD patients testing positive for high levels of chlamydia antibodies.

CONCLUSION

The pharmacologic therapy of intermittent claudication encompasses a vast armamentarium of drugs, only a few of which have demonstrated clinically relevant efficacy in improving exercise capacity and quality of life in patients seriously affected by the disease. Although exercise therapy remains a cornerstone in the management of patients with PAD, drugs such as cilostazol, because of their favorable safety profile and dramatic effects on ambulatory capacity, are quickly becoming front line agents in the treatment of intermittent claudication. The potential of other agents, including oral prostaglandins, gene therapy, and antibiotic drugs in select patients, is at the present time an exciting but unfulfilled vision. The salutary effects of risk factor modification and the benefits of antiplatelet drug therapy in decreasing the global cardiovascular risk in these patients cannot be overemphasized. It is only through the judicious use, often in combination of these various complementary modalities, that meaningful modification of the natural history of PAD and intermittent claudication can be realized.

REFERENCES

1. Samlaska CP, Winfield, EA. Pentoxifylline. *J Am Acad Dermatol.* 1994;30:603-621.

2. Porter JM, Cutler BS, Lee BY, et al. Pentoxifylline efficacy in the treatment of intermittent claudication: multicenter controlled double-blind trial with objective assessment of chronic occlusive arterial disease patients. *Am Heart J.* 1982;80:1549-1556.

3. Lindgarde F, Jelnes R, Bjorkman H, et al. Conservative drug treatment in patients with moderately severe chronic occlusive peripheral arterial disease. *Circulation.* 1989;80:1549-1556.

4. Dawson DL, Cutler BS, Hiatt WR, et al. A comparison of cilostazol and pentoxifylline for treating intermittent claudication. *Am J Med.* 2000;109:523-530.

5. Girolami B, Bernardi E, Prins MH, et al. Treatment of intermittent claudication with physical training, smoking cessation, pentoxifylline, or nafronyl: a meta-analysis. *Arch Intern Med.* 1999;159:337-345.

6. Gillings DB. Pentoxifylline and intermittent claudication: review of clinical trials and cost-effectiveness analyses. *Cardiovasc Pharmacol.* 1995;25(Suppl 2)S44-S50.

7. Stergachis A, Sheingold S, Luce BR, Psaty BM, Revicki DA. Medical care and cost outcomes after pentoxifylline treatment for peripheral arterial disease. *Arch Intern Med.* 1992;152:1220-1224.

8. Hirsch AT, Haskal ZJ, Hertzer NR, et al. ACC/AHA 2005 practice guidelines for the management of patients with peripheral arterial disease (lower extremity, renal, mesenteric, and abdominal aortic): Executive Summary. *Circulation.* 2006;113:463-654.

9. Sorkin EM, Markham A. Cilostazol: new drug profile. *Drugs Aging.* 1999;14:63-71.

10. Hiatt WR. Medical treatment of peripheral arterial disease and claudication. *N Engl J Med.* 2001;344:1608-1621.

11. Dawson DL, Cutler BS, Meissner MH, Strandness DE. Cilostazol has beneficial effects in treatment of intermittent claudication: results from a multicenter, randomized, prospective, double-blind trial. *Circulation.* 1998;98:678-686.

12. Money SR, Herd JA, Isaacsohn JL, et al. Effect of cilostazol on walking distances in patients with intermittent claudication caused by peripheral vascular disease. *J Vasc Surg.* 1998;27:267-274.

13. Beebe HG, Dawson DL, Cutler BS, et al. A new pharmacological treatment for intermittent claudication: results of a randomized, multicenter trial. *Arch Intern Med.* 1999;159:2041-2050.

14. Dawson DL, DeMaioribus CA, Hagino RT, et al. The effect of withdrawal of drugs treating intermittent claudication. *Am J Surg.* 1999;178:141-146.

15. Elam MB, Heckman J, Crouse JR, et al. Effect of the novel antiplatelet agent cilostazol on plasma lipoproteins in patients with intermittent claudication. *Arterioscler Thromb Vasc Biol.* 1998;18:1942-1947.

16. Cheng KS, Mikhailidis DP, Hamilton G, Seifalian AM. A review of the carotid and femoral intima-media thickness as an indicator of the presence of peripheral vascular disease and cardiovascular risk factors. *Cardiovas Res.* 2002;54(3):528-538.

17. Bramer SL, Forbes WP. Effect of hepatic impairment on the pharmacokinetics of a single dose of cilostazol. *Clin Pharmacokin.* 1999;37(Suppl 2):25-32.

18. Mallikaarjun D, Forbes WP, Bramer SL. Effect of renal impairment on the pharmacokinetics of cilostazol and its metabolites. *Clin Pharmacokin.* 1999;37(Suppl 2):33-40.

19. Wilhite DB, Comerota AJ, Schnieder FA, Throm RC, Gaughan JP, Rao AK. Managing PAD with multiple platelet inhibitors: the effect of combination therapy on bleeding time. *J Vasc Surg.* 2003;38(4):710-713.

20. Packer M, Carver JR, Rodenheffer RJ, et al. Effect of oral milrinone on mortality in severe congestive heart failure. *N Engl J Med.* 1991;325:1468-1475.

21. Hiatt WR. Medical treatment of claudication: IV: Morbidity of PAD: medical approaches to claudication. In: Hirsh AT, Hiatt WR, eds. An Office-Based Approach to the Diagnosis and Treatment of Peripheral Arterial Disease. Continuing Education Monograph Series from the American Journal of Medicine, Bellemead, NJ: Excerpta Medica; 1999:6-15.

22. Hiatt WR, Wolfel EE, Regensteiner JG, Brass EP. Skeletal muscle carnitine metabolism in patients with unilateral peripheral arterial disease. *Appl Physiol.* 1992;73:346-353.

23. Brevetti G, Perna S, Sabba C, Martone VD, Condorelli M. Superiority of L-propionyl carnitine vs. L-carnitine in improving walking capacity in patients with peripheral vascular disease: an acute, intra-venous, double-blind, cross-over study. *Eur Heart.* 1992;13:251-255.

24. Brevetti G, Perna S, Sabba C, Martone VD, Condorelli M. Propionyl-L-carnitine in intermittent claudication: double-blind, placebo-controlled, dose titration, multicenter study. *J Am Coll Cardiol.* 1995;26:1411-1416.

25. Brevetti G, Diehm C, Lambert D. European multicenter study on propionyl-L-carnitine in intermittent claudication. *J Am Coll Cardiol.* 1999;34:1618.

26. Clyne CA, Galland RB, Fox MJ, Gustave R, Jantet GH, Jamieson CW. A controlled trial of naftidrofuryl (Praxilene) in the treatment of intermittent claudication. *Brit J Surg.* 1980; 67:347-348.

27. Adhoute G, Bacourt F, Barral M, et al. Naftidrofuryl in chronic arterial disease. Results of a six month controlled multicenter study using naftidrofuryl tablets 200 mg. *Angiology.* 1986;37: 160-169.

28. Kriessman A, Neiss A. Demonstration of the clinical effectiveness of naftidrofuryl in the intermittent claudication. *VASA.* 1988;24:27-32.

29. Trübestein G, Bohme H, Heidrich H, et al. Naftidrofuryl in chronic arterial disease. Results of a controlled multicenter study. *Angiology.* 1984;35:701-708.

30. Moody AP, al-Khaffaf HS, Lehert P, Harris PL, Charlesworth D. An evaluation of patients with severe intermittent claudication and the effect of treatment with naftidrofuryl. *Cardiovasc Pharmacol.* 1994;23(Suppl 3):S44-S47.

31. Trübestein G, Balzer K, Bisler H, et al. Buflomedil in arterial occlusive disease: results of a controlled multicenter study. *Angiology.* 1984;35:500-505.

32. Chacon-Quevedo A, Eguaras MG, Calleja F, et al. Comparative evaluation of pentoxifylline, buflomedil, and nifedipine in the treatment of intermittent claudication of the lower limbs. *Angiology.* 1994;45:647-653.

33. Scheffler P, de la Hamette D, Gross J, Mueller H, Schieffer H. Intensive vascular training in stage IIb of peripheral arterial occlusive disease: the additive effects of intravenous prostaglandin E1 or intravenous pentoxifylline during training. *Circulation.* 1994;90:818-822.

34. Belch JJ, Bell PR, Creissen D, et al. Randomized, double-blind, placebo-controlled study evaluating the efficacy and safety of AS-013, a prostaglandin E1 prodrug, in patients with intermittent claudication. *Circulation.* 1997;95:2298-2302.

35. Lievre M, Azoulay S, Lion L, Morand S, Girre JP, Boissel JP. A dose–effect study of beraprost sodium in intermittent claudication. *Cardiovasc Pharm.* 1996;27:788-793.

36. Mohler III ER, Hiatt WR, Olin JW, et al. Treatment of intermittent claudication with beraprost sodium, an orally active prostaglandin I$_2$ analogue: a double-blinded, randomized, controlled trial. *J Am Coll Cardiol.* 2003;41(10):1679-1686.

37. Boger RH, Bode-Boger SM, Thiele W, Creutzig A, Alexander K, Frolich JC. Restoring vascular nitric oxide formation by L-arginine improves the symptoms of intermittent claudication in patients with peripheral arterial occlusive disease. *J Am Coll Cardiol.* 1998;32:1336-1344.

38. Maxwell AJ, Anderson B, Cooke JP. Nutritional therapy for peripheral arterial disease: a double-blind, placebo-controlled, randomized trial of HeartBar®. *Vasc Med.* 2000; 5:11-19.

39. Baumgartner I, Isner JM. Somatic gene therapy in the cardiovascular system. *Annu Rev Phys.* 2001;63:427-450.

40. Comerota AJ, Throm RC, Miller KA, et al. Naked plasmid DNA encoding fibroblast growth factor type 1 for the treatment of end-stage unreconstructible lower extremity ischemia: Preliminary results of a phase I trial. *J Vasc Surg.* 2002; 35:930-936.

41. Rajagopalan S, Shah M, Luciano A, Crystal R, Nabel EG. Adenovirus-mediated gene transfer of VEGF121 improves lower-extremity endothelial function and flow reserve. *Circulation.* 2001;104:753-755.

42. Baumgartner I, Pieczek A, Manor O, et al. Constitutive expression of phVEGF165 after intramuscular gene transfer promotes collateral vessel development in patients with critical limb ischemia. *Circulation.* 1998;97:1114-1123.

43. Tsurumi Y, Takeshita S, Chen D, et al. Direct intramuscular gene transfer of naked DNA encoding vascular endothelial growth factor augments collateral development and tissue perfusion. *Circulation.* 1996;94:3281-3290.

44. Rajagopalan S, Trachtenberg J, Mohler E, et al. Phase I study of direct administration of a replication deficient adenovirus vector containing the vascular endothelial growth factor cDNA (CI-1023) to patients with claudication. *J Am Coll Cardiol.* 2002;90;5:512-516.

45. Lazarous DF, Unger EF, Epstein SE, et al. Basic fibroblast growth factor in patients with intermittent claudication: results of a phase I trial. *J Am Coll Cardiol.* 2000;36:1239-1244.

46. Lederman RT. TRAFFIC (Therapeutic Angiogenesis with rFGF-2 for Intermittent Claudication). Presentation at the American College of Cardiology 50th Scientific Session. Progress in Clinical Trials. *Clin Cardiol.* 2001;24:481.

47. Ferrari PA. Defibrotide versus placebo in the treatment of intermittent claudication: a meta-analysis. *Drug Invest.* 1994;7: 157-160.

48. Strano A, Fareed J, Sabba C, et al. A double-blind, multicenter, placebo-controlled, dose comparison study of orally administered defibrotide: preliminary results in patients with peripheral arterial disease. *Semin Thromb Hemost.* 1991; 17(Suppl 2):228-234.

49. Libretti A, Catalano M. Treatment of claudication with dipyridamole and aspirin. *Int J Clin Pharm Res.* 1986;6:59-60.

50. Giansante C, Calabrese S, Fisicaro M, Fiotti N, Mitri E. Treatment of intermittent claudication with antiplatelet agents. *J Int Med Res.* 1990;18:400-407.

51. Balsano F, Coccheri S, Libretti A, et al. Ticlopidine in the treatment of intermittent claudication: a 21-month double-blind trial. *J Lab Clin Med.* 1989;114:84-91.

52. Arcan JC, Panak E. Ticlopidine in the treatment of peripheral occlusive arterial disease. *Sem Thromb Hemost.* 1989;15:167-170.

53. Jackson MR, Clagett GP. Antithrombotic therapy in peripheral arterial occlusive disease. *Chest.* 2001;119:(Suppl): 283S-299S.

54. De Cree J, Leempoels J, Geukens H, Verhaegen H. Placebo-controlled, double-blind trial of ketanserin in treatment of intermittent claudication. *Lancet.* 1984;2:775-779.

55. Thulesius O, Lundvall J, Kroese A, et al. Ketanserin in intermittent claudication: effect on walking distance, blood pressure, and cardiovascular complications. *Cardiovasc Pharm.* 1987;9:728-733.

56. Hamilton M, Wilson GM, Armitage P, Boyd JT. The treatment of intermittent claudication with Vitamin E. *Lancet.* 1953;1:367-370.

57. Livingston PD, Jones, C. Treatment of intermittent claudication with Vitamin E. *Lancet.* 1958;2:602-604.

58. The Heart Outcome Prevention Evaluation Study Investigators. Vitamin E supplementation and cardiovascular events in high-risk patients. *N Engl J Med.* 2000;342:154-160.

59. Guldager B, Jelnes R, Jorgensen SJ, et al. EDTA treatment of intermittent claudication: a double-blind, placebo-controlled study. *J Intern Med.* 1992;231:261-267.

60. Price JF, Leng GC. Steroid sex hormones for lower limb atherosclerosis. *Cochrane Data Syst Rev.* 2000:CD000188.

61. Donald JF. A multicenter general practice study of cinnarizine in the treatment of peripheral vascular disease. *J Int Med Res.* 1979;7:502-506.

62. Kiff RS, Quick CRG. Does inositol nicotinate (hexapol) influence intermittent claudication? A controlled trial. *Br J Clin Pract.* 1988;42:141-145.

63. Bagger JP, Helligsoe P, Randsback F, Kimose HH, Jensen BS. Effect of Verapamil in intermittent claudication: a randomized, double-blind, placebo-controlled, cross-over study after individual dose-response assessment. *Circulation.* 1997;95:411-414.

64. Mannarino E, Pasqualini L, Innocente S, et al. Efficacy of low-molecular-weight heparin in the management of intermittent claudication, *Angiology.* 1991;42:1-7.

65. Picano E, Testa R, Pogliani M, Lattanzi F, Gaudio V, L'Abbate A. Increase of walking capacity after acute amino-phylline administration in intermittent claudication. *Angiology.* 1989;40:1035-1039.

66. Brass EP, Anthony R, Cobb FR, Koda I, Jiao J, Hiatt WR. The novel phosphodiesterase inhibitor NM-702 improves claudication-limited exercise performance in patients with peripheral arterial disease. *J Am Coll Cardiol.* 2006;48;(12):2539-2545.

67. Pittler MH, Ernst, E. Ginko biloba extract for the treatment of intermittent claudication: a meta-analysis of randomized trials. *Am J Med.* 2000;108:276-281.

68. Grayston JT, Campbell L, Crouse III JR, Hiatt WR. Infectious contributions to atherosclerosis and vascular disease: do we really know the answer? *Vasc Dis Manag.* 2006;3:287-296.

69. Krayenbuehl P, Wiesli P, Maly FE, Vetter W, Schulthess G. Progression of peripheral arterial occlusive disease is associated with chlamydia pneumoniae seropositivity and can be inhibited by antibiotic treatment. *Atherosclerosis.* 2005;179:103-110.

70. Wiesli P, Wolfgang C, Meniconi A, et al. Roxithromycin treatment prevents progression of peripheral arterial occlusive disease in chlamydia pneumoniae seropositive men. A randomized, double-blind, placebo-controlled trial. *Circulation.* 2002;105:2646-2652.

chapter 35

Approach to the Patient with Critical Limb Ischemia of the Lower Extremities: Chronic Peripheral Arterial Disease

Christy M. Lawson, MD / *Oscar Grandas, MD*

● INTRODUCTION

Chronic ischemia of the lower extremities is extremely prevalent in Western societies and accounts for a significant amount of morbidity and mortality. Atherosclerosis, although not the only cause of chronic lower extremity ischemia, is, by far, the most common. Together with critical ischemia of the heart, brain, and abdominal organs, atherosclerotic peripheral vascular disease constitutes the leading cause of death in the United States.[1] As the mean age of the population increases, the number of individuals with atherosclerotic lesions of the lower extremities also rises. Patients with peripheral arterial disease (PAD) are at significantly higher risk of death compared to healthy controls from cardiovascular morbidity and mortality, as well as at increased risk of impaired functional status.[2] A basic understanding of the pathogenesis, presentation, diagnosis, and treatment of chronic peripheral vascular disease is an integral part of medical and surgical practice in the United States.

● EPIDEMIOLOGY

In order to gauge the prevalence of PAD in asymptomatic subjects, several epidemiological studies have been done using ankle–brachial index (ABI) as a measure of arterial stenosis. ABI is obtained using a standard blood pressure cuff placed just above the ankle. A Doppler is used to measure the systolic pressure of posterior tibial and dorsalis pedis arteries of each leg. The higher of the systolic pressures in each leg (DP vs. PT) is divided by the higher systolic pressure of either arm. An ABI of ≤ 0.90 indicates hemodynamically significant stenosis. The National Health and Nutritional Examination Survey included 2174 asymptomatic subjects aged ≥ 40 years. The prevalence of PAD, defined by an ABI of ≤ 0.90, ranged from 2.5% in people aged 50 to 59 years to 14.5% in people aged > 70 years.[3] All told, PAD affects a total of around 10 million people. This translates to around 3% to 10% of the general population, with this percentage increasing to 15% to 20% in people older than 70 years (Figure 35-1).[4–6]

Despite aggressive screening policies with ABI, studies show that the number of people in the general population with PAD is grossly underestimated. This is, in part, because of the limitations of ABI alone in diagnosing PAD in some patients.[7] This underestimation could indicate that the prevalence of this already widespread disease is actually much higher. Exercise testing in a noninvasive vascular laboratory setting should be considered in patients for whom the clinical suspicion of PAD is high, yet they have a normal or indeterminate ABI.[8]

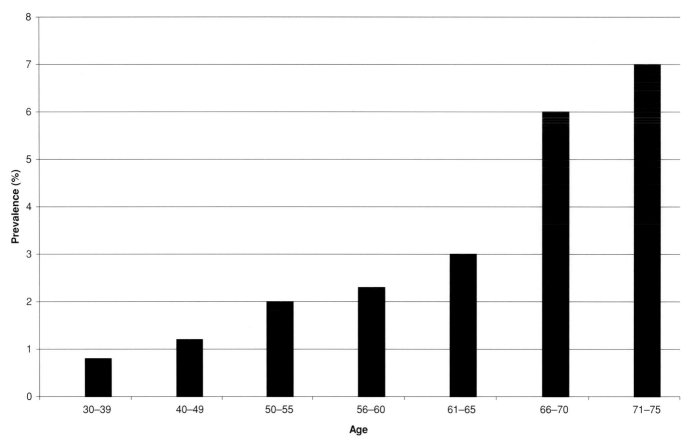

● **FIGURE 35-1.** Mean prevalence of symptomatic PAD in population-based studies.

Data from TransAtlantic Intersociety Consensus (TASC).

● BASIC CONSIDERATIONS AND RISK FACTORS

Atherosclerosis is a chronic inflammatory condition that affects the intima of elastic and muscular arteries of the body in a segmental fashion. Atherosclerosis is evident from early childhood in susceptible populations, and lesions progress through a series of stages before manifesting with clinically significant symptomatology later in life.

Risk factors for PAD are similar to those for heart disease. Most factors have been proven only to have an association with disease, not a true causal relationship.

Increasing age has been found to be associated with increased risk of PAD. Because atherosclerosis is a process related to aging, there is a stepwise increase in the incidence of PAD with each decade of age. This is demonstrated clearly in epidemiological studies.[6]

Male gender is a risk that slightly increases the incidence of PAD, with a ratio of 2:1 when compared to females, especially in younger age brackets. However, some studies conflict these data, illustrating a 1:1 ratio, or even a slightly higher percentage of women with chronic critical limb ischemia in postmenopausal populations.[6]

The GENOA study (Genetic Epidemiology Network of Arteriopathy) showed that PAD was more common in non-Hispanic blacks than in whites, with percentages of 7.8% and 4.4%, respectively. This increased prevalence is not explained by a difference in classical risk factors for atherosclerosis and is, therefore, considered an independent risk factor.[9]

Perhaps the most widely recognized risk factor for PAD is its relationship to cigarette smoke. In fact, it has been suggested that the association between smoking and PAD is even greater than that between smoking and coronary artery disease. A diagnosis of PAD is often made earlier in smokers than in nonsmokers, up to a decade earlier. Cigarette smoking increases the severity of PAD in both men and women proportionally to the number of cigarettes smoked, with heavy smokers having a fourfold increased risk of developing intermittent claudication than nonsmokers.[10]

Diabetes has also been shown to have a significant relationship with the development of PAD. Intermittent claudication is approximately twice as common among diabetic patients as nondiabetic patients.[6] For every 1% increase in hemoglobin A1C, there is a 26% increased risk of PAD.[11] Even in nondiabetic patients, insulin resistance is shown to carry an increased risk for the development of limb ischemia.[12] PAD in diabetic patients is also more aggressive than that found in nondiabetic patients, with early large vessel disease combined with peripheral neuropathy.[6] This translates to a 5 to 10 times higher risk for amputation. Currently, the American Diabetes Association recommends that diabetic patients have ABI screening every 5 years.[13]

Hypertension, shown to be associated with all forms of cardiovascular disease, increases the risk of symptom development as much as 2.5-fold in men and 3.9-fold in women in some studies. However, the relative risk of PAD is less for hypertension than diabetes or smoking.[6,14,15]

Dyslipidemia has also been implicated in the development of PAD. In the Framingham study, a fasting total cholesterol level of greater than 270 mg/dL was shown to correlate with a doubling of the incidence of intermittent claudication.[6] Patients with PAD have significantly higher levels of serum triglycerides, very low-density lipoproteins, intermediate-density lipoproteins, and lower levels of high-density lipoproteins than controls.[16] Cigarette smoking and dyslipidemia may actually have a synergistic effect in the development of PAD.

Other risk factors such as hyperfibrinogenemia, elevated C-reactive protein, hypercoagulable states, and hyperhomocysteinemia have also been implicated in the development of PAD.[2,6,17] The recognition and modification of these risk factors are essential in the diagnosis and treatment of chronic lower extremity ischemia. Guidelines for risk factor modification are published and updated by the American Heart Association.

Atherosclerosis accounts for most cases of peripheral arterial occlusive disease; however, there are other conditions that cause chronic limb ischemia. These include popliteal artery entrapment, mucinous cystic degeneration, Burger disease (thomboangiitis obliterans), abdominal aortic coarctation, fibrodysplasia, and primary arterial tumors.[18]

PATHOPHYSIOLOGY

Atherosclerosis is a chronic, progressive disease of the intima. Many factors are involved in the development of atheromatous plaques, the common denominator between them all being endothelial injury. The most likely model for atherosclerosis points to intimal injury and the subsequent repair process leading to the formation of fibrous plaques. Factors contributing to this model of intimal injury are multifactorial and can include shear stress, hyperlipidemia, and cigarette smoking.[19]

The earliest manifestation of atherosclerosis is the fatty streak, which is identifiable in children as young as 10 years of age. The fatty streak consists of lipid-laden macrophages superimposed over lipid-laden smooth muscle cells of the arterial intima. These occur at the same places where subsequent fibrous plaques are most often found, namely, at bifurcations or bends where decreased shear stress, turbulence, and stasis are known to occur. Increased surface involvement of fatty streaks has been shown to precede the development of fibrous plaques, supporting the idea that the fatty streak is the precursor to fully developed fibrous plaques.[20]

The "response to injury" model of atherosclerosis demonstrates the clustering of monocytes on arterial endothelium. Activated monocytes, induced by IL-1 released in response to endothelial injury, adhere to the intimal lining and migrate to a subendothelial position and become activated macrophages.[21] The receptors for low-density lipoproteins found on the surface of monocytes allow them to absorb lipids and transform into the so-called foam cells. These activated macrophages release chemoattractants (IL-1, TNF-α, and transforming growth factor-β), which serve to recruit more macrophage and smooth muscle cells, as well as lymphocytes and other inflammatory cells, to the developing plaque. The recruited smooth muscle cells will also migrate to the subendothelial position and convert into foam cells. The accumulation of these foam cells distorts the endothelial lining, leading to platelet deposition and the formation of a fibrous cap. Platelets also contribute to the recruitment of more precursors to plaque development by the release of platelet-derived growth factor. Platelet-derived growth factor is a potent stimulus for the migration and proliferation of smooth muscle cells. This process repeats itself, leading to a progressively larger plaque with progressive inflammation and luminal narrowing.[20]

The inflammatory response initiated by the release of cytokines from recruited macrophages and lymphocytes is the driving force behind thrombosis and subsequent arterial occlusive disease. Inflammation leads to increased levels of C-reactive protein, matrix metalloproteinases, and other enzymes that, once released by the recruited macrophages and smooth muscle cells, weaken the connective tissue matrix of the fibrous cap. This leads to plaque instability and rupture. Rupture of the plaque leads to plaque hemorrhage and thrombus formation.[20]

PRESENTATION

Because chronic lower extremity ischemia develops slowly over time, a good portion of patients will have had time to adapt to a compromised arterial system and will present with minimal symptoms in the face of hemodynamically significant stenoses or occlusions. Collaterals will often form and vasodilation will be maximized, bypassing areas of atherosclerosis and minimizing symptoms. In addition, the patient's activity level will sometimes be severely limited by coronary disease or other processes, allowing symptoms to remain undetected for some time.[22]

The patient with lower extremity pain, classically described as a reproducible cramping pain, which is elicited by exercise and relieved only by rest, is said to have intermittent claudication. The pain usually occurs in the muscle group immediately below the level of arterial disease. For example, patients with calf claudication usually have superficial femoral arterial disease, while patients with buttock claudication will have iliac disease. Intermittent claudication is the most common presentation of short segmental disease.[18] For patients with multiple sequential segments of disease affecting the aortoiliac level and the superficial femoral and popliteal levels, or one of these segments combined with severe infrapopliteal disease will more frequently present with disabling intermittent claudication, or rest pain, defined as constant, severe pain in the foot, often at the metatarsophalangeal joint, which is relieved only by dependency, or tissue necrosis. It is important to note that there is no evidence to support that patients with symptoms of PAD progress more frequently or rapidly to critical limb ischemia than those without symptoms; in fact, the presence or absence of symptoms has more to do with the activity level of a patient rather than the severity of disease. Several studies demonstrate only a 1% to 7% amputation rate among claudicants at 5 to 10 years, and only one out of four patients will complain of escalating symptoms for more than 5 years.[23,24]

Critical limb ischemia is defined as inadequate arterial blood flow to accommodate the metabolic needs of resting tissue.[18] With critical limb ischemia, tissue necrosis and ulceration will often be present. The determination of the cause of ulcerating lesions on the ankle and foot becomes an important part of the presentation of PAD. Typical arterial or ischemic ulcers are exquisitely painful and are associated with other physical features of ischemia, including cool, dusky lower extremities, skin and nail changes, and hair loss. Usually they are located at an area of chronic pressure, such as over the malleoli, and their bases usually have a more necrotic appearance. Venous ulcers occur with the stigmata of associated chronic venous disease, including venous stasis dermatitis and edema, and usually improve with compression and elevation. Venous ulcers are also usually less painful than arterial ulcers.

One of the difficulties in evaluating the patient who presents with complaints of lower extremity pain is elucidating whether that pain comes from true limb ischemia or other etiologies. The incidence of PAD increases with every decade of age, as does the incidence of other conditions leading to lower extremity pain, such as osteoarthritis, degenerative joint disease of the spine, and other spine or nerve disorders. Careful history and physical examination, combined with selective diagnostic strategies, help to determine whether PAD is responsible for the patient's symptoms or not.

● STAGING OF LIMB ISCHEMIA

Chronic lower extremity ischemia exists on a clinical spectrum. The Fontaine classification system for lower extremity arterial occlusive disease organizes patients by symptoms.

1. Asymptomatic
2. Claudication present after walking <1 block; no physical changes
3. Ischemic rest pain, atrophy, cyanosis, and dependent rubor
4. Ischemic ulceration/necrosis

Despite the existence of this classification system, many patients do not fit into these groupings. For every one patient who meets the criteria for intermittent claudication, there are an estimated three to four patients with PAD who do not meet these criteria.[25–27] For example, many patients who are considered "asymptomatic" will have some element of exertional lower extremity pain, but not the classic symptoms of claudication. Also, patients with ischemic ulceration and pedal necrosis are extremely variable with respect to the extent of pedal involvement, severity of the necrosis, and underlying etiology (i.e., trauma or pressure necrosis in the face of preexisting ischemia).

To accurately stage limb ischemia objectively and develop a reasonable treatment strategy, diagnostic testing combined with functional assessment remains the most effective way of stratifying the disease (Table 35-1). Results of ABI and selected noninvasive studies have been shown to correlate with risk of limb loss and cardiovascular mortality.[28–30] Walking distance in patients with symptoms of claudication will provide an indication of their functional status. This can be assessed by exercise testing in the noninvasive vascular laboratory. Exercise testing involves recording an ABI at rest, followed by having the patient walk on a treadmill at 3.5 km/h at a 12% incline until claudication symptoms begin. An ABI is then repeated. If there is a significant decrease, this indicates a vascular etiology. If there

---

TABLE 35-1. Clinical Staging of Limb Ischemia

Fontaine Stage	Clinical Symptoms	Noninvasive Results
I	Asymptomatic	Normal treadmill test
IIa	Mild claudication	Normal treadmill test
IIb	Moderate claudication	Completes treadmill exercise; AP after exercise >50 mm Hg, but >20 mm Hg lower than resting value
IIb	Severe claudication	Completes treadmill exercise; AP after exercise >50 mm Hg, but >20 mm Hg lower than resting value
III	Ischemic rest pain	Resting AP <60 mm Hg, ankle or metatarsal PVR flat or barely pulsatile, TP <40 mm Hg
IV	Minor tissue loss	Resting AP <60 mm Hg, ankle or metatarsal PVR flat or barely pulsatile, TP <40 mm Hg
IV	Ulceration or gangrene	Resting AP <60 mm Hg, ankle or metatarsal PVR flat or barely pulsatile, TP <40 mm Hg

AP, ankle pressure; PVR, pulse volume recording; TP, toe pressure.

is not a significant decrease, a nonvascular etiology is likely.[8] These parameters are commonly used to evaluate patients for treatment options.

As a general rule, patients with stage III and IV disease are those whose limbs are imminently threatened and who have disease at multiple levels. Invasive diagnostic procedures and aggressive revascularization interventions are easily justified in these patients.[6] For patients with stage I and most patients with stage II disease, analgesia, risk factor modification, graded exercise programs, and reassurance with observation are more reasonable options. Without treatment, 10% to 15% of stage I patients will improve during 5 years and 60% to 70% do not progress further. The remaining 10% to 15% who do progress are best treated with therapeutic interventions after their disease progresses rather than before.

● TREATMENT

General Considerations

Treatment for PAD is aimed at limb preservation when possible (Table 35-2). A majority of patients with critical limb ischemia will receive some form of active treatment, whether that is revascularization or amputation, although medical management is still recommended as the first approach for non-limb-threatening ischemia. Approximately 25% of patients with chronic limb ischemia will receive medical treatment only, 50% eventually receive a revascularization procedure, and the remaining 25% will have a primary amputation. Figure 35-2 illustrates the 1-year outcomes of these patients after their respective treatments.[6]

Medical Therapy

Before surgical intervention should be pursued, medical treatment of lower extremity ischemia must first be attempted. No truly effective therapy is available; however, the principles of risk factor modification, graded exercise programs, smoking cessation, and prevention of local tissue

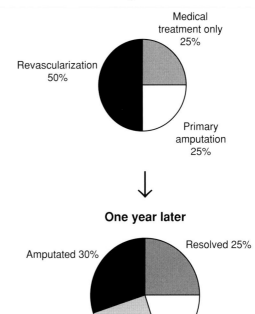

FIGURE 35-2. Fate of patients presenting with critical limb ischemia.

Data from TASC.

trauma and infection in the foot can prolong and sometimes even prevent the need for surgical revascularization.

Risk Factor Modification. The first step in medical therapy of the patient with chronic lower extremity peripheral vascular disease should be risk factor modification. The risk factors associated with the development and progression of PAD, discussed earlier, are largely ones that can be reduced or eliminated by proper patient education, treatment of associated disease processes, and patient compliance. The

---

TABLE 35-2. Summary of Evaluation and Treatment Strategy for PAD

Recognizing At-Risk Patients	*Workup and Medical Management*
History	• PAD screening (ABI/exercise testing)
• Previous diagnosis of PAD	• Evaluation of perfusion on physical examination
• Claudication/walking impairment	• Documentation of ABI
• Risk factors for PAD	• Skin protection from pressure and shear forces
• Renal failure	• Wound management
• Diabetes	
• Acute and chronic heart disease	
Physical findings	Surgical therapy
• Absent pulses	• Endarterectomy
• Abnormal ABI	• Bypass
• Abnormal Exercise test	• Catheter directed atherectomy
• Skin changes/tissue loss	• Balloon angioplasty
	• Stents

Inter-Society Consensus for the Management of Peripheral Arterial Disease (TransAtlantic Intersociety Consensus [TASC] II) provides specific recommendations for risk factor modification.

Smoking. One of the more important steps in nonoperative therapy of PAD is complete cessation of cigarette smoking. Studies show that less than half of patients understand the relationship between peripheral vascular disease and smoking.[31] Physicians should encourage the cessation of smoking regularly, as studies have also demonstrated a higher incidence of abstinence in patient populations encouraged by their physician to quit, as opposed to those who received no counseling from a health care provider.[32] Physicians should also provide nicotine replacement therapies as well as medications such as bupropion, fluoxetine, or varenicline, which can help decrease craving and physiological symptoms of withdrawal. The best success rates are achieved when these modalities are used together in conjunction with group counseling sessions.[6]

Diabetes. Diabetes is a strong risk factor for the development of peripheral vascular disease. Although strict control of blood glucose has been shown to have beneficial effects on other related complications like coronary artery disease, it has not been shown to slow the progression of PAD.[33] Preventive foot care in diabetic patients is of paramount importance in the nonoperative treatment of PAD in diabetic patients. Current recommendations advise aggressive control of blood sugars with a hemoglobin A1c goal of <7%.[6]

Hyperlipidemia. Studies have demonstrated that lipid-reducing strategies designed to increase HDL levels and decrease low-density lipoprotein and triglyceride levels have led to stabilization and sometimes regression of peripheral atherosclerosis. The Heart Protection Study also found that maintaining patients on lipid-lowering agents can reduce the need for surgical revascularization.[34] Physicians should obtain a fasting lipid profile on patients with PAD and initiate therapy when warranted. Dietary modification should be the initial intervention, with lipid-lowering agents started if this is ineffective. Target low-density lipoprotein levels are <100 mg/dL, target HDL levels are >35 mg/dL in men and >45 mg/dL in women, and target triglyceride levels are <150 mg/dL. If patients with PAD have a history of vascular disease in other locations, it is advisable to lower low-density lipoprotein levels to <70 mg/dL.[6]

Hypertension. Although hypertension is a major risk factor in the development of PAD, no data currently exist to prove that blood pressure control would alter the outcome of the disease.[35] β-Blockers are frequently given to patients with PAD in the preoperative period to reduce the incidence of myocardial infarction. Currently, it is recommended that patients with PAD should have blood pressure controlled to <140/90 mm Hg, or <130/80 mm Hg if

in conjunction with diabetes and/or renal insufficiency, as per the JNC VII guidelines.[6]

Homocysteine. Elevated homocysteine levels, which are damaging to the vascular endothelium, have been shown to increase the risk of PAD by speeding the development of atherosclerosis.[36] No studies have shown that reduction of homocysteine levels affects outcomes. Although supplementation with B-vitamins and/or folate has been shown to decrease homocysteine levels, no data have demonstrated a benefit in patients with PAD or other cardiovascular disease and therefore is not recommended.[6]

Exercise Conditioning. If collateral pathways exist around a focal segment of atherosclerotic disease, often the symptoms of ischemia leading to the need for surgical revascularization are minimized. Although several pharmacologic treatments for claudication exist, the best stimulus to increase exercise conditioning seems to be a regular program of physical activity. The most effective exercise programs include supervised walking at least three times a week, for 60 minutes or more.[37] This has been shown to improve claudication symptoms and increase in exercise tolerance by 200 meters. Unless exercise is continued indefinitely, the benefits fade and symptoms return.

Pharmacologic Agents. Several agents exist for the treatment of claudication symptoms, although these have not been proven to change the eventual need for surgical revascularization in patients with advanced symptoms. Pentoxifylline (Trental) and cilostazol (Pletal) are two drugs currently available in the United States. Both have been shown to increase exercise tolerance, with cilostazol having a statistically significant advantage over pentoxifylline in some studies. A 3- to 6-month trial of cilostazol is currently recommended in patients with PAD and claudication symptoms.[6,38]

In addition to the above medications, the use of antiplatelet therapy is also recommended in patients with PAD. A large amount of data exists to support the routine use of antiplatelet agents to decrease the risk of cardiovascular morbidity and mortality.[39] Aspirin/ASA should be routinely given to patients with PAD in conjunction with either coronary or cerebral artery disease.[40] Clopidogrel has also been shown to reduce cardiovascular events in patients with PAD.[41]

Prevention of Local Tissue Damage. Because of the impact of ischemia and reduced blood flow on wound healing, local foot care and the prevention of tissue trauma and infection are extremely important to the nonoperative management of PAD. A comprehensive wound management strategy emphasizing the principles of pressure relief, debridement, infection control, and moist wound healing increases wound closure rates without the need for revascularization.[42] Trauma and infection are often the inciting events leading to gangrene and tissue necrosis, and the ultimate need for revascularization or amputation.

Surgical Consideration

Surgical correction of arterial occlusive disease should be considered in patients who have exhausted medical therapy and lifestyle limiting symptomatic ischemic disease, as well as in patients with limb-threatening ischemia. Unless the ischemia has progressed to gangrene with involvement of deeper tissues of the foot and leg, or the patient is unable to ambulate, communicate, and provide self-care or is otherwise severely disabled and bedridden, limb salvage should be attempted. Patients who are not candidates for surgical revascularization secondary to severe gangrene/necrosis or whose quality of life will remain unaffected by limb salvage should undergo primary above- or below-knee amputation. Medical optimization of comorbidities, such as cardiac, renal, and diabetic disease, should be undertaken prior to proceeding with arteriography and surgical intervention.

● SURGICAL THERAPY

General Principles

The most common sites for chronic arterial occlusive disease are the infrarenal abdominal aorta and the iliac arteries.[43] Because atherosclerosis is a generalized disease process, aortoiliac disease often coexists with atherosclerotic disease in other locations, including the infrainguinal vessels. Segments of disease are usually short and focal, and, therefore, surgical strategies for revascularization are easily implemented, even in patients with multilevel disease. Diagnostic evaluation, including noninvasive studies and arteriography, should be implemented prior to proceeding with surgical revascularization in order to localize and determine the extent of the diseased segments, plan a surgical approach, and determine whether or not the patient is a candidate for surgical intervention at all. In addition, these studies will also help determine which patients are suitable for endovascular-based interventions.

The TASC has developed a classification system to stratify vascular lesions and guide decision making as to the most appropriate therapeutic intervention (Figure 35-3). TASC A lesions represent those that have excellent results with endovascular therapy. TASC B lesions still have good results with endovascular therapy and should be treated with such an approach unless an open revascularization is required for other lesions in the same anatomic area. TASC C lesions have superior results with open revascularization and should be treated in this manner except in patients with high operative risk. TASC D lesions do not achieve good results with endovascular therapy. With TASC B and C lesions, the patient's comorbidities and the long-term success rates of the surgeon of record are taken into consideration when deciding what therapeutic strategy to use (Table 35-3).[6]

Graft Material

The choice of graft material for the management of infrainguinal occlusive disease is one which has resulted in much debate for the past three decades. Prior to the introduction of tubular expanded polytetrafluoroethylene (ePTFE), reversed autogenous saphenous vein grafts (ASV) were the material of choice. Once ePTFE grafts were introduced in the 1970s, practitioners were quick to side with one material type over the other. The first major comparison study of ASV and ePTFE grafts was published by Veith et al. in 1986. In this study, ASV and ePTFE grafts were compared in 845 infrainguinal bypass procedures: 485 to the popliteal and 360 to the infrapopliteal vessels. At 4 years, the primary patency rates between the two groups became significantly different, 68% for ASV vs. 47% for ePTFE.[44] Although this difference was not apparent in the above-knee group, the difference was striking in the infrapopliteal procedures, with 76% primary patency for ASV vs. 45% for ePTFE. This study failed to support the routine use of ePTFE for infrainguinal procedures. However, the authors did conclude that ePTFE was a viable bypass conduit in high-risk patients, especially in those patients without an autogenous vein source or in those patients with above-knee lesions. In 1992, Mcfarland et al. described using a composite bypass graft of ePTFE with a vein cuff in those patients without an adequate autogenous source. At 5 years, the primary patency rate of composite bypass grafts is slightly better than ePTFE alone.[45] Numerous alternatives to ePTFE have been proposed, including the human umbilical vein graft (HUV). Although randomized comparisons between HUV and ePTFE showed promising results, HUV seems to have a high rate of aneurysmal degeneration and should be used with caution.[18] Recently HUV has gained attention as a possible material in composite grafts with autogenous veins. The primary patency rate at 4 years in patients with an HUV composite bypass was 53%, similar to composite ePTFE grafts. While autogenous vein should be used as the bypass conduit of choice whenever possible, up to 40% of patients will have a small (<3 mm), fibrotic, or insufficient saphenous vein. In these cases, it is much better to proceed with an ePTFE graft rather than compromising the procedure with an inadequate autogenous graft.[18]

Aortoiliac Disease

General Considerations. The infrarenal abdominal aorta and the iliac arteries are the most common place for symptomatic chronic atherosclerotic disease to occur. Most patients who have distal arterial occlusive disease severe enough to require surgical revascularization will have some degree of aortoiliac disease as well. Patients who have several levels of infrainguinal occlusive disease often have significant relief of symptoms simply from correction of the hemodynamic impairment of the aortoiliac arterial inflow. In addition, if surgical correction of infrainguinal lesions is pursued without assessment of the adequacy of the inflow system, it is often difficult to achieve symptom relief and durable results. Presentation is usually claudication involving the muscles of the thigh, hip, and buttock, varying in severity. In all, 30% to 50% of men with aortoiliac disease will have complaints of impotence.[46] Complete

Type A lesions

• Unilateral or bilateral stenoses of CIA
• Unilateral or bilateral single short (≤3 cm) stenosis of EIA

Type B lesions

• Short (≤3 cm) stenosis of infrarenal aorta
• Unilateral CIA occlusion
• Single or multiple stenosis totaling 3–10 cm involving the EIA not extending into the CFA
• Unilateral EIA occlusion not involving the origins of internal iliac or CFA

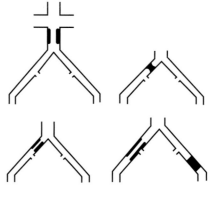

Type C lesions

• Bilateral CIA occlusions
• Bilateral EIA stenoses 3–10 cm long not extending into the CFA
• Unilateral EIA stenosis extending into the CFA
• Unilateral EIA occlusion that involves the origins of internal iliac and/or CFA
• Heavily calcified unilateral EIA occlusion with or without involvement of origins of internal iliac and/or CFA

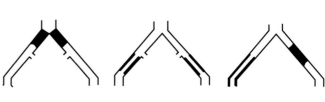

Type D lesions

• Infrarenal aortoiliac occlusion
• Diffuse disease involving the aorta and both iliac arteries requiring treatment
• Diffuse multiple stenoses involving the unilateral CIA, EIA, and CFA
• Unilateral occlusions of both CIA and EIA
• Bilateral occlusions of EIA
• Iliac stenoses in patients with AAA requiring treament and not amenable to endograft placement or other lesions requiring open aortic or iliac surgery

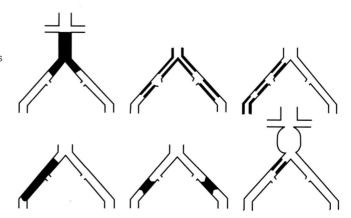

● **FIGURE 35-3.** Morphologic classification of iliac lesions.

Source: Reprinted with permission from Elsevier in Norgren L, Hiatt WR, Dormandy JA, et al. Inter-Society Consensus for the Management of Peripheral Arterial Disease (TASC II). J Vasc Surg 2007;45(1):S5-S67. (continued)

aortoiliac occlusion, or Leriches's syndrome, is characterized by impotence, buttock and thigh claudication, and absent femoral pulses.[6]

The parameters defined by the TASC criteria provide a framework for the decision of how to approach the correction of aortoiliac disease. Type A lesions are focal, short (≤3 cm), unilateral, or bilateral lesions of the common iliac artery or external iliac artery and are generally amenable to endovascular therapy. Because type A lesions are so localized, the potential for the development of collater-

als around the diseased segment is very high. Collateral pathways can be derived from both visceral and parietal routes, including the internal mammary artery to the inferior epigastric artery, the intercostals and lumbar arteries to the circumflex iliac and hypogastrics, the hypogastrics and gluteals to the common femoral and profunda femoris, and the superior mesenteric to inferior mesenteric and superior hemorrhoidals through the marginal artery of Drummond. These collateral pathways can allow a patient to remain asymptomatic until more severe disease evolves.

Type A lesions

- Single stenosis ≤10 cm in length
- Single occlusion ≤5 cm in length

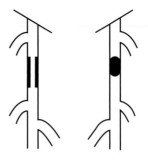

Type B lesions

- Multiple lesions (stenoes or occlusions), each ≤5 cm
- Single stenosis or occlusion ≤15 cm not involving the infrageniculate popliteal artery
- Single or multiple lesions in the absence of continuous tibial vessels to improve inflow for a distal bypass
- Heavily calcified occlusion ≤5 cm in length
- Single popliteal stenosis

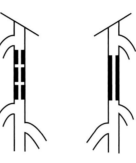
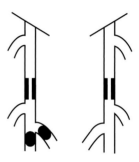

Type C lesions

- Multiple stenoses or occlusions totaling >15 cm with or without heavy calcification
- Recurrent stenoses or occlusions that need treatment after two endovascular interventions

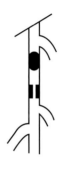

Type D lesions

- Chronic total occlusions of CFA or SFA (>20 cm, involving the popliteal artery)
- Chronic total occlusion of popliteal artery and proximal trifuraction vessels

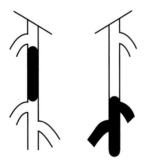

● **FIGURE 35-3.** (*continued*) TASC II classification of lesions. A-aorto-iliac B-femoropoliteal.

Source: Reprinted with permission from Elsevier in Norgren L, Hiatt WR, Dormandy JA, et al. Inter-Society Consensus for the Management of Peripheral Arterial Disease (TASC II). J Vasc Surg 2007;45(1):S5-S67.

Type B lesions are short (≤3 cm) stenoses of the infrarenal aorta, unilateral common iliac artery occlusion, single or multiple stenoses equaling a total of 3 to 10 cm of the external iliac without extension into the common femoral artery (CFA), or unilateral external iliac artery occlusion without involvement of the internal iliac or CFA. Type B lesions are generally still treatable with endovascular therapy, unless there are multiple other lesions within the same area that collectively would make the overall presentation more amenable to open surgical revascularization.

Type C lesions are bilateral common iliac artery occlusions, bilateral external iliac artery stenoses equaling a total of 3 to 10 cm without extension into the CFA, unilateral external iliac artery occlusion that involves the origin of the internal iliac and/or CFA, or heavily calcified unilateral external iliac artery occlusion with or without involvement of the internal iliac or common femoral. Unless a patient has multiple comorbidities imparting unacceptable surgical risk, Type C lesions should be treated with open surgical therapy.[47,48]

TABLE 35-3. TASC Classification

Type A	• Single stenosis ≤10 cm • Single occlusion ≤5 cm
Type B	• Multiple lesions, each ≤5 cm • Single stenosis or occlusion <15 cm not involving infrageniculate popliteal artery • Single or multiple lesions without continuous vessels for distal bypass • Heavily calcified occlusion <5 cm • Single popliteal stenosis
Type C	• Multiple stenoses or occlusions totaling >15 cm with or without heavy calcification • Recurrent stenoses or occlusions that need treatment after two endovascular procedures
Type D	• Chronic, total occlusions >20 cm involving popliteal artery • Chronic, total occlusions of popliteal artery and proximal trifurcation

Type D lesions are infrarenal aortoiliac occlusion; diffuse disease involving the aorta and both iliac arteries and diffuse, multiple, unilateral stenoses of the common iliac artery, the external iliac, and the common femoral, unilateral occlusions of the common iliac and external iliac; bilateral occlusions of the external iliac; or iliac stenoses in patients with AAA requiring treatment that is not amenable to endograft repair or with other lesions that require open aortic or iliac surgery. Type D lesions do not have good success rates with endovascular therapy.

Type C and D lesions are the most prevalent, accounting for 65% of patients. Often referred to as "combined segment" or "multilevel" disease, these patients are typically older at presentation and are more often male than female. Usually, they have multiple comorbidities such as hypertension and diabetes and have atherosclerotic disease involving cerebral and coronary arteries as well. These patients are also more likely to have progression of their disease than the other types. Because of this, most patients with Type C and D disease will present with signs of advanced ischemia and have significantly decreased life expectancies compared to patients with more localized aortoiliac disease.

Indications for operative therapy of aortoiliac disease include patients who have optimized medical therapy and are still significantly symptomatic, as well as patients with ischemic rest pain, tissue necrosis, or distal atheromatous emboli from proximal ulcerated plaques. Short-segment disease or patients who are poor candidates for surgical revascularization should be considered for endovascular therapy. If a patient has been determined to be a surgical candidate, several techniques exist and must be tailored to the extent and location of the diseased segment.

Aortoiliac Endarterectomy. For patients with truly localized disease, aortoiliac endarterectomy may be considered. The advantages of endarterectomy are that no prosthetic material is used, infection rates are lower, and it may provide better inflow to the hypogastrics, which could decrease impotence rates in men. The segment of disease should be limited to the distal aorta and common iliacs and must end at or just beyond the bifurcation of the common iliacs so that the surgeon has an end point that does not extend into the external iliac.[18]

To perform an aortoiliac endarterectomy, an arteriotomy is typically made at the distal aorta, with smaller arteriotomies in both of the common iliacs at the level where the diseased segment terminates. The endarterectomy plane is developed at the level of the external elastic lamina, and the plaque is removed. Tacking sutures may or may not be required to achieve a secure end point. Generally, arteriotomies can be closed primarily; however, if necessary, a patch can be used.[49,50]

Endarterectomy is contraindicated in patients with evidence of aneurysmal change of the involved segment, with total aortic occlusion to the level of the renal arteries, and in patients who have extension of the disease process into the external iliacs or distal vessels. The external iliac artery is not as amenable to endarterectomy because of its smaller size, longer length, and more muscular medial layer. The rates of early thrombosis and late failure are unacceptably high, thus making bypass grafting a more suitable approach.[18]

Aortoiliac Bypass

General Principles. When the decision to proceed with bypass grafting of an aortoiliac segment has been made, careful evaluation of the diseased segment with arteriography must be undertaken preoperatively. This will identify whether or not the patient has concomitant aneurysmal disease, the anatomy of the aorta and takeoff of the renal arteries, and the extent of the diseased segment. In addition, an operative strategy for proximal and distal anastomosis of the bypass graft can be developed. Also, assessment of adequate graft outflow at the level of the femoral artery anastomosis is extremely important to optimize early and late graft results. The orifice of the profunda femoris must be visualized on arteriography. Femoral endarterectomy of the profunda femoris may be required if the vessel is extensively diseased and impairs the outflow of the graft in any way.[51,52]

Operative Technique. The "gold standard" for the treatment of aortoiliac occlusive disease is the aortobifemoral graft. Direct aortic grafting is the most durable and effective revascularization technique available for aortoiliac disease. The day before surgery, the patient must undergo bowel preparation. Clear liquid diet with mechanical preparation via stool softeners and enemas are generally recommended. Prophylactic antibiotics should be given 1 to 2 hours preoperatively. Some studies recommend continuing these antibiotics for 24 to 48 hours postoperatively.[18]

Once the patient has been positioned in the operative suite and placed under general anesthesia, the entire abdomen, up to the level of the nipple, and both groins are prepared with a sterile solution and draped in a standard fashion. Often, an adhesive iodophor-impregnated drape is placed over the operative field to reduce contamination of the bypass graft by skin flora. Bilateral groin incisions should be made to expose both femoral arteries from just above the level of the inguinal ligament to below the femoral bifurcation. Care should be taken to identify the landmarks of the inguinal ligament prior to making the groin incision, as many obese patients have a groin crease that lies several centimeters below the inguinal ligament. The common femoral, superficial femoral, and profunda femoral arteries should be identified and isolated. It is helpful at this point in the procedure to begin creation of a retroperitoneal tunnel tract beneath the inguinal ligament and superficial to the femoral and external iliac arteries to accommodate the femoral limb of the bypass graft. For the purposes of this discussion, we will first focus on the transperitoneal approach to the aortobifemoral bypass and later discuss the alternative retroperitoneal approach. A midline incision should be made to allow for adequate visualization of the operative field. Once in the peritoneal cavity, the transverse colon should be retracted superiorly. The ligament of Treitz is then divided to mobilize the duodenum medially. The small bowel should be packed superiorly and medially, with the descending and sigmoid colon packed and retracted laterally and inferiorly. There are numerous self-retaining retractors that are helpful for this propose. The peritoneum over the aorta is then opened with care to preserve the hypogastric nerve plexus to prevent long-term sexual dysfunction postoperatively. This peritoneal dissection is carried down to below the aortic bifurcation. The ureters should be identified to avoid injury, particularly in the area of the common iliac arteries. Once the aorta has been adequately dissected from below the renal arteries to the common iliac arteries, the patient is given a heparin infusion and clamps are placed proximally and distally. A decision must then be made as to the type of proximal anastomosis. The two choices are an end-to-side and an end-to-end anastomosis. The end-to-end anastomosis is the classically described proximal anastomosis and has several potential benefits. Firstly, this anastomosis provides for better flow patterns than the end-to-side alternative with better long-term patency rates. Secondly, the end-to-end anastomosis allows for the graft to lie within the retroperitoneal aortic bed with less chance for aortoenteric fistula formation. Alternatively, the end-to-side anastomosis should be considered in younger patients who have bilateral external iliac occlusive disease and inadequate flow to the pelvic vessels. In these patients, interrupted pelvic collateralization with an end-to-end anastomosis risks impotence postoperatively.[53] We will now focus on the end-to-end anastomosis. The aorta should be divided just distal to the renal vessels in a segment of the artery without disease. The proximal limb of the graft should be appropriately measured, usually 16 mm for occlusive disease. The proximal anastomosis is created using a continuous polypropylene suture. The first suture should be placed from outside to inside of the graft at the

3-o'clock position and then inside to outside on the aortic wall. The posterior portion of the anastomosis is completed to the area around the 9-o'clock position. The anastomosis is then completed anteriorly. After completion of the anastomosis, the proximal aortic clamp should be removed and the graft flushed. The suture line should be inspected for areas of leak. The distal aortic stump should then be oversewn with a running locking polypropylene suture.

Both femoral limbs are then tunneled beneath the inguinal ligament and brought into the femoral dissection field. Although an anastomosis is feasible at the level of the external iliac arteries, this procedure is more technically demanding and has a higher rate of failure over time. An anastomosis at the femoral level ensures adequate runoff and profunda femoral outflow. The femoral vessels are controlled proximally and distally and an arteriotomy is made over the CFA. The graft is appropriately trimmed for the anastomosis with a broad hood. The heel of the hood is anastomosed to the proximal arteriotomy with polypropylene suture, and the anastomosis is created in a circumferential fashion. In patients with superficial femoral disease, outflow through the profunda femoral artery must be assured for long-term graft patency. Any stenosis at the level of the profunda femoral artery should be recognized by the surgeon and corrected with an endarterectomy and patch angioplasty using the toe of the femoral graft. Once hemostasis is assured at the proximal and distal anastomosis sites, the peritoneum is closed over the aortic graft to reduce the risk for aortoenteric fistula formation. At the completion of the procedure, restoration of distal flow should be assured via palpation of distal pulses or Doppler signals.

Long-term patency of aortobifemoral reconstructions are extremely good with 5-year patency rates of up to 90% and 10-year patency rates of up to 75% (Figure 35-4). However, survival rates remain lower than age-related controls, mostly owing to atherosclerotic heart disease. Twenty-five percent of patients will have died at 5 years and up to 60% are dead at 10 years.[54,55]

Complications. Short-term complications from aortobifemoral bypass include graft thrombosis and limb ischemia, renal failure, and colonic ischemia.[18] Graft thrombosis and distal embolization can be minimized by ensuring systemic anticoagulation at the time of surgery and adequate flushing of the graft prior to performing the distal anastomosis.[56] In any patient with limb ischemia postoperatively, the patient should be returned to the operating room and thrombectomy of the graft performed. This complication is usually related to kinking of the graft in the retroperitoneal tunnel or technical error at the distal anastomosis. In cases of inadequate runoff as a cause for graft thrombosis, a distal bypass may be required to preserve flow in the aortofemoral graft. Renal failure following aortobifemoral bypass occurs in approximately 4.6% of cases and is usually a result of acute tubular necrosis or embolization with suprarenal clamping.[57] This complication can be avoided by minimizing suprarenal cross-clamp time, avoiding hypotension with

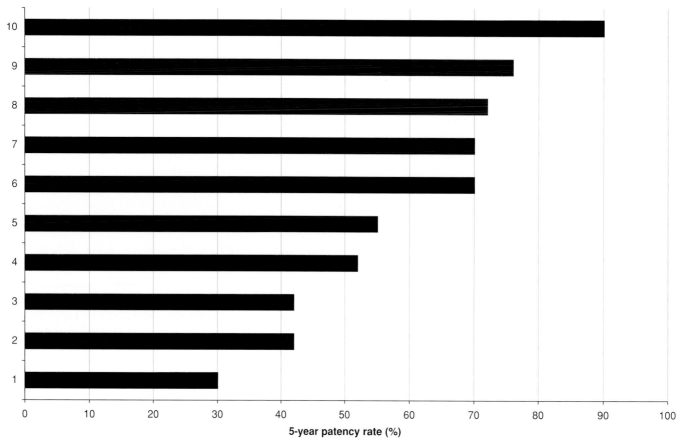

FIGURE 35-4. Average results for surgical treatment.

removal of the clamp, and providing appropriate fluid resuscitation postoperatively.[18] Colonic ischemia occurs in approximately 2% of cases and results from loss of the collateral flow through the inferior mesenteric artery.[58] Any patient with bloody stools or severe metabolic acidosis postoperatively should be evaluated with sigmoidoscopy to evaluate mucosal ischemia. These patients should be treated with bowel rest and intravenous antibiotics. Should the patient's clinical status deteriorate, prompt surgical intervention should be pursued. Nonviable bowel should be resected and a proximal colostomy with distal Hartmann's pouch performed. Care should be taken to avoid exposing the aortic graft. Mortality rates are high if the patient population is high and can range up to 75%.[56]

Late complications include graft occlusion, impotence, infection, and aortoenteric fistula. Graft occlusion and thrombosis is the most common late complication of aortic bypass surgery, occurring in 10% of patients at 5 years.[59] Most commonly this affects one limb of the graft with preserved flow in the contralateral limb, resulting in unilateral limb ischemia. This complication can usually be managed with thrombectomy of the affected limb with a Fogarty thromboembolectomy catheter (Figure 35-5). During the procedure, the profunda femoral artery should

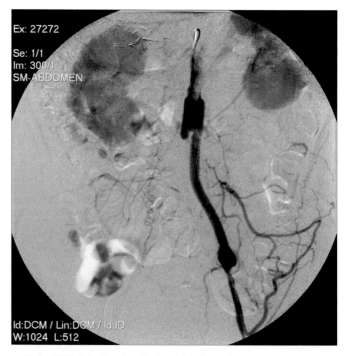

FIGURE 35-5. Aortic Graft Limb occlusion.

be examined and profundaplasty performed in cases of advanced atherosclerotic disease. In those patients with chronic thrombosis of one limb of the bypass graft, a femoral–femoral bypass is a reasonable approach to restoring flow. Total graft occlusion is usually caused by ongoing atherosclerotic disease, especially in patients who continue to smoke postoperatively.[60,61] These patients should be managed with either a repeat aortobifemoral bypass or an extra-anatomic bypass.[62]

Postoperative sexual dysfunction can occur in up to 25% of male patients following aortic surgery.[63] This complication can be minimized by limiting the aortic dissection on the lateral wall of the aorta and to the right of the aortic bifurcation where autonomic nerve fibers travel into the pelvis.[64] Additional maneuvers to preserve flow to the hypogastric arteries, including an end-to-side proximal graft anastomosis, seem to help diminish postoperative sexual complications.[65]

Graft infection, while fortunately rare with an incidence of 1% or less, is a dreaded complication of aortic surgery and carries a significant risk of morbidity and mortality.[66] It is believed that bacterial contamination occurs at the time of graft implantation and may not become clinically apparent for many months to years. *Staphylococcus aureus* is the most common causative organism.[67] Rates of graft infection can be minimized by the use of perioperative antibiotics and meticulous sterile technique at the time of surgery. Once diagnosed, the graft infection should be treated with graft excision, antibiotics, and extra-anatomic bypass.[68]

Aortoenteric fistula can occur as a late complication of aortic surgery when there is inadequate peritoneal coverage over the bypass graft. These patients present with massive gastrointestinal hemorrhage as a result of graft erosion into adjacent viscera. This erosion usually occurs between the proximal anastomotic line and the second or third portions of the duodenum. Once the diagnosis has been established, these patients are treated with graft excision, repair of the affected hollow viscous, and extra-anatomic bypass. Despite these efforts, mortality and limb loss rates remain high, approaching 50% in some studies.[56]

Extra-anatomic Bypass Procedures

Axillofemoral Bypass. In those patients who cannot tolerate an open aortic procedure, or who have an infected or otherwise compromised aortic graft, axillofemoral bypass is well suited. The recovery time from the procedure is quicker than with a laparotomy and the hemodynamic stress significantly reduced. This procedure requires tunneling a graft between the right axillary artery and the right CFA and then between each femoral artery. Because occlusive disease is less common in the right innominate than in the left subclavian artery, the right axillary artery is chosen as the inflow vessel.

To perform the procedure, the patient is positioned in a supine position and the right chest, arm, and both groins are prepped into the sterile field. The axillary artery is dissected through a horizontal incision measuring approximately

6 cm just inferior to the clavicle. The pectoralis muscle fibers are bluntly separated to expose the axillary vein, which is retracted caudally. The axillary artery lies just inferior to the vein. The artery is freed from the surrounding tissues, with care to avoid injuring the underlying brachial plexus. Both femoral arteries are then exposed through standard groin incisions. A graft of ePTFE measuring 80 to 100 cm in length and 8 to 10 mm in diameter is then tunneled from the axillary incision, down the flank, to the ipsilateral groin incision; a counter incision in the midaxillary line at the seventh intercostals space will aid in tunneling the graft. Distally, the graft should be tunneled along the flank, over the iliac crest just anterior to the anterior-superior iliac spine and into the groin. A second tunnel is made between the groin incisions anterior to the pubis to allow for the femoral portion of the graft. Once the grafts are positioned, the patient should be systemically anticoagulated with heparin. The axillary artery is controlled proximally and distally, and a longitudinal arteriotomy is performed. The proximal anastomosis is created in an end-to-side fashion. The anastomosis must be positioned medial to the pectoralis minor muscle to prevent traction on the graft with arm abduction. Flow is then restored to the arm once the proximal anastomosis is completed. The right CFA and its branches are controlled, and a longitudinal arteriotomy is performed down to the superficial femoral artery. The distal anastomosis is created in an end-to-side fashion. The crossover graft is then anastomosed proximally to the hood of the axillofemoral graft and distally to the contralateral femoral artery in an end-to-side configuration.[69,70]

Femorofemoral Bypass. In those patients with unilateral iliac occlusion with preserved contralateral flow, a femoro-femoral crossover graft is a reasonable alternative to aortobifemoral bypass. The bypass is performed essentially the same way as mentioned above for the axillofemoral crossover bypass.[71]

Femorofemoral bypass and axillobifemoral bypass have expected 5-year patency rates of 70% to 75% and 60% to 85%, respectively. Some studies suggest that long-term anticoagulation, particularly in patients with an axillobifemoral bypass, may improve graft survival. Long-term patency seems to be most impacted by concurrent superficial femoral artery disease.[70,72]

Infrainguinal Disease

General Considerations. The mainstay of treatment for lower extremity limb-threatening ischemia involving the infrainguinal vessels is the infrainguinal bypass, which comprises several treatment strategies. Autologous vein bypass of diseased segments for limb salvage has become the standard of care, prosthetic materials are used only when autologous vein is not available. As techniques have improved, surgeons have pushed the limits of distal bypass to include distal tibial and tarsal vessels. These more distal procedures have provided a new treatment strategy, which, in the hands of experienced surgeons, can provide good results. Nevertheless, with any bypass procedure, lower extremity bypass should only be offered to appropriate surgical candidates. Those patients with deep tarsal gangrene who are nonambulatory or who have long-standing dementia should be offered primary amputation rather than bypass.

Preoperative Evaluation. All patients should be assessed with a thorough history and physical examination to evaluate the extent of peripheral vascular disease. It is important to note any history of prior vascular surgeries and the severity of the patient's ischemic symptoms. In addition, physical signs of arterial disease should be noted including decreased pulses, diminished skin temperature, rubor, and pain that is relieved with dependent positioning of the extremity.

Noninvasive testing should be performed in all patients. ABI can provide an assessment of baseline circulation. As mentioned earlier, an ABI of 0.5 to 0.9 is indicative of claudication and less than 0.5 of limb-threatening ischemia. This procedure is limited in those patients with highly calcified vessels (i.e., end-stage renal disease and diabetic patients). The ABI is falsely elevated in this patient population secondary to the inability to compress the vessels.

Duplex ultrasound scanning can be extremely helpful in evaluating lower extremity PVD. Numerous studies have shown that duplex scanning is quite sensitive in detecting iliac and infrainguinal stenosis and can predict the point of distal reconstitution. Duplex scanning should be considered in those patients who have calcified vessels as a means of determining the extent of disease prior to undergoing angiography.[73,74]

Arteriography remains the gold standard for the surgical planning of PVD. This procedure allows for evaluation of the entire arterial tree and potentially offers therapeutic options with the advent of endovascular surgery. Arteriography also allows the surgeon to determine the type of bypass procedure and distal bypass targets, which might best suit the patient's disease. Typically, arteriography has a complication rate of 1.5% to 3%, with complications including hematoma, dissection, thrombosis, embolization, and pseudoaneurysm.[18] This procedure should be used with caution in those patients with preexisting renal dysfunction and, in particularly, the elderly. The patients should be adequately hydrated pre and post procedure and should be given oral acetylcysteine, which has been shown to diminish the risk of contrast nephropathy. Newer technologies such as magnetic resonance angiography and CT angiography with 3-D reconstruction have the potential to supplant arteriography in the future. These modalities are noninvasive and provide excellent imaging of the distal lower-extremity vessels with specificities that approach standard angiography. However, until these modalities become more readily available, contrast arteriography will remain the gold standard.

Femoropopliteal Bypass. In those patients with superficial femoral or popliteal artery occlusion and a patent distal popliteal artery, consideration should be given to femoropopliteal bypass. The patient should have an adequate popliteal target, usually greater than 7 mm, and preserved distal runoff through at least one of the distal vessels, even if that vessel is occluded at the foot. In all other situations, consideration should be made for a distal or a sequential bypass.[75]

Above-Knee Bypass. The patient is positioned supine with the knee flexed to 30 degrees to allow for exposure of the femoral and popliteal artery as well as the saphenous vein. The greater saphenous vein is harvested through either continuous or interrupted incisions starting in the groin and proceeding distally toward the knee. The interrupted technique is preferred by some surgeons as a result of presumed decreased postoperative pain and diminished risk for skin necrosis or infection. The most proximal incision is made at the groin. This incision can be used for the femoral artery exposure. The saphenofemoral junction is identified and mobilized. The vein should be ligated as close to this junction as possible. Dissection continues distally where all tributaries are identified and ligated with 3-0 silk sutures. Once an adequate length of vein has been mobilized, the vein is ligated and removed from the field. The graft should be placed in a heparinized saline solution. Prior to performing the anastomosis, the vein should be tested for leaks by placing a cannula at the distal end of the graft and irrigating the vein. Any leaks should be identified and repaired.

As mentioned earlier, the incision for saphenous vein harvest can be used for exposing the femoral artery. The lymphatics overlying the artery should be avoided and retracted medially. Any lymphatic leaking should be controlled at this point. Self-retaining retractors should be placed in the wound to aid visualization. The fascia overlying the femoral artery is then opened. The common and superficial femoral arteries are identified and isolated with Silastic vessel loops. The profunda femoral artery is then identified by retracting the common femoral and superficial femoral vessels superiorly. The profunda femoral lies lateral and posterior to the CFA. The vessel should be mobilized with care and isolated with vessel loops. Attention is then given to the popliteal vessels. An incision is made in the lower thigh just medial to the sartorius muscle and extending down to the level of the knee. The sartorius muscle is retracted posteriorly to expose the underlying popliteal artery as it emerges from the adductor hiatus. It may be necessary to divide the adductor magnus tendon to expose the most proximal portion of the popliteal artery. The overlying fascia is divided and the neurovascular bundle identified. The arterial sheath is opened, and the popliteal artery is dissected free from the adjacent tissues. Care must be taken to avoid injuring the popliteal vein, which lies in close proximity to the artery. A length of 3 to 4 cm is usually adequate for the distal anastomosis. A tunnel for the graft is then created just deep to the sartorius muscle by using a tunneling device or large aortic clamp. The patient is then given heparin (100 units/kg), and vascular clamps are placed on the femoral vessels. The saphenous vein graft is brought into the field and reversed for the proximal anastomosis. The graft is opened along the posterior wall and trimmed to create a hood. A longitudinal arteriotomy is then made on the femoral artery approximately twice the diameter of the vessel. Using a double-armed polypropylene suture the heel of the graft is anastomosed to the arteriotomy, with the sutures passing from outside to inside the graft and inside to outside the arteriotomy. This process is repeated for the toe of the graft. The graft is then approximated to the arteriotomy in a continuous running fashion, starting at the toe and moving toward the heel to a point at the middle portion of the anastomosis. Equal portions of all tissue layers should be taken on both the graft and the artery. This process is repeated from the heel toward the toe of the graft. The sutures are tied at the midpoint of the anastomosis. The clamps are removed and the anastomosis inspected for hemostasis. The graft is then marked to prevent twisting and brought through the tunnel for the distal anastomosis. The graft is trimmed as it was for the femoral anastomosis. Clamps are placed on the popliteal artery, and a longitudinal arteriotomy is made. The anastomosis is created using two double-armed polypropylene sutures just as the proximal anastomosis was. The clamps are removed and the distal anastomosis inspected for hemostasis. All wounds are then irrigated. The subcutaneous tissues are then closed in three layers using an absorbable suture. Skin incisions are closed with skin staples. Prior to closure, distal perfusion should be ensured by manual palpation of the pedal vessels or Doppler signal.[18]

Below-Knee Bypass. In certain situations, the proximal portion of the popliteal artery is occluded or markedly stenotic and thus cannot be used for a distal anastomosis. In these cases, the distal popliteal artery, which is usually free of atherosclerotic disease, should be used for the distal anastomosis. In addition to being relatively free of atherosclerotic disease, the distal popliteal artery has few branches and the arterial wall is often more suitable for anastomosis than the proximal artery. To expose the distal popliteal artery, the patient's knee is flexed and a roll is placed beneath the leg for elevation. An incision is made, measuring approximately 10 cm just posterior to the posteromedial aspect of the tibia. If it has not already been harvested for the graft, the greater saphenous vein must be identified to prevent damage. The crural fascia is identified and divided along the fibers. The gracilis and semitendinous tendons are separated from the crural fascia and retracted; in some cases, it is necessary to divide these tendons to provide adequate visualization. The gastrocnemius and soleus muscles are retracted posteriorly to expose the underlying vascular bundle as it crosses the popliteus muscle. The popliteal artery is free from the vascular bundle, and vessel loops are placed around the artery. The femoral artery exposure and saphenous vein harvest are carried out exactly as these would be for an above-knee bypass. The tunnel for the graft is passed through Hunter's canal, through the popliteal space, and behind the popliteus muscle. The proximal and distal anastomoses and placement of the graft within the tunnel are created in a similar fashion to the above-knee bypass (Figure 35-6).

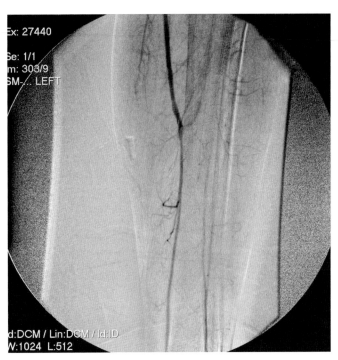

● **FIGURE 35-6.** Open revascularization: Infrainguinal bypass.

Outcomes. In general, above-knee bypass has a better long-term patency than below-knee bypass.[76] Reversed saphenous vein grafts have an excellent long-term patency rate, with 5-year primary and secondary patency rates of 75% and 80%, respectively, and limb salvage rates of 90%.[77] Polytetrafluoroethylene grafts have similar patency and limb salvage rates above the knee, but success drops significantly below the knee.[75,77,78] In light of this, most surgeons recommend using autologous tissue for the most lower extremity bypass procedures and reserving polytetrafluoroethylene grafts for above-the-knee bypass and bypasses in those patients without adequate autologous options.[79]

An alternative to the reversed saphenous vein graft is using the greater saphenous vein in its in situ position for the anastomosis.[77] In order for this approach to be successful, the competent valves within the vein must be disrupted with a valvulotome to allow for antegrade flow down the vein. This procedure offers several theoretical advantages over the reversed vein graft. First, leaving the vein in situ allows for a better size match for both the proximal and the distal anastomoses. Also, the in situ technique preserves the vasa vasorum and endothelium of the vein graft, although this has never been proven to improve graft patency. Despite these advantages, most studies show that in situ saphenous vein bypass has patency rates equivalent to reversed saphenous vein bypass.[77]

Infrapopliteal Bypass. With advances in surgical techniques, bypasses to the infrapopliteal arteries have become more widely accepted. These procedures are technically difficult and should only be performed when a femoropopliteal bypass is contraindicated. Bypasses can be performed, in order of preference, to the posterior tibial, anterior tibial, and peroneal arteries. The least advantageous bypass is one to the peroneal artery. This bypass procedure should only be performed if the peroneal artery has one or both of its terminal branches in continuity with foot vessels.[80,81]

Operative Technique. The dissection for inflow vessels and graft anastomosis for infrapopliteal bypass are the same as described previously. For the purposes of discussion, we will address each bypass exposure separately. It should be noted that all these bypasses should be performed with autologous tissue, either reversed or in situ saphenous vein graft.[82,83]

Posterior Tibial Artery Exposure. The posterior tibial artery is exposed through an incision similar to the below-the-knee popliteal incision. The crural fascia is divided and the gastrocnemius muscle retracted posteriorly. The soleus muscle must be divided from its tibial origin. The artery is found in the underlying vascular bundle. The more proximal posterior tibial artery is more difficult to isolate. The more distal posterior tibial artery can be found by incising along the posterior margin of the distal tibia and dividing the posterior tibialis muscle. The artery is found just deep to the posterior tibialis muscle. Creating a tunnel for the proximal posterior tibial artery is the same as for the below-knee popliteal bypass. A tunnel for the more distal artery must pass deep to the posterior tibialis muscle.

Anterior Tibial Artery Exposure. The anterior tibial artery is exposed through an anterolateral incision between the tibia and the fibula. The dissection is carried down through the deep fascia. The anterior tibial and extensor digitorum longus muscles are identified and separated to uncover the underlying vascular bundle. The anterior tibial artery should be freed from the adjacent veins and dissected proximally to the interosseous membrane. The interosseous membrane should be opened to allow for passage of the bypass graft. A tunnel can then be created between the popliteal fossa and the anterior tibial artery via blunt dissection. The distal anterior tibial artery is exposed through a similar anterolateral incision placed approximately 6 cm above the lateral malleolus. Tunneling for this more distal bypass requires running the graft deep to the fascial layers. With the more distal bypass, it may be necessary to divide tendons that run in proximity to the graft and may cause compression of the graft. This should be noted at the time of anastomosis and appropriately corrected.

Peroneal Artery Exposure. The peroneal artery is the hardest of the infrapopliteal vessels to isolate and the least appropriate for distal bypass. It should only be used when the anterior and posterior tibial arteries are not adequate for bypass. The proximal peroneal artery can be exposed through the same incision described above for the posterior tibial artery. The artery is located medial to the fibula. Distally, the artery can be more difficult to isolate. A lateral incision is made over the fibula, and dissection is carried down onto the bone. This requires extensive dissection of the fibular muscle attachments to isolate the bone. Using blunt dissection, the medial edge of the fibula is freed with care to avoid the adjacent peroneal vessels. The bone is then divided with a saw. The peroneal vessels are just medial to the fibula, and the artery can thus be isolated and anastomosis performed. A tunnel is created for the graft by blunt dissection medially and superiorly to the popliteal fossa.

Outcomes. Infrapopliteal bypasses have a 5-year primary patency rate of approximately 60%, with limb salvage rates of approximately 70%.[84–86] All patients with distal bypass grafts should have close follow-up and graft surveillance with duplex imaging to diminish complications and graft failure.

Graft Surveillance. For any patient with infrainguinal bypass, graft surveillance has proven to be critical in assuring long-term graft patency. A third of bypass grafts will develop intimal hyperplasia within the first 2 years following bypass.[87,88] In addition, atherosclerotic lesions can develop over time at inflow and outflow points on the graft. These lesions can be easily identified on duplex imaging.[89] Current recommendations are to utilize vein graft surveillance via duplex imaging for all autologous vein grafts. However, no benefit, when compared to cost analysis, has been proven in prosthetic grafts.[90,91]

Autotransplantation of the omentum has been used by some for cases without nonamputation alternatives, including patients with Buerger disease. Although not commonly performed, published reports appear promising for ulcer healing and symptom relief.

● ENDOVASCULAR SURGERY AND CHRONIC LOWER EXTREMITY ISCHEMIA

General Principles

The advent of endovascular surgery has revolutionized the management of chronic lower extremity ischemia. This approach provides a minimally invasive, low-morbidity alternative for the treatment of chronic vascular disease. Other advantages include the following: percutaneous interventions can be repeated if necessary, general anesthesia can often be avoided, and patients may experience less systemic stress with fewer complications than open surgery.[92] In addition, the catheter and stent systems currently in use provide a lower cost alternative to open surgical procedures. Modern endovascular surgery is based on the used of catheters, guidewires, percutaneous transluminal angioplasty balloons (PTA), and stents to treat atherosclerotic lesions. This technology is dependent on contrast arteriography with fluoroscopy. In recent years, the medium of angiography has been improved through digital subtraction arteriography. Digital subtraction arteriography allows for a higher-resolution image, smaller contrast loads, intraoperative road mapping, and image manipulation. Most interventions would not be possible without the use of digital subtraction arteriography.[93]

As technologies advance, new endovascular alternatives are sure to become available. However, there are limitations to the applications of endovascular therapies. Little is known about the long-term results of many cutting-edge interventions because of the ever-changing technologies in the endovascular armamentarium. Also, as endovascular skills have improved, clinicians are beginning to tackle more complex lesions in an attempt to supplant open procedures, but with poorer results. Nevertheless, there is little doubt that endovascular surgery is a valid treatment option and should be offered to select patients.

Patient Selection

Patent selection is a key to endovascular surgery as it is to any procedure. Patients should be evaluated for the severity of their symptoms, the risk of general anesthesia, the risk of limb loss, and the expectation of long-term survival. In general, patients who are medically able to undergo open procedures are also candidates for endovascular therapies. Also, patients whose medical conditions prohibit open procedures may, in fact, be candidates for minimally invasive alternatives. Regardless of the patient, the benefits of the minimally invasive approach must be balanced by the fact that endovascular surgery is often less durable than arterial reconstruction.[92,94]

A thorough history and physical examination must be performed in all patients. Patients should be asked about prior vascular procedures, anticoagulant use, and any history of renal insufficiency or contrast agent allergies. Often, physical examination and patient history are sufficient to determining the extent of lower extremity atherosclerotic disease. Nevertheless, all patients should be evaluated with noninvasive testing prior to endovascular intervention. These tests include lower extremity segmental arterial pressures and duplex ultrasound mapping. Pressure gradients between two arterial segments greater than 20 mm Hg are highly suggestive of arterial stenosis within the segment.[95] While segmental pressures are helpful in patients with single-level disease, this test is limited in patients with multilevel stenotic segments and in patients with medial arterial calcification, which limits arterial compression. Duplex ultrasound mapping can be quite helpful in identifying lesions that may be amenable to endovascular intervention. Duplex mapping localizes diseased segments prior to arteriography, allows for the differentiation of stenotic and occluded segments, and provides a baseline for the severity of ischemia. Arteriography should only be considered once it has been determined that the patient is suitable for operative intervention.[93]

Prior to any endovascular interventions, baseline laboratory data should be obtained in all patients. Patients with a serum creatinine concentration greater than 1.5 should be placed on a renal protection protocol consisting of *N*-acetylcysteine 600 mg orally twice a day for a total of four doses starting 12 prior to the planned procedure and intra-venous hydration with normal saline or a sodium bicarbonate drip both prior to and following the procedure. In patients with chronic renal insufficiency, alternative contrast agents should be used. To prevent bleeding complications, the patient should have an international normalized ratio lower than 1.4 and a platelet count higher than 50 000.[92]

There are several factors that influence the success of endovascular therapies, including location of the lesion, stenosis versus occlusion, lesion length, the pattern of atherosclerotic disease, and runoff status.[6] In general, the larger the caliber of the vessel, the better the long-term patency of PTA with or without stenting. Common iliac artery angioplasty has superior patency rates compared to external iliac artery angioplasty: 65% versus 48% at 4 years.[95,96] Patency rates decline as vessel caliber decreases with 5-year patency rates of only 38% for femoropopliteal artery PTA.[92,97] Stenotic segments are more likely to be amenable to endovascular treatment than occluded segments, with fewer technical failures. Shorter lesions, less than 9 cm, have a greater patency rate than longer lesions.[98] Multisegment disease is an independent risk for endovascular failure.[6] Finally, poor runoff decreases patency rates by more than one-half.[92] In addition, the patient's clinical picture can greatly influence outcomes. Patients with claudication alone typically have better outcomes from endovascular intervention than those patients with limb-threatening ischemia. Also, patients who have failed endovascular surgery with recurrent stenosis are more likely to require an open procedure.[94]

The TASC Working Group classification system is helpful in determining the most appropriate therapeutic intervention. In general, TASC A lesions should be treated with endovascular therapy and TASC D lesions treated with open surgery. Debate continues around TASC B and C lesions and the role of endovascular therapy. As technologies and endovascular skills improve, it is likely that endovascular surgery will supplant open surgery for these more complex lesions.

Basic Lower Extremity Angiography and Interventions

Diagnostic Angiography. For lower extremity angiography, vascular access should be obtained in the CFA contralateral to the affected extremity. The CFA provides an easily accessible target, which is easily compressible and can be used to study and treat most lower extremity arterial diseases. In cases where the CFA cannot be used, the brachial and axillary arteries provide alternative access sites, but at the cost of higher complications.[94]

The patient is positioned for fluoroscopy, and the CFA is palpated just below the inguinal ligament. The CFA typically lies approximately 4 cm lateral to the pubic tubercle over the medial third of the femoral head. The artery should be punctured in the area over the femoral head to allow for compression following the procedure. In patients with a pulseless CFA, fluoroscopy can be used to identify calcifications and bony landmarks to aid in puncture. In addition, ultrasonography can also be useful in identifying the CFA.

Once the CFA has been accessed, a 0.035-in guidewire is passed under fluoroscopic guidance into the CFA and up to the level of the visceral aorta. The needle is then removed and a 4 or 5 French diagnostic sheath is placed over the wire to secure the access site. A 4 or 5 French diagnostic catheter, usually a pigtail multiside hole catheter, is then placed over the wire and positioned at the level of the renal arteries. Aortic films are obtained at this level. The catheter is then brought down to the aortic bifurcation to obtain pelvic images. At this point, the aortic bifurcation is crossed by changing out the diagnostic catheter for a curved catheter and passing a 0.035-in guidewire into the iliac system and positioned in the CFA. The curved catheter is advanced into the external iliac artery. Digital subtraction arteriography should then be employed to evaluate the lower extremity vessels. These images are then used as a "roadmap" for any planned intervention.[93,94]

Iliac Interventions. In general, lesions within the common iliac artery 1 cm or more distal to the aortic bifurcation and lesions within external iliac artery can be treated with unilateral PTA with or without stenting[99] (Figure 35-7). In this setting, a retrograde transfemoral approach is usually most feasible, although crossover techniques can be used for more distal lesions. The previously placed diagnostic sheath should be exchanged for a larger sheath to accommodate the balloon catheter. The dilation balloon is sized to match or slightly exceed the normal vessel diameter. The patient is then given 5000 units of heparin to help prevent thrombosis. Once positioned, the balloon is inflated to a pressure of 6 to 8 atm. This dilatation creates a local dissection within the plaque. Completion angiography

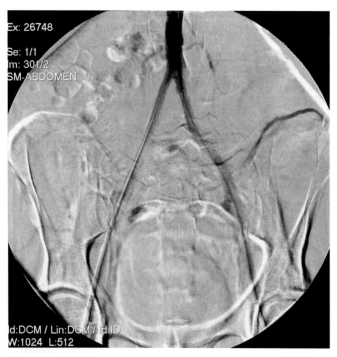

● **FIGURE 35-7.** Percutaneous iliac revascularization: Bilateral Iliac Stenting.

should then be performed. If a stenosis persists, the dissection extends to normal artery, or, in the case of an occluded segment, a stent should be placed according to normal vessel size with up to 10% oversizing. Typically, the choice of stent is based on location of the lesion. For lesions above the inguinal ligament, balloon expandable stents are usually used owing to their greater hoop strength, which resists vessel recoil.[100]

In the case of more proximal iliac lesions, a "kissing" technique should be used to prevent contralateral occlusion. This procedure involves the simultaneous placement of bilateral PTA balloons or stents that traverse the ostia of each common iliac artery. Stents should be placed in parallel to ensure that flow within one stent is not hindered by the other.[94]

Results of iliac artery balloon angioplasty and PTA have been well documented. Becker et al. reported a 5-year patency of 72% for iliac lesions treated with PTA alone, while Tegtemeyer et al. reported a single institution experience with a 5-year patency of 85% for PTA alone.[94,101] Primary patency rates with stenting indicate a 5-year patency rate of up to 80%, with secondary patency rates of up to 90%.[98] In light of these findings, endovascular procedures have assumed a dominant role in the treatment of aortoiliac atherosclerotic disease.

Femoropopliteal Interventions. Advances in endovascular techniques have led clinicians to pursue treatment of femoropopliteal lesions by endovascular means. Unfortunately, the results of endovascular interventions for infrainguinal lesions have been quite disappointing. PTA can be performed in the femoropopliteal vessels with an initial success rate of up to 90%.[102] Nevertheless, primary patency rates drop from around 50% at 1 year to 30% at 5 years.[98] Many factors seem to play a role in the failure of PTA. First, longer lesions tend to fare worse than shorter lesions, usually less than 5 cm. Occlusions have a higher failure rate than stenotic lesions. Patients with limb-threatening ischemia fare worse than those with claudication. Finally, poor outflow seems to adversely affect outcome. The addition of stent placement for these lesions seems to only marginally improve outcome with primary patency rates of 54% to 86% at 1 year and 29% to 48% at 3 years.[102] Recently, ePTFE-covered stents have been used with some success in the superficial femoral and popliteal arteries, with 2-year primary patency rates being reported to reach 87%.[103] The best results of PTA and stenting for SFA lesions appear to be in those patients with TASC A and B lesions, with an overall 6-year patency rate of 52% in them.[6] In light of these findings, much debate has now centered on the appropriate means for endovascular treatment of infrainguinal disease. Some argue that the poor outcomes of PTA and stenting for femoropopliteal disease indicate that it should not be used as a first-line therapy and should only be used in patients who are not candidates for open surgery. At our institution, we tend to favor endovascular therapies as a first-line approach and then move to open surgery once a patient has failed endovascular intervention.

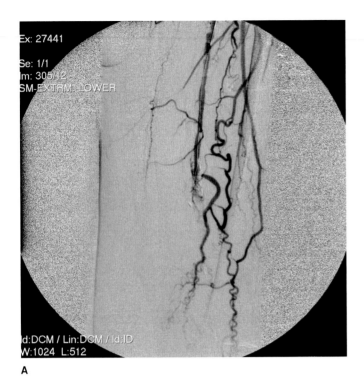 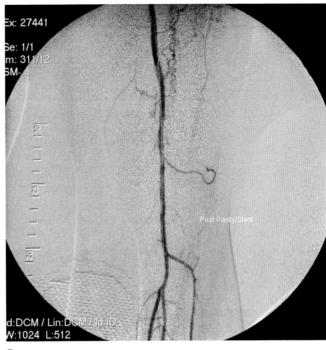

A   **B**

● **FIGURE 35-8.** Percutaneous management of Chronic Total Occlusion: a- Subintimal recanalization b. Successful stenting and revascularization.

Techniques for endovascular interventions for the femoropopliteal arteries are similar to those for the iliac system. As mentioned above, diagnostic images should be obtained through an access site in the contralateral femoral artery. After performing diagnostic angiography, the diagnostic catheter is removed over a wire and the diagnostic sheath is exchanged for a larger stiff sheath, usually 6 Fr, which is curved to allow for crossing over the aortic bifurcation. The tip of the catheter is usually positioned within the external iliac artery. Once the sheath is positioned, a hydrophilic J-tipped 0.035 in glide wire is used, through an end-hole guide catheter, to cross the lesion of interest. For occluded segments, a subintimal plane may have to be created. To do this, the guidewire is pushed forward across the guide catheter near the proximal portion of the lesion, creating a loop deformity in the wire (Figure 35-8A and 35-8B). The wire is advanced until access is gained in the true lumen. In some cases, access into the true lumen can prove difficult, requiring intravascular ultrasound or even reentry devices such as the Outback catheter (LuMend, Redwood City, CA). Once the lesion is crossed, plans are made for intervention. Angioplasty should be performed first, with completion angiogram to determine the need for stent placement. In most cases, self-expanding stents are used below the inguinal ligament because of the ability to cover larger areas with the stent and the innate ability of the stent to withstand deformation.[94]

Tibial Interventions. At the present time, the debate about endovascular interventions for tibial disease remains unsettled. Patients with tibial disease tend to be older with mul-

tiple comorbidities, which increases their risk for complications related to open surgery. In general, the use of endovascular modalities for the tibial vessels is reserved for those patients at high risk of surgery and as a "bailout" procedure to potentially avoid amputation.[104,105] The technique for intervention is the same as for femoropopliteal disease, with the only difference being the need for smaller guidewires, i.e., 0.014-in guidewire. Angioplasty is preferred as the primary treatment owing to the risk for thrombosis with stent placement. Results of endovascular interventions for tibial disease are limited. However, most data would suggest that PTA provides a means of treatment of critical limb ischemia in this patient population, with prolonged time to open intervention or amputation.[106]

Complications in Endovascular Surgery

Hematoma at the access site remains the most common complication of endovascular surgery. Other access site complications include pseudoaneurysm and arteriovenous fistula formation. The incidence of hematoma and other access site-related complications can be reduced by using the smallest acceptable sheath, allowing clotting times to normalize post procedure, and holding manual compression on the site for 30 minutes after the procedure. Although numerous vessel closure devices are available, none of these devices appears to reduce the incidence of access site complications.[107]

Complications arising during an endovascular procedure can be quite challenging and should be understood by the clinician. Complications often encountered are arterial dissections, vessel perforation, vessel thrombosis, and various stent complications.[94]

Arterial dissections, both flow-limiting and non-flow-limiting, are not uncommon following angioplasty. When recognized, the angioplasty balloon should be reinflated over the dissection for 5 to 10 minutes, to allow the dissection to appose to the vessel wall. If this maneuver is unsuccessful, a stent should be placed across the dissection.[108,109]

Vessel perforation can occur with wire manipulation or during angioplasty. Small perforations as a result of wire manipulation can be observed. Large perforations with evidence for extravasation of contrast can be managed either with balloon tamponade or with covered stent placement.[109]

Occasionally, thrombosis will occur within the vessel following angioplasty or stenting. If thrombosis occurs following angioplasty, a stent can usually be placed across the thrombosed segment. However, if this measure fails or if the thrombosis occurs after stent deployment, thrombolysis should be performed. This can be achieved via either rheolytic catheters or infusion of a thrombolytic agent across a catheter. In patients with persistent thrombosis, the thrombolytic catheter may be left for up to 24 hours or consideration can be given to a covered stent placement.[109]

Stent placement provides its own unique set of complications. Stent dislodgement, although rare with modern stent deployment systems, can occur and should be managed by maneuvering the dislodged stent into a safe area with a partially inflated balloon and deployed. It is more likely that stent failure will occur as a result of the stent becoming lodged within a heavily calcified lesion, more commonly with self-expanding stents. In this case, a series of balloons should be used to sequentially deploy the stent.[92]

Newer Interventions

Endovascular surgery is a field that seems to be evolving daily. While this provides for exciting new technologies, it also creates a field with numerous treatment modalities with little long-term data. Nevertheless, it is worthwhile to mention a few modalities that are being used with increased frequency.

Directional atherectomy devices are being used for chronic atherosclerotic lesions. These devices debulk the atherosclerotic plaque to improve flow across the lesion through enlarging the luminal diameter. Several such devices are available on the market; the most commonly used device employs a catheter over a 0.014-in guidewire with a revolving blade at the tip. The catheter shaves the plaque and stores the shavings within the catheter tip. Once the storage device is full, the catheter can be removed, cleaned, and reused. Although initial results appear promising, the multicenter trial for this device is ongoing.[92,110,111]

Cryoplasty balloons are being used in some centers in the place of PTA. These balloons use nitrous oxide to induce a cold thermal injury to the plaque. It is believed that this process creates a controlled dissection and promotes cell death, which, over time, will reduce the inflammatory response to the angioplasty and further reduce the rate of restenosis. At present, this device is only being used for lesions within the SFA. Initial reports for the device appear promising, but long-term results are limited.[92]

● CONCLUSION

Chronic lower extremity ischemia is a widely prevalent disease that is underdiagnosed and presents unique treatment challenges. Patient screening including thorough history and physical examination to address risk factors, signs and symptoms of PAD, and the utilization of noninvasive vascular tests should be a ready part of any primary-care physician's armamentarium. Medical therapy remains a mainstay of treatment, combining risk factor modification, exercise therapy, and limited use of oral agents. When medical therapy fails, many options for endovascular and open surgical revascularization exist, depending on the extent and location of the lesion in question. With proper surgical technique and adequate postoperative surveillance, the morbidity and mortality of surgical therapy can be reduced.

REFERENCES

1. Belkin M, et al. Peripheral arterial occlusive disease. In: Townsend CM, Beuchamp RD, Evers BM, Mattox KL, eds. *Sabiston Textbook of Surgery*. Philadelphia, PA: Elsevier; 2004:1989-2027.

2. Selvin E, Erlinger TP. Prevalence of and risk factors for peripheral arterial disease in the United States: results from the National Health and Nutrition Survey 1999–2000. *Circulation*. 2004;110(6):738-743.

3. Lane JS, Vittinghoff E, Lane KT, Hiramoto JS, Messina LM. Risk factors for premature peripheral vascular disease: results for the National Health and Nutritional Survey, 1999–2002. *J Vasc Surg*. 2006;44(2):319-324.

4. Criqui MH, Fronek A, Barrett-Connor E, Klauber MR, Gabriel S, Goodman D. The prevalence of peripheral arterial disease in a defined population. *Circulation*. 1985;71(3): 510-551.

5. Hiatt WR, Hoag S, Hamman RF. Effect of diagnostic criteria on the prevalence of peripheral arterial disease. The San Luis Valley Diabetes Study. *Circulation*. 1995;91(5):1472-1479.

6. TASC. Management of Peripheral Arterial Disease (PAD). TransAtlantic Inter-Society Consensus (TASC). *J Vasc Surg*. 2000;31:S1-S287.

7. Stein R, Hrljac JL, Gustavson SM, et al. Limitation of the resting ankle-brachial index in symptomatic patients with peripheral arterial disease. *Vasc Med*. 2006;11(1):29-33.

8. Gahtan V. The noninvasive laboratory. *Surg Clin North Am*. 1998;78:507-518.

9. Kullo IJ, Bailey KR, Kardia SL, Mosley TH Jr, et al. Ethnic differences in peripheral arterial disease in the NHLBI Genetic Epidemiology Network of Arteriopathy (GENOA) study. *Vasc Med.* 2003;8(4):237-242.

10. Fowkes FG, Housley E, Cawood EH, Macintyre CC, et al. Edinburgh Artery Study; prevalence of asymptomatic and symptomatic peripheral arterial disease in the general population. *Int J Epidemiol.* 1991;20(2):384-392.

11. Bhatt D, Steg P, Ohman E, et al. International prevalence, recognition, and treatment of cardiovascular risk factors in outpatients with atherothrombosis. *JAMA.* 2006;295:180-189.

12. Muntner P, Wildman RP, Reynolds K, Desalvo KB, et al. Relationship between HbA1c level and peripheral arterial disease. *Diabetes Care.* 2005;26(12):1981-1987.

13. ADA Peripheral arterial disease in people with diabetes. *Diabetes Care.* 2003;26(1):3333-3341.

14. Kannel WB, McGee DL. Update on some epidemiological features of intermittent claudication. *J Am Geriatr Soc.* 1985;33:13-18.

15. Fowkes GR, Housley E, Riemersa RA, et al. Smoking, lipids, glucose intolerance, and blood pressure as risk factors for peripheral atherosclerosis compared with ischemic heart disease in the Edinburgh Artery Study. *Am J Epidemiol.* 1992;135:331-340.

16. Senti M, Nogues X, Pedro-Botet J, et al. Lipoprotein profile in men with peripheral vascular disease. Role of intermediate density lipoproteins and apoprotein E phenotypes. *Circulation.* 1992;85(1):30-36.

17. Taylor LM Jr, Moneta GL, Sexton GJ, Schuff RA, Porter JM. Prospective blinded study of the relationship between plasma homocysteine and progression of symptomatic peripheral arterial disease. *J Vasc Surg.* 1999;29(1):8-19.

18. Johnston KW, et al. Management of chronic ischemia of the lower extremities. In: Rutherford RB, et al., eds. *Vascular Surgery.* 6th ed. Philadelphia, PA: Elsevier; 2005:1077-1269.

19. Schoen FJ. Blood vessels. In: Robbins SL, Cotran RS, et al., eds. *Pathologic Basis of Disease.* Philadelphia, PA: Elsevier; 2005:511-554.

20. Ouriel K, Green RM. In: Schwartz SI, et al., eds. *Principles of Surgery.* 8th ed. New York, NY: McGraw-Hill; 2001:931-1001.

21. Nasir K, Guallar E, et al. Relationship of monocyte count and peripheral arterial disease: results from the National Health and Nutrition Examination Survey 1999–2002. *Arterioscler Thromb Vasc Biol.* 2005;25(9):1966-1971.

22. Hiatt WR, Hoag S, Hamman RF. Effect of diagnostic criteria on the prevalence of peripheral arterial disease. The San Luis Valley Diabetes Study. *Circulation.* 1995;91:1472-1479.

23. Dormandy JA, Murray GD. The fate of the claudicant—a prospective study of 1969 claudicants. *Eur J Vasc Surg.* 1991;5:131-133.

24. O'Riordan DS, O'Donnell JA. Realistic expectations for the patient with claudication. *Br J Surg.* 1991;78:861-863.

25. Criqui MH, Denenberg JO, Bird CE, et al. The correlation between symptoms and non-invasive test results in patients referred for peripheral arterial disease testing. *Vasc Med.* 1996;1:65-71.

26. McDermott MM, Mehta S, Greenland P. Exertional leg symptoms other than intermittent claudication are common in peripheral arterial disease. *Arch Int Med.* 1999;159:387-393.

27. McDermott MM, Fried L, Simonsick E, et al. Asymptomatic peripheral arterial disease is independently associated with impaired lower extremity functioning: the Women's Health and Aging Study. *Circulation.* 2000;101:1007-1012.

28. Newman AB, Naydeck BL, Sutton-Tyrrell K, et al. The role of comorbidity in the assessment of intermittent claudication in older adults. *J Clin Epidemiol.* 2001;54:294-300.

29. Hooi JD, Stoffers HE, Kester AD, et al. Peripheral arterial occlusive disease: prognostic value of signs, symptoms, and the ankle-brachial index. *Med Decis Making.* 2002;22:99-107.

30. Criqui MH. Peripheral arterial disease and subsequent cardiovascular mortality: a strong and consistent association. *Circulation.* 1990;82:2246-2247.

31. Clyne CA, Arch PJ, Carpenter D, et al. Smoking, ignorance, and peripheral vascular disease. *Arch Surg.* 1982;117:1062-1065.

32. Krupski WC, Nguyen HT, Jones DN, et al. Smoking cessation counseling: a missed opportunity for general surgery trainees. *J Vasc Surg.* 2002;36:257-262.

33. Effect of intensive diabetes management on macrovascular events and risk factors in the Diabetes Control and Complications Trial. *Am J Cardiol.* 1995;75:894-903.

34. MRC/BHF Heart Protection Study of cholesterol lowering with simvastatin in 20,536 high risk individuals: a randomized placebo-controlled trial. *Lancet.* 2002;360:7-22.

35. The sixth report of the Joint National Committee on Preventing, Detection, Evaluation, and Treatment of High Blood Pressure. *Arch Intern Med.* 1997;157:2413-2446.

36. Graham IM, Daly LE, Refsum HM, et al. Plasma homocysteine as a risk factor for vascular disease. The European Concerted Action Project. *JAMA.* 1997;277:1775-1781.

37. Nehler MR, Hiatt WR. Exercise therapy for claudication. *Ann Vasc Surg.* 1999;13:109-114.

38. Dawson DL, Cutler BS, Hiatt WR, et al. A comparison of colostazol and pentoxifylline for treating intermittent claudication. *Am J Med.* 2000;109:523-530.

39. Lechat P, Priollet P. Prevention of major ischemic events in lower limb arterial disease: does aspirin play a role? *J Mal Vasc.* 2006;31(3):129-134.

40. Clagett P, Sobel M, Jackson M, et al. Antithrombotic therapy in peripheral arterial disease: the Seventh ACCP Conference on Antithrombotic and Thrombolytic Therapy. *Chest.* 2004;126:S609-S626.

41. CAPRIE. A randomized, blinded, trial of clopidogrel versus aspirin in patients at risk of ischemic events (CAPRIE). CAPRIE Steering Committee. *Lancet.* 1996;348(9038):1329-1339.

42. Marston WA, Davies SW, et al. Natural history of limbs with arterial insufficiency and chronic ulceration treated without revascularization. *J Vasc Surg.* 2006;44(1):108-114.

43. DeBakey ME, Lawrie GM, Glaeser DH. Patterns of atherosclerosis and their surgical significance. *Ann Surg.* 1985;201:115.

44. Veith FJ, Gupta SK, et al. Six-year prospective multicenter randomized comparison of autologous saphenous vein and expanded polytetraflouroethylene grafts in infrainguinal arterial reconstructions. *J Vasc Surg.* 1986;3:104-114.

45. McFarland RJ, et al. Improved technique for polytetrafluoroethylene bypass grafting: long-term results using anastamotic vein patches. *Br J Surg.* 1982;79(4):348-354.

46. Brewster DC. Clinical and anatomical considerations for surgery in aortoiliac disease and results of surgical treatment. *Circulation.* 1991;83(suppl 1):I42.

47. Mozersky DJ, Sumner DS, et al. Long-term results of reconstructive aortoiliac surgery. *Am J Surg.* 1972;123:503.

48. Malone JM, Moore WS, Goldstone J. Life expectancy following aortofemoral arterial grafting. *Surgery.* 1977;81:551.

49. Inahara T. Evaluation of endarterectomy for aortoiliac and aortoiliac femoral occlusive disease. *Arch Surg.* 1975;110:1458.

50. Van der Akker PJ, van Schilfaarde R. Long term results of prosthetic and non-prosthetic reconstruction for obstructive aorto-iliac disease. *Eur J Vasc Surg.* 1992;6:53.

51. Bernhard VM, Ray LI, Militello JP. The role of angioplasty of the profunda femoris artery in revascularization of the ischemic limb. *Surg Gynecol Obstet.* 1976;142:840.

52. Malone JM, Goldstone J, Moore WS. Autogenous profundaplasty: The key to long-term patency in secondary repair of aortofemoral graft occlusion. *Ann Surg.* 1978;188:817.

53. Dunn DA, Downs AR, et al. Aortoiliac reconstruction for occlusive disease: comparison of end-to-end and end-to-side proximal anastamoses. *Can J Surg.* 1982;25:382.

54. Nash T. Aortoiliac occlusive vascular disease: a prospective study of patients treated by endarterectomy and bypass procedures. *Aust N Z J Surg.* 1979;49:223.

55. de Vries SO, Hunink MG. Results of aortic bifurcation grafts for aortoiliac occlusive disease: a meta-analysis. *J Vasc Surg.* 1997;26:558.

56. Brewster DC. Complications of aortic and lower extremity procedures. In: Strandness DE Jr, van Breda A, eds. *Vascular Diseases: Surgical and Interventional Therapy.* New York, NY: Churchill Livingstone; 1994:1151-1177.

57. Diehl JT, Cali RJ, Hertzer NR, et al. Complications of abdominal aortic reconstruction: an analysis of perioperative risk factors in 557 patients. *Ann Surg.* 1983;197:50.

58. Ernst CB. Prevention of intestinal ischemia following abdominal aortic reconstruction. *Surgery.* 1983;92:102.

59. Brewster DC, Meier GH, Darling RC, et al. Reoperation for aortofemoral graft limb occlusion: optimal methods and long term results. *J Vasc Surg.* 1987;5:363.

60. Nevelsteen A, et al. Graft occlusion following aortofemoral Dacron bypass. *Ann Vasc Surg.* 1991;5:32.

61. Brewster DC. Aortic graft limb occlusion. In: Ernst CB, Stanley JC, eds. *Current Therapy in Vascular Surgery.* 3rd ed. St Louis, MO: Mosby-Year Book; 1995:419-426.

62. Dick LS, Brief DK, et al. A twelve year experience with femorofemoral crossover grafts. *Arch Surg.* 1980;115:1359.

63. Flanigan DP, Schuler JJ, Keifer T, et al. Elimination of iatrogenic impotence and improvement of sexual function after aortoiliac revascularization. *Arch Surg.* 1982;117:544.

64. DePalma RG, Levine SB, Feldman S. Preservation of erectile function after aortoiliac reconstruction. *Arch Surg.* 1978;113:958.

65. Queral LA, Whitehouse WM Jr, Flinn WR, et al. Pelvic hemodynamics after aortoiliac reconstruction. *Surgery.* 1979;86:799.

66. Moore WS, Cole CW. Infection in prosthetic vascular grafts. In: Moore WS, ed. *Vascular Surgery: A Comprehensive Review.* 3rd ed. Philadelphia, PA: WB Saunders; 1991:598-609.

67. Bandyk DF. Aortic graft infection. *Semin Vasc Surg.* 1990;3:122.

68. O'Hara PJ, Hertzer NR, Beven EG, et al. Surgical management of infected abdominal aortic grafts: review of a 25-year experience. *J Vasc Surg.* 1986;3:725.

69. Passman MA, Taylor LM, Moneta GL, et al. Comparison of axillofemoral and aortofemoral bypass for aortoiliac occlusive disease. *J Vasc Surg.* 1996;23:263.

70. Martin D, Katz SG. Axillofemoral bypass for aortoiliac occlusive disease. *Am J Surg.* 2000;180:100.

71. Criado E, Burnham SJ, Tinsley EA Jr, et al. Femorofemoral bypass graft: analysis of patency and factors influencing long-term outcome. *J Vasc Surg.* 1993;18:495.

72. Langsfeld M, Nupute J, Hershey FB, et al. The use of deep duplex scanning to predict hemodynamically significant aortoiliac stenosis. *J Vasc Surg.* 1988;7:395.

73. Ascher E, Mazzariol F, Hingorani A, et al. The use of duplex ultrasound arterial mapping as an alternative to conventional arteriography for primary and secondary infrapopliteal bypasses. *Am J Surg.* 1999;178:162.

74. Veith FJ, Gupta SK, Samson RH, et al. Progress in limb salvage by reconstructive arterial surgery combined with new or improved adjunctive procedures. *Ann Surg.* 1980;194:386.

75. Veith FJ, Gupta SK, Samson RH, et al. Superficial femoral and popliteal arteries as inflow site for distal bypasses. *Surgery.* 1981;90:980.

76. Kram HB, Gupta SK, Veith FJ, et al. Late results of two hundred seventeen femoropopliteal bypasses to isolated popliteal artery segments. *J Vasc Surg.* 1991;14:386.

77. Wengerter KR, Veith FJ, Gupta SK, et al. Prospective randomized multi center comparison of in situ and reversed vein infrapopliteal bypasses. *J Vasc Surg.* 1991;13:189.

78. Rosenbloom JS, Walsh JJ, Schuler JJ, et al. Long-term results of infragenicular bypasses with autogenous vein originating from the distal superficial femoral and popliteal arteries. *J Vasc Surg.* 1988;7:691.

79. Veith FJ, Gupta SK, Daly V. Femoropopliteal bypass to the isolated popliteal segment: is polytetrafluoroethylene graft acceptable? *Surgery.* 1981;89:296.

80. Ascer E, Veith FJV, Gupta SK. Bypasses to plantar arteries and other tibial branches: an extended approach to limb salvage. *J Vasc Surg.* 1988;8:434.

81. Andros G. Bypass grafts to the ankle and foot: a personal perspective. *Surg Clin North Am.* 1995;75:715.

82. Lyon RT, Veith FJ, Marsan BU, et al. Eleven-year experience with tibiotibial bypass: an unusual but effective solution to distal tibial artery occlusive disease and limited autologous vein. *J Vasc Surg.* 1994;17:1128.

83. Schneider JR, Walsh DB, McDaniel MD, et al. Pedal bypass versus tibial bypass with autogenous vein: a comparison of outcome and hemodynamic results. *J Vasc Surg.* 1993; 17:1029.

84. Biancari F, Alback A, Kantonen I, et al. Predictive factors for adverse outcome of pedal bypasses. *Eur J Vasc Endovasc Surg.* 1999;18:138.

85. Kram HB, Gupta SK, Veith FJ, et al. Late results of two hundred seventeen femoropopliteal bypasses to isolated popliteal artery segments. *J Vasc Surg.* 1991;14:386.

86. Wengerter KR, Yang PM, Veith FJ, et al. A twelve-year experience with the popliteal-to-distal artery bypass: the significance and management of proximal disease. *J Vasc Surg.* 1992;15:143.

87. Szilagyi DE, Elliot J, Hageman JH, et al. Biologic fate of autogenous vein implants as arterial substitutes: clinical, angiographic, and histo-pathological observations in femoro-popliteal operations for atherosclerosis. *Ann Surg.* 1973;178:232-246.

88. Mills JL. Mechanisms of vein graft failure: the location, distribution, and characteristics of lesions that predispose to graft failure. *Semin Vasc Surg.* 1993;6:78-91.

89. Mills JL, Wixon CL, James DC, et al. The natural history of intermediate and critical vein graft stenosis: recommendations for continued surveillance or repair. *J Vasc Surg.* 2001;33:273-280.

90. Dunlop P, Sayers RD, Naylor AR, et al. The effect of a surveillance program on the patency of synthetic infrainguinal bypass grafts. *Eur J Vasc Endovasc Surg.* 1996;11:441-445.

91. Lalak NJ, Hanel KC, Hunt J, Morgan A. Duplex scan surveillance of infrainguinal prosthetic bypass grafts. *J Vasc Surg.* 1994;20:637-641.

92. Moore WS, Ahn SS. *Endovascular Surgery.* 3rd ed. Philadelphia, PA: WB Saunders 2001.

93. Loewe C, Schoder M, Rand T, et al. Peripheral vascular occlusive disease: evaluation with contrast-enhanced moving-bed MR angiography versus digital subtraction angiography in 106 patients. *AJR Am J Roentgenol.* 2002;179:1013.

94. Valji K. *Vascular and Interventional Radiology.* Philadelphia, PA: WB Saunders 1999.

95. Gray BH, Sullivan TM. Aortoiliac occlusive disease: surgical versus interventional therapy. *Curr Interv Cardiol Rep.* 2001;3:109.

96. TASC Working Group Management of peripheral arterial disease (PAD). Transatlantic Inter-Society Consensus (TASC). *Eur J Vasc Endovasc Surg.* 2000;19:S1.

97. Murphy TP, Khwaja AA, Webb MS. Aortoiliac stent placement in patients treated for intermittent claudication. *J Vasc Interv Radiol.* 1998;9:421.

98. Back MR, Novotney M, Roth SM, et al. Utility of duplex surveillance following iliac artery angioplasty and primary stenting. *J Endovasc Ther.* 2001;8:629.

99. Karch LA, Mattos MA, Henretta JP, et al. Clinical failure after percutaneous transluminal angioplasty of the SFA and popliteal arteries. *J Vasc Surg.* 2000;31: 880.

100. Hood DB, Hodgson KJ. Percutaneous transluminal angioplasty and stenting for iliac artery occlusive disease. *Surg Clin North Am.* 1999;79:575.

101. Henry M, Clonaris C, Amor M, et al. Which stent for which lesion in peripheral interventions? *Texas Heart Inst J.* 2000;27:119.

102. Becker GJ, Palmaz JC, Rees CR, et al. Angioplasty-induced dissections in human iliac arteries: management with Palmaz balloon expandable intraluminal stents. *Curr Opin Radiol.* 1992;176:31-38.

103. Davies MG, Waldman DL, Pearson TA. Comprehensive endovascular therapy for femoropopliteal arterial atherosclerotic occlusive disease. *J Am Coll Surg.* 2005;201:275.

104. Vroegindeweij D, Vos LD, Buth J, et al. Balloon angioplasty combined with primary stenting versus balloon angioplasty alone in femoropopliteal obstructions: a comparative randomized study. *Cardiovasc Intervent Radiol.* 1997;20: 420.

105. Schwarten DE. Clinical and anatomical considerations for nonoperative therapy in tibial disease and the results of angioplasty. *Circulation.* 1991;83(suppl I):86.

106. Saab MH, Smith DC, et al. Percutaneous transluminal angioplasty of the tibial arteries for limb salvage. *Cardiovasc Intervent Radiol.* 1992;15:211-216.

107. Buckingham TM, Loh A, Dormandy JA, et al. Infrapopliteal angioplasty for limb salvage. *Eur J Vasc Surg.* 1993;7: 21-25.

108. Pentecost MJ, Criqui MH, Dorros G, et al. Guidelines for peripheral percutaneous transluminal angioplasty of the abdominal aorta and lower extremity vessels. *Circulation.* 1994;89:511-531.

109. Fransson SG, Nylander E. Vascular injury following catheterization, coronary angiography, and coronary angioplasty. *Eur Heart J.* 1994;15:232-235.

110. Baltacioglu F, Cimsit NC, Cil B, et al. Endovascular stent graft applications in iatrogenic vascular injuries. *Cardiovasc Intervent Radiol.* 2003;26:434-439.

111. Zeller T, Rastan A, Schwarzwalder U, et al. Percutaneous peripheral atherectomy of femoropopliteal stenosis using a new-generation device: six-month results from a single-center experience. *J Endovasc Ther.* 2004;11: 676.

chapter 36

Acute Limb Ischemia

Brian Reed, MD / *Mitchell H. Goldman, MD*

● ACUTE LIMB ISCHEMIA

Acute arterial occlusion is one of the most devastating diseases in vascular surgery, resulting in limb loss, long-term morbidity, and death. Early recognition of symptoms of limb ischemia is necessary in order to salvage limb function and prevent an increased risk of mortality. Patients with acute limb ischemia often present soon after the onset of symptoms and are able to describe the exact moment symptoms began. This process should be differentiated from chronic limb ischemia, which occurs over a prolonged period of time with progression of symptoms. Severity of symptoms is dependent on the amount of arterial collateralization around the site of occlusion which can often reflect underlying chronic vascular disease.

The aim of this chapter is to discuss the diagnosis, etiology, pathophysiology, and treatment of patients with acute limb ischemia.

Pathophysiology

Acute arterial ischemia occurs as a result of embolization, thrombosis, trauma, or vasculitis (Figures 36-1 and 36-2). A central source can be found in the vast majority of patients with macroembolic disease (Table 36-1). These patients are likely to have atrial arrhythmias or recent myocardial infarction. The presentation of embolization is sometimes difficult to distinguish from thrombosis. Patients with arterial emboli typically have a discrete onset of symptoms, have a history of or are at risk of emboli, have no history of claudication, and have preserved flow in the contralateral extremity. In contrast, patients with arterial thrombosis are more likely to have preexisting vascular disease and a history of claudication and physical findings of disseminated disease or previous extremity bypass (Table 36-2).

Factors affecting the clinical outcome of embolic disease include the size of the affected vessel, the amount of collateral flow, and the degree of obstruction. In patients with underlying atherosclerotic vascular disease, an embolus may have little clinical significance because of preexisting collaterals. However, embolization to a healthy artery will create significant ischemia because of lack of collateralization. Once embolization occurs, events that follow must be abrogated to prevent irreversible ischemia. Clot propagation occurs once emboli lodge within the affected vessel and an environment of stasis develops allowing further clot formation and propagation. Limb ischemia may be made worse by distal migration of clot fragments and debris. Venous thrombosis may occur because of the low flow state created by the embolus and resultant ischemia. This phenomenon is clinically significant in that it may make revascularization more difficult, increase the patient's risk for pulmonary emboli, and may result in compartment syndrome after revascularization.

Regardless of the causes, the ischemia resulting from arterial occlusion follows a relatively similar course. The extremities are more resistant to ischemia than other tissues and can tolerate up to 5 to 6 hours of ischemia depending on the amount of collateralization. Each of the tissues within the extremity has different vulnerabilities. Nerves are the most sensitive, resulting in paresthesia as an early sign of ischemia, while skin and bone are the most resistant. Paresis and paralysis represent severe and limb-threatening ischemia. Skeletal muscle comprises the largest and most metabolically active constituent of the lower extremity. As such, skeletal muscle plays a significant role in the morbidity and mortality of acute limb ischemia and resulting reperfusion injury. The lactic acidosis, hyperkalemia, and myoglobulinuria, which occurs when ischemic muscle is reperfused, can result in systemic dysfunction and renal failure.

Cellular membrane function is impaired by severe ischemia from direct membrane damage as well as damage to the membrane transport proteins, including adenosine triphosphatase (ATPase). This results in a loss of normal

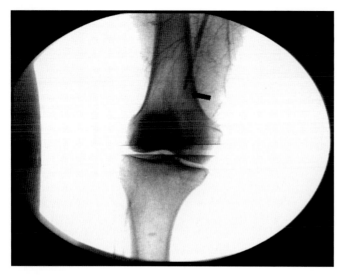

● FIGURE 36-1. Embolus to the popliteal artery in a patient with atrial fibrillation (arrow).

TABLE 36-1. Sources of Peripheral Embolization

Cardiac (80%–90%)
    Atrial fibrillation
    Valvular heart disease
    Myocardial infarction
    Endocarditis
    Ventricular aneurysm
Noncardiac
    Aneurysmal disease
    Proximal artery
    Paradoxic embolus

cellular barriers and transport with resulting intracellular edema. Interstitial edema occurs secondary to increased basement membrane permeability to ions and proteins. The amount of interstitial edema depends on the length of ischemia; as length of ischemia increases, interstitial edema increases, especially in patients without adequate collateralization. The effects of interstitial edema are most evident in fascial compartments after revascularization. As interstitial edema increases, compartment pressures increase beyond capillary perfusion pressures, usually around 30 mm Hg and compartment syndrome develops. In the setting of compartment syndrome, fasciotomy must be performed in addition to revascularization to allow for adequate tissue perfusion.

As ischemia develops, the sarcolemma plasma membrane becomes disrupted, resulting in intracellular swelling. Once flow is reestablished, the damaged sarcolemma membrane cannot maintain a normal cellular barrier. Intracellu-

lar ions, proteins, and enzymes are released into the circulation, resulting in the myonephropathic or reperfusion syndrome. Myoglobin, once released systemically, is cleared by the kidney. As myoglobin casts deposit in the renal tubules, acute renal failure may ensue. Myoglobin and creatinine phosphokinase levels can be elevated for up to 4 days following reperfusion. Also, hyperkalemia, from release of intracellular potassium stores, can cause myocardial depression and dysrhythmias.

In addition to systemic effects of ischemia and reperfusion, there are numerous events that occur at the tissue level, which are incompletely understood. As ischemia develops, cellular oxygen delivery becomes hampered, normal cellular ionization becomes disrupted, and cellular membrane permeability increases, as described above. With reperfusion, injury can continue to occur at the cellular level, despite adequate oxygen delivery. As oxygen delivery returns to the tissues, neutrophils within damaged tissue take up oxygen, converting the molecule via univalent reduction into free radical species, including superoxide radicals, hydrogen peroxide, and hydroxyl radicals. Free radicals are typically generated through an nicotinamide adenine dinucleotide phosphate (NADPH) oxidase enzyme located on the cellular membranes of neutrophils. Once formed, these compounds are highly unstable, usually overwhelm the body's natural scavenging system, and begin to attack the phospholipid cellular membrane, primarily through reduction of fatty acids, resulting in continued cellular damage.[1]

Diagnosis

In light of the potentially life-threatening effects of untreated ischemia, early diagnosis of acute limb ischemia is important. The diagnosis of acute limb ischemia is usually a clinical one, made by history and physical examination. It is important when obtaining the history of extremity pain to include duration of symptoms, intensity, and location. In general, patients with acute arterial occlusion from embolic sources present soon after onset of symptoms with complaints of severe lower extremity pain and can document a discrete onset. The past history should include prior

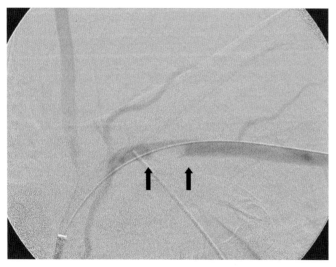

● FIGURE 36-2. Intimal injury of the subclavian artery from blunt trauma as the source of distal emboli.

TABLE 36-2. Distinguishing Embolic Disease from Thrombosis

	Embolism	*Thrombosis*
Timeline	Acute, discrete onset	Usually develops over a period of days
Claudication and PVD	Rarely	Frequently
Physical examination findings	Preserved contralateral pulses	Evidence of peripheral, vascular disease bilaterally
Angiographic findings	Meniscus sign, paucity of collateralization	Diffuse atherosclerotic changes; collateral flow around occlusion

vascular surgeries, cardiac history (myocardial infarction or arrhythmias), history of claudication, history of coagulation disorders, and known aortic aneurysms. Risk factors for atherosclerotic disease should be ascertained as well, including diabetes, hypertension, hyperlipidemia, and smoking history.

Physical examination can often localize the point of arterial occlusion. The classic mnemonic for arterial occlusion is the "six Ps": pain, pulselessness, pallor, paralysis, paresthesia, and poikilothermia. The affected limb, as well as contralateral extremity, should be examined for pulses. The affected extremity may be pale and cool. Patients complain of a constant pain or pain with simple passive movement. As ischemia progresses, the patient may develop numbness or neuromuscular dysfunction, foot drop, indicating damage to nerves and muscles. As a rule, patients with "two Ps," paralysis and paresthesia, require immediate intervention to prevent limb loss.

The Rutherford classification system has been developed to define the extent of ischemia.[2,3] The system is divided into three classes:

- Class 1: a viable extremity that has no ischemic pain and no neurologic deficits, is with clearly audible Doppler flow, and does not require intervention.
- Class 2a: limbs that are threatened to have mild neurologic deficits and ischemic pain with no clear Doppler flow but do not require immediate intervention.
- Class 2b: limbs that are threatened and require immediate intervention.
- Class 3: limbs with irreversible ischemia, profound motor and sensory loss, absent capillary flow, and skin marbling; these limbs are not salvageable.

Distal embolization can be difficult to distinguish from in situ thrombosis, particularly in the setting of underlying vascular disease. Patients presenting with limb ischemia who do not have paralysis or paresthesia may, as time allows, undergo echocardiography, electrocardiography, cardiac assays, and thrombophilia workup to evaluate for possible embolic sources. Imaging modalities have been developed and refined to help determine the cause of acute limb ischemia.

The standard for identifying arterial occlusion remains contrast arteriography. It allows for accurate diagnosis and operative planning. Angiography can help differentiate an embolus from in situ thrombosis. On arteriogram, emboli appear as a filling defect with a meniscus sign in an otherwise normal vessel. In addition, patients with embolization typically have sparse collateral flow without the presence of other arterial disease. Finally, a vessel with multiple filling defects should raise the suspicion of embolization. In acute in situ thrombosis, patients will typically have multilevel atheromatous changes and diffuse collaterals. From a therapeutic standpoint, arteriography offers an opportunity for thrombolytic therapy and endovascular approaches for treating ischemia. However, arteriography is not without risks, including contrast nephrotoxicity, and antiphylaxis and should be reserved for patients for whom a surgical intervention is planned.

Noninvasive modalities as an alternative to arteriography include duplex ultrasound, Magnetic resonance (MR) angiography, and computed tomography (CT) scan angiography. Duplex ultrasound has been shown to be quite useful in evaluating the patency of bypass grafts and single arterial segments, but it has not proven as effective as arteriography in planning for operative intervention. MR angiography is gaining popularity in some centers, as its sensitivity and specificity are greater than duplex ultrasonography and the risks of contrast nephropathy are significantly reduced through the use of gadolinium as a contrast agent. MR is useful for identifying possible bypass targets in the distal extremity. CT scan angiography with 3D reconstruction has also become a popular noninvasive imaging modality, with sensitivity and specificity rivaling MR angiography. It is associated with a large contrast load.[4] Despite imaging advances, for those patients in whom therapeutic interventions are planned, or in patients when the delay of intervention may have adverse consequences, contrast arteriography remains the standard of care.

Whenever embolic or thrombotic events occur, thrombophilia must be considered as an etiology, or at least a contributing factor (Table 36-3). Up to 15% of the population may have an acquired or genetic propensity to clot. In addition to the disorders listed in the table, in patients who have been previously treated for cardiovascular disease, new onset of embolic or thrombotic events may be a harbinger of heparin-associated antibodies or thrombosis. Thrombolytic disorders should be considered and treated in conjunction with relieving the ischemia presented. Antithrombin III deficiency should be suspected in patients who require large doses of heparin. In general, a family history of

TABLE 36-3. Routine Tests for Hypercoagulable State
• Antithrombin III
• Protein C and protein S
• Factor V Leiden mutation
• Prothrombin gene mutation 20210A
• PAI inhibitor
• MT HFR
• Fibrinogen
• ANA
• Antiphospholipid antibodies
• Platelet count
• Factor VIII
• Factor VII

PAI, plasminogen activator inhibitor; MTHFR, 5,10-methylene-tetrahydrofolate reductase; ANA, antinuclear antibody.

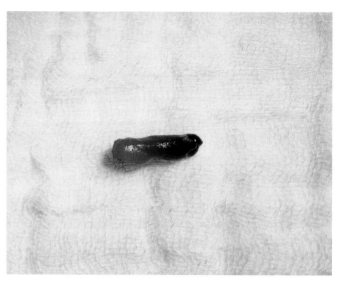

● **FIGURE 36-3.** Arterial embolism with organized fibrous portion.

thrombotic events can raise a suspicion for hereditary genetic disorders.

● ARTERIAL THROMBOEMBOLISM

Arterial thromboembolism has long been a problematic disease in vascular surgery. Prior to the existence of catheter-based interventions and synthetic grafts, removing embolic material was difficult. The landmark introduction of the Fogarty catheter, a balloon embolectomy device, allowed for easy arterial access and retrieval of embolic material without significant damage to the native vessel. Since that time many changes have occurred in the treatment of acute arterial thromboembolism. The introduction of thrombolytic agents and newer minimally invasive techniques has significantly changed the field of vascular surgery. Despite these advances, mortality rates from acute peripheral arterial occlusion have changed only slightly, averaging 10% to 25%.[5] Medical comorbidities and concurrent chronic vascular disease have kept the morbidity and mortality constant, even in light of technological advances. Part of the difficulty in the treatment of peripheral thromboembolism is the change in etiology from previous decades. Prior to the advent of antibiotics, rheumatic heart disease, and peripheral embolization from mitral valve vegetations were the most common causes for thromboembolic phenomena. Today a plethora of etiologies exist, including atherosclerotic heart and vascular disease, dysrhythmias, and iatrogenic catheter manipulation.[6]

Arterial emboli are classified on the basis of size, origin, and content. This classification allows for a uniform treatment and understanding of the natural history of embolic phenomena. For the purposes of discussion, we will divide emboli into macro- and microemboli. These are clearly two separate entities with different clinical presentations and treatment options.

Macroemboli

Macroemboli most commonly occur as a result of valvular plaques or mural thrombus breaking off and causing large vessel occlusion (Figure 36-3). Although etiologies have shifted over time, the heart is the source for acute arterial embolization in greater than 80% of cases. In past decades, rheumatic heart disease with mitral valvular vegetations was the most common source for emboli. Today, rheumatic heart disease accounts for only 5% of cases of acute vessel occlusion. Atrial fibrillation and myocardial infarction have surpassed rheumatic valvular disease, accounting for almost 90% of cardiac sources. Clot embolizing from atrial fibrillation typically forms in the left atrium as a result of stasis. This location has made diagnosis extremely difficult. Transthoracic echocardiography has been disappointing in accurate visualization of atrial thrombus. Even transesophageal echocardiography, although more sensitive, cannot thoroughly rule out atrial thrombus. Nevertheless, all patients with acute thromboembolism should undergo electrocardiogram, 24-hour arrhythmia monitoring, and echocardiogram to evaluate for cardiogenic sources for embolization.

Myocardial infarction has been associated with an increasing number of cases of peripheral arterial embolization and is second to atrial fibrillation as a cardiac source. Although less than 5% embolize, left ventricular thrombus formation is a common finding in anterior transmural myocardial infarction.[7] In this patient population, symptoms of limb ischemia typically develop 2 to 4 weeks following myocardial infarction, although silent myocardial infarction presenting with limb ischemia from embolization is not uncommon. Therefore, any patient suspected of acute limb ischemia should have cardiac enzyme assays drawn as well as electrocardiography. Mortality rates are significantly higher in this patient population because of the risk of intervention in the presence of acute myocardial injury.

While rheumatic valvular disease may be on the decline, valvular replacement procedures and prosthetic valvular devices have become common practice and are a common source of emboli. Prosthetic valves are more thrombogenic than biosynthetic valves, owing to their mechanics, where thrombus formation is common at low flow sites and mechanical hinges. To prevent embolic complications, these patients should be on chronic anticoagulation therapy.

Rarer causes of cardiac embolization, such as intracardiac tumors and myxomas, should be suspected if emboli retrieved at surgery have an unusual appearance. All specimens should be sent for pathologic evaluation for accurate diagnosis. Another rare cause for embolization is septic emboli from endocarditis. Intravenous drug use has increased greatly in recent decades and with it rates of endocarditis. These emboli usually lodge in smaller vessels and result in septic complications. This diagnosis should be suspected in younger patients with no underlying cardiac history. Pathologic evaluation of the clot is often diagnostic.

Noncardiogenic emboli are much rarer, but no less significant. These are largely from atherosclerotic lesions from proximal vessels. In this scenario, mural erosion from atherosclerotic plaque embolizes to smaller vessels. The source of embolization is broad and can range from thoracic, aortoiliac, femoral, or popliteal sources. Aneurysms of the abdominal aorta, iliac, and popliteal arteries should be considered as possible sources. Aneurysmal changes can be evaluated by CT scan, MRI, or ultrasound. In addition, upper extremity emboli can result from diseased arterial walls as a consequence of longstanding thoracic outlet syndrome and aneurysmal degeneration. These emboli present in a similar fashion to their cardiac counterparts. All patients with acute limb ischemia should be evaluated for possible arterial sources by evaluating for bruits and obtaining a history of underlying vascular disease.

Rarely, arterial emboli can result from venous sources through a patent foramen ovale of the heart.[8] This process, known as paradoxic embolization, should be suspected in patients with concurrent deep venous thrombosis or pulmonary emboli. In the presence of a cardiac murmur, evaluation of the legs by duplex scanning is appropriate.

In less than 10% of cases, a source for embolization cannot be identified. This process is known as cryptogenic emboli. This diagnosis should only be reached after a thorough history and physical examination and after all diagnostic testing fails to identify a source for peripheral embolism. These patients are often anticoagulated because the suspicion is that the embolus is cardiac in origin.

Sites of Embolization

Although the axial limbs are the most common site of peripheral embolization, the effects of cerebral and visceral embolization should not be underestimated. The lower extremity is affected in 75% of cases. Owing to changing diameters, emboli typically lodge at branch points in vessels. The most common site of lower extremity embolization is the femoral bifurcation, with the popliteal artery being the second most common. These numbers have changed little in recent years, although patients are much more likely to have underlying peripheral vascular disease. This fact makes diagnosis of embolization more difficult, particularly when emboli lodge within atherosclerotic lesions at or away from arterial bifurcations. With the increasing incidence of aortoiliac atherosclerotic disease, aortoiliac emboli are becoming more common. In a healthy vessel, most emboli are too small to lodge within the aorta or iliac vessels. With vessel narrowing from atherosclerotic plaques, emboli can lodge within these larger vessels. The upper extremities are affected in 10% of cases, with emboli lodging typically at the brachial artery bifurcation.

Treatment (Figure 36-4)

Early intervention is the key to limb salvage in patients with acute limb ischemia. Systemic anticoagulation should

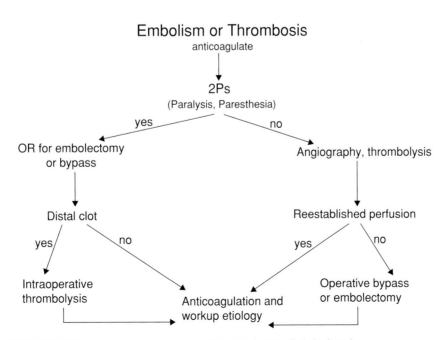

● **FIGURE 36-4.** Algorithm for the treatment of acute limb ischemia.

be instituted immediately upon making the diagnosis. This is accomplished through a bolus of unfractionated heparin with a maintenance infusion of heparin to maintain a therapeutic partial thromboplastin time (pTT). Not only anticoagulation is effective at decreasing propagation, but it also prevents ongoing embolization. Often, heparin improves perfusion such that time is gained to pursue diagnostic testing. In most circumstances, treatment of the threatened limb should supersede investigations as to the underlying cause for ischemia. However, patients with suspected embolization should ultimately undergo a cardiac evaluation to search for a central source for embolization.

Therapeutic options for acute limb ischemia are based around the Rutherford criteria and the patients' overall medical status. Patients who do not have limb-threatening ischemia (Rutherford class 1 and 2A) are candidates for anticoagulation alone, with plans for revascularization as an elective procedure. In patients with class 2B ischemia, contrast arteriography should be obtained as urgently as possible, as they will require some form of early intervention. After angiographic images are obtained, there are two basic treatment modalities: percutaneous or open surgical revascularization. Percutaneous intervention can be performed at the time of angiography.

Traditionally, open surgical repair was universally accepted as the treatment of choice for acute limb ischemia. Open repair is performed either as a balloon catheter thromboembolectomy for embolic disease or as a bypass graft for atherosclerotic occlusion. Angioplasty and stenting may be performed if, after thrombectomy is completed, a stenosis is seen on completion angiography. Open surgical procedures are not without significant risk of morbidity and mortality. Historically, mortality rates for open surgical interventions were as high as 30%, with most individuals succumbing to myocardial infarction, cardiac arrhythmias, or pneumonia. Most centers now quote perioperative mortality rates between 10% and 20%.

In an attempt to decrease mortality rates related to limb ischemia, thrombolytic therapy was developed as an alternative to open surgical procedures. Fibrinolytic drugs help dissolve clot via stimulated conversion of plasminogen to plasmin. The most commonly used agents have been tissue plasminogen activator (tPA) and urokinase, although urokinase is currently not available in the United States. Attempts have been made to use these drugs both regionally and systemically in acute embolic events as well as acute venous thrombosis. Regional administration of thrombolytics is preferred over systemic administration because of the lower risk of bleeding complications. Thrombolysis is achieved via an angiographically placed catheter just proximal to or within the clot. A bolus of thrombolytic is infused followed by a maintenance dose until the clot has cleared. Systemic anticoagulation with unfractionated heparin is administered throughout thrombolytic therapy to prevent the risk for new thrombus formation near or around the infusion catheter. Many patients require 48 hours of infusion time and should be monitored carefully in an intensive care unit for possible bleeding events with

evaluation every 6 to 12 hours for evidence of worsening ischemia.

Early studies comparing thrombolytic therapy to open surgical techniques suggested better perioperative mortality rates with thrombolytics with limb salvage rates similar to operative intervention.[9–11] Yet, these improvements have not been proven definitively at this point, as several follow-up studies failed to show significant survival benefits for thrombolysis.[12–14] Nevertheless, thrombolysis can and should be used in patients for whom open surgical techniques would carry greater perioperative risks. Patients for whom thrombolytic therapy is chosen should be advised of the risk of systemic bleeding. In patients with history of recent surgery, gastrointestinal bleeding, trauma, stroke, or pregnancy, thrombolytic therapy should not be used. Absolute contraindications to thrombolytic therapy include dissecting aortic aneurysm, pericarditis, stroke, or neurosurgical procedures within 6 months or known intracranial neoplasm. To decrease risk of bleeding, baseline fibrinogen levels should be obtained and followed throughout therapy. A drop in fibrinogen to less than 50% of baseline or less than 100 mg/dL is essentially a systemic lytic state and raises the risk for major bleeding episode.

In addition to bleeding risks, all patients should be evaluated for severity of ischemia prior to initiation of thrombolytic therapy. Those patients with significant neuromotor deficits or advancing ischemia should be treated with open surgical procedures because of the increased risk for limb loss and postischemia morbidity associated with the longer time it takes to reestablish perfusion with lytic therapy. Despite its risks, thrombolytic therapy remains a viable treatment modality for acute limb ischemia, particularly in appropriately selected patients.

As endovascular surgical procedures have advanced to the forefront of modern vascular surgery, new devices have been developed for use in acute thromboembolic states. These percutaneous mechanical thrombectomy devices were initially developed for use in clotted dialysis grafts.[15] The benefits of mechanical thrombectomy include a minimally invasive procedure, minimal duration and dose of thrombolytic administration, and decreased operative time with rapid restoration of flow.

The systems make use of the Venturi effect by creating a negative pressure zone behind the high-velocity jet, which acts to evacuate the fragmented clot with minimal arterial wall injury, or local dispersion and infusion therapy using balloons for localized thrombolysis and mechanical thrombolysis. These procedures are not without risks as distal embolization of microfragments can occur. Several studies have been developed to compare mechanical thrombectomy with open surgery, although none with a randomized prospective comparison.[16–18] These studies suggest that the mechanical thrombectomy, in conjunction with thrombolytic therapy, may be an effective adjuvant modality in the treatment of acute limb ischemia. When using the mechanical thrombectomy in native vessels, a distal protection device should be used to prevent downstream emboli. Also, there is a risk of pancreatitis associated with the use of mechanical thrombectomy devices. Early data on these devices are limited but suggest that these may be effective modalities, particularly in synthetic bypass graft occlusion.[17]

Thrombosis

It is important to distinguish embolic events from thrombosis occurring as an inevitable consequence of atherosclerotic disease progression. Differentiation may help in planning intervention, as thrombotic events may not be amenable solely to embolectomy or thrombolysis. A history of claudication and physical signs of chronicity such as absence of hair, presence of onychogryphosis, absence of contralateral pulses, or presence of contralateral popliteal aneurysm may provide clues to the presence of underlying disease, which may lead to thrombosis. If the degree of ischemia permits, the longer time it takes for thrombolytic therapy and angiography may expose underlying stenosis or disease, which may be treated with angioplasty, atherectomy, or with or without stenting. If the presence of paresthesia and paralysis mandates immediate relief of ischemia, operative angiography in conjunction with catheter embolectomy may be quicker and may help define whether intraoperative angioplasty, atherectomy, or stenting may be useful or whether bypass is necessary. Under these circumstances, the patient should be prepared and draped so that all potential inflow and outflow sites are available. For the lower extremity, it is prudent also to make sure that the ipsilateral vein is available and has not been used for previous vascular or cardiac procedures. If it is absent, the contralateral leg or the arm should be prepared.

Surgical Intervention

Once the diagnosis of arterial thromboembolism is established, plans must be made for reestablishing flow to the affected limb. Regardless of therapy, timely reestablishment of flow is what will have the greatest effect on overall morbidity and mortality. While each therapy has its advantages and disadvantages, therapeutic interventions should be based on the clinician's comfort level with various interventions, the patient's overall medical condition, and the status of the ischemic extremity. For the purposes of this chapter, we will approach surgical interventions based on the location of embolization.

Iliac and Femoral Thromboemboli. A groin incision is the incision of choice for the management of femoral and iliac emboli. This incision allows for exposure and control of the distal external iliac, the common, superficial, and profunda femoral arteries. A transverse arteriotomy is made in healthy arteries to allow for primary closure without luminal narrowing. In the case of diseased arteries, a longitudinal arteriotomy is sufficient, but the arteriotomy should be closed with a patch to prevent further narrowing of the vessel.

Once the arteriotomy is performed, and the patient systemically anticoagulated, an appropriately sized embolectomy catheter is passed proximally to reestablish inflow. With femoral vessel embolism, a no. 3 or 4 mm balloon catheter should suffice. Care should be taken to avoid overinflating the catheter balloon, as intimal damage and arterial disruption may ensue. If the surgeon experiences difficulty in catheter passage, angiography with image retention can assist in embolectomy. Intraoperative fluoroscopy allows for visualization of catheter passage, and several "over-the-wire" embolectomy catheters have been developed to allow for accurate positioning of the embolectomy catheter and to improve embolectomy results.

The catheter should be passed until no further debris is noted and pulsatile flow is restored in the inflow vessel. Once inflow is established, this procedure should be repeated for the distal vessels. This can prove difficult as the vessel anatomy can be quite difficult to navigate with the embolectomy catheter. Here again, a guide-wire with intraoperative angiography and fluoroscopy will aid the surgeon in correct catheter positioning. Also, accessing the distal vessels at the ankle and retrograde embolectomy will ensure distal flow. A venous patch often is used to close the distal site.

After completion of thromboembolectomy, the surgeon must verify that adequate flow has been reestablished. Completion arteriograms must be performed to document restored flow.[19] The presence of backflow of blood does not establish that all material has been removed, as collateral flow a short distance from the arteriotomy site may mask more distal emboli. These studies can be complicated by postprocedure vasospasm. The primary means of verifying distal flow should be through angiography, Doppler signals, and clinical examination of the extremity. Where there is residual clot in small distal vessels, adjunctive thrombolytics may be infused through angiographically placed catheters.

Aortic Occlusion. Acute aortic occlusion from thromboembolism can be treated with balloon catheter embolectomy. The clinician must be prepared for potential bypass procedures and prepare the patient accordingly. Access for embolectomy is performed through both femoral arteries. Systemic anticoagulation is begun, and large no. 5 or 6 mm Fogarty catheter is placed sequentially up each femoral artery and the clot removed. The contralateral femoral artery should be occluded during embolectomy to prevent distal embolization. The procedure is repeated on the contralateral side. If emboli cannot be satisfactorily removed, aortobifemoral bypass or extra-anatomic bypass may be needed.

Once flow is reestablished, the patient is at risk of decompensation from acidosis and hyperkalemia. Metabolic products from the ischemia state are returned to the circulation and result in cardiac arrhythmia or decompensation. Also, the peripheral vasodilation that occurs as a result of prolonged ischemia may cause hypotension upon release of flow to the extremities. This can be overcome by adequate hydration prior to release of flow.

Popliteal Thromboemboli. There are two approaches to popliteal emboli, a transfemoral and direct popliteal arteriotomy. The transfemoral approach embolectomy has a success rate of 49%. A small embolectomy catheter is passed into the distal vessels through a femoral arteriotomy. The peroneal artery will be preferentially cannulated as a result of the anatomy of the popliteal trifurcation. If this occurs, "over the wire" techniques with fluoroscopy may be used to access the anterior and posterior tibial arteries. Also, the popliteal artery can be exposed below the knee to direct the catheter into the branch vessels. Finally, a popliteal arteriotomy can be performed and the branch vessels cannulated directly. The best results occur when all branches of the popliteal artery are cleared of clot.

Distal Thromboemboli. Distal tibial thromboemboli present a unique challenge to the vascular surgeon. It is not uncommon to have residual thrombus within the tibial vessels following proximal embolectomy. These delicate vessels are more sensitive to occlusion and manipulation than proximal vessels. While embolectomy can be performed with no. 2 Fogarty catheters in the tibioperoneal artery through a small arteriotomy, these vessels are quite sensitive to wall damage and subsequent thrombosis following arteriotomy closure. A reasonable alternative to embolectomy is catheter-directed regional thrombolytic therapy. Distal embolization that is not cleared can result in loss of digits or even the whole foot.

Upper Extremity Emboli. Upper extremity emboli typically lodge in the brachial artery at the radial and ulnar bifurcation (Figure 36-5). This is the most common cause of hand ischemia, with most emboli arising from the heart. Other sources of emboli include atherosclerotic lesions, iatrogenic manipulation, subclavian aneurysms, and thoracic outlet syndrome, and often thrombectomy of upper arm dialysis access. Upper extremity emboli can be approached through an antecubital incision for exposure of the brachial artery. Once exposed, a no. 2 or 3 Fogarty embolectomy catheter can be used to facilitate removal of clot. Upper ex-

tremity emboli are usually well tolerated and carry a lower risk for limb loss than their lower extremity counterparts.

Results of Therapeutic Modalities

The debate between open surgical interventions and minimally invasive procedures continues to rage and is not likely to be settled soon. Technological advances continue to bring forth new inventions and treatment modalities in an attempt to improve patient survival and outcomes. Mortality rates from open interventions remain high, between 10% and 20%, largely because of medical comorbidities, which complicate postoperative care. When applied early, limb salvage rates of open surgery approach 93%, decreasing to 78% when instituted after 8 hours of ischemia.

Thrombolytic therapy does appear to offer a short-term survival advantage over open surgical therapies, but at the cost of increased bleeding risk and possible poorer functional outcome, if the clot cannot be removed expeditiously. In addition, endovascular modalities such as Trellis and AngioJet are proving to be as effective as open surgery, especially in patients with graft thrombosis. As technology advances, it is likely that newer devices will be introduced, which have the potential of surpassing open surgery in effectiveness.

Nevertheless, just as technology is changing, the patient population with embolic disease is changing as well. Patients are now more likely to be older and have underlying atherosclerotic disease and previous vascular surgery. With these changes, the focus of the clinician should be not only the best way to treat the acute embolus, but also how to best approach the patient's underlying medical conditions. Only through this approach can the high mortality of macroembolic disease be diminished.

Microembolization

Microembolization occurs in the setting of advanced atherosclerotic disease and is often referred to as atheromatous embolization or "blue toe syndrome" (Figure 36-6). Advanced atherosclerotic plaques are at risk of rupture and distal embolization. Once plaques rupture, the core of the plaque, rich in cholesterol crystals and platelet-fibrin aggregates, embolizes downstream to small vessels. This should be differentiated from macroemboli, which may result from atherosclerotic plaques as well but consist mainly of the large fibrous cap or clots forming in ulcerations and platelet debris. The cholesterol crystals within the microemboli travel downstream and lodge within smaller vessels, where these incite an immune response. Eosinophils and neutrophils flood the affected area and set the stage for a chronic inflammatory response. As inflammatory cells invade the area, fibrin is deposited and endothelial proliferation occurs. This leads to luminal narrowing and occlusion with end-organ dysfunction. The process of cholesterol crystal embolization is typically seen in infrarenal aortic disease. Microemboli can also contain fibrin and platelet aggregates, which can also occlude distal vessels, resulting in ischemia. Atheroembolization can occur from any arterial

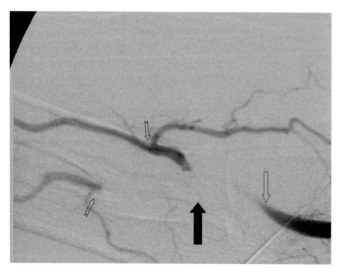

● **FIGURE 36-5.** Arterial embolism to the bifurcation of the brachial artery occluding both radial and ulnar arterial runoff.

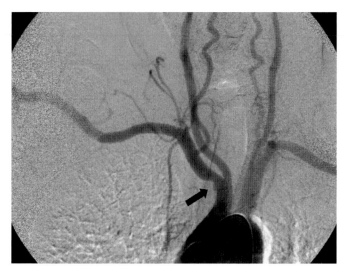

● **FIGURE 36-6.** Subclavian artery irregular plaque as a source of microemboli to the fingers.

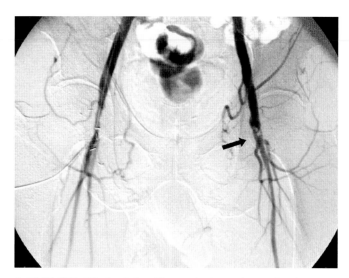

● **FIGURE 36-8.** Intimal hyperplasia or clot at distal anastomosis of an aortofemoral bypass graft after thrombolysis needing further revision.

source from the aorta to the popliteal artery. Microemboli have a strong association with popliteal aneurysms. Any patient with diffuse atherosclerotic disease is at a risk of atheroembolization. Coral reef aorta must be considered as an etiology as well. Coral reef aorta is an unusual entity that typically occurs in the suprarenal aorta. In this condition, a heavily calcified polypoid plaque develops along the posterior surface of the suprarenal aorta. This calcification can become extensive enough to cause aortic occlusion. Patients with this condition may present with blue toe syndrome, visceral ischemia, or, in extreme cases, visceral, renal, and lower extremity ischemia from embolization of large amounts of atherosclerotic material. This lesion should be approached through a retroperitoneal thoracoabdominal incision with endarterectomy. In some patients, replacement of the aortic segment may be required.

In the clinical setting, microemboli typically lodge within the digital vessels, resulting in the blue toe syndrome (Figure 36-7). Patients usually complain of a painful digit,

with a bluish discoloration in the distribution of the affected vessel. The pain can be severe and last for weeks. There are often palpable pedal pulses in the presence of gangrenous changes of the digits. Once recognized, the clinician should evaluate the patient for obvious causes for microemboli and make plans for definitive management. In addition, the involved digit may have to be amputated to relieve pain. Workup for blue toe syndrome should include both thoracic and abdominal CT scan to look for "shaggy" changes in the aorta and iliac vessels, and arteriography of the lower extremities to evaluate the peripheral arteries for ulcerations.

● **GRAFT THROMBOSIS**

Graft thrombosis occurs commonly after open vascular bypass procedures (Figure 36-8). This condition should be divided into early and late thrombosis. Early graft thrombosis is usually secondary to a technical defect. This is treated by reexploring both anastomoses and intraoperative angiography, which allows visualization of twist, kinks, or retained valves. Late thrombosis occurs weeks following the procedure, and intervention should be based on the degree of ischemia. Class 1 and 2a patients can be treated with lytic therapy, which allows for lesions to be unmasked and repaired with graft revision. Once lytic therapy is completed, these patients should undergo follow-up angiography with either endovascular or open repair of the graft. Class 2b patients should undergo urgent operative intervention, with plans for thrombectomy or revision of the bypass.

● **THORACIC AORTIC ATHEROSCLEROSIS**

Atherosclerosis of the thoracic aorta, particularly proximal to the left subclavian ostium, carries a significant risk for cerebral and peripheral vascular emboli. Several studies have concluded that patients with atherosclerotic plaques

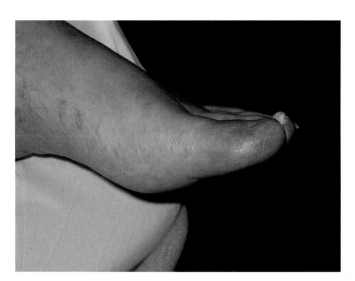

● **FIGURE 36-7.** Microemboli to the toes causing "blue toe syndrome".

measuring >4 mm carry an annual risk of major embolic event of ~30%. In light of these findings, the American College of Chest Physicians now recommends that patients with aortic plaques greater than 4 mm or mobile atheromas measured on transesophageal echocardiography should be managed with warfarin therapy. Surgery for thoracic atherosclerotic lesions can prove quite challenging and carries a significant risk of stroke and paraplegia. Therefore, aortic endarterectomy should be reserved for those patients with ongoing embolic phenomena despite medical treatment.

● SUMMARY

Acute limb ischemia occurs when a distal extremity experiences hypoperfusion as a result of sudden arterial or bypass graft occlusion. This should be a clinical diagnosis based on the patients' history and physical examination findings, with diagnostic testing to help plan for appropriate intervention. Delay in diagnosis or treatment increases the risk for limb loss. Treatment should be instituted in a timely fashion with plans for open surgical, thrombolytic therapy, or minimally invasive procedures. Despite advances in technologies, mortality rates remain high in acute limb ischemia, largely owing to multiple medical comorbidities, which complicate the posttherapy course. Successful management of patients with acute limb ischemia depends on accurate diagnosis, early restoration of blood flow, and correcting the underlying cause for the ischemic event. As technology advances, new devices will certainly be introduced in an effort to decrease the invasiveness of open surgery and perioperative mortality. These efforts should be made in conjunction with efforts to understand and treat the underlying causes of acute limb ischemia to possibly prevent the event from occurring.

REFERENCES

1. Bulkley GB. Pathophysiology of free radical-mediated reperfusion injury. *J Vasc Surg.* 1987;5:512-517.

2. Rutherford RB, Baker JD, Ernst C, et al. Recommended standards for reports dealing with lower extremity ischemia: revised version. *J Vasc Surg.* 1997;26:517-538.

3. Rutherford RB, et al. *Vascular Surgery.* 6th ed. Philadelphia, PA: Elsevier Saunders; 2005.

4. Rubin GD, Dake MD, Semba CP. Current status of three-dimensional spiral CT scanning for imaging the vasculature. *Radiol Clin North Am.* 1995;33:51-70.

5. Becquemin J, Kovarsky S. Arterial emboli of the lower limbs: analysis of risk factors for mortality and amputation. *Ann Vasc Surg.* 1995;9:S32.

6. Sharma P, Babu S, Shah P, Nassoura Z. Changing patterns of atheroembolism. *Cardiovasc Surg.* 1996;4:573.

7. Keeley E, Hillis L. Left ventricular mural thrombus after acute myocardial infarction. *Clin Cardiol.* 1996;19:83.

8. Ward R, Jones D, Haponik E. Paradoxical embolism: an underrecognized problem. *Chest.* 1995;108:549.

9. Ouriel K, Veith FJ, Sasahara AA. Thrombolysis or peripheral arterial surgery: phase I results. TOPAS Investigators. *J Vasc Surg.* 1996;23:64-73.

10. Parent N, Bernhard V, Pabst T, et al. Fibrinolytic treatment of residual thrombus after catheter embolectomy for severe lower limb ischemia. *J Vasc Surg.* 1989;9:153.

11. Ricotta JJ, Green RM, DeWeese JA. Use and limitations of thrombolytic therapy in the treatment of peripheral arterial ischemia: results of a multi-institutional questionnaire. *J Vasc Surg.* 1987;6:45-50.

12. Korn P, Khilnani NM, Fellers JC, et al. Thrombolysis for native arterial occlusions of the lower extremities: clinical outcome and cost. *J Vasc Surg.* 2001;33:6.

13. Ouriel K, Veith FJ, Sasahara AA. A comparison of recombinant urokinase with vascular surgery as initial treatment for acute arterial occlusion of the legs. Thrombolysis or Peripheral Arterial Surgery (TOPAS) Investigators. *N Engl J Med.* 1998;338:1105-1111.

14. Singh S, Ackroyd R, Lees T, et al. Thrombo-embolectomy and thrombolytic therapy in acute lower limb ischemia: a five-year experience. *Int Angiol.* 1996;15:6.

15. Castaneda F, Cragg A, Wyffels P, et al. New thrombolytic brush catheter in thrombosed polytetrafluoroethylene dialysis grafts: preliminary animal study. *Radiology.* 1994;193:324.

16. Gunther R, Vorweck D. Aspiration catheters for percutaneous thrombectomy: clinical results. *Radiology.* 1990;175:271.

17. Kasirajan K, Gray B, Beavers FP, et al. Rheolytic thrombectomy in the management of acute and subacute limb-threatening ischemia. *J Vasc Interv Radiol.* 2001;12:413-421.

18. Sharafuddin M, Hicks M, Jenson M, et al. Rheolytic thrombectomy with the AngioJet-F105 catheter: preclinical evaluation of safety. *J Vasc Interv Radiol.* 1997;8:939.

19. Crolla RM, van de Pavoordt ED, Moll FL. Intraoperative digital subtraction angiography after thromboembolectomy: preliminary experience. *J Endovasc Surg.* 1995;2:168-171.

chapter 37

Lower Extremity Revascularization for Atherosclerotic Occlusive Disease

John B. Chang, MD / Robert W. Chang, MD / L. Michael Graver, MD

● NATURAL HISTORY

During the past half century, vascular specialists have made major progress in treating vascular diseases with chronic ischemia of the lower extremities. Peripheral arterial occlusive disease (PAOD) presents a clinical spectrum from asymptomatic, intermittent claudication, or critical ischemic change.

The TransAtlantic Inter-Society Consensus (TASC) conference defined critical limb ischemia (CLI) as persistent recurring ischemic rest pain requiring opiate analgesia for at least 2 weeks, ulceration or gangrene of the foot or toes, and ankle systolic pressure <50 mm Hg or toe systolic pressure <30 mm Hg (or absences of pedal pulses in patients with diabetes).

Most patients with rest pain or tissue necrosis have limb loss. Small ulcers may heal with aggressive local management and intermittent rest pain or night pain may improve with the development of collaterals or improvement of cardiac hemodynamics. The mortality rate associated with patients who have claudication is 50% at 5 years, and for patients with CLI, the rate is 70%. This high mortality rate is most commonly associated with cardiac disease, and is generally unrecognized by clinicians. Consequently, the opportunity for risk factors or cardiac intervention maybe overlooked.[1]

● NONOPERATIVE TREATMENT

Atherosclerosis is a systemic disease that is most frequently associated with fatal and nonfatal myocardial infarction (MI), stroke and disease of the aorta, and lower extremities. Peripheral arterial disease (PAD), atherosclerosis in the arteries of the lower extremities; whether it is asymptomatic or symptomatic is a common disorder in the general population. The prevalence of PAD increases with age and presence of vascular risk factors. The estimated overall prevalence of PAD among people of 55 years of age or older varies between 9% and 23%.[2] The incidence of PAD measured in an open population is 9.9 per 1000 people per year.[3] Because of aging population in Western societies, the prevalence of PAD will rise and the medical treatment will become increasingly important.

The majority of patients with PAD is asymptomatic or has leg symptoms other than classic intermittent claudication, which is defined as leg pain usually involving one or both calves that arises by walking and is relieved by rest only. It is estimated that only 22% of patients with PAD have these symptoms.[4] Elderly male patients with diabetes are especially more likely to have asymptomatic PAD.[5] The overall annual incidence of symptomatic PAD, with typical intermittent claudication is 1.5 to 2.6 per 1000 men and 1.2 to 3.6 per 1000 women.[6]

Of the patients with asymptomatic PAD, only 5% to 10% will develop symptomatic PAD in a period of over 5 years.[7] The majority of patients with intermittent claudication as the clinical symptoms of PAD can remain stable over many years. Approximately 15% of these patients develop critical leg ischemia (with ulceration and rest pain) and a high risk for amputation. The annual incidence of CLI is estimated to be 0.25 to 0.45 per 1000 persons.[8,9] Of the patients with

CLI, between approximately 20% and 45% will require an amputation of the leg.[10]

Approximately 30% of the symptomatic patients will die within 5 years because of vascular diseases and 5% to 10% because of a nonvascular cause.[11–13] There is even a trend toward an increased total as well as cardiovascular mortality in patients with asymptomatic PAD.[7,14,15]

Risk Factor Modification

Smoking Cessation. Smoking behavior is associated with a considerably increased risk of symptomatic PAD.[16] Symptoms of PAD arise approximately a decade earlier in smokers than in nonsmokers, whereas smokers with PAD have amputation rates twice as high as those who have never smoked.[10] There are suggestions that smoking cessation will decrease the risk for critical leg ischemia and reduce the mortality in patients with PAD.[17,18] Smoking cessation is considered to be critical step in the risk factor management. Although smoking cessation probably reduces the severity of claudication, a meta-analysis concluded that it did not significantly improve the walking distance or walking capacity.[19] There are several possible strategies to support the cessation of smoking, including nicotine replacement,[20–24] and bupropion, an antidepressant drug.[25–29] A combination of pharmacology and counseling achieves the highest rate of smoking cessation,[29] although there are other modalities including hypnotherapy, acupuncture, aversive smoking.[20,30–32]

Hypertension. It is recommended that patients with PAD acquire a blood pressure of <130/85 mm Hg,[33,34] although there is no data available to suggest that hypertension treatment alters the arising of intermittent claudication or progression of the disease in the peripheral circulation.

ACE inhibitors showed significantly greater hemodynamic improvement in the extremity in which baseline blood flow is decreased by limb arterial atherosclerosis compared with either or beta-blockers,[35,36] although there is no evidence that beta-blockers are particularly culpable as has been suggested previously.[37,38]

Diabetes Mellitus. Diabetes mellitus is highly associated with PAD and its progression.[39,40]

Hyperlipidemia. Lipid modification is associated with stabilization and even regression of femoral atherosclerosis.[41–44] Although diet and exercise have been found to alter the lipid profile toward a less atherogenic type, many patients require lipid-lowering medications. Statins are effective at reducing low-density lipoprotein (LDL)-cholesterol levels, causing a significant reduction in all-cause mortality from 14.7% to 12.9% with the use of simvastatin compared to placebo. For the first occurrence of a major vascular event, a relative reduction of 24% (in absolute terms from 25.2% to 19.8%) was found in the Heart Protection Study.[45]

Lowering the total cholesterol and LDL by 25% with a statin reduces cardiovascular mortality and morbidity in patients with PAD by approximately 25% (relative), irrespective of age, sex, or baseline cholesterol concentration.[45] In one study,[46] simvastatin significantly reduces the incidence of new intermittent claudication by 38% compared with placebo (in absolute terms from 3.6% to 2.3%) over 6 years in patients with hypercholesterolemia and coronary heart disease. Both simvastatin and atorvastatin significantly increased the pain-free walking distance after 1 year of treatment with 63%, compared with placebo.[47,48] This effect is most likely to be independent of the effects of serum lipid measurements because of statin use.[47,48]

Other lipid-lowering agents including bezafibrate, nicotinic acid, and cilostazol, which have proved to be beneficial in lowering nonfatal coronary events or cardiovascular morbidity and mortality and decreasing plasma triglycerides.[49–53]

Hyperhomocyteinemia. This condition has a strong association between the increases in plasma homocysteine concentration and PAD.[54,55] There is no current trial available on the treatment of hyperhomocyteinemia in patients with PAD.[56] An increased level of homocysteine is associated with an increased risk of death from cardiovascular causes.[55]

Antiplatelet Therapy. Antiplatelet therapy with aspirin in patients with PAD showed a significant reduction of 23% (in absolute from 7.1% to 5.8% over an unspecified period) in subsequent serious cardiovascular events, with similar benefit among patients with intermittent claudication.[57,58]

Aspirin. Antiplatelet therapy is to be considered in the management of PAD. There is strong evidence that antiplatelet agents reduce major cardiovascular events over an average of 2 years compared with controlled treatment.[57,58] Based on the available evidence, the first line of antiplatelet therapy should be aspirin or clopidogrel.[59]

Clopidogrel. Clopidogrel is a thienopyridyne antiplatelet and associated with less gastrointestinal hemorrhage and upper gastrointestinal upset compared with aspirin.[60] Although there is little evidence, a combination of antiplatelet therapy with aspirin and clopidogrel could be initiated if a patient experiences a second vascular event while receiving monotherapy.[59,61] However, potential risk of a prolonged bleeding time during this combination of antiplatelet therapy is a concern.[62]

Dipyridamole. There is no evidence that dipyridamole, as monotherapy or combined with other antiplatelet agents, reduces the risk of vascular death, although it may reduce the risk of further vascular event.[63]

Anticoagulant Therapy. There is no evidence to support the routine use of warfarin in patients with intermittent claudication who show regular sinus rhythm.[64]

Management of PAD.

Exercise. Exercise for the treatment of PAD is highly effective.[65] With exercise therapy, there is an overall improvement of maximum walking distance of approximately 150% (ranges from 68% to 230%).[65] Supervised exercise therapy program has significant effect in prolonged maximum walking distance of approximately 300 m after 6 months.[66,67]

Pentoxifylline. Pentoxifylline has a small effect on walking ability, although the available data are insufficient to support its widespread use.[19,68–70] Several reports were not able to reveal consistent benefit of pentoxifylline versus placebo.[71–74]

Cilostazol. The treatment with drug has shown an increase of the maximum walking distance of approximately 28% to 100%.[74–79] The use of cilostazol was also associated with improvements in physical performance and functional status.[76,77] Cilostazol treatment for up to 12 weeks maybe needed before improvements are experienced, but a favorable response maybe seen as early as 2 to 4 weeks after initiating the therapy.[79] Cilostazol is contraindicated if symptoms of heart failure are present.

Naftidrofuryl. Several studies with this drug revealed greater efficacy in improving walking distances compared with pentoxifylline and buflomedil by approximately 50% to 80%,[80–82] although another study showed no significant difference.[83] In other studies, this drug also improved the quality of life of the patient with intermittent claudication.[84] However, in our routine practice, this drug has not been used as a routine drug.

Other Agents. Both statins and ACE inhibitors are associated with the pain-free walking distance.[36,85–88] Several meta-analyses of studies evaluating the Ginkgo biloba special extract, EGb 761, showed a clinically relevant benefit for the treatment of patients with PAD, with significant increase of the pain-free walking distance compared with placebo.[89–91] There is insufficient evidence of effective of treatment of propionyl L-carnitine, ozonated autohemotherapy, and chelation therapy in patients with intermittent claudication to recommend its use.[92–94] In addition, buflomedil, beraprost, ketanserin, nifedipine, fish oil supplementation, vasodilators, calcium channel antagonists, and alpha-adrenergic blocking agents have shown to be ineffective in the treatment of intermittent claudication.[95]

Prostanoids. This may have beneficial effects on wound healing, limb loss, and survival in patients with CLI.[10] The currently available data support the use of iloprost in patients who are unsuitable for any procedure or in whom revascularization attempts have failed.[10]

Antiplatelets and Anticoagulants. Long-term treatment with aspirin and ticlopidine has been shown to reduce the progression of femoral atherosclerosis.[96] Anticoagulant treatment with low-molecular-weight heparin showed positive results with a decrease in rest pain and an improvement in healing of ulcers previously resistant to treatment.[97] No clinical trials have been published on the use of unfractionated heparin for critical limb loss or CLI.

Gene-Based Therapy. Therapeutic angiogenesis is suggested to be effective in the treatment of CLI, improving collateral vessel development with subsequent significant improvement in tissue loss, resolution of rest pain, and lowering the level of amputation.[98–100] The efficacy was associated with the clinical objective findings of an improved ankle-brachial index (ABI) with a difference of approximately 0.14,[100] a significant increase in pain-free walking time (from 2.5 to 3.8 min) at an average of 13 weeks after gene therapy ($p = 0.043$), and blood flow on magnetic resonance angiography.[98,100]

Vascular endothelial growth factor (VEGF)-induced angiogenic gene therapy in patients with PAD showed clinical efficacy including resolution of resting pain, and healing of ischemic ulcers, associated with objective findings of improved ABI, and blood flow on angiography, on phase I study with intramuscular VEGF gene transfer in their study.[101]

There is a large volume of literature available on the use of the VEGF gene in ischemic animal limb models. The first group to describe this technique was Takeshita et al.[102,103] who administered plasmids coding for VEGF by the intra-arterial route after ligation of the femoral artery in rabbits and documented an augmentation in collateral circulation through angiography and an increase in capillary density through histology. Using the same model, the authors[104] obtained similar results with an intramuscular injection plasmids coding VEGF 165 (500 μg).

In a recent phase I trial involving treatment of 20 patients (7 with stage IV PAD and 10 with stage III PAD) with 4000 μg of plasmids coding for VEGF, after a 6-month follow-up period, the investigators noted a nonsignificant increase in systolic pressure index with healing of trophic lesions. Angiomagnetic resonance imaging demonstrated increased collateral circulation in all cases. Limb salvage was achieved in three patients. After amputation in one patient, immunohistochemical examination of the ischemic muscle showed intense proliferation of endothelial cells. No systemic complications were observed. The only side effect was treatable lower extremity edema secondary to the increased capillary patency induced by VEGF.[105] Another report showed similar results on the feasibility, efficacy, and safety of VEGF plasmid therapy.[106]

Experimental data reported by Ohara et al.[107] showed that the angiographic criteria and capillary density were significantly higher in the treatment group than in the control group after adenovirus-mediated transfer of fibroblast growth factor (FGF) via the intra-arterial route in rabbit ischemic hind limb model. This study suggests that transinfection had a beneficial effect.

There are two studies now underway to evaluate the use of FGF for treatment of patients with occlusive arterial disease. One uses a plasmid coding FGF-1 and the other an adenovirus coding for FGF-4, result of which has not been published.[108]

Another alternative for using therapeutic angiogenesis is bone marrow mononuclear cell therapy. The bone marrow cells have a natural ability to supply endothelial progenitor cells and to secrete various angiogenic factors or cytokines. In a small randomized trial, the ABI significantly improved with a difference of 0.09 (95% CI: 0.06–0.11), the transcutaneous oxygen pressure increased from 28.8 to 46.3, and pain-free walking distance significantly improved by approximately 3.5 min 24 weeks after injection with bone marrow mononuclear cells. Besides these ischemic status, improvements also rest pain was resolved in 16 out of 20 treated patients, which all was maintained during 24 weeks follow-up.[99]

Pain Relief. A recent meta-analysis about spinal cord stimulation showed that the additional use of spinal cord stimulation to the standard conservative treatment is better than the standard conservative treatment alone.[109] Pooled data showed a significant beneficial effect in terms of limb salvage with a relative risk of 0.71 (95% CI: 0.56–0.90) after 12 months of treatment. Beside pain relief and ulcer healing it may also improve walking ability, and also enhance local circulation.

Thrombolysis. In acute limb ischemia, an acute onset because of an embolic or thrombotic occlusion, thrombolysis is indicated. Two meta-analysis in patients with acute limb ischemia concluded that there is an equal mortality (RR 1.24; 95% CI: 0.80–1.90) and amputation rate (RR 0.89; 95% CI: 0.58–1.38) between patients treated with thrombolysis or surgery. The need for open major surgical procedures on the contrary is reduced after thrombolysis, although with a higher rate of bleeding (RR 2.9; 95% CI: 1.1–7.9) and distal embolization (OR 8.4; 95% CI: 4.5–15.6).[110,111] Urokinase and recombinant tissue-type plasminogen activator are most widely used agents. Both agents reported a similar efficacy and safety level in the STILE study,[112] although thrombolysis using low doses of tissue plasminogen activator has a shorter duration and therefore provides a significant overall cost reduction.[113]

Additional Agents. The combination of eptifibatide and tenecteplase showed to be a viable option in the treatment of acute limb ischemia. In a study, a high immediate clinical and technical success was demonstrated, as well as an acceptable 3-month clinical outcome, without any case of death, intracranial hemorrhage, or remote-site bleeding.[114]

Another adjunctive therapy using abciximab, which prevents the binding of fibrinogen, and by this means inhibiting platelet aggregation.[115] This treatment was associated with a reduced need for hospitalization, interventions, and amputations and also markedly shortened the duration of clot lysis in comparison with aspirin.[116] It is reported that thrombolysis occurred faster using a combination of urokinase and abciximab compared with urokinase alone, although with a higher rate of nonfatal major bleeding.[117]

In conclusion, all patients with PAD should be treated with the best possible medical modality and risk reduction. When the best medical management and risk reduction management fails to control the problem, the next management plan should be in place including interventional procedure or surgical revascularization. Medical, cardiac, renal, and endocrine optimization of the PAD patient will lead to a successful vascular intervention and surgical revascularization.

● SURGICAL MANAGEMENT OF PAD—LOWER EXTREMITIES

Endovascular Procedures

Aortoiliac Occlusive Disease. In 2000 and again in 2007, the release of the TASC statement on treatment of peripheral vascular disease gave stratification by length and morphology of lesions and reinforced the concept of treating short, focal stenoses through endovascular techniques. Long-segment occlusions have been treated using surgical revascularization.

TASC-B lesions include unilateral common iliac artery occlusions only. TASC-C iliac lesions include unilateral external iliac occlusions that do not extend into the common femoral artery, or bilateral common iliac occlusions. TASC-D lesions are bilateral external iliac occlusions, ipsilateral common and external iliac artery occlusions, or diffuse disease of the aorta and both iliac arteries. Endovascular procedures are thought to be the treatment of choice for type A lesions (stenoses <3 cm only), and open surgical therapy is thought to be the procedure of choice for type D lesions. According to the TASC statement, more evidence is needed for type B and C lesions, with a preference for endovascular methods for the former and surgical methods for the latter.[118]

Several studies have documented the outcomes in the treatment of more complex iliac occlusions of the TASC-C and TASC-D lesions. Review of the data published since 1995 reveals that primary patency ranges from 69% to 76% at 2 years, with a secondary patency rate of 85% to 95% at 2 years.[119–122] Furthermore, overall complication rates were lower in recent series (1.4% to 4.8%), likely because of improvements in technique and device technology. In a series of 212 patients with chronic iliac occlusions, successful recanalization was accomplished in nearly 90% of patients, with marked clinical improvement in the vast majority of patients.[123] The primary patency at 4 years was 75% in that series.

In the Cleveland Clinic, a total of 89 patients underwent 92 procedures for symptomatic iliac occlusions using endovascular techniques. Recanalization and percutaneous

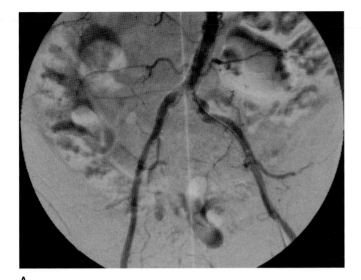

A

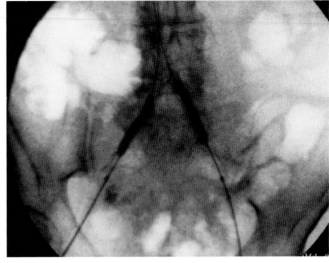

B

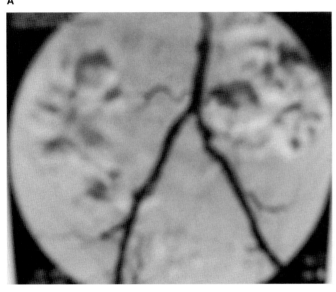

C

● FIGURE 37-1. (A) Patient with patient bilateral common iliac artery stenosis (*arrows*). (B) Balloon angioplasty being performed (*arrows*; inflated balloons, in both proximal and common iliac arteries). (C) Angiogram after completion of balloon angioplasty and kissing stent for bilateral proximal iliac artery stenosis.

transluminal angioplasty (PTA)-stenting was successful in 82 (91%) of 89 patients, with success rate of 95% and 94% in patients with TASC-B and -C lesions, respectively, as opposed to 86% in TASC-D lesions (not significant).

The inability to completely cross the occluded segment or reenter the distal native artery safely, led to the technical failures. The mean ABI increased from 0.45 to 0.83 after successful treatment.[124] In their series, intraoperative complications included flow-limiting dissection ($n = 5$), which was resolved with prolonged balloon angioplasty and stent placement in all cases. Extravasation was seen in two patients and was also treated with prolonged balloon inflation and additional stent placement. Postoperative complications included pseudoaneurysm formation at the access site in two patients treated successfully with thrombin injection. Two patients had distal embolization during the recanalization procedure. One patient required a below-knee amputation and eventually died. The additional patient had embolization that required a minor toe am-

putation. An additional two perioperative deaths occurred (total $n = 3; 3.4\%$) from cardiac arrest and respiratory arrest.

The primary patency for the complete cohort was 76% at 36 months. Primary patency did not vary significantly ($p = 0.99$) with TASC stratification and ranged from 73% to 80%. The secondary patency rate for all patients was 90% at 3 years. Patients with TASC-B and TASC-C lesions had secondary patency rates of 95% and 93%, respectively, whereas TASC-D patients had a secondary rate of 83%. However, this difference was not statistically significant ($p = 0.86$) (Figures 37-1 and 37-2).

Femoral and Distal Arterial Occlusive Disease. PTA is increasingly replacing bypass surgery in the treatment of chronic limb ischemia without compromising patient survival or limb salvage rate. In a study of 57 patients who previously untreated with 71 limbs having chronic arteriosclerotic superficial femoral artery (SFA) occlusion with

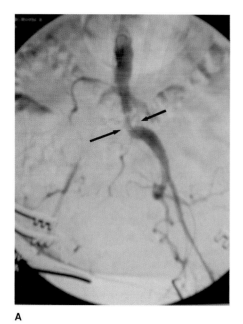
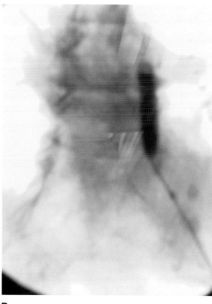
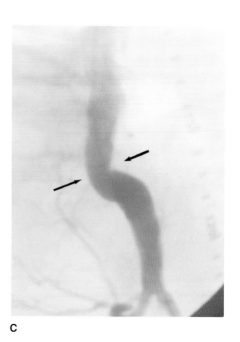

A   B   C

● FIGURE 37-2. (A) Angiogram showing completely occluded right common iliac artery as well as external iliac artery, with high-grade stenosis at left common iliac artery, proximally. (B) Balloon angioplasty and stent being performed (*arrows* indicating inflated balloon catheter). (C) A completed angiogram showing successful restoration of arterial lumen at the left proximal common iliac artery which was severely stenotic (*arrows*). This patient underwent left femoral–right femoral artery bypass graft at the same sitting.

suprageniculate reconstitution and patent tibial runoff, with critical ischemia (Society for Vascular Surgery category, 4–6), showed 1- and 3-year patency rates of 54.6% ± 6.3% and 29.9% ± 6.6% in primary patency; assisted primary 72.3% ± 5.6% and 59.0% ± 6.8%; and secondary, 81.6% ± 4.8% and 68.3% ± 6.5%. Three-year secondary patency when preprocedural thrombolysis was required was 35.7% ± 12.5% compared with 70.6% ± 7.4% for limbs not requiring periprocedural thrombolysis ($p = 0.02$); the differences in occlusion length and severity of ischemia were not significant between these two groups. In that study group, length of occlusion was 14.4 ± 9.9 cm, with the mean length of stented artery was 24.3 ± 11.1 cm (mean ± SD). ABIs increased from 0.59 ± 0.14 to 0.86 ± 0.16. PTA and stenting yielded higher patency rates than historical controls undergoing PTA alone. When periprocedural thrombolysis is required, subsequent patency appeared to be significantly worse.[125]

The patencies observed in this study do suggest better results, more comparable to those achieved with bypass, may eventually be achievable with devices such as coated stents[126–130] or possibly with addition of adjunctive brachytherapy.[131,132] Ultimately, as endovascular devices and methods improve and mature, good prospective trials comparing conservative, endovascular, and surgical therapy will be needed to understand the optimum roles of each of these management technologies. PTA is increasing replacing bypass surgery in the treatment of chronic limb ischemia, without compromising patient survival or limb salvage rate[113] (Figure 37-3).

A large perspective cohort study of patients, confirm the poor progress of chronic limb ischemia. The overall mortality rate at 12 months was 19.1%, indicating that the prognosis is similar to that of MI and stroke. The suitability and practicability of revacularization profoundly affected the prognosis of the patients. Compared with patients for whom revascularization was deemed unnecessary, the risk of dying within 6 or 12 months was double among patients considered unsuitable for intervention.[134]

In a randomized study of 104 patients comparing primary stent implantation or angioplasty had severe claudication or chronic limb ischemia because of stenosis or occlusion of the SFA, the intermediate term, treatment of SFA disease by primary implantation of a self-expanding nitinol stent yielded results that were superior to those with the currently recommended approach of balloon angioplasty with optional secondary stenting.[135]

There was a multicenter and randomized controlled trial on bypass versus angioplasty in severe ischemia of the leg (BASIL). The randomized 452 patients who presented to 27 UK hospitals, with severe limb ischemia caused by infrainguinal disease, were to receive a surgery-first ($n = 228$) or an angioplasty-first ($n = 224$) strategy. The primary endpoint was amputation (of trial leg) free survival. Analysis was by intention to treat. The BASIL trial is registered with National Research Registrar (NRR) and is an

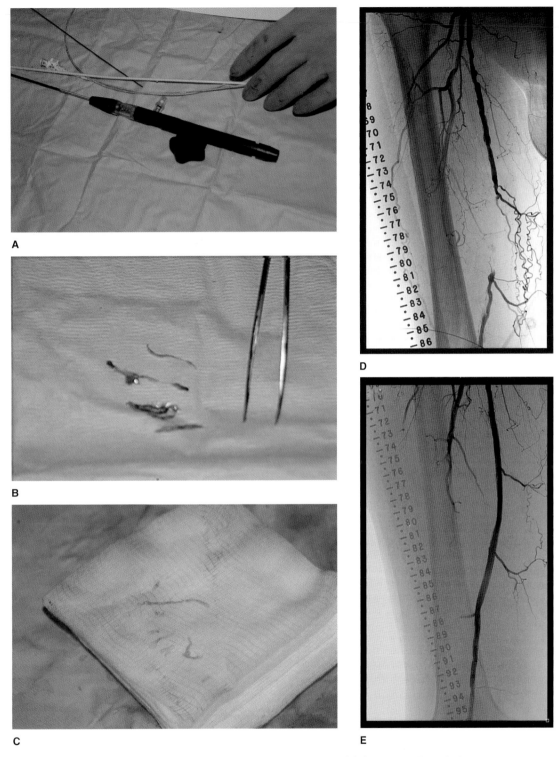

● **FIGURE 37-3.** (A) Silver Hawk device being used. (B) Some specimen being collected. (C) More specimens collected. (D) Preoperative angiogram showing complete occlusion of the right SFA. (E) Same patient—postprocedure completion angiogram. (*continued*)

International Standard Randomized Controlled Trial, number ISRCTN45398889.

The trial ran for 5.5 years, and follow-up finished when the patients reached an endpoint (amputation of trial leg above the ankle or death). In their findings, after 6 months, the two strategies did not differ significantly in amputation-free survival (48 vs. 60 patients; unadjusted hazard ratio 1.07, 95% CI: 0.72–1.6; adjusted hazard ratio 0.73, 0.49–1.07). There was no difference in health-related quality of life between the two strategies, but for the first year,

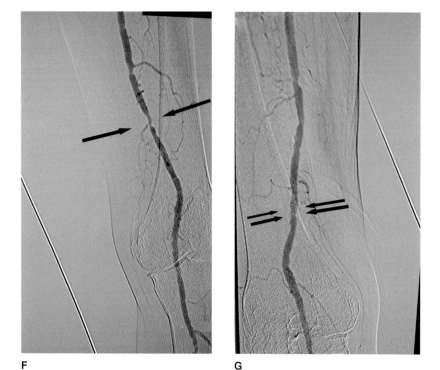
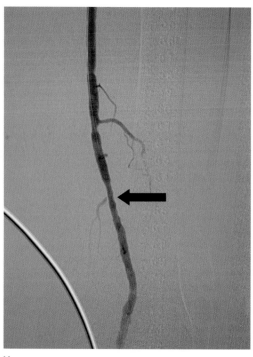

F   G   H

● **FIGURE 37-3.** (*Continued*) (F) Another patient with severe stenosis at the mid SFA (*arrow*). (G) Completion angiogram showing patency of the stenotic lesion after procedure (*double arrows*). (H) Closeup view of completion angiogram of the lesion corrected as shown in 12G (*arrow*).

the hospital costs associated with a surgery-first strategy were approximately one-third higher than those with an angioplasty-first strategy[136] (Figure 37-4).

They have summarized their trial as follows; severe limb ischemia imposes a very high human cost as well as a major economic burden on health and social care, not only in developed countries, but also increasingly in developing countries. It is their hope that BASIL trial data will help the clinician advise, and obtain fully informed consent from, their patients in the knowledge that the decision-making process is based on level 1 evidence regarding the relative risks and benefits of strategies of bypass surgery first and balloon angioplasty first. The medium-term result of the BASIL trial indicates that patients presenting with severe limb ischemia caused by infrainguinal atherosclerosis and who seem technically suitable for both treatments can reasonably be treated with either method in the first instance, depending on individual characteristics and local expertise. However, notwithstanding the high failure and reintervention rate associated angioplasty, patients who are expect to live less than 1 to 2 years and have significant comorbidity should probably, when possible, be offered angioplasty first. Thus, even if the procedure fails, the patient may not be disadvantaged in the short term and can go on to have surgery if regarded as appropriate. Angioplasty also seems to be a much less expensive option than surgery, at least in the short term. By contrast, in patients expected to live more than 2 years and who are relatively fit, the apparent

durability and reduced reintervention rate of surgery could outweigh the short-term considerations of increased morbidity and cost. Long-term follow-up and a detailed analysis of the BASIL trial dataset will probably allow these provisional recommendations to be refined in the future.[136]

The number of diseased vessels in the treated limb was found to predict long-term limb salvage according to multivariate analysis: limbs with one to five diseased vessels diagnosed on preoperative angiography had a better prognosis than limbs with six or more diseased vessels. Factors that have previously been associated with limb salvage according to multivariate analyses are the number of diseased vessels, the number of treated lesions, the type of treated lesions, the state postprocedural peripheral runoff,[137] renal insufficiency, and lack of angiographic improvement achieved by PTA at the site of most severe ischemia.[138] The limb salvage rates were worse at all time periods when surgical revascularizations were included. More than half the limbs that required repeat surgical operations had already undergone repeat endovascular operations. Therefore, profound ischemia and the presence of severe trophic lesions may have affected these findings.

The survival rate of cases in one study showed 72%, 26%, and 14% at 1, 5, and 10 years.[139] The similar findings were reported in other series.[140] Therefore, chronic limb ischemia is a serious threat to patient's lives and limbs.[141] Despite the progression of PAD to the end stage in these patients, aggressive systemic risk factor modification

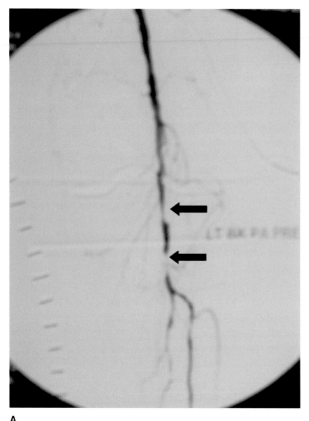

A

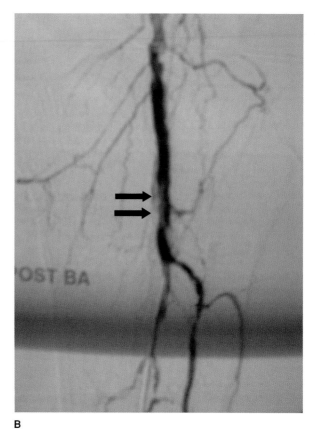

B

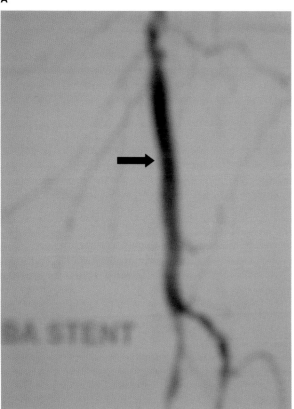

C

● **FIGURE 37-4.** (A) Angiogram on a patient with extremely high surgical risk, and failed previous multiple bypasses, without available autogenous vein in the lower or upper extremities. This angiogram shows multiple stenoses at the popliteal artery down to the distal artery proximal to ATA origin (*arrows*). (B) The same patient after balloon angioplasty, the patient developed a dissection (*arrows*). (C) The same patient, this dissection was treated with a stent procedure. The patient was discharged with limb salvage.

is still warranted to decrease morbidity and mortality in patients with chronic limb ischemia.[142] In a population of patients with unrevascularized chronic limb ischemia, only 28% were alive without amputation of their affected limb at 1 year[143] compared with 53%.[139] Further randomized studies maybe necessary to compare crucial and final outcome of PTA with other surgical revascularizations.

Open Surgical Management

Aortoiliac Arterial Occlusive Disease

Aortofemoral Bypass. When patients present with ischemia requiring revascularization, caused by occlusive disease limited to the aortoiliac segment, the vascular surgeon has only to deal various surgical options available for the treatment of aortoiliac occlusive disease and need not be concerned about the treatment of infrainguinal occlusive disease.

There are three types of lesions:

1. *Type I*, or truly segmental aortoiliac disease, occurs in only in 5% to 10% of the patients. These patients are commonly younger and smokers. Half are women, and they frequently have elevated blood lipids. With localized bifurcation disease, they characteristically have symptoms of thigh or buttock claudication. Impotence is common in male (Leriche's syndrome).

2. *Type 2*, with atherosclerotic involvement of the distal aorta and iliac arteries, comprises an additional group of approximately 25% of the patients. Involvement is still confined to the abdomen without significant distal disease. As a result of collateral circulation in the pelvis, claudication is most common presenting symptom in such patients and advanced distal ischemia is unusual.

3. *Type 3*, with diffuse, multilevel disease, comprises 65% to 75% of the patients. It involves the infrainguinal arterial tree as well as the aortoiliac system. Associated occlusive disease in these patients most commonly involves the SFA, popliteal or runoff vessels, and/or the profunda origin. There is clearly male predominance (7 to 1) in this group. Many of the patients have diabetes and hypertension as well as other sites of atherosclerotic involvement such as in the carotid and coronary vessels. Symptoms of more advanced ischemia, including rest pain and tissue necrosis, often are the presenting complaints in this category.[144]

Aortofemoral Dacron reconstruction for aortoiliac occlusive disease was instituted over 40 years ago. Following the original publications, its efficacy was soon recognized and it became probably the most widely employed arterial reconstruction.[145–152]

One large series of aortobifemoral bypass graft procedures had late patency rate of 74% and 70% after 10 and 15 years, respectively.[153] Operative mortality rates of 2%, 2.9%, and 4.5% have been reported.[153–155]

One study showed that aortobifemoral bypass is the preferred operation for extensive iliac artery occlusive disease that is hemodynamically significant only on the symptomatic side unless specifically contraindicated by prohibitive risk or abdominal disease. This is particularly true in the face of SFA occlusion.[156]

Transabdominal Approach. This approach is most commonly used for the aortofemoral bypass procedure in our practice, as well as many other surgeons. A midline incision is made, extending from the xiphoid process down to the pubic bone, removing the umbilicus, at the time of midline incision, in order to eliminate a potential source of contamination from the umbilicus. Dissection is carried out with sharp dissection at the midline. Following abdominal exploration, the transverse colon and small intestines are eviscerated onto the right side of the abdominal wall or within the right side of the abdominal cavity using self-retaining retractor devices. The retroperitoneal space is entered. The abdominal aorta proximal to the disease and slightly below the renal artery is routinely used for proximal anastomosis. In the event the proximal aorta has extensive disease and/or juxtarenal aortic occlusive process, temporary aortic clamping is done above the renal artery origin for infrarenal aortic endarterectomy. Following the infrarenal or juxtarenal endarterectomy, aortic clamps are then safely moved on the infrarenal aorta for the proximal anastomosis. It is the author's practice to do proximal anastomosis at the most proximal end at the infrarenal portion of the proximal aorta.

In most cases, particularly with extensive proximal disease, the proximal aorta is transected for true end-to-end anastomosis. However, if there are good segments of proximal aorta in a young male patient, the author prefers to do end-to-side proximal anastomosis.

The distal anastomoses are chosen, most of the time, on the femoral arteries. At the time of femoral artery anastomosis, if the patient has occlusive or stenotic disease at the profunda femoral artery with an occluded SFA system, the author's preferred choice would be profundaplasty at the time of distal anastomosis with or without endarterectomy. At the time of endarterectomy, we use liberal dissection into the distal profunda femoral artery beyond the disease point to insure that proper reconstruction is accomplished.

In most cases, double velour Dacron Y graft, No. 18, is used. In the small aorta, particularly in female patients, No. 16 polytetrafluoroethylene Y graft has been utilized. The prosthesis is completely covered using vascularized pedicle of omentum[157] (Figure 37-5).

Retroperitoneal Approach. Retroperitoneal aortic reconstruction has been performed successfully since the report by Rob[158] on 500 aortic reconstructions performed through the retroperitoneal approach in 1962. They listed benefits to be less ileus, less atelectasis and pain, reduced incidence of wound dehiscence, easier anesthesia, a shorter stay in bed and in the hospital, and faster return to work.

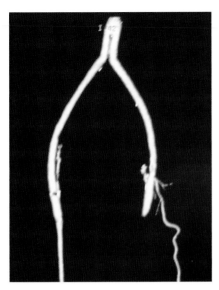

● **FIGURE 37-5.** Reconstructed CTA showing patent aortofemoral bypass graft after 18 years, even though there was extensive distal, particularly of the left lower extremity arterial system.

Certain pitfalls of retroperitoneal aortic reconstruction deserve comment. These include injury to the vena cava, which is very difficult to manage through the retroperitoneal approach. Vigorous retraction in the upper aspect of the operative field may lead to unrecognized splenic trauma. This should be minimized using self-retaining retractors. The lumbar branch of the left renal vein must be identified not only because it serves as a marker to the left renal artery, but to avoid injuring it as well.

Similarly, although rarely, a retroaortic left renal vein or circumaortic left renal vein may cause problems, if not recognized. During mobilization of the retroperitoneum, it is important to identify the left gonadal vein so that, during the course of sweeping the retroperitoneum anteriorly, the gonadal vein is not avulsed from the left renal vein. A left pneumothorax may occur and be unrecognized, particularly if the left 11th intercostal space incision is not made carefully. Both the inferior mesenteric artery and the left renal artery are swept anteriorly when retrorenal dissection is performed and must be identified to prevent injury.

Proper positioning of the patient is important. The left thorax is elevated 45 to 60 degrees, while the hips should lie as flat as possible to allow access to the right groin should that become necessary. The patient's position is secured by placement on a vacuum Styrofoam been bag. The midpoint between the patient's left costal margin and iliac crest is centered over the table flexion point, so that flexing the operating table causes the incision to spiral open. Wound closure is facilitated by flatting the operating table. The surgeon stands to the left of the patient. Rotation of the table away from the surgeon facilitates retroperitoneal dissection, while rotation toward the surgeon facilitates groin dissection.

An oblique left flank incision is used starting midway between the umbilicus and symphysis pubis and extending from the lateral margin of the left rectus sheath into the 11th intercostal space for 8 to 10 cm. The abdominal wall and intercostal muscles are divided in the line of the incision, taking care not to injure the 11th and 12th dorsal neurovascular bundles. Damage to these nerves denervates the abdominal wall, leading to muscle weakness, manifest as an asymmetric abdominal contour with unsightly bulging.

The retroperitoneal space is entered at the tip of the 12th rib, and with blunt dissection, the anterior peritoneum is dissected away from the transversalis fascia as far as the rectus sheath. Dissection medial to the rectus is not necessary for exposure. Also, this prevents tearing the peritoneum where it is firmly attached at the lateral border of the rectus.

Posterior laterally, the plan of the flank musculature, psoas, and diaphragm are followed as the peritoneal sac and its contents are dissected and retracted anteromedially. This plane is developed along the lumbodorsal fascia behind the left kidney and ureter anteriorly. Alternatively, dissection can be performed anterior to the left kidney and ureter, but an advantage of the retroperitoneal approach is lost, since the left renal vein obscured the juxtarenal aorta. However, dissection anterior to the kidney is useful when exposure of the superior mesenteric artery beyond its origin is required for endarterectomy or when endarterectomy of the pararenal aorta is anticipated.

The aorta is easily exposed from above the renal artery to the aortic bifurcation. To prevent injury to the left renal artery, its identification is important. The artery can usually be identified behind the lumbar branch of the left renal vein, which is a fairly constant structure. Ligation of this lumbar branch, which crosses over the aorta, provides good exposure of the aorta and origin of the left renal artery.

Lymphatics and fat overlying the aorta are ligated to minimized lymphorrhea. Blunt dissection of the aorta, anteriorly and posteriorly, either above or below the renal artery, is performed to allow placement of the proximal clamp. Circumferential aortic dissection is not required as long as the tip of the clamp can reach beyond the aortic wall. Inferior vena cava injury is not a concern, as it is not immediately adjacent to the aorta at this level.

If suprarenal aortic control is required, dissection is carried out cephalad, with longitudinal division of the diaphragmatic crus. Suture ligation of the areolar tissue surrounding the origin of the superior mesenteric artery minimizes potential lymphatic leaks. With the need for supraceliac exposure, dissection proceeds further cephalad. Investing fascia around the aorta is incised and blunt dissection anteriorly and posteriorly creates tunnels to accommodate the jaws of an aortic clamp. Supraceliac control is often easier to obtain the juxtarenal control because of the relative paucity of lymphatics and fat at the para celiac level. If juxtarenal or supraceliac aortic clamping is anticipated preoperatively, a ninth or tenth intercostal space incision is recommended.

Distal exposure of the iliac arteries is accomplished by blunt dissection of the peritoneal sac out of the iliac fossa. The left iliac artery can be exposed easily over its entire length. Exposure of the right iliac artery is more challenging. Minimal dissection of the distal aorta is required when managing occlusive disease and the inferior mesenteric artery is preserved.

Anastomoses to the right distal common iliac or external iliac arteries are difficult through the left retroperitoneal approach. Some authors have advocated extending the abdominal incision across the midline into the right lower quadrant to facilitate right iliac arterial exposure. A right lower quadrant counterincision a few centimeters above the inguinal ligament with extraperitoneal dissection of the iliac vessels provides excellent exposure for right external iliac artery anastomoses. This avoids groin dissection with its small but real risk of infection even though one should not hesitate to make a groin incision if necessary.[155–159]

A meta-analysis published in 1997 on 23 studies that met the inclusion criteria. The aggregated operative mortality risk in the older studies (started before 1975) was 4.6%, as compared with 3.3% in the more recent groups ($p = 0.01$).

This study was based on a MEDLINE® search based on the literature published between 1970 and 1996. Studies were included if (1) they reported patency rates based on life tables and the number at risk was provided at yearly intervals and (2) patients and study characteristics were reported in sufficient detail. Mortality and morbidity risks were reported using a fixed-effects model. The patency data were combined using a technique that enables adjustment for differences across studies in patient characteristics or reporting methods. In the current analysis, they corrected for the symptomatic status of the patients at the time of surgery (claudication vs. ischemia) and the unit of observation used in the report the patency (limb vs. patient).

The aggregated systemic morbidity risk was 13.1% in the older studies and 8.3% in the more recent studies ($p < 0.001$). Limb-based patency rates for patients with claudication or 91% and 86.8% at 5 and 10 years, respectively, as compared with 87.5% and 81.8% for patients with ischemia. Patency rates reported in the older studies were markedly similar to those of more recent studies ($p = 0.58$). The conclusion of this meta-analysis is that the studies suggest the mortality and systemic morbidity rates of aortic bifurcation graft procedures have dropped since 1975, whereas patency rates seem to be fairly constant over the years.[160] Type III pattern is the most common form of occlusive disease, ranging 50% to 75% of the time in the literature, as far as our experience.[161–165] In this group of patients, proximal reconstruction may fail to achieve satisfactory relief of ischemic symptoms in up to one-third.[163,166–174] Careful preoperative assessment using hemodynamic studies and clinical evaluation including ischemic pattern of distal portion of the limb may predict a need of a simultaneous distal bypass or revascularization to achieve a successful outcome of a combined procedure.

Associated Visceral or Renal Artery Lesions. The dilemma of whether or not to attempt simultaneous correction of both abdominal aortic and visceral lesions is frequently encountered and difficult to resolve.[175,176] In our practice, preoperative evaluation is given to those incidental findings and an individual decision is made including preoperative angioplasty of the distal vessels or renal artery lesions, if so indicated with a careful assessment. In rare incidences, and on an individual basis, it is necessary to combine the procedure at the time of aortic surgery.

In carefully selected patients, combined reconstruction of associated renal artery disease can give a reasonable outcome.[177–181] Simultaneous aortic operation and renal artery revascularization has increased morbidity and mortality[177,178] (Figure 37-6).

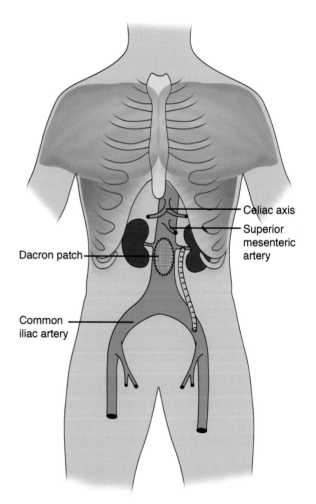

● FIGURE 37-6. Patient who had bilateral renal angioplasty in the past, presented with severe ischemic symptoms involving the lower extremities. Further studies including angiogram, showed complete occlusion of juxta aorta extending to suprarenal as well as infrarenal aorta, and with a complete occluded, previously stented, left renal artery. This patient was treated with supra and juxtarenal aortic endarterectomy and Dacron patch angioplasty using medial visceral rotation with supraceliac aortic clamp, temporarily. At the same sitting, left common iliac artery–left renal artery bypass was performed using PTFE graft (*arrow*).

Complications

Early Complications

HEMORRHAGE: With the current reliable prosthetic graft and suture material, early postoperative bleeding is unusual (1% to 2%). The most common cause of postoperative bleeding is technical error or abnormality of the coagulation mechanism.[182] Meticulous techniques and proper hydration and limiting blood loss are essential keys to prevent these complications.

LIMB ISCHEMIA: This is caused by thrombosis of the graft or more commonly distal embolization.[182] Besides technique, careful layout of the graft is essential to prevent this complication. Acute thrombosis of an aortofemoral bypass graft limb is extremely rare, ranging 1% to 3% in practice and/or literature.[183]

INTESTINAL ISCHEMIA: This complication occurs in 1% to 2% of the cases.[184–186] Most common site of ischemia is the rectosigmoid colon. The cause of these complications is multifactorial including critical loss of blood flow to the involved intestinal segment or thromboembolic complications during the manipulation of blood vessels during surgery.

Postoperatively, high index suspicion is the key for early diagnosis. If clinical suspicion of intestinal ischemia exists, prompt sigmoidoscopy or colonoscopy is indicated. Initial management should be supported care with gastrointestinal tract decompression and intravenous antibiotics. However, if the patient develops any clinical deterioration indicating the need for prompt operative intervention, there should be no waste of time for best protection and lifesaving. During the reexploration, care should be taken to avoid graft exposure. This event of complication has significant mortality ranging from 50% to 75% in many series.[182,185]

ACUTE RENAL FAILURE: Acute renal failure is a rare complication ranging from 1% to 8% with overall mortality of 40%. However, if emergency aortic surgery is indicated, the incidence of acute renal failure is higher with 50% to 90% mortality.[187] To prevent or minimize this complication, careful monitoring intraoperatively to minimize risk of hypovolemia or decrease in cardiac output, particularly during the declamping procedure. The incidence of declamping complications is less in aortic occlusive disease than aortic aneurysm, because the aorta has been chronically occluded, giving less of a hemodynamic impact in cross-clamping. During the cross-clamping for juxtarenal aortic renal occlusion, it is safer to cross-clamp at supraceliac rather suprarenal in some cases, in order to avoid atheroembolic insult to renal arteries.

Late Complications

GRAFT OCCLUSION: Five to ten percent of patients within the first 5 years after operation and in 15% to 30% of patients in 10 years or more postoperatively,[188–190] the most common occlusion affects one limb of the graft with a patent contralateral graft limb. Depending upon the situation and individual basis, there are a variety of techniques including extra-anatomic bypass, thoracic aortofemoral bypass, femoral–femoral bypass, or other intervention.

ANASTOMOTIC FALSE ANEURYSM: With excellent suture material and grafts, this complication is extremely rare, ranging from 1% to 5%.[164] Recognition of femoral anastomotic aneurysm is usually simple. Detection of retroperitoneal or at the aortic anastomosis maybe difficult unless graft surveillance is available or CT scan is done. Management is individualized depending upon the location.

Once the anastomotic false aneurysm is diagnosed, it is advisable to correct the aneurysm to prevent thromboembolic complications or rupture. This fearful complication is extremely rare with modern graft and suture material and techniques as well as prophylactic antibiotics. However, this incidence is reported to be approximately 1% or less in many series.[181,182,191,192]

INFECTION: Graft excision is usually required, and revascularization via remote uncontaminated routes or use of autogenous methods of anatomic revascularization is often necessary to maintain limb viability.[193–198] If the patient's condition is stable and diagnosis of graft infection is established, extra-anatomic revascularization preceding graft excision appears to give a better outcome.[199,200]

Another approach to the treatment of entirely infected aortofemoral grafts consist of graft excision and in situ graft replacement, sometimes with "neoaortoiliac systems" constructed from autogenous superficial femoral veins.[201] This rare and formidable complication is best treated with early diagnosis with a high index of suspicion. When the patient has episode of gastrointestinal hemorrhage with a history of aortic graft in place, high index suspicion should prompt the diagnosis using upper gastrointestinal radiographic evaluation or endoscopic examination.

AORTOENTERIC FISTULA: An acceptable method of treatment for aortoenteric fistula generally requires removal of all prosthetic material, closure of the infrarenal abdominal aorta, repair of the gastrointestinal tract, and revascularization by means by an extra-anatomic bypass graft.[202–205]

Symptomatic atherosclerosis in young adults has been reported in the literature as a poor prognostic finding because of multiple vascular bed involvement and accelerated nature of the disease process.[206–209] Some reports indicated that younger patients have more localized aortic atherosclerosis.[210] In a study which directly compared 45 patients of less than 50 years of age with groups from 50 to 59 years of age ($n = 93$) and of more than 60 years of age ($n = 146$) and found that younger patients had significantly inferior patency rate, with a 66% 5-year cumulative patency rate compared with 96% in the older age group ($p < 0.05$).[211] In that study, the age and aortic size were important predictors for graft failure. There were a no appreciable differences in patency when looking at construction of the proximal anastomosis or gender.

The findings of inferior long-term patency in young adults are consistent with other studies,[212] which showed a 65% 3-year cumulative graft patency rate, and 34% of younger patients in other studies that need further intervention to maintain long-term patency after aortobifemoral bypass.[213]

Patients with smaller aortas had poorer long-term patency rate, consistent with other studies.[206–210,212–215] It appears that risk factors for graft occlusion have no gender difference in various studies.[212,216]

Aortoiliac angioplasty, with or without stenting, is the preferred treatment for patients with segmental aortoiliac disease. Perhaps patients with severe multifocal disease and occlusions (TASC C and D patients)[217] are generally considered better candidates for surgical reconstruction.[211]

Reasonable results have been reported with aggressive applications of endovascular therapy in these patients.[218,219] In one study, they found acceptable primary assisted patency rates of 72% at 3 years with a reintervention rate of 29% at a mean time of 10 ± 3 months in patients undergoing angioplasty and stenting of multisegment of iliac occlusive disease.[220]

Aortoiliac Endarterectomy. Thoughtful selection of patients for patients of aortoiliac endarterectomy is crucial. This procedure should be considered primarily in the 5% to 10% of patients in whom diseases is localized to the aortic bifurcation (type 1). Although the procedure is technically demanding, it offers several advantages. No prosthetic material is used, so the infection rate is virtually nil. Inflow to the hypogastric arterial network may be better preserved than with a bypass method; it may even be increased. Improved hypogastric inflow in turn may better maintain or restore erectile function in the male population.[144,221]

Technical success of aortoiliac endarterectomy depends on the proper plane of the dissection at the level of the external elastic lamina. This dissection can be done in even in the presence of extensive calcification in the wall of the aorta or the proximal common iliac arteries. A secure endpoint to prevent flaps in subintimal dissection is necessary. One or more tacking sutures of 5-0 or 6-0 Prolene placed in a mattress fashion across the distal end point are often required to hold the distal intima in place. When disease is localized to larger common iliac vessels, this is possible under direct vision. Endarterectomy becomes a suboptimal procedure when atherosclerotic disease extends beyond the bifurcation of the common iliac vessels. Extension of endarterectomy distally into the external iliac artery makes the operation longer and more difficult. It is often technically less satisfactory, because of the more difficult exposure, the small size of the external iliac artery, and adherence of the intima to the more muscular vessel. Distal extension of aortoiliac endarterectomy is associated with a decrease in long-term patency, with the late failure rate climbing 25% at 5 years.[154]

The most common cause of failure after endarterectomy is progression of disease distal to the endarterectomy segment.[148,154,222] It is important to remember, that angiographic evidence or an operative finding of occlusive disease extending beyond the iliac bifurcation favors bypass favors bypass grafting. Moreover, endarterectomy is frankly contraindicated whenever there is evidence of aneurysmal disease, because the endarterectomized vessel is prone to continued aneurysmal degeneration. Similarly, total occlusion of the infrarenal aorta is best handled by simple transection of the aorta within several centimeters of the renal arteries, with thrombectomy of the aorta cuff and subsequent graft insertion. This is more expedient then endarterectomy and is associated with better long-term function.[223]

The follow-up results of aortoiliac endarterectomy, accumulated and tabulated in the same manner as described for the bypass procedure, disclosed a patency rate of 88.8% at the end of the first year of observation. Thereafter, the rate showed deterioration closely comparable to that seen for the bypass operations, namely a deterioration of nearly 3% per year. Again, the 15-year patency rate was just below 50%, and the late cumulative mortality rate was 36.8%.[224]

In one study of 15-year duration of aortoiliac endarterectomy, there was no operative mortality and an early patency rate of approximately 98% with a 66% 15-year patency rate. Limb salvage was 92% and 79% at the fifth and tenth years, respectively.[224]

At the present time, aortoiliac endarterectomy is infrequently used by many vascular surgeons. Most patients have more diffuse disease than is suitable for endarterectomy, and few surgeons practiced in the past few decades have had adequate experience and training to be comfortable and confident with this technique, which is generally acknowledged to be more technically demanding than bypass grafting. Most important, PTA, stents, and other endovascular techniques have evolved, and usually consider this first-line treatment in current practice for the relatively focal aortoiliac occlusive disease,[225–227] formally treatment by endarterectomy. However, the technique of endarterectomy remains an important technical adjunctive in the management of aortoiliac occlusive disease.

Ascending Aortofemoral Bypass. This author has published the first successful case on a 49-year-old male with ischemic symptoms. The study showed an occluded abdominal aorta with abdominal surgery and failed renal bypass, left hemiparesis with possible need for left nephrectomy. Left axillofemoral grafting was not considered to be suitable. Right axillofemoral grafting was not possible because of the right subclavian artery with diffuse disease. This patient underwent a successful, and uneventful ascending aorta–bifemoral bypass[228] (Figures 37-7 and 37-8). Since this publication, we have found patients who require this type of bypass procedure without complications. Others[229] have also reported technique of ascending aortofemoral bypass.

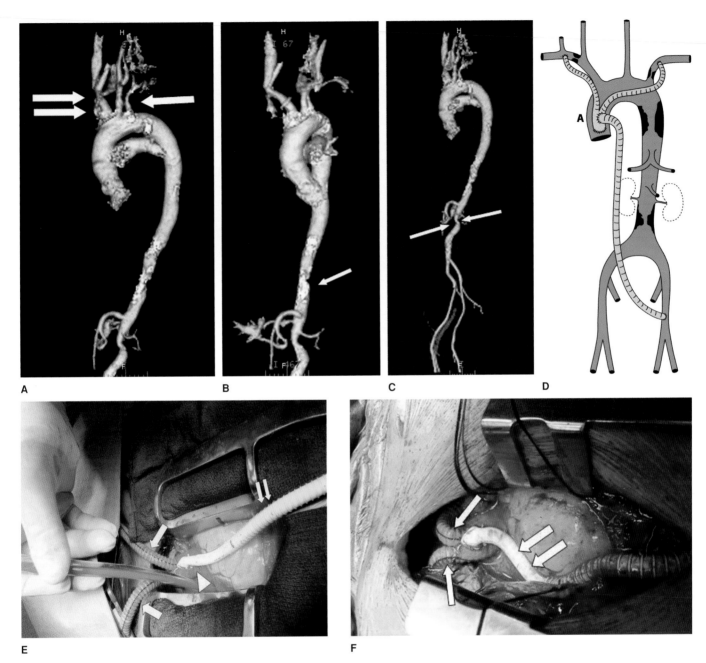

● **FIGURE 37-7.** A 55-year-old female patient who is working as a medical technologist, developed severe ischemic symptoms in the left hand with claudication of the right upper arm, and severe claudication of both lower extremities. Further (A) cardiovascular evaluation including cardiac catheterization and angiogram showed complete occlusion of innominate artery, "*double arrows*" and high-grade stenosis at the left subclavian common artery (*single arrow*). On the aortic pressure measurement, her thoracic aortic pressure measure 230 with right brachial pressure of 90 and left brachial pressure of 80. (B) Further evaluation showed coarctation of the descending thoracic aorta (*arrow*) with a significant pressure gradient above and below on the same patient. (C) The same patient had significant coarctation with heavy calcification at the infrarenal aorta with a further drop of pressure. With this complex multilevel vascular occlusive disease, further careful cardiovascular workup was performed which revealed no evidence of arthritis. (D) Patient underwent complex reconstructive surgery. With a mini sternotomy, the ascending aortobilateral subclavian artery bypass was performed using a No. 18 Hemashield Dacron Y graft. During the same sitting, a 10-mm PTFE graft was anastomosed to the side of the Dacron graft, and was then tunneled under the sternum and peritoneally to the left external iliac artery for distal anastomosis. Following this operation, her blood pressure at the upper extremity with is normal at 120/70 bilaterally, with complete restoration of symptoms (*continued*)

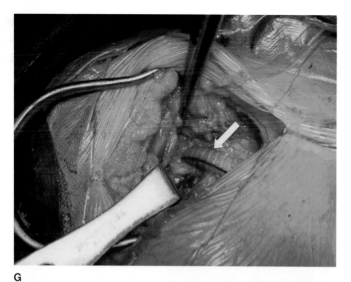

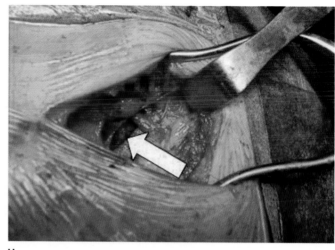

H

G

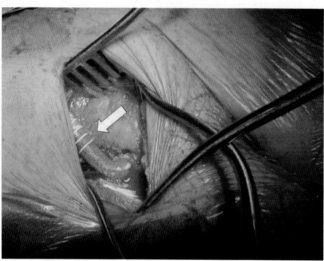

I

● **FIGURE 37-7.** (*Continued*) involving both upper and lower extremities. In this patient, cardiac catheterization showed normal coronary arterial system. (E) Operative picture with upper portion of sternum has been opened and retracted. The patient's head is to the left. Using side-bitting clamp at the ascending aorta end-to-side anastomosis was made between the proximal and the Dacron Y graft and side of ascending aorta (*triangle arrow*). By using this technique, the ascending aorta did not need to be cross-clamped or require cardiac pulmonary bypass. Then the right and left limbs of the Dacron Y graft is extended to bilateral subclavian arteries using second intercostal space. The subclavian arteries are exposed infraclavicularly to lay down the graft naturally. (F) Operative picture showing completion of the surgery in the chest. Two ascending limbs (*arrow*) leading to bilateral subclavian arteries through intercostal spaces. PTFE graft (*double arrows*) leading under the sternum down to left external iliac artery. (G) Operative picture showing distal anastomosis at the left subclavian artery, infraclavicular (*arrow*). (H) Operative picture showing distal anastomosis at the right subclavian artery of the chest (*arrow*). Patient's head is on the left side. (I) Operative picture showing distal anastomosis of PTFE to left external iliac artery (*arrow*). Patient's head is on the left side.

Descending Thoracic Aortofemoral Bypass. In a good surgical risk patient with hostile abdominal condition for standard aortofemoral bypass grafting, this approach is useful with good long-term graft patency.[230,231] The proximal anastomosis can be done at the lower portion of the descending thoracic aorta in end-to-side fashion using partial clamping without the need of total cross-clamping. By do-

ing it this way, renal blood flow is preserved during proximal anastomosis. Then the grafts to both the femoral or iliac arteries, in which some cases the graft can be anastomosed to the ipsilater iliac or femoral artery, and then crossed-over to the contralateral iliac or femoral artery. This is another good alternative method in the treatment of aortoiliac occlusive disease with hostile abdominal condition from

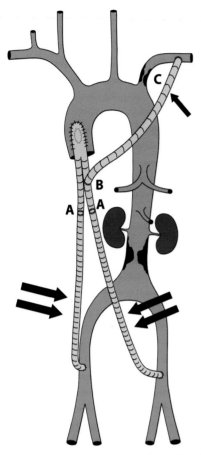

● **FIGURE 37-8.** An artist's sketch of complex reconstructive surgery. A 60-year-old female patient with a history of heaving smoking and COPD had complete occlusion of aortobifemoral bypass graft which was formally inserted at an outside institute. The patient now presented with ischemic symptoms in the lower extremities, in addition to symptomatic left subclavian steal syndrome. These were documented and a duplex scan, MRA, and angiogram (not shown here) were given. After a previous abdominal aortobifemoral bilateral femoral artery bypass, the patient developed a massive wound infection, Bentyl hernia requiring abdominal wall reconstruction and mash. Because of COPD, the left thoracotomy for the descending thoracic aorta, bilateral femoral artery bypass was deemed unwise. Therefore, a mini sternotomy was performed using a side-bitting clamp at the ascending aorta, end-to-side anastomosis was made between proximal end of a No. 18 Hemashield Dacron graft and to the side of aorta. Then the Dacron graft limbs were extended using a No. 8 PTFE graft with rings. This graft was tunneled under the sternum then preperitoneally, subcutaneously down to both femoral artery systems for distal anastomosis. At the same sitting, a bypass graft was extended to the left subclavian artery from the Dacron graft within the chest (*arrow*).

multiple previous procedures, potential sepsis, radiation therapy, abdominal stoma, or other conditions prohibiting the abdominal approach as a safe method.

Extra-Anatomic Bypass.

AXILLOFEMORAL BYPASS: Since 1963, when Blaisdell[232] introduced axillofemoral bypass as an alternative reconstruc-

tive procedure or aortoiliac occlusive disease, a number of techniques have been described. The primary purposes of the extra-anatomic bypasses are to reduce operative risks, to overcome the problem with infection at the primary surgical site, or to achieve other medical and surgical aims. The author and his group have reported their experience with axillofemoral bypass, as a form of extra-anatomic bypass,[233–235] and the current state of extra-anatomic bypass was published in 1986.[236]

This bypass graft is an essential tool in treating infected aorta or prosthetic arterial graft,[237] although alternatives have been proposed even for these patients.[238,239] It is essential that the side of the axillary artery for proximal anastomosis to be checked carefully to be sure that artery has no proximal stenosis. We do an extensive preoperative vascular evaluation to rule out possible proximal disease. In the event there is no proximal disease, we select one side for bypass if blood pressure is higher than the other side. In addition to noninvasive vascular studies, we utilized MRA or CTA for evaluation of aortic arch and proximal arterial trees before final selection of the site for proximal anastomosis.

The author prefers doing axillobifemoral bypass even though ipsilateral ischemic change is predominant with less or mild symptoms on the contralateral side with proximal occlusion. It is our observation that axillobilateral femoral bypass graft has a much better long-term patency, contrary axillounilateral femoral bypass.

A transverse incision is made on the anterior chest wall, approximately two fingerbreadths below the clavicle and parallel to the clavicle. The incision is deepened by sharp and blunt dissection, splitting the pectoris major muscle along the direction of the muscle fibers. The pectoris minor muscle is retracted laterally. Care should be taken to avoid any other injury to the vein or brachial praxis during the dissection and placement of retractors.

We normally use 8-mm-ringed PTFE grafts, with proximal anastomosis is oblique fashion and avoid tension from the shoulder or upper extremity movement. We normally put arms on the side of patient at the time of preparation. Then depending on the condition of the groin, such as previous scars, we sometimes make a transverse incision at the level or slightly above the inguinal ligament to expose fresh artery of proximal common femoral or distal external iliac artery, avoiding dissection at the previously operated on groin.

In a situation where the external iliac artery is exposed, avoiding previous surgical scar and groin, we can use a similar incision on the contralateral side. The graft is tunneled under the pectoris major muscle and along the anterior lateral chest wall to the lower margin of rib cage where the graft is then brought out subcutaneously and along the anterior lateral of the abdominal wall, and medial to the anterior iliac crest into the target vessels, external iliac artery, common femoral artery or deep femoral artery, depending upon the anatomic situation.

If there is disease at the deep femoral artery system, we extend the arteriotomy from the common femoral artery to the deep femoral artery beyond the disease with profundaplasty at the time of anastomosis, with/without necessary endarterectomy of the deep femoral artery system. In the event the distal target vessels are external iliac artery, we make a side-to-side anastomosis at the ipsilateral external iliac artery, and then bring the graft subcutaneous over the pubic bone into contralateral iliac vessel. By using this technique, we minimize the extra number of anastomoses.

In the situation, when ipsilateral femoral anastomosis is extensive, then we take a separate graft in end-to-side fashion to the ipsilateral femoral artery or distal end of the axilla–ipsilateral femoral artery graft. The second piece of the PTFE graft is tunneled over the pubic bone in S- or inverted U-shape to prevent tension. Once the tunnel is made, we use systemic heparin during the vascular procedure, then neutralize with protamine at the end of the vascular anastomosis. The 5-year secondary patency rate was superior for the axillobifemoral grafting compared to axillounifemoral grafting, 74% versus 37% in one series,[240] and similar findings were noted in other studies.[232,233,241]

When axillofemoral bypass grafting was performed for acute vascular occlusion, there was a higher incidence of perioperative complications (63% vs. 26%, $p = 0.001$), perioperative mortality (26% vs. 3%, $p < 0.05$), lower graft patency after 1 year (60% vs. 90%, $p < 0.05$), lower rate of patent from reoperation in the first year (50% vs. 82%, $p < 0.01$), and lower rates of limb salvage (76% vs. 94%, $p < 0.05$) than patients undergoing axillofemoral bypass grafting for chronic symptoms or occlusion. These two groups did not differ in any other risk factors or perioperative characteristics. Therefore, the authors of this study concluded that axillofemoral bypass grafting performed for indications other than acute vascular occlusion is associated with acceptable morbidity, mortality, graft patency, and limb salvage rate.[242]

By the mid to late 1970s, some reports advocated extending these procedures to more patients and in some cases advocated axillofemoral bypass as the procedure of choice for all but the youngest and healthiest of patients when anatomy allowed. Many surgeons were strongly influenced by some favorable results reported.[243–245] But some feel that the favorable experiences reported in these articles may have been as a result of the characteristics of the patients reported and the approach to patency reporting[246] (Figures 37-9 to 37-12).

FEMORAL–FEMORAL ARTERY BYPASS GRAFT: Since Vetto[247] reported in 1962, there have been reports of favorable results.[248–250] The long-term patency rate of this bypass graft was 85% at 5 years and 75% at 10 years in our own series.[236]

With the proper indication and sound surgical technique, this bypass procedure will give optimum results.[247,251–254] To achieve successful results, it is crucial that the patient be evaluated preoperatively with noninvasive vascular and other studies including MRA, CTA, and/or angiographic studies. One of the major contraindications to

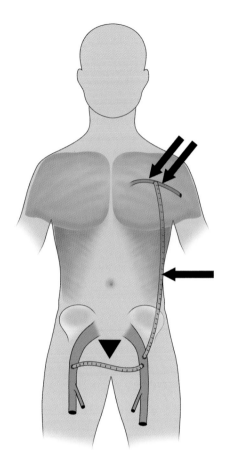

● **FIGURE 37-9.** Artistic drawing for typical left axillo-bilateral femoral artery bypass on virgin territories. Using eight ringed PTFE grafts from left axillary artery to left femoral artery (*arrow*). The anastomosis at the axillary artery needed to be performed in an oblique manner, with the left upper extremity on the side of patient. The graft was then tunneled under the pectoris major muscle, then subcutaneously at the level of the lower rib cage, then subcutaneously down to the femoral artery, anterior to anterior iliac crest. The femoral artery and femoral artery bypass graft is laid subcutaneously above the pubic bone, in SU or inverted U shape, in order to minimize tension and movement of the hip joint (*triangular arrow*). Elderly patients with a high surgical comorbidity developed severe ischemic symptoms and ischemic change in the lower extremities. For this study, we included a MRA, the juxtarenal showed an aortic occlusion (*arrow*). This patient had a stent in the femoral arterial systems, including deep femoral artery and SFA, bilaterally (not shown here).

this procedure used to be stenotic lesion at the donor side of the iliac artery. The new improvements in technology using endovascular procedures, angioplasty and other modalities, some limited cases with extreme high risk, we combine the procedure with an ipsilateral percutaneous or endovascular procedure to correct the proximal disease and use as a donor site for femoral–femoral bypass grafting with successful outcome. Distal extension of the bypass has to be based on the condition of the individual patient. It is advisable to extend distal bypass grafting in multilevel disease with tissue necrosis at the foot. It is our policy to revascularize

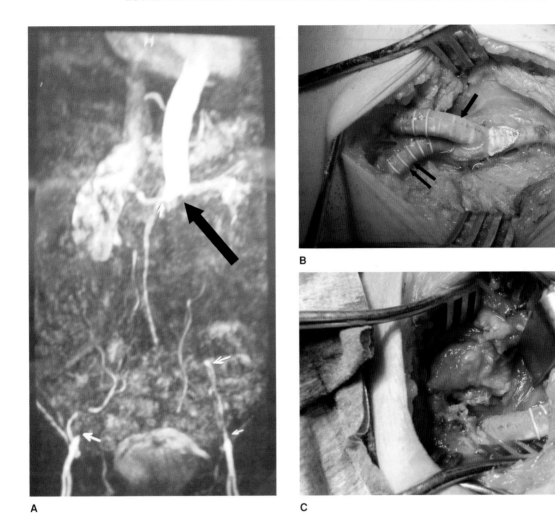

● **FIGURE 37-10.** (A) MRA film showing juxtarenal aortic occlusion (*arrow*), including both iliac arteries. (B) Operative picture showing distal anastomosis of PTFE graft at the femoral artery (*arrow*), which is coming down from the left axillary artery. Then a separate end-to-side anastomosis was made. A proximal or distal on this case, his case proximal, using an 8-mm ringed graft for left-femoral right-femoral bypass (*double arrows*). (C) Operative picture showing end-to-side anastomosis between the distal end of the PTFE graft coming from left femoral artery to the side of the right common femoral artery (*arrow*). Patient's head is on the left hand side. *Note:* The PTFE graft is anastomosed in an oblique fashion since the graft has helped under the tunnel in S-shaped, curving up toward the proximal femoral artery in order to make oblique anastomosis without tension.

in maximum degree for limb salvage purposes in cases with multilevel occlusive process and tissue necrosis.

A tunnel is made subcutaneously over pubic bone in inverted U shape or S shape, in order to prevent tension to the graft on joint movement. Therefore, we avoid straight grafting in T shape (Figure 37-13).

ILIOFEMORAL ARTERY BYPASS GRAFT: Ipsilateral iliofemoral bypass through a retroperitoneal incision maybe preferable to femorofemoral artery bypass if the occlusive disease is limited to the external iliac artery because it can avoid violating the opposite groin and a normal femoral artery.[258] Ipsilateral iliofemoral bypass, with or without distal extension, had been one of the preferred choices in aortoiliac occlusive disease management in our experience.[144]

CONCLUSION: The management of aortoiliac occlusive disease has been challenging for vascular surgeons. With the new technological advances, including endovascular procedures and catheter based endoluminal techniques, and a variety of anatomic and extra-anatomic bypass procedures, the surgeon now has in his armament multiple choices. By understanding alternatives, and careful patient evaluation, we are able to provide safe procedures to individual patients giving proper and a long-term successful outcome with less or least surgical or procedural related morbidity or mortality.

Femoral and Popliteal Occlusive Disease. The patient requiring infrainguinal bypass frequently has medical comorbidities, including coronary artery heart disease,

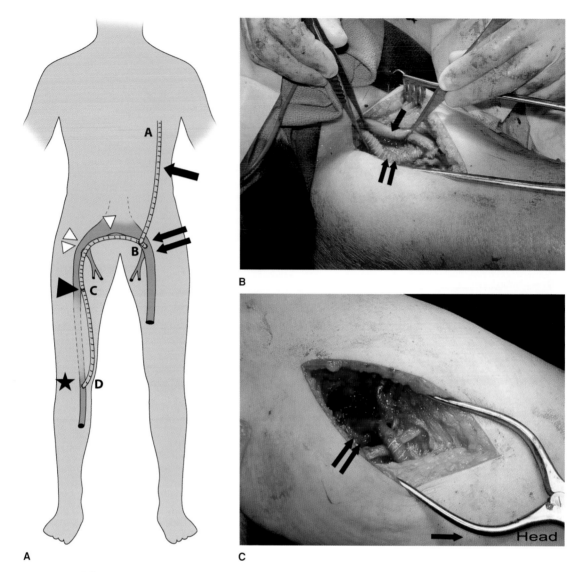

● **FIGURE 37-11.** (A) This drawing illustrates axillobifemoral bypass, with a distal extension to the popliteal artery. This patient had severe ischemic change in right lower extremity with ischemic lesions and severe claudication. Both extremities were disabling. An angiogram confirmed complete occlusion of the infrarenal aorta and bilateral iliac artery system, with an obstruction of the right SFA. Left common femoral artery anastomosis was made with an 8-mm PTFE graft (*double arrows*). The graft was then passed through the tunnel to the right common femoral artery in side-to-side fashion (*double open triangle*). A side-to-side anastomosis was made between the PTFE graft and the right common femoral artery. Then the same PTFE graft was extended further by anastomosing a new 6-mm PTFE graft at point C. When this anastomosis is done between 8-mm and 6-mm PTFE grafts, the anastomosis was made after appropriate spatulation to minimize the size mismatch (*black triangle arrow*). The new 6-mm PTFE graft was extended down to the right above knee popliteal artery for distal anastomosis (D*). The left axillofemoral artery bypass graft was shown as A (*arrow*). (B) On the same patient, end-to-side anastomosis between the descending limb of the left axillofemoral artery bypass graft (*arrow*), and left femoral–right femoral artery bypass graft (*double arrow*). (C) Operative picture of the same patient at the distal anastomosis between the 6-mm PTFE graft and above-knee left popliteal artery (*arrows*). The patient's head is on the right side.

diabetes mellitus, chronic obstructive pulmonary disease, and renal insufficiency. The incidence of perioperative MI ranges from 2% to 6.5% following lower extremity arterial reconstruction; approximately 70% of both perioperative and late mortality in these patients is caused by concomi-tant coronary artery heart disease.[256] In a major study in which preoperative coronary arteriography was performed in 1000 consecutive patients undergoing evaluation for PAD, severe coronary artery heart disease (>70% steno-sis of at least one coronary artery) in 25% of patients and

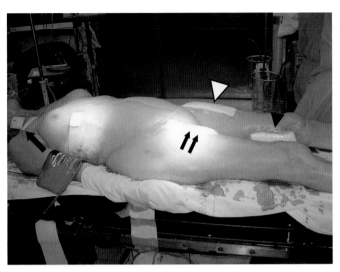

● **FIGURE 37-12.** Typical picture of the completion of right axillo (*arrow*) right femoral artery (*double arrows*), left femoral artery (*open triangle*), left above-knee popliteal artery (*black triangle*), sequential bypass for limb salvage purpose.

severe inoperative coronary artery disease in 6% of such individuals were identified.[257] Similar data has been found by other investigators.[256]

All PAD patients require a detailed history and physical examination as well as a baseline electrocardiogram (ECG). Important risk factors (modified from Detsky,[258] Goldman,[259] and Eagle[260]) to delineate the presence or absence of angina are previous MI, congestive heart failure (CHF), ventricular ectopy requiring treatment, the presence of valvular heart disease; particularly aortic stenosis, and ischemic findings on ECG.

Perioperative blood pressure control, antianginal regimens, and treatment for CHF are optimized, and based on level 1 data,[261] perioperative beta-blockade is employed if there are no contraindications.[262,263] Careful preoperative medical, cardiac, renal, and endocrine evaluations are necessary. In selective cases, invasive coronary intervention should be considered. Chronic limb ischemic patients are best treated with meticulous perioperative medical and cardiac optimization, and expeditious lower extremity reconstruction to minimize perioperative morbidity and mortality, and achieve successful limb revascularization for limb salvage purpose, minimizing amputation risk.

A meta-analysis of femoropopliteal bypass grafts for lower extremity arterial insufficiency, with extensive review of the literature, the background of that study is to analyze the long-term outcome of saphenous vein graft and prosthetic graft materials. Studies published from 1986 through 2004 were identified from electronic databases and references lists; 73 articles contributed one or more series that used survival analysis, assessed femoropopliteal bypasses in one of the foregoing configurations, reported a 1-year graft patency rate, and included at least 30 bypasses. The series with a predominance of claudicant patients were included in meta-analysis C, and the series in which critical ischemia predominated were included in meta-analysis CI. Pooled survival curves of graft patency were constructed.

In the results; in meta-analysis C, the pooled primary graft patency was 57.4% for above-knee PTFE, 77.2% for above-knee vein, and 64.8% for below-knee vein at 5 years; there was a significant difference between above-knee grafts at 3, 4, and 5 year ($p < 0.05$). The corresponding pooled secondary graft patency was 73.2%, 80.1%, and 79.7%,

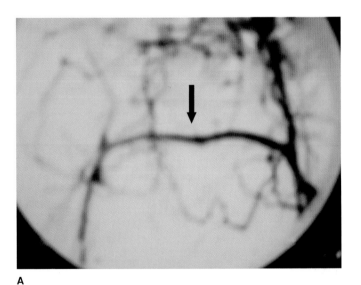

A

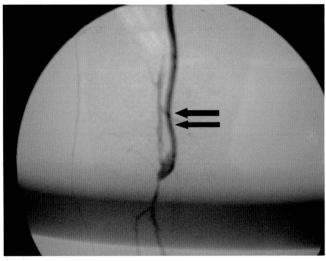

B

● **FIGURE 37-13.** (A) Angiogram showing patent left femoral–right femoral bypass graft 18 years post operatively. (B) Same patient, after 18 years, he developed further ischemic deterioration in the right lower extremity requiring distal bypass to above knee popliteal artery using a PTFE (*double arrow*).

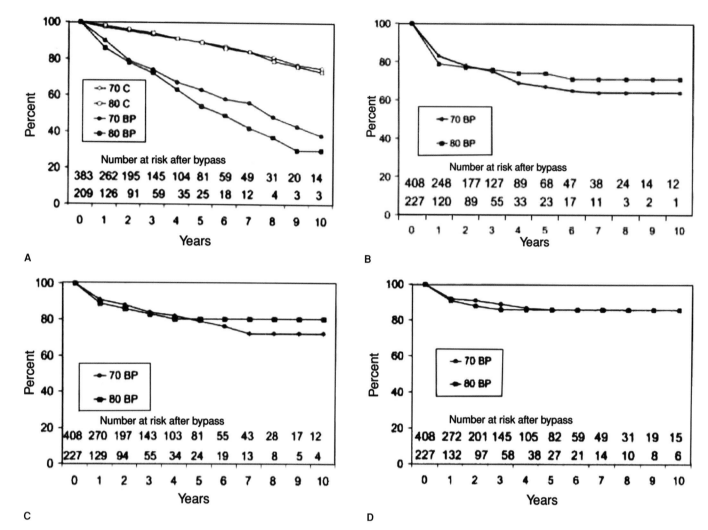

● **FIGURE 37-14.** (A) Cumulative life-table survival after femoropopliteal and femorotibial bypass grafts in 209 octogenarians (80 *BP*) and 383 septuagenarians (70 BP) and of 1514 octogenarian controls (80 C) and 2001 septuagenarian controls who had mild–moderate atherosclerosis and no revascularization. Survival in controls was higher ($p < 0.0001$) compared with either bypass group, or survival among bypass groups was lower ($p < 0.025$) in octogenarians. Number of patients at risk after bypass graft at beginning of each time interval is shown; number of octogenarians listed below number of septuagenarians. (B) Cumulative life-table primary patency rates after femoropopliteal and femorotibial bypass grafts in 227 limbs of 209 octogenarians (80 BP) and 408 limbs of 1383 septuagenarians (70 BP). Number of limbs at risk after bypass graft at beginning of each time interval is shown; number for octogenarians is listed below number for septuagenarians. (C) Cumulative life-table secondary patency rates after femoropopliteal and femorotibial bypass grafts in 227 limbs of 209 octogenarians (80 BP) and 408 limbs of 383 septuagenarians (70 BP). Number of limbs at risk after bypass graft at beginning of each time interval is shown; number for octogenarians is listed below number for septuagenarians. (D) Cumulative life-table limb salvage rates after femoropopliteal and femorotibial bypass grafts in 227 limbs of 209 octogenarians (80 BP) and 408 limbs of 383 septuagenarians (70 BP). Number of limbs at risk after bypass graft at beginning of each time interval is shown; number for octogenarians is listed below number for septuagenarians.

Reproduced with permission from Chang JB, Stein TA. Infrainguinal revascularizations in octogenarians and septuagenarians. J Vasc Surg. 2001;34:133-138.

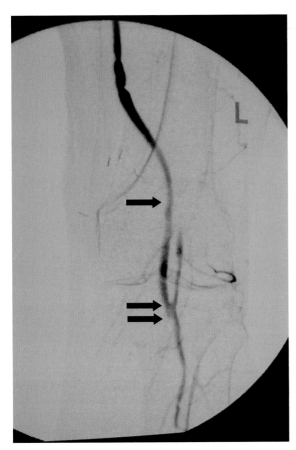

● **FIGURE 37-15.** An angiogram showing patent left femoral–popliteal vein graft after 5 years (*arrow*). Double arrows are at the distal anastomosis.

respectively ($p > 0.05$). In meta-analysis CI, the pooled primary graft patency was 48.3% for above-knee PTFE, 69.4% for above-knee vein, and 68.9% for below-knee vein at 5 years; there was a significant difference between above-knee grafts until 4 years ($p < 0.05$). The corresponding pooled secondary graft patency was 54.0%, 71.9%, and 77.8%, respectively, with a significant difference above-knee grafts at 2, 3, and 4 years ($p < 0.05$).

In conclusion, the great saphenous vein performs better than PTFE in femoropopliteal bypass grafting and should be used whenever possible.[264] Furthermore, the absence of suitable saphenous vein remains and acceptable invitation for above-knee PTFE, at least until the potential of other alternatives are fully established.

One of another alternative, peripheral atherectomy can achieve good early clinical and hemodynamic success in patients with TASC C lesions and CLI. However, midterm restenosis rates are high in this challenging cohort of patients.[265] We have determined the long-term efficacy of composite grafts, autogenous vein grafts, and PTFE grafts for limb salvage. Between 1975 and July 1998, 781 patients had 1025 arterial revascularization procedures, with the proximal anastomosis at the femoral artery level and the distal anastomosis below the knee. Patients were followed from 0 to 16 years. More than one bypass was performed in 19.7% of the patients. There were 52 femoropopliteal com-

posite graft bypasses in 50 patients, 279 femoropopliteal greater saphenous vein graft bypasses in 258 patients, and 186 femoropopliteal PTFE graft bypasses in 165 patients. There were also 135 femorotibial composite graft bypasses in 113 patients, 337 femorotibial greater saphenous vein graft bypasses in 313 patients, and 36 femorotibial PTFE graft bypasses in 36 patients. In most patients, the greater saphenous vein was used for initial bypasses.[264] When the vein could not be used, PTFE grafts were the second choice for femoropopliteal bypasses and composite grafts were the second choice for femorotibial bypasses. Patients who required multiple bypasses had composite sequential bypass grafts to bridge occlusions.

All patients had ischemic rest pain and some also had gangrene and/or ischemic ulcers. Claudication only was not considered an indication for a bypass procedure. Surgery was indicated by a limb-threatening ischemia and was determined by the criteria of the Society for Vascular Surgery and the International Society for Cardiovascular Surgery.[267] Before operation, patients had Doppler spectral images determined at all levels, pulse volume recordings, and segmental pressure measurements to determine the site of occlusion. The mean ankle–brachial systolic pressure index was <0.4. Some patients with diabetes had incompressible arteries, and at metatarsal and toe pressures, pulse volume recordings were obtained to determine the severity of the disease. The coexistence of other vascular diseases such carotid artery disease, aortoiliac disease, and aneurysmal disease was determined by Doppler and duplex scans. Conventional angiography or digital subtraction angiography was used to determine the distal runoff to the foot. Magnetic resonance angiography has also been suggested in the literature for the preoperative evaluation of these patients.[268,269]

Femoropopliteal Artery Bypass. The first choice for a graft was the greater saphenous vein. Reverse greater saphenous vein segments were used for most (72%) vein femoropopliteal procedures and the in situ greater saphenous vein for others. After the location of the occlusion was determined, the SFA and deep femoral artery should be evaluated for the inflow source. The common femoral artery should be considered when these arteries are inadequate, and the iliac artery may even be used if necessary. The great saphenous vein was anastomosed to the donor artery end-to-side in pure vein grafts and with composite grafts; PTFE was used for femoropopliteal bypasses only when distal runoff was good. The size of the PTFE graft was selected on the basis of the distal runoff and the size of the donor and receiving arteries. Although PTFE sizes ranged from 6 to 10 mm, the most common size was 6 mm. A tunnel was made along Hunter's canal, and the graft was pulled through which is to be anastomosed to the popliteal artery. Patients with occlusive disease in the SFA with limited runoff at the remaining popliteal segment from thrombosis had a thrombectomy and thrombolysis therapy with urokinase or sometimes streptokinase before completion of the bypass procedure.

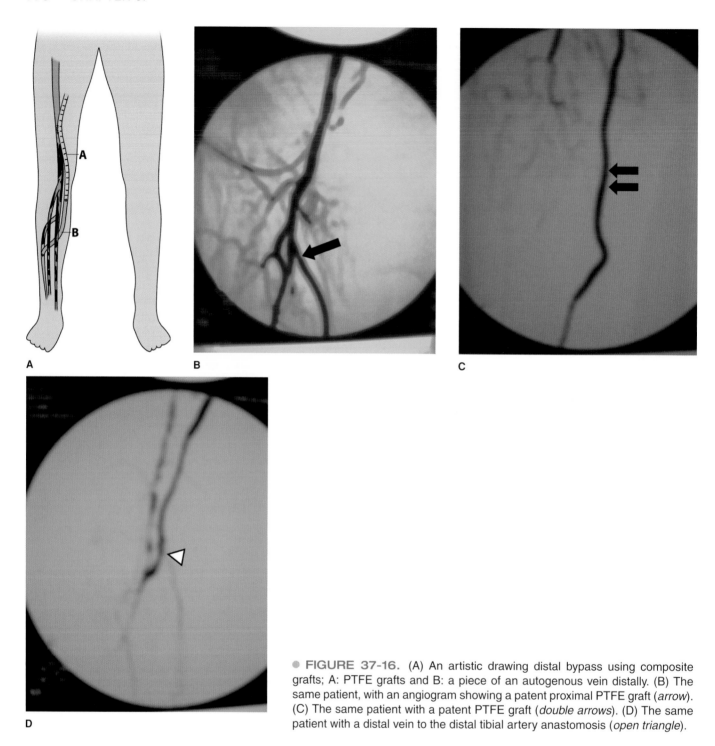

● **FIGURE 37-16.** (A) An artistic drawing distal bypass using composite grafts; A: PTFE grafts and B: a piece of an autogenous vein distally. (B) The same patient, with an angiogram showing a patent proximal PTFE graft (*arrow*). (C) The same patient with a patent PTFE graft (*double arrows*). (D) The same patient with a distal vein to the distal tibial artery anastomosis (*open triangle*).

Femorotibial Artery Bypass. The best choice for the femorotibial bypass graft is also the autogenous greater saphenous vein. The in situ greater saphenous vein was used for most (68%) of our vein femorotibial grafts. An end-to-side anastomosis was made between the graft and the best inflow artery. The conventional femorotibial bypass graft was usually passed through a subcutaneous tunnel and the distal graft was anastomosed to a tibial artery with good runoff. For these long distal bypasses, the greater saphenous vein is frequently unavailable for the entire length,

and a composite graft is constructed of a proximal segment of the greater saphenous vein to a distal segment of PTFE. Femorotibial bypasses with PTFE alone were performed only as a last resort to prevent amputation, because these grafts have had poor long-term results[270] (Figure 37-14).

Profundaplasty. The profunda femoral artery in this situation with SFA, popliteal artery, or both are severely diseased or occluded, serves as the primary collateral channel from the iliac and common femoral artery to the distal extremity.

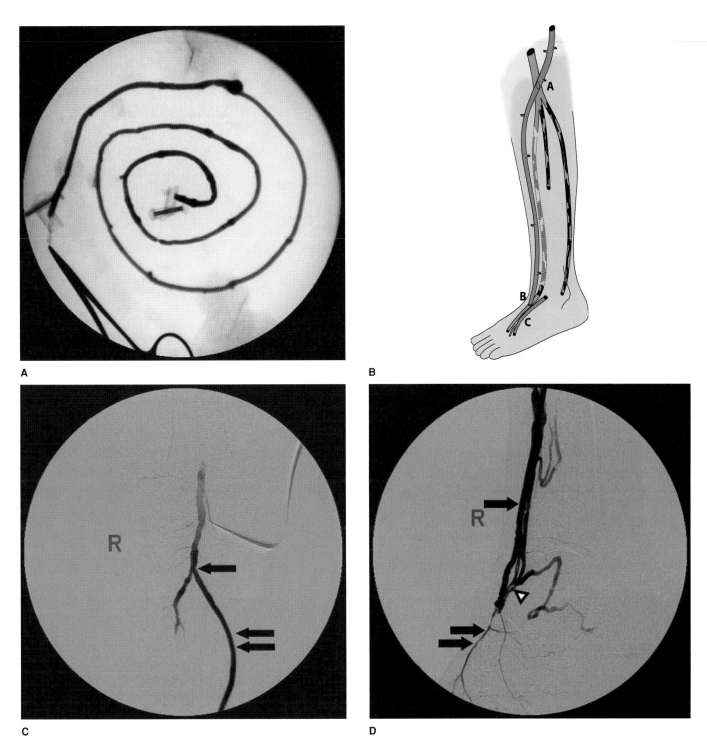

● **FIGURE 37-17.** (A) This is an ex vivo angiogram of a harvested left greater saphenous vein. We have begun using an ex vivo angiogram of the harvested vein graft for examination of the integrity of the vein graft before implanting it into the patient. In this particular patient, an elderly lady, who had multiple bypasses in the past, and which failed and resulted in severe ischemic change in the right foot, with poor distal runoff. She also developed a gangrenous left foot with ischemic rest pain. Because of the previous surgeries on the right lower extremity several times, she does not have an autogenous vein in the right lower extremity. Therefore, the entirely of the left greater saphenous vein was harvested for simultaneous distal bypass in both limbs. (B) Artistic drawing showing bypass distally after dorsalis pedis artery (**B**) with the creation of distal AV fistula (**C**), between distal DPA and DPV, in order to increase distal flow. (C) Completion angiogram showing proximal anastomosis at the right popliteal artery (*arrow*) with a patent vein graft (*double arrow*). (D) Completion angiogram showing patent vein graft (*arrow*), DPA (*double arrows*), DPV (*open triangle*), reverse filling into vein system from distal AVF. (*continued*)

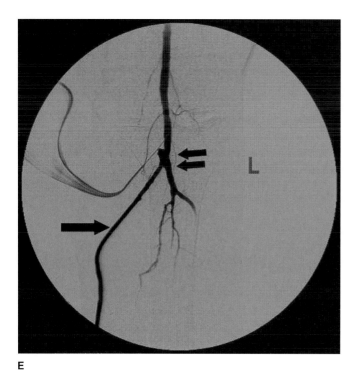

E

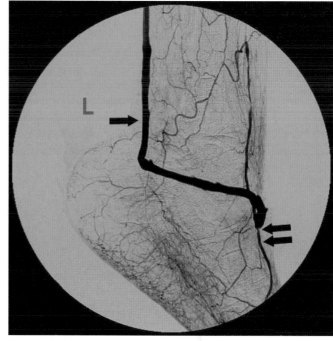

F

● **FIGURE 37-17.** (*Continued*) (E) Completion angiogram of the same patient, at the same sitting, showing proximal anastomosis between the left popliteal artery (*double arrow*), and the remaining vein graft (*arrow*), which is patent. (F) Completion angiogram of the same patient showing patent left popliteal-left DPA bypass graft (*arrow*), with a patent distal anastomosis at the DPA (*double arrows*).

Profundaplasty has proven to be an effective alternative to distal bypass in some selected patients with critical ischemia.[271,272] Most common use of profundaplasty in our practice is in combination to distal bypass and/or in conjunction with aortofemoral reconstruction.

Exposure. A standard vertical groin incision is made for common femoral artery exposure. The common femoral artery is exposed at the level of the inguinal ligament. Distal dissection is carried out to expose the proximal SFA. Then the SFA is gently retracts medially using vessel loops. At the point of origin of SFA and reduced diameter of distal common femoral artery, the profunda femoral artery originates slightly posteriorly and laterally to SFA. Further distal dissection can be carried out along the anterior surface of the profunda femoral artery, ligating and dividing the crossing-over vein branches. Care should be taken to preserve side branches of the profunda femoral artery. Careful dissection can be carried out further distally, beyond the point of the diseased endpoint. The profundaplasty then can be carried out using a vein patch, prosthetic patch, or part of on-lay patch anastomosis or proximal or distal destiny of that anastomosis. This could be a vessel anastomosis from proximal arterial source or could be proximal anastomosis from the distal bypass purpose[273-275] (Figures 37-15 to 37-17).

We have reported on infrainguinal revascularization in octogenarians and septuagenarians. Death and cardiovascular events are higher after revascularization in octogenarians

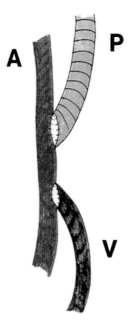

● **FIGURE 37-18.** Composite graft with the patent segment of an artery (**A**) interposed between the proximal PTFE grafts (**P**) and the distal vein graft (**V**).

Reproduced with permission from Chang JB, Stein TA. Composite graphs for limb salvage. In: Chang JB, ed. Textbook of Angiology. New York, NY: Springer; 2000:835-845.

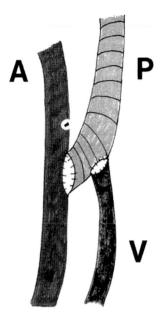

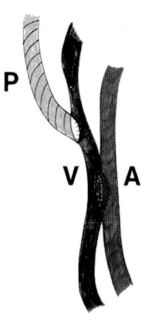

● **FIGURE 37-19.** Composite graft with the proximal PTFE graft (**P**) anastomosed to a short, patent segment of an artery (**A**) and the distal vein graft (**V**) anastomosed to the distal portion of the PTFE graft.

Reproduced with permission from Chang JB, Stein TA. Composite graphs for limb salvage. In: Chang JB, ed. Textbook of Angiology. New York, NY: Springer; 2000:835-845.

● **FIGURE 37-21.** Composite graft with a proximal PTFE graft (**P**) anastomosed end to side to a tibial vein (**V**) distally the vein is anastomosed side to side to the tibial artery (**A**).

Reproduced with permission from Chang JB, Stein TA. Composite graphs for limb salvage. In: Chang JB, ed. Textbook of Angiology. New York, NY: Springer; 2000:835-845.

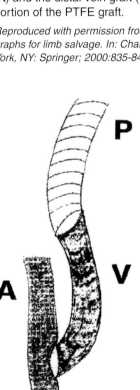

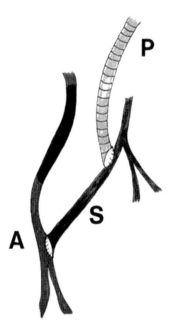

● **FIGURE 37-20.** Composite graft with a single distal anastomosis into the artery (**A**). The proximal PTFE graft (**P**) is anastomosed end to end to the vein graft (**V**).

Reproduced with permission from Chang JB, Stein TA. Composite graphs for limb salvage. In: Chang JB, ed. Textbook of Angiology. New York, NY: Springer; 2000:835-845.

● **FIGURE 37-22.** Composite graft utilizing an in situ segment of a saphenous vein (**S**) remnant to receive the proximal PTFE graft (**P**) and for a distal end-to-side anastomosis with a tibial artery (**A**).

Reproduced with permission from Chang JB, Stein TA. Composite graphs for limb salvage. In: Chang JB, ed. Textbook of Angiology. New York, NY: Springer; 2000:835-845.

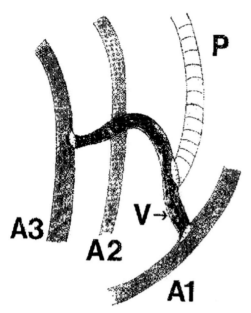

● **FIGURE 37-23.** Multiple sequential composite graft with a proximal PTFE graft (**P**) anastomosed end to side to a vein graft (**V**) that has the proximal end anastomosed to the posterior tibial artery (**A1**), the middle segment anastomosed side to side to the peroneal artery (**A2**), and the distal end anastomosed to the side of the anterior tibial artery (**A3**).

Reproduced with permission from Chang JB, Stein TA. Composite graphs for limb salvage. In: Chang JB, ed. Textbook of Angiology. New York, NY: Springer; 2000:835-845.

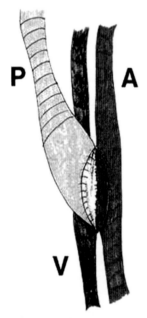

● **FIGURE 37-24.** Composite graft with the proximal PTFE graft (**P**) comprising the anterior wall of the anastomosis with the tibial artery (**A**) and the tibial vein (**V**) and a side-to-side anastomosis between the posterior walls of the artery and vein.

Reproduced with permission from Chang JB, Stein TA. Composite graphs for limb salvage. In: Chang JB, ed. Textbook of Angiology. New York, NY: Springer; 2000:835-845.

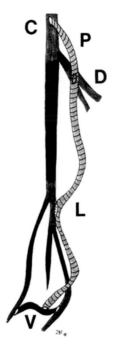

● **FIGURE 37-25.** Multiple sequential composite graft with the PTFE graft (**P**) having a proximal anastomosis with the common femoral artery (**C**), a side-to-side anastomosis with the deep femoral artery (**D**), a side-to-side anastomosis with the distal popliteal artery (**L**) and a terminal end-to-side anastomosis with a short segment of vein graft (**V**).

Reproduced with permission from Chang JB, Stein TA. Composite graphs for limb salvage. In: Chang JB, ed. Textbook of Angiology. New York, NY: Springer; 2000:835-845.

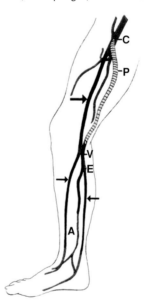

● **FIGURE 37-26.** Diagram showing the presence of occlusions (*arrows*) in the arterial system and location of the composite bypass graft. A PTFE graft (**P**) extends from the common femoral artery (**C**) and is anastomosed end to end to a vein graft (**V**) that has been used to form an angioplasty graft after an extended endarterectomy (**E**) of the popliteal artery (**A**), tibioperoneal trunk, and A: peroneal artery.

Reproduced with permission from Chang JB, Stein TA. Composite graphs for limb salvage. In: Chang JB, ed. Textbook of Angiology. New York, NY: Springer; 2000:835-845.

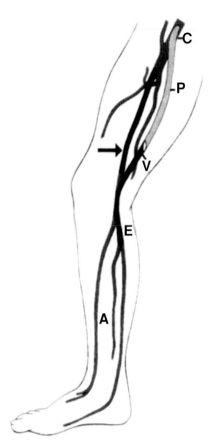

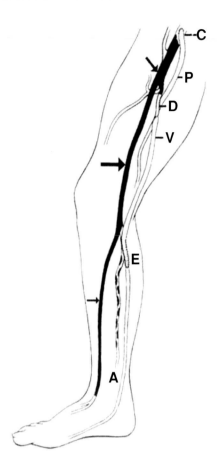

● **FIGURE 37-27.** Diagram showing the presence of occlusion (*arrow*) in the arterial system and location of the composite bypass graft. The distal end of a PTFE graft (**P**) extends from the common femoral artery (**C**) and is anastomosed end to end to the proximal end of a vein graft (**V**) whose distal end has been used for an angioplasty patch after an extended endarterectomy (**E**) to the proximal tibial arteries (**A**).

Reproduced with permission from Chang JB, Stein TA. Composite graphs for limb salvage. In: Chang JB, ed. Textbook of Angiology. New York, NY: Springer; 2000:835-845.

● **FIGURE 37-28.** Diagram showing the presence of occlusions (*arrows*) in the arterial system and location of the composite bypass graft. A PTFE graft (**P**) extends from the common femoral artery (**C**) and is anastomosed end to side to the deep femoral artery (**D**). A vein graft (**V**) extends from the deep femoral artery to form an angioplasty graft after an extended endarterectomy (**E**) of the popliteal artery, tibioperoneal trunk, and posterior tibial artery (**A**).

Reproduced with permission from Chang JB, Stein TA. Composite graphs for limb salvage. In: Chang JB, ed. Textbook of Angiology. New York, NY: Springer; 2000:835-845.

and septuagenarians, compared with controls, are related to the severity of arteriosclerosis and not age. Patency rates are excellent and similar. Limb salvage procedure should be considered for most octogenarians, as concluded in that study.[276]

We have analyzed the long-term value of composite graft for limb salvage. The 8-year primary and secondary patency rates were 56% and 62% for femoropopliteal procedures with composite grafts, respectively, and 53% and 59% for autogenous vein grafts, respectively. The secondary patency rate for PTFE was 35% and was less ($p < 0.05$) than the rate for vein grafts. Secondary patency rates for femorotibial procedures were 66% for the vein grafts, 56% for single outflow composite grafts, and 52% for dual outflow composite grafts. Limb salvage rates for femoropopliteal procedures were 73% for composite grafts, 63% for PTFE, and 82% vein grafts, and for femorotibial procedures were 53% for single outflow composite grafts, 65% dual outflow composite grafts, and 86% for vein grafts. In that study, we concluded

that composite grafts achieve long-term preservation of ischemic limbs in patients who are facing limb loss because of poor runoff and insufficient autogenous vein for graft.[277]

A multicenter randomized perspective trial compared a precuffed PTFE graft to vein cuffed PTFE for infrainguinal arterial bypass. This study showed similar primary and secondary graft patency and limb salvage rate with use of precuffed ePTFE grafts or a vein cuffed PTFE grafts for infragenicular arterial bypasses. This clinical experience lends more support to the concept anastomotic engineering; the distal graft geometric configuration may have a protective effect by decreasing anastomotic intimal hyperplasia. However, as they concluded, clearly further clinical experience with a larger number of patients and longer follow-up is required to better access the true benefit precuffed grafts.[278] Reasonable patency with femoropopliteal and femorodistal bypass with vein graft has been established in our early studies.[279]

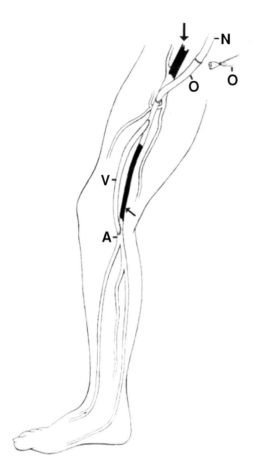

● **FIGURE 37-29.** Diagram showing the presence of occlusions (*arrows*) in the arterial system and location of the composite bypass graft. Occluded graft (**O**) is ligated and divided, and a new graft (**N**) is anastomosed to the thrombectomized endo of the old graft. A vein graft (**V**) is then anastomosed proximally to the patent portion of the SFA and distally to the distal portion of the popliteal artery (**A**).

Reproduced with permission from Chang JB, Stein TA. Composite graphs for limb salvage. In: Chang JB, ed. Textbook of Angiology. New York, NY: Springer; 2000:835-845.

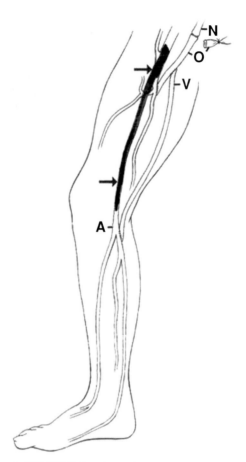

● **FIGURE 37-30.** Diagram showing the presence of occlusions (*arrows*) in the arterial system and location of the composite bypass graft. An occluded graft (**O**) is ligated and divided. A new graft (**N**) is anastomosed to the thrombectomized end of the old graft. A vein graft (**V**) is then anastomosed proximally to the distal portion of the graft and distally to the distal portion of popliteal artery (**A**).

Reproduced with permission from Chang JB, Stein TA. Composite graphs for limb salvage. In: Chang JB, ed. Textbook of Angiology. New York, NY: Springer; 2000:835-845.

Development of pseudoaneurysm in our observation was rare.[280] In a large series, anastomotic pseudoaneurysm was reported to be 1.7%, and the most common cause was the structural deficiency of the host artery. Other factors were arterial hypertension, mechanical stress, defective graft material, noninfective healing complications, possibly endarterectomy as a factor weakening the arterial wall and suture defect.[281]

To determine the functional outcome after revascularization for CLI and the analysis of 1000 consecutive interventions were accessed. In conclusion, the functional outcome for patients undergoing intervention for CLI is not solely determined by the traditional measures of reconstruction patency and limb salvage, but also by intrinsic patient comorbidities at the time of presentation. These findings question the benefit of our current approach to CLI and functionally impaired, chronically ill patients; patients

who undoubtedly will be more prevalent as our population ages.[282]

A multicenter, randomized trial of edifoligide for the prevention of vein graft failure in lower extremity bypass surgery was performed. In this prospective, randomized, placebo-controlled clinical trial, ex vivo treatment of the lower extremity vein grafts with edifoligide did not confer protection from reintervention for graft failure.[283]

In conclusion of this study, this prospective randomized clinical trail failed to demonstrate a reduction in vein graft failure in CLI patients treated with a single ex vivo administration of a normal molecular agent, edifoligide. Although the primary result were disappointing, PREVENT III has demonstrated that large multicenter trials of intraoperative genetic intervention designed to moderate the vascular injury response can be executed safely with high surgical and scientific quality. It is hoped that future investigators informed by the design and outcome of this study, will continue to explore targeted molecular

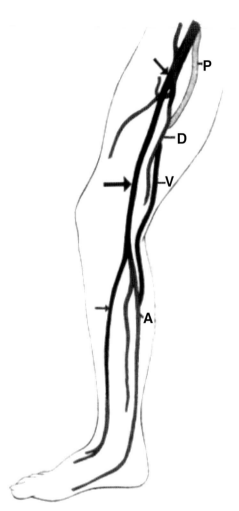

● **FIGURE 37-31.** Diagram showing the presence of occlusions (*arrows*) in the arterial system and location of the composite bypass graft. A PTFE graft (**P**) is anastomosed to the deep femoral artery (**D**), and a vein graft (**V**) extends from the deep femoral artery to the posterior tibial artery (**A**).

Reproduced with permission from Chang JB, Stein TA. Composite graphs for limb salvage. In: Chang JB, ed. Textbook of Angiology. New York, NY: Springer; 2000:835-845.

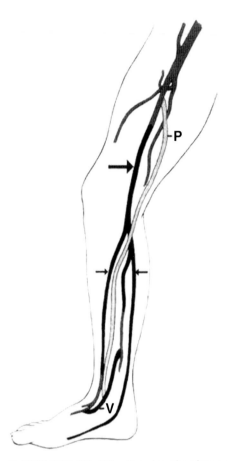

● **FIGURE 37-32.** Drawing showing a composite graft. This type of patient had multiple bypasses in the past with no available vein. Furthermore, the patient had extremely poor distal runoff. Thus, many times we use composite grafts, which consist of PTFE graft (**P**) and autogenous vein (**A**), from the legs or arms.

Reproduced with permission from Chang JB, Stein TA. Composite graphs for limb salvage. In: Chang JB, ed. Textbook of Angiology. New York, NY: Springer; 2000:835-845.

therapies to improve outcomes for patients undergoing vascular reconstruction.[283]

A comparative analysis of autogenous infrainguinal bypass graft in African Americans and Caucasians concluded that autogenous infrainguinal bypass surgery in African Americans is associated with poor primary graft patency and limb salvage rate, compared with those of Caucasians. This may partially account for the higher rate of limb loss in African Americans with arterial occlusive disease.[284]

Crural artery revascularization reduces the number of primary amputation by 50%. Literature data state that crural and pedal artery revascularization is a feasible, effective, and durable procedure. Revascularization therefore, is more cost-effective than primary amputation for the management of advanced limb ischemia.[285]

In a meta-analysis of popliteal-to-distal vein bypass graft for critical ischemia, the conclusion was the popliteal to

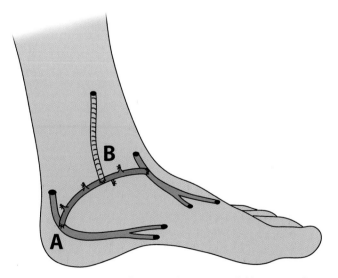

● **FIGURE 37-33.** Compression sequential bypass using arm vein from PTA (**A**) to DPA (**B**), then PTFE graft into the midportion of the arm vein, making the sequential bypass technique.

distal vein is a tool of high efficiency in the treatment of severe, chronic, critical ischemia in the lower extremity. In that study, the 5-year pooled estimate ± standard error was 63.1% ± 4.3% for primary patency, 70.7% ± 4.6% for secondary patency, and 77.7% ± 4.3% for foot preservation. There was a superiority trend favoring reversed vein graft and tibial bypass that became more apparent in sensitivity analysis. No publication bias was detected. Cost-utility analysis of treating severe PAOD has been reported.[286]

In practice, the therapy of PAOD always consists of a multiplicity of interventions that should work curing mortality, because the patients are acutely threatened. The question is how far this model represents reality. In judging this aspect, the calculated life expectancy of patients aged between 65 and 75 years, who were included into the model as a hypothetical cohort, and the real epidemiological data can be compared. Ten years after reconstructing the femoropopliteal vessel segment, 95% of the patients

with PAOD in Stage IV died as well as 80% in Stage 3.[287] The model calculation shows that approximately 80% of the patients died within the treatment strategies with bypass as the initial measure. The other treatment strategies, the modality probabilities are approximately between 85% and 95%. A study from Finland shows the average life expectancy after arterial reconstruction is 4.2 years.[288] The calculation with model variation leads to value between 4.44 and 4.70 years according to the selection of the second line therapy. Despite the different information in epidemiological studies, these comparisons can be regarded as signs that realistic assumptions about the transition probabilities met in the model. The comparison of the results with other model calculations referring to PAOD is difficult.[289–292] For a better estimation of treatment cost and impact on quality of life of the different therapy options for patients with PAOD, further comparative data must be collected. The presented analysis suggests the inclusion of conservative treatment in future research[286] (Figures 37.18 to 37.33).

REFERENCES

1. Johnston KW. Management of chronic ischemia of the lower extremities. In: Rutherford RB, ed. *Vascular Surgery*. 6th ed. Philadelphia, PA: Elsevier Saunders; 2005;1077-1082.

2. Rutgers D, Meijer WT, Hoes AW, et al. Prevalentie van perifere arteriële vaatziekte en claudicatio intermittens bij personen van 55 jaar en ouder: het ERGO-onderzoek. *NTVG* 1988;142:2851-2856.

3. Hooi JD, Kester AD, Stoffers HE, et al. Incidence of and risk factors for asymptomatic peripheral arterial disease: a longitudinal study. *Am J Epidemiol*. 2001;153:666-672.

4. Stoffers HEJH, Rinkens PELM, Kester ADM, et al. The prevalence of asymptomatic and unrecognized peripheral arterial occlusive disease. *Int J Epidemiol*. 1996;25:282-290.

5. McDermott MM, Mehta S, Greenland P. Exertional leg symptoms other than intermittent claudication are common in peripheral arterial disease. *Arch Intern Med*. 1999; 159:387-392.

6. Kannel WB, McGee DL. Update on some epidemiological features of intermittent claudication. *J Am Geriatr Soc*. 1985;33:13-18.

7. Hooi JD, Stoffers HEJH, Knotterus JA, et al. The prognosis of non-critical limb ischemia: A systemic preview of population-based evidence. *Br J Gen Prac*. 1999;49:49-55.

8. Catalano M. Epidemiology of critical limb ischemia: Northern Italian data. *Eur J Med*. 1993;2:11-14.

9. Ebskov L, Schroeder T, Holstein P. Epidemiology of leg amputation: the influence of vascular surgery. *Br J Surg*. 1994;81:1600-1603.

10. Dormandy JA, Rutherford RB. Management of peripheral arterial disease. TASC Working Group. Trans-Atlantic Inter-Society Consensus (TASC). *J Vasc Surg*. 2000;31:S1-S296.

11. Dormandy JA, Heeck L, Vig S. The natural history of claudication: risk to life and limb. *Semin Vasc Surg*. 1999;12:123-137.

12. Aquino R, Johnnides C, Makaroun M, et al. Natural history of claudication: long-term serial follow-up study of 1244 claudicants. *J Vasc Surg*. 2001;34:962-970.

13. Hooi JD, Stoffers HE, Kester AD, et al. Peripheral arterial occlusive disease: prognostic value of signs, symptoms, and the ankle–brachial pressure index. *Med Decis Making*. 2002;22:99-107.

14. Kornitzer M, Dramaix M, Sobolski J, et al. Ankle/arm pressure index in asymptomatic middle-aged males: an independent predictor of ten-year coronary heart disease mortally. *Angiology*. 1995;46:211-219.

15. Leng GC, Lee AJ, Fowkes FGR, et al. Incidence, natural history and cardiovascular events in symptomatic and asymptomatic peripheral arterial disease in the general population. *Int J Epidemiol*. 1996;25:1172-1181.

16. Willigendael EM, Teijink JAW, Bartelink MEL, et al. Influence of smoking on incidence and prevalence of peripheral arterial disease. *J Vasc Surg*. 2004;40:1158-1165.

17. Quick CRG, Cotton LT. The measured effect of stopping smoking on intermittent claudication. *Br J Surg*. 1982; 69:S24-S26.

18. Jonason T, Bergstron R. Cessation of smoking in patients with intermittent claudication. *Acta Med Scan*. 1987;221:253-260.

19. Girolami B, Bernardi E, Prins MH, et al. Treatment of intermittent claudication with physical training, smoking cessation, pentoxifylline, or nafronyl: a meta-analysis. *Arch Intern Med*. 1999;159:337-345.

20. Gey DC, Lesho EP, Manngold J. Management of peripheral arterial disease. *Am Fam Phys*. 2004;69:525-532.

21. Fiore MC, Smith SS, Jorenby De, et al. The effectiveness of the nicotine patch for smoking cessation: a meta-analysis. *JAMA*. 1994;271:1940-1947.

22. Hays JT, Croghan IT, Schroeder DR, et al. Over-the-counter nicotine patch therapy for smoking cessation: results from

a randomized, double-blind, placebo-controlled, and open label trials. *Am J Public Health*. 1999;89:1701-1707.

23. Joseph AM, Norman SM, Ferry LH, et al. The safety of transdermal nicotine as an aid to smoking cessation in patients with cardiac disease. *New Eng J Med*. 1996;335:1792-1798.

24. Silagy C, Lancaster T, Stead L, et al. Nicotine replacement therapy for smoking cessation.*Cochrane Database Syst Rev*. 2004;(3):CD000146. doi: 10.1002/14651858.CD000146.

25. Fiore M. *Treating Tobacco Use and Dependence*. Rockville MD: US Dept of Health and Human Services, Public Health Service; 2000.

26. Lancaster T, Stead LF. Individual behavioural counselling for smoking cessation. *Cochrane Database Syst Rev*. 2002;(3):CD001007. doi: 10.1002/14651858.CD001292.

27. Stead LF, Lancaster T. Group behaviour therapy programmes for smoking cessation.*Cochrane Database Syst Rev*. 2002;(2):CD001007. doi: 10.1002.14651858.CD001007.

28. Power L, Brown NS, Makin GS. Unsuccessful outpatient counseling to help patients with peripheral vascular disease to stop smoking. *Ann Royal Coll Surg Engl*. 1992;74:31-34.

29. Jorenby DE, Leischow SJ, Nides MA, et al. A controlled trial of sustained-release bupropion, a nicotine patch, or both for smoking cessation. *N Engl J Med*. 1999;340:685-691.

30. Abbot NC, Stead LF, White AR, et al. Hypnotherapy for smoking cessation.*Cochrane Database Syst Rev*. 1998;(2):CD001008. doi: 10.1002/14651858.CD001008.

31. Hajek P, Stead LF. Aversive smoking for smoking cessation.*Cochrane Database Syst Rev*. 2004;(3):CD000546. doi: 101002/14651858.CD000546.

32. White AR, Rampes H, Ernst E. Acupuncture for smoking cessation. *Cochrane Database Syst Rev*. 2002;(2): CD000009. doi: 10.1002/14651858.CD000009.

33. Anonymous. The sixth report of the Joint National Committee on Prevention, Detection, Evaluation and Treatment of High Blood Pressure. *Arch Intern Med*. 1997;157:2413-2446.

34. Doyle J, Creager MA. Pharmacotherapy and behavioural interventions for peripheral arterial disease. *Rev Cardiovasc Med*. 2003;4:18-24.

35. Roberts DH, Tsao Y, Linge K, et al. Double-blind comparison of captopril with nifedipine in hypertension complicated by intermittent claudication. *Angiology*. 1992;43:748-756.

36. Roberts DH, Tsao Y, McLoughlin GA, et al. Placebo-controlled comparison of captopril, atenolol, labetalol, and pindolol in hypertension complicated by intermittent claudication. *Lancet*. 1987;2:650-653.

37. Heintzen MP, Strauer BE. Peripheral vascular effects of beta-blockers. *Eur Heart J*. 1994;15:2-7.

38. Lip GYH, Makin AJ. Treatment of hypertension in peripheral arterial disease. *Cochrane Database Syst Rev*. 2002; (2):CD003075. doi: 10.1002/146517858. CD003285.

39. Gordon T, Kannel WB. Predisposition to atherosclerosis in the head, heart, and leg: the Framingham Study. *JAMA*. 1972;221:661-666.

40. Fowkes FG, Housley E, Riemersma RA, et al. Smoking, lipids, glucose intolerance and blood pressure as risk factors for peripheral atherosclerosis compared with ischemic heart disease in the Edinburgh Artery Study. *Am J Epidemiol*. 1992;135:331-340.

41. Olsson AG, Ruhn G, Erikson U. The effect of serum lipid regulation on the development of femoral atherosclerosis in hyperlipidemia: a non-randomized controlled study. *J Intern Med*. 1990;227:381-390.

42. Duffield RGM, Lewis B, Miller NE, et al. Treatment of hyperlipidemia retards progression on symptomatic femoral atherosclerosis: a randomized controlled trial. *Lancet*. 1983;2:639-642.

43. Anonymous. The Lipid Research Clinics Coronary Primary Prevention Trial Results. I: Reduction in incidence of coronary heart disease. *JAMA*. 251:351-364.

44. De Groot E, Jukema JW, van Boven AJ, et al. Effect of pravastatin on progression and regression of coronary atherosclerosis and vessel wall changes in carotid and femoral arteries; a report for the Regression Growth Evaluation Statin Study. *Am J Cardiol*. 1995;76:40C-46C.

45. Heart Protection Study Collaborative Group. MRC/BHF Heart Production Study of cholesterol lowering with simvastatin in 20,536 high-risk individuals: a randomized placebo-controlled trial. *Lancet*. 2002;360:7-22.

46. Pedersen TR, Kjekshus J, Pyörälä K, et al. Effect of simvastatin on ischemic signs and symptoms in the Scandinavian Simvastatin Survival Study (4S). *Am J Cardiol*. 1998;81: 333-335.

47. McDermott MM, Guralnik JM, Greeland P, et al. Statin use and leg functioning in patients with and without lower-extremity peripheral arterial disease. *Circulation*. 2003; 107:57-61.

48. Mondillo S, Ballo P, Barbati R, et al. Effects of simvastatin on walking performance and symptoms of intermittent claudication in hypercholesterolemic patients with peripheral vascular disease. *Am J Med*. 2003;114:359-364.

49. Meade T, Zuhrie R, Cook C, et al. Bezafibrate in men with lower extremity arterial disease: randomized controlled trial. *BMJ*. 2002;325:1139-1141.

50. Canner PL, Berge KG, Wenger NK, et al. Fifteen year mortality in Coronary Drug Project patients: long-term benefit with niacin. *J Am Coll Cardiol*. 1986;8:1245-1255.

51. Brown G, Albers JJ, Fisher LD, et al. Regression of coronary artery disease as a result of intensive lipid lowering therapy in men with high levels of apolipoprotein B. *N Engl J Med*. 1990;323:1289-1298.

52. Elam MB, Hunninghake DB, Davis KB, et al. Effect of niacin on lipid and lipoprotein levels and glycemic control in patients with diabetes and peripheral arterial disease. The ADMIT Study: a randomized trial. *JAMA*. 2000;284:1263-1270.

53. Elam MB, Heckman JR, Crouse JF, et al. Effect of the novel antiplatelet agent cilostazol on plasma lipoproteins in patients with intermittent claudication. *Arterioscler Thromb Vasc Biol*. 1998;18:1942-1947.

54. Clarke R, Daly L, Robinson K, et al. Hyperhomocysteinemia: an independent risk factor for vascular disease. *N Eng J Med*. 1991;324:1149-1155.

55. Graham IM, Daly LE, Refsum HM, et al. Plasma homocysteine as a risk factor for vascular disease. The European Concerted Action Project. *JAMA*. 1997;277:1775-1781.

56. Hansrani M, Stansby G. Homocysteine lowering interventions for peripheral arterial disease and bypass grafts. *Cochrane Database Syst Rev.* 2002;(3):CD003285. doi: 10.14651858.CD003285.

57. Robles P, Mikhailidis DP, Stansby G. Systemic review of antiplatelet therapy for the prevention of myocardial infarction, stroke or vascular death in patients with peripheral vascular disease. *Br J Surg.* 2001;88:787-800.

58. Antithrombotic Trialists' Collaboration. Collaborative meta-analysis or randomized trials of antiplatelet therapy for prevention of death, myocardial infarction and stroke in high risk patients. *BMJ.* 2002;324:71-86.

59. Tran H, Anand SS. Oral antiplatelet therapy in cerebrovascular disease, coronary artery disease, and peripheral artery disease. *JAMA.* 2004;292:1867-1874.

60. Hankey GJ, Sudlow CLM, Dunbabin DW. Thienopyridine derivatives (Ticlopidine, Clopidogrel) versus aspirin for preventing stroke and other serious vascular events in high vascular risk patients.*Cochrane Database Syst Rev.* 1999;(4):CD001246. doi: 10.1002/14651858.CD001246.

61. Anonymous. Medical Economics Company. PDR® entry for Plavix tablets (Sanofi-Synthelabo). *Physician's Desk Reference.* Montvale, NJ: Medical Economics Company, Inc; 2001.

62. Wilhite DB, Comerota AJ, Schmieder, FA, et al. Managing peripheral arterial disease with multiple platelet inhibitors: the effect of combination therapy on bleeding time. *J Vasc Surg.* 2003;38:710-713.

63. De Schryver ELLM, Algra A, van Gijn J. Dipyridamole for preventing stroke and other vascular events in patients with vascular disease. *Cochrane Database Syst Rev.* 2002; (2):CD000990. doi: 10.1002/14651858. CD001820.

64. Cosmi B, Conti E, Coccheri S. Anticoagulants (heparin, low molecular weight heparin and oral anticoagulants) for intermittent claudication. *Cochrane Database Syst Rev.* 2000:CD000990. doi: 10.1002/14651858. CD001820.

65. Leng GC, Fowler B, Ernst E. Exercise for intermittent claudication. *Cochrane Database Syst Rev.* 2000: CD000990. doi: 10:1002/14651858. CD000990.

66. Patterson RB, Pinto B, Marcus B, et al. Value of a supervised exercise program for the therapy of arterial claudication. *J Vasc Surg.* 1997;25:312-319.

67. Cheetham DR, Burgess L, Ellis M, et al. Does supervised exercise offer adjuvant benefit over exercise alone for the treatment of intermittent claudication? A randomized trial. *Eur J Vasc Endovasc Surg.* 2004;27:17-23.

68. Hood SC, Moher D, Barber GG. Management of intermittent claudication with pentoxifylline: a meta-analysis of randomized controlled trials. *CMAJ.* 1996;155:1053-1039.

69. Ernst E. Pentoxifylline for intermittent claudication: a critical review. *Angiology.* 45:339-345.

70. Radack K, Wyderski RJ. Conservative management of intermittent claudication. *Ann Intern Med.* 1990;113:135-146.

71. Porter JM, Cutler BS, Lee BY, et al. Pentoxifylline efficacy in the treatment of intermittent claudication: multicenter controlled double-blind trial with objective assessment of chronic occlusive arterial disease patients. *Am Heart J.* 1982;194:66-72.

72. Gallus AS, Gleadow F, Dupont P, et al. Intermittent claudication: a double-blind crossover trial of pentoxifylline. *Aust NZ J Med.* 1985;5:402-409.

73. Reilly DT, Quinton DN, Barrie WW. A controlled trial of pentoxifylline (Trental 400) in intermittent claudication: clinical haemostatic and rheological effects. *Aust NZ J Med.* 1987;100:445-447.

74. Dawson DL, Cutler BS, Hiatt WR, et al. A comparison of cilostazol and pentoxifylline for treating intermittent claudication. *Am J Med.* 2000;109:523-530.

75. Dawson DL, Cutler BS, Meissner MH, et al. Cilostazol has beneficial effect in treatment of intermittent claudication: results from a multicenter, randomized prospective, double-blind trial. *Circulation.* 1998;98:678-686.

76. Money SR, Herd JA, Isaacsohn JL, et al. Effect of cilostazol on walking distances in patients with intermittent claudication caused by peripheral vascular disease. *J Vasc Surg.* 1998;27:267-275.

77. Beebe HG, Dawson DL, Cutler BS, et al. A new pharmacological treatment for intermittent claudication: results of a randomized, multicenter trial. *Arch Intern Med.* 1999; 159:2041-2050.

78. Regensteiner JG, Ware JE Jr, McCarthy WJ, et al. Effect of cilostazol on treadmill walking, community-based walking ability, and health-related quality of life in patients with intermittent claudication due to peripheral arterial disease: meta-analysis of six randomized controlled trials. *J Am Geriatr Soc.* 2002;50:1939-1946.

79. Anonymous. *Pletal (Package Insert).* Gaithersburg, MD: Otsuka Pharmaceuticals; 1999.

80. Spengel F, Brown TM, Poth J, et al. Naftidrofuryl can enhance the quality of life in patients with intermittent claudication. *VASA.* 1999;28:207-212.

81. Kieffer E, Bahnini A, Mouren X, et al. A new study demonstrates the efficacy of naftidrofuryl in the treatment of intermittent claudication. Findings of the Naftidrofuryl Clinical Ischemia Study (NCIS). *Int Angiol.* 2001;20:58-65.

82. Lehert P, Riphagen FE, Gamand S. The effect of Naftidrofuryl on intermittent claudication: a meta-analysis. *J Cardiovasc Pharmacol.* 1990;16:81-86.

83. Trübestein G, Bohme H, Heidrich H, et al. Naftidrofuryl in chronic arterial disease: results of a controlled multicenter study. *Angiology.* 1994;35:701-708.

84. Spengel F, Clement D, Boccalon H, et al. Findings of the Naftidrofuryl in Quality of Life (NIQOL) European study program. *Int Angiol.* 2002;21:20-27.

85. Aronow WS, Nayak D, Woodworth S, et al. Effect of simvastatin versus placebo on treadmill exercise time until the onset of intermittent claudication in older patients with peripheral arterial disease at six months and at one year after treatment. *Am J Cardiol.* 2003;92:711-712.

86. Mohler ER, Hiatt WR, Creager MA. Cholesterol reduction with atorvastatin improves walking distance in patients with peripheral arterial disease. *Circulation.* 2003;108:1481-1486.

87. Novo S, Abrignani MG, Pavone G, et al. Effects of captopril and ticlopidine, alone or in combination, in hypertensive patients with intermittent claudication. *Int Angiol.* 1996;15:169-174.

88. Ven van de LL, van Leeuwen JT, Smit AJ. The influence of chronic treatment with beta-blockade and converting enzyme inhibition on peripheral blood flow in hypertensive patients with and without concomitant intermittent claudication. *Vasa*. 1994;23:357-362.

89. Horsch S, Walther C. Ginkgo biloba special abstract EGb 761 in the treatment of peripheral arterial occlusive disease (PAOD)—a review based on randomized, controlled studies. *Int J Clin Pharm Ther*. 2004;42:63-72.

90. Pittler MH, Ernst E. Ginkgo biloba extract for the treatment of intermittent claudication: a meta-analysis of randomized trials. *Am J Med*. 2000;108:276-281.

91. Heidrich H, Trampisch HJ, Röhmel J. Prüfrichtlinien für Therapiestudien im Fontaine-Stadium II-IV bei peripherer arterieller Verschlusskrankheit. *VASA*. 1995;24:107-113.

92. Brevetti G, Diehm C, Lambert D. European multicenter study on propionyl-L-carnitine in intermittent claudication. *J Am Coll Cardiol*. 1999;34:1618-1624.

93. Biedunkiewicz B, Tylicki L, Nieweglowski T, et al. Clinical efficacy of ozonated autohemotherapy in hemodialyses patients with intermittent claudication: an oxygen-controlled study. *Int J Artif Organs*. 2004;27:29-34.

94. Villaruz MV, Dans A, Tan F. Chelation therapy for atherosclerotic cardiovascular disease. *The Cochrane Database Syst Rev*. 2002;(4):CD002785. doi: 10.1002/14641858.

95. Bendermacher BLW, Willigendael EM, Teijink JAW, et al. Medical management of peripheral arterial disease. *J Thromb Haemost*. 2005;3:1628-1637.

96. Hess H, Mietaschk A, Deichsel G. Drug-induced inhibition of platelet function delays progression in peripheral occlusive arterial disease: a prospective double-blind arteriographically controlled trial. *Lancet*. 1985;1:41-49.

97. Gauthier O. Efficacy and safety of CY216 in the treatment of specific leg ulcers. In: Breddin K, Fareed J, Samama M, eds. *Faxiparine. Analytic and Structural Data, Pharmacology, Clinical Trials*. Stuttgart: Schattauer; 1987:21.

98. Baumgartner I, Pieczek A, Manor O, et al. Constitutive expression of phVEGF165 after intramuscular gene transfer promotes collateral vessel development in patients with critical limb ischemia. *Circulation*. 1998;97:1114-1123.

99. Tateishi-Yuyama E, Matsubara H, Murohara T, et al. Therapeutic angiogenesis for patients with limb ischemia by autologous transplantation of bone-marrow cells: a pilot study and a randomized controlled trial. *Lancet*. 2002;360:427-435.

100. Shyu KG, Chang H, Wang BW, et al. Intramuscular vascular endothelial growth factor gene therapy in patients with chronic critical leg ischemia. *Am J Med*. 2003;359:2053-2058.

101. Kim H-J, Jang SY, Park J-I, et al. Vascular endothelial growth factor-induced angiogenic gene therapy in patients with peripheral artery disease. *Exp Mol Med*. 2004;36:336-344.

102. Takeshita S, Tsurumi Y, Couffinhal T, et al. Gene transfer of naked DNA encoding for three isoforms, of vascular endothelial growth factor stimulates collateral development in vivo. *Lab Invest*. 1996;75:487-501.

103. Takeshita S, Zheng LP, Brogi E, et al. Therapeutic angiogenesis: a single intra-arterial bolus of vascular endothelial growth

104. factor augments revascularization in a rabbit ischemic hind limb model. *J Clin Invest*. 1994;93:662-670.

104. Takeshita S, Wier L, Chen D, et al. Therapeutic angiogenesis following arterial gene transfer of vascular endothelial growth factor in a rabbit model of hind limb ischemia. *Biochem Biophys Res Commun*. 1996;227:628-635.

105. Baumgartner I, Pieczek A, Manor O, et al. Constitutive expression of phVEGF165 after intramuscular gene transfer promotes collateral vessel development in patients with critical limb ischemia. *Circulation*. 1999;99:3188-3198.

106. Shyu KG, Chang H, Wang BW, et al. Intramuscular vascular endothelial growth factor gene therapy in patients with chronic critical leg ischemia. *Am J Med*. 2003;114:85-92.

107. Ohara N, Koyama H, Miyata T, et al. Adenovirus-mediated ex vivo gene transfer of basic fibroblast growth factor promotes collateral development in a rabbit model of hind limb ischemia. *Gene Ther*. 2001;8:837-845.

108. Barandon L, Leroux L, Dufourcq P, et al. Gene therapy for chronic peripheral arterial disease: what role for the vascular surgeon? *Ann Vasc Surg*. 2004;18:758-765.

109. Ubbink DT, Vermeulen H, Spincemaille GHJJ, et al. Systemic review and meta-analysis of controlled trials assessing spinal cord stimulation of inoperable critical leg ischemia. *Eur J Vasc Endovasc Surg*. 2004;28:9-23.

110. Palfrayman SJ, Booth A, Michaels JA. A systemic review of intra-arterial thrombolytic therapy for lower limb ischemia. *Eur J Vasc Endovasc Surg*. 2000;19:143-157.

111. Berridge DC, Kessel D, Robertson I. Surgery versus thrombolysis for initial management of acute limb ischemia. *Cochrane Database Syst Rev*. 2002;(1):CD002784. doi: 10.1002/14651858.

112. The STILE Investigators. Results of a prospective randomized trial evaluating surgery versus thrombolysis for ischemia of the lower extremity: the STILE Trial. *Ann Surg*. 1994;220:251-268.

113. Sugimoto K, Hofmann LV, Fazavi MK, et al. The safety, efficacy, and pharmacoeconomics of low-dose alteplase compared with urokinase for catheter-directed thrombolysis of arterial and venous occlusions. *J Vasc Surg*. 2003;37:512-517.

114. Burkart DJ, Borsa JJ, Anthony JP, et al. Thrombolysis of acute peripheral arterial and venous occlusions with tenecteplase and eptifibatide: a pilot study. *J Vasc Interv Radiol*. 2003;14:729-733.

115. Lefkovits J, Plow E, Topol E. Mechanisms of disease: platelet glycoprotein IIb/IIIa receptors in cardiovascular medicine. *N Engl J Med*. 1995;332:1553-1559.

116. Schweizer J, Kirch W, Koch R, et al. Short- and long-term results of abciximab versus aspirin in conjunction with thrombolysis for patients with peripheral occlusive arterial disease and arterial thrombosis. *Angiology*. 2000;51:913-923.

117. Duda SH, Tepe G, Luz O, et al. Peripheral artery occlusion: treatment with abciximab plus urokinase versus urokinase alone: a randomized pilot trial (the PROMPT study). *Radiology*. 2001;221:689-696.

118. Management of peripheral arterial disease (PAD). TransAtlantic Inter-Society Consensus (TASC). *J Vasc Surg*. 2000; 31 (suppl):1-296.

119. Dyer JF, Gaines PA, Nicholson AA, et al. Treatment of chronic iliac artery occlusions by means of endovascular stent placement. *J Vasc Interv Radiol.* 1997;3:349-353.

120. Henry M, Amor M, Ethervenot G, et al. Percutaneous endoluminal treatment of iliac occlusions: long-term follow-up in 105 patients. *J Endovasc Surg.* 1998;5:228-233.

121. Uher P, Nyman U, Lindh M, et al. Long-term results of stenting chronic iliac artery occlusions. *J Endovasc Ther.* 2002; 9:67-75.

122. Carnevale FC, De Blas M, Merino S, et al. Percutaneous endovascular treatment of chronic iliac artery occlusion. *Cardiovasc Intervent Radiol.* 2004;27:447-452.

123. Scheinert D, Schroeder M, Ludwig J, et al. Stent-supported recanalization of chronic iliac occlusions. *Am J Med.* 2001;110:708-715.

124. Leville CD, Kashyap, VS, Clair DG, et al. Endovascular management of iliac artery occlusions: extending treatment to TransAtlantic Inter-Society Consensus class C and D patients. *J Vasc Surg.* 2006;43:32-39.

125. Gordon IL, Conroy RM, Arefi M, et al. Three-year outcome of endovascular treatment of superficial femoral artery occlusion. *Arch Surg.* 2001;136:221-228.

126. Kearney M, Pieczek A, Haley L, et al. Histopathology of in-stent restenosis in patients with peripheral artery disease. *Circulation.* 1997;95:1998-2002.

127. Gray B, Olin JW. Limitations of percutaneous transluminal angioplasty with stenting for femoropopliteal arterial occlusive disease. *Semin Vasc Surg.* 1997;10:8-16.

128. Cikrit DF, Dalsing MC. Lower-extremity arterial endovascular stenting. *Surg Clin North Am.* 1998;78:617-629.

129. Hussain FM, Kopchuck G, Heilbron M, et al. Wall-graft endoprothesis: initial canine evaluation. *J Am Surg.* 1998; 64:1002-1006.

130. Matin ML, Veith FJ, Cynamon J, et al. Human transluminally placed endovascular stented grafts: preliminary histopathologic analysis of healing grafts in aortoiliac and femoral artery occlusive disease. *J Vasc Surg.* 1995;21:595-604.

131. Minar E, Porkrajac B, Ramazanali A, et al. Brachytherapy for prophylaxis of restenosis after long-segment femoropopliteal angioplasty: pilot study. *Radiology.* 1998;208:173-179.

132. Lierman DD, Bauernaschs R, Schopohl B, et al. Five-year follow-up after brachytherapy for restenosis in peripheral arteries. *Semin Intervent Cardiol.* 1997;2:133-137.

133. Nasr MK, McCarthy RJ, Hardman J, et al. The increasing role of percutaneous transluminal angioplasty in the primary management of critical limb ischemia. *Eur J Vasc Endovasc Surg.* 2002;23:398-403.

134. Bertele V, Roncaglioni MC, Pangrazzi J, et al. Clinical outcome and its predictors in 1560 patients with critical leg ischemia. Chronic Critical Leg Ischemia Group. *Eur J Vasc Endovasc Surg.* 1999;18:401-410.

135. Schillinger M, Sabeti S, Loewe C, et al. Balloon angioplasty versus implantation of nitinol stents in the superficial femoral artery. *N Engl J Med.* 2006;354:1879-1888.

136. BASIL Trial Participants. Bypass versus angioplasty in severe ischemia of the leg (BASIL): multicentre, randomized controlled trial. *Lancet.* 2005;366:1925-1934.

137. Matsi PJ, Manninen HI, Suhonen MT, et al. Chronic critical lower-limb ischemia: prospective trial of angioplasty with 1-36 months follow-up. *Radiology.* 1993;188:381-387.

138. Soder HK, Manninen HI, Jaakkola P, et al. Prospective trial of infrapopliteal artery balloon angioplasty for critical limb ischemia: angiographic and clinical results. *J Vasc Interv Radiol.* 2000;11:1021-1031.

139. Jämsén T, Manninen H, Tulla H, et al. The final outcome of primary infrainguinal percutaneous transluminal angioplasty in 100 consecutive patients with chronic critical limb ischemia. *J Vasc Interv Radiol.* 2002;13:455-463.

140. Walker SR, Yusuf SW, Hopkinson BR. A 10-year follow-up of patients presenting with ischaemic rest pain of the lower limbs. *Eur J Vasc Endovasc Surg.* 1998;15:478-482.

141. A prospective epidemiological survey of the natural history of chronic critical leg ischaemia. The I.C.A.I. Group (gruppo di studio dell'ischemia cronica critica degli arti inferior). *Eur J Vasc Endovasc Surg.* 1996;11:112-120.

142. Management of peripheral arterial disease (PAD). Trans Atlantic Inter-Society Consensus (TASC). Section D: chronic critical limb ischaemia. *Eur J Vasc Endovasc Surg.* 2000;19 (suppl A):S144-S243.

143. Lepantalo M, Matzke S. Outcome of unreconstructed chronic critical leg ischeamia. *Eur J Vasc Endovasc Surg.* 1996;11:153-157.

144. Chang JB. Surgical management of aortoiliac occlusive disease. In: Chang JB, ed. *Modern Vascular Surgery.* Vol 6. New York, NY: Springer-Verlag; 1994:306-333.

145. Szilagyi DE. Ten years experience with aortoiliac and femoropopliteal arterial reconstruction. *J Cardiovasc Surg.* 1964;5:502-509.

146. Hansteen V, Lorensten E, Sivertsseb E, et al. Long-term follow-up of patients with peripheral arterial obliterations treated with arterial surgery. *Acta Chir Scand.* 1975; 141:725-730.

147. Malone JM, Moore WS, Goldstone J. The natural history of bilateral aortofemoral bypass grafts for ischemia of the lower extremities. *Arch Surg.* 1975;110:1300-1306.

148. Brewster DC, Darling RC. Optimal methods of aortoiliac reconstruction. *Surgery.* 1978;84:739-748.

149. Nevelsteen A, Suy R, Daenen W, et al. Aortofemoral grafting: factors influencing late results. *Surgery.* 1980;88:642-653.

150. Crawford ES, Bomberger RA, Glaeser DH, et al. Aortoiliac occlusive disease: factors influence survival and function following reconstructive operation over a twenty-five-year period. *Surgery.* 1981;90:1055-1067.

151. Poulias GE, Polemis L, Skoutas B, et al. Bilateral aorta-femoral bypass in the presence of aorta–iliac occlusive disease and factors determining results: experience and long-term follow-up with 500 consecutive cases. *J Cardiovasc Surg.* 1985;26:527-538.

152. Szilagyi DE, Elliott JP, Smith RF, et al. A thirty-year survey of reconstructive surgical treatment of aortoiliac occlusive disease. *J Vasc Surg.* 1986;3:421-436.

153. Nevelsteen A, Wouters L, Suy R. Aortofemoral Dacron reconstruction for aorta–iliac occlusive disease: a 25-year survey. *Eur J Vasc Surg.* 1991;5:19-186.

154. Von Gryska P, Brewster DC. Surgical treatment of aortoiliac occlusive disease. Surgical pitfalls. In: Chang JB, ed. *Modern Vascular Surgery*. Vol 2. New York, NY: PMA Publishing Corp; 1987;54-68.

155. Tollefson DFJ, Ernst CB. Retroperitoneal aortic reconstruction: indications and pitfalls. In: Chang JB, ed. *Modern Vascular Surgery*. Vol 5. New York, NY: Springer-Verlag; 1992: 126-131.

156. Piotrowski JJ, Pearce WH, Jones DN, et al. Aortobifemoral bypass: the operation of choice of unilateral iliac occlusion? *J Vasc Surg*. 1988;8:211-218.

157. Chang JB. Surgical treatment of aorta–iliac artery disease. *Angiology*. 1981;32:73-105.

158. Rob C. Extraperitoneal approach to the abdominal aorta. *Surgery*. 1963;3:53-87.

159. Sicard GA, Freeman MB, VanderWoude JC, et al. Comparison between the transabdominal and retroperitoneal approach for reconstruction of the intrarenal abdominal aorta. *J Vasc Surg*. 1987;5:19.

160. deVries SO, Hunink MGM. Results of aortic bifurcation grafts for aortoiliac occlusive disease: a meta-analysis. *J Vasc Surg*. 1997;2:558-569.

161. Brewster DC, Darling RC. Optimal methods of aortoiliac reconstruction. *Surgery*. 1978;84:739.

162. Crawford ES, Bomberger RA, Glaeser DH, et al. Aortoiliac occlusive disease: factors influencing survival and function following reconstructive operation over a twenty-five year period. *Surgery*. 1981;90:1555.

163. Malone JM, Moore WS, Goldstone J. The natural history of bilateral aortofemoral bypass grafts for ischemia of the lower extremities. *Arch Surg*. 1975;110:1300.

164. Szilagyi DE, Hageman JH, Smith RF, et al. A thirty-year survey of the reconstructive surgical treatment of aortoiliac occlusive disease. *J Vasc Surg*. 1986;3:421.

165. Nevelsteen A, Wouters L, Suy R. Aortofemoral Dacron reconstruction for aortoiliac occlusive disease: a 25-year survey. *Eur J Vas Surg*. 1991;5:179.

166. Mozersky DJ, Sumner DS, Strandness DE. Long-term results of reconstructive aortoiliac surgery. *Am J Surg*. 1972; 123:503.

167. Eagle KA, Coley CM, Newell JB, et al. Combining clinical and thallium data optimizes preoperative assessment of cardiac risk before major vascular surgery. *Ann Intern Med*. 1989;110:859-866.

168. Mulcare RJ, Royster TS, Lynn RA, et al. Long-term results of operative therapy for aortoiliac disease. *Arch Surg*. 1978; 113:601.

169. Rutherford RB, Jones DN, Martin MS, et al. Serial hemodynamic assessment of aortobifemoral bypass. *J Vasc Surg*. 1986;4:428.

170. Martinez BD, Hertzer NR, Beven EG. Influence of distal arterial occlusive disease on prognosis following aortobifemoral bypass. *Surgery*. 1980;88:795.

171. Sumner DS, Strandness DE Jr. Aortoiliac reconstruction in patients with combined iliac and superficial femoral arterial occlusion. *Surgery*. 1978;84:348.

172. Hill DA, McGrath MA, Lord RSA, et al. The effect of superficial femoral artery occlusion on the outcome of aortofemoral bypass for intermittent claudication. *Surgery*. 1980;87:133.

173. Galland RB, Hill DA, Gustave R, et al. The functional result of aortoiliac reconstruction. *Br J Surg*. 1980;67:344.

174. Jones AF, Kempczinski RF. Aortofemoral bypass grafting: a reappraisal. *Arch Surg*. 1981;16:301.

175. Tollefson DFJ, Ernst CB. Natural history of atherosclerotic renal artery stenosis associated with aortic disease. *J Vasc Surg*. 1991;14:327.

176. Zierler RE, Bergelin RO, Isaacson JA, et al. Natural history of atherosclerotic renal artery stenosis: a prospective study with duplex ultrasonography. *J Vasc Surg*. 1994;19(2): 250.

177. Dean RH, Keyser JE III, Dupont WD, et al. Aortic and renal vascular disease: factors affecting the value of combined procedures. *Ann Surg*. 1984;200:336.

178. Tarazi RY, Hertzer NR, Beven EG. Simultaneous aortic reconstruction and renal revascularization: risk factors and late results in eighty-nine patients. *J Vasc Surg*. 1987;5:707.

179. Brewster DC, Buth J, Darling RC, et al. Combined aortic and renal artery reconstruction. *Am J Surg*. 1976;131:457.

180. Cambria RP, Brewster DC, L'Italien G, et al. Simultaneous aortic and renal artery reconstruction: evaluation of an eighteen-year experience. *J Vasc Surg*. 1995;21:916.

181. Chaikof EL, Smith RB III, Salam AA, et al. Empirical reconstruction of the renal artery: long-term outcome. *J Vasc Surg*. 1996;24:406.

182. Brewster DC. Complications of aortic and lower extremity procedures. In: Strandness DE Jr, van Breda A, eds. *Vascular Diseases: Surgical and Interventional Therapy*. New York, NY: Churchill Livingstone; 1994:1151-1177.

183. Brewster DC. Reoperation for aortofemoral graft limb occlusion. In: Veith F, ed. *Current Critical Problems in Vascular Surgery*. St. Louis, MO: Quality Medical; 1989:341-351.

184. Ernst CB. Prevention of intestinal ischemia following abdominal aortic reconstruction. *Surgery*. 1983;93:102.

185. Brewster DC, Franklin DP, Cambria RP, et al. Intestinal ischemia complicating abdominal aortic surgery. *Surgery*. 1981;109:447.

186. Bjorck M, Bergqvist D, Troeng T. Incidence and clinical presentation of bowel ischemia after aortoiliac surgery: 2930 operations from a population-based registry in Sweden. *Eur J Vasc Endovasc Surg*. 1996;12:139.

187. Castronuovo JJ, Flanigan DP. Renal failure complicating vascular surgery. In Bernhard VM, Towne JB, eds. *Complications in Vascular Surgery*. Orlando: Grune & Stratton, 1985;258-274.

188. Brewster DC, Meier GH, Darling RC, et al. Reoperation of aortofemoral graft limb occlusion: optimal methods and long-term results. *J Vasc Surg*. 1987;5:363.

189. Brewster DC. Surgery of late aortic graft occlusion. In Bergan JJ, Yao JST, eds. *Aortic Surgery*. Philadelphia, PA: WB Saunders; 1989:519-538.

190. Nevelsteen A, Suy R. Graft occlusion following aortofemoral Dacron bypass. *Ann Vasc Surg*. 1991;5:32.

191. Moore WS, Cole CW. Infection in prosthetic vascular grafts. In Moore WS, ed. *Vascular Surgery: A Comprehensive Review*. 3rd ed. Philadelphia, PA: WB Saunders; 1991:598-609.

192. O'Hara PJ, Hertzer NR, Beven EG, et al. Surgical management of infected abdominal aortic grafts: review of a 25-year experience. *J Vasc Surg.* 1986;3:725.

193. Piotrowski JJ, Bernhard VM. Management of vascular graft infections. In Bernhard VM, Towne JB, eds. *Complications in Vascular Surgery.* St. Louis, MO: Quality Medical; 1991: 235-258.

194. Reilly LM, Altman H, Lusby RJ, et al. Late results following surgical management of vascular graft infection. *J Vasc Surg.* 1984;1:36.

195. Quinones-Baldrich WJ, Hernandez JJ, Moore WS. Long-term results following surgical management of aortic graft infection. *Arch Surg.* 1991;126:507.

196. Yeager RA, Moneta GL, Taylor LM, et al. Improving survival and limb salvage in patients with aortic graft infection. *Am J Surg.* 1990;159:466.

197. Schmitt DD, Seabrook GR, Bandyk DF, et al. Graft excision and extra-anatomic revascularization: the treatment of choice for the septic aortic prosthesis. *J Cardiovasc Surg.* 1990;31:327.

198. Sharp WJ, Hoballah JJ, Mohan CR, et al. The management of the infected aortic prosthesis: a current decade of experience. *J Vasc Surg.* 1994;19:844.

199. Reilly LM, Stoney RJ, Goldstone J, et al. Improved management of aortic graft infection: the influence of operation sequence and staging. *J Vasc Surg.* 1987;5:421.

200. Trout HH III, Kozloff L, Giordano JM. Priority of revascularization in patients with graft enteric fistulas, infected arteries, or infected arterial prostheses. *Ann Surg.* 1984;199:669.

201. Clagett GP, Valentine RJ, Hagino RT. Autogenous aortoiliac/femoral reconstruction from superficial femoral–popliteal veins: feasibility and durability. *J Vasc Surg.* 1997;25:255.

202. Bernhard VM. Aortoenteric fistula. In: Bernhard VM, Towne JB, eds. *Complications in Vascular Surgery.* Orlando: Grune & Stratton; 1985:513-525.

203. Connolly JE, Kwann JHM, McCart PM, et al. Aortoenteric fistula. *Ann Surg.* 1981;194:402.

204. Perdue GD Jr, Smith RB III, Ansley JD, et al. Impending aortoenteric hemorrhage: the effect of early recognition on improved outcome. *Ann Surg.* 1980;192:237.

205. Reilly LM, Ehrenfeld WK, Goldstone J, et al. Gastrointestinal tract involvement by prosthetic graft infection: the significance of gastrointestinal hemorrhage. *Ann Surg.* 1985;202:342.

206. Nunn DB. Symptomatic peripheral arteriosclerosis of patients under age 40. *Am Surg.* 1973;39:224-228.

207. Mingoli A, Sapienza P, Feldhaus RJ, et al. Aortoiliofemoral bypass grafts in young adults: long-term results in a series of sixty-eight patients. *Surgery.* 1997;121:646-653.

208. Jensen BV, Egeblad K. Aortoiliac arteriosclerotic disease in young human adults. *Eur J Surg.* 1990;4:583-586.

209. Levy PJ, Hornung CA, Haynes JL, et al. Lower extremity ischemia in adults younger than 40 years of age: a community-wide survey of premature atherosclerotic arterial disease. *J Vasc Surg.* 1994;19:873-881.

210. Cronenwett JL, Davis JT, Gooch JB, et al. Aortoiliac occlusive disease in women. *Surgery.* 1980;88:775-784.

211. Reed AB, Conte MS, Donaldson MC, et al. The impact of patient age and aortic size on the results of aortobifemoral bypass grafting. *J Vasc Surg.* 2003;37:1219-1225.

212. Valentine RJ, Hansen ME, Myers SI, et al. The influence of sex and aortic size on late patency after aortofemoral revascularization in young adults. *J Vasc Surg.* 1995;88:775-784.

213. Olsen PS, Gustafsen J, Rasmussen L, et al. Long-term results after arterial surgery for atherosclerosis of the lower limbs in young adults. *Eur J Vasc Surg.* 1988;2:15-18.

214. DeLaurentis DA, Friedmann P, Wolferth CC, et al. Atherosclerosis and the hypoplastic aortoiliac system. *Surgery.* 1978;83:27-37.

215. Caes F, Cham B, Van den Brande P, et al. Small artery syndrome in women. *Surg Gynecol Obstet.* 1985;161:165-170.

216. Schneider JR, Zwolak RM, Walsh DB, et al. Lack of diameter effect on short-term patency of size-matched Dacron aortobifemoral grafts. *J Vasc Surg.* 1991;13:785-791.

217. TransAtlantic Inter-Society Consensus (TASC). Management of peripheral arterial disease (PAD). *J Vasc Surg.* 2000;31(part 2):50-54.

218. Strecker EP, Boos IBL, Hagen B. Flexible tantalum stents for the treatment of iliac artery lesions: long-term patency, complications, and risk factors. *Radiology.* 1996;199:641-647.

219. Henry M, Amor M, Ethevenot G, et al. Palmaz stent in iliac and femoropopliteal arteries: primary and secondary patency in 310 patients with 2–4 year follow-up. *Radiology.* 1995;197:170-174.

220. Powell RJ, Fillinger M, Bettmann M, et al. The durability of endovascular treatment of multisegment iliac occlusive disease. *J Vasc Surg.* 2000;31:1178-1184.

221. Wylie EJ, Olcott C IV, String ST. Aortic thromboendarterectomy. In: Varco RL, Delaney JP, eds. *Controversy in Surgery.* Philadelphia, PA: WB Sauders; 1976:437-350.

222. Crawford ES, Manning LG, Kelly TF. "Redo" surgery after operations for aneurysm and occlusion of the abdominal aorta. *Surgery.* 1977;81:41-52.

223. Corson JD, Brewster DC, Darling RC. The surgical management of infrarenal aortic occlusion. *Surg Gynecol Obstet.* 1982;155:369.

224. Imparato AM, Riles TS, Weintraub N. Aortoiliac femoral endarterectomy: a reappraisal. *Circulation.* 1984;70:136.

225. d'Othee BJ, Haulon S, Mounier-Vehier C, et al. Percutaneous endovascular treatment for stenoses and occlusions of infrarenal aorta and aortoiliac bifurcation: midterm results. *Eur J Vasc Endovasc Surg.* 2002;24:516.

226. Elkouri S, Hudon G, Demers P, et al. Early and long-term results of a percutaneous transluminal angioplasty of the lower abdominal aorta. *J Vasc Surg.* 199;30:679.

227. Hood DB, Hodgson KJ. Percutaneous transluminal angioplasty and stenting for iliac artery occlusive disease. *Surg Clin North Am.* 1999;79:575.

228. Chang JB, Rao GN, Thomson NB Jr. Ascending aorta to bilateral femoral artery graft. *Vasc Surg.* 1979;13:202-206.

229. Baird RJ, Ropchan GV, Oates TK, et al. Ascending aorta to bifemoral bypass—a ventral aorta. *J Vasc Surg.* 1986;3:405.

230. Criado E, Johnson G Jr, Burnham SJ, et al. Descending thoracic aorta-to-iliofemoral artery bypass as an alternative to aortoiliac reconstruction. *J Vasc Surg.* 1992;15:550.

231. McCarthy WJ, Mesh CL, McMillian WD, et al. Descending thoracic aorta-to-femoral artery bypass: ten years' experience with a durable procedure. *J Vasc Surg.* 1993;17: 336.

232. Blaisdell FW, Hall AD. Axillary-femoral artery bypass for lower extremity ischemia. *Surgery.* 1963;54:563-568.

233. Chang JB, Chan F. Axillobifemoral bypass. *Vasc Surg.* 1986;20:27-35.

234. Chang JB. Extracranial revascularization. In: Chang JB, ed. *Vascular Surgery.* New York, NY: Spectrum Publications; 1985:31-83.

235. Chang JB. Extra-anatomic bypasses and their long-term results. In: Chang JB, ed. *Modern Vascular Surgery.* Vol 2. New York, NY: PMA Publishing Corp; 1987:45-53.

236. Chang JB. Current state of extra-anatomic bypasses. *Am J Surg.* 1986;152:202-205.

237. Seeger JM, Pretus HA, Welborn MB, et al. Long-term outcome after treatment of aortic graft infection with staged extra-anatomic bypass grafting and aortic graft removal. *J Vasc Surg.* 2000;32:451-461.

238. Clagett BP, Valentine RJ, Hagino RT. Autogenous aortoiliac/femoral reconstruction from superficial femoral–popliteal veins: feasibility and durability. *J Vasc Surg.* 1997; 25:255-270.

239. Bandyk DF, Novotney ML, Johnson BL, et al. Use of rifampin-soaked gelatin-sealed polyester grafts for in situ treatment of primary aortic and vascular prosthetic infections. *J Surg Res.* 2001;95:44-49.

240. LoGerfo FW, Johnson MC, Corson, JD, et al. A comparison of the late patency rates of axillobilateral femoral and axillounilateral femoral grafts. *Surgery.* 1977;81:33-40.

241. Eugene J, Goldstone J, Moore WS. Fifteen-year experience with subcutaneous bypass grafts for lower extremity ischemia. *Ann Surg.* 1977;186:177-183.

242. Agee KM, Kron IL, Flanagan T, et al. The risks of axillofemoral bypass grafting for acute vascular occlusion. *J Vasc Surg.* 1991;14:190-194.

243. Ray LI, O'Connor JB, Davis CC, et al. Axillofemoral bypass: a critical reappraisal of its role in the management of aortoiliac disease. *Surgery.* 1979;138:117-128.

244. Johnson WC, LoGerfo FW, Vollman RW, et al. Is axillobilateral femoral graft an effective substitute for aortic-bilateral iliac/femoral graft? An analysis of ten years' experience. *Ann Surg.* 1977;186:123-129.

245. LoGerfo FW, Johnson WC, Corson JD, et al. A comparison of the late patency rates of axillobilateral femoral and axillounilateral femoral grafts. *Surgery.* 1977;81:33-40.

246. Schneider JR. Extra-anatomic bypass. In: Rutherford, RB, ed. *Vascular Surgery.* 6th ed. Philadelphia, PA: Elsevier Saunders; 2005:1137-1153.

247. Vetto RM. The treatment of unilateral iliac artery obstruction with a transabdominal, subcutaneous femorofemoral graft. *Surgery.* 1962;52:342-345.

248. Chang JB. Surgical treatment of aorta–iliac artery disease. *Angiology.* 1981;32:73-105.

249. Deruyter L, Caes F, Van den Brande P, et al. Femorofemoral bypass grafting in high-risk patients. *Acta Chir Belg.* 1986;86:271-276.

250. Fahal AH, McDonald AM, Marston A. Femorofemoral bypass in unilateral iliac artery occlusion. *Br J Surg.* 1989; 76:22-25.

251. Blaisdell FW. Extraanatomical bypass procedures. *World J Surg.* 1988;12:798-804.

252. Rutherford RB, Patt A, Pearce WH. Extra-anatomic bypass: a closer view. *J Vasc Surg.* 1987;6:437-446.

253. Hepp W, deJonge K, Pallua N. Late results following extra-anatomic bypass procedures for chronic aortoiliac disease. *J Cardiovasc Surg.* 1988;29:181-185.

254. Pietri P, Pancrazio F, Adovasio R, et al. Long-term results of extra-anatomical bypasses. *Int Angiol.* 1987;6:429-433.

255. Rutherford RB. Management of aortoiliac disease with and without infrainguinal occlusion: indications and technique. In: Chang JB, ed. *Modern Vascular Surgery.* Vol 3. New York, NY: PMA Publishing Corp; 1989:201-204.

256. Marek JM, Mills JL. Risk factor assessment and indications for reconstruction. In Mills JL, ed. *Management of Chronic Lower Limb Ischemia.* London: Arnold; 2000:30-44.

257. Hertzer NR, Beven EG, Young JR, et al. Coronary artery disease in peripheral vascular patients. A classification of 1000 coronary angiograms and results of surgical management. *Ann Surg.* 1984;199:223-233.

258. Detsky AS, Abrams HB, Foburth N, et al. Cardiac assessment for patients undergoing noncardiac surgery: a multifactorial clinical risk index. *Arch Intern Med.* 1996;146:2131-2134.

259. Goldman L, Caldera DL, Nessbaum SR, et al. Multifactorial index of cardiac risk in noncardiac surgical procedures. *N Engl J Med.* 1977;297:845-853.

260. Eagle KA, Coley CM, Newell JB, et al. Combining clinical and thallium data optimizes preoperative assessment of cardiac risk before major vascular surgery. *Ann Intern Med.* 1989;110:859-866.

261. Cook DJ, Guyatt GH, Laupacis A, et al. Rules of evidence and clinical recommendations on the use of antithrombotic agents. *Chest.* 1992;102(suppl):305S-311S.

262. Mangano DT, Layug E, Wallace A, et al. Effect of atenolol on mortality and cardiovascular morbidity after noncardiac surgery. *N Engl J Med.* 1996;335:1713-1720.

263. Poldermans D, Boersma E, Bax JJ, et al. The effect of bisoprolol on perioperative mortality and myocardial infarction in high-risk patients undergoing vascular surgery. Dutch Echocardiographic Cardiac Risk Evaluation Applying Stress Echocardiography Study Group. *N Eng J Med.* 1999;341:1789-1794.

264. Pereira CE, Albers M, Romiti M, et al. Meta-analysis of femoropopliteal bypass grafts for lower extremity arterial insufficiency. *J Vasc Surg.* 2006;44:510-517.

265. Yancey AE, Minion DJ, Rodriguez C, et al. Peripheral atherectomy in TransAtlantic InterSociety Consensus type C femoropopliteal lesions for limb salvage. *J Vasc Surg.* 2006;44:503-509.

266. Chang JB, Stein TA. The long-term value of composite grafts for limb salvage. *J Vasc Surg.* 1995;22:25-31.

267. Ad Hoc Committee on Reporting Standards, Society for Vascular Surgery, and the International Society for Cardiovascular Surgery. Standards for reports dealing with lower extremity ischemia. *J Vasc Surg.* 1986;4:80-94.

268. Hoch JR, Tullis MJ, Kennell TW, et al. Use of magnetic resonance angiography for the preoperative evaluation of patients with infrainguinal arterial occlusive disease. *J Vasc Surg.* 1996;23:792-801.

269. Chang JB. Popliteal and tibial artery revascularization. In: Chang JB, ed. *Vascular Surgery.* New York, NY: Spectrum Publications; 1985:194-229.

270. Whittemore AD, Kent KC, Donaldson MC, et al. What is the proper role of polytetrafluoroethylene grafts in infrainguinal reconstruction? *J Vasc Surg.* 1989;10:299-305.

271. David TE, Key JA. Profundaplasty for limb salvage. *Can J Surg.* 1978;21:107-109.

272. David TE, Drezner AD. Extended profundaplasty for limb salvage. *Surgery.* 1978;84:758-763.

273. Tweedie JH, Ballantyne KC, Callum KG. Direct arterial pressure measurements during operation to assess adequacy of arterial reconstruction in lower limb ischemia. *Br J Surg.* 1986;73:879-881.

274. Hansen AK, Billie S, Nielsen PH, et al. Profundaplasty as the only reconstructive procedure in patients with severe ischemia of the lower extremity. *Surg Gynecol Obstet.* 1990;171:47-50.

275. Kalman PG, Johnston KW, Walker PM. The current role of isolated profundaplasty. *J Cardiovasc Surg.* 1990;31:107-111.

276. Chang JB, Stein TA. Infrainguinal revascularizations in octogenarians and septuagenarians. *J Vasc Surg.* 2001;34:133-138.

277. Chang JB, Stein TA. The long-term value of composite grafts for limb salvage. *J Vasc Surg.* 1995;22:25-31.

278. Panneton JM, Hollier LH, Hofer JM. Multicenter randomized prospective trial comparing a pre-cuffed polytetrafluoroethylene graft to a vein cuffed polytetrafluoroethylene graft for infragenicular arterial bypass. *Ann Vasc Surg.* 2004;18:199-206.

279. Chang JB. Popliteal and tibial artery bypasses for limb salvage. *Vasc Surg.* 1985;19:137-146.

280. Chang JB, Borrero E. Peripheral pseudoaneurysms: an eleven year experience. *Vasc Surg.* 1986;20:166-174.

281. Szilagy DE, Smith RF, Elliott JP, et al. Anastomotic aneurysms after vascular reconstruction: Problems of incidence, etiology, and treatment. *Surgery.* 1975;78:800-816.

282. Taylor SM, Kalbaugh CA, Blackhurst DW, et al. Determinants of functional outcome after revascularization for critical limb ischemia: an analysis of 1000 consecutive vascular interventions. *J Vasc Surg.* 2006;44:747-756.

283. Conte MS, Bandyk DF, Clowes AW, et al. Results of PREVENT III: a multicenter randomized trial of edifoligide for the prevention of vein graft failure in lower extremity bypass surgery. *J Vasc Surg.* 2006;43:742-751.

284. Chew DK, Nguyen LL, Owens CD, et al. Comparative analysis of autogenous infrainguinal bypass in African Americans and Caucasians: the association of race with graft function and limb salvage. *J Vasc Surg.* 2005;42:695.

285. Van Damme H. Crural or pedal artery revascularization for limb salvage: is it justified? *Acta Chir Belg.* 2004;104:148-157.

286. Holler D, Claes C, Matthias Graf von der Schulenburg J. Cost-utility analysis of treating severe peripheral arterial occlusive disease. *Int J Angiol.* 2006;15:25-33.

287. Cutler BS, Thompson JE, Kleinsasser LJ, et al. Autologous saphenous vein femoropopliteal bypass: analysis of 298 cases. *Surgery.* 1976;79:325-331.

288. Luther M. Treatment of chronic critical leg ischemia—a cost benefit analysis. *Ann Chir Gynaecol.* 1997;213 (suppl):1-142.

289. Bosch JL, Tetteroo E, Mali WP, et al. Iliac arterial occlusive disease: cost-effectiveness analysis of stent placement versus percutaneous transluminal angioplasty. Dutch Iliac Stent Trial Study Group. *Radiology.* 1998;208:641-648.

290. Hunink MG, Wong JB, Donaldson MC, et al. Revascularization for femoropopliteal disease. A decision and cost-effective analysis. *JAMA.* 1995;274:165-171.

291. Laurilla J, Brommels M, Stadertskjold-Nordenstam CG, et al. Cost-effectiveness of percutaneous transluminal angioplasty (PTA) versus vascular surgery in limb-threatening ischaemia. *Int J Angiol.* 2000;9:214-219.

292. Sculpher M, Michaels J, McKenna M, et al. A cost-utility analysis of laser-assisted angioplasty for peripheral arterial occlusions. *Int J Technol Assess Health Care.* 1996;12:104-125.

chapter 38

Endovascular Therapies in Peripheral Arterial Disease

Michael H. Lebow, MD / *Scott L. Stevens, MD*

IN THE BEGINNING

In 1929, a 25-year-old intern named Werner Forssman was dissatisfied with the available methods of evaluating cardiac function at his hospital in Berlin. His appeals to his supervising physicians for permission to test a cardiac catheterization technique he had envisioned were flatly denied. Secretly, Forssman enlisted the help of a nurse and conducted the experiment on himself. Threading a rubber catheter through a vein in his left arm to the level of his heart and injecting dye, Forssman completed the first successful cardiac catheterization. Upon discovery of his experiment, he was promptly fired from his job and ostracized by the medical community. It was not until 27 years later, in 1956, that Forssman was awarded the Nobel Prize in physiology and medicine for his achievement.

Several other great medical inventions made their debut around the time Forssman received the Nobel Prize. John Gibbons revealed his heart–lung machine, and Michael Debaky successfully performed open heart surgery and created the artificial arterial conduit Dacron. The field of cardiovascular surgery was at the forefront of new medical technologies. During the same period, when the medical community was enchanted with open surgery, minimally invasive techniques were quietly being developed.

In 1953, a 32-year-old Swedish radiologist named Sven Seldinger developed a percutaneous technique in which a wire, threaded through a needle into a vessel, is exchanged for a catheter. The "Seldinger technique" is ubiquitous in medicine today and makes a surgical incision unnecessary for catheter-based therapies. Another important, although less well-known, contribution of Seldinger's was the design of a U-shaped catheter tip for selective catheterizations. By placing a wire through a straight catheter and bending both together over the steam of a coffee pot before cooling them rapidly, Seldinger fabricated a bent tipped catheter that could be straightened by advancing the wire through the lumen. This model, common today, makes selective arterial catheterization feasible for physicians of average dexterity. The Seldinger technique was widely practiced in Sweden soon after its description, but it took more than a decade and the endorsement by radiologist Charles Dotter from the University Of Oregon Health Sciences for the technique to catch on in the United States.

A SWITCH TO INTERVENTIONS

In 1958, Mason Sones, a pediatric cardiologist at the Cleveland Clinic, made a landmark discovery. At that time, the current practice for obtaining coronary angiograms involved a large-volume contrast injection into the aortic arch to opacify the coronary arteries. It was thought that selectively coronary cannulation would cause fatal arrhythmias. While attempting a left ventricular image, Sones inadvertently cannulated the right coronary and produced a selective arteriogram with 30 cc of Hypaque contrast. Initially horrified, when the patient suffered only a transient rhythm disturbance and recovered quickly, Sones realized that selective coronary angiography could be tolerated. In 1962, he published his technique of slowly hand injecting 3 to 6 cc of contrast and using an image intensifier to obtain high-quality coronary angiograms with high success and minimal contrast.

The ability to selectively cannulate vessels along with improvements in fluoroscopy and the development of rapid film changers and power injectors greatly improved the quality of arteriographic images. Using the Seldinger technique and shaped catheters, it became possible to accurately visualize almost any named vessel without making an incision. As the quality of images improved, radiologists became increasingly valuable diagnosticians to the medical community and their prestige grew accordingly.

In 1964, the same year Debakey successfully completed the world's first coronary artery bypass graft, Charles Dotter was the first nonsurgeon to cross into the realm of arterial remodeling. He used catheters of increasing diameter to open the iliac artery of an 82-year-old woman with an ischemic foot to complete the first percutaneous arterial angioplasty.[1] *Time Life Magazine* chronicled this achievement with a series of vivid intraoperative photographs in August 1964. Dotter's toothy grin and elated facial expressions shown in these pictures earned him the nickname "Crazy Charlie." Dotter built his own guidewires using anything from a guitar string to a Volkswagon speedometer cable and catheters using Teflon tubing and a blow torch. He is considered by many to be the founding father of interventional radiology.

Europeans coined the phrase "dottering" to describe the opening of a stenosis by passing serial coaxial dilating catheters of increasing diameter. Dotter's technique was the method of choice worldwide until the 1970s. There were limitations to this method, including a limitation to small-diameter lesions, because the largest dilating catheter had to fit through the access arteriotomy and the fact that the stiff catheters could not be maneuvered to branch vessels. Even in his original publication, Dotter foresaw the development of radially expanding dialating catheters.

A collaborative effort between Dotter, Forssman, and others to develop a balloon dialating catheter became a primary focus of their efforts. Their models were based on the concept of an inflatable balloon-tipped catheter pioneered by a cardiovascular surgeon, Thomas Fogarty, nearly a decade earlier. Fogarty, using his boyhood Fly-tying kit and the fingertip of a latex glove, had designed an inflatable balloon-tipped catheter capable of removing intravascular thrombus by passing it through an open artery. Fogarty's balloon catheter made its debut as an embolectomy catheter but had been used for balloon angioplasty as early as 1965, making it the first successful technology of this type.

Early models of angioplasty balloons by Dotter and Forssman were "caged" or "corseted" balloons made of Teflon. The outer size-restricting component was used to ensure that the balloon would not overinflate and rupture the vessel being treated. Despite early success, these catheters were not highly successful because of problems with inflexibility and thrombogenicity. It was not until a young German physician, Andreas Gruentzig, used polyvinyl chloride to build a balloon-tipped, double-lumen catheter that had the handling characteristics of modern-day catheters. Gruentzig presented his initial animal research results at the American Heart Association meeting in 1976 and was largely met with skepticism. One year later in 1977, when he presented the results of his first four human coronary angioplasties at the American Heart Association meeting, the audience burst into applause and provided him with a standing ovation. It was clear that a medical revolution had taken place.

● ANGIOPLASTY TODAY

In the 1980s, public awareness of percutaneous arterial interventions soared. Patients who wanted their coronary vessels treated without a sternotomy embraced PTCA, and celebrity patients increased awareness of alternatives to open surgery. Johnny Carson, after choosing peripheral angioplasty over surgery for claudication, joked with Ed Mc-man on the *Tonight Show* about his "balloon job." Meanwhile, in the medical community, the reality of restenosis became evident.

From the beginning, studies have documented the increased rate of restenosis of angioplasty compared to surgery, but this has not slowed the progression of catheter-based interventions. The battle against restenosis is a primary focus of physicians and industries today.

Multiple techniques from atherectomy to stenting have been used, but none are as durable as surgery. Currently, dozens of stents with various materials and sizes are available from a number of manufacturers. Balloon expandable drug-eluting stents have been the most effective in intermediate-length trials. Industry-sponsored trials of the first coronary drug-eluting stents showed a reduction of restenosis rates into the single digits for the first time (33% of the bare metal stents restenosed), but recent analysis suggests that these are more predisposed to late thrombosis than their bare metal counterparts and may be overused. Other emerging technologies such as cryoplasty, cutting balloon angioplasty, and stent brachytherapy are also areas of active research.

What started as a cottage industry, with catheters being developed by physicians in their basements and attics, grew into a multibillion dollar industry dominated by major corporations. One emerging dilemma is that the physicians who are most qualified to evaluate new products often have financial interests in the results. In addition, concerns about the economic impact on our health care system are rising as the use of expensive technology increases. Drug-eluting stents, in particular, because of their high price, have been criticized in a "societal cost–benefit analysis" through multiple studies. The sudden emergence of endovascular therapy into medicine has magnified philosophical dilemmas within our field. Issues such as "cost containment vs. individual benefit" and the emerging partnerships between physicians and industry with their inherent conflict of interest are two such examples.

● ABDOMINAL AORTIC ANEURYSM

The historically standard method for the surgical repair of abdominal aortic aneurysms involves a transperitoneal approach, clamping the aorta proximally and distally, incising the aneurysm anteriorly, sewing in an interposition graft, and finally closing the aneurysm sac around the graft to prevent an aortoenteric fistula. This method replaced nonresective approaches such as ligation, thrombosis, and aneurysm wrapping, which produced unacceptable rates of rupture and mortality. A shortcoming of the open repair is the detrimental impact of a transperitoneal operation and aortic cross-clamping in patients with significant comorbidities. These high-risk patients were the original candidates for endovascular repair because the less invasive nature of endovascular abdominal aortic aneurysm repair (EVAR) shifted the risk–benefit ratio in their favor.

In 1987, J.C. Palmaz, inventor of the Plamaz stent, revealed that he and Jaun Parodi, an Argentinean vascular surgeon, had conceptualized the use of a covered stent to exclude an abdominal aortic aneurysm. Three years later, Parodi used a Dacron graft handsewn into a Palmaz stent to complete the first successful EVAR via a common femoral artery approach. Soon afterward, in November 1991, Parodi, Palmaz, and Barone published a series of five high-risk patients treated successfully with EVAR in *The Annals of Vascular Surgery* and brought to international attention the feasibility of a catheter-based repair. One year after Parodi's benchmark paper, Frank Veith, with Parodi and a team of coworkers from Buenos Aires, performed the first EVAR in the United States at Montefiore medical center in New York, on November 23, 1992.

During the next decade, multiple studies showed both the limitations and the benefits of EVAR. Parodi himself published an 80% initial failure rate in his first 15 patients. But as devices and techniques become more refined, the data are being accumulated in support of EVAR. The first FDA-approved trials of the Ancure endograft showed an equivalent perioperative mortality between open and endovascular repair, but, by 2004, there was growing level 1 data showing benefit to EVAR. Well-designed trials published in the *Lancet* and *The New England Journal of Medicine* show that patients with EVAR suffer significantly fewer perioperative complications and lower rates of 30-day mortality.[2,3] Stent-graft patients do, however, have an increased need for secondary interventions and require lifelong surveillance to screen for graft migration and, more commonly, continued aneurysm expansion owing to endoleaks.

While critics of EVAR cite the necessary surveillance and the lack of long-term data as justification for open surgery, the trend toward EVAR predominance is clearly underway. The proportion of patients who are considered eligible for EVAR has risen from approximately 20% to 80% in recent years. Current indications for EVAR are the same as those for open repair, size >5.5 cm in asymptomatic patients, but in future years the lower morbidity and mortality of EVAR may make the repair of smaller aneurysms a safe option. As technology continues to expand and devices become more advanced, it is inevitable that many of the current hurdles will be crossed. One example is a recently developed pressure-sensing device that can be deployed into the aneurysm sac at the time of graft deployment and monitored easily in the clinical setting, potentially minimizing the need for serial contrast-based imaging. Other horizons include the ability to repair currently prohibitive anatomy, such as juxtarenal aneurysms, with fenestrated grafts that allow simultaneous stetting of major aortic branches.

● EXTRACRANIAL CAROTID ARTERY

The consequences of carotid arterial disease were observed by physicians centuries ago, but carotid interventions did not begin in earnest until the 1950s. The word carotid is derived from the Greek *karotide* or*karos* meaning stupefy or put to sleep. Hippocrates described intermittent neurosensory deficits as a precursor to stroke in early medical literature, but attempts to treat carotid disease were not recorded until centuries later. Willis described the intercerebral vasculature and the circular system of collaterals at the base of the brain in 1665, and, in 1856, Virchow linked carotid occlusion to ipsilateral blindness in one of his patients. By the turn of the 19th century, Chiari described embolizing atherosclerotic debris from the carotid plaques as an etiology for stroke, and, in 1914, a neurologist, Hunt, coined the phrase "cerebral claudication" referring to what we would now consider a transient ischemic attack. In 1927, a French radiologist, Egas Moniz, imaged the carotid arteries with angiography, and the era of modern diagnostic cerebral vascular imaging was born.

The advent of digital subtraction angiography 10 years later refined angiography, and images of nonocclusive carotid lesions in symptomatic patients challenged the predominant theory that the majority of strokes were caused by aberrancies in the cerebral vasculature. Fisher delineated between partial and total carotid occlusions and conceptualized the diverting of blood flow through or around carotid blockages. The first documented case of surgically corrected carotid artery stenosis came from Dr. Carrea and coworkers in Buenos Aires, who performed an external to internal carotid artery bypass in a patient with a symptomatic stenosis. Surgical techniques of the extracranial carotid artery continued to progress through the 1950s, and the concept of extracranial atherosclerotic disease-causing stroke and transient ischemic attack became well accepted. In 1951, Wylie introduced the concept of thromboendarterectomy of the aortoiliac system, and 2 years later the first carotid endarterectomy (CEA) was performed in the United States. Since that time, CEA has been one of the most commonly performed operations of vascular surgeons and also the most studied. Refinements to the original technique such as patch closure to widen the artery and the monitoring of cerebral ischemia with selective shunting have resulted in a safe operation with minimal recurrence. It is critical that the morbidity and mortality in carotid surgery be very low because it is performed on tens of thousands asymptomatic patients each year.

Several large, well-designed, multicenter trials have been performed to evaluate CEA, and their results have served as guidelines for vascular surgeons around the world. Furthermore, the results generated by these trials are now the standards to which carotid artery stenting (CAS) is being measured against. Because of this, it is essential for all physicians treating vascular disease to understand the studies comparing CEA to medical management and to apply that background in the analysis of studies comparing CAS to CEA.

The fact that CEA has been so thoroughly studied is a testament to the fact that its benefits over medical management are not overtly apparent. In fact, the preemptive nature of asymptomatic carotid intervention, stopping an event before it occurs, makes the benefit of CEA more subtle than that of operations designed to correct a symptomatic state. The effectiveness of medical management for asymptomatic states further narrows the therapeutic window for CEA, and it should be remembered that the landmark trials comparing surgery to medical management for carotid stenosis preceded the advent of HMG-CoA reductase inhibitors and the newer antiplatelet medications.

The first two randomized trials of CEA in the 1980s failed to show benefit over medical therapy.[4] As a response to these studies, and the fact that more than 100 000 CEAs were being performed annually without proven benefit, The North American Symptomatic Carotid Endarterectomy Trial (NASCET) was designed in 1991. NASCET proved the superiority of surgery with medical management over medical management alone for the treatment of symptomaticpatients with ipsilateral carotid stenosis of 70% to 99%. The rate of major ipsilateral stroke at 2 years was 13.1% in the medical group compared to 2.5% in the surgical group with a low surgical stroke and death rates of 2.1% and 0.6%. Two similar trials, The European Carotid Surgery Trial and the Veterans Administration Symptomatic Surgery Trial, followed NASCET and supported its results.

NASCET results are applicable to patients younger than 80 years old, experiencing only minor fluctuating neurologic symptoms, when operations are performed by experienced carotid surgeons. Patients with recent major cerebral event, stroke in evolution, poor cardiac function, or unfavorable plaque morphology have a higher risk of complications. NASCET also found women to have less favorable outcomes, but Mattos et al. have since challenged the concept of female sex being an independent risk factor. Critics of the NASCET trial cite its low rate of complications as a confounding factor. NASCET's favorable stroke and death rates have failed to be reproduced by multiple smaller studies carried out since then, including recent studies comparing CAS to CEA.

The logical progression following NASCET was to study CEA in asymptotic patients, and the Asymptomatic Carotid Atherosclerosis Study (ACAS) trial was designed with this goal. Similar to NASCET, several of the trials preceding ACAS failed to show benefit to surgery. In fact, The Mayo Asymptomatic Carotid Endarterectomy Trial was terminated early because surgical patients not taking aspirin were having a prohibitively high rate of perioperative myocardial infarction. The studies preceding ACAS are generally considered to have methodological flaws, and ACAS, published in 1995, is, by far, the most accepted study analyzing treatment for asymptomatic stenosis.

In ACAS, 1662 patients were randomized to aspirin 325 mg daily or surgery plus aspirin and followed for 5 years. By the end of the study period, the medical group had an ipsilateral stroke or death rate of 11% compared to 5.1% for the surgical group for a relative risk reduction of 53%. These findings in the setting of a 0.14% operative mortality and 1.5% stroke rate provide evidence supporting CEA for asymptomatic lesions greater than 60%. In practice, however, many institutions have not been able to duplicate the low stoke and death rates of ACAS, and the risk of complications are generally considered too high to justify intervening on a 60% asymptomatic lesion. Most vascular surgeons delay intervention until asymptomatic lesions reach at least 75% to 80%.

One reason for the high operative risk for CEA is the strong association between carotid artery and coronary artery atherosclerosis. Up to 40% of patients with transient ischemic attack or stroke have been shown to have previously unrecognized flow limiting coronary disease by provocative tests.[5] Cervical block anesthesia has been used to reduce perioperative cardiac complications with some success, but many surgeons find operating on awake patients less desirable. CAS is associated with less surgical stress, and postoperative pain and may reduce the risk of perioperative myocardial infarction.

Carotid artery angioplasty made its début in 1980, but early studies showed a high rate of periprocedural stroke. The first randomized study of carotid artery angioplasty vs. endarterectomy was terminated early because of a dismal 71% stroke rate in the angioplasty arm.[6] Three years later, a trial comparing CAS with the Wallstent to CEA was terminated for similar reasons. Both the studies were small and the expertise of the participating interventionalists has been questioned. The Carotid Artery and Vertebral Artery Transluminal Angioplasty Study (CAVATAS) was the first large, multicenter, randomized trial designed to definitively compare the two techniques. Unfortunately, the results of CAVATAS raised more questions and doubts about treating carotid artery disease than it answered.

In CAVATAS, 504 patients were randomized to endovascular or surgical treatment arms. Stents were placed in 26% of the angioplasty group. The results of the two techniques were similarly poor for both groups. The stroke and death rate was 10% for the endovascular group and 9.9% for CEA. CAVATAS failed to support angioplasty and stenting of carotid stenosis and simultaneously showed complication rates for CEA, which exceeded those of NASCET, ACAS, and the safety guidelines set by the American Heart Association. CAVATAS preceded the advent of embolic protection devices (EPDs), which have become a widely accepted means to reduce the effects of embolic debris during angioplasty and stenting. EPDs, originally in the form of occlusion balloons and more recently as filtering devices, are quickly becoming the standard of care despite a lack of level 1 data to support their use.

The largest clinical trials evaluating CEA to CAS with EPDs to date have been industry-sponsored registries. The Stenting and Angioplasty with Protection in Patients at

High Risk for Endarterectomy trial sponsored by Cordis and conducted at the Cleveland Clinic randomized 334 high-risk symptomatic and asymptomatic patients into CEA and CAS arms. Additionally, 406 nonrandomized patients who were not candidates for surgery underwent CAS and seven nonrandomized patients not candidates for CAS underwent CEA. The patients were followed for 2 years, and end points of stroke, death, and myocardial infarction were measured with intent to prove that CAS was not inferior to CEA. A primary end point was reached in 20 patients with CAS and 32 who underwent CEA, and the authors concluded that CAS with distal protection is not inferior to CEA. Patients with CAS also benefited from no cranial nerve injury, while 5% of the CEA group had such an injury although most of these injuries were transient neurapraxias and not permanently debilitating. Perioperative non-Q wave MI accounted for a large portion of the cardiac events in the surgical arm, a fact that may represent bias in favor of stenting since these events are of questionable clinical significance. Importantly, more than half of the patients in Stenting and Angioplasty with Protection in Patients at High Risk for Endarterectomy trial were reoperations. In this circumstance, it is likely that smooth neointimal hyperplasia rather than atherosclerotic plaque is the cause of restenosis resulting in a lower risk of embolization and possibly biases the study in favor of CAS. Incidentally, the lead investigator in the study was also the inventor of the distal protection device being used, and 11 of the 15 authors acknowledged financial support from the manufacturing company.[7] Clearly, there is room for improvement study designs comparing CEA and CAS with EPDs.

Nonetheless, Stenting and Angioplasty with Protection in Patients at High Risk for Endarterectomy trial does not stand alone in its finding that CAS with distal protection is a safe alternative to CEA in selected patients. Several industry-sponsored registries developed by stent manufacturers to track the safety and efficacy of their devices support the safety of CAS with EPDs. Acculink's ARCHER, Boston Scientific's CABERNET, and Abbot's SECuRITY are examples of such registries. While the agenda of these registries is to demonstrate the advantages of a particular device and gain FDA approval, they do provide new data on stroke rates for CAS with EPDs. Data from registries suggest that use of EPD in conjunction with the fact that surgeons are becoming more experienced with CAS (specifically learning what to avoid, e.g., tortuosity, calcifications, and ulcerated lesions) has reduced periprocedural stroke rates to an acceptable level in some industry-sponsored trials.[8]

Two controlled, prospective, randomized trials comparing CEA to CAS with EPDs have been completed. The first, Endarterectomy Versus Stenting in Patients with Symptomatic Severe Carotid Stenosis (EVA-3S), was conducted in France and published in *The New England Journal* in October 2006. Like in NASCET, an independent neurologist examined all enrolled patients. Primary end point of 30-day stroke and death rate was reached in 3.9% in the CEA group, compared to 9.6% following CAS. An unprece-

dented 91% of the CAS were performed with EPDs. At 6-month follow-up, stroke and death was 6.1% following CEA and 11.7% after CAS. The trial's safety committee stopped enrollment after the inclusion of 527 patients because of significantly better outcomes in the surgery arm. The second is the SPACE trial (Stent-Protected Angioplasty Versus Carotid Endarterectomy in Symptomatic Patients) published in *Lancet*. In this study, 1200 symptomatic patients were randomized to CAS or CEA. The primary end points were stroke or death within 30 days of the procedure. The rate of death or stroke was 6.84% in the CAS group and 6.34% in the CEA group. The final conclusion drawn from this study is that CAS failed to be the noninferiority when compared with CEA (*p*-value of 0.09) and that the widespread use of CAS should not replace CEA.

Other similar trials are underway in Europe and the United States. The Carotid Revascularization Endarterectomy Versus Stenting trial is a multicenter trial comparing CAS with EPDs to CEA in symptomatic and asymptomatic patients currently enrolling. Supported by the National Institute of Health and the National Institute of Neurologic Disorders and Stroke, the Carotid Revascularization Endarterectomy Versus Stenting trial will compare the incidence of stroke, myocardial infarction, and death in CAS and CEA performed by credentialed operators. Carotid Revascularization Endarterectomy Versus Stenting trial will use aspirin and plavix as medical therapy, and an independent neurologist will evaluate patients pre- and postprocedurally.

For now, CEA continues to be the mainstay of therapy for most of the medical community, and, until convincing level 1 evidence shows CAS to be noninferior, most surgeons, neurologists, and internists will likely stick to traditional referral patterns. Currently, there are defined anatomic and physiologic criteria set by Medicare that define which patients will receive reimbursement for CAS. So today, outside of registries and clinical trials, only patients with anatomy unfavorable to surgery (previous ipsilateral neck operation, contralateral vocal cord paralysis, high lesions, and neck irradiation) and those unfit for surgery (severe COPD, CRI, or cardiac disease) are eligible for CAS.

● ILIAC ARTERIES

Since the mid-1990s, catheter-based interventions have been the preferred method of treating most lesions of the iliac arteries. Multiple studies have documented high technical success rates and long-term patency following iliac angioplasty and stenting. Limb salvage rates of up to 97% have been reported.[9] In recent years, even chronic occlusions of the iliacs have been successfully treated using subintimal angioplasty and stenting.[10] The feasibility and durability of iliac angioplasty has reduced the number of aortobifemoral bypass operations performed for iliac occlusive disease.

There has been debate on whether angioplasty is as durable as angioplasty and stenting in the iliac arteries. In

1998, The Dutch Iliac Stent Trial Study Group randomized 279 patients with claudication to receive angioplasty with or without routine stenting for iliac artery stenosis. The angioplasty arm received stents only when residual pressure gradients >10 mm Hg persisted following dilatation and the other group received stents routinely. At 2 years, they found no difference in patency or degree of symptoms and concluded that selective stenting is an effective approach to iliac stenosis. Other studies since then have duplicated these results, but the practice of selective stenting is not uniformly accepted.[11] Today, surgeons and interventionalists frequently treat complex lesions, which routinely require stenting for optimum outcomes.

In September 2006, The TransAtlantic Inter-Society Consensus (TASC) published their second consensus recommendations for treatment of aortailiac and infrainguinal occlusive disease. Patterns of disease were graded from A to D, and the recommendations for treatment were based on lesion classification (Figure 35-3 and Table 35-3). Endovascular therapy is recommended for TASC A lesions and surgery for TASC D. Endovascular therapy is preferred for TASC B lesions and surgery is preferred for TASC C lesions in good-risk patients. The changes to the TASC guidelines are representative of recent advances in technology and physician experience.

● LOWER EXTREMITY

Below the inguinal ligament, the success of endovascular therapy has been more limited than in other vascular beds. The femoral arteries are a frequent site of atherosclerosis, but, traditionally, SFA angioplasty has been plagued by high restenosis rates. The infrapopliteal arteries are especially difficult. Several newer techniques such as cutting or laser atherectomy devices and drug-eluting stents are being used with cautious optimism in the treatment of tibioperoneal disease.

Lower extremity occlusive vascular disease can be broadly divided into claudication and critical limb ischemia (CLI). Interventions for intermittent claudication are generally performed for lifestyle improvement, while treatment for CLI focuses on limb salvage. Only approximately 5% of claudicants will progress to CLI, and even less, roughly 2%, progress to amputation.[12] Up to half of patients with CLI report having no symptoms 6 months prior to presentation.[12] The first-line therapy for claudication is lifestyle modification with cessation of smoking and a structured exercise regimen. When these regimens are followed, an increase in walking distance by up to 33% in 6 months can be achieved without intervention. Claudicants are an unhealthy population, with up to 60% of patients with PAD also having significant coronary or cerebral vascular disease. In fact, the 5-, 10-, and 15-year mortality for claudicants approximates those with Duke B colon cancer at 30%, 50%, and 70%.[12] The gold standard operation for lifestyle limiting claudication is the femoral to popliteal artery bypass. The 5-year patency of a femoral–popliteal bypass is 70% to 80% with vein and 60% to 70% with PTFE.

In May 2006, a well-designed trial comparing angioplasty to angioplasty and stenting of the SFA followed patients for 1 year. At 12 months, the angioplasty group has a 37% patency rate compared to 63% in the stent group.[13] These findings suggest that stenting increases durability compared to angioplasty alone but that neither treatment achieves the durability of bypass grafting. Self-expanding SMART stents eluting sirolimus have failed to show superior patency when compared to bare metal stents in the lower extremity.[14] Nonetheless, there is still a role for percutaneous intervention of SFA disease in many patients. For patients with severe coexisting conditions, such as cardiopulmonary disease, stenting is an effective alternative to surgical revascularization. Additionally, for patents who do not have adequate vein, the 12-month patency for stenting and artificial conduit bypass is similar with stenting offering less pain and complications and a shorter hospital stay.

Endovascular techniques have been more widely studied for CLI than for claudication. Amputation rates for CLI are higher than claudication and there is evidence that these can be lowered by early intervention. Several European studies have shown a reduction in amputation rates by 22% to 54%, with patients older than 65 years showing the most benefit.[12] There are several small trials of angioplasty and stenting with 2- to 3-year follow-up, which show encouraging results in the setting of limb salvage.[15–17] Generally, percutaneous interventions are less durable than vein bypass but can be effective for wound healing, limb salvage, and temporary relief of rest pain. The BASIL trial, Bypass Versus Angioplasty in Severe Ischemia of the Leg, compared angioplasty to surgery in 452 patients with CLI. The study ran for 5 years with primary end points of amputation or death. Amputation rates between the two methods were not statistically different in the short term, but, for patients who lived for more than 2 years without amputation (55%), the surgery group had lower rates of subsequent amputation and death.[5]

There is a large array of devices and techniques available to the interventionalist treating lower extremity occlusive disease. While there is a lack of consistent long-term data to support most of these techniques, experienced operators have been able to use those with success in specific circumstances. The "cryo" balloon freezes to −10° while inflating, with the theoretical advantage of inducing apoptosis of endothelial and smooth muscle cells and decreasing neointimal hyperplasia. A cutting balloon actually makes small incisions in the lesion as it expands and may be useful in reducing recoil and intimal hyperplasia. An atherectomy device cut out plaque, but data are conflicting regarding the degree of inflammation and restenosis following this procedure.

While there certainly is a role for peripheral percutaneous interventions, there is a paucity of level 1 data supporting the use of many commonly employed techniques. Available data on endovascular treatment of lower extremity PAOD have consisted of small comparative studies with relatively short follow-up and retrospective series. One problem has been the glut of new techniques available in the last decade and the tendency of second-generation devices to outpace the ability of investigators to thoroughly evaluate what is current.

REFERENCES

1. Dotter C, Judkins M. Transluminal treatment of atherosclerotic obstruction. *Circulation*. 1964;30:654-670.

2. Greenhalgh RM, et al. Comparison of endovascular aneurysm repair with open repair in patients with abdominal aortic aneurysm, 30-day operative mortality results: randomized controlled trial. *Lancet*. 2004;364(9437):818-820.

3. Prinssen, et al. A randomized trial comparing conventional and endovascular repair of abdominal aortic aneurysms. *NEJM*. 2004;14(16):351.

4. Fields WS, Lemark NA. *A History of Stroke*. Oxford University Press; 1989.

5. Rutherford R. *Vascular Surgery*. 6th ed. Elsevier Saunders.

6. Naylor R, et al. Randomized study of carotid angioplasty and stenting versus carotid endarterectomy: a stopped trial. *JVS*. 1998;28(2).

7. Thomas. Protected carotid artery stenting versus endarterectomy in high-risk patients reflections from SAPPHIRE. *Stroke*. 2005;36(4):912-913.

8. Schonholz CJ, et al. Is there evidence that cerebral protection is beneficial? *J Cardiovasc Surg*. 2006;47:137-141.

9. Leville CD, et al. Endovascular management of iliac artery occlusions: extending treatment to TASC C and D patients. *JVS*. 2006;43:32-39.

10. Carnevale FC, et al. Percutaneous endovascular treatment of chronic iliac artery occlusion. *Cardiovasc Intervent Radiol*. 2004;27(5):447-452.

11. Toshifumi K, et al. Long-term outcomes and predictors of iliac angioplasty with selective stenting. *JVS*. 2005;3(42):466.

12. TASC guidelines. *JVS*. 31(1) part 2.

13. Martin S. Balloon angioplasty versus implantation of nitinol stents in the superficial femoral artery. *NEJM*. 2006;354(18).

14. Duda SH, et al. Drug-eluting and bare nitinol stents for the treatment of atherosclerotic lesions in the superficial femoral artery: long-term results of the SIROCCO trial. *J Endovasc Surg*. 2006;13(6):7012-7010.

15. Surowiec SM, et al. Percutaneous angioplasty and stenting of the superficial femoral artery. *JVS*. 2005;4(42):822-824.

16. Lipsitz EC, et al. Does subintimal angioplasty have a role in the treatment of severe lower extremity ischemia? *JVS*. 2003;2(37):386-391.

17. Treiman GS, et al. Results of percutaneous subintimal angioplasty using routine stenting. *JVS*. 2006;3(43):513-519.

18. Thompson J. The evolution of surgery for the treatment and prevention of stroke. *Stroke*. 1996;27:1427-1434.

19. Mattos MA, Summer DS, Bohannon WT, et al. Carotid endarterectomy in women: challenging the results from ACAS and NASET. *Ann Surg*. 2001;234:438-446.

20. Bradbury A. Bypass versus angioplasty in severe ischemia of the leg (BASIL): multicenter, randomized controlled trial. *Lancet*. 2005;366:1925-1934.

21. Castriota F, et al. Impact of cerebral protection devices on the outcome of carotid stenting. *J Endovasc Ther*. 2002;9:786-792.

22. TASC-II Inter society consensus on peripheral arterial disease. *Eur J Vasc Endovasc Surg*. 2007;33(suppl 1).

23. Schonholz CJ, et al. Is there evidence that cerebral Protection is beneficial? *J Cardiol Vasc Surg*. 2006;47:137-141.

24. Yadav JS, et al. Protected carotid artery stenting versus endarterectomy in high risk patients. *NEJM*. 2004;351:1493-1501.

chapter 39

The Vascular Biology and Clinical Efficacy of Drug-Eluting Stents for the Treatment of Peripheral Arterial Disease

Robert S. Dieter, MD, RVT / *Leonardo Clavijo, MD, PhD* / *Scott L. Stevens, MD* /
John R. Laird, MD

Nearly 10% of the population older than 65 years has atherosclerotic lower extremity peripheral arterial disease. Older patients and those with risk factors may have up to a 25% incidence of lower extremity peripheral arterial disease.[1] Percutaneous vascular interventions are rapidly emerging as a less invasive therapy for symptomatic lower extremity occlusive arterial disease.[2-4] Despite recent advances, restenosis remains a significant problem with catheter-based revascularization. By delivering high local doses, drug-eluting stents have the potential to overcome the limitations of restenosis and advance stent-based therapies for lower extremity peripheral arterial disease (Table 39-1).

There is interest in the applicability of drug eluting stent (DES) in other arterial beds as well. Most studies and case series have focused on the efficacy in the renal arteries, intracranial circulation, and extracranial carotid or vertebral arteries. To date, the bulk of clinical studies have been in the evaluation of drug-eluting stents to reduce restenosis in the coronary arteries, with dramatic results, which are simultaneously changing the treatment paradigm for multivessel coronary artery disease and raising long-term safety concerns.

● MECHANISM OF BALLOON ANGIOPLASTY AND STENTING

Balloon angioplasty of occlusive arterial disease results in a lumen diameter gain through several mechanisms. Angioplasty compresses the atherosclerotic plaque, shifting it laterally and axially, as well as causing a "controlled" intimal and medial dissection.[5] Angioplasty is, however, limited by the acute elastic recoil properties of the arterial wall with up to a 40% loss in lumen area.[5,6] Flow-limiting dissections can occur and may lead to acute or subacute vessel closure.[7] As a scaffold, stents improve the initial results of percutaneous interventions by increasing the arterial lumen and tacking up intimal flaps between the stent and the vessel wall. The scaffolding properties of stents virtually eliminate acute arterial recoil and reduce the subsequent risk of acute or subacute vessel closure.[5,7-9]

● RESTENOSIS PATHOPHYSIOLOGY

Restenosis is characterized by three processes: acute vessel recoil, late vessel remodeling (negative/constrictive remodeling), and neointimal hyperplasia.[5,7,10] Stents effectively

> **TABLE 39-1.** Challenges of Stent-Based Drug Delivery
>
> - Formulation and processing
> - Mechanical integrity
> - Drug loading
> - Sterilization
> - Release kinetics

eliminate acute vessel recoil and negative vessel remodeling. In-stent restenosis is, therefore, almost entirely owing to neointimal hyperplasia.[8,11,12] Compared to balloon angioplasty, stents can cause more tissue proliferation by virtue of greater chronic injury to the vessel wall. The long-term effectiveness of stents is mitigated by this "late loss" of the arterial lumen because of tissue proliferation within the stent.

The pathophysiology of vascular repair mechanisms after angioplasty and stenting has been extensively studied in a variety of experimental models. Angioplasty and stenting cause local vascular injury, including disruption of the intima, denudation of the endothelium, and penetration of the media.[6–8] Disruption of the endothelium and exposure of the contents of the subintimal space such as collagen, von Willebrand factor, and the lipid core result in vessel inflammation, the activation of platelets, and the release of growth factors, oxygen-derived free radicals, cytokines, adhesion molecules, and macrophage chemotactic factors.[5–7,13] Fibrin deposition and thrombus formation at the injury site can provide a matrix for cellular migration and proliferation.[6] The degranulation of platelets and stimulation of inflammatory cells trigger the release of mitogens and further cellular activation and proliferation.[8,11,14,15] Subsequently, there is the migration and proliferation of vascular smooth muscle cells and fibroblasts into the area of injury. The final component of the tissue response to injury is extracellular matrix deposition of collagen and proteoglycan.[7,8] The neointima of in-stent restenosis has a limited cellularity, primarily vascular smooth muscle cells, and is mostly composed of collagen, proteoglycans, and extracellular material.[6,8,13]

The time course of the vascular proliferative response following stenting has been well established in experimental restenosis models and has been confirmed in human atherosclerotic lesions. Earlier, following stent implantation, there is deposition of platelets, fibrin, and acute inflammatory cells around the stent struts. Within a few weeks after stent implantation, the stent is covered by an immature neointima consisting of macrophages and alpha-actin negative spindle cells. This is followed by smooth muscle cell differentiation and proliferation and extracellular matrix formation. The final step in the healing process is re-endothelialization, which occurs within several weeks to a couple of months following stent implantation.

OVERVIEW OF THE CELL CYCLE AND REGULATORY COMPONENTS (FIGURE 39-1)

Current pharmacologic approaches to inhibit restenosis target key steps in the cell cycle. The cell cycle describes the sequence of events that regulate cellular growth and ultimately cell division. During Gap 1 (G1) the cell is regulated by external stimuli with gene expression and protein synthesis in preparation for the synthesis (S) phase. The nuclear content doubles during the S phase. The Gap 2 (G2) is characterized by increased protein synthesis and cellular growth. G2 phase further prepares the cell for mitosis (M phase). During mitosis, the cell undergoes cytokinesis (producing two daughter cells). The daughter cells can then enter a quiescent phase (G0) or enter G1.

Regulatory pathways of the cell cycle are complex and still being elucidated. Cyclin and cyclin-dependent kinases are involved in the regulation of cellular progression through the cell cycle. p53, a tumor suppressor, inhibits cell-cycle progression if DNA is damaged (or induces apoptosis if there is severe DNA damage). p27 binds cyclin and cyclin-dependent kinase, blocking progression to the S phase of the cell cycle. Phosphorylation of the retinoblastoma protein (pRb) is involved in the regulation of the cell entering the S phase and, subsequently, the G2 phase.

ELUTION KINETICS

In order to have maximal vascular inhibitory effects on restenosis, yet minimize injury and delay of re-endothelialization, it is necessary to determine the optimal elution kinetics for each candidate molecule. This requires an understanding of the therapeutic window for each molecule, the optimal inhibitory concentration, rate and duration of release, as well as polymer interactions.

Polymers

To establish a predictable release of drugs, polymer coatings are utilized as a reservoir for controlled elution. With the exception of some compounds, such as paclitaxel, which are lipophilic and can be dip coated onto stents, a polymeric coating is necessary.[15] In order for drug-eluting stents to be successful, the polymeric vehicle must not induce inflammation and subsequent in-stent restenosis. Several biodegradable and nonbiodegradable polymers have been tested as candidate vehicles for drug-eluting stents. Van der Giessen et al.[16] demonstrated that a variety of biodegradable polymers (polyglycolic acid/polylactic acid, polycaprolactone, polyhydroxybutyrate valerate, polyorthoester, and polyethyleneoxide/polybutylene terephthalate) and nonbiodegradable polymers (polyurethane, silicone, and polyethylene terephthalate) are not inert and can induce extensive inflammatory responses. Several other polymers have been tested, including chondroitin sulfate A/gelatin, polyacrylate plastic sleeves, and polyethylenevinylacetate/polybutylmethacrylate, with varying success.[7,17,18]

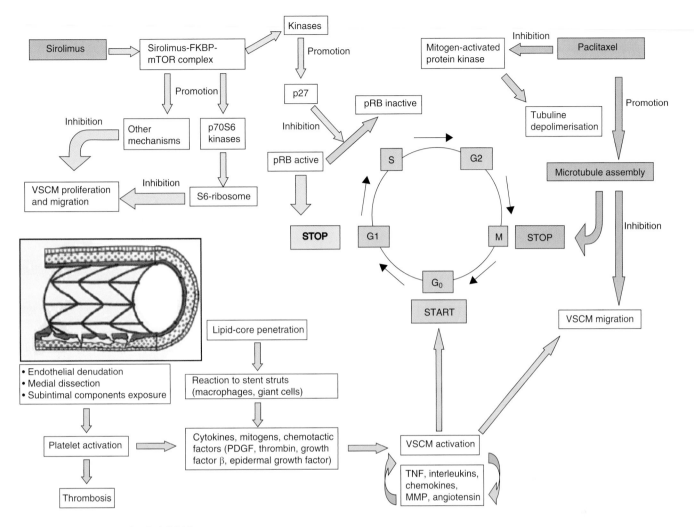

Drug-eluting stents: mitosis inhibition

VSCM=vascular smooth muscle cell, MMp=matrix metalloproteinase, FKBP=tacrolimus binding protein, mTOR=mammalian target of sirolimus.

● **FIGURE 39-1.** Overview of the cell cycle and points of inhibition.

Reprinted with permission from Fattori R, Piva T. Drug-eluting stents in vascular intervention. Lancet 2003;361:247-249.

Release Rates

Clinical studies of paclitaxel-coated stents in coronary arteries have evaluated nonpolymer bonding and a variety of polymers and elution kinetics. Park et al.[19] evaluated the efficacy of two doses of non-polymer-based paclitaxel elution for coronary stenting. They found that in-stent intimal hyperplasia was reduced in a dose-dependent manner. TAXUS II evaluated two separate polymer-based elution regimens in the coronary arteries. Both formulations were designed to have an initial bolus release for the first 48 hours post implantation and a slower release during the next 10 days. The TAXUS-SR (slow release) stent had eight times less drug released than the TAXUS-MR (moderate release) stent. Six-month angiography revealed significantly less in-stent restenosis in both TAXUS-SR and TAXUS-MR arms (5.5% and 8.6%, respectively) compared to their respective controls (20.1% and 23.8%).[20]

Similar elution kinetic studies have been performed on sirolimus-coated stents. Two principal release formulations have been tested for sirolimus—both in the coronary and in the peripheral arteries. A ratio of approximately 30:70 sirolimus to copolymer is utilized. The polymer is a 50:50 combination of polyethylenevinylacetate and polybutylmethacrylate.[7] Stents are coated with a basecoat copolymer and sirolimus; in order to achieve a slower elution, a top-coat diffusion barrier is applied. The fast-release formulation allows for drug release in <15 days, whereas the slow-release allows for a ≥28-day release.[21] In general, there has been similar results for the slow- and fast-release sirolimus stents, although there may be an advantage in in-stent late loss for the slow-release formulation.[22]

● STENT DESIGN (TABLE 39-2)

There is evidence in the coronary literature and emerging data in the periphery to suggest that stent design may have an impact on restenosis.

Lasers are generally used to cut patterns into either metal tubes or sheets, which are subsequently welded together,

TABLE 39-2. Factors Influencing Intimal Hyperplasia after Drug-Eluting Stent Implantation

- Stent design
  - Strut thickness
  - Strut spacing
- Pharmacological agent
- Polymer
- Reservoir-based platforms

TABLE 39-3. Candidate Drugs

Antineoplastic
  Actinomycin-D
  Methotrexate
  Paclitaxel
  Paclitaxel derivative (QP-2)
  Vincristine
Antithrombins
  Glycoprotein IIb/IIIa inhibitors
  Heparin
  Hirudin
  Iloprost
Immunosuppressants
  Cyclosporine
  Dexamethasone
  Sirolimus (rapamycin)
  Everolimus
  Tacrolimus (FK506)
  Tranilast
Collagen synthetase inhibitor/enhance healing/
  promote endothelial function
  17-β-Estradiol
  Angiopeptin V
  C-proteinase inhibitors
  Matrix metalloproteinase inhibitors
  VEGF

to manufacture stents.[23] Stents can be broadly classified by the cell design. Open-cell design allows for the cell area to change during flexion, while closed-cell stents maintain a relatively fixed cell area. Each design allows for trade-offs between deliverability, plaque covering, apposition, and access to side branches.[24] Stent design also has an impact on local drug delivery. Hwang et al.[25] demonstrated that the local tissue concentration of eluted drugs is dependent, in part, on strut spacing—more so for hydrophilic than for hydrophobic drugs. Inhomogeneity in strut spacing may also be significant for drugs with a narrow therapeutic window.[24]

The ISAR-STEREO trial evaluated the effect of stent strut thickness on angiographic restenosis in coronary arteries. Patients were randomized to receive the ACS RX Multi-Link stent (Guidant/Advanced Cardiovascular Systems, Santa Clara, CA) with a strut thickness of either 50 or 140 μm. The primary end point of angiographic restenosis ≥50% was seen in 15% of those receiving the thin strut and in 25.8% receiving the thick strut stent, a 42% risk reduction.[26] A follow-up study (ISAR-STEREO-2) compared the ACS RX Multi-Link stent with a strut thickness of 50 μm and a strut width of 100 μm to the BX Velocity (Cordis Corporation, Miami, FL) with a strut thickness of 140 μm and strut width of 130 μm. The ACS RX Multi-Link stent has an interconnected ring design, whereas the BX Velocity is a closed-cell design (both stainless steel). The primary end point of angiographic restenosis ≥50% was seen in 17.9% of the thin-strut and 31.4% of the thick-strut stent—a 43% risk reduction, suggesting that thinner strut thickness, regardless of stent design, results in less angiographic restenosis.[27]

● IDEAL DRUG TO INHIBIT RESTENOSIS (TABLE 39-3)

The complexity of the cell cycle underscores the challenge in designing a drug that inhibits neointimal hyperplasia and restenosis. Because there are multiple pathways by which neointimal formation is stimulated, a drug that has a highly specialized and focused mechanism of action will likely fail in preventing restenosis.[5] Furthermore, the ideal agent would be anti-inflammatory and inhibit vascular smooth muscle cell activation yet allow endothelial paving for a

quiescent vessel.[11,28] Such a drug would also lack systemic side effects. Finally, the carrier polymer to facilitate drug attachment to the stent needs to be inert. In fact, early attempts at polymer design demonstrated that some carrier polymers were proinflammatory, stimulating cellular proliferation.[8,11,13]

● SYSTEMIC VERSUS LOCAL DRUG DELIVERY (TABLE 39-4)

Animal experiments and limited human studies have shown some reduction in neointimal formation with systemically administered drugs such as vascular permeability factor (VEGF), cilostazol, troglitazone, paclitaxel, FK506, and everolimus.[13,29–32] However, correlation between animal models and human clinical trials is not always concordant. Despite advances in preventing acute stent thrombosis with systemically administered agents, particularly

TABLE 39-4. Factors Influencing Local Drug Delivery

- Biocompatibility of polymer
- Elution kinetics
- Solubility of pharmacologic agent
- Local drug concentration

antiplatelet and antithrombotic drugs, systemically administered drugs have nearly universally failed to prevent restenosis and neointimal proliferation in humans.[13,33] The likely explanation for the failure of systemically administered drugs to inhibit restenosis is the inability to achieve adequate local tissue concentrations of the drug at site of vessel injury.[7,11,34] Furthermore, the dose of systemically administered drugs needed to achieve local inhibitory concentrations required to prevent the activation and cascade of restenosis may cause systemic toxicity.[7] Although many of the studied agents failed when given systemically, encouraging results are being demonstrated when these agents are delivered locally on a stent-based platform.

● OVERVIEW OF CANDIDATE MOLECULES FOR DRUG-ELUTING STENTS

Neointimal proliferation has several biological similarities to tumor physiology and injury repair processes.[13] The search for candidate drugs, which will impact restenosis, when delivered locally at the site of arterial injury and inflammation, has therefore focused upon immunosuppressive and antitumor agents.[8,13] To date, the bulk of clinical studies have been in the evaluation of drug-eluting stents to reduce restenosis in the coronary arteries, with dramatic results, which are changing the treatment paradigm for multivessel coronary artery disease. Similarly, studies involving drug-eluting stents for the treatment of peripheral arterial disease are beginning to emerge, with encouraging results.[35]

The two most promising candidate drugs for the use on peripheral stents are paclitaxel and sirolimus.

Paclitaxel

A derivative of the Pacific yew, *Taxus brevifolia*, paclitaxel, has been used as an antineoplastic drug. Paclitaxel, and related taxane compounds, reversibly bind to the beta subunit of tubulin, resulting in the production of abnormal tubulin and resultant stable polymerization of microtubules, which blocks disassembly.[17,36] By interfering with normal microtubule production, paclitaxel affects multiple pathways in the cell cycle (blocking progression from G2 to M and interference with the mitotic spindle apparatus), signal transduction, and migration of vascular smooth muscle cells.[5,13,36–38] 7-Hexanoyltaxol, an esterified taxane analog with caproic acid, has been developed to alter elution kinetics and slow its release from the stent polymer.[36] The lipophilic properties of paclitaxel are ideally suited for its uptake into injured vascular tissue.[5,39]

Results with taxane-based drug-eluting stents in the coronary arteries are promising.[13] Long-term follow-up has generally demonstrated reduced neointimal formation and binary restenosis. As with other therapies, which limit vessel healing after injury, dose-dependent inhibition of endothelialization has been observed along with positive remodeling, raising the concern of increased stent thrombogenicity by persistent exposure of circulating cells to bare

metal and unhealed vessel wall.[5,37,40] Furthermore, long-term follow-up is necessary to determine if the beneficial effects are persistent or if the restenosis process is merely delayed.[17]

Sirolimus (Rapamycin)

Sirolimus, a macrocyclic lactone, is a weak antibiotic produced by *Streptomyces hygroscopicus*, found in the soil of Easter Island (Rapa Nui). Although a weak antibiotic, it is a strong immunosuppressant. This agent has been approved by the FDA since 1999 as an adjunctive treatment for renal allograft rejection.

Sirolimus is structurally similar to tacrolimus (FK506), and both molecules share the same intracellular receptor, FK-binding protein 12. The ternary complex formed by this bond contributes to the separate intracellular actions of sirolimus and FK506. Whereas FK506 prevents the transition from G0 to G1, sirolimus blocks progression from G1 to the S phase, normally stimulated by cytokines, such as IL-2.[7]

The binding of sirolimus to its intracellular receptor protein, FK-binding protein 12, interacts with the mammalian target of rapamycin (mTOR, also known as FRAP or RAFT1). Through the interaction and inhibition of mTOR, an essential regulatory kinase, sirolimus has multiple targets: S6 protein kinase p70 (S6 regulates translation of pathways critical to the cell cycle), the eukaryotic initiation factor eIF-4F, G1 controlling cyclin-dependent kinases, p27, and pRb (reduced phosphorylation).[5,7,8,13,41] Ultimately, the cell cycle is blocked from entering the S phase. Sirolimus prevents the cytokine activation of T-cells and the stimulation and migration of vascular smooth muscle cells. It has been suggested that sirolimus stimulates a cellular survival process similar to that observed during nutrient deprivation, resulting in autophagy—releasing intracellular amino acids and thus blocking transition from G1 to S.[42]

Based on the multiple mechanisms of suppression of the cell cycle and inhibitory response to inflammatory signals, sirolimus has been studied as a candidate for drug-eluting stents to prevent restenosis. Clinical trials using sirolimus eluting coronary stents have been promising, demonstrating a 270-day 8.9% in-segment (3.2% in-stent) restenosis within the sirolimus-treated stent compared to a 36.3% in-segment (35.4% in-stent) restenosis in the bare-metal stent-treated segment.[43] Other studies, including intravascular ultrasound examinations up to 2 years post-stent implantation, have confirmed the dramatic clinical superiority of sirolimus-eluting stents compared to bare-metal stents in the coronary artery circulation.[22,44–47] Analogs and derivatives of sirolimus are also being evaluated as candidate molecules. There are mixed data in the coronary literature whether sirolimus is superior to paclitaxel in higher-risk patients such as diabetic patients. Everolimus is an analog of sirolimus. Although there are no trials evaluating the efficacy of everolimus stents in the peripheral arterial system, data in the coronary literature suggest that this agent is efficacious in reducing neointimal hyperplasia and will likely be evaluated for its applicability in the peripheral arterial system.

Trials of Sirolimus-Coated Stents in the SFA

Trials of sirolimus-eluting stents in the periphery are encouraging. The early results from the SIROCCO feasibility study compared sirolimus-coated nitinol SMART stents to uncoated SMART stents for the treatment of chronic limb ischemia in 36 patients with occlusive femoral artery disease. Eighteen patients were randomized to each arm (slow release, five; fast release, 13; and bare metal, 18). Lesions up to 20 cm were treated, and there were 57% total occlusions. Angiography at 6 months demonstrated 0% binary in-lesion restenosis in the sirolimus arm and 23.5% in-lesion restenosis in the uncoated arm. The mean lumen diameter within the stent was significantly greater in the sirolimus-coated stents than in the bare-metal stents (4.95 vs. 4.31 mm, $p = 0.047$).[48] Twenty-four-month SIROCCO I follow-up, however, demonstrated a late attrition rate for in-stent restenosis: 40% (slow elution), 44.4% (fast elution), and 47.1% (placebo).

SIROCCO II compared the sirolimus slower elution kinetics stent in 29 patients to the bare-metal SMART stent in 28 patients. Patients had stenosis or total occlusions from 7 to 14.5 cm. Six-month angiographic results showed a mean stent diameter of 4.94 mm in the sirolimus group and 4.76 mm in the control group. The late loss was 0.38 mm in the sirolimus arm compared with 0.68 mm in the bare-metal arm, with no restenosis in the sirolimus group, whereas there was 7.7% restenosis in the bare SMART stent arm. Although the short-term results appeared very favorable for both DES and BMS, the long-term results were essentially equivalent with a restenosis rate of approximately 25%.

Other Potential Candidates for Drug-Eluting Stents

A variety of other compounds have been investigated in order to limit neointimal formation after stent implantation. Actinomycin-D is an antibiotic produced by *Streptomyces antibioticus*. Structurally, actinomycin-D contains a phenoxazone ring system with cyclic pentapeptides. By intercalating between DNA base pairs, actinomycin-D prevents complimentary DNA strand separation, inhibiting transcription of DNA by RNA polymerase, thus blocking cellular proliferation. Although actinomycin-D has the potential to inhibit restenosis, initial clinical trials have been disappointing, paradoxically with a higher incidence of restenosis in those receiving the actinomycin-D-coated stents.[13]

Animal models have demonstrated that 17 beta-estradiol-coated stents may reduce the in-stent intimal area.[49] Re-endothelialization seems to occur relatively early after the use of 17 beta-estradiol-coated stents, which may have several advantages.[49] Local delivery of a nitric oxide donor (sodium nitroprusside) have demonstrated the ability to upregulate cGMP but failed to reduce the neointimal area.[50] Stents with adsorbed antibody to glycoprotein IIb/IIIa have been evaluated to prevent restenosis in animal models.[51] Animal models of dexamethasone-coated stents have had mixed results in the reduction of neointimal hyperplasia and in-stent restenosis.[52,53]

● DES FOR OTHER ARTERIAL BEDS

In the renal artery, rates of restenosis following stent implantation are approximately 10% to 20%, depending on the vessel diameter, patient comorbidities, and the study design. The GREAT trial attempted to evaluate the efficacy of using a sirolimus-based Palmaz stent for primary reduction in angiographic restenosis. Compared to the bare-metal arm, the restenosis rates were reduced from 14% to 7%. The utility of DES for the primary treatment of renal artery stenosis will likely be limited as a result of the inherently low restenosis rates (particularly since most renal arteries are 5–6 mm in diameter) and cost of a DES platform.[54]

The use of drug-eluting stents in the intracranial circulation, extracranial carotid artery, and vertebrobasilar arteries has not been adequately studied in prospective and randomized trials. However, there are case series of using coronary-based platforms (paclitaxel and sirolimus) in the treatment of intracranial artery stenosis. Historically, the 6-month restenosis rate for bare-metal stents placed intracranially is approximately 35%. Short-term (average 4 months) follow-up demonstrated a restenosis rate of less than 10% with DES. Late stent thrombosis in the intracranial circulation has been reported and should temper the use of DES intracranially prior to well-controlled trials and long-term follow-up.[55] DES have also been employed in both the extracranial and cervical internal carotid artery. Since the currently available DES are all balloon expandable coronary stents (none indicated for non-coronary interventions), there is concern over both using an undersized stent and a stent deformity. The use of balloon expandable stents has been all but abandoned in areas where there is potential for extrinsic compression because of concerns over stent deformation (especially the cervical carotid artery). Long-term effects of the elution of the drug on the cerebrovasculature are unknown.

● FUTURE DIRECTIONS

Long-term outcomes with the use of drug-eluting stents are not available. Potential local or systemic toxicities have yet to be seen. Perhaps, the most concerning are late stent malapposition, positive arterial remodeling, and delayed re-endothelialization of the stent.[33,40,44,56] All these raise the risk for delayed stent thrombosis from exposed bare stent struts and unhealed vessels. Consequently, appropriate duration and type of oral antiplatelet therapy have not been determined. Furthermore, the initial cost of drug-eluting stents will be much greater than bare-metal stents. The impact of this on our already economically threatened health-care system is uncertain.[57] Clinical statements for the use of drug-eluting coronary stents are already formulated, and there will likely be similar discussions for the use of drug-eluting peripheral stents.

The use of locally delivered drugs for the prevention of restenosis is in its infancy, particularly in the treatment of peripheral arterial disease. At present, the most promising molecules for the use in the peripheral arterial system are sirolimus (and its analogs) and paclitaxel. Drug-eluting stents to primarily prevent neointimal proliferation and restenosis may allow the greater use of percutaneous therapy for the treatment of peripheral arterial disease and significantly expand the indications for percutaneous revascularization with stents.

REFERENCES

1. Dieter RS, Chu WW, Pacanowski JP Jr, McBride PE, Tanke TE. The significance of lower extremity peripheral arterial disease. *Clin Cardiol.* 2002;25:3-10.

2. Gray BH, Laird JR, Ansel GM, Shuck JW. Complex endovascular treatment for critical limb ischemia in poor surgical candidates: a pilot study. *J Endovasc Ther.* 2002;9:599-604.

3. Timaran CH, Stevens SL, Freeman MB, Goldman MH. External iliac and common iliac artery angioplasty and stenting in men and women. *J Vasc Surg.* 2001;34:440-446.

4. Timaran CH, Stevens SL, Freeman MB, Goldman MH. Infrainguinal arterial reconstructions in patients with aortoiliac occlusive disease: the influence of iliac stenting. *J Vasc Surg.* 2001;34:971-978.

5. Bennett MR. In-stent stenosis: pathology and implications for the development of drug eluting stents. *Heart.* 2003;89:218-224.

6. Fattori R, Piva T. Drug-eluting stents in vascular intervention. *Lancet.* 2003;361:247-249.

7. Regar E, Sianos G, Serruys PW. Stent development and local drug delivery. *Br Med Bull.* 2001;59:227-248.

8. Schwertz DW, Vaitkus P. Drug-eluting stents to prevent reblockage of coronary arteries. *J Cardiovasc Nurs.* 2003;18:11-16.

9. Ozaki Y, Violaris AG, Serruys PW. New stent technologies. *Prog Cardiovasc Dis.* 1996;39:129-140.

10. Sidawy AN, Weiswasser JM, Waksman R. Peripheral vascular brachytherapy. *J Vasc Surg.* 2002;35:1041-1047.

11. Hehrlein C, Arab A, Bode C. Drug-eluting stent: the "magic bullet" for prevention of restenosis? *Basic Res Cardiol.* 2002;97:417-423.

12. Inoue S, Koyama H, Miyata T, Shigematsu H. Pathogenetic heterogeneity of in-stent lesion formation in human peripheral arterial disease. *J Vasc Surg.* 2002;35:672-678.

13. Lemos PA, Regar E, Serruys PW. Drug-eluting stents in the treatment of atherosclerotic coronary heart disease. *Ind Heart J.* 2002;54:212-216.

14. Neville RF, Sidawy AN. Myointimal hyperplasia: basic science and clinical considerations. *Semin Vasc Surg.* 1998;11:142-148.

15. Heldman AW, Cheng L, Jenkins GM, et al. Paclitaxel stent coating inhibits neointimal hyperplasia at 4 weeks in a porcine model of coronary restenosis. *Circulation.* 2001;103:2289-2295.

16. van der Giessen WJ, Lincoff AM, Schwartz RS, et al. Marked inflammatory sequelae to implantation of biodegradable and nonbiodegradable polymers in porcine coronary arteries. *Circulation.* 1996;94:1690-1697.

17. Liistro F, Stankovic G, Di Mario C, et al. First clinical experience with a paclitaxel derivate-eluting polymer stent system implantation for in-stent restenosis immediate and long-term clinical and angiographic outcome. *Circulation.* 2002;105:1883-1886.

18. Farb A, Heller PF, Shroff S, et al. Pathological analysis of local delivery of paclitaxel via a polymer-coated stent. *Circulation.* 2001;104:473-479.

19. Park SJ, Shim WH, Ho DS, et al. A paclitaxel-eluting stent for the prevention of coronary restenosis. *N Engl J Med.* 2003;348:1537-1545.

20. Colombo A, Drzewiecki J, Banning A, et al.; TAXUS II Study Group. Randomized study to assess the effectiveness of slow- and moderate-release polymer-based paclitaxel-eluting stents for coronary artery lesions. *Circulation.* 2003;108:788-794.

21. Sousa JE, Costa MA, Abizaid A, et al.. Lack of neointimal proliferation after implantation of sirolimus-coated stents in human coronary arteries: a quantitative coronary angiography and three-dimensional intravascular ultrasound study. *Circulation.* 2001;103(2):192-195.

22. Sousa JE, Costa MA, Sousa AGMR, et al. Two-year angiographic and intravascular ultrasound follow-up after implantation of sirolimus-eluting stents in human coronary arteries. *Circulation.* 2003;107:381-383.

23. McClean DR, Eigler NL. Stent design: implications for restenosis. *Rev Cardiovasc Med.* 2003;3(suppl 5):S16-S22.

24. Rogers CDK. Drug-eluting stents: role of stent design, delivery vehicle, and drug selection. *Rev Cardiovasc Med.* 2002;3(suppl 5):S10-S15.

25. Hwang C-W, Wu D, Edelman ER. Physiological transport forces govern drug distribution for stent-based deliver. *Circulation.* 2001;104:600-605.

26. Kastrati A, Mehilli J, Dirschinger J, et al. Intracoronary stenting and angiographic results: strut thickness effect on restenosis outcome (ISAR-STEREO) trial. *Circulation.* 2001;103:2816-2821.

27. Pache J, Kastrati A, Mehilli J, et al. Intracoronary stenting and angiographic results: strut thickness effect on restenosis outcome (ISAR-STEREO-2) trial. *J Am Coll Cardiol.* 2003;41:1283-1288.

28. Stevens SL, Stern D, Levy J. Introduction of Interleukin-6 following balloon injury in rats. *Circ Suppl.* 1991;84:1365.

29. Takagi T, Akasaka T, Yamamuro A, et al. Troglitazone reduces neointimal tissue proliferation after coronary stent implantation in patients with non-insulin dependent diabetes

mellitus: a serial intravascular ultrasound study. *J Am Coll Cardiol.* 2000;36:1529-1535.

30. Farb A, John M, Acampado E, Kolodgie FD, Prescott MF, Virmani R. Oral everolimus inhibits in-stent neointimal growth. *Circulation.* 2002;106:2379-2384.

31. Kolodgie FD, John M, Khurana C, et al. Sustained reduction of in-stent neointimal growth with the use of a novel systemic nanoparticle paclitaxel. *Circulation.* 2002;106:1195-1198.

32. Hilgarth K, Trachtenbert J, Choi E, Stevens SL, Callow AD. The inhibitory effects of FK-506 on intimal hyperplasia. *FASEB J.* 1992;6:A1029.

33. Virmani R, Farb A, Kolodgie FD. Histopathologic alterations after endovascular radiation and antiproliferative stents: similarities and differences. *Herz.* 2002;27:1-6.

34. Jenkins NP, Prendergast BD, Thomas M. Drug eluting coronary stents may sound the death knell for restenosis. *Br Med J.* 2002;325:1315-1316.

35. Karamanoukian HL. What will be the impact of drug-eluting stents on hybrid coronary revascularization. *Heart Surg Forum.* 2002;5:e24-e27.

36. Kataoka T, Grube E, Honda Y, et al.; for the SCORE Investigators. 7-hexanoyltaxol-eluting stent for prevention of neointimal growth an intravascular ultrasound analysis from the study to compare restenosis rate between quest and quads-qp2 (SCORE). *Circulation.* 2002;106:1788-1793.

37. Grube E, Silber S, Hauptmann KE, et al. TAXUS I six- and twelve-month results from a randomized, double-blind trial on a slow-release paclitaxel-eluting stent for de novo coronary lesions. *Circulation.* 2003;107:38-42.

38. Tanabe K, Serruys PW, Grube W, et al. TAXUS III trial in-stent restenosis treated with stent-based delivery of paclitaxel incorporated in a slow-release polymer formulation. *Circulation.* 2003;107:559-564.

39. Virmani R, Liistro F, Stankovic G, et al. Mechanism of late in-stent restenosis after implantation of a paclitaxel derivate-eluting polymer stent system in humans. *Circulation.* 2002;106:2649-2651.

40. Hong M-K, Mintz GS, Lee CW, et al. Paclitaxel coating reduces in-stent intimal hyperplasia in human coronary arteries a serial volumetric intravascular ultrasound analysis from the Asian paclitaxel-eluting stent clinical trial. *Circulation.* 2003;107:517-520.

41. Stanislaw M. Stepkowski (2000) Molecular targets for existing and novel immunosuppressive drugs. *Exp Rev Mol Med.* 21 June. http://www.ermm.cbcu.cam.ac.uk/00001769h.htm.

42. Kamada Y, Funakoshi T, Shintani T, Nagano K, Ohsumi M, Ohsumi Y. Tor-mediated induction of autophagy via an Apg1 protein kinase complex. *J Cell Biol.* 2000;150:1507-1513.

43. Moses JW, Leon MB, Popma JJ, et al.; for the SIRIUS Investigators. Sirolimus-eluting stents versus standard stents in patients with stenosis in a native coronary artery. *N Engl J Med.* 2003;349:1315-1323.

44. Serruys PW, Degertekin M, Tanabe K, et al.; for the RAVEL Study Group. Intravascular ultrasound findings in the multi-center, randomized, double-blind RAVEL trial. *Circulation.* 2002;106:798-803.

45. Sousa JE, Costa MA, Abizaid A, et al. Sirolimus-eluting stent for the treatment of in-stent restenosis a quantitative coronary angiography and three-dimensional intravascular ultrasound study. *Circulation.* 2003;107:24-27.

46. Sousa JE, Costa MA, Abizaid AC, et al. Sustained suppression of neointimal proliferation by sirolimus-eluting stents one year angiographic and intravascular ultrasound follow-up. *Circulation.* 2001;104:2007-2011.

47. Degertekin M, Serruys PW, Foley DP, et al. Persistent inhibition of neointimal hyperplasia after sirolimus-eluting stent implantation long-term (up to 2 years) clinical, angiographic, and intravascular ultrasound follow-up. *Circulation.* 2002;106:1610-1613.

48. Duda SH, Pusich B, Richter G, et al. Sirolimus-eluting stents for the treatment of obstructive superficial femoral artery disease. *Circulation.* 2002;106:1505-1509.

49. New G, Moses JW, Roubin GS, et al. Estrogen-eluting, phosphorylcholine-coated stent implantation is associated with reduced neointimal formation but no delay in vascular repair in a porcine coronary model. *Catheter Cardiovasc Interv.* 2002;57:266-271.

50. Yoon J, Wu C-J, Homme J, et al. Local delivery of nitric oxide from an eluting stent to inhibit neointimal thickening in a porcine coronary injury model. *Yonsei Med J.* 2002;43:242-251.

51. Aggarwal RK, Ireland DC, Azrin MA, Exekowitz MD, de Bono DP, Gershlick AH. Antithrombotic potential of polymer-coated stents eluting platelet glycoprotein IIb/IIIa receptor antibody. *Circulation.* 1996;94:3311-3317.

52. Strecker E-P, Gabelmann A, Boos I, et al. Effect on intimal hyperplasia of dexamethasone released from coated metal stents compared with non-coated stents in canine femoral arteries. *Cardiovasc Intervent Radiol.* 1998;21:487-496.

53. Lincoff AM, Furst JG, Ellis SG, Tuch RJ, Topol EJ. Sustained local delivery of dexamethasone by a novel intravascular eluting stent to prevent restenosis in the porcine coronary injury model. *J Am Coll Cardiol.* 1997;29:808-816.

54. Zeller T, Rastan A, Rothenpieler U, Muller C. Restenosis after stenting of atherosclerotic renal artery stenosis: is there a rationale for the use of drug eluting stents? *Catheter Cardiovasc Interv.* 2006;68:125-130.

55. Gupta R, Al-Ali F, Thomas AJ, et al. Safety, Feasibility, and short-term follow-up of drug-eluting stent placement in the intracranial and extracranial circulation. *Stroke.* 2006;37:2562-2566.

56. Shah VM, Mintz GS, Apple S, Weissman NJ. Background incidence of late malapposition after bare-metal stent implantation. *Circulation.* 2002;106:1753-1755.

57. Sharma S, Bhambi B, Nyitray W. Sirolimus-eluting coronary stents (letter). *N Engl J Med.* 2002;347:1285.

chapter 40

Gene Therapy for Peripheral Arterial Disease

Daniel R. Guerra, MD / Brian H. Annex, MD

● INTRODUCTION

Peripheral arterial disease (PAD) caused by atherosclerotic occlusions that impair blood flow to the lower extremity is now recognized as a major health care problem. Despite the growing enthusiasm and improvements in both surgical and percutaneous techniques to improve blood flow to ischemic lower extremities in PAD,[1,2] a sizeable portion of patients with PAD, and especially those with critical limb ischemia (CLI), cannot benefit from these procedures because of diffuse atherosclerotic disease, poor distal conduits, or co-morbid conditions that make them poor revascularization candidates. Angiogenesis can be defined as the growth and proliferation of blood vessels from existing vascular structures, while therapeutic angiogenesis is an investigational method designed to employ the growth of new blood vessels to improve the vascular supply of ischemic tissues.[3,4] The purpose of this chapter is to review the evolution of gene therapy as a method to induce therapeutic angiogenesis in patients with PAD. To that end, we will review the mechanisms of new blood vessel growth, gene therapy vectors and delivery techniques, and human clinical trials that have used this technology to date. Finally, we discuss the recent studies of novel gene therapy approaches to therapeutic angiogenesis.

● BIOLOGY OF NEW BLOOD VESSEL FORMATION

Angiogenesis, Arteriogenesis, and Vasculogenesis

In the adult organism, blood vessel number is under tight biologic control. New blood vessel formation, or neovascularization, is an extremely complex process that is tightly reg-ulated, both temporally and spatially, and involves the production and interaction of numerous cytokines and signaling molecules. Neovascularization can be categorized into three distinct components: angiogenesis, arteriogenesis, and vasculogenesis (Figure 40-1). Although the term *angiogenesis* is frequently used to describe the process of new blood vessel growth in general, it specifically denotes the sprouting of new capillaries from existing vascular structures.[5] These capillary networks consist of only endothelial cell tubes and lack additional stabilizing components in the vessel wall. Angiogenesis can significantly expand the capillary bed, but the growth of larger vessels is often required to produce a significant increase in total blood flow. Tissue hypoxia or ischemia is considered the most important stimulus for angiogenesis.

Arteriogenesis refers to the maturation of existing collateral conduits, or perhaps de novo growth of new vessels, frequently large enough to be visualized angiographically (greater than 130 μm in diameter). Because this process leads to the formation of arterial conduits, arteriogenesis can significantly increase distal blood flow.[6,7] It is thought that local shear stress and inflammation are the primary processes that stimulate arteriogenesis.[8,9]

Once thought to occur only during embryonic development, *vasculogenesis* denotes the in situ formation of blood vessels from circulating endothelial progenitor cells (EPCs).[10,11] EPCs are CD34+ stem cells of bone marrow origin that are thought to migrate to areas of neovascularization and fuse with other EPCs and capillaries, leading to the local expansion of the vascular network. Recent studies, however, call into question the exact origin of so-called EPCs[12,13] and challenge the notion that these cells truly promote angiogenesis by incorporating into vessel walls.[14] Despite these uncertainties, it appears likely that all three

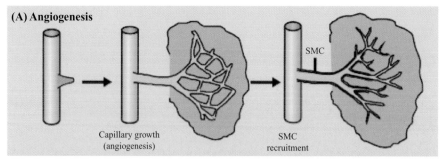

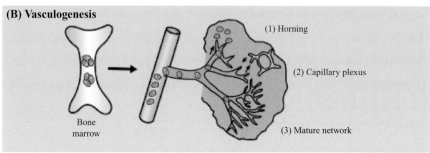

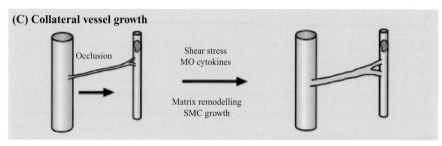

● **FIGURE 40-1.** Mechanisms of neovascularization in the adult. (A) Angiogenesis describes the sprouting of new capillaries from existing structures. Smooth muscle cells (SMCs) and other stabilizing components of the vessel wall are necessary to produce mature vessels. (B) Vasculogenesis refers to the recruitment of EPCs from the bone marrow to areas of neovascularization. These cells may become incorporated into nascent capillaries or stimulate vessel growth via the local release of proangiogenic factors. (C) Arteriogenesis, or collateral vessel growth, denotes the maturation of existing collateral conduits upon occlusion of a supply vessel (e.g., by a thrombus). Sheer stress and monocyte recruitment are thought to result in the local production of cytokines that drives arteriogenesis.

Figure reproduced with permission from Carmeliet P. Manipulating angiogenesis in medicine. J Intern Med. 2004;255:538-561, and Carmeliet P. Mechanisms of angiogenesis and arteriogenesis. Nat Med. 2000;6:389-95.

components of new blood vessel growth contribute to neo-vascularization in the adult organism.

Stimuli, Mechanisms, and Growth Factors in Neovascularization

Hypoxia and Angiogenesis. Tissue hypoxia, inflammation, and mechanical forces such as shear stress are all thought to play critical roles in neovascularization. Of these, tissue hypoxia-induced angiogenesis is the best understood. Tissue hypoxia of the lower extremity occurs during exertion in patients with intermittent claudication (IC) and is constant in the setting of CLI. Hypoxia induces numerous processes at the local and systemic levels aimed at maintaining tissue homeostasis and viability. These pro-tective mechanisms include local angiogenesis to enhance blood flow, erythropoesis to increase oxygen carrying capacity and delivery, and local alterations in metabolism to favor glycolysis for local energy production over oxidative metabolism.[15] The hypoxia-inducible factor (HIF) system is an example of a "master genetic program" that regulates many of these processes in the tissue.

HIF-1 is a heterodimeric transcription factor composed of the HIF-1α and HIF-1β proteins that bind specifically to a hypoxia-responsive element (HRE) in more than 40 hypoxia-inducible genes.[16] HIF-1β (also known as aryl hy-drocarbon receptor nuclear transporter or ARNT) is a stable subunit that is constitutively expressed under most conditions. HIF-1α, in contrast, has a half-life of less than 5 minutes during normoxic conditions because of the ongoing degradation via the ubiquitin proteosome pathway. Immediately following translation, the HIF-1α protein is tagged for degradation by prolyl hydroxylase-containing enzymes that require oxygen as a cofactor.[17] This pathway is impaired in the setting of hypoxia, which causes a rapid increase in the intracellular levels of HIF-1α and subsequent heterodimerization with HIF-1β to form the stable HIF-1 complex. Numerous genes induced by HIF-1 are directly involved in angiogenesis, including the vascular endothelial growth factor (VEGF) family of genes, the angiopoitins, matrix metalloproteinases (MMPs), and others.[16] The most salient of these with regards to angiogenic growth factor therapy are the VEGF family of genes.

The VEGF family contains five closely related genes: VEGF-A, -B, -C, -D, and placental growth factor (PIGF).[18] Of these, the progangiogenic effects of VEGF-A (hereafter referred to as VEGF) have been most extensively studied. In the adult human, the VEGF mRNA transcript undergoes alternative splicing that results in the expression and secretion of at least four functional isoforms that are named based on the number of amino acid residues in the mature protein (the murine orthologs are each shorter by one residue): $VEGF_{121}$, $VEGF_{165}$, $VEGF_{189}$, and $VEGF_{206}$.[18,19] The larger splice variants (165, 189, and 206) include exons that code for heparin-binding sequences. Whereas $VEGF_{121}$ is freely diffusible in the extracellular environment, $VEGF_{165}$ (the most highly expressed isoform) is partially circulating and partially bound to heparan sulfate proteoglycans in the extracellular matrix. The largest isoforms (189 and 206) remain fixed in the extracellular matrix. Because both $VEGF_{121}$ and $VEGF_{165}$ can be delivered systemically as soluble, recombinant proteins or by various gene transfer techniques, initial therapeutic angiogenesis trials of VEGF tested the effects of these isoforms. However, numerous studies suggest that the larger heparin-bound VEGF isoforms are important to angiogenesis in vivo.[20–22]

VEGF exerts its angiogenic effects via binding to two closely related tyrosine kinase receptors, VEGFR-1 (Flt-1) and VEGFR-2 (KDR/Flk-1), which are located primarily on the surface on endothelial cells.[18] VEGF is required for normal embryonic vascular development[23,24] and is a potent inducer of endothelial cell mitogenesis, chemotaxis, and survival, all of which are necessary for angiogenesis in the adult organism.[18] VEGF also stimulates recruitment of blood-borne inflammatory cells, such as macrophages and T-lymphocytes, which are vital to initiating and maintaining the process of neovascularization.[25,26]

Arteriogenesis. Arteriogenesis describes the growth of functional collateral arteries from preexisting arterio-arteriolar anastomoses that occur as a result of arterial occlusion.[27] Unlike angiogenesis, the primary stimulus for arteriogenesis is not likely to be hypoxia. The initial trigger for arteriogenesis is thought to be changes in wall stress or shear stress that occur within a collateral arteriole after an increase in blood flow. These forces cause local endothelial cell activation, which induces the expression of multiple genes involved in chemoattraction and cell–cell

adhesion.[28,29] As with angiogenesis, numerous cytokines have been implicated in arteriogenesis. The members of fibroblast growth factor (FGF) family are perhaps the best characterized arteriogenic growth factors, and like VEGF have been studied extensively in preclinical and human trials.

The FGFs are a family of more than 20 structurally related growth factors that exert their proangiogenic effects through interactions with numerous high-affinity tyrosine kinase receptors (FGFRs) on the surface of target cells. FGFs 1 (acidic FGF), 2 (basic FGF), 4, and 5 have the most pronounced angiogenic effects, and like VEGF are potent inducers of endothelial cell proliferation, migration, and activation.[30] Unlike VEGF, which acts primarily on endothelial cells, FGFs are capable of stimulating numerous cell types involved in vessel formation and maturation. These include pericytes, fibroblasts, and myoblasts, which are essential for muscularization of nascent capillaries.[31,32] Also unlike VEGF, whose activity is determined at the level of growth factor expression, the biologic effects of FGF are regulated predominantly by the amount of FGF receptor expression and activation in target tissues.[33,34]

● GROWTH FACTOR DELIVERY

The rationale for the use of exogenous growth factors in PAD is that supplementation with growth factors can overcome the endogenous deficit of cytokines and produce a therapeutic angiogenic response.[35] It should be noted, however, that little direct evidence exists to support the notion that cytokine growth factors are truly deficient in ischemic tissues. Despite this controversy, exogenous cytokine growth factor delivery is an accepted method to induce therapeutic angiogenesis and has been widely utilized. Cytokines can be delivered by direct administration of recombinant human protein or via gene transfer into target tissues, which results in subsequent protein production by transfected cells. Each method of growth factor delivery has its advantages and disadvantages. For example, although the transfer of protein cannot technically be classified as gene therapy, early attempts at angiogenic growth factor therapy utilized the delivery of recombinant protein to ischemic tissues. The primary advantage of protein therapy is the ability to deliver a known quantity of growth factor, and thus construct precise pharmacokinetic and dose–response relationships.[36] However, the limited tissue half-life of angiogenic proteins may be insufficient to produce the sustained activation necessary for a robust and complete angiogenic response.[37] The advent of gene therapy, which results in the prolonged expression of the protein of interest by transfected cells, circumvents this limitation. Gene transfer methods can be roughly divided into two categories: nonviral and viral.

Nonviral Vectors

The most basic method of nonviral gene transfer is direct incubation with unmodified plasmid DNA, often called "naked" DNA. The use of naked DNA is simple and well-tolerated because of its low toxicity and immunogenicity,[38] but there are several factors that limit the efficacy of this method. The small amount of naked DNA taken into a cell generally leads to low gene transfer efficiency,[39] although naked plasmids have been reported to induce relatively high levels of gene expression in muscle tissue.[40] Naked plasmid DNA is also rapidly degraded after intravenous injection, which necessitates direct delivery into tissue, usually by intramuscular injection. A clear advantage of this approach is the ability to administer repeated doses of DNA.

Numerous methods have been used to enhance transmission efficiency of plasmid DNA. One is the coupling of plasmid DNA to carrier molecules such as liposomes or polymer complexes, which facilitate transport of the DNA across cell membranes.[41] Cell targeting with DNA–liposome complexes can be achieved by conjugating specific proteins to the complex, which results in the liposome preferentially entering cells with the appropriate cell surface receptors.[42,43] The use of ultrasound energy and microbubble echocontrast agents has also been used to enhance transfer of naked DNA. This technique increases cell membrane permeability by producing transient small holes through which DNA is rapidly translocated, and has been shown to enhance transgene expression in cell culture and animal models.[44–46] One advantage of plasmid and carrier molecule-based therapy is their relative ease of production, especially when compared to viral vectors.

Viral Vectors

Because of the relatively low gene transfer efficiency of plasmid-based techniques, numerous viral vectors have been used in therapeutic angiogenesis. Replication-defective adenovirus systems are the most commonly used viral vectors and are approximately 1000 times more efficient in transfecting cells than plasmid DNA.[47] Adenoviruses can transfect both dividing and nondividing cells. The viruses enter the cells directly through the Coxsackie-adenovirus receptor (CAR)[48] and through specific integrins.[49] Once internalized, the adenovirus can escape from the endosome and release its transgene into the cytoplasm. The adenovirus remains extrachromosomal and provides transient expression of the transgene for 1 to 2 weeks.[50] In human trials, adenoviral vectors have caused inflammatory reactions, transient fevers, increases in liver transaminases, and one highly publicized death.[51] Despite this, the safety profile of adenoviral vectors is well established and their use in clinical trials has by and large been free of severe adverse events. Other limitations of adenoviral vector use include the lack of sustained gene expression (since the virus remains extrachromosomal), the antigenicity of viral proteins, and the lack of tissue specificity.[38]

Other viral vectors that have been studied for angiogenic gene therapy include adeno-associated viruses (AAVs), lentiviruses, and retroviruses, all of which integrate into the host genome and can induce long-lasting transgene expression.[39,52] AAVs can efficiently transduce skeletal muscle, myocardium, and blood vessels[53,54] and cause a diminished inflammatory response compared to adenovirus.[55] However, the utility of vectors that induce long-term transgene expression in the treatment of PAD is unclear, especially since prolonged and unregulated expression of potent growth factors may cause unwanted and deleterious side-effects. Thus, the transient growth factor expression produced by extrachromosomal adenoviral or plasmid vectors may be ideal in the PAD setting.[56]

Route of Administration

There are several routes of vector delivery that have been used in human angiogenesis trials. Plasmid DNA is rapidly degraded in the bloodstream and therefore is usually administered locally by direct intramuscular injection. Since systemic delivery of adenoviral vectors results in liver uptake and expression, local delivery via intramuscular injection is also preferred when viral vectors are used. In the setting of proximal arterial occlusion, which is often present in PAD, direct injection into tissues may be the only feasible delivery method. Angiogenic proteins can be delivered systemically into the bloodstream, although physical targeting via catheter-mediated intra-arterial delivery is generally preferred.[57]

● HUMAN CLINICAL TRIALS

The literature is filled with studies that detail the use of cytokine growth factors, especially VEGF and FGF, to induce therapeutic angiogenesis in preclinical models of PAD. A systematic review of those data is beyond the scope of this chapter. Instead, we will focus on published phase I and phase II human clinical trials of cytokine growth factor therapy for PAD (Table 40-1). In humans, $VEGF_{165}$ has been used in one published case report, two phase I uncontrolled, nonrandomized trials, and two phase II randomized, double blind, placebo-controlled trials. $VEGF_{121}$ has been tested in two phase I trials and one large phase II randomized, double blind, placebo-controlled trial. FGF-2 has been investigated in one phase I and one large phase II trial, while one human phase I study with FGF-1 has been published. The human trials reviewed below can be described as the first "phase" of studies that examined the role of gene therapy in PAD. A second, more recent phase of human trials (both completed and ongoing) using novel cytokine growth factors and gene therapy constructs will be discussed later.

Human Trials with $VEGF_{165}$

Initial Case Report. In 1996, Isner et al.[58] published the first case report that described the use of gene transfer to treat PAD in a human subject. In this pioneering case, a 71-year-old woman patient with diabetes suffering from toe gangrene caused by multiple atherosclerotic arterial occlusions was treated with site-specific gene transfer of plasmid DNA encoding $VEGF_{165}$ ($phVEGF_{165}$). This plasmid consisted of a eukaryotic PUC 118 expression vector into which cDNA encoding $VEGF_{165}$ has been inserted, and

TABLE 40-1. Published Phase I and Phase II Human Clinical Trials of Cytokine Growth Factor Therapy for PAD

	Author/Name of Trial	Disease	Treatment	N	Comments
Phase I	Baumgartner et al.[60]	CLI	Intramuscular phVEGF$_{165}$	9	Improvement in perfusion by angiography and MRA
	Shyu et al.[62]	CLI	Intramuscular phVEGF$_{165}$	21	Improvement in ABI and perfusion by MRA
	Rajagopalan, et al.[65]	IC	Intramuscular AdVEGF$_{121}$	15	Trend toward improvement in ABI and peak walking time
	Mohler et al.[66]	CLI	Intramuscular AdVEGF$_{121}$	13	Demonstrated safety
	Lazarous et al.[76]	IC	Intra-arterial FGF-2 protein	19	Demonstrated safety
	Comerota et al.[77]	CLI	Intramuscular FGF-1 plasmid	51	Improvement in symptoms, ABI, and ulcer healing
Phase II	Mäkinen et al.[63]	IC and CLI	Intra-arterial VEGF$_{165}$ via plasmid and adenoviral vectors	54	Delivered VEGF$_{165}$ post-angioplasty; demonstrated increased vascularity
	Kusamanto et al.[64]	CLI	Intramuscular phVEGF$_{165}$	54	Diabetic patients; improvements in wound healing and hemodynamics
	TRAFFIC[78]	IC	Intra-arterial FGF-2 protein	190	Improvement in peak walking time
	RAVE[67]	IC	Intramuscular AdVEGF$_{121}$	105	No difference in primary or secondary end points

CLI, critical limb ischemia; IC, intermittent claudication; ph, plasmid; Ad, adenoviral; MRA, magnetic resonance angiography; ABI, ankle-brachial blood pressure index.

contains a cytomegalovirus promoter/enhancer to drive production. Gene transfer was achieved by the use of a hydrogel-coated balloon angioplasty catheter system that the same investigators had successfully tested in animal models.[59] A sterile pipette was used to apply 2000 μg of plasmid DNA to the external hydrogel coating of the balloon. Under fluoroscopic guidance, this balloon catheter was inflated in the distal popliteal artery, proximal to occlusions of the peroneal, anterior tibial, and posterior tibial arteries.

Digital subtraction angiography (DSA) 4 and 12 weeks after gene transfer revealed increased collateral vessels in the treated limb at the knee, midtibial, and ankle levels (Figure 40-2). The investigators also noted increased intra-arterial Doppler flow measurements after gene transfer. In addition, magnetic resonance angiography at 4 and 12 weeks showed improved flow distal to the preexisting arterial occlusions. Approximately 7 days after gene transfer, the patient developed edema of the treated limb and three spider angiomas were noted over the medial and dorsal forefoot. The edema subsided within 4 weeks of treatment, and after excision of one angioma, the remaining two regressed by week 8 posttreatment. The investigators attributed all these findings to successful gene transfer of VEGF and subsequent gene expression in ischemic tissues. Despite an apparent improvement in this patient's blood flow, she eventually required a below-the-knee amputation of the treated limb. This landmark study not only demonstrated that gene

transfer with VEGF could promote angiogenesis in patients with PAD, but also highlighted the potential deleterious effects of VEGF gene transfer, specifically edema resulting from new blood vessel growth or enhanced vascular permeability.

Phase I Trials with VEGF$_{165}$

Baumgartner et al.[60] Approximately 14 months after Isner's initial report, the same group published a phase I non-randomized human trial that used phVEGF$_{165}$ in patients with chronic CLI. In this study, a total of nine patients (10 limbs) with nonhealing ulcers (7/10 limbs) and/or ischemic rest pain (10/10) who were not revascularization candidates were treated with intramuscular injection of phVEGF$_{165}$. Hemodynamic criteria included a rest ankle-branchial index (ABI) <0.6 and/or toe brachial index (TBI) <0.3 in the affected limb on two consecutive examinations at least 1 week apart. Each patient received a total of 2000 μg of plasmid DNA (4 aliquots of 500 μg each) by direct intramuscular injection into the ischemic limb. Injection sites were chosen arbitrarily based on available muscle mass and sites were both above and below the knee. Patients received a second 2000 μg dose 4 weeks after the initial injections, and all injections were well tolerated. There was no evidence of tumor development or worsening retinopathy during the follow-up period of the study (the average length of follow-up was 6 ± 3 months).

● **FIGURE 40-2.** Selective digital subtraction angiography of the lower leg immediately before (*left*) and 4 weeks after (*right*) phVEGF$_{165}$ gene transfer. New collateral vessels are visible.

Reproduced with permission from Isner JM, Pieczek A, Schainfeld R, et al. Clinical evidence of angiogenesis after arterial gene transfer of phVEGF165 in patient with ischaemic limb. Lancet. 1996;348(9024):370–374.

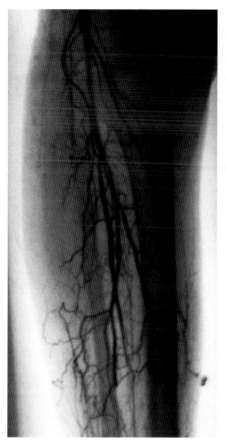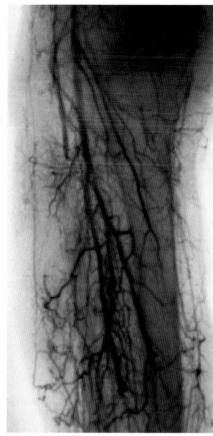

In this report, the investigators provided what was felt to be direct and indirect evidence of successful gene transfer. Serum (not plasma) levels of VEGF (determined by enzyme-linked immunosorbent assay (ELISA)) peaked 1 to 3 weeks after gene transfer in the seven of nine patients from whom blood was collected, which demonstrated transgene expression at the protein level. Six of the nine patients developed clinically evident edema after gene transfer, and the edema was bilateral (although more severe in the treated limb) in two patients. Immunohistochemical staining of tissue obtained from one amputee 10 weeks after gene therapy treatment revealed proliferating endothelial cells, which is rare in normal arteries. Polymerase chain reaction (PCR) performed on the same tissue revealed DNA fragments unique to phVEGF$_{165}$ in several tissue samples both near and remote from the sites of injection. In addition, Southern blot analysis of tissue obtained from two other treated amputees (8 and 10 weeks after treatment) confirmed the presence of DNA fragments unique to phVEGF$_{165}$.

The authors reported several striking physiologic benefits of phVEGF$_{165}$ treatment. DSA demonstrated newly visible collateral vessels at the knee, calf, and ankle levels in 7 of 10 treated limbs, and follow-up angiograms did not reveal evidence of collateral regression. Serial magnetic resonance angiograms of the ischemic limbs revealed qualitative evidence of improved distal flow in eight limbs. Absolute systolic ankle or toe pressure increased in eight limbs and was unchanged in one limb, and exercise performance improved in all five patients who were able to perform graded

treadmill exercise. All patients also experienced a statistically significant increase in pain-free walking time (2.5 ± 1.1 minutes before gene therapy versus 3.8 ± 1.5 minutes after gene therapy), which was measured an average of 13 weeks after treatment. In addition, the frequency of ischemic rest pain, defined as nights with pain per week, decreased significantly (5.9 ± 2.1 nights/week at baseline versus 1.5 ± 2.8 nights/week) after therapy. Nine of ten treated limbs had an improvement in limb status based on the Rutherford criteria,[61] with moderate improvement reported in five limbs. The investigators cautiously concluded that this study supported the strategy of intramuscular gene therapy with VEGF$_{165}$ to induce therapeutic angiogenesis in selected patients with PAD.

Shyu et al.[62] A second study of phVEGF$_{165}$ in patients with chronic CLI was performed by Shyu et al.[62] from Shin Kong Wu Ho-Su Memorial Hospital in Taipei, Tiawan. Patient selection and inclusion were similar to the study by Baumgartner et al.,[60] and patients were treated with intramuscular (IM) injections of the VEGF$_{165}$ plasmid in the same manner. This study sought to establish the minimal effective dose of phVEGF$_{165}$ in a Chinese patient population. Gene transfer was performed in 24 limbs of 21 patients with rest pain, some of which also had nonhealing ulcers (*n* = 16). Doses ranging from 400 to 2000 μg were given at the beginning of the study, and the same dose was given 4 weeks later. A total of five patients received an additional 2000 μg "booster" injection 2 to 3 months after the second injection.

Mean plasma levels of VEGF increased significantly 2 weeks after the initial treatment, but the authors were unable to demonstrate a statistically significant dose–response curve. Transient edema occurred in 6/24 limbs, but only in patients treated with 1600 or 2000 μg injections. Rest pain resolved completely in 12 limbs and improved significantly in 8 limbs, and 12 of 16 limbs with nonhealing wounds had improved tissue integrity. Treatment failure was more frequent in patients treated with lower doses of plasmid. The mean ankle-brachial blood pressure index increased significantly from 0.58 ± 0.24 before treatment to 0.72 ± 0.28 ($P < 0.001$) 4 weeks after completing two injections. The increase in ABI in patients receiving 1600 μg of plasmid was significantly higher than patients treated with 400 or 800 μg of phVEGF$_{165}$, but there was no apparent benefit seen with the 2000 μg dose. The mean magnetic resonance angiographic score also increased after treatment. Compared to the study by Baumgartner et al.,[60] Shyu et al.[62] noted a lower complication rate (predominantly due to less lower extremity edema) and a higher failure rate, which the authors attributed to the lower treatment doses of plasmid. The investigators concluded benefits of treatment with phVEGF$_{165}$ required at least two 1200 μg injections.

Phase II Trials with VEGF$_{165}$

Mäkinen et al.[63] In 2002, Mäkinen et al.[63] published a randomized, placebo-controlled, double blinded phase-II study that investigated the utility of local catheter-mediated VEGF$_{165}$ gene therapy after percutaneous transluminal angioplasty (PTA) of stenotic lower-limb arteries.[63] Patients with angiographically proven atherosclerotic infrainguinal stenosis or occlusion suitable for PTA were included in the study. Forty patients suffered from IC and 14 patients had CLI. Patients were randomized into one of three study groups: (1) VEGF$_{165}$ gene transfer using a replication-deficient adenoviral vector (VEGF-Ad) ($n = 18$); (2) VEGF$_{165}$ plasmid/liposomse complex (VEGF-P/L) gene transfer ($n = 17$); or (3) control group treated with Ringer's lactate ($n = 19$). The adenoviral VEGF vector and VEGF plasmid contained the same VEGF$_{165}$ expression cassette. The dose of VEGF-Ad was 2×10^6 colony forming units (CFUs), and that of VEGF P/L was 2000 μg of plasmid complexed with 2000 μL of DOTMA:DOPE liposome. Following PTA, the study agent was infused over 10 minutes at the site of PTA with one of two specialized balloon catheters (depending on the anatomic location and vessel diameter at the PTA site). The primary end point of the study was the change in vascularity as assessed by DSA at 3 months. Secondary clinical end points included restenosis rates, change in Rutherford class, and ABI at 3 months. DSA was performed prior to PTA, immediately following study agent infusion, and at 3 months. Two radiologists blinded to clinical information read all of the angiograms and classified each study as either unchanged/decreased vascularity or increased vascularity.

VEGF gene transfer was well-tolerated in general, without any observed hemodynamic effects during infusion or marked edema after treatment. Several patients in all treatment groups (including placebo) experienced mild edema, but this resolved spontaneously without specific treatment in all cases. An increase in antiadenovirus antibodies appeared in 11 of the VEGF-Ad treated patients, and transient febrile reactions occurred in one VEGF-Ad and three VEGF-P/L treated patients. Visually-assessed peripheral vascularity distal to the site of gene transfer increased significantly in both VEGF treatment groups as compared to control patients. The authors also reported that the VEGF-Ad group showed increased vascularity in the area of the most severe ischemia (this area was determined clinically, i.e., nonhealing ulcers or other trophic changes). No statistically significant differences in major amputations, ulcer healing, or resolution of rest pain were observed in the VEGF-treated groups. There was no difference in restenosis rates among the three groups, and statistically significant improvements in ABI and Rutherford class occurred in all the three groups. The authors concluded that gene transfer therapy with either VEGF-Ad or VEGF-P/L at the time of PTA produced an increase in distal vascularity and was well tolerated. However, this study did not demonstrate a clear clinical benefit of either treatment modality in this setting.

Kusamanto et al.[64] A recent placebo-controlled double blind randomized trial from the Netherlands evaluated phVEGF$_{165}$ treatment among patients with CLI and type 1 or 2 diabetes mellitus.[64] Patients with rest pain and/or nonhealing ulcers despite a minimum of 2 weeks of conventional therapy who were unsuitable candidates for either surgical or percutaneous revascularization were considered for this study. Patients in whom blood pressure could be obtained had resting ankle systolic BP of <50 mm Hg or resting toe systolic BP of <30 mm Hg. Patients randomized to the VEGF group were treated with IM injections of 2000 μg of phVEGF$_{165}$ (obtained from Isner's group) at the beginning of study followed by a second injection of 2000 μg 4 weeks later. At each treatment, patients received four injections of 500 μg/mL of plasmid, with two injections into the calf and two into the thigh of the ischemic limb. Patients assigned to placebo received four injections of 1 mL 0.9 % NaCl, which was physically indistinguishable from the phVEGF$_{165}$ injections. The primary endpoint was the major amputation rate, defined as an amputation above the ankle, at 100 days. Secondary end points were a 15% increase in pressure indices (ABI and TBI), clinical end points (ulcer healing, pain, and quality of life score), and safety. A total of 54 adult patients were included in the study (27 in each group). This is the number of patients the authors calculated would be necessary to demonstrate the expected decrease in amputations from 50% to 25% (power, 0.85, $p = 0.05$). Between February 2000 and January 2004, 97 patients were screened to find the 54 eligible patients.

In this study, phVEGF$_{165}$ treatment was well tolerated. There were no changes in blood pressure observed with treatment. Patients in both groups experienced an increase in baseline edema ($n = 21$) or new edema ($n = 7$), but this occurred equally in both groups. Unexplained hypoglycemia did occur in two phVEGF$_{165}$ treated patients in the first 2 to 3 weeks after treatment, but there were no other documented adverse reactions.

By day 100, a major amputation had been performed in six of the control patients compared to three of the phVEGF$_{165}$-treated patients ($p =$ NS). Hemodynamic parameters improved in 7 of 21 evaluable patients in the treatment group compared to 1 of 17 evaluable patients in the control group ($p = 0.05$). Improvement was defined as an absolute increase in ABI or TBI of >15% on at least two separate occasions. Seven of twenty-one patients with ischemic ulcers showed clinical improvement after treatment, compared to 0 patients in the control group ($p = 0.01$). Overall, the authors identified a total of 17 responders; 14 in the treatment group and three in the control group ($p = 0.003$). There was no demonstrable difference in pain scores between the two groups. Although the overall quality of life assessment was the same in both groups, clinical and/or hemodynamic responders reported improved physical functioning, social functioning, and health as compared with nonresponders. Although this study did not meet its primary end point, the authors point out that the actual rate of amputation in the control group (22%) was much lower than the expected rate (50%) and therefore decreased their ability to detect a significant difference. The study did demonstrate significant improvements in wound healing and hemodynamic insufficiency, which can be considered important clinical findings.

Human Trials with VEGF$_{121}$.

Phase I Trials with VEGF$_{121}$.

Rajagopalan et al.[65] The first human clinical trial that investigated the use of VEGF$_{121}$ was published by Rajagopalan et al.[65] in 2002. In this trial, the investigators studied the safety and efficacy of an adenovirus encoding VEGF$_{121}$ (AdVEGF$_{121}$) in patients with advanced claudication symptoms caused by infrainguinal atherosclerotic PAD. The AdVEGF$_{121}$ is an adenoviral construct based on the replication-deficient adenovirus type 5 vector that carries the VEGF$_{121}$ transgene. The study was initially designed as a double blind, placebo-controlled, dose-escalation study in patients with CLI and IC, but the CLI cohort results were reported separately.[66] The total doses in each group ranged from 4×10^8 to 4×10^{10} particle units (pu) proceeding in half-log increments. In each of the first three dose groups, one patient received the carrier and served as a control while three patients received AdVEGF$_{121}$. However, after the third dosing cohort, the protocol was changed to an open-label format without placebo because patients refused to enroll in placebo treatment. A total of three patients received placebo, while 15 received the study agent. Inclusion criteria included age >40 years, patent aortoiliac segments, angiographic evidence of >35% stenosis involving infrageniculate vessels, disabling unilateral claudication, rest ABI < 90% and/or exercise ABI < 75%. The total dose of the AdVEGF$_{121}$ was divided into 20 one mL aliquots, and direct intramuscular injection of all aliquots

was performed in one setting. The investigators chose areas of potential collateralization based on angiographic findings (e.g., the thigh for patients with predominant superficial femoral/popliteal artery disease and thigh and calf for patients with infrapopliteal disease). The investigators evaluated safety parameters at days 1 to 7, 15, 30, 90, 180, and 360 after enrollment. As a measurement of efficacy, walking time to maximum claudication pain was determined at days 30, 90, 180, and 360.

All patients tolerated initial treatment well. Seven patients in total developed either localized edema at injection sites or more extensive limb swelling that resolved spontaneously by day 23 posttreatment. Two treated patients experienced mild hypersensitivity reactions. In the AdVEGF$_{121}$ group, there was one death due to necrotizing pancreatitis at day 160, and one early stage bladder carcinoma was discovered in a 70-year-old man on day 274. Among the 38% of subjects who had neutralizing anti-adenovirus antibodies at baseline, 70% had a doubling of their titers by day 7. The investigators reported nonsignificant trends toward improvement in ABIs and peak walking time among patients treated with AdVEGF$_{121}$, but definitive conclusions on efficacy were not possible. This study did demonstrate the safety of AdVEGF$_{121}$ in patients with PAD and IC.

Mohler III et al.[66] Along with the patients enrolled in the study by Rajagopalan et al.[65] described above, a total of 15 patients suffering from CLI due to atherosclerotic PAD were treated with the AdVEGF$_{121}$ ($n = 13$) or placebo ($n = 2$).[66] Patients in the CLI cohort were aged 35 years or older, had angiographic evidence of >50% infrainguinal stenosis, and had ongoing rest pain or tissue loss. Patients were not thought to be revascularization candidates at the time of enrollment. The dosage amounts, dosing schedule, technique of study agent administration, and safety follow-up schedule were the same as in the IC cohort. With regards to safety, the investigators focused specifically on events such as worsening of disease, development of gangrene, or amputation. Rest ABIs were also measured in all patients.

There were no serious complications related to study agent injection. Only one patient had injection site edema, which started on day 1 and resolved by day 7. Of the 11 patients for whom safety data was obtained through day 360 (1 control and 10 treated patients), a total of 10 surgical bypass procedures and 9 amputations were performed between days 30 and 360 posttreatment. The authors concluded that use of AdVEGF$_{121}$ in patients with CLI was safe and well-tolerated. However, there did not appear to be any clinical benefit to AdVEGF$_{121}$ administration, which is illustrated by the number of necessary amputations and attempts at surgical revascularization among treated patients.

The RAVE Trial with VEGF$_{121}$. The encouraging results from the phase I AdVEGF$_{121}$ trial in patients with IC prompted the completion of a larger phase II randomized, double blind, controlled study. The Regional Angiogenesis with Vascular Endothelial Growth Factor in Peripheral Arterial Disease (RAVE) trial[67] was designed to test the efficacy and safety of intramuscular delivery of $AdVEGF_{121}$ to the lower extremities of patients with unilateral PAD and exercise-limiting claudication. The primary end point was changed from baseline in peak walking time at 12 weeks after treatment. Secondary efficacy end points included change in peak walking time at 26 weeks, claudication onset time at 12 and 26 weeks, resting and postexercise ABI in the treated limb at 12 and 26 weeks, and quality of life (using the Physical Component Summary Scale of the SF-36 survey and the Walking Impairment Questionaire). Men and women aged 40 to 80 years with PAD (resting ABI $<$ 0.8 in the affected limb) and chronic, stable, predominantly unilateral IC of $\geq$6 months duration were recruited for the study. In addition, study participation required preserved proximal arterial inflow, $>$50% femoropopliteal stenosis (determined by conventional or magnetic resonance angiography, or by duplex ultrasound), and at least one patent infrapopliteal artery. A total of 105 subjects were randomized to either placebo ($n = 33$), low-dose $AdVEGF_{121}$ (4×10^9 PU, $n = 32$), or high-dose $AdVEGF_{121}$ (4×10^9 PU, $n = 40$) treatment. Study drug was administered by direct intramuscular injection as previously described.[65,68]

Patients tolerated treatment well. Similar to prior studies with VEGF, edema of the injected extremity occurred in $AdVEGF_{121}$-treated patients and was more common in the high-dose group (3/33 patients in the placebo group, 6/32 patients in the 4×10^9 PU group, and 11/48 patients in the 4×10^{10} PU group). However, since systemic levels of VEGF were not measured or reported, it is unclear if the increase in edema was due to an increase in VEGF expression or the local effects of the adenoviral vector. There were no other major safety issues, including excess malignancy, retinal neovascularization, or an increase in cardiovascular events, at 1 year of follow-up. Data was reported using a modified intention-to-treat analysis, which excluded missing data and data collected after revascularization or treatment with cilostazol. Circulating $AdVEGF_{121}$ was noted in 75% (six of eight patients in whom this was measured) of patients treated with high-dose $AdVEGF_{121}$ 24 hours after dosing, but was not seen in any patients in the low-dose or placebo groups. All groups demonstrated improvements in the primary efficacy end point (change in peak walking time at 12 weeks), but there was no difference between groups. Likewise, there was no difference in claudication onset time or ABI in the $AdVEGF_{121}$ groups compared with control at either 12 or 26 weeks. Results of intention-to-treat analysis were no different. All groups also reported improvement in quality of life as assessed by the questionnaires, but there was no difference among the groups. The authors concluded that a single unilateral intramuscular administration of $AdVEGF_{121}$ did not improve exercise performance or quality of life in these patients, and therefore could not support its use as a treatment strategy in patients with unilateral PAD.

The investigators cited several potential causes for the lack of efficacy of VEGF seen in this study. One unexpected finding was the amount of improvement in the study end points seen in placebo-treated patients, which may have limited the ability to discern a benefit of $AdVEGF_{121}$. Another possibility cited by the authors is that one-time dosing of $AdVEGF_{121}$ did not produce sufficient transgene expression to induce physiologically pertinent neovascularization. In addition, the authors questioned whether the adenoviral gene transfer system is appropriate in this setting given the relative difficulty transfecting skeletal muscle.[69–72]

Human Trials with FGF

Phase I Trials with FGF.

Lazarous et al.[76] By 1996, several investigators had demonstrated that treatment with FGF-2 (basic FGF) improved collateral development in animal models of hind limb ischemia.[73–75] Given these findings, Lazarous et al.[76] evaluated the safety, tolerability, and pharmacokinetics of intra-arterial FGF-2 in patients with atherosclerotic PAD and IC.[76] Patients included in the study were 40 years of age or older, had a history of IC symptoms for $>$6 months, and had an ABI of $<$0.8 either at rest or after exercise. A total of 19 patients were randomized in a 2:1 fashion to either escalating doses of intra-arterial FGF-2 protein (10 μg/kg once, $n = 4$; 30 μg/kg once, $n = 5$; or 30 μg/kg on two consecutive days, $n = 4$) or placebo ($n = 6$). After determining which limb was more ischemic (based on ABI), the femoral artery was percutaneously cannulated with an 18-gauge catheter and the study agent was infused intra-arterially over 15 minutes.

The investigators attempted to answer several questions regarding the safety of FGF-2 treatment. The first subject randomized to FGF-2 treatment experienced a significant transient drop in blood pressure after receiving the 10 μg/kg dose over 2 minutes. The protocol was subsequently modified to increase the infusion time, and no other subjects experienced significant hypotension during study drug infusion. Two potential deleterious effects of FGF treatment, retinal neovascularization and proteinuria, were not observed in this small patient group during the follow-up period of the trial.

Although the primary goals of the study were to ascertain the safety and pharmacokinetics of intra-arterial FGF-2 protein administration, the investigators did measure resting calf blood flow by strain gauge plethysmography in the two higher-dose treatment groups. The investigators recorded initial flow immediately before treatment, at 1 month, and at 3 to 7 months following treatment (median time-point = 6 months). There was no significant increase in flow seen in the six placebo patients, but both higher dose treatment groups experienced a statistically significant increase in calf blood flow. It should be noted that the trial was not specifically designed to assess efficacy. Only one of the four patients in the placebo arm reported marked improvement in symptoms at 1 month, compared to six of nine patients in the two higher dose groups. Based on the results of this double blind, placebo-controlled phase I trial, the investigators concluded that intra-arterial administration of bFGF protein was well-tolerated and may have a beneficial effect in patients with PAD and IC.

Comerota et al.[77] In 2001, Comerota et al.[77] published a phase I open-label, dose escalation trial that evaluated the safety and efficacy of DNA encoding FGF-1 (NV1FGF) treatment in patients with CLI. The NV1FGF plasmid contains a fusion gene between the human fibroblast interferon secretion signal peptide and the naturally occurring truncated form of FGF-1. Patients were considered for enrollment if they had nonrevascularizable CLI with ischemic rest pain or evidence of ulceration and/or tissue loss. Objective evidence of PAD defined by ABI < 0.4, TBI < 0.3, or abnormal metatarsal pulse volume recording (PVR) was present in all patients. Angiography was performed to confirm arterial occlusion. A total of 51 patients received single (500, 1000, 2000, 4000, 8000, or 16 000 µg) or repeated (2 × 500, 2 × 1000, 2 × 2000, 2 × 4000, or 2 × 8000 µg) injections of NV1FGF into the distal thigh and distal leg muscles. The repeated doses were given 2 weeks apart. Of the 51 total patients treated, only 15 were available for evaluation of biologic activity and clinical outcomes (treatment doses ranged from 500 to 4000 µg). All 51 patients had safety data recorded.

There were no serious adverse events attributed to NV1FGF administration, and aside from local irritation, pain, and one instance of edema the injections were tolerated well. The authors reported that NV1FGF was present in the plasma transiently and resolved within 4 weeks of injection. No plasmid was detected in the urine. Among the 15 patients on whom clinical data was collected, the investigators noted statistically significant decreases in reported pain from baseline starting at week 8 and continuing to week 24 of the study. ABI, TBI, and ulcer healing (measured as a decrease in aggregate ulcer size among the nine patients with ulcers at enrollment) also improved significantly from baseline. It should be noted, however, that the absolute increase in ABI (0.08) was quite small. This study demonstrated the safety of NV1FGF in this patient population and suggested possible beneficial physiologic effects. Two phase-II randomized clinical trial testing NV1FGF have been completed (one in Europe and one in the United States), but the results are not yet published.

TRAFFIC Study with Recombinant FGF-2 Protein. The Therapeutic Angiogenesis with Recombinant Fibroblast Growth Factor-2 for Intermittent Claudication (TRAFFIC) trial was a placebo-controlled, double blinded, randomized trial that compared one or two intra-arterial infusions of recombinant FGF-2 (rFGF-2) with placebo in patients with IC.[78] The rFGF-2 used was a 146 amino acid, nonglycosylated, monomeric, 16.5 kDa protein produced in genetically engineered yeast. The rFGF-2 dose used (30 µg/kg) was the maximum dose tolerated in phase I studies of intracoronary infusion[79,80] and was tolerated in the phase I

PAD study by Lazarous et al.[76] Patients older than 40 years with exercise-induced IC were eligible for this study. All patients had a peak walking time between 1 and 12 minutes, evidence of infrainguinal obstructive atherosclerosis (≥70% stenosis of femoral, popliteal, or tibial arteries on angiography) and a resting ABI of <0.8 on the most affected limb. One hundred and ninety such patients were randomized in a 1:1:1 fashion to bilateral intra-arterial infusions of placebo on days 1 and 30 ($n = 63$), rFGF-2 on day 1 and placebo on day 30 (single-dose, $n = 66$), or rFGF-2 on days 1 and 30 (double-dose, $n = 61$). The primary outcome was change from baseline in 90-day peak walking time. Secondary outcomes included change in 180-day peak walking time, claudication onset time at 90 and 180 days, ABI change at 90 and 180 days, change in quality of life, and safety.

Study drug was administered after contrast angiography. Equal amounts of study drug were administered into each common femoral artery, usually via unilateral femoral artery puncture with iliac crossover to the contralateral artery. A bolus of heparin (40 U/kg) was given intravenously 10 to 20 minutes before study drug infusion. Exercise performance was measured with a standard treadmill protocol, and patients were instructed to exercise until they "absolutely had to stop." Patients were excluded from the trial if they stopped exercise for some reason other than claudication symptoms (e.g., angina, fatigue, joint pain, dyspnea, etc.) or if they had peak walking times that varied by more than 20% on two consecutive tests (>24 hours but <2 weeks apart).

One hundred and seventy-four of the 190 patients originally enrolled were available for treadmill assessment at 90 days. Compared with baseline, patients in the placebo group increased peak walking time by 0.60 minute (34%), patients in the single-dose increased this time by 1.77 minutes (34%), and patients in the double-dose group showed an increase of 1.54 minutes (20%). By ANOVA, log-transformed data for the 174 patients did not differ significantly ($p = 0.075$), but results of intention-to-treat analysis (which included all 190 patients) showed a significant difference between the three groups ($p = 0.034$). Pairwise analysis showed a statistically significant increase in peak walking time in the single-dose versus the placebo group ($p = 0.026$), but not in the placebo versus the double-dose group ($p = 0.45$). A small improvement in ABI was seen in both the single-dose and double-dose groups compared to baseline at 90 days. This increase seemed to persist at 180 days but was not statistically significant. There was no difference in the change in quality of life measures among the groups. Both doses of rFGF-2 seemed to be well tolerated. Transient hypotension was uncommon but occurred more frequently in the rFGF-2 groups (two patients in the placebo group; four in the single-dose group, and five in the double-dose group). Proteinuria was also infrequent but likewise arose more often in patients treated with rFGF-2 (two in the placebo group, six in the single-dose group, and seven in the double-dose group). There was no evidence of increased mortality, cardiovascular events, or acceleration of PAD in patients treated with rFGF-2. The TRAFFIC study successfully demonstrated that intra-arterial rFGF-2 improvement in peak walking time at 90 days and ABI in patients with IC. Although both dosing regimens showed improvement, there was no statistical benefit of two versus one dose of 30 μg/kg. The investigators concluded that the results provided evidence of clinically therapeutic angiogenesis after rFGF-2 treatment.

Safety Considerations

Deleterious effects of therapeutic angiogenesis remain an area of great concern. Peripheral edema due to increased vascular permeability is a common side effect seen in clinical trials, especially when single isoforms of VEGF are used. A notable disadvantage of virally mediated gene transfer is the inflammatory and immunologic reactions that often occur.[81,82] Another theoretical concern is that angiogenic growth factor therapy could enhance the growth of unrecognized tumors,[83] hence the careful screening for possible malignancy of patients enrolled in angiogenesis trials. The possibility of significant abnormal blood vessel growth is highlighted by the observation that direct injection of VEGF-expressing myoblasts induced hemangioma formation in mouse myocardium.[84,85] Despite these observations, there is no evidence of an increased risk of malignancy or deleterious blood vessel growth among patients enrolled in randomized clinical trials during the follow-up period of those trials.

● NEW DIRECTIONS

Despite the often dramatic benefits that were observed in early phase I clinical trials, larger randomized phase II studies achieved only modest success in attaining their stated clinical end points. The reasons for this apparent lack of efficacy are varied, and include patient and end point selection, placebo effect, the duration and level of transgene expression, the dose and method of delivery of angiogenic factors, and the choice of angiogenic agents tested.[9] Perhaps the most glaring potential flaw of the first phase of clinical trials in angiogenesis is the "monogene" approach. Given the complexity inherent in the regulation of neovascularization, it seems improbable that treatment with a single agent can induce the production of a robust vascular network capable of alleviating ischemia. Recent efforts in the field of therapeutic angiogenesis have focused on methods to induce the simultaneous expression of multiple angiogenic growth factors. Two noteworthy techniques are the use of engineered transcription factors and the delivery of "master switch" genes that are capable of initiating the neovascular cascade.[86]

Engineered Zinc Finger Protein Transcription Factors

As noted earlier in the chapter, the human VEGF gene is differentially spliced to produce at least four functional isoforms in vivo, $VEGF_{121}$, $VEGF_{165}$, $VEGF_{189}$, and $VEGF_{206}$.

Although $VEGF_{165}$ is thought to possess optimal angiogenic properties due to its combination of diffusibility and heparin binding, one would expect that expression of all isoforms of VEGF would lead to more physiological angiogenic effects. Whitlock et al.[87] investigated this possibility in a murine model of hindlimb ischemia. The investigators compared the ability of an adenoviral vector that encoded all three major murine isoforms of VEGF (120, 164, and 188, AdVEGF-All) with vectors that encoded each isoform separately. They found that AdVEGF-All treatment resulted in significantly improved recovery from hind limb ischemia compared to each isoform separately. An alternative approach to express multiple VEGF isoforms simultaneously involves the use of an engineered zinc fingered protein (ZFP) transcription factor to drive the expression of the endogenous VEGF gene in target cells.

ZFP transcription factors are composed of zinc finger DNA-binding domains that bind to specific DNA sequences within gene regulatory domains. If the sequencing data for a given gene's promoter region is known, individual ZFPs can be engineered to bind that promoter. This ZFP can then be matched with a transcription activation or repression domain from another protein, resulting in a new fusion protein that selectively activates or represses the gene of interest. Using this technique, Liu et al.[88] generated several VEGF-activating ZFPs (VEGF-ZFPs) that can bind to the promoter region of the human and mouse VEGF gene and induce transcription. Furthermore, delivery of the VEGF-ZFP construct using either an adenoviral vector or plasmid DNA results in expression of all major isoforms of VEGF.[88–90] Rebar et al.[89] were the first to study the effects of a murine-specific VEGF-ZFP construct in vivo. The investigators demonstrated that adenoviral delivery of the VEGF-ZFP to the skin in an ear angiogenesis model led to a significant increase in blood vessel density (Figure 40-3). Mice treated with an adenovirus encoding only $VEGF_{164}$ developed focal hemorrhage and edema, whereas the VEGF-ZFP-mediated angiogenesis occurred without these unwanted effects.

To test the ability of the VEGF-ZFP to induce therapeutic angiogenesis, our research group examined the effects of a VEGF-ZFP-containing plasmid (Figure 40-4) on skeletal muscle perfusion recovery and capillary density following the induction of hind limb ischemia in a rabbit model.[90] The VEGF-ZFP plasmid construct makes direct injection of the VEGF-ZFP into the ischemic muscle bed possible, resulting in targeted expression of the VEGF isoforms. Intramuscular injection of the VEGF-ZFP plasmid induced expression of all three major VEGF splice variants, which resulted in increased capillary density and perfusion recovery in the ischemic limb. The beneficial effects of the VEGF-ZFP plasmid have also been shown in hypercholesterolemic $ApoE^{-/-}$ mice,[91] which have impaired perfusion recovery and angiogenesis compared to wild-type mice. A human phase I clinical trial to evaluate the safety of the VEGF-ZFP plasmid in patients with CLI is currently underway.

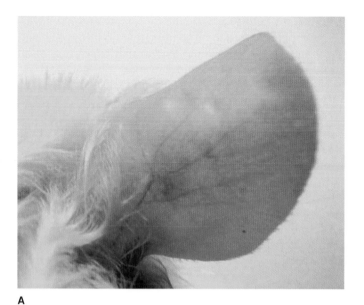
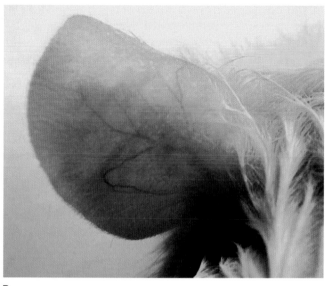

A
B

● **FIGURE 40-3.** Increase in vessel density 3 days after adenoviral delivery of ZFP-VEGF in a mouse ear model. (A) Ear injected with a GFP-encoding (control) adenoviral vector. (B) Contralateral ear on the same animal injected with the ZFP-VEGF-encoding vector. The authors reported an approximately 2.5-fold increase in visible vessels in a 40 × microscopic field.

Figure reproduced with permission from Rebar EJ, et al. Induction of angiogenesis in a mouse model using engineered transcription factors. Nat Med. 2002;8:1427–1432.

HIF-1α/VP16 Hybrid Transcription Factor

Another approach to induce the expression of multiple endogenous growth factors, including VEGF, PIGF, Ang-2, and Ang-4,[92] is to harness the natural response to tissue

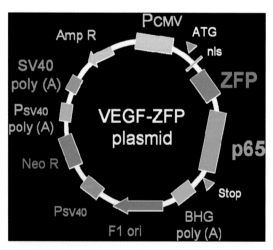

● **FIGURE 40-4.** Schematic representation of the ZFP-VEGF plasmid. The plasmid encodes an engineered three-finger ZFP DNA binding domain (ZFP), the nuclear translocation signal from SV40 large T antigen (nls), and the transactivation domain from the p65 subunit of human nuclear factor-kB (p65) in the pVAX1 plasmid (Invitrogen). Expression is under the control of the CMV immediate early promoter (P_{CMV}).

Figure courtesy of Gregory K. Lam, M.D.

hypoxia via the HIF system. An engineered transcription factor construct that contains the DNA binding and dimerization domains from HIF-1α fused to a herpes virus VP16 transactivation domain (HIF-1α/VP16) has been developed and tested in preclinical models of PAD. Using the rabbit hind limb ischemia model, Vincent et al.[93] demonstrated an increase in limb blood pressure, capillary density, and maximal blood flow following intramuscular delivery of plasmid DNA encoding the HIF-1α hybrid transcription factor. In addition, the HIF-1α/VP16 DNA produced superior results compared to treatment with a plasmid encoding human VEGF$_{165}$.

Very recently, Rajagopalan et al.[65] published the results of a phase I human trial that evaluated the safety and clinical effects of treatment with an adenoviral vector containing the constitutively active HIF-1α hybrid (Ad2/HIF-1α/VP16).[94] In this study, a total of 34 patients with CLI and no options for revascularization were treated with escalating doses of the study agent, ranging from 1×10^8 to 2×10^{11} viral particles. No serious adverse events were attributable to the study agent, but vision disorders (associated with minor retinal findings) and flu-like symptoms were more common in treated patients. The authors were unable to arrive at any conclusions regarding clinical outcomes due to the small number of patients enrolled. However, they did report complete resolution of rest pain in 14 of 32 patients and ulcer healing in 5 of 18 patients at 1 year. In general, treatment with the Ad2/HIF-1α/VP16 construct was well tolerated, but further randomized studies will be needed to evaluate its clinical efficacy.

Hepatocyte Growth Factor

Hepatocyte growth factor (HGF), along with HIF-1α, is an attractive "master switch" gene that is currently being studied in humans with PAD. HGF induces the expression of multiple proteins involved in angiogesis, including VEGF, the VEGFR-2 receptor, and proteins involved in matrix degradation.[95,96] The proangiogenic effects of HGF are primarily mediated by the induction of the transcription factor ets-1.[95] HGF administration has been shown to promote angiogenesis in animal models of both myocardial infarction[97] and hind limb ischemia.[98,99] Based on these preclinical results, the HGF-STAT trial was designed to test the ability intramuscular injections of an HGF-containing plasmid to improve perfusion in patients with unrevascularizable CLI.[100] The results of this trial were recently published.[101] In the HGF-STAT trial, 106 patients with rest pain or ischemic ulcers and a transcutaneous oxygen tension (TcPO$_2$) of less than 40 mm Hg and/or a toe pressure of less than 50 mm Hg were randomized to receive intramuscular injections of either placebo or three different doses of HGF plasmid (low, middle, and high dose; randomized in a 1:1:1:1 manner). The primary objective of the study was to assess the safety and tolerability of the HGF plasmid at 12 months. Limb perfusion was assessed as a change TcPO$_2$, ABI, and TBI at six months after enrollment. Ulcer healing was also assessed.

At 6 months, patients treated with the high dose regimen of HGF plasmid had a significant increase in TcPO$_2$ compared to the other treatment groups. There was no difference among the groups in ABI, TBI, pain relief, wound healing, or major amputation at 6 months. It should be noted that the study was not adequately powered to assess differences in these secondary endpoints. Importantly, there was no evidence of adverse events attributable to the use of the HGF plasmid at 12 months. The HGF-STAT trial established the safety of the HGF plasmid as a possible treatment for CLI, but larger studies with the HGF plasmid are needed to determine if the increase seen in TcPO$_2$ translate into improved clinical outcomes in patients with CLI.

● CONCLUSION

Despite the initial enthusiasm and enormous potential of gene therapy for the treatment of PAD, the results of human trials published to date have been disappointing. These trials, however, contain serious flaws, the most significant of which may be the use of single growth factors as a means to induce therapeutic angiogenesis. Newer treatment modalities designed to induce more "physiologic" neovascularization, such as engineered transcription factors and HIF-1α hybrid constructs, could prove to be an important step in the field of therapeutic angiogenesis. Several other gene therapy techniques, including the use of PlGF alone[102] or as a chimera gene with VEGF-E[103] have been tested in animal models and appear to be effective. Other potential agents for therapeutic angiogenesis undoubtedly will come to light as our knowledge of the basic molecular mechanisms involved in neovascularization grows. Taken as a whole, gene therapy in the treatment of PAD is an ever-expanding field that still holds great promise.

REFERENCES

1. Schillinger M, Sabeti S, Loewe C, et al. Balloon angioplasty versus implantation of nitinol stents in the superficial femoral artery. *N Engl J Med.* 2006;354(18):1879-1888.

2. Adam DJ, Beard JD, Cleveland T, et al. Bypass versus angioplasty in severe ischaemia of the leg (BASIL): multicentre, randomised controlled trial. *Lancet.* 2005;366(9501):1925-1934.

3. Ferrara N, Alitalo K. Clinical applications of angiogenic growth factors and their inhibitors. *Nat Med.* 1999;5(12):1359-1364.

4. Melillo G, Serino F, Cirielli C, Capogrossi MC. Gene therapy in peripheral artery disease. *Curr Drug Targets Cardiovasc Haematol Disord.* 2004;4(3):295-300.

5. Carmeliet P. Mechanisms of angiogenesis and arteriogenesis. *Nat Med.* 2000;6(4):389-395.

6. Schaper W, Buschmann I. Arteriogenesis, the good and bad of it. *Cardiovasc Res.* 1999;43(4):835-837.

7. Helisch A, Schaper W. Arteriogenesis: the development and growth of collateral arteries. *Microcirculation.* 2003;10(1):83-97.

8. Resnick N, Einav S, Chen-Konak L, Zilberman M, Yahav H, Shay-Salit A. Hemodynamic forces as a stimulus for arteriogenesis. *Endothelium.* 2003;10(4-5):197-206.

9. Simons M. Angiogenesis: where do we stand now? *Circulation.* 2005;111(12):1556-1566.

10. Asahara T, Murohara T, Sullivan A, et al. Isolation of putative progenitor endothelial cells for angiogenesis. *Science.* 1997;275:964-967.

11. Asahara T, Masuda H, Takahashi T, et al. Bone marrow origin of endothelial progenitor cells responsible for postnatal vasculogenesis in physiological and pathological neovascularization. *Circ Res.* 1999;85(3):221-228.

12. Schmeisser A, Garlichs CD, Zhang H, et al. Monocytes coexpress endothelial and macrophagocytic lineage markers and form cord-like structures in Matrigel under angiogenic conditions. *Cardiovasc Res.* 2001;49(3):671-680.

13. Rehman J, Li J, Orschell CM, March KL. Peripheral blood "endothelial progenitor cells" are derived from monocyte/macrophages and secrete angiogenic growth factors. *Circulation.* 2003;107(8):1164-1169.

14. Ziegelhoeffer T, Fernandez B, Kostin S, et al. Bone marrow-derived cells do not incorporate into the adult growing vasculature. *Circ Res.* 2004;94(2):230-238.

15. Ke Q, Costa M. Hypoxia-inducible factor-1 (HIF-1). *Mol Pharmacol.* 2006;70(5):1469-1480.

16. Hirota K, Semenza GL. Regulation of hypoxia-inducible factor 1 by prolyl and asparaginyl hydroxylases. *Biochem Biophys Res Commun.* 2005;338(1):610-616.

17. Ivan M, Kondo K, Yang H, et al. HIFalpha targeted for VHL-mediated destruction by proline hydroxylation: implications for O2 sensing. *Science.* 2001;292(5516):464-468.

18. Ferrara N. Vascular endothelial growth factor: basic science and clinical progress. *Endocr Rev.* 2004;25(4):581-611.

19. Robinson CJ, Stringer SE. The splice variants of vascular endothelial growth factor (VEGF) and their receptors. *J Cell Sci.* 2001;114(pt 5):853-865.

20. Carmeliet P, Ng YS, Nuyens D, et al. Impaired myocardial angiogenesis and ischemic cardiomyopathy in mice lacking the vascular endothelial growth factor isoforms VEGF164 and VEGF188. *Nat Med.* 1999;5(5):495-502.

21. Dor Y, Djonov V, Abramovitch R, et al. Conditional switching of VEGF provides new insights into adult neovascularization and pro-angiogenic therapy. *Embo J.* 2002;21(8):1939-1947.

22. Ruhrberg C, Gerhardt H, Golding M, et al. Spatially restricted patterning cues provided by heparin-binding VEGF-A control blood vessel branching morphogenesis. *Genes Dev.* 2002;16(20):2684-2698.

23. Carmeliet P, Ferreira V, Breier G, et al. Abnormal blood vessel development and lethality in embryos lacking a single VEGF allele. *Nature.* 1996;380:435-439.

24. Ferrara N, Carver-Moore K, Chen H, et al. Heterozygous embryonic lethality induced by targeted inactivation of the VEGF gene. *Nature.* 1996;380:439-442.

25. Sullivan GW, Sarembock IJ, Linden J. The role of inflammation in vascular diseases. *J Leukoc Biol.* 2000;67(5):591-602.

26. Arras M, Ito WD, Scholz D, Winkler B, Schaper J, Schaper W. Monocyte activation in angiogenesis and collateral growth in the rabbit hindlimb. *J Clin Invest.* 1998;101(1):40-50.

27. Heil M, Eitenmuller I, Schmitz-Rixen T, Schaper W. Arteriogenesis versus angiogenesis: similarities and differences. *J Cell Mol Med.* 2006;10(1):45-55.

28. Lee CW, Stabile E, Kinnaird T, et al. Temporal patterns of gene expression after acute hindlimb ischemia in mice: insights into the genomic program for collateral vessel development. *J Am Coll Cardiol.* 2004;43(3):474-482.

29. Heil M, Schaper W. Influence of mechanical, cellular, and molecular factors on collateral artery growth (arteriogenesis). *Circ Res.* 2004;95(5):449-458.

30. Presta M, Dell'Era P, Mitola S, Moroni E, Ronca R, Rusnati M. Fibroblast growth factor/fibroblast growth factor receptor system in angiogenesis. *Cytokine Growth Factor Rev.* 2005;16(2):159-178.

31. Papetti M, Herman IM. Mechanisms of normal and tumor-derived angiogenesis. *Am J Physiol Cell Physiol.* 2002;282(5):C947-970.

32. Madeddu P. Therapeutic angiogenesis and vasculogenesis for tissue regeneration. *Exp Physiol.* 2005;90(3):315-326.

33. Cao R, Brakenhielm E, Pawliuk R, et al. Angiogenic synergism, vascular stability and improvement of hind-limb ischemia by a combination of PDGF-BB and FGF-2. *Nat Med.* 2003;9(5):604-613.

34. Simons M. Integrative signaling in angiogenesis. *Mol Cell Biochem.* 2004;264(1-2):99-102.

35. Henry TD, Abraham JA. Review of preclinical and clinical results with vascular endothelial growth factors for therapeutic angiogenesis. *Curr Interv Cardiol Rep.* 2000;2(3):228-241.

36. Freedman SB, Isner JM. Therapeutic angiogenesis for coronary artery disease. *Ann Intern Med.* 2002;136(1):54-71.

37. Post MJ, Laham R, Sellke FW, Simons M. Therapeutic angiogenesis in cardiology using protein formulations. *Cardiovasc Res.* 2001;49(3):522-531.

38. Bobek V, Taltynov O, Pinterova D, Kolostova K. Gene therapy of the ischemic lower limb–Therapeutic angiogenesis. *Vascul Pharmacol.* 2006;44(6):395-405.

39. Yla-Herttuala S, Martin JF. Cardiovascular gene therapy. *Lancet.* 2000;355(9199):213-222.

40. Tripathy SK, Svensson EC, Black HB, et al. Long-term expression of erythropoietin in the systemic circulation of mice after intramuscular injection of a plasmid DNA vector. *Proc Natl Acad Sci U S A.* 1996;93(20):10876-10880.

41. Simberg D, Danino D, Talmon Y, et al. Phase behavior, DNA ordering, and size instability of cationic lipoplexes. Relevance to optimal transfection activity. *J Biol Chem.* 2001;276(50):47453-47459.

42. Legendre JY, Szoka FC, Jr. Cyclic amphipathic peptide-DNA complexes mediate high-efficiency transfection of adherent mammalian cells. *Proc Natl Acad Sci U S A.* 1993;90(3):893-897.

43. Puyal C, Milhaud P, Bienvenue A, Philippot JR. A new cationic liposome encapsulating genetic material. A potential delivery system for polynucleotides. *Eur J Biochem.* 1995;228(3):697-703.

44. Lawrie A, Brisken AF, Francis SE, Cumberland DC, Crossman DC, Newman CM. Microbubble-enhanced ultrasound for vascular gene delivery. *Gene Ther.* 2000;7(23):2023-2027.

45. Taniyama Y, Tachibana K, Hiraoka K, et al. Development of safe and efficient novel nonviral gene transfer using ultrasound: enhancement of transfection efficiency of naked plasmid DNA in skeletal muscle. *Gene Ther.* 2002;9(6):372-380.

46. Taniyama Y, Tachibana K, Hiraoka K, et al. Local delivery of plasmid DNA into rat carotid artery using ultrasound. *Circulation.* 2002;105(10):1233-1239.

47. Teiger E, Deprez I, Fataccioli V, et al. Gene therapy in heart disease. *Biomed Pharmacother.* 2001;55(3):148-154.

48. Bergelson JM, Cunningham JA, Droguett G, et al. Isolation of a common receptor for Coxsackie B viruses and adenoviruses 2 and 5. *Science.* 1997;275(5304):1320-1323.

49. Wickham TJ, Mathias P, Cheresh DA, Nemerow GR. Integrins alpha v beta 3 and alpha v beta 5 promote adenovirus internalization but not virus attachment. *Cell.* 1993;73(2):309-319.

50. Yang Y, Nunes FA, Berencsi K, Furth EE, Gonczol E, Wilson JM. Cellular immunity to viral antigens limits E1-deleted adenoviruses for gene therapy. *Proc Natl Acad Sci U S A.* 1994;91(10):4407-4411.

51. Lehrman S. Virus treatment questioned after gene therapy death. *Nature.* 1999;401(6753):517-518.

52. Kootstra NA, Verma IM. Gene therapy with viral vectors. *Annu Rev Pharmacol Toxicol.* 2003;43:413-439.

53. Svensson EC, Marshall DJ, Woodard K, et al. Efficient and stable transduction of cardiomyocytes after intramyocardial injection or intracoronary perfusion with recombinant adeno-associated virus vectors. *Circulation.* 1999;99(2):201-205.

54. Monahan PE, Samulski RJ. Adeno-associated virus vectors for gene therapy: more pros than cons? *Mol Med Today.* 2000;6(11):433-440.

55. Khan TA, Sellke FW, Laham RJ. Gene therapy progress and prospects: therapeutic angiogenesis for limb and myocardial ischemia. *Gene Ther.* 2003;10(4):285-291.

56. Yla-Herttuala S, Alitalo K. Gene transfer as a tool to induce therapeutic vascular growth. *Nat Med.* 2003;9(6):694-701.

57. Hughes GC, Annex BH. Angiogenic therapy for coronary artery and peripheral arterial disease. *Expert Rev Cardiovasc Ther.* 2005;3(3):521-535.

58. Isner JM, Pieczek A, Schainfeld R, et al. Clinical evidence of angiogenesis after arterial gene transfer of phVEGF165 in patient with ischaemic limb. *Lancet.* 1996;348(9024):370-374.

59. Riessen R, Rahimizadeh H, Blessing E, Takeshita S, Barry JJ, Isner JM. Arterial gene transfer using pure DNA applied directly to a hydrogel-coated angioplasty balloon. *Hum Gene Ther.* 1993;4(6):749-758.

60. Baumgartner I, Pieczek A, Manor O, et al. Constitutive expression of phVEGF165 after intramuscular gene transfer promotes collateral vessel development in patients with critical limb ischemia. *Circulation.* 1998;97(12):1114-1123.

61. Rutherford RB, Baker JD, Ernst C, et al. Recommended standards for reports dealing with lower extremity ischemia: revised version. *J Vasc Surg.* 1997;26(3):517-538.

62. Shyu KG, Chang H, Wang BW, Kuan P. Intramuscular vascular endothelial growth factor gene therapy in patients with chronic critical leg ischemia. *Am J Med.* 2003;114(2):85-92.

63. Mäkinen K, Manninen H, Hedman M, et al. Increased vascularity detected by digital subtraction angiography after VEGF gene transfer to human lower limb artery: a randomized, placebo-controlled, double-blinded phase II study. *Mol Ther.* 2002;6(1):127-133.

64. Kusamanto YH, van Weel V, Mulder NH, et al. Treatment with intramuscular vascular endothelial growth factor gene compared with placebo for patients with diabetes mellitus and critical limb ischemia: a double-blind randomized trial. *Hum Gene Ther.* 2006;17(6):683-691.

65. Rajagopalan S, Trachtenberg J, Mohler E, et al. Phase I study of direct administration of a replication deficient adenovirus vector containing the vascular endothelial growth factor cDNA (CI-1023) to patients with claudication. *Am J Cardiol.* 2002;90(5):512-516.

66. Mohler ER, III, Rajagopalan S, Olin JW, et al. Adenoviral-mediated gene transfer of vascular endothelial growth factor in critical limb ischemia: safety results from a phase I trial. *Vasc Med.* 2003;8(1):9-13.

67. Rajagopalan S, Mohler ER, III, Lederman RJ, et al. Regional angiogenesis with vascular endothelial growth factor in peripheral arterial disease: a phase II randomized, double-blind, controlled study of adenoviral delivery of vascular endothelial growth factor 121 in patients with disabling intermittent claudication. *Circulation.* 2003;108(16):1933-1938.

68. Rajagopalan S, Mohler E, III, Lederman RJ, et al. Regional angiogenesis with vascular endothelial growth factor (VEGF) in peripheral arterial disease: design of the RAVE Trial. *Am Heart J.* 2003;145(6):1114-1118.

69. Tomko RP, Xu R, Philipson L. HCAR and MCAR: the human and mouse cellular receptors for subgroup C adenoviruses and group B coxsackieviruses. *Proc Natl Acad Sci U S A.* 1997;94(7):3352-3356.

70. Bergelson JM, Krithivas A, Celi L, et al. The murine CAR homolog is a receptor for coxsackie B viruses and adenoviruses. *J Virol.* 1998;72(1):415-419.

71. Thirion C, Larochelle N, Volpers C, et al. Strategies for muscle-specific targeting of adenoviral gene transfer vectors. *Neuromuscul Disord.* 2002;12 (suppl 1):S30-S39.

72. O'Hara AJ, Howell JM, Taplin RH, et al. The spread of transgene expression at the site of gene construct injection. *Muscle Nerve.* 2001;24(4):488-495.

73. Yang HT, Deschenes MR, Ogilvie RW, Terjung RL. Basic fibroblast growth factor increases collateral blood flow in rats with femoral arterial ligation. *Circ Res.* 1996;79(1):62-69.

74. Chleboun JO, Martins RN, Mitchell CA, Chirila TV. bFGF enhances the development of the collateral circulation after acute arterial occlusion. *Biochem Biophys Res Commun.* 1992;185(2):510-516.

75. Baffour R, Berman J, Garb JL, Rhee SW, Kaufman J, Friedmann P. Enhanced angiogenesis and growth of collaterals by in vivo administration of recombinant basic fibroblast growth factor in a rabbit model of acute lower limb ischemia: dose-response effect of basic fibroblast growth factor. *J Vasc Surg.* 1992;16(2):181-191.

76. Lazarous DF, Unger EF, Epstein SE, et al. Basic fibroblast growth factor in patients with intermittent claudication: results of a phase I trial. *J Am Coll Cardiol.* 2000;36(4):1239-1244.

77. Comerota AJ, Throm RC, Miller KA, et al. Naked plasmid DNA encoding fibroblast growth factor type 1 for the treatment of end-stage unreconstructible lower extremity ischemia: preliminary results of a phase I trial. *J Vasc Surg.* 2002;35(5):930-936.

78. Lederman RJ, Mendelsohn FO, Anderson RD, et al. Therapeutic angiogenesis with recombinant fibroblast growth factor-2 for intermittent claudication (the TRAFFIC study): a randomised trial. *Lancet.* 2002;359(9323):2053-2058.

79. Laham RJ, Chronos NA, Pike M, et al. Intracoronary basic fibroblast growth factor (FGF-2) in patients with severe ischemic heart disease: results of a phase I open-label dose escalation study. *J Am Coll Cardiol.* 2000;36(7):2132-2139.

80. Unger EF, Goncalves L, Epstein SE, et al. Effects of a single intracoronary injection of basic fibroblast growth factor in stable angina pectoris. *Am J Cardiol.* 2000;85(12):1414-1419.

81. Leiden JM. Human gene therapy: the good, the bad, and the ugly. *Circ Res.* 2000;86(9):923-925.

82. Verma IM. A tumultuous year for gene therapy. *Mol Ther.* 2000;2(5):415-416.

83. Epstein SE, Kornowski R, Fuchs S, Dvorak HF. Angiogenesis therapy: amidst the hype, the neglected potential for serious side effects. *Circulation.* 2001;104(1):115-119.

84. Carmeliet P. VEGF gene therapy: stimulating angiogenesis or angioma-genesis? *Nat Med.* 2000;6(10):1102-1103.

85. Lee RJ, Springer ML, Blanco-Bose WE, Shaw R, Ursell PC, Blau HM. VEGF gene delivery to myocardium: deleterious effects of unregulated expression. *Circulation.* 2000; 102(8):898-901.

86. de Muinck ED, Simons M. Re-evaluating therapeutic neo-vascularization. *J Mol Cell Cardiol.* 2004;36(1):25-32.

87. Whitlock PR, Hackett NR, Leopold PL, Rosengart TK, Crystal RG. Adenovirus-mediated transfer of a minigene expressing multiple isoforms of VEGF is more effective at inducing angiogenesis than comparable vectors expressing individual VEGF cDNAs. *Mol Ther.* 2004;9(1):67-75.

88. Liu PQ, Rebar EJ, Zhang L, et al. Regulation of an endogenous locus using a panel of designed zinc finger proteins targeted to accessible chromatin regions. Activation of vascular endothelial growth factor A. *J Biol Chem.* 2001; 276(14):11323-11334.

89. Rebar EJ, Huang Y, Hickey R, et al. Induction of angiogenesis in a mouse model using engineered transcription factors. *Nat Med.* 2002;8(12):1427-1432.

90. Dai Q, Huang J, Klitzman B, et al. Engineered zinc finger-activating vascular endothelial growth factor transcription factor plasmid DNA induces therapeutic angiogenesis in rabbits with hindlimb ischemia. *Circulation.* 2004; 110(16):2467–2475.

91. Xie D, Li Y, Reed EA, Odronic SI, Kontos CD, Annex BH. An engineered vascular endothelial growth factor-activating transcription factor induces therapeutic angiogenesis in ApoE knockout mice with hindlimb ischemia. *J Vasc Surg.* 2006;44(1):166-175.

92. Yamakawa M, Liu LX, Date T, et al. Hypoxia-inducible factor-1 mediates activation of cultured vascular endothelial cells by inducing multiple angiogenic factors. *Circ Res.* 2003;93(7):664-673.

93. Vincent KA, Shyu KG, Luo Y, et al. Angiogenesis is induced in a rabbit model of hindlimb ischemia by naked DNA encoding an HIF-1alpha/VP16 hybrid transcription factor. *Circulation.* 2000;102(18):2255-2261.

94. Rajagopalan S, Olin J, Deitcher S, et al. Use of a constitutively active hypoxia-inducible factor-1alpha transgene as a therapeutic strategy in no-option critical limb ischemia

patients: phase I dose-escalation experience. *Circulation.* 2007;115(10):1234-1243.

95. Tomita N, Morishita R, Taniyama Y, et al. Angiogenic property of hepatocyte growth factor is dependent on upregulation of essential transcription factor for angiogenesis, ets-1. *Circulation.* 2003;107(10):1411-1417.

96. Wojta J, Kaun C, Breuss JM, et al. Hepatocyte growth factor increases expression of vascular endothelial growth factor and plasminogen activator inhibitor-1 in human keratinocytes and the vascular endothelial growth factor receptor flk-1 in human endothelial cells. *Lab Invest.* 1999;79(4): 427-438.

97. Aoki M, Morishita R, Taniyama Y, et al. Angiogenesis induced by hepatocyte growth factor in non-infarcted myocardium and infarcted myocardium: up-regulation of essential transcription factor for angiogenesis, ets. *Gene Ther.* 2000;7(5):417-427.

98. Taniyama Y, Morishita R, Hiraoka K, et al. Therapeutic angiogenesis induced by human hepatocyte growth factor gene in rat diabetic hind limb ischemia model: molecular mechanisms of delayed angiogenesis in diabetes. *Circulation.* 2001;104(19):2344-2350.

99. Taniyama Y, Morishita R, Aoki M, et al. Therapeutic angiogenesis induced by human hepatocyte growth factor gene in rat and rabbit hindlimb ischemia models: preclinical study for treatment of peripheral arterial disease. *Gene Ther.* 2001;8(3):181-189.

100. Powell RJ, Dormandy J, Simons M, Morishita R, Annex BH. Therapeutic angiogenesis for critical limb ischemia: design of the hepatocyte growth factor therapeutic angiogenesis clinical trial. *Vasc Med.* 2004;9(3):193-198.

101. Powell RJ, et al. Results of a double-blind placebo controlled study to assess the safety of intramuscular injection of hepatocyte growth factor plasmid to improve limb perfusion in patients with critical limb ischemia. *Circulation.* 2008:11;58-65.

102. Li W, Shen W, Gill R, et al. High-resolution quantitative computed tomography demonstrating selective enhancement of medium-size collaterals by placental growth factor-1 in the mouse ischemic hindlimb. *Circulation.* 2006; 113(20):2445-2453.

103. Inoue N, Kondo T, Kobayashi K, et al. Therapeutic angiogenesis using novel vascular endothelial growth factor-E/human placental growth factor chimera genes. *Arterioscler Thromb Vasc Biol.* 2007;27(1):99-105.

chapter 41

Peripheral Arterial Brachytherapy

Ron Waksman, MD

With the growing popularity of peripheral vascular medicine, identifying a reliable treatment to the plaguing recurrence of restenosis will increase and augment the benefits of vascular intervention. Investigators have shown that the endovascular delivery of radiation therapy is one such treatment. Combating restenosis in the peripheral vascular system is contingent upon understanding the processes, mechanisms, and potential targets affected by using brachytherapy. The successful outcome of clinical trials in the coronary arteries facilitated recognition of vascular brachytherapy (VBT) to become standard of care for the treatment of in-stent restenosis (ISR). Expansion of the indications to de novo lesions identified the potential but also limitations of the technology (late thrombosis and edge effect). Simultaneously, investigators embarked on a series of studies utilizing VBT as adjunct therapy for intervention in peripheral arteries.

As patients in the baby boomer generation near their 60s, the full impact of peripheral and coronary atherosclerosis in the United States is apparent. Whereas coronary vascular procedures increase at a rate of 8% per year, there is greater growth in the frequency of peripheral procedures, estimated at 19% per year. Despite new advances such as drug-eluting stents, atherectomy devices, thrombectomy, and endoluminal grafts, the restenosis rate after peripheral artery intervention continues to compromise the overall success of these procedures.

Restenosis is still considered the "Achilles heel" of percutaneous endovascular intervention.[1-8] Among the approaches for restenosis prevention and treatment in the peripheral arterial system (PAS), only VBT is reported to be safe and effective in this select group of patients. This article reviews the status of VBT, the available systems and dosimetry for use, and provides a summary of the latest reports from the clinical trials utilizing VBT to prevent or treat restenosis in the PAS.

RADIATION SYSTEMS FOR THE PERIPHERAL VASCULAR SYSTEM

The vessel size of the PAS favored the use of gamma radiation because of the penetration characteristics of the emitter. The majority of investigational work performed in the PAS used Ir-192 in doses of 14 to 18 Gy prescribed at 2 mm from the source center.

Understanding Gamma Radiation

Gamma rays are photons that originate from the center of the nucleus, as opposed to X-rays, which originate from the orbital outside of the nucleus. Gamma rays have deeply penetrating energies between 20 keV and 20 MeV, which require an excess of shielding, as compared to beta and X-ray emitters. The only gamma-ray isotope currently in use is Ir-192. Other isotopes which emit both gamma- and X-rays are Iodine-125 (I-125) and Palladium-103 (Pd-103), which have lower energies and require higher activities to deliver the prescribed dose in an acceptable dwell time (<20 min). The latter isotopes are either not available in such activities or too expensive for this application. The dosimetry of Ir-192 is well understood and as a result of the lesser fall-off in dose compared with beta emitters, the dose gradient at the area of interest is acceptable. Ir-192 is available in activities of up to 10 Ci, but because of the high penetration, the average shielding of a catheterization laboratory will not be able to handle more than 500-mCi source in activity. This limitation is associated with dwell times >12 minutes for doses >15 Gy when prescribed at 2-mm radial distance from the source.

Understanding Beta Radiation

Beta rays are high-energy electrons emitted by nuclei and contain too many or too few neutrons. These negatively charged particles have a wide variety of energies including transition energy, particularly between parent-daughter cells, and have a wide variety of half-lives, from several minutes (Cu-62) to 30 years (Sr/Y-90). Beta emitters rapidly lose their energy to the surrounding tissue and their range is within 1 cm of tissue. Therefore, they are associated with a higher gradient to the near wall. The use of beta sources for vascular application is attractive from both the radiation exposure and safety points of view.

External Radiation

External beam radiation is a viable option for the treatment of peripheral vessels because it allows a homogenous dose distribution with the possibility of fractionation.

External radiation is currently used in a few centers for the treatment of ISR of the superficial femoral artery (SFA). Preliminary reports are encouraging, although caution should be applied to this strategy because of the potential for radiation injury to the nerve, vein, and the skin. Preliminary attempts with external radiation for the treatment of arteriovenous dialysis grafts failed to reduce the restenosis rate. This unsuccessful attempt was attributed to the conservative use of low doses and thrombosis of these grafts. Using sterotactic techniques to localize the radiation to the target area may improve the results of this approach.

In their study, Therasse et al.[9] tested the theory that external beam radiation would be more practical to administer than VBT after percutaneous transluminal angioplasty (PTA) in reducing restenosis. After femoropopliteal PTA without stent placement, 99 patients were randomly assigned to 0 Gy (placebo; $n = 24$), 7 Gy ($n = 24$), 10.5 Gy ($n = 26$), or 14 Gy ($n = 25$) of external beam radiation of the PTA site (with a 3-cm margin at both extremities) in 1 session 24 hours after PTA. Restenosis >50% was present in 50%, 65%, 48%, and 25% of patients, for the 0-, 7-, 10.5-, and 14-Gy groups, respectively ($p = 0.072$). At 18 months, repeated revascularizations were required in 25% of patients in the 0-Gy group versus 12% of patients in the 14-Gy group ($p = 0.24$). It was found that a single session of external beam radiation of 14 Gy of the femoropopliteal angioplasty site significantly reduced restenosis at 1 year.[9]

Catheter-Based Gamma Systems

The most common catheter-based system used for SFA application is the MicroSelectron HDR system (Nucletron-Odelft, Delft, Netherlands), which uses a computerized, high-dose rate afterloader system that delivers a 3-mm stepping, 10 Ci activity of Ir-192 into a closed-lumen radiation catheter (Figure 41-1). The Peripheral Brachytherapy Centering Catheter (Paris; Guidant Corporation, Indianapolis, IN) is a 7-F, double-lumen catheter with multiple centering balloons near its distal tip that enable the catheter to be in the center of the lumen of large peripheral vessels during inflation. The Paris catheter is no longer available. The only closed-end lumen catheter available is that used for oncology applications.

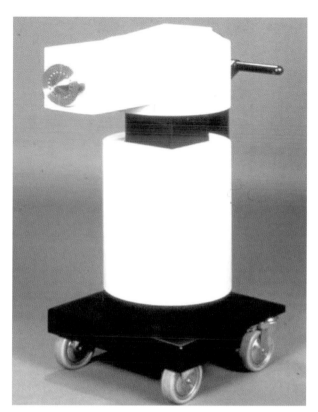

● **FIGURE 41-1.** MicroSelectron high dose rate automatic afterloader.

Courtesy of Nucletron-Odelft, Delft, Netherlands.

Catheter-Based Beta Systems

The only catheter-based beta system available is the Beta-Cath system, with a source train of up to 60 mm, which can be pulled back to allow coverage of long lesions (Figure 41-2). The main limitation of the system is the penetration of the beta emitter, which is weakened significantly beyond 5 mm. This system can be used for below-the-knee applications or for other small vessels, including in-stent renal stenosis. It is recommended to perform the radiation prior to the intervention to ensure better centering and a higher dose to the treated proliferating tissue.

Other innovative catheter-based radiation system developments have been halted because of the declining interest in the VBT field or slow recruitment into clinical trials. Included among these halted developments was the Radiance balloon system (Radiance Medical Systems; Irvine, CA), which was particularly attractive for peripheral applications because it is associated with apposition of a solid beta P-32 source attached to the inner balloon surface into the surface of the vessel wall. Another approach was the use of low X-ray energy delivered intraluminally via a catheter. The emitter was 5 mm in length and 1.25 to 2.0 mm in diameter and could be administered distally to the lesion and pulled back to cover the entire lesion length.

The Corona system, a modification of the BetaCath system, was used to accommodate beta systems with the Sr/Y-90 emitter in the peripheral system. In this system, the balloon was filled with CO_2, allowing centering and preventing dose attenuation. A clinical study in SFA for ISR

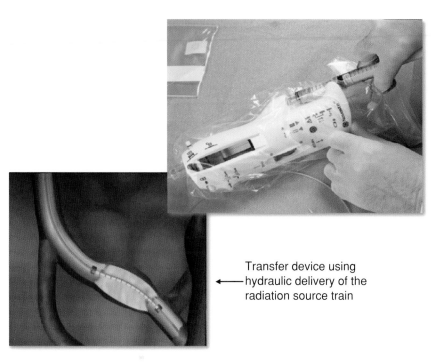

● **FIGURE 41-2.** Novoste BetaCath system.

Courtesy of Novoste, Best Vascular, Inc, Norcross, GA.

Transfer device using ←hydraulic delivery of the radiation source train

lesions entitled MOBILE was terminated because of poor enrollment. The Corona system was also used in the BRAVO study for patients with AV dialysis grafts.

● CLINICAL TRIALS

Liermann and Schopohl were the first to perform VBT for the treatment of ISR in the peripheral arteries. Known as the Frankfurt Experience, this pilot study was conducted in 30 patients with ISR in their SFAs.[10–13] Patients underwent atherectomy and PTA followed by endovascular radiation using the MicroSelectron HDR afterloader and a noncentering catheter with Ir-192. No adverse effects from the radiation treatment were reported at up to 7-year follow-up. The 5-year patency rate of the target vessel was 82%, with only 11% stenosis within the treated segment reported. Late total occlusion developed in 7% of the treated vessels after 37 months (Table 41-1).

The Vienna Experience

A series of studies was conducted at the University of Vienna. The majority were randomized studies targeting the SFA with or without stents using the MicroSelectron HDR afterloader with or without a centering catheter utilizing different doses.

Vienna I was a pilot study with an indication of radiation safety after PTA that showed only 60% patency at 1 year.[14] The Vienna II trial had 113 patients with de novo or recurrent femoropopliteal lesions who were randomized to PTA + brachytherapy ($n = 57$) or PTA alone ($n = 56$). The primary end point of cumulative patency rate at 12 month follow-up was higher in the PTA + brachytherapy group (63.6%) compared to the PTA group (35.3%). The patients from this study were followed-up to 36 months and demonstrated durability of the results[15] (Figure 41-3). In Vienna III, a centering catheter that was used for the

TABLE 41-1. SFA Radiation Trials

Study	No. of Patients	Randomized	Center Cath	Dose	@ mm	Patency Control (%)	Patency VBT (%)
Frankfurt	40	—	—	12 Gy	3	—	82
Vienna I	10	—	No	12 Gy	3	—	60
Vienna II	113	Yes	No	12 Gy	r + 0	—	72
Vienna III	134	Yes	Yes	18 Gy	r + 2	46	77
Vienna IV	33	No	Yes	14 Gy	r + 2	—	79
Vienna V	98	Yes	Yes	14 Gy	r + 2	45	88*
PARIS pilot	40	No	Yes	14 Gy	r + 2	—	88
PARIS randomized	300	Yes	Yes	14 Gy	r + 2	80	76
Swiss 4-arm study	346	Yes	Yes	12 Gy	r + 2	58	83

*Excluding thrombosis cases.

Restenosis free survival curves

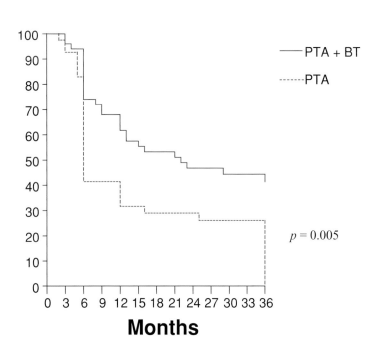

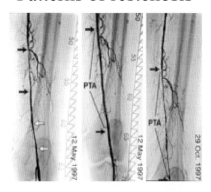

Placebo

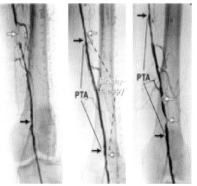

Radiation

Patterns of restenosis

$p = 0.005$

● **FIGURE 41-3.** Results from Vienna II.

same patient population with a dose of 18 Gy showed a restenosis rate of 23.4% in the irradiated group compared to 53.3% in the placebo arm.[16] Vienna IV was a pilot study examining radiation with stenting of the SFA; and Vienna V was a randomized study for similar indications. Both Vienna IV and V demonstrated an increase rate of subacute and late thrombosis when stents were combined with radiation, with up to 16.7% in the radiation group versus 4.3% in the control stenting without radiation. Once thrombosis was controlled, the radiation group had less restenosis.[17]

To summarize, the Vienna trials demonstrated efficacy of gamma radiation in reduction of restenosis following PTA to the SFA. However, these studies also demonstrated late catch-up of restenosis and late thrombosis in arteries that underwent stenting and radiation therapy.

The PARIS Trials

The Paris Radiation Investigational Study (PARIS) is the first FDA-approved, multicenter, randomized, double-blind, controlled study involving 300 patients following PTA to SFA stenosis using a gamma radiation Ir-192 source. Utilizing the MicroSelectron HDR afterloader, a treatment dose of 14 Gy was delivered via a centered segmented end-lumen balloon catheter. The primary objectives of this study were to determine angiographic evidence of patency and a reduction of >30% of the restenosis rate of the treated

lesion at 6 months. A secondary end point aimed to determine the clinical patency at 6 and 12 months by treadmill exercise and by the ankle-brachial index (ABI). In the feasibility phase of PARIS, 40 patients with claudication were enrolled. The mean lesion length was 9.9 ± 3.0 cm with a mean reference vessel diameter of 5.4 ± 0.5 mm. The 6-month angiographic follow-up was completed on 30 patients; 13.3% of them had evidence of clinical restenosis.[18]

Because of poor enrollment, only 203 patients with claudication and femoropopliteal disease were enrolled in the study. After successful PTA, a segmented centering balloon catheter was positioned to cover the PTA site. The patients were transported to the radiation oncology suite and randomized to receive either radiation therapy using the MicroSelectron HDR afterloader with Ir-192 at a dose of 14 Gy at 2 mm into the vessel wall (105 patients), or treatment with a sham control in 98 patients. Patients were followed for 12 months, with clinic visits at 1, 6, and 12 months and follow-up angiography at 12 months. The restenosis rate at follow-up was similar in both groups (28.6% brachytherapy vs. 27.5% placebo). There was no significant difference in minimal lumen diameter, late loss, or the number of total occlusions. Exercise ABI, resting ABI, and maximum walking time were not different between treatment groups. For patients older than 65 years, maximum walking times at 6 and 12 months were better in the brachytherapy group. In the subgroups of patients with diabetes, male patients, or patients receiving clopidogrel or who have a proximal/medial lesion, maximum walking time in the brachytherapy group was better than in the placebo at 6 months but not different at 12 months.

More studies to support the effectiveness of gamma radiation for ISR were recently published by Krueger et al.[19] In this study, 30 patients who underwent PTA for de novo femoropopliteal stenoses were randomly assigned to undergo 14 Gy centered endovascular irradiation (irradiation group, $n = 15$) or no irradiation (control group, $n = 15$). Intra-arterial angiography was performed 6, 12, and 24 months after treatment; and duplex ultrasonography was performed the day before and after PTA and at 1, 3, 6, 9, 12, 18, and 24 months later. Baseline characteristics did not differ significantly between the two groups. Mean absolute individual changes in degree of stenosis, compared with the degrees of stenosis shortly after PTA in the irradiation group versus in the control group were $10.6\% \pm 22.3$ versus $39.6\% \pm 24.6$ ($p < 0.001$) at 6 months, $2.0\% \pm 34.2$ versus $40.6\% \pm 32.6$ ($p = 0.002$) at 12 months, and $7.4\% \pm 43.2$ versus $37.7\% \pm 34.5$ ($p = 0.043$) at 24 months. The rates of target lesion restenosis at 6 months ($p = 0.006$) and 12 months ($p = 0.042$) were significantly lower in the irradiation group. The authors concluded that endovascular radiation was effective for patients who were treated with angioplasty for de novo femoropopliteal lesions.

Restenostic Lesions and VBT

The effectiveness of VBT for restenotic SFA lesions was examined in another randomized study reported by Zehnder et al.[20] In this study, gamma radiation was used at a dose of 12 Gy. The primary endpoint was >50% restenosis at 12 months assessed by duplex Doppler. The recurrence rate in the radiation arm was 23% versus 42% in the PTA alone group.[20] This study demonstrated that VBT can be effective in restenotic lesions.

Brachytherapy and Probucol

In another randomized, four-arm study for patients with PTA lesions, patients were randomized to VBT, VBT and probucol, probucol alone, or placebo. The recurrence rate in the radiation arm alone was 17%, VBT and probucol was 20%, probucol alone was 27%, and the placebo group was 42%. This study confirms prior observations regarding the effectiveness of VBT for the treatment of SFA lesions without additional benefit of probucol when compared to PTA alone.[21]

AV Dialysis Studies

An initial study at Emory University in 1994 to treat patients who had failed PTA of arteriovenous dialysis grafts using the MicroSelectron HDR afterloader reported 40% patency rate at 44 weeks[22]; however, the long-term results of this study were similar to stand alone PTA without radiation. Similar disappointing results were reported by Parikh et al. from a pilot study utilizing external radiation doses of

12 Gy and 18 Gy for AV dialysis shunts in 10 patients.[23] At 6 months, target lesion revascularization was 40%, but at 18 months all grafts failed and required intervention. Cohen et al.[24] randomized 31 patients to PTA or stent placement alone followed by external radiation of 14 Gy in two 7-Gy fractions and reported restenosis rates of 45% versus 67% in the irradiated and control groups, respectively, at 6 months. New studies are currently underway using low-dose external radiation to reduce restenosis of vascular access for AV grafts in hemodialysis patients, as are other studies using a centering device to deliver an accurate homogenous dose of radiation after PTA. The BRAVO (Beta Radiation following balloon angioplasty for improving life span of recurrent failed ArterioVenous fistulae) was a pilot study utilizing the Corona system with an Sr/Y90 beta emitter. In the study of 10 patients with an average of 3.9 previous angioplasties to their AV graft, there was 60% primary patency and cumulative patency of 80% at 12-month mean follow-up.[25]

VBT for ISR of Renal Arteries

The incidence of ISR after renal artery stenting is 12% to 21%, yet there is no standard treatment method for this problem. VBT is not approved for this indication but several studies aimed to look into the efficacy of gamma brachytherapy for the treatment of ISR in renal arteries. Kuchulakanti et al.[26] studied 11 patients who presented with renal ISR documented by selective renal angiography and who were assigned to treatment with γ-BT using Ir-192, followed by balloon angioplasty, laser, or restenting (Figure 41-4). The patients were followed clinically at 1, 3, 6, and 9 months, and duplex ultrasound was conducted at 9 months. Procedural success was 100% and free of complications. Clinical follow-up was available in all patients and duplex ultrasound in 10 patients. No significant

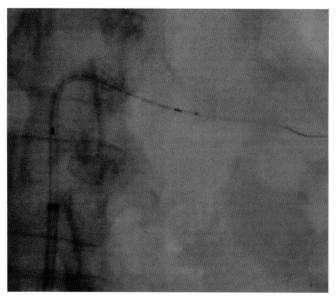

● **FIGURE 41-4.** Active Ir-192 source across the ISR lesion at the ostium of left renal artery.

changes in blood urea nitrogen, serum creatinine, creatinine clearance, or the number of antihypertensive medications were observed at follow-up. One patient (9.1%) required target lesion revascularization at 9 months. It was found that gamma brachytherapy as adjunct therapy for the treatment of renal artery ISR appears safe and feasible. However, the clinical benefit of this therapy has to be proven in a large randomized clinical trial. Smaller renal arteries with ISR can utilize the BetaCath system that is currently used for ISR in coronary arteries; however, the dose should be adjusted to the vessel size.

Limitations to Brachytherapy

Although clinical trials using VBT for both coronary and peripheral applications have demonstrated positive results in reducing restenosis rates, these trials have also identified two major complications related to the technology—late thrombosis, especially in the presence of stents, and edge stenosis. Late thrombosis is probably because of the delay in healing associated with radiation. It has been demonstrated that late thrombosis can be remedied through the prolonged administration of antiplatelet therapy after intervention. The main explanation for the occurrence of edge effect is a combination of low doses at the edges of the radiation source and an injury created by the device for intervention that is not covered by the radiation source. It has been shown that wider margins of radiation treatment to the intervening segment significantly reduce the edge effect.

With the growing popularity of peripheral vascular medicine, identifying a reliable treatment for the plaguing recurrence of restenosis will increase and augment the benefits of vascular intervention. Investigators have shown that the endovascular delivery of radiation therapy is one such treatment. Combating restenosis in the peripheral vascular system is contingent upon understanding the processes, mechanisms, and potential targets affected by brachytherapy use. The successful outcome of clinical trials in the coronary arteries facilitated recognition of VBT to become standard of care for the treatment of ISR. Expansion of the indications to de novo lesions identified the potential, but also the limitations, of the technology. Simultaneously, investigators embarked on a series of studies utilizing VBT as adjunct therapy for intervention in peripheral arteries. The outcome of these trials will determine the future role of VBT as a tool for prevention of restenosis in the peripheral vascular system.

REFERENCES

1. Murray RR Jr, Hewews RC, White RI Jr, et al. Long-segment femoro-popliteal stenoses: is angioplasty a boon or a bust? *Radiology.* 1987;162:473-476.

2. Vroegindeweij D, Kemper FJ, Teilbeek AV, et al. Recurrence of stenosis following balloon angioplasty and Simpson atherectomy of the femoropopliteal segment. A randomized comparative. 1 year follow-up study using color flow duplex. *Eur J Vasc Surg.* 1992;6:164-171.

3. Rees CR, Palmaz JC, Becker GJ, et al. Palmaz stent in atherosclerotic stenosis involving the ostia of the renal arteries: preliminary report of a multicenter study. *Radiology.* 1991;181:507-514.

4. Hunink MFM, Magruder CD, Meyerovitz MF, et al. Risks and benefits for femoropopliteal percutaneous balloon angioplasty. *J Vasc Surg.* 1993;17:183-194.

5. White GF, Liew SC, Waugh RC, et al. Early outcome of intermediate follow-up of vascular stents in the femoral and popliteal arteries without long term anticoagulation. *J Vasc Surg.* 1995;21:279-281.

6. Dolmath BL, Gray RJ, Horton KM, et al. Treatment of anastomotic bypass graft stenosis with directional atherectomy: short term and intermediate-term results. *J Vasc Int Radiol.* 1995;6:105-113.

7. Johnston KW. Femoral and popliteal arteries: Reanalysis of results of angioplasty. *Radiology.* 1987;162:473-476.

8. Haude M, Erbel R, Issa H, et al. Quantitative analysis of elastic recoil after balloon angioplasty and after intracoronary implantation of balloon-expandable Palmaz-Schatz stents. *J Am Coll Cardiol.* 1993;21:26-34.

9. Therasse E, Donath D, Lesperance J, et al. External beam radiation to prevent restenosis after superficial femoral artery balloon angioplasty. *Circulation.* 2005;111:3310-3315.

10. Liermann DD, Bottcher HD, Kollath J, et al. Prophylactic endovascular radiotherapy to prevent intimal hyperplasia after stent implantation in femoropopliteal arteries. *Cardiovasc Intervent Radiol.* 1994;17:12-16.

11. Bottcher HD, Schopohl B, Liermann D, et al. Endovascular irradiation—a new method to avoid recurrent stenosis after stent implantation in peripheral arteries: technique and preliminary results. *Int J Rad Oncol Biol Phys.* 1994;29:183-186.

12. Liermann D, Kirchner J, Schopohl B, et al. Brachytherapy with iridium-192 HDR to prevent restenosis in peripheral arteries: an update. *Herz.* 1998;23:394-400.

13. Sidawy AN, Weiswasse JM, Waksman R. Peripheral vascular brachytherapy. *J Vasc Surg.* 2002;35:1041-1047.

14. Minar E, Pokrajac B, Ahmadi R, et al. Brachytherapy for prophylaxis of restenosis after long-segment femoropopliteal angioplasty: pilot study. *Radiology.* 1998;208:173-179.

15. Minar E, Pokrajac B, Maca T, et al. Endovascular brachytherapy for prophylaxis of restenosis after femoropopliteal angioplasty: results of a Prospective Randomized Study. *Circulation.* 2000;102:2694-2699.

16. Pokrajac B, Schmid R, Poetter R, et al. Endovascular brachytherapy prevents restenosis after femoropopliteal angioplasty: results of the Vienna-3 multicenter study. *Int J Radiat Oncol Biol Phys.* 2003;57(suppl):S250.

17. Wolfram RM, Pokrajac B, Ahmadi R, et al. Endovascular brachytherapy for prophylaxis against restenosis after

long-segment femoropopliteal placement of stents: initial results. *Radiology.* 2001;220:724-729.

18. Waksman R, Laird JR, Jurkovitz CT, et al. Intravascular radiation therapy after balloon angioplasty of narrowed femoropopliteal arteries to prevent restenosis: results of the PARIS feasibility clinical trial. *J Vasc Interv Radiol.* 2001; 12:915-921.

19. Krueger K, Zaehringer M, Bendel M, et al. De novo femoropopliteal stenoses: endovascular gamma irradiation following angioplasty—angiographic and clinical follow-up in a prospective randomized controlled trial. *Radiology.* 2004;231:546-554.

20. Zehnder T, von Briel C, Baumgartner I, et al. Endovascular brachytherapy after percutaneous transluminal angioplasty of recurrent femoropopliteal obstructions. *J Endovasc Ther.* 2003;2:304-311.

21. Gallino A, Do DD, Alerci M, et al. Effects of probucol versus aspirin and versus brachytherapy on restenosis after femoropopliteal angioplasty: the PAB randomized multicenter trial. *J Endovasc Ther.* 2004;11:595-604.

22. Waksman R, Crocker IA, Kikeri D, et al. Long term results of endovascular radiation therapy for prevention of restenosis in the peripheral vascular system. *Circulation.* 1996;94(8)1-300,1745.

23. Parikh S, Nori D, Rogers D, et al. External beam radiation therapy to prevent postangioplasty dialysis access restenosis: a feasibility study. *Cardiovasc Radiat Med.* 1999;1:36–41.

24. Cohen GS, Freeman H, Ringold MA. External beam irradiation as an adjunctive treatment in failing dialysis shunts. *JVIR.* 2000;11:1364.

25. Bonan R. BRAVO. Presented at Cardiovascular Revascularization Therapies 2004.

26. Waksman R, Kuchulakanti PK, Laird JR, et al. Gamma Brachytherapy for the Treatment of In-Stent Restenosis of Renal Arteries. *Vasc Dis Manag.* 2006;3(1):178-183.

chapter 42

Diabetic Peripheral Arterial Disease

James M. Scanlon, MD / *Robyn A. Macsata, MD* / *Richard F. Neville, MD* /
Anton N. Sidawy, MD

Diabetes mellitus is among the leading causes of mortality and major morbidity in the United States. It continues to plague society with an additional 800 000 new cases diagnosed each year.[1] Consequently, the cost of treating the associated complications such as cardiovascular death, end-stage renal failure, and major amputations has created a growing economic burden on U.S. health care systems. Fifty percent of diabetics will be affected by a manifestation of diabetic foot (neuropathy, ischemia, or infection) and 15% of diabetics will experience a foot ulcer in their lifetime.[2,3] Diabetic foot problems are among the leading causes of hospitalization for diabetics; the cost of caring for diabetic foot ulcers is estimated as high as $13 billion annually, a figure that is approximately 27% of the total cost of diabetes care.[4] Its seriousness cannot be overstated; 20% of those affected with a foot ulcer will progress to an amputation, a lower extremity amputation rate of 4.1 per 1000 diabetics per year.[1,5] This confers an amputation relative risk 40 times greater for diabetics and a reamputation rate of more than 60% at 5 years.[3,6]

The pathophysiology of the diabetic foot is a multifactorial problem including neuropathy, ischemia, and infection. Treatment is based on a multidisciplined approach and requires control of infection, evaluation of ischemia, arterial reconstruction, and ultimate wound closure.

● PATHOPHYSIOLOGY OVERVIEW

The diabetic foot is a result of the synergistic derangements affecting the peripheral nerves, peripheral vasculature, and host defenses. The contribution each makes to a particular clinical situation may vary, but the underlying changes in physiology and function of these three systems are chiefly responsible for the cascade of events that lead to an insensate foot, ulceration, bone and joint destruction, infection, ischemia, and possibly limb loss (Figure 42-1).[7] An understanding of these primary processes is essential to treating a patient with diabetic foot.

Diabetic Peripheral Neuropathy

An estimated 15% to 50% of diabetics have some degree of peripheral neuropathy.[4] The importance of neuropathy as a contributory cause to foot ulceration was confirmed in a large multicenter study from Europe and North America that reported a 7% annual risk of ulceration in neuropathic patients. Previous evidence had suggested that the risk in non-neuropathic patients is less than 1%.[8] Diabetic neuropathy is a result of segmental demyelination and axonal and neuronal degeneration. The nerve cell transmits afferent signals (pain, temperature, proprioception) along the axon to the neuron body and transmits efferent signals (motion, reflexes) in the opposite direction "down" the axon. Signal conduction is a complex process of electrical potential changes conducted along the axon. This conductance depends on the highly metabolic axon's ability to generate and maintain electrical action potentials (electrical gradients) across its membrane and also on the support of the myelin sheath that surrounds the axon as both an insulator and conductor. This myelin sheath is produced by the metabolically active Schwann cells that line the axon. Hyperglycemia and/or hyperinsulinemia cause defects in neuron and Schwann cell metabolism that result in cellular dysfunction and subsequent impaired signal conduction. There are several well-studied theories of how diabetes causes this neuronal dysfunction. Evidence suggests that a combination of metabolic derangements with microvascular dysfunction (discussed below) lead to creation of oxidative stress, alteration of cellular energy and substrate handling, production of abnormally glycosylated proteins, and creation of an environment of "nerve hypoxia."[9,10]

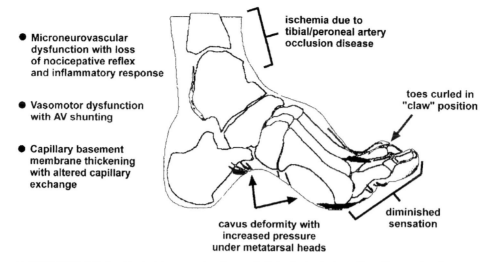

- Microneurovascular dysfunction with loss of nocicepative reflex and inflammatory response

- Vasomotor dysfunction with AV shunting

- Capillary basement membrane thickening with altered capillary exchange

ischemia due to tibial/peroneal artery occlusion disease

toes curled in "claw" position

diminished sensation

cavus deformity with increased pressure under metatarsal heads

● FIGURE 42-1. Underlying mechanisms of diabetic foot ulceration. Sensorimotor neuropathy leads to diminished sensation and small muscle atrophy in foot, resulting in flexed metatarsals, metatarsal head prominence, and clawing of toes. Altered architecture of foot, coupled with ischemia and microvascular dysfunction, ultimately leads to ulceration.

Reproduced with permission from Akbari CM, LoGerfo FW. Diabetes and peripheral vascular disease. J Vasc Surg. 1999;30:373–384.

Oxidative stress occurs when the production of free radical moieties exceeds the antioxidant capacity of a cell or system. Free radicals attack and damage the proteins, lipids, and nucleic acids. These oxidized or nitrosylated products have decreased biological activity, leading to loss of energy metabolism, cell signaling, transport, and other major functions. Free radicals in the form of reactive oxygen species (such as superoxide, hydrogen peroxide, and nitric oxide) are byproducts of the glycolytic pathway. Under normal conditions, their presence can be controlled by antioxidant systems. However, under conditions of hyperglycemia these radicals are overproduced and damage cellular proteins, DNA, and disrupt energy pathways. The damage can be far reaching within each cell, and in the case of neurons and Schwann cells the critical process of signal conduction is hindered.[11,12] Increasing the oxidative stress level within cells also causes a proinflammatory state and induces the process of apoptosis and cell death.

Altered energy and substrate pathways also lead to cellular damage. One well-described pathway, the polyol pathway, has been implicated in diabetic neuropathy. The enzyme aldose reductase converts toxic aldehydes to inactive alcohols. Glucose is a poor substrate for aldose reductase, but in hyperglycemia this enzyme coverts glucose to sorbitol, initiating the polyol pathway of glucose conversion to fructose. Increased aldose reductase activity in response to hyperglycemia, in turn, has been shown to result in several deleterious effects. It causes a decrease in nitric oxide (NO) synthase activity with reduced production of nitric oxide—a potent vasodilator and effector of vascular smooth muscle cells (VSMCs). It consumes and depletes the intracellular supply of the cofactor NADPH, this interferes with several cellular pathways and increases the oxidative stress level within a cell. It also impairs myo-inositol uptake by the Schwann cell. Myo-inositol is the precursor in the inositol containing phospholipids which are essential to myelin production and nerve conduction.[13]

Hyperglycemic conditions lead to the nonenzymatic glycolation of proteins. These products are termed advanced glycation endproducts—AGEs. Formation of AGEs may damage cells by inducing modifications of extracellular or intracellular proteins. Modification of an extracellular protein such as collagen causes alterations in its structure, strength, and electrical charge. This results in basement membrane thickening which represents a poorly functioning barrier between tissues and the intracellular environment. This barrier is critical in the maintenance of signaling, transportation of cellular products, and local homeostasis. Modification of intracellular proteins causes nonspecific binding to a family if IgG related transmembrane receptors (RAGEs) that produces a cascade of cellular signaling events. One of these, the activation of the mitogen-activated protein kinase (MAP kinase) causes dysfunction of pathways involved with gene expression, mitosis, and apoptosis.[10] Disruption of the pathway that controls sodium–potassium adenosine triphosphatase expression and activity leads to an inability to maintain adequate membrane electrical potentials. This results in the loss of electrical conduction in neural tissue and segmental demyelination of the axon.[14]

Another cause for diabetic neuropathy is localized "nerve hypoxia." This is a result of pathologic blood shunting and increased vascular resistance (discussed below under autonomic dysfunction) leading to decreased endoneurial blood flow.[15,16] Poor endoneurial blood flow is made worse by the metabolic derangements of hyperglycemia and hyperinsulinemia on NO production by the endothelial cells of the nerve blood supply—the vasa vasorum.[17] Decreased NO production leads to VSMC dysfunction that can result in an occlusive-like process of these nutrient vessels. The end result of all these injurious processes manifests itself microscopically as basement membrane thickening, breakdown of the myelin sheath into separate conglomerates, and axon degeneration. The nerves of the distal part of the leg are more affected than the proximal nerves and the cell bodies themselves mirror a pattern of injury involving the distal segments of the spinal cord first.[18] The clinical manifestation is delayed nerve conduction velocity that seems to affect initially unmyelinated or thinly myelinated nociceptive sensory nerve fibers but gradually involves all nerve types. Clinically, these do result in a neuropathy involving all three neural systems—sensory, motor, and autonomic—that contribute to ulceration.

The loss of sensation leads to a loss of the protective nature of pain perception. The onset is usually insidious and often unrecognized by the patient. Some patients may complain of uncomfortable, painful, and paresthetic symptoms in a symmetrical, "stocking" distribution, but just as commonly there will be no symptoms. Another manifestation of sensory neuropathy also involves autonomic nerves and is called the axon reflex. Injury stimulating a nociceptive fiber not only conducts to the spinal cord but also in a local arc to adjacent fibers and other axon branches near the site of stimulation. One function of this axon reflex is to stimulate secretion of several active peptides, such as substance P and calcitonin gene-related peptide, which directly and indirectly (through mast cell release of histamine) cause vasodilation and increased permeability—allowing for the delivery of cells and other factors involved in inflammation and healing. Because of sensory nerve dysfunction and delayed signal conduction in diabetes, this neurogenic vasodilatory response is impaired thereby blunting the hyperemic response when it is most needed under conditions of injury and inflammation.[19]

The clinical presentation of motor nerve dysfunction is wasting of the small muscles in the feet and absent ankle reflexes. This chronic motor denervation results in malfunction of the intrinsic muscles of the foot that distorts foot architecture. Chronic metatarsal flexion, extensor subluxation of the toes, proximal migration of the metatarsal fat pad and an imbalance in the action of the toe flexors and extensors leads to a claw foot deformity. More importantly, with dislocation of the metatarsophalangeal joints the heads of the metatarsals become more prominent and become the striking surface during ambulation. Other bony prominences become abnormal pressure points as well and combined with a loss of pain sensation the overlying skin is subject to repeated injury and ulceration.

Sympathetic autonomic neuropathy leads to a loss of sympathetic tone and increased arteriovenous shunting in the foot. This can mistakenly give the impression of a warm, well-perfused foot, but effective nutrient and oxygen delivery is actually impaired. Autonomic denervation of the skin leads to reduced sweating, dry skin, and development of cracks and fissures which predispose to skin breakdown. Blood flow to the bone becomes unregulated and the increased flow causes osteopenia and "bone washout" which may also contribute to osteoarthropathy and decreased joint mobility. Continued ambulation on an insensate joint, combined with muscle imbalance and atrophy from motor neuropathy and limited joint mobility, leads to joint instability, loss of joint architecture, and ultimately bone and joint destruction.[20] This process, leading to collapse of the ankle mechanism and collapse of the plantar arch, results in the deformity known as Charcot's foot.

Peripheral Arterial Disease

The incidence of lower extremity arterial disease is roughly four times greater among patients with diabetes compared to nondiabetics. Moreover, diabetics with peripheral arterial disease (PAD) carry a two- to threefold excess risk of intermittent claudication.[21] Of the numerous risk factors for PAD, diabetes is one of the two strongest factors (smoking is the other.) For diabetics the risk of developing PAD is related to age, duration of diabetes, and presence of neuropathy.[22] Diabetics are also more likely to present with a more severe form of ischemia and more likely to progress quicker to critical limb ischemia.[23] The impact of PAD is quite significant, approximately 27% of PAD patients demonstrate progression of symptoms over a 5-year period with limb loss occurring in approximately 4%. During this same 5-year period there is a 20% stroke or myocardial infarction risk and a 30% mortality rate.[24] For those with critical limb ischemia the outcomes are worse: 30% will have amputations and 20% will die within 6 months.[25] The natural history of PAD in diabetics has not specifically been studied longitudinally, but it is known from prospective clinical trials of risk interventions that the cardiovascular event rates in patients with PAD and diabetes are higher than those of their nondiabetic counterparts.[22]

Arterial disease in diabetes may be summarized as an alteration in vascular function at both the microvascular and macrovascular levels.[7] The microvascular component is best described as a nonocclusive microcirculatory impairment. This should not be confused with the term "small vessel disease" which refers to the common misconception of an untreatable occlusive lesion in the microcirculation. Dispelling the notion of "small vessel disease" has been fundamental to diabetic limb salvage, because arterial reconstruction is almost always possible and successful in these patients.[3] Whereas there is no occlusive disease in the microcirculation, multiple structural and physiologic abnormalities result in a functional microvascular impairment.[26] Endothelial cell dysfunction as a result of hyperglycemia and hyperinsulinemia has been well studied and shown to play a major role in this functional defect.[27] NO is the main vasodilator released by the endothelium and causes vasodilation by diffusing into the adjacent VSMCs and stimulating cyclic guanosine 3′,5′-monophosphate mediated relaxation. NO is synthesized in the endothelial cell through the action of an endothelial specific NO synthase (ecNOS). The expression of ecNOS has been shown to be reduced in response to hyperglycemic and hyperinsulinemic conditions.[27] Also, loss of NO homeostasis at the microcirculatory level creates a proinflammatory environment with liberation of damaging oxygen free radical species into the vasculature and surrounding tissues.

Another effect of hyperglycemia is the nonspecific glycosylation of proteins, so-called ts (AGEs). AGEs impair the actions of NO by stimulating the formation of free oxygen radicals that react with NO and convert it to a pro-oxidant. AGEs also displace disulfide cross-linkages in collagen proteins thereby diminishing the charge in the capillary basement membrane and altering its diffusion properties.[28] These basement membrane alterations contribute to increased vascular permeability and inflammation. AGEs activate and upregulate the expression of endothelial AGE receptors—these add to the local inflammatory state by increasing leukocyte chemotaxis and transformation into foam cells which contribute to increasing local oxidative stress.[22] One result of this increase in inflammation is an increase in C-reactive protein which is strongly related to widespread acceleration of atherosclerosis and promotion of endothelial cell apoptosis.[29] These and other mechanisms result in the impaired microvasculature marked by a characteristic thickening of the capillary basement membrane which does not affect arteriolar luminal diameter or blood flow but does impair nutrient and substrate flow into the adjacent tissues. This, coupled with autonomic dysfunction at the capillary level described earlier, severely hinders the hyperemic response to injury, inflammation, and infection.

The macrovascular component of PAD in diabetics is caused by atherosclerosis. The atheromatous changes occur in a similar fashion as in nondiabetics, but in an accelerated way. This acceleration could be because of the previously described diabetes-driven increases in inflammation that worsen the course of "normal" plaque pathophysiology, changes in platelet and coagulation system function, and the high coincidence of hypertension among diabetics caused by diabetic nephropathy.

Another common finding among diabetics is extensive medial calcification of the arteries. This is a process that can occur either at or separate from sites of atheromatous plaque, and in diabetics is characteristically found throughout the arteries of the legs. There are several different disease states and proposed pathways for this abnormal calcification of the media; in diabetics both hyperinsulinemia and hyperglycemia are implicated. Both have been shown to alter gene and protein expression in endothelial and VSMC that directly result in "osteoblast-like" activity of the VSMC and perictye cells of the artery.[30] An example is the abnormal expression of proteins like osteopontin by these cells. Osteopontin coupled with an environment of chronic inflammation, high presence of oxygen free radicals, and C-reactive protein within the vessel wall lead to the deposition of calcium phosphate complexes that mineralize within the media. Although this is generally a nonobstructive lesion it leads to noncompliant arteries unable to augment flow in response to increased demand and, depending on the lu-minal diameter of the vessel, long segmental stenoses that disturb normal blood flow.

As mentioned before, the formation of atheromatous plaques in diabetics is similar in most regards to nondiabetics, but the pattern of involvement has a unique characteristic in diabetics. Despite sometimes the presence of widespread calcinosis are found, the larger iliofemoral arteries are commonly spared of hemodynamically significant disease. However, in diabetics the popliteal and infrapopliteal vessels are more frequently involved than the larger arteries and more frequently diseased compared to nondiabetics.[31] The foot vessels are relatively spared in diabetics, even in the face of severe tibial level disease, which is important to the success of revascularization.[32]

In addition to the effects on the endothelium and VSMC, diabetes also leads to a hypercoagulable state through alterations in platelet function, coagulation, and blood rheology. Platelet uptake of glucose is unregulated in hyperglycemia and results in increased oxidative stress which enhances platelet aggregation. These platelets also have increased expression of glycoprotein Ib and IIb/IIIa receptors which are important in thrombosis and adhesion. The coagulation system is affected by diabetic-related increases in tissue factor expression by VSMC and endothelial cells, and increases in plasma concentrations of Factor VII. Hyperglycemia is also associated with a decreased concentration of antithrombin and protein C, impaired fibrinolytic function, and excess plasminogen activator inhibitor-1.[33] Blood rheology is altered as a consequence of an increase in viscosity and fibrinogen content caused by hyperglycemia.

In summary, the effects of PAD in diabetics confer alterations in the microvascular functioning and macrovascular supply that lead to ischemia. Because of the synergistic consequences of both processes, the actual degree of ischemia can be greater than suspected and even relatively minor trauma or infection can be made worse because of vascular insufficiency. The contribution of neuropathy with even moderate levels of ischemia is particularly worrisome as these "neuroischemic" feet are more prone to ulceration and infection.[34,35]

Infection

The presence of infection in a diabetic foot is usually a consequence of the neuropathy and ischemia already described (i.e., it typically follows an ulcer) and the impaired host defenses brought upon by hyperglycemia and hyperinsulinemia. Skin breakdown and ulceration allow a portal of entry for bacteria. Inadequate blood flow, blunted hyperemic response, and dysfunctional delivery of nutrients and immunologic cells create an environment ideally suited for bacterial overgrowth. Foot wounds are the most common diabetes-related cause for hospitalization. Infected diabetic foot wounds precede two-thirds of lower extremity amputations, and diabetics have at least a 10-fold greater risk of being hospitalized for soft tissue and bone infections of the foot than individuals without diabetes.[36] Among diabetics the risk for developing an infection is related to

---

TABLE 42-1. Effect of Hyperglycemia on Immune System Function

Immune System Component	Effect
Phagocytosis	Impaired phagocytosis by neutrophils
Chemotaxis	Impaired migration by neutrophils
Apoptosis	Increased neutrophil apoptosis after LPS challenge
ROS generation	Reduced generation of ROS, reduced killing
Adhesion/transmigration	Increased expression of adhesion molecules on endothelium and leukocytes
Complement cascade	Increased plasma level of complement products; Decreased complement function
Cytokine network	Increased early proinflammatory cytokine levels (TNF-α, Il-1β, IL-6)—*this effect reversed in hyperinsulinemia*

LPS, lipopolysaccharide; ROS, reactive oxygen species; TNF, tumor necrosis factor; IL, interleukin.

---

control of diabetes, presence of neuropathy, presence of PAD, chronicity of wound (>30 days), a recurrent wound, and a traumatic wound.[35,37]

The hyperglycemic state enhaces conditions that promote infection in diabetic patients. Studies have shown that nearly every component of the immunological system is negatively affected by hyperglycemia[38] (Table 42-1). For example, leukocyte adhesion and transmigration to the site of injury is impaired by poor chemotaxis signaling and receptor activity. The intracellular signaling necessary for bactericidal and phagocytic activity is also interrupted. When glucose levels exceed 200 mg/dL, tissue glycosylation occurs, which impairs wound healing by increasing the collagenase activity that reduces the collagen content at the site of tissue injury. Poor vascular supply and oxygenation provides a fertile environment for development of a synergistic microbial infection. Tight blood glucose control, especially in ill and infected patients, has been shown to reduce morbidity and mortality and should be viewed as an important component in the management of diabetic foot infections.[39,40]

The microbiology of diabetic foot infections is unique, gram-positive, gram-negative, and anaerobes can be responsible (Table 42-2). Staphylococci and streptococci are the most common pathogens. However, infection caused by gram-negative and anaerobic organisms occurs in approximately 50% of patients and quite often infection is polymicrobial (>3 organisms).[37] *S. aureus* is the most common organism, and methicillin-resistant *Staphylococcus aureus* (MRSA) is increasingly found in infected ulcers. Because of the poor immune response to infection and inflammation even bacteria regarded as skin commensals may cause severe tissue damage. These include gram-negative organisms such as *Citrobacter, Serratia, Pseudomonas*, and *Acinetobacter* species. Proper evaluation and antimicrobial treatment will be covered below, but it is advisable to send swabs or tissue for culture after initial debridement in all patients with deep ulcers or any evidence of local infection (warmth, swelling, cellulitis, foul smelling drainage, pus). Deeper wounds should raise the possibility of more than a soft tissue infection and osteomyelitis should be considered. In osteomyelitis, superficial swab cultures do not reliably

---

TABLE 42-2. Pathogens Associated with Various Diabetic Foot Infection Scenarios

Foot-Infection Scenario	Pathogens
Cellulits without an open skin wound*	β-Hemolytic streptococcus and *Staphylococcus aureus*
Infected ulcer and antibiotic naive*	*S. aureus* and β-hemolytic streptococcus
Infected ulcer that is chronic or was previously treated with antibiotic therapy[†]	*S. aureus* (includes MRSA) and β-hemolytic streptococcus, and Enterobacteriaceae
Ulcer that is macerated because of soaking[†]	*Pseudomonas aeruginosa* (often in combination with other organisms)
Long-duration nonhealing wounds with prolonged, broad-spectrum antibiotic therapy[†,‡]	Aerobic gram-positive cocci (*S. aureus*, MRSA, coagulase-negative staphylococci, and enterococci), Enterobacteriaceae, *Pseudomonas* spp.,*Acinetobacter* spp., *Stenotrophomonas* spp., fungi
"Fetid foot": extensive necrosis, gangrene, malodorous[†]	Mixed, aerobic gram-positive cocci, *Peptostreptococcus*, nonfermenting gram-negative rods, *Escherichia coli, Citrobacter, Proteus, Serratia, Bacteroides*

Often monomicrobial, especially in first time ulcers or early presentation.
[†] *Usually polymicrobial. Average of 2.1 isolates in nonlimb threatening infections, 4.1 to 5.8 isolates in limb threatening infections.*
[‡] *Increasing incidence of antibiotic-resistant species (MRSA, vancomycin resistant enterococcus, extended spectrum beta-lactamase producing gram-negative rods).*

identify bone bacteria, but percutaneous bone biopsy seems to be safe for patients with diabetic foot osteomyelitis.[37] Necrotizing soft tissue infections are also more common in diabetics, and an understanding of the anatomy and muscular compartments of the foot is essential in understanding the pattern of spread and control.

● EVALUATION

The clinical evaluation of the diabetic foot hinges on assessing the presence and degree of neuropathy, ischemia, and infection. Several scoring systems have been devised to describe the state of a diabetic foot, although they have their differences, all address these three facets as each one is critical to treatment planning (Table 42-3).

Neuropathy

Neuropathy should be assessed in every diabetic patient whether the foot is "at risk" or not. Protective sensation may be assessed at various points on the foot using a Semmes-Weinstein 5.07 strength monofilament: inability to feel the monofilament when pressed to the skin correlates well with increased risk of foot ulceration.[34] Visual inspection of the foot can also reveal evidence of the osteoarthropathy and foot deformity that result in abnormal pressure points. These pressure points, namely, the metatarsal heads and margins of the feet should be carefully inspected for any evidence of trauma, irritation, or ulceration.

Ischemia

Assessment of arterial perfusion is critical to the diabetic foot evaluation. Owing to the presence of both micro- and macrovascular abnormalities it can be challenging to discern the contribution of both, therefore it is wise to assume that a macrovascular problem (the one that can be corrected) exists until proven otherwise. A careful physical examination of all peripheral pulses and extremities is the cornerstone to a vascular evaluation. Muscle atrophy, hair loss, thinned skin, dependent rubor, and coolness can all be assessed clinically and suggest arterial insufficiency. But, as mentioned above, the diabetic foot can sometimes appear warm and well perfused and harbor critical ischemia nonetheless. With any sign of gangrene or tissue loss it can be assumed that critical ischemia exists that requires revas-

cularization for salvage regardless of how the rest of the foot appears. Degrees of infection lesser than overt gangrene or wounds that are slow to heal warrant a thorough evaluation of arterial perfusion as the diabetic foot requires maximal perfusion to heal. Absence of a palpable pedal pulse is also a strong indicator of critical ischemia that will require revascularization to restore pulsatile flow to the foot.

While clinical judgment and examination remain critical to assessment, as discussed previously, often the diabetic foot presents confounding "data." This can also be the case with noninvasive testing. Ankle-brachial indices (ABI) can be erroneous the presence of medial calcinosis that renders the arteries in leg and ankle noncompressible. In fact, an ABI that is grossly elevated (≥ 1.3) should be taken as evidence of calcinosis and does not indicate adequate arterial flow. The lower degrees of calcinosis in the toe vessels support the use of toe systolic pressures, but their use often is limited by the proximity of the foot ulcer to the cuff site. Pulse volume recordings and segmental duplex systolic velocities are unaffected by calcinosis, but evaluation of these waveforms is primarily qualitative and not quantitative. The waveforms may be affected by peripheral edema and the presence of ulceration can affect adequate cuff placement. Exercise testing or reactive hyperemia testing can also be used if an abnormality is suspected but not demonstrated on the above tests. Transcutaneous oximetry (TcO_2) has been shown to reliably predict healing of ulcers and amputation levels. It is not affected by calcinosis but can be affected by edema and concurrent smoking. The abnormal arteriovenous shunting in diabetes can actually cause a "falsely" increased TcO_2 reading. Compared with toe pressures, TcO_2 better predicted healing, but positive predictive values for both were only 67% and 79%, respectively.[41]

If noninvasive testing or clinical judgment suggests arterial insufficiency an arteriogram should be obtained. Arteriography has been shown to detect clinically significant disease even in the presence of normal noninvasive testing.[42] Concern about contrast-induced renal dysfunction in the presence of diabetes should not mitigate against the performance of a high-quality arteriogram of the entire distal circulation. Several prospective studies have demonstrated that the incidence of contrast-induced nephropathy is not higher in the diabetic patient without preexisting renal disease, particularly with the judicious use of hydration and

---

TABLE 42-3. Staging of the Diabetic Foot

Stage 1	Normal foot	Absence of neuropathy, ischemia, deformity, callus and edema
Stage 2	At-risk foot	Presence of neuropathy, ischemia, deformity, callus and edema
Stage 3	Ulcerated foot	Neuropathic ulcer on plantar or pressure surface, neuroischemic ulcer on foot margins
Stage 4	Infected foot	Localized ulcer infection, cellulitis, lymphangitis, osteomyelitis
Stage 5	Necrotic foot	Wet necrosis in the neuropathic foot or dry necrosis in the neuroischemic foot

Source: Reproduced with permission from Edmonds M. Diabetic foot ulcers: Practical treatment recommendations. Drugs. 2006;66:913–929.

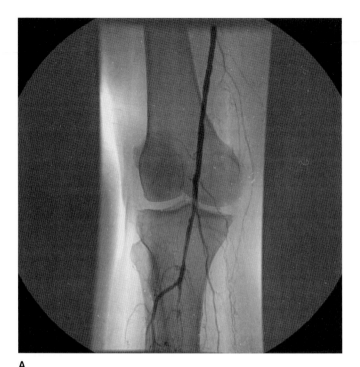

A

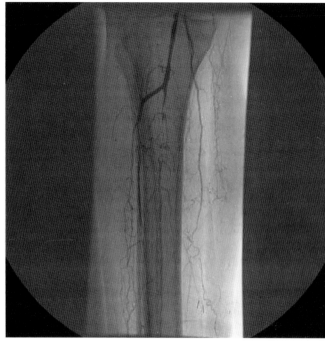

B

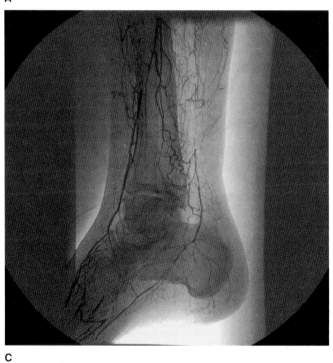

C

● **FIGURE 42-2.** Typical angiographic findings of tibial-peroneal disease. Digital subtraction angiography in a diabetic patient with a nonhealing foot ulcer. The iliac and femoral inflow was normal, in (A) the popliteal artery is essentially normal but the anterior tibial artery, peroneal artery, and posterior tibial artery are severely diseased. (B) Image shows the extent of involvement in the mid-calf. (C) Image shows reconstitution of a dorsalis pedis artery and posterior tibial artery at the level of the ankle. This patient underwent superficial femoral artery to dorsalis pedis bypass with autogenous vein with restoration of pulsatile flow to the foot and subsequent healing of the ulcer.

renal protective agents.[3] Particular emphasis must be paid on imaging the infrapopliteal arteries and the pedal arteries. The expected pattern of disease involving primarily the tibial arteries can be readily assessed with arteriography, as can inflow source and, more importantly, adequacy of outflow vessel, if lateral and anterior views of the foot are obtained (Figure 42-2). Noninvasive imaging such as MRA has made significant technological strides, but imaging of the smaller infrapopliteal arteries is of limited quality. Although the use of contrast enhanced MRA does carry a lower risk of inducing renal failure than the iodinated agents used in angiogra-

phy, this risk is greatest in those with diabetic nephropathy and low glomerular filtration rates.[43]

Infection

In general, any finding of infection must be taken into context of the entire foot and the patient's status. A thorough search for infection and its sequelae must be a part of the diabetic foot evaluation. This especially includes "hidden" spaces (toe web spaces, under callouses, or encrusted areas) and pressure points. It should be remembered that often the appearance of the infected diabetic foot will be underwhelming, and knowledge of this fact should enter into any examiner's thought process. The diabetic patient may not manifest pain or erythema or even chills, leukocytosis, and fever in up to two-thirds of cases.[3] The most minor finding is cellulitis, presenting as warmth and erythema of the skin without a defect in the skin. However, diabetic foot infections that are deeper (fasciitis, osteomyelitis) may manifest first as an area of cellulitis or a sinus tract that belies the seriousness of the underlying infection. Ulcers should be unroofed of necrotic crusts or debris to assess the base. Purulence, foul odor, or surrounding erythema of an ulcer indicates infection. Cultures should be obtained from ulcer bases to avoid culturing only skin-colonizing organisms. Charcot's osteoarthropathy can present as an "acute foot" with symptoms of pain and findings of edema, warmth, and generalized erythema without any evidence of skin ulceration or infection as the cause. Radiographs will show fractures and inflammation. This state is actually one of active bone inflammation and destruction and is very rarely caused by a primary infectious etiology.

Osteomyelitis is usually associated with ulceration and cellulitis. In the initial stages, radiographs may be normal but MRI can detect early changes.[44] Clinically, it can be diagnosed if a sterile probe inserted into the ulcer penetrates to bone. This test has a sensitivity of 66%, specificity of 85%, and positive predictive value of 89%.[45] This simple procedure can save on obtaining specialized and costly radiographic tests.

● TREATMENT

Treatment is based primarily upon the results of the clinical evaluation of the diabetic foot taking into account the pathogenic processes of neuropathy, ischemia, and infection outlined above. Use of a staging system is helpful in managing and coordinating care that can involve several disciplines (Table 42-4). Regardless of the stage of involvement it is important that the basic principles of prevention, infection control, revascularization, and wound closure/secondary procedures be closely monitored in order to ensure proper healing and prevent ulcer progression. Also, central to diabetic foot management is patient education and compliance. Identification of the "at-risk foot" before ulcer development, proper ulcer treatment before infection occurs, or prompt recognition of infection before necrosis sets in are possible intervention points where prevention strategies can yield improved outcomes.[46]

Prevention

Glucose control should be a prominent goal for all diabetics, strategies to improve patient compliance with diet, medications and monitoring must be emphasized and taught to these patients. The other common risk factors, such as hypertension, hyperlipidemia, and tobacco usage should also be aggressively treated since the synergistic effects of all four conspire to cause and worsen atherosclerosis. Patients with symptoms of claudication should undergo noninvasive testing and placement on an increased walking distance program along with consideration for treatment with cilostazol and/or clopidogrel.

Patients with evidence of neuropathy or foot deformities caused by osteoarthropathy are at risk for ulcer development at sites of abnormal pressure. These patients need education on foot hygiene and daily self-inspection of their feet. Proper footwear should be used that does not put any mechanical friction or force on the toes. Because peak plantar pressures are highest in the forefoot, it is essential that footwear properly supports this area and allows extra room in the toe box for the existing deformities such as claw toes, etc.[47] Pressure offloading means the redistribution of load bearing on the plantar surface of the foot and is critical once an area of ulceration has occurred. Increased padding, placement of orthoses to support the plantar arch or relieve the forefoot or heel of pressure are initial measures toward offloading. Failing in this application, the most effective way one could use is the application of some form of cast such as a total-contact cast or other commercially available devices such as Aircast Walker™, Scotchcast™ boot, etc. These devices allow the patient to be treated as an outpatient and can be used in combination with some wound dressings if needed. Total contact casting is also employed in the management of Charcot's foot, complete pressure offloading to allow the foot to "cool down" from active bone destruction as a step in preserving tissue and function. Simple bed rest and elevation is also recommended when an ulcer is complicated by serious infection requiring systemic antibiotics and hospitalization and for the acute phase of Charcot's foot.

Infection Control

Because infection is directly related to increased rates of amputation and increased morbidity and mortality from sepsis, infection control should be first and foremost of the treatment imperatives.[35] While no uniform antimicrobial treatment algorithm exists, knowledge of the patient's history, likely microorganisms involved, and assessment of the foot allow for general guidelines for insightful use of antibiotics (Table 42-5). Topical antibiotics such as mupirocin can be recommended in patients with areas of broken skin or early skin breakdown.

In the patient with a clinically noninfected ulcer no widely agreed practice on the place of antimicrobials has been established. Studies done to compare using oral antibiotics in this setting showed no difference in outcome compared to placebo with the exception that patients with a noninfected but ischemic ulcer that was culture-positive did benefit from antibiotic treatment.[37] Patients with ulceration and signs of local infection—namely, surrounding cellulitis—require ulcer debridement with culturing and can be treated with an oral antibiotic with gram-positive and gram-negative coverage for 10 to 14 days. Agents that have been used include: cephalosporins, amoxicillin-clavulanate, fluoroquinolones, dicloxacillin, clindamycin, or trimethoprim/sulfamethoxazole.[48]

TABLE 42-4. Multidisciplinary Management of the Diabetic Foot

Stage	Mechanical Control	Wound Control	Infectious Control	Vascular Control	Metabolic Control	Education
1: Normal foot	Encourage suitable footwear				Control glucose, blood pressure, lipids	Teach patient foot self-examination
2: At-risk foot	Accommodate deformity, remove callus			Statins and antiplatelet agents	Smoking cessation	Teach signs of early sensory/tissue loss
3: Ulcerated foot	Offload ulcers, consider orthopedic procedures*	Debridement dressings	Assess for early signs of infection Antibacterials: oral/topical	Evaluation and revascularization	Treat impaired renal and cardiac function	Teach ulcer care and early signs of infection
4: Infected foot	Acute stage: bed rest Chronic stage: casts to offload the foot, orthopedic procedures	Surgical debridement, advanced dressings and adjunct healing measures†	Assess for local extent or systemic spread Antibacterials: intravenous	Evaluation and revascularization	Tight glucose control, optimize cardiac and renal function	Teach patients to observe for signs of infection
5: Necrotic foot	Acute stage: bed rest Chronic stage: casts to offload the foot	Surgical debridement, advanced dressings and adjunct healing measures†	Assess for local extent or systemic spread Antibacterials: intravenous	Evaluation and revascularization	Tight glucose control, optimize cardiac and renal function	Teach patients care of necrotic toes Rehabilitation

*See text for specific procedures.
†Biological dressings. vacuum-assisted dressings. topical growth factors. hyperbaric oxygen therapy.
Source: Reproduced with permission from Edmonds M. Diabetic foot ulcers: practical treatment recommendations. Drugs. 2006;66:913-929.

TABLE 42-5. Suggested Empirical Antibiotic Regimens (Based on Clinical Severity)*

Route and Agent(s)	Mild	Moderate	Severe
Advised route	Oral for most	Oral or parenteral, based on clinical situation and agent selected	Intravenous
Dicloxacillin	Yes	—	—
Clindamycin	Yes	—	—
Cephalexin	Yes	—	—
Trimethoprim-sulfamethoxazole	Yes	Yes	—
Amoxicillin/clavulanate	Yes	Yes	—
Levofloxacin	Yes	Yes	—
Cefoxitin	—	Yes	—
Ceftriaxone	—	Yes	—
Ampicillin/sulbactam	—	Yes	—
Linezolid (with or without aztreonam)	—	Yes	—
Daptomycin (with or without aztreonam)	—	Yes	—
Ertapenem	—	Yes	—
Cefuroxime (with or without metronidazole)	—	Yes	—
Ticarcillin/clavulanate	—	Yes	—
Piperacillin/tazobactam	—	Yes	Yes
Levofloxacin (or ciprofloxacin) with clindamycin	—	Yes	Yes
Imipenem-cilastatin	—	—	Yes
Vancomycin and ceftazidime (with or without metronidazole)	—	—	Yes

*Severity grades: Mild—local evidence of inflammation (purulence, erythema, pain/tenderness, warmth, induration) but no spread beyond 2 cm of ulcer, confined to skin or superficial subcutaneous tissues and no systemic illness. Moderate—inflammation beyond 2 cm of ulcer, lymphangitic streaking, deep tissue abscess, gangrene, involvement of muscle, tendon, joint or bone, but patient is systemically well and metabolically stable. Severe—above signs of local inflammation in a patient with systemic toxicity or metabolic instability (e.g., fever, chills, tachycardia, hypotension, leukocytosis, acidosis, severe hyperglycemia).

Hospitalization and initiation of broad-spectrum intravenous antibiotics are indicated in any patient with evidence of systemic sepsis, significant metabolic derangements, tissue necrosis, or gangrene. Because these infections can become life and/or limb-threatening it is recommended that gram-positive, gram-negative, anaerobes, and possibly resistant organisms be covered until culture results are obtained. A variety of intravenous antibiotics such as ampicillin/sulbactam, imipenem/cilastin, meropenem, ertapenem, piperacillin/tazobactam, daptomycin, levofloxacin, moxifloxacin, or a combination of metronidazole and aztreonam have all been used effectively.[48–51]

It deserves mentioning that debridement is also crucial for effective infection control and should be done early in the treatment of a patient with local or systemic signs of infection and particularly in the setting of wet or dry gangrene. In order to properly assess an existing ulceration or expose areas beneath callus formation it is imperative that debridement be done to remove all necrotic tissue and debris. In uninfected and nongangrenous feet this can commonly be done in the outpatient setting. Determining any areas of undermining or deep penetration to bone are key to the goals of debridement as well.

More extensive debridement involving dry gangrenous toe removal or larger heel ulcers will usually require operating room services in order to effectively remove all devitalized tissue. Taking care to remove any poorly vascularized tissue encountered, such as cartilage, tendon, or sesamoid bones removes potential sites for bacterial growth. Knowledge of the fascial planes dividing the plantar muscle compartments is necessary. As the important muscle groups and vasculature are contained within the plantar space, it is advisable to avoid incisions of the dorsum unless direct involvement of the skin there is present. The medial plantar compartment and central plantar compartment can usually be accessed via a medial longitudinal incision, the lateral compartment can be similarly approached through a longitudinally based lateral incision. Web space infections may be approached and drained through the plantar aspect of the foot. The direction and location of incisions should take into account likely levels of amputation, likely planned bypass incisions, and type of wound closure. In the acute setting it is generally advised to leave drainage wounds open to allow some period of observation and continued drainage. Life-threatening sepsis caused by a foot infection may preclude the use of debridement, antibiotics, and time, and is best treated by guillotine amputation.

Revascularization

Arterial insufficiency should be ruled out in any patient, with evidence of an ischemic ulcer, a nonhealing ulcer or significant infection of the foot—particularly when extensive debridement or amputation is planned. After physical examination, the initial step is noninvasive testing. An abnormal ABI, either low in the presence of diseased noncalcified arteries or high in the presence of calcified arteries should be followed with testing to assess the level and extent of involvement. Segmental pressures are usually employed next with either pulse volume recordings or arterial duplex velocities used to identify the level and quantify the degree of insufficiency. Angiography is typically employed when an attempt, surgical or endovascular, is planned to improve hemodynamically significant stenoses. Hemodynamically significant arterial insufficiency should be corrected, if possible, with the goal of restoring a palpable pedal pulse. This usually involves restoration of direct in-line flow to the pedal arteries and can be accomplished either with endovascular or open procedures, or a combination of both.

Endovascular therapy has the attraction of less morbidity related to a lesser degree of invasiveness, but historically the durability is typically less as well. These interventions are well suited for discrete, small (<5 cm) lesions of the iliac and femoral arteries. However, since the distribution of diabetic PAD often involves the tibial arteries the results of percutaneous interventions in these small arteries is suboptimal, especially given that the disease is usually very extensive in that location. Angioplasty alone is associated with a high restenosis rate and therefore an increased need for reintervention.[52] Advanced techniques such as atherectomy and use of stents in the tibial arteries have improved upon the results of angioplasty alone, but these smaller arteries with multiple lesions can result in lengthy procedures in order to obtain an angiographically acceptable result. In addition, there is a small but present risk of causing vessel occlusion as a result of the procedure and thereby render a viable foot ischemic necessitating emergent bypass. Small studies employing techniques ranging from angioplasty alone, laser or cutting atherectomy, stenting, or a combination of any of these have 1-year primary patency rates from 13% to 80% and average near 50% at 2 years.[53] Limb salvage rates at 1 year can range from 70% to 88%. Most of the literature in this area comprise small, heterogenous patients or procedures with limited follow-up, and easy comparison with open surgical bypass is difficult to make.[54,55] It seems reasonable to assume that while endovascular therapies are improving, treating the typical diffuse involvement of smaller tibial arteries with the goal of restoring pulsatile flow in the foot is more successfully done with bypass. A related consideration is that some interventions that are unsuccessful, or likely to be unsuccessful, can have the unintended consequence of negatively affecting future bypasses. Injury or alteration to the target inflow or outflow vessel can necessitate a longer conduit—this may introduce the need for a groin incision and/or synthetic graft—both with higher rates of infectious complications. Nonetheless, in the patient without an adequate outflow vessel or comorbidities that preclude an open bypass, angioplasty may allow for time for wound healing or amputation healing.

The pattern of PAD in diabetics as outlined above allows for distal bypass procedures to be quite successful in patients with adequate outflow.[32] A meta-analysis of 31 studies on open bypass patients illustrates the favorable outcomes of bypass surgery to the distal tibial and pedal arteries.[56] Primary patency at 1 and 5 years was 85% and 69% for tibial bypasses and 78% and 57% for pedal bypasses. Secondary patency, at 5 years, was 76% for tibial and 66% for pedal bypasses. Overall limb salvage at 5 years was 80% for tibial bypasses and 76% for pedal bypasses. The vein graft in distal bypasses can be prepared as an in situ, reversed, or nonreversed translocated graft without significant difference in outcome.[57] The choice of conduit in these locations favors use of autogenous vein over prosthetics for improved patency, reduced secondary procedures, and improved salvage rates.[32,56,57]

With the goal of restoring maximal perfusion and a palpable pulse, efforts to ensure high success rate of surgical bypass should be made to keep the bypass length as short as possible to restore direct flow to the longest patent tibial vessel. The inflow source can be the common femoral, superficial femoral, or even popliteal artery so long as the inflow is adequate. Bypassing to very distal vessels is quite common in diabetics, and bypass to the dorsalis pedis artery has become one of the most commonly performed procedures because of its well established durability and effectiveness in some medical centers.[3,37,57] Fundamental to the success of the dorsalis pedis artery bypass graft is meticulous technique and its appropriate use. It should be performed when no other vessel has continuity with the foot, particularly in cases with tissue loss of the forefoot. It can be used to heal ulcers of the heel;[58] however, in that location ulcers best heal with bypasses to the posterior tibial artery bypass if it is patent and continuous to the foot. Dorsalis pedis bypass is unnecessary when a more proximal bypass graft will restore foot pulses and should not be done if there is an inadequate length of very good quality autogenous vein. Instances where the dorsum of the foot is extensively infected lead to the recommendation of bypass to the peroneal artery if it is of adequate quality. Active infection of the foot is not a contraindication to autogenous vein bypass grafting, as long as the infectious process is controlled and away from the proposed incision area.[59] In the absence of autogenous vein to perform a distal bypass to the peroneal or tibial arteries and because of the inferior patency of prosthetic bypasses to those target vessels, investigators devised adjunct procedures or treatment to improve their patency. Anticoagulation with coumadin has been used to improve such patency with varying results. Adjuvant surgical techniques in the form of distal arteriovenous fistula to improve the outflow rate and thus improve patency.[60] In addition, the use of autogenous venous tissue between the prosthetic graft and the distal tibial artery in the form of a cuff or patch has been popularized by investigators to improve patency and limb salvage rates of these grafts[61] (Figure 42-3). Such autogenous tissue placement is designed to improve the hemodynamics at the distal anastomosis to lessen the chance of formation of intimal hyperplasia in that location. However, such a function is yet to be proven. A more possible explanation is that placement of distal cuff or patch

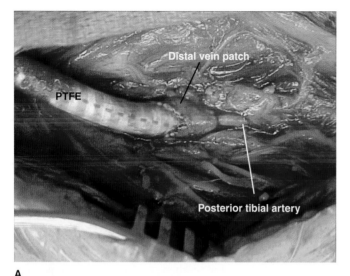

A

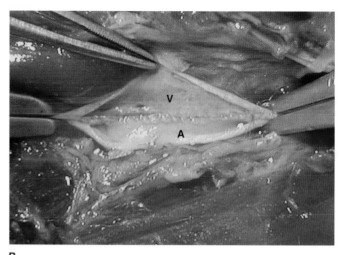

B

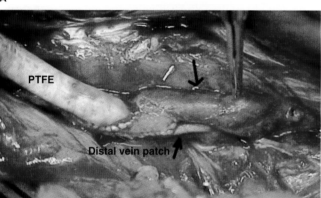

C

● **FIGURE 42-3.** Different techniques in distal anastomosis. Image (A) is an intraoperative picture of a completed synthetic graft to posterior tibial artery bypass using a distal vein patch (comprising of a segment of greater saphenous vein) at the distal anastomosis. Image (B) is an intraoperative picture of the creation of an arteriovenous fistula between the posterior tibial artery (**A**) and adjacent vein (**V**). In image (C), the fistula has been closed with a vein patch and the synthetic graft (PTEF) is anastomosed to the distal vein patch covering the artery (*solid arrow*) and vein (*open arrow*) fistula.

would markedly increase the space at the distal anastomosis, which would require a larger amount of hyperplastic lesion to occlude the outflow. Supporting evidence to this explanation lies in the finding that with the addition of the distal autogenous tissue, the intimal hyperplastic lesion forms at the graft/autogenous venous tissue interface instead of the graft/distal artery interface, which is rather small.

Wound Closure/Secondary Procedures

Ultimately the goal of treatment is to control the infection and wounds that can threaten a patient's limb or life. Once revascularization has been established the management shifts to wound closure and/or secondary procedures to treat the acute or underlying problem. Major debridement or minor amputations of the foot, in the setting of dry gangrene or the nonseptic patient, have better outcomes when done after successful revascularization as opposed to before.[62] It is recommended that a period of 7 to 10 days after revascularization be allowed for tissue recovery and demarcation. This allows for preservation of as much tissue as possible. The appropriate level of amputation is usually based upon clinical factors such as gross extent of necrotic or infected tissue, state of revascularization, and anticipated level of functioning. TcPO$_2$ measurements can aid in iden-

tifying an amputation level with adequate healing potential. An amputation level that preserves ambulatory function should be sought particularly in younger patients and high-functioning older patients so long as adequate healing conditions are not compromised.

Wounds of the diabetic foot require the same considerations to healing that any other wounds do. Wounds must be kept noninfected, free of necrotic debris, and well vascularized. Keeping in mind the diabetic foot pathophysiology, these conditions can be more difficult to attain and maintain. A strategy that includes close monitoring and in particular, frequent wound size measurement, is more likely to result in wound closure.[47] As mentioned, pressure offloading is a fundamental step. Keeping the wound moist helps in keeping the wound "clean" and better able to heal by promoting epidermal cell migration. Topical antibiotics have a role in wounds with healthy appearing granulation tissue, silver-containing compounds are very effective and do not hinder wound healing. There are many dressings options, the optimal one can vary on location, size and depth of the wound.

Advances in wound care including biologic dressings, growth factors, hyperbaric oxygen, and vacuum-assisted drainage that have all been shown to be beneficial and effective in certain scenarios—underscoring the importance of close monitoring in order to assess when these advanced therapies are indicated.[47,63-65]

Since revascularization does not address neuropathy or microvascular alterations these adjuncts may be helpful in overcoming the difficulties in healing. More extensive or difficult open wounds may require plastic reconstructive surgical consultation to assess for the feasibility of tissue flap or skin substitutes in order to attain closure. Orthopedic/podiatric surgical consultation is also important in order to assess for possible interventions that reduce pressure-induced skin ulceration. Dorsiflexion osteotomy or resection of the metatarsal head to address forefoot deformities can be effective. Bone and joint fusions may be indicated in order to correct alignment and prevent arch destruction. Achilles' tendon lengthening procedures are also employed in order to relieve the forces of plantar flexion contributing to arch collapse.

● SUMMARY

The problems presented in the management of the diabetic foot are multifactorial and require an understanding of the pathophysiologic derangements brought upon by diabetes. The salient contributions of peripheral neuropathy, PAD and altered host defenses must be appreciated through a careful assessment of each patient. Proper evaluation and treatment rests upon recognizing the need for infection control, debridement, pressure off-loading, revascularization, amputation, and wound closure. Given the enormous economic impact of caring for the complications of a diabetic foot it is equally important that strategies to prevent these complications be utilized as well. Patient and practitioner education on foot care, frequent foot examinations, glucose control, and control of hyperlipidemia, hypertension and tobacco use can all contribute to preserving life and limb.

REFERENCES

1. United States Department of Health and Human Services: National Diabetes Information Clearinghouse. http://diabetes.niddk.nih.gov/dm/pubs/overview. Accessed September 2008.

2. Millington JT, Ellenzweig J. The comprehensive therapy of diabetic foot ulcers. *Comp Ther.* 2005;31:50.

3. Akbari CM, Macsata R, Smith BM, et al. Overview of the diabetic foot. *Semin Vasc Surg.* 2003;16:3.

4. Gordois A, Scuffham P, Shearer A, et al. The health care costs of diabetic peripheral neuropathy in the U.S. *Diabetes Care.* 2003;26:1790.

5. Boulton AJ, Kirsner RS, Vileikyte L. Neuropathic diabetic foot ulcers. *N Engl J Med.* 2004;351:48.

6. Izumi Y, Satterfield K, Lee S, et al. Risk of reamputation in diabetic patients stratified by limb and level of amputation: a 10-year observation. *Diabetes Care.* 2006;29:566.

7. Akbari CM, LoGerfo FW. Diabetes and peripheral vascular disease. *J Vasc Surg.* 1999;30:373.

8. Abbott CA, Vileikyte L, Williamson S, et al. Multicentre study of the incidence of and predictive risk factors for diabetic neuropathic foot ulceration. *Diabetes Care.* 1998;21:1071.

9. Vincent AM, Russell JW, Low P, et al. Oxidative stress in the pathogenesis of diabetic neuropathy. *Endocr Rev.* 2004;25:612.

10. Sheetz MJ, King GL. Molecular understanding of hyperglycemia's adverse effects for diabetic complications. *JAMA.* 2002;288:2579.

11. Pfeifer MS, Schumer MP. Clinical trials of diabetic neuropathy: past, present, and future. *Diabetes.* 1995;44:1355.

12. Young Mj, Veves A, Boulton AJM. The diabetic foot: aetiopathogenesis and management. *Diabetes Metab Rev.* 1993;9:109.

13. Gillon KR, Hawthorne JN. Transport of *myo*-inositol into endoneurial preparations of sciatic nerve from normal and streptozotocin-diabetic rats. *Biochem J.* 1983;210:775.

14. Greene DA, Lattimer SA, Sima AA. Sorbitol, phosphoinositides, and sodium–potasssium ATPase in the pathogenesis of diabetic complications. *N Engl J Med.* 1987;316:599.

15. Tuck RR, Schmelzer JD, Low PA. Endoneurial blood flow and oxygen tension in the sciatic nerves of rats with experimental diabetic neuropathy. *Brain.* 1984;107:935.

16. Tesfaye S, Harris N, Jakubowski JJ, et al. Impaired blood flow and arterio-venous shunting in human diabetic neuropathy: a novel technique of nerve photography and flourescin angiography. *Diabetologia.* 1993;36:1266.

17. Gupta S, Sussman I, McArthur CS, et al. Endothelium-dependent inhibition of $Na^+-K^{\pm}$ATPase activity in rabbit aorta by hyperglycemia: Possible role of endothelium-derived nitric oxide. *J Clin Invest.* 1992;90:727.

18. Olsson Y, Save-Soderbergh J, Sourander P, et al. A patho-anatomical study of the central and peripheral nervous system in diabetics of early onset and long duration. *Pathol Eur.* 1968;3:62.

19. Parkhouse N, LeQueen PM. Impaired neurogenic vascular response in patients with diabetes and neuropathic foot lesions. *N Engl J Med.* 1988;318:1306.

20. Frykberg RG, Kozak GP. The diabetic Charcot foot. In: Kozak GP, Campbell DR, Frykberg RG, et al, eds. *Management of Diabetic Foot Problems.* 3rd ed. Philadelphia, PA: WB Saunders; 1995:88.

21. Brand FN, Abbott RD, Kannel WB. Diabetes, intermittent claudication, and risk of cardiovascular events. The Framingham Study. *Diabetes.* 1989;38:504.

22. Sheehan P. The Consensus Panel of the American Diabetes Association. Peripheral arterial disease in people with diabetes. *Diabetes Care.* 2003;26;3335.

23. Dormandy JA, Heeck L, Vig S. Predicting which patients will develop chronic critical leg ischemia. *Semin Vasc Surg.* 1999;12:138.

24. Weitz JI, Byrne J, Clagett GP, et al. Diagnosis and treatment of chronic arterial insufficiency of the lower extremities: a critical review. *Circulation.* 1996;94:3026.

25. Dormandy JA, Rutherford BB. Management of peripheral arterial disease (PAD): TASC working group: TransAtlantic Inter-Society Concensus (TASC). *J Vasc Surg*. 2000;31: S1.

26. LoGerfo FW. Vascular disease, matrix abnormalities, and neuropathy: implications for limb salvage in diabetes mellitus. *J Vasc Surg*. 1987;5:793.

27. Veves A, Akbari CM, Primavera J, et al. Endothelial dysfunction and the expression of endothelial nitric oxide synthatase in diabetic neuropathy, vascular disease, and foot ulceration. *Diabetes*. 1998;47;457.

28. Brownlee M, Cerami A, Vlassare H. Advanced glycosylation end products in tissue and the biochemical basis of diabetic complications. *N Engl J Med*. 1988;318:1315.

29. Ridker PM, Cushman M, Stampfer MJ, et al. Plasma concentration of C-reactive protein and risk of developing peripheral vascular disease. *Circulation*. 1998;97:425.

30. Hayden MR, Tyagi SC, Kolb L, et al. Vascular ossification-calcification in metabolic syndrome, type 2 diabetes mellitus, chronic kidney disease, and calciphylaxis-calcific uremic arteriolopathy: the emerging role of sodium thiosulfate. *Cardiovasc Diabetol*. 2005;4:4.

31. Menzoian JO, LaMorte WW, Paniszyn CC, et al. Symptomatology and anatomic patterns of peripheral vascular disease; Differing impact of smoking and diabetes. *Ann Vasc Surg*. 1989;3:224.

32. Akbari CM, Pomposelli FB, Gibbons GW, et al. Revascularization in diabetes: late observations. *Arch Surg*. 2000;135:452.

33. Schneider DL, Sobel BE. Diabetes and thrombosis. In: Johnstone MT, Veves A, eds. *Diabetes and Cardiovascular Disease*. Totowa, NJ: Humana Press; 2001:149.

34. Boyko EJ, Ahroni JH, Cohen V, et al. Prediction of diabetic foot ulcer occurrence using commonly available clinical information. *Diabetes Care*. 2006;29:1202.

35. Lavery LA, Armstrong DG, Wunderlich RP, et al. Risk factors for foot infections in individuals with diabetes. *Diabetes Care*. 2006;29:1288.

36. Boyko EJ, Lipsky BA. Infection and diabetes mellitus. In: Harris MI, ed. *Diabetes in America*. 2nd ed. Washington, DC: National Institutes of Health; 1995:485.

37. Edmonds M. Diabetic foot ulcers-practical treatment recommendations. *Drugs*. 2006;66:913.

38. Turina M, Fry DE, Polk HC. Acute hyperglycemia and the innate immune system: clinical, cellular and molecular aspects. *Crit Care Med*. 2005;33:1624.

39. Van Den Berghe G, Wouters P, Weekers F, et al. Intensive insulin therapy in the critically ill patient. *N Engl J Med*. 2001;345:1359.

40. Dronge AS, Perkal MF, Kancir S, et al. Long-term glycemic control and postoperative infectious complications. *Arch Surg*. 2006;141:375.

41. Kalani M, Brismar K, Fagrell B, et al. Transcutaneous oxygen tension and toe blood pressure as predictors for outcomes of diabetic foot ulcers. *Diabetes Care*. 1999;22:147.

42. Faglia E, Favales F, Quarantiello A, et al. Angiographic evaluation of peripheral arterial occlusive disease and its role as a prognostic determinant for major amputation in diabetic subjects with foot ulcers. *Diabetes Care*. 1998;21:625.

43. Ergun I, Keven K, Uruc I, et al. The safety of gadolinium in patients with stage 3 and 4 renal failure. *Neph Dial Transplant*. 2006;21:697.

44. Morrison WB, Schweitzer ME, Batte WG, et al. Osteomyelitis of the foot: relative importance of primary and secondary MR imaging signs. *Radiology*. 1998;207:625.

45. Grayson ML, Gibbons GW, Balogh K, et al. Probing to bone in infected pedal ulcers: a clinical sign of underlying osteomyelitis in diabetic patients. *JAMA*. 1995;273:721.

46. McCabe CJ, Stevenson RC, Dolan AM. Evaluation of a diabetic foot screening and protection programme. *Diabet Med*. 1998;15:80.

47. Brem H, Sheehan P, Rosenberg HJ, et al. Evidence-based protocol for diabetic foot ulcers. *Plast Reconstr Surg*. 2006; 117:193S.

48. Temple ME, Nahata MC. Pharmacotherapy of lower limb diabetic ulcers. *J Am Geriatr Soc*. 2000;48:822.

49. Oberdorfer K, Swoboda S, Hamam A, et al. Tissue and serum levofloxacin concentration in diabetic foot infection patients. *J Antimicrob Chemother*. 2004;54:836.

50. Edmiston CE, Krepel CJ, Seabrook GR, et al. *In vitro* activities of moxifloxacin against 900 aerobic and anaerobic isolates from patients with intra-abdominal and diabetic foot infections. *Antimicrob Agents Chemother*. 2004;48:1012.

51. Lipsky BA, Stoutenburgh U, et al. Daptomycin for treating infected diabetic foot ulcers: evidence from a randomized, controlled trial comparing daptomycin with vancomycin or semi-synthetic penicillins for complicated skin and skin-stucture infections. *J Antimicrob Chemother*. 2005;55:240.

52. Soder HK, Manninen HI, Jaakola P, et al. Prospective trial of infrapopliteal artery balloon angioplasty for critical limb ischemia: angiographic and clinical results. *J Vasc Intervent Rad*. 2000;11:1021.

53. Tsetis D, Belli AM. The role of infrapopliteal angioplasty. *Br J Rad*. 2004;77:1007.

54. Feiring AJ, Wesolowski AA, Lade S. Primary stent-supported angioplasty for treatment of below-knee critical limb ischemia and severe claudication. *J Am Coll Card*. 2004;44:2307.

55. Jahnke T, Link J, Muller-Hulsbeck S, et al. Treatment of infrapopliteal occlusive disease by high = speed rotational atherectomy: initial and mid-term results. *J Vasc Intervent Rad*. 2001;12:221.

56. Albers M, Romiti M, Brochado-Neto FC, et al. Meta-analysis of popliteal-to-distal vein bypass grafts for critical limb ischemia. *J Vasc Surg*. 2006;43:498.

57. Pomposelli FB, Jepsen SI, Gibbons GW, et al. A flexible approach to infrapopliteal vein grafts in patients with diabetes mellitus. *Arch Surg*. 1991;126:724.

58. Bercelli SA, Chan AK, Pomposelli FB, et al. Efficacy of dorsal pedal artery bypass in limb salvage for ischemic heel ulcers. *J Vasc Surg*. 1999;30:499.

59. Tannenbaum GA, Pomposelli FB Jr, Marcaccio EJ, et al. Safety of vein bypass grafting to the dorsal pedal artery in diabetic patients with foot infections. *J Vasc Surg*. 1992;15:982.

60. Dardik H, Impeduglia TM. Distal arteriovenous fistulas in prosthetic distal bypasses. In: Sidawy AN, ed. *Diabetic Foot: Lower Extremity Arterial Disease and Limb Salvage*. 1st ed. Philadelphia, PA: Lippincott Williams & Wilkins; 2005:245.

61. Neville RF. Vein cuffs, patches and boots in prosthetic distal bypasses. In: Sidawy AN, ed. *Diabetic Foot: Lower Extremity Arterial Disease and Limb Salvage.* 1st ed. Philadelphia, PA: Lippincott Williams & Wilkins; 2005:255.

62. Sheahan MG, Hamdan AD, Veraldi JR, et al. Lower extremity minor amputation: the roles of diabetes mellitus and timing of revascularization. *J Vasc Surg.* 2005;42:476.

63. Kranke P, Bennett M, Roeckl-Wiedmann I, et al. Hyperbaric oxygen therapy for chronic wounds. *Cochrane Database Sys Rev.* 2006;4:125.

64. Hong JP, Jung HD, Kim YW. Recombinant human epidermal growth factor (EGF) to enhance healing for diabetic foot ulcers. *Ann Plast Surg.* 2006;56:394.

65. Caputo GM, Cavanaugh PR, Ulbrecht JS, et al. Current concepts: assessment and management of foot disease in patients with diabetes. *N Engl J Med.* 1994;331:854.

chapter 43

Wound Care

David G. Stanley, MD

INTRODUCTION

Chronic wounds and ulcers are frequently encountered in patients with peripheral vascular disease (PVD) who often have insufficient distal arterial perfusion for wound healing. If the obstructed or stenosed inflow arteries can be bypassed or dilated, the wounds usually heal. However, the wound itself must be addressed surgically and medically along with revascularization. Until recently, wound care has not always been adequately emphasized in undergraduate medical programs.

This chapter addresses much of the current wound treatment available today. How one may incorporate these methods in one's practice and when referral to a wound treatment center (WTC) may be appropriate for problem wounds will vary with each clinician and his practice environment.

BASIC HEALING PROCESS

Wound repair and regeneration following acute injury begins within minutes with spasm of blood vessels, coagulation of bleeding surfaces, and accumulation of platelets on the damaged cells. A fibrinous layer derived from activated fibrinogen, collagen, and other trapped cells fills the injured surface. Factors released from platelets activate monophages and leucocytes which remove debris and bacteria. This debris is ingested or destroyed using peroxidase, which is oxygen-dependent. The necessary proliferation of fibroblasts, leucocytes, and keratinocytes, as well as collagen production by fibroblasts also requires sufficient oxygen. If microvascular profusion of oxygen and nutrients is insufficient, the wound will not heal.

Most surgical incisions or other wounds heal rapidly in less than 30 days. Clinical treatment of wounds in healthy patients usually requires only cleaning with saline or antiseptic solutions and sterile wound coverage. If there is significant inflammation clinically associated with the wound one may add topical zinc oxide, or silver in addition to systemic antibiotics.[1]

PROBLEM WOUNDS

Wounds that fail to heal or to progress normally toward healing over a 30-day period may be defined as "chronic" or "problem" wounds. There are multiple factors that combine in most patients to cause problem wounds. These factors may be local or systemic. Photography or measurement of wounds allows for an objective method to analyze wound evolution.

Local factors involve the tissue immediately surrounding the wound. Examples of local factors include scars from past trauma, fractures, pressure points, diabetic neuropathy with sensory loss and foot deformity, arthritis, and bunions of feet. Fibrotic changes related to radiation, lupus, venous hypertension, and lymphedema may be present as well. Patients may have chronic ischemia from peripheral arterial disease (PAD) or acute ischemia of embolic nature to fingers, toes, and other areas of the body. Bacterial infection of the wound with inadequate or inappropriate treatment allows accumulation of necrotic infected biofilm or eschar. Lack of sharp or enzymatic debridement, poor choice of topical agents, inappropriate dressings, or inadequate tissue cultures are local factors related to inadequate medical care or patient neglect.

Systemic factors include malnutrition, poorly controlled diabetes, renal, or liver failure, age, chemotherapy, steroids, morbid obesity, congestive heart failure (CHF) with generalized edema, inadequate oxygen delivery including chronic obstructive pulmonary disease (COPD), and large-vessel arterial disease. Socioeconomic, spiritual, and psychosocial factors may include lack of transportation, insufficient supplies, poor family support, sedentary lifestyle, morbid obesity, and alcohol or drug addiction. Noncompliance with dressing changes, inattention to weight-bearing protocols, and missed office visits are frequently a problem. Autoimmune disorders, vitamin and mineral deficiencies, inadequate diet, and failure to "quit smoking" may contribute to nonhealing wounds.

Problem wounds affect patients and their physicians in a negative way. These wounds are costly, painful, unattractive, and malodorous creating a social embarrassment and a nuisance to the patient, the patient's family, and even the treating physicians. Patients frequently spend 1.5 to 2 hours a day thinking about and caring for nonhealing wounds.[2] Limitation in activity is frustrating and depressing. Deterioration of health in patients with chronic wounds is very significant, especially in older patients.[3]

It is clear that good medical treatment of "problem wounds' must include significant time, resources, and diagnostic skill from the physician. The frustration of a nonhealing wound to the treating physician is significant. The "guilt feeling" of unsuccessful treatment may result in unintentional projected anger or blame toward the patient. The problem wound presenting in the midst of a busy office day can be a significant inconvenience and frustration.[4]

Referral of patients with problem wounds to a specialized WTC may be a welcome and logical plan of action for both physician and patient.

BASIC DIFFERENCES IN HEALING WOUNDS AND PROBLEMS WOUNDS

Over the past decade, the understanding of the molecular, cellular, and biologic problems found in chronic wounds has led to rapid changes in the recommended treatment of problem wounds. Prolonged inflammation in the nonhealing wound results in elevated levels of cytokines, matrix metalloproteinases (MMP), neutrophil elastase, decreased levels of growth factors, and poorly responding or senescent wound cells.[5-7]

With proper local wound treatment, and attention to critical local and general factors necessary to support healing, the molecular and biologic cellular profile of the chronic wound becomes similar to the acute wound and healing is observed.[8]

WOUND CARE

Debridement

We know that one reason chronic, infected wounds do not heal is because of bioburden. Bioburden includes bacteria, dead tissue, and senescent cells on wound margins with decreased mitogenic, and protease activity and a proinflammatory cytokine environment. Clean wounds with adequate arterial and venous flow usually heal. After appropriate cultures of the wound, the bioburden and senescent cells must be removed. Debridement to a healthy wound bed and skin margins turns a nonhealing chronic wound into an actively healing, clean, acute wound.

The clinician should understand that sharp or enzymatic debridement of ischemic wounds or dry gangrene will only damage marginally perfused tissue leading to more rapid and progressive necrosis. One must first improve local tissue health by addressing contributing general health factors and arterial and venous circulation. Chronic wounds close secondarily from the edges by epithelialization and contraction. This process requires excision of necrotic tissue, callous, and overhanging wound edges. Pressure points and movement of wound edges during patient activity disrupts new skin growth and must be addressed. Surgeons tend to use sharp debridement while other physicians may favor enzymatic or mechanical measures. Often unsuspected foreign objects are found in the depths of a wound during sharp debridement. Until all foreign material is removed, a wound will not heal. Plain films may be helpful in assessing for the presence of a foreign body.

Types of Debridement

For years, wet-to-dry has been the most common dressing used by physicians and involves moistened gauze that is placed on the wound and then removed after drying. It is commonly assumed that removing the dry gauze and replacing it with wet gauze is an effective way to debride the wound. However, if left dry too long, healthy cells may become desiccated and necrotic. Unfortunately, during removal of the dry gauze, healthy new cells may be torn off the wound along with eschar. Wet-to-dry gauze is labor-intensive requiring multiple changes daily.

Autolytic debridement by covering the wound with an occlusive sheet of hydrocolloid changed every 3 days is slow, but very selective in removing dead tissue and avoiding injury to healthy cells. Enzymatic therapy is faster, but may be painful and may injure surrounding skin if applied too liberally. Blunt debridement with moist gauze may be used to carefully clean the wound. More recently "pulse lavage" with 8 to 10 psi or less has been utilized in some wound centers.

Necrotic tissue may be pulled bluntly from the wound if directed from the wound edge toward the center to avoid injury to the wound edges. Sharp debridement with knife or curette is fast and effective in the hands of a skilled vascular specialist. However, it is the most harmful if used indiscriminately. One must generally avoid sharp debridement over grafts, tendons, bones, joints, or very vascular tissue. Gauze moistened with 4% lidocaine applied 15 minutes before debridement will help control pain. Bleeding may be controlled with pressure, elevation, silver nitrate sticks, Monsel's solution (ferric sulfate), or electrocautery.

Dressings

Over the last 50 years, wound care has evolved along with other advances in medicine. This has been especially true in the last two decades. In the 1950s and 1960s, wounds were left open or betadine and dry dressings applied. Wet-to-dry dressing for debridement or application of gauze impregnated with antibiotic under dry gauze was also common. As the benefits of a moist wound environment became known, adhesive, semipermeable dressings, and hydrocolloids were used. Hydrocolloids are now used to hydrate wounds and reduce pain. Foams and alginates can absorb secretions in venous stasis ulcers and may be used under compression dressings. Alginates may be impregnated with silver to control bacterial load. Collagen dressings normalize cellular activity and stimulate wound matrix activity. Collagen may promote epithelial growth.

Large, irregular, or deep wounds and wounds with overhanging skin edges are difficult management problems. The vacuum assisted closure device (VAC; Kinetic Concepts, Inc San Antonio, TX) has gained wide acceptance as an effective dressing for these complex wounds.

A VAC foam dressing is cut to fit the contour of the wound approximating the edge, but not overlying healthy skin. Several pieces of foam may be used for irregular wounds. The evacuation tube is pushed through a small cut in the foam so that the vent openings are inside the foam. An adhesive film supplied with the VAC is placed over the foam dressing and the tube. The film should extend at least 3.5 cm peripherally over surrounding healthy skin and be airtight. The open end of the tubing is connected to the vacuum pump and the proper suction (50–125 mm Hg) selected. The foam is usually reapplied every 2 to 4 days depending on the type of wound.

The benefits of VAC dressings include faster contraction and healing of the wounds with more effective bacterial and exudate clearance, accelerated growth of granulation tissue, contraction of the wound, and increased oxygen tension. The VAC may be used to prepare wounds for skin grafts and also used immediately after applying the grafts.

Large, acute, and surgical wounds, pressure ulcers, venous ulcers, drained abscess cavities, and diabetic foot ulcers have responded favorably when treated with the VAC.[9–12]

There are several thousand wound care products and dressings available. The choice of dressings is influenced by the need to remove eschar and debride (if not done surgically), to keep the wound moist, and to avoid excessive exudate accumulation that will macerate the tissue. Dressings must also protect the wound from further injury. The relative cost of various wound care products is also very important to the physician and facility.

HYPERBARIC OXYGEN & PROBLEM WOUNDS

Many dedicated WTCs may effectively utilize hyperbaric oxygen (HBO) in some chronic wounds such as diabetic ulcers, deep ischemic wounds with osteomyelitis, failing skin grafts or flaps, and nonhealing wounds in previously irradiated tissue (Figure 43-1). These problem wounds may have continuing ischemia despite appropriate vascular evaluation and treatment.

Transcutaneous oximetry (TCOM, $TcPO_2$) has been utilized to predict appropriate levels of limb amputation for years and now has become popular in predicting

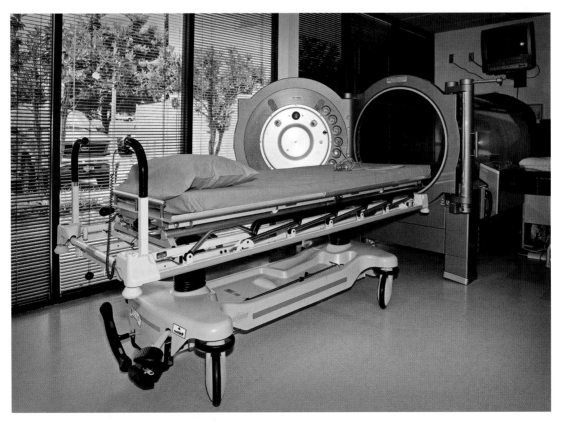

● **FIGURE 43-1.** A commonly used acrylic monoplace chamber designed for 100% oxygen at a pressure up to 3 ATA. Most "dives" are at 2 ATA or 2.4 ATA for 60 to 90 min.

the likelihood of wound healing. Diabetic patients with TCOMs (TcPO$_2$) below 40 mm Hg (nondiabetic patients <30 mm Hg), while breathing room air have a very poor chance of healing caused by severe tissue hypoxia. If TCOM (TcPO$_2$) values in the skin proximal to the ulcer increase on 100% oxygen mask breathing for 10 minutes at >100 mm Hg or to >200 mm Hg in a HBO chamber at two atmospheres absolute, healing is likely with the assistance of HBO.[13]

Patients treated with HBO must stop smoking for best results.[14] TCOMs (TcPO$_2$) are repeated after 15 treatments and then every 10 treatments. When TCOMs (TcPO$_2$) are >40 mm Hg on room air with clinical evidence of healing, HBO can usually be discontinued while the wound continues to heal. HBO promotes angiogenesis via a steep oxygen gradient between the ischemic wound and the surrounding tissue. HBO also enhances leukocyte killing and bacterial clearance and stimulates fibroblast proliferation and collagen synthesis.[15]

● DIABETIC FOOT ULCERS

Foot ulcers are present in approximately 15% of all diabetics. The annual incidence of foot ulcers is 2% of diabetics. Forty-six percent of hospital admissions for foot ulcers are diabetic patients.[16,17] Diabetic ulcers are caused by several factors including vascular disease, neuropathy, intrinsic foot deformity, and repeated trauma on pressure points. Vascular disease is 20 times more common in diabetics and more commonly involves the femoral, popliteal, tibioperoneal arteries, the pedal arch, and the digital arteries. Evaluation and treatment of arterial perfusion with surgical, endovascular, or medical measures is very important in wound healing and should be addressed early.

Neuropathy evaluation including the use of a 10-g monofilament is important in determining the prognosis and treatment. The loss of protective pain response, poor joint mobility, and foot deformity with secondary callus formation leads to repeated trauma at pressure points and results in ulcers developing under the metatarsal heads, toes, and heels.

Infection is usually secondary to deep tissue trauma or ulceration and is diagnosed clinically by fever, warmth, erythema, tenderness, pus, and leukocytosis.[18] If significant infection is suspected, a deep-tissue culture rather than a swab, is more likely to isolate the infecting organism. Two weeks of antibiotics should be used for soft-tissue infections and treatment for 6 weeks or longer in conjunction with surgical excision of infected bone if ostomylitis is present. HBO should be considered if osteomyelitis does not respond to surgery and antibiotics.

Osteomyelitis may be present in up to two-thirds of diabetic foot ulcers. Plain x-rays of the foot are helpful for evaluation of foot deformity, pressure points, and osteomyelitis. If bone can be probed with a blunt probe, one study demonstrated an 89% incidence of osteomyelitis.[19] While culture of a bone biopsy is the gold standard, white-cell scans or MRI can assist in diagnosing osteomyelitis.

Glucose control, cessation of smoking, and good nutrition are very important in healing the diabetic foot ulcer. Diabetic renal failure is associated with a high incidence of amputation. For best results, sharp debridement with removal of callus, necrotic tissue, infected material, and senescent cells should be performed weekly. Pressure should be removed from the ulcerated area with casts, boots, sole inserts, sandals, or other measures. Consultation with a podiatrist may be helpful. Patients living at home have been demonstrated to wear protective shoes or removable casts only 28% of the time. Nonremovable total contact casts are more effective, but must be changed each week.[20,21]

If a diabetic foot ulcer has not decreased in size after 4 to 6 weeks of therapy, reevaluation and other treatment may be considered.

Platelet-derived growth factor (Regranex, Ortho-McNeill) has been approved by the Food and Drug Administration and a recent review concluded that it may be helpful in stimulating healing in chronic diabetic ulcers that have not responded to aggressive treatment.[22]

Cultured living dermis and sequentially cultured epidermis derived from neonatal foreskin (Apligraf, Organogenesis) is associated with increased healing and less osteomyelitis. Dermis from human fibroblasts (Dermagraft, Smith, and Nephew) was reported to heal 30% of diabetic wounds compared to 18% healing in the control patients.[23]

Low-intensity ultrasound (US) has been reported to stimulate healing cell activity in chronic wounds. US acts as a thermal stimulus but acts primarily by increasing the permeability of cell membranes to calcium ions. Cells in the path of low-intensity US are stimulated to increase their healing activity. Illustrations of this activity include leukocytes ingesting debris, fibroblasts synthesizing matrix material, and endothelial cells multiplying and migrating into the wound. US, when combined with aggressive wound care, may significantly decrease healing time. One must be educated in the different US therapeutic devices available and the proper therapeutic frequencies.[24]

Case Report

This 70-year-old diabetic male presented with a history of walking barefoot on rough concrete. He developed a bruise and then a Wagner 3 ulcer on the right great toe under the callus (Figure 43-2). The ulcer enlarged while he treated it at home for 3 weeks with warm soaks and Neosporin ointment. General risk factors included peripheral vascular disease with angioplasty and stent procedures of the right superficial femoral artery twice over the previous 2 years, COPD, arthritis, and diabetes. Local risk factors included flexion contracture of the right great toe, diabetic neuropathy, and callus over the pressure point from the toe contracture. He was initially treated with sharp debridement of necrotic tissue and callus, Augmentin 875 mg bid, accuzyme dressings daily, and off loading shoe and glucose control. As healthy granulation developed, he was treated with Panafil packing daily and evaluation at the WTC with minor debridement every 2 weeks. Complete healing at

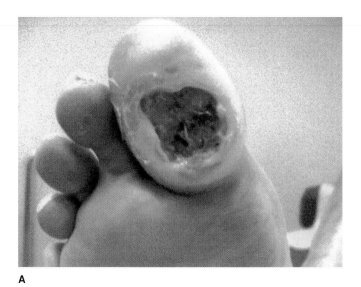

A

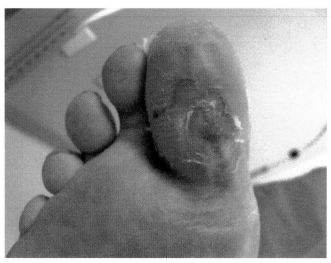

B

● **FIGURE 43-2.** A 70-year-old diabetic man with an ulcer on the right great toe. (A). Initial wound. (B). Most recent wound.

59 days was followed by long-term diabetic shoes to prevent pressure.

● VENOUS STASIS ULCERS

Venous stasis ulcers are usually chronic and/or recurrent ulcers of the legs secondary to venous hypertension in the skin and subcutaneous tissue. The incidence of venous stasis ulcers in the United States is approximately 400 000 to 600 000 at any time. Recurrent ulceration is 37% to 48% over 3 to 5 years.[25]

Venous hypertension is positional and is usually secondary to venous valvular incompentency or deep venous obstruction. The majority of patients also have severe varicose veins or "frozen valves" from previous deep venous thrombosis (DVT) of the lower extremities. The most difficult ulcers to heal may be associated with PAD, poor mobility, sitting with legs dependant, and infrequent "calf muscle pump activity" in patients with other comorbidities.

Investigation of the microcirculation around venous ulcers suggests "white cell trapping" which may release toxins causing tissue injury, fibrolytic dysfunction, and fibrin obstruction to oxygen diffusion.

Complications of venous stasis include dermatitis with hyperpigmentation, fibrosis, and contraction of subcutaneous tissue and skin. Fibrous contraction of skin and subcutaneous tissue progresses to secondary erythema, blistering, weeping, scaling, crusting, and secondary bacterial infection. Severe itching is followed by ulceration and severe pain. Ulcers may also occur suddenly after mild trauma or be secondary to surgical or other wounds.

The physician must not only treat the ulcer but also determine the contributing cause(s). Ankle-brachial index (ABIs) and pulse volume recordings must be obtained in all patients. TBIs may be necessary if the ulcer location does not permit ABIs. Abnormal ABIs (>1.1 or <0.9) should lead to a complete lower extremity arterial duplex study

and consultation to optimize arterial oxygen perfusion. Standing venous duplex evaluation for incompetent varicose veins and perforating veins is very important. Incompetent perforating veins and varicose veins can be corrected by subcutaneous ligation or endovascular ablation with improvement in the venous hypertension. This is of critical importance if one hopes to avoid frequent recurrent ulcerations and long-term morbidity.

Wound treatment for stasis ulcers should include debridement of necrotic tissue and biofilm to decrease infection and to stimulate senescent cells. Topical dressings with calcium dexomer iodine[26] or silver products[27] followed by compression dressings with two layers (20 TORR) or four layer (40 TORR) elastic bandages are applied. If significant infection is present with >10^5 organisms per gm on deep tissue culture, appropriate oral or intravenous antibiotics are important. Topical vitamin A and zinc are helpful in healing chronic ulcers. In resistant ulcers, Apligraft may accelerate healing with the addition of live keratinocytes and fibroblasts.[28]

After healing of stasis ulcers, fitted support hose and lifestyle changes are critical to avoid recurrence.

Case Report

A 50-year-old male was referred to the WTC with multiple recurrent ulcers on the lower extremities that appeared to be venous stasis ulcers. He had only a few months over the last 10 years without these painful lesions and was considering bilateral amputations. He complained of severe burning and itching pain in both legs, recurrent fever, loss of work, and social isolation. He would not wear support hose or compression dressings as directed because of itching when the legs were covered.

Systemic risk factors for problem wounds included CAD, congestive heart failure, atrial fibrillation, anticoagulation, COPD, chronic bronchitis, cigarette smoking, sleep

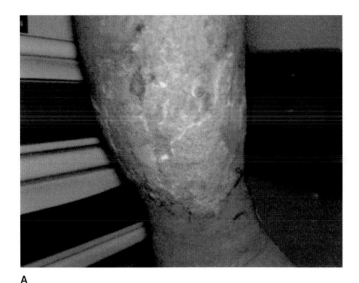

A

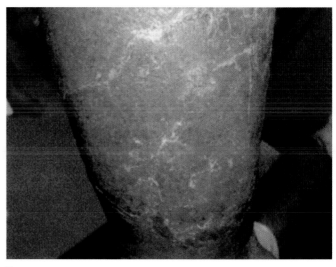

B

● **FIGURE 43-3.** A 50-year-old man with multiple ulcers on the lower extremities. (A). Initial wound. (B). Most recent wound.

apnea, diabetes, and malnutrition. Physical examination revealed multiple inflamed, weeping ulcerations on both legs with chronic fibrosis, hyperpigmentation, edema, and cellulites (Figure 43-3). No varicose veins were visible. He had no palpable pedal pulses but Doppler flow sounds were present.

Duplex lower extremity arterial examination was reported as normal arterial flow from aorta to tibial arteries with tibial and pedal arch disease. The TCOM ($TcPO_2$) report indicated low normal (40–50 mm Hg) central and peripheral levels. Limited compression dressing of 20 to 30 TORR to avoid ischemia were applied. Standing venous duplex examination revealed normal bilateral deep veins with competent valves. There were greater saphenous vein (GSV) varicosities with incompetent valves as well as incompetent bilateral perforating veins. Combined arterial and venous insufficiency was thus diagnosed. This case highlights the importance of evaluating the arterial pressures prior to the application of compression stockings which could potentially exacerbate arterial insufficiency; in some cases ankle pressures alone are sufficient, in some settings toe pressures are required for complete precompression evaluation.

Culture and sensitivity of the ulcers revealed methicillin resistant *Staph aureus* (MRSA) and *Pseudomonas auriginosa*. He was placed on protein supplements, multivitamins, leg elevation 3 times daily for 30 minutes, appropriate systemic antibiotics and weekly visits to the WTC for sharp debridement of necrotic biofilm, as well as the application of topical vitamin A, silver calcium alginate with foam, and two layer compression dressings. Dressings were changed every 2 or 3 days by visiting nurses. Appointments were made with his internists and other specialists for treatment of his systemic risk factors. He refused to quit smoking, lose weight, or to allow treatment of his sleep apnea. Six of the leg ulcerations healed within 90 days and complete healing was accomplished by 126 days. He was referred to vascular surgery for endovascular laser ablation of the greater saphenous veins and ligation of perforating veins. Unna boot treatment was continued until the vein ablation procedure. He has had no recurrent ulcerations over the last year.

● PRESSURE ULCERS

Pressure ulcers or "bed sores" are frequently seen by vascular specialists. Patients may present with pressure ulcers or develop them after admission to the hospital. The most common anatomic sites are the sacrum and heels. They may also be found on the elbows, toes, ischial tuberosities, trochanters, and knees.

The primary cause of these ulcers is unrelieved compression exceeding capillary pressure of 12 to 32 mm Hg for over 2 hours. Other causes included shearing, where skin remains in place while underlying tissue is pulled downward such as prolonged high Fowler's position. Friction of skin against bed sheets in mentally or emotionally ill patients and moisture from incontinence or other drainage may lead to ulcers. Malnutrition, aging, thin skin, paralysis, neuropathy, obesity, and amputation may be significant factors.

Critical care patients on standard beds versus air mattresses have been reported to have a much higher incidence of pressure ulcers. Heel ulcers are reported in patients enduring long operative procedures.

Pressure ulcers should be staged at the time of diagnosis:

Stage I—Nonblanchable erythema of intact skin
Stage II—Partial-thickness skin loss involving epidermis, dermis, or both
Stage III—Full-thickness skin loss with destruction of all or part of the subcutaneous layer down to but not through underlying fascia
Stage IV—Skin and subcutaneous tissue loss associated with damage to muscle, bone, or facial layers

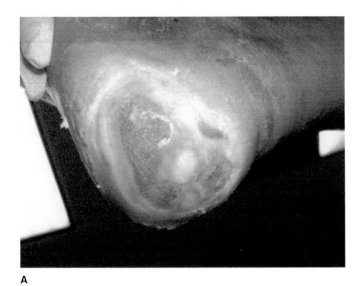

A

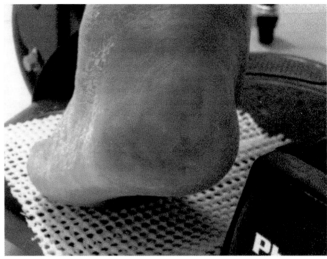

B

● FIGURE 43-4. A 68-year-old man with a pressure ulcer on the left heel. (A). Initial wound. (B). Most recent wound.

undermining and sinus tracts also may be associated with stage IV pressure ulcers

Wound care of pressure ulcers is similar to care of other chronic wounds with careful attention to pressure reduction.

Case Report

A 68-year-old man was referred to the WTC with a pressure ulcer on the left heel and a recent right BKA (Figure 43-4). He was treated with Accuzyme, a protective semipermeable dressing and foam heel protectors. General risk factors were PAD, diabetes, COPD, hypertension, chronic renal disease, and malnutrition. TCOM (TcPO$_2$) revealed >50 mm Hg O$_2$ proximal to the heel ulcer on

room air. He had a daily dressing change by nurses at home and weekly evaluation at the WTC. Complete healing was documented at 6 weeks.

● OTHER WOUNDS

There are many other acute and problem wounds that the vascular specialist may encounter in clinical practice. These wounds may include partial loss of skin grafts or necrotic areas on anterior, or posterior amputation flaps.

Surgical incisions in irradiated areas of the body following mastectomy for breast cancer, head and neck cancers, and abdominal malignancies may not heal and usually become problem wounds. The vascular specialist may seek help from the plastic surgeon or from wound specialty clinics in healing these wounds.

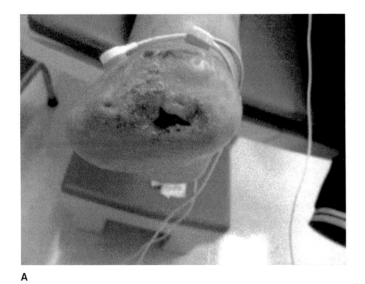

A

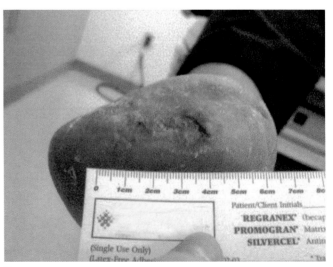

B

● FIGURE 43-5. A 62-year-old man with a nonhealing amputation. (A). Initial wound. (B). Most recent wound.

Addition of HBO may salvage some of these wounds with marginal arterial perfusion confirmed by TCOMs (TcPO$_2$) <40 mm Hg on room air. Nurses specializing in ostomy and wound care can be a very valuable asset to the surgeon in the hospital, home health care settings, and nursing homes. These specialists should be utilized for help with timely and proper wound care and dressing changes.

Case Report

A 62-year-old man was referred to the WTC after a right transmetatarsal amputation (TMA) 2 years earlier that had not healed despite proper wound care, skin grafts, and supportive treatment by his vascular surgeon (Figure 43-5). Below knee amputation had been suggested. General risk factors included PAD, diabetes, neuropathy, and colon cancer with chemotherapy beginning at the time of referral. TCOM (TcPO$_2$) revealed 33 mm Hg O$_2$ at the dorsum of the foot on room air increasing to >100 mm Hg O$_2$ with 100% O$_2$ mask. X-rays revealed osteomyelitis of the sec-

ond and third distal metatarsal bones. At the WTC sharp debridement of the necrotic soft tissue and bone was performed. The wound was covered daily with silver hydrogel and semipermeable dressing. Addition of HBO at 2.4 ATA for 14 days resulted in significant improvement with increased sensation, healthy granulation tissue, and TCOM (TcPO$_2$) of 68 mm Hg proximal to the wound. After 15 more HBO treatments and weekly wound care he completely healed.

● SUMMARY

When a wound is not healing as expected, it should be given timely and complete reevaluation and an aggressive treatment plan followed using the many resources now available to us. It is not acceptable to give wound treatment less than our best effort. In the vascular specialist's practice, amputations should be less common than in the past and be recommended only if we have exhausted the many resources now available to us for wound healing.

REFERENCES

1. Agren MS, Ostenfeld N, Kallehave F, et al. *Wound Repair Regen.* 2006;14(5):526-535.

2. Baharestani MM. *Wound Care Essentials.* Ambler, PA: Lipponcott Williams &Wilkins; 2004:2-18.

3. Franks PJ, Moffatt CJ, Doherty CD, et al. *Wound Repair Regen.* 2006;14(5):536-541.

4. Franks PJ, Moffatt CJ, Doherty DC. Longer-term changes in quality of life in chronic leg ulceration. *Wound Repair Regen.* 2006;14:536-541.

5. Gillitzer R, Goebeler M. Chemokines in cutaneous wound healing. *J Leukoc Biol.* 2001;69:513-521.

6. Bhushan M, Young HS, Brenchley PE, Griffiths CE. Recent advances in cutaneous angiogenesis. *Br J Dermatol.* 2002;147: 418-425.

7. O'Toole EA. Extracellular matrix and keratinocyte migration. *Clin Exp Dermatol.* 2001;26:525-530.

8. Baker EA, Leaper DJ. Proteinases, their inhibitors, and cytokine profiles in acute wound fluid. *Wound Repair Regen.* 2000;8:392-392.

9. Argenta LC, Morykwas MJ. Vacuum-assisted closure: a new method for wound controal and treatment: clinical experience. *Ann Plast Surg.* 1997;38:563.

10. Mullner T, et al. The use of negative pressure to promote the healing of tissue defects: a clinical trial using the vacuum seal technique. *Br J Plast Surg.* 1997;50:194.

11. Joseph E, et al. A prospective randomized trial of vacuum assisted closure versus standard therapy of chronic non-healing wounds. *Wounds.* 2000;12:60.

12. McCallon SK, et al. Vacuum assisted closure versus saline-moistened gauze in the healing of postoperative diabetic foot wounds. *Ostomy Wound Manage.* 2000;46:28.

13. Fife CE, Buyukcakir C, Otto GH, et al. The predictive value of transcutaneous oxygen tension measurement in diabetic lower extremity ulcers treated with hyperbaric oxygen therapy: a retrospective analysis of 1144 patiens. *Wound Rep Reg.* 2002;10:198-207.

14. Oren S, Isakov I, Golzman B, et al. The influence of smoking cessation on hemodynamics and arterial compliance. *Angiology.* 2006;57:564-568.

15. Gimbel M, Hunt T. Wound healing and hyperbaric oxygenation. In: Kindwall EP, Whelam HT, eds. *Hyperabaric Medicine Practice.* Rev ed. Flagstaff, AZ: Best Publishing; 1999:1969-2004.

16. Consenus Development Conference on Diabetic Foot Wound Care: 7–8 April 1999, Boston, MA. *Diabetes Care.* 1999;22: 157-162.

17. Abbott CA, Carrington AL, Ashe H, et al. The North-West Diabetes Foot Care Study: incidence of, and risk factors for, new diabetic foot ulceration in a community-based patient cohort. *Diabet Med.* 2002;19:377-384.

18. Lipsky BA, Berendt AR. Principles and practice of antibiotic therapy of diabetic foot infections. *Diabetes Metab Res.* 2000;16(suppl 1):S42-S46.

19. Grayson ML, Gibbon GW, Balogh K, et al. Probing to bone in infected pedal ulcers: a clinical sign of underlying osteomyelitis in diabetic patients. *JAMA.* 1995;272:721-723.

20. Armstrong DG, Hguyen HC. Improvement in healing with aggressive edema reduction after debridement of foot infection in person with diabetes. *Arch Surg.* 2000;135:1405-1409.

21. Armstrong DG, Lavery LA, Kimbriel HR, et al. Activity patterns of patients with diabetic foot ulceration: patients with active ulceration may not adhere to a standard pressure off-loading regimen. *Diabetes Care.* 2003;26:2595-2597.

22. Bennett SP, Griffiths GD, Schor AM, et al. Growth factors in the treatment of diabetic foot ulcers. *Br J Surg.* 2003;90:133-149.

23. Marston WA, Hanft J, Norwood P, et al. The efficacy and safety of Dermagraft in improving the healing of chronic diabetic foot ulcers: results of a prospective randomized trial. *Diabetes Care.* 2003;26:1701-1705.

24. Sussman C, Dyson M. Therapeutic and diagnostic ultrasound. In: Sussman C, Bates-Jenson BM, eds. *Wound Care: A Collaborative Manual for Physical Therapists and Nurses.* Gaithersburg, MD: Aspen Publishers; 1998;427-445.

25. Valencia IC, Falabella A, Kirsner RS, et al. Chronic venous insufficiency and venous leg ulceration. *J Am Acad Dermatol.* 2001;44:401-424.

26. Zhou LH, Nahm WK, Badiavas E, et al. Slow release iodine preparation and wound healing: in vitro effects consistent with lack of in vivo toxicity in human chronic wounds. *Br J Dermatol.* 2002;146:365-374.

27. Thomas S, McCubbin P. A comparison of the antimicrobial effects of four silver-containing dressings on three organisms. *J Wound Care.* 2003;12:101-107.

28. Brem H, Tomic-Canic M, Tarnovskaya A, et al. Healing of elderly patients with diabetic foot ulcers, venous stasis ulcers, and pressure ulcers. *Surg Technol Int.* 2003;11:161-167.

chapter 44

Erectile Dysfunction

Ryan Payne, MD / *Peter Langenstroer, MD, MS*

● INTRODUCTION

Since the introduction of oral therapy, erectile dysfunction (ED) has become a widely publicized disease. These agents have revolutionized the management of ED and helped identify patients at risk for developing ED and other associated medical conditions. Since the erectile bodies of the penis are nothing more than a complex vascular structure, it has become evident that ED dysfunction may represent a local manifestation of widely systemic disease. Evaluation and management of the patient with ED may have a global impact on the overall health. With that in mind, this chapter represents a review of the current status of ED diagnosis, evaluation, and management.

● ANATOMY

General Anatomy

The penis is composed of three main functional structures; two dorsal erectile bodies and one ventral urethra. The urethra functions to allow for the egress of urine and ejaculate. Whereas erectile bodies are vital biologic functions, they are not required for erectile functioning. Despite the anatomic association and proximity of the erectile bodies, urination, orgasm, emission, and erectile function can occur independently.

The corporal bodies are the functional units for penile tumescence. These two parallel structures are anchored proximally at the inferior puboischial rami. Initially, they are separate but fuse in the midline as the penis extends from the perineum. This proximal separation allows for the urethra to assume its position in the ventral midline by passing beneath the crus of the proximal corporal bodies. As the penis extends from the body, it is supported by the suspensory ligament of the penis. This ligament offers erectile support and facilitates directed penetration. The erectile bodies terminate distally beneath the glans penis which acts as a cap over the distal end. The glans penis is contiguous with the corpus spongiosum or spongy sinusoids that surround the penile urethra.

Tunica Albuginea

Another important and underestimated anatomic component for erectile function is the tunica albuginea of the cavernous body. This bilaminar casing has functionality based on its elasticity and pliability. In the flaccid state, the tunica albuginea is soft and relaxed. This allows for open venous drainage to the cavernous sinusoids. In contrast, during tumescence the longitudinal and circular fibers of the tunica albuginea occlude of the emissary veins restricting venous outflow. This leads to corporal filling during the erectile response and ultimately penile rigidity. If the tunica albuginea loses its elasticity, the occlusive process fails and venous leak ED ensues.

Arterial Supply

The primary arterial supply originates from the terminal branch of the internal iliac artery. This vessel, the internal pudendal artery, passes through Alcock's canal and divides to give rise to the penile artery. The penile artery branches into the bulbar, urethral, and cavernous arteries. The cavernous artery provides the main arterial inflow to the corporal body. However, perforating branches of the dorsal artery can provide additional blood flow. This artery arises from the superficial branch of the inferior external pudendal artery.

Venous Drainage

Venous drainage of the erectile bodies originates from the emissary veins that perforate the tunica albuginea of the corporal bodies. These veins drain to the deep dorsal vein of the penis, which passes through the pelvic floor and into the prostatic venous plexus. This plexus will drain into the internal iliac venous system bilaterally.

Nervous Innervation

Neurologic control of vascular inflow is heavily mediated by nonadrenergic noncholinergic (NANC) nerves from the cavernous nerves. These nerves supply the nitric oxide (NO) that leads to the profound vasodilation resulting in tumescence. The cavernous nerves arise from the pelvic plexus on the lateral aspect of the rectum. This plexus is a consolidation of the cholinergic, adrenergic, and NANC nerves supplying the pelvic and genital organs. The cavernous nerve arises from this plexus to penetrate the pelvic floor that is posterolateral to the urethra. It terminates in the corporal body. Injury to this nerve during pelvic surgery leads to ED.

● EMBRYOLOGY OF THE PENIS

Penile development requires two separate but overlapping organ systems to develop simultaneously. Both systems, genital and urinary, are needed for a fully functional male penis. Penile development is orchestrated by a complex interplay of developmental timing, hormonal regulation, and tissue interactions. The initiation of development of the external genitalia is the same in both males and females. During the fifth week of development, a pair of swellings develops on either side of the cloacal membrane. The cloacal folds meet just anterior to the cloacal membrane and form a midline swelling called the genital tubercle. In the seventh week, there is fusion of the urorectal septum with the cloacal membrane creating the primitive perineum. This divides the posterior anal membrane to form the urogenital membrane anteriorly. The cloacal fold flanking the urogenital membrane is now called the urethral fold (also known as the genital or urogenital fold). The new labioscrotal swellings appear after the urethral fold. During the sixth week, the cavity of the urogenital sinus extends onto the enlarging genital tubercle and becomes the urethral groove. This groove is temporarily filled by the urethral plate, which as the phallus grows recanalizes to form an even deeper urethral groove. The urogenital membrane ruptures during the seventh week opening the cavity of the urogenital sinus to the amniotic fluid. The genital tubercle elongates to form the penis. The coronary sulcus on the genital tubercle demarcates the primordial glans penis from the phallic shaft. The adult derivatives of these embryonic structures are listed in Table 44-1.[1,2]

The most popular hypothesis of external genital and urethral development was proposed by Glenister[3] in 1954. At the start of the fourth month, the effects of androgens (especially dihydrotestosterone [DHT]) on the male external genitalia become apparent. The perineum elongates and the labioscrotal folds fuse in the midline to form the scrotum. As the penis elongates, the urethral folds grow toward the midline and enclose the penile urethra by 14-week gestation.[3] The penile urethra is initially blind ending as the

TABLE 44-1. Development of External Genital Structures

Primordial Structure	Structure in Adult Male
Genital tubercle	Glans penis and corpus cavernosa
Urogenital sinus	Penile urethra
Urethral fold	Corpus spongiosum surrounding penile urethra
Labioscrotal fold	Scrotum

urethral groove that does not extend onto the glans penis which originated from the distal part of the genital tubercle. There is an ectodermal invagination from the tip of the glans that then completes the terminal portion of the penile urethra.

● PHYSIOLOGY OF ERECTIONS

Neurophysiology

In the flaccid penis, the smooth musculature of the arterial and arteriolar walls of the corpora cavernosa is tonically contracted, allowing only a small amount of arterial flow for nutritional purposes.[4,5] This state of moderate contraction is maintained by a combination of three main factors: intrinsic myogenic activity; endothelium-derived contracting factors such as prostaglandin I_2, prostaglandin $F_{2\alpha}$, thromboxane A_2, and endothelins; and α-adrenergic receptors on the arteries, arterioles, and cavernous trabeculae are stimulated by norepinephrine (NE) from sympathetic nerve endings.[6–9]

Sexual stimulation triggers release of neurotransmitters, principally NO, from the cavernous nerve terminals. NO released from NANC nerve endings and from the endothelium diffuses into smooth muscle cells activating guanylyl cyclase. This increases the production of intracellular cyclic guanosine monophosphate (cGMP) causes increased phosphorylation of myosin light-chain kinase resulting in dissociation of myosin and actin, which in turn results in relaxation of cavernous smooth muscle. Potassium influx is also induced through cGMP depended potassium channels and NO simulation of the Na-K ATPase. This increased potassium influx causes hyperpolarization, which leads to closure of voltage depended calcium channels and a decrease in intracellular calcium. Acetylcholine and vasointestinal peptide (VIP) likely play some role in cavernous smooth muscle relaxation during erections, but this seems to be secondary to the role of NO.[8,10–14]

Hemodynamics

The development and maintenance of erection is a complex mechanism dependent on smooth muscle relaxation involving both arterial dilation and sinusoidal relaxation causing venous compression.[15,16] Dilation of the cavernous smooth muscle increases blood flow to the corporal bodies which initiates a well-studied cascade of events resulting in an erection.

The initial event is dilation of the arteries and arterioles increasing blood flow to the cavernous sinusoids. The resultant expansion of the cavernous sinusoids traps the incoming blood. Compression of the subtunical venous plexuses, peripheral sinusoids, and emissary veins from tunical stretching increases the intracavernous pressure to approximately 100 mm Hg and establishing a full erection. Contraction of the ischiocavernosus muscles leads to a further increase in pressure.

Detumescence after erection is likely is in part because of a combination of cessation of NO release and the breakdown on cGMP by phosphodiesterases. However, the sympathetic discharge during ejaculation is extremely important for return to the flaccid state. Norepinepherine's action on α-receptors in the cavernous trabeculae and arteries seems to be the principal neurotransmitter in detumescence. Three hemodynamic phases of detumescence have been reported.[17] First, a smooth muscle contraction initiated by norepinephrine against a closed venous system causes a transient intracorporeal pressure increase. Second, the resumption of basal arterial flow and a slow reopening of the venous channels result in a slow pressure decrease. Finally, a fully restored venous outflow capacity results in a fast pressure decrease and return of the penis to the flaccid state.

EPIDEMIOLOGY

The prevalence of ED increases with age. The Massachusetts Male Aging Study (MMAS) is the only longitudinal study conducted in the United States. This study reports that the overall prevalence increases from about 40% of men in their forties to about 70% of men aging 70 years.[18] The National Health and Social Life Survey (NHSLS) also estimated the prevalence of ED in men. This study reported dysfunction in 7% of men aging from 18 to 29 years, 9% for ages 30 to 39 years, 11% for ages 40 to 49 years, and 18% for ages 50 to 59 years.[19] There were 24 international studies looking at the prevalence of ED between 1993 and 2003. All showed a rising prevalence when stratified by age, but the absolute prevalence varied widely. Almost all of the studies reported rates of less than 10% for men younger than 40 years and rates of 50% to 75% or higher for men older than 70 years.

The crude incidence rate in the United States was estimated by the Massachusetts Male Aging Study to be 25.9 cases per 1000 man-years. Incidence was also shown to be a function of age with the annual incidence rate increasing with each decade. Using these data, it is estimated that there would be over 600 000 new cases of ED in white men between the ages of 40 and 69 each year in the United States.[20] Studies in South America and Europe also suggest incidence rates between 25 and 30 per 1000 man-years.[21,22]

TABLE 44-2. Common Side Effects of PDE5 Inhibition

Headache	13%
Flushing	10%
Sinus congestion	10%
Dyspepsia	5%
Blue vision (sildenafil)	10%
Myalgias (tadalafil)	12%

ETIOLOGY OF ED

Organic

The risk factors of ED are varied and include age, general health status, diabetes mellitus, cardiovascular disease, genitourinary disease, psychiatric or psychologic disorders, sociodemographic conditions, smoking, medications, hormonal factors, neurologic diseases, and other chronic diseases. Diabetes is associated with decreased libido, orgasmic dysfunction, and ED. Endothelial dysfunction is a common pathway for many cases of ED and is a manifestation of many of the above conditions.

Many classifications have been proposed based on the cause (diabetic, traumatic, iatrogenic, etc.) or mechanism (neurogenic, arterial, venous, etc.). The International Society of Impotence Research recommended a classification system in 1999 that is the most widely used classification scheme (Table 44-2).[23] It is unlikely that any individual patient's impotence is derived from a single source, and many cases have a significant psychologic component (Figure 44-1).

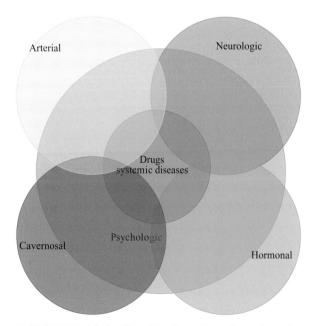

● **FIGURE 44-1.** Classification of impotence in patients is rarely because of a single source, and most patients have some degree of psychologic component.

Psychogenic

In the 1970s, this was believed to be the most common cause of ED and was thought to affect 90% of impotent men;[24] however, it is now understood that ED is typically a mixed condition that is predominantly function or physical.

Centrally, erections are controlled by the hypothalamus, limbic system, and cerebral cortex. The spinal erection centers are controlled by these higher centers. The proposed mechanisms for psychogenic ED involve excessive direct inhibition of the spinal erection center by the higher centers and or excessive sympathetic outflow mediating an increase in penile smooth muscle tone.[25–28]

Neurogenic

The medial preoptic area, paraventricular nucleus, and hippocampus are important integration centers for both sex drive and erection. Any pathologic state in these areas, such as Parkinson disease, stroke, encephalitis, epilepsy, trauma, or dementia, is frequently associated with ED.[29,30]

The innervation to the penis is both autonomic and somatic. The somatic nerves are primarily responsible for sensation and contraction of the bulbocavernosus and ischiocavernosus muscles. The parasympathetic innervation arises from the intermediolateral cell columns in the second, third, and fourth sacral cord segments and travels into the pelvic plexus. The sympathetic innervation originates from the 11th thoracic to 2nd lumbar spinal segments and passes to the sympathetic chain ganglia through the lumbar splanchnic nerves, inferior mesenteric, and superior mesenteric plexus to the hypogastric plexus. From there they travel to the pelvic plexus where they join the parasympathetic fibers and form the cavernous nerves.[31] The location and extent of a spinal cord injury will largely determine the degree of the resultant erectile function. Although the thoracolumbar pathway may be compensatory, the sacral parasympathetic neurons mediate reflexogenic erections. Reflex erections are preserved in 95% of men with complete upper cord lesions, but only 25% of men with complete lower cord injuries.[32,33]

The cavernous nerves arise from the pelvic plexus and travel to innervate the penis. These nerves can be easily damaged during pelvic surgery, and a clear understanding of the course of these nerves is essential in order to preserve their function and prevent neurogenic ED after pelvic surgery.[34,35] A more complete understanding of these pathways has resulted in a dramatically decreased incidence of ED following radical pelvic surgery for cancer.[4]

Arteriogenic

Any resistance to blood flow through the hypogastric-cavernosal arterial tree can decrease perfusion pressure and blood flow into the sinusoidal spaces. This leads to increased time to maximal erection and decreased rigidity. In the majority of patients, this is a single component of a more generalized atherosclerotic process. Vascular disease of penis is a local manifestation of more systemic disease. Common

risk factors for penile arterial insufficiency and ED include hypertension, hyperlipidemia, cigarette smoking, diabetes mellitus, pelvic irradiation, and pelvic or perineal trauma. Many studies have shown that the patient age and incidence of ED parallel other arterial and atherosclerotic disease processes, especially coronary artery disease.[18,36–38] In vasculogenic ED, corporal oxygen tension is decreased from baseline, and decreased from that seen in psychogenic ED.[39] Formation of PGE_2 is oxygen dependent, and chronic decreases in oxygen tension leads to lower levels of PGE_2, and may diminish the corporal trabecular smooth muscle content and induce collagen synthesis leading to diffuse venous leakage.[40–43] Endothelium-dependent release of NO and resultant smooth muscular vasodilatation has been shown to be further suppressed in patients with endothelial dysfunction due essential hypertension, elevated low-density lipoproteins, or diabetes.[16,44] This leads to further suppression of penile blood flow with erectile stimulation independent of structural vascular changes.

Traumatic injury to the hypogastric, penile, or cavernosal arteries can result in chronic focal stenosis of the injured vessel. This is most commonly associated with young patients who have sustained blunt pelvic or perineal trauma, however, it has also been reported in long-distance cycling, through the pressure placed on the hypogastric and common penile artery traversing Alcock's canal from the bicycle seat.[45,46]

Veno-Occlusive

Failure of adequate venous occlusion to develop and maintain an erection is a common cause of ED and results from a variety of processes. Degenerative changes of the tunica albuginea or subtunical architecture can impair compression of the subtunical and emissary veins. This can be as a result of a diffused process throughout the corpora, as seen with aging or diabetes, or can be caused by focal areas of inelasticity such as prior penile trauma or Peyronie disease.[47–50] ED can also result from the creation of cavernosal spongiosal shunts formed after traumatic injuries or surgical manipulation for urethral stricture disease.[51]

Furthermore, structural or functional abnormalities in the fibroelastic, smooth muscle, or endothelium of the trabeculae of the corpora may result in venous leakage. This may occur as a result of systemic disease, resultant chronic changes, or excessive androgen tone in anxious individuals or patients with psychogenic ED. This is frequently associated with a relative decrease in corporal NO and an increase in α-adenoreceptor tone, and it can be modified by increasing corporal NO.[6] It has been shown that stripping the deep dorsal vein, thereby dramatically reducing the vascular outflow, that venogenic ED can be partially corrected.[52]

Endocrinologic

Hypogonadism is a prevalent finding in men with ED. Mulligan and Schmitt performed a review of articles on male hypogonadism from 1975 until 1992 and concluded that androgens are important for sexual interest, increase the frequency of sexual acts, and increase the frequency of nocturnal erections. However, testosterone has little if any effect on fantasy or visually stimulated erections.[53] In multiple animal models, castration has been shown to decrease arterial flow and induce venous leakage and reduce the erectile response to stimulation of the cavernous nerve, as well as decreasing nitric oxide synthase (NOS) activity and increasing cavernosal cellular apoptosis in these animals.[4] It is clinically well established that men who are castrated or receive androgen ablative therapy for prostate cancer report poor libido and ED. Also any disruption of the hypothalamic-pituitary-gonadal axis, such as hyperprolactinemia, hyper- or hypothyroidism, mumps orchitis, surgery, tumor, or trauma can result in decrease circulating levels of testosterone and ED. Diabetes mellitus is the most common endocrine disorder associated with ED, but its mechanism is though a combination of vascular, endothelial, and neurogenic mechanism, and will be discussed further in those sections.

Drug-Induced

Many older male patients are on medication for conditions that are themselves risk factors for ED. Untreated systemic disease, such as hypertension, diabetes, depression, or cardiovascular diseases, often pose a greater threat to erectile function than the medications used to treat them.

Multiple antihypertensive agents have been associated with ED. Thiazide diuretics have shown an increased incidence of ED when compared to placebo in multiple large historic trials on antihypertensive treatments.[54,55] These findings were reproduced in the Treatment of Mild hypertension Study, where the thiazide arm reported ED at double the rate of the placebo arm after 2 years. However, the rate of ED in the placebo group had approached the rate of the thiazide group by 4 years, which could be caused by the vascular effects of poorly treated hypertension.[56] Nonselective β-antagonists have been shown to produce more ED than placebo. This is felt to be due to some β_2 receptor-mediated smooth muscle relaxation in the corporal tissue. These results have not been reproduced when testing the newer cardio-selective agents. Calcium channel blockers have not been shown to cause ED at any rate greater than placebo. α-Blockers and angiotensin-converting enzyme inhibitors do not induce ED and have tended to improve sexual function when compared against placebo.[56]

Multiple psychotropic medications have been associated with sexual dysfunction, but as with hypertension it is difficult to distinguish the effects of the medication from the effects of the disease. Selective serotonin reuptake inhibitors (SSRI) are the most common drug used to treat depression. The estimated incidence of sexual side effects from this class of medication is reported to be 50%.[57,58] However, there have been randomized controlled trials suggesting that the improved sexual function from treatment of depression can outweigh any negative effects from the medicine.[59] Selective serotonin reuptake inhibitors exert their antidepressant effect by inhibiting reuptake of 5-HT into central nervous system (CNS) neurons. Their sexual side effects are likely partly because of the 5-HT$_2$ and 5-HT$_3$ receptors in the spinal cord are believed to be inhibitors of erectogenic pathways. They also have some inhibitory effects of NOS. Multiple other psychotropic medications including antipsychotics, tricyclic antidepressants, monoamine oxidase inhibitors, and anxiolytics have also been associated with sexual side effects and ED.

Antiandrogens are another major class of pharmacologic agents associated with sexual side effects. 5-α-reductase inhibitors have minimal effect on circulating testosterone, but block its conversion to the more potent androgen DHT. There is some evidence that DHT is important for maintaining NOS activity in penile tissue.[60] The 5-α-reductase inhibitor finasteride had a 5% rate compared to 1% with placebo.[61] More complete ablation of the androgen effects produces more pronounced sexual side effects. Androgen receptor blockers such as flutamide and bicalutamide cause a significant reduction in sexual desire, but are less likely to effect erectile function than castration.[62] Luteinizing hormone-releasing hormone (LHRH) agonist treatment, which decreases circulating testosterone levels to castrate values cause a profound decrease in sexual desire and a high incidence of ED.[62,63]

Nicotine containing products, especially cigarette smoking, is strongly associated with ED. Nicotine is a vasoconstrictor that reduces penile blood flow. The contractile effect on the corporal smooth muscle also leads to venous leakage and impaired erections. Alcohol in small amounts improves erections and sexual drive through a combination of vasodilatory and anxiolytic properties. However, large amounts of alcohol consumption cause CNS depression, decreased libido, and ED. Chronic alcoholism leads to decreased levels of circulating testosterone, increased estrogen, and peripheral neuropraxia, all of which can lead to ED.[4]

Aging

A variety of studies has shown a progressive decline in erectile function in "healthy" men as they age. Masters and Johnson were the first to note many of these changes in aging men including greater latency to erection, less turgidity, less forceful erection, and longer refractory periods.[64] Multiple authors have proposed a number of mechanisms to explain these changes, but it is most likely because of a combination of physiologic changes that occur with normal aging including decreased testosterone, increased vascular muscle tone, increased corporal muscle tone, and decreased relaxation to acetylcholine resulting in decreased penile NO.

Primary ED

Primary ED refers to a lifelong inability develop or maintain an erection, beginning with the first attempt at a sexual encounter. This can be caused by developmental abnormalities, physical causes, or psychologic causes. The largest series of patients with primary ED describes 67 patients, 11 (16%) had a predominantly psychologic cause with the remaining because of a variety of structural, arterial, neurologic, or veno-occlusive dysfunction. However, an additional 39 of the 57 patients (68%) had a significant psychologic component in addition to some organic abnormalities.[65] Primary ED with a normal phallus is exceedingly rare, but several structural abnormalities of the corpora or vascular anomalies have been reported.[4]

● EVALUATION AND DIAGNOSTIC TESTING

In modern clinical practice, the mainstay of evaluation for ED is a thorough history and physical examination. Invasive or advanced testing is only occasionally indicated. The patient-centered or goal-directed approach is an important concept in the evaluation and the eventual treatment of patients with ED. The treating physician should not only incorporate the biologic factors about the disease, but also incorporate the patient's individual beliefs and goals when providing care in both the workup and eventual treatment of sexual dysfunction.[66]

History

A detailed medical, psychosocial, and sexual history is the cornerstone in the evaluation of patients with ED. The style of interview is as important as the questions, and it is important to maintain a nonjudgmental attitude of comfort and flexibility. The medical history should be conducted with the goal of identifying medical conditions, prior operations, medications, and psychogenic issues that may be important to the diagnosis of ED. Sexual history should be performed to ascertain the severity, onset, and duration of the problem. It is important to attempt to distinguish functional problems with erections from the other sexual issues including desire, ejaculation, or orgasm, and to take an opportunity to discuss partner-related issues along with diagnostic and treatment goals with the patient. Psychosocial history should be assessed as sexual dysfunction frequently has a detrimental effect on patients' self-esteem and coping mechanisms. It is also important to realize that the psychogenic factors frequently coexist in patients with organic ED.[66,67]

There are many validated sexual function and ED questionnaires. These have the most benefit in clinical trials, but can occasionally be helpful in attempting to quantify the severity of sexual dysfunction in a given patient. The most commonly referenced include the International Index of Erectile Function (IIEF), the Brief Male Sexual Function Inventory (BMSFI), and the ED Inventory for Treatment Satisfaction (EDITS), but many other questionnaires exist.[68–70] The IIEF is a 15-item questionnaire that attempts to quantify erectile function, orgasmic function, sexual desire, intercourse satisfaction, and overall satisfaction. A five question version of the IIEF, known as the Sexual Health Inventory for Men (SHIM) has been developed with the hope of providing a quick tool in the office that would allow physicians to quickly assess ED. This tool incorporates four items on erectile function and one item

on overall satisfaction.[71] All questionnaires have significant limitations in the clinical setting and should not take the place of a good case history.

Physical Examination

The physical examination frequently does not identify the pathology in patients complaining of sexual dysfunction. However, it is important to evaluate and assess cardiovascular and neurologic systems, including regular blood pressure screening. A thorough genital examination is also indicated. Occasionally, an obvious cause is identified (e.g., Peyronie plaque, hypogonadism, chordee) which can direct further diagnostic studies or treatment.[67]

Laboratory Testing

Screening fasting glucose and lipids are important screening parameters for all men complaining of ED. Also, hormonal studies can be helpful in certain patients with complaints of decreased libido or decreased energy, or in patients with clinical signs of hypogonadism. Additional laboratory tests including thyroid screening, prolactin levels, or prostate-specific antigen screening should be implemented at the discretion of the treating physician. Prostate-specific antigen testing should be performed prior to hormonal supplementation in men with hypogonadism.[66,67]

Diagnostic Testing

Nocturnal Penile Tumescence. Measurement of nocturnal erections (nocturnal penile tumescence [NPT]) was originally proposed in 1940 by Halverson, and in 1966 NPT was demonstrated to occur during rapid eye movement sleep.[72] The number and duration of nocturnal erections peak at puberty and decrease throughout life. Many methods have been used to measure NPT including the stamp test and snap gauges, but the most effective and well studied is the RigiScan, introduced in 1985.[73] This was the first portable device that allowed the monitoring of tumescence, rigidity, number, and duration of erectile events. NPT has the major advantages of relative freedom from psychologic influence when testing the neurovascular axis, and the ability to detect sleep-related abnormalities. However, the few normal values that exist for aging men and the wide range of data that exists for normal young subjects makes data difficult to interpret. These factors limit the clinical usefulness of NPT in the routine evaluation for patients with ED.[66] It remains an important study in specific circumstances such as suspected sleep disorders, obscure causes of ED, or suspected purely psychogenic ED.[74]

Intracavernous Injection. A commonly performed screening test for patients with ED is combined intracavernous injection and stimulation (CIS). It involves direct intracavernosal injection of a vasodilating agent and audiovisual stimulation, followed by assessment of the erection by an observer.[75,76] This test provides a direct assessment of the penile vascular status by bypassing neural and endocrine influences. It is also beneficial in the study that accurately predicts response to injection therapy as a treatment option for ED. The most commonly used vasodilators are alprostadil, papaverine, and phentolamine, either alone or in combination. There are four commercially available formulations: alprostadil alone (Caverject or Edex), papaverine and phentolamine combination (Bimix), or all three in combination (Trimix). These agents can also be compounded in combination at specialized pharmacies. Comparisons with other hemodynamic evaluations suggest that this test is better associated with normal venous occlusion, but false-negative studies are reported in up to 20% of patients.[77] The possible side effects include priapism which has been reported at rates ranging from 0% to 35% when using injection therapy for treatment of ED, although in a review of the published literature Linet reported an overall priapism rate of 1.3% after injection therapy, and most believe it is lower when used diagnostically in an office setting.[78–81]

Ultrasonography. In some circumstances, further evaluation of penile blood flow is indicated such as patients with prior penile or perineal trauma or other complex patients. The most reliable and least invasive test is color duplex ultrasound in combination with combined intracavernous injection and stimulation. Arterial flow velocities and erectile quality are measured at baseline and 5 to 10 minutes after injection. Analysis of the symmetry of arterial flow bilaterally, Doppler waveform and peak systolic velocity (PSV) correlate to vascular erectile disease. The Mayo Clinic series reported that PSV of less than 25 cm/s predicted an abnormal pudendal arteriography with a sensitivity of 100% and a specificity of 95%.[82] Multiple other studies suggest that the PSV consistently increases to above 25 cm/s in patients without arteriogenic ED.[83–86] Veno-occlusive dysfunction can be diagnosed by examining the PSV, end diastolic velocity (EDV), and resistive index (RI). RI is defined by the equation: $RI = (PSV - EDV)/PSV$. As the penile pressure approaches diastolic pressure during full erection, the RI will approach 1.[87] Naroda et al.[88] found that a RI was associated with normal cavernous function in 90% of the subjects and an RI was associated with venogenic ED in 95% of subjects.

Arteriography and Cavernosometry. Penile arteriography is performed by selective cannulation of the internal pudendal artery, intracavernous injection of a vasodilating agent, and injection of radiographic contrast. This directly evaluates the anatomy of the pudendal and penile arterial tree. This test is invasive and is superior for diagnosing anatomic rather than functional information. The main indications are young patients with ED secondary to traumatic arterial injury to provide anatomic information prior to attempted surgical revascularization, or patients with traumatic high-flow priapism as a roadmap to endovascular treatment. There is limited clinical value in most other patients with ED. Cavernosometry which involves infusion of radiographic contrast into the corporal body after injection of a vasodilating agent can directly identify areas of venous leak in patients with venous leak ED. As with arteriography, its clinical usefulness is reserved for young patients who are candidates for vascular operations to treat their ED.

● TREATMENT OPTIONS

The treatment options for ED encompass a broad range of treatment types. This spectrum spans from medical management to surgical implantation. As the treatments become more complex patient education, expectations and understanding are critical to achieving a satisfactory outcome. Frequently, patients do not wish to actively pursue management of their ED if it involves more than taking oral medication. For the motivated individual or couple for whom sexual intimacy remains as an important aspect of their lives and more aggressive treatment for the ED is indicated even if it involves surgical implantation.

The unique aspect of ED management is the treatment simplicity and ubiquity. In most cases, the etiology of the disease does not alter the treatment algorithm or the diagnostic evaluation. Some would argue that the aggressive diagnostic testing is not indicated for most patients with ED since it does not alter the treatment pathway. Thus, extensive testing such as penile Doppler studies, as described earlier in this chapter, are not performed on most patients. Finally, it critical to ensure that the patient has enough cardiovascular reserve to tolerate the physical activity of intercourse prior to initiating therapy. It is estimated that sexual intercourse utilizes four METS of activity.

● TREATMENT PYRAMID

The management of ED can be broken down into three tiers (Figure 44-2). The first tier and the foundation of modern ED management are oral agents. They reside alone in the first tier based on their simplicity, safety, noninvasiveness, and patient acceptance. The second tier involves three techniques: injection therapy, vacuum erection devices, or urethral suppositories. These require more involvement by

Tier 3
Penile implants

Tier 2
Vacuum devices,
Urethral suppository
Injection therapy

Tier 1
Oral agent, PDE5 inhibitors

● **FIGURE 44-2.** Illustration of the three tiered pyramid for the management of ED. Escalating the pyramid fewer patients are interested in pursuing ED treatment as they become more invasive. The foundation and mainstay for ED management remains the oral agents.

the patient in order to achieve adequate treatment for their ED. They are selected for patients with a contraindication, lack of efficacy, or intolerable side effects with the oral agents. The third tier represents surgical implantation. This requires the greatest degree of motivation by patient as it is a formal surgical procedure. The patient must be a suitable surgical candidate in order for this to be a viable option.

Oral Agents

Currently, there are three FDA-approved oral agents for the management of ED: tadalafil (Cialis), vardenafil (Levitra), and sildenafil (Viagra). These agents all work via the same pharmacologic mechanism, which is inhibition of PDE5. Inhibition of this phosphodiesterase prolongs the effect of NO-mediated vasodilation in the corporal vascular smooth muscle. Fortunately, PDE5 is relatively specific to the corporal bodies resulting in a very tolerable side effect profile for this class of medications. All three drugs are very well tolerated and have an excellent safety profile. The side effects common to this class of drugs is listed in Table 44-2. Headache, flushing, and sinus congestion are the most common complaints. Discolored vision secondary to cross-reactivity with PDE6 is most typical for patients taking sildenafil, whereas myalgias are most common for patients taking tadalafil due in part to PDE11 cross-reactivity.[89] The main and absolute contraindication for this class of agents is nitrates. Any nitrate or nitroglycerin type agent is strictly contraindicated do to a profound hypotension that can ensue when taken simultaneously. α-Blockers can be taken concurrently but a precautionary warning should be given to the patient.

Quality comparative studies with these agents are lacking, but patient preference studies have been performed with varying results and significant design flaws.[90] However, patients appreciate the opportunity to try all three agents in order to establish a personal preference pattern. Factors affecting preference include, efficacy, side effects, duration of action, duration to onset, sexual frequency, and spontaneity. Moreover, nonresponders to one agent may be salvaged with another. A therapeutic trial with all three agents may be indicated before considering the patient a nonresponder. Neurologic conditions that have impacted cavernous nerve function have universally poor efficacy. Nonetheless, numerous studies have demonstrated efficacy with these agents in a broad range of patients and pathologies including cardiovascular disease.[91] Table 44-3 represents a pharmacologic comparison of these agents.

Urethral Suppository

The medicated urethral suppository (MUSE) is a product that was promoted as the first needle free medical treatment for ED. Its active compound is prostaglandin E_1 or alprostadil. This medication is placed into the urethra and causes direct cavernosal and vascular smooth muscle relaxation by penetrating the corporal bodies via communicating veins with the urethra. This product has limited use because of penile pain, urethral pain, and limited efficacy.[92]

Injection Therapy

Injection therapy is a very efficacious method for treating ED in patients who are refractory to oral agents. It allows for the right medications to be in the right place (corporal body) at the right time. This product comes in a number of forms. The agent or agents used is tailored by the prescribing physician. Two proprietary products are available on the market both of which are alprostadil (EDEX and Caverject).[93] Alprostadil acts as a direct smooth-muscle vasodilator when it is injected into the corporal body via a precontained syringe in dose ranges from 5 to 40 μg. This product can be compounded by specialized pharmacies for considerably less price. Additionally, other products such as Trimix have been compounded by hospital and compounding pharmacies as an alternative to pure alprostadil. In 30% of patients, alprostadil can cause intracavernosal discomfort following injection. By decreasing the quantities of alprostadil and adding other agents to the mixture, this side effect can be minimized. Trimix is a combination of papaverine, phentolamine, and alprostadil. The exact mixture of these agents can be varied to improve efficacy.[94] A major advantage of the compounded products is cost, whereas the advantage of the proprietary products is portability and availability.

A significant hurdle for the patient who is initiating injection therapy is the penile injection itself. Whereas it is virtually painless, patients need to overcome the psychologic hurdle of injecting a medication directly in their penis. Some elect not to try this therapy.

Vacuum Erection Device

Vacuum erection devices (VED) are very common and available devices. This option is attractive to patients who wish to avoid pharmacologic therapies. They can be purchased from a variety of different sources including men's health magazines, the internet, and medical grade devices

---

TABLE 44-3. Pharmacologic Comparison of PDE5 Inhibitors

	Sildenafil	Vardenafil	Tadalafil
Half-life (h)	3.7	4.6	17.5
Onset (h)	1 (0.5–2)	0.8 (0.3–2)	2 (0.2–12)
PDE cross-reactivity	PDE6	Minimal PDE6	PDE11

from ED clinics. A cylinder is placed over the penis which draws blood into the penis by suction. As the penis engorges with blood, an elastic band is placed at the base of the penis to maintain the erection. These devices give most men a functional erection. Some complain of penile petechiae, hinging of the penis proximal to the ring, coolness to the glans, and discomfort when applying the constrictor band. Long-term use with these devices is less than that of other treatment modalities. Approximately 65% of the patients with these devices are no longer using them long-term.[95]

Penile Implantation

Penile implants remain the main stay for patients who are refractory to all other treatments. It represents a third tier of ED management. This option requires patients to undergo a surgical procedure to reestablish sexual functioning.[96–98] Penile implants are available in two basic types, malleable and inflatable. The malleable prosthesis represents two bendable rods fixed in length and girth that are placed inside the corporal bodies. The penis is bent downward for concealment and is then straightened for sexual activity. They provide adequate axial rigidity for penetration. The disadvantage of this type is that there is no length or girth expansion. The advantages of this device are its simplicity, its ease of placement, and ease of functionality. Patients with limited manual dexterity can use this device.

The inflatable penile prosthesis is available in a variety of styles. The most widely used penile prosthesis is a three piece penile prosthesis. This device has a reservoir, a scrotal pump, and two cylinders placed in the corporal bodies. The reservoir is placed through the inguinal canal into the retropubic space that is just behind the pubic bone. A small piece of tubing exits from the reservoir into the scrotum and is attached to the pump. The pump is preconnected to two cylinders which sit within the corporal bodies. The device is filled with 0.9% saline for functionality. When an erection is desired, the scrotal pump is palpated and activated. This will transfer fluid from the reservoir to the cylinders and establish penile rigidity for intercourse. A deflation button on the pump is activated to return the penis to the flaccid state. The advantages of this device are in its concealment and expansion. In the flaccid state, the penis is normal in appearance, soft, and pliable. In the erect state, it allows for girth expansion and a minimal amount of length expansion. The device can be inflated and deflated as frequently as necessary and it will remain inflated until it is manually deflated. Thus this device allows for spontaneity, adequate rigidity for intercourse, and cosmetically a very satisfactory appearance. Patients are required to have manual dexterity in order to function the intrascrotal pump. The patient–partner satisfaction with these devices can be as high as 90%.

Thus, the available treatment options for ED allow most patients desirous of returning to sexual functioning that opportunity. The motivated patient who is willing to step through the appropriate tiers to return to intimacy is virtually always satisfied with the outcome.

REFERENCES

1. Larson WJ. Development of the urogenital system. In: Larsen WJ, ed. *Human Embryology*. New York, NY: Churchill Livingstone; 1997:261-309.

2. Park JM. Normal development of the urogenital system. In: Walsh PC, et al., eds. *Campbell-Walsh Urology*. Philadelphia, PA: Saunders; 2007:3121-3148.

3. Glenister TW. The origin and fate of the urethral plate in man. *J Anatomy*. 1954;88:413-424.

4. Lue TF. Physiology of penile erection and pathophysiology of erectile dysfunction. In: Walsh PC, et al., eds. *Campbell-Walsh Urology*. Philadelphia, PA: Saunders; 2007:718-749.

5. Sattar AA, Salpigidis G, Schulman CC, et al. Relationship between intrapenile O_2 lever and quantity of intracavernous smooth muscle fibers: current physiopathological concept. *Acta Urologica Belgica*. 1995;63:53-59.

6. Christ GJ, Maayani S, Valcic M, Melman A. Pharmacologic studies of heman erectile tissue: characteristics of spontaneous contractions and alterations in alpha-adrenoceptor responsiveness with age and disease in isolated tissues. *Br J Pharmacol*. 1990;101:375-381.

7. Traish AM, Netsuwan N, Daley J, et al. A heterogenous population of alpha 1 adrenergic receptors mediates contraction of human corpus cavernosum smooth muscle to norepinephrine. *J Urol*. 1995;153:222-227.

8. Andersson KE, Wagner G. Physiology of penile erection. *Physiol Rev*. 1995;75:191-236.

9. Diederichs W, Stief CG, Lue TF, Tanagho EA. Norepinephrine involvement in penile detumescence. *J Urol*. 1990;43(6):1264-1266.

10. Kim N, Azadzoi KM, Goldstein I, et al. A nitric oxide–like factor mediates nonadrenergic noncholinergic neurogenic relaxation of penile corpus cavernosum smooth muscle. *J Clin Invest*. 1991;88:112-118.

11. Trigo-Rocha F, Aronson WJ, Hohenfellner M, et al. Nitric oxide and cGMP: mediators of pelvic nerve-stimulated erection in dogs. *Am J Physiol*. 1993;264:H419-H422.

12. Burnett AL, Lowenstein CJ, Bredt DS, et al. Nitric oxide: a physiologic mediator of penile erection. *Science*. 1992;257:401-403.

13. Trigo-Rocha F, Hsu GL, Donatucci CF, et al. The role of cyclic adenosine monophosphate, cyclic guanosine monophosphate, endothelium and nonadrenergic, noncholinergic neurotransmission in canine penile erection. *J Urol*. 1993;149:872-877.

14. Rajfer J, Aronson WJ, Bush PA, et al. Nitric oxide as a mediator of relaxation of the corpus cavernosum in response to nonadrenergic, noncholinergic neurotransmission. *N Engl J Med*. 1992;326:90-94.

15. Lue TF, Takamura T, Schmidt RA, et al. Hemodynamics of erection in the monkey. *J Urol.* 1983;130:1237-1241.

16. Saenz de Tejada I, Goldstein I, Azadzoi K, et al. Impaired neurogenic and endothelium mediated relaxation of penile smooth muscle from diabetic men with impotence. *N Engl J Med.* 1989;320:1025-1030.

17. Bosch RJ, Benard F, Aboseif SR, Stief CG, Lue TF, Tanagho EA. Penile detumescence: characterization of three phases. *J Urol.* 1991;146(3):867-871.

18. Johannes CB, Araujo AB, Feldman HA, et al. Incidence of erectile dysfunction in men 40 to 69 years old: longitudinal results from the Massachusetts Male Aging Study. *J Urol.* 2000;163:460-463.

19. Laumann EO, Paik A, Rosen RC. Sexual dysfunction in the United States: prevalence and predictors. *J Am Med Assoc.* 1999;281:537-544.

20. Lewis RW, Hatzichristou D, Laumann E, McKinlay J. Epidemiology and natural history of erectile dysfunction; risk factors including iatrogenic and aging. In: Jardin A, Wagner G, Khoury S, Giuliano F, eds. *Proceedings of First International Consultation on Erectile Dysfunction.* Plymbridge, UK: Health Publication; 2000:21-51.

21. Moreira ED Jr, Lbo CF, Diament A, et al. Incidence of erectile dysfunction in men 40 to 69 years old: results from a population-based cohort study in Brazil. *Urology.* 2003; 61:431-436.

22. Schouten BW, Bosch JL, Bernsen RM, et al. Incidence rates of erectile dysfunction in the Dutch general population. Effects of definition, clinical relevance and duration of followup in the Krimpen Study. *Int J Impot Res.* 2005;17:58-62.

23. Lizza EF, Rosen RC. Definition and classification of erectile dysfunction: report of the Nomenclature Committee of the International Society of Impotence Research. *Int J Impot Res.* 1999;11:141-143.

24. Masters WH, Johnson VE. *Human Sexual Response.* Boston, MA: Little, Brown; 1970.

25. Steers WD. Neural control of penile erection. *Semin Urol.* 1990;8:66-79.

26. Diederichs W, Stief CG, Benard F, et al. The sympathetic role as an antagonist of erection. *Urol Res.* 1991;19:123-126.

27. Diederichs W, Stief CG, Lue TF, et al. Sympathetic inhibition of papaverine induced erection. *J Urol.* 1991;146:195-198.

28. Kim SC, Oh MM. Norepinephrine involvement in response to intracorporeal injection of papaverine in psychogenic impotence. *J Urol.* 1992;147:1530-1532.

29. Sachs BD, Meisel RL. The physiology of male sexual behavior. In: Knobil E, Neill JD, Ewing LL, et al., eds. *The Physiology of Reproduction.* New York, NY; Raven Press; 1988:1393-1423.

30. Wermuth L, Stenager E. Sexual aspects of Parkinson's disease. *Semin Neurol.* 1992;12:125-127.

31. de Groat WC, Booth A. Neural control of penile erection. In: Maggi CA, ed. *The Autonomic Nervous System.* London, UK: Harwood; 1993:465-513.

32. Eardley I, Kirby R. Neurogenic impotence. In: Kirby RS, Carson CC, Webster GD, eds. *Impotence: Diagnosis and Management of Male Erectile Dysfunction.* Oxford, UK: Butterworth-Heinemann; 1991:227-231.

33. Courtois FJ, Macdougall JC, Sachs BD. Erectile mechanism in paraplegia. *Physiol Behav.* 1993;53:721-726.

34. Walsh PC, Donker PJ. Impotence following radical prostatectomy: insight into etiology and prevention. *J Urol.* 1982;128:492-497.

35. Walsh PC, Brendler CB, Chang T, et al. Preservation of sexual function in men during radical pelvic surgery. *Md Med J.* 1990;39(4):389-393.

36. Michal V, Ruzbarsky V. Histological changes in the penile arterial bed with aging and diabetes. In: Zorgniotti AW, Rossi G, eds. *Vasculogenic Impotence: Proceedings of the First International Conference on Corpus Cavernosum Revascularization.* Springfield, Ill: Charles C Thomas; 1980:113-119.

37. Feldman HA, Goldstein I, Hatzichristou DG, et al. Impotence and its medical and psychosocial correlates: results of the Massachusetts Male Aging Study. *J Urol.* 1994;151:54-61.

38. Kaufman JM, Hatzichristou DG, Mulhall JP, et al. Impotence and chronic renal failure: a study of the hemodynamic pathophysiology. *J Urol.* 1994;151:612-618.

39. Tarhan F, Kuyumcuoglu U, Kolsuz A, et al. Cavernous oxygen tension in the patients with erectile dysfunction. *Int J Impot Res.* 1997;9:149-153.

40. Nehra A, Azadzoi KM, Moreland RB, et al. Cavernosal expandability is an erectile tissue mechanical property which predicts trabecular histology in an animal model of vasculogenic erectile dysfunction. *J Urol.* 1998;159:2229-2236.

41. Nehra A, Gettman MT, Nugent M, et al. Transforming growth factor-beta1 (TGF-beta1) issufficient to induce fibrosis of rabbit corpus cavernosum in vivo. *J Urol.* 1999;162:910-915.

42. Moreland RB, Albadawi H, Bratton C, et al. O_2-dependent prostanoid synthesis activates functional PGE receptors on corpus cavernosum smooth muscle. *Am J Physiol.* 2001;281:H552-H558.

43. Sáenz de Tejada IJ, Angulo JS, Cellek S, et al. Physiology of erectile function and pathophysiology of erectile dysfunction. In: Lue TF, Basson R, Rosen R, et al., eds. *Sexual medicine: Sexual Dysfunctions in Men and Women.* Paris, France: Health Publications; 2004.

44. Panza JA, Quyyumi AA, Brush JE Jr, et al. Abnormal endothelium-dependent vascular relaxation in patients with essential hypertension. *N Engl J Med.* 1990;323:22-27.

45. Levine FJ, Greenfield AJ, Goldstein I. Arteriographically determined occlusive disease within the hypogastric-cavernous bed in impotent patients following blunt perineal and pelvic trauma. *J Urol.* 1990;144:1147-1153.

46. Andersen KV, Bovim G. Impotence and nerve entrapment in long distance amateur cyclists. *Acta Neurol Scand.* 1997;95:233-240.

47. Kugiyama K, Kerns SA, Morrisett JD, et al. Impairment of endothelium-dependent arterial relaxation by lysolecithin in modified low-density lipoproteins. *Nature.* 1990;344:160-162.

48. Metz P, Ebbehoj J, Uhrenholdt A, et al. Peyronie's disease and erectile failure. *J Urol.* 1983;130:1103-1104.

49. Iacono F, Barra S, de Rosa G, et al. Microstructural disorders of tunica albuginea in patients affected by impotence. *Eur Urol.* 1994;26:233-239.

50. Iacono F, Barra S, de Rosa G, et al. Microstructural disorders of tunica albuginea in patients affected by Peyronie's disease with or without erection dysfunction. *J Urol.* 1993;150:1806-1809.

51. Graversen PH, Palle R, Colstrup H. Erectile dysfunction following direct vision internal urethrotomy. *Scand J Urol Nephrol.* 1991;25:175-178.

52. Chen SC, Hsieh CH, Hsu GL, et al. The progression of the penile vein: could it be recurrent? *J Androl.* 2005;26:53-60.

53. Mulligan T, Schmitt B. Testosterone for erectile failure. *J Gen Int Med.* 1993;8:517-521.

54. Chang SW, Fine R, Siegel D, et al. The impact of diuretic therapy on reported sexualfunction. *Arch Intern Med.* 1991;151:2402-2408.

55. Medical Research Council Working Party on Mild to Moderate Hypertension. Adverse reactions to bendrofluazide and propranolol for the treatment of mild hypertension. *Lancet.* 1981;2:539-543.

56. Grimm RH Jr, Grandits GA, Prineas RJ, et al. Long-term effects on sexual function of five antihypertensive drugs and nutritional hygienic treatment in hypertensive men and women. Treatment of Mild Hypertension Study (TOMHS). *Hypertension.* 1997;29:8-14.

57. Keltner NL, McAfee KM, Taylor CL. Mechanisms and treatments of SSRI-induced sexual dysfunction. *Perspect Psychiatr Care.* 2002;38:111-116.

58. Rosen RC, Lane RM, Menza M. Effects of SSRIs on sexual function: a critical review. *J Clin Psychopharmacol.* 1999;19:67-85.

59. Michelson D, Schmidt M, Lee J, et al. Changes in sexual function during acute and six month fluoxetine therapy: a prospective assessment. *J Sex Marital Ther.* 2001;27:289-302.

60. Lugg JA, Rajfer J, Gonzalez-Cadavid NF. Dihydrotestosterone is the active androgen in the maintenance of nitric oxide–mediated penile erection in the rat. *Endocrinology.* 1995;136:1495-1501.

61. Gormley GJ, Stoner E, Bruskewitz RC, et al. The effect of finasteride in men with benign prostatic hyperplasia. The Finasteride Study Group. *N Engl J Med.* 1992;327:1185-1191.

62. Iversen P, Melezinek I, Schmidt A. Nonsteroidal antiandrogens. A therapeutic option forpatients with advanced prostate cancer who wish to retain sexual interest and function. *BJU Int.* 2001;87:47-56.

63. Basaria S, Lieb J II, Tang AM, et al. Long-term effects of androgen deprivation therapy in prostate cancer patients. *Clin Endocrinol.* 2002;56:779-786.

64. Masters WH, Johnson VE. Sex after sixty-five. *Reflections.* 1977;12:31-43.

65. Stief CG, Bähren W, Scherb W, Gall H. Primary erectile dysfunction. *J Urol.* 1989;141(2):315-319.

66. Lue TF, Broderick GA. Evaluation and nonsurgical management of erectile dysfunction and premature ejaculation. In: Walsh PC, et al., eds. *Campbell-Walsh Urology.* Philadelphia, PA: Saunders; 2007:750-787.

67. Rosen RC, Hatzichristou D, Broderick G, et al. Clinical evaluation and symptom scales: sexual dysfunction assessment in men. In: Lue TF, Basson R, Rosen R, et al., eds. *Sexual Medicine: Sexual Dysfunctions in Men and Women.* Paris, France: Health Publications; 2004:173-220.

68. Rosen RC, Riley A, Wagner G, et al. The international index of erectile function (IIEF): a multidimensional scale for assessment of erectile dysfunction. *Urology.* 1997;49:822-830.

69. O'Leary MP, Fowler FJ, Lenderking WR, et al. A brief male sexual function inventory for urology. *Urology.* 1995;46:697-706.

70. Althof SE, Corty EW, Levine SB, et al. EDITS. Development of questionnaires for evaluating satisfaction with treatments for erectile dysfunction. *Urology.* 1999;53:793-799.

71. Rosen RC, Capelleri JC, Smith MD, et al. Development and evaluation of an abridged, 5-item version of the International Index of Erectile Function (IIEF-5) as a diagnostic tool for erectile function. *Int J Impot Res.* 1999;11:319.

72. Karacan I, Goodenough DR, Shapiro A. Erection cycle during sleep in relation to dream anxiety. *Arch Gen Psychiatry.* 1966;15:183-189.

73. Bradley WE, Timm GW, Gallagher JM, et al. New method for continuous measurement of nocturnal penile tumescence and rigidity. *Urology.* 1985;26:4-9.

74. Heaton JP, Morales A. Facts and controversies of the application of penile tumescence and rigidity: recording for erectile dysfunction. In: Hellstrom WJG, ed. *Male Infertility and Sexual Dysfunction.* New York, NY: Springer-Verlag; 1997:579.

75. Donatucci CF, Lue TF. The combined intracavernous injection and stimulation test: diagnostic accuracy. *J Urol.* 1992;148:61-62.

76. Katlowitz NM, Albano GJ, Morales P, et al. Potentiation of drug-induced erection with audiovisual sexual stimulation. *Urology.* 1993;41:431-434.

77. Pescatori ES, Hatzichristou DG, Namburi S, et al. A positive intracavernous injection test implies normal veno-occlusive but not necessarily normal arterial function: a hemodynamic study. *J Urol.* 1994;151:1209-1216.

78. Linet OI, Neff LL. Intracavernous prostaglandin E1 in erectile dysfunction. *J Clin Invest.* 1994;72:139-149.

79. Linet OI, Ogrinc FG. Efficacy and safety of intracavernosal alprostadil in men with erectile dysfunction. The Alprostadil Study Group. *N Engl J Med.* 1996;334:873-877.

80. Abdallah HM. Comparison of Alprostadil (Caverject) and a combination of vasoactive drugs as local injections for the treatment of erectile dysfunction. *Int Urol Nephrol.* 1998;30(5):617-620.

81. Barada JH, McKimmy RM. Vasoactive pharmacotherapy. In: Bennett AH, ed. *Impotence: Diagnosis and Management of Erectile Dysfunction.* Philadelphia, PA: WB Saunders; 1994.

82. Lewis RW, King BF. Dynamic color Doppler sonography in the evaluation of penile erectile disorders. *Int J Impot Res.* 1994;6:30.

83. Benson CB, Vickers MA. Sexual impotence caused by vascular disease: diagnosis with duplex sonography. *Am J Roentgenol.* 1989;153:1149-1153.

84. Lue TF, Hricak H, Marich KW, et al. Vasculogenic impotence evaluated by high-resolution ultrasonography and pulsed Doppler spectrum analysis. *Radiology.* 1985;155:777-781.

85. Mueller SC, Lue TF. Evaluation of vasculogenic impotence. *Urol Clin North Am.* 1988;15:65-76.

86. Shabsigh R, Fishman IJ, Shotland Y, et al. Comparison of penile duplex ultrasonography with nocturnal penile tumescence monitoring for the evaluation of erectile impotence. *J Urol.* 1990;143:924-927.

87. Planiol T, Pourcelot L. Doppler effect study on the carotid circulation. In: de Vlieger M, White DN, McCready VR, eds. *Ultrasonics in Medicine.* Amsterdam, the Netherlands: Excerpta Medica; 1974:104-111.

88. Naroda T, Yamanaka M, Matsushita K, et al. Evaluation of resistance index of the cavernous artery with color Doppler ultrasonography for venogenic impotence. *Int J Impot Res.* 1994;6:D62.

89. Shabsigh R, Seftel AD, Rosen R, et al. Review of time of onset and duration of clinical efficacy of phosphodiesterase type 5 inhibitors in treatment of erectile dysfunction. *Urology.* 2006;68(4):689-696.

90. Moore RA, Derry S, McQuay HJ. Indirect comparison of interventions using published randomized trials: systematic review of PDE-5 inhibitors for erectile dysfunction. *BMC Urol.* 2005;5:18.

91. Kloner RA, Mullin SH, Shook T, et al. Erectile dysfunction in the cardiac patient: how common and should we treat. *J Urol.* 2003;170(2, pt 2):S46-S50.

92. Mulhall JP, Jahoda AE, Ahmed A, Parker M. Analysis of the consistency of intraurethral prostaglandin E(1) (MUSE) during at-home use. *Urology.* 2001;58(2):262-266.

93. Colli E, Calabro A, Gentile V, Mirone V, Soli M. Alprostadil sterile powder formulation for intercavernous treatment of erectile dysfunction. *Eur Urol.* 1996;29(1):59-62.

94. Seyam R, Mohamed K, Akhras AA, Rashwan H. A prospective randomized study to optimize the dosage of trimix ingredients and compare its efficacy and safety with prostaglandin E1. *Int J Impot Res.* 2005;17(4)346-353.

95. Dutta TC, Eid JF. Vacuum constriction devices for erectile dysfunction: a long-term prospective study of patients with mild, moderate and severe dysfunction. *Urology.* 1999;54(5):891-893.

96. Jain S, Terry TR. Penile prosthetic surgery and its role in the treatment of end-stage erectile dysfunction—an update. *Ann R Coll Surg Engl.* 2006;88(4):343-348.

97. Montague DK, Angermeier KW. Current status of penile prosthesis implantation. *Curr Urol Rep.* 2000;1(4):291-296.

98. Moncada I, Martinez-Salamanca JI, Allona A, Hernadez C. Current role of penile implants for erectile dysfunction. *Curr Opin Urol.* 2004;14(6):375-380.

chapter 45

Embolic Disorders of the Pulmonary Artery

Tina M. Dudney, MD / *Michael T. McCormack, MD* / *Jeffrey H. Freihage, MD*

● INTRODUCTION

As the initial recipient of the venous circulation, the pulmonary vascular bed is uniquely positioned to filter diverse particulates within the venous circulatory system. The etiology of these circulating particles may be thrombotic, as seen in pulmonary thromboembolism, or nonthrombotic, as encountered in a number of uncommon syndromes including embolism from air, amniotic fluid, fat, tumors, septic foci, and other miscellaneous sources. The pathophysiologic sequelae of these emboli are related to both mechanical occlusion of the pulmonary vasculature and inflammatory mediated damage to the pulmonary microvasculature resulting in capillary leak and pulmonary edema. The intent of this chapter is to describe the incidence, pathophysiology, and clinical features of these varied embolic phenomena and to provide a rational approach to the diagnosis and treatment of these disorders.

● PULMONARY EMBOLISM

Introduction

Pulmonary embolism (PE) is a commonly occurring condition associated with significant morbidity and mortality. Although there is a well-established and decreased incidence of PE with appropriate prophylaxis and a significant improvement in patient outcome associated with the prompt institution of appropriate therapy, prophylaxis and therapy for venous thromboembolic disease continue to be underused, thereby contributing to the morbidity, mortality, and high costs associated with the condition. In the United States, it is estimated that more than 500 000 cases of PE occur each year[1] with a mortality rate of greater than 15% in the first 3 months after diagnosis.[2] Despite our increased knowledge about the condition and ever-increasing technological sophistication, mortality rates associated with PE remain high and relatively unchanged over the past half century.[3] Additionally, autopsy studies continue to demonstrate that the diagnosis of PE is made less than 50% of the time prior to death.[4] While specific risk factors have been identified for the occurrence of PE and numerous effective prophylactic regimens have been demonstrated, recent studies show that appropriate prophylactic regimens continue to be significantly underused.[5]

Pathophysiology

PE results from the detachment and migration of thrombi fragments, which lodge within and obstruct blood flow to a single or multiple areas of the pulmonary vascular bed (Figure 45-1). Pulmonary emboli generally detach from deep venous thromboses (DVTs) of the proximal lower extremities.[6] Less commonly, deep pelvic veins or proximal upper extremity DVTs associated with central venous catheters can be the source of pulmonary emboli.[7] PE is, therefore, a part of the continuum of venothromboembolism (VTE). Thrombi, from which pulmonary emboli may arise, occur, in the majority of cases, when one or more components of Virchow's classic triad is/are present: Venous stasis, hypercoagulability, and/or intimal injury.

A cascade of pathophysiologic mechanisms ensues with the pulmonary embolic event, which can lead to hypoxemia and cardiovascular compromise. The reduction of the cross-sectional area of the pulmonary arterial bed caused by the embolism has been shown to correlate with the degree of physiologic impairment. Pulmonary arterial pressure generally begins to rise with a 25% to 30% occlusion of the pulmonary vascular bed in otherwise normal heart

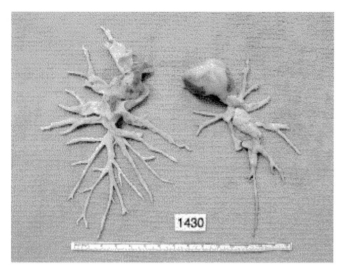

● **FIGURE 45-1.** Endarterectomy specimen demonstrating obstruction of pulmonary vascular bed.

Reproduced, with permission, from Jamieson SW, Kapelanski DP, Sakakibara N, et al. Pulmonary endarterectomy: experience and lessons learned in 1500 cases. Ann Thorac Surg. 2003;76: 1457-1464.

and lungs,[8] while greater than 50% obstruction is generally present before a clinically significant elevation occurs. Increased right ventricular afterload can cause right ventricular dilatation, hypokinesis, tricuspid regurgitation, and eventual right heart failure.[9] A normal right ventricle can fail with acute increases of the pulmonary arterial pressure to 40 to 50 mm Hg when obstruction of the pulmonary vascular bed approaches 75%. Patients with PE and preexisting cardiopulmonary disease may experience more severe physiologic impairment with lesser degrees of pulmonary vascular obstruction.[10] The increase in pulmonary vascular resistance, which occurs with PE, can impede cardiac right ventricular outflow and diminish left ventricular preload to cause an acute decrease in forward cardiac output and, ultimately, hemodynamic collapse. Hypoxic pulmonary vascular vasoconstriction and the release of neurohumeral factors incited by the embolic event are additional factors, contributing to increases in pulmonary vascular resistance and the resultant adverse hemodynamic consequences.[11]

Hypoxemia results from pulmonary emboli by a number of mechanisms. PE creates a redistribution of pulmonary blood flow to alter ventilation–perfusion characteristics in the lung, thereby decreasing the efficiency of alveolar gas exchange.[12] Atelectasis may also occur and contribute to altered ventilation–perfusion relationships and gas exchange impairment.[9] A right-to-left shunt may develop with PE by the intrapulmonary passage of blood through unventilated gas exchange units and/or intracardiac shunting of blood through a patent foramen ovale associated with increases in right atrial pressure occurring with PE.[11] The inability to correct arterial hypoxemia with supplemental oxygen suggests the existence of intrapulmonary and/or intracardiac right-to-left shunting of blood. Additionally, decreased cardiac output and hypoxemia can lead to a low

venous blood oxygen tension, which may amplify gas exchange impairment through lung gas exchange units with poor ventilation–perfusion characteristics.

While arterial hypoxemia and an increased alveolar–arterial oxygen gradient are the most common abnormalities of gas exchange, hyperventilation is common with PE and can cause hypocapnia and respiratory alkalosis. However, PE can increase both anatomic and physiologic dead space, thus impairing carbon dioxide removal. Hypercapnia associated with PE suggests underlying obstructive airway disease or a massive clot burden.[13]

Risk Factors

One or more elements of Virchow's triad (stasis, hypercoagulability, and intimal injury) are present in the vast majority of patients with VTE.[14] General risk factors for VTE include age, immobility, surgical procedures, congestive heart failure, stroke and paralysis, trauma, malignancy, and hypercoagulable states. However, numerous clinical circumstances associated with an increased risk for the development of VTE have been identified (Table 45-1). Most patients with PE have more than one risk factor.[14] Various degrees of risk have been defined for individual risk factors, with some patient populations having a greater than 50% incidence of VTE.[15] Knowledge of these risk factors and a thorough patient history investigation for these factors are needed in order to develop an efficient and rational approach to the evaluation, diagnosis, and treatment of PE for the individual patient, particularly since presenting clinical signs and symptoms are insensitive and nonspecific for the diagnosis of PE.

Clinical Presentation

Symptoms and physical examination findings have been consistently shown to be insensitive and nonspecific for the diagnosis of VTE.[16–19] Classic clinical findings of DVT include pain and swelling of the affected extremity, warmth and superficial venous dilatation, a thrombosed venous cord, and pain upon passive dorsiflexion of the foot (Homan's sign). Patients with PE frequently present with dyspnea, tachypnea, tachycardia, and/or chest pain.[20] Cough and hemoptysis may also be present. Lightheadedness, syncope, and hypotension can occur and may indicate a greater clot burden. Patients with massive PE may present with shock, refractory hypoxemia, or cardiopulmonary arrest.[21] Patients with underlying cardiopulmonary disease can develop more severe pathophysiologic consequences of PE with less clot burden.[22]

The initial laboratory evaluation has also been shown to be insensitive and nonspecific for the diagnosis of PE.[23] Most patients with PE have abnormal, but nonspecific, chest radiograph findings.[24] Atelectasis, pleural effusions, pulmonary infiltrates, and/or hemidiaphragm elevation have been commonly found on chest radiographs in patients presenting with PE, but these findings are also observed with numerous other conditions. Hampton's hump and Westermark's sign are considered to be suggestive of

Environmental
Long-haul air travel
Obesity
Cigarette smoking
Hypertension
Immobility
Natural
Increasing age
Women's health
Oral contraceptives, including progesterone-only and
    especially third-generation pills
Pregnancy
Hormone replacement therapy
Medical illness
Previous PE or DVT
Cancer
Congestive heart failure
Chronic obstructive pulmonary disease
Diabetes mellitus
Inflammatory bowel disease
Antipsychotic drug use
Chronic indwelling central venous catheter
Permanent pacemaker
Internal cardiac defibrillator
Stroke with limb paresis
Nursing-home confinement or current or repeated
    hospital admission
Varicose veins
Surgical
Trauma
Orthopaedic surgery, especially total hip replacement,
    total knee replacement, hip fracture surgery, knee
    arthroscopy
General surgery, especially for cancer
Gynaecological and urological surgery, especially for
    cancer
Neurosurgery, especially craniotomy for brain tumour
Thrombophilia
Factor V Leiden mutation
Prothrombin gene mutation
Hyperhomocysteinaemia (including mutation in
    methylenetetrahydrofolate reductase)
Antiphospholipid antibody syndrome
Deficiency of antithrombin III, protein C, or protein S
High concentrations of factor VIII or XI
Increased lipoprotein (a)
Nonthrombotic
Air
Foreign particles (e.g., hair, talc, as a consequence of
    intravenous drug misuse)
Amniotic fluid
Bone fragments, bone marrow
Fat
Cement

PE, pulmonary embolism; DVT, deep venous thromboses.
Reprinted, with permission, from Goldhaber SZ. Pulmonary embolism
Lancet. 2004;363:1295-1305.

PE, though they are present infrequently. A normal chest radiograph in a patient with dyspnea and hypoxemia without bronchospasm or evidence of anatomic cardiac shunt suggests a high likelihood of PE.[25]

Arterial blood gas analysis, as well, cannot confirm or exclude the diagnosis of PE. As discussed, arterial blood gas abnormalities commonly found in the setting of PE include arterial hypoxemia, increased alveolar–arterial oxygen gradient, hypocapnea, and respiratory alkalosis. Hypercapnia and respiratory acidosis are signs of underlying cardiopulmonary disease or a massive PE. A normal arterial oxygen pressure and, less commonly, a normal alveolar–arterial oxygen gradient may be present, particularly in patients who are young with otherwise normal lungs.[26] While arterial blood gas analysis has been shown to be neither sensitive nor specific for the diagnosis of PE, correlation has been demonstrated between the extent of the clot burden and the degree of the alveolar–arterial oxygen gradient.[23]

Electrocardiogram (ECG) abnormalities are seen in up to 80% to 90% of cases of PE; however, a wide variety of abnormalities can be observed, and these findings are not sensitive or specific for the diagnosis of PE.[27] A major limitation of studies on ECG abnormalities and PE is that most studies have been done on patients after the diagnosis of PE has been confirmed. Tachycardia and incomplete right bundle branch block have been found more often in confirmed than suspected cases.[28] S1Q3T3 is a nonspecific and infrequent finding that may suggest right heart strain from a massive or submassive PE. ECG analysis may be most useful to identify or exclude diagnoses other than PE.

D-dimer is a degradation product present in the circulation, which is produced by endogenous fibrinolysis of cross-linked fibrin. A number of different methods have been developed as assays for D-dimer. Enzyme-linked immunosorbent assay (ELISA), enzyme-linked fluorescent assay (ELFA), and newer generation latex agglutination assays have been shown to have a high sensitivity for PE, and when used in conjunction with a clinical scoring system, these have been demonstrated in some studies to have sufficient negative predicative value to rule out the diagnosis of PE in the emergency department setting.[29] The specificity of these assays, however, is poor, as D-dimer levels have been found to be elevated with many conditions.[30] Additionally, D-dimer assays have been found to be less accurate in hospitalized patients.[31] Therefore, D-dimer assays are not useful in confirming the diagnosis of PE or in ruling out the diagnosis of PE for hospitalized patients.

Confirmatory Tests

As reviewed above, PE can present with a variety of symptoms, signs, and initial diagnostic studies, though it is unusual to be able to confirm or exclude the diagnosis of PE based on these findings. Initial evaluation based on these data, therefore, is generally most useful in assigning a probability of PE in a particular patient. Additionally, specific quantitation of this probability cannot be determined because of differences in patient populations and discrepancies in study results. However, a qualitative assessment of the probability of PE can usually be determined on the basis of the initial presentation data, which can then be used to guide the subsequent approach to further diagnostic evaluation and therapy. The initial presenting data should be used to determine a qualitative pretest probability for further diagnostic testing as well as to consider when evaluating the potential risks and benefits of therapeutic options.

Ventilation–perfusion (V/Q) scanning has been used frequently as a diagnostic study for the evaluation of acute PE and, under the appropriate clinical circumstances, may yield results that the clinician can use to confirm or exclude the diagnosis of PE. However, V/Q scanning is nondiagnostic for PE in the majority of cases.[32,33] The collaborative Prospective Investigation of Pulmonary Embolism Diagnosis (PIOPED) helped shape consensus on the interpretation of V/Q scans. Important information determined from this investigation included the finding that the degree of pretest clinical suspicion is crucial in determining the probability of PE when V/Q scanning is used. It was found that a low probability V/Q scan was associated with PE in 40% of patients with a high clinical suspicion of PE, and that a high probability scan was associated with only a 56% incidence of PE in patients with a low clinical suspicion of PE.[34] However, a normal or near normal perfusion scan was found to be associated with a low incidence of PE in all clinical risk groups studied, and a low probability V/Q scan for patients with a low clinical probability was associated with a very low incidence of PE (4%).[34] Additionally, a high probability scan in patients with a high clinical suspicion was associated with a 96% incidence of PE.[34]

Helical or spiral computed axial tomography (helical or spiral CT) requiring the administration of a contrast agent has been developed to evaluate for the presence of PE. Some studies have reported high sensitivity (>95%) and specificity (>95%) for acute PE,[35] though more recent and larger studies have reported less sensitivity for this study, suggesting that a negative CT may not be useful to rule out PE.[36–39] Subsegmental pulmonary artery emboli are less readily appreciated by spiral CT, though subsegmental pulmonary emboli are found in a minority of patients presenting with acute PE and their clinical significance is uncertain. Improvements in spiral CT technique for the evaluation of PE are ongoing and include thinner sectioning and three-dimensional reformation, which may improve the sensitivity and specificity of this diagnostic study. Spiral CT has the additional advantage of being able to evaluate for the presence of other potential cardiopulmonary conditions including tumors, lymphadenopathy, emphysema, pleural, and/or pericardial disease. Spiral CT is an increasingly used study to evaluate for the diagnosis of acute PE. While a high specificity has been demonstrated with spiral CT, sufficient sensitivity has not yet been well enough established to exclude the diagnosis of acute PE independent of a low pretest probability. Spiral CT of the thorax with intravenous contrast should, therefore, be considered a confirmatory, rather than screening, test for acute PE.

Magnetic resonance imaging (MRI) and magnetic resonance angiography (MRA) are newer methods of evaluating for acute PE. MRI and MRA have not been studied as extensively as other methods to diagnose PE, though some studies have reported a high sensitivity and specificity for the diagnosis of PE.[40] MRI and MRA techniques continue to evolve, and these diagnostic methods show a number of potential advantages over more traditionally employed methods of testing for PE. MRI/MRA is noninvasive, uses a noniodinated intravenous contrast agent, and can demonstrate both perfusion and ventilation characteristics of the lungs. Also, MRI venography has been found to be highly sensitive (97%) and specific (98%) for the detection of DVT, and it can be used to demonstrate pelvic deep vein thrombosis, which cannot be detected by ultrasound.[41,42]

Echocardiography is a potentially rapidly available method that is insensitive for the diagnosis of acute PE, though it may add information useful in the setting where the diagnosis is suspected. Transthoracic echocardiography (TTE) may rarely allow for direct visualization of emboli in transit to the pulmonary vascular bed or large emboli located in the main, right, or proximal left pulmonary arteries.[11] Additionally, TTE may show indirect evidence of acute PE through the demonstration of right ventricular dysfunction in association with right ventricular pressure overload.[11] TTE in the setting of acute PE may demonstrate right ventricular dilatation and/or hypokinesis, paradoxical interventricular motion, tricuspid regurgitation, and pulmonary hypertension. Regional right ventricular dysfunction with apex sparing, severe free wall hypokinesis is an echocardiographic finding considered specific for PE.[43] In a normotensive patient with PE, TTE may reveal right ventricular hypokinesis, which may be an independent risk factor for early death. Some studies have suggested that normotensive patients who have acute PE and demonstrate evidence of right ventricular strain and dysfunction by echocardiography might benefit from the administration of thrombolytic therapy.[11]

Transesophageal echocardiography (TEE) expands the limited acoustic window, which limits TTE. Studies have reported a 60% to 80% sensitivity and 95% to 100% specificity for acute PE, and a 90% to 95% sensitivity and 100% specificity for central PE using TEE.[11,44] TEE, similar to TTE, can also demonstrate indirect evidence of acute PE suggested by right ventricular abnormalities, though these echocardiographic findings must be interpreted cautiously, as numerous cardiopulmonary conditions may be associated with abnormalities of right ventricular anatomy and function. While TEE has been shown to offer advantages over TTE in the diagnosis of acute PE, the use of TEE is more limited because it requires a higher level of training to perform and interpret the study and also requires conscious sedation of a patient who may have hemodynamic or respiratory compromise.

Pulmonary angiography continues to be considered the gold standard for the diagnosis of PE; however, it is being used less frequently because the diagnosis of PE is being confirmed or excluded to the satisfaction of treating

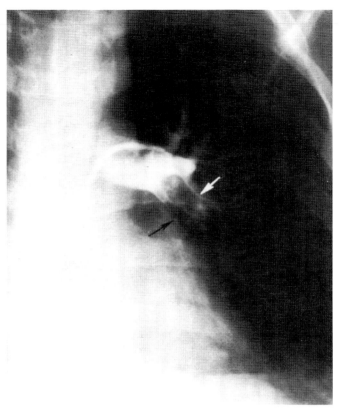

● **FIGURE 45-2.** Pulmonary angiogram demonstrating large left pulmonary artery filling defect.

Reproduced, with permission, from Moser KM. Pulmonary embolism. In: Baum GL, Wolinsky E, eds. Textbook of Pulmonary Diseases. Vol 2. 4th ed. Philadelphia: Lippincott Williams & Wilkins; 1989:1163-1180.

clinicians by less invasive and resource intensive studies (Figure 45-2). An alternative perspective is that pulmonary angiography has historically been underused in the diagnosis of PE and that it continues to be a useful method in the evaluation of acute PE, particularly for those patients who have a high clinical probability of PE and for whom other methods of evaluation have not sufficiently confirmed the diagnosis. Pulmonary angiography has a significant complication rate, which should be considered when deciding about the use of the study. It requires the administration of an iodinated intravenous contrast agent and, therefore, can induce renal failure. PIOPED reported a 0.3% rate of renal failure requiring dialysis associated with pulmonary angiography. It also reported cardiopulmonary compromise requiring intubation or cardiopulmonary resuscitation in 0.4% of the patients undergoing the procedure and an incidence of 0.2% of groin hematoma requiring blood transfusion.[45] The death rate associated with the procedure reported by PIOPED was 0.5%. Severely ill patients, such as those in intensive care units, have been shown to have a higher incidence of complications associated with the procedure. Additionally, while pulmonary angiography has been considered the gold standard for the diagnosis of PE, significant interobserver disagreement may occur with the interpretation of the study. Pulmonary angiography remains a potentially useful study for the evaluation of PE

despite these issues because of the high diagnostic accuracy of the procedure for PE as well as the ability of the procedure to facilitate the inclusion of hemodynamic data and/or catheter-directed therapy. Once again, however, pulmonary angiography should be considered a confirmatory study, the use of which is based on the pretest probability of the condition as well as the inherent risks and potential benefits of the procedure.

PE may be insufficiently confirmed or excluded on the basis of the available studies previously reviewed. In these instances, it may be useful to proceed with studies to evaluate for the presence of proximal DVT. Proximal DVT is the source for PE and, if DVT is found, can serve as a basis for the institution of therapy with anticoagulation, which is also therapeutic for acute PE. A number of methods with a high sensitivity and/or specificity are available for the diagnosis of proximal DVT including: Doppler ultrasound, impedance plethysmography, contrast venography, MRI, and CT. In cases where proximal DVT has been demonstrated and PE remains a high clinical suspicion without the ability to confirm or exclude the diagnosis of PE, anticoagulant therapy may be administered to treat both conditions. However, under these circumstances, the absence of a definitive diagnosis or exclusion of PE may interfere with the ability to make more informed decisions about future diagnostic strategies and therapy for the affected patient.

Treatment of Acute Pulmonary Embolism

The objective of therapy for acute PE is to prevent thrombus extension, as well as early and late DVT and PE. Treatment of uncomplicated PE consists of anticoagulation and/or inferior vena caval filter placement. Therapeutic anticoagulation has generally been achieved in the setting of acute PE with the use of unfractionated heparin (UFH) or low molecular weight heparin (LMWH) preparations. These agents achieve a prompt antithrombotic effect by accelerating the action of antithrombin III to prevent propagation of thrombus.[10] These compounds do not dissolve thromboemboli; rather, they allow endogenous fibrinolytic mechanisms to proceed unopposed. Because a significant improvement in outcome is associated with quickly achieving a therapeutic level of anticoagulation for acute PE,[46] therapeutic anticoagulation should be instituted promptly and aggressively with the diagnosis or strong suspicion of acute PE. However the potential benefit of therapy should be weighed against the risk of complications.

UFH is administered as an intravenous bolus to attempt to achieve immediate anticoagulation. Therapeutic anticoagulation is subsequently maintained by the administration of UFH as a continuous intravenous infusion titrated to achieve an activated partial thromboplastin time of 2 to 3 times the upper normal limit (60–80 s). Algorithms using weight-based nomograms have been shown to achieve and maintain therapeutic anticoagulation better than nonstandardized methods.[47] Adverse reactions associated with UFH anticoagulation include bleeding and heparin-induced thrombocytopenia (HIT), which may be associated with thrombosis. Major episodes of bleeding occur in approximately 2% of patients treated with UFH.[48] Risk factors for the development of UFH associated bleeding complications include advanced age, recent surgery, trauma, concurrent use of aspirin, and thrombolytic therapy. HIT is a potential complication, which occurs by the action of heparin-dependent IgG antibodies that activate platelets through their Fc receptors.[49] HIT usually develops 5 or more days after the administration of heparin and occurs in approximately 5% of patients treated with UFH.[50]

LMWH preparations are being more commonly used as the agent of choice to achieve therapeutic anticoagulation for patients with acute PE. These agents have been demonstrated to have comparable safety and efficacy to UFH for the treatment of acute PE, and they may offer some advantages over therapy with UFH.[51–54] LMWHs have a longer half-life, greater bioavailability, and a more predictable dose response than UFH.[55] Additionally, LMWHs are subcutaneously administered based on weight and generally do not require laboratory monitoring. In contrast to hepatically cleared UFH, LMWHs are renally cleared and thus require dose adjustments or alternative anticoagulant use for patients with significant renal insufficiency. HIT can be seen with LMWH as well as UFH; however, the incidence of HIT has been found to be less for LMWH.[56]

Newer agents have been developed to achieve therapeutic anticoagulation. Fondaparinux, a synthetic pentasaccharide and selective inhibitor of activated clotting factor X, has been shown to be safe and effective for the treatment of acute PE[57] and is approved by the U.S. Food and Drug Administration (FDA) for this purpose. Fondaparinux is administered as a once daily subcutaneous injection and does not require laboratory monitoring. It is also renally cleared and must be dose adjusted in patients with renal insufficiency. Argatroban and lepirudin are direct thrombin inhibitors approved by the FDA for the treatment of VTE complicated by HIT. Argatroban is hepatically metabolized and is contraindicated in patients with significant hepatic dysfunction, while lepirudin is cleared by renal mechanisms and requires dosage modifications for renal insufficiency. The oral agent ximelagatran and hirudin, which is derived from leech saliva, are direct thrombin inhibitors, which are showing promise in ongoing studies as agents to achieve therapeutic anticoagulation.

Definitive anticoagulation requires the depletion of factor II (thrombin) and takes approximately 5 days to achieve.[10] Treatment with UFH or LMWH is, therefore, generally recommended for a minimum of 5 days. Oral vitamin K antagonists, such as warfarin, are usually instituted for continuing outpatient therapy of VTE. Oral therapy with warfarin can be instituted once therapeutic levels of anticoagulation are achieved with UFH or LMWH. Warfarin therapy is then overlapped for a period of 5 days of heparin therapy and until a therapeutic level of anticoagulation is achieved with warfarin, as determined by measurement of the prothrombin international normalized ratio. The target international normalized ratio for the majority of patients being treated for PE is between 2.0 and 3.0.

Variation in anticoagulant effect with warfarin therapy can occur due to interactions of the agent with many foods and drugs as well as due to genetic variations in warfarin metabolism.[58] The duration of anticoagulation depends on the continuing risk of recurrent VTE versus the risk of complications, generally bleeding, with continued anticoagulant therapy.

In some patients with acute PE, inferior vena cava (IVC) filters may be indicated. IVC filters are used where anticoagulation is contraindicated, in patients with recurrent PE despite therapeutic levels of anticoagulation, and in those patients undergoing surgical embolectomy. While IVC filters do nothing to decrease thrombus formation and have actually been associated with increased rates of DVT,[59] they reduce the incidence of clinically significant embolization of thrombi to the pulmonary vasculature and decrease mortality associated with VTE.[60] Retrievable IVC filters have been developed and may be useful in patients with a reversible, short-term increased risk of acute PE.[61]

The use of thrombolytic therapy has been shown to achieve greater initial resolution of thrombus and lower residual pulmonary vascular resistance than therapy with UFH for the treatment of acute PE. However, because of the high rate of bleeding complications associated with thrombolytic therapy, it has not been conclusively demonstrated to offer an advantage over conventional anticoagulation for patients with acute PE and stable hemodynamics.[62] However, evidence suggests that thrombolytic therapy for the treatment of massive PE causing hypotension, which otherwise treated may have a mortality rate as high as 30%,[63] may result in improved outcomes compared to therapy with heparin.[64,65] Additionally, there is ongoing debate as to whether patients with acute PE and stable hemodynamics but with echocardiographic evidence of cardiac right ventricular strain, might benefit from the administration of thrombolytic therapy.[66] FDA approved regimens exist for the use of alteplase, streptokinase, and urokinase for the therapy of acute PE. Catheter-directed methods of thrombolytic administration are being developed to attempt to improve efficacy and decrease complication rates, but data are insufficient to make recommendations about the specific role of these methods in the management of acute PE.

Pulmonary embolectomy can be used to relieve pulmonary vascular obstruction caused by acute PE and is considered for patients with massive PE when thrombolytic therapy is contraindicated or ineffective. High morbidity and mortality rates have historically been associated with the procedure; however, procedural techniques have undergone refinement with reports of improved outcomes. A 2002 publication of a study conducted at Brigham and Women's Hospital on 29 patients presenting with acute PE treated with surgical embolectomy reported an 89% 1-month survival.[67] Catheter thrombectomy and/or clot fragmentation are other potential alternatives to attempt to relieve cardiac right ventricular failure and cardiogenic shock associated with massive PE.[68–71] Many patients presenting with massive PE have contraindications to the administration of fibrinolytics, and few hospitals are able to have constant availability of personnel and resources to perform surgical embolectomy. Catheter-directed methods may, therefore, become a feasible approach in the management of acute, massive PE, though additional studies are needed to define their safety and efficacy.

Prophylaxis

Appropriate prophylaxis has been well established to decrease the incidence of VTE in a wide variety of patients and clinical settings; however, VTE prophylaxis remains grossly underused. Mechanical and/or pharmacologic methods are available to reduce patient's risk for PE. A thorough investigation for risk factors should be conducted to determine the specific prophylactic measures employed. Mechanical prophylactic devices include graduated compression stockings, intermittent pneumatic stockings, and IVC filter placement. Pharmacologic agents used to reduce the risk of VTE include subcutaneous UFH, LMWH, warfarin, and fondaparinux. UFH at a dosage of 5000 units subcutaneously every 8 hours has been shown to be an effective means to decrease the incidence of VTE in patients at low to moderate risk for VTE.[72] LMH is comparable to UFH in efficacy and complications for VTE prophylaxis[73] and has been shown to be more effective than UFH in specific high-risk patient populations, including hip and knee replacement patient and multitrauma patient populations.[73,74] Very high-risk patients may benefit from combined mechanical and pharmacologic prophylactic interventions. Comprehensive consensus guidelines exist to guide VTE prophylaxis for specific patient populations.[75] Computer-assisted VTE prophylaxis protocols have been shown to improve rates of appropriate prophylaxis administration and reduce the risk of VTE[76] and are coming into common hospital usage.

● NONTHROMBOTIC PULMONARY EMBOLI

Venous Air Embolism

Venous air embolism (VAE) as a cause of mortality was initially described in animals by the Italian naturalist Redi in 1667.[77] It was reported in humans by Morgagni in 1769 based on postmortem findings,[78] and subsequently by Beauchesne (1818) and Magendie (1821), both reports in association with neck tumor excision.[79] VAE occurs in a variety of circumstances, including diagnostic and therapeutic medical and surgical interventions and their complications. These circumstances include but are not limited to neurosurgical procedures, particularly in the sitting position[80–82]; intracardiac pacemaker placement,[83,84] orthopedic and general surgical procedures[85]; obstetrical/gynecologic cases[86–91]; trauma[92,93]; diving/decompression accidents[94,95]; positive pressure ventilation[96]; percutaneous lung biopsy[97–99]; penetrating lung injury[100,101]; vascular cannulation[102–111]; hemodialysis[112,113]; mechanical ventilation[96,114,115]; epidural catheter insertion[116]; and contrast injection[117–119] (Table 45-2).

Distinction is made between venous, or pulmonary air embolism, and arterial air embolism, as their pathologic and clinical manifestations, as well as therapeutic interventions, may differ.[120] In VAE, air enters the venous circulation and passes into the right heart and lungs. The deleterious effects in this circumstance are generally exerted in the pulmonary[121] and cardiovascular systems. It is possible that the filtering capacity of the lungs may be exceeded, allowing air to pass into the arterial system,[122–125] and causing an arterial air embolus, even in the absence of an intracardiac defect.[126,127] Arterial air embolism may also be the result of air that enters the venous circulation and passes through a patent foramen ovale, which may occur in up to 30% of the population based on autopsy studies.[128–131] This phenomenon is referred to as a paradoxical embolism, and more commonly has manifestations affecting the heart and central nervous system. Either venous or arterial embolism may result in death.

The incidence of VAE in multiple studies varies depending on the patient population observed and the method of detection employed. The highest incidence of VAE occurs in neurosurgical patients undergoing surgery in the sitting, or Fowler's, position. This approach was previously used more commonly,[81] but is used now primarily in high midline, posterior fossa procedures.[82] The incidence of VAE in retrospective and prospective studies of neurosurgical patients has ranged from 2% to 58% (Table 45-3)[80]; however, with the introduction of TEE, the incidence has been reported to be as high as 76%.[132] Many of these VAE are small, but may herald the advent of a larger and clinically more significant event.[133]

The pathophysiology of VAE includes mechanical effects resulting from obstruction as well as inflammatory mediated events resulting from the release of thromboxane and free radicals with subsequent endothelial damage and increased capillary permeability.[83,134–138] Air can enter the venous system at a communication between a gas (usually the atmosphere) and the open venous system where the ingress of gas is favored by a pressure gradient.[106] The air can either be injected under pressure, or it may move along a gradient of atmospheric to subatmospheric pressure. The former situation is seen in the setting of an injection of air via a syringe or pressurized infusion device. The latter mechanism occurs in the setting of surgery or other invasive procedures, where veins above the level of the heart are exposed to the atmosphere. This second mechanism may be a particular problem in the presence of increased negative intrathoracic pressure, such as in patients with obstructive lung disease. Once air enters the pulmonary circulation, it causes an increase in pulmonary pressure because of obstruction and reflex pulmonary vasoconstriction.[139] This increase in pulmonary vasoconstriction leads to an increase in right ventricular end-diastolic pressure and right atrial pressure. Additionally, this vascular obstruction causes an increase in dead space leading to hypercapnia and a decrease in end-tidal carbon dioxide ($ETCO_2$).[140,141]

The adverse effects of VAE cannot be attributed solely to vascular obstruction by air bubbles and vasoconstriction.

TABLE 45-2. Surgical and Medical Settings in Which Venous Air Embolism May Occur

Surgical

Neurosurgery
  Craniotomies
  Laminectomies
  Pin holder placement
  Shunt placement

Cardiac surgery
  Vein harvesting

General surgery
  Thoracic trauma
  Head and neck trauma
  Craniofacial surgery
  Transplantation
  Pneumoperitoneum from ruptured viscus

Obstetrics/Gynecology
  Caesarian section
  Hysteroscopy
  Laparoscopy
  Orogenital sex during pregnancy
  Epidural catheter insertion

Orthopedics
  Pulse lavage of fractures
  Arthroscopy
  Total hip arthroplasty
  Spine surgery in prone position

Dentistry
  Root canal procedures

Medical

Cardiology
  Pericardiocentesis
  Pacemaker placement
  Cardiac catheterization

Nephrology
  Hemodialysis

Critical care medicine
  Placement/maintenance/removal of central venous/PA catheters
  Mechanical ventilation
  Diving/decompression accidents

Radiology
  Contrast injection
  Arthrography
  Percutaneous lung biopsy

Gastroenterology
  Air entry into veins during upper/lower endoscopy
  Air entry into veins during ERCP

PA, pulmonary artery; ERCP, endoscopic retrograde cholangiopancreatography.

In experimental animals, a complex interaction of air and blood occurs in the right heart as air and blood are whipped together, creating a network of air bubbles, fibrin stands, erythrocytes, fat globules, and platelet aggregates.[142,143] This fibrin mesh is then ejected into the terminal branches of the pulmonary arteries. The role of the neutrophil in VAE-induced lung injury has been investigated by numerous authors.[83,135,137,142–148] Neutrophils are sequestered in the lungs during VAE, and in the experiments by Albertine et al. were shown to clump around air bubbles and

TABLE 45-3. Incidence of Venous Air Embolism During Neurosurgical Procedures Conducted with the Patient in the Sitting Position

Authors	Year	Type of Study	No. of Cases	Incidence (%)	Method of Detection
Bithal et al.[495]	2004	Prospective	334	28	Capnography
Young et al.[496]	1986	Retrospective	255	30	Capnography or Doppler
Papadopoulos et al.[132]	1994	Prospective	62	76	TOE
Michenfelder et al.[497]	1972	Prospective	69	32	Doppler
Slbin et al.[498]	1976	Retrospective	180	25	Doppler
Voorhies et al.[499]	1983	Prospective	81	50	Doppler
Standefer et al.[500]	1984	Retrospective	488	7	Doppler
Matjasko et al.[501]	1985	Prospective and retrospective	554	23	Doppler
Black et al.[502]	1988	Retrospective	333	45	Doppler

TOE, transoesophageal echocardiography.
Reprinted, with permission, from Leslie K, Hui R, Kaye AH. Venous air embolism and the sitting position: a case series. J Clin Neurosci. 2006;13: 419-422.

attach to the endothelium of the pulmonary arterioles, distorting the microvascular architecture, and producing endothelial cell gaps.[137] This disruption of the endothelium led to increased lung lymph flow and protein flux. The cascade of events initiated by the release of thromboxane and leukotrienes causes increased alveolar–capillary permeability with resultant edema and a dose-dependent inactivation of surfactant.[83] All of these factors may lead to an increase in intrapulmonary shunting, decreased arterial oxygen tension, and decreased pulmonary compliance.[149]

A classic study of VAE done by Durant et al.[150] in 1947 demonstrated that mortality during VAE was associated with the amount of air embolized, the speed at which it entered the body and the body position at the time it occurred. A fatal dose is considered to be 300 to 500 mL of air at a rate of 100 mL/s, which can be achieved with a 14-gauge needle and a pressure gradient of only 5 cm H_2O between air and venous blood.[106,107] In the critically ill and unstable patient, smaller volumes of air may also be fatal.[151] A grading system has been developed for VAE in the neurosurgical patient population based on emboli size, monitoring device detection, and physiologic changes occurring in the operating theatre. A large embolus (>50 mL) may require abandonment of the surgical procedure if any concern exists for recurrence of the VAE.[82]

The clinical manifestations of VAE may be nonspecific and require vigilance with a high index of suspicion to promptly identify the occurrence of VAE. The symptoms associated with VAE may mimic a variety of other disorders. Faintness, chest pain, lightheadedness, and a feeling of impending doom have been reported[106,152]; and in one series, 100% of patients had the onset of sudden dyspnea.[153] A classic "gasp" reflex caused by acute hypoxemia[106,107] has been described. Physical examination findings are also nonspecific. The typical mill wheel murmur is a splashing auscultatory sound heard over the precordium because of the presence of gas in the cardiac chambers and great vessels, although it is a late finding.[119,150] More commonly, a harsh systolic murmur or normal heart sounds are heard.[154] Chest examination may reveal rales or wheezing, and abnormal mental status or neurologic findings are relatively common. Kashuk et al.[153] reported a 42% incidence of central nervous system manifestations in a series of 24 cases of air embolism with abnormalities ranging from altered mental status to coma. Tachypnea, tachycardia, and hypotension may also occur, heralding the onset of further hemodynamic compromise.[120] Central nervous system manifestations may develop secondary to hypoxemia and hypoperfusion as a result of hemodynamic compromise or as a result of cerebral arterial embolism via intracardiac or intrapulmonary shunts.

Similar to the clinical findings associated with VAE, routine laboratory analysis in this disorder may be nonspecific. Arterial blood gas analysis may show hypoxemia of varying severity as well as hypercapnia.[155] Review of electrocardiographic data may demonstrate sinus tachycardia, right heart strain, and myocardial ischemia.[156–158] Chest radiography is most commonly normal, but may exhibit a variety of ad-

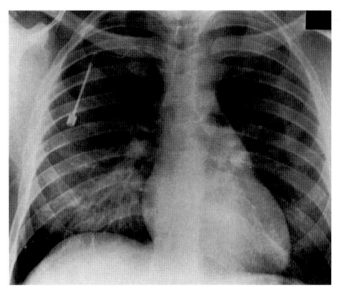

● **FIGURE 45-3.** Anteroposterior chest radiograph. Main pulmonary artery demonstrates characteristic bell, or cone-shaped, air collections. Additionally, focal oligemia is suggested in the left upper lobe.

Reproduced, with permission, from Kizer KW, Goodman PC. Radiographic manifestations of venous air embolism. Radiology. 1982;144:35-39.

ditional findings such as pulmonary edema, characteristic bell or cone shaped air collections in the main pulmonary artery (Figure 45-3), enlarged pulmonary arteries, focal pulmonary edema, atelectasis, intracardiac air, and air in the hepatic venous circulation.[159] CT of the chest may be of diagnostic value by demonstrating air in the vasculature and cardiac chambers,[118] and has also been implicated as a cause of VAE during the administration of intravenous contrast. Knowledge of the most frequent anatomic locations for air emboli to collect may help the radiologist in differentiating between air embolism and other phenomena[117,118,160] (Figure 45-4). Central nervous system imaging may be performed if cerebral air embolism as a complication of VAE is suspected. However, CT of the brain is rarely diagnostic in this setting, as the CT must be obtained immediately after the event because of the rapid resorption of air from cerebral arterioles.[161] A restricted diffusion pattern on MRI may be seen in cerebral air embolism, but further evaluation of this MRI pattern as characteristic for cerebral air embolism is required.[83,162]

Echocardiography, both transthoracic (TTE) and transesophageal (TEE), is well documented as a valuable tool for monitoring and detecting VAE.[108,163] Precordial Doppler remains an essential noninvasive first-line tool for monitoring patients during high-risk surgical procedures because of its availability and high sensitivity.[164–166] Additionally, echo detects VAE well before the earliest evidence of physiologic changes.[167] Proper probe positioning and verification of accurate positioning is crucial to its efficacy, and left parasternal positioning is as sensitive as right parasternal.[168,169] However, TEE is the most sensitive method of detection of VAE and is considered the gold standard.[106,107,127,151] Its

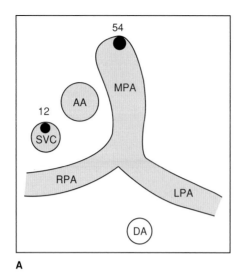
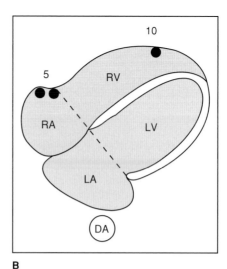

A **B**

FIGURE 45-4. Diagrams show frequent locations of air emboli (depicted as large black dots) observed on axial CT scans in (A) vessels and (B) cardiac chambers after insertion of an intravenous cannula or injection of contrast agent. The numbers indicate the frequency of air emboli at the corresponding locations in 677 CT examinations with contrast material enhancement. In six patients, air embolism was found in the subclavian or brachiocephalic vein, which are not shown on the figure.

AA, ascending aorta; DA, descending aorta; LA, left atrium; LPA, left pulmonary artery; LV, left ventricle; MPA, main pulmonary artery; RA, right atrium; RPA, right pulmonary artery; RV, right ventricle; SVC, superior vena cava.

Reproduced, with permission, from Groell R, Schaffler GJ, Rienmueller R, et al. Vascular air embolism: location, frequency, and cause on electron-beam CT studies of the chest. Radiology. 1997;202:459-462.

use is limited primarily by cost and the advanced level of training required to attain operator expertise in study performance and interpretation.[119,170] In institutions where TEE is used, the procedure allows additional information to be obtained including an assessment for the presence of a patient foramen ovale when the probe is placed prior to beginning the surgical procedure.

Other forms of monitoring and detection during surgical procedures include capnography, pulmonary artery catheters, air aspiration via a central venous catheter, pulse oximetry, arterial blood gas analysis, and mass spectrometry. VAE results in a decrease in $ETCO_2$, and is always significant when detected by this method.[82] Pulmonary artery catheter monitoring is invasive, but has similar sensitivity to capnography[82] and can demonstrate an increase in pulmonary arterial pressure with VAE when employed as a monitoring device. The pressure gradient measured between the left and right atria may also help in assessing the potential for paradoxical air embolism. Pulmonary artery catheters are of no use in aspirating air if a VAE is detected,[166] but an appropriately placed central venous catheter may aspirate air and confirm VAE.[107,140,171] Mass spectrometry to measure end-tidal nitrogen may be used to diagnose VAE, but is not available at most institutions.[82]

Treatment of VAE begins with methods to prevent and detect its occurrence, followed by supportive care and standard resuscitation. Measures to prevent the occurrence of VAE should be undertaken in any circumstance where the risk for VAE exists. These measures include the previously reviewed monitoring during surgical procedures at risk for VAE. Additionally, volume loading to reduce negative venous pressure at the wound level should be employed preemptively, with some authors recommending colloid over crystalloid because of a more prolonged increase in vascular volume.[82] If VAE is suspected to have occurred, the surgical field should be irrigated so that no further entrainment of air can occur, and the surgical site should be lowered below the level of the heart if possible.[119] Neck tourniquets may be used to increase cerebral venous pressure either during periods of high risk for VAE or during episodes of recorded VAE. However, care should be taken to ensure that the pressure generated by the tourniquet is in the venous and not arterial range, and that the potential complications of increased cerebral edema or carotid plaque disruption are considered. If a central venous catheter is appropriately located at the superior vena cava-right atrial junction, air may be aspirated via the catheter, with multiorifice catheters being more effective than single lumen catheters in aspirating air.[82,172,173] Even with appropriate positioning of the catheter, studies have shown that only approximately 50% of the air will be successfully aspirated.[107,149] In addition to prevention, detection, and aspiration of air, supportive therapies such as volume expansion, vasopressors to support organ perfusion, and 100% FiO_2 to facilitate the washout of nitrogen from the air bubble should be employed. Nitrous oxide should be avoided as an anesthetic agent, but if being used, should be stopped if VAE is suspected. The deleterious effects of nitrous oxide are due to the differential solubilities of nitrous oxide and nitrogen, which allow nitrous oxide to replace nitrogen in the blood, potentially increasing the gas bubble volume and rendering lethal what might have otherwise been an innocuous air bubble.[140,174,175] The patient should be moved to the left lateral decubitus position to prevent air lock at the pulmonary outflow tract.[176] Closed chest cardiac massage has been used successfully in the resuscitation of patients with VAE,[177] and was found to improve survival to the same degree as left lateral decubitus positioning and air aspiration in the canine model.[178] Left lateral decubitus positioning reduced mortality in one series of 93 cases of air embolism from 88% to 33%.[79] If evidence for cerebral air embolism exists, arrangements should be made promptly for hyperbaric oxygen therapy in an attempt to decrease the size of the air emboli and allow passage into smaller vessels perfusing smaller areas of the brain.[179,180] Expeditious transport should be arranged, and ground transport for short trips is preferred due to the potential for worsening of a patient's condition in the setting of bubble expansion with a decrease in atmospheric pressure as a result of an increase in altitude. If long-distance transport is required, aircraft should be pressurized to 1.0 ata. If helicopter transport is used, maintaining an altitude of 300 to 500 feet, volume loading, and 100% FiO_2 are all recommended.[181]

Amniotic Fluid Embolism

Amniotic fluid embolism (AFE) is a catastrophic complication of pregnancy, which classically presents with hypoxemia, cardiopulmonary collapse, and disseminated intravascular coagulation during labor or in the immediate postpartum period. Initially described by Meyer[182] in 1926 and further clarified in the early 1940s by Steiner and Lushbaugh,[183] AFE has generated intense interest and has been widely reported and reviewed in the obstetric, anesthesia, pulmonary, and critical care literature over the ensuing years. More than 400 cases have been reported in the literature, and yet the incidence, mortality, and diagnostic criteria are still controversial.

The reported incidence of AFE has varied, with many authors citing ranges from 1 in 8000 to 1 in 80 000.[183–189] Albeit rare, AFE is a significant disorder because of the high associated maternal mortality and morbidity. An early review of 272 cases reported in the English literature cited a maternal mortality rate of 86%.[190] Later data from the U.S. National Registry demonstrated a maternal mortality of 61%, but included significant additional maternal morbidity with only 15% of patients surviving neurologically intact.[185] In a population-based study of 1 094 248 deliveries from California, a frequency of 1 in 20 646 deliveries was reported with a maternal mortality of 26%.[184] However, a subsequent case–fatality rate in a large Canadian cohort of patients was only 13%.[186] The United Kingdom Amniotic Fluid Embolism Registry reported an incidence of 1 in 120 000 cases and a maternal mortality of 37%.

AFE is a significant cause of maternal mortality in the United States, United Kingdom, and Australia and has accounted for approximately 7.5% to 10% of all maternal deaths in various long-term analyses.[185,191–195] Fifty percent of AFE-related mortality occurs acutely within the first hour of presentation, requiring a proactive and informed response to the acute presentation.[86,196–198] Fetal mortality is also high, approaching 40% in some studies.[185,199] There is no consensus on the occurrence of AFE in subsequent pregnancies owing to its significant maternal morbidity and mortality, but several cases of uncomplicated pregnancies after AFE are reported in the literature.[194,200–205] It is apparent that in spite of years of AFE case compilations and established AFE registries, the incidence and mortality of AFE have not been clearly defined.

Multiple factors contribute to the difficulty in determining the true incidence and mortality of AFE. These factors include inaccuracies in reporting causes of maternal deaths,[191,206,207] reliance upon multiple case reviews and small patient series, variations in diagnostic criteria and study design among case series and registries,[184,185] and publication bias owing to selective reporting of severe cases.[186] Additionally, AFE may occur with disparate clinical presentations and is difficult to specifically diagnose in subclinical or nonfatal cases.[207–209] The more recent findings of lower reported maternal mortalities than those seen in earlier case reports and case series may reflect both advancements in intensive care medicine and supportive therapies for patients treated for AFE over the last few decades as well as recognition that subclinical or milder cases of the disorder exist.[184,185,193,210]

The pathophysiology of AFE remains poorly understood because of its low incidence and difficulties in duplicating the event in animal studies. Amniotic fluid increases from 50 to 1000 mL at term and contains multiple vasoactive materials, as well as various elements of fetal origin including: fetal squamous cells (squames), lanugo hairs, vernix caseosa, gut-derived mucin, and occasionally, bile containing meconium.[190,211] While the pathophysiology of AFE is not clearly delineated, it is presumed that amniotic fluid containing fetal debris enters the maternal circulation via uterine venous sinuses within the endometrium or endocervix.[184] The constituents of the amniotic fluid then travel to the pulmonary vascular bed and cause acute right heart failure followed by left heart failure, an assumption based primarily on data derived from animal models. There are no case reports in humans where central hemodynamic monitoring was in place prior to the onset of AFE to document this presumed hemodynamic response,[212] and there are only rare instances of normative hemodynamic data documented in the gravid female.[213] The currently available animal and human hemodynamic data suggest a biphasic pathophysiology for AFE,[214] with initial right heart failure secondary to pulmonary vasoconstriction and vascular occlusion, followed by left heart failure because of inadequate filling and coronary ischemia in the setting of hypoxemia.[197,214] In animal studies with documented central hemodynamic data, severe acute right heart failure was not prominent, but the animals had previously undergone intubation and general anesthesia, which may have blunted their response to the acute insult of amniotic fluid introduction into the pulmonary circulation.[199] However, it does appear that the most severe cardiopulmonary response occurred in the groups with meconium stained amniotic fluid, which supports observations in both animals[199] and humans. Another criticism of many animal studies is that heterologous versus autologous amniotic fluid was infused, which would not mimic true AFE.[215] The infusion of autologous amniotic fluid in two primate studies failed to demonstrate the dramatic clinical syndrome of AFE seen in other animal studies.[216,217] Overall, results of available animal studies are conflicting and difficult to compare because of differing experimental designs and interspecies variation in clinical response to experimental AFE.[218]

Originally, the cascade of events causing AFE was felt to be caused by mechanical occlusion of the pulmonary vasculature in the setting of tumultuous labor with a large volume of amniotic fluid infused under pressure. However, the contribution of tumultuous labor and large volume infusion cannot explain the documented occurrence of AFE early in pregnancy, when the volume of amniotic fluid is small. The presumption of tumultuous labor intuitively also leads to a concern for an increased risk of AFE with uterine stimulants in the induction or augmentation of labor. In Morgan's early series[190] and the later National Registry data,[185] the authors dispute that tumultuous labor and uterine hyperstimulation as a result of labor induction are associated with AFE. Instead, Clark proposes that the uterine hypertonicity seen in AFE is a result of the cardiopulmonary compromise associated with the disorder, rather than the cause of the insult. Wagner strongly criticized the statistical methods used by these authors as well as the validity of their assertions, and called for greater scientific scrutiny of maternal deaths and the association of AFE with uterine stimulants for induction or augmentation of labor.[219] A recent large population-based cohort[186] did show an association of AFE with the use of uterine stimulants, leaving the question of uterine stimulants as a predisposing factor in the development of AFE controversial. Multiple attempts have been made to determine other risk factors for AFE. The best data at this point suggest the strongest associations for the following risk factors: advanced maternal age, meconium stained amniotic fluid, placental abruption, placenta previa, fetal death, and multiparity.[184,186,220–222]

Similarities in clinical characteristics of AFE to anaphylaxis and sepsis have led Clark and others to propose an "anaphylactoid" syndrome of pregnancy, with small volumes of amniotic fluid precipitating a vasoactive procoagulant cascade leading to pulmonary edema, vascular thrombosis in situ and coagulopathy[183–185,206,223] (Figure 45-5). An anaphylactoid theory is supported by data from the National Registry, which demonstrated that AFE was more common in association with male fetuses, and in patients who reported a history of atopy. It is important to recognize, however, that other symptoms associated with anaphylaxis were not present to the same degree in AFE, notably bronchospasm and urticaria.[224] Bronchospasm was seen in only 15% of the National Registry patients, and in 1% of the patients in Morgan's early analysis, but is seen in approximately 40% of patients with anaphylaxis.[225] The association of male fetuses and AFE noted by Clark (67%) was also not identified in a large population–based study of AFE, where 49% of the fetuses were female.[184]

The diagnosis of AFE is largely clinical, with a classic presentation of hypoxemia, hemodynamic instability, altered mental status, and disseminated intravascular coagulation occurring during active labor and delivery or in the immediate postpartum period. AFE has additionally been reported as a consequence of abdominal trauma, amniocentesis, and first and second trimester abortions.[120,196]. The presenting features of AFE in the National Registry were seizure or seizure-like activity (30%), dyspnea (27%), fetal bradycardia (17%), and hypotension (13%). However, during the course of the disease, 100% of patients had hypotension and fetal distress, with 93% experiencing pulmonary edema or acute respiratory distress syndrome (ARDS) and 87% having cardiopulmonary arrest, 37% of those within 5 minutes of symptom onset. Coagulopathy was associated with AFE in 40% of patients.[185] In contrast to the National Registry data, 51% of patients in Morgan's series presented with respiratory distress. Dyspnea may be more difficult to define in the pregnant patient, as up to 60% of pregnant women may develop the dyspnea of pregnancy during the first trimester, even before the mechanical effects of the gravid uterus on the diaphragm are apparent.[226] However, the presentation of AFE, particularly in fatal cases, is generally dramatic with sudden rather than gradual onset of symptoms, including dyspnea. This rapid onset of symptoms seen in most patients with AFE prompted Benson to include sudden onset of symptoms as a key feature in his proposed criteria for diagnosis of AFE.[209]

The finding of fetal squamous cells in the maternal circulation was previously felt to be pathognomic for the condition, but the significance of this finding has been refuted because of the high false-positive rate of squamous cells seen in the maternal circulation of patients without AFE, and because of the difficulty in differentiating between maternal and fetal squamous cells.[206,227–231] A key observation may be that the squamous cells seen in patients with AFE, unlike those in patients without AFE, are coated with leukocytes in many cases; this finding may suggest a maternal reaction to a foreign (fetal) antigen. Additionally, the squames in patients with documented AFE may also be seen pathologically in association with other fetal debris.[207,227]

Serologic studies have more recently been proposed to assist in the diagnosis of AFE, including serum tryptase levels to assess for mast cell degranulation,[232,233] and a monoclonal antibody (TKH2) that recognizes the sialyl Tn structure characteristically found in meconium and amniotic fluid.[234,235] Serum tryptase may be useful in both antemortem and postmortem diagnosis of AFE given its more prolonged serum half-life,[233,236] although some dispute the postmortem significance of an elevated tryptase level.[237] Other investigators have found associated low levels of

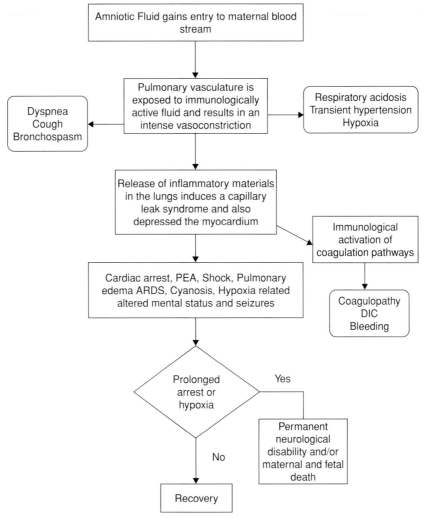

● **FIGURE 45-5.** Proposed mechanism for the pathogenesis of amniotic fluid embolism. ARDS, acute respiratory distress syndrome; PEA, pulseless electrical activity.

Reproduced, with permission, from Aurangzeb I, George L, Raoof S. Amniotic fluid embolism. Crit Care Clin. 2004;20:643-650.

complement in patients with AFE,[238,239] elevated zinc coproporphyrin levels,[239,240] and increases in tissue factor[241] in amniotic fluid versus in maternal serum. None of these tests has been validated in a series of AFE patients, and all have limited practical utility at present. Currently, the finding of fetal debris in the pulmonary circulation at autopsy with a compatible clinical scenario defines the diagnosis of AFE, although routine hematoxylin and eosin staining may be insufficient to demonstrate fetal elements and special stains may be required.[211,242]

Clinical findings suggest the diagnosis in nonfatal cases, with laboratory and imaging studies providing supportive evidence. The normal arterial blood gas in the pregnant patient demonstrates a mild chronic respiratory alkalosis with compensatory metabolic acidosis.[226] In the pregnant patient with respiratory distress and shock, the arterial blood gas may show development of acute respiratory alkalosis and acute metabolic acidosis in addition to the chronic acid base changes associated with pregnancy. In those patients

with AFE who develop coagulopathy, numerous coagulation abnormalities may be seen. These include thrombocytopenia, increased fibrinopeptide A, increased D-dimer, decreased antithrombin III, decreased fibrinogen, increased fibrin degradation products, and increased prothrombin and partial thromboplastin times.

The majority of imaging studies documented in patients with AFE are those that can be done at the bedside. Chest radiographs obtained in the patient with AFE are nonspecific. The radiograph may be normal or may demonstrate bilateral pulmonary infiltrates consistent with either cardiogenic or noncardiogenic pulmonary edema.[86,243,244] Ventilation–perfusion scans may show multiple perfusion defects, which is a nonspecific finding and can also be seen in pulmonary thromboembolism, a disorder for which pregnant patients are also at high risk. Because of the dramatic presentation of AFE in many cases and the associated hemodynamic instability, extensive radiographic imaging to include CT with PE protocol is usually impractical acutely.

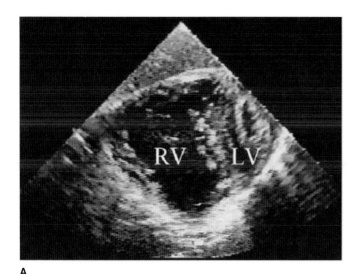

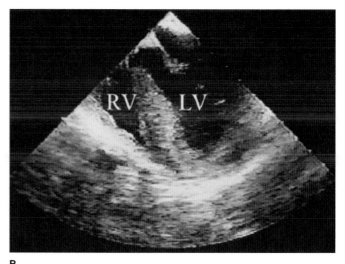

A

B

● **FIGURE 45-6.** (A) Transesophageal echocardiogram view taken with 10 minutes of acute amniotic fluid embolus, demonstrating dilated right ventricle (RV) and small left ventricle (LV). (B) Transesophageal echocardiogram reflecting a return to normal size and function of the right and left ventricles after intervention including cardiopulmonary bypass.

Reproduced, with permission, from Stanten RD, Iverson LIG, Daugharty TM, Lovett SM, Terry C, Blumenstock E. Amniotic fluid embolism causing catastrophic pulmonary vasoconstriction: diagnosis by transesophageal echocardiogram and treatment by cardiopulmonary bypass. Obstetr Gynecol. 2003;102:496-498.

There is no data on characteristic CT findings in AFE or CT methods to distinguish AFE from PE. TTE and TEE, however, can be done at the bedside and may be useful in the short-term diagnosis of AFE.[245,246] Two case reports used TEE acutely in the abrupt decompensation of a patient in labor—one within 10 minutes of decompensation after elective caesarean section,[247] and one within 30 minutes of caesarean section for fetal distress.[245] In both cases, acute right heart failure with normal left ventricular ejection fraction was seen on TEE (Figure 45-6). Neither case demonstrated evidence of acute pulmonary artery thromboembolism, either by Doppler examination of the pulmonary arteries in the first case[245] or by direct surgical exploration of the pulmonary arteries during cardiopulmonary bypass in the second case.[247] Autopsy findings in the first case revealed pulmonary edema with extensive microvascular plugging of pulmonary capillaries by fetal squamous epithelial cells, and the second patient had an uneventful recovery. These reports are intriguing, as they may provide evidence for the right heart failure postulated as the initial phase of hemodynamic response to AFE in humans, and could have therapeutic implications as well. In most instances, however, the echocardiogram will demonstrate left ventricular failure unless done immediately during the acute decompensation. The electrocardiographic findings are nonspecific in AFE, but may include evidence of ischemia or right heart strain.

The astute intensivist must possess an understanding of the differences in physiology of the pregnant patient in order to optimally support the patient with AFE. The cardiac output and plasma volume are markedly increased in the pregnant patient at term, in combination with a relative decrease in colloid oncotic pressure, which may predispose to the development of pulmonary edema. These cardiovascular physiologic changes, coupled with hormonal changes in pregnancy, also promote increased mucosal edema. This increase in mucosal edema mandates downsizing both nasogastric and endotracheal tubes and increases the risk for a difficult airway.[248] Minute ventilation increases as pregnancy advances owing to changes in metabolic rate, changes in respiratory mechanics, and increases in serum progesterone. Progesterone has a direct respiratory stimulant effect on the respiratory center, and increases in minute ventilation as pregnancy progresses correlate with increasing maternal serum progesterone concentrations.[226,249] Functional residual capacity decreases as pregnancy advances as a result of decreases in expiratory reserve volume and residual volume. The combination of decreased functional residual capacity and increased minute ventilation leads to an overall decrease in maternal oxygen reserve. Progesterone also causes smooth muscle relaxation and decreases lower esophageal sphincter tone, which is further decreased by stomach displacement as pregnancy advances, contributing to aspiration risk. The glomerular filtration rate and creatinine clearance are also increased in pregnancy, and renal compromise may be present and should be considered at lower levels of BUN/Cr.

The treatment of AFE is largely supportive, with the goal in fulminant cases of providing cardiopulmonary support, including Advanced Cardiac Life Support; reversing hypoxemia with intubation and mechanical ventilation; reversing shock with volume resuscitation, pressor agents, and inotropic therapy as needed; using blood products as indicated to treat hemorrhage and reverse coagulopathy;

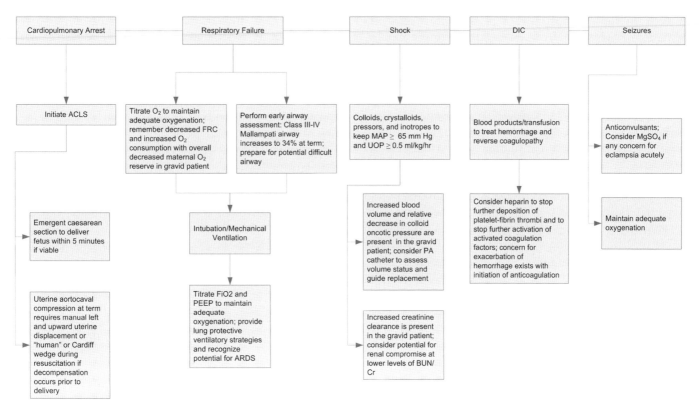

● **FIGURE 45-7.** A multidisciplinary approach to the treatment of amniotic fluid embolism.

and treating with anticonvulsants and airway management to control seizures. A multidisciplinary approach to the treatment of AFE, with close collaboration between the intensivist, obstetrician, and hematologist or neurologist as indicated, is imperative in ensuring an optimal outcome (Figure 45-7).

Cardiac arrest may occur abruptly in patients with AFE, and should follow standard resuscitation algorithms with a few modifications, including lateral displacement of the uterus, early airway assessment, and consideration for emergent caesarian section. The Cardiff resuscitation wedge was developed specifically for CPR in the pregnant patient, but may not be available in all critical care units. In those settings where it is not available, alternative measures may be used to relieve aortocaval compression, including manual displacement of the uterus upward and to the left, placing a wedge under the right hip to achieve an angle of 27 degrees, or using a "human" wedge where one rescuer kneels with the woman's back positioned against his or her thighs.[250] Early airway assessment and rapid control of the airway is also recommended because of the increased risk of aspiration in the pregnant patient and her decrease in oxygen reserve. In the acute decompensation seen with AFE, urgent placement of a secure airway is vital, and should be performed by the most experienced airway management provider present. In the most recent practice guidelines for the management of a "cannot intubate, cannot ventilate" (CVCI) airway situation, a laryngeal mask airway is the tool of choice followed by further difficult airway management as indicated.[248] Adequate maternal oxy-

genation with a $PaO_2 \geq 60$ mm Hg should be achieved as rapidly as possible by titrating FiO_2 and PEEP. The potential for the development of ARDS should be recognized and lung protective ventilatory strategies employed.[224] Emergent caesarean section is recommended as soon as possible after maternal cardiac arrest, although fetal neurologic injury may be present even in those infants delivered within 5 minutes of maternal arrest.[251] Caesarian section may both rescue the infant and aid in maternal resuscitation, as the blood volume returned to the maternal circulation after delivery increases cardiac output by 30% of the prelabor values.[208,250]

The cardiovascular physiologic changes seen in pregnancy may predispose to the pulmonary edema and ARDS seen in AFE, and should lead to consideration of pulmonary artery catheter placement to guide fluid management.[86,224,238,252] However, significant debate currently exists in regards to the risks and benefits of pulmonary artery catheters in the management of critically ill patients.[253–258] Pressor agents should be used to maintain mean arterial pressure (MAP) ≥65 and urine output (UOP) ≥0.5 mL/kg/h. Digitalization, afterload reduction and diuresis have been suggested as potentially beneficial therapies in those patients with severe left ventricular dysfunction and adequate preload.[86,259]

In conjunction with providing the basics of airway and circulatory support, the intensivist must also manage the other sequelae of AFE, including seizures and coagulopathy. Anticonvulsants should be administered to treat and control seizures, with consideration of $MgSO_4$

if concern for eclampsia exists in the short-term presentation. Aggressive airway management to prevent hypoxemia is an adjunct in the control of seizures. Some authors have suggested heparin to manage disseminated intravascular coagulation and prevent further deposition of platelet–fibrin thrombi and generation of activated coagulation factors.[252,259–262] However, aggravation of hemorrhage is a potential risk of this approach, and multiple authors have concluded that routine heparinization is not warranted.[86,120,198,244] Since no absolute transfusion guidelines for blood product treatment of this bleeding diathesis exist, replacement of blood products and consideration of heparin infusion would best be guided by coagulation studies and in conjunction with the expertise of an experienced hematologist. If uterine atony and hemorrhage develop, oxytocin and sometimes hysterectomy are required.[263]

A variety of other more controversial treatment strategies have been proposed in AFE and are open to further investigation. These include inhaled nitric oxide,[264] high dose corticosteroids,[185,224] plasma exchange transfusions,[265] inhaled prostacyclin,[266] serum protease inhibitors,[207] continuous hemofiltration,[267] cell salvage combined with blood filtration, antithrombin III infusion,[224] uterine artery embolization, intra-aortic balloon counterpulsation, and extracorporeal membrane oxygenation.[224,268] One case of cardiopulmonary bypass performed in the setting of AFE and acute right heart failure circumvented the catastrophic cardiovascular collapse seen with this disorder and allowed for complete patient recovery.[247] Cardiopulmonary bypass with pulmonary thrombectomy was reported as therapeutic in an additional patient with AFE.[269] The utilization of cardiopulmonary bypass and/or embolectomy in this setting is fraught with difficulties and would require further evaluation before it could be universally recommended as a treatment for AFE.

In spite of recent advances in our knowledge of AFE, the syndrome is still poorly understood and associated with significant maternal and fetal morbidity and mortality. The National Registries in the United States and United Kingdom have been closed, but the United Kingdom Obstetric Surveillance System continues to collect cases, and with additional data collection from that group and others, a more precise determination of risk factors may be possible.[270] Additionally, further investigations of potential causative mediators in amniotic fluid may provide more definitive diagnostic markers as well as a more complete understanding of the underlying pathophysiology of the disease. AFE is best identified and managed by clinicians who maintain a high index of clinical suspicion in the appropriate clinical setting. An optimal outcome is then dependent on prompt diagnosis coupled with proactive, aggressive resuscitative measures undertaken in a multidisciplinary fashion.

Fat Embolism

Fat embolism (FE) is another form of nonthrombotic embolism which has been reported for many years, having first been described histologically in the postmortem of lung by

Zenker in 1862 and then detailed pathologically in a series of cases by von Bergeman in 1865. The first clinical recognition of fat embolism syndrome (FES) occurred in 1873.[120,271] The classic presentation is of a trauma patient with long bone or pelvic fracture who develops respiratory failure, neurologic impairment, hematologic abnormalities, and a petechial rash within 72 hours of injury. However, a spectrum of manifestations of FE exists, and the diagnosis of the disorder may be difficult because of the multiple confounding injuries often occurring in the trauma patient and to the lack of specific tests for differentiating the disorder from other disease processes.

The incidence of FE is varied, with studies reporting incidences as low as 1% to as high as 20%.[272–275] Clinically significant disease is reported in 5%, with the higher mortality rates noted in the older literature progressively decreasing with the advent of specialized intensive care units.[276–278] FES may be acute and fulminant, with severe physiologic impairment within hours of injury described in the fulminant form.[279,280] A subacute form of FES also exists with milder manifestations,[281] and the occurrence of embolism of fat globules without clinical FES has been widely reported. Palmovic noted that 90% of patients had FE after major trauma.[282] The incidence of FES has been reported to decrease in those fractures operatively repaired within 24 hours of injury versus those with delayed repair.[279,283–286] While the majority of fat emboli occur in association with trauma, with 95% in the setting of long bone fractures, the syndrome has also been reported in a number of other clinical situations,[201,271] including: nontraumatic orthopedic procedures,[287–292] burns,[293] soft tissue injuries,[294] pancreatitis,[295,296] osteomyelitis,[297] diabetes,[298] liposuction,[299–303] bone tumor lysis,[304] bone marrow harvest[305] and transplantation,[306] alcoholic liver disease,[307,308] lipid infusion,[309] steroid therapy,[310–313] sickle cell hemoglobinopathies,[314,315] extracorporeal circulation,[316,317] blood transfusion,[316] and in association with cyclosporine A solvent.[318,319]

The pathophysiology of FE has two proposed mechanisms of injury: Mechanical and physiochemical.[201,320–323] The mechanical mechanism has extensive experimental support and is related to bone marrow disruption at the site of injury, with embolization of fat globules and obstruction of flow in the pulmonary circulation, leading to right heart failure in fulminant cases.[283,324,325] The pulmonary microvessels effectively filter 80% of the fat globules, with the majority of fat globules becoming lodged in vessels of less than 75 μm.[283,326,327] As little as 20 cm^3 of bone marrow fat can temporarily occlude the pulmonary microvasculature.[201] The second mechanism of injury is tissue damage caused by the release of free fatty acids. Neutral fat does not seem to injure pulmonary parenchyma, however, and the current theory is that endothelial-derived lipoprotein lipase causes fatty acid release and subsequent local tissue damage.[328–331] This delay in free fatty acid release presumably explains the time that elapses between the onset of injury to development of the clinical manifestations of the syndrome.

The diagnosis of FE remains a clinical diagnosis, with a triad of respiratory insufficiency, neurologic alteration, and petechial rash frequently occurring in conjunction with fever. Respiratory impairment occurs in all patients with FES, with hypoxemia accompanied by dyspnea and tachypnea being the most common findings.[332] Hypoxemia is caused by ventilation–perfusions mismatch and intrapulmonary shunting.[330,333–338] Investigations of pulmonary gas exchange in animals and humans have also shown increased dead space ventilation consistent with pulmonary vascular occlusion, vasoconstriction, and decreased alveolar perfusion.[328,333–338] Diminished arterial oxygen concentration is the most consistent laboratory finding.[330] Neurologic abnormalities occur in up to 85% of patients who die with FES,[339] with variable occurrence in survivors of the syndrome. When neurologic alteration exists, it is typically an impairment of consciousness that may proceed to stupor, coma, seizures, and focal neurologic deficits.[339,340] Fortunately, in spite of initial severe impairment, permanent deficits in survivors are infrequent. Skin manifestations in the appropriate clinical setting are nearly pathognomic for the disorder.[341] However, the petechial rash, which is typically distributed over the head, neck, anterior thorax, and axillae, only occurs in 20% to 50% of cases[201] (Figure 45-8).

Trauma patients have numerous other etiologies for the respiratory insufficiency and neurologic dysfunction seen with FES, and thus various criteria for the diagnosis have been proposed (Tables 45-4 to 45-6). Although FES remains a clinical diagnosis, none of these proposed criteria has been validated as the gold standard by which to diagnose the disorder.[342–344] There are likewise no specific diagnostic laboratory studies, which define FES. The presence of serum fat globules is neither sensitive nor specific for the clinical syndrome. Serum fat has been demonstrated in a variety of circumstance where clinical FE syndrome did not develop, and even in those circumstances where FES

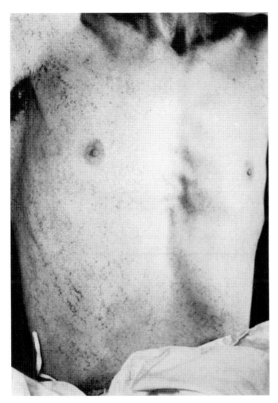

● **FIGURE 45-8.** Photograph depicting the characteristic distribution of petechiae.

Reproduced with permissionfrom Gurd AR, Wilson RI. The fat embolism syndrome. J Bone Joint Surg (Br). 1974;56B:408-416.

TABLE 45-4. Gurd and Wilson Criteria for Diagnosis of Fat Embolism*

Major features
    Respiratory insufficiency
    Cerebral involvement
    Petechial rash
Minor features
    Pyrexia
    Tachycardia
    Retinal changes
    Jaundice
    Renal changes
Laboratory features
    Anemia
    Thrombocytopenia
    Elevated erythrocyte sedimentation rate
    Fat macroglobulinemia

*A positive diagnosis requires one major feature plus four minor features and fat macroglobulinemia.
Reprinted from Dudney TM, Elliott CG. Pulmonary embolism from amniotic fluid, fat, and air. Prog Cardiovasc Dis. 1994;36:447–474, with permission from Elsevier. Table text reproduced with permission and copyright © of the British Editorial Society of Bone and Joint Surgery from the Journal of Bone and Joint Surgery (Br.), Vol. 56B; Gurd AR, Wilson RI; The fat embolism syndrome; 408-16, 1974.

TABLE 45-5. Schonfeld et al. Criteria for Diagnosis of Fat Embolism*

Symptom	Score
Petechiae	5
Diffuse alveolar infiltrates	4
Hypoxemia (arterial PO$_2$ <70 mm Hg)	3
Confusion	1
Fever ≥38°C	1
Heart rate ≥120/min	1
Respiratory rate ≥30/min	1

*A positive diagnosis has a cumulative score ≥5.
Reprinted from Dudney TM, Elliott CG. Pulmonary embolism from amniotic fluid, fat, and air. Prog Cardiovasc Dis. 1994;36:447-474, with permission from Elsevier. Table text reproduced with permission from the American College of Physicians from Schonfeld SA, Ploysongsang Y, DiLisio R, et al. Fat embolism prophylaxis with corticosteroids: a prospective study in high-risk patients. Ann Intern Med. 1983;99:438-443.

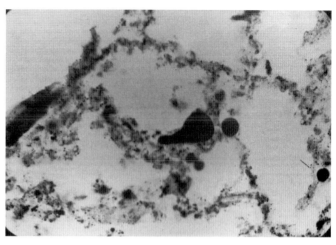

● **FIGURE 45-9.** Oil red O stain (original magnification X 200) demonstrating fat globules in pulmonary capillary arterial bed is shown.

Reproduced, with permission, from Dudney TM, Elliott CG. Pulmonary embolism from amniotic fluid, fat, and air. Prog Cardiovasc Dis. 1994;36;447-474.

does occur, the globules may not remain in the circulation at the time clinical symptoms appear. Evaluation of urine and sputum stainable fat are also insensitive.[287,345] Bronchoalveolar lavage fluid stained with Oil red O for fat was additionally proposed as a potential diagnostic tool in the evaluation of FES, but follow-up studies did not substantiate this early hypothesis[346,347] (Figure 45-9).

Radiologic imaging studies are frequently employed in the evaluation of the patient with suspected FES. While they are not specific for the disorder, they may provide supportive evidence to substantiate clinical suspicion or may serve to exclude other potential etiologies for the clinical

manifestations.[348] The chest radiograph is usually normal initially in the absence of other thoracic abnormalities but may progress over a period of 48 hours to develop a diffuse infiltrative or "snowstorm" pattern consistent with the clinical picture of ARDS[276,332,349,350] (Figure 45-10). The chest radiographic abnormalities generally resolve over a period of 2 weeks.[273,323,351] Ventilation–perfusion scans in

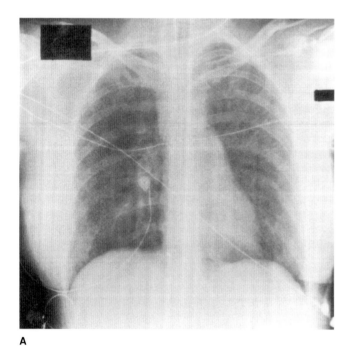

A

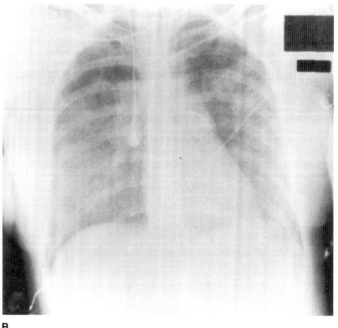

B

● **FIGURE 45-10.** (A) Initial nearly normal chest radiograph in an obtunded patient with a femoral fracture who develops mild respiratory insufficiency. (B) Subsequent progressive coma and moderate ARDS with diffuse infiltrates developed in the ensuing 48 hours in the absence of petechiae.

Reproduced, with permission, from King MB, Harmon KR. Unusual forms of pulmonary embolism. Clin Chest Med. 1994;15:561-580.

FES demonstrate a mottled pattern of subsegmental perfusion defects with normal ventilation, even in the absence of radiographic abnormalities.[352,353] Findings on high resolution CT of the chest may include focal areas of consolidation or ground glass opacities and nodules, predominantly in the non-dependent and peripheral portions of the upper lungs.[354,355] In one case report with pathologic correlation, the ground glass opacities on CT were shown to be the result of diffuse pulmonary hemorrhage.[356] One autopsy series over a 20-year period showed fat globules, edema, and alveolar hemorrhage in the lung initially, followed by hyaline membranes, ARDS, and pneumonia.[357] In patients with neurologic abnormalities, CT of the brain may show either low-density areas in the white matter consistent with infarction or increased density consistent with hemorrhage.[358,359] MRI may have a greater sensitivity in identifying white matter lesions in the central nervous system in the circumstance where the CT of the brain is normal.[360,361] Paradoxical cerebral embolization through a venous to arterial circulation shunt has been studied in elective orthopedic surgery and proposed as a mechanism for the neurologic deficits in FES and is also postulated to be one etiology of postoperative confusion complicating major surgery.[362] A patent foramen may exist in 20% to 34% of the general population[128] and may be the source of systemic emboli (Figure 45-11).

The treatment of FES remains largely supportive, with fairly good prognosis in those patients who meet strict diagnostic criteria for the disorder.[277] The incidence of FES has been shown to be decreased in patients treated with operative versus nonoperative, conservative treatment of long bone and pelvic fractures.[272] The timing of operative intervention would appear to favor early intervention based on both prospective and retrospective analyses, and acute immobilization is recommended.[284,285,363–365] The use of prophylactic steroids has been proposed to decrease the incidence and severity of hypoxemia in patients at risk for FES.[366–368] However, given the low incidence of the disorder, the overall good clinical outcome, and the documentation of a death from infectious complications in one patient treated with steroids for FES, steroid treatment cannot be universally recommended at this time.[343,369–372]

Tumor Embolism

Embolism from malignant cells occurs from a variety of etiologies and can be acute or subacute in its presentation. The first case of tumor embolization to the lungs was reported by Schmidt in 1897,[373,374] with numerous case reports and several autopsy series described over the next century.[373,375–392] The disorder remains an underdiagnosed and likely underappreciated cause of morbidity and mortality in the cancer patient.

The lung is the most common site for malignant metastasis as a result of the potential for intravascular circulation of neoplastic cells.[393] Malignant cells may access the venous circulation by active invasion of small veins, and their subsequent course may result in a picture consistent with thromboembolic disease or with evolving parenchymal metastasis. However, most tumor cells are destroyed by the shear forces of the microcirculation or by effector cells of the immune system, with less than 1% of cells surviving the passage through the lung.[394] Of the cells that do survive, experimental studies have shown that only 20% of emboli evolve into parenchymal metastatic deposits. Acute pulmonary tumor emboli and acute cor pulmonale[395] may result if large tumor emboli obstruct the pulmonary vasculature (Figure 45-12); however, this appears to be a much less common entity than microscopic emboli.[396] Subacute cor pulmonale and associated pulmonary hypertension occur when the tumor emboli lodge in the lumen of the arterioles with subsequent thrombus formation causing endarteritis.[397] Pathologically, Soares et al.[392] described a pulmonary hypertensive arteriopathy consisting of a proliferative endarteritis with hypertrophy and fibrosis of the media and splitting of the elastic lamina in the majority of patients with arterial tumor embolism, in contrast to patients with carcinomatous lymphangitis. They suggest the pathogenesis of the pulmonary hypertensive arteriopathy is therefore due to arrest of the tumor emboli and subsequent damage to the vascular endothelium. Hypertrophy and dilatation of the right ventricle were likewise more common in the patient with arterial tumor embolism,[392] with right ventricular hypertrophy estimated to occur after approximately 2 months of increased right ventricular pressure.[396,398]

Tumor embolism has been documented to occur from a variety of primary sources, including breast, ovaries, lung, choriocarcinoma, stomach, liver, pancreas, prostate,

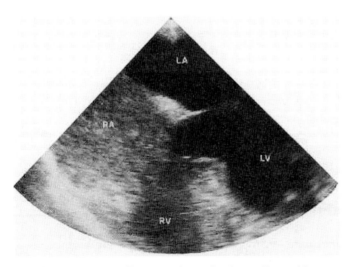

● **FIGURE 45-11.** Transesophageal echocardiographic four-chamber view demonstrates multiple fat emboli in the right atrium (RA) and right ventricle (RV) during intramedullary manipulation. Both right atrium and right ventricle are completely opacified with embolic material.
LA, left atrium; LV, left ventricle.

Reproduced, with permission, from Pell AC, Hughes D, Keating J, et al. Brief report: fulminating fat embolism syndrome caused by paradoxical embolism through a patent foramen ovale. N Engl J Med. 1993;329: 926-929.

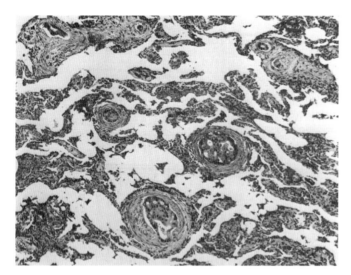

● **FIGURE 45-12.** Autopsy material from patient with primary adenocarcinoma of the lung demonstrates massive tumor embolization in small muscular pulmonary arteries with occlusion by tumor cell clumps and reactive obliterative intimal fibrosis (H & E, X120).

This material is reproduced with permission of Wiley-Liss, Inc., a subsidiary of John Wiley & Sons, Inc. Material is taken from the following article: Gonzalez-Vitale JC, Garcia-Bunuel R. Pulmonary tumor emboli and cor pulmonale in primary carcinoma of the lung. Cancer. 1976;38(5):2105-2110. Copyright © 1976 American Cancer Society.

and kidney.[373,396,399–402] The incidence in retrospective autopsy reviews and a prospective analysis of consecutive autopsies in cancer patients has varied from 0.9% to 26%,[373,392,396,400,403] with tumor embolism thought to be a significant causal factor in the patient's death in 1% to 8% of cases. The incidence has recently been shown in a retrospective review of postmortem examinations to vary according to tumor histopathology and tumor site.[404] In spite of the relatively common occurrence of tumor embolism in autopsy series, the diagnosis is infrequently made antemortem.

The presenting signs and symptoms of tumor embolism are nonspecific and include dyspnea, tachypnea, and tachycardia in association with hypoxemia and respiratory alkalosis. Chest X-rays and ECGs are normal in more than 50% of cases.[394] Tumor embolism generally occurs in the patient with known carcinoma, but has also been reported as the initial presentation of metastatic carcinoma.[401,402,405,406] Acute and subacute cor pulmonale have also been reported.[407,408]

Radiologic studies are frequently employed in the evaluation of a patient who presents with complaints of dyspnea, with or without a known diagnosis of malignancy. Chest radiography is frequently normal in tumor embolism as previously mentioned, or may show signs of primary or metastatic lung cancer. Perfusion scans have shown a characteristic segmental contour pattern[409] in which numerous small defects outline the pulmonary fissures and bronchopulmonary segments; multiple case reports have described a pattern of numerous small, peripheral, or sub-

segmental perfusion defects with normal ventilation, emphasizing the need for consideration of tumor embolization in the differential diagnosis of V/Q mismatch[394,410–415] (Figure 45-13). CT may reveal dilated, beaded peripheral pulmonary arteries or peripheral wedge shaped opacities suggestive of pulmonary infarcts.[416,417] Pulmonary angiography may be unrevealing or may show delayed filling of segmental arteries with pruning and tortuosity of the third to fifth order vessels and occasional subsegmental filling.[418] Tree-in-bud opacities on thin-section CT of the chest have also been reported as manifestations of tumor embolism.[419]

The diagnosis of tumor embolism requires lung biopsy, either transbronchial or by open lung biopsy. There is no clear evidence that early diagnosis alters mortality, although unnecessary anticoagulation could be avoided or appropriate oncologic treatment instituted if there were a simple diagnostic test to differentiate tumor embolism from pulmonary thromboembolism.[420] Geschwind et al.[421] describe a case in which a patient with previously diagnosed breast carcinoma was treated for a presumed pulmonary embolus with both systemic and intra-arterial thrombolytic therapy; subsequent biopsy of the intra-arterial mass demonstrated adenocarcinoma of the breast, which responded to systemic chemotherapy with complete resolution of symptoms.[421] Tumor emboli are an incidental finding at autopsy in anywhere from 18% to 68% of patients, and both macroscopic and microscopic tumor emboli are often diagnosed in patients with previously unknown malignancies.[422] In some instances of tumor embolism, the primary tumor site cannot be determined.[423,424] As in other unusual forms of embolism, a high clinical suspicion is needed to reach the appropriate diagnosis.

Septic Embolism

Septic pulmonary embolism (SPE) historically was a complication of septic pelvic thrombophlebitis caused by septic abortion and postpartum uterine infection,[425] or from appendiceal, prostatic, or diverticular abscesses. More recently, the incidence and etiologies of SPE have changed owing to increases in intravenous drug use, invasive catheters for diagnostic or therapeutic purposes, and the use of immunosuppressive chemotherapeutic agents.[133,201,417,426–434]

Septic phlebitis is an admixture of purulent material and fibrin thrombus, which obstructs small pulmonary vessels, but has as its major consequence pulmonary parenchymal infection. Infections arising from abdominal and pelvic sources are generally anaerobic, with bacteroides and anaerobic streptococci being notable in their invasion of the venous circulation. Septic emboli also result from endocarditis and ventricular septal defects, with the predominant organisms in this instance generally being streptococcus or staphylococcus.[435–438] Pulmonary symptoms tend to predominate in intravenous drug abuse (IVDA) patients with tricuspid valve endocarditis (TVE) and SPE, and these organisms tend to be particularly virulent.[436,439] The increased incidence of SPE with IVDA has been shown in

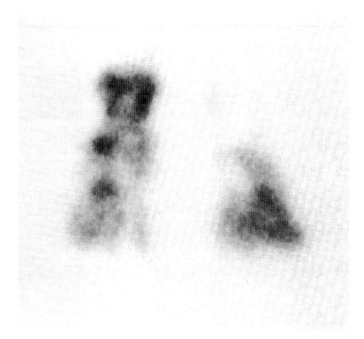
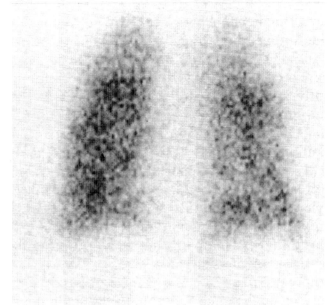

● **FIGURE 45-13.** Posterior view of a ventilation–perfusion scan of a patient with tumor emboli. Multiple bilateral unmatched subsegmental defects are seen in the perfusion scan on the left, with a large defect noted in the right upper lobe. The ventilation scan on the right is normal.

Reproduced, with permission, from Bassiri AG, Haghighi B, Doyle RL, et al. Pulmonary tumor embolism. Am J Respir Crit Care Med. 1997;155:2089-2095.

multiple patient cohorts of intravenous drug users.[440–442] A decrement in SPE associated with IVDA in later studies has been speculated to be related to improved needle hygiene practices[443] and possibly, to less intravenous drug use as a consequence of increased awareness of HIV complications associated with IVDA.[435] Septic pulmonary emboli also arise as a complication of Lemierre's syndrome, which is septicemia arising from inflammatory lesions in tissue cavities where anaerobic organisms exist physiologically, including the pharynx, oral/periodontal areas, middle ear, and the mastoid sinuses. The infection is associated with internal jugular vein thrombosis,[444–448] and subsequent septic pulmonary emboli occur in 97% of cases of Lemierre's syndrome.[449,450] Internal jugular vein thrombosis may also be seen with trauma, head and neck malignancies, hemodialysis shunts, and central venous catheter or Swan-Ganz catheter cannulation of the internal jugular vein. This internal jugular vein thrombosis, if infected, may also lead to SPE.[440,445,451] In cancer patients, Ghanem et al.[431] reported that catheter-related *Staphylococcus aureus* bacteremia with septic thrombosis is more common in those patients with solid tumors, but extravascular complications including septic pulmonary emboli were more common in patients with hematologic malignancies. Central venous catheters in cancer patients have a catheter thrombosis rate as high as 71%, due in part to the hypercoagulable state seen in patients with underlying malignancies.[431] Septic pulmonary emboli have also been detected in infected indwelling long-term catheters and pacemaker

wires.[452] Early diagnosis and aggressive treatment of SPE is imperative, as mortality rates of SPE have been reported to be up to 73% for infected cavitating pulmonary infarcts.[453,454]

Clinical manifestations of SPE may include signs and symptoms of sepsis, fever, cough, purulent sputum, pleuritic chest pain, and hemoptysis. Fever is the most common manifestation, occurring in up to 93% of patients in one study.[426] Predisposing factors for SPE include TVE with or without IVDA, alcoholism, skin infections, immune deficiencies, lymphoma,[33] and septic thrombophlebitis. Depending on the etiology of the septic pulmonary emboli, differing clinical manifestations may be evident. A cardiac murmur may be present in patients with TVE, although this is less commonly noted in TVE in addicts.[436,442] The most specific physical examination finding in septic pelvic thrombophlebitis is a rope or sausage-shaped tender abdominal mass; however, this is a rare finding.[455] Jaundice may occur in SPE in patients with hepatic involvement.[456] In Lemierre's syndrome, tonsillar or peritonsillar abscesses may be noted, as well as tenderness along the sternocleidomastoid muscle and angle of the mandible. Cellulitis, trismus, and dysphagia may also be present in Lemierre's syndrome.[457]

The diagnosis of SPE is generally suspected when appropriate clinical symptoms exist in the presence of clinical risk factors. Fever is commonly present, and a complete blood count and blood cultures should be obtained to assess for leukocytosis and bacteremia, and to guide subsequent

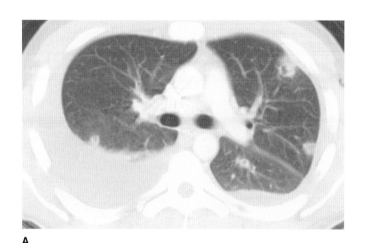

A

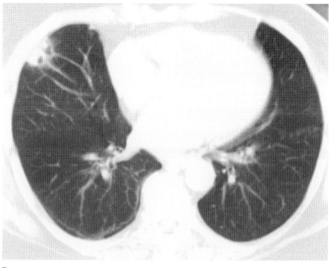

B

● **FIGURE 45-14.** (A) CT of the chest demonstrating four lung nodules, some of which are cavitary, in a patient with Lemierre's syndrome and SPE. Bilateral pleural effusions, a possible complication of SPE, are also present. (B) CT of the chest in a patient with perinephric abscess and SPE, demonstrating a subpleural opacity with cavitations and feeding vessels in the right lung.

Reproduced, with permission, from Cook RJ, Ashton RW, Aughenbaugh GL, et al. Septic pulmonary embolism: presenting features and clinical course of 14 patients. Chest. 2005;128:162-166.

antimicrobial coverage. Clinical signs and symptoms such as fever and cough also dictate review of a chest radiograph, which may be nonspecific, but can include small scattered areas of consolidation or bronchopneumonia with multiple rapidly extending round or wedge shaped peripherally located pulmonary infiltrates.[458] These infiltrates may develop cavitation over a period of hours to a few days,[459] and in some instances, coalesce to form lung abscesses or extend to pleural space involvement with resultant empyema, bronchopleural fistula, or pneumothorax.[460]

CT of the chest is more specific than plain chest radiography in identifying SPE, and reveals multiple nodular opacities with peripheral distribution and both thick and thin walled cavities[452,461–464] (Figure 45-14A). Kwon et al.[465] additionally defined detailed CT characteristics of nodules related to causative organisms, however these characteristics would require further validation before being used to dictate treatment.[465] A "feeding vessel" (Figure 45-14b) has been described as a characteristic CT sign in some studies,[452,462,463] but not in others.[426] A series of patients with SPE who underwent high-resolution multiplanar digital reconstruction (HRMDT) actually showed that the feeding vessel in question was either a pulmonary vein or that the vessel actually coursed around and not into the nodule.[466] The use of ventilation–perfusion scans in SPE is limited, although a "reverse mismatch" pattern has been reported in some instances.[467]

Echocardiography is also useful as a diagnostic tool in patients with SPE[468] and should be performed to screen for endocarditis, valvular insufficiency, perivalvular abscesses, or congestive heart failure.[469] TEE is superior for assessing small vegetations or abscesses,[470–472] and is preferred as a more accurate diagnostic tool in the evaluation of prosthetic valves.[430]

Imaging studies such as abdominal/pelvic CT and MRI are also used in the diagnosis of septic pelvic thrombophlebitis as a potential source for SPE.[455] CT of the neck may be indicated if Lemierre's syndrome is the inciting event in SPE. Ultrasound of the neck is inexpensive and may be used, although it provides poor imaging posterior to the mandible and does not detect intracerebral propagation of clot.[473,474]

The treatment of SPE involves identifying the source of underlying infection and treating accordingly. In patients with cavitary lung lesions, the lack of blood flow in the affected cavity may preclude adequate antibiotic penetration, and in some cases, surgical resection of the cavity may be necessary.[440,459] An infected indwelling catheter as the source of infection should be promptly removed,[133,434] particularly in the presence of fungal infection.[427] If septic pelvic thrombophlebitis is the etiology of the septic emboli, heparin and antibiotics are generally used, and surgical ligation of the IVC or involved pelvic veins, once the treatment of choice, is not now considered necessary.[455,475,476] Infected jugular thrombosis in Lemierre's syndrome likewise rarely requires surgical intervention, with the exception of drainage of an abscess and occasional resection of the vessel in head and neck malignancies. The use of anticoagulants, however, remains controversial in all etiologies of septic thrombophlebitis,[455,475,477–482] and, if used in the presence of septic pulmonary emboli, could lead to increased morbidity and mortality owing to tissue infarction and hemoptysis.

In patients with infective endocarditis as the precursor to SPE, surgical intervention has been suggested as an adjunct to medical therapy when the valvular vegetation was of significant size (>1.0 cm).[468,483–488] The benefit of intervention based on vegetation size has not clearly been demonstrated in other studies, or in the isolated TVE with SPE.[438,489,490] However, Hecht et al.[439] did note an increase in mortality in patients with TVE and vegetations of greater than 2 cm. In the IVDA population with TVE, the tricuspid valve is not always replaced because of concerns for reinfecting a prosthetic valve in the setting of ongoing IVDA. This patient population may later require valve replacement, but in some instances the time elapsing between the initial endocarditis and subsequent valve replacement may allow time for cessation of drug use and improved

outcomes.[491] While the infection in right-sided endocarditis is generally eradicated by antibiotics alone, excision may be required in the setting of persistent bacteremia, ongoing septic pulmonary emboli, congestive heart failure in the absence of left sided valvular involvement, or in the presence of fungal valvular infections.[439,484,491,492]

Miscellaneous Nonthrombotic Emboli

A variety of other miscellaneous causes of nonthrombotic emboli are recorded in the literature, but their description is beyond the scope of this chapter. These emboli may originate from the parasitic sources, most notably *Echinococcus* and *Schistosomiasis*[201,493,494] as well as from invasive diagnostic and therapeutic procedures. Examples of the latter include embolic phenomenon from catheter fragments, particulate matter such as talc in IVDA, iodinated oil, metallic mercury, and methyl methacrylate.[33]

REFERENCES

1. Dalen JE, Alpert JS. Natural history of pulmonary embolism. *Prog Cardiovasc Dis.* 1975;17:259-270.
2. Goldhaber SZ, Visani L, De Rosa M. Acute pulmonary embolism: clinical outcomes in the international cooperative pulmonary embolism registry (ICOPER). *Lancet.* 1999;353:1386-1389.
3. Heit JA. The epidemiology of venous thromboembolism in the community: implications for prevention and management. *J Thromb Thrombolysis.* 2006;21:23-29.
4. Stein PD, Henry JW. Prevalence of acute pulmonary embolism among patients in a general hospital and at autopsy. *Chest.* 1995;108:978-981.
5. Goldhaber SZ, Tapson VF; DVT FREE Steering Committee. A prospective registry of 5451 patients with ultrasound-confirmed deep vein thrombosis. *Am J Cardiol.* 2004;93:259-262.
6. Sevitt S, Gallagher N. Venous thrombosis and pulmonary embolism. A clinico-pathological study in injured and burned patients. *Br J Surg.* 1961;48:475-489.
7. Haire WD. Arm vein thrombosis. *Clin Chest Med.* 1995;16:341-351.
8. McIntyre KM, Sasahara AA. The ratio of pulmonary arterial pressure to pulmonary vascular obstruction: index of preembolic cardiopulmonary status. *Chest.* 1977;71:692-697.
9. Goldhaber SZ, Elliott CG. Acute pulmonary embolism: part I: epidemiology, pathophysiology, and diagnosis. *Circulation.* 2003;108:2726-2729.
10. Tapson VF. Acute pulmonary embolism. *Cardiol Clin.* 2004;22:353-365, v.
11. Rahimtoola A, Bergin JD. Acute pulmonary embolism: an update on diagnosis and management. *Curr Probl Cardiol.* 2005;30:61-114.
12. Itti E, Nguyen S, Robin F, et al. Distribution of ventilation/perfusion ratios in pulmonary embolism: an adjunct to the interpretation of ventilation/perfusion lung scans. *J Nucl Med.* 2002;43:1596-1602.
13. Wood KE. Major pulmonary embolism: review of a pathophysiologic approach to the golden hour of hemodynamically significant pulmonary embolism. *Chest.* 2002;121:877-905.
14. Piazza G, Goldhaber SZ. Acute pulmonary embolism: part I: epidemiology and diagnosis. *Circulation.* 2006;114:e28-e32.
15. Geerts WH, Code KI, Jay RM, Chen E, Szalai JP. A prospective study of venous thromboembolism after major trauma. *N Engl J Med.* 1994;331:1601-1606.
16. Cranley JJ, Canos AJ, Sull WJ. The diagnosis of deep venous thrombosis. Fallibility of clinical symptoms and signs. *Arch Surg.* 1976;111:34-36.
17. Landefeld CS, McGuire E, Cohen AM. Clinical findings associated with acute proximal deep vein thrombosis: a basis for quantifying clinical judgment. *Am J Med.* 1990;88:382-388.
18. Wells PS, Hirsh J, Anderson DR, et al. Accuracy of clinical assessment of deep-vein thrombosis. *Lancet.* 1995;345:1326-1330.
19. Miniati M, Prediletto R, Formichi B, et al. Accuracy of clinical assessment in the diagnosis of pulmonary embolism. *Am J Respir Crit Care Med.* 1999;159:864-871.
20. Langan CJ, Weingart S. New diagnostic and treatment modalities for pulmonary embolism: one path through the confusion. *Mt Sinai J Med.* 2006;73:528-541.
21. Hirsh J, Hoak J. Management of deep vein thrombosis and pulmonary embolism. A statement for healthcare professionals. Council on thrombosis (in consultation with the council on cardiovascular radiology), American Heart Association. *Circulation.* 1996;93:2212-2245.
22. Goldhaber SZ. Pulmonary embolism. *N Engl J Med.* 1998;339:93-104.
23. Fedullo PF, Morris TA. Pulmonary thromboembolism. In: Mason RJ, Broaddus VC, Murray JF, Nadel JA, eds. *Murray and Nadel's Textbook of Respiratory Medicine.* Vol 2. 4th ed. Philadelphia, PA: Elsevier Saunders; 2005:1425-1458.

24. Worsley DF, Alavi A, Aronchick JM, Chen JT, Greenspan RH, Ravin CE. Chest radiographic findings in patients with acute pulmonary embolism: observations from the PIOPED study. *Radiology.* 1993;189:133-136.

25. Tapson VF, Carroll BA, Davidson BL, et al. The diagnostic approach to acute venous thromboembolism. Clinical practice guideline. American Thoracic Society. *Am J Respir Crit Care Med.* 1999;160:1043-1066.

26. Stein PD, Terrin ML, Hales CA, et al. Clinical, laboratory, roentgenographic, and electrocardiographic findings in patients with acute pulmonary embolism and no pre-existing cardiac or pulmonary disease. *Chest.* 1991;100:598-603.

27. Stein PD, Dalen JE, McIntyre KM, Sasahara AA, Wenger NK, Willis PW III. The electrocardiogram in acute pulmonary embolism. *Prog Cardiovasc Dis.* 1975;17:247-257.

28. Rodger M, Makropoulos D, Turek M, et al. Diagnostic value of the electrocardiogram in suspected pulmonary embolism. *Am J Cardiol.* 2000;86:807-809, A10.

29. Dunn KL, Wolf JP, Dorfman DM, Fitzpatrick P, Baker JL, Goldhaber SZ. Normal D-dimer levels in emergency department patients suspected of acute pulmonary embolism. *J Am Coll Cardiol.* 2002;40:1475-1478.

30. Sadosty AT, Boie ET, Stead LG. Pulmonary embolism. *Emerg Med Clin North Am.* 2003;21:363-384.

31. Schrecengost JE, LeGallo RD, Boyd JC, et al. Comparison of diagnostic accuracies in outpatients and hospitalized patients of D-dimer testing for the evaluation of suspected pulmonary embolism. *Clin Chem.* 2003;49:1483-1490.

32. Sostman HD, Coleman RE, DeLong DM, Newman GE, Paine S. Evaluation of revised criteria for ventilation-perfusion scintigraphy in patients with suspected pulmonary embolism. *Radiology.* 1994;193:103-107.

33. Han D, Lee KS, Franquet T, et al. Thrombotic and non-thrombotic pulmonary arterial embolism: spectrum of imaging findings. *Radiographics.* 2003;23:1521-1539.

34. Value of the ventilation/perfusion scan in acute pulmonary embolism. Results of the prospective investigation of pulmonary embolism diagnosis (PIOPED). The PIOPED Investigators. *JAMA.* 1990;263:2753-2759.

35. Remy-Jardin M, Remy J, Wattinne L, Giraud F. Central pulmonary thromboembolism: diagnosis with spiral volumetric CT with the single-breath-hold technique—comparison with pulmonary angiography. *Radiology.* 1992;185:381-387.

36. Sostman HD, Layish DT, Tapson VF, et al. Prospective comparison of helical CT and MR imaging in clinically suspected acute pulmonary embolism. *J Magn Reson Imaging.* 1996; 6:275-281.

37. Drucker EA, Rivitz SM, Shepard JA, et al. Acute pulmonary embolism: assessment of helical CT for diagnosis. *Radiology.* 1998;209:235-241.

38. Perrier A, Howarth N, Didier D, et al. Performance of helical computed tomography in unselected outpatients with suspected pulmonary embolism. *Ann Intern Med.* 2001;135:88-97.

39. Laack TA, Goyal DG. Pulmonary embolism: an unsuspected killer. *Emerg Med Clin North Am.* 2004;22:961-983.

40. Erdman WA, Clarke GD. Magnetic resonance imaging of pulmonary embolism. *Semin Ultrasound CT MR.* 1997;18: 338-348.

41. Stern JB, Abehsera M, Grenet D, et al. Detection of pelvic vein thrombosis by magnetic resonance angiography in patients with acute pulmonary embolism and normal lower limb compression ultrasonography. *Chest.* 2002;122:115-121.

42. Fraser DG, Moody AR, Davidson IR, Martel AL, Morgan PS. Deep venous thrombosis: diagnosis by using venous enhanced subtracted peak arterial MR venography versus conventional venography. *Radiology.* 2003;226:812-820.

43. McConnell MV, Solomon SD, Rayan ME, Come PC, Goldhaber SZ, Lee RT. Regional right ventricular dysfunction detected by echocardiography in acute pulmonary embolism. *Am J Cardiol.* 1996;78:469-473.

44. Leibowitz D. Role of echocardiography in the diagnosis and treatment of acute pulmonary thromboembolism. *J Am Soc Echocardiogr.* 2001;14:921-926.

45. Stein PD, Athanasoulis C, Alavi A, et al. Complications and validity of pulmonary angiography in acute pulmonary embolism. *Circulation.* 1992;85:462-468.

46. Hirsh J, Raschke R. Heparin and low-molecular-weight heparin: the seventh ACCP conference on antithrombotic and thrombolytic therapy. *Chest.* 2004;126:188S-203S.

47. Bernardi E, Piccioli A, Oliboni G, Zuin R, Girolami A, Prandoni P. Nomograms for the administration of unfractionated heparin in the initial treatment of acute thromboembolism—an overview. *Thromb Haemost.* 2000;84:22-26.

48. Tran H, McRae S, Ginsberg J. Anticoagulant treatment of deep vein thrombosis and pulmonary embolism. *Clin Geriatr Med.* 2006;22:113-134, ix.

49. McRae SJ, Ginsberg JS. Initial treatment of venous thromboembolism. *Circulation.* 2004;110:I3-I9.

50. Chong BH. Heparin-induced thrombocytopenia. *J Thromb Haemost.* 2003;1:1471-1478.

51. Gould MK, Dembitzer AD, Doyle RL, Hastie TJ, Garber AM. Low-molecular-weight heparins compared with unfractionated heparin for treatment of acute deep venous thrombosis. A meta-analysis of randomized, controlled trials. *Ann Intern Med.* 1999;130:800-809.

52. Dolovich LR, Ginsberg JS, Douketis JD, Holbrook AM, Cheah G. A meta-analysis comparing low-molecular-weight heparins with unfractionated heparin in the treatment of venous thromboembolism: examining some unanswered questions regarding location of treatment, product type, and dosing frequency. *Arch Intern Med.* 2000;160:181-188.

53. Hull RD, Raskob GE, Brant RF, et al. Low-molecular-weight heparin vs heparin in the treatment of patients with pulmonary embolism. American-Canadian Thrombosis Study Group. *Arch Intern Med.* 2000;160:229-236.

54. Simonneau G, Sors H, Charbonnier B, et al. A comparison of low-molecular-weight heparin with unfractionated heparin for acute pulmonary embolism. The THESEE Study Group. Tinzaparine ou heparine standard: evaluations dans l'embolie pulmonaire. *N Engl J Med.* 1997;337:663-669.

55. Weitz JI. Low-molecular-weight heparins. *N Engl J Med.* 1997;337:688-698.

56. Warkentin TE, Greinacher A. Heparin-induced thrombocytopenia: recognition, treatment, and prevention: the seventh ACCP conference on antithrombotic and thrombolytic therapy. *Chest.* 2004;126:311S-337S.

57. Buller HR, Davidson BL, Decousus H, et al. Subcutaneous fondaparinux versus intravenous unfractionated heparin in the initial treatment of pulmonary embolism. *N Engl J Med.* 2003;349:1695-1702.

58. Piazza G, Goldhaber SZ. Acute pulmonary embolism: part II: treatment and prophylaxis. *Circulation.* 2006;114:e42-e47.

59. Decousus H, Leizorovicz A, Parent F, et al. A clinical trial of vena caval filters in the prevention of pulmonary embolism in patients with proximal deep-vein thrombosis. Prevention du risque d'embolie pulmonaire par interruption cave study group. *N Engl J Med.* 1998;338:409-415.

60. Kucher N, Rossi E, De Rosa M, Goldhaber SZ. Massive pulmonary embolism. *Circulation.* 2006;113:577-582.

61. Millward SF, Oliva VL, Bell SD, et al. Gunther Tulip Retrievable Vena Cava Filter: results from the Registry of the Canadian Interventional Radiology Association. *J Vasc Interv Radiol.* 2001;12:1053-1058.

62. Anderson DR, Levine MN. Thrombolytic therapy for the treatment of acute pulmonary embolism. *CMAJ.* 1992;146:1317-1324.

63. Dalen JE, Alpert JS, Hirsh J. Thrombolytic therapy for pulmonary embolism: is it effective? Is it safe? When is it indicated? *Arch Intern Med.* 1997;157:2550-2556.

64. Goldhaber SZ, Haire WD, Feldstein ML, et al. Alteplase versus heparin in acute pulmonary embolism: randomised trial assessing right-ventricular function and pulmonary perfusion. *Lancet.* 1993;341:507-511.

65. Konstantinides S, Geibel A, Olschewski M, et al. Association between thrombolytic treatment and the prognosis of hemodynamically stable patients with major pulmonary embolism: results of a multicenter registry. *Circulation.* 1997;96:882-888.

66. Konstantinides S, Geibel A, Heusel G, Heinrich F, Kasper W; Management Strategies and Prognosis of Pulmonary Embolism-3 Trial Investigators. Heparin plus alteplase compared with heparin alone in patients with submassive pulmonary embolism. *N Engl J Med.* 2002;347:1143-1150.

67. Aklog L, Williams CS, Byrne JG, Goldhaber SZ. Acute pulmonary embolectomy: a contemporary approach. *Circulation.* 2002;105:1416-1419.

68. Brady AJ, Crake T, Oakley CM. Percutaneous catheter fragmentation and distal dispersion of proximal pulmonary embolus. *Lancet.* 1991;338:1186-1189.

69. De Gregorio MA, Gimeno MJ, Mainar A, et al. Mechanical and enzymatic thrombolysis for massive pulmonary embolism. *J Vasc Interv Radiol.* 2002;13:163-169.

70. Schmitz-Rode T, Gunther RW. New device for percutaneous fragmentation of pulmonary emboli. *Radiology.* 1991;180:135-137.

71. Sze DY, Carey MB, Razavi MK. Treatment of massive pulmonary embolus with catheter-directed tenecteplase. *J Vasc Interv Radiol.* 2001;12:1456-1457.

72. Prevention of fatal postoperative pulmonary embolism by low doses of heparin. An international multicentre trial. *Lancet.* 1975;2:45-51.

73. Koch A, Ziegler S, Breitschwerdt H, Victor N. Low molecular weight heparin and unfractionated heparin in thrombo-sis prophylaxis: meta-analysis based on original patient data. *Thromb Res.* 2001;102:295-309.

74. Geerts WH, Heit JA, Clagett GP, et al. Prevention of venous thromboembolism. *Chest.* 2001;119:132S-175S.

75. Geerts WH, Pineo GF, Heit JA, et al. Prevention of venous thromboembolism: the seventh ACCP conference on antithrombotic and thrombolytic therapy. *Chest.* 2004; 126:338S-400S.

76. Kucher N, Koo S, Quiroz R, et al. Electronic alerts to prevent venous thromboembolism among hospitalized patients. *N Engl J Med.* 2005;352:969-977.

77. Larson CP. Venous air embolism; report of four cases; suggested method of treatment. *Am J Clin Pathol.* 1951;21:247-250.

78. Mansour A, AbdelRaouf S, Qandeel M, Swaidan M. Acute coronary artery air embolism following CT-guided lung biopsy. *Cardiovasc Intervent Radiol.* 2005;28:131-134.

79. Gottlieb JD, Ericsson JA, Sweet RB. Venous air embolism: a review. *Anesth Analg.* 1965;44:773-779.

80. Leslie K, Hui R, Kaye AH. Venous air embolism and the sitting position: a case series. *J Clin Neurosci.* 2006;13:419-422.

81. Domaingue CM. Neurosurgery in the sitting position: a case series. *Anaesth Intensive Care.* 2005;33:332-335.

82. Domaingue CM. Anaesthesia for neurosurgery in the sitting position: a practical approach. *Anaesth Intensive Care.* 2005;33:323-331.

83. van Hulst RA, Klein J, Lachmann B. Gas embolism: pathophysiology and treatment. *Clin Physiol Funct Imaging.* 2003;23:237-246.

84. Gottdiener JS, Papademetriou V, Notargiacomo A, Park WY, Cutler DJ. Incidence and cardiac effects of systemic venous air embolism. Echocardiographic evidence of arterial embolization via noncardiac shunt. *Arch Intern Med.* 1988; 148:795-800.

85. Spiess BD, Sloan MS, McCarthy RJ, et al. The incidence of venous air embolism during total hip arthroplasty. *J Clin Anesth.* 1988;1:25-30.

86. Gei AF, Vadhera RB, Hankins GD. Embolism during pregnancy: thrombus, air, and amniotic fluid. *Anesthesiol Clin North America.* 2003;21:165-182.

87. Lew TW, Tay DH, Thomas E. Venous air embolism during cesarean section: more common than previously thought. *Anesth Analg.* 1993;77:448-452.

88. Kaiser RT. Air embolism death of a pregnant woman secondary to orogenital sex. *Acad Emerg Med.* 1994;1:555-558.

89. McGrath BJ, Zimmerman JE, Williams JF, Parmet J. Carbon dioxide embolism treated with hyperbaric oxygen. *Can J Anaesth.* 1989;36:586-589.

90. Lowenwirt IP, Chi DS, Handwerker SM. Nonfatal venous air embolism during cesarean section: a case report and review of the literature. *Obstet Gynecol Surv.* 1994;49:72-76.

91. Stoloff DR, Isenberg RA, Brill AI. Venous air and gas emboli in operative hysteroscopy. *J Am Assoc Gynecol Laparosc.* 2001;8:181-192.

92. Start RD, Cross SS. Acp. Best practice no 155. Pathological investigation of deaths following surgery, anaesthesia, and medical procedures. *J Clin Pathol.* 1999;52:640-652.

93. Bricker MB, Morris WP, Allen SJ, Tonnesen AS, Butler BD. Venous air embolism in patients with pulmonary barotrauma. *Crit Care Med.* 1994;22:1692-1698.

94. Valic Z, Duplancic D, Bakovic D, et al. Diving-induced venous gas emboli do not increase pulmonary artery pressure. *Int J Sports Med.* 2005;26:626-631.

95. Boussuges A, Pinet C, Thomas P, Bergmann E, Sainty JM, Vervloet D. Haemoptysis after breath-hold diving. *Eur Respir J.* 1999;13:697-699.

96. Kane G, Hewins B, Grannis FW Jr. Massive air embolism in an adult following positive pressure ventilation. *Chest.* 1988;93:874-876.

97. Tolly TL, Feldmeier JE, Czarnecki D. Air embolism complicating percutaneous lung biopsy. *AJR Am J Roentgenol.* 1988;150:555-556.

98. Kodama F, Ogawa T, Hashimoto M, Tanabe Y, Suto Y, Kato T. Fatal air embolism as a complication of CT-guided needle biopsy of the lung. *J Comput Assist Tomogr.* 1999;23:949-951.

99. Arnold BW, Zwiebel WJ. Percutaneous transthoracic needle biopsy complicated by air embolism. *AJR Am J Roentgenol.* 2002;178:1400-1402.

100. Thomas AN, Stephens BG. Air embolism: a cause of morbidity and death after penetrating chest trauma. *J Trauma.* 1974;14:633-638.

101. Estrera AS, Pass LJ, Platt MR. Systemic arterial air embolism in penetrating lung injury. *Ann Thorac Surg.* 1990;50:257-261.

102. Moorthy SS, Tisinai KA, Speiser BS, Cikrit DF, Dierdorf SF. Cerebral air embolism during removal of a pulmonary artery catheter. *Crit Care Med.* 1991;19:981-983.

103. Halliday P, Anderson DN, Davidson AI, Page JG. Management of cerebral air embolism secondary to a disconnected central venous catheter. *Br J Surg.* 1994;81:71.

104. Heckmann JG, Lang CJ, Kindler K, Huk W, Erbguth FJ, Neundorfer B. Neurologic manifestations of cerebral air embolism as a complication of central venous catheterization. *Crit Care Med.* 2000;28:1621-1625.

105. Kuhn M, Fitting JW, Leuenberger P. Acute pulmonary edema caused by venous air embolism after removal of a subclavian catheter. *Chest.* 1987;92:364-365.

106. Orebaugh SL. Venous air embolism: clinical and experimental considerations. *Crit Care Med.* 1992;20:1169-1177.

107. Palmon SC, Moore LE, Lundberg J, Toung T. Venous air embolism: a review. *J Clin Anesth.* 1997;9:251-257.

108. Maddukuri P, Downey BC, Blander JA, Pandian NG, Patel AR. Echocardiographic diagnosis of air embolism associated with central venous catheter placement: case report and review of the literature. *Echocardiography.* 2006;23:315-318.

109. Brouns R, De Surgeloose D, Neetens I, De Deyn PP. Fatal venous cerebral air embolism secondary to a disconnected central venous catheter. *Cerebrovasc Dis.* 2006;21:212-214.

110. Putterman C. Central venous catheterization. Indications, techniques, complications, management. *Acute Care.* 1986;12:219-234.

111. Seidelin PH, Stolarek IH, Thompson AM. Central venous catheterization and fatal air embolism. *Br J Hosp Med.* 1987; 38:438-439.

112. Dunbar EM, Fox R, Watson B, Akrill P. Successful late treatment of venous air embolism with hyperbaric oxygen. *Postgrad Med J.* 1990;66:469-470.

113. Yu AS, Levy E. Paradoxical cerebral air embolism from a hemodialysis catheter. *Am J Kidney Dis.* 1997;29:453-455.

114. Ulyatt DB, Judson JA, Trubuhovich RV, Galler LH. Cerebral arterial air embolism associated with coughing on a continuous positive airway pressure circuit. *Crit Care Med.* 1991;19:985-987.

115. Marini JJ, Culver BH. Systemic gas embolism complicating mechanical ventilation in the adult respiratory distress syndrome. *Ann Intern Med.* 1989;110:699-703.

116. Naulty JS, Ostheimer GW, Datta S, Knapp R, Weiss JB. Incidence of venous air embolism during epidural catheter insertion. *Anesthesiology.* 1982;57:410-412.

117. Husain S, Ahmed L, Al-Sawwaf M. Venous air embolism from intravenous CT contrast administration. *J Am Coll Surg.* 2006;202:197.

118. Groell R, Schaffler GJ, Rienmueller R, Kern R. Vascular air embolism: location, frequency, and cause on electron-beam CT studies of the chest. *Radiology.* 1997;202:459-462.

119. Marco AP, Furman WR. Anesthetic problems. Venous air embolism, airway difficulties, and massive transfusion. *Surg Clin North Am.* 1993;73:213-228.

120. Dudney TM, Elliott CG. Pulmonary embolism from amniotic fluid, fat, and air. *Prog Cardiovasc Dis.* 1994;36:447-474.

121. Fraser RG, Pare JAP, Pare PD, et al., eds. Embolic and thrombotic diseases of the lung. In: *Diagnosis and Diseases of the Chest.* Vol 3. 2nd ed. Philadelphia, PA: Saunders; 1990:1791-1794.

122. Heinemann HO, Fishman AP. Non-respiratory functions of the mammalian lung. *Physiol Rev.* 1969;49:1-47.

123. Marquez J, Sladen A, Gendell H, Boehnke M, Mendelow H. Paradoxical cerebral air embolism without an intracardiac septal defect. Case report. *J Neurosurg.* 1981;55:997-1000.

124. Butler BD, Hills BA. The lung as a filter for microbubbles. *J Appl Physiol.* 1979;47:537-543.

125. Butler BD, Hills BA. Transpulmonary passage of venous air emboli. *J Appl Physiol.* 1985;59:543-547.

126. Black M, Calvin J, Chan KL, Walley VM. Paradoxic air embolism in the absence of an intracardiac defect. *Chest.* 1991;99:754-755.

127. Thackray NM, Murphy PM, McLean RF, deLacy JL. Venous air embolism accompanied by echocardiographic evidence of transpulmonary air passage. *Crit Care Med.* 1996;24:359-361.

128. Hagen PT, Scholz DG, Edwards WD. Incidence and size of patent foramen ovale during the first 10 decades of life: an autopsy study of 965 normal hearts. *Mayo Clin Proc.* 1984;59:17-20.

129. Penther P. Patent foramen ovale: an anatomical study. Apropos of 500 consecutive autopsies. *Arch Mal Coeur Vaiss.* 1994;87:15-21.

130. Schneider B, Zienkiewicz T, Jansen V, Hofmann T, Noltenius H, Meinertz T. Diagnosis of patent foramen ovale by transesophageal echocardiography and correlation with autopsy findings. *Am J Cardiol.* 1996;77:1202-1209.

131. Foster PP, Boriek AM, Butler BD, Gernhardt ML, Bove AA. Patent foramen ovale and paradoxical systemic embolism: a bibliographic review. *Aviat Space Environ Med.* 2003;74:B1-64.

132. Papadopoulos G, Kuhly P, Brock M, Rudolph KH, Link J, Eyrich K. Venous and paradoxical air embolism in the sitting position. A prospective study with transoesophageal echocardiography. *Acta Neurochir (Wien).* 1994;126:140-143.

133. McGee DC, Gould MK. Preventing complications of central venous catheterization. *N Engl J Med.* 2003;348:1123-1133.

134. Flick MR, Hoeffel JM, Staub NC. Superoxide dismutase with heparin prevents increased lung vascular permeability during air emboli in sheep. *J Appl Physiol.* 1983;55:1284-1291.

135. Flick MR, Perel A, Staub NC. Leukocytes are required for increased lung microvascular permeability after microembolization in sheep. *Circ Res.* 1981;48:344-351.

136. Ohkuda K, Nakahara K, Binder A, Staub NC. Venous air emboli in sheep: reversible increase in lung microvascular permeability. *J Appl Physiol.* 1981;51:887-894.

137. Albertine KH, Wiener-Kronish JP, Koike K, Staub NC. Quantification of damage by air emboli to lung microvessels in anesthetized sheep. *J Appl Physiol.* 1984;57:1360-1368.

138. Wang D, Li MH, Hsu K, Shen CY, Chen HI, Lin YC. Air embolism-induced lung injury in isolated rat lungs. *J Appl Physiol.* 1992;72:1235-1242.

139. Kealey GP, Brody MJ. Studies on the mechanism of pulmonary vascular responses to miliary pulmonary embolism. *Circ Res.* 1977;41:807-814.

140. Munson ES. Pathophysiology and treatment of venous air embolism—a review. *Middle East J Anesthesiol.* 1988;9:315-325.

141. Petts JS, Presson RG Jr. A review of the detection and treatment of venous air embolism. *Anesthesiol Rev.* 1992;19:13-21.

142. Hartveit F, Lystad H, Minken A. The pathology of venous air embolism. *Br J Exp Pathol.* 1968;49:81-86.

143. Warren BA, Philp RB, Inwood MJ. The ultrastructural morphology of air embolism: platelet adhesion to the interface and endothelial damage. *Br J Exp Pathol.* 1973;54:163-172.

144. Staub NC, Schultz EL, Albertine KH. Leucocytes and pulmonary microvascular injury. *Ann N Y Acad Sci.* 1982;384:332-343.

145. Jerome EH, Bonsignore MR, Albertine KH, et al. Timing of corticosteroid treatment. Effect of lung lymph dynamics in air injury in awake sheep. *Am Rev Respir Dis.* 1990;142:872-879.

146. Pfitzner J, Petito SP, McLean AG. Hypoxaemia following sustained low-volume venous air embolism in sheep. *Anaesth Intensive Care.* 1988;16:164-170.

147. Perschau RA, Munson ES, Chapin JC. Pulmonary interstitial edema after multiple venous air emboli. *Anesthesiology.* 1976;45:364-368.

148. Lam KK, Hutchinson RC, Gin T. Severe pulmonary oedema after venous air embolism. *Can J Anaesth.* 1993;40:964-967.

149. Adornato DC, Gildenberg PL, Ferrario CM, Smart J, Frost EA. Pathophysiology of intravenous air embolism in dogs. *Anesthesiology.* 1978;49:120-127.

150. Durant TM, Long J, Oppenheimer MJ. Pulmonary (venous) air embolism. *Am Heart J.* 1947;33:269-281.

151. Sviri S, Woods WP, van Heerden PV. Air embolism—a case series and review. *Crit Care Resusc.* 2004;6:271-276.

152. O'Quin RJ, Lakshminarayan S. Venous air embolism. *Arch Intern Med.* 1982;142:2173-2176.

153. Kashuk JL, Penn I. Air embolism after central venous catheterization. *Surg Gynecol Obstet.* 1984;159:249-252.

154. Michenfelder JD, Martin JT, Altenburg BM, Rehder K. Air embolism during neurosurgery. An evaluation of right-atrial catheters for diagnosis and treatment. *JAMA.* 1969;208:1353-1358.

155. English JB, Westenskow D, Hodges MR, Stanley TH. Comparison of venous air embolism monitoring methods in supine dogs. *Anesthesiology.* 1978;48:425-429.

156. Mendieta JM, Roy TM, Denny DM, Ossorio M. Venous air embolism associated with removal of central venous catheters. *J Ky Med Assoc.* 1988;86:169-173.

157. Green HL, Nemir P Jr. Air embolism as a complication during parenteral alimentation. *Am J Surg.* 1971;121:614-616.

158. Dasher WA, Weiss W, Bogen E. The electrocardiographic pattern in venous air embolism. *Dis Chest.* 1955;27:542-546.

159. Kizer KW, Goodman PC. Radiographic manifestations of venous air embolism. *Radiology.* 1982;144:35-39.

160. Cuvelier A, Muir JF. Images in clinical medicine. Venous air embolism. *N Engl J Med.* 2006;354:e26.

161. Wijman CA, Kase CS, Jacobs AK, Whitehead RE. Cerebral air embolism as a cause of stroke during cardiac catheterization. *Neurology.* 1998;51:318-319.

162. Caulfield AF, Lansberg MG, Marks MP, Albers GW, Wijman CA. MRI characteristics of cerebral air embolism from a venous source. *Neurology.* 2006;66:945-946.

163. Fitchet A, Fitzpatrick AP. Central venous air embolism causing pulmonary oedema mimicking left ventricular failure. *BMJ.* 1998;316:604-606.

164. Chang JL, Albin MS, Bunegin L, Hung TK. Analysis and comparison of venous air embolism detection methods. *Neurosurgery.* 1980;7:135-141.

165. Cucchiara RF, Nugent M, Seward JB, Messick JM. Air embolism in upright neurosurgical patients: detection and localization by two-dimensional transesophageal echocardiography. *Anesthesiology.* 1984;60:353-355.

166. Souders JE. Pulmonary air embolism. *J Clin Monit Comput.* 2000;16:375-383.

167. Gildenberg PL, O'Brien RP, Britt WJ, Frost EA. The efficacy of Doppler monitoring for the detection of venous air embolism. *J Neurosurg.* 1981;54:75-78.

168. Schubert A, Deogaonkar A, Drummond JC. Precordial Doppler probe placement for optimal detection of venous air embolism during craniotomy. *Anesth Analg.* 2006;102:1543-1547.

169. Craft RM, Weglinski MR, Perkins WJ, Losasso TJ. Precordial Doppler probe placement for detecting venous air embolism reassessed. *Anaesthesia.* 1994;81:A230.

170. Muth CM, Shank ES. Gas embolism. *N Engl J Med.* 2000;342:476-482.

171. Marshall WK, Bedford RF. Use of a pulmonary-artery catheter for detection and treatment of venous air embolism: a prospective study in man. *Anesthesiology.* 1980;52:131-134.

172. Colley PS, Artru AA. Bunegin-albin catheter improves air retrieval and resuscitation from lethal venous air embolism in dogs. *Anesth Analg.* 1987;66:991-994.

173. Bunegin L, Albin MS, Helsel PE, Hoffman A, Hung TK. Positioning the right atrial catheter: a model for reappraisal. *Anesthesiology.* 1981;55:343-348.

174. Munson ES. Effect of nitrous oxide on the pulmonary circulation during venous air embolism. *Anesth Analg.* 1971; 50:785-793.

175. Munson ES. Transfer of nitrous oxide into body air cavities. *Br J Anaesth.* 1974;46:202-209.

176. Ordway CB. Air embolus via CVP catheter without positive pressure: presentation of case and review. *Ann Surg.* 1974; 179:479-481.

177. Ericsson JA, Gottlieb JD, Sweet RB. Closed-chest cardiac massage in the treatment of venous air embolism. *N Engl J Med.* 1964;270:1353-1354.

178. Alvaran SB, Toung JK, Graff TE, Benson DW. Venous air embolism: comparative merits of external cardiac massage, intracardiac aspiration, and left lateral decubitus position. *Anesth Analg.* 1978;57:166-170.

179. Layon AJ. Hyperbaric oxygen treatment for cerebral air embolism—where are the data? *Mayo Clin Proc.* 1991;66: 641-646.

180. Fowler MJ Jr, Thomas CE, Koenigsberg RA, Schwartzman RJ, Kantharia BK. Diffuse cerebral air embolism treated with hyperbaric oxygen: a case report. *J Neuroimaging.* 2005;15: 92-96.

181. Thom SR. Barotrauma, decompression sickness, and air embolism. In: Carlson RW, Geheb MA, eds. *Principles and Practice of Medical Intensive Care.* Philadelphia, PA: Saunders; 1993:907-911.

182. Meyer JR. Embolis pulmonary caseosa. *Bras Med.* 1926;1: 301-303.

183. Steiner PE, Lushbaugh CC. Landmark article, Oct. 1941: Maternal pulmonary embolism by amniotic fluid as a cause of obstetric shock and unexpected deaths in obstetrics. By Paul E. Steiner and C. C. Lushbaugh. *JAMA.* 1986;255:2187-2203.

184. Gilbert WM, Danielsen B. Amniotic fluid embolism: decreased mortality in a population-based study. *Obstet Gynecol.* 1999;93:973-977.

185. Clark SL, Hankins GD, Dudley DA, Dildy GA, Porter TF. Amniotic fluid embolism: analysis of the National Registry. *Am J Obstet Gynecol.* 1995;172:1158-1167; discussion 1167-1169.

186. Kramer MS, Rouleau J, Baskett TF, Joseph KS; Maternal Health Study Group of the Canadian Perinatal Surveillance System. Amniotic-fluid embolism and medical induction of labour: a retrospective, population-based cohort study. *Lancet.* 2006;368:1444-1448.

187. Liban E, Raz S. A clinicopathologic study of fourteen cases of amniotic fluid embolism. *Am J Clin Pathol.* 1969;51:477-486.

188. Barno A, Freeman DW. Amniotic fluid embolism. *Am J Obstet Gynecol.* 1959;77:1199-1210.

189. Abouleish E. Amniotic fluid embolism: report of a fatal case. *Anesth Analg.* 1974;53:549-553.

190. Morgan M. Amniotic fluid embolism. *Anaesthesia.* 1979;34: 20-32.

191. Kaunitz AM, Hughes JM, Grimes DA, Smith JC, Rochat RW, Kafrissen ME. Causes of maternal mortality in the United States. *Obstet Gynecol.* 1985;65:605-612.

192. Moore J, Baldisseri MR. Amniotic fluid embolism. *Crit Care Med.* 2005;33:S279-S285.

193. Tuffnell DJ. Amniotic fluid embolism. *Curr Opin Obstet Gynecol.* 2003;15:119-122.

194. Burrows A, Khoo SK. The amniotic fluid embolism syndrome: 10 years' experience at a major teaching hospital. *Aust N Z J Obstet Gynaecol.* 1995;35:245-250.

195. Tuffnell DJ. United Kingdom amniotic fluid embolism register. *BJOG.* 2005;112:1625-1629.

196. Chatelain SM, Quirk JG Jr. Amniotic and thromboembolism. *Clin Obstet Gynecol.* 1990;33:473-481.

197. Clark SL. Amniotic fluid embolism. *Crit Care Clin.* 1991;7: 877-882.

198. Clark SL, Montz FJ, Phelan JP. Hemodynamic alterations associated with amniotic fluid embolism: a reappraisal. *Am J Obstet Gynecol.* 1985;151:617-621.

199. Hankins GD, Snyder RR, Clark SL, Schwartz L, Patterson WR, Butzin CA. Acute hemodynamic and respiratory effects of amniotic fluid embolism in the pregnant goat model. *Am J Obstet Gynecol.* 1993;168:1113-1129; discussion 1129-1130.

200. Clark SL. Successful pregnancy outcomes after amniotic fluid embolism. *Am J Obstet Gynecol.* 1992;167:511-512.

201. King MB, Harmon KR. Unusual forms of pulmonary embolism. *Clin Chest Med.* 1994;15:561-580.

202. Dashow EE, Cotterill R, Benedetti TJ, Myhre S, Kovanda C, Sarrafan A. Amniotic fluid embolus. A report of two cases resulting in maternal survival. *J Reprod Med.* 1989;34:660-666.

203. Gregory MG, Clayton EM Jr. Amniotic fluid embolism. *Obstet Gynecol.* 1973;42:236-244.

204. Lumley J, Owen R, Morgan M. Amniotic fluid embolism. A report of three cases. *Anaesthesia.* 1979;34:33-36.

205. Resnik R, Swartz WH, Plumer MH, Benirschke K, Stratthaus ME. Amniotic fluid embolism with survival. *Obstet Gynecol.* 1976;47:295-298.

206. Masson RG. Amniotic fluid embolism. *Clin Chest Med.* 1992;13:657-665.

207. Davies S. Amniotic fluid embolus: a review of the literature. *Can J Anaesth.* 2001;48:88-98.

208. Fletcher SJ, Parr MJ. Amniotic fluid embolism: a case report and review. *Resuscitation.* 2000;43:141-146.

209. Benson MD. Nonfatal amniotic fluid embolism. Three possible cases and a new clinical definition. *Arch Fam Med.* 1993;2:989-994.

210. Clutton-Brock T. Maternal deaths from anaesthesia. An extract from why mothers die 2000-2002, the confidential

enquiries into maternal deaths in the United Kingdom: trends in intensive care. *Br J Anaesth*. 2005;94:424-429.

211. Attwood HD. The histological diagnosis of amniotic-fluid embolism. *J Pathol Bacteriol*. 1958;76:211-215.

212. Clark SL, Cotton DB, Gonik B, Greenspoon J, Phelan JP. Central hemodynamic alterations in amniotic fluid embolism. *Am J Obstet Gynecol*. 1988;158:1124-1126.

213. Clark SL, Cotton DB, Lee W, et al. Central hemodynamic assessment of normal term pregnancy. *Am J Obstet Gynecol*. 1989;161:1439-1442.

214. Clark SL. Amniotic fluid embolism. *Clin Perinatol*. 1986;13: 801-811.

215. Clark SL. Amniotic fluid embolism and leukotrienes. *Am J Obstet Gynecol*. 1988;158:681.

216. Adamsons K, Mueller-Heubach E, Myers RE. The innocuousness of amniotic fluid infusion in the pregnant rhesus monkey. *Am J Obstet Gynecol*. 1971;109:977-984.

217. Stolte L, van Kessel H, Seelen J, Eskes T, Wagatsuma T. Failure to produce the syndrome of amniotic fluid embolism by infusion of amniotic fluid and meconium into monkeys. *Am J Obstet Gynecol*. 1967;98:694-697.

218. Clark SL. Arachidonic acid metabolites and the pathophysiology of amniotic fluid embolism. *Semin Reprod Endocrinol*. 1985;3:253-257.

219. Wagner M. From caution to certainty: hazards in the formation of evidence-based practice—a case study on evidence for an association between the use of uterine stimulant drugs and amniotic fluid embolism. *Paediatr Perinat Epidemiol*. 2005;19:173-176.

220. Drife J. Amniotic fluid embolism. In: Editorial Board of the Confidential Enquiries into Maternal Deaths in the United Kingdom, ed. *Why Mothers Die 1997-1999. Fifth Report of the Confidential Enquiries into Maternal Deaths in the United Kingdom*. London: RCOG Press; 2001. http://www.Cemd.Org.uk/reports/c5.Pdf. Accessed January 8, 2007.

221. Dorfman SF. Maternal mortality in new york city, 1981-1983. *Obstet Gynecol*. 1990;76:317-323.

222. Peterson EP, Taylor HB. Amniotic fluid embolism. An analysis of 40 cases. *Obstet Gynecol*. 1970;35:787-793.

223. Graham HK. Amniotic fluid embolism. *Am J Obstet Gynecol*. 1955;70:657-659.

224. Aurangzeb I, George L, Raoof S. Amniotic fluid embolism. *Crit Care Clin*. 2004;20:643-650.

225. Harboe T, Benson MD, Oi H, Softeland E, Bjorge L, Guttormsen AB. Cardiopulmonary distress during obstetrical anaesthesia: attempts to diagnose amniotic fluid embolism in a case series of suspected allergic anaphylaxis. *Acta Anaesthesiol Scand*. 2006;50:324-330.

226. Chesnutt AN. Physiology of normal pregnancy. *Crit Care Clin*. 2004;20:609-615.

227. Clark SL. New concepts of amniotic fluid embolism: a review. *Obstet Gynecol Surv*. 1990;45:360-368.

228. Clark SL, Pavlova Z, Greenspoon J, Horenstein J, Phelan JP. Squamous cells in the maternal pulmonary circulation. *Am J Obstet Gynecol*. 1986;154:104-106.

229. Lee W, Ginsburg KA, Cotton DB, Kaufman RH. Squamous and trophoblastic cells in the maternal pulmonary

circulation identified by invasive hemodynamic monitoring during the peripartum period. *Am J Obstet Gynecol*. 1986; 155:999-1001.

230. Fava S, Galizia AC. Amniotic fluid embolism. *Br J Obstet Gynaecol*. 1993;100:1049-1050.

231. Plauche WC. Amniotic fluid embolism. *Am J Obstet Gynecol*. 1983;147:982-983.

232. Farrar SC, Gherman RB. Serum tryptase analysis in a woman with amniotic fluid embolism. A case report. *J Reprod Med*. 2001;46:926-928.

233. Nishio H, Matsui K, Miyazaki T, Tamura A, Iwata M, Suzuki K. A fatal case of amniotic fluid embolism with elevation of serum mast cell tryptase. *Forensic Sci Int*. 2002;126:53-56.

234. Kobayashi H, Ohi H, Terao T. A simple, noninvasive, sensitive method for diagnosis of amniotic fluid embolism by monoclonal antibody TKH-2 that recognizes NeuAc alpha 2-6GalNAc. *Am J Obstet Gynecol*. 1993;168:848-853.

235. Benson MD, Lindberg RE. Amniotic fluid embolism, anaphylaxis, and tryptase. *Am J Obstet Gynecol*. 1996;175:737.

236. Aguilera LG, Fernandez C, Plaza A, Gracia J, Gomar C. Fatal amniotic fluid embolism diagnosed histologically. *Acta Anaesthesiol Scand*. 2002;46:334-337.

237. Fineschi V, Gambassi R, Gherardi M, Turillazzi E. The diagnosis of amniotic fluid embolism: an immunohistochemical study for the quantification of pulmonary mast cell tryptase. *Int J Legal Med*. 1998;111:238-243.

238. Karetzky M, Ramirez M. Acute respiratory failure in pregnancy. An analysis of 19 cases. *Medicine (Baltimore)*. 1998;77: 41-49.

239. Benson MD, Kobayashi H, Silver RK, Oi H, Greenberger PA, Terao T. Immunologic studies in presumed amniotic fluid embolism. *Obstet Gynecol*. 2001;97:510-514.

240. Kanayama N, Yamazaki T, Naruse H, Sumimoto K, Horiuchi K, Terao T. Determining zinc coproporphyrin in maternal plasma—a new method for diagnosing amniotic fluid embolism. *Clin Chem*. 1992;38:526-529.

241. Lockwood CJ, Bach R, Guha A, Zhou XD, Miller WA, Nemerson Y. Amniotic fluid contains tissue factor, a potent initiator of coagulation. *Am J Obstet Gynecol*. 1991;165:1335-1341.

242. Attwood HD. Fatal pulmonary embolism by amniotic fluid. *J Clin Pathol*. 1956;9:38-46.

243. Fidler JL, Patz EF Jr, Ravin CE. Cardiopulmonary complications of pregnancy: radiographic findings. *AJR Am J Roentgenol*. 1993;161:937-942.

244. Green BT, Umana E. Amniotic fluid embolism. *South Med J*. 2000;93:721-723.

245. James CF, Feinglass NG, Menke DM, Grinton SF, Papadimos TJ. Massive amniotic fluid embolism: diagnosis aided by emergency transesophageal echocardiography. *Int J Obstet Anesth*. 2004;13:279-283.

246. Girard P, Mal H, Laine JF, Petitpretz P, Rain B, Duroux P. Left heart failure in amniotic fluid embolism. *Anesthesiology*. 1986;64:262-265.

247. Stanten RD, Iverson LI, Daugharty TM, Lovett SM, Terry C, Blumenstock E. Amniotic fluid embolism causing catastrophic pulmonary vasoconstriction: diagnosis by

transesophageal echocardiogram and treatment by cardiopulmonary bypass. *Obstet Gynecol.* 2003;102:496-498.

248. Munnur U, Suresh MS. Airway problems in pregnancy. *Crit Care Clin.* 2004;20:617-642.

249. Garcia-Rio F, Pino JM, Gomez L, Alvarez-Sala R, Villasante C, Villamor J. Regulation of breathing and perception of dyspnea in healthy pregnant women. *Chest.* 1996;110:446-453.

250. Mallampalli A, Powner DJ, Gardner MO. Cardiopulmonary resuscitation and somatic support of the pregnant patient. *Crit Care Clin.* 2004;20:747-761, x.

251. Dildy GA, Clark SL. Cardiac arrest during pregnancy. *Obstet Gynecol Clin North Am.* 1995;22:303-314.

252. McDougall RJ, Duke GJ. Amniotic fluid embolism syndrome: case report and review. *Anaesth Intensive Care.* 1995; 23:735-740.

253. Bernard GR, Sopko G, Cerra F, et al. Pulmonary artery catheterization and clinical outcomes: National Heart, Lung, and Blood Institute and Food and Drug Administration workshop report. Consensus statement. *JAMA.* 2000;283:2568-2572.

254. Connors AF Jr, Speroff T, Dawson NV, et al. The effectiveness of right heart catheterization in the initial care of critically ill patients. SUPPORT investigators. *JAMA.* 1996;276:889-897.

255. Pinsky MR, Vincent JL. Let us use the pulmonary artery catheter correctly and only when we need it. *Crit Care Med.* 2005;33:1119-1122.

256. Richard C, Warszawski J, Anguel N, et al. Early use of the pulmonary artery catheter and outcomes in patients with shock and acute respiratory distress syndrome: a randomized controlled trial. *JAMA.* 2003;290:2713-2720.

257. Rhodes A, Cusack RJ, Newman PJ, Grounds RM, Bennett ED. A randomised, controlled trial of the pulmonary artery catheter in critically ill patients. *Intensive Care Med.* 2002; 28:256-264.

258. Shah MR, Hasselblad V, Stevenson LW, et al. Impact of the pulmonary artery catheter in critically ill patients: meta-analysis of randomized clinical trials. *JAMA.* 2005;294: 1664-1670.

259. Bick RL. Syndromes of disseminated intravascular coagulation in obstetrics, pregnancy, and gynecology. Objective criteria for diagnosis and management. *Hematol Oncol Clin North Am.* 2000;14:999-1044.

260. Bick RL. Disseminated intravascular coagulation. Objective criteria for diagnosis and management. *Med Clin North Am.* 1994;78:511-543.

261. Brandjes DP, Schenk BE, Buller HR, ten Cate JW. Management of disseminated intravascular coagulation in obstetrics. *Eur J Obstet Gynecol Reprod Biol.* 1991;42(suppl):S87-S89.

262. Kent KJ, Cooper BC, Thomas KW, Zlatnik FJ. Presumed antepartum amniotic fluid embolism. *Obstet Gynecol.* 2003; 102:493-495.

263. Locksmith GJ. Amniotic fluid embolism. *Obstet Gynecol Clin North Am.* 1999;26:435-444, vii.

264. Tanus-Santos JE, Moreno H Jr. Inhaled nitric oxide and amniotic fluid embolism. *Anesth Analg.* 1999;88:691.

265. Dodgson J, Martin J, Boswell J, Goodall HB, Smith R. Probable amniotic fluid embolism precipitated by amniocentesis and treated by exchange transfusion. *Br Med J (Clin Res Ed).* 1987;294:1322-1323.

266. Van Heerden PV, Webb SA, Hee G, Corkeron M, Thompson WR. Inhaled aerosolized prostacyclin as a selective pulmonary vasodilator for the treatment of severe hypoxaemia. *Anaesth Intensive Care.* 1996;24:87-90.

267. Kaneko Y, Ogihara T, Tajima H, Mochimaru F. Continuous hemodiafiltration for disseminated intravascular coagulation and shock due to amniotic fluid embolism: report of a dramatic response. *Intern Med.* 2001;40:945-947.

268. Hsieh YY, Chang CC, Li PC, Tsai HD, Tsai CH. Successful application of extracorporeal membrane oxygenation and intra-aortic balloon counterpulsation as lifesaving therapy for a patient with amniotic fluid embolism. *Am J Obstet Gynecol.* 2000;183:496-497.

269. Esposito RA, Grossi EA, Coppa G, et al. Successful treatment of postpartum shock caused by amniotic fluid embolism with cardiopulmonary bypass and pulmonary artery thromboembolectomy. *Am J Obstet Gynecol.* 1990;163:572-574.

270. Knight M, Kurinczuk JJ, Tuffnell D, Brocklehurst P. The UK obstetric surveillance system for rare disorders of pregnancy. *BJOG.* 2005;112:263-265.

271. Evarts CM. The fat embolism syndrome: a review. *Surg Clin North Am.* 1970;50:493-507.

272. Riska EB, Myllynen P. Fat embolism in patients with multiple injuries. *J Trauma.* 1982;22:891-894.

273. Mellor A, Soni N. Fat embolism. *Anaesthesia.* 2001;56:145-154.

274. Fabian TC, Hoots AV, Stanford DS, Patterson CR, Mangiante EC. Fat embolism syndrome: prospective evaluation in 92 fracture patients. *Crit Care Med.* 1990;18:42-46.

275. Bulger EM, Smith DG, Maier RV, Jurkovich GJ. Fat embolism syndrome. A 10-year review. *Arch Surg.* 1997;132: 435-439.

276. Fat embolism syndrome. *West J Med.* 1984;141:501-505.

277. Guenter CA, Braun TE. Fat embolism syndrome. Changing prognosis. *Chest.* 1981;79:143-145.

278. Pollak R, Myers RA. Early diagnosis of the fat embolism syndrome. *J Trauma.* 1978;18:121-123.

279. Carr JB, Hansen ST. Fulminant fat embolism. *Orthopedics.* 1990;13:258-261.

280. Hagley SR. The fulminant fat embolism syndrome. *Anaesth Intensive Care.* 1983;11:162-166.

281. McCarthy B, Mammen E, Leblanc LP, Wilson RF. Subclinical fat embolism: a prospective study of 50 patients with extremity fractures. *J Trauma.* 1973;13:9-16.

282. Palmovic V, McCarroll JR. Fat embolism in trauma. *Arch Pathol.* 1965;80:630-635.

283. Byrick RJ, Kay JC, Mullen JB. Capnography is not as sensitive as pulmonary artery pressure monitoring in detecting marrow microembolism. Studies in a canine model. *Anesth Analg.* 1989;68:94-100.

284. Johnson KD, Cadambi A, Seibert GB. Incidence of adult respiratory distress syndrome in patients with multiple musculoskeletal injuries: effect of early operative stabilization of fractures. *J Trauma.* 1985;25:375-384.

285. Riska EB, von Bonsdorff H, Hakkinen S, Jaroma H, Kiviluoto O, Paavilainen T. Prevention of fat embolism by early internal fixation of fractures in patients with multiple injuries. *Injury.* 1976;8:110-116.

286. Tachakra SS, Potts D, Idowu A. Early operative fracture management of patients with multiple injuries. *Br J Surg.* 1990;77:1194.

287. Herndon JH, Bechtol CO, Crickenberger DP. Fat embolism during total hip replacement. A prospective study. *J Bone Joint Surg Am.* 1974;56:1350-1362.

288. Hagley SR, Lee FC, Blumbergs PC. Fat embolism syndrome with total hip replacement. *Med J Aust.* 1986;145:541-543.

289. Caillouette JT, Anzel SH. Fat embolism syndrome following the intramedullary alignment guide in total knee arthroplasty. *Clin Orthop Relat Res.* 1990;(251):198-199.

290. Orsini EC, Richards RR, Mullen JM. Fatal fat embolism during cemented total knee arthroplasty: a case report. *Can J Surg.* 1986;29:385-386.

291. Galdermans D, Coolen D, Neetens I, Bultinck J, Parizel G. Pulmonary fat embolism presenting as chronic respiratory failure. *Eur Respir J.* 1989;2:185-187.

292. Edwards KJ, Cummings RJ. Fat embolism as a complication of closed femoral shortening. *J Pediatr Orthop.* 1992;12:542-543.

293. Pollak S, Vycudilik W. Pulmonary lipids in fatal burns (author's transl). *Wien Klin Wochenschr.* 1981;93:111-117.

294. Nichols GR II, Corey TS, Davis GJ. Nonfracture-associated fatal fat embolism in a case of child abuse. *J Forensic Sci.* 1990;35:493-499.

295. Lynch MJ. Nephrosis and fat embolism in acute hemorrhagic pancreatitis. *AMA Arch Intern Med.* 1954;94:709-717.

296. Guardia SN, Bilbao JM, Murray D, Warren RE, Sweet J. Fat embolism in acute pancreatitis. *Arch Pathol Lab Med.* 1989;113:503-506.

297. Broder G, Ruzumna L. Systemic fat embolism following acute primary osteomyelitis. *JAMA.* 1967;199:150-152.

298. Cuppage FE. Fat embolism in diabetes mellitus. *Am J Clin Pathol.* 1963;40:270-275.

299. Laub DR Jr, Laub DR. Fat embolism syndrome after liposuction: a case report and review of the literature. *Ann Plast Surg.* 1990;25:48-52.

300. Dillerud E. Re: fat embolism after liposuction. *Ann Plast Surg.* 1991;26:293.

301. Ross RM, Johnson GW. Fat embolism after liposuction. *Chest.* 1988;93:1294-1295.

302. Christman KD. Death following suction lipectomy and abdominoplasty. *Plast Reconstr Surg.* 1986;78:428.

303. Boezaart AP, Clinton CW, Braun S, Oettle C, Lee NP. Fulminant adult respiratory distress syndrome after suction lipectomy. A case report. *S Afr Med J.* 1990;78:693-695.

304. Menendez LR, Bacon W, Kempf RA, Moore TM. Fat embolism syndrome complicating intraarterial chemotherapy with cis-platinum. *Clin Orthop Relat Res.* 1990;(254):294-297.

305. Baselga J, Reich L, Doherty M, Gulati S. Fat embolism syndrome following bone marrow harvesting. *Bone Marrow Transplant.* 1991;7:485-486.

306. Lipton JH, Russell JA, Burgess KR, Hwang WS. Fat embolization and pulmonary infiltrates after bone marrow transplantation. *Med Pediatr Oncol.* 1987;15:24-27.

307. Durlacher SH, Meier JR, Fisher RS, Lovitt WV. Sudden death due to pulmonary fat embolism in chronic alcoholics with fatty liver. *Acta Med Leg Soc (Liege).* 1958;11:229-230.

308. Lynch MJ, Raphael SS, Dixon TP. Fat embolism in chronic alcoholism; control study on incidence of fat embolism. *AMA Arch Pathol.* 1959;67:68-80.

309. McCracken M. Fat embolism after lipid emulsion infusion. *Lancet.* 1991;337:983.

310. Jones JP Jr, Engleman EP, Najarian JS. Systemic fat embolism after renal homotransplantation and treatment with corticosteroids. *N Engl J Med.* 1965;273:1453-1458.

311. Hill RB. Fatal fat embolism from steroid-induced fatty liver. *N Engl J Med.* 1961;265:318-320.

312. Rosen JM, Braman SS, Hasan FM, Teplitz C. Nontraumatic fat embolization. A rare cause of new pulmonary infiltrates in an immunocompromised patient. *Am Rev Respir Dis.* 1986;134:805-808.

313. Hulman G. Pathogenesis of non-traumatic fat embolism. *Lancet.* 1988;1:1366-1367.

314. Graber S. Fat embolization associated with sickle cell crisis. *South Med J.* 1961;54:1395-1398.

315. Garza JA. Massive fat and necrotic bone marrow embolization in a previously undiagnosed patient with sickle cell disease. *Am J Forensic Med Pathol.* 1990;11:83-88.

316. Miller JA, Fonkalsrud EW, Latta HL, Maloney JV Jr. Fat embolism associated with extracorporeal circulation and blood transfusion. *Surgery.* 1962;51:448-451.

317. Adams JE, Owens G, Mann G, Headrick JR, Munoz A, Scott HW Jr. Experimental evaluation of pluronic F68 (A nonionic detergent) as a method of diminishing systemic fat emboli resulting from prolonged cardiopulmonary bypass. *Surg Forum.* 1960;10:585-589.

318. Hoefnagels WA, Gerritsen EJ, Brouwer OF, Souverijn JH. Cyclosporin encephalopathy associated with fat embolism induced by the drug's solvent. *Lancet.* 1988;2:901.

319. Krupp P, Busch M, Cockburn I, Schreiber B. Encephalopathy associated with fat embolism induced by solvent for cyclosporin. *Lancet.* 1989;1:168-169.

320. Peltier LF. Fat embolism. A perspective. *Clin Orthop Relat Res.* 1988;(232):263-270.

321. Lehman EP, Moore RM. Fat embolism; including experimental production without trauma. *Arch Surg.* 1927;14:621.

322. Gauss H. The pathology of fat embolism. *Arch Surg.* 1924;9:593.

323. Shier MR, Wilson RF. Fat embolism syndrome: traumatic coagulopathy with respiratory distress. *Surg Annu.* 1980;12:139-168.

324. Byrick RJ, Forbes D, Waddell JP. A monitored cardiovascular collapse during cemented total knee replacement. *Anesthesiology.* 1986;65:213-216.

325. Pell AC, Hughes D, Keating J, Christie J, Busuttil A, Sutherland GR. Brief report: fulminating fat embolism syndrome caused by paradoxical embolism through a patent foramen ovale. *N Engl J Med.* 1993;329:926-929.

326. Gossling HR, Pellegrini VD Jr. Fat embolism syndrome: a review of the pathophysiology and physiological basis of treatment. *Clin Orthop Relat Res.* 1982;(165):68-82.

327. Masson RG, Ruggieri J. Pulmonary microvascular cytology. A new diagnostic application of the pulmonary artery catheter. *Chest.* 1985;88:908-914.

328. Bruecke P, Burke JF, Lam KW, Shannon DC, Kazemi H. The pathophysiology of pulmonary fat embolism. *J Thorac Cardiovasc Surg.* 1971;61:949-955.

329. Fonte DA, Hausberger FX. Pulmonary free fatty acids in experimental fat embolism. *J Trauma.* 1971;11:668-672.

330. Riseborough EJ, Herndon JH. Alterations in pulmonary function, coagulation and fat metabolism in patients with fractures of the lower limbs. *Clin Orthop Relat Res.* 1976;(115):248-267.

331. Peltier LF. Fat embolism. III. The toxic properties of neutral fat and free fatty acids. *Surgery.* 1956;40:665-670.

332. Lepisto P, Alho A. Diagnostic features of the fat embolism syndrome. *Acta Chir Scand.* 1975;141:245-250.

333. Sevitt S. The significance and pathology of fat embolism. *Ann Clin Res.* 1977;9:173-180.

334. Prys-Roberts C, Greenbaum R, Nunn JF, Kelman GR. Disturbances of pulmonary function in patients with fat embolism. *J Clin Pathol Suppl (R Coll Pathol).* 1970;4:143-149.

335. Ross AP. The fat embolism syndrome: with special reference to the importance of hypoxia in the syndrome. *Ann R Coll Surg Engl.* 1970;46:159-171.

336. Benoit PR, Hampson LG, Burgess JH. Respiratory gas exchange following fractures: the role of fat embolism as a cause of arterial hypoxemia. *Surg Forum.* 1969;20:214-216.

337. Gossling HR, Donohue TA. The fat embolism syndrome. *JAMA.* 1979;241:2740-2742.

338. Weisz GM, Steiner E. The cause of death in fat embolism. *Chest.* 1971;59:511-516.

339. Jacobson DM, Terrence CF, Reinmuth OM. The neurologic manifestations of fat embolism. *Neurology.* 1986;36:847-851.

340. Dorr LD, Merkel C, Mellman MF, Klein I. Fat emboli in bilateral total knee arthroplasty. Predictive factors for neurologic manifestations. *Clin Orthop Relat Res.* 1989;(248):112-118; discussion 118-119.

341. Garner JH Jr, Peltier LF. Fat embolism. The significance of provoked petechiae. *JAMA.* 1967;200:556-557.

342. Gurd AR, Wilson RI. The fat embolism syndrome. *J Bone Joint Surg Br.* 1974;56B:408-416.

343. Schonfeld SA, Ploysongsang Y, DiLisio R, et al. Fat embolism prophylaxis with corticosteroids. A prospective study in high-risk patients. *Ann Intern Med.* 1983;99:438-443.

344. Lindeque BG, Schoeman HS, Dommisse GF, Boeyens MC, Vlok AL. Fat embolism and the fat embolism syndrome. A double-blind therapeutic study. *J Bone Joint Surg Br.* 1987;69:128-131.

345. Rokkanen P, Lahdensuu M, Kataja J, Julkunen H. The syndrome of fat embolism: analysis of thirty consecutive cases compared to trauma patients with similar injuries. *J Trauma.* 1970;10:299-306.

346. Chastre J, Fagon JY, Soler P, et al. Bronchoalveolar lavage for rapid diagnosis of the fat embolism syndrome in trauma patients. *Ann Intern Med.* 1990;113:583-588.

347. Vedrinne JM, Guillaume C, Gagnieu MC, Gratadour P, Fleuret C, Motin J. Bronchoalveolar lavage in trauma patients for diagnosis of fat embolism syndrome. *Chest.* 1992;102:1323-1327.

348. Ravenel JG, Heyneman LE, McAdams HP. Computed tomography diagnosis of macroscopic pulmonary fat embolism. *J Thorac Imaging.* 2002;17:154-156.

349. Feldman F, Ellis K, Green WM. The fat embolism syndrome. *Radiology.* 1975;114:535-542.

350. Levy D. The fat embolism syndrome. A review. *Clin Orthop Relat Res.* 1990;(261):281-286.

351. Muangman N, Stern EJ, Bulger EM, Jurkovich GJ, Mann FA. Chest radiographic evolution in fat embolism syndrome. *J Med Assoc Thai.* 2005;88:1854-1860.

352. Milstein D, Nusynowitz ML, Lull RJ. Radionuclide diagnosis in chest disease resulting from trauma. *Semin Nucl Med.* 1974;4:339-355.

353. Park HM, Ducret RP, Brindley DC. Pulmonary imaging in fat embolism syndrome. *Clin Nucl Med.* 1986;11:521-522.

354. Arakawa H, Kurihara Y, Nakajima Y. Pulmonary fat embolism syndrome: CT findings in six patients. *J Comput Assist Tomogr.* 2000;24:24-29.

355. Heyneman LE, Muller NL. Pulmonary nodules in early fat embolism syndrome: a case report. *J Thorac Imaging.* 2000;15:71-74.

356. Choi JA, Oh YW, Kim HK, Kang KH, Choi YH, Kang EY. Nontraumatic pulmonary fat embolism syndrome: radiologic and pathologic correlations. *J Thorac Imaging.* 2002;17:167-169.

357. Dines DE, Burgher LW, Okazaki H. The clinical and pathologic correlation of fat embolism syndrome. *Mayo Clin Proc.* 1975;50:407-411.

358. Beers GJ, Nichols GR, Willing SJ, Reiss SJ. CT demonstration of fat-embolism-associated hemorrhage in the anterior commissure. *AJNR Am J Neuroradiol.* 1988;9:212-213.

359. Sakamoto T, Sawada Y, Yukioka T, Yoshioka T, Sugimoto T, Taneda M. Computed tomography for diagnosis and assessment of cerebral fat embolism. *Neuroradiology.* 1983;24:283-285.

360. Kawano Y, Ochi M, Hayashi K, Morikawa M, Kimura S. Magnetic resonance imaging of cerebral fat embolism. *Neuroradiology.* 1991;33:72-74.

361. Takahashi M, Suzuki R, Osakabe Y, et al. Magnetic resonance imaging findings in cerebral fat embolism: correlation with clinical manifestations. *J Trauma.* 1999;46:324-327.

362. Riding G, Daly K, Hutchinson S, Rao S, Lovell M, McCollum C. Paradoxical cerebral embolisation. An explanation for fat embolism syndrome. *J Bone Joint Surg Br.* 2004;86:95-98.

363. Svenningsen S, Nesse O, Finsen V, Hole A, Benum P. Prevention of fat embolism syndrome in patients with femoral fractures—immediate or delayed operative fixation? *Ann Chir Gynaecol.* 1987;76:163-166.

364. Behrman SW, Fabian TC, Kudsk KA, Taylor JC. Improved outcome with femur fractures: early vs. delayed fixation. *J Trauma.* 1990;30:792-797; discussion 797-798.

365. Bone LB, Johnson KD, Weigelt J, Scheinberg R. Early versus delayed stabilization of femoral fractures. A prospective randomized study. *J Bone Joint Surg Am*. 1989;71:336-340.

366. Ashbaugh DG, Petty TL. The use of corticosteroids in the treatment of respiratory failure associated with massive fat embolism. *Surg Gynecol Obstet*. 1966;123:493-500.

367. Taviloglu K, Yanar H. Fat embolism syndrome. *Surg Today*. 2007;37:5-8.

368. Gossling HR, Ellison LH, Degraff AC Jr. Fat embolism. The role of respiratory failure and its treatment. *J Bone Joint Surg Am*. 1974;56:1327-1337.

369. Shier MR, Wilson RF, James RE, Riddle J, Mammen EF, Pedersen HE. Fat embolism prophylaxis: a study of four treatment modalities. *J Trauma*. 1977;17:621-629.

370. Kallenbach J, Lewis M, Zaltzman M, Feldman C, Orford A, Zwi S. 'Low-dose' corticosteroid prophylaxis against fat embolism. *J Trauma*. 1987;27:1173-1176.

371. ten Duis HJ. The fat embolism syndrome. *Injury*. 1997;28:77-85.

372. Richards RR. Fat embolism syndrome. *Can J Surg*. 1997;40:334-339.

373. Winterbauer RH, Elfenbein IB, Ball WC Jr. Incidence and clinical significance of tumor embolization to the lungs. *Am J Med*. 1968;45:271-290.

374. Schmidt MB. Ueber krebszellenembolien in den lungenarterien. *Zentralbl allg Path*. 1897;8:860.

375. Hughes JE. A case of hydatidiform mole with multiple small syncytial infarctions of the lungs. *Proc R Soc Med*. 1930;23:1157.

376. Mason DG. Subacute cor pulmonale. *Arch Intern Med*. 1940;66:1221.

377. Marcuse PM. Pulmonary syncytial giant cell embolism; report of maternal death. *Obstet Gynecol*. 1954;3:210-213.

378. Trotter RF, Tieche HL. Maternal death due to pulmonary embolism of trophoblastic cells. *Am J Obstet Gynecol*. 1956;71:1114-1118.

379. Arnold HA, Bainborough AR. Subacute cor pulmonale following trophoblastic pulmonary emboli. *Can Med Assoc J*. 1957;76:478-482.

380. Fahrner RJ, McQueeney AJ, Mosely JM, Petersen RW. Trophoblastic pulmonary thrombosis with cor pulmonale. *JAMA*. 1959;170:1898.

381. Bagshawe KD, Brooks WD. Subacute pulmonary hypertension due to chorionepithelioma. *Lancet*. 1959;1:653-658.

382. Durham JR, Ashley PF, Dorencamp D. Cor pulmonale due to tumor emboli; review of literature and report of a case. *JAMA*. 1961;175:757-760.

383. Acosta-Sison H. Fatal complications of hydatidiform mole before evacuation of the uterus. *Am J Obstet Gynecol*. 1962;84:1425-1426.

384. Lipp RG, Kindschi JD, Schmitz R. Death from pulmonary embolism associated with hydatidiform mole. *Am J Obstet Gynecol*. 1962;83:1644-1647.

385. Storey PB, Goldstein W. Pulmonary embolization from primary hepatic carcinoma. *Arch Intern Med*. 1962;110:262-269.

386. Case records of the Massachusetts general hospital. *N Engl J Med*. 1962;266:1110.

387. Giertsen JC, Hansen ES. Pulmonary carcinomatous thrombo-embolism. *Acta Pathol Microbiol Scand*. 1964;60:164-172.

388. DeVita VT, Trujillo NP, Blackman AH, Ticktin HE. Pulmonary manifestations of primary hepatic carcinoma. *Am J Med Sci*. 1965;250:428-436.

389. De Hendrickse JP, Willis AJ, Evans KT. Acute dyspnoea with trophoblastic tumours. *J Obstet Gynaecol Br Commonw*. 1965;72:376-383.

390. Dyke PC, Fink LM. Latent choriocarcinoma. *Cancer*. 1967;20:150-154.

391. Altemus LR, Lee RE. Carcinomatosis of the lung with pulmonary hypertension. Pathoradiologic spectrum. *Arch Intern Med*. 1967;119:32-38.

392. Soares FA, Pinto AP, Landell GA, de Oliveira JA. Pulmonary tumor embolism to arterial vessels and carcinomatous lymphangitis. A comparative clinicopathological study. *Arch Pathol Lab Med*. 1993;117:827-831.

393. Orr FW, Buchanan MR, Weiss L, eds. *Microcirculation in Cancer Metastasis*. Boca Raton, FL: CRC Press Inc; 1991.

394. Bassiri AG, Haghighi B, Doyle RL, Berry GJ, Rizk NW. Pulmonary tumor embolism. *Am J Respir Crit Care Med*. 1997;155:2089-2095.

395. Odeh M, Oliven A, Misselevitch I, Boss JH. Acute cor pulmonale due to tumor cell microemboli. *Respiration*. 1997;64:384-387.

396. Kane RD, Hawkins HK, Miller JA, Noce PS. Microscopic pulmonary tumor emboli associated with dyspnea. *Cancer*. 1975;36:1473-1482.

397. Saphir O. The fate of carcinoma emboli in the lung. *Am J Pathol*. 1947;23:245-253.

398. Thompson WP, White PD. The commonest cause of hypertrophy of the right ventricle: left ventricular strain and failure. *Am Heart J*. 1936;12:641-649.

399. Gonzalez-Vitale JC, Garcia-Bunuel R. Pulmonary tumor emboli and cor pulmonale in primary carcinoma of the lung. *Cancer*. 1976;38:2105-2110.

400. Veinot JP, Ford SE, Price RG. Subacute cor pulmonale due to tumor embolization. *Arch Pathol Lab Med*. 1992;116:131-134.

401. Lambert-Jensen P, Mertz H, Nyvad O, Christensen JH. Subacute cor pulmonale due to microscopic pulmonary tumour cell embolization. *J Intern Med*. 1994;236:597-598.

402. Montero A, Vidaller A, Mitjavila F, Chivite D, Pujol R. Microscopic pulmonary tumoral embolism and subacute cor pulmonale as the first clinical signs of cancer. *Acta Oncol*. 1999;38:1116-1118.

403. Goldhaber SZ, Dricker E, Buring JE, et al. Clinical suspicion of autopsy-proven thrombotic and tumor pulmonary embolism in cancer patients. *Am Heart J*. 1987;114:1432-1435.

404. Sakuma M, Fukui S, Nakamura M, et al. Cancer and pulmonary embolism: thrombotic embolism, tumor embolism, and tumor invasion into a large vein. *Circ J*. 2006;70:744-749.

405. Gutierrez-Macias A, Barandiaran KE, Ercoreca FJ, De Zarate MM. Acute cor pulmonale due to microscopic tumour

embolism as the first manifestation of hepatocellular carcinoma. *Eur J Gastroenterol Hepatol.* 2002;14:775-777.

406. Koskinas J, Betrosian A, Kafiri G, Tsolakidis G, Garaziotou V, Hadziyannis S. Combined hepatocellular-cholangiocarcinoma presented with massive pulmonary embolism. *Hepatogastroenterology.* 2000;47:1125-1128.

407. Nakamura H, Adachi H, Sudoh A, et al. Subacute cor pulmonale due to tumor embolism. *Intern Med.* 2004;43:420-422.

408. Abbondanzo SL, Klappenbach RS, Tsou E. Tumor cell embolism to pulmonary alveolar capillaries. Cause of sudden cor pulmonale. *Arch Pathol Lab Med.* 1986;110:1197-1198.

409. Sostman HD, Brown M, Toole A, Bobrow S, Gottschalk A. Perfusion scan in pulmonary vascular/lymphangitic carcinomatosis: the segmental contour pattern. *AJR Am J Roentgenol.* 1981;137:1072-1074.

410. Boudreau RJ, Lisbona R, Sheldon H. Ventilation-perfusion mismatch in tumor embolism. *Clin Nucl Med.* 1982;7:320-322.

411. Bulas DI, Thompson R, Reaman G. Pulmonary emboli as a primary manifestation of wilms tumor. *AJR Am J Roentgenol.* 1991;156:155-156.

412. Yutani C, Imakita M, Ishibashi-Ueda H, Katsuragi M, Yoshioka T, Kunieda T. Pulmonary hypertension due to tumor emboli: a report of three autopsy cases with morphological correlations to radiological findings. *Acta Pathol Jpn.* 1993;43:135-141.

413. Schriner RW, Ryu JH, Edwards WD. Microscopic pulmonary tumor embolism causing subacute cor pulmonale: a difficult antemortem diagnosis. *Mayo Clin Proc.* 1991;66:143-148.

414. Crane R, Rudd TG, Dail D. Tumor microembolism: pulmonary perfusion pattern. *J Nucl Med.* 1984;25:877-880.

415. Chan CK, Hutcheon MA, Hyland RH, Smith GJ, Patterson BJ, Matthay RA. Pulmonary tumor embolism: a critical review of clinical, imaging, and hemodynamic features. *J Thorac Imaging.* 1987;2:4-14.

416. Shepard JA, Moore EH, Templeton PA, McLoud TC. Pulmonary intravascular tumor emboli: dilated and beaded peripheral pulmonary arteries at CT. *Radiology.* 1993;187:797-801.

417. Rossi SE, Goodman PC, Franquet T. Nonthrombotic pulmonary emboli. *AJR Am J Roentgenol.* 2000;174:1499-1508.

418. Chakeres DW, Spiegel PK. Fatal pulmonary hypertension secondary to intravascular metastatic tumor emboli. *AJR Am J Roentgenol.* 1982;139:997-1000.

419. Franquet T, Gimenez A, Prats R, Rodriguez-Arias JM, Rodriguez C. Thrombotic microangiopathy of pulmonary tumors: a vascular cause of tree-in-bud pattern on CT. *AJR Am J Roentgenol.* 2002;179:897-899.

420. Egermayer P. The lung scan appearances of tumor embolization. *Chest.* 1998;113:562-563.

421. Geschwind JF, Dagli MS, Vogel-Claussen J, Seifter E, Huncharek MS. Metastatic breast carcinoma presenting as a large pulmonary embolus: case report and review of the literature. *Am J Clin Oncol.* 2003;26:89-91.

422. Jakel J, Ramaswamy A, Kohler U, Barth PJ. Massive pulmonary tumor microembolism from a hepatocellular carcinoma. *Pathol Res Pract.* 2006;202:395-399.

423. Mutlu GM, Factor P. Pulmonary tumor embolism of unknown origin. *Mayo Clin Proc.* 2006;81:721.

424. Ha JW, Kim SK, Chang BC. Pulmonary tumour embolism. *Lancet.* 2002;359:2158.

425. Collins CG, Nelson EW, Collins JH, Weinstein BB, MacCallum EA. Suppurative pelvic thrombophlebitis. II. Symptomatology and diagnosis; a study of 70 patients treated by ligation of the inferior vena cava and ovarian veins. *Surgery.* 1951;30:311-318.

426. Cook RJ, Ashton RW, Aughenbaugh GL, Ryu JH. Septic pulmonary embolism: presenting features and clinical course of 14 patients. *Chest.* 2005;128:162-166.

427. Clarke DE, Raffin TA. Infectious complications of indwelling long-term central venous catheters. *Chest.* 1990;97:966-972.

428. Klug D, Lacroix D, Savoye C, et al. Systemic infection related to endocarditis on pacemaker leads: clinical presentation and management. *Circulation.* 1997;95:2098-2107.

429. Cacoub P, Leprince P, Nataf P, et al. Pacemaker infective endocarditis. *Am J Cardiol.* 1998;82:480-484.

430. Karchmer AW, Longworth DL. Infections of intracardiac devices. *Infect Dis Clin North Am.* 2002;16:477-505, xii.

431. Ghanem GA, Boktour M, Warneke C, et al. Catheter-related *Staphylococcus aureus* bacteremia in cancer patients: high rate of complications with therapeutic implications. *Medicine (Baltimore).* 2007;86:54-60.

432. Julander I. Staphylococcal septicaemia and endocarditis in 80 drug addicts. Aspects on epidemiology, clinical and laboratory findings and prognosis. *Scand J Infect Dis Suppl.* 1983;41:49-55.

433. Longhi A, Rimondi E, Loro L, et al. Pulmonary nodules in osteosarcoma patients: differential diagnosis of central venous catheter-related infections in the lungs. *Radiol Med (Torino).* 2006;111:192-201.

434. Pittet D, Hulliger S, Auckenthaler R. Intravascular device-related infections in critically ill patients. *J Chemother.* 1995;7(suppl 3):55-66.

435. Saccente M, Cobbs CG. Clinical approach to infective endocarditis. *Cardiol Clin.* 1996;14:351-362.

436. Reisberg BE. Infective endocarditis in the narcotic addict. *Prog Cardiovasc Dis.* 1979;22:193-204.

437. Hoen B, Alla F, Selton-Suty C, et al. Changing profile of infective endocarditis: results of a 1-year survey in france. *JAMA.* 2002;288:75-81.

438. Mouly S, Ruimy R, Launay O, et al. The changing clinical aspects of infective endocarditis: descriptive review of 90 episodes in a French teaching hospital and risk factors for death. *J Infect.* 2002;45:246-256.

439. Hecht SR, Berger M. Right-sided endocarditis in intravenous drug users. Prognostic features in 102 episodes. *Ann Intern Med.* 1992;117:560-566.

440. MacMillan JC, Milstein SH, Samson PC. Clinical spectrum of septic pulmonary embolism and infarction. *J Thorac Cardiovasc Surg.* 1978;75:670-679.

441. O'Donnell AE, Pappas LS. Pulmonary complications of intravenous drug abuse. Experience at an inner-city hospital. *Chest.* 1988;94:251-253.

442. Chambers HF, Korzeniowski OM, Sande MA. *Staphylococcus aureus* endocarditis: clinical manifestations in addicts and nonaddicts. *Medicine (Baltimore)*. 1983;62:170-177.

443. O'Donnell AE, Selig J, Aravamuthan M, Richardson MS. Pulmonary complications associated with illicit drug use. An update. *Chest*. 1995;108:460-463.

444. Lemierre A. On certain septicaemias due to anaerobic organisms. *Lancet*. 1936;1:701-703.

445. Gormus N, Durgut K, Ozergin U, Odev K, Solak H. Lemierre's syndrome associated with septic pulmonary embolism: a case report. *Ann Vasc Surg*. 2004;18:243-245.

446. Shiota Y, Arikita H, Horita N, et al. Septic pulmonary embolism associated with periodontal disease: reports of two cases and review of the literature. *Chest*. 2002;121:652-654.

447. Mattar CS, Keith RL, Byrd RP Jr, Roy TM. Septic pulmonary emboli due to periodontal disease. *Respir Med*. 2006;100:1470-1474.

448. Russi EW, Dazzi H, Gaumann N. Septic pulmonary embolism due to periodontal disease in a patient with hereditary hemorrhagic telangiectasia. *Respiration*. 1996;63:117-119.

449. Sinave CP, Hardy GJ, Fardy PW. The Lemierre syndrome: suppurative thrombophlebitis of the internal jugular vein secondary to oropharyngeal infection. *Medicine (Baltimore)*. 1989;68:85-94.

450. Koay CB, Heyworth T, Burden P. Lemierre syndrome—a forgotten complication of acute tonsillitis. *J Laryngol Otol*. 1995;109:657-661.

451. Merrer J, De Jonghe B, Golliot F, et al. Complications of femoral and subclavian venous catheterization in critically ill patients: a randomized controlled trial. *JAMA*. 2001;286:700-707.

452. Huang RM, Naidich DP, Lubat E, Schinella R, Garay SM, McCauley DI. Septic pulmonary emboli: CT-radiographic correlation. *AJR Am J Roentgenol*. 1989;153:41-45.

453. Murin S, Romano PS, White RH. Comparison of outcomes after hospitalization for deep venous thrombosis or pulmonary embolism. *Thromb Haemost*. 2002;88:407-414.

454. Libby LS, King TE, LaForce FM, Schwarz MI. Pulmonary cavitation following pulmonary infarction. *Medicine (Baltimore)*. 1985;64:342-348.

455. Garcia J, Aboujaoude R, Apuzzio J, Alvarez JR. Septic pelvic thrombophlebitis: diagnosis and management. *Infect Dis Obstet Gynecol*. 2006;2006:15614.

456. Gibson GJ, Geddes DM, Costabel U, Sterk PJ, Corrin B, eds. *Respiratory Medicine*. 3rd ed. Philadelphia, PA: Saunders Ltd; 2003:1749.

457. Charles K, Flinn WR, Neschis DG. Lemierre's syndrome: a potentially fatal complication that may require vascular surgical intervention. *J Vasc Surg*. 2005;42:1023-1025.

458. Lee SJ, Cha SI, Kim CH, et al. Septic pulmonary embolism in korea: microbiology, clinicoradiologic features, and treatment outcome. *J Infect*. 2007;54:230-234.

459. Butler MD, Biscardi FH, Schain DC, Humphries JE, Blow O, Spotnitz WD. Pulmonary resection for treatment of cavitary pulmonary infarction. *Ann Thorac Surg*. 1997;63:849-850.

460. Jaffe RB, Koschmann EB. Septic pulmonary emboli. *Radiology*. 1970;96:527-532.

461. Kuhlman JE, Fishman EK, Teigen C. Pulmonary septic emboli: diagnosis with CT. *Radiology*. 1990;174:211-213.

462. Wong KS, Lin TY, Huang YC, Hsia SH, Yang PH, Chu SM. Clinical and radiographic spectrum of septic pulmonary embolism. *Arch Dis Child*. 2002;87:312-315.

463. Iwasaki Y, Nagata K, Nakanishi M, et al. Spiral CT findings in septic pulmonary emboli. *Eur J Radiol*. 2001;37:190-194.

464. Lee KH, Lee JS, Lynch DA, Song KS, Lim TH. The radiologic differential diagnosis of diffuse lung diseases characterized by multiple cysts or cavities. *J Comput Assist Tomogr*. 2002;26:5-12.

465. Kwon WJ, Jeong YJ, Kim KI, et al. Computed tomographic features of pulmonary septic emboli: comparison of causative microorganisms. *J Comput Assist Tomogr*. 2007;31:390-394.

466. Dodd JD, Souza CA, Muller NL. High-resolution MDCT of pulmonary septic embolism: evaluation of the feeding vessel sign. *AJR Am J Roentgenol*. 2006;187:623-629.

467. Spencer RP. Ventilation/perfusion reverse mismatch in septic pulmonary emboli. *Clin Nucl Med*. 1996;21:328-329.

468. Ginzton LE, Siegel RJ, Criley JM. Natural history of tricuspid valve endocarditis: a two dimensional echocardiographic study. *Am J Cardiol*. 1982;49:1853-1859.

469. Scarvelis D, Malcolm I. Embolization of a huge tricuspid valve bacterial vegetation. *J Am Soc Echocardiogr*. 2002;15:185-187.

470. Mylonakis E, Calderwood SB. Infective endocarditis in adults. *N Engl J Med*. 2001;345:1318-1330.

471. Sachdev M, Peterson GE, Jollis JG. Imaging techniques for diagnosis of infective endocarditis. *Infect Dis Clin North Am*. 2002;16:319-337, ix.

472. Sexton DJ, Spelman D. Current best practices and guidelines. Assessment and management of complications in infective endocarditis. *Infect Dis Clin North Am*. 2002;16:507-521, xii.

473. Shadowen RD, Trevor RP. Lemierre's postanginal septicemia: internal jugular vein thrombosis related to pharyngeal infection. *South Med J*. 1989;82:1583-1584.

474. Shaham D, Sklair-Levy M, Weinberger G, Gomori JM. Lemierre's syndrome presenting as multiple lung abscesses. *Clin Imaging*. 2000;24:197-199.

475. Brown CE, Stettler RW, Twickler D, Cunningham FG. Puerperal septic pelvic thrombophlebitis: incidence and response to heparin therapy. *Am J Obstet Gynecol*. 1999;181:143-148.

476. Dunnihoo DR, Gallaspy JW, Wise RB, Otterson WN. Postpartum ovarian vein thrombophlebitis: a review. *Obstet Gynecol Surv*. 1991;46:415-427.

477. Plemmons RM, Dooley DP, Longfield RN. Septic thrombophlebitis of the portal vein (pylephlebitis): diagnosis and management in the modern era. *Clin Infect Dis*. 1995;21:1114-1120.

478. Aslam AF, Aslam AK, Thakur AC, Vasavada BC, Khan IA. *Staphylococcus aureus* infective endocarditis and septic pulmonary embolism after septic abortion. *Int J Cardiol*. 2005;105:233-235.

479. Morizono S, Enjoji M, Sonoda N, et al. Lemierre's syndrome: porphyromonas asaccharolytica as a putative pathogen. *Intern Med*. 2005;44:350-353.

480. Falagas ME, Vardakas KZ, Athanasiou S. Intravenous heparin in combination with antibiotics for the treatment of deep vein septic thrombophlebitis: a systematic review. *Eur J Pharmacol.* 2007;557:93-98.

481. Armstrong AW, Spooner K, Sanders JW. Lemierre's syndrome. *Curr Infect Dis Rep.* 2000;2:168-173.

482. Lin D, Reeck JB, Murr AH. Internal jugular vein thrombosis and deep neck infection from intravenous drug use: management strategy. *Laryngoscope.* 2004;114:56-60.

483. Robbins MJ, Frater RW, Soeiro R, Frishman WH, Strom JA. Influence of vegetation size on clinical outcome of right-sided infective endocarditis. *Am J Med.* 1986;80:165-171.

484. Chan P, Ogilby JD, Segal B. Tricuspid valve endocarditis. *Am Heart J.* 1989;117:1140-1146.

485. Wong D, Chandraratna AN, Wishnow RM, Dusitnanond V, Nimalasuriya A. Clinical implications of large vegetations in infectious endocarditis. *Arch Intern Med.* 1983;143:1874-1877.

486. Buda AJ, Zotz RJ, LeMire MS, Bach DS. Prognostic significance of vegetations detected by two-dimensional echocardiography in infective endocarditis. *Am Heart J.* 1986;112:1291-1296.

487. Gilbert BW, Haney RS, Crawford F, et al. Two-dimensional echocardiographic assessment of vegetative endocarditis. *Circulation.* 1977;55:346-353.

488. Durack DT, Beeson PB. Experimental bacterial endocarditis. II. Survival of a bacteria in endocardial vegetations. *Br J Exp Pathol.* 1972;53:50-53.

489. Lutas EM, Roberts RB, Devereux RB, Prieto LM. Relation between the presence of echocardiographic vegetations and the complication rate in infective endocarditis. *Am Heart J.* 1986;112:107-113.

490. Manolis AS, Melita H. Echocardiographic and clinical correlates in drug addicts with infective endocarditis. Implications of vegetation size. *Arch Intern Med.* 1988;148:2461-2465.

491. Barbour DJ, Roberts WC. Valve excision only versus valve excision plus replacement for active infective endocarditis involving the tricuspid valve. *Am J Cardiol.* 1986;57:475-478.

492. Yee ES, Ullyot DJ. Reparative approach for right-sided endocarditis. Operative considerations and results of valvuloplasty. *J Thorac Cardiovasc Surg.* 1988;96:133-140.

493. Lioulias A, Kotoulas C, Kokotsakis J, Konstantinou M. Acute pulmonary embolism due to multiple hydatid cysts. *Eur J Cardiothorac Surg.* 2001;20:197-199.

494. Kardaras F, Kardara D, Tselikos D, et al. Fifteen year surveillance of echinococcal heart disease from a referral hospital in greece. *Eur Heart J.* 1996;17:1265-1270.

495. Bithal PK, Pandia MP, Dash HH, et al. Comparative incidence of venous air embolism and associated hypotension in adults and children operated for neurosurgery in the sitting position. *Eur J Anaesthesiol.* 2004;21:517-522.

496. Young ML, Smith DS, Murtagh F, et al. Comparison of surgical and anesthetic complications in neurosurgical patients experiencing venous air embolism in the sitting position. *Neurosurgery.* 1986;18:157-161.

497. Michenfelder JD, Miller RH, Gronert GA. Evaluation of an ultrasonic device (Doppler) for the diagnosis of venous air embolism. *Anesthesiology.* 1972;36:164-167.

498. Slbin MS, Babinski M, Maroon JC, et al. Anesthetic management of posterior fossa surgery in the sitting position. *Acta Anaesthesiol Scand.* 1976;20:117-128.

499. Voorhies RM, Fraser RA, Van Poznak A. Prevention of air embolism with positive end expiratory pressure. *Neurosurgery.* 1983;12:503-506.

500. Standefer M, Bay JW, Trusso R. The sitting position in neurosurgery: a retrospective analysis of 488 cases. *Neurosurgery.* 1984;14:649-658.

501. Matjasko J, Petrozza P, Cohen M, et al. Anesthesia and surgery in the seated position: analysis of 554 cases. *Neurosurgery.* 1985;17:602-695.

502. Black S, Ockert DB, Oliver WC Jr, et al. Outcome following posterior fossa craniectomy in patients in the sitting or horizontal positions. *Anesthesiology.* 1988;69:49-56.

chapter 46

Nonembolic Disorders of the Pulmonary Artery

Jeffrey H. Freihage, MD / Tina M. Dudney, MD / Michael T. McCormack, MD

● INTRODUCTION

The pulmonary artery (PA) functions as a low resistance conduit for blood to travel from the right heart to the systemic circulation. However, to view the PA as a passive conduit is to underestimate the complex physiologic interactions between the neurohormonal control of vascular tone, environmental factors (including infectious agents, toxins, and prolonged hypoxia), and congenital abnormalities that may occur within the PA. An understanding of the normal PA physiology is of paramount importance in understanding the clinical course of pathologic disease states. Although the acute PA response to a congenital abnormality or an environmental insult may be beneficial in the short term, prolonged response may lead to a severely debilitating and life-shortening pathologic condition. Recognition of pathologic conditions within the PA and the role of altered PA physiology is the focus of this chapter.

The following sections attempt to provide a detailed discussion of the common and rare congenital and acquired abnormalities affecting the PA. The presentation, etiology, and clinical course of pathologic PA conditions are outlined. In order to provide guidance on the delivery and timing of optimal and appropriate therapy, the diagnostic workup and data on medical, surgical, and percutaneous treatments are presented. Also discussed are "clinical pearls" that should lead the clinician to consider a rare PA abnormality over a more common disease process.

● ANATOMY, EMBRYOLOGY, AND PHYSIOLOGY OF THE PULMONARY ARTERY

The precursors to the adult pulmonary arterial system become recognizable by day 27 of fetal development. The main PA forms from the division of the truncus arteriosus by the aorticopulmonary septum (Figure 46-1).[1] The right and left sixth aortic arches, known as the pulmonary arches, form the proximal right and left pulmonary arteries, respectively. By day 29 of embryologic development, the sixth aortic arches are continuous with the pulmonary trunk. The distal portion of the left sixth arch forms the ductus arteriosus, and the distal part of the right sixth arch involutes.[2] Buds from the sixth arch arteries grow into primitive lungs and anastomose with the primitive pulmonary circulation.[3]

The absence of a PA (PA interruption) and anomalous left PA (pulmonary sling) are two rare conditions resulting from abnormal embryologic development of the PA.[2] The absence of a PA is most likely the result of involution of the proximal sixth aortic arch with a corresponding reduction in lung size on the affected side. The blood supply to the affected lung is usually supplied through collateral vessels such as the bronchial or intercostal arteries. The anomalous left PA (Figure 46-2) is because of involution of the left sixth aortic arch with the blood supply being from a vessel of the right PA coursing between the trachea and esophagus toward the left.[4]

In the adult, the main PA exits the base of the right ventricle anterior and left of the aorta. The main PA then ascends posterior and medial for 4 to 5 cm until it divides into the right and left main pulmonary arteries. The left main PA (mean diameter 26.4 mm) continues in the same posterior direction until reaching the left main bronchus at which point it arches over the left main bronchus and descends posterior to it. The right main PA (mean diameter 23.4 mm) courses in a horizontal direction posterior to the aorta, superior to the vena cava, and anterior to the right main bronchus before further subdividing. While the course of the main pulmonary arteries is predictable,

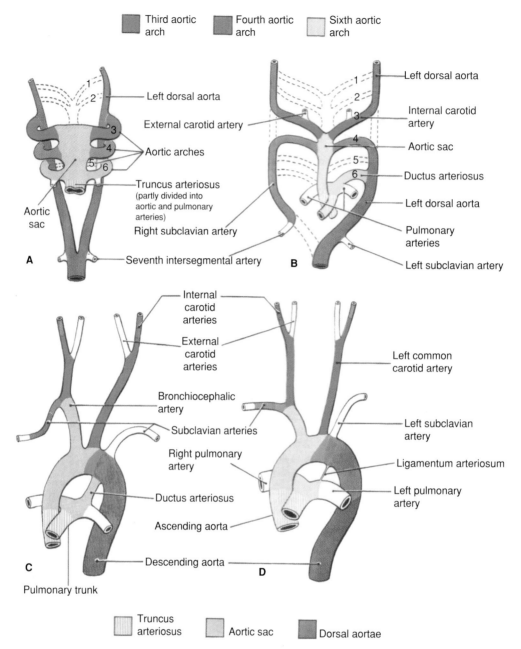

● **FIGURE 46-1.** Embryologic transformation of aortic arches into the adult arterial system. (A) Aortic arches at 6 weeks of development demonstrating disappearance of the first and second arches. (B) Aortic arches at 7 weeks of development demonstrating further transformation with the disappearance of parts of the dorsal aorta and the fifth aortic arch. (C) Aortic arches at 8 weeks of development demonstrating patency of the ductus arteriosus. (D) Arterial system at 6 months after birth.

Reproduced, with permission, from The cardiovascular system. In: Moore KL, Persaud TVN, eds. The Developing Human: Clinically Oriented Embryology. 3rd ed. Philadelphia, PA: WB Saunders; 1993:304-353.

the branching patterns of lobar and segmental arteries demonstrate considerable variability.[5] After passing over the left main bronchus, the left main PA usually continues to descend posterior in a vertical direction to form the left interlobar artery, from which the segmental arteries to the upper and lower lobes arise. However, the left main PA may give off an ascending branch that divides into the segmental branches of the upper lobe after passing over the left main bronchus.[6] The right main PA divides into the ascending and descending branches anterior to the right main bronchus. The ascending artery usually further divides into segmental branches that supply the right upper lobe, while the descending branch further subdivides into the segmental arteries of the middle and lower lobes of the right lung.[6] Although lobar and segmental branching demonstrate considerable variability, the branching pattern

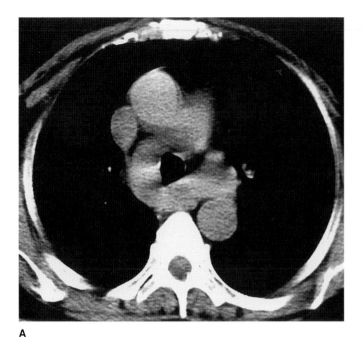

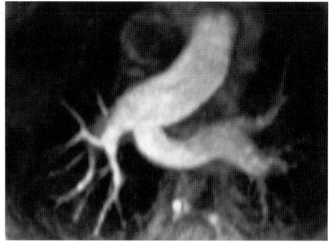

● **FIGURE 46-2.** Anomalous left PA arising from the right. (A) CT scan and (B) MR angiogram demonstrate the course of the anomalous left PA originating from the right PA and passing posterior to the trachea.

Case courtesy of Eva Castaner, MD, Hospital Parc Jauli, Sabadell, Spain. Reproduced, with permission, from Zylak CJ, Eyler WR, Spizarny DL, et al.; Developmental lung anomalies in the adult: radiologic-pathologic correlation. Radiographics. 2002:22;S25-S43.

is intimately related to bronchial branching; a branch always accompanies the adjacent airway down to the level of the distal respiratory bronchiole.[7] Furthermore, multiple "supernumerary" branches outnumber conventional branches and directly penetrate the lung parenchyma.[7]

Histologically, the pulmonary arteries can be divided into elastic, muscular, and arteriolar arteries.[7] The elastic arteries include the main PA and its branches down to the level of the bronchi–bronchiolar junction. The elastic arteries are usually greater than 1 mm and function as a reservoir for right ventricular output. The muscular arteries are 1.0 to 0.1 mm in diameter and have a well-developed medial smooth muscle layer that thins progressively until it becomes arterioles. The arteriolar arteries are less than 0.1 mm in diameter and are made up of only a thin intima and a single elastic lamina. The pulmonary vasculature has been shown to undergo age-related changes similar to the systemic circulation such as decreased distensibility of elastic arteries, development of fatty streaks and atherosclerotic plaques, and progressive intimal fibrosis.[8–10]

The normal pulmonary vascular bed is a low-pressure system in which resistance is less than one-tenth that of the systemic bed. During exercise, the normal pulmonary bed is able to accommodate a large increase in pulmonary blood flow with minimal rise in PA pressures as a result of recruitment of under-perfused segments. Alternatively, in response to hypoxia, blood flow is reduced to underventilated segments in order to improve ventilation perfusion matching.

The rapid and dynamic changes in pulmonary vascular tone result from a complex interplay between the endothelium, smooth muscle, platelets, and vasoactive mediators. The endothelium plays a central role in maintaining appropriate tone via the balanced production of vasoactive mediators. Such endothelial mediators are prostacyclin (PGI_2), nitric oxide (NO), and endothelin (ET-1). PGI_2 and NO are potent vasodilators, whereas ET-1 and serotonin (produced from platelets) act as vasoconstrictors. Through complex cellular pathways, many vasoactive mediators also have mitogenic functions in which they either inhibit or promote proliferation of endothelial and smooth muscle cells, as well as activation of platelets. In general, NO and PGI_2 can be thought of as vasodilators which inhibit both platelet activation, as well as proliferation of endothelial and smooth muscle cells. ET-1 and serotonin, on the other hand, promote cellular proliferation. While the mediators of vascular tone function to preserve health in the acute setting (i.e., vasoconstriction as a response to acute hypoxia), prolonged response or imbalance can have deleterious effects.

● **PULMONARY ARTERY CATHETER**

The pulmonary artery catheter (PAC), or Swan-Ganz catheter, was introduced into clinical practice in the 1970s in order to enhance the treatment of critically ill patients. The diagnostic procedure was rapidly embraced by many clinicians because of the ability of the PAC to provide hemodynamic information that was unavailable through

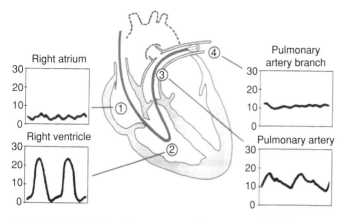

● **FIGURE 46-3.** Pressure waveforms recorded during insertion of a PA catheter.

Reproduced, with permission, from Marino PL. The pulmonary artery catheter. In: The ICU Book, 2nd ed, Philadelphia: Lippincott Williams & Wilkins. 1998;154-165.

other clinical tools. Clinicians reasoned that better treatment would be provided through the direct measurement of right-sided pressures (Figure 46-3), estimation of cardiac index and cardiac output via thermodilution techniques, and calculation of systemic and pulmonary vascular resistances. The use of the PAC was further supported by studies demonstrating the inability of clinician to estimate reliably these hemodynamic variables on clinical examination in the intensive care unit (ICU) setting.[11–13]

During 1980s and 1990s, in spite of the lack of data from randomized controlled trials evaluating PAC efficacy, PACs were commonly used in surgical, trauma, advanced heart failure, and acute myocardial infarction patients, as well as in patients admitted to the ICU with sepsis and/or acute respiratory distress syndrome. It was widely believed that the information obtained from PACs improved mortality. Consequently, physicians were unwilling to randomize patients in clinical trials. However, the data obtained from large observational studies suggested that PACs had either no influence or a negative impact on mortality.[14–18] The SUPPORT investigators provided alarming data on the aggressive use of PACs within the first 24 hours of admission to the ICU.[14] Using a propensity score, a statistical method of adjusting for treatment bias, these investigators found the 30-day mortality to be higher in patients who received a PAC than those managed without a PAC. This study raised concern over the widespread use of PACs, although the observational nature of this study was called into question because of the potential for confounding variables, lack of uniformity in treatment styles, and data interpretation. In 1997, the National Heart, Lung, and Blood Institute conducted the Pulmonary Artery Catheterization and Clinical Outcomes workshop to develop recommendations regarding actions to improve PAC utility and safety.[19] The two major outcomes of this workshop were the recognition of a need for randomized clinical trials assessing the efficacy of PACs in certain high risk patient populations and a need for standardized training in obtaining and interpreting PAC-derived information.

As a result of the National Heart, Lung, and Blood Institute workshop, multiple randomized controlled trials evaluating the effect of the PAC on mortality have been conducted.[20–27] These studies have demonstrated neither an increased mortality nor improved survival associated with PAC use in heart failure,[20] ICU,[21–23] elective vascular surgery,[24–26] or high risk general surgery[27] populations. Despite the lack of mortality benefit demonstrated in these randomized trials, proponents of the PAC do not believe sufficient evidence exists for a moratorium on the PAC.[28] These proponents argue that the PAC is a diagnostic, not therapeutic, modality requiring proper data interpretation. Furthermore, they claim that the lack of PAC benefit is because of the shortage of specific therapies to treat the underlying conditions.[29] The PAC may exhibit a benefit when coupled with a treatment plan that is known to improve outcomes.[28,30] Despite the controversy, approximately one million PACs are used annually in the United States.[31]

The indications for PAC insertion, like any diagnostic test, are difficult to define. In general, the decision to place a PAC should be based on the need for information that will guide therapy and that is not available from a noninvasive modality. Furthermore, PACs should only be used by health care providers experienced in PAC management and interpretation, because of the potential for patient harm if data is misinterpreted. In general, the physician must weigh the risks versus the benefits of the PAC prior to placement.

● PULMONARY ARTERIAL HYPERTENSION

Pulmonary hypertension (PH) is defined as a mean PA pressure greater than 25 mm Hg at rest or 30 mm Hg with exercise. Elevations in pulmonary vascular pressure can be caused by an isolated increase in pulmonary arterial pressure or by an increase in both pulmonary arterial and pulmonary venous pressure (precapillary vs. postcapillary). Because of the diverse etiologies, the World Health Organization proposed a classification scheme in 2003 to organize PH into categories (Table 46-1) that share similarities in pathophysiologic mechanisms, clinical presentation, and therapeutic options.[32]

Pulmonary arterial hypertension (PAH) is a World Health Organization classification scheme subset in which patients have PH (mean PA pressure >25 mm Hg at rest) with a normal pulmonary capillary wedge pressure (<15 mm Hg).[33] However, because patients with lung disease or embolic disease may also have PH with a normal pulmonary capillary wedge pressure, PAH should be viewed as PH that is limited predominantly to constriction, proliferation, and in situ thrombosis within the arterial component of the pulmonary vasculature.[34] PAH can occur in the absence of a demonstrable cause (idiopathic PAH [IPAH] or familial PAH [FPAH]) or in relation to another condition, such as collagen vascular disease, congenital systemic-to-pulmonary shunt, HIV infection, portal hypertension, or drug toxicity.

TABLE 46-1. Clinical Classification of Pulmonary Hypertension (Venice 2003)

1. PAH
   1.1 IPAH
   1.2 FPAH
   1.3 Associated with (APAH):
      1.3.1 Collagen vascular disease
      1.3.2 Congenital systemic-to-pulmonary shunts**
      1.3.3 Portal hypertension
      1.3.4 HIV infection
      1.3.5 Drugs and toxins
      1.3.6 Other (thyroid disorders, glycogen storage disease, Gaucher disease, hereditary hemorrhagic telangiectasia, hemoglobinopathies, myeloproliferative disorders, splenectomy)
   1.4 Associated with significant venous or capillary involvement
      1.4.1 Pulmonary veno-occlusive disease
      1.4.2 Pulmonary capillary hemangiomatosis
   1.5 Persistent pulmonary hypertension of the newborn
2. Pulmonary hypertension with left heart disease
   2.1 Left-sided atrial or ventricular heart disease
   2.2 Left-sided valvular heart disease
3. Pulmonary hypertension associated with lung diseases and/or hypoxemia
   3.1 Chronic obstructive pulmonary disease
   3.2 Interstitial lung disease
   3.3 Sleep-disordered breathing
   3.4 Alveolar hypoventilation disorders
   3.5 Chronic exposure to high altitude
   3.6 Developmental abnormalities
4. Pulmonary hypertension caused by chronic thrombotic and/or embolic disease
   4.1 Thromboembolic obstruction of proximal pulmonary arteries
   4.2 Thromboembolic obstruction of distal pulmonary arteries
   4.3 Nonthrombotic pulmonary embolism (tumor, parasites, foreign material)
5. Miscellaneous
   5.1 Sarcoidosis, histiocytosis X, lymphangiomatosis, compression of pulmonary vessels (adenopathy, tumor, fibrosing mediastinitis)

Source: Reprinted from Simonneau G, Galiè N, Rubin LJ, et al. Clinical classification of pulmonary hypertension. J Am Coll Cardiol. 2004;43:5S-12S.

Clinical Presentation

The presence of PH can come to clinical attention as a result of symptoms, screening in an at-risk population, or as an incidental finding.[35] A delay in the diagnosis is not uncommon, as the nonspecific symptoms of dyspnea and fatigue in patients with PH are often attributed to normal aging or weight gain. Dyspnea, the most common symp-tom, first presents with exertion because of an exagger-ated increase in PA pressures with exercise. With disease progression, patients may develop angina, lower extremity edema or syncope. Angina is caused by decreased coronary blood flow secondary to hypertrophy of the right ventricle. With progressive right ventricular failure, lower extremity edema from venous congestion occurs. Near-syncope and syncope result from the exercise-induced right ventricular failure that is caused by an increase in PA pressures with exercise. Patients with PAH very rarely have symptoms of hemoptysis, orthopnea, or paroxysmal nocturnal dyspnea.

Diagnostic Evaluation

The importance of a thorough and accurate diagnostic work-up can not be overemphasized, as the etiology of PH is paramount to treatment and prognosis.[36] The goal in evaluation of the patient with PH is to define the hemo-dynamic abnormality and underlying disease state, deter-mine prognosis, and develop a therapeutic plan.[34] A de-tailed medical history and physical examination should be performed to elucidate the presence of a family history of PH or any disease states or exposures that would place the patient at risk for PH. Figure 46-4 outlines a reasonable diagnostic algorithm for PH, with an emphasis on noninva-sive testing initially. The transthoracic Doppler echocardio-gram is an invaluable noninvasive tool in screening for PH, because of the strong correlation with invasive assessment of PA pressures.[37] The echocardiogram also allows evalua-tion of right and left ventricular function, valvular function, and evidence of intracardiac shunting from congenital heart disease. Caution must be taken in attributing PH to a col-lagen vascular disease based on serologic studies alone, as up to 40% of patients with IPAH have an abnormal sero-logic study.[38] Many patients will ultimately require cardiac catheterization to confirm the presence of PH, establish the etiology, assess severity, and guide therapy.[39]

Pathophysiology of PAH

PAH comprises a group of disorders in which the vas-culature of the PA develops vascular constriction, cellu-lar proliferation, and in situ thrombosis. Histologically, the lung tissue demonstrates intimal fibrosis, increased medial thickness, pulmonary arteriolar occlusion, and plexiform lesions.[40] The mechanism which accounts for the struc-tural alterations in the pulmonary arterial vasculature is not known. However, evidence exists that a complex interac-tion between a permissive genetic substrate, environmen-tal factors, and alterations in the production of vasoactive mediators contribute to the development of PAH.[41–48] A multihit theory has been suggested in which an individ-ual with a genetic predisposition encounters additional in-sults before the disease manifests.[42,43] Although the exact mechanism by which PAH occurs has not been elucidated, an association between certain molecular abnormalities and particular clinical types of PAH has been identified.

Genetic studies have demonstrated that mutations in two receptors of the transforming growth factor-beta

● **FIGURE 46-4.** Evaluation of pulmonary hypertension.
BNP, brain natriuretic peptide; CBC, complete blood count; CT, computed tomography; HIV, human immunodeficiency virus; HRCT, high-resolution computed tomography; LFTs, liver function tests; PH, pulmonary hypertension; RHC, right heart catheterization; SaO₂, systemic arterial oxygen saturation; TEE, transesophageal echocardiography; VD, vasodilator; V/Q, ventilation/perfusion.

Reproduced, with permission, from Barst RJ, McGoon M, Torbicki A, et al. Diagnosis and differential assessment of pulmonary arterial hypertension. J Am Coll Cardiol. 2004;43: 40S-47S.

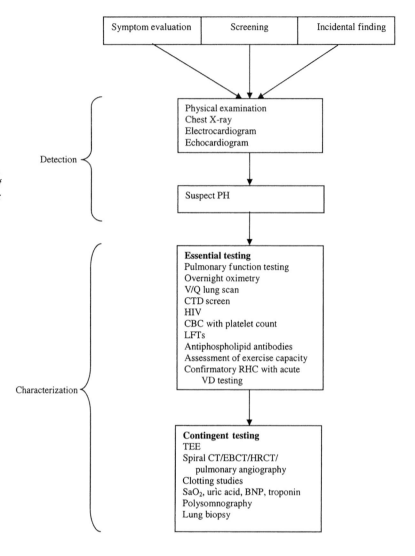

(TGF-β) family[49] and a serotonin transporter[50] provide the genetic substrate for the development of PAH in certain disease states. Bone morphogenetic protein receptor II (BMPR2) is a TGF-β receptor that functions to suppress the growth of vascular cells. Mutations within the BMPR2 gene result in altered signal transduction favoring vascular cell proliferation. BMPR2 gene mutations have been most strongly associated with FPAH.[44,51,52] However, mutations have also been observed in cases of IPAH,[53] as well as in patients in whom PAH develops after exposure to fenfluramine.[54] Activin-like kinase type-1 receptor (ALK1) is another TGF-β receptor family member that is believed to promote vascular growth after gene mutations through a similar aberrant signaling pathway as BMPR2 mutations.[55] Mutations in ALK1 have been observed in patients with hereditary hemorrhagic telangiectasia and PAH.[56] Finally, increased expression of an allelic variant of the serotonin transporter (5-HTT) gene, a promoter of PA smooth muscle cell proliferation, has been demonstrated to be present in a greater percentage of patients with IPAH compared with controls (65% vs. 27%).[50]

In addition to a permissive genetic substrate, complex interactions between the mediators of vascular tone, the PA endothelium, smooth muscle cells, and platelets manifest and contribute to the development of PAH.[41] Whether the involvement of each individual factor is a cause or a consequence in the development of PAH has not been entirely elucidated. Endothelial cell dysfunction, as a result of hypoxia, shear stress, inflammation, and toxic exposures, plays a central role in the promotion of the homeostatic imbalance that occurs within the pulmonary arterial system of patients with PAH.[34,41,42] Abnormal and disorganized endothelial proliferation results in the formation of the plexiform lesion. Injury to the endothelium affects its ability to perform appropriate homeostatic functions with regard to coagulation and the production of growth factors and vasoactive agents. Endothelial dysfunction promotes platelet activation and the creation of a prothrombotic state through elevated levels of von Willebrand factor and plasminogen activator type-1. The interaction between the dysfunctional endothelium and activated platelets leads to in situ thrombosis and platelet release of procoagulant, vasoactive, and mitogenic mediators.[41,57]

Multiple perturbations in the pathways which maintain appropriate pulmonary arterial tone have been discovered (Table 46-2). Nitric oxide, a potent vasodilator, is

TABLE 46-2. Mediators of Pulmonary Vascular Responses in PAH

Vasoconstriction	Cell Proliferation	Thrombosis
Increased TxA$_2$	Increased VEGF	Increased TxA$_2$
Decreased PGI$_2$	Decreased PGI$_2$	Decreased PGI$_2$
Decreased NO	Decreased NO	Decreased NO
Increased ET-1	Increased ET-1	
Increased 5-HT	Increased 5-HT	Increased 5-HT
Decreased VIP	Decreased VIP	Decreased VIP

TxA$_2$, thromboxane A$_2$; PGI$_2$, prostaglandin I$_2$ (prostacyclin); NO, nitric oxide; ET-1, endothelin-1; 5-HT, 5-hydroxytryptamine (serotonin); VEGF, vascular endothelial growth factor; VIP, vasoactive intestinal peptide.
Source: Reproduced with permission from Farber HW, Loscalzo J. Pulmonary arterial hypertension. N Engl J Med. 2004;351:1655-1665.

produced locally by endothelial cells within the PA. Decreased nitric oxide synthase expression leading to vasoconstriction has been demonstrated in patients with PAH.[46] The metabolism of arachidonic acid to prostacyclin (PGI$_2$) and thromboxane is also altered by reduced endothelial expression of prostacyclin synthase in patients with PAH.[45] Reduced prostacyclin synthase activity results in decreased prostacyclin and increased thromboxane. The net effect is a loss of prostacyclin's vasodilatory and antiproliferative properties, with a concomitant increase in vasoconstriction and platelet activation by thromboxane. Endothelin (ET-1) is a peptide with potent vasoconstrictor and mitogenic effects via endothelin receptor A (PA smooth muscle cells) and endothelin receptor B (PA smooth muscle cells and endothelial cells). ET-1 levels are elevated in patients with PAH of various etiologies.[48] Vasoactive intestinal peptide (VIP) has been shown to be a pulmonary vasodilator and inhibitor of platelet activation and vascular smooth muscle cell proliferation.[58-60] VIP has been implicated as having a role in progression of PAH because of the evidence of decreased VIP levels in patients with PAH.[61] Finally, serotonin (5-HT), a mediator of vasoconstriction, smooth muscle cell proliferation and platelet activation, has been suggested to have a role in the development of PAH as a result of elevated plasma levels of 5-HT and depleted platelet 5-HT in this population.[62]

Classification of PAH

PAH has been further subclassified into the following groups of disorders.

Idiopathic Pulmonary Arterial Hypertension. IPAH, formerly called primary PAH, is a distinct form of PAH which must be distinguished from other forms of PAH because of its unique clinical features, age of onset, and clinical course. This rare disease has an incidence of 2 to 5 per million per year.[34,63] National Registry Data has shown that most patients are diagnosed in the fourth decade of life (mean age

37 years) with a female to male ratio of 1.7:1.[38] Other forms of PAH must be excluded in order to make the diagnosis of IPAH.

Familial Pulmonary Arterial Hypertension. FPAH is a form of IPAH in which genetic transmission of the disease state occurs. FPAH accounts for at least 6% of all cases of PAH. Mutations in the BMPR2 gene are believed to be the causative agent of FPAH.[44,52] Unique features of the transmission of FPAH include incomplete penetrance and genetic anticipation and development of a more severe phenotype at a younger age. Because the BMPR2 gene mutation has been identified in 25% of patients with IPAH and both diseases have similar clinical and pathologic features, IPAH and FPAH are thought to be related diseases.

Diseases Associated with PAH

Multiple disease processes have been associated with the development of PAH. The associated disease may be regarded as one of the "hits" leading to the development of PAH.[34]

Collagen Vascular Disease. Collagen vascular disorders associated with the development of PAH include scleroderma, systemic lupus erythematosus (SLE), mixed connective tissue disease (MCTD), and rheumatoid arthritis. Of the collagen vascular disorders, scleroderma is the most common cause of PAH.[63] Autopsy studies have demonstrated evidence of PAH in up to 70% of scleroderma patients, with a higher prevalence in limited, rather than diffuse, scleroderma.[64,65] The presence of PAH portends a worse prognosis relative to scleroderma patients without PAH.[66] In multiple studies, Doppler echocardiogram has demonstrated the presence of PAH despite the lack of respiratory symptoms in a high percentage (23%–35%) of patients with scleroderma.[65,67] Thus, routine screening for PAH in the scleroderma population has been recommended. A strong association between PAH and Raynaud's phenomenon has also been observed.[68]

Congenital Systemic to Pulmonary Shunts. Congenital systemic to pulmonary shunts are a well recognized cause of PAH. Lesions with a left to right shunt (such as atrial septal defect, ventricular septal defect, patent ductus arteriosus, and truncus arteriosus) lead to chronically elevated pulmonary blood flow and mechanical stress on the pulmonary endothelium. If a significant left to right shunt (pulmonary flow/systemic flow >1.5) is not corrected, reversal of flow (Eisenmenger syndrome) may result. Children with congenital systemic to pulmonary shunts should be evaluated and followed by pediatric cardiologists experienced in the treatment of congenital heart defects. Of the conditions associated with the development of PAH, congenital heart disease has the best prognosis.

Portal Hypertension. Portopulmonary hypertension (PPHTN) is defined as PAH in the setting of underlying portal hypertension (portal pressure >10 mm Hg).[69] Of the patients diagnosed with PAH, 9% have portal hypertension.[70] Cirrhosis is not necessary for the development of PAH, as evidenced by cases of PPHTN in which portal hypertension was caused by nonhepatic causes.[71] The prevalence of PAH in patients with portal hypertension is 2% to 5%.[72,73] However, the risk of developing PAH increases with the duration of portal hypertension.[73] On average, PPHTN is diagnosed in the fifth decade with an even male to female distribution.[69,74,75] The mean survival after diagnosis is 15 months with a median survival of 6 months.[74] The factors initiating endothelial injury and leading to the development of PAH are not known but appear to be more complicated than shear stress from increased pulmonary blood flow.[76] Finally, in patients undergoing lung transplantation, the presence of moderate or severe PAH is known to increase mortality and morbidity.[77,78]

HIV Infection. HIV infection as a causative agent in the development of PAH is supported by a higher prevalence of PAH in HIV infected patients than in the general population (0.5% vs. 0.02%).[79] Direct viral action on endothelial and smooth muscle cells has been dismissed as a possible mechanism as a result of the lack of viral material in lung tissue and lack of data showing that endothelial cells are capable of supporting growth of HIV.[80,81] Furthermore, monkeys infected with the simian immunodeficiency virus developed PAH similar to that seen in humans, but viral material was not identified within the lung tissue.[82] Alterations in pulmonary endothelial cell homeostasis or an autoimmune mechanism is now believed to be the most logical mechanism for PAH.[83,84] The development of PAH is not related to the degree of immunosuppression or the CD4 cell count.[85] PAH in patients infected with HIV portends a poor prognosis, with median survival of 6 months after diagnosis of PH.[84] Controversy exists with regard to the impact of treatment of HIV on progression of PAH.[84,86,87]

Drugs and Toxins. Several appetite suppressants (anorexic drugs) are well known to increase risk for the development of PAH. Aminorex, fenfluramine, and dexfenfluramine have all been withdrawn from clinical use by the U.S. Food and Drug Administration (FDA) because of the increase risk of PAH is associated with consumption.[88,89] Fenfluramine has been shown to increase the odd of developing PAH by a factor of 6.3. The risk increases to a factor of 23.1 when exposed for greater than 3 months. The mechanism by which anorexic drugs lead to PAH is thought to be related to inhibition of voltage gated potassium channels (vasoconstriction because of the increased intracellular calcium) and depressed basal nitric oxide production.[90,91]

PAH Associated with Venous or Capillary Involvement

PAH associated with venous or capillary involvement consists of two rare disorders: pulmonary veno-occlusive disease and pulmonary capillary hemangiomatosis. Histologi-

cally, these disease entities resemble other forms of PAH. However, the vasculopathy involves not only the precapillary vasculature but also the capillaries, venules, and veins. Clinically, these disease entities can be difficult to distinguish from IPAH. Development of pulmonary edema after initiation of medical therapy with calcium channel blocker and epoprostenol has been reported.[92,93] Patients should be referred promptly to a lung transplant center for evaluation early in the course of the disease.

Persistent Pulmonary Hypertension of the Newborn

Persistent pulmonary hypertension of the newborn (PPHN) exist in three forms: hypertrophic, hypoplastic, and reactive. The hypertrophic form results in hypertrophied muscular tissue of the pulmonary arteries as a result of chronic fetal distress. Hypoplastic PPHN involves underdevelopment of the pulmonary arteries because of either congenital diaphragmatic hernia or amniotic fluid leakage. The reactive form has normal lung tissue but vasoconstriction because of an imbalance of vasoactive mediators.

Prognosis

The natural history and prognostic variables in patients with PAH is best studied in the IPAH population. The National Institute of Health (NIH) registry on the natural history of IPAH has demonstrated that the median survival is 2.8 years with a 1-, 3-, and 5-year survival rates of 68%, 48%, and 34%, respectively.[94] Relative to IPAH, PAH in association with either HIV or collagen vascular disease has a worse prognosis, whereas patients with PAH in the setting of congenital heart disease fare better.[95]

Clinical factors that predict a favorable outcome in patients PAH have been elucidated.[95] Functional class (Table 46-3), exercise tolerance (6-minute walk test [6MWT]), presence of a pericardial effusion, and hemodynamic variables have shown correlation with clinical outcome. Multiple studies have demonstrated that the NYHA Functional Class (NYHA-FC) is associated with improved survival and can be used as a predictor of mortality.[95] For example, the median survival of IPAH patients with NYHA-FC I or II is 6 years versus 2.5 years for patients with NYHA-FC-III and 6 months for NYHA-FC-IV.[94] Furthermore, IPAH patients with NYHA-FC IV have a significantly higher risk of death relative to patients with NYHA-FC I, II, or III when receiving similar medical therapy.[96,97] Finally, IPAH patients who are in NYHA-FC III or IV and who fail to respond after 3 months of treatment have worse survival relative to those whose symptoms improve.[98]

The 6MWT is an easy, safe, and reproducible test for the assessment of exercise capacity in patients with PAH. Multiple studies have demonstrated that baseline distance during the 6MWT is predictive of survival.[99–101] However, comparison of different distances and treatments modalities in each study limit the ability to assign a predicted survival to a distance walked. Echocardiography studies in patient with IPAH have found that the presence and severity of a pericardial effusion is an independent predictor of

TABLE 46-3. Functional Classification of Pulmonary Arterial Hypertension (PAH)

Class	Description
I	PAH without a resulting limitation of physical activity. Ordinary physical activity does not cause undue dyspnoea or fatigue, chest pain or near-syncope.
II	PAH resulting in a slight limitation of physical activity. The patient is comfortable at rest, but ordinary physical activity causes undue dyspnoea or fatigue, chest pain or near-syncope.
III	PAH resulting in a marked limitation of physical activity. The patient is comfortable at rest, but less than ordinary activity causes undue dyspnoea or fatigue, chest pain or near-syncope.
IV	PAH resulting in an inability to carry out any physical activity without symptoms. The patient has signs of right heart failure. Dyspnoea, fatigue or both may be present even at rest, and discomfort is increased by any physical activity.

Source: Reprinted with permission from Hoeper MM. Drug treatment of pulmonary arterial hypertension: current and future agents. Drugs. 2005;65;1337-1354.

poor outcome in patients with IPAH.[102,103] The negative effect of a pericardial effusion on exercise tolerance is as a result of impairment of right heart function. In individual studies, multiple different hemodynamic variables have been shown to predict outcome in IPAH patients.[94,104–106] However, mean right atrial pressure (mRAP) and cardiac index have most consistently demonstrated predictive value, with mRAP being the most powerful hemodynamic predictor of survival.[95]

Treatment

The leading cause of death in patients with PAH is progressive right heart failure. Thus, treatment of patients with PAH is aimed at improving or halting the progression of right heart failure, in order to improve symptoms and functional class as well as prolong life and delay the potential need for lung transplantation. A delay in the diagnosis of PAH of months to years is not uncommon as the nonspecific symptoms early in the course of the disease are often attributed to normal aging or weight gain. Unfortunately, 70% to 90% of patients have developed NYHA-FC III or IV symptoms by the time the correct diagnosis is made.[36] As such, most clinical trials have focused on NYHA-FC III or IV patients with little data on the benefits and risks of treating patients who are less symptomatic or have only mildly elevated PA pressures.[34,36] Patients should be referred to a specialized medical center experienced in the treatment of PAH to receive appropriate tailored therapy. Medical therapies for the treatment of patients with PAH

can be divided into lifestyle alterations, conventional therapies, and vasodilator therapy. Finally, most available data is from studies of patients diagnosed with IPAH.

Lifestyle Alterations

Patients with PAH must be educated as to activities which are potentially hazardous to their well being. In general, any activity that has the potential to cause hypoxemia, pulmonary vasoconstriction, or syncope must be avoided.[39] In patients with PAH who have cardiac arrest, resuscitation has demonstrated limited success (6% at 90 days).[107] High altitude and air travel may not be well tolerated because of the potential for hypoxia, pulmonary vasoconstriction, and worsening of right-sided heart failure. Decongestants and appetite suppressants must also be avoided because of the risk of worsening PH. Also, heavy exertion increases the risk for syncope, cardiopulmonary arrest, and death. However, low-dose exercise may be beneficial to patients with PAH.[108] Patient should be advised to receive immunization against influenza and pneumococcal pneumonia. Pregnancy should be discouraged as the hemodynamic changes during pregnancy impose a significant stress on women with PAH, with a resultant mortality rate of 30% to 50%.[109] Finally, elective surgery should be approached with caution because of high risk for vasovagal events which can rapidly lead to syncope, cardiopulmonary arrest, and even death.[36]

Conventional Therapies

Anticoagulation with warfarin for patients with IPAH has demonstrated a survival benefit in two small trials.[110,111] Based on these findings and the known role of in situ thrombosis in the pathogenesis of IPAH, warfarin therapy is generally recommended in the absence of contraindications, although the optimal INR is not known. As a result of the vasoconstrictor effects of hypoxia, oxygen supplementation is recommended to maintain oxygen saturation greater than 90%. Diuretics are indicated for the management of volume overload from right-sided heart failure. Digoxin has been used in the presence of right heart failure[112] and for rate control in patients with atrial fibrillation or atrial flutter. However, limited data is available on the efficacy of digoxin in PAH.

Vasodilator Therapy

Several medications with pulmonary arterial vasodilatory effects have been approved by the FDA and are available for clinical use in patients with PAH. Figure 46-5 outlines the therapeutic approach to NYHA-FC III and IV patients with PAH. The therapeutic agent to be chosen depends upon the results of acute vasodilator testing and NYHA functional class. Acute reversibility to vasodilator therapy is defined as a drop in mean PAP by at least 10 mm Hg to less than 40 mm Hg with either an increase or no change in cardiac output. Inhaled nitric oxide, intravenous epoprostenol, and intravenous adenosine are all short-acting pulmonary vasodilators which are acceptable for use in testing for reversibility. Patients with NYHA-FC IV

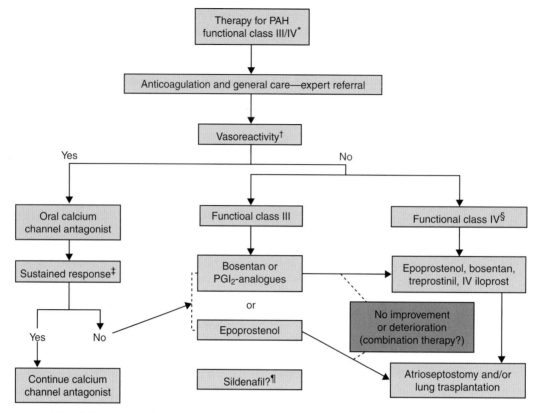

● **FIGURE 46-5.** Current treatment algorithm for PAH.
PGI$_2$, prostaglandin I$_2$.

*The algorithm is restricted to patients in functional class III or IV because very few data are available for functional class I/II patients, and class III/IV patients represent the largest population among PAH patients. All treatments have been evaluated mainly in sporadic PAH and in PAH associated with scleroderma. Extrapolation of these recommendations to the other PAH subgroups should be made with caution.

†A positive acute response to vasodilators is defined as a drop in mean PA pressure by at least 10 mm Hg to <40 mm Hg, in the presence of a normal cardiac output during acute challenge with inhaled nitric oxide, intravenous (IV) epoprostenol, or IV adenosine.

‡Sustained response to calcium channel antagonists is defined as patients being in functional class I or II with normal or near normal haemodynamics after several months of treatment.

§According to most experts, patients in functional class IV who present in a haemodynamically unstable condition should be treated immediately with IV epoprostenol.

¶Because of the lack of data from randomised controlled trials, the exact position of sildenafil has not been assigned.

Reproduced, with permission, from Hoeper MM. Drug treatment of pulmonary arterial hypertension: Current and future agents. Drugs. 2005;65:1337-1354.

symptoms or overt right heart failure probably should not undergo vasodilator testing, as they are not candidates for calcium channel blocker (CCB) therapy and the risks of the test outweigh the benefit.[34]

Calcium Channel Blockers. Patient who will derive a survival benefit from long-term therapy with calcium channel blockers (CCBs) can be identified by vasodilator testing.[111,113] Unfortunately, only a small percentage of patients (12.8%) demonstrate a positive response to vasodilator testing and only half of those patients (6.8%) will have a favorable long-term response.[114] However, because of the potential for drastic improvement in functional class

(NYHA-FC I or II) over a prolonged period and the relative ease of therapy relative to other treatment regimens, nearly all patients should be evaluated for CCB therapy. After initiation of therapy with an oral CCB (nifedepine, diltiazem, or amlodopine), patients must be assessed regularly to ensure a sustained response. If the patient does not achieve NYHA-FC I or II with near normal hemodynamics during the first year of follow-up, treatment with an alternative agent should be pursued.[34,115]

Prostacyclin. Prostacyclin (PGI$_2$) is a potent vasodilator, inhibitor of smooth muscle cell proliferation, and inhibitor of platelet activation. Prostacyclin is available in intravenous (epoprostenol, treprostinil, iloprost), subcutaneous (treprostinil), and inhaled (iloprost) forms in the United States. Beraprost, an oral prostacyclin, is available in Japan but not the United States because of the lack of data supporting long-term efficacy.[116] All forms of PGI_2 have short half lives requiring either continuous infusion or frequent administration. Continuous epoprostenol infusion is approved by the FDA for NYHA-FC III and IV patients with IPAH because of its positive impact on exercise tolerance, hemodynamics, and long-term survival.[98,101] Epoprostenol should be considered first line therapy for patients with NYHA-FC IV symptoms as a result of the proven survival benefit.[98] Epoprostenol also has FDA approval for PAH patients with scleroderma. Because epoprostenol administration requires continuous infusion through an indwelling central venous catheter, concern over line infection, catheter associated thrombus, and rebound PH with interruption of therapy add to the complexity of epoprostenol therapy. Treprostinil (subcutaneous and intravenous) is a more stable prostacyclin which has FDA approval for NYHA-FC II, III, and IV patients because of its ability to improve 6MWD and hemodynamic parameters.[117,118] Intravenous treprostinil is only approved for patients who develop intolerable pain and erythema at the subcutaneous infusion site. Although the longer half-life of treprostinil (4 hours) relative to epoprostenol is advantageous, epoprostenol is the only vasodilator proven to prolong survival. Inhaled iloprost has demonstrated improvement with regard to 6MWD, NYHA-FC, and hemodynamic variables.[119,120] Iloprost is approved for patient with NYHA-FC III of IV symptoms. However, because of a short half-life, iloprost require six to nine inhalations per day.

Endothelin Receptor Antagonists. Endothelin-1 (ET-1) is a potent vasoconstrictor and smooth muscle mitogen. ET-1 works through endothelin receptor A (ETA), present on PA smooth muscle cells, and endothelin receptor B (ETB), present on PA smooth muscle cells and endothelial cells. Activation of ETA and ETB receptors on smooth muscle cells leads to vasoconstriction and proliferation of vascular smooth muscle, whereas endothelial ETB receptor activation leads to vasodilatation via endothelial release of nitric oxide and prostacyclin. Bosentan is a dual ETA/ETB receptor antagonist approved by the FDA for NYHA-FC III and IV patients as a result of improvement in 6MWD, NYHA-FC, and hemodynamic variables.[121,122] Because of a theoretical advantage of selective ETA receptor antagonism, selective ETA receptor agents are currently under investigation.

Phosphodiesterase-5 Inhibitors. The vasodilatory response to nitric oxide is dependent upon the presence of cyclic guanosine monophosphate (cGMP). Phosphodiesterases (PDEs) function to inactivate cGMP. Thus, inhibition of PDE-5, an isoform found in the lung, has the potential to augment the pulmonary vascular response to nitric oxide.[123] Sildenafil, a PDE-5 antagonist, is approved

by the FDA for treatment of PAH because of the beneficial impact of sildenafil on exercise capacity, NYHA-FC, and hemodynamics.[124]

Combination Therapy. The different mechanisms of action of the various drugs currently available make combination therapy an intriguing option. Studies are currently ongoing to determine if combination therapy will be of clinical benefit.

Atrial Septostomy and Lung Transplantation

In atrial septostomy, a right to left intraatrial shunt is created in order to decompress the failing right heart and increase filling of the left-sided heart chambers. Atrial septostomy has substantial risk and is offered only as palliation or as a bridge to lung transplantation. The primary indication for lung transplantation in patients with PAH is clinical deterioration despite optimal medical therapy. Survival at 1 year for PAH is approximately 70%.[125]

● PA ANEURYSM

Aneurysms of the PA have been defined pathologically as localized vascular dilatations with deterioration of one or more layers of the vessel wall.[126] Clinically, PA aneurysms (PAAs) are radiologically demonstrable blood-filled sacs formed by dilatation of the walls of the artery.[127] Dissecting aneurysm refers to blood tracking within the arterial wall as a result of a tear in the intimal layer. Pseudoaneurysms or false aneurysms result from a breach in all layers of the vessel wall but with contained blood from compression by surrounding structures and clotting.

PA aneurysms are quite rare. The largest review found only eight cases of PAA in 109 571 autopsies performed—an incidence of one in 13 696.[128] Previous classification schemes have grouped PAAs as congenital or acquired,[129] large vessel or medium/small vessel,[130] and those with and without associated arteriovenous communications.[127] These classification schemes are limited because of the diverse etiology, poor understanding of the pathophysiology, and the probable interplay of multiple factors leading to the development of PAAs. The conditions known to be associated with the development of PAAs include (Table 46-4): infection (mycotic), congenital heart disease, PH, inherent weakness in the arterial wall and trauma. The primary factor leading to the development of a PAA is often difficult to elucidate as many patients have more than one condition; that is, congenital heart disease with PH[131] or congenital heart disease and endocarditis.[132]

Infection plays a significant role in the development of PAAs. In the past, syphilis and tuberculosis (Rasmussen's aneurysm) were the most common causative agents. Autopsy studies have demonstrated an incidence of PAAs of at least 4% in patients with untreated tuberculosis.[133] However, with the development of antibiotics and public health screening programs, PAAs from syphilis and tuberculosis are now rarely seen in developed countries. Pyogenic bacteria (i.e., *Staphylococcus aureus*, *Streptococcus* spp., and

---

TABLE 46-4. Conditions Associated with the Development of PA Aneurysms

Infection
    Tuberculosis (Rasmussen's aneurysm)
    Syphilis
    Pyogenic bacteria
    Fungal infection

Congenital heart disease
    Patent ductus arteriosus
    Atrial or ventricular septal defect
    Pulmonary valve agenesis
    Tetralogy of fallot

Pulmonary hypertension

Inherent weakness in the arterial wall
    Marfan syndrome
    Behcet's syndrome
    Hughes-Stovin syndrome
    Polyarteritis nodosa

Trauma
    Swan-Ganz catheterization
    Penetrating chest wall injuries

---

corynebacterium diphtheriae) and fungal species (*Candida albicans* and *Aspergillus flavus*) play a more prominent role. Whereas syphilis and tuberculosis alone can lead to the development of a PAA,[127] mycotic aneurysms associated with bacterial and fungal infections often occur in association with concomitant congenital heart disease, PH, or right-sided endocarditis.[134] Three mechanisms account for the development of mycotic aneurysms. In tuberculosis, the mechanism of aneurysm formation is caused by the external destruction of the vessel wall, replacement with granulation tissue and ultimately vessel weakness with aneurysm formation or rupture. PAAs from syphilis result in weakening of the vessel wall and atherosclerotic changes due infection of the vasa vasorum by *Treponema pallidum*.[135] The development of PAAs in patients with bacterial and fungal infections is from direct invasion of the intima of the pulmonary vessel at the site of septic embolism.[134]

While the association of congenital heart disease with PAAs is firmly established, the pathogenesis is not clearly understood. Although structural abnormalities of the arterial wall are often observed, it is unknown if these abnormalities are inherent or acquired.[136] Acquired lesions could result from increased pulmonary blood flow resulting in the development of PH,[127] abnormal high velocity vascular jets,[137] or an association with endocarditis.[138] Patent ductus arteriosus is the most common congenital anomaly associated with PAA formation. Atrial septal defect, ventricular septal defect, tetralogy of Fallot and transposition of the great vessels have also been associated. While the above congenital conditions of PAAs often occur in patients with PH, congenital pulmonary stenosis, and congenital pulmonary regurgitation are worthy of mention because of their occurrence in patients with normal pulmonary pressures. The proximal PAA that forms in patients with pulmonary valve abnormalities probably results from abnormal valve opening and asymmetric jet of blood flow (stenosis) and abnormal stress from increased stroke volume (regurgitation) leading to weakening of the vessel wall.[139]

Although case reports exist of patients with PAAs in which PH was the only identified pathogenic factor,[140] other factors are usually present. The role of PH in the development of PAAs is because of the presence of atheromatous disease (cystic medial necrosis) which leads to weakness within the wall of the vessel.[141] Patients with Marfan's syndrome are at risk for development of PAAs as a result of inherent vessel wall weakness from fibrillin deficiency and the presence of cystic medial necrosis.[142] Vasculitis, most notably Bechet disease,[143–145] can also affect the pulmonary arteries and lead to the development of PAAs via weakness in the vessel walls. Other vasculitis associated with PAAs includes giant cell arteritis[146] and microscopic polyangiitis.[147] Hugh-Stovin syndrome (aneurysms of the PA, thrombosis of peripheral veins and dural sinuses) is thought to share a common mechanism with Bechet disease.[148]

Trauma can lead to PAAs either from intravascular (Swan-Ganz catheter) or external (chest wall or surgical) injury. The majority of traumatic PAAs is actually pseudoaneurysms and will be discussed separately.

PAAs are often overshadowed by the underlying medical condition and often only come to medical attention because of an abnormality on a routine chest radiogram (CXR). PAAs must be considered in the work-up of a pulmonary nodule because of the potential morbidity and mortality of percutaneous needle biopsy of an aneurysm.[149] Symptoms of a PAA include hemoptysis, precordial pain caused by dissection, dyspnea, or cough. Of patients who present with hemoptysis, 3% to 6% is accounted for by PAAs.[150] The most life-threatening complications of PAAs are rupture and dissection. Other complications of PAAs are because of the compression of adjacent structures: coronary artery,[151] pulmonary vein,[151] and bronchus.[152]

While angiography is still considered the "gold standard" for diagnosis of PAAs, invasive imaging can be reserved until intervention is planned (Figure 46-6). Computed tomography (CT), magnetic resonance imaging (MRI) and echocardiography are reasonable first-line diagnostic tests.[130]

Other than treatment of the underlying etiology of the aneurysm, the optimal management strategy for PAAs is not known. Factors that are believed to increase risk of dissection or rupture are the presence of PH[153] and hemoptysis.[127] Because of the increased wall stress with any change in size (LaPlace's law), many advocate for an aggressive approach in all patients with a PAA. Certainly, the presence or absence of PH must be assessed. Although at least one case report exists in which a patient with severe PH is alive several years after diagnosis of a "giant" (greater than 5 cm) aneurysm,[154] a more aggressive approach is warranted. Because of increased surgical risk in patients with PH, endovascular stenting[155] and embolization with coils[156] is an alternative that may become the

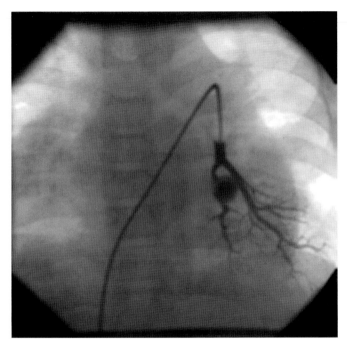

● **FIGURE 46-6.** Selective pulmonary angiogram of the left lower PA demonstrating mycotic aneurysm in a 9-year-old female with infective endocarditis and a patent ductus arteriosus.

Reproduced, with permission, from Lertsapcharoen P, Chottivittayatarakorn P, Benjacholamas V. Mycotic aneurysms of the pulmonary arteries. Heart. 2002;88:524.

preferred therapy. In patients with Behcet disease (BD), improved survival has been demonstrated in patients who received embolization therapy versus those who underwent surgery.[157] Patients without PH or pulmonic valve pathology can follow more conservative management as they have confirmed late survival.[158]

● PA PSEUDOANEURYSMS

Pseudoaneurysms or false aneurysms of the PA result from a breach in all layers of the vessel wall but with contained blood from compression by surrounding structures and clotting. Pseudoaneurysms may result from trauma (intravascular or extravascular), malignant lung tumors, infections, and rarely, in primary PH.[159] Intravascular trauma occurs mostly in association with placement of intravascular catheters (i.e., Swan-Ganz catheter). Extravascular trauma from chest tube placement,[160] penetrating chest wall injury, surgery in the thorax (i.e., Glenn operation),[161] or blunt trauma[162] can result in pseudoaneurysm formation. Malignant tumors that have been reported to lead to the development of pseudoaneurysms include metastatic angiosarcoma,[163] bronchial carcinoma,[164] squamous cell carcinoma,[165] and pulmonary leiomyosarcoma.[166]

The incidence of pseudoaneurysm formation from placement of a PA catheter is 1 per 1600 cases.[167] While the mechanism by which the PA catheter causes pseudoaneurysm formation has not been elucidated, plausible mechanisms include pressure from the expanded balloon exceeding the tensile strength of vessel wall,[168] "spearing" of the vessel wall by the catheter tip,[169] retraction of the wedged balloon and flushing of the wedged catheter.[170] Risk factors for pseudoaneurysm formation include anticoagulation, older than 60 years of age, improper balloon inflation, improper catheter positioning, cardiopulmonary bypass with catheter in place,[170] and chronic steroid administration.[171] Conflicting data exist over the contribution of PH to pseudoaneurysm formation.[172]

Rupture of a PA with compression by lung parenchyma and clot formation is the nidus for pseudoaneurysm formation. Most pseudoaneurysms present as hemoptysis during the inciting event.[173] However, some patients remain asymptomatic and only come to clinical attention years later.[174] In either case, treatment is warranted as a result of the high mortality associated with an observational approach.[175] While spiral is a useful noninvasive modality for diagnosis of pseudoaneurysms, angiography remains the gold standard (Figure 46-7). Angiography not only allows imaging of the pseudoaneurysm but also allows for immediate treatment of the abnormality. Embolization with coils is the treatment of choice for most PA pseudoaneurysms because of high success rate and limited morbidity compared to surgical resection.[173]

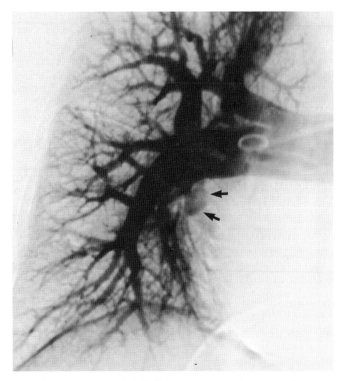

● **FIGURE 46-7.** A right PA arteriogram demonstrating a pseudoaneurysm arising form the right middle lobe PA.

Reproduced, with permission, from Poplausky MR, Rozenblit G, Rundback JH, Crea G, Maddineni S, Leonardo R. Swan-Ganz catheter-induced pulmonary artery pseudoaneurysm formation: three case reports and a review of the literature. Chest. 2001;120: 2105-2111.

● PULMONARY ARTERIOVENOUS MALFORMATIONS

Pulmonary arteriovenous malformations (PAVMs) are abnormal direct communications between a branch of the PA and pulmonary vein which may be small telangiectasias or associated with an aneurysm. Because these anomalies lack an intervening capillary bed, direct communication exists between the pulmonary and systemic circulations. Hypoxemia may result (right-to-left shunt), as well as polycythemia. Fifty percent of patients remain asymptomatic,[176] although significant hypoxemia may be present. However, even in patients without hypoxemia or symptoms, a substantial risk for paradoxical emboli exists.[177]

PAVMs are usually congenital but can be acquired. Congenital causes include hereditary hemorrhagic telangiectasia (HHT), that is, Osler-Weber-Rendu disease and Fanconi syndrome. The most common congenital cause of PAVMs is HHT, which accounts for more than 80% of congenital cases[178] and at least 60% of all cases.[179] Acquired causes of PAVMs include postthoracic surgery, trauma, hepatic cirrhosis, metastatic carcinoma, mitral stenosis, systemic amyloidosis, bronchiectasis, and infections (tuberculosis, actinomycosis, and schistosomiasis).[180–186]

Hereditary hemorrhagic telangiectasia (HHT) consists of a classic triad of epistaxis, telangiectasias, and a family history of the disorder. Because most PAVMs occur in patients with HHT, it is important to consider this disease entity in patients with a PAVM. In order to increase diagnostic accuracy of HHT, four criteria have been developed: spontaneous recurrent nose bleeds, mucocutaneous telangiectasia, visceral involvement, and an affected first-degree relative.[187] Definite HHT is present when patients have three criteria, suspected HHT if two criteria are present, and unlikely HHT when only one criterion is present.

HHT is inherited in an autosomal dominant fashion. The disease has been shown to be associated with mutations in at least two genes: endogolin on chromosome 9 and activin receptor-like kinase 1 (ALK-1) on chromosome 12, termed HHT1 and HHT2, respectively.[188,189] Both of these genes encode proteins which are part of the transforming growth factor-β (TGF-β) superfamily and are involved in vascular development and homeostatis.[176] HHT is believed to develop because of aberrant TGF-β signaling during vascular development and homeostatis.[190]

The clinical manifestations of PAVMs result from the capillary free communication of the PA and the systemic circulation leading to a right-to-left (R-L) shunt, as well as a route for emboli to reach the systemic circulation, most notably the cerebral circulation. Despite the presence of a R-L shunt, cardiac hemodynamics are usually within normal limits.[191] Furthermore, if PH is discovered during the work-up of a PAVM, other causes should be investigated, as PAVMs rarely contribute to elevated pulmonary pressures.[190] The complications of PAVMs can be divided into respiratory and neurological. While half of patients are asymptomatic from a respiratory standpoint, 47%

of patients report dyspnea on exertion.[176] The severity of dyspnea and the degree of hypoxemia are directly related to the magnitude of the shunt. Eleven percent of patients develop hemoptysis[176] which can be life threatening. However, most episodes are from bronchial telangiectasias in association with concomitant HHT. Neurologic complications result from paradoxical emboli. The rate of neurologic events is significant: stroke (18%), transient ischemic attack (37%), cerebral abscess (9%), migraine (43%), and seizure (8%).[192] Reportedly, 75% of patients with PAVMs have detectable abnormalities on physical examination,[193] most commonly a bruit (49%) but also cyanosis (30%) and clubbing (36%).[176] The bruit can be made more prominent by inspiration and the Muller maneuver (inspiration with a closed glottis). Some patients also exhibit platypnea orthodeoxia[194] because of the basilar location of most PAVMs.

The diagnostic work-up of PAVMs consists of demonstration of a right to left shunt, as well as imaging studies consistent with the finding of a PAVM. The tests used to determine the presence of a R-L shunt are the 100% oxygen method, contrast echocardiography and radionuclide imaging. The 100% oxygen method is a reasonable first test because of low cost, ease of performance,[186] and high sensitivity (exceeding 95% in multiple studies).[195,196] Thus, the 100% oxygen method is considered the gold standard for noninvasive estimation of shunt size.[176] After the patient breathes 100% oxygen for 15 to 20 minutes, a shunt fraction is calculated. The normal physiologic shunt is 5%, and any value that exceeds this threshold is considered abnormal.

Contrast echocardiography consists of injecting agitated saline into a peripheral vein. In normal subjects, air bubbles will appear only in the right-sided cardiac chambers, as they are unable to pass through the pulmonary capillary network. However, in patients with a R-L shunt, bubbles appear in the left atrium within 1 to 2 beats in the presence of an intracardiac shunt and 3 to 5 beats if the shunt is within the pulmonary circulation. However, contrast echocardiography is limited by the inability to determine the degree of the shunt, as well as being too sensitive for routine clinical use.

Radionuclide imaging consists of injecting technetium-99 m labeled albumin. The activity over the lung and the right kidney are measured by a gamma camera which allows for comparison between the amounts of tracer reaching the systemic circulation with the total received.[197] While sensitive for detection of R-L shunt, this method is unable to differentiate between an intracardiac versus an intrapulmonary shunt.[198]

The classic chest radiograph (CXR) (Figure 46-8) finding is a sharply defined round or oval mass of uniform density that ranges in size from 1 to 5 cm in diameter and is often associated with band-shaped shadows because of feeding and draining vessels.[191] While some authors report CXR abnormalities in up to 90% of patients with PAVMs,[179,199] the abnormal findings are often very subtle.[190] Thus, a normal CXR does not rule out the presence of PAVMs.[200]

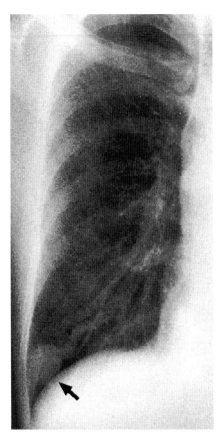

● **FIGURE 46-8.** Chest radiograph demonstrating a pulmonary arteriovenous malformation in the right lower lobe.

Reproduced, with permission, from Guttmacher AE, Marchuk DA, White RI. Hereditary hemorrhagic telangiectasia. N Engl J Med. 1995;333:918-924.

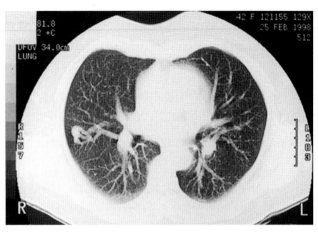

● **FIGURE 46-9.** CT of a pulmonary arteriovenous malformation in the right middle lobe.

Reproduced, with permission, from Shovlin CL, Letarte M. Hereditary haemorrhagic telangiectasia and pulmonary arteriovenous malformations: issues in clinical management and review of pathogenic mechanisms. Thorax. 1999;54:714-729.

formed, multiple studies have demonstrated that the natural history of untreated malformations leads to considerable PAVM related morbidity (15%–31%)[179,200,204] and mortality (8%–25%).[179,200,204,205] Because of the development of percutaneous embolization techniques, surgical resection is now performed only when embolization therapy has failed or is contraindicated. Percutaneous embolization therapy consists of placing detachable but retrievable stainless steel coils and/or balloons into the feeding artery of the PAVM. The thrombogenic foreign objects lead to blood stagnation

Both contrast enhanced CT and 3-D helical CT have been employed for diagnosis and visualization of PAVMs (Figure 46-9). Contrast enhanced CT has proven to be significantly better for diagnosis of PAVMs than pulmonary angiography (98% vs. 60%).[201] Whereas contrast enhanced CT allows for detection of PAVMs, 3-D helical CT is required for defining the angioarchitecture. In comparison to pulmonary angiography, 3-D helical CT combined with transverse sections allow for accurate assessment of 95% of PAVMs versus 32% with unilateral pulmonary angiography.[202] The disadvantage of 3-D helical CT is false positive diagnosis, especially of vascular tumors.[203] While pulmonary angiography remains the gold standard for diagnosis of PAVMs (Figure 46-10), angiography can be reserved for patients in whom therapy is being contemplated in order to better define the feasibility prior to intervention on an individual PAVM. MRI is rarely used for the diagnosis of PAVM mostly because of limited availability, relative expense and the need of highly specialized staff for interpretation.[191]

The optimal management strategy for patients with PAVMs has not been established.[191] While no randomized study comparing treatment to observation has been per-

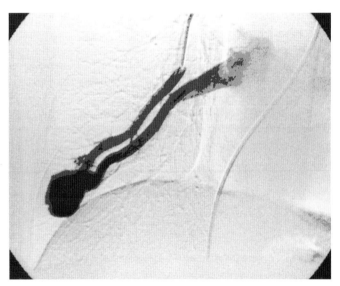

● **FIGURE 46-10.** Selective pulmonary angiogram of solitary pulmonary arteriovenous malformation in the right lower lobe.

Reproduced, with permission, from Guttmacher AE, Marchuk DA, White RI. Hereditary hemorrhagic telangiectasia. N Engl J Med. 1995;333:918-924.

and thrombus formation which obliterates the communication. Some authors have advocated for embolization therapy in patients with symptomatic PAVMs and also for prophylaxis when the feeding artery is >3 mm in diameter.[186] The largest series of embolization therapy (Baltimore-Yale series[192,194,206–208] and Hammersmith series[209–211]) report no mortality related to the procedure. The most common complication is pleurisy, which can occur in 7% to 31% of patients. The cause of pleurisy has not been elucidated but does not appear related to pulmonary infarction. Paradoxical embolization can occur but does not appear to exceed 4% in the more recent series. Despite apparent successful therapy, a residual shunt may persist and recanalization may occur, in which case reembolization may be indicated.

Screening for PAVMs should be done in all patients with HHT[186] as well as family members of patients with HHT.[212] Screening after embolization therapy should be performed at 1 month and 1 year to assess for residual shunt.[186] Screening with 3-D helical CT is recommended every 3 to 5 years to assess for the development of new PAVMs.[208]

Antibiotic prophylaxis is recommended, even after treatment of a PAVM, for any procedure in which bacteremia is expected, that is, dental and surgical interventions.[213] Female patients with PAVMs should be counseled as to the risk of PAVM growth and rupture during pregnancy.[214]

● PULMONARY ARTERY STENOSIS

Pulmonary artery stenosis (PAS) is most often found in association with congenital heart disease or as a complication of congenital heart disease treatment. Historically, PAS has been treated primarily by pediatric specialists. However, because of the advances in the treatment of congenital heart disease, congenital heart disease patients now commonly live into adulthood and may be encountered by physicians who treat adults.

The etiology of PAS is categorized as congenital, postsurgical, and acquired.[215] PAS occurs in 2% to 3% of patients with congenital heart disease[216] and has been associated with nearly every congenital heart disease, including pulmonary valve stenosis, aortic valve stenosis, atrial septal defect, ventricular septal defect, patent ductus arteriosus, transposition of the great vessels, and the tetralogy of Fallot.[217] Congenital PAS occurs in isolation 40% of the time.[218] It has also been associated with very rare congenital syndromes, including Williams Beuren syndrome,[219,220] Alagille syndrome,[221] and total generalized lipodystrophy.[222] Postsurgical PAS can occur after either lung transplantation or correction of a congenital heart disease. Postlung transplant PAS is not common but carries a poor prognosis.[223] Because of scarring at the site of anastomoses,[215,224,225] PAS has been reported following the Blalock-Taussig, Waterston-Cooley, Potts, Glenn, and Fontan procedures. Indeed, any surgical manipulation of the PA may lead to scarring and stenosis.[215] Acquired causes of PAS include Takayasu's arteritis (TA) and rubella. Furthermore, external compression of the PA leading to

stenosis has been reported in intrathoracic malignancy, fibrosing mediastinitis, silicosis, and sarcoidosis.[226,227]

PAS occurs in four morphologic forms.[218] Type I has a single constriction in the main right or left PA. Type II lesions are located at the bifurcation of the distal main PA and the origin of the right or left PA. Type III lesions are defined as stenosis at the ostium of multiple segmental pulmonary arteries with associated poststenotic dilatation and sparing of the main PA and proximal branch arteries. Type IV lesions are multiple stenoses involving both the segmental and central pulmonary arteries.

Right-sided heart failure caused by pulmonary hypertension is the most serious potential complication of untreated PAS. Patients with hemodynamically significant PAS may present with dyspnea from pulmonary hypertension or signs and symptoms of right-sided heart failure. Pulmonary angiography remains the gold standard for diagnosis and preintervention evaluation of PAS. However, CT and MRI may be of benefit in some conditions. Patients with PAS and evidence of pulmonary hypertension may be misdiagnosed and treated for chronic pulmonary thromboembolic disease because of a similar appearance on ventilation perfusion imaging.[228]

Treatment of PAS is generally indicated when patients have significantly elevated right ventricular pressure, hypertension in the unaffected segments of the PA, marked decrease in flow in the affected segment of the lung, right ventricular dysfunction, or symptoms.[216,229] Most data on the outcome of treatment modalities are limited to the pediatric population, since PAS is predominantly a pediatric disease. However, case reports do exist of successful treatment of PAS in the adult population. Stent implantation has become the preferred treatment modality, although surgery and balloon dilation are treatment options in some cases.[230] Surgical repair of PAS is reserved for supravalvular pulmonary stenosis and stenosis at the bifurcation of branch pulmonary arteries.[217] Proximal lesions of the PA should be addressed when a patient is undergoing surgical repair of a cardiac lesion.[217] Surgical treatment of PAS in the peripheral PA is best avoided because of the high rates of restenosis (50%–60% at 5 years) and a higher rate of complications relative to other treatment options.[230,231] Prior to the development of stents, balloon angioplasty was utilized as a less invasive alternative to surgery.[232,233] Balloon angioplasty was found to be acutely successful in 50% to 60% of patients with a restenosis rate of 15% and a complication rate of 5% to 10%.[234,235] The development of high pressure inflation (17–20 atmospheres) improved immediate success rates from 50% to 81% but with an increased rate of complications (13%).[236] Complications from balloon angioplasty include transient pulmonary edema, PA dissection, aneurysm, rupture, and death.

PA stenting has demonstrated both immediate (up to 96%) and sustained long-term success.[237–241] Stent implantation has proven to improve significantly the pressure gradient across the lesion (from severe to mild), double the PA diameter at the site of the stenosis (5–6 mm present to 11 mm poststent), and increase ipsilateral lung

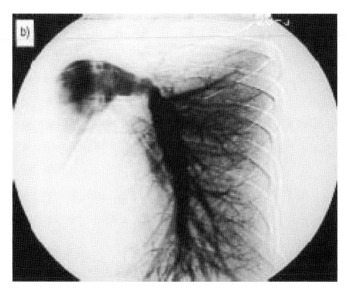

● **FIGURE 46-11.** Successful stent implantation in patient with pulmonary atresia and ventricular septal defect.

Reproduced, with permission, from O'Laughlin MP. Catheterization treatment of stenosis and hypoplasia of pulmonary arteries. Pediatr Cardiol. 1998;19:48-56.

perfusion[237–239] (Figure 46-11). The success of stent implantation compared to balloon angioplasty relates to the reduction in vessel recoil by providing a scaffold for the PA. Furthermore, the intimal tear that is required for successful balloon dilation is not needed with stent implantation.[215] After stent implantation, all stents demonstrate some degree of tissue in growth.[240] However, significant restenosis is rare and, when present, is nearly always treatable with redilation.[215,238,240] Other complications of stent implantation include ventricular arrhythmias, thrombus formation, compromise of arterial side branches, intimal flaps with or without arterial rupture, and the misplacement and migration of stents.[242,243] However, with increased clinical experience, morbidity, and mortality have improved.[241] Although most series report data on interventions in patients with congenital lesions, multiple reports of successful stenting for external compression (i.e., malignancy) are available.[226,227,244] Finally, stenting has proven to be a more cost-effective treatment for PAS than either surgery or balloon dilation.[230]

● **VASCULITIS**

Vasculitis, inflammation of blood vessels, not only affects the systemic vasculature but also may involve the pulmonary vascular bed. Pulmonary vasculitis can be divided into those disease entities affecting the large to medium sized pulmonary arteries and those involving primarily the small vessels (i.e., arterioles, venules, and alveolar capillaries). Vasculitides affecting the large to medium sized pulmonary arteries usually manifest as either aneurysms or stenosis,[245] whereas small vessel vasculitis leads to capillaritis and possibly diffuse alveolar hemorrhage (DAH).

Large to Medium Vessel Vasculitis of the PA

TA, BD, and its variant, Hughes-Stovin syndrome, are the predominant vasculitides affecting the large to medium sized arteries of the lung.

Takayasu's Arteritis. TA is a chronic, idiopathic, and inflammatory disease affecting primarily large vessels, such as the aorta and its main branches.[246] Although TA has been observed worldwide, most cases present in women of reproductive age, with the highest prevalence in individuals of Asian descent.[247] The predominant clinical manifestations are from systemic arterial stenosis and occlusion, but aneurismal dilatation can occur. The clinical presentation relates to the systemic arteries involved: Subclavian (93%); aorta (65%); common carotid (58%); renal (38%); vertebral (35%); innominate (27%); axillary (20%); celiac (18%); superior mesenteric (18%); and common iliac (17%).[246]

Although originally thought to be rare, PA involvement occurs in 50% or more of cases when specifically investigated (Figure 46-12).[248] It is often overlooked, however, as patients focus on systemic manifestations of TA and deny pulmonary symptoms even in the presence of moderate to severe pulmonary hypertension.[249] No correlation exists between the extent of PA involvement and systemic arteritis.[250] Rarely, the PA can be affected in the absence of systemic involvement,[251–255] with patients reporting dyspnea, chest pain, or hemoptysis. In the absence of systemic arterial involvement, the diagnosis of TA may be difficult to establish and may be mistaken for chronic pulmonary embolism because of the similar appearance on ventilation perfusion scan and pulmonary angiography.[254] An elevated erythrocyte sedimentation rate may not be present even in active disease,[246] and reliance on clinical, angiographic, and pathologic data is required for diagnosis.[254] The classification scheme for TA originally involved three varieties: Type I or Shimizu-Sano (aortic arch and branches), Type II or Kimoto (thoracic aorta and branches) and Type III or Inada (feature of Type I and II).[255] However, the addition of Type IV or Oota has been advocated for those patients with PA involvement.[249]

The clinical impact of TA PA involvement on patient outcome is not known. Current treatment focuses predominantly on systemic involvement and consists of glucocorticoids with the addition of cytotoxic agents when glucocorticoids fail to arrest progression or patients relapse with glucocorticoid taper. Thus, the affect of treatment on pulmonary vasculature and pulmonary hypertension (when present) is not known.

Behcet Disease. BD is a multisystem and chronic inflammatory disorder of unknown etiology. It is characterized by recurrent oral and genital ulcerations, ocular manifestations, and additional clinical manifestations in multiple organ systems.[256] The diagnostic criteria proposed by the International Study Group of BD relies upon the presence of recurrent oral ulcerations, as well as any two of the following: Recurrent genital ulceration, eye lesions, skin

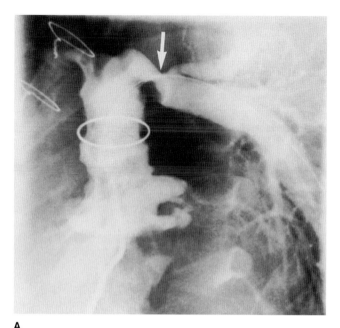

A

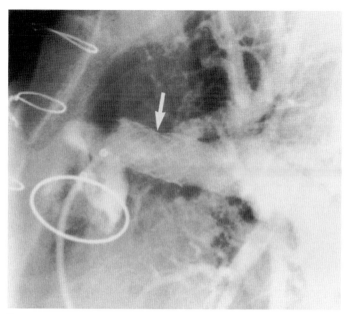

B

● FIGURE 46-12. (A and B) Pulmonary angiogram demonstrating pulmonary arterial stenosis.

Brugiere O, Mal H, Sleiman C, Groussard O, Mellot F, Fournier M. Isolated pulmonary arteries involvement in a patient with Takayasu's arteritis. Eur Respir J. 1998;11:767-770.

lesions, and a positive pathergy test (the development of an aseptic erythematous nodule or pustule 24 to 48 hours after skin prick with a sterile needle).[257] The onset of symptoms is usually in the third or fourth decade of life,[258] with equal prevalence in both males and females.[259] Although seen worldwide, the highest prevalence is in Turkey, with a clustering along the Silk Road, the ancient route of silk trade extending from eastern Asia to the Mediterranean basin.[258] Male sex and onset of symptoms before 25 years of age are very strong prognostic indicators of disease severity.[260]

Pulmonary artery aneurysms (PAA), pulmonary arterial and venous thrombosis, and pulmonary infarction are noninfectious pulmonary manifestations of BD (Figure 46-13).[259] Vasculitis in the pulmonary vasculature is the common mechanism responsible for PAA, thrombosis, and infarction in BD. Inflammation of the vasa vasorum leads to degeneration of the elastic lamina, in situ thrombus formation, and thickening and weakening of the vessel wall.[256,261] The prevalence of thoracic involvement in BD is estimated to be 5% to 10%; however, studies are limited by small sample size and retrospective data in which patients came to attention secondary to symptoms.[262–264]

BD is thought to be the most common cause of PAAs.[265] Patients who have BD and a PAA are mostly young males (89% male with a mean age of 30.1 years).[266] Thrombophlebitis may also be associated with PAAs in patients with BD.[263] On average, more than 5 years elapse between the diagnosis of BD and the manifestation of a PAA.[266] Multiple PAAs are most commonly observed, but some patients present with a solitary aneurysm.[261]

The presence of PAAs in patients with BD is a very poor prognostic sign[261,267] and may be the leading cause of death.[264] Retrospective data has shown that the 1 year and 5 years survival after the recognition of a PAA is 57% and 39%, respectively.[266] In one series, the mean length

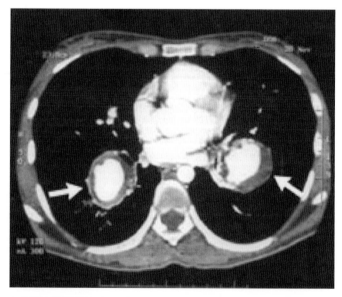

● FIGURE 46-13. Computed tomographic scan of the chest demonstrating bilateral PA aneurysms.

Reproduced, with permission, from Lohani S, Niven R. Images in clinical medicine. Bilateral pulmonary-artery aneurysms in Behcet's syndrome. N Engl J Med. 2005;353:400.

of survival of patients who presented with hemoptysis was 10 months.[263] Alarmingly, hemoptysis is the most common presenting symptom of PAAs.[256] The mechanism of hemoptysis is thought to be due to the rupture of the aneurysm with erosion into a bronchus.[259] This theory is supported by the observation of an air-filled cavity on CT after embolization of a ruptured PAA.[268] Other mechanisms of hemoptysis in patients with BD include angiodysplastic bronchial arteries and pulmonary embolism with infarction.[269]

Because of the high mortality associated with PAAs, a screening chest X-ray with a follow-up spiral CT scan has been advocated for patients with BD.[262] Spiral CT is preferred over magnetic resonance angiography because of the ability of the CT to assess lung parenchyma and vasculature.[256] Furthermore, angiography should be used with caution, as an aneurysm may not be visualized because of the organized thrombus within the lumen of the vessel.[261] Furthermore, in patients with BD, the risk for thrombosis at venous puncture sites and aneurysm formation at arterial puncture sites is increased.[256]

The management of PAAs in patients with BD includes medical therapy (steroids and immunosuppressive medications), percutaneous embolization, and surgical resection. Medical therapy with steroids and immunosuppressive medications is thought to be best if instituted when aneurysms are small and before irreversible arterial wall damage has occurred.[270] Disappearance of PAAs has been reported with both steroids[267,271] and immunosuppressive medications.[272] Anticoagulation is not recommended, even in the presence of thrombi, because of the increased mortality most likely secondary to increased bleeding with PA rupture.[258,266] Furthermore, in BD, thrombi form in situ in the pulmonary vasculature and are organized. In the presence of hemoptysis or an enlarging aneurysm, embolization is recommended.[266,273] If embolization is not available, surgical intervention should be considered.[273] However, caution should be used when considering surgical intervention, as rupture of a contralateral aneurysm has occurred after surgical resection, possibly related to increased flow through the contralateral lung.[274]

Hughes-Stovin Syndrome. Hughes-Stovin syndrome is a very rare disorder in which patients develop deep venous thrombosis (usually caval veins) and single or multiple PA aneurysms.[275] This syndrome predominately affects young males in the second to fourth decade of life and is thought to be a variant of BD, because of similar clinical, angiographic (Figure 46-14), and histologic features, that is, inflammation of the vasa vasorum.[276] Hughs-Stovin syndrome is treated in a manner similar to BD, with steroids and immunosuppressants.[277] However, the effectiveness of treatment is in doubt because of the high mortality associated with the syndrome, even when treated.[276] Massive pulmonary hemorrhage caused by aneurysm rupture is a frequent terminal event.[278]

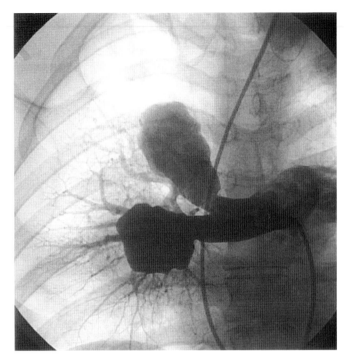

● FIGURE 46-14. Angiogram of a pulmonary arterial aneurysm.

Reproduced, with permission, Kindermann M, Wilkens H, Hartmann W, et al. Images in cardiovascular medicine: Hughes-Stovin syndrome. Circulation. 2003;108;e156.

Small Vessel Vasculitis of the PA

Small vessel vasculitis of the pulmonary vasculature can involve the arterioles, venules, and/or alveolar capillaries. This disease is often termed capillaritis, a necrotizing inflammatory process that can lead to destruction of the interstitium and the alveolar capillary basement membrane. If destruction of the basement membrane allows red blood cells to enter the alveolar space, DAH may ensue.

In capillaritis, the neutrophil plays a central role in the inflammatory and destructive process within the alveolar capillary. Histologically, capillaritis is characterized by an edematous interstitium infiltrated by neutrophils undergoing leukocytoclasis (fragmentation). The fragmented neutrophils lead to fibrinoid necrosis and loss of integrity of the alveolar capillary membrane, thereby allowing red blood cells to enter the alveolar space.[279] While it is recognized that the infiltration and activation of neutrophils lead to release of proteolytic enzymes responsible for necrosis and the loss of integrity of the interstitium and alveolar capillary basement membrane, the stimuli which attract, prime, and activate the neutrophils are not known.[280] Antineutrophil cytoplasmic autoantibodies (ANCA)[281] and immune complex deposition[282] may play a role in some diseases.

Patients with capillaritis most often come to clinical attention as a result of the symptoms related to DAH. Hemoptysis is the most common clinical manifestation. However, even in the presence of significant alveolar bleeding, more than 30% of patients do not develop

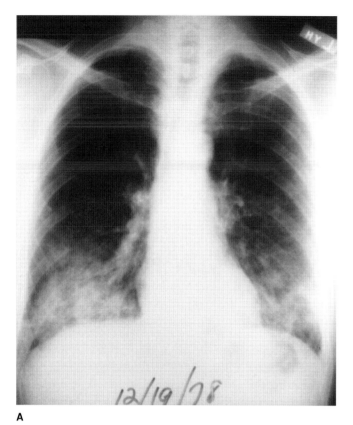

A

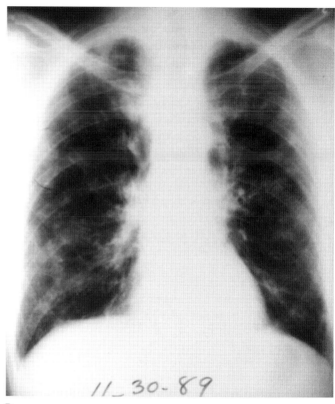

B

● **FIGURE 46-15.** Chest x-ray demonstrating DAH.

Reproduced, with permission, from Schwarz MM, Brown KK. Small vessel vasculitis of the lung. Thorax. 2000;55:502-510.

hemoptysis.[280] Patients may also develop dyspnea, anemia, low-grade fever, and diffuse, bilateral alveolar infiltrate on chest radiograph (Figure 46-15). Approximately 50% of patients with DAH require assisted ventilation.[280] Although capillaritis accounts for 80% of the cases of DAH, other etiologies including bland pulmonary hemorrhage and diffuse alveolar damage, which must be considered because of the differences in treatment and prognosis.[283] Whereas the diagnosis of DAH is clinical, capillaritis requires a pathologic specimen for diagnosis. However, DAH can be assumed to be capillaritis in the presence of an associated disease condition.

Capillaritis most commonly occurs in isolation, that is, isolated pauci-immune capillaritis. The ensuing discussion will divide capillaritis as follows (Table 46-5): (1) Isolated pauci-immune capillaritis; (2) Capillaritis in the setting of systemic vasculitis; (3) Capillaritis in the setting of collagen vascular disease; and (4) Miscellaneous conditions associated with autoantibody production.[280]

Isolated Pauci-Immune Capillaritis. Isolated pauci-immune capillaritis is small vessel vasculitis limited to the lung without systemic involvement.[282] The disease can present with and without the presence of serum p-ANCA. Isolated pauci-immune capillaritis without p-ANCA is the most common form of pulmonary capillaritis and DAH in one series.[282] When treated with corticosteroids

and cyclophosphamide, the prognosis was generally good. p-ANCA positive isolated pauci-immune capillaritis has been reported; however, long-term follow-up to determine if these patients developed a systemic disease is not available.[284] Finally, concern has been raised that patients with isolated pauci-immune vasculiti s may have been misdiagnosed as having idiopathic pulmonary hemosiderosis in the past.[280]

Capillaritis in the Setting of Systemic Vasculitis.

Wegener's Granulomatosis. Wegener's granulomatosis (WG) is a syndrome consisting of a triad of necrotizing granulomatous inflammation of the upper and lower respiratory tract, necrotizing glomerulonephritis, and small vessel vasculitis. The presence of the full triad is not necessary for the WG diagnosis. In limited forms, c-ANCA is particularly helpful because of the strong association between c-ANCA and WG.[285] Capillaritis is a common finding, occurring in up to 40% of patients.[286,287] However, DAH occurs in less than 10% of patients with WG.[287,288] Hemoptysis in patients with WG is usually caused by nodules and/or infiltrates than DAH.[289] Patients who have WG and develop DAH usually have a more fulminant course in which DAH is the initial manifestation of their disease.[289,290] Whereas patients with WG generally have a good prognosis, those with DAH have a very high mortality (up to 66%) even

TABLE 46-5. Aetiology of Small Vessel Vasculitis of the Lungs (Pulmonary Capillaritis) in Order of Relative Frequency

Isolated pauci-immune pulmonary capillaritis
Pulmonary allograft rejection
SLE
Wegener's granulomatosis
Microscopic polyangiitis
Goodpasture's syndrome
Rheumatoid arthritis
Polymyositis
Primary antiphospholipid syndrome
Scleroderma
Idiopathic pauci-immune glomerulonephritis
Henoch-Schoenlein purpura
IgA nephropathy
Behcet's syndrome
Hypersensitivity vasculitis
   PTU
   Diphenylhydantoin
Churg-Strauss syndrome
Essential cryoglobulinaemia
Acquired immune deficiency syndrome
Myasthenia gravis
Ulcerative colitis
Retinoic acid syndrome
Autologous bone marrow transplantation

Source: Reprinted, with permission, from Schwarz MM, Brown KK. Small vessel vasculitis of the lung. Thorax. 2000;55:502-510.

with aggressive medical treatment of corticosteroids and cyclophosphamide.[283]

Microscopic Polyangiitis. Microscopic polyangiitis is a pauci-immune necrotizing vasculitis that affects small blood vessel (venules, arterioles and capillaries) of predominantly the kidneys and lungs with or without involvement of medium-sized vessels.[291] Microscopic polyangiitis has a strong association with p-ANCA[292] and is considered to be the small vessel variant of polyarteritis nodosa.[280] These conditions are differentiated by the lack of small vessel, renal, and lung involvement in polyarteritis nodosa. Capillaritis and DAH can occur 10% to 30% of patients with microscopic polyangiitis.[293,294] Capillaritis may be the only evidence of small vessel involvement that allows differentiation from other disease states.[295] The mortality associated with the first episode of DAH is up to 25%, with recurrence expect in survivors.[280]

Goodpasture's Syndrome. Goodpasture's syndrome is a disease associated with antibasement membrane antibodies (ABMA) direct against the noncollagenous carboxyl-terminal region of type IV basement membrane collagen molecule in the kidney and the lung.[296] Rare cases of capillaritis associated with DAH have been reported; however,

DAH in Goodpasture's syndrome is more frequently because of bland hemorrhage.[297]

Churge-Strauss Syndrome. Churge-Strauss syndrome (allergic granulomatosis and angiitis) is a systemic necrotizing vasculitis of small vessels in patients with asthma and eosinophilia. Asthma is the most common form of respiratory tract involvement preceding onset of vasculitis by 3 to 8 years. Fifty percent of patients have the presence of serum p-ANCA. Chest radiograph abnormalities are usually because of eosinophilic pneumonitis. However, alveolar hemorrhage has been reported, albeit rarely.[298]

Henoch-Schonlein Purpura. Henoch-Schonlein Purpura (HSP) is a small vessel vasculitis characterized by palpable purpura, arthritis, abdominal pain, and renal involvement. HSP is predominantly a disease of children;[299] however, adults can be affected.[300] The deposition of IgA immune complexes in and around the walls of small vessels is the hallmark of HSP. Capillaritis and DAH, with histologic confirmation of IgA immune complex deposition, have been reported in HSP.[301,302] However, the incidence of lung involvement is low, up to 6.5%, in HSP.[303]

IgA Nephropathy. IgA Nephropathy (Berger disease) is a mesangial proliferative glomerulonephritis that is the most common nephropathy worldwide. Because of similar serologic abnormalities, IgA nephropathy is thought to be a spectrum of HSP. Capillaritis with fatal hemorrhage and IgA confirmation by biopsy has been reported in IgA nephropathy.[304]

Behcet Disease (BD). The details of BD have been discussed previously in the context of large to medium vessel vasculitis. While PA aneurysm is the predominant form of lung involvement in BD, small vessel involvement (capillaritis) can occur.[305]

Mixed Cryoglobulinemia. Mixed cryoglobulinemia is a small vessel vasculitis manifesting with palpable purpura, arthritis, glomerulonephritis, and hepatitis.[306] A very strong association to infection with the hepatitis C virus has been observed. Interstitial lung disease is the most common form of pulmonary involvement, with only isolated case reports of capillaritis and DAH in mixed cryoglobulinemia.[307,308]

Capillaritis in the Setting of Collagen Vascular Disease

Systemic Lupus Erythematosus. SLE is an autoimmune disorder of unknown etiology with diverse clinical manifestations characterized by the production of antibodies to components of the cell nucleus, that is, antinuclear antibodies (ANA). Lung manifestations include pneumonitis, pulmonary hypertension, pulmonary embolism with infarction, DAH with or without capillaritis, and pleural effusions.[309,310] Capillaritis and DAH occur in approximately 4% of patients with SLE.[311] Capillaritis is believed to be the most common cause of DAH in SLE, although bland hemorrhage and diffuse alveolar damage are other etiologies.[311,312] Acute lupus pneumonitis is the initial manifestation of SLE in 50% of cases,[313] whereas DAH is rarely the initial manifestation and occurs later in the course in association with active glomerulonephritis.[311,314] However, reports do exist of DAH as the initial manifestation of SLE.[312] The mortality associated with DAH in SLE is 50%, which is the highest of any of the causes of DAH.[280] On histologic examination, immune complex deposition in the walls of the small arteries and the alveolar interstitium is often but not always observed.[315,316]

Rheumatoid Arthritis. Rheumatoid arthritis is a systemic inflammatory disorder that predominantly manifests in the synovial membrane of diarthrodial joints. DAH in patients with rheumatoid arthritis can be due to bland pulmonary hemorrhage[317] or capillaritis.[318,319] Furthermore, vasculitis can be limited to the lung[318] or part of systemic vasculitis, that is, glomerulonephritis.[319]

Mixed Connective Tissue Disease. MCTD is a variant of SLE. Several case reports of DAH in patients with MCTD exist.[318,320,321] Most reports of DAH have associated glomerulonephritis.[320,321] However, vasculitis may remain isolated to the lungs.[318]

Polymyositis. Polymyositis is an idiopathic inflammatory myopathy which affects the muscles of the shoulder and pelvic girdle most severely. Capillaritis with DAH has been reported to occur simultaneously with muscle involvement in patients with polymyositis.[322]

Scleroderma. Scleroderma is a multisystem disease characterized by functional and structural abnormalities of small blood vessels, fibrosis of the skin and internal organs, immune system activation, and autoimmunity. Capillaritis and DAH have been reported to complicate scleroderma.[323,324]

Antiphospholipid Syndrome. Antiphospholipid syndrome is a syndrome in which patients develop arterial and venous thrombosis, thrombocytopenia, and placental insufficiency resulting in fetal loss. Two case reports exist in the literature describing DAH with capillaritis in patients with antiphospholipid syndrome.[325]

Miscellaneous Conditions Associated with Autoantibody Production. Capillaritis and DAH can also occur in various conditions or treatments in which autoantibodies may be produced. Acute pulmonary allograft rejection presenting as capillaritis with DAH weeks to months after transplantation is a life threatening complication requiring immediate recognition and treatment.[326] Myasthenia gravis, ulcerative colitis, Crohn disease, autoimmune hepatitis, acquired immune deficiency syndrome, and bone marrow transplantation are other conditions in which capillaritis and DAH have been reported.[280,327]

Several medications have also been reported to cause capillaritis and DAH. Propylthiouracil (PTU) has been demonstrated to be the etiologic factor for capillaritis with DAH through p-ANCA mediated vasculitis.[328,329] Diphenylhydantoin is believed to have induced a hypersensitivity vasculitis leading to capillaritis in one patient.[330] DAH has been reported in patients being treated with penicillamine for several medical conditions.[331,332] Although immune complex deposition has never been demonstrated in the capillaries of the lungs, many believe that the presence of circulating immune complexes and concomitant glomerulonephritis is evidence enough for the diagnosis of capillaritis from penicillamine.[280,331] Finally, retinoic acid used for the treatment of acute promyelocytic leukemia has been reported to cause capillaritis with DAH.[333,334]

Diagnosis of Capillaritis. Capillaritis with DAH can present with or without hemoptysis. Patients may also present with dyspnea, anemia, low-grade fever, and diffuse, bilateral alveolar infiltrate on chest radiograph. For any patient presenting with DAH, it is crucial to aggressively exclude infection, often with bronchoscopy and bronchoalveolar lavage.[280] Once the diagnosis of DAH is established, the clinician must determine if DAH is from capillaritis, bland hemorrhage, or diffuse alveolar damage. Strictly speaking, capillaritis is a histopathologic diagnosis in which biopsy is not always feasible because of mechanical ventilation or coagulopathy.[280] In these cases, a thorough medical history and physical examination can often lead to clues of the underlying condition. Laboratory work-up should begin with a urinalysis looking for active urine sediment in order to diagnose active glomerulonephritis. Furthermore, ANCA, ANA, and ABMA are serologic tests which may direct the diagnostic work-up and treatment. The sensitivity and specificity of ANCA are best for Wegener's granulomatosis.[285] ANA is particularly helpful for the diagnosis of SLE, whereas ABMA is virtually diagnostic of Goodpasture's syndrome.[296] Table 46-6 outlines other tests which may be useful.

Treatment of Capillaritis. Once the diagnosis of capillaritis is established, aggressive treatment should be initiated promptly owing to the potential for continued rapid deterioration. Because of the limited data on the efficacy of therapy, most experts agree that corticosteroids and cyclophosphamide are the mainstays of therapy.[280,335,336] This regimen has proven to be effective for the treatment of Wegener's granulomatosis,[335] MPA,[293] and Goodpasture's syndrome.[337] Because capillaritis in other conditions is mostly reported as individual cases, randomized data may never be available for direct comparison, and thus corticosteroids and cyclophosphamide should be given as first line therapy because of their efficacy in other conditions. Azathioprine, instead of cyclophosphamide, has proven efficacy in MPA[338] and can also maintain remission in Wegener's granulomatosis after induction of remission by cyclophosphamide.[335] Plasmapheresis should be considered when corticosteroids and cyclophosphamide

TABLE 46-6. Ancillary Diagnostic Studies in Pulmonary Capillaritis

Laboratory studies
    ANCA
        Cytoplasmic
        Perinuclear
    ANA
    Anti-dsDNA antibodies
    Complement levels
    Rheumatoid factor
    Antiglomerular basement membrane antibodies
    Cryoglobulins
    Erythrocyte sedimentation rate
Other studies
    Assay for circulating immune complexes
    Urinalysis with microscopic examination for erythrocyte
        casts
    Radiologic examination of the sinuses
    Renal biopsy for necrotizing glomerulonephritis
    Skin biopsy for leukocytoclastic vasculitis

Source: Reprinted from Green RJ, Ruoss SJ, Kraft SA, et al. Pulmonary capillaritis and alveolar hemorrhage: update on diagnosis and management. Chest. 1996;110:1305-1316.

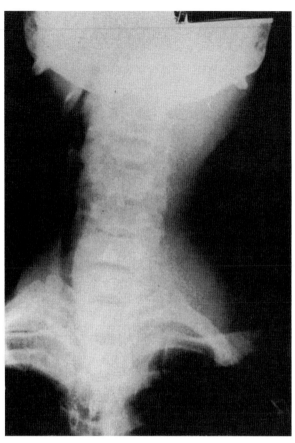

● **FIGURE 46-16.** Spiral CT scan—large filling defect in the right main PA.

Reproduced, with permission, from Loredo JS, Fedullo PF, Piovella F, et al. Digital clubbing associated with pulmonary artery sarcoma. Chest. 1996;109:1651-1653.

fail.[280,339] However, except for observed clinical benefit in Goodpasture's syndrome, the efficacy of plasmapheresis in other conditions is not known.[280] Prophylaxis against *Pneumocystis carinii* with Bactrim DS is recommended for all patients.[280] Finally, broad spectrum antibiotic should also be considered upon presentation until infection is definitively excluded.[283]

● **PA NEOPLASM**

PA neoplasms are extremely rare. In a Mayo Clinic review of patient records of more than a 30-year time period, only nine cases of PA neoplasm, all of which were sarcomas, were identified.[340] Because of a paucity of literature on other forms of PA malignancy, only sarcomas are discussed further.

Sarcomas in the PA arise most often from the dorsal area of the pulmonary trunk near the pulmonary valve.[341] Rarely, PA sarcomas can be located at the bifurcation of the main PA or within the right or left PA. More distal locations are unusual. The sarcoma is believed to arise from the mesenchymal cells of the muscle anlage of the bulbus cordis.[342]

Histologically, PA sarcomas are classified as undifferentiated (34%), fibrosarcoma or fibromyxosarcoma (21%), leiomyosarcoma (20%), rhabdomyosarcoma (6%), mesenchymoma (6%), chondrosarcoma (4%), angiosarcoma (4%), osteosarcoma (3%), and malignant fibrous histiocytoma (2%).[343] However, differentiation is not thought to be of clinical or prognostic utility.[340]

Patients with PA sarcoma come to clinical attention at a mean age of 52 years (range 13 to 86 years).[344–346] A slight female preponderance exists. Unfortunately, the disease is generally asymptomatic until the development of significant obstruction of right ventricular outflow, at which time patients may report symptoms of dyspnea, chest pain, syncope, or palpitations.[347] Chest pain is thought to be secondary to emboli to the distal pulmonary circulation.[348] Syncope and even sudden death are because of the progressive occlusion and obstruction of the PA by the tumor mass. Findings on chest radiograph include a hilar mass, an enlarged PA, pulmonary nodule, or pulmonary infiltrates.[349,350] CT and MRI are noninvasive modalities which have demonstrated utility in the diagnosis of PA sarcoma (Figure 46-16).[346,351,352] Because of similar symptoms and findings on ventilation perfusion scan, many patients with PA sarcoma have been initially misdiagnosed and treated for a pulmonary embolism, with the correct diagnosis being discovered postmortem.[340,353–356] PA sarcoma should be considered in patients whose condition does not improve or worsens while receiving anticoagulation for a pulmonary embolism.[340,353] The lack of risk factors for venous thrombosis, unilateral absence of blood flow on perfusion scan, elevated erythrocyte sedimentation rate, fevers, and weight loss are other features that should raise suspicion of PA sarcoma.[340,353] Differentiation of a tumor mass from a thrombus may be enhanced by use of Gd-DPTA on MRI.[357] On CT, PA sarcoma should be suspected if the mass expands the artery or extends into the mediastinum or lungs.[358]

Patients with PA sarcoma often present with advanced disease because of a prolonged asymptomatic course. The mean survival after diagnosis without treatment is 1.5 months[352] and only slightly better (several months) with therapy.[350,359] However, long-term survival has been reported in patients with a tumor confined to the PA.[359] Thus, early diagnosis and management are paramount. Metastasis, most commonly within the lung but to other parts of the body as well, can occur.[360] Surgical resection for cure and/or palliation is the mainstay of therapy. Because of the rarity of PA sarcoma, data on the efficacy of chemotherapy and radiation therapy is not available.

REFERENCES

1. Sadler TW. Cardiovascular system. In: Langman J, Sadler TS, eds. *Langman's Medical Embryology*. 7th ed. Baltimore, MD: Williams & Wilkins; 1995:183-231.

2. Davies M, Guest PJ. Developmental abnormalities of the great vessels of the thorax and their embryological basis. *Br J Radiol*. 2003;76:491-502.

3. Moore KL. The circulatory system. In: Moore KL, ed. *The Developing Human: Clinically Oriented Embryology*. 3rd ed. Philadelphia, PA: WB Saunders; 1982:298-338.

4. Arey JB. Malformations of the aorta and aortic arches. In: Arey JB, ed. *Cardiovascular Pathology in Infants and Children*. Philadelphia, PA: WB Saunders; 1984:242-244.

5. Cory RA, Valentine EJ. Varying patterns of the lobar branches of the pulmonary artery. A study of 524 lungs and lobes seen at operation of 426 patients. *Thorax*. 1959;14:267-280.

6. Jefferson KE. The pulmonary vessels in the normal pulmonary angiogram. *Proc R Soc Med*. 1965;58:677-681.

7. Fraser RF, Muller NL, Colman N, et al. The pulmonary and bronchial vascular systems. In: Fraser RF, Muller NL, Colman N, Pare PD, eds. *Fraser and Pare's Diagnosis and Diseases of the Chest*. 4th ed. Philadelphia, PA: WB Saunders; 1999:71-125.

8. Mackay EH, Banks J, Sykes B, Lee G. Structural basis for the changing physical properties of human pulmonary vessels with age. *Thorax*. 1978;33:335-344.

9. Brinkman GL. Ultrastructure of atherosclerosis in the human pulmonary artery. *Am Rev Respir Dis*. 1972;105:351-357.

10. Fernie JM, Lamb D. Effects of age and smoking on intima of muscular pulmonary arteries. *J Clin Pathol*. 1986;39:1204-1208.

11. Forrester JS, Diamond GA, Swan HJ. Correlative classification of clinical and hemodynamic function after acute myocardial infarction. *Am J Cardiol*. 1977;39:137-145.

12. Eisenberg PR, Jaffe AS, Schuster DP. Clinical evaluation compared to pulmonary artery catheterization in the hemodynamic assessment of critically ill patients. *Crit Care Med*. 1984;12:549-553.

13. Connors AF Jr, McCaffree DR, Gray BA. Evaluation of right-heart catheterization in the critically ill patient without acute myocardial infarction. *N Engl J Med*. 1983;308:263-267.

14. Connors AF Jr, Speroff T, Dawson NV, et al. The effectiveness of right heart catheterization in the initial care of critically ill patients. SUPPORT investigators. *JAMA*. 1996;276:889-897.

15. Yu DT, Platt R, Lanken PN, et al. Relationship of pulmonary artery catheter use to mortality and resource utilization in patients with severe sepsis. *Crit Care Med*. 2003;31:2734-2741.

16. Blumberg MS, Binns GS. Swan-Ganz catheter use and mortality of myocardial infarction patients. *Health Care Financ Rev*. 1994;15:91-103.

17. Zion MM, Balkin J, Rosenmann D, et al. Use of pulmonary artery catheters in patients with acute myocardial infarction. Analysis of experience in 5841 patients in the SPRINT Registry. SPRINT Study Group. *Chest*. 1990;98:1331-1335.

18. Gore JM, Goldberg RJ, Spodick DH, Alpert JS, Dalen JE. A community-wide assessment of the use of pulmonary artery catheters in patients with acute myocardial infarction. *Chest*. 1987;92:721-727.

19. Bernard GR, Sopko G, Cerra F, et al. Pulmonary artery catheterization and clinical outcomes: National Heart, Lung, and Blood Institute and Food and Drug Administration workshop Report. Consensus Statement. *JAMA*. 2000;283:2568-2572.

20. Binanay C, Califf RM, Hasselblad V, et al. Evaluation study of congestive heart failure and pulmonary artery catheterization effectiveness: the ESCAPE Trial. *JAMA*. 2005;294:1625-1633.

21. Harvey S, Harrison DA, Singer M, et al. Assessment of the clinical effectiveness of pulmonary artery catheters in management of patients in intensive care (PAC-man): a randomised controlled trial. *Lancet*. 2005;366:472-477.

22. Rhodes A, Cusack RJ, Newman PJ, Grounds RM, Bennett ED. A randomised, controlled trial of the pulmonary artery catheter in critically ill patients. *Intensive Care Med*. 2002;28:256-264.

23. Richard C, Warszawski J, Anguel N, et al. Early use of the pulmonary artery catheter and outcomes in patients with shock and acute respiratory distress syndrome: a randomized controlled trial. *JAMA*. 2003;290:2713-2720.

24. Bender JS, Smith-Meek MA, Jones CE. Routine pulmonary artery catheterization does not reduce morbidity and mortality of elective vascular surgery: results of a prospective, randomized trial. *Ann Surg*. 1997;226:229-236; discussion 236-237.

25. Valentine RJ, Duke ML, Inman MH, et al. Effectiveness of pulmonary artery catheters in aortic surgery: a randomized trial. *J Vasc Surg*. 1998;27:203-211; discussion 211-212.

26. Bonazzi M, Gentile F, Biasi GM, et al. Impact of perioperative haemodynamic monitoring on cardiac morbidity after major vascular surgery in low risk patients. A randomised pilot trial. *Eur J Vasc Endovasc Surg*. 2002;23:445-451.

27. Sandham JD, Hull RD, Brant RF, et al. A randomized, controlled trial of the use of pulmonary-artery catheters in high-risk surgical patients. *N Engl J Med.* 2003;348: 5-14.

28. Pinsky MR, Vincent JL. Let us use the pulmonary artery catheter correctly and only when we need it. *Crit Care Med.* 2005;33:1119-1122.

29. Matthay MA, Chatterjee K. Bedside catheterization of the pulmonary artery: risks compared with benefits. *Ann Intern Med.* 1988;109:826-834.

30. Shah MR, Hasselblad V, Stevenson LW, et al. Impact of the pulmonary artery catheter in critically ill patients: meta-analysis of randomized clinical trials. *JAMA.* 2005; 294:1664-1670.

31. Chalfin DB. The pulmonary artery catheter: economic aspects. *New Horiz.* 1997;5:292-296.

32. Simonneau G, Galie N, Rubin LJ, et al. Clinical classification of pulmonary hypertension. *J Am Coll Cardiol.* 2004;43:5S-12S.

33. Barst RJ, McGoon M, Torbicki A, et al. Diagnosis and differential assessment of pulmonary arterial hypertension. *J Am Coll Cardiol.* 2004;43:40S-47S.

34. McLaughlin VV, McGoon MD. Pulmonary arterial hypertension. *Circulation.* 2006;114:1417-1431.

35. Chemla D, Castelain V, Herve P, Lecarpentier Y, Brimioulle S. Haemodynamic evaluation of pulmonary hypertension. *Eur Respir J.* 2002;20:1314-1331.

36. Hoeper MM. Drug treatment of pulmonary arterial hypertension: current and future agents. *Drugs.* 2005;65:1337-1354.

37. Currie PJ, Seward JB, Chan KL, et al. Continuous wave doppler determination of right ventricular pressure: a simultaneous doppler-catheterization study in 127 patients. *J Am Coll Cardiol.* 1985;6:750-756.

38. Rich S, Dantzker DR, Ayres SM, et al. Primary pulmonary hypertension. A national prospective study. *Ann Intern Med.* 1987;107:216-223.

39. Rubin LJ, Badesch DB. Evaluation and management of the patient with pulmonary arterial hypertension. *Ann Intern Med.* 2005;143:282-292.

40. Rubin LJ. Primary pulmonary hypertension. *N Engl J Med.* 1997;336:111-117.

41. Humbert M, Morrell NW, Archer SL, et al. Cellular and molecular pathobiology of pulmonary arterial hypertension. *J Am Coll Cardiol.* 2004;43:13S-24S.

42. Farber HW, Loscalzo J. Pulmonary arterial hypertension. *N Engl J Med.* 2004;351:1655-1665.

43. Yuan JX, Rubin LJ. Pathogenesis of pulmonary arterial hypertension: the need for multiple hits. *Circulation.* 2005;111:534-538.

44. Machado RD, James V, Southwood M, et al. Investigation of second genetic hits at the BMPR2 locus as a modulator of disease progression in familial pulmonary arterial hypertension. *Circulation.* 2005;111:607-613.

45. Christman BW, McPherson CD, Newman JH, et al. An imbalance between the excretion of thromboxane and prostacyclin metabolites in pulmonary hypertension. *N Engl J Med.* 1992;327:70-75.

46. Giaid A, Saleh D. Reduced expression of endothelial nitric oxide synthase in the lungs of patients with pulmonary hypertension. *N Engl J Med.* 1995;333:214-221.

47. Tuder RM, Cool CD, Geraci MW, et al. Prostacyclin synthase expression is decreased in lungs from patients with severe pulmonary hypertension. *Am J Respir Crit Care Med.* 1999;159:1925-1932.

48. Giaid A, Yanagisawa M, Langleben D, et al. Expression of endothelin-1 in the lungs of patients with pulmonary hypertension. *N Engl J Med.* 1993;328:1732-1739.

49. Newman JH, Trembath RC, Morse JA, et al. Genetic basis of pulmonary arterial hypertension: current understanding and future directions. *J Am Coll Cardiol.* 2004;43:33S-39S.

50. Eddahibi S, Humbert M, Fadel E, et al. Serotonin transporter overexpression is responsible for pulmonary artery smooth muscle hyperplasia in primary pulmonary hypertension. *J Clin Invest.* 2001;108:1141-1150.

51. Deng Z, Morse JH, Slager SL, et al. Familial primary pulmonary hypertension (gene PPH1) is caused by mutations in the bone morphogenetic protein receptor-II gene. *Am J Hum Genet.* 2000;67:737-744.

52. Newman JH, Wheeler L, Lane KB, et al. Mutation in the gene for bone morphogenetic protein receptor II as a cause of primary pulmonary hypertension in a large kindred. *N Engl J Med.* 2001;345:319-324.

53. Thomson JR, Machado RD, Pauciulo MW, et al. Sporadic primary pulmonary hypertension is associated with germline mutations of the gene encoding BMPR-II, a receptor member of the TGF-beta family. *J Med Genet.* 2000;37:741-745.

54. Humbert M, Deng Z, Simonneau G, et al. BMPR2 germline mutations in pulmonary hypertension associated with fenfluramine derivatives. *Eur Respir J.* 2002;20:518-523.

55. Heldin CH, Miyazono K, ten Dijke P. TGF-beta signalling from cell membrane to nucleus through SMAD proteins. *Nature.* 1997;390:465-471.

56. Trembath RC, Thomson JR, Machado RD, et al. Clinical and molecular genetic features of pulmonary hypertension in patients with hereditary hemorrhagic telangiectasia. *N Engl J Med.* 2001;345:325-334.

57. Herve P, Humbert M, Sitbon O, et al. Pathobiology of pulmonary hypertension. The role of platelets and thrombosis. *Clin Chest Med.* 2001;22:451-458.

58. Soderman C, Eriksson LS, Juhlin-Dannfelt A, Lundberg JM, Broman L, Holmgren A. Effect of vasoactive intestinal polypeptide (VIP) on pulmonary ventilation-perfusion relationships and central haemodynamics in healthy subjects. *Clin Physiol.* 1993;13:677-685.

59. Cox CP, Linden J, Said SI. VIP elevates platelet cyclic AMP (cAMP) levels and inhibits in vitro platelet activation induced by platelet-activating factor (PAF). *Peptides.* 1984;5: 325-328.

60. Maruno K, Absood A, Said SI. VIP inhibits basal and histamine-stimulated proliferation of human airway smooth muscle cells. *Am J Physiol.* 1995;268:L1047-L1051.

61. Petkov V, Mosgoeller W, Ziesche R, et al. Vasoactive intestinal peptide as a new drug for treatment of primary pulmonary hypertension. *J Clin Invest.* 2003;111:1339-1346.

62. Herve P, Launay JM, Scrobohaci ML, et al. Increased plasma serotonin in primary pulmonary hypertension. *Am J Med.* 1995;99:249-254.

63. Mitchell H, Bolster MB, LeRoy EC. Scleroderma and related conditions. *Med Clin North Am.* 1997;81:129-149.

64. D'Angelo WA, Fries JF, Masi AT, Shulman LE. Pathologic observations in systemic sclerosis (scleroderma). A study of fifty-eight autopsy cases and fifty-eight matched controls. *Am J Med.* 1969;46:428-440.

65. Battle RW, Davitt MA, Cooper SM, et al. Prevalence of pulmonary hypertension in limited and diffuse scleroderma. *Chest.* 1996;110:1515-1519.

66. Steen V, Medsger TA Jr. Predictors of isolated pulmonary hypertension in patients with systemic sclerosis and limited cutaneous involvement. *Arthritis Rheum.* 2003;48:516-522.

67. Wigley FM, Lima JA, Mayes M, McLain D, Chapin JL, Ward-Able C. The prevalence of undiagnosed pulmonary arterial hypertension in subjects with connective tissue disease at the secondary health care level of community-based rheumatologists (the UNCOVER study). *Arthritis Rheum.* 2005;52:2125-2132.

68. Peacock AJ. Primary pulmonary hypertension. *Thorax.* 1999; 54:1107-1118.

69. Mandell MS, Groves BM. Pulmonary hypertension in chronic liver disease. *Clin Chest Med.* 1996;17:17-33.

70. The International Primary Pulmonary Hypertension Study Group. The International Primary Pulmonary Hypertension Study (IPPHS). *Chest.* 1994;105:37S-41S.

71. Cohen MD, Rubin LJ, Taylor WE, Cuthbert JA. Primary pulmonary hypertension: an unusual case associated with extrahepatic portal hypertension. *Hepatology.* 1983;3:588-592.

72. Yang YY, Lin HC, Lee WC, et al. Portopulmonary hypertension: distinctive hemodynamic and clinical manifestations. *J Gastroenterol.* 2001;36:181-186.

73. Hadengue A, Benhayoun MK, Lebrec D, Benhamou JP. Pulmonary hypertension complicating portal hypertension: prevalence and relation to splanchnic hemodynamics. *Gastroenterology.* 1991;100:520-528.

74. Robalino BD, Moodie DS. Association between primary pulmonary hypertension and portal hypertension: analysis of its pathophysiology and clinical, laboratory and hemodynamic manifestations. *J Am Coll Cardiol.* 1991;17:492-498.

75. Kuo PC, Plotkin JS, Johnson LB, et al. Distinctive clinical features of portopulmonary hypertension. *Chest.* 1997;112:980-986.

76. Budhiraja R, Hassoun PM. Portopulmonary hypertension: a tale of two circulations. *Chest.* 2003;123:562-576.

77. Krowka MJ, Plevak DJ, Findlay JY, Rosen CB, Wiesner RH, Krom RA. Pulmonary hemodynamics and perioperative cardiopulmonary-related mortality in patients with portopulmonary hypertension undergoing liver transplantation. *Liver Transpl.* 2000;6:443-450.

78. Ramsay MA, Simpson BR, Nguyen AT, Ramsay KJ, East C, Klintmalm GB. Severe pulmonary hypertension in liver transplant candidates. *Liver Transpl Surg.* 1997;3:494-500.

79. Speich R, Jenni R, Opravil M, Pfab M, Russi EW. Primary pulmonary hypertension in HIV infection. *Chest.* 1991; 100:1268-1271.

80. Mette SA, Palevsky HI, Pietra GG, et al. Primary pulmonary hypertension in association with human immunodeficiency virus infection. A possible viral etiology for some forms of hypertensive pulmonary arteriopathy. *Am Rev Respir Dis.* 1992;145:1196-1200.

81. Beilke MA. Vascular endothelium in immunology and infectious disease. *Rev Infect Dis.* 1989;11:273-283.

82. Chalifoux LV, Simon MA, Pauley DR, MacKey JJ, Wyand MS, Ringler DJ. Arteriopathy in macaques infected with simian immunodeficiency virus. *Lab Invest.* 1992;67:338-349.

83. Humbert M, Monti G, Fartoukh M, et al. Platelet-derived growth factor expression in primary pulmonary hypertension: comparison of HIV seropositive and HIV seronegative patients. *Eur Respir J.* 1998;11:554-559.

84. Mehta NJ, Khan IA, Mehta RN, Sepkowitz DA. HIV-related pulmonary hypertension: analytic review of 131 cases. *Chest.* 2000;118:1133-1141.

85. Petitpretz P, Brenot F, Azarian R, et al. Pulmonary hypertension in patients with human immunodeficiency virus infection: comparison with primary pulmonary hypertension. *Circulation.* 1994;89:2722-2727.

86. Opravil M, Pechere M, Speich R, et al. HIV-associated primary pulmonary hypertension: a case control study: Swiss HIV cohort study. *Am J Respir Crit Care Med.* 1997;155:990-995.

87. Pellicelli AM, Palmieri F, D'Ambrosio C, et al. Role of human immunodeficiency virus in primary pulmonary hypertension—case reports. *Angiology.* 1998;49:1005-1011.

88. Rich S, Rubin L, Walker AM, Schneeweiss S, Abenhaim L. Anorexigens and pulmonary hypertension in the united states: results from the surveillance of north american pulmonary hypertension. *Chest.* 2000;117:870-874.

89. Abenhaim L, Moride Y, Brenot F, et al. Appetite-suppressant drugs and the risk of primary pulmonary hypertension: International Primary Pulmonary Hypertension Study Group. *N Engl J Med.* 1996;335:609-616.

90. Weir EK, Reeve HL, Huang JM, et al. Anorexic agents aminorex, fenfluramine, and dexfenfluramine inhibit potassium current in rat pulmonary vascular smooth muscle and cause pulmonary vasoconstriction. *Circulation.* 1996; 94:2216-2220.

91. Archer SL, Djaballah K, Humbert M, et al. Nitric oxide deficiency in fenfluramine- and dexfenfluramine-induced pulmonary hypertension. *Am J Respir Crit Care Med.* 1998;158:1061-1067.

92. Humbert M, Maitre S, Capron F, Rain B, Musset D, Simonneau G. Pulmonary edema complicating continuous intravenous prostacyclin in pulmonary capillary hemangiomatosis. *Am J Respir Crit Care Med.* 1998;157:1681-1685.

93. Okumura H, Nagaya N, Kyotani S, et al. Effects of continuous IV prostacyclin in a patient with pulmonary veno-occlusive disease. *Chest.* 2002;122:1096-1098.

94. D'Alonzo GE, Barst RJ, Ayres SM, et al. Survival in patients with primary pulmonary hypertension. Results from a national prospective registry. *Ann Intern Med.* 1991;115:343-349.

95. McLaughlin VV, Presberg KW, Doyle RL, et al. Prognosis

of pulmonary arterial hypertension: ACCP evidence-based clinical practice guidelines. *Chest.* 2004;126:78S-92S.

96. Kuhn KP, Byrne DW, Arbogast PG, Doyle TP, Loyd JE, Robbins IM. Outcome in 91 consecutive patients with pulmonary arterial hypertension receiving epoprostenol. *Am J Respir Crit Care Med.* 2003;167:580-586.

97. Appelbaum L, Yigla M, Bendayan D, et al. Primary pulmonary hypertension in israel: a national survey. *Chest.* 2001; 119:1801-1806.

98. Sitbon O, Humbert M, Nunes H, et al. Long-term intravenous epoprostenol infusion in primary pulmonary hypertension: prognostic factors and survival. *J Am Coll Cardiol.* 2002;40:780-788.

99. Raymond RJ, Hinderliter AL, Willis PW, et al. Echocardiographic predictors of adverse outcomes in primary pulmonary hypertension. *J Am Coll Cardiol.* 2002;39:1214-1219.

100. Miyamoto S, Nagaya N, Satoh T, et al. Clinical correlates and prognostic significance of six-minute walk test in patients with primary pulmonary hypertension. Comparison with cardiopulmonary exercise testing. *Am J Respir Crit Care Med.* 2000;161:487-492.

101. Barst RJ, Rubin LJ, Long WA, et al. A comparison of continuous intravenous epoprostenol (prostacyclin) with conventional therapy for primary pulmonary hypertension. The Primary Pulmonary Hypertension Study Group. *N Engl J Med.* 1996;334:296-302.

102. Hinderliter AL, Willis PW, IV, Long W, et al. Frequency and prognostic significance of pericardial effusion in primary pulmonary hypertension. PPH Study Group. Primary pulmonary hypertension. *Am J Cardiol.* 1999;84:481-484, A10.

103. Eysmann SB, Palevsky HI, Reichek N, Hackney K, Douglas PS. Two-dimensional and doppler-echocardiographic and cardiac catheterization correlates of survival in primary pulmonary hypertension. *Circulation.* 1989;80:353-360.

104. Sandoval J, Bauerle O, Palomar A, et al. Survival in primary pulmonary hypertension. Validation of a prognostic equation. *Circulation.* 1994;89:1733-1744.

105. Okada O, Tanabe N, Yasuda J, et al. Prediction of life expectancy in patients with primary pulmonary hypertension. A retrospective nationwide survey from 1980–1990. *Intern Med.* 1999;38:12-16.

106. Rajasekhar D, Balakrishnan KG, Venkitachalam CG, et al. Primary pulmonary hypertension: natural history and prognostic factors. *Indian Heart J.* 1994;46:165-170.

107. Hoeper MM, Galie N, Murali S, et al. Outcome after cardiopulmonary resuscitation in patients with pulmonary arterial hypertension. *Am J Respir Crit Care Med.* 2002;165:341-344.

108. Mereles D, Ehlken N, Kreuscher S, et al. Exercise and respiratory training improve exercise capacity and quality of life in patients with severe chronic pulmonary hypertension. *Circulation.* 2006;114:1482-1489.

109. Weiss BM, Zemp L, Seifert B, Hess OM. Outcome of pulmonary vascular disease in pregnancy: a systematic overview from 1978 through 1996. *J Am Coll Cardiol.* 1998;31:1650-1657.

110. Fuster V, Steele PM, Edwards WD, Gersh BJ, McGoon MD, Frye RL. Primary pulmonary hypertension: natural history and the importance of thrombosis. *Circulation.* 1984; 70:580-587.

111. Rich S, Kaufmann E, Levy PS. The effect of high doses of calcium-channel blockers on survival in primary pulmonary hypertension. *N Engl J Med.* 1992;327:76-81.

112. Rich S, Seidlitz M, Dodin E, et al. The short-term effects of digoxin in patients with right ventricular dysfunction from pulmonary hypertension. *Chest.* 1998;114:787-792.

113. Sitbon O, Humbert M, Jagot JL, et al. Inhaled nitric oxide as a screening agent for safely identifying responders to oral calcium-channel blockers in primary pulmonary hypertension. *Eur Respir J.* 1998;12:265-270.

114. Sitbon O, Humbert M, Jais X, et al. Long-term response to calcium channel blockers in idiopathic pulmonary arterial hypertension. *Circulation.* 2005;111:3105-3111.

115. Humbert M, Sitbon O, Simonneau G. Treatment of pulmonary arterial hypertension. *N Engl J Med.* 2004;351:1425-1436.

116. Barst RJ, McGoon M, McLaughlin V, et al. Beraprost therapy for pulmonary arterial hypertension. *J Am Coll Cardiol.* 2003;41:2119-2125.

117. Simonneau G, Barst RJ, Galie N, et al. Continuous subcutaneous infusion of treprostinil, a prostacyclin analogue, in patients with pulmonary arterial hypertension: a double-blind, randomized, placebo-controlled trial. *Am J Respir Crit Care Med.* 2002;165:800-804.

118. Tapson VF, Gomberg-Maitland M, McLaughlin VV, et al. Safety and efficacy of IV treprostinil for pulmonary arterial hypertension: a prospective, multicenter, open-label, 12-week trial. *Chest.* 2006;129:683-688.

119. Olschewski H, Simonneau G, Galie N, et al. Inhaled iloprost for severe pulmonary hypertension. *N Engl J Med.* 2002;347: 322-329.

120. Hoeper MM, Schwarze M, Ehlerding S, et al. Long-term treatment of primary pulmonary hypertension with aerosolized iloprost, a prostacyclin analogue. *N Engl J Med.* 2000;342:1866-1870.

121. Channick RN, Simonneau G, Sitbon O, et al. Effects of the dual endothelin-receptor antagonist bosentan in patients with pulmonary hypertension: a randomised placebo-controlled study. *Lancet.* 2001;358:1119-1123.

122. Rubin LJ, Badesch DB, Barst RJ, et al. Bosentan therapy for pulmonary arterial hypertension. *N Engl J Med.* 2002;346: 896-903.

123. Cohen AH, Hanson K, Morris K, et al. Inhibition of cyclic 3′-5′-guanosine monophosphate-specific phosphodiesterase selectively vasodilates the pulmonary circulation in chronically hypoxic rats. *J Clin Invest.* 1996;97:172-179.

124. Galie N, Ghofrani HA, Torbicki A, et al. Sildenafil citrate therapy for pulmonary arterial hypertension. *N Engl J Med.* 2005;353:2148-2157.

125. Mendeloff EN, Meyers BF, Sundt TM, et al. Lung transplantation for pulmonary vascular disease. *Ann Thorac Surg.* 2002;73:209-217; discussion 217-219.

126. Boyd LJ, McGavack TH. Aneurysm of the pulmonary artery: a review of the literature and report of two new cases. *Am Heart J.* 1939;18:562-578.

127. Bartter T, Irwin RS, Nash G. Aneurysms of the pulmonary arteries. *Chest.* 1988;94:1065-1075.

128. Deterling RAJ, Clagett OT. Aneurysm of the pulmonary artery: review of the literature and report of a case. *Am Heart J.* 1947;34:471-499.

129. Williams TE Jr, Schiller M, Craenen J, Hosier DM, Sirak HD. Pulmonary artery aneurysm: successful excision and replacement of the main pulmonary artery. *J Thorac Cardiovasc Surg.* 1971;62:63-67.

130. Mason RJ, Broaddus VC, Murray JF, Nadel JA. *Murray and Nadel's Textbook of Respiratory Medicine.* 4th ed. Philadelphia, PA: Elsevier Saunders; 2005.

131. Cevik C, Izgi C, Boztosun B. A rare consequence of uncorrected atrial septal defect: diffuse pulmonary artery aneurysms. *Tex Heart Inst J.* 2004;31:328-329.

132. Lertsapcharoen P, Chottivittayatarakorn P, Benjacholamas V. Mycotic aneurysms of the pulmonary arteries. *Heart.* 2002;88:524.

133. Auerbach O. Pathology and pathogenesis of pulmonary artery aneurysm in tuberculous cavities. *Am Rev Tuberc.* 1939;39:99-115.

134. Benveniste O, Bruneel F, Bedos JP, et al. Ruptured mycotic pulmonary artery aneurysm: an unusual complication of right-sided endocarditis. *Scand J Infect Dis.* 1998;30:626-629.

135. Warthin AS. Syphilis of the pulmonary artery: sayphilitic aneurysm of the left upper division: demonstration of spirochete pallida in wall of artery and aneurismal sac. *Am J Syph.* 1917;1:693-711.

136. Niwa K, Perloff JK, Bhuta SM, et al. Structural abnormalities of great arterial walls in congenital heart disease: light and electron microscopic analyses. *Circulation.* 2001;103:393-400.

137. Patent ductus arteriosus. In: Perloff JK, ed. *Clinical Recognition of Congenital Heart Disease.* 2nd ed. Philadelphia, PA: WB Saunders; 1978:524-560.

138. Kauffman SL, Lynfield J, Hennigar GR. Mycotic aneurysms of the intrapulmonary arteries. *Circulation.* 1967;35:90-99.

139. Veldtman GR, Dearani JA, Warnes CA. Low pressure giant pulmonary artery aneurysms in the adult: natural history and management strategies. *Heart.* 2003;89:1067-1070.

140. Luchtrath H. Dissecting aneurysm of the pulmonary artery. *Virchows Arch A Pathol Anat Histol.* 1981;391:241-247.

141. Khattar RS, Fox DJ, Alty JE, Arora A. Pulmonary artery dissection: an emerging cardiovascular complication in surviving patients with chronic pulmonary hypertension. *Heart.* 2005;91:142-145.

142. Tung HL, Liebow AA. Marfan's syndrome; observations at necropsy: with special reference to medionecrosis of the great vessels. *Lab Invest.* 1952;1:382-406.

143. Uzun O, Akpolat T, Erkan L. Pulmonary vasculitis in Behcet disease: a cumulative analysis. *Chest.* 2005;127:2243-2253.

144. Lohani S, Niven R. Images in clinical medicine: bilateral pulmonary-artery aneurysms in Behcet's syndrome. *N Engl J Med.* 2005;353:400.

145. Ozge C, Calikoglu M, Yildiz A, Tursen U, Tamer L. Bilateral pulmonary artery aneurysms with protein C and protein S deficiency in a patient with Behcet's disease. *Scand J Rheumatol.* 2004;33:52-54.

146. Dennison AR, Watkins RM, Gunning AJ. Simultaneous aortic and pulmonary artery aneurysms due to giant cell arteritis. *Thorax.* 1985;40:156-157.

147. Ortiz-Santamaria V, Olive A, Holgado S, Muchart J. Pulmonary aneurysms in microscopic polyangiitis. *Clin Rheumatol.* 2003;22:498-499.

148. Durieux P, Bletry O, Huchon G, Wechsler B, Chretien J, Godeau P. Multiple pulmonary arterial aneurysms in Behcet's disease and Hughes-Stovin syndrome. *Am J Med.* 1981;71:736-741.

149. Eisenberg D, Gordon RL, Weineman EE, Romanoff H. Pulmonary artery aneurysm presenting as a peripheral coin lesion–the danger of needle biopsy. *Cardiovasc Intervent Radiol.* 1984;7:280-282.

150. Remy J, Lemaitre L, Lafitte JJ, Vilain MO, Saint Michel J, Steenhouwer F. Massive hemoptysis of pulmonary arterial origin: diagnosis and treatment. *AJR Am J Roentgenol.* 1984;143:963-969.

151. Decuypere V, Delcroix M, Budts W. Left main coronary artery and right pulmonary vein compression by a large pulmonary artery aneurysm. *Heart.* 2004;90:e21.

152. Dransfield MT, Johnson JE. A mycotic pulmonary artery aneurysm presenting as an endobronchial mass. *Chest.* 2003;124:1610-1612.

153. Senbaklavaci O, Kaneko Y, Bartunek A, et al. Rupture and dissection in pulmonary artery aneurysms: incidence, cause, and treatment—review and case report. *J Thorac Cardiovasc Surg.* 2001;121:1006-1008.

154. Smalcelj A, Brida V, Samarzija M, Matana A, Margetic E, Drinkovic N. Giant, dissecting, high-pressure pulmonary artery aneurysm: case report of a 1-year natural course. *Tex Heart Inst J.* 2005;32:589-594.

155. Wilson N, McLeod K, Hallworth D. Images in cardiology. Exclusion of a pulmonary artery aneurysm using a covered stent. *Heart.* 2000;83:438.

156. Santelli ED, Katz DS, Goldschmidt AM, Thomas HA. Embolization of multiple rasmussen aneurysms as a treatment of hemoptysis. *Radiology.* 1994;193:396-398.

157. Hamuryudan V, Yurdakul S, Moral F, et al. Pulmonary arterial aneurysms in Behcet's syndrome: a report of 24 cases. *Br J Rheumatol.* 1994;33:48-51.

158. Casselman F, Meyns B, Herygers P, Verougstraete L, Van Elst F, Daenen W. Pulmonary artery aneurysm: is surgery always indicated? *Acta Cardiol.* 1997;52:431-436.

159. Hiraki T, Kanazawa S, Mimura H, et al. Transcatheter embolization of pulmonary artery false aneurysm associated with primary pulmonary hypertension. *Cardiovasc Intervent Radiol.* 2004;27:186-189.

160. Podbielski FJ, Wiesman IM, Yaghmai B, Owens CA, Benedetti E, Massad MG. Pulmonary artery pseudoaneurysm after tube thoracostomy. *Ann Thorac Surg.* 1997;64:1478-1480.

161. Vaidyanathan B, Kannan BR, Kumar RK. Images in cardiovascular medicine. Catheter closure of pseudoaneurysm of the main pulmonary artery. *Circulation.* 2004;110:e322-e323.

162. Fuller J, Clark TC. Repair of traumatic aneurysm of the

pulmonary artery with arteriovenous fistula. *Minn Med.* 1987;70:521-522.

163. Agarwal PP, Dennie CJ, Matzinger FR, Peterson RA, Seely JM. Pulmonary artery pseudoaneurysm secondary to metastatic angiosarcoma. *Thorax.* 2006;61:366.

164. Oliver TB, Stevenson AJ, Gillespie IN. Pulmonary artery pseudoaneurysm due to bronchial carcinoma. *Br J Radiol.* 1997;70:950-951.

165. Gomez-Jorge J, Mitchell SE. Embolization of a pulmonary artery pseudoaneurysm due to squamous cell carcinoma of the lung. *J Vasc Interv Radiol.* 1999;10:1127-1130.

166. Ablett MJ, Elliott ST, Mitchell L. Case report: pulmonary leiomyosarcoma presenting as a pseudoaneurysm. *Clin Radiol.* 1998;53:851-852.

167. Shah KB, Rao TL, Laughlin S, El-Etr AA. A review of pulmonary artery catheterization in 6245 patients. *Anesthesiology.* 1984;61:271-275.

168. Fletcher EC, Mihalick MJ, Siegel CO. Pulmonary artery rupture during introduction of the Swan-Ganz catheter: mechanism and prevention of injury. *J Crit Care.* 1988;3:116-121.

169. Shin B, Ayella RJ, McAslan TC. Pitfalls of Swan-Ganz catheterization. *Crit Care Med.* 1977;5:125-127.

170. Kearney TJ, Shabot MM. Pulmonary artery rupture associated with the Swan-Ganz catheter. *Chest.* 1995;108:1349-1352.

171. Lois JF, Takiff H, Schechter MS, Gomes AS, Machleder HI. Vessel rupture by balloon catheters complicating chronic steroid therapy. *AJR Am J Roentgenol.* 1985;144:1073-1074.

172. Poplausky MR, Rozenblit G, Rundback JH, Crea G, Maddineni S, Leonardo R. Swan-Ganz catheter-induced pulmonary artery pseudoaneurysm formation: three case reports and a review of the literature. *Chest.* 2001;120:2105-2111.

173. Ray CE Jr, Kaufman JA, Geller SC, Rivitz SM, Kanarek DJ, Waltman AC. Embolization of pulmonary catheter-induced pulmonary artery pseudoaneurysms. *Chest.* 1996;110:1370-1373.

174. Donaldson B, Ngo-Nonga B. Traumatic pseudoaneurysm of the pulmonary artery: case report and review of the literature. *Am Surg.* 2002;68:414-416.

175. Dieden JD, Friloux LA III, Renner JW. Pulmonary artery false aneurysms secondary to Swan-Ganz pulmonary artery catheters. *AJR Am J Roentgenol.* 1987;149:901-906.

176. Shovlin CL, Letarte M. Hereditary haemorrhagic telangiectasia and pulmonary arteriovenous malformations: issues in clinical management and review of pathogenic mechanisms. *Thorax.* 1999;54:714-729.

177. Westermann CJ, Rosina AF, De Vries V, de Coteau PA. The prevalence and manifestations of hereditary hemorrhagic telangiectasia in the afro-caribbean population of the netherlands antilles: a family screening. *Am J Med Genet A.* 2003;116:324-328.

178. Shovlin CL, Jackson JE. In: Peacock A, Ruin L, eds. *Pulmonary Circulation.* 2nd ed. London, UK: Arnold; 2004:589-599.

179. Dines DE, Arms RA, Bernatz PE, Gomes MR. Pulmonary arteriovenous fistulas. *Mayo Clin Proc.* 1974;49:460-465.

180. Symbas PN, Goldman M, Erbesfeld MH, Vlasis SE. Pulmonary arteriovenous fistula, pulmonary artery aneurysm, and other vascular changes of the lung from penetrating trauma. *Ann Surg.* 1980;191:336-340.

181. Manganas C, Iliopoulos J, Pang L, Grant PW. Traumatic pulmonary arteriovenous malformation presenting with massive hemoptysis 30 years after penetrating chest injury. *Ann Thorac Surg.* 2003;76:942-944.

182. Pierce JA, Reagan WP, Kimball RW. Unusual cases of pulmonary arteriovenous fistulas, with a note on thyroid carcinoma as a cause. *N Engl J Med.* 1959;260:901-907.

183. Kamei K, Kusumoto K, Suzuki T. Pulmonary amyloidosis with pulmonary arteriovenous fistula. *Chest.* 1989;96:1435-1436.

184. Kopf GS, Laks H, Stansel HC, Hellenbrand WE, Kleinman CS, Talner NS. Thirty-year follow-up of superior vena cava-pulmonary artery (Glenn) shunts. *J Thorac Cardiovasc Surg.* 1990;100:662-670; discussion 670-671.

185. Srivastava D, Preminger T, Lock JE, et al. Hepatic venous blood and the development of pulmonary arteriovenous malformations in congenital heart disease. *Circulation.* 1995;92:1217-1222.

186. Iqbal M, Rossoff LJ, Steinberg HN, Marzouk KA, Siegel DN. Pulmonary arteriovenous malformations: a clinical review. *Postgrad Med J.* 2000;76:390-394.

187. Shovlin CL, Guttmacher AE, Buscarini E, et al. Diagnostic criteria for hereditary hemorrhagic telangiectasia (Rendu-Osler-Weber syndrome). *Am J Med Genet.* 2000;91:66-67.

188. McAllister KA, Grogg KM, Johnson DW, et al. Endoglin, a TGF-beta binding protein of endothelial cells, is the gene for hereditary haemorrhagic telangiectasia type 1. *Nat Genet.* 1994;8:345-351.

189. Johnson DW, Berg JN, Baldwin MA, et al. Mutations in the activin receptor-like kinase 1 gene in hereditary haemorrhagic telangiectasia type 2. *Nat Genet.* 1996;13:189-195.

190. Shovlin CL, Jackson JE, Hughes JM. Pulmonary arteriovenous malformations and other pulmonary vascular abnormalities. In: Mason B, Murray N, eds. *Murray and Nadel's Textbook of Respiratory Medicine.* 4th ed. Philadelphia, PA: Saunders; 2005:1480-1490.

191. Khurshid I, Downie GH. Pulmonary arteriovenous malformation. *Postgrad Med J.* 2002;78:191-197.

192. White RI Jr, Lynch-Nyhan A, Terry P, et al. Pulmonary arteriovenous malformations: techniques and long-term outcome of embolotherapy. *Radiology.* 1988;169:663-669.

193. Puskas JD, Allen MS, Moncure AC, et al. Pulmonary arteriovenous malformations: therapeutic options. *Ann Thorac Surg.* 1993;56:253-257; discussion 257-258.

194. Terry PB, White RI Jr, Barth KH, Kaufman SL, Mitchell SE. Pulmonary arteriovenous malformations. Physiologic observations and results of therapeutic balloon embolization. *N Engl J Med.* 1983;308:1197-1200.

195. Kjeldsen AD, Oxhoj H, Andersen PE, Elle B, Jacobsen JP, Vase P. Pulmonary arteriovenous malformations: screening procedures and pulmonary angiography in patients with hereditary hemorrhagic telangiectasia. *Chest.* 1999;116:432-439.

196. Lee WL, Graham AF, Pugash RA, et al. Contrast echocardiography remains positive after treatment of pulmonary arteriovenous malformations. *Chest.* 2003;123:351-358.

197. Chilvers ER, Peters AM, George P, Hughes JM, Allison DJ. Quantification of right to left shunt through pulmonary arteriovenous malformations using 99 Tcm albumin microspheres. *Clin Radiol*. 1988;39:611-614.

198. Whyte MK, Peters AM, Hughes JM, et al. Quantification of right to left shunt at rest and during exercise in patients with pulmonary arteriovenous malformations. *Thorax*. 1992;47:790-796.

199. Dines DE, Seward JB, Bernatz PE. Pulmonary arteriovenous fistulas. *Mayo Clin Proc*. 1983;58:176-181.

200. Sluiter-Eringa H, Orie NG, Sluiter HJ. Pulmonary arteriovenous fistula. Diagnosis and prognosis in noncomplainant patients. *Am Rev Respir Dis*. 1969;100:177-188.

201. Remy J, Remy-Jardin M, Wattinne L, Deffontaines C. Pulmonary arteriovenous malformations: evaluation with CT of the chest before and after treatment. *Radiology*. 1992;182:809-816.

202. Remy J, Remy-Jardin M, Giraud F, Wattinne L. Angioarchitecture of pulmonary arteriovenous malformations: clinical utility of three-dimensional helical CT. *Radiology*. 1994;191:657-664.

203. Halbsguth A, Schulze W, Ungeheuer E, Hoer PW. Pitfall in the CT diagnosis of pulmonary arteriovenous malformation. *J Comput Assist Tomogr*. 1983;7:710-712.

204. Stringer CJ, Stanley AL, Bates RC, Summers JE. Pulmonary arteriovenous fistula. *Am J Surg*. 1955;89:1054-1080.

205. Yater WM, Finnega J, Giffin HM. Pulmonary arteriovenous fistula. *J Am Med Assoc*. 1949;141:581-589.

206. Barth KH, White RI Jr, Kaufman SL, Terry PB, Roland JM. Embolotherapy of pulmonary arteriovenous malformations with detachable balloons. *Radiology*. 1982;142:599-606.

207. Pollak JS, Egglin TK, Rosenblatt MM, Dickey KW, White RI Jr. Clinical results of transvenous systemic embolotherapy with a neuroradiologic detachable balloon. *Radiology*. 1994;191:477-482.

208. Lee DW, White RI Jr, Egglin TK, et al. Embolotherapy of large pulmonary arteriovenous malformations: long-term results. *Ann Thorac Surg*. 1997;64:930-939; discussion 939-940.

209. Jackson JE, Whyte MK, Allison DJ, Hughes JM. Coil embolization of pulmonary arteriovenous malformations. *Cor Vasa*. 1990;32:191-196.

210. Hartnell GG, Allison DJ. Coil embolization in the treatment of pulmonary arteriovenous malformations. *J Thorac Imaging*. 1989;4:81-85.

211. Dutton JA, Jackson JE, Hughes JM, et al. Pulmonary arteriovenous malformations: results of treatment with coil embolization in 53 patients. *AJR Am J Roentgenol*. 1995;165:1119-1125.

212. Haitjema T, Disch F, Overtoom TT, Westermann CJ, Lammers JW. Screening family members of patients with hereditary hemorrhagic telangiectasia. *Am J Med*. 1995;99:519-524.

213. Chan P. Antibiotic prophylaxis for patients with hereditary hemorrhagic telangiectasia. *J Am Acad Dermatol*. 1992;26:282-283.

214. Shovlin CL, Winstock AR, Peters AM, Jackson JE, Hughes JM. Medical complications of pregnancy in hereditary haemorrhagic telangiectasia. *QJM*. 1995;88:879-887.

215. O'Laughlin MP. Catheterization treatment of stenosis and hypoplasia of pulmonary arteries. *Pediatr Cardiol*. 1998;19:48-56; discussion 57-58.

216. Trivedi KR, Benson LN. Interventional strategies in the management of peripheral pulmonary artery stenosis. *J Interv Cardiol*. 2003;16:171-188.

217. Bacha EA, Kreutzer J. Comprehensive management of branch pulmonary artery stenosis. *J Interv Cardiol*. 2001;14:367-375.

218. Gay BB Jr, French RH, Shuford WH, Rogers JV Jr. The roentgenologic features of single and multiple coarctations of the pulmonary artery and branches. *Am J Roentgenol Radium Ther Nucl Med*. 1963;90:599-613.

219. Williams JC, Barratt-Boyes BG, Lowe JB. Supravalvular aortic stenosis. *Circulation*. 1961;24:1311-1318.

220. Beuren AJ, Apitz J, Harmjanz D. Supravalvular aortic stenosis in association with mental retardation and a certain facial appearance. *Circulation*. 1962;26:1235-1240.

221. Alagille D, Estrada A, Hadchouel M, Gautier M, Odievre M, Dommergues JP. Syndromic paucity of interlobular bile ducts (alagille syndrome or arteriohepatic dysplasia): review of 80 cases. *J Pediatr*. 1987;110:195-200.

222. Uzun O, Blackburn ME, Gibbs JL. Congenital total lipodystrophy and peripheral pulmonary artery stenosis. *Arch Dis Child*. 1997;76:456-457.

223. Clark SC, Levine AJ, Hasan A, Hilton CJ, Forty J, Dark JH. Vascular complications of lung transplantation. *Ann Thorac Surg*. 1996;61:1079-1082.

224. Somerville J, Barbosa R, Ross D, Olsen E. Problems with radical corrective surgery after ascending aorta to right pulmonary artery shunt (Waterston's anastomosis) for cyanotic congenital heart disease. *Br Heart J*. 1975;37:1105-1112.

225. Sreeram N, Saleem M, Jackson M, et al. Results of balloon pulmonary valvuloplasty as a palliative procedure in tetralogy of Fallot. *J Am Coll Cardiol*. 1991;18:159-165.

226. Fierro-Renoy C, Velasquez H, Zambrano JP, Ridha M, Kessler K, Schob A. Percutaneous stenting of bilateral pulmonary artery stenosis caused by malignant extrinsic compression. *Chest*. 2002;122:1478-1480.

227. Mahnken AH, Breuer C, Haage P. Silicosis-induced pulmonary artery stenosis: demonstration by MR angiography and perfusion MRI. *Br J Radiol*. 2001;74:859-861.

228. Kreutzer J, Landzberg MJ, Preminger TJ, et al. Isolated peripheral pulmonary artery stenoses in the adult. *Circulation*. 1996;93:1417-1423.

229. Baker CM, McGowan FX Jr, Keane JF, Lock JE. Pulmonary artery trauma due to balloon dilation: recognition, avoidance and management. *J Am Coll Cardiol*. 2000;36:1684-1690.

230. Trant CA Jr, O'Laughlin MP, Ungerleider RM, Garson A Jr. Cost-effectiveness analysis of stents, balloon angioplasty, and surgery for the treatment of branch pulmonary artery stenosis. *Pediatr Cardiol*. 1997;18:339-344.

231. Stamm C, Friehs I, Zurakowski D, et al. Outcome after reconstruction of discontinuous pulmonary arteries. *J Thorac Cardiovasc Surg*. 2002;123:246-257.

232. Lock JE, Castaneda-Zuniga WR, Fuhrman BP, Bass JL. Balloon dilation angioplasty of hypoplastic and stenotic pulmonary arteries. *Circulation*. 1983;67:962-967.

233. Rocchini AP, Kveselis D, Dick M, Crowley D, Snider AR, Rosenthal A. Use of balloon angioplasty to treat peripheral pulmonary stenosis. *Am J Cardiol*. 1984;54:1069-1073.

234. Hosking MC, Thomaidis C, Hamilton R, Burrows PE, Freedom RM, Benson LN. Clinical impact of balloon angioplasty for branch pulmonary arterial stenosis. *Am J Cardiol*. 1992;69:1467-1470.

235. Zeevi B, Berant M, Blieden LC. Midterm clinical impact versus procedural success of balloon angioplasty for pulmonary artery stenosis. *Pediatr Cardiol*. 1997;18:101-106.

236. Gentles TL, Lock JE, Perry SB. High pressure balloon angioplasty for branch pulmonary artery stenosis: early experience. *J Am Coll Cardiol*. 1993;22:867-872.

237. Mendelsohn AM, Bove EL, Lupinetti FM, et al. Intraoperative and percutaneous stenting of congenital pulmonary artery and vein stenosis. *Circulation*. 1993;88:II210-II217.

238. O'Laughlin MP, Slack MC, Grifka RG, Perry SB, Lock JE, Mullins CE. Implantation and intermediate-term follow-up of stents in congenital heart disease. *Circulation*. 1993; 88:605-614.

239. Nakanishi T, Kondoh C, Nishikawa T, et al. Intravascular stents for management of pulmonary artery and right ventricular outflow obstruction. *Heart Vessels*. 1994;9: 40-48.

240. Fogelman R, Nykanen D, Smallhorn JF, McCrindle BW, Freedom RM, Benson LN. Endovascular stents in the pulmonary circulation. Clinical impact on management and medium-term follow-up. *Circulation*. 1995;92:881-885.

241. McMahon CJ, El Said HG, Vincent JA, et al. Refinements in the implantation of pulmonary arterial stents: impact on morbidity and mortality of the procedure over the last two decades. *Cardiol Young*. 2002;12:445-452.

242. O'Laughlin MP, Perry SB, Lock JE, Mullins CE. Use of endovascular stents in congenital heart disease. *Circulation*. 1991;83:1923-1939.

243. Hosking MC, Benson LN, Nakanishi T, Burrows PE, Williams WG, Freedom RM. Intravascular stent prosthesis for right ventricular outflow obstruction. *J Am Coll Cardiol*. 1992;20:373-380.

244. Muller-Hulsbeck S, Bewig B, Schwarzenberg H, Heller M. Percutaneous placement of a self-expandable stent for treatment of a malignant pulmonary artery stenosis. *Br J Radiol*. 1998;71:785-787.

245. Seo JB, Im JG, Chung JW, et al. Pulmonary vasculitis: the spectrum of radiological findings. *Br J Radiol*. 2000;73:1224-1231.

246. Kerr GS, Hallahan CW, Giordano J, et al. Takayasu arteritis. *Ann Intern Med*. 1994;120:919-929.

247. Lande A, Bard R, Rossi P, Passariello R, Castrucci A. Takayasu's arteritis. A worldwide entity. *N Y State J Med*. 1976;76:1477-1482.

248. Sharma S, Kamalakar T, Rajani M, Talwar KK, Shrivastava S. The incidence and patterns of pulmonary artery involvement in Takayasu's arteritis. *Clin Radiol*. 1990;42:177-181.

249. Lupi E, Sanchez G, Horwitz S, Gutierrez E. Pulmonary artery involvement in Takayasu's arteritis. *Chest*. 1975; 67:69-74.

250. Yamato M, Lecky JW, Hiramatsu K, Kohda E. Takayasu arteritis: radiographic and angiographic findings in 59 patients. *Radiology*. 1986;161:329-334.

251. Nakabayashi K, Kurata N, Nangi N, Miyake H, Nagasawa T. Pulmonary artery involvement as first manifestation in three cases of Takayasu arteritis. *Int J Cardiol*. 1996;54(suppl):S177-S183.

252. Hayashi K, Nagasaki M, Matsunaga N, Hombo Z, Imamura T. Initial pulmonary artery involvement in Takayasu arteritis. *Radiology*. 1986;159:401-403.

253. Ferretti G, Defaye P, Thony F, Ranchoup Y, Coulomb M. Initial isolated Takayasu's arteritis of the right pulmonary artery: MR appearance. *Eur Radiol*. 1996;6:429-432.

254. Brugiere O, Mal H, Sleiman C, Groussard O, Mellot F, Fournier M. Isolated pulmonary arteries involvement in a patient with Takayasu's arteritis. *Eur Respir J*. 1998;11:767-770.

255. Ueno A, Awane Y, Wakabayashi A, Shimizu K. Successfully operated obliterative brachiocephalic arteritis (Takayasu) associated with the elongated coarctation. *Jpn Heart J*. 1967;8:538-544.

256. Hiller N, Lieberman S, Chajek-Shaul T, Bar-Ziv J, Shaham D. Thoracic manifestations of Behcet disease at CT. *Radiographics*. 2004;24:801-808.

257. Criteria for diagnosis of Behcet's disease: International Study Group for Behcet's disease. *Lancet*. 1990;335:1078-1080.

258. Sakane T, Takeno M, Suzuki N, Inaba G. Behcet's disease. *N Engl J Med*. 1999;341:1284-1291.

259. Erkan F, Gul A, Tasali E. Pulmonary manifestations of Behcet's disease. *Thorax*. 2001;56:572-578.

260. Yazici H, Tuzun Y, Pazarli H, et al. Influence of age of onset and patient's sex on the prevalence and severity of manifestations of Behcet's syndrome. *Ann Rheum Dis*. 1984;43:783-789.

261. Numan F, Islak C, Berkmen T, Tuzun H, Cokyuksel O. Behcet disease: pulmonary arterial involvement in 15 cases. *Radiology*. 1994;192:465-468.

262. Gunen H, Evereklioglu C, Kosar F, Er H, Kizkin O. Thoracic involvement in Behcet's disease and its correlation with multiple parameters. *Lung*. 2000;178:161-170.

263. Hamuryudan V, Yurdakul S, Moral F, et al. Pulmonary arterial aneurysms in Behcet's syndrome: a report of 24 cases. *Br J Rheumatol*. 1994;33:48-51.

264. Raz I, Okon E, Chajek-Shaul T. Pulmonary manifestations in Behcet's syndrome. *Chest*. 1989;95:585-589.

265. Grenier P, Bletry O, Cornud F, Godeau P, Nahum H. Pulmonary involvement in Behcet disease. *AJR Am J Roentgenol*. 1981;137:565-569.

266. Uzun O, Akpolat T, Erkan L. Pulmonary vasculitis in Behcet disease: a cumulative analysis. *Chest*. 2005;127:2243-2253.

267. Stricker H, Malinverni R. Multiple, large aneurysms of pulmonary arteries in Behcet's disease. Clinical remission and radiologic resolution after corticosteroid therapy. *Arch Intern Med*. 1989;149:925-927.

268. Ahn JM, Im JG, Ryoo JW, et al. Thoracic manifestations of Behcet syndrome: radiographic and CT findings in nine patients. *Radiology.* 1995;194:199-203.

269. Greene RM, Saleh A, Taylor AK, et al. Non-invasive assessment of bleeding pulmonary artery aneurysms due to Behcet disease. *Eur Radiol.* 1998;8:359-363.

270. Tuzun H, Hamuryudan V, Yildirim S, et al. Surgical therapy of pulmonary arterial aneurysms in Behcet's syndrome. *Ann Thorac Surg.* 1996;61:733-735.

271. Lohani S, Niven R. Images in clinical medicine. Bilateral pulmonary-artery aneurysms in Behcet's syndrome. *N Engl J Med.* 2005;353:400.

272. Tunaci M, Ozkorkmaz B, Tunaci A, Gul A, Engin G, Acunas B. CT findings of pulmonary artery aneurysms during treatment for Behcet's disease. *AJR Am J Roentgenol.* 1999;172:729-733.

273. Cil BE, Turkbey B, Canyigit M, Kumbasar OO, Celik G, Demirkazik FB. Transformation of a ruptured giant pulmonary artery aneurysm into an air cavity after transcatheter embolization in a Behcet's patient. *Cardiovasc Intervent Radiol.* 2006;29:151-154.

274. de Montpreville VT, Macchiarini P, Dartevelle PG, Dulmet EM. Large bilateral pulmonary artery aneurysms in Behcet's disease: rupture of the contralateral lesion after aneurysmorrhaphy. *Respiration.* 1996;63:49-51.

275. Hughes JP, Stovin PG. Segmental pulmonary artery aneurysms with peripheral venous thrombosis. *Br J Dis Chest.* 1959;53:19-27.

276. Herb S, Hetzel M, Hetzel J, Friedrich J, Weber J. An unusual case of Hughes-Stovin syndrome. *Eur Respir J.* 1998; 11:1191-1193.

277. Bowman S, Honey M. Pulmonary arterial occlusions and aneurysms: a forme fruste of Behcet's or hughes-stovin syndrome. *Br Heart J.* 1990;63:66-68.

278. Kindermann M, Wilkens H, Hartmann W, Schafers HJ, Bohm M. Images in cardiovascular medicine. Hughes-stovin syndrome. *Circulation.* 2003;108:e156.

279. Mark EJ, Ramirez JF. Pulmonary capillaritis and hemorrhage in patients with systemic vasculitis. *Arch Pathol Lab Med.* 1985;109:413-418.

280. Schwarz MI, Brown KK. Small vessel vasculitis of the lung. *Thorax.* 2000;55:502-510.

281. Jennette JC, Falk RJ. Pathogenic potential of anti-neutrophil cytoplasmic autoantibodies. In: Gross WL, ed. *ANCA-Associated Vasculitides: Immunological and Clinical Aspects.* New York, NY: Plenum Press; 1993:7-15.

282. Jennings CA, King TE Jr, Tuder R, Cherniack RM, Schwarz MI. Diffuse alveolar hemorrhage with underlying isolated, pauciimmune pulmonary capillaritis. *Am J Respir Crit Care Med.* 1997;155:1101-1109.

283. Green RJ, Ruoss SJ, Kraft SA, Duncan SR, Berry GJ, Raffin TA. Pulmonary capillaritis and alveolar hemorrhage. Update on diagnosis and management. *Chest.* 1996;110:1305-1316.

284. Bosch X, Font J, Mirapeix E, Revert L, Ingelmo M, Urbano-Marquez A. Antimyeloperoxidase autoantibody-associated necrotizing alveolar capillaritis. *Am Rev Respir Dis.* 1992; 146:1326-1329.

285. Rao JK, Weinberger M, Oddone EZ, Allen NB, Landsman P, Feussner JR. The role of antineutrophil cytoplasmic antibody (c-ANCA) testing in the diagnosis of Wegener granulomatosis. A literature review and meta-analysis. *Ann Intern Med.* 1995;123:925-932.

286. Myers JL, Katzenstein AL. Wegener's granulomatosis presenting with massive pulmonary hemorrhage and capillaritis. *Am J Surg Pathol.* 1987;11:895-898.

287. Travis WD, Hoffman GS, Leavitt RY, Pass HI, Fauci AS. Surgical pathology of the lung in Wegener's granulomatosis. Review of 87 open lung biopsies from 67 patients. *Am J Surg Pathol.* 1991;15:315-333.

288. DeRemee RA. Pulmonary vasculitis. In: Fishman AP, Elias JA, Fishman JA, Grippi MA, Kaiser LR, Senior RM, eds. *Fishman's Pulmonary Diseases and Disorders.* 3rd ed. New York, NY: McGraw-Hill; 1998:1357-1374.

289. Leatherman JW, Davies SF, Hoidal JR. Alveolar hemorrhage syndromes: diffuse microvascular lung hemorrhage in immune and idiopathic disorders. *Medicine (Baltimore).* 1984;63:343-361.

290. Stokes TC, McCann BG, Rees RT, Sims EH, Harrison BD. Acute fulminating intrapulmonary haemorrhage in Wegener's granulomatosis. *Thorax.* 1982;37:315-316.

291. Jennette JC, Falk RJ, Andrassy K, et al. Nomenclature of systemic vasculitides. Proposal of an international consensus conference. *Arthritis Rheum.* 1994;37:187-192.

292. Gross WL, Csernok E. Immunodiagnostic and pathophysiologic aspects of antineutrophil cytoplasmic antibodies in vasculitis. *Curr Opin Rheumatol.* 1995;7:11-19.

293. Savage CO, Winearls CG, Evans DJ, Rees AJ, Lockwood CM. Microscopic polyarteritis: presentation, pathology and prognosis. *Q J Med.* 1985;56:467-483.

294. Guillevin L, Durand-Gasselin B, Cevallos R, et al. Microscopic polyangiitis: clinical and laboratory findings in eighty-five patients. *Arthritis Rheum.* 1999;42:421-430.

295. Bosch X, Lopez-Soto A, Mirapeix E, Font J, Ingelmo M, Urbano-Marquez A. Antineutrophil cytoplasmic autoantibody-associated alveolar capillaritis in patients presenting with pulmonary hemorrhage. *Arch Pathol Lab Med.* 1994;118:517-522.

296. Wilson CB. Immunologic diseases of the lung and kidney (Goodpasture's syndrome). In: Fishman AP, ed. *Pulmonary Diseases and Disorders.* Vol 1. 2nd ed. New York, NY: McGraw-Hill; 1988:675-681.

297. Lombard CM, Colby TV, Elliott CG. Surgical pathology of the lung in anti-basement membrane antibody-associated Goodpasture's syndrome. *Hum Pathol.* 1989;20:445-451.

298. DeRemee RA. Pulmonary vasculitides. In: Lanzer P, Topol EJ, eds. *PanVascular Medicine: Integrated Clinical Management.* New York, NY: Springer Verlag; 2002:1599-1609.

299. Saulsbury FT. Henoch-Schonlein purpura in children. Report of 100 patients and review of the literature. *Medicine (Baltimore).* 1999;78:395-409.

300. Watts RA, Carruthers DM, Scott DG. Epidemiology of systemic vasculitis: changing incidence or definition? *Semin Arthritis Rheum.* 1995;25:28-34.

301. Kathuria S, Cheifec G. Fatal pulmonary Henoch-Schonlein syndrome. *Chest.* 1982;82:654-656.

302. Markus HS, Clark JV. Pulmonary haemorrhage in Henoch-Schonlein purpura. *Thorax.* 1989;44:525-526.

303. Leavitt RY, Fauci AS. Pulmonary vasculitis. *Am Rev Respir Dis.* 1986;134:149-166.

304. Lai FM, Li EK, Suen MW, Lui SF, Li PK, Lai KN. Pulmonary hemorrhage. A fatal manifestation in IgA nephropathy. *Arch Pathol Lab Med.* 1994;118:542-546.

305. Gamble CN, Wiesner KB, Shapiro RF, Boyer WJ. The immune complex pathogenesis of glomerulonephritis and pulmonary vasculitis in Behcet's disease. *Am J Med.* 1979; 66:1031-1039.

306. Lamprecht P, Gause A, Gross WL. Cryoglobulinemic vasculitis. *Arthritis Rheum.* 1999;42:2507-2516.

307. Bombardieri S, Paoletti P, Ferri C, Di Munno O, Fornal E, Giuntini C. Lung involvement in essential mixed cryoglobulinemia. *Am J Med.* 1979;66:748-756.

308. Gomez-Tello V, Onoro-Canaveral JJ, de la Casa Monje RM, et al. Diffuse recidivant alveolar hemorrhage in a patient with hepatitis C virus-related mixed cryoglobulinemia. *Intensive Care Med.* 1999;25:319-322.

309. Brasington RD, Furst DE. Pulmonary disease in systemic lupus erythematosus. *Clin Exp Rheumatol.* 1985;3:269-276.

310. Haupt HM, Moore GW, Hutchins GM. The lung in systemic lupus erythematosus. Analysis of the pathologic changes in 120 patients. *Am J Med.* 1981;71:791-798.

311. Zamora MR, Warner ML, Tuder R, Schwarz MI. Diffuse alveolar hemorrhage and systemic lupus erythematosus. Clinical presentation, histology, survival, and outcome. *Medicine (Baltimore).* 1997;76:192-202.

312. Myers JL, Katzenstein AA. Microangiitis in lupus-induced pulmonary hemorrhage. *Am J Clin Pathol.* 1986;85:552-556.

313. Matthay RA, Schwarz MI, Petty TL, et al. Pulmonary manifestations of systemic lupus erythematosus: review of twelve cases of acute lupus pneumonitis. *Medicine (Baltimore).* 1975;54:397-409.

314. Santos-Ocampo AS, Mandell BF, Fessler BJ. Alveolar hemorrhage in systemic lupus erythematosus: presentation and management. *Chest.* 2000;118:1083-1090.

315. Rodriguez-Iturbe B, Garcia R, Rubio L, Serrano H. Immunohistologic findings in the lung in systemic lupus erythematosus. *Arch Pathol Lab Med.* 1977;101:342-344.

316. Desnoyers MR, Bernstein S, Cooper AG, Kopelman RI. Pulmonary hemorrhage in lupus erythematosus without evidence of an immunologic cause. *Arch Intern Med.* 1984;144:1398-1400.

317. Torralbo A, Herrero JA, Portoles J, Barrientos A. Alveolar hemorrhage associated with antineutrophil cytoplasmic antibodies in rheumatoid arthritis. *Chest.* 1994;105:1590-1592.

318. Schwarz MI, Zamora MR, Hodges TN, Chan ED, Bowler RP, Tuder RM. Isolated pulmonary capillaritis and diffuse alveolar hemorrhage in rheumatoid arthritis and mixed connective tissue disease. *Chest.* 1998;113:1609-1615.

319. Naschitz JE, Yeshurun D, Scharf Y, Sajrawi I, Lazarov NB, Boss JH. Recurrent massive alveolar hemorrhage, crescentic glomerulonephritis, and necrotizing vasculitis in a patient with rheumatoid arthritis. *Arch Intern Med.* 1989;149:406-408.

320. Sanchez-Guerrero J, Cesarman G, Alarcon-Segovia D. Massive pulmonary hemorrhage in mixed connective tissue diseases. *J Rheumatol.* 1989;16:1132-1134.

321. Germain MJ, Davidman M. Pulmonary hemorrhage and acute renal failure in a patient with mixed connective tissue disease. *Am J Kidney Dis.* 1984;3:420-424.

322. Schwarz MI, Sutarik JM, Nick JA, Leff JA, Emlen JW, Tuder RM. Pulmonary capillaritis and diffuse alveolar hemorrhage. A primary manifestation of polymyositis. *Am J Respir Crit Care Med.* 1995;151:2037-2040.

323. Griffin MT, Robb JD, Martin JR. Diffuse alveolar haemorrhage associated with progressive systemic sclerosis. *Thorax.* 1990;45:903-904.

324. Kallenbach J, Prinsloo I, Zwi S. Progressive systemic sclerosis complicated by diffuse pulmonary haemorrhage. *Thorax.* 1977;32:767-770.

325. Gertner E, Lie JT. Pulmonary capillaritis, alveolar hemorrhage, and recurrent microvascular thrombosis in primary antiphospholipid syndrome. *J Rheumatol.* 1993;20:1224-1228.

326. Badesch DB, Zamora M, Fullerton D, et al. Pulmonary capillaritis: a possible histologic form of acute pulmonary allograft rejection. *J Heart Lung Transplant.* 1998;17:415-422.

327. Fullmer JJ, Langston C, Dishop MK, Fan LL. Pulmonary capillaritis in children: a review of eight cases with comparison to other alveolar hemorrhage syndromes. *J Pediatr.* 2005;146:376-381.

328. Dhillon SS, Singh D, Doe N, Qadri AM, Ricciardi S, Schwarz MI. Diffuse alveolar hemorrhage and pulmonary capillaritis due to propylthiouracil. *Chest.* 1999;116:1485-1488.

329. Pirot AL, Goldsmith D, Pascasio J, Beck SE. Pulmonary capillaritis with hemorrhage due to propylthiouracil therapy in a child. *Pediatr Pulmonol.* 2005;39:88-92.

330. Yermakov VM, Hitti IF, Sutton AL. Necrotizing vasculitis associated with diphenylhydantoin: two fatal cases. *Hum Pathol.* 1983;14:182-184.

331. Louie S, Gamble CN, Cross CE. Penicillamine associated pulmonary hemorrhage. *J Rheumatol.* 1986;13:963-966.

332. Sternlieb I, Bennett B, Scheinberg IH. D-penicillamine induced Goodpasture's syndrome in wilson's disease. *Ann Intern Med.* 1975;82:673-676.

333. Raanani P, Segal E, Levi I, et al. Diffuse alveolar hemorrhage in acute promyelocytic leukemia patients treated with ATRA—a manifestation of the basic disease or the treatment. *Leuk Lymphoma.* 2000;37:605-610.

334. Jung JI, Choi JE, Hahn ST, Min CK, Kim CC, Park SH. Radiologic features of all-trans-retinoic acid syndrome. *AJR Am J Roentgenol.* 2002;178:475-480.

335. Fauci AS, Haynes BF, Katz P, Wolff SM. Wegener's granulomatosis: prospective clinical and therapeutic experience with 85 patients for 21 years. *Ann Intern Med.* 1983;98:76-85.

336. Lynch JP III, McCune WJ. Immunosuppressive and cytotoxic pharmacotherapy for pulmonary disorders. *Am J Respir Crit Care Med.* 1997;155:395-420.

337. Johnson JP, Moore J Jr, Austin HA III, Balow JE, Antonovych TT, Wilson CB. Therapy of anti-glomerular basement membrane antibody disease: analysis of prognostic significance of clinical, pathologic and treatment factors. *Medicine (Baltimore).* 1985;64:219-227.

338. Schwarz MI, Mortenson RL, Colby TV, et al. Pulmonary capillaritis: the association with progressive irreversible airflow limitation and hyperinflation. *Am Rev Respir Dis.* 1993; 148:507-511.

339. Lewis EJ, Hunsicker LG, Lan SP, Rohde RD, Lachin JM. A controlled trial of plasmapheresis therapy in severe lupus nephritis: the Lupus Nephritis Collaborative Study Group. *N Engl J Med.* 1992;326:1373-1379.

340. Parish JM, Rosenow EC III, Swensen SJ, Crotty TB. Pulmonary artery sarcoma: clinical features. *Chest.* 1996;110: 1480-1488.

341. Burke AP, Virmani R. Sarcomas of the great vessels. A clinicopathologic study. *Cancer.* 1993;71:1761-1773.

342. Baker PB, Goodwin RA. Pulmonary artery sarcomas. A review and report of a case. *Arch Pathol Lab Med.* 1985;109:35-39.

343. McGlennen RC, Manivel JC, Stanley SJ, Slater DL, Wick MR, Dehner LP. Pulmonary artery trunk sarcoma: a clinicopathologic, ultrastructural, and immunohistochemical study of four cases. *Mod Pathol.* 1989;2:486-494.

344. Britton PD. Primary pulmonary artery sarcoma: a report of two cases, with special emphasis on the diagnostic problems. *Clin Radiol.* 1990;41:92-94.

345. Pagni S, Passik CS, Riordan C, D'Agostino RS. Sarcoma of the main pulmonary artery: an unusual etiology for recurrent pulmonary emboli. *J Cardiovasc Surg (Torino).* 1999;40:457-461.

346. Smith WS, Lesar MS, Travis WD, et al. MR and CT findings in pulmonary artery sarcoma. *J Comput Assist Tomogr.* 1989;13:906-909.

347. Shmookler BM, Marsh HB, Roberts WC. Primary sarcoma of the pulmonary trunk and/or right or left main pulmonary artery—a rare cause of obstruction to right ventricular outflow: report on two patients and analysis of 35 previously described patients. *Am J Med.* 1977;63:263-272.

348. Berg GA, Hamid BN, Kenyon WE, Drakeley MJ. Primary pulmonary artery sarcoma: intra-operative similarity to pulmonary embolus. *Postgrad Med J.* 1987;63:389-391.

349. Moffat RE, Chang CH, Slaven JE. Roentgen considerations in primary pulmonary artery sarcoma. *Radiology.* 1972;104:283-288.

350. Rafal RB, Nichols JN, Markisz JA. Pulmonary artery sarcoma: diagnosis and postoperative follow-up with gadolinium-diethylenetriamine pentaacetic acid-enhanced magnetic resonance imaging. *Mayo Clin Proc.* 1995;70:173-176.

351. FitzGerald PM. Primary sarcoma of the pulmonary trunk: CT findings. *J Comput Assist Tomogr.* 1983;7:521-523.

352. Kotooka N, Nagaya N, Tanaka R. Pulmonary artery sarcoma. *Heart.* 2003;89:1388.

353. Loredo JS, Fedullo PF, Piovella F, Moser KM. Digital clubbing associated with pulmonary artery sarcoma. *Chest.* 1996;109:1651-1653.

354. Kauczor HU, Schwickert HC, Mayer E, Kersjes W, Moll R, Schweden F. Pulmonary artery sarcoma mimicking chronic thromboembolic disease: computed tomography and magnetic resonance imaging findings. *Cardiovasc Intervent Radiol.* 1994;17:185-189.

355. Varriale P, Chryssos B. Pulmonary artery sarcoma: another cause of sudden death. *Clin Cardiol.* 1991;14:160-164.

356. Delany SG, Doyle TC, Bunton RW, Hung NA, Joblin LU, Taylor DR. Pulmonary artery sarcoma mimicking pulmonary embolism. *Chest.* 1993;103:1631-1633.

357. Weinreb JC, Davis SD, Berkmen YM, Isom W, Naidich DP. Pulmonary artery sarcoma: evaluation using gd-DTPA. *J Comput Assist Tomogr.* 1990;14:647-649.

358. Yi CA, Lee KS, Choe YH, Han D, Kwon OJ, Kim S. Computed tomography in pulmonary artery sarcoma: distinguishing features from pulmonary embolic disease. *J Comput Assist Tomogr.* 2004;28:34-39.

359. Mattoo A, Fedullo PF, Kapelanski D, Ilowite JS. Pulmonary artery sarcoma: a case report of surgical cure and 5-year follow-up. *Chest.* 2002;122:745-747.

360. Bleisch VR, Kraus FT. Polypoid sarcoma of the pulmonary trunk: analysis of the literature and report of a case with leptomeric organelles and ultrastructural features of rhabdomyosarcoma. *Cancer.* 1980;46:314-324.

chapter 47

Steal Syndromes

Raymond A. Dieter, Jr., MD, MS / George B. Kuzycz, MD

When one discusses vascular diseases, a number of problems or situations may develop and require the patient to seek medical assistance. Most such problems may be readily recognized and many may be treated conservatively and successfully with little effort or risk. Some situations, however, may produce vague or confusing symptoms and thus may be very difficult to sort out or to diagnose. These patients may then see numerous physicians and have extensive evaluation before the correct diagnosis or therapy is appropriately delineated. Such a diagnostic and therapeutic challenge for physicians may be a patient with a steal syndrome (SS).

Patients present with the more classic, cerebral steal symptomatology in which the diagnosis was readily proven or established. We have also seen a number of individuals with vague, perplexing symptoms for evaluation and in whom eventually a steal syndrome was diagnosed. Those patients who have an established, symptomatic steal syndrome need to be provided the therapeutic options, including major invasive procedures or corrective surgery. Patients with asymptomatic incidentally encountered steal findings present a different situation. Many of these situations require little or no treatment and close periodic follow-up. Avoidance of major interventions and their potential complications may thus be minimized. The severely debilitating or acute life-threatening "steal" developments may require urgent or emergent intervention and the accompanying risk to preserve life or limb. Multiple considerations affect the ultimate therapy and prognosis for the patient (Table 47-1).

DEFINITION

What is the definition of a steal syndrome? Different authors may ascribe different definitions or characteristics to this syndrome. A simple definition might be the taking of a blood supply from its usual direction and organ to another area as a result of a change in pressure gradient. This phenomenon can then occur in a number of situations. The classic example is where an artery is obstructed and the blood flow is then reversed in a vessel taking origin distal to the obstruction. The flow then travels around the obstruction and into the distal obstructed artery to serve the tissues distal to the obstruction. This may particularly occur when a greater need is recognized distally because of increased exercise or usage.

When this occurs, the blood, which originally flows away from the vessel obstructed, now flows toward the obstructed vessel and reverses the flow of blood into the circuitous route. This then redirects blood away from the original end-organ and provides the blood and nutrients to the ischemic or needy tissues. Thus, the original end-organ may receive a smaller supply of blood or nutrients. If the patient has findings on vascular study of blood flow redirection, or reversal, and the patient is asymptomatic, the process is called a "steal phenomenon" (SP). If the patient becomes symptomatic as a result of their obstruction and flow reversal, the diagnosis of a steal syndrome (SS) is established.

In essence, a steal occurs when blood is syphoned off from one area to another when a demand for blood or tissue nutrition presents at the second site. When this diversion occurs, the patient may develop symptoms relative to the area from which blood is diverted or stolen. The severity of the patient's problem will then define how severe the steal and thus the steal syndrome. The organ or structure from which blood is stolen from may initiate symptoms such as dizziness, pain, syncope, or weakness.

ETIOLOGY AND CLASSIFICATION

There are a number of causes for the development of the "steal" in a patient (Table 47-2). The most commonly recognized and understood steal situation develops as a result of arteriosclerotic, occlusive disease. This usually develops in

---

TABLE 47-1. Steal Syndrome Considerations

I. Etiology
II. Anatomy and physiology
III. Diagnosis
   A. Testing
   B. Symptoms
   C. Type of steal
IV. Therapy
   A. Risks
V. Prognosis

TABLE 47-3. End-Organ Stolen From

I. Brain
   A. Brain stem
II. Heart
   A. Coronary artery
III. Gastrointestinal tract
IV. Extremity
   A. Lower
   B. Upper to hand

---

elderly patients who have a propensity to form arteriosclerotic (cholesterol) plaque build up within an artery, which may lead to occlusion of a major vessel. Most commonly, this will involve the cerebral central nervous system (CNS) vasculature-carotid and subclavian arteries. The classic example is the left subclavian artery occlusion with vertebral vessel flow redirection. However, the arteriosclerotic process may also cause obstruction of other vessels such as the iliac arteries, which may lead to the development of a steal. Such a phenomenon may become particularly evident during the correction of an obstructing lesion. Coronary symptoms may even develop as a result of an occlusive process postcoronary bypass using the internal mammary artery.

Atherosclerotic occlusive disease is not the only etiology for a steal development. Iatrogenic causes include vascular surgery for congenital heart lesions, which may obstruct the normal subclavian routing and lead to CNS problems or symptoms. These patients may develop the SP but not the SS for years and their problems may thus be difficult to recognize. Arterial shunting of blood from a high-flow or high-pressure system to a low-resistance vessel may also lead to the steal occurring, e.g., the iliac steal postvascular repair of the iliac occlusion. Another iatrogenic cause is seen by the nephrologists who have noted a steal in a number of their fistula or shunt dialysis patients. When severe, these patients have required additional surgery to correct the problem and prevent tissue loss. Traumatic vascular lesions may also lead to steal through vascular occlusion or fistula formation. Such lesions may require extensive difficult surgical intervention.

Further classification according to the end-organ stolen from is well illustrated (Table 47-3). The end-organ affected may be the brain/brain stem in the subclavian steal. However, the coronary artery and heart may develop ischemia when the subclavian artery occludes postcoronary bypass utilizing the left internal mammary artery. The distal organ "stolen from" may include the hand, gastrointestinal system, or lower extremity and thus the end-organ classification.

Multiple vessels may be involved in the development of the SP. These vessels are usually larger vessels which carry a large volume of blood. Thus, when these vessels occlude, symptoms may be expected. Vessels that may be listed or involved in a "steal" include not only the larger readily recognized but also the smaller tributaries and capillaries (Table 47-4). Some of these steal situations may be

---

TABLE 47-2. Etiology of a Steal

I. Arteriosclerotic occlusive disease
   A. Takayasu's disease
II. Traumatic
III. Iatrogenic
   A. Dialysis access
   B. Congenital heart surgery
      1. Blaloch-Taussig ligation subclavian artery
   C. Postoperative procedures
   D. Ligation anomalous origin subclavian artery
IV. Spontaneous

TABLE 47-4. Types of Steal and Vessels Involved (Usually Arteries)

I. Cerebral
   A. Subclavian
   B. Vertebral
II. Abdominal
   A. Mesenteric
   B. Aorta
   C. Vena cava
   D. Iliac
III. Extremity
   A. Lower extremity
      1. Femoral
      2. Posterior tibial
   B. Upper extremity-dialysis access
      1. Brachial
      2. Radial
      3. Accompanying veins
IV. Coronary
   A. Subclavian

recognized by their vessel names, e.g., subclavian or coronary steal.

First described in 1960 by Contorni, a number of additions to our knowledge took place in a short time.[1] The subclavian steal phenomenon (SSP) was shown to be a result of severe stenosis or occlusion of the subclavian artery. One year later, Ravitch demonstrated that the subclavian artery occlusion could be associated with neurologic symptoms.[2] Fisher then called cerebrally symptomatic patients with subclavian flow reversal the subclavian steal syndrome (SSS).[3] Brainstem ischemia could thus be considered a result of the SSS. It should be noted that the SSS occurs only when the subclavian artery occlusion is proximal to the vertebral artery origin and the vertebral artery is patent.

The cerebral-subclavian steal is the most commonly recognized steal in which the subclavian artery becomes occluded and the flow is reversed in the left vertebral artery. This then changes the directional flow so that blood from the circle of Willis flows outward through the vertebral artery to the left upper extremity on demand. In the abdominal (mesenteric) steal, the blood is redirected from one organ to serve another during occlusion of the visceral vessels, or on aortic occlusion, into the iliac system. The dialysis access steal is seen particularly when the brachial artery or large radial artery fistulas are created and the arterial blood flows away from the hand.

Another steal example is the coronary artery steal (CAS). This occurs when the proximal left subclavian artery occludes and the left internal mammary artery has been used to revascularize the coronary vessels. A possible iatrogenic cause may develop when the Blalock-Taussig operation is performed for congenital heart disease. During this surgery, division of the distal left subclavian artery, proximal to the origin of the left vertebral artery, may create a potential SP. With growth and aging, these individuals may develop symptoms, including headaches, as a result of an iatrogenic induced subclavian steal. Cerebral lesions and other anatomic lesions should be sought in order to be sure of the diagnosis, the anatomy, and the possible treatment. With time and growth, collateral circulation may then develop through multiple vessels to provide appropriate tissue nourishment.

● ANATOMY AND PHYSIOLOGY

The anatomic location of the disease process and the number of lesions varies from patient to patient. When the subclavian artery acutely becomes severely stenotic, such that flow is reduced or totally occluded, the arm distally may become symptomatic caused by ischemia. When the stenosis occurs over a long period of time, collateral circulation may develop and maintain the viability of the distal extremity with or without symptoms. Netter's textbook of anatomy delineates the cerebral arterial system simply and graphically.[4] The developing collaterals will include the vertebral artery, arterial branches to the chest wall, the circle of Willis, the carotid artery, and other collateral vessels

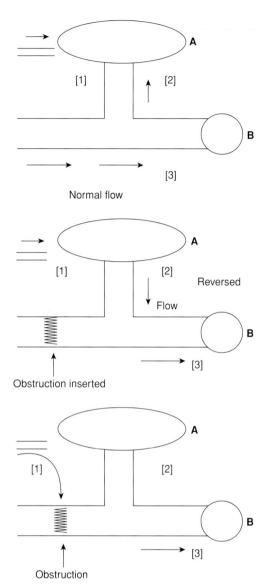

Normal flow

Reversed Flow

Obstruction inserted

Obstruction

Rerouting after obstruction: A has supply diminished to prefeve B.

● **FIGURE 47-1.** Flow direction with resistance change: such a situation in which either (I) resistance increases (at **A**) or (II) resistance decreases (at **B**) will lead to less flow to organ (**A**) and more to organ (**B**). Technically, one might argue against this being a steal phenomenon, but we have considered this to be the practical case.

(Figure 47-1). The blood flow for the subclavian steal will usually take place through the right innominate into the right carotid and the circle of Willis [1]. The blood will then flow down the left vertebral [2] to the distal left subclavian artery [3] and then out to the brachial vessels and the arm and hand (B). Increased arm exercise will demand more circulation through the brachial vessels to the left upper extremity. During this period of time, vertebral basilar and other symptomatology may develop. Some individuals, however, have felt that such symptoms may not be because of a reduction in cerebral blood flow (A). This, however, is not the usual consideration. Of interest is the fact that many patients with the SP remain totally asymptomatic.

We have seen patients with multiple etiologies for what is felt to be a subclavian steal. This includes the individual with Takayasu's disease, as well as the typical elderly arteriosclerotic obliterans process. However, traumatic occlusion of the subclavian artery as well as the iatrogenic causes for subclavian artery disease have been noted, including those patients who have had an anomalous right subclavian artery originating from the left descending thoracic aorta. Subsequent to ligation or division of the anomalous subclavian artery, patients may develop the SSS years later. After extensive arm usage they may pass out or develop syncope with no other anatomic abnormality except the ligated right subclavian artery.

The steal syndrome may also develop when a blood flow circuit is modified or changed. Such may occur when an obstruction or new connection (bypass) reroutes the blood away from the usual distal end-organ and into a different pathway. When this occurs, the blood may literally take a shortcut and follow the path of least resistances as exemplified in Figure 47-1.

At low flow or reduced need, both organs or areas normally perfused may not initiate any symptoms despite an obstruction, flow reversal, or change in distal resistance. Oxygen and nutrient supply are adequate at this point in time. But with increased demand by the end-organ (B) and decreased flow to organ (A), the blood may be shunted or "stolen" away from the usual recipient of the normally directed blood flow to organ (A). This decreased flow to (A) may then initiate hypoxic and hypovolemic symptoms referral to organ (A) in addition to decreased nutrient symptoms from organ (B).

A parallel phenomenon occurs when a large vessel normally serves both a high-and low-resistance area. The blood will flow away from the higher-resistance area when no obstruction is present to the lower-resistance area or the obstruction has been removed.

● DIAGNOSIS

Many of the patients found to have a SP are asymptomatic and the steal is found only during diagnostic studies for other reasons. Such asymptomatic findings are unexpected in most patients and are usually not treated. When symptoms do develop, the type and severity depends on the organ or structures involved. The SSS patients may have both arm and cerebral symptoms, but the arteriovenous (A-V) access patients usually will not have cerebral symptoms. Suspicion and awareness in the symptomatic patient will lead to a more concentrated physical examination and subsequent appropriate diagnostic testing. Weakened or absent pulses, an auscultatory bruit, and blood pressure variance from extremity to extremity may all be clues to the problem.

Diagnosis of this syndrome relies primarily on the awareness and then the performance of the appropriate diagnostic studies. These studies include a good physical examination. When considering a SSS, the physical examination should include comments regarding the presence or absence of the radial and carotid pulses, the blood pressure in both upper extremities, and if a bruit is present. Diagnostic studies may include a number of imaging techniques, including the colored Doppler studies, angiography, and magnetic resonance angiography.[5] Standard x-ray examinations usually will yield no benefit. More recently, CT scan angiography is being utilized to diagnose and delineate vascular problems. False-positive and false-negative studies must be guarded against and further delineated.

Angiography, utilizing the standard injection of contrast dye, has been the mainstay in diagnosing extracranial and intracranial, vascular disease. Initially, direct needle vascular puncture and injection of iodine based contrast material was utilized. Carotid and brachial artery puncture with appropriate timing produced good quality radiographs. These studies required multiple access sites and retrograde injection when utilizing the brachial artery. With the development of the catheter angiographic techniques, especially through the groin, multiple injections and multiple vessels could be studied with single vessel access. Smaller catheters, flexible guidewires, power injectors, and introducer sheaths, all added to the increased angiographic techniques aided by safer contrast materials. Thus, stenotic as well as forward and reverse flow studies were readily accepted and performed. Currently, when intraarterial angiography is necessary, a retrograde transfemoral catheter approach is preferred unless the groin presents a contraindication such as occlusive disease, infection, or previous graft concerns.

In addition, the noninvasive studies may include the vascular ultrasound, magnetic resonance imaging (MRI) and angiography (MRA), and positron emission tomography (PET) scanning techniques. Duplex ultrasonography of carotid, vertebral, and subclavian arteries may be very revealing in screening for stenosis, occlusion, and flow. Flow direction in the subclavian and vertebral artery may be evaluated at the same time. Provactive maneuvers and the "bunny" waveform evaluation may further define the steal process. Invasive studies including arch angiography and selective carotid and subclavian studies will all assist in the diagnosis. If the patient is asymptomatic, most of the time the steal phenomena will be diagnosed only coincidentally. In the past, digital subtraction angiography has been utilized to a great extent, but has a lesser value with the advent of the more modern studies.

The question of evaluating these patients and their cerebral blood flow utilizing the PET (exercise thallium-201 stress imaging) scan has been raised by Mase et. al.[6] They found a dramatic decrease of cerebral blood flow on PET study in the steal syndrome. Their patient had complained of headache and dizziness. Extensive evaluation included cranial MRI, oxygen-labeled gases, oxygen extraction fraction, and regional metabolic rate for oxygen. They suggested that PET scanning could possibly be a study to assist in the evaluation of an individual and whether or not the steal syndrome was significant. In response to this, Steve Powel questions the value of performing a PET scan in these individuals.[7] He stated that vascular surgeons have known for years that a history of upper extremity claudication, a subclavian bruit, and a diminished blood pressure in the affected arm are diagnostic in most patients. Watson et. al, however, felt that this technique could become a valuable study in the future.[8]

● SPECIFIC STEAL PATIENTS

Subclavian Steal

Subclavian steal occurs on an infrequent basis but represents the most frequent of the steal diagnoses. The patients may be totally asymptomatic and the problem found incidentally during other studies. However, when the symptoms do develop, the patients are now felt to have the steal syndrome as compared to the SP. The symptoms vary from patient to patient but, in general, are related to the central nervous system and to the upper extremity. The most common symptoms are dizziness, syncope, headache, and weakness—all manifestations of vertebral basilar insufficiency.[9] Other such central nervous system problems may include blurred vision, nausea, vomiting, and drop attacks as well as auditory phenomenon. On occasion chest pain may develop and produce symptoms suggesting angina. The upper extremity may present with ulceration of the fingertips, paresthesias, and painful symptomatology both at rest or with exercise. Stroke or hemiparesis as well as hemisensory dysfunction are less common and might suggest carotid disease as compared to subclavian difficulties. Less commonly, lower extremity claudication and gastrointestinal complaints such as distention, pain, and shock may be seen. These patients when examined may be totally normal on examination or there may be obvious physical findings such as differential blood pressure in the right and left upper extremity, carotid bruits, absence of left radial pulsation, as well as digital ulceration and discoloration of the upper extremity. Most of our patients have not had major symptoms or have been asymptomatic. It should be noted that some individuals feel that the reversal of flow in the vertebral system and the flow away from the circle of Willis may actually cause no symptomatology. In the younger individual in whom subclavian artery stenosis or occlusion is present, headaches seem to be one of the main presenting difficulties.

The examination of these patients utilizing noninvasive techniques such as duplex ultrasound, CT scan angiography, and magnetic resonance angiography all may further delineate and confirm the diagnosis. The patient's collateral circulation may be extensive and through multiple routes including the internal or external carotid, the vertebral artery, the thyrocervical and costocervical trunk, as well as transcervical anastomosis between the inferior thyroid vessels and indirect communications (Table 47-5). Arch angiography will delineate the major vessels coming off of the arch with a single injection and hopefully avoid selective angiography and the potential complications of such.

TABLE 47-5. Subclavian Artery Occlusion Collaterals

I. Vertebral communication via circle of Willis from the internal carotid artery

II. Anastomoses between the inferior thyroid arteries and transcervical vessels

III. Indirect vertebral to vertebral-spinal branch anastomosis

IV. Vertebral collateralization from the external carotid and the thyrocervical and the costocervical trunks

V. Internal thoracic or aorta internal thoracic artery communication through the intercostals

---

We have seen a number of patients with congenital aortic arch and anomalous subclavian artery abnormalities. Years ago patients with the anomalous subclavian origin difficulty were treated primarily with ligation and division of the anomalous vessel and no reattachment to the aorta anterior to the esophagus. When we first saw these patients, diagnostic angiography and symptomatology led us to total operative correction and avoidance of potential future subclavian steal symptoms.[10,11] The same consideration has been given to the patient with congenital cardiac abnormalities requiring transfer of the subclavian artery and distal ligation. The question then becomes relevant as to whether a bypass to the distal subclavian artery should be considered with the appearance of symptoms or whether the vertebral artery could have been ligated at the initial surgery.

The three major SSSs include the subclavian, the innominate, and the carotid steal (Table 47-6). The subclavian steal is the most frequent and the other two are very uncommon and questioned as to their diagnoses. In the subclavian steal, vertebral basilar insufficiency, vertigo, transient blindness, and syncopal episodes are the most common patient complaints (Table 47-7). Blood pressure changes greater than 20 mm Hg between the right and left arm may be very suggestive. Further, the differential diagnosis must be considered in those who have normal blood pressure in both arms with symptomatology suggestive of the steal. Bilateral subclavian steal would be very uncommon, and care with placement of diagnostic catheters to avoid erroneous data is required. Patients who have concomitant carotid disease

---

TABLE 47-6. Types of Subclavian Steal Syndromes (SSS) or Phenomenon (SSP)

I. Subclavian steal

II. Innominate steal (right side only)

III. Carotid basilar steal

IV. External carotid to vertebral steal

V. Coronary subclavian steal (CSS) via mammary artery graft

TABLE 47-7. Subclavian Steal Syndrome (SSS) Symptomatology

I. Upper extremity
   A. Pain: rest or claudication
   B. Paresthesias
   C. Ulceration or gangrene
II. Central nervous system
   A. Headache
   B. Dizziness/vertigo
   C. Syncopal or drop attacks
   D. Nausea and vomiting
   E. Ataxia
III. Vision
   A. Blurred
   B. Diplopic
IV. Auditory
V. Cardiac
   A. Angina or chest pain
VI. Hemiparesis: uncommon
VII. Gastrointestinal: uncommon

TABLE 47-8. Therapeutic Options for Treatment of the Subclavian Steal Syndrome

I. Observation
II. Correction
   A. Lipid abnormality
   B. Blood pressure
   C. Diabetes mellitus
   D. Smoking cessation
III. Percutaneous approach
   A. Angioplasty +/− stent placement.
   B. Endovascular atherectomy.
IV. Intrathoracic
   A. Endarterectomy with patch graft of subclavian or vertebral artery
   B. Complete correction of congenital aortic arch abnormalities
   C. Ligation of vertebral artery and its branches
   D. Aortosubclavian bypass
   E. Aortoinnominate bypass
V. Extrathoracic
   A. Endarterectomy of stenotic or occluded vessels (subclavian, brachiocephalic, vertebral, or thyrocervical).
   B. Grafting (vein or synthetic material)
      1. Carotid—axillary
      2. Carotid—subclavian
      3. Subclavian—subclavian
      4. Femoral—axillary
      5. Carotid—vertebral
      6. Axillary—axillary
   C. Direct anastomoses
      1. Vertebral to carotid
      2. Subclavian to carotid

at the same time as a steal syndrome will usually require carotid surgery prior to correction of the steal.

Morbidity from this syndrome is usually low, but severely debilitated patients may be seen with episodes of arm and intracranial ischemic symptoms. The finding of extracranial arterial occlusion during angiographic studies has been reported as high as 15% to 17% in studied patients. Many of these will have concomitant obstructive findings in the carotid system and, as many as 5% of the patients may have an asymptomatic subclavian SP. However, this usually is around 1% or less. SSS does occur more commonly in males and particularly in the older Caucasian population. The Takayasu arteritis symptoms, however, may occur in the younger female individual.

Treatment of the SSP is usually not required as these patients are asymptomatic and the lesion is an incidental finding. When the SSP patient progresses to the SSS, therapy must then be considered. When possible, correcting the blood pressure, diabetes, and activity (especially arm usage) level may all reduce the need for intervention. However, when intervention requires surgery, the patient's surgical approach should restore antegrade vertebral artery flow, increase the cerebral arterial flow, and hopefully relieve the cerebral symptomatology (Table 47-8).

We have preferred avoiding a major thoracotomy if possible, particularly when the SSS is found in the older individuals. Most patients with the finding of a subclavian steal have not required surgery. Many of the patients will have a carotid stenosis along with the steal. In these individuals, a carotid endarterectomy may be the best approach. On occasion, however, this surgery may either exacerbate or not relieve the steal syndrome and the patient may then require a second surgery. The consideration for surgery should take into account the phrenic nerve, the scalenus anticus muscle, and the recurrent laryngeal nerve. We have performed both extrathoracic as well as the intrathoracic procedures with success in the appropriate clinical situation. One should be aware, however, that the subclavian artery may be very friable and difficult to suture. Various bypass procedures include the subclavian-subclavian bypass via the supraclavicular approach, an axillo-axillary bypass (may be a safer approach), and a femoral axillary bypass with a tunneled graft. We prefer to avoid the latter. Patients must be cautioned to notify physicians of the graft, especially when a midsternotomy is to be performed.

In our experience, midsternotomy has not been required for the treatment of most of these patients. However, some authors have reported utilization of this approach, particularly in Takayasu's syndrome, where additional vessels may require bypass. The transfemoral catheter angioplasty approach may be utilized in a number of these patients, particularly the ones with a stenosis as compared to a complete obstruction. Restenosis, a consideration in the transformal patients, requires periodic prospective patient monitoring.

In patients with congenital vascular abnormalities, we have attempted to perform total correction, with respect to the aberrant retroesophageal right subclavian artery. Combining various techniques in some patients may be more appropriate than a single, more complicated, and potentially higher-risk procedure.

Complications of these procedures certainly do occur. One must be aware of the potential for thrombosis and rethrombosis of the graft or anastomosis.[12] When this does occur, the risk to the patient includes a stroke and hemiplegia. Thoracic duct injury may lead to a lymph fistula. Laryngeal or phrenic nerve injuries may occur while performing subclavian or innominate surgical procedures. Adequacy of the graft without injury to the other structures will avoid postoperative symptoms such as dyspnea caused by diaphragmatic palsy and Horner's syndrome. The correction of these patients' problems without morbidity and mortality may be a challenge to the most adept. Other considerations, including the medicolegal pitfalls, may also be a concern.

Therapy for these patients is varied and requires considerable evaluation prior to a definitive approach.[13] Certainly, one needs to know whether the patient is symptomatic, and whether the symptoms are felt to be a result of the steal, or whether the symptoms could be because of another etiology. Multiple causes of arm claudication may be present. If there is an indication for another diagnosis, evaluation for such should be taken into consideration prior to any surgery. Symptoms thought to be caused by the steal syndrome may mimic those caused by a thoracic outlet syndrome, a carpal tunnel compression, or other processes that create pain in the arm, especially with usage of that extremity. There may be multiple types of steal present, and this therefore requires the appropriate diagnosis. With multiple types of steal, it is pertinent to define the correct anatomic and functional flow abnormality. Flow abnormalities in the vertebral artery may be divided into three categories: stage 1, reduced antegrade flow; stage 2, exercise-induced reversal of flow; stage 3, permanent reversal of flow. Knowing the characteristics of the obstruction and symptomatology, the correct diagnosis and the patient's limitations one can then develop the best approach for treatment, whether medical or surgical.

● CORONARY SUBCLAVIAN STEAL

A separate subclavian steal occurance has been described in patients having coronary artery surgery. This syndrome has been variously classified as a SSS, an internal thoracic artery steal syndrome, and a coronary subclavian steal (CSS). It has occurred in individuals who have had occlusive coronary disease requiring coronary bypass procedures. As experience has progressed, the internal mammary bypass has been utilized to a greater degree as a donor vessel. When the left internal mammary artery is anastomosed to a coronary artery, the patients have a situation where occlusion of the subclavian artery may create symptomatology suggestive of both recurrent coronary disease as well as the CNS symptoms of subclavian artery occlusion. The development of angina in these individuals should be studied with both noninvasive and invasive considerations to evaluate the potential for an occluded subclavian artery with coronary circulation hypoperfusion because of a steal into the upper extremity, especially with exercise.

If the subclavian artery is stenotic but not totally occluded, angioplastic procedures with or without stent placement has relieved a number of these patients. Transfemoral, percutaneous, and directional atherectomy has also been utilized for the treatment of the occlusion and relief of the coronary anginal symptomatology. If this is not feasible, subclavian, or axillary bypass grafting (Gore-Tex) has been utilized for treatment of these individuals. Pocar and Ferges et al. have discussed the incidence of perioperative internal thoracic artery steal syndrome following coronary bypass surgery.[14,15] The flow reversal in the LIMA graft has been demonstrated to be the explanation for the repeat chest pain and symptoms in these individuals. When possible, a noncardiac extrathoracic approach should be considered for the treatment of these individuals.[16] There have been reports stating that as long as coronary perfusion is maintained, isoflurane does not cause coronary steal or ischemia. Teo and Koe, however, have reported where this was not the case and where isoflurane did not have myocardial protective properties in their patients.[17] The patient requiring coronary surgery should thus be considered for arch angiography, particularly when there is a discrepancy in the blood pressure between the two upper extremities. Elian et al. had seven patients who presented with recurrent angina because of subclavian artery stenosis.[18] In each of these, the internal mammary graft was open and, in their studies, they did not see a true steal mechanism. However, stent angioplasty and stenting of the subclavian artery resulted in immediate disappearance of the angina.

● HEMOACCESS STEAL

Patients with chronic renal failure and elevated blood urea nitrogen (BUN) and creatinine are a frequent medical problem in the community. Because of this, renal dialysis and renal dialysis centers have continued to develop throughout North America and the world. With the finding of these nephrotic or prenephrotic patients who require dialysis, a decision must be made whether they will have peritoneal dialysis or hemodialysis. If the patients are to have hemodialysis, appropriate hemoaccess procedures are required. Acutely ill patients may be treated with temporary hemodialysis procedures through the subclavian, internal jugular, or femoral veins. Those patients requiring long-term dialysis may be then converted to other more convenient chronic long-term access modalities. The most common such procedures include A-V anastomatic access using the radial artery or loop grafting (gortex, vein, bovine) at the elbow using the brachial artery and vein. The creation of the hemodialysis fistula at or just above the wrist may proceed well with a good flow and little symptomatology once the patient's wound has healed and matured. However, a number of these patients may have a high flow through the fistula and develop symptoms distal to the anastomosis of swelling, painful edema, loss of function, and discoloration of the extremity and hand. Ulceration of the fingers and numbness have been seen. In these individuals additional surgery may be required to ligate the distal end of the fistula to hopefully avoid and reduce the steal symptomology. However, the most common difficulties noted in the creation of brachial/radial A-V access is not the steal but the small vein, low flow, and thrombotic considerations. Studies have been carried out to evaluate the patient as to the potential for developing the steal concern and the risk factors such as hypertension, race, diabetes, smoking, and coronary disease.[19] Diabetic patients, people of aboriginal race, and women may develop more steal symptoms compared to men. If complications or infection develop, repeated surgery as well as a risk to the extremity viability may be seen, possibly requiring further surgery.

Patients having more proximal procedures such as a brachial artery to vein anastomosis, a proximal radial artery to vein anastomosis or a prosthetic graft procedure, may have an increased risk of developing the SP. Patients with the more proximal procedure are more apt to develop a steal than the ones with the distal procedure according to Davidson et al.[19] They demonstrated an approximate 6% overall rate of steal in these proximal renal dialysis access patients. The best patient access procedure is performed when good distal vessels, both arterial and venous, exist and when the patient otherwise has a good palpable distal pulse. If they require a more central shunt, then the risks would certainly be enhanced. The arterial steal syndrome in the brachial artery-based procedure has, on occasion, led to loss of distal function, but with close observation this should be minimized. The brachiocephalic as well as the A-V grafts may all develop the steal syndrome. Femoral-femoral grafting and potential steal is very uncommon.

Various techniques have been proposed as to the best approach to resolve the patient's difficulty when a steal syndrome is considered (Table 47-9). Angiography may assist in the decision as to whether surgical intervention is required to alleviate the symptoms or the findings and whether there are other accompanying abnormalities leading to or enhancing the problem.[20] Individual techniques to

---

TABLE 47-9. Treatment Modalities for Upper Extremity Hemoaccess Steal Syndrome

I. Arteriography
II. Distal ligation
III. Lengthening of graft
IV. Circular constriction
V. Take down access— move to new site
VI. Correction of proximal stenosis

---

reduce the incidence of steal or the symptomatology as a result have been utilized. These have included the ligation of distal vessels, the graft lengthening procedures to increase the resistance in a graft, the placement of a stricture, or band on a graft subsequent to noninvasive as well as invasive studies. This banding technique has also been used for distal venous aneurysm formation post-A-V access. The individuals with a cold hand that is painful at rest and during dialysis more commonly will require further consideration and surgical intervention to avoid destructive arthropathy and reflex sympathetic dystrophy. An additional finding of angiography in some individuals may be a significant arterial stenosis. Thus, angiography is warranted to select the proper course of treatment for these individuals. Preferably, modification of the fistula or graft will resolve the problem rather than complete removal of the fistula or graft.

AORTOILIAC (MESENTERIC ARTERIAL) STEAL

Trippel et al. discussed the incidence of this syndrome 35 years ago and mentioned that it was originally described several years prior to their presentation by Dr. DeBakey.[21] Occasionally, patients are seen with total obstruction of the subrenal aorta and absence or diminished femoral, popliteal, or pedal pulses because of occlusive disease of the aorta and iliac vessels. These individuals will have large, collateral, circulatory changes through connecting vessels. The collateral vessels may include the celiac, the inferior mesenteric, the superior mesenteric artery, and the distal iliac or femoral vessels. In these circumstances when aortofemoral bypass grafting is accomplished, the patient may develop severe abdominal pain with an intraabdominal crisis. Symptomatic individuals may progress rapidly to gangrene of the bowel and massive sepsis. Exploratory laparotomy will usually demonstrate no inappropriately placed ligatures or twists. The patient may, however, have a mesenteric vessel stenosis and a meandering mesenteric artery. Reconstruction with perfusion of the distal extremities relieves the pressure and high flow to the mesenteric vessels and may lead to decreased flow in the mesenteric system, increased leg flow, and death of the bowel.[22] It has been our experience that when this occurs, no other revascularization technique has assisted these individuals. However, the enlarged, central, anastomotic artery on angiography may demonstrate and suggest a potential compromise of the mesenteric circulation as well as a stenosis or stricture of two or three of the mesenteric vessels.

SPLANCHNIC STEAL

A separate, splanchnic steal syndrome has also been described. Keswani et al reported a patient that they felt had a splanchnic steal syndrome.[23] Their patient developed light-headedness, right-sided numbness, and weakness after eating along, with slurred speech. Following evaluation, the patient was found to have internal carotid stenosis and poor collateral flow to the left hemisphere. Subsequent to correction of her internal carotid stenosis, her postprandial weakness disappeared and she no longer had difficulty after large meals. They discussed the incidence of postprandial hypotension in wheelchair-bound elderly individuals and hypothesized that this postprandial drop in blood pressure may be caused by inadequate sympathetic response in the elderly. They further demonstrated how their patient was relieved of symptomatology because of diminished gastrointestinal flow and cerebral hypoxia. They reduced the "splanchnic steal" by having the patient eat smaller and more frequent meals and by correcting the carotid stenosis, thus relieving the patients symptoms.

OTHER

Other potential steal syndromes may be present or considered in patients but to a much lesser degree and lesser understanding of the process. We have seen patients with posterior tibial artery to vein fistulae who had audible bruits and palpable thrills. These individuals complained of pain and coldness in the extremity distal to this area. With cor-

rection of the fistula or with spontaneous healing of the traumatic lesion, the patient's symptoms improved and disappeared. It has been our feeling that this represented a localized, traumatic, posterior, tibial artery steal syndrome. This process has also been noted following balloon angioplasty.

Another group of patients that have been considered to have a potential for a steal syndrome have been the patients with an aortocaval fistula. In these individuals, the aortic blood flow may be diverted from a higher blood pressure into a lower pressure system (the vena cava) and when this occurs, diminished blood flow to the lower extremities and to the pelvic organs may occur. Most of these patients will be seen prior to complaining of severe distal pain because of other more central symptomatology. However, the flow from the high to the low pressure system and the diversion of blood seems to be aperfect setup for the creation of a SP or syndrome. Correction of the lesion should reduce both the distal and central symptoms if there is no distal obstruction. If there is an obstruction distally, correction of the fistula along with distal bypass should relieve the symptomatology.

REFERENCES

1. Contorni L. Il circola collateral vertebraovertebrale nell obliterazionne iell' arterio subclavia all sua origine. *Minerva Chir.* 1960;15:268-271.

2. Reivich M, Holling HE, Roberts B, et al. Reversal of blood flow through the vertebral artery and it's effect on cerebral circulation. *N Eng J Med.* 1961;265:878-885.

3. Fisher CM. Editorial comment: a new vascular syndrome—the subclavian steal. *N Engl J Med.* 1961;265:912-913.

4. Netter FH. *Atlas of Human Anatomy.* 3rd ed. Univ of Rochester School of Medicine and Dentistry. Rochester NY, Teterboro, NJ: Icon Learning Systems; 2003.

5. Kalaria VG, Jacob S, Irwin W, Schainfeld RM. Duplex ultrasonography of vertebral and subclavian arteries. *J Amer Soc Echocardiogr.* 2005;18(10):1107-1111.

6. Mase M, Yamada K, Matsumoto T, Fujimoto S, Lida A. Cerebral blood flow and metabolism of steal syndrome evaluated by PET. *Neurology.* 1999;52(7):1515-1516.

7. Powell S. Response to determine functional significance of subclavian artery stenosis using exercise thallium 201 stress imaging. [Letters to the Editor]. *South Med J.* 2005;98(12):1223.

8. Watson S, Bedi S, Singh S. Determining functional significance of subclavian artery stenosis using exercise thallium-201 stress imaging. *South Med J.* 2005;98:559-560.

9. Dieter RA Jr, Maganini RO, Dieter R. Subclavian steal syndrome. In: John C, ed. *Text Book of Angiology.* New York, NY: Springer; 2000:629-634.

10. Piffare R, Dieter RA Jr, Niedballa RG. Definitive surgical treatment of the aberrant retroesophageal right subclavian artery in the adult. *Thorac Cardiovasc Surg.* 1971;61:154-159.

11. Dieter RA Jr, Kuzycz G. The steal syndrome: iatrogenic causes. *Internat Surg.* 1998;83:355-357.

12. Thrombosis of the subclavian arteries in the steal syndrome, complications of extracranial cerebrovascular procedures. In: Baum S, ed. *Abrams Angiography. Vascular and Interventional Radiology.* Vol 1. 4th ed. Boston, MA: Little, Brown & Co; 164-165, 287-291.

13. Brophy DP. Subclavian Steal Syndrome, e Medicine Journal [serial online]. Knowledge Resource Library. http://www.emedicine.com/radio/topic 663.htm. February 15, 2006:1-9.

14. Pocar M, Moneta A, Passolunjhi D, Mattioli R, Clerissi J, Donatelli F. Perioperative internal thoracic artery steal syndrome after coronary bypass surgery. *J Thor Cardiovasc Surg.* 2005;130:562-563.

15. Fergus T, Pacanowski JP Jr, Fasseas P, Nanjundappa A, Ahmed MH, Dieter RS. Coronary subclavian steal: presentation and management: two case reports. *Angiol.* 2006;57:T1-T4.

16. Kern KB, Warner NE, Sulek CA, Osaki K, Lobato EB. Angina as an indication for noncardiac surgery: the case of the coronary subclavian steal syndrome. *Anesthesiol.* 2000;92(2):610-612.

17. Teo A, Koh KF. Isoflurane in coronary steal. *Anesthes.* 2003;58:95-96.

18. Elian D, Gerniak A, Guetta V, et al. Subclavian coronary steal syndrome, and obligatory common fate between subclavian artery, internal mammary graft and coronary circulation. *Cardiol.* 2002;97:175-179.

19. Davidson D, Louridas G, Guzman R, et al. Steal syndrome

complicating upper extremity hemoaccess procedures, incidence and risks factors. *Canad Surg.* 2003;46(6):408-412.

20. Asif A, Leon C, Merrill D, et al. Arterial steal syndrome secondary to dialysis: a modest proposal for an old paradigm. *Amer J Kidney Dis.* 2006;48(1):88-97.

21. Trippel OH, Juraj MN, Midell AI. The aortoiliac steal, a review of this syndrome and a report of one additional case. *Ann Surg.* 1972;175(3):454-457.

22. Connolly JE, Stemmer EA. Intestinal gangrene as the result of mesenteric anterial steal. *Am J Surg.* 1973;12:197-204.

23. Keswini SC, Wityk R. A case of steal syndrome. *Lancet Neurol.* 2003;2:379.

chapter 48

Hemodialysis Access

John B. Chang, MD / Robert W. Chang, MD / Lorena De Marco Garcia, MD

● INTRODUCTION

Patients with acute and chronic renal failure require dependable access for dialysis. Dialysis access failure has been reported to be one of the most frequent causes of hospitalization among patients with end-stage renal disease (ESRD).[1] With our ability to treat ESRD, improving the longevity of our patient population has been steadily increasing.

The Kidney Dialysis Outcomes Quality Initiative (DOQI),[2] as published by the National Kidney Foundation, sets forth recommendations as part of a national consensus that parishioners avoid percutaneous-catheter based arteriovenous (AV) hemodialysis access in favor of autogenous access (AA), followed by prosthetic access (PA), as a second preference. With vascular access (VA) complications accounting for 15% of hospital admissions among hemodialysis patients,[3,4] and Medicare costs approximating $182 million in 2003,[4] the population of patients requiring hemodialysis access is expected to increase by 10% per year from a group which exceeded 345 000 patients in 2000.[5]

The current DOQI recommendations for practice patterns are the insertion of an AA in 50% of long-term access patients. However, some centers have had trouble achieving this goal as a result of vein mapping results or availability of forearm basilic vein.[6] The DOQI guidelines-recommended surgical referral pattern should begin when a patient exhibits a creatinine clearance of less than 25 mL/min or a serum creatinine greater than 4 mg/dL or when AV access is anticipated within 1 year.[2]

The introduction of hemodialysis as routine treatment of ESRD made it necessary to find a simple form of repeated access to the vascular system. It was only after the introduction of external silastic cannulae by Quinton and Scribner[7] in 1960 that extracorporeal treatment could be established. Several years later, Brescia and Cimino[8] devised the AV fistula, which overcame the limitations of frequent infections and thrombosis. In the 1970s the implantation of grafts was introduced,[9–11] which permitted renal replacement therapy in patients devoid of venous vessels.

Currently, complications of VA (i.e., dysfunction, thrombosis, or infection) are a major cause of hospital admission. They affect the quality of life. For this there are objective reasons (they make it difficult to administer sufficient dose of dialysis) and subjective ones (anxiety because of uncertainty about correct functioning).[12] Furthermore, they give rise to frustration in health care personnel.[13–15] Recently, repeated VA failure has been identified as a risk factor for mortality.[16] Finally, VA failure causes high economic costs, accounting for up to one-third of ESRD expenditure.[17]

The radiocephalic AV fistula is the preferred VA because of its low complication rates, its long survival, and its ease of puncture once it has matured.[18–20] Nevertheless, its establishment on the wrist or in the anatomical snuffbox of the nondominant arm is potentially inconvenient for two reasons: (1) Four to eight weeks are necessary until the venous wall has arterialized and (2) a high rate, 8% to 30% of initial failure or insufficient development is observed, necessitating the use of other modalities of VA.[21] Recently, AV fistulae higher up in the forearm and on the upper arm have been put forward as acceptable alternatives. Some studies have documented primary patency rate >80% in the first 2 years of observation,[22] but there is no information on the long-term outcome for this type of AV fistula.

The second mode of permanent VA are grafts, the use of which has increased in recent years, and in numerous centers it is today the most frequently used type of VA.[23] This tendency has been related to recent demographic changes in the hemodialysis population, the scarcity of transplants with the consecutive increased time on hemodialysis treatment, and increase comorbidity of patients beginning renal replacement therapy. In fact the median age of incident patients is actually around 60 years, more than half of the patients have at least two comorbid conditions, and 20% to 40% are diabetic patient—all factors that could affect the success of the VA.[17,24] On top of this, patients are not infrequently referred to the nephrologists in the terminal stages of renal failure or during an episode of acute deterioration of pre-existing renal failure. In these circumstances, it is frequently impossible to create a VA in time.[25]

● ACUTE ACCESS

For patients who require immediate dialysis access, that is, those requiring hemodialysis of less than 3-week duration, a double-lumen cuffed or noncuffed catheter should be inserted into the femoral, internal jugular, or subclavian vein.[26] The most common catheter for this purpose is the Quinton catheter, which can be placed at the bedside and must be able to support a flow rate of 250 mL/min.[27] In case of femoral vein catheter insertion, the catheter should not remain longer than 5 days, because of the high propensity for infection or dislodgment with ambulation.[28] Most importantly, the subclavian position should be avoided if the patient is to be considered for an ipsilateral arm access procedure because the incidence of subclavian vein stenosis or thrombosis or both increases steadily with the presence of a catheter in this position, rendering the extremity useless for insertion of a permanent access.[29,30]

● SUBACUTE ACCESS

For the patient who requires hemodialysis for more than 3-week duration, insertion of a cuffed, tunneled, double-lumen catheter should be considered. The preference of location would be the internal jugular vein. The right internal jugular vein is preferred because of its proximity to the atrial-caval junction (allowing for better flow), but with the added emphasis of placing the catheter in the right internal jugular.

Aside from complications associated with insertion, (hemothorax and pneumothorax), the tunneled cuffed catheter can be relied on to function for an average of 6 months, after which infection, fibrin sheath formation, or thrombosis may curtail usage.[31] Using endoluminal therapy or percutaneous mechanical techniques, prolonged usage can be obtained up to 12.7 months as reported in a study.[32] Local infection and sepsis,[31] and infection elsewhere[33] are typical reasons for removal of the catheter.

● CHRONIC ACCESS AUTOGENOUS

Snuffbox Fistula

These consist of end-to-side anastomosis between the distal cephalic vein and the thenar branch of the radial artery, the pulse of which is usually palpable through the floor of the anatomic snuffbox, created through the one incision. In one European study over a 12-year period, 11% thrombosed within 24 hours of creation, and 80% had matured for hemodialysis within 6 weeks. The 1- and 5-year patency rates were 65% and 45%. Of the fistulae

that thrombosed, ipsilateral wrist angio access was successfully constructed in 45%.[34] Similar results were obtained in another study,[35] which reported on 139 patients who underwent snuffbox fistula creation with and without diabetic nephropathy. After 57 months, 87% of patients without diabetic nephropathy had patent access, whereas 72% were patent among patients with diabetic nephropathy, and they concluded that patients with diabetic nephropathy may not arterialize their accesses as well as patients without diabetic nephropathy (Figure 48-1).

Radial-Cephalic

Direct autogenous radial artery-cephalic vein fistula was first described in 1966.[36] This access has also been called the *Cimino fistula* or the *wrist fistula*. Different configurations of anastomosis have been employed with varying results as far as development of a steal phenomenon or speed of maturation,[37] although the cephalic vein end-to-side configuration seems to be the most popular. Cephalic veins of less than 1.6 mm in diameter have been associated with early failure[38] (Figures 48-2 and 48-3).

Results of the Cimino fistula have been generally good, with 6-, 12-, and 36-month patency rate of 80%, 71%, and 64%, respectively.[39] In a series, reported factors suspected to have influence on AV fistula included age, BUN, blood pressure at the time of operation, serum cholesterol, and creatinine levels. The 1-year patency rate was 59.8% and 40.8% at 5 years.[40]

Other reports suggest that early failure is considered one of the major determinants affecting the long-term patency, because, after 1 year, the rate of access failure was slow, steady, and near the same regardless of the type of surgery of the fistula.[41]

Our routine practice of creating a fistula technique is as follows:

1. One incision at the wrist between the distal radial artery and cephalic vein under local anesthesia.
2. Between the distal radial artery and the cephalic vein.
3. Divide the distal end of the cephalic vein, after the patient is heparinized.
4. Bring the end of the cephalic vein to the site of the radial artery in an end-to-side fashion with an arteriotomy of 5 to 8 mm in length.
5. With the radial artery cross-clamped proximally after the arteriotomy is made, release the distal clamp of the radial artery. If pulsatile backflow is observed, we then ligate the radial artery distal to the end-to-side anastomosis. This pulsatile flow indicates complete palmar arcade.

By doing these techniques, we are able to improve on the following important points:

1. Maturation is fast.
2. Minimize early thrombosis because of flow-related problems.

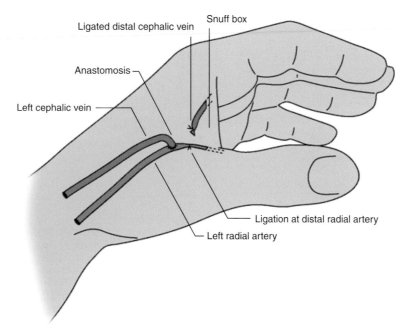

● **FIGURE 48-1.** A snuffbox AV fistula. A small vertical incision is made on the snuffbox at the area of the pulsating distal radial artery. The distal cephalic vein is dissected and ligated. The distal end of the cephalic vein is brought to the side of the radial artery. An end-to-side anastomosis is made using 7.0 Prolene sutures. If the patient has a good pulsatile back flow from the distal radial artery, with the proximal being cross-clamped, indicating complete palmar arcade, the distal radial artery, distal to the anastomosis can be ligated in order to convert from anatomic end-to-side anastomosis to functional end-to-end anastomosis.

3. Minimize distal venous hypertension if you want to construct side-to-side anastomosis.
4. Minimize distal ischemic change because of reversal of the flow from the distal radial artery into the vein at the later stage when the venous system becomes enlarged.

● **BRACHIAL–CEPHALIC ACCESS**

Anastomosis of the antecubital veins with the brachial artery can be accomplished with good results. Despite favorable results, the fistula has a higher incidence of steal, especially with long donor arteriotomies. In one study, the antecubital vein fistula had a primary patency rate of 80% at a medium follow-up of 36 months, compared with 66% of brachial–cephalic fistulae at 24 months.[42] This study suggests that the brachial–cephalic fistula was a favorable alternative in elderly patients, women, and diabetic patients. In another study, 74% 1-year patency rate was accomplished.[43]

● **BASILIC VEIN TRANSPOSITION**

Brachial–Radial at Forearm

Hakaim et al.[44] showed superior patency and maturation rates of primary brachial–basilic vein with transposition, compared with 78% and 79% for brachial–basilic and transposed brachial–basilic access.

Brachial–Basilic at Upper Arm

This procedure was first described in 1976.[45] The procedure involved mobilization, distal division, and superficial tunneling and transposition of the basilic vein with distal end-to-side anastomosis with the brachial artery. The technical alternatives and modification include elevating the basilic vein rather than rerouting it[46] or superficializing the basilic vein as part of a staged procedure.[47] Others employed endoscopic techniques as a means of reducing the incision length.[48]

In a large study, the long-term follow-up for patients having undergone the procedure were, 1-year patency of 84%, 73% at 3 and 5 years, and 52% at 10 years.[49] Also, less favorable results were reported in other studies.[50]

● **LOWER EXTREMITY AA**

In a rare incidence, lower extremity AA can be done. This technique involved dissection and mobilization of the entire superficial femoral vein, with transposition into a superficial position in the thigh, and end-to-side anastomosis.[51] In a retrospective analysis of 25 patients for more than 2 years, cumulative patency was 78% and 73% for 6 and 12 months follow-up. Steal syndrome necessitated further intervention in 40%, and of those, 80% required another procedure to treat steal. Major wound complications affected 28%, and one patient required above-knee amputation after developing a compartment syndrome. Therefore,

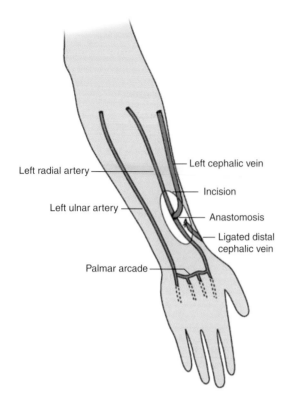

● **FIGURE 48-2.** Primary AVF. A small vertical incision is made on the radial aspect of the wrist on the nondominant hand if at all possible. Preoperative cephalic vein map of the area with a duplex scan may help in evaluation of the quality of the cephalic vein. After dissection of the distal cephalic vein, distal end is ligated. The distal end of the proximal cephalic vein is brought to the radial artery, which can be dissected out through the same incision. End-to-side anastomosis is made between the distal ends of the cephalic vein to the side of the radial artery using 7.0 prolene sutures. At the time of arterial anastomosis, the palmar arcade can be checked by confirming pulsatile back flow from the distal radial artery with proximal radial artery being cross-clamped. If the patient has complete palmar arcade with pulsatile back flow the radial artery distal to the anastomosis can be ligated. In this way, the patient has an anatomical end-to-side anastomosis with a functional end-to-end anastomosis.

it has been suggested not to undertake this technique without serious evaluation, such as good-risk patients who have no other possible sites for fistula creation.

● **PROSTHETIC ACCESS**

There are currently 2 major manufacturers of expanded polytetrafluoroethylene (PTFE) for use in hemodialysis access; Gore-Tex (W. L. Gore & Associates, Flagstaff, AZ) and Impra (Impra, Inc., Tempe, AZ). Although manufacturer claim that each of these are having distinct patency and cost advantages over the other, this has not been borne out comparative investigations of either product.[52,53]

Stenosis of the venous outflow, generally as a result of neointimal hyperplasia, remains the sentinel cause of graft failure, accounting for approximately 80% of graft failure.[54] Measurement of the outflow tract have been correlated

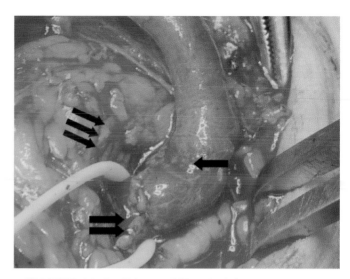

● **FIGURE 48-3.** Primary AVF at the left wrist. An anastomic end vein, topside arterial anastomosis. This can then be converted to a function end-do-side anastomosis by ligating the clipping with wet clips of the radial artery, distal to the anastomosis. This can be done if the patient has pulsatile back flow at the radiotomy with proximal cross-clamp indicating an intact palmar arcade. A distal cephalic vein indicated by *one arrow*; distal radial artery, distal to the anastomosis is indicated by *two arrows*; and the proximal radial artery, proximal to the anastomosis is indicated by *three arrows*.

with graft patency: lesions that account for less than 30% stenosis were associated with a less than 30% thrombosis rate at 6 months, whereas lesions that accounted for greater than 50% of the outflow were associated with an almost 100% failure rate at 6 months.[55] As a result of the association of turbulent flow at the anastomosis with the formation of neointimal hyperplasia,[56,57] investigators designed expanded PTFE grafts that incorporated a cuffed geometry of the venous anastomosis site, a design that had shown bench utility in minimizing shear stress.[58] This configuration was studied prospectively in 48 patients, although overall primary patency was not affected, secondary patency was increased from 32% to 64% at 12 months.[59]

There are many varieties of prosthetic angio access graft procedures.

Forearm, Loop (U-Shaped)

Technique. A small transverse incision is made on the upper portion of the forearm, approximately 2 fingerbreadths distal to the antecubital vein. The superficial vein and antecubital vein are isolated. Depending upon the condition of the antecubital vein, sometimes one has to use the basilic portion or a separate portion proximally, or at the antecubital vein. Using the same incision, the brachial artery is isolated. Then a subcutaneous tunnel is made distally to the distal forearm near the wrist curving back to the antecubital incision in a U-shape. Small counted incisions at the distal forearm are made to facilitate the tunnelling procedure with the ease of bringing the graft into the tunnel. After appropriate heparinization, we normally make an end-to-side

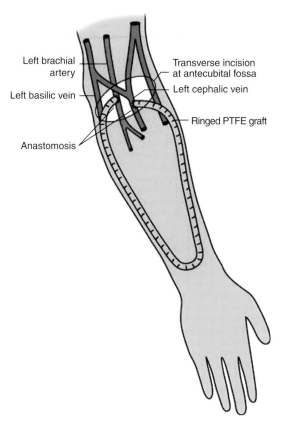

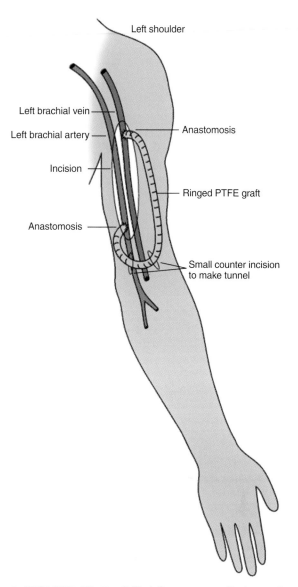

● **FIGURE 48-4.** Forearm loop AVG. A transverse incision is made on the proximal portion of the forearm, slightly distal to the elbow joint. The brachial artery and antecubital vein is freed. If the quality of the antecubital vein at the same incision is good, then the vein can be used. The brachial artery is freed through the same incision. An end-to-side anastomosis is made between the ends of a 6-mm PTFE graft and to the side of the antecubital vein using 6.0 or 7.0 PTFE sutures. Then a subcutaneous tunnel is made in a U-shape, making a 2-count incision distally to facilitate the curvature of the tunnel. The graft is passed through the tunnel back to the antecubital incision. The other end of the PTFE graft is then anastomosed to the side of the brachial artery using 6.0 or 7.0 PTFE sutures.

anastomosis on the venous side first, using either 6.0 or 7.0 PTFE sutures. The graft is then passed through the tunnel into the antecubital incision. At this point, an arterial anastomosis is made in an end-to-side fashion. Following the completion of the procedure, we either neutralize the heparin or leave the heparin on board with careful hemostasis (Figure 48-4).

Forearm, Straight Graft

Using the brachial artery or the radial artery and the antecubital vein or distal cephalic vein, the graft is placed in the subcutaneous tunnel.

Upper Arm, Loop (C-Shaped)

In patients who had failed or nonaccessible forearm angio access with a graft, we use the upper arm. A longitudinal small incision is made on the inner aspect of the upper arm

● **FIGURE 48-5.** AVG, left upper arm, C-shape. A vertical incision is made on the medial aspect of the upper thigh at the area of the brachial artery. Through the same incision, the brachial artery and vena comitantes (brachial vein) is freed. An end-to-side anastomosis is made between the side of the vein and the end of the PTFE graft using 6.0 or 7.0 PTFE sutures. The graft is passed through a tunnel which is made in a C-shape, using a small count incision. After the graft is passed through the tunnel, the other end of the graft is anastomosed with the brachial artery in an end-to-side fashion using PTFE sutures.

to expose the brachial artery and vein. From that incision, a tunnel is made curving down distally, laterally then upwardly on the lateral aspect of the upper arm, then curving medially and downward into the incision. Following heparinization, end-to-side anastomosis is made between the PTFE graft and the vein. The graft is then passed through the tunnel distally, laterally, upwardly, and then medially into the incision. The other end of the PTFE graft is anastomosed to the arterial side in an end-to-side fashion. The reason for this type of anastomosis is to make thrombectomy

● **FIGURE 48-6.** A loop AVG using axillary artery and ipsilateral axillary vein. An anastomosis is made through a single transverse incision in the left anterior chest wall below the clavicle. Through the same incision, the axillary vein can be freed. Following venous anastomosis, the graft is tunneled subcutaneously down the distal end of the upper arm, then curving back to the shoulder in a loop-shape. The other end of the PTFE is anastomosed to the axillary artery.

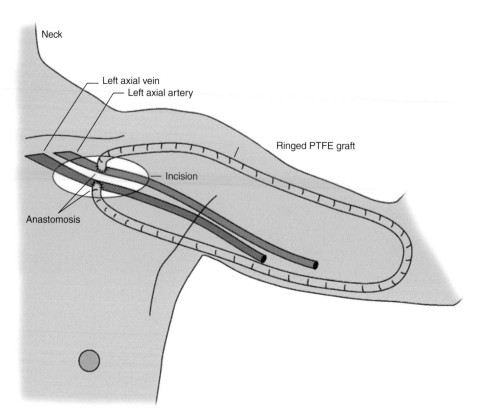

easy at a later date. Following the completion of the procedure, the heparin is either neutralized or left on board without neutralization (Figure 48-5).

Axillary Artery-Ipsilateral Axillary Vein, U-Shaped (or C-Shaped)

This technique is utilized on the patient who has exhausted the site at the ipsilateral forearm and upper arm, by making a small transposition on the ipsilateral anterior chest wall, approximately 2 fingerbreadths below the clavicle and parallel to the clavicle. The pectoris major muscle is split along the direction of the muscle fiber. The pectoris minor muscle is retracted laterally. The axillary artery and vein are freed and isolated. Using either a U-shape or C-shape, a tunnel is made on the ipsilateral shoulder and chest wall, to create an arterial-venous graft (Figure 48-6).

Axillary Artery-Contralateral Axillary Vein Access (U- or C-Shaped)

This is an alternative choice when the ipsilateral vein or artery is not suitable for the same side, the artery and veins were isolated from two separate incisions in the chest wall (Figure 48-7).

Femoral Artery-Greater Saphenous Vein Graft (U-Shaped)

The superficial femoral artery is exposed through a vertical incision. Through the same incision, the proximal greater saphenous vein is freed. Using a subcutaneous tunnel created distally in a U-shape, an anastomosis can be made on the vein side then to the other side (Figure 48-8).

Femoral Artery-Femoral Vein (U-Shaped)

Incisions made in a vertical fashion on the upper portion of the body, the superficial artery and vein are isolated, using a subcutaneous tunnel in U-shape.

There is much other variety of choices, which can be made (Figure 48-9).

● COMPLICATION AND MANAGEMENT

Acute Thrombosis

The patency of hemodialysis access grafts is compromised primarily by areas of intimal fibromuscular hyperplasia in perivenous fibrosis that develops in response to turbulence and shear stress. The events affect the venous outflow, primarily at the graft-to-vein anastomosis.[60-62] Numerous studies have demonstrated the effectiveness of balloon angioplasty, but this procedure is associated with a high rate of recurrent loss of patency. As a result of this, acute thrombosis occurs. The three main principles in the management of acutely thrombosed grafts are complete thrombus removal, total graft imaging, and identification and correction of all significant stenoses. We prefer open or percutaneous thrombectomy. In the case of open thrombectomy, in order to achieve complete thrombectomy, we make a transverse incision over the suitable site

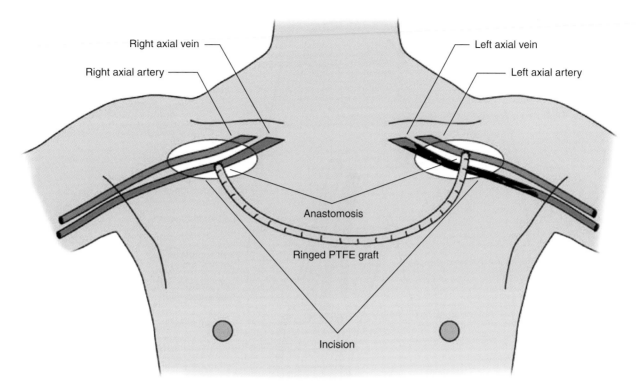

● **FIGURE 48-7.** AVG, using axillary artery and contralateral axillary vein. In a situation where the ipsilateral vein or artery is not sufficient because of the prior surgery or other problems, then the artery and vein can be used in either side. In this drawing, a transverse incision is made on the right anterior chest wall, 2 fingerbreadths below the clavicle and parallel to the clavicle. The axillary vein is then freed. With a similar technique, an incision is made on the left anterior chest wall, and the contralateral axillary artery is freed. An end-to-side anastomosis is first made to the vein, then a gentle U-shape subcutaneous tunnel is made over the sternum, and graft is then passed through the tunnel to the contralateral axillary artery for anastomosis.

of the graft and make a transverse incision at the graft using No. 3 and No. 4 Fogarty catheters. Following complete thrombectomy, an on-table angiogram should be performed to identify any underlying stenoses. If this is identified, this is corrected either by balloon angioplasty or stent, or open revision. If the venous anastomosis site is not salvageable with this technique, then we extend the graft further to the proximal suitable vein site.

After angioplasty, the 6-month primary patency rate is only 31% to 64%.[62–65] The outcomes are further adversely affected by preexisting graft thrombosis,[66,67] and repeated treatments.[62] Angioplasty is also jeopardized by elastic recoil and venous rupture.

In view of these restrictions, investigators have primarily studied the Wallstent, as first reported more than 15 years ago.[68] Various indications for stent use have been studied; including elastic recoil/dissection after angioplasty,[69–74] rapid recurrences after PTA,[75,76] venous rupture after PTA,[77,78] and prophylaxis against recurrent stenosis.[79–81]

Nitinol stents are gaining greater acceptance in their application in other anatomic regions, especially the carotid and superficial femoral arteries. A retrospective study showed 6-month primary access patency rates of 51% in patients treated with the nitinol SMART (shape memory alloy recoverable technology) stent (Cordis, Miami Lakes, FL).[82] Further application of this SMART stent have been reported better patency rates than PTA alone.[83]

Aneurysms (Pseudoaneurysms)

1. At the graft
2. At the vein
3. At the artery

(Figures 48-10 to 48-14).

Pseudoaneurysms are associated with an increase risk of graft thrombosis, pain, cosmetic problems, infection, bleeding, and difficulty accessing the graft.[84]

Pseudoaneurysms formation in PTFE AV grafts is relatively uncommon, but well documented, occurring in 2% to 10% of grafts.[85] Management of pseudoaneurysms of the graft is by segmental resection and bypassing the graft with a newer graft.

Several series have been reported repairing pseudoaneurysms by using covered stents.[84,86] The pseudoaneurysm at the arterial anastomosis can be repaired surgically. A pseudoaneurysm at the venous anastomosis or venous system can be repaired surgically, and in some instances with a covered stent.

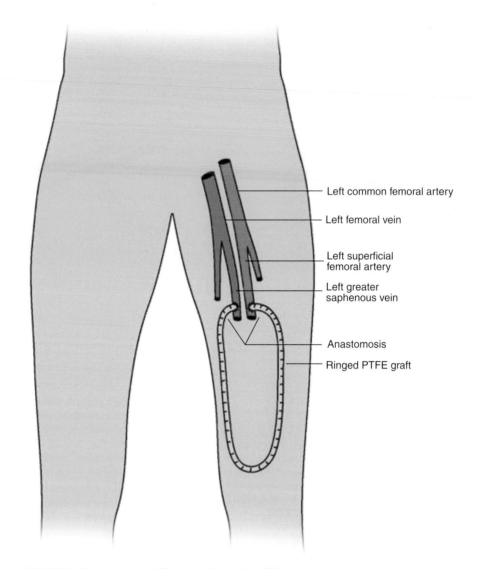

● **FIGURE 48-8.** Loop AVG at the thigh using SFA and proximal greater saphenous vein or SFV. A small vertical incision is made on the medial aspect of the upper thigh. Either the proximal greater saphenous vein or SFV can be freed although the same incision as the SFA. A loop-type of tunnel is made distally back to the groin incision. An end-to-side anastomosis is made between the vein and graft. The graft is then placed through the tunnel back to the groin incision. The other end of the graft is anastomosed to the SFA.

Stenosis

Stenosis at the venous anastomosis can be treated surgically or with PTA and stent procedure as described above in the management of acute thrombosis. Stenosis at the arterial anastomosis can be treated by angioplasty, if not feasible with angioplasty, it may require surgical repair.

Infection

Infection is common in prosthetic hemodialysis access but is also seen in autogenous venous access.[87] Infection is the second leading cause for access loss and can cause significant morbidity or even mortality. Infectious complications of all types are the second leading cause of death in dialysis patients, accounting for 15% to 36%.[88–91] Impaired humoral

and cellular immunity, nutritional deficiencies, and type of VA are thought to be among the major determinants.[92] The severity of infection can be graded as follows[93]:

Grade 0: None
Grade 1: Resolved with antibiotic treatment
Grade 2: Loss of AV access because of ligation, removal of bypass
Grade 3: Loss of limb

The bacteriology of hemodialysis-related infections shows a predominance of gram-positive organisms, with *Staphylococcus aureus* being he most common isolate. Gram-negative organisms account for roughly another 25%, and a smaller percentage are polymicrobial.[94,95] Two reports exist of infection with *Clostridium perfringens.*[96,97]

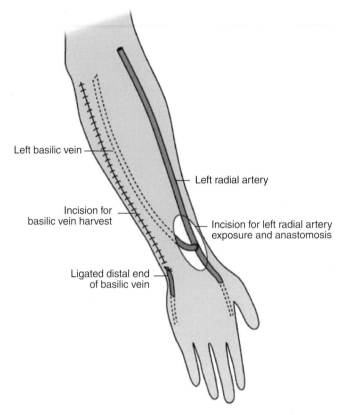

● **FIGURE 48-9.** Basilic vein transposition. A longitudinal incision is made over the course of the basilic vein, which can be started and mapped preoperatively using a duplex scan. The basilic vein is then transposed subcutaneously to the side of the radial artery, which can be exposed through a small vertical incision on the radial aspect of the wrist. An end-to-side anastomosis is made between the distal end of the basilic vein and the side of the radial artery using 7.0 Prolene sutures. If the patient has a good pulsatile back flow with the proximal radial artery being cross-clamped, indicating intact palmar arcade, the radial artery distal to the anastomosis can be ligated to convert from anatomic end-to-side anastomosis to functional end-to-end anastomosis.

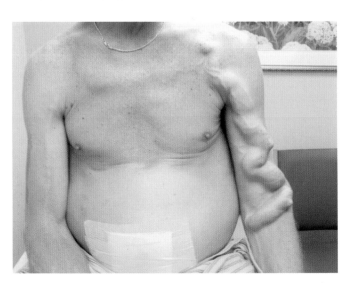

● **FIGURE 48-10.** Aneurysmal degradation of left cephalic vein system. A huge aneurysmal degradation of the left cephalic vein system after primary AVS.

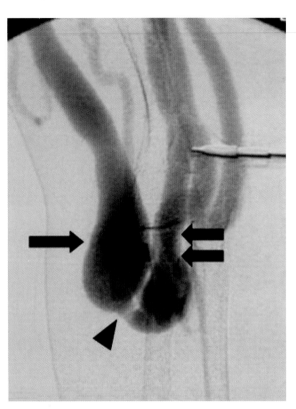

● **FIGURE 48-11.** Angiogram of aneurysmal dilatation of the cephalic vein. An angiogram showing an aneurysmal dilatation of the cephalic vein (*arrow*), and dilatation of the brachial artery (*two arrows*), with no distal flow beyond the anastomosis (*triangle*), indicating steal.

Steal

Steal after an AV access was first described in 1969 following Bescia-Cimino hemodialysis access.[98] It has been documented in 73% of autogenous AV access and 91% PA had a form of steal. Despite the frequency of demonstrable alterations in flow, a symptomatic steal syndrome is much less common. After proper diagnostic evaluation on symptomatic steal, treatment options are as follows[99]:

1. Banding or reducing the flow.
2. Ligation.
3. Extending the graft further to increase overall resistance.

Banding with suture plication of a proximal portion of the access and monitoring the first option.[100] Others obtained similar results using a band around the access and tightening it until the desired result is achieved.[101] The banding procedure involves narrowing the lumen of the conduit more than 1 cm or more rather than simple suture stenosis. Making the band wider is the thought to allow more accurate adjustments in flow with possibly less turbulent flow, and minimize acute thrombosis.

Venous Hypertension

Venous hypertension manifested by minimal arm swelling is quite common in hemodialysis patients with upper

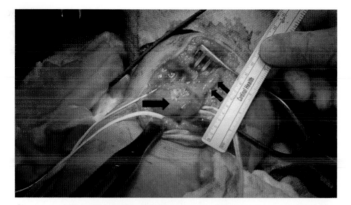

A

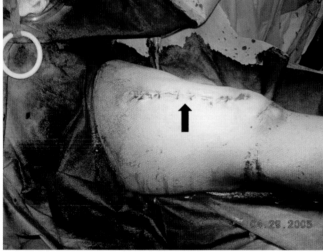

C

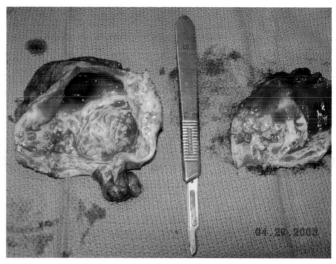

B

● **FIGURE 48-12.** (A) Large aneurysm. This is an operative picture showing a large aneurysm at the vein distal to the anastomosis (*one arrow*); and the proximal brachial artery proximal to the anastomosis (*two arrows*). (B) Large-sized aneurysm. This figure is a gross specimen, showing the large size of the aneurysm of Figure 12A. (C) Skin following aneurysm repair. This figure is following the aneurysm repair with the skin incision closed (*arrow*).

extremity access. The reporting standard document recommends the severity from Grade 0 to 3, as follows:

Grade 0: None
Grade 1: Mild (minimal symptoms, discoloration, minimal extremity swelling)—no treatment needed

Grade 2: Moderate (intermittent discomfort, severe swelling)—intervention usually needed
Grade 3: Severe (persistent discomfort with hyperpigmentation, persistent swelling, severe or massive, venous ulceration)—intervention mandatory

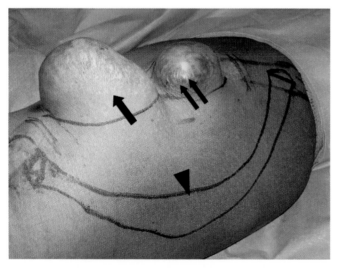

● **FIGURE 48-13.** Multiple large graft aneurysms. This figure shows a patient with multiple large graft aneurysms (*one and two arrows*), which was resected and replaced with a new graft (*triangle*).

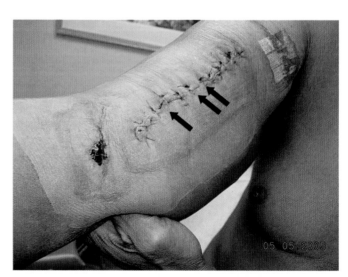

● **FIGURE 48-14.** Repair of multiple large graft aneurysms. This figure shows the patient after completion of aneurysm repair and skin closure at the right upper arm (*arrow*).

A variety of surgical techniques have been described to alleviate the symptoms from the central venous obstruction. The first venous reconstruction described for central venous obstruction came in 1976 by Doty and Baker, who described a reconstruction of the inferior vena cava using a spiraled saphenous vein graft.[102] Others have described using a prosthetic graft from subclavian vein to the right atrium. One report even cited the use of the femoral vein as an outflow vessel.[103] Fortunately most patients can be managed by procedures that do not require entering the thoracic cavity or lengthy extra-anatomic bypasses. For lesions of the subclavian medial to the internal jugular vein an autologous internal jugular to internal jugular vein crossover technique has been described.[104] For the more common stenosis seen lateral to the internal jugular, an ipsilateral internal jugular turn-down technique can be used,[105] or we find a technically easier procedure that preserves the internal jugular to be a subclavian-to-ipsilateral internal jugular bypass using 6 mm PTFE. This can be done under local anesthesia and, with a functioning AV access, has had a very satisfactory long-term patency.[106]

Neuropathy

Neuropathy is a common finding among hemodialysis patients. The Reporting Standard document[107] sets out four gradations of severity to describe neuropathy related to hemodialysis access as follows:

Grade 0: No symptoms
Grade 1: Mild, intermittent sensory changes (pain/paresthesia/numbness with sensory deficit)
Grade 2: Moderate, persistent sensory changes

Grade 3: Severe, sensory changes and progressive loss of motor function (movement/strength/muscle wasting)

The major causes of neuropathy in the hemodialysis patient include uremic neuropathy, diabetic neuropathy, mononeuropathies from anatomic compression such as occurs in carpal tunnel syndrome, and the uncommon but important ischemic monomanic neuropathy (IMN) that can occur acutely after access creation. Hand pain and numbness are not uncommon with long-standing dialysis fistulae or shunts.[108] It is seen in 50% to 70% of patients on long-term hemodialysis.[109,110] Several studies have demonstrated that initiation of dialysis tends to improve but not necessarily eliminate the symptoms over time. The nerve conduction velocities tend to stabilize but not improve.[109-113] Worsening of the symptoms over time is an indication of inadequate dialysis.

Carpal tunnel syndrome occurs with greater frequency in dialysis patients than in the general population.

IMN is a distinctive syndrome of nerve injury resulting from acute vascular compromise in an extremity.[114] The pathogenesis of IMN is likely related to preexisting marginal distal tissue perfusion in some diabetic patients. The additional flow requirements imposed by a proximal shunt cannot be compensated, leading to ischemia of the nerves. The ischemia is transient or insufficient to cause muscle or skin necrosis but results in severe ischemic nerve injury.

Because IMN represents a form of steal, treatment of the syndrome must include either ligation of the access or correction of the steal physiology. Even with early access closure, paralysis and pain may be permanent or only partially reversible.[115-118]

REFERENCES

1. Eknoyan G, Levin NW, Schwab S, et al. NKF-DOQI clinical practice guidelines for vascular access. *Am J Kid Dis.* 1997; 30:S148-S191.

2. NKF-K/DOQI. Clinical practice guidelines for vascular access: update 2000. *Am J Kid Dis.* 2001;37:S137-S181.

3. Chazan JA, London MR, Pono LM. Long-term survival of vascular accesses in a large chronic hemodialysis population. *Nephron.* 1995;69:228-233.

4. Feldman HI, Held PJ, Hutchinson JT, et al. Hemodialysis vascular access morbidity in the United States. *Kidney Int.* 1993;43:1091-1096.

5. United States Renal Data System (USRDS) Coordinating Center, National Institute of Diabetes and Digestive and Kidney Disease (NIDDK). 2002 ADR Atlas, table K-4, 532. http://www.usrds.org.

6. Fullerton JK, McLafferty RB, Ramsey DE, et al. Pitfalls in achieving the dialysis outcome quality initiative guidelines for hemodialysis access? *Ann Vasc Surg.* 2002;16:613-617.

7. Quinton WE, Dillard DH, Scribner BH. Cannulation of blood vessels for prolonged hemodialysis. *Trans Am Soc Artif Intern Organs.* 1960;6:104-113.

8. Brescia MJ, Cimino JE, Appel K, et al. Chronic hemodialysis using venipuncture and a surgically created arteriovenous fistula. *N Engl J Med.* 1996;275:1089-1092.

9. Flores-Izquierdo G, Vivero RR, Exaire E, et al. Autoinjerto venoso para hemodialysis. *Arch Inst Cardiol Mex.* 1969; 39:255-266.

10. Dunn I, Frumkin E, Forte R, et al. Dacron velour vascular prosthesis for hemodialysis. *Proc Clin Dial Transplant Forum.* 1972;2:85.

11. Baker LD, Johnson JM, Goldfarb D. Expanded polytetrafluoroethylene (PTFE) subcutaneous arteriovenous conduit: an improved vascular access for chronic hemodialysis. *Trans Soc Artif Intern Organs.* 1976;22:382-387.

12. Rodriguez JA, Armadans L, Ferrer E, et al. The function of permanent vascular access. *Nephrol Dial Transplant.* 2000; 15:402-408.

13. Fan PY, Schawab SJ. Vascular access: concepts for the 1990s. *J Am Soc Nephrol.* 1992;3:1-11.

14. Himmelfarb J, Saad T. Hemodialysis vascular access: emerging concepts. *Curr Opin Nephrol Hypertens.* 1996;5:485-491.

15. Hakim R, Himmelfarb J. Hemodialysis access failure: a call to action. *Kidney Int.* 1998;54:1029-1040.

16. Almeida E, Dias L, Teixeira F, et al. Survival in hemodialysis: is there a role for vascular access? *Nephrol Dial Transplant.* 1997;12:852.

17. Feldman HL, Kobin S, Wasserstein A. Hemodialysis vascular access morbidity. *J Am Soc Nephrol.* 1996;7:523-535.

18. Kinnaert P, Vereerstraeten P, Taussaint C, et al. Nine years' experience with internal arteriovenous fistulas for hemodialysis: a study of some factors influencing the results. *Br J Surg.* 1977;64:242-246.

19. Reilly DT, Wood RFM, Bell PRF. Prospective study of dialysis fistulas: problem patients and their treatment. *Br J Surg.* 1982;69:549-553.

20. Windus DW. Permanent vascular access: a nephrologist's view. *Am J Kidney Dis.* 1993;21:457-471.

21. Winset OE, Wolmn FJ. Complications of vascular access for hemodialysis. *South Med J.* 1985;66:23-28.

22. Bender MH, Bruininckx CM, Gerlag PG. The brachial cephalic elbow fistula: a useful alternative angioaccess for hemodialysis. *J Vasc Surg.* 1994;20:808-813.

23. Kaufmann JL. The decline of autogenous hemodialysis access site. *Semin Dial.* 1995;8:59-61.

24. United States Renal Data System (USRDS). 1998 Annual Data Report. Bethesda, MD: National Institute of Diabetes and Digestive and Kidney Disease (NIDDK); 1998. http://www.usrds.org.

25. Obrador GT, Brian GG, Pereira DM. Early referral to the nephrologist and timely initiation of renal replacement therapy: a paradigm shift in the management of patients with renal failure. *Am J Kidney Dis.* 1998;31:398-417.

26. Bander SJ, Schwab SJ. Central venous angioaccess for hemodialysis and its complications. *Semin Dial.* 1992;5:121-128.

27. Quinton W, Dillar D, Schribner B. Cannulation of blood vessels for prolonged hemodialysis. *Trans Am Soc Artif Intern Organs.* 1960;6:104-113.

28. Kelber J, Delmez JA, Windus DW. Factors affecting delivery of high-efficiency dialysis using temporary vascular access. *Am J Kidney Dis.* 1993;22:24-29.

29. Schwab SJ, Quarles LD, Middleton JP, et al. Hemodialysis-associated subclavian vein stenosis. *Kidney Inst.* 1988;33:1156-1159.

30. Spinowitz BS, Galler M, Golden RA, et al. Subclavian vein stenosis as a complication of subclavian catheterization for hemodialysis. *Arch Intern Med.* 1987;147:305-307.

31. Schwab SJ, Buller GL, McCann RL, et al. Prospective evaluation of a Dacron cuffed hemodialysis catheter for prolonged use. *Am J Kidney Dis.* 1988;11:166-169.

32. Suchoki P, Conlon P, Knelson M, et al. Silastic cuffed catheters for hemodialysis vascular access: thrombolytic and mechanical correction of HD catheters malfunction. *Am J Kidney Dis.* 1996;28:379-386.

33. Kovalik EC, Raymond JR, Albers FA, et al. A clustering of epidural abscesses in chronic hemodialysis patients: risks of salvaging access catheters in cases of infection. *J Am Soc Nephrol.* 1996;7:2264-2267.

34. Wolowczyk L, Williams AJ, Donovan KL, et al. The snuffbox arteriovenous fistula for vascular access. *Eur J Vasc Endovasc Surg.* 2000;19:70-76.

35. Horimi H, Kusano E, Hasegawa T, et al. Clinical experience with an anatomic snuff box arteriovenous fistula in hemodialysis patients. *ASAIO J.* 1996;42:177-180.

36. Brescia M, Cimino J, Appel K, et al. Chronic hemodialysis using venipuncture and a surgically created arteriovenous fistula. *N Engl J Med.* 1966;275:1089-1092.

37. Rutherford R, ed. *Vascular Surgery.* 5th ed. Philadelphia, PA: WB Saunders; 2000.

38. Wong V, Ward R, Taylor J, et al. Factors associated with early failure of arteriovenous fistulae for hemodialysis access. *Euro J Vasc Endovasc Surg.* 1996;12:207-213.

39. Kherlakian GM, Roedersheimer LR, Arbaugh JJ, et al. Comparison of autogenous fistula versus expanded polytetrafluoroethylene graft fistula for angioaccess in hemodialysis. *Am J Surg.* 1986;152:238-243.

40. Cho WH, Kim YS, Kim HC. Factors influencing the patency of arteriovenous fistulae in patients with chronic renal failure. In: Chang JB, ed. *Vascular Surgery.* Vol 6. New York, NY: Springer-Verlag; 1994:577-586.

41. Kim YS, Choo SH, Park K. Arteriovenous fistula for hemodialysis. Early failure or complications according to different criteria for patient selection and surgical procedures. In: Chang JB, ed. *Vascular Surgery.* Vol 6. New York, NY: Springer-Verlag; 1994:587-592.

42. Sparks SR, Vanderlinden JL, Gnanadev DA, et al. Superior patency of perforating antecubital vein arteriovenous fistulae for hemodialysis. *Ann Vasc Surg.* 1997;11:165-167.

43. Revanur VK, Jardine AG, Hamilton DH, et al. Outcome for arteriovenous fistula at the elbow for hemodialysis. *Clin Transplant.* 2000;14:318-322.

44. Hakaim AG, Nalbandian M, Scott T. Superior maturation and patency of primary brachiocephalic and transposed basilic vein arteriovenous fistulae in patients with diabetes. *J Vasc Surg.* 1998;27:154-157.

45. Dagher F, Gelber R, Ramos E, et al. The use of basilic vein and brachial artery as an A-V fistula for long-term hemodialysis. *J Surg Res.* 1976;20:373-376.

46. Davis JN, Howell CG, Humphries AL. Hemodialysis access: elevated basilic vein arteriovenous fistula. *J Pediatr Surg.* 1986;21:1182-1183.

47. Zielinski CM, Mittal SK, Anderson P, et al. Delayed superficialization of brachiobasilic fistula: technique and initial experience. *Arch Surg.* 2001;136:929-932.

48. Hayakawa K, Tsuha M, Aoyagi T, et al. A new method to create arteriovenous fistula in the arm with an endoscopic technique. *J Vasc Surg.* 2002;36:635-638.

49. Humphries AL, Col born GL, Wynn JJ. Elevated basilic vein arteriovenous fistula. *Am J Surg.* 1999;177:489-491.

50. Murphy GJ, White SA, Knight AJ, et al. Long-term results of arteriovenous fistulas suing transposed autologous basilic vein. *Br J Surg.* 2000;87:819-823.

51. Gradman WS, Cohen W, Massoud HA. Arteriovenous fistula construction in the thigh with transposed superficial femoral vein: our initial experience. *J Vasc Surg.* 2001;33:968-975.

52. Hurlbert SN, Mattos MA, Henretta JP, et al. Long-term patency rates, complications and cost-effectiveness of polytetrafluoroethylene (PTFE) grafts for hemodialysis access:

a prospective study that compares Impra versus Gore-tex grafts. *Cardiovasc Surg.* 1998;6:652-656.

53. Kaufman JL, Garb JL, Berman JA, et al. A prospective comparison of two expanded polytetrafluoroethylene grafts for linear forearm hemodialysis access: does the manufacturer matter? *J Am Coll Surg.* 1997;185:74-79.

54. Roberts A, Valji K, Bookstein J, et al. Pulse-spray pharmacomechanical thrombolysis for the treatment of thrombosed dialysis access grafts. *Am J Surg.* 1983;166:221-226.

55. Strauch B, O'Connell R, Geoly K, et al. Forecasting thrombosis of vascular access with Doppler color flow imaging. *Am J Kidney Dis.* 1992;19:554-557.

56. Stehbens W, Karmody A. Venous atherosclerosis associated with arteriovenous fistulas for hemodialysis. *Arch Surg.* 1975;110:176-180.

57. Scholz H, Zanow J, Petzold K, et al. Five years' experience with an arteriovenous patch prosthesis as access for hemodialysis. In: Henry M, ed. *Vascular Access for Hemodialysis IV.* Chicago, IL: Precept Press; 1999:241-254.

58. Escobar FI, Schwartz S, Aboulijoud M, et al. A preliminary study comparing a new "hooded" vs. conventional ePTFE graft in hemodialysis patients. *Proceedings of Vascular Access for Hemodialysis, IV.* Miami, FL, 1998.

59. Sorom A, Hughes CB, McCarthy J, et al. Prospective, randomized evaluation of a cuffed expanded polytetrafluoroethylene graft for hemodialysis vascular access. *Surgery.* 2002;132:135-140.

60. Swedberg SH, Brown BG, Sigley R, et al. Intimal fibromuscular hyperplasia at the venous anastomosis of PTFE grafts in hemodialysis patients. *Circulation.* 1989;80:1726-1736.

61. Saed M, Newman GE, McCann RL, et al. Stenoses in dialysis fistulas: treatment with percutaneous angioplasty. *Radiology.* 1987;164:693-697.

62. Kanterman RY, Vesely TM, Pilgrim TK, et al. Dialysis access grafts: anatomic location of venous stenosis and results of angioplasty. *Radiology.* 1995;195:135-139.

63. Glanz S, Gordon DH, Butt KMH, et al. The role of percutaneous angioplasty in the management of chronic hemodialysis fistulas. *Ann Surg.* 1987;206:777-781.

64. Valji K, Bookstein JJ, Roberts AC, et al. Pharmacomechanical thrombolysis and angioplasty in the management of clotted hemodialysis grafts: early and late clinical results. *Radiology.* 1991;178:243-247.

65. Beathard GA. Percutaneous transluminal angioplasty in the treatment of vascular access stenosis. *Kidney Int.* 1992; 42:1390-1397.

66. Cohen MAH, Kumpe DA, Durham JD, et al. Improved treatment of thrombosed hemodialysis access sites with thrombolysis and angioplasty. *Kidney Int.* 1994;46:1375-1380.

67. Gmelin E, Winterhoff R, Rinast E. Insufficient hemodialysis access fistulas: late results of treatment with percutaneous balloon angioplasty. *Radiology.* 1989;171:657-660.

68. Gunther RW, Vorwerk D, Bohndorf K, et al. Venous stenoses in dialysis shunts: treatment with self-expanding metallic stents. *Radiology.* 1989;170:401-405.

69. Gunther RW, Vorwerk D, Bohndorf K, et al. Follow-up results after stent placement in failing arteriovenous shunts:

a three year experience. *Cardiovasc Intervent Radiol.* 1991; 14:285-289.

70. Patel RI, Peck SH, Cooper SG, et al. Patency of Wallstents placed across the venous anastomosis of hemodialysis grafts after percutaneous recanalization. *Radiology.* 1998;209:365-370.

71. Kolakowski S, Dougherty MJ, Calligaro KD. Salvaging prosthetic dialysis fistulas with stents; forearm grafts vs upper arm grafts. *J Vasc Surg.* 2003;38:719-723.

72. Gray RJ, Horton KM, Dolmatch BL, et al. Use of Wallstents for hemodialysis access-related venous stenoses and occlusions untreatable with balloon angioplasty. *Radiology.* 1995;195:479-484.

73. Vesley TM, Hovsepian DM, Pilgram TK, et al. Upper extremity central venous obstruction in hemodialysis patients: treatment with Wallstents. *Radiology.* 1997;204:343-348.

74. Vorwerk D, Guenther RW, Mann H, et al. Venous stenosis and occlusion in hemodialysis shunts: follow-up results of stent placement in 65 patients. *Radiology.* 1995;195:140-146.

75. Turmel-Rodrigues L, Pengloan J, Blanchier D, et al. Insufficient dialysis shunts: improved long-term patency rates with close hemodynamic monitoring, repeated percutaneous balloon angioplasty, and stent placement. *Radiology.* 1993;187:273-278.

76. Turmel-Rodrigues L, Blanchard D, Pengloan J, et al. Wallstents and Craggstents in hemodialysis grafts and fistulas: results for selective indications. *J Vasc Interv Radiol.* 1997;8:975-982.

77. Raynaud AC, Angel CY, Sapoval MR, et al. Treatment of hemodialysis access rupture during PTA with Wallstent implantation. *J Vasc Interv Radiol.* 1998;9:437-442.

78. Rajan DK, Clark TW. Patency of Wallstents placed at the venous anastomosis of dialysis grafts for salvage of angioplasty-induced rupture. *Cardiovasc Intervent Radiol.* 2003;26:242-245.

79. Hoffer EK, Shahnaz S, Herskowitz MM, et al. Prospective randomized trial of a metallic intravascular stent in hemodialysis graft maintenance. *J Vasc Interv Radiol.* 1997;8:965-973.

80. Mickley V, Gorich J, Rilinger N, et al. Stenting of central venous stenoses in hemodialysis patients: long-term results. *Kidney Int.* 1997;51:277-280.

81. Haage PH, Vorwerk DV, Piroth W, et al. Treatment of hemodialysis-related central venous stenosis or occlusion: results of primary Wallstent placement and follow-up in 50 patients. *Radiology.* 1999;212:175-180.

82. Vogel PM, Parise C. SMART stent for salvage of hemodialysis access grafts. *J Vasc Interv Radiol.* 2004;15:1051-1060.

83. Vogel PM, Parise C. Comparison of SMART stent placement for arteriovenous graft salvage versus successful graft PTA. *J Vasc Interv Radiol.* 2005;16:1619-1626.

84. Ryan JM. Using a covered stent (Wallstent) to treat pseudoaneurysms of dialysis grafts and fistulas. *AJR Am J Radiol.* 2002;180:1067-1071.

85. Najibi S, Bush RL, Terremani TT, et al. Covered stent exclusion of dialysis access pseudoaneurysms. *J Surg Res.* 2002; 106:15-19.

86. Hausegger KA, Tiessenhausen K, Klimpfinger M, et al. Aneurysms of hemodialysis access grafts: treatment with covered stents—a report of three cases. *Cardiovasc Intervent Radiol*. 1998;21:334.

87. NIH, US Renal Data System. *USRDS 1999 Annual Data Report*. Bethesda, MD: National Institutes of Health, National Institute of Diabetes and Digestive and Kidney Diseases; 2002. http://www.usrds.org.

88. Morbidity and Mortality of Dialysis. *NIH Consensus Statement*. Washington, DC: National Institutes of Health; 1993:1-3.

89. Butterly DW, Schwab SJ. Dialysis access infections. *Curr Opin Nephrol Hypertens*. 2000;9:631-635.

90. Maillous LU, Bellucci AG, Wilkes BM, et al. Mortality in dialysis patients: analysis of the causes of death. *Am J Kidney Dis*. 1991;18:236-235.

91. Stevenson KB, Hannah EL, Lowder CA, et al. Epidemiology of hemodialysis vascular access infections from longitudinal infection surveillance data: predicting the impact of NKF-DOQI Clinical Practice Guidelines for Vascular Access. *Am J Kidney Dis*. 2002;359:549-555.

92. Jaar BG, Hermann JA, Furth SL, et al. Septicemia in diabetic hemodialysis patients: comparison on incidence, risk factors, and mortality with non-diabetic hemodialysis patients. *Am J Kidney Dis*. 2000;35:282-292.

93. Adams ED, Sidaway AN. Non thrombotic complications of arteriovenous access for hemodialysis. In: Rutherford RB, ed. *Vascular Surgery*. Vol 2. 6th ed. Philadelphia, PA: Elsevier-Saunders; 2005:1692-1606.

94. Marr KA, Sexton DJ, Conlon PJ, et al. Catheter-related bacteremia and outcome of attempted catheter salvage in patients undergoing hemodialysis. *Ann Intern Med*. 1997;127: 275-280.

95. Saad TF. Bacteremia associated with tunneled, cuff hemodialysis catheters. *Am J Kidney Dis*. 1999;34:1114-1124.

96. Claeys LGY, Matamoros R. Anaerobic cellulitis as the result of *Clostridium perfringens*: a rare cause of vascular access graft infection. *J Vasc Surg*. 2002;35:1287-1288.

97. Oliveras A, Orfila A, Inigo V. *Clostridium perfringens*: an unusual pathogen infecting arteriovenous shunts for dialysis. *Nephron*. 1998;80:479.

98. Storey BG, George CR, Stewart JH, et al. Embolic and ischemic complications after anastomosis of radial artery to cephalic vein. *Surgery*. 1969;66:325-327.

99. West JC, Evans RD, Kelley SE, et al. Arterial insufficiency in hemodialysis access procedures: reconstruction by an interposition PTFE conduit. *Am J Surg*. 1987;153:300-301.

100. Rivers SP, Scher LA, Veith FJ. Correction of steal syndrome secondary to hemodialysis access fistulas: a simplified quantitative technique. *Surgery*. 1992;112:593-597.

101. Mattson WJ. Recognition and treatment of vascular steal secondary to hemodialysis prostheses. *Am J Surg*. 1987;154: 198-201.

102. Doty DB, Baker WH. Bypass of superior vena cava with spiral vein graft. *Ann Thorac Surg*. 1976;22:490-493.

103. Ayarragaray JEF. Surgical treatment of hemodialysis-related central venous stenosis or occlusion: another option to maintain vascular access. *J Vasc Surg*. 2003;37:1043-1046.

104. Hoballah JJ, Eid GM, Nazzal MM, et al. Contralateral internal jugular vein interposition for salvage of a functioning arteriovenous fistula. *Ann Vasc Surg*. 2000;14:679-682.

105. Puskas JD, Gertler JP. Internal jugular to axillary vein bypass for subclavian vein thrombosis in the setting of brachial arteriovenous fistula. *J Vasc Surg*. 1994;19:939-942.

106. Currier CB Jr, Widder S, Ali A, et al. Surgical management of subclavian and axillary vein thrombosis in patients with a functioning arteriovenous fistula. *Surgery*. 1985;100:25-28.

107. Sidaway AN, Gray R, Besarab A, et al. Recommended standards for reports dealing with arteriovenous hemodialysis access. *J Vasc Surg*. 2002;35:603-610.

108. Rutherford RB. The value of noninvasive testing before and after hemodialysis access in the prevention and management of complications. *Semin Vasc Surg*. 1997;10:157-161.

109. Pirzada NA, Morgenlander JC. Peripheral neuropathy in patients with chronic renal failure: a treatable source of discomfort and disability. *Postgrad Med*. 1997;102:249-261.

110. Burn DJ, Bates D. Neurology and the kidney. *J Neurol Neurosurg Psychiatry*. 1998;65:810-821.

111. Ogura T, Makinodan A, Kubo T, et al. Electrophysiological course of uremic neuropathy in hemodialysis patients. *Postgrad Med J*. 2001;77:451-454.

112. Nielson VK. The peripheral nerve function in chronic renal failure: VIII. Longitudinal course during terminal renal failure and regular hemodialysis. *Acta Med Scand*. 1974;195: 155-162.

113. Bolton CF, Lindsay RM, Linton AL. The course of uremic neuropathy during chronic hemodialysis. *Can J Neurol Sci*. 1975;2:332-333.

114. Kaku DA, Malamut RI, Frey DJ, et al. Conduction block as an early sign of reversible injury in ischemic monomelic neuropathy. *Neurology*. 1993;43:1126-1130.

115. Hye RJ, Wolf YG. Ischemic monomelic neuropathy: an unrecognized complication of hemodialysis access. *Ann Vasc Surg*. 1994;8:578-582.

116. Wytrzes L, Markley HG, Fisher M, et al. Brachial neuropathy after brachial artery-antecubital vein shunts for chronic hemodialysis. *Neurology*. 1987;37:1398-1400.

117. Miles AM. Vascular steal syndrome and ischemic monomelic neuropathy: two variants of upper limb ischemia after hemodialysis vascular access surgery. *Nephrol Dial Transplant*. 1999;14:297-300.

118. Redfern AB, Zimmerman NB. Neurologic and ischemic complications of upper extremity vascular access for dialysis. *J Hand Surg*. 1995;20A:199-204.

chapter 49

Vascular Trauma

Brian J. Daley, MD / J. Fernando Aycinena, MD / Ali F. Mallat, MD / Dana A. Taylor, MD

The world of surgery is constantly changing as new and novel technologies are applied to diagnosis and treatment modalities. Over just the last few years, vascular surgery has seen a major paradigm shift following the endovascular explosion and the minimally invasive trends established in general surgery and gynecology. The reductions in surgical stress, shortened lengths of stay and of convalescence, and equivalent or improved outcomes have made endovascular operations and minimally invasive surgery a standard of care.

Minimally invasive vascular surgery, however, poses even a new set of anatomic and physiologic hurdles beyond even the technical challenges of endovascular surgery. Dealing with not only the injury or disease itself, minimally invasive vascular techniques must be technically sound as to avoid loss of vascular control, sufficiently brief so as to avoid interruption of tissue oxygenation and immediately safe from the devastating vascular complications possible such as embolism or thrombosis.

It is likely that endovascular techniques will replace open surgical techniques (if they have not already replaced) because of the benefits of the minimally invasive approach. Over the next few years, the practice of vascular trauma will likely bear this out and not the scientific outcome parameters. The problem is that the therapeutic interventions are changing at a rapid pace, the surgeons are becoming more facile with the techniques, and the endovascular equipment arena is constantly changing.

The final chapter is unlikely to be written for some time, and in trauma, as always, will never be validated by strict evidence-based medicine. Also looming on the horizon for vascular disease is the possibility of avoiding surgery altogether with gene manipulation. Unfortunately, this modality is unlikely to be temporally adequate to deal with the topic of this chapter, and there will always be a need for immediate vascular intervention in trauma, yet the reconstructions may be manipulated postrepair to assure patency.

● HISTORY

Experience with vascular injuries predates any recorded history as our species developed from not only the gatherers but also the hunters. Understanding vascular anatomy for a quick and successful kill is still passed on orally in non-Western and nonliterate cultures. Understanding vascular anatomy is essentially for appropriate dressing of the carcass and understanding vascular anatomy for the harvesting of blood as a renewable food resource in some cultures is necessary. Lastly, the reality of war has driven the knowledge of vascular anatomy not only for killing one's opponent but also for the salvage of the injured combatant.

The first medical discussions of vascular injury are found in the Edwin Smith Papyrus from approximately 3000 BC. Galen may be the best resource for his descriptions of arterial and venous injuries in the wounds seen by the gladiators. He advises ligature for arterial injuries and styptic for venous wounds. Galen and his remaining theories remained in practice through the Dark Ages, when surgical care was left to the barbers and other tradesman. Through the Napoleonic Age and into the 19th century, vascular surgery was comprised solely of amputation as no other therapy existed. Suffice it to say, any large vessel vascular injury was fatal, and only peripheral extremity injuries would be the vascular trauma that survived to the surgeon's table. One needs to bear in mind this was the same therapy for open fractures or large soft tissue injury as well. Arteriovenous fistulas (AVFs), which were the sequelae of survivable injuries, were frequent and surgical treatment constituted the literature of this age.

Despite the case reports of Carrel and Hunter, the application of vascular reconstruction for injuries would wait until late in the 20th century. During the Civil War, *The Practice of Surgery* by Samuel Cooper[1] (the text of choice for the South) and Samuel D. Gross's *A Manual of Military Surgery*[2] (North) both elaborate immediate amputation of any extremity injury with ligation of the artery and often the vein to avoid hemorrhage, gangrene and/or sepsis, and death. The exhaustive reports during World War I by Makins[3] and World War II by DeBakey and Simeone[4] are unfortunate testimonials of logistics and the lack of standard techniques resulting in virtually the same outcomes. Control of life-threatening bleeding and avoiding gangrene and sepsis took preference over limb salvage, exactly the same as the last 2000 years.

Despite the capability of arterial suturing for direct injury, the key problem in trauma during this time period remained finding a suitable vascular replacement. During the Korean War and through today's latest conflicts, vascular grafts from autogenous vein have been used with documented limb salvage.[5–7] Unfortunately, the scourge of interpersonal violence in American cities has had probably more to do with shaping current techniques and therapies for vascular trauma than mankind's long military experience.[8]

The are no subtle differences in the comparisons of military versus civilian vascular trauma—types of weapons, projectile velocity, transport times, and availability of diagnostic and therapeutic resources are but a few. While the civilian trauma systems may have had their basis in the military, modern vascular treatments are primarily based on that urban experience. Whereas, the majority of survivable war related injuries involve extremity injuries or wounds with devastating soft-tissue trauma as well, the modern "knife and gun club" presents with far more isolated injuries, with injuries that would not be survivable with prolonged transport or delayed resuscitation and in settings where resources are virtually unlimited.

Lastly, a new classification of vascular injuries must be named. With the burgeoning growth of interventional and endovascular techniques, iatrogenic injuries are increasing in frequency. This is not new,[9,10] but now only we see more with the rapidly expanding volume in the diagnostic and therapeutic setting. Also, we see the subsequent need for secondary interventions as medical care improves and allows patients to live longer and with severe disease.[11] While many of these injuries are related to the treatment for vascular disease, others are for diagnosis, monitoring, or nonvascular disease therapies and performed by practioners without vascular surgical skills.

● CURRENT ISSUES

Three key issues in the management of the trauma patient suffering vascular injury have come to light recently. We seem to be capable of learning from our past and the laboratory and carrying this to the bedside with improved outcomes. The first is the concept of directed resuscitation—fashioned and now carried down to basic physiologic principles. The second is the concept of the damage control procedure. Short abbreviated interventions reduce the second hit of surgical intervention, and allow restoration of normal physiology between stresses. Lastly, there is a rebirth of delayed repair—temporizing often with "damage

control" until definitive intervention is possible—a concept that most often seen with blunt aortic injury (BAI), but applicable to virtually any injury or anatomic region.

The standard resuscitation model was challenged by many researchers seeking to reduce the purely iatrogenic problems of Adult Respiratory Distress Syndrome seen after aggressive resuscitation. Shock is inadequate end-organ perfusion. In today's molecular nomenclature, however, this amounts to cellular or even subcellular hypoxia. Resuscitation is the restoration of organ perfusion and the restoration of molecular level oxygenation. Aggressive fluid administration was borne out of the wartime experiences, where the renal failure from hypovolemia in World War II and Korea was traded for ARDS or the Da Nang Lung of Vietnam. The choice of crystalloid, colloids, and/or hypertonic solutions remains the constant and current battlefield for the surgical researchers seeking the Holy Grail of resuscitation.

Bickell et al.[12] challenged resuscitation dogma on a different level and demonstrated that preoperative resuscitation of the trauma patient was not to be guided by rigid protocols, but rather by common sense and simple standard markers. Their study marked a "delay" in resuscitation to avoid overzealous fluid until the bleeding could be surgically stopped with improved outcome. Until the arterial injury/venous injury/bleeding is stopped, it makes little sense to pour fluid and resources to the patient until operation can be performed simply to reach an arbitrary physiologic parameter. Such misdirected resuscitation leads to further bleeding and a loss of endogenous clotting factors.

As documented now, most accepted clinical parameters such as blood pressure and pulse are not good indicators of occult hypoperfusion. Many authors have sought the single marker of adequate resuscitation. In the Eastern Association for the Surgery of Trauma's (EAST) Practice Guideline on the Endpoints of Resuscitation,[13] it is scientifically supported to monitor lactate and/or base deficit and to gauge adequate resuscitation by the correction of this molecular/cellular level acidosis. Once the vascular injury is fixed, salvage depends more on correcting this physiology rather than technical aplomb.[14]

Stemming from both these concepts has been the rebirth of what has been termed "damage control."[15] In order to again reduce overzealous and futile resuscitative efforts, abbreviated procedures are performed in fitting with the patient's physiology. Rather than carrying on in the face of the fatal triad of coagulopathy, hypothermia, and acidosis, the arterial bleeding is stopped, often by ligation, the venous bleeding is controlled by packing and enteric soilage is limited. The operative wound is not formally closed, but temporized for reduction of heat and fluid losses, to allow tissue edema without creating a compartment syndrome, and as a window to the area of concern. Many employ some technique, which is homemade or commercially available, that creates a water-tight, compressive temporary closure with great success. The patient is then returned for resuscitation to restore normal physiology—correct hypothermia,[16] restore clotting capacity and reverse the acidosis. This process can be applied anywhere—the chest, the abdomen, and even the extremities.[17]

Once the patient's physiology has been corrected, the patient is returned for definitive procedures—arterial reconstruction, restoration of bowel continuity, osteosynthesis, or whatever. It should be noted that there is a substantial set of these patients in whom the physiologic derangements will not be corrected and the patient will expire. From our experience, this number is approximately 50%.

Traumatic injury is unlike elective surgery in that the patient has already suffered a major systemic stress, and is now faced with secondary stress from surgery. With the realization that there are such risks to emergent operative repair—i.e., the cure is worse than the disease, delayed repair has not only been applied in extremis, but for the stable patient. The best example of this has been BAI.[18–21]

The diagnosis of BAI is derived mostly from the high index of suspicion of the causative mechanism as well as incidental findings on screening radiographs. The diagnosis is confirmed by aortography, today either direct intra-aortic contrast injection, or from rapid acquisition computed tomography (CT),[22,23] which allows evaluation of other key thoracic anatomy as well.[24–26]

BAI is the result of a rapid acceleration or deceleration, and therefore not exclusive to any particular mechanism or any particular direction of force. The aorta is disrupted usually just distal to the left subclavian artery.[27] The incidence of BAI is greater than seen by the clinician as most victims exsanguinate and die at the scene. The fortunate few in whom the adventitia remains intact enter the emergency department with near normal blood pressures.

Findings that are worrisome on the initial chest radiograph during the initial evaluation are widened mediastinum, the loss of the aortic knob, left apical cap, nasogastric tube deviation, or even large left hemothorax.[28] These nondiagnostic findings should be followed by diagnostic testing, from obtaining an erect chest radiograph to aortography. With the new generation of CT scanners available, contrasted CT of the chest is a rapid, sensitive and specific test to ascertain if BAI or some other injury is present.[29] For many centers, this has replaced aortogram as the diagnostic test of choice and carries with it a sensitivity of 97% to 100%, negative predictive value of 100%, and specificity of 83% to 99%.[23,25]

The second interesting facet of BAI is the timing of repair. The natural history of this injury is rapid exsanguinations once the adventia is disrupted. Formerly, this mandated immediate repair, before this nonsurvivable event occurred. Several anecdotal reports of survivors without repair, of increased mortality in the elderly with trauma and thoracotomy, as well as the blossoming concept of maximizing resuscitation altered the immediate repair plan of care. More recently, with the multiply injured patient, in whom a thoracotomy represents a taxing metabolic and physiologic stress, BAI therapy has been delayed. Resuscitation is guided by correcting the immediate life-threatening in-

juries, restoring perfusion and avoiding hypertension.[23,30] The repair of the stable BAI is turned into an elective procedure and can even be accomplished by endovascular technique to further reduce the surgical insult.[31–35] For open procedures, the debate continues over the use of bypass[36,37]; it remains as an operator-dependent surgical decision based on associated injuries.[38,39]

This concept of reducing or delaying additional surgical stresses after acute injury can be applied not only to life-threatening abdominal or thoracic injury, but to other devastating injuries, such as extremity vascular and/or skeletal injuries, or massive soft tissue injuries. The goal remains to restore normal physiology, and use operation as a means to and not an end of resuscitation.

● DIAGNOSIS

The diagnosis of vascular trauma is generally quite simple—it is based on the clinical manifestations on the physical examination: After the initial assessment, a thorough palpation of all major pulses (radial/ulnar, brachial, dorsalis pedis/posterior tibial, popliteal, femoral, and carotid) is performed as part of the secondary survey. Palpable pulses are sufficient to determine if further testing is needed.[39] A thorough history taking is of paramount importance especially in the aging population as vascular disease may have already altered pulses or present reconstructed anatomy. The expectation should be palpable pulses in all sites. Any alteration in pulses is concern for an injury and should be investigated further, with operation and/or confirmatory testing. The decision making for operative exploration depends mostly on the physiologic state of the patient. If they are hypotensive, and the pathway to resuscitation involves stopping the bleeding from the vascular injury, further diagnostic and therapeutic intervention should occur in the operating room (OR). If the patient is physiologically stable, other modes of diagnosis may be employed.

Louis Pasteur is quoted "in the field of observation, chance favors the prepared mind." The diagnosis of vascular injury also depends on the clinician's index of suspicion. The clinical manifestations are usually dependent on the mechanism, the location, the time since the injury and the overall severity of the injury, yet there are injuries that have no such manifestations, or the manifestations of such injuries are delayed but devastating. A vascular injury may exist with palpable pulses, so the physician must be acutely aware of such circumstances to reliably diagnose occult injury. Not surprisingly, the outcome of these injuries is often excellent.[40]

Blunt trauma patients are more prone to intimal injury and dissection then full thickness transection injury from penetrating trauma. This type of injury usually involves large vessels like thoracic aorta in a deceleration injury or carotid injury from a direct blow where the elasticity of each layer of the vessel reacts differently.[41] Extremity vessels are more commonly involved in penetrating trauma but may also be injured because of the blunt mechanisms such as fractures and/or dislocations. A knee dislocation is especially worrisome for popliteal injury, which may present as the spectrum of vascular injury, from total occlusion to AVFs.[32,42]

Penetrating trauma can present with other clinical manifestations beside pulse alterations, such as external or internal bleeding, pulsatile hematoma, or distal ischemia. The injury may present only as end-organ malperfusion such as altered neurologic states from carotid injury or limb ischemia from superficial femoral artery injuries. On the other hand, other injuries may not cause any clinical signs because of the collaterals such as with the profunda femoris artery. The time of occurrence of the injury should be documented since it directly impacts both the diagnosis and management. The duration of time since injury can dictate the amount of blood loss as well as ischemia time to prevent permanent injury.[44] The correctable defect in the trauma patient is hypoperfusion and stems either from hypovolemia or impairment of cardiac function. All trauma patients should be treated as having a vascular injury until the physical examination or further testing rules this out. For vascular injuries, further tailoring of the examination can be done to the location of injury and specific clinical signs. We describe the main points of diagnosis and management based on the location of injury for convenience. Both arterial and/or venous injuries are detailed.

● DIAGNOSTIC ADJUNCTS

Other than the physical examinations, diagnostic adjuncts such as ultrasound and angiography are used to help diagnose vascular injury. Again, the unstable patient with suspected vascular injury needs to be in the operating room. These modalities should be employed only in the stable patient within time constraints for ischemia or potential ischemia. The role of both modalities is changing rapidly as technologic advances are made and now that these same approaches can now offer therapeutic roles as well.

● ULTRASOUND

The use of sound energy to detect and describe blood flow and blood vessels is a fundamental part of vascular diagnosis outside of trauma.[45] It only makes sense that this modality, which is easy, mobile, painless, interpretable by the surgeon and repeatable, would be applied to the trauma victim. The two forms of ultrasound, Doppler flow and B-mode imaging now have been combined within a graphic format of color imaging which makes interpretation intuitive. The details of this modality are covered in depth elsewhere, but the use of ultrasound is playing a larger role in vascular diagnosis. It, however, is limited and has not yet reached "gold standard" applicability for any disease process.[46]

● ANGIOGRAPHY

Angiography has advanced technologically to be an excellent diagnostic tool to a means of therapy with reduced complications.[47] Again the in-depth review of the principle and techniques is described elsewhere. Delineation of the vascular system was formerly accomplished by filling the vessel in question with radio-opaque contrast material and obtaining at the least biplanar radiographs to assess continuity, intimal integrity and anatomy. Today, with advances in technology, contrast angiography can be direct, i.e., with contrast media directly in the vessel, or indirect, i.e., using intrinsic properties of the imaging modality and blood vessels to differentiate the above goals.[48]

Today, digital subtraction angiography offers clear images with lower contrast doses to provide this information with minimal risks of radiation and contrast.[49] Rapid spiral CT with increasing numbers of detectors now offers a similar digital image that is amenable to computer manipulations to give high quality imaging in three dimensions. Today, these multidetector images are encroaching on the gold standards of contrast angiography.

Magnetic resonance angiograms may also be performed with a noniodinated contrast, gadolinium, and without ionizing radiation. Currently, however, these MRAs are not as accurate for lesions, although if the past development of CT is a comparator, MRA imaging quality will also be improved to produce reliable diagnostic images.[50]

● TREATMENT OVERVIEW AND OUTCOME

Vascular injuries are managed by four primary techniques:

1. Observation: Best for nonocclusive injuries found on diagnostic evaluation.
2. Direct repair (arteriorrhaphy/venorrhaphy): Amenable in only roughly 10% of cases.
3. Patch or interposition grafts: The majority of modern repairs.
4. Ligation.

This applies to open, endovascular, and minimally invasive techniques as well, in which only the technical approach is different. The choice of management technique is fluid and depends on the clinical status of the patient, the extremity, and the resources available. Time is perhaps the greatest factor and must be accounted for in every therapeutic plan. Just as our history reminds us, the goal is survival—life over limb. Restoring blood volume, reducing further blood loss and reestablishing flow are the priorities.

Today's outcomes from vascular trauma are marvelous. An overall survival of 93% and limb salvage rate of 98% are quoted.[51] These figures are the product of time, frequency, and location of injury. While even a common but relatively minor injury can be fatal, there are virtually fatal injuries that are fortunately infrequent. The surgeon facing any vascular injury, however, must be ready for even the most devastating of injuries, prolonged presentation, and abnormal physiology and rapidly fashion a plan of care that is based upon these goals.

● HEAD TRAUMA

Blunt

Trauma to the scalp comes from unnamed vessels but with significant blood flow that failure to stop bleeding can cause significant hemorrhage, shock, hypothermia, and disseminated intravascular coagulation (DIC) or even death. Temporal artery injury is usually manifested by active bleeding or expanding hematoma on the side of the head. Nonexpanding hematomas and smaller size hematomas although may occur with temporal artery injury are more frequently associated with venous injury. Bleeding from the scalp may be exacerbated when patient is coagulopathic as a result of the significant blood loss or hypothermia. Control of bleeding is the main treatment and is generally effected by suturing the wound closed and direct pressure. The single named vessel which may bleed is the superficial temporal artery and is treated uniformly with ligation. Evacuation of the hematoma prior to intervention reduces infection and deformity as well as exposes bleeding vessels needing direct ligation or clipping. Since the scalp is heavily vascularized, one should not be concerned about ischemic changes form ligation of these vessels, but one must be sure to debride any nonviable tissue prior to definitive closure.

Vascular injuries to the face are usually ligated with the rich collateral flow available from the branches of the external carotid and jugular system.

Basilar skull fracture can be associated with carotid injury. Basilar skull fracture is a clinical diagnosis and suspected when a patient presents with raccoon eyes, hemotympanum and/or Battle's sign (mastoid contusion). Carotid injury must also be expected after significant force that results in mandibular or Le Fort type fractures.[52] Blunt carotid injury (BCI) can be from a partial occlusion because of a hematoma in the arterial wall, an intimal flap or a local thrombus as well as wall disruption.

Because of the specific course of the internal carotid artery inside a bony compartment, a fixed point is created and again a difference in elasticity or stretch of the arterial walls is possible. Occlusion from external compression or thrombosis after intimal injury is the rule and presents as significant neurologic deficits unexplained by other anatomic injuries.[54,55] Therefore, internal carotid injury at the skull base level is suspected when focal neurologic impairment is identified. After blunt trauma significant carotid disruption is rare and therefore local hemorrhage or expanding hematomas are very rare or rapidly fatal before definitive diagnosis or repair are made.

Controversy exists in the screening regimen for blunt carotid injury. Although quite rare by some accounts (0.5%–0.004% of trauma victims),[54] BCI can have devastatingly poor outcomes.[55] Quite logically, these poor outcomes are reduced by aggressive screening, but the utility of such widespread screening for large populations with such a low incidence of injury remains problematic. Furthermore, generally the treatment for BCI is anticoagulation, which may be difficult or precluded by neurologic bleeding or

other associated injuries present in the multisystem trauma victim, and currently experimental methods may be employed based on atherosclerotic therapies.[56]

Penetrating scalp injuries are treated similarly. Large lacerations require expeditious control and injuries from gunshot wounds are generally sufficiently small so as not to require any therapy other than debridement and local wound care. Intracranial vascular injuries are the purview of the neurosurgeon, although embolization may be a useful adjunct for lifesaving control.

● NECK INJURIES

Blunt

Blunt vascular injury in the neck although rare can be fatal or even worse, result in a devastating neurologic insult and result from even minimal trauma.[57–59] Unfortunately, physical examination may miss many cases because of lack of physical signs or the clinical result is neurologically irreversible. Inspection may show ecchymosis, abrasions, or a seat belt sign at the base of the neck. A large hematoma may cause tracheal compression and deviation, as well as facial swelling caused by impaired venous return. Even a small size hematoma when deep and paratracheal can cause laryngospasm and become a major airway threat. It is always prudent to intubate a patient with a neck hematoma before tracheal compression occurs. Auscultation may reveal a carotid murmur when there is a partial occlusion of the carotid artery because of an intimal flap or dissection, but as in atherosclerotic disease, a near complete occlusion of the carotid artery may not manifest a murmur on auscultation.

A thorough neurologic examination is mandatory for any trauma patient. This is important for isolated neck injuries as well. Finding altered function secondary to an embolic or an occlusive event, i.e., fitting a stroke like pattern initiates the evaluation and treatment for BCI. Vertebral artery injury is associated with cervical vertebral fractures and would be very hard to diagnose on physical examination if one omits the neurologic examination. When arterial injury is suspected, even based on mechanisms alone, physical examination should always be supplemented by Doppler ultrasound or CT angiogram of the neck. Presently, arteriogram is the gold standard to rule out vascular injury,[60,61] but CT technology is likely to eclipse this in the near future.[62,63]

One must also be wary of carotid injury from iatrogenic mechanisms as well. Diagnostic angiography, endovascular therapies for virtually any problem at/or above the arch vessels, or cardiac catheterization with or without coronary manipulation places the carotid system at risk. Similarly, the diagnosis my not be evident until neurologic changes have occurred.[64–66]

BCI can occur more proximally than the base of the skull. Using CT angiography or 4 vessel angiography are the gold standards for diagnosis. Injuries to the carotid around the bifurcation and in the common carotid are also generally managed with anticoagulation unless an easily repairable intimal flap is seen.[67,68] Vertebral injuries are also managed with anticoagulation or embolization.[69] It is important to note that vascular injuries to the neck in blunt trauma have a very low incidence and the frequency of such diagnosis has been on the rise probably because of the aggressive screening in the recent years.[55,69–71] While a constellation of associated injuries are noted in BCI (Seatbelt mark, cervical spine fractures, mandible fracture) routine screening for patients with these injuries is hotly debated.[72–75] New endovascular alternatives are described frequently.[76,77] Despite this, the outcome is often devastating.[78,79] Vertebral artery injuries are very amenable to angiographic or endovascular treatment with good outcomes.[80]

Injury to the jugular vein can cause an expanding hematoma and may not be controlled by simple compression because of the amount of swelling and bleeding. The development of a hematoma in the neck is worrisome more for potential airway compromise than exsanguination, and early airway control is advisable. Although a constant; jugular vein injury is not differentiated from arterial neck injury by color of the blood, lack of arterial pulsations by palpating a pulsatile mass in the later. If the patient is stable and the hematoma is not expanding or impinging on the airway, nonoperative therapy is possible, otherwise operative ligation is needed.

AVFs are a consequence of injury of both vessels or of failed surgical repair. AVFs were probably more frequent before aggressive surgical repair, and the historical reports spend a great deal of discussion over the only available therapy then of ligation. Classically, the diagnosis is made by a thrill or bruit in the area of injury. High flow vessels may lead to venous congestion, either manifest as edema or even near congestive heart failure. Physical examination reveals a pulsatile mass and confirms the thrill.

Today, AVFs either recognized at the time of injury and repaired or unrecognized until presenting late are managed with both arterial and venous reconstruction. Current management options are dependent on location, as endovascular procedures avoid some very morbid surgical approaches. Beside open repair or ligation, endovascular stenting (both arterial and venous), or embolization are feasible and readily performed.[52,81]

Penetrating

Penetrating injury to the neck may present a major threat to life because of the hemorrhage or airway compromise. As with any trauma patient the airway should be secured, breathing maintained and shock treated. Airway control is paramount—it is easier to extubate the uninjured patient than to delay and be faced with a very difficult airway and a potentially impossible surgical airway. Bleeding control is obtained by simple pressure until further definitive treatment can be accomplished in the operating room.

The dynamics of injury is an integral part of the history—a high-velocity missile will cause different injuries than a penknife. On inspection, one should assess the location, the depth, and extent of the injury. Long lacerations made with a knife in a suicide attempt tend to be superficial to the platysma and would cause only superficial bleeding which is easy to control, whereas injuries penetrating the platysma require operative exploration and proximal and distal vascular control. High-velocity projectiles may not only create vascular injuries but result in airway, esophageal, nervous, or bony injuries as well and can be managed in damage control fashion, including the use of shunts.[82] Operative exploration for trauma is conducted in a similar technical fashion to elective carotid surgery to avoid those iatrogenic injuries intrinsic to the surgical approach such as cranial nerve injuries.

The standard approach to the carotid sheath is the common incision along the anterior border of the sternocleidomastoid muscle. The muscle is retracted laterally and the carotid sheath is visible beneath. Opening the sheath exposed the internal jugular vein medially and the vagus nerve posteriorly as well.

There are clinical manifestations that are an immediate indication for surgical exploration. Such signs and symptoms are active arterial bleeding, expanding hematomas, thrill, or bruit and diminished or absent distal carotid sounds or pulse. Neurologic impairment with a focal deficit is also an indication for exploration. Other signs that constitute an indication for exploration are related to airway injury such as subcutaneous air, stridor, hoarseness, dysphagia, and hemoptysis.

Palpation is useful to assess the extent and size of the hematoma as well as to identify the location of the trachea if swelling occurs. If the wound is not actively bleeding, it is prudent not to probe or expose the wound until definitive control can be established in the operating room.

The location of the injury determined during the physical examination directs the subsequent management. Anatomically the neck can be initially divided into two simple triangles: anterior and posterior triangles divided by the sternocleidomastoid muscle. All major vessels are contained in the anterior triangle. The platysma constitutes the superficial border of the anterior triangle and if not violated a major vessel injury is far less likely.

The neck is also divided into three zones from inferior to superior. Zone I, or the thoracic inlet, extends from the sternal notch to the cricoid cartilage. The proximal location of this zone signifies that the great vessels in the chest or at the base of the neck are injured and prudent planning for the operative approach to assure proximal control is very important. When patient is stable, an arteriogram or high resolution CT angiogram is indicated to identify the extent of the injury.[83] When unstable, patient should be explored to control bleeding and a combined median sternotomy and anterior neck approach is best. Most surgeons would begin with the neck incision and extend inferiorly as needed for control. If the arch vessels are involved a thoracic extension into the second rib interspace (i.e., the trap-door incision) is performed.

Zone II, or the midzone, extends from the cricoid cartilage to the angle of the mandible. An injury at this zone is fairly easy to identify by physical examination and the management is dependent on the symptoms. If any of the above signs, the so-called hard signs, is present then exploration is indicated. When no hard signs are present and patient is stable an arteriogram or CT angiogram may be done. This may obviate operation[84] and the ensuing complications. Additional testing is performed for other structures in the neck such as bronchoscopy and esophagoscopy, to rule out as associated injury.

Zone III is between the angle of the mandible and the skull base. Symptoms and physical examination findings can be very subtle at this location.[68] An onsite Doppler ultrasound may not rule out injury at this location because of bony structures. Carotid arteriogram or a high resolution CT angiogram employed to determine injury. Because distal control is often impossible, ligation, embolization, or packing of the foramen lacerum with sternocleidomastoid muscle may be the only recourse. The unfortunate outcome is often survival but with a dense neurologic insult for the younger patient without collateralization. Exposure at this location may require a mandibular disarticulation, although endovascular techniques offer both diagnostic accuracy and interventional therapy.

Injury to the neck may not be limited to one zone and may involve two or three zones at the same time especially in gunshot wounds or high-velocity missile injury. When arterial injury is suspected by proximity or mechanism, exploration or arteriogram is indicated to rule out or define the extent of the injury. Recently, CT angiography of the neck defines vascular as well as other system injuries quickly and assists in therapeutic planning. With the newly found interventional skills, adopted from embolization as well as endovascular treatment for carotid occlusive disease, the use of the angiography/endovascular suite is particularly appealing.[85] For injuries to the vertebral system an area in which the surgical options for approach are virtually impossible and even the open therapy involves ligation, the endovascular route is ideal.[86]

● CHEST VASCULAR INJURIES

Blunt

History taking again should focus on the mechanism of injury. Blunt injury should be classified between a deceleration injury and a direct impact to heighten the surgeon's index of suspicion for BAI. Unfortunately, physical examination can be very limited in these types of injuries and not be helpful to identify the location or the extent of the injured vessel. After securing the airway and ventilation, a vascular injury is suspected when a patient is hypotensive or shows signs of shock. Major vascular injuries must always be considered, but usually solid organ injuries are the cause and identified at the time of abdominal exploration. The evaluation for the hypotensive patient undergoing active resuscitation includes a chest radiograph to show if hemothorax, BAI, or pneumothorax is present and Focused Assessment with Sonography for Trauma (FAST) examination of the abdomen to evaluate for free fluid. Each pertinent issue is addressed immediately as it is identified

to restore normal physiologic parameters. When stable, patients are evaluated with CT scanning.

On inspection, abrasion, ecchymoses, and "seat belt signs" should be noted. Palpation may reveal crepitus, chest wall instability, or subcutaneous emphysema. Distended jugular veins may indicate a tension hemothorax or pericardial tamponade. Decreased or muffled breath sounds on auscultation may lead to a diagnosis of hemothorax. Unequal blood pressures or pulses in the extremities may indicate an innominate artery injury. Palpable fracture of the sternum is another signs that should raise the suspicion of an innominate artery injury. Some commonly noted signs in patients with BAI are pseudocoarctation and intrascapular murmur.[87–89] Unfortunately, physical examination can be very limited as to identify the location or the extent of the injured vessel but represent sufficient energy transfer to create such an injury. A negative finding on physical examination should not rule out aortic injury if suspected by the history.[90,91]

Similarly, there may be no external signs of injury and yet an injury may exist. A thoracic vascular injury may not be detected until a chest tube is placed; a CT scan is performed or worse until a hemorrhagic shock has occurred. The presence or absence of restraints does not appear to affect the incidence of BAI.[92] In the chest, the vessels more prone to injury after a blunt trauma include the thoracic aorta most commonly, followed by innominate artery, pulmonary veins and vena cava. Aortic injuries constitute up to 15% of immediate deaths after a motor vehicle crash with the proximal descending aorta disruption in up to 65% of the cases.[93,94]

An initial rush of blood of more than 1500 mL on insertion of chest tube or ongoing hemorrhage of more than 200 mL/h is an indication for exploratory thoracotomy since major vessel injury is clinically suspected and bleeding control is lifesaving. Serial monitoring of chest tube output is also necessary, as continued outputs in excess of 200 mL/h also warrant exploration. As with any trauma patient there must be a concerted effort to maintain end-organ perfusion, maintain euthermia and avoid coagulopathy. When stable, patients can be diagnosed with major thoraco–abdominal vascular injuries by routine contrasted trauma CT scan.[95–98]

Other than BAI, virtually any thoracic vessel can be injured by a blunt mechanism.[99–101] Similar to BAI, any free rupture likely leads to rapid death, and only the victims who have contained hematoma or intact adventia survive to hospital. Because of this particular fact, they are amenable again to evaluation with rapid sequence helical acquisition CT with contrast and endovascular repair; venous injuries are diagnosed and treated similarly.[99,100,102,103] Because these injuries are infrequent, there are no prospective management series, and endovascular or open techniques become interchangeable regardless of mechanism.

Thoracic vena cava injury is very rare but carries a mortality rate greater than 60%. Such injury may be suspected after hemopericardium and cardiac tamponade. Pulmonary vein injury when associated with bronchus disruption may lead to a systemic air embolism when intrabronchial pressure increases to above 60 Torr.[104] As above this usually manifest as mental status changes, seizures, and cardiac arrest.

On the other hand, penetrating injury can have different outcomes depending on the mechanism and location of the injury. Again the type of weapon used, the trajectory of the projectile and the time since injury are all pertinent to the evaluation and therapeutic plans.[105] Approximately 85% of gunshot wounds to the chest on reaching the hospital will require only tube thoracostomy for evacuation of blood and air, and restoration of normal physiologic parameters from bleeding and disruption of lung tissue integrity. For those patients who do not resuscitate or have the same signs of massive ongoing bleeding, major vascular injury is suspected and those patients mandate exploration.

Simply "connecting the dots" between wounds or tracing the presumed trajectory of the missile; either by visual inspection or chest radiography diagnoses the presumed anatomic injury. This is crucial for surgical planning, primarily choosing the incision that is most expedient for control and definitive repair.

The standard thoracotomy must be a mastered skill for any general and vascular surgeon. The transverse incision is made over the inframammary crease starting at the lateral sternal border of the concerned side and extending to the anterior axillary line. The pectoralis and intercostals muscles are divided and the fifth intercostals space is entered. The internal mammary artery and vein are near the lateral border of the sternum so care must be taken to not injure them. The lung is collapsed and a rib spreader is inserted. The lung is retracted upward and the inferior pulmonary ligament is divided. On the left, the descending thoracic aorta is visualized in the posterior mediastinum. The mediastinal pleura is incised. Vascular control is obtained with blunt dissection of the aorta being careful not to injure the esophagus which is anterior to the aorta. The vascular clamp is placed around the aorta to occlude it just above the diaphragm. On the right, access to the superior vena cava, azygos system, inferior vena cava (IVC), and esophagus are subpleural in the posterior mediastinum.

The "cardiac box" is the topographic anatomy that predicts cardiac and major vascular injury. Any penetrating wound within the parallelogram defined by connecting the midclavicular lines at the clavicles and the costal margins is worrisome. Ultrasonography (echocardiography) is a rapid and repeatable noninvasive method to diagnose pericardial fluid. If the patient is hemodynamically unstable, pericardial fluid is present or both are present, median sternotomy is the best approach for control of cardiac and most major vascular injuries. This box applies post trauma as well.

Median sternotomy is the rapid and best approach for most major vascular injuries of the arch and distal vessels—heart, ascending and aortic arch, innominate, carotids and proximal subclavian vessels, vena cava, and jugular veins as well. Sternotomy is performed by incising the skin from the sternal notch to just below the xiphoid process. Blunt finger dissection develops the pretracheal space superiorly and the subxiphiod space inferiorly to allow the power saw or Lebschke knife to cut the sternum vertically. Both halves are retracted laterally and the pericardial sac and great vessels are in plain view.

The sternotomy may be extended into the neck for more distal injuries to the carotids or subclavian vessels. A suspected injury to the more distal left subclavian vessels should be approached by thoracotomy and sternotomy extended up the neck for the right side. If the injury suspected is distal to the arch, a left thoracotomy is the best approach for descending aortic injury. Pulmonary hilar injuries are best controlled through a thoracotomy on the side of suspected injury.

Repair of the injury can be accomplished with continuous size appropriate monofilament suture or interposition grafts. The decision point is extent of the vascular injury and the ability to mobilize uninjured segments together for a tensionless anastomosis. This requires that there be a ready supply of vascular graft material available. The technique of clamp and sew is employed most frequently as the additional time for initiating cardiopulmonary bypass is prohibitive; anticoagulation is inappropriate because of additional injuries or both. Autogenous graft material is also infrequently used because of availability, size mismatch, and time constraints.

The operating team, especially the anesthesiology team, must be ready for the potential massive blood loss encountered when opening and exposing the injury and the changes in physiology resulting from control before repair is effected. Over resuscitation can result in cardiac strain and the anesthesiologist must be ready to rapidly shift from massive transfusion to vasodilating therapy virtually in a heartbeat. Concomitantly, other concerns must be shared. If the left subclavian artery is clamped, blood pressure monitoring is inaccurate on the left side, if the pulmonary hilum is to be clamped, ventilatory adjustments must be made, but most of all, someone must be watching the clock. Hypothermia, coagulopathy, and even likely neurologic injury are time dependent, and with the success of damage control procedures and the aggressive intensive are unit resuscitative capabilities, the initial procedure must be limited. For our patients in extremis, undergoing massive resuscitation, we limit operating room time to 60 minutes—door to door.

Emergency Department Thoracotomy

Emergency department thoracotomy (EDT) is a dramatic surgical display that factually rarely results in salvage.[106] The procedure can consume vast resources and is not without substantial healthcare provider risk,[107] nevertheless, its results can truly be awesome, and it does have role within very strict guidelines. Clear indications for which patient and which practioner performs EDT are facility dependent. First and foremost, there must be the immediately available resources to care for the patient with their chest open and cross clamps in place, and there must be clear decision points for terminating interventions if normal physiology is not reestablished. Well-defined algorithms have been published.[108] For our Trauma Center, even where an operating room, surgeons, anesthesiologists, and laboratory resources are immediately available, we strictly limit EDT based upon our Center's outcome data. For penetrating chest injury only, we perform EDT only if ECG monitor electrical activity is present, FAST examination shows cardiac motion of any kind and no abdominal fluid, and there have been signs of life within 10 minutes of arrival.

The goal of EDT is to restore sufficient circulation for immediate operation. This is accomplished by relieving cardiac tamponade, cross clamping the descending aorta to restore circulating volume quickly to maintain perfusion, and rapidly controlling active thoracic bleeding until the patient is rapidly transported to the operating room. EDT is simply a left anterolateral thoracotomy. It is performed by making an incision from the midsternum across the chest horizontally just below the nipple to the table. The chest is rapidly entered at the fourth interspace and the surgeon's hand enters the chest to evacuate hematoma, gain access to the pericardium and find the aorta. The pericardium is opened on the anterior surface and care is taken to preserve the phrenic nerve which runs for superior to inferior along the lateral border of the pericardial sac. The pericardium is tough and difficult to grasp so often it is easier to incise a centimeter size hole with the knife, and then use the scissors to fully open the pericardium and evacuate any clots. Bleeding from the heart or great vessels is controlled by a finger, simple sutures, clamps, temporary ligation, or any other method that allows resuscitation to progress. Open cardiac massage to revive the heart is done, and to try to preserve blood flow to the brain.

Clamping the descending aorta will decrease the volume needed to restore perfusion to the brain and is accomplished by the surgeon hand sliding along the posterior thoracic wall, up onto the vertebral column. The aorta is generally flaccid and feels like a penrose drain; passing a nasogastric tube makes aortic identification easier as the tube can be felt to the right of the aorta. The cross clamp is applied by breaking through the pleura and applying the clamp across all the structures on top of the vertebral column. An injury to the left lung hilum is controlled by simply cross clamping the entire hilum. If no blood is found in the left thorax, the thoracotomy can be extended across the sternum to open the right chest in similar fashion for immediate control of bleeding.

TRANSMEDIASTINAL GUNSHOT WOUNDS

Transmediastinal gunshot wounds are particularly worrisome for major vascular injury. They are also worrisome for aerodigestive tract injury and/or neurologic injury as well. As discussed frequently, the unstable patient needs operation. Current management of the stable patient includes helical CT.[92,109–112] Despite normal or easily corrected vital signs, significant major vascular injury may still exist with transmediastinal gunshots.[113]

SUBCLAVIAN INJURIES

The subclavian vessels broach the neck, the thorax, and the extremity. The surgeon must be prepared to deal with any region and be expected to gain control rapidly and without delay. For the stable patient, arteriography is crucial for operative strategy.[114,115] Endovascular techniques are superior to open procedures which risk multiple incisions, complex approaches and dangerous dissections. Nervous structures at risk for injury include vagus, phrenic, and the brachial plexus. Because of the proximity of these structures to the vessels, preoperative examination is imperative to document the deficits from the injury.

Exposure for the subclavian vessels is different for the right and the left side. On the right, median sternotomy with a cervical extension offers the best approach. On the left, however, a left thoracotomy and potential supraclavicular incision offer the exposure for control. The incisions may be combined through the sternum in the so called trap-door approach. Because of the bony structures and fixed position of the arch, there is insufficient mobility to fashion a tension-free anastomosis and interposition grafts are employed; because of the caliber of the vessel, polytetraflouroethylene (PTFE) grafts are most commonly used.[116]

SUMMARY

In summary, major vascular injuries that reach the hospital; either blunt or penetrating are managed with similar schema—hypotensive patients go to the operating room and stable patients are evaluated with helical CT. Thoracic injuries are particularly amenable to endovascular techniques because of the current technology and surgeon increasing experience. It is beneficial to the patient to avoid thoracotomy as the second insult, temporizing with damage control and definitive repair when the patient is warm, fluid replete, and not coagulopathic.

ABDOMINAL VASCULAR INJURIES

The data from civilian trauma centers reveal that the incidence of abdominal vascular trauma is significantly higher than that in military injuries, because of the logistics of devastating injuries making it alive to medical care. The Ben Taub General Hospital in Houston published a 30-year review in 1989 that documented civilian inner city abdominal vascular injuries at 33.8%.[117] The military, abdominal vascular injury experience demonstrates only an incidence of 2% in the paper by DeBakey and Simeone in 1946,[4] of 2.3% in Korean conflict[6] and Rich et al.[7] reported an incidence of 2.9% in Vietnam due primarily to logistics, and ballistics. The high-velocity, repeating weapons (projectile velocity greater than 2000 feet/s) and other weapons designed to fragment as compared to the single shot low-velocity weapons being used by the civilian population transfer greater injury. The projectiles are designed for stopping power, a military objective, rather than accuracy.

Despite remarkable improvements in prehospital care in theater, the simple fact remains that the individual is injured in a "hostile" environment. Intercity violence has forced prehospital system improvements that have resulted in shorter transport times and earlier surgical intervention.

The incidence of abdominal vascular injury sustained after blunt trauma is 5% to 10% while penetrating stab wounds to the abdomen similarly have a low incidence of vascular injury.[117,118] The most commonly injured abdominal vessels were the IVC (25%), the aorta (21%), the iliac arteries (20%), the iliac veins (17%), the superior mesenteric vein (SMV) (11%), and the SMA (10%).[119]

Iatrogenic injuries to abdominal vessels are caused by laparoscopy (primarily trocar injuries), angiography, cardiac catheterization, abdominal procedures (pelvic and retroperitoneal dissections), and spinal procedures.[120–124] Injuries created are similar to stab wounds and the only caveat for the operating surgeon is that a major vascular injury has been described even during the most mundane cases.[125] Early diagnosis and a high index of suspicion must always be maintained when sharp objects are manipulated in proximity to vascular structures. Repair is dependent on the clinical status of the patient and endovascular and minimally invasive techniques are acceptable in the stable patient.[126,127] Patients in extremis require immediate control by whatever means are most expedient.[128]

Diagnosis

Physical examination is relatively inconclusive; decision for operation is made largely depending on the amount of hemorrhage and associated shock, or the presence of peritoneal signs. The usefulness of the physical examination is limited in the trauma patients who are intubated, have altered consciousness or who have other distracting injuries. The physical findings also depend on the location of the injury—contained within the retroperitoneum or intraperitoneal injury/hemorrhage. Contained hematomas may present with a hypotension which responds to a fluid bolus. Active free hemorrhage presents with shock that transiently responds or is refractory to resuscitation. Although there is considerable hemorrhage within the peritoneum there may not be either a distended abdomen or peritoneal signs.

Inspection of the bluntly injured patient may identify a seat belt sign, abrasion or ecchymosis. The EAST practice management guidelines for the evaluation of blunt abdominal trauma recommended that patients with seatbelt sign should be admitted for observation and serial physical examination.[129] Auscultation is rarely useful, and palpation can elicit peritonitis. When hemorrhage is contained retroperitoneally or in the lesser sac, the patient may show signs of transient hypotension that is usually corrected with fluid resuscitation. In this case hypotension may be delayed, or not seen until the time of exploration. Patients with abdominal vascular injuries, a systolic blood pressure in the emergency department of more than 100 mm Hg

and a base deficit of more than −7.2 have been shown to have favorable survival rate of 96.2%.[130] Equivocal physical examination findings or altered mental status constitute an indication for objective diagnostic measures like CT scan, FAST, etc. FAST offers immediate information that is repeatable and simple. It requires no ionizing radiation and many of the ultrasound machines are portable and lightweight. Because of its high accuracy when used to evaluate hypotensive patients who present with blunt abdominal trauma, every abdominal physical examination should be complemented with FAST when possible. Detection of intraperitoneal fluid is best made by this surgeon performed examination.[131–133]

In the hemodynamically stable blunt trauma patient, FAST is performed and may be complemented with CT scan. CT offers several additional data to detect injury (retroperitoneum, contrast studies, osseous anatomy) and plan therapeutic maneuvers. Hemodynamically unstable patients may be evaluated initially with FAST to ascertain if the hemorrhage is indeed within the abdomen. The hemodynamically unstable patient with abdominal hemorrhage needs to be taken to the operating room as quickly as possible.

In the emergency department the ATLS regimen is initiated as quickly as is possible—high flow intravenous access, crystalloid and O-negative blood infusion and an active attempt to prevent hypothermia.[134] Although the only important decision is if and when take the patient to the operating room, being prepared for other contingencies is necessary—assuring the availability of blood and blood products for massive hemorrhage, quickly administering antibiotic/tetanus prophylaxis, and preparing the operating room and associated personnel for impending arrival are crucial system issues. The precise diagnosis is made at operation with the most likely source coming from a solid organ injury, but full exploration is needed to fully evaluate all organs and vessels.

Nonoperative therapy for solid organ injury is now standard. There are cases in which angiographic or endovascular techniques are employed to stop bleeding in the liver and spleen[135,136] identified on CT. These interventions avoid laparotomy and its associated morbidity but are not wholly innocuous.[137]

If the FAST or a CT scan detects free fluid, and there is no evidence of a solid organ injury (spleen or liver) in a patient mandates either deep peritoneal lavage to determine the nature of the fluid or exploratory laparotomy. Laparoscopy in experienced hand may also be an alternative in selected stable patients. The concern here is for hollow viscus injury, but mesenteric injury that devitalizes an intestinal segment, or creates a potential defect for bowel herniation. Hematuria, although is nonspecific, it may be a sign of retroperitoneal injury especially when associated with the pelvic fractures. An unstable pelvic fracture can be associated with pelvic vascular disruption. The control of pelvic hemorrhage associated with pelvic fractures is embolization. There have been reports of packing of the pelvic fractures most recently,[138] a challenge to the strict policy of never opening a contained retroperitoneal or preperitoneal hemorrhage from a pelvic fracture. Currently, this practice is best left to the experienced surgeons who routinely employ this technique.

Penetrating abdominal vascular injuries are evaluated with physical examination looking for entrance and exit wounds from the nipples to the upper thighs. Other findings on physical findings worrisome for intra-abdominal injury are hematuria and loss of femoral pulses. The trajectory of the missile or stab wound predicts the organ or vessel injured. As in the blunt vascular trauma the physical examination depends on whether the hematoma is contained or active hemorrhage is present. A FAST may be performed to evaluate for cardiac tamponade from cardiac injury. A chest X-ray and an abdominal X-ray are of diagnostic value in revealing a hemothorax and the trajectory of the missile.

In penetrating injury, the location and the number of lacerations or entry points are noted. For most gunshot wounds, intra-abdominal injury occurs frequently, and exploration is generally the next step.[139] There are some injuries that miss the peritoneum, and for the stable patient evaluation with CT to track the course of the projectile is acceptable and avoids nontherapeutic laparotomy and its consequences.[140] There is a subset of patients with gunshot wounds to the abdomen who can be evaluated with CT and observed despite intra-abdominal injuries.[141,142]

For knife wounds, violation of the abdominal wall fascia is a key in decision making. Unlike the cavitary distribution of energy from guns that creates a conical blast injury in the tissue of adjacent organs; only fascial penetration creates the potential for penetrating abdominal injury with sharp objects. If this is not obvious from peritonitis or evisceration, a local wound exploration in a stable patient using local anesthesia may determine the depth of the laceration. Again, selective exploration is performed to avoid unneeded laparotomy. Laparoscopy is often used at our center, not only for diagnosis, but therapy as well. Repair of intra-abdominal injuries requires advanced laparoscopic skills.[143,144]

Management

Virtually, an EDT is never indicated to cross clamp the aorta in cases of imminent or cardiac arrest for abdominal injuries. A large series by Feliciano et al.[145] revealed only one of 59 patients with isolated penetrating wounds to the abdomen survived after an EDT. Determining the patients and situations for which this dramatic intervention is undertaken is paramount to performing it.

The management of both penetrating and blunt abdominal vascular trauma depends on the location of the injury. Hematoma when identified by CT scan or at operative exploration are explored for penetrating injury and observed intraoperatively for blunt mechanisms. If the hematoma is expanding, it too is explored to control the bleeding point. The abdomen has been divided into 3 zones to classify the vessel or vessels injured and to help the surgeon in operative

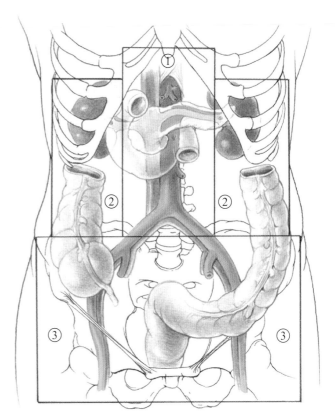

● **FIGURE 49-1.** Retroperitoneal zones. Zone 1: Midline retroperitoneum; Zone 2: Upper lateral retroperitoneum; Zone 3: Pelvic retroperitoneum.

Reproduced, with permission, from Valentine RJ. Abdominal aorta. In: Thal ER, Weigelt JA, Carrico CJ, eds. Operative Trauma Management: An Atlas. 2nd ed. New York, NY: McGraw-Hill; 2002:302-315.

decision making: (1) Zone I include the midline retroperitoneum, (2) Zone II include the upper retroperitoneum with renal artery and vein, and (3) Zone III or pelvic retroperitoneum (Figure 49-1 and Table 49-1).

TABLE 49-1. Anatomic Location of Intra-Abdominal and Retroperitoneal Vasculature

Zone 1: Midline retroperitoneum subdivided into supramesocolic and inframesocolic areas
  Supramesocolic area—Suprarenal abdominal aorta, celiac axis, proximal SMA, proximal renal artery, and superior mesenteric vein (either supramesocolic or retromesocolic)
  Inframesocolic area—Infrarenal abdominal aorta and infrahepatic IVC

Zone 2: Upper lateral retroperitoneum
  Renal artery and renal vein

Zone 3: Pelvic retroperitoneum
  Iliac artery and iliac vein

Portal–retrohepatic area
  Portal vein, hepatic artery, and retrohepatic vena cava

Pathophysiology

Vascular injuries from blunt trauma are associated with rapid deceleration in motor vehicle crashes and falls. The forces can avulse branches from major vessels at their fixation points, such as the major visceral arteries. Blunt forces may create intimal injuries with thrombosis which has been seen in the renal arteries, or crush injury from a direct blow. A direct blow may completely disrupt the layers of the vessel and cause local hematoma or even massive hemorrhage if there is loss of containing tissue planes. Lastly, blunt injury can create penetrating injury by lacerating vessels from bone fragments, probably seen commonly with high-energy pelvic fractures.

Penetrating injuries produce blast injuries, intimal flaps and thrombosis, disrupt the wall, or completely transect the vessel. An AVF may be produced. Understanding that the large amount of energy transferred from guns is dissipated in the soft tissue means that penetrating injuries than can also create vascular injury from blunt forces as well. Formerly, a gunshot in proximity to any vessel required angiography. This policy is now refined by evidence-based study and discussed in the peripheral vascular injury section.

The question of reducing the hypercoaguable state following traumatic injury and repair is always at question. Very often, there is a contraindication to anticoagulant therapy because of associated injuries. Others conjecture there has been the intervening development of a coagulopathy that "effectively" offers early protection. Whereas anticoagulation has been demonstrated to be of benefit in BCI, nontrauma vascular stents,[146] and peripheral arterial venous repairs,[147] there is no conclusive evidence that anticoagulation after thoracic or abdominal vascular repair improves patency, limb salvage, or survival.[148]

Operating Room

Once in the operating room the patient is prepped and draped from the chin to the lower thighs. This is performed to gain distal vascular control, for vein harvests, and immediate access to the chest cavity if needed for a thoracic injury and proximal aortic control. A midline abdominal incision is made and the peritoneal cavity is entered. Clotted and nonclotted blood is evacuated. If needed, an aortic compression device may be used to compress the aorta at the aortic hiatus.[149] This quick measure allows the surgeon to better localize the source and to plan the next steps in the conduct of the operation. All four quadrants of the abdomen are packed with laparotomy pads. This allows anesthesia to catch up with blood products and fluid resuscitation. The bleeding must be controlled by direct pressure or packing during these initial steps so that an adequate exploration may performed.

The exploration is best done in an orderly fashion. We prefer to start at the aorta at the diaphragm and work clockwise to be sure to evaluate all areas. The packs are removed and a rapid inspection is done for active bleeding, expanding hematomas, and contamination. When bleeding is encountered, it is stopped. Active bleeding from solid organs maybe packed. A splenectomy maybe performed if this is expeditious, or simply clamping the hilum may suffice to stop active hemorrhage. Arterial injuries maybe controlled with direct pressure with fingers, laparotomy pads, or sponge sticks. Proximal and distal control is the goal but immediate control is performed with the former. Major venous control is obtained with finger pressure, laparotomy pads, sponge sticks, or vascular clamps.

If exsanguinating hemorrhage persists, aortic control is obtained at the nearest easily accessible level—the diaphragmatic hiatus is easily performed, especially if one has used direct pressure with fingers or T-bar (aortic compression device) at the beginning of the operation. An atraumatic vascular clamp must be used for prolonged control. Once the hemorrhage is under control the contamination is controlled with applying Babcock clamps, noncrushing intestinal clamps, or stapling devices. Small injuries to the intestines with soilage may be controlled with a simple running suture.

Each quadrant of the abdomen is palpated and visually inspected. Solid organs are mobilized if needed, the bowel is evaluated from diaphragmatic hiatus to rectum, and the lesser sac and upper retroperitoneum are investigated. When the entire abdominal cavity and the retro peritoneum have been evaluated, the injuries identified, a surgical plan is developed based greatly on the physiologic state of the patient. Modern surgical planning for major vascular injuries now includes aggressive resuscitation, temporizing measures before definitive repair, and the use of noninvasive or less invasive modalities such as angiography, embolization, and endovascular repair.

The surgeon must anticipate the ongoing physiologic processes in the patient with a major vascular injury, including the development of abdominal compartment syndrome (ACS). Simply, the interstitial fluid that accumulates from both injury and resuscitation creates swelling. If this swelling occurs in a closed space, intracompartmental hypertension is created. This is true in the brain, in the extremities, and in the intraperitoneal spaces as well. The syndrome of increased abdominal hypertension which leads to organ dysfunction has been named ACS.[150]

ACS involves abdominal pressures greater than 25 cm of water and is generally measured by intravesicular pressures. For ACS to be present there must be an impact on ventilation (increased peak pressures, low tidal volumes, etc.), decreased venous return (hypotension, ongoing volume needs, elevated central venous pressures, etc.) and/or decreased urine output. The treatment of ACS is release of the compartment, as is performed with other elevated compartment pressures in other locations. There may be initial success with intragastric decompression or neuromuscular blockade, however, ACS generally involves opening (or re opening) the abdominal fascia. Temporary closure is obtained with watertight vacuum dressings. After the initial resuscitation is completed, and the physiologic response to injury abates, the abdominal fascia is reapproximated (see subsection on Damage Control below).

Hemorrhage and hematomas from abdominal vascular injuries are localized by their anatomic zones. Zone 1, midline retroperitoneum; Zone 2, upper lateral retroperitoneum; Zone 3, pelvic retroperitoneum; and the portal–retrohepatic area. These zones have been described earlier.

Zone 1—Midline Supramesocolic Injuries

A hematoma or active bleeding in Zone 1 mandates an exploration for both penetrating and blunt injuries. The supramesocolic area is superior to the transverse mesocolon. A hematoma or bleeding in this region may indicate an injury to the suprarenal aorta, celiac axis, proximal superior mesenteric artery (SMA), or proximal renal artery.

Proximal aortic control should be obtained prior to opening the supramesocolic hematoma as a result of the difficulty in exposure of the vessels in this area. There are several techniques for obtaining proximal control of the aorta. If the injury is supraceliac, intrathoracic control may be needed at the descending thoracic aorta via a left anterior thoracotomy. Another technique to gain access to the aorta is by left medial visceral rotation.

The left colon is mobilized by incising the left lateral peritoneal attachments from the splenic flexure to the distal sigmoid. The splenophrenic and splenorenal ligaments are divided and the spleen, fundus of the stomach, tail of the pancreas, and kidney are mobilized by blunt dissection (Figure 49-2). This will expose the entire abdominal aorta, left iliac system, suprarenal aorta, celiac axis, proximal SMA, and left renal arteries. The kidney does not need to be included in the rotation to expose the celiac axis but if it performed, it allows access to the posterior wall of the aorta. An alternate approach is to leave the kidney and rotate the spleen, pancreas, and left colon (Figure 49-3).

Another approach that is quicker than the medial visceral rotation is to incise the left triangular ligament and retract the left lobe of the liver. The hepatogastric ligament is incised just to the right of the esophagus and extended along the lesser curvature of the stomach. The stomach and esophagus are retracted to the left. The posterior peritoneum is excised and the right crus of the diaphragm is exposed (Figure 49-4A). The aorta is posterior to the right crus and exposed by blunt dissection. The surgeon's index and middle fingers are placed on either side of the aorta and used to guide the clamp into position (Figure 49-4B).[151]

Most injuries to the suprarenal aorta may be repaired with a lateral arteriorrhaphy with a 3-0 or 4-0 polypropylene suture after adequate debridement of the edges. The surgeon must be sure the closure is tension free. Generally an end-to-end anastomosis can be performed if the defect is less than 2 cm in length. If tension is present, or the defect is larger, a patch angioplasty or an interposition graft of Dacron or PTFE is used. Patch angioplasty is also indicated when there is a large defect that will cause luminal compromise if the wound is repaired in a simple running fashion.

The graft is oversewn with 3–0 or 4–0 polyproplene, the repair flushed by briefly opening the proximal clamp, and the distal clamp is removed. Prior to removal of the proximal clamp, the surgeon must notify anesthesia to prepare to infuse fluid. The proximal clamp is then removed slowly. Long clamp times produce profound acidosis from the ischemic lower extremities and warrant prophylactic administration of intravenous bicarbonate.[152]

When there is gross contamination it is preferred to use saphenous vein or hypogastric artery interposition grafts over prosthetic material.[153] Enteric spillage is not a contraindication for prosthetic graft.[154,155] The abdominal cavity should be irrigated well and the enteric spillage controlled prior to the repair.

Injuries to the celiac artery and branches are also difficult to expose because of the dense neural plexus and lymphatic tissue which cover this region of the aorta. Exposure here requires time consuming dissection which the patient in extremis may not have. Fortunately if the injury is distal the celiac axis, i.e., the left gastric and splenic arteries, they may be ligated because of the extensive collateral circulation that exists between the celiac and superior mesenteric systems. The common hepatic artery may also be ligated proximal to the gastroduodenal artery based on similar redundant blood supply. The liver will receive adequate blood supply from the portal vein and gastroduodenal artery.

It may be feasible to repair the hepatic artery if the patient is stable. The repair may be done by whichever method offers the best technical repair—lateral arteriorrhaphy, end-to-end anastomosis, or saphenous vein interposition graft. If the patient is unstable with other injuries one must not hesitate to ligate the common hepatic artery. Although the same approach can be applied to injuries of the celiac axis, the larger size of the common hepatic artery generally makes this technically easier. If the patient is unstable, ligation is performed and the consequences are dealt with when the patient is resuscitated; rewarmed; and not coagulopathic. In stable patients with minimal injuries repair may be performed with an interposition saphenous vein graft.

Proceeding just inferiorly along the aorta, the SMA is the next anterior structure the surgeon encounters. The SMA gives off the inferior pancreaticoduodenal artery, the middle colic artery, the jejunal arterial arcade with multiple intestinal branches, the right colic artery, and the ileocolic artery in sequence. SMA injuries are divided into four zones:

- Zone 1: Between the origin and the inferior pancreaticoduodenal artery
- Zone 2: Between the inferior pancreaticoduodenal artery and the middle colic artery
- Zone 3: Distal to the middle colic artery
- Zone 4: The segmental intestinal branches

Ligation of Zone 1 or 2 of the SMA in a patient that has been in hemorrhagic shock will result in small bowel and right colon ischemia caused by vasoconstriction of the collateral vessels.[156] Ligation of Zone 3 and 4 may result in localized segments of ischemia of the small bowel.

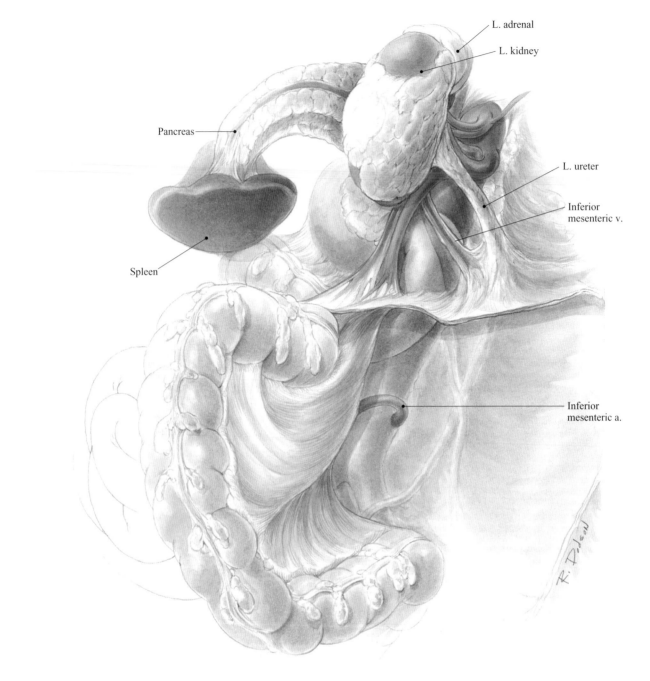

● **FIGURE 49-2.** Left medial visceral rotation.

Reproduced, with permission, from Valentine RJ. Abdominal aorta. In: Thal ER, Weigelt JA, Carrico CJ, eds. Operative Trauma Management: An Atlas. 2nd ed. New York, NY: McGraw-Hill; 2002: 302-315.

SMA injuries may also be divided into two zones: the short retropancreatic segment and the segment that emerges from under the body of the pancreas, over the uncinate process and the third portion of the duodenum.[157–159]

Exposure of the SMA is performed with a left medial rotation as previously described. The kidney does not need to be rotated medially. If an injury to the posterior wall of the aorta is suspected, then medial rotation of the kidney is necessary to fully expose the posterior wall. Alternatively, the surgeon may expose this area by opening the lesser sac and approaching the aorta directly. The SMA resides at the inferior border of the pancreas and falls inferiorly over the third portion of the retroperitoneal duodenum.

To expose Zone 1 of the SMA, the pancreas may be transected through its neck if there is extensive bleeding and rapid control is needed. This is done easily and quickly with a linear stapler. If there is extensive damage to this area and potential injury to the pancreas, the SMA should be ligated, and if the patient is stable a jump graft of saphenous vein or PTFE from the distal infrarenal aorta is safest, as it is away from injured pancreas. The choice of anastomosis in this repair is inconsequential and depends on how best the vessel

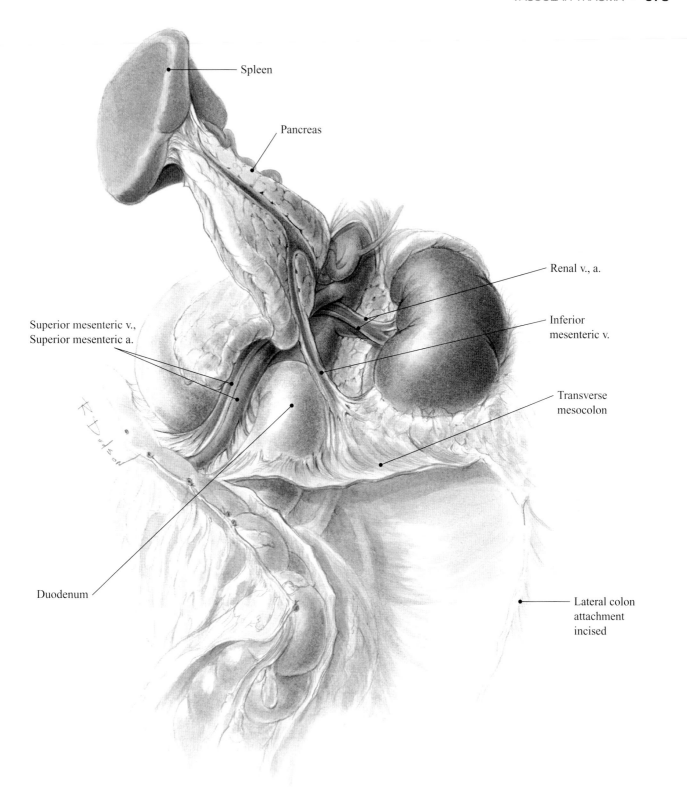

● **FIGURE 49-3.** Left medial visceral rotation with kidney left *in situ*.

Reproduced, with permission, from Valentine RJ. Abdominal aorta. In: Thal ER, Weigelt JA, Carrico CJ, eds. Operative Trauma Management: An Atlas. 2nd ed. New York, NY: McGraw-Hill; 2002:302-315.

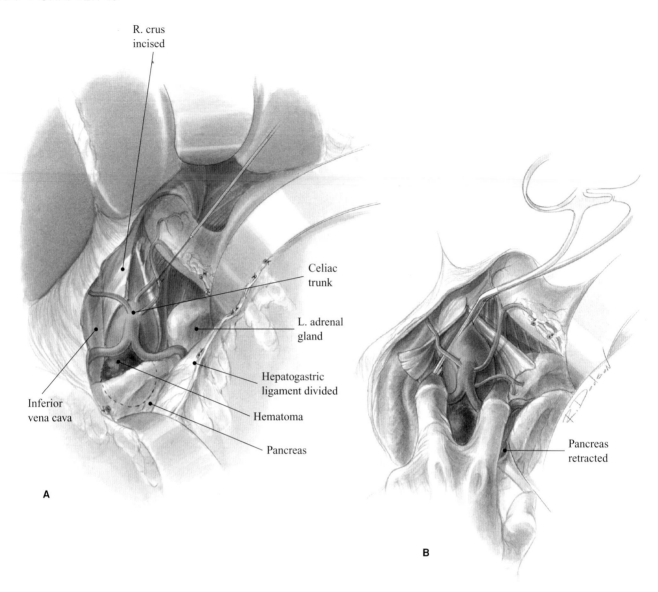

R. crus
incised

Celiac
trunk

L. adrenal
gland

Hepatogastric
ligament divided

Inferior
vena cava

Hematoma

Pancreas

A

Pancreas
retracted

B

● **FIGURE 49-4.** Superior mesenteric artery exposure. (A) Lesser sac approach.
(B) Transected pancreas approach.

*Reproduced, with permission, from Valentine RJ. Abdominal aorta. In: Thal ER, Weigelt JA, Carrico
CJ, eds. Operative Trauma Management: An Atlas. 2nd ed. New York, NY: McGraw-Hill; 2002:
302-315.*

and graft lay in apposition. It may be an end to end to the distal transected portion of the SMA or an end to side, the anterior, or lateral side to the SMA. The repair must be a tension-free and the aortic suture line needs to be covered with soft tissue to prevent the formation of an aortoenteric fistula postoperatively. If the patient is unstable a temporary intraluminal shunt may even be placed and definitive repair deferred to until after the patient is resuscitated in the critical care unit for 24 to 48 hours.[160] Nevertheless, SMA injury is lethal in 40% of cases and this is increased in proximal injuries.

Zone 2 injuries may be exposed by dividing the ligament of Treitz and mobilizing the duodenum laterally (Figure 49-5). The middle colic artery is identified and traced to its origin, the SMA. For more exposure, the inferior border of the pancreas can be retracted cephalad. Zone 2 injuries are repaired similarly to Zone 1 injuries.

Zone 3 and 4 injuries are approached directly through the mesentery of the small intestine. Attempts should be made to restore continuity of the vessels involved in these injuries if the patient is stable. Ligation in these segments will result in ischemic bowel and need for resection, whereas ligation of more proximal vessels are fed by collateral flow from either the celiac or inferior mesenteric arteries.

Injuries to the SMV are difficult to manage because of the location posterior to the pancreas and to the right of the SMA. As with the injuries to the SMA, the pancreas may need to be transected to gain control. If the injury is visible below the inferior border the pancreas, digital pressure should be applied and a repair is accomplished with a running 5-0 polypropylene suture. An end-to-end tension-free anastomosis may be performed for a transected SMV.

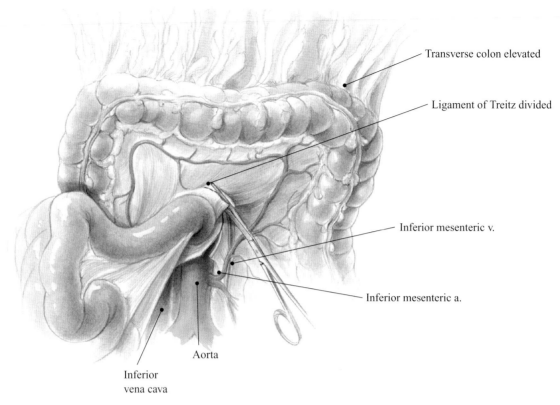

Transverse colon elevated

Ligament of Treitz divided

Inferior mesenteric v.

Inferior mesenteric a.

Aorta

Inferior
vena cava

FIGURE 49-5. Zone 2 exposure.

Reproduced, with permission, from Valentine RJ. Abdominal aorta. In: Thal ER, Weigelt JA, Carrico CJ, eds. Operative Trauma Management: An Atlas. 2nd ed. New York, NY: McGraw-Hill; 2002: 302-315.

Penetrating posterior injuries may be difficult to expose because of the numerous collaterals. Care must be taken to ligate these collaterals for proper exposure to be achieved and to avoid further bleeding.

When extensive vascular and abdominal injuries are present the SMV may be ligated. There are reports in young patients with survival rates of 85% after ligation of the SMV. Stone and associates emphasized aggressive fluid resuscitation after ligation of the SMV because of splanchnic hypervolemia that leads to peripheral hypovolemia. This hypovolemia may last for several days. Because of the venous congestion and swelling of the intestines the abdomen should not be closed and a temporary closure be performed and the patient monitored closely for ACS. A second look should be performed in 24 to 48 hours to evaluate the bowel for ischemia.[160]

Injuries to the inferior mesenteric artery are routinely ligated, as there is collateral flow to supply the colon.

RENOVASCULAR INJURIES

The proximal renal arteries may be exposed by retracting the transverse colon superiorly and the small bowel to the right. The retroperitoneum is incised directly over the aorta. The left renal vein is identified and retracted superiorly to expose the renal arteries. The vena cava may need to be retracted to the right. Proximal control is best obtained with vessel loops. Additionally, the entire right renal artery can be exposed by a right medial rotation of the colon and an extensive Kocher maneuver. This will mobilize the duodenum and head of the pancreas to the midline so as to identify the vena cava and the right renal vein. To fully expose the entire renal artery the vena cava and the right renal vein are retracted. Similarly, medial visceral rotation on the left gives access to the left kidney and its hilum.

Repair should be attempted if the patient is stable, bilateral injuries, or if a single kidney is present. Time limits the return of functional renal tissue. It is recommended revascularization be attempted in a stable patient within 4 to 6 hours of the injury; revascularization up to 20 hours is possible for patients with bilateral injuries or a single kidney.[162,163] A nephrectomy should be performed if the patient is unstable, there is prolonged ischemia, or has extensive injuries. Nonoperative treatment is an option if the diagnosis is delayed, and the patient is not actively bleeding from the kidney. These patients need to be monitored for the development of hypertension in the future. Repairs may be done by simple closure, patch angioplasty, resection and anastomosis, or interposition graft.

Iatrogenic injuries, especially from transplantation must be dealt with quickly, but the physiologic state of these patients and isolated vascular injuries is more amenable to endovascular techniques.[164]

Renal vein injuries may be repaired by lateral venorrhaphy or by ligation in extensive injuries. A nephrectomy should be concomitantly performed after ligation of the right renal vein. The left renal vein may be ligated and the kidney survives as a result of the collateral drainage through the left gonadal vein, the left adrenal vein, and the lumbar veins.

Blunt injury to the renal artery resulting in thrombosis may not present early enough to consider auto transplantation although some have reported success.[165] Most surgeons would opt for operation only if both kidneys are totally involved. Endovascular stents are more commonly employed today.[166]

Zone 1: Midline Inframesocolic Injuries

The inframesocolic area is described as the space inferior to the transverse mesocolon. Hemorrhage or bleeding in this region may indicate an injury to the infrarenal abdominal aorta or infrahepatic IVC. To expose the infrarenal aorta, the transverse colon is elevated cephalad and the small bowel is packed to the right. The posterior peritoneum is incised superiorly and the structures exposed from the left renal vein and inferiorly to the aortic bifurcation. The superior incision includes the ligament of Treitz and the third and fourth portions of the duodenum are then retracted to the right. Care must be taken not to injure the inferior mesenteric vessels just left to the aorta. Direct pressure with a digit or sponge stick allows proximal and distal control of the aorta. All surfaces of the aorta must be visualized including the posterior wall, to locate all injuries and their extent for determining proper definitive care.

The edges of the wound are debrided and approximated with a running polypropylene 3-0 or 4-0 suture. Most wounds may be approximated with a simple lateral arteriorrhaphy. A patch angioplasty is indicated when there is a large defect that will cause luminal compromise. End-to-end anastomosis may be performed if the aorta is mobilized to create a tension-free anastomosis. If greater than 2 cm of the aorta is damaged then an interposition graft of PTFE or Dacron should be placed to create a tension-free repair. One must be wary of long clamp times which can produce profound acidosis from the ischemic lower extremities and warrant prophylactic bicarbonate.

When there is gross contamination it is preferred but not mandatory to use saphenous vein or hypogastric artery over prosthetic material. If there is gross contamination from colon injuries extra-anatomic bypass may be an additional option to reestablish perfusion to the lower extremities. The ends of the aorta are oversewn and an extra-anatomic bypass is performed. Bypass techniques depend on the location and complexity of the injury present—axillofemoral inflow, either bilaterally or unilaterally with femorofemoral bypass are possible. It may be preferable to perform a unilateral axillofemoral bypass graft with an end-to-end iliac artery anastomosis.[167,168]

If a vena cava injury is suspected a right medial visceral rotation will expose the vena cava and the aorta. The lateral peritoneal attachments from the cecum to the hepatic flexure are incised. The right colon is reflected to the right by blunt dissection in a plane anterior to Gerota's fascia. The duodenum and head of pancreas are mobilized by incising the hepatoduodenal ligament and the retroperitoneum. This allows visualization to the vena cava and access to the vasculature of the right kidney. The aortic bifurcation and iliac arteries are exposed by extending the incision inferiorly along the root of the small bowel mesentery.[169]

The cava wall is tenuous and great care must be taken or further injury can result. Proximal and distal control are best obtained with gentle digital pressure or sponge sticks. Again, full evaluation of the cava must be performed, and it may be easier to assess the integrity of the vessel by further opening the traumatic venotomy to visualize the posterior of lateral walls. Venorrhaphy of these injuries may be accomplished by 3-0 or 4-0 polypropylene suture intravascularly, and then the anterior venotomy closed similarly. Ligation is again an option of last resort, but there have been reports of salvage.[170,171] For those facile with total hepatic isolation from transplant experience, this also provides an option for repair of caval injuries.[172]

Aortic and cava injuries are devastating and survival hovers approximately 50%.[173] While a subtle exsanguinations intraoperatively the majority die from multisystem failure. Caval flow after repair can be demonstrated by ultrasound.[174]

Zone 2: Upper Lateral Retroperitoneum

Hematoma or hemorrhage in Zone 2 may indicate injury to the renal artery, the renal vein, or the kidney. Penetrating trauma mandates exploration. Blunt trauma with a nonexpanding hematoma does not mandate exploration. Exposure and repair options are described in renovascular injuries in zone 1. Late complications such as AVF are successfully dealt with endovascularly.[175]

Zone 3: Pelvic Retroperitoneum

Hematoma or hemorrhage in Zone 3 may indicate injury to the iliac artery, iliac vein, or both. Hematomas from blunt trauma need to be exposed only if there is hemorrhage intraperitoneally, or a rapidly expanding hematoma, or absent or diminished femoral pulses. Prior teaching was absolute about not opening pelvic hematomas, as the large area, venous plexus and open bone marrow was felt to be uncontrollable. There are reports of packing and damage control procedures, but this is not commonplace. All hematomas should be explored in penetrating injuries.

While obtaining proximal and distal control, digital pressure against the bone is very effective until definitive vascular clamps can be applied. The common iliac arteries are exposed by retracting the small bowel superiorly and to the right. The retroperitoneum over the aorta is incised exposing the aorta and the common iliac arteries. Care must be taken when dissecting distally not to injure the ureter that crosses over the bifurcation of the common iliac artery. For injuries in this region it is best to fully demonstrate the ureter to assure its safety and determine if there is concomitant injury.

When obtaining arterial control, one must be cautious not to injure the veins lying posterior to the arteries. Once proximal control is obtained, distal control of the external iliac artery is obtained at the pelvic brim. If there is difficulty obtaining control of the external iliac artery a transverse lower abdominal incision or a longitudinal incision over the groin with division of the inguinal ligament may be needed. Control of the internal iliac artery is essential to control back bleeding. Vessel loops are ideal for control in this location, as clamps may be hard to apply or cumbersome during repair efforts.

Common and external iliac arteries injuries need to be repaired. The common and the external iliac arteries should not be ligated. Ligation will lead to ischemia of the lower extremity. The internal iliac artery, however, may be ligated.[176]

As with other major vessels, small injuries are debrided and repaired with a lateral arteriorrhaphy. Again care must be taken not to narrow the lumen—a venous or PTFE patch may be necessary. Similarly, more extensive injuries are debrided and repaired by an end-to-end anastomosis, saphenous vein or PTFE graft. If resuscitation efforts are ongoing, or other time issues present themselves, temporary shunting can be utilized. Implanting the common iliac to the opposite common iliac artery, or using the internal iliac as an interposition graft are autologous repairs that may helpful in the stable patient to avoid prosthetic material.[173]

Extensive injuries with enteric contamination are a vexing problem. Options discussed previously dividing the artery proximal to the injury, oversewing with a double row of sutures, and covering with peritoneum. If the extremity appears to be ischemic, an extra-anatomic femoral–femoral crossover graft is performed. Other options are controlling the enteric contamination, washing the cavity extensively and proceeding with the repair, even using PTFE.[177]

Iliac vein injuries are difficult to expose. The vein may be compressed with fingers or sponge sticks for immediate control and injury assessment. Some authors recommend temporary division of the iliac artery to gain access to the vein; every attempt should be made to carefully dissect and retract the artery before adding an additional anastomosis and increasing ischemia. One should recall that to better mobilize the common iliac artery, the internal iliac artery may be divided and not repaired. Repairs are done by lateral venorrhaphy with a technique to avoid narrowing the vein. Ligation may be performed and we have had some personal success with this without devastating ipsilateral venous insufficiency. Survival from iliac injuries also ranges at 60%.[176,179]

Portal–Retrohepatic Area

Hematoma or hemorrhage in the portal area may indicate injury to the portal vein, hepatic artery, or common bile duct. If a hematoma is present with no active hemorrhage, proximal and distal control of the porta hepatis is obtained with vascular clamps. If there is active hemorrhage finger compression (Pringle maneuver) is applied until the anatomy is clear enough for vascular clamps to be applied. Once control is obtained, the structures are carefully dissected and inspected.

Hepatic artery injuries may be repaired with lateral arteriorrhaphy or may be ligated if beyond the origin of the gastroduodenal artery. If the right hepatic artery is ligated, a cholecystectomy must be performed as this represents interruption of the end artery to the gall bladder. Reconstruction is usually not performed because of the severity of associated injuries to the liver and surrounding organs. Intrahepatic arterial bleeding is likewise controlled with hepatic artery ligation or embolization. There remains sufficient oxygen in the portal system to prevent hepatic ischemia.[180,181]

Portal vein injuries in the hepatoduodenal ligament are approached in the same fashion as the hepatic artery injuries. The structures of the porta hepatis are dissected carefully and isolated. An extensive Kocher maneuver with mobilization of the common bile duct to the left and the cystic duct superior allows visualization of the suprapancreatic and posterior portal vein.

Retropancreatic portal vein injuries are difficult to isolate. An extensive Kocher maneuver is performed. The same avascular plane that determines resectability in malignancy is exploited for control. This space is developed between the pancreatic head and the portal vein gingerly with a clamp and then the pancreas is divided between two clamps or with a stapler device. Small injuries may be repaired primary with lateral venorrhaphy after applying a partially occluding vascular clamp. The repair is performed with a 4-0 or 5-0 polypropylene suture. More extensive injuries must be repaired by tension-free end-to-end anastomosis, and prostheses have been employed.[182] Many of the newer techniques are borrowed from transplantation and include interposition venous grafting or PTFE.[183–185]

If the patient is unstable with an extensive injury to the portal vein ligation should be an option. The ends of the portal vein are oversewn with a nonabsorbable suture. Hypovolemia as seen with SMV ligation mandates aggressive resuscitation because of the splanchnic fluid sequestration. The abdomen needs to be vacuum packed as a result of the intestinal edema and for a second-look in 24 to 48 hours to evaluate the viability of the bowel.

Ligation to the portal vein and the hepatic artery is not compatible with life. This is a situation where reconstruction of the portal vein should be performed. The reconstruction may be done with a saphenous vein graft. Injury to lobar branches of the portal vein and hepatic artery will create an ischemic lobe which can be resected "electively" at second look.

Hematoma or hemorrhage in the retrohepatic area may indicate injury to the retrohepatic vena cava, a hepatic vein or renal vessel. Injuries to the IVC in this area challenge the surgeon and have a high mortality rate. The challenge is to avoid opening a stable and self-tamponaded injury, even from a penetrating injury. Such "nonoperative" treatment may prevent likely loss of control and exsanguniation in exchange for the potential of delayed complications. Damage control dogma strongly supports this train of thought. Nonexpanding and contained retrohepatic hematomas should be packed with laparotomy pads and a second look performed in 24 to 48 hours.

If the hematoma is expanding or ruptured with massive venous bleeding, a temporizing procedure is to compress the liver posteriorly and the Pringle maneuver is applied. The surgical team, anesthesiologist, and the blood bank are notified for a massive transfusion. Gaining access to and controlling these retrohepatic caval injuries is intense. The surgeon must bring to bear every potential resource to stop the bleeding.

If available, endovascular or interventional techniques using occlusive balloon catheters within the cava, aorta, or both, can isolate the injury and avoid further blood loss,[136] a second incision/thoracotomy and ensuing coagulopathies.[186] Similarly, there is no dishonor in asking for the surgical expertise of hepatic and/or transplant surgeons who may be available for this infrequent injury. Unfortunately, both of these call for resources which may not be readily available.

To visualize and repair retro hepatic injuries, the liver is mobilized by incising the triangular and anterior coronary ligaments and rotating the liver anteriorly and medially. Once rotated, if the wound is visible, it can quickly be controlled by grasping with forceps or an Allis clamp. It may be possible then for a Satinsky clamp to be applied for definitive control. If one is unable to visualize the wound because of massive hemorrhage, it is unlikely to be better on multiple attempts and another technique must be tried.

The atriocaval shunt was described by Schrock in 1968. The shunt traverses the hepatic veins and is positioned after sternotomy, right atriotomy, and passage of the shunt (either an endotracheal tube or chest thoracosotmy tube) is positioned across the injury. Further control is established with Rommel ties at the diaphragm and suprarenally on the cava to force blood through the shunt. This is is technically challenging, two teams are needed and basically mentioned only for historical interest. Today, hepatic vascular isolation with a Pringle maneuver and infrahepatic and suprahepatic caval clamping is borrowed from elective hepatic surgery and is more likely to be known to the surgeon. The last approach is direct transhepatic approach by transecting the liver to expose the injury. Damage control and packing the liver may be an option for limited injuries.

Repairs of the vena cava are done with continuous 4-0 polypropylene sutures. Roughly one-third of retrohepatic caval injuries survive operation.

Damage Control

The "damage control" laparotomy is part of every trauma surgeon's armamentarium. Although a historical tenet that was buried beneath surgical hubris as bigger and longer operations were technically possible, it was concisely modernized and codified by Rotondo.[15] The focus is no longer on definitive repair at any cost and/or in one sitting, but on the physiologic status of the patient. Rotondo[15] defined "damage control" as:

1. Initial control of hemorrhage and contamination.
2. Intraperitoneal packing and rapid closure, allowing for aggressive resuscitation in the intensive care unit.
3. Subsequent definitive reexploration.

In "damage control," intestinal reanastomosis may be delayed until reexploration. Arterial injuries may be shunted and extensive venous injuries packed or ligated. Any diffuse retroperitoneal or pelvic bleeding may be tightly packed. The patient is resuscitated in the intensive care unit and returns to the operating room after acidosis, hypothermia, and coagulopathy are returned to normal (24–48 hours). During this resuscitation, adjusts such as embolization if solid organs or end arteries may be employed to help vascular control.[187]

Angiography and embolization is also an adjunct to nonoperative therapy for solid organ injuries- primarily liver and spleen. Avoiding the additional physiologic stress of laparotomy is beneficial not only in the isolated injury but the multiply injured patient. There is a unique set of complications that may arise hepatic or splenic necrosis are the most obvious and can lead to bile leaks, infections, persistent fevers, and pelvic effusions which must factor into the decision in utilizing these modalities.[188]

Angiography is also used for pelvic bleeding. With the aggressive and ubiquitous use of CT scanning, arterial pelvic bleeding is readily diagnosed. Pelvic stabilization is accomplished by a simple pelvic binder or tying a sheet around the pelvis between the anterior superior iliac crests and greater trochanters. Arterial bleeding is very amenable to embolization.[189]

● PERIPHERAL VASCULAR INJURIES

Vascular trauma in the extremities results from both penetrating and blunt injuries, although in today's violent society, young men with penetrating trauma constitute the vast majority of injuries. The most common clinical presentation is acute limb ischemia and the most common injuries are complete transections and partial lacerations from penetrating wounds. Although peripheral vascular injuries are more common in upper extremities in civilian trauma patients, the same are seen more frequently in the lower extremities among the military patients.

The historical context of peripheral vascular trauma is notable for the fact that only recently has there been the surgical environment to allow primary repair. The classic history until the late 20th century was of nonoperative therapy for injuries that did not require immediate ligation and allow the natural history of such wounds to progress to aneurysm, AVF, or gangrene.

Complete transections usually allow the vessel to retract and the normal hemostatic events to occur with vasoconstriction and initial thrombus formation. The hallmark is loss of distal pulses. Partial lacerations may be insidious and present as an ischemic limb because of an occlusion by dissection or distal thrombus. Blunt trauma as well as low velocity gunshot wounds and stab wounds are associated with acute ischemia; on the other hand, high-velocity missiles or crushing mechanisms cause massive soft tissue loss around the injured vessel and eliminate the tamponade effect of these investing structures, thus increase the chance of extensive, but obvious external bleeding.

There have always been vascular injuries associated with blunt mechanisms. Today, with the array of diagnostic and therapeutic options available, there is an ever-improving limb salvage rate—again the limiting factor is always duration of ischemia. With the concomitant increase in invasive diagnostic and therapeutic procedures, there has been an expected rise in vascular complications from interventional coronary procedures, elective endovascular, and angiographic approaches and long tern venous access. Such events rarely present with the same threatening manner as acute trauma, although there are cases in which limb survival and even patient survival are at risk.

Diagnosis

Prehospital information is a very important in extremity vascular trauma. When a complete vessel transection occurs, the initial bleeding is brisk and pulsatile until vascular contraction and initial thrombus occur. Thrombus formation is also enhanced by the ensuing lower blood pressure. After resuscitation with adequate volume expansion and restoration of a normal blood pressure, rebleeding may occur if this key clue to a major extremity vascular injury was overlooked. During history taking, details from emergency medical personnel or bystanders about on-scene active arterial bleeding, the amount quality, and color should be elicited.

Secondly, the timing of injury is paramount, especially when the limb shows signs of ischemia. Presence or absence of pulse at the injury scene and information about associated injury to muscles, tendons, bones, and nerves can help differentiate a primary injury to these structures versus a progression of the ischemic process. Although muscle is moderately tolerant of ischemia, delays greater than 6 hours portend limb loss. Any delay increases the risks of ischemia, its sequelae, as well as reperfusion injury and the devastating effects of compartment syndrome.

After the primary survey is completed, bleeding is stopped and resuscitation is ongoing, the secondary physical examination focuses on the injured extremity. Bleeding which was identified early and controlled with direct pressure or clamping, is examined to determine where best to restore blood flow and how to get this accomplished as quickly as possible. Again, the best place for an actively bleeding vascular injury is the operating room. Fortunately, today's modern operative suites are amenable to radiological or endovascular procedures and the administrative personnel must be made aware of the need for those specialized services at any time.[190]

The clinical manifestations of ischemia are remembered by rote as the 5 P's: Pain, Paralysis, Paresthesia, Pallor, and Pulselessness. The pain of ischemia is excruciating, especially for the naïve extremity. Therefore, pain out of proportion to physical findings is the indicator of a vascular injury until proven wrong. In the unconscious or neuromuscularly blocked patients, these signs cannot be elicited and the surgeon must default to demonstrating that there is not an injury. The demonstration by the physical examination is sufficient to rule out a significant vascular injury. Conversely, any deviation from the normal examination must be investigated. Of note pallor is a very nonspecific signs that is present when patient is hypothermic or the extremity is exposed during transport. Comparison to the contralateral side helps isolate specific findings from global events.

Physical examination is not only important in the diagnosis but also in the management. A comprehensive examination also helps to carry out the decision about the futility of the arterial repair in an extremity that has no neurologic function or is unusable because of significant soft tissue or bone loss. Specific scoring systems have been developed to assist in determining when an ablative procedure is the best choice—Mangled extremity score (MESS) and the Gustillo classification are a few of the better known and validated systems.[191–193] Although scoring systems are present, each case must be individualized, especially if amputation is considered primarily.[194] Another simple example of employing physical examination for deciding on repair is the identification of a good palmar flow using Allen test in a setting of ulnar or radial artery injury. If there is a sufficient collateral flow, further revascularization offers no gain but risks surgical complications.

In such cases of combined trauma, vascular repair should be accomplished quickly, even if temporized by shunting, before skeletal repair. Avoiding ischemia and preventing further reperfusion injury allows the limb to survive immediately, and before the full effects of the injury are known on nervous injury and functional outcome. If revasculatization cannot be accomplished, then no further intervention other than amputation is needed.[195,196]

There are associated injuries that should raise the likelihood of a specific arterial injury: Fracture–dislocation of the posterior portion of the first rib and subclavian artery injury, brachial plexus and subclavian artery or vein injury with neck hyperextension, brachial artery injuries and supracondylar fractures of the humerus, and knee dislocation and popliteal artery injury. Since knee dislocation has been associated to popliteal artery injury, arteriogram of the involved extremity had been a common practice. A recent study has shown that the mere presence of a palpable pulse distal to the extremity can obviate arteriography, an examination though very useful has its own set of complications and may delay further treatment of other injuries in a setting where time is a critical matter.[197]

Classically, any extremity vascular injury has been described to have either hard signs, meaning a finding that demands immediate exploration or soft signs, a finding that requires investigation. Hard signs include external bleeding, a pulseless limb distal to the injury, distal ischemia and a pulsatile hematoma. Soft signs are location of the injury and its proximity to a large vessel, the presence of a decreased or diminished distal pulses as well as associated hypotension.

In the extremities and in contrast to vascular injury of the chest and abdomen, the history and physical examination can locate the injured vessel and the level of the injury in the majority of the cases. Inspection alone offers a good assessment of the location of the injury, sites of the injury, presence of active bleeding, expanding hematoma and distal pallor. When possible, the patient should move the involved extremity voluntarily to rule out paralysis. Palpation also assesses the patient for paresthesias and numbness. Numbness portends early ischemic complications, a "hard" sign that should urge an immediate restoration of blood flow before paralysis occurs; a sign that usually indicate irreversible ischemia.

Auscultation helps the examiner identify the presence of a pseudoaneurysm or AVF by hearing a bruit or feeling a thrill. Auscultation via ultrasound is usually sufficient to identify the acute signs of ischemia through the ankle–brachial index (ABI). Briefly, the distal systolic Doppler pressure of the extremity is measured and divided by the brachial systolic pressure of the uninjured extremity. An ABI less than 1.0 (0.9) is indicative of arterial injury and should prompt further diagnostic investigation. Again, comparison to the opposite extremity can help distinguish preexisting vascular insufficiency as its prevalence becomes greater in our aging population.

The ABI is also important to monitor the status of the distal circulation over time in patients with life-threatening injuries in other body areas that require operative intervention (craniotomy, thoracotomy, or laparotomy) or in patients who are too unstable to undergo exploration of the arterial system. As in blunt traumatic knee dislocation, physical examination alone has been considered as a replacement for arteriography in penetrating extremity injury to rule out vascular injury. Frykberg et al.[39] found it to be a very reliable way to exclude vascular injury with a diagnostic accuracy of 99.5% and a false negative rate of only 0.8%. Gonzalez and Falimirski[198] reported an equivalent result with a diagnostic accuracy of 98.7% in 460 patients. Using only the presence or absence of hard signs should be used as a reliable method to avoid delays in treatment and reduce the cost of any further diagnostic testing especially in a critically injured trauma patient.

Noninvasive methods have been reportedly employed in the evaluation of trauma using the standard arterial pressure ratio between normal pressure and extremity pressure the ratio can help determine if a arterial injury is present or absent. Unfortunately the use of Doppler offers no therapeutic benefit and only helps to determine if further testing is necessary. The use of duplex ultrasonography that is real time mode scanning with pulse Doppler flow indication can determine the velocity spectra in that vessel. These color flow images of an area of injury can also be used as a screen for trauma; however, the same caveats apply and require a highly sophisticated technician and machine.

Therapy

As the era of endovascular surgery blossoms the use of angiography with both diagnostic and therapeutic effects is present. It is likely that this will replace virtually every other mode both of confirming diagnosis and therapeutic intervention. Addressing extremity vascular injuries is similar to any other injury. The area of injury is localized; control of inflow and outflow is obtained. The injury may be repaired, patched, bridged with an interposition graft, or ligated. Unique to extremity injuries is the addition of thrombectomy to assure outflow, and the instillation of heparin into the distal vessels to prevent further thrombosis while the repair is affected.

Completion Angiography/Ultrasonography

After completion of an extremity vascular repair it is paramount to document flow by either a completion angiogram, or demonstration of adequate flow by ultrasound. The large conducting vessels in the chest and abdomen rarely clot, but the supply vessels of the extremities are prone to spasm, embolism, and thrombosis. Embolectomy is a crucial part of restoring peripheral flow, and completion arteriography documents patent vessels or directs further therapy to reestablish flow.[199]

● VENOUS INJURY

Venous injuries usually present as dark nonpulsatile bleeding if the wound is open or more commonly as hematoma or contusion. Venous injury is usually contained by the surrounding tissue because of the low pressure in the venous system. There may be associated arterial injuries and then the venous injury is diagnosed at the time of exploration. The superficial femoral vein is the most commonly injured major vein and the popliteal vein is the second most common.[200] In the thigh when blunt injury has created venous bleeding, hypotension might occur even before a large size hematoma becomes clinically apparent. Ecchymosis, abrasions, and thigh deformity may be the only clue for the diagnosis.

● COMPARTMENT SYNDROME

Compartment syndrome can occur with any traumatic injury to the extremity. The compartment syndrome may arise from the initial injury from ischemia from a vascular injury from thrombosis form a venous injury or from reperfusion injury after flow is reestablished. A high index of suspicion must be maintained at all times for the development of this syndrome,[201] but uniform fasciotomy for any arterial injury is not indicated.[202]

The pathophysiology has been well established but in simplistic terms a vicious cycle of injury leading to edema leading to increase compartment pressure is leading to further ischemia and further injury and edema eventually leads to the cessation of oxygenated blood getting in tissues.[203] This can occur in the face of all of the above mentioned injuries; it often occurs when there are palpable pulses present as the injury occurs primarily from obstruction of venous capillary flow. Treatment involves releasing the containing structures of the particular compartment. Compartment injury should be assumed in all injuries and fasciotomy should be preformed virtually when ever the diagnosis is entertained on physical findings, or when the patient is unable to describe symptoms.

The use of compartment pressure monitors confirms the clinical suspicion. An elevated pressure with 20 mm Hg of the diastolic pressure or 20 mm Hg below mean arterial pressure is the lower limit for threatened limb ischemia and should provoke fasciotomy.[204]

Fasciotomy is performed most commonly through two incisions—one medially and one laterally to open all four compartments—the lateral incision made parallel to the fibula and a fingerbreadth anteriorly opens the anterior and lateral compartments. The medial incision made parallel to the tibia and a fingerbreadth posteriorly to the bony edge is used to open the deep and superficial posterior compartments. The lateral incision and fasciotomy must avoid the peroneal nerve as it passes the fibular neck. Liberal and expedient fasciotomy is limb saving.[201,205]

FEMORAL INJURIES

The femoral artery is the most frequently injured extremity artery.[206,207] Roughly one-third of the time there is an associated venous injury and a quarter of the time an associated nervous injury. The frequency of the femoral site likely is increased by its frequency for an access site for diagnostic and endovascular and cardiovascular procedures. For most of history a femoral arterial wound was fatal, or lead to the development of AVF. The older literature is replete with the diagnosis and care of AVF (i.e., ligation), today's leading cause is iatrogenic and the repair involves both artery and vein.[11,208,209]

As with other vascular injuries, an unstable patient is best evaluated, resuscitated and repaired in the operating room. Germane to extremity trauma, is the complete exposure of the entire limb, not only for evaluation of distal pulses, but the harvest of potential endogenous conduits, and thrombectomy and fasciotomy. Prepping another source of autogenous vein is always helpful—usually the uninjured contralateral limb. Direct pressure is the best method for control until proximal and distal exposure and vascular clamping can be effected. The most common incision is the longitudinal groin and thigh incision directly over the course of the femoral artery.

Once control is gained, and in the groin this may require exposure above the inguinal ligament, which can be divided for just such a need. Distally the profunda femoris as well as the superficial femoral artery require control. If more proximal control is needed, a retroperitoneal approach to the external iliac artery can be made through a separate oblique incision in the flank.

After gaining proximal and distal control, repair is affected. Because of the mobility available form proximal and distal dissection, sufficient length can be gained for primary end-to-end anastomosis frequently. About as frequently, interposition grafting is performed to avoid tension, using saphenous vein harvested distally from the same extremity, or from the uninjured limb.[210]

Iatrogenic hematomas are frequent with the number of femoral lines and with its prominence as an access for most invasive radiologic and cardiac procedures. A hematoma or leak may spread out of sight into the retroperitoneum. Similarly, AVF may be created and require repair. A good repair without impinging on the caliber of the lumen of the artery and vein is necessary, and may require a patch to avoid narrowing the lumen(s). Interposing tissue between the vessels protects the fistula from reoccurring. AVF in this region are amenable to endovascular intervention.[211–213]

POPLITEAL INJURIES

The popliteal artery is the only vessel to the shank and must be preserved if the calf and foot are to be salvaged. Severe blunt injuries or wartime injuries may mangle the limb, destroy bone and nerves which lead to amputation. Most penetrating injuries are reconstructable and the limb salvageable.[214] Anticoagulation after repair of popliteal injuries is beneficial.[215]

Popliteal injuries arise from both mechanisms, but concern arises with posterior knee dislocations, which may relocate spontaneously or be relocated without continued vigilance of the popliteal artery. While angiography is not universally indicated, aggressive monitoring of the physical examination is needed. Missed injuries may result in AVF.[216] Currently, repair is performed via endovascular techniques if at all possible.[217]

Exploration of the popliteal fossa is begun by a sigmoid incision with a transverse arm across the back of the knee to avoid a debilitating contracture. Virtually repair is always by interposition grafting and vein is the conduit of choice in this location.[218] When there are combined venous and arterial injuries, outcomes are improved if both vessels are repaired.[219] Vascular inflow should be established first in combined orthopedic and vascular injuries, even if it is temporary.[220]

DISTAL LOWER EXTREMITY INJURIES

Injuries to the distal lower extremity vessels are controversial as there is little new literature to guide decision making.[221,222] Liberal use of angiography is paramount. Whereas the anatomy is often variable, the operative decision making has been as well. The demonstration of sufficient collateral flow is important is deciding which distal vessel to target. Simply, the peroneal is insufficient to assure limb salvage. If there is an isolated injury to one of the three vessels ligation is acceptable. If there is injury to the anterior tibial or posterior tibial, or both, reconstruction should be performed. If all three vessels are injured, reconstruction to either the anterior or posterior tibial artery is needed. Most reconstructions will be extra-anatomic, and vein, harvested from the uninjured limb is used. Again, any mechanism, including surgical misadventures can cause injury.[223]

SUMMARY

An evidence based summary of lower extremity arterial and venous injuries has been completed by the EAST in the practice guideline format.[224,225] While a lot of that literature has been referred to in the above paragraphs, the assessment of the data following rigorous review is best summarized in that there is no overwhelming scientific support (i.e., a Level 1 recommendation) for the diagnosis and management of such injuries.

AXILLARY AND BRACHIAL INJURIES

Axillary artery injuries are infrequent, but complex because of associated injuries of the brachial plexus. Repair follows the same principles and salvage rates are high.[226] Brachial injuries are the most common site of injury in the upper extremity, accounting for approximately half of all injuries seen in penetrating wounds, and the majority of iatrogenic injuries requiring intervention. Although there are collaterals, the majority of brachial artery injuries are easy to diagnose by ischemia and pulselessness. Repair is necessary and end-to-end anastomosis or vein interpositions are preferred. The median nerve is intimately associated with the artery and must be inspected for injury. Care must be taken to avoid the nerve during operative exposure. Ligation results in an unacceptable high rate of amputation.[4] Endovascular repair is well known and very successful.[227,228]

DISTAL UPPER EXTREMITY INJURIES

Radial and ulna artery injury rates are poorly known, probably because of the ability to ligate either the radial or ulnar artery after demonstrating adequate collateral flow from the other vessel. Repair is indicated if there is insufficient flow or both vessels are injured vide infra shank injuries and the military history of amputation with combined injuries.[4]

Radial arteries are cannulated almost with impunity and complications are infrequent. Radial artery thrombosis likely fails to manifest symptoms unless there is inadequate flow through the ulnar connection to the palmar arch. Ischemia after arterial line placement is generally cured by removal of the line. If this is unsuccessful, anticoagulation and arteriography are performed. AVF aneurysms form commonly and can be treated by ligation.

VENOUS INJURY

Venous injury in the extremities is most often associated with arterial injury, and often of small clinical consequence as history has supported ligation as an acceptable clinical course, and complications are infrequent, however, in the stable patients there is benefit to repair.[224] Hemodynamically compromised patients should under ligation as the expedient procedure. Several locations should mandate attempt at venous repair—especially femoral and politeal to avoid not only limb loss but long tern venous insufficiency. Even a repair with thromboses days later is not met

when the same concerns. Overall patience for venous repair is 60%.[229] Patients with venous repair have less edema, and most repairs remain patent after a modest initial failure rate.[230,231] Concerns over thromboembolism are unfounded.

ENDOVASCULAR CONSIDERATIONS

Therapeutic Interventions

The first description about the use of intraluminal prosthesis in humans by Parodi et al.[232] was for degenerative aortic disease. The first stents used in these situations were made out of Dacron and since then a number of alternatives are available for the current management of vascular pathology.[232] Marked improvements in technique and equipment have allowed the introduction of such interventions to the care of the trauma patient. There are a number of case reports on the treatment of iatrogenic or traumatic vascular lesions, namely pseudoaneurysms, AVFs, arterial ruptures, perforations, and occlusions.[233–238]

Vascular trauma has increased over the past decade, either in the form of arterial or venous and generally results from complications of interventional procedures and civilian or military blunt or penetrating injuries. Trauma is now the third leading cause of death and the No. 1 killer of people younger than 45 years. Vascular injuries compromise 3% of all civilian traumas[239] and penetrating trauma accounts for approximately 90% of arterial injuries.[233] Reuben et al.[240] identified an overall utilization of endovascular procedures in over 12,000 vascular injuries in a 9-year interval nationwide retrospective study of 2.2%. Newer diagnostic and therapeutic modalities improve patient outcome, but arteriography remains the diagnostic study of choice and operative intervention is still considered the gold standard for vascular trauma until more data is obtained from endovascular approaches.

Trauma patients frequently have multiple injuries which may compromise routine vascular repairs. Endovascular stent–graft placement offers a new and less invasive technique for the treatment of acute traumatic vascular injuries.[233] It has the advantages that it can be performed under local anesthesia, is well tolerated by the patient, and is associated with a shorter hospitalization time than that of surgery.[234] This less invasive method seems to be associated with less blood loss and requirement for anesthesia. If successfully applied, the endovascular approach offers the advantage of simplicity and decreased operative time[238,241] which in the severely traumatized patient with risks of coagulopathy, acidosis, and hypothermia or in the patient with multiple comorbidities seems to be a reasonable option. The endovascular approach allows arteriography at the same intervention, adding diagnostic advantages over an open procedure. It allows embolization of active bleeding vessels (i.e., pelvic fractures) and to obtain proximal.[239]

As any other intervention, the endovascular procedures carry their own risks and complications such as stent

---

TABLE 49-2. Indications for Endovascular Technique

Inaccesibility of the vascular lesion (central vessel involvement)

Contaminated field (access site remote from injured area)

Anatomic distortion creating venous hypertension with excessive bleeding

Severe medical comorbidities

---

deformation and kinking, difficult access, thrombosis, loss of vessel branches after placement, and the formation of intimal hyperplasia at the junction of the artery and the stent–graft. The Palmaz stent has been associated with only minimal inflammatory reaction and hyperplasia.[235,237,239,244] A serious and often lethal complication associated with endovascular procedures is the potential microembolization of aneurysmal contents[239] but seldom reported in trauma patients.

It has been approximately 30 years since an endovascular technique to control traumatic hemorrhage was first described and such should be an essential part of vascular trauma management, but yet is rarely considered as part of frontline management for vascular trauma.[242] Endoluminal approaches may be beneficial in those circumstances in which operative therapy may be limited (Table 49-2).

Patients with vascular trauma who present with hemodynamic instability, signs of active bleeding or ischemia (hard signs of vascular injury) should have operative intervention. Patients who have endovascular repairs tend to have higher revised trauma scores implying better hemodynamic stability.[240] At present, surgery is considered the gold standard approach and is not until enough level one data has been published about the safety and efficacy of endovascular techniques to recommend it as initial management for vascular injuries.

Several endovascular device options are available for the treatment of an injured vessel.[239,244,245] The most common used device is a self expandable stent rendered nonporous with an outer covering which can be Dacron, PTFE, vein (saphenous or jugular), or other material. The composition of the covering does not appear to make a difference in outcome.[246] The most widely used stents for vascular injury are the Palmaz stent, Corvita stent–graft, Wallgraft, and the Hemobahn graft. Heparin is used during insertion but the use of long term anticoagulation is not needed[239] although some advocate the use of clopidogrel for a short period of time postoperatively and acetylsalicylic acid for life.[234]

The efficacy of endovascular therapies for cerebrovascular injuries remains unclear. While there is a clear role of endovascular coiling for intracranial aneurysms[242] its role in trauma is still experimental.[248] Case reports had been published in the setting of closed head injury.[249,250]

One of the areas in which endovascular interventions have been widely applied is in penetrating or blunt cervi-

cal trauma. Internal carotid injuries may complicate percutaneous procedures as central line or hemodyalisis access placement. Even asymptomatic lesions pose a significant risk of stroke or hemorrhage warranting their treatment[251] and stent or graft placement is gaining acceptance for this purpose. Dissections, intimal hyperplasias and specially AVFs of the carotid or vertebral arteries and jugular veins have been successfully treated with this approach and its use is of great significance when the lesions are near the skull base allowing the surgeon to avoid mandible disarticulation.[81,239,252–257]

Thoracic outlet injuries may be associated with subclavian and axillary vessels, innominate artery and brachiocephalic injuries all of which have been successfully controlled with coiling and stents.[102,233,239,258–260] Mechanism of injury may include penetrating trauma, compression with contusion, avulsion and traction form rotational stress. The incisions used to approach and repair such vessels require clavicular resection, sternotomy or thoracotomy and each one of them may be associated with increased morbidity[239,241] which may be avoided with a percutaneous approach. The technical success reported for endovascular stent–graft repair of axillary or subclavian artery injury is 94%.[261]

Cardiac catheterization may be complicated with coronary artery injury such as dissections and perforations. The placement of covered stents has been described and allows treatment of those iatrogenic injuries during the same procedure decreasing the need for additional anesthesia or additional operative interventions.[262,263]

Aortic stent–grafts are frequently used for aneurysms, ulcers and fistulas but may be indicated in the posttraumatic aortic rupture or descending dissections following trauma.[264,265] The initial management of the latter is medical control of the blood pressure with nitrates or beta blockers, but the option of endovascular repair must be entertained specially in patients who are poor surgical candidates. Description of the use of aortic extender cuffs emergently or electively for the treatment of blunt (stenosis, pseudoaneuysms)[266] and penetrating abdominal aortic trauma (aortocaval fistulas) have been described.[267] Injuries to other intraabdominal vessels (renal, portal vein, IVC) or active bleeding from solid organs (spleen, liver) using this technique is reported elsewhere.[268–271]

The use of endovascular techniques for peripheral trauma has increased as consequence of the rising percutaneous diagnostic and therapeutic invasive procedures. Vascular access for cardiac catheterization accounts for the vast majority of the case reports in the literature. The relative occurrence and severity of iatrogenic arterial injury compared with those of penetrating and blunt vascular trauma is unknown.[11] Covered stents are preferred for major peripheral vascular injuries but the use of Dacron plugs and embolization has been use with successful outcomes.[211] The most common site for iatrogenic vascular injury seen is in the femoral artery (58%)[43] but iliac vessels[272] and popliteal

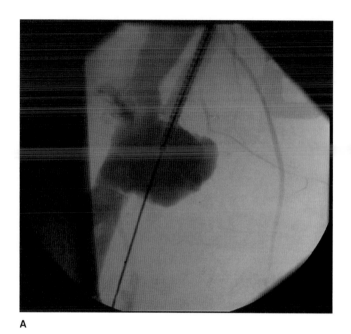

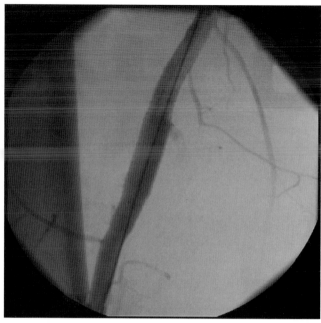

A

B

● **FIGURE 49-6.** Arteriograms of a traumatic lower extremity AVF after a gunshot wound to the thigh. (A) The guidewire is seen in the superficial femoral artery and contrast filling the femoral vein. (B) In the same patient a covered Viabahn stent is placed to exclude femoral vessel traumatic AVF.

Images courtesy of Dr. Scott Stevens from University of Tennessee Medical Center, Knoxville.

lesions[217,273] are also seen and they can be repaired with endoprocedures in appropriately selected patients (Figure 49-6).

The most common application for endovascular therapy in the trauma patient is in the setting of pelvic fractures with active extravasation. Frequently used for coiling of hypogastric artery branches in polytraumatized patients who are not candidates for operative intervention providing a minimally invasive therapeutic option to control potential life-threatening hemorrhage.[274–276]

REFERENCES

1. Samuel C. The practice of surgery. http://www.sonofthesouth. net/leefoundation/amputation.htm. Accessed November 20, 2006.

2. Samuel D. Gross. A manual of military surgery. http://jdc.jefferson.edu/milsurgusa/. Accessed November 20, 2006.

3. Makins GH. *On Gunshot wounds to the Blood Vessels*. Bristol, England: John Wright and Sons; 1919.

4. DeBakey ME, Simeone FA. Battle injuries of the arteries in World War II: an analysis of 2471 cases. *Ann Surg*. 1946; 123:534-579.

5. Janhke EJ Jr, Howard JM. Primary repair of major arterial injuries. *Arch Surg*. 1953;66:646-649.

6. Hughes CW. Acute vascular trauma in Korean War causalities. An analysis of 180 cases. *Surg Gynecol Obstet*. 1954;99:91-100.

7. Rich NM, Baugh JH, Hughes CW. Acute arterial injuries in Vietnam: 1000 cases. *J Trauma*. 1970;10:359-367.

8. Mattox KL, Feliciano DV, Burch J, et al. 5760 cardiovascular injuries in 4459 patients: epidemiologic evolution 1958–1987. *Ann Surg*. 1989;209:698-705.

9. Rich NM, Hobson RW II, Fedde CW. Vascular trauma secondary to diagnostic and therapeutic procedures. *Am J Surg*. 1974;128:715-722.

10. Younkey JR, Clagett GP, Rich NM, et al. Vascular trauma secondary to diagnostic and therapeutic procedures.: 1974 to 1982. *Am J Surg*. 1983;146:788-795.

11. Giswold ME, Landry GJ, Taylor LM, et al. Iatrogenic arterial injury is an increasingly important cause of arterial trauma. *Am J Surg*. 2004;187(5):590-592.

12. Bickell WH, Wall MJ, Pepe PE, et al. Immediate versus delayed fluid resuscitation for hypotensive patients with penetrating torso injuries. *New Engl J Med*. 1994;331:1105-1109.

13. Tischerman SA, Barie P, Bokhari F, et al. Clinical practice guideline: endpoints of resuscitation. *J Trauma*. 2004;57: 898-912.

14. Kaplan LJ, Kellum JA. Initial pH, base deficit, lactate, anion gap, strong ion difference, and strong ion gap predict outcome from major vascular injury. *Crit Care Med*. 2004;32 (5):1120-1124.

15. Rotondo MF, Schwab CW, Mcgonigal MD, et al. Damage

control: an approach for improved survival in exsanguinating penetrating abdominal injury. *J Trauma*. 1993;35(3):375-383.

16. Arthurs Z, Cuadrado D, Beekley A, et al. The impact of hypothermia on trauma care at the 31st Combat Support Hospital. *Am J Surg*. 2006;191(5):610-614.

17. Fox CJ, Gilespie DL, O'Donnell SD, et al. Contemporary management of wartime vascular trauma. *J Vasc Surg*. 2005; 41(4):638-644.

18. Symbas PN, Sherman AJ, Silver JM, et al. Traumatic rupture of the aorta: immediate or delayed repair? *Ann Surg*. 2002; 235(6):796-802.

19. Santaniello JM, Miller PR, Croce MA, et al. Blunt aortic injury with concomitant intra-abdominal solid organ injury: treatment priorities revisited. *J Trauma*. 2002;53(3):442-445; discussion 445.

20. Simeone A, Freitas M, Frankel HL. Management options in blunt aortic injury: a case series and literature review. *Am Surg*. 2006;72(1):25-30.

21. Nzewi O, Dkight RD, Zamvar V. Management of blunt thoracic aortic injury. *Eur J Vasc Endovasc Surg*. 2006;31(1):18-27.

22. Dyer DS, Moore EE, Ilke DN, et al. Thoracic aortic injury: how predictive is mechanism and is chest computed tomography a reliable screening tool? A prospective study of 1561 patients. *J Trauma*. 2000;48:673-682.

23. Fabian TC, Davis KA, Gavant ML, et al. Prospective study of blunt aortic injury: helical CT is diagnostic and antihypertensive therapy reduced rupture. *Ann Surg*. 1998;227:666-676.

24. Wicky S, Capasso P, Meuli R, et al. Spiral CT aortography: an efficient technique for the diagnosis of traumatic aortic injury. *Eur Radiol*. 1998;8:828-833.

25. Fabian TC, Richardson JD, Croce MA, et al. Prospective study of blunt aortic injury: multicenter trial of the American association for the surgery of trauma. *J Trauma*. 1997;42:374-380.

26. Biquet JF, Dondelinger RF, Roland D. Computed tomography of thoracic aortic trauma. *Eur Radiol*. 1996;6:25-29.

27. Carter Y, Meissner M, Bulger E, et al. Anatomical considerations in the surgical management of blunt thoracic aortic injury. *J Vasc Surg*. 2001;34(4):628-633.

28. Krish MM, Sloan M. Blunt chest trauma. *General Principles of Vascular Management*. Little, Brown; 1977.

29. Trupka A, Waydhas C, Hallfeldt KK, et al. Value of computed tomography in the first assessment of severely injured patients with blunt chest trauma: results of a prospective study. *J Trauma*. 1977;43(3):405-411.

30. Hirose H, Gill IS, Malangoni MA. Nonoperative management of traumatic aortic injury. *J Trauma*. 2006;60(3):597-601.

31. Berthet JP, Marty-Ane CH, Veerapen R, et al. Dissection of the abdominal aorta in blunt trauma; endovascular or conventional surgical management. *J Vas Surg*. 2003;38(5):997–1003; discussion 1004.

32. Lawlor DK, Ott M, Forbes TL, et al. Endovascular management of traumatic thoracic aortic injuries. *Can J Surg*. 2005;48(4):293-297.

33. Ott MC, Stewart TC, Lawlor DK, et al. Management of blunt thoracic aortic injuries: endovascular stents versus open repair. *J Trauma*. 2004;56(3):565-570.

34. Amabile P, Collart F, Gariboldi V, et al. Surgical versus endovascular treatment of traumatic thoracic aortic rupture. *J Vas Surg*. 2004;40(5):873-879.

35. Lebl DR, Dicker RA, Spain DA, et al. Dramatic shift in the primary management of traumatic thoracic aortic rupture. *Arch Surg*. 2006;141(2):177-180.

36. Miller PR, Kortesis BG, McLaughlin CA, et al. Complex blunt aortic injury or repair: beneficial effects of cardiopulmonary bypass use. *Ann Surg*. 2003;237(6):877-883; discussion 883-884.

37. Cook J, Salerno C, Krishnadasan B, et al. The effect of changing presentation and management on the outcome of blunt rupture of the thoracic aorta. *J Thorac Cardiovasc Surg*. 2006;131(3):594-600.

38. Langanay T, Verhoye JP, Corbineau H, et al. Surgical treatment of acute traumatic rupture of the thoracic aorta a timing reappraisal? *Eur J Cardiothorac Surg*. 2002;21(2):282-287.

39. Frykberg ER, Denis JW, Bishop K, et al. The reliability of physical examination the evaluation of penetrating extremity trauma for vascular injury results at one year. *J Trauma*. 1991;31:502-511.

40. Frykberg ER, Vines FS, Alexander RH. The natural history of clinically occult arterial injuries a prospect evaluation. *J Trauma*. 1989;29:577-584.

41. Baker WE, Wassermann J. Unsuspected vascular trauma: blunt arterial injuries. *Emerg Med Clin North Am*. 2004; 22(4):1081-1098.

42. Rowe VL, Salim A, Lipham J, et al. Shank vessel injuries. *Surg Clin North Am*. 2002;82(1):91-104.

43. Frykberg ER. Popliteal vascular injuries. *Surg Clin North Am*. 2002;82(1):67-89.

44. Perry MO, Paul T, Shires GT. Management of arterial injuries. *Ann Surg*. 1971;173:404-411.

45. Davidsin BD, Polak JF. Arterial injuries: a sonographic approach. *Radiol Clin North Am*. 2004;42(2):383-396.

46. Gagne PJ, Cone JB, Macfarland MS, et al. Proximity penetrating extremity trauma: the role of duplex ultrasound in the detection of occult venous injuries. *J Trauma*. 1995;39:1157-1193.

47. Bladuf LM, Langsfeld M, Marek JM, et al. Complication rates of diagnostic angiography performed by vascular surgeons. *Vasc Endovasc Surg*. 2002;36(6):439-445.

48. Nicholson AA. Vascular radiology in trauma. *Cardiovasc Intervent Radiol*. 2004;27(2):105-120.

49. Berg M, Zhang Z, Ikonen A, et al. Multidetector row CT angiography in the assessment of carotid artery disease in symptomatic patients: comparison with rotational angiography and digital subtraction angiography. *Am J Neuroradiol*. 2005;26(5):1022-1034.

50. Lapeyre M, Kobeiter H, Desgrandes P, et al. Assessment of critical limb ischemia in patients with diabetes: comparison of MR angiography and digital subtraction angiography. *Am J Roentegenol*. 2005;185(6):1641-1650.

51. Frykberg E. Commentary on peripheral vascular injuries. In Mattox KL, Feliciano DV, Moore EE, eds. *Trauma*. McGraw Hill; 2000:1045-1046.

52. Singh RR, Barry MC, Ireland A, et al. Current diagnosis and management of blunt internal carotid artery injury. *Eur J Vasc Endovasc Surg*. 2004;27(6):577-584.

53. Cothren CC, Moore EE. Blunt cerebrovascular injuries. *Surg Clin*. 2005;60(6):489-496.

54. Cuff RF, Thomas JH. Pediatric blunt carotid injury from low-impact trauma: a case report and review of the literature. *J Trauma*. 2005;58(3):620-623.

55. Biffl WL. Diagnosis of blunt cerebrovascular injuries. *Curr Opin Crit Care*. 2003;9(6):530-534.

56. Berne JD, Norwood SH, McAuley CE, et al. The high morbidity of blunt cerebrovascular injury in an unscreened population: more evidence of the need for mandatory screening protocols. *J Am Coll Surg*. 2001;192(3):314-321.

57. Fateri F, Groebli Y, Rufenacht DA. Intraarterial thrombolysis and stent placement in the acute phase of blunt internal carotid artery trauma with subocclusive dissection and thromboembolic complication: case report and review of the literature. *Ann Vasc Surg*. 2005;19(3):434-437.

58. Agner C, Weig SG. Arterial dissection and stroke following child abuse: case report and review of the literature. *Childs Nerv Syst*. 2005;21(5):416-420.

59. DeBehnke DJ, Brady W. Vertebral artery dissection due to minor neck trauma. *J Emerg Med*. 1994;12:27.

60. Hollingworth W, Nathens AB, Kanne JP, et al. The diagnostic accuracy of computed tomography angiography for traumatic or atherosclerotic lesions of the carotid and vertebral arteries: a systematic review. *Eur J Radiol*. 2003;48(1):88-102.

61. Berne JD, Reuland KS, Villarreal DH, et al. Sixteen-slice multi-detector computed tomographic angiography improves the accuracy of screening for blunt cerebrovascular injury. *J Trauma*. 2006;60(6):1204-1209.

62. Bub LD, Hollingworth W, Jarvik JG, et al. Screening for blunt cerebrovascular injury: evaluating the accuracy of multidetector computed tomographic angiography. *J Trauma*. 2005;59(3):691-697.

63. Eastman AL, Chason DP, Perez CL, et al. Computed tomographic angiography for the diagnosis of blunt cervical vascular injury: is it ready for primetime? *J Trauma*. 2006;60(5):925-929.

64. Burger T, Tautenhahn J, Grote R, et al. Diagnosis and management of trauma and iatrogenic induced arteriovenous fistulas in the neck. *Vasa*. 1999;28(4):297-300.

65. Yu NR, Eberhardt RT, Menzoian JO, et al. Vertebral artery dissection following intravascular catheter placement: a case report and review of the literature. *Vasc Med*. 2004;9(3):199-203.

66. Iatrogenic carotid artery injury in neurosurgery. *Neurosurg Rev*. 2005;28(4):239-247. discussion 248.

67. Cothren CC, Moore EE, Biffl WL, et al. Anticoagulation is the gold standard therapy for blunt carotid injuries to reduce stroke rate. *Arch Surg*. 2004;139(5):540-545.

68. Wahl WL, Brandt MM, Thompson BG, et al. Antiplatelet therapy: an alternative to heparin for blunt carotid injury. *J Trauma*. 2002;52(5):896-901.

69. Eachempati SR, Vaslef SN, Sebastian MW, et al. Blunt vascular injuries of the head and neck: is heparinization necessary? *J Trauma*. 1998;45:997.

70. Miller PR, Fabian TC, Croce MA, et al. Prospective screening for blunt cerebrovascular injuries: analysis of diagnostic modalities and outcomes. *Ann Surg*. 2002;236(3):386-393.

71. Schneidereit NP, Simons R, Nicolaou S, et al. Utility of screening for blunt vascular neck injuries with computed tomographic angiography. *J Trauma*. 2006;60(1):209-215.

72. Rozycki GS, Tremblay L, Feliciano DV, et al. A prospective study for the detection of vascular injury in adult and pediatric patients with cervicothoracic seat belt signs. *J Trauma*. 2002;52(4):618-623.

73. Lew SM, Frumiento C, Wald SL. Pediatric blunt carotid injury: a review of the National Pediatric Trauma Registry. *Pediatr Neurosurg*. 1999;30(5):239-244.

74. Berbe JD, Norwood SH, McAuley CE, et al. The high morbidity of blunt cerebrovascular injury in an unscreened population: more evidence of the need for mandatory screening protocols. *J Am Coll Surg*. 2001;192(3):314-321.

75. Cothren CC, Moore EE, Biffl WL, et al. Cervical spine fracture patterns predictive of blunt vertebral artery injury. *J Trauma*. 2003;55(5):811-813.

76. Cothren CC, Moore EE, Ray CE, et al. Carotid artery stents for blunt cerebrovascular injury: risks exceed benefits. *Arch Surg*. 2005;140(5):480-485.

77. Fusonie GE, Edwards JD, Reed AB. Covered stent exclusion of blunt traumatic carotid artery pseudoaneurysm: case report and review of the literature. *Ann Vasc Surg*. 2004;18(3):376-379.

78. Martin MJ, Mullenix PS, Steel SR, et al. Functional outcome after blunt and penetrating carotid artery injuries: analysis of the National Trauma Data Bank. *J Trauma*. 2005;59(4):860-864.

79. Biffl WL, Moore EE, Elliott JP, et al. The devastating potential of blunt vertebral arterial injuries. *Ann Surg*. 2000;231(5):672-681.

80. Inamasu J, Guiot BH. Vertebral artery injury after blunt cervical trauma: an update. *Surg Neurol*. 2006;65(3):238-245.

81. O'Shaughnessy BA, Bendok BR, Parkinson RJ, Shaibani A, Batjer HH. Transarterial coil embolization of a high-flow vertebrojugular fistula due to penetrating craniocervical trauma: case report. *Surg Neurol*. 2005;64(4):335-340.

82. Fox CJ, Gillespie DL, Weber MA, et al. Delayed evaluation of combat-related penetrating neck trauma. *J Vasc Surg*. 2006;44(1):86-93.

83. Baumgartner FJ, Rayhanabad J, Bongard FS, et al. Central venous injuries of the subclavian–jugular and innominate–caval confluenced. *Tex Heart Inst J*. 1999;26(3):177-181.

84. Woo K, Magner DO, Wilson MT, et al. CT angiography in penetrating neck trauma reduces the need for operative neck exploration. *Am Surg*. 2005;71(9):754-758.

85. Ferguson E, Dennis JW, Vu JH, et al. Redefining the role of arterial imaging in the management of penetrating zone 3 neck injuries. *Vascular*. 2005;13(3):158-163.

86. Mwipatayi BP, Jeffery P, Beningfield SJ, et al. Management of extra-cranial vertebral artery injuries. *Eur J Vas Endovasc Surg.* 2004;27(2):157-162.

87. Mattox KL, Pickard L, Allen MK, Garcia-Rinaldi R. Suspecting thoracic aortic transection. *JACEP.* 1978;7:12-15.

88. Richardson RL, Khandekar A, Moseley PW. Traumatic rupture of the thoracic aorta. *South Med J.* 1979;72:300-301.

89. DeMeules JE, Cramer G, Perry JF. Rupture of aorta and great vessels due to blunt thoracic trauma. *J Thorac Cardiovasc Surg.* 1971;61:438-442.

90. Kram HB, Appel PL, Wohlmuth DA, Shoemaker WC. Diagnosis of traumatic thoracic aortic rupture: a 10-year retrospective analysis. *Ann Thorac Surg.* 1989;47:282-286.

91. Lee J, Harris JH, Duke JW, Williams JS. Noncorrelation between thoracic skeletal injuries and acute traumatic aortic tear. *J Trauma.* 1997;43:400-404.

92. Horton TG, Cohn SM, Heid MP, et al. Identification of trauma patients at risk of thoracic aortic tear by mechanism of injury. *J Trauma.* 2000;48:1008-1014.

93. Kaytal D, McLellan BA, Brenneman FD, et al. Lateral impact motor vehicle collisions: significant cause of blunt traumatic rupture of the thoracic aorta. *J Trauma.* 1997;42:769-772.

94. Williams JS, Graff JA, Uku JM, Steining JP. Aortic injury in vehicular trauma. *Ann Thorac Surg.* 1994;57:726.

95. Wintermark M, Wicky S, Schnyder P. Imaging of acute traumatic injuries of the thoracic aorta. *Eur Radiol.* 2002;12(2):431-442.

96. Vignon P, Boncoeur MP, Rambaud G, et al. Comparison of multiplane transesophageal echocardiography and contrast-enhanced helical CT in the diagnosis of blunt traumatic cardiovascular injuries. *Anesthesiology.* 2001;94(4):615-622.

97. Scaglione M, Pinto F, Romano L, et al. Role of contrast-enhanced helical CT in the evaluation of acute thoracic aortic injuries after blunt chest trauma. *Eur Radiol.* 2001;11(12):2444-2448.

98. Bruckner BA, DiBardino DJ, Cumbie TC, et al. Critical evaluation of chest computed tomography scans for blunt descending thoracic aortic injury. *Ann Thorac Surg.* 2006;81(4):1339-1346.

99. Chu MW, Myers ML. Traumatic innominate artery disruption and aortic valve rupture. *Ann Thorac Surg.* 2006;82(3):1095-1097.

100. Kepros J, Angood P, Jaffe CC, Rabinovici R. Aortic intimal injuries from blunt trauma: resolution profile in nonoperative management. *J Trauma.* 2002;52(3):475-478.

101. Ray CE Jr, Bauer JR, Cothren CC, et al. Occult mediastinal great vessel trauma: the value of aortography performed during angiographic screening for blunt cervical vascular trauma. *Cardiovasc Intervent Radiol.* 2005;28(4):422-425.

102. Werre A, van der Vilet JA, Biert J, et al. Endovascular management of a gunshot wound injury to the innominate artery and brachiocephalic vein. *Vascular.* 2005;13(1):58-61.

103. Jeroukhimov I, Altshuler A, Peer A, et al. Endovascular stent–graft is a good alternative to traditional management of subclavian vein injury. *J Trauma.* 2004;57(6):1329-1330.

104. Graham JM, Beall AC Jr, Mattox KL, et al. Systemic air embolism following penetrating trauma to the lung. *Chest.* 1977;72:449.

105. Demetriades D, Velmahos GC. Penetrating injuries of the chest: indications for operation. *Scand J Surg.* 2002;91(1):41-45.

106. Rhee PM, Acosta J, Bridgeman A, et al. Survival after emergency department thoracotomy; review of published data from the last 25 years. *J Am Coll Surg.* 2000;190:288.

107. Caplan ES, Preas MA, Kerns T, et al. Seroprevalence of human immunodeficiency virus, hepatitis B virus, hepatitis C virus, and rapid plasma reagin in a trauma population. *J Trauma.* 1995;39:533.

108. ACS-COT Subcommittee on Outcomes. Practice management guidelines for emergency department thoracotomy. *J Am Coll Surg.* 2001;193:303.

109. Renz B, Cava RA, Feliciano DV, Rozycki GS. Transmediastinal gunshot wounds: a prospective study. *J Trauma.* 2000;48(3):416-421.

110. Stassen NA, Lukan JK, Spain DA, et al. Reevaluation of diagnostic procedures for transmediastinal gunshot wounds. *J Trauma.* 2002;53(4):635-638.

111. Grossman MD, May AK, Schwab CW, et al. Determining anatomic injury with computed tomography in selected torso gunshot wounds. *J Trauma.* 1998;45(3):446-456.

112. Ibirogba S, Nichol AJ, Navsaria PH. Screening helical computed tomographic scanning in haemodynamic stable patients with transmediastinal gunshot wounds. *Injury.* 2007;38(1):48-52.

113. Nagy KK, Roberts RR, Smith RF, et al. Trans-mediasinal gunshot wounds: are "stable" patients really stable? *World J Surg.* 2002;26(10):1247-1250.

114. Gasparri MG, Lorelli DR, Kralovich KA, et al. Physical examination plus chest radiography in penetrating periclavicular trauma: the appropriate trigger for angiography. *J Trauma.* 2000;49(6):1029-1033.

115. Gonzalez RP, Falimirski ME. The role of angiography in periclavicular penetrating trauma. *AM Surg.* 1999;65(8):711-713.

116. Demetriades D, Asensio JA. Subclavian and axillary vascular injuries. *Surg Clin North Am.* 2001;81(6):1357-1373.

117. Rapaport A, Feliciano DV, Mattox KL. An epidemiologic profile of urban trauma in America—Houston style. *Tex Med.* 1982;78:44.

118. Cox CF. Blunt abdominal trauma. A 5-year analysis of 870 patients requiring celiotomy. *Ann Surg.* 1984;199:467.

119. Feliciano DV, Burch JM, Spjut-Patrinely V, et al. Abdominal gunshot wounds: an urban trauma center's experience with 300 consecutive patients. *Ann Surg.* 1988;208:362.

120. Asensio TA, Chahwan S, HanpeterD, et al. Operative management and outcomes of 302 abdominal vascular injuries. *Ann Surg.* 2000;180:528-534.

121. Chandler JG, Corson SL, Way LW. Three spectra of laparoscopic entry access injuries. *J Am Coll Surg.* 2001;192(4):478-490.

122. Moore Cl, Vasquez NF, Lin H, Kaplan LJ. Major vascular injury after laparoscopic tubal ligation. *J Emerg Med.* 2005;29(1):67-71.

123. Battaglia L, Bartolucci R, Berni A, et al. Major vessel injuries during laparoscopic cholecystectomy: a case report. *Chir Ital.* 2003;55(2):291-294.

124. Oskouian RJ Jr, Johnson JP. Vascular complications in anterior thoracolumbar spinal reconstruction. *J Neurosurg.* 2002; 96(1 suppl):1-5.

125. Saville LE, Woods MS. Laparoscopy and major retroperitoneal vascular injuries (MRVI). *Surg Endosc.* 1995;9(10): 1096-1100.

126. Owen RJ, Rose JD. Endovascular treatment of a portal vein tear during TIPSS. *Cardiovasc Intervent Radiol.* 2000;23(3): 230-232.

127. Zhou W, Bush RL, Terramani TT, et al. Treatment options of iatrogenic pelvic vein injuries: conventional operative versus endovascular approach—case report. *Vas Endovasc Surg.* 2004;38(6):569-573.

128. Oderich GS, Panneton JM, Hofer J, et al. Iatrogenic operative injuries of abdominal and pelvic veins: a potentially lethal complication. *J Vas Surg.* 2004;39(5):931-936.

129. Eastern Association for the Surgery of Trauma. EAST practice management guidelines for the evaluation of blunt abdominal trauma. East.org/pg161untabd.pdc. Accessed April 3, 2007.

130. Gushman JG, Feliciano DV, Renz BM, et al. Iliac vessel injury: operative physiology related to outcome. *J Trauma.* 1997;42(6):1033-1040.

131. Sisley AC, Rozycki GS, Ballard RB, et al. Rapid detection of traumatic effusion using surgeon-performed ultrasonography. *J Trauma.* 1998;44:291.

132. Rozycki GS, Feliciano DV, Davis TP. Ultrasound as used in thoracoabdominal trauma. *Surg Clin North Am.* 1998;78: 295.

133. Rozycki GS, Ballard RB, Feliciano DV, et al. Surgeon-performed ultrasound for the assessment of truncal injuries. Lessons learned from 1540 patients. *Ann Surg.* 1998;228: 557.

134. Committee on Trauma, American College of Surgeons. *Advanced Trauma Life Support.* 7th ed. Chicago, IL: American College of Surgeons; 2005.

135. Liu PP, Lee WC, Cheng YF, et al. Use of splenic artery embolization as an adjunct to nonsurgical management of blunt splenic injury. *J Trauma.* 2004;56(4):768-772.

136. Wahl WL, Ahrns KS, Brandt MM, et al. The need for early angiographic embolization in blunt liver injuries. *J Trauma.* 2002;52(6):1097-1101.

137. Haan J, Scott J, Boyd-Kranis RL, et al. Admission angiography for blunt splenic injury: advantages and pitfalls. *J Trauma.* 2001;51(6):1161-1165.

138. Smith WR, Moore EE, Agudelo JF, et al. Retroperitoneal packing as a resuscitation technique for hem dynamically unstable patients with pelvic fractures: report of two representative cases and a description of technique. *J Trauma.* 2005;59(6):1510-1514.

139. McCarthy MC, Lowdermilk GA, Canal DF, Broadie TA. Prediction of injury caused by penetrating wounds to the abdomen, flank and back. *Arch Surg.* 1991;126:962-966.

140. Renz BM, Feliciano DV. Unnecessary laparotomies for trauma; a prospective study of morbidity. *J Trauma.* 1995;38: 350-356.

141. Velmahos GC, Demetriades D, Toutouzas KG, et al. Selective non-operative management in 1856 patients with abdominal gunshot wounds: should routine laparotomy still be the standard of care? *Ann Surg.* 2001;234:395-402.

142. Demetriades D, Hadjizacharia P, Constantinou C, et al. Selective nonoperative management of penetrating abdominal solid organ injuries. *Ann Surg.* 2006;244(4):620-628.

143. Miles EJ, Dunn E, Howard D, Mangram A. The role of laparoscopy in penetrating abdominal trauma. *JSLS.* 2004; 8(4):304-309.

144. Iannelli A, Fabiani P, Karimsje E, et al. Therapeutic Laparoscopy for blunt abdominal trauma with bowel injuries. *J Laparoendosc Adv Surg Tech A.* 2003;13(3):189-191.

145. Feliciano DV, Bitondo CG, Cruse PA, et al. Liberal use of emergency center thoracotomy. *Am J Surg.* 1986;152:654.

146. The Dutch Study Group. Efficacy of oral anticoagulants compared with aspirin after infrainguinal bypass surgery (The Dutch Bypass Oral Anticoagulants or Aspirin Study): a randomized trial. *Lancet.* 2000;355(9201):346-351.

147. Melton SM, Croce MA, Patton JH, et al. Popliteal artery trauma. Systemic anticoagulation and intraoperative thrombolysis improves limb salvage. *Ann Surg.* 1997;225(5):518-527.

148. Assadian A, Senekowitsch C, Assadian O, et al. Antithrombotic strategies in vascular surgery: evidence and practice. *Eur J Vasc Endovasc Surg.* 2005;29(5):516-521.

149. Mahoney BD, Gerdes D, Roller B, et al. Aortic compressor for aortic occlusion in hemorrhagic shock. *Ann Emerg Med.* 1984;13:29.

150. Meldromd R, Moore FA, Moore EE, et al. Prospective characterization and selective management of the abdominal compartment syndrome. *Am J Surg.* 1997;174(6):667-672.

151. Veith FJ, Gupta S, Daly V. Technique for occluding the supraceliac aorta through the abdomen. *Surg Gynecol Obstet.* 1980;151:426.

152. Accola KD, Feliciano DV, Mattox KL, et al. Management to injuries to the suprarenal aorta. *Am J Surg.* 1987;154:613-618.

153. Mullins RJ, Huckfeldt R, Trunkey DD. Abdominal vascular injuries. *Surg Clin North Am.* 1996;76:813-832.

154. Shah DM, Leather RP, Colson JD, Karmory AM. Polytetrafluoroethylene grafts in the reconstruction of acute contaminated peripheral vascular injuries. *Am J Surg.* 1984; 148(2):229-233.

155. Shah PM, Ito K, Claus RH et al. Expanded microporous polytetrafluoroethylene (ptfe) grafts in contaminated wounds: experimental and clinical study. *J Trauma.* 1983;23(12): 1030-1322.

156. Oyama M, McNamara JJ, Surhiro GT, et al. The effects of thoracic aortic cross-clamping and declamping on visceral organ blood flow. *Ann Surg.* 1983;197:459.

157. Mullins RJ, Huckfeldt R, Trunkey DD, et al. Complex and challenging problems in trauma surgery: abdominal vascular injuries. *Surg Clin North Am.* 1996;76:813-832.

158. Asensio JA, Berne JD, Chahwan S, et al. Traumatic injury to the superior mesenteric artery. *Am J Surg.* 2000;178(3):235-239.

159. Demetriades D. Abdominal vascular injuries. In: Rutherford R. ed. *Vascular Surgery.* 6th ed. Philadelphia, PA: Elsevier Sanders; 2005;1028-1044.

160. Asensio JA, Britt LD, Bulzotta A, et al. Multiinstitutional experience with the management of superior mesenteric artery injuries. *J Am Coll Surg.* 2001;193(4):354-365.

161. Sutton E, Bochicchio GV, Bochicchio K, et al. Long term impact of damage control surgery: a preliminary prospective study. *J Trauma.* 2006;61(4):831-836.

162. Carroll PR, McAninch JW, Klosterman P, Greenblatt M. Renovascular trauma: risk assessment, surgical management, and outcome. *J Trauma.* 1990;30:547.

163. Maggio AJ, Brosman S. Renal artery trauma. *Urology.* 1978; 11:125.

164. Dorffner R, Thurnher S, Prokesch R, et al. Embolization of iatrogenic vascular injuries of renal transplants: immediate and follow-up results. *Cardiovasc Intervent Radiol.* 1998; 21(2):129-134.

165. Grenholz SK, Moore EE, Peterson NE, et al. Traumatic bilateral renal artery occlusions: successful outcomes without surgical intervention. *J Trauma.* 1997;42:330.

166. Sprouse LR, Hamilton IN Jr. The endovascular treatment of a renal arteriovenous fistula: placement of a covered stent. *J Vasc Surg.* 2002;36(5):1066-1068.

167. Feliciano DV. Approach to major abdominal vascular injury. *J Vasc Surg.* 1988;7:730.

168. Feliciano DV. Heroic procedures in vascular injury management: the role of extra-anatomic bypasses. *Surg Clin North Am.* 2002;82(1):115-124.

169. Coimbra R, Hoyt D, Winchell R, et al. The ongoing challenge of retroperitoneal vascular injuries. *Am J Surg.* 1996; 172(5):541-544.

170. Ivy ME, Possenti P, Atweh M, et al. Ligation of the suprarenal vena cava after a gunshot wound. *J Trauma.* 1998;45(3):630-632.

171. Bucek RA, Schneider G, Ahmadi A, et al. Penetrating abdominal vena cava injuries. *Eur J Vasc Endovasc Surg.* 2005; 30(5):499-503.

172. Khaneja SC, Pizzi WF, Barie PS, et al. Management of penetrating juxtahepatic inferior vena cava injuries under total vascular occlusion. *J Am Coll Surg.* 1997;184(5):469-474.

173. Asensio JA, Chahwan S, Hanpeter D, et al. Operative management and outcome of 302 abdominal vascular injuries. *Am J Surg.* 2000;180(6):528-533.

174. Porter JM, Ivatury RR, Islam SZ, et al. Inferior vena cava injuries: noninvasive follow-up of venorrhaphy. *J Trauma.* 1997;42(5):913-917; discussion 917-918.

175. Lupattelli T, Garaci FG, Manenti G, et al. Giant high-flow renal arteriovenous fistula treated by percutaneous embolization. *Urology.* 2003;61(4):837-838.

176. Carrillo EH, Spain DA, Wilson MA, et al. Alternatives in the management of penetrating injuries to the iliac vessels. *J Trauma.* 1998;44(6):1024-1029.

177. Zamir G, Berlatxky Y, Anner H, et al. Results of reconstruction in major pelvic and extremity venous injuries. *J Vasc Surg.* 1998;28(5):901-908.

178. Tyburski JG, Wilson RF, Dente C, et al. Factors affecting mortality rates in patients with abdominal vascular injuries. *J Trauma.* 2001;50:1020.

179. Asensio JA, Petrone P, Roldan G, et al. Analysis of 185 iliac vessel injuries: risk factors and predictors of outcome. *Arch Surg.* 2003;138(11):1187-1193.

180. Pearl J, Chao A, Kennedy S, et al. Traumatic injuries to the portal vein: case study. *J Trauma.* 2004;56(4):779-782.

181. Coimbra R, Filho AR, Nesser RA, et al. Outcome from traumatic injury of the portal and superior mesenteric veins. *Vasc Endovasc Surg.* 2004;38(3):249-255.

182. Buckman RF, Pathak AS, Badellino MM, et al. Portal vein injuries. *Surg Clin North Am.* 2001;81(6):1449-1462.

183. Hashimoto K, Shimada M, Suehiro T, et al. Gore-Tex jump graft for portal vein thrombosis following living donor transplantation. *Hepaticogastroenterology.* 2003;50(52):1146-1148.

184. Sugawar Y, Makuuchi M, Tamaru S, et al. Portal Vein reconstruction in adult living donor transplantation using cryopreserved vein grafts. *Liver Transpl.* 2006;12(8):1233-1236.

185. Prakash K, Regimbeau JM, Belghiti J. Reconstruction of portal vein using hepatic vein patch after combined hepatectomy and portal vein resection. *Am J Surg.* 2003;185(3):230-231.

186. Hagiwara A, Murata A, Matsuda T, et al. The usefulness of transcatheter arterial embolization for patients with blunt polytrauma showing transient response to fluid resuscitation. *J Trauma.* 2004;57(2):271-276.

187. Kusjimoto S, Arai M, Aiboshi J, et al. The role of interventional radiology in patients requiring damage control laparotomy. *J Trauma.* 2003;54(1):171-176.

188. Mohr AM, Lavery RF, Barone A, et al. Angiographic embolization for liver injuries: low mortality, high morbidity. *J Trauma.* 2003;55(6):1077-1081.

189. Stephen DJ, Kreder HJ, Day AC, et al. Early detection of arterial bleeding in acute pelvic trauma. *J Trauma.* 1999; 47(4):638-642.

190. Conrad MF, Patton JH, Parikshak M, et al. Evaluation of vascular injury in penetrating extremity trauma: angiographers stay home. *Am Surg.* 2002;68(3):269-274.

191. Howe HR, Poole GV, Hansen KJ, et al. Salvage of lower extremities following combined orthopedic and vascular trauma. A predictive salvage index. *Am Surg.* 1987;53(4):205-208.

192. McNamara MG, Heckman JA, Colley FG. Severe open fractures of the lower extremity: a retrospective evaluation of the mangled extremity score (MESS). *J Orthop Trauma.* 1994; 8(2):81-87.

193. Giannoudis PV, Papakostidis N, Roberts C. A review of the management of open fractures of the tibia and femur. *J Bone Joint Surg Br.* 2006;88(3):281-289.

194. Durham RM, Mistry BM, Mazuski JE, et al. Outcome and utility of scoring systems in the management of the mangledextremity. *Am J Surg.* 1996;172:569.

195. Barros D'Sa AA, Markin DW, Blair PN, et al. The Belfast approach to managing complex lower limb vascular injuries. *Eur J Vasc Endovasc Surg.* 2006;32(3):246-256.

196. Huynh TT, Pham M, Griffin LW, et al. Management of distal femoral and popliteal arterial injuries. An update. *Am J Surg.* 2006;192(6):773-778.

197. Hollis JD, Daley BJ. 10-year review of knee dislocation: is arteriography necessary? *J Trauma.* 2005;59:672-676.

198. Gonzalez RP, Falimirski ME. The utility of physical examination in proximity penetrating extremity trauma. *Am Surg.* 1999;65:784.

199. Pash AR, Bishara RA, Lim LT, et al. Optimal limb salvage in penetrating civilian vascular trauma. *J Vasc Surg.* 1986;3:189.

200. Meyer J, Walsh J, Schuler J, et al. The early fate of venous repair after civilian vascular trauma. *Ann Surg.* 1987;206:458.

201. Abouezzi Z, Nassoura Z, Ivatury RR, et al. A critical reappraisal of indications for fasciotomy after extremity vascular trauma. *Arch Surg.* 1998;133(5):547-551.

202. Finkelstein JA, Hunter GA, Hu RW. Lower limb compartment syndrome: course after delayed fasciotomy. *J Trauma.* 1996;40:342.

203. Velmahos GC, Toutouzas KG. Vascular trauma and compartment syndrome. *Surg Clin North Am.* 2002;82(1):125-141.

204. Olson SA, Glasgow RR. Acute compartment syndrome in lower extremity musculoskeletal trauma. *J Am Acad Orthop Surg.* 2005;13(7):436-444.

205. Rich NM. Complications of vascular injury management. *Surg Clin North Am.* 2002;82(1):143-174.

206. Asensios A, Kuncur EJ, Garcia LM, Petrone P. Femoral vessel injuries: analysis of factors predictive of outcomes. *J Am Coll Surg.* 2006;203(4):512-570.

207. Carrillo EH, Spain DA, Miller FB, et al. Femoral vessel injuries. *Surg Clin North Am.* 2002;82(1):49-65.

208. Ierardi RP, Rich N, Kerstein MD. Peripheral venous injuries: a collective review. *J Am Coll Surg.* 1996;183(5):531-540.

209. Kaufman J, Moglia R, Lacy C, Dinerstein C, Moreyra A. Peripheral vascular complications from percutaneous transluminal coronary angioplasty: a comparison with trans femoral cardiac catheterization. *Am J Med Sci.* 1989;297(1):22-25.

210. Rozycki GS, Tremblay LN, Feliciano DV, et al. Blunt vascular trauma in the extremity: diagnosis, management, and outcome. *J Trauma.* 2003;55(5):814-824.

211. Deshpande A, Denton M. Endovascular treatment of a post-traumatic femoral vein-profunda femoris artery fistula. *J Endovasc Surg.* 1999;6(3):301-303.

212. Uppot RN, Garcia M, Nguyen H, et al. Traumatic common iliac vein disruption treated with an endovascular stent. *AJR Am J Roentgenol.* 2001;177(3):606.

213. Compton C, Rhee R. Peripheral vascular trauma. *Perspect Vasc Surg Endovasc Ther.* 2005;17(4):297-307.

214. Padberg FT, Rubelowsky JJ, Hernandez-Maldanado JJ et al. Infrapopliteal arterial injury prompt revascularization affords optimal limb salvage. *J Vasc Surg.* 1992;16:877.

215. Melton SM, Croce MA, Patton JH, et al. Popliteal artery trauma. Systemic anticoagulation and intraoperative thrombolysis improves limb salvage. *Ann Surg.* 1997;225(5):518-527.

216. Ilijevski N, Radak D, Radevic B, et al. Popliteal traumatic arteriovenous fistulas. *J Trauma.* 2002;52(4):739-744.

217. Tielliu IF, Verhoeven EL, Prins TR, et al. Stent–graft of a recurrent popliteal arteriovenous fistula. *J Endovasc Ther.* 2002;9(3):375-378.

218. Dorweiler B, Neufang A, Schmiedt W, et al. Limb trauma with arterial injury: long-term performance of venous interposition grafts. *Thorac Cardiovasc Surg.* 2003;51(2):67-72.

219. Mullenix PS, Steele SR, Andersen CA, et al. Limb salvage and outcomes among patients with traumatic popliteal vascular injury. An analysis of national trauma data bank. *J Vasc Surg.* 2006;44(1):94-100.

220. McHenry TP, Holcomb JB, Aoki N, Lindsey RW. Fractures with major vascular injury from gunshot wounds: implications of surgical sequence. *J Trauma.* 2002;53(4):717-721.

221. Thomas DD, Wilson RF, Wiencek RG. Vascular injury about the knee: improved outcome. *Am Surg.* 1989;55(6):370-377.

222. Padberg FT, Rubelowsky JJ, Hernandez-Maldonado JJ, et al. Infrapopliteal arterial injury: prompt revascularization affords optimal limb salvage. *J Vasc Sueg.* 1992;16:877-885.

223. Ramsheyi A, Soury P, Saliou C, et al. Inadvertent arterial injury saphenous vein stripping: three cases and therapeutic strategies. *Arch Surg.* 1998;133(10):1120-1123.

224. Eastern Association for the Surgery of Trauma. Practice management guidelines for evaluation and management of lower extremity venous injuries from penetrating trauma. http://east.org/pg. Accessed January 15, 2007.

225. Practice management guidelines for diagnosis and management of lower extremity isolated arterial injuries from penetrating trauma. http://east.org/pg. Accessed January 15, 2007.

226. Fields CE, Latifi R, Ivatury RR. Brachial and forearm vessel injuries. *Surg Clin North Am.* 2002;82(1):105-114.

227. Zanchetta M, Rigatelli G, Dimopoulos K, et al. Endoluminal repair of axillary artery and vein rupture after reduction of shoulder dislocation. A case report. *Minerva Cardioangiol.* 2002;50(1):69-73.

228. Onki T, Veith FJ, Latz E, at al. Endovascular therapy for upper extremity injury. *Semin Vasc Surg.* 1998;11(2):106-115.

229. Parry NG, Feliciano DV, Burke RM, et al. Management and short-term patency of lower extremity venous injuries with various repairs. *Am J Surg.* 2003;186(6):631-635.

230. Bermudez KM, Knudson MM, Nelken NA, et al. Long-term results of lower-extremity venous injuries. *Arch Surg.* 1997;132(9):963-967.

231. Smith LM, Block EF, Buechter KJ, et al. The natural history of extremity venous repair performed for trauma. *Am Surg.* 1999;65(2):116-120.

232. Parodi JC, Palmaz JC, Barone HD. Transfemoral intraluminal graft implantation for abdominal aortic aneurysms. *Ann Vasc Surg.* 1991;5(6):491-499.

233. Stecco K, Meier A, Seiver A, Dake M, Zarins C. Endovascular stent–graft placement for treatment of traumatic penetrating subclavian artery injury. *J Trauma.* 2000;48(5):948-950.

234. Onal B, Ilgit ET, Kosar S, Akkan K, Gumus T, Akpek S. Endovascular treatment of peripheral vascular lesions with stent–grafts. *Diagn Interv Radiol.* 2005;11(3):170-174.

235. Baltacioglu F, Cimsit NC, Cil B, Cekirge S, Ispir S. Endovascular stent–graft applications in iatrogenic vascular injuries. *Cardiovasc Intervent Radiol.* 2003;26(5):434-439.

236. Thalhammer C, Kirchherr AS, Uhlich F, Waigand J, Gross CM. Postcatheterization pseudoaneurysms and

arteriovenous fistulas: repair with percutaneous implantation of endovascular covered stents. *Radiology.* 2000;214(1): 127-131.

237. Nyman U, Uher P, Lindh M, Lindblad B, Brunkwall J, Ivancev K. Stent–graft treatment of iatrogenic iliac artery perforations: report of three cases. *Eur J Vasc Endovasc Surg.* 1999; 17(3):259-263.

238. Aytekin C, Boyvat F, Yildirim E, Coskun M. Endovascular stent–graft placement as emergency treatment for ruptured iliac pseudoaneurysm. *Cardiovasc Intervent Radiol.* 2002; 25(4):320-322.

239. McArthur CS, Marin ML. Endovascular therapy for the treatment of arterial trauma. *Mt Sinai J Med.* 2004;71(1): 4-11.

240. Reuben BR, Whitten MG, Sarfatu MR, Kraiss LW. Increasing utilization of endovascular therapy in trauma: analysis of the National Trauma Bank. University of Utah, Salt Lake City. Abstract presented at: Annual Vascular Meeting 2006, Baltimore, Maryland. 2006.

241. Xenos ES, Freeman M, Stevens S, Cassada D, Pacanowski J, Goldman M. Covered stents for injuries of subclavian and axillary arteries. *J Vasc Surg.* 2003;38(3):451-454.

242. Beregi JP, Prat A, Willoteaux S, Vasseur MA, Boularand V, Desmoucelle F. Covered stents in the treatment of peripheral arterial aneurysms: procedural results and midterm follow-up. *Cardiovasc Intervent Radiol.* 1999;22(1):13-19.

243. Nicholson AA. Vascular radiology in trauma. *Cardiovasc Intervent Radiol.* 2004;27(2):105-120.

244. Marin ML, Veith FJ. Clinical application of endovascular grafts in aortoiliac occlusive disease and vascular trauma. *Cardiovasc Surg.* 1995;3(2):115-120.

245. Marin ML, Veith FJ, Panetta TF, et al. Transluminally placed endovascular stented graft repair for arterial trauma. *J Vasc Surg.* 1994;20(3):466-472.

246. Marin ML, Veith FJ. Endovascular stents and stented grafts for the treatment of aneurysms and other arterial lesions. *Adv Surg.* 1996;29:93-109.

247. Sluzewski M. Procedural morbidity and mortality of elective coil treatment of unruptured intracranial aneurysms. *AJNR Am J Neuroradiol.* 2006;27(8):1678-1680.

248. Biffl WL, Moore EE, Elliott JP, Brega KE, Burch JM. Blunt cerebrovascular injuries. *Curr Probl Surg.* 1999;36(7):505-599.

249. Kuether TA, O'Neill O, Nesbit GM, Barnwell SL. Endovascular treatment of traumatic dural sinus thrombosis: case report. *Neurosurgery.* 1998;42(5):1163-1166.

250. Suzuki S, Endo M, Kurata A, et al. Efficacy of endovascular surgery for the treatment of acute epidural hematomas. *AJNR Am J Neuroradiol.* 2004;25(7):1177-1180.

251. Hurst RW, Haskal ZJ, Zager E, Bagley LJ, Flamm ES. Endovascular stent treatment of cervical internal carotid artery aneurysms with parent vessel preservation. *Surg Neurol.* 1998;50(4):313-317.

252. Naesens R, Mestdagh C, Breemersch M, Defreyne L. Direct carotid-cavernous fistula: a case report and review of the literature. *Bull Soc Belge Ophtalmol.* 2006;299:43-54.

253. Inamasu J, Guiot BH. Iatrogenic carotid artery injury in neurosurgery. *Neurosurg Rev.* 2005;28(4):239-247.

254. Chang EF, Claus CP, Vreman HJ, Wong RJ, Noble-Haeusslein LJ. Heme regulation in traumatic brain injury: relevance to the adult and developing brain. *J Cereb Blood Flow Metab.* 2005;25(11):1401-1417.

255. Hung CL, Wu YJ, Lin CS, Hou CJ. Sequential endovascular coil embolization for a traumatic cervical vertebral AV fistula. *Catheter Cardiovasc Interv.* 2003;60(2):267-269.

256. Duncan IC, Fourie PA. Percutaneous management of concomitant post-traumatic high vertebrovertebral and carotico-jugular fistulas using balloons, coils, and a covered stent. *J Endovasc Ther.* 2003;10(5):882-886.

257. Sanabria A, Jimenez CM. Endovascular management of an exsanguinating wound of the right internal jugular vein in zone III of the neck: case report. *J Trauma.* 2003;55(1):158-161.

258. Jeroukhimov I, Altshuler A, Peer A, Bass A, Halevy A. Endovascular stent–graft is a good alternative to traditional management of subclavian vein injury. *J Trauma.* 2004; 57(6):1329-1330.

259. Kumar V. Endovascular treatment of penetrating injury of axillary vein with Viabahn endoprosthesis. *J Vasc Surg.* 2004; 40(6):1243-1244.

260. Zanchetta M, Rigatelli G, Dimopoulos K, Pedon L, Zennaro M, Maiolino P. Endoluminal repair of axillary artery and vein rupture after reduction of shoulder dislocation. A case report. *Minerva Cardioangiol.* 2002;50(1): 69-73.

261. Rich NM, Hobson RW, Jarstfer BS, Geer TM. Subclavian artery trauma. *J Trauma.* 1973;13(6):485-496.

262. Rogers JH, Lasala JM. Coronary artery dissection and perforation complicating percutaneous coronary intervention. *J Invasive Cardiol.* 2004;16(9):493-499.

263. Tortoledo F, Izaguirre L, Trujillo MH, Tortoledo MA. Endovascular repair of accidental ligation of the right coronary artery during cardiorrhaphy for penetrating heart wound. *Cardiol Rev.* 2003;11(6):303-305.

264. Thomson I, Muduioa G, Gray A. Vascular trauma in New Zealand: an 11-year review of NZVASC, the New Zealand Society of Vascular Surgeons' audit database. *N Z Med J.* 2004;117(1201):U1048.

265. Teruya TH, Bianchi C, Abou-Zamzam AM, Ballard JL. Endovascular treatment of a blunt traumatic abdominal aortic injury with a commercially available stent graft. *Ann Vasc Surg.* 2005;19(4):474-478.

266. Sigler L, Gutierrez-Carreno R, Martinez-Lopez C, Lizola RI, Sanchez-Fabela C. Aortocava fistula: experience with five patients. *Vasc Surg.* 2001;35(3):207-212.

267. Mejia JC, Myers JG, Stewart RM, Dent DL, Connaughton JC. A right renal vein pseudoaneurysm secondary to blunt abdominal trauma: a case report and review of the literature. *J Trauma.* 2006;60(5):1124-1128.

268. Benson DA, Stockinger ZT, McSwain NE Jr. Embolization of an acute renal arteriovenous fistula following a stab wound: case report and review of the literature. *Am Surg.* 2005;71 (1):62-65.

269. Owen RJ, Rose JD. Endovascular treatment of a portal vein tear during TIPSS. *Cardiovasc Intervent Radiol.* 2000;23(3): 230-232.

270. Castelli P, Caronno R, Piffaretti G, Tozzi M. Emergency endovascular repair for traumatic injury of the inferior vena cava. *Eur J Cardiothorac Surg*. 2005;28(6):906-908.

271. Buckman RF, Pathak AS, Badellino MM, Bradley KM. Injuries of the inferior vena cava. *Surg Clin North Am*. 2001; 81(6):1431-1447.

272. Lee JT, Bongard FS. Iliac vessel injuries. *Surg Clin North Am*. 2002;82(1):21-48.

273. Verhoeven EL, Prins TR, van Det M, van den Dungen JJ. Stent–graft repair of a recurrent popliteal arteriovenous fistula. *J Endovasc Ther*. 2002;9(3):375-378.

274. Starnes BW, Arthurs ZM. Endovascular management of vascular trauma. *Perspect Vasc Surg Endovasc Ther*. 2006;18(2): 114-129.

275. Zhou W, Bush RL, Terramani TT, Lin PH, Lumsden AB. Treatment options of iatrogenic pelvic vein injuries: conventional operative versus endovascular approach— case reports. *Vasc Endovascular Surg*. 2004;38(6):569-573.

276. Howells GA, Janczyk RJ. *Principles of Vascular Trauma. Mastery of Vascular and Endovascular Surgery*. Lippincott Williams & Wilkins; 2006.

chapter 50

Primary Vascular Tumors

Samuel L. Johnston, MD / *Terrence C. Demos, MD* / *Edward J. Keuer, MD* /
Mamdouh Bakhos, MD / *Robert S. Dieter, MD, RVT*

● INTRODUCTION

Peripheral vascular tumors are rare, yet some physicians encounter patients with these tumors regularly and most physicians encounter them at least several times in the course of their practice. The clinical significance of vascular tumors ranges from trivial to cosmetically and psychosocially burdensome to life threatening. Some have characteristic clinical manifestations while many are found incidentally but have characteristic imaging findings. However, rare lesions and variable clinical presentations can result in delayed or misdiagnosis. This chapter will provide an overview of primary vascular tumors, emphasizing those affecting arteries and capillaries.

● CLASSIFICATIONS

Primary vascular neoplasms are defined as those arising from vascular elements, such as endothelial cells and pericytes. Most involve the microvasculature and manifest in the skin, but others affect deep structures and occasionally manifest in large vessels.

Historically, clinicians and pathologists have used conflicting descriptions and schemes in classifying vascular tumors and vascular malformations (VM). In some cases, different labels have been used to describe the same disease while in other cases the same label has been applied to vastly different diseases.

In 1982, Mulliken and Glowacki[1] published a classification system based on endothelial characteristics and biologic behavior, in part to address this confusion (Table 50-1). A subsequent revision of their classification system broadened the category of vascular tumors of infancy to include pyogenic granuloma, tufted angioma, kaposiform hemangioendothelioma (KH), and hemangiopericytoma.[2] This revised classification has become the standard for distinguishing hemangiomas from VM and is the official classification schema of the International Society for the Study of Vascular Anomalies.

Despite the current acceptance of this standard, imprecise terminology remains widespread in the scientific literature.[3] Furthermore, pathologists, who are often unaware of a patient's clinical presentation, still use histopathologic diagnoses and classify vascular lesions by the type of vessel that predominates (arterial, venous, or lymphatic). In contrast, clinicians often make the diagnosis without relying on biopsy or histopathology.

● BENIGN NEOPLASMS

Hemangioma

Hemangiomas are benign tumors of vascular endothelium and, by far, the most common form of primary vascular tumor. They most commonly affect the skin, but can occur in nearly any organ (Table 50-2). Hemangiomas are often without clinical significance, but they can cause complications such as disfigurement, ulceration, bleeding, organ failure, and death. Most hemangiomas present early in life. In some cases, hemangiomas are inherited as part of rare syndromes. Newly diagnosed superficial hemangiomas are uncommon after 30 years of age, but deep hemangiomas are often discovered incidentally in adults during imaging studies.

Hemangiomas have often been confused with VM.[1] The clinical distinction between hemangiomas and VM is not always initially apparent, but the diagnosis usually becomes clear with time. There are several features that distinguish hemangiomas from VM. Hemangiomas are more common in Caucasians than other races, more common in females than males, have early growth that is disproportionate to that of the patient, are composed of immature hyperplastic

TABLE 50-1. Classification of Primary Vascular Tumors

Benign neoplasms
    Hemangioma
    Capillary
    Cavernous
    Pyogenic granuloma (lobular capillary hemangioma)
    Glomus tumor
    Tufted angioma (Angioblastoma of Nakagawa)
Intermediate-grade neoplasms
    Kaposiform hemangioendothelioma
    Kaposi sarcoma
Malignant neoplasms
    Angio sarcoma
    Hemangiopericytoma

Adapted from Mulliken JB, Glowacki J. Hemangiomas and vascular malformations in infants and children: a classification based on endothelial characteristics. Plast Reconstr Surg. 1982;69(3):412-422 and Cotran RS, et al. Robbins Pathologic Basis of Disease. 6th ed. Philadelphia: PA: Saunders; 1999.

TABLE 50-3. Differentiating Vascular Anomalies

Hemangiomas	*Vascular Malformation*
Endothelial cell hyperplasia	Dysplastic vessels with normal endothelial turnover
Small or absent at birth	Present at birth
Rapid growth during infancy	Growth proportional to child
Involution phase during childhood	No regression

Adapted from Mulliken JB, Glowacki J. Hemangiomas and vascular malformations in infants and children: a classification based on endothelial characteristics. Plast Reconstr Surg. 1982;69(3):412-422.

endothelial cells, have increased numbers of mast cells, and have upregulated expression of proliferative cell markers (see Pathophysiology below) (Table 50-3).

In contrast to hemangiomas: VM have equal sex distribution, are often present and fully formed at birth, grow proportionately with the child, are composed of mature and often combined arterial, venous, or lymphatic vascular elements, have normal numbers of mast cells, have no

TABLE 50-2. Distribution of 570 Hemangiomas

Location	No. of Cases
Cutaneous or mucosal	370
Oral cavity	80
Face	75
Arm	60
Leg	50
Scalp	46
Vulva or scrotum	5
Other	54
Liver	109
Central nervous system	43
Heart	16
Bone	12
GI tract, kidney, mesentery	10
Muscle	10
Total	570

Adapted from Geshickter CF, Keasbey LE. Tumors of blood vessels. Am J Cancer. 1935;23:568.

increase in proliferative cell markers, and unlike hemangiomas, endothelial cells from VM do not grow in tissue culture.

Pathophysiology. Although theories abound, the etiology of hemangiomas and the mechanisms that control their proliferation and involution are not well understood. At least four general theories predominate, as discussed below.

Chorionic Villi. There is strong evidence of a relationship between hemangiomas and placental chorionic villi. The gene expression profiles of hemangiomas and placentae are similar and they share a tissue-specific marker called *GLUT-1*.[4] It has been hypothesized that hemangiomas represent the embolization of placental tissue to the fetus.[5] However, contrary to popular belief, it has recently been shown that chorionic villous sampling is probably not a contributing factor to the development of hemangiomas.[6]

Angiogenesis. Hemangiomas have long been thought to represent a localized derangement of *angiogenesis* (the growth of new vessels from existing vessels). As evidence for this theory, proliferating hemangiomas have upregulated expression of angiogenic factors, such as vascular endothelial growth factor (VEGF), basic fibroblast growth factor (BFGF), fibroblast growth factor (FGF), and type-IV collagenase.[7–9] Furthermore, therapy directed at inhibiting angiogenesis, such as corticosteroids and interferons, is often effective in causing involution of hemangiomas.

Vasculogenesis. More recently, however, some have argued that hemangiomas are mediated not by angiogenesis, but instead, by an error in *vasculogenesis* (the formation of blood vessels from angioblasts). This theory postulates that hemangiomas represent an incomplete maturation of the endothelial component of the fetal vasculature. The supporters of this theory point to the clonality of proliferating hemangioma endothelial cells.[10,11]

Immune-Mediated. Immunohistochemical staining suggests a causal role for hematopoietic cells of myeloid origin.[12] Expression of specific clusters of differentiation (CD83, CD32, CD14, CD15), possibly triggered by local tissue hypoxia, have been demonstrated in hemangioma endothelial cells.

The evidence for these differing putative mechanisms suggests either a multifactorial process or the presence of different disease entities under the umbrella diagnosis of "hemangioma."

Pathologic Classifications. Hemangiomas are classified by pathologists as being *capillary, cavernous,* or *pyogenic*

granuloma (lobular capillary hemangioma).[13] However, the American Academy of Dermatology refers to capillary hemangiomas as "superficial hemangiomas" and cavernous hemangiomas as "deep hemangiomas."[14] Hemangiomas that involve both superficial and deep tissue are called *combined* (or compound) lesions.

Capillary Hemangioma. Capillary ("strawberry") hemangiomas represent the major common form of hemangioma. Most often, they are located in the skin or subcutaneous tissue. Grossly, these lesions appear red to purple in color (Figure 50-1). Histologically, one sees a proliferation of capillary-sized vessels surrounding a feeder vessel

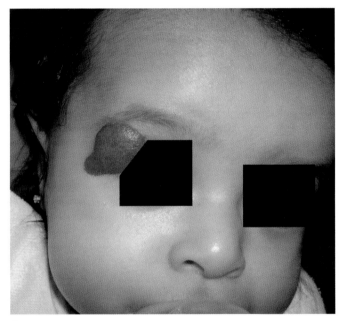

A

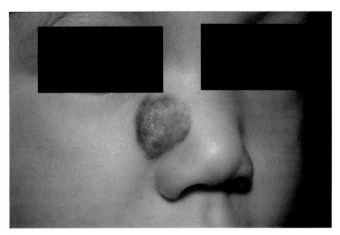

B

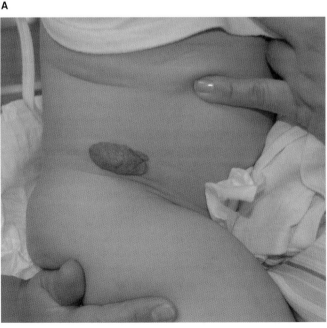

C

● FIGURE 50-1. Capillary (superficial) Hemangioma. (A) Periorbital. (B) Nasal (late state of resolution). (C) Hip (early stage of resolution).

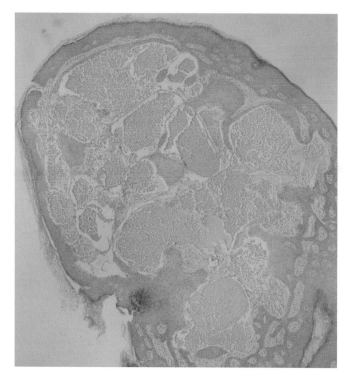

● **FIGURE 50-2.** Capillary hemangioma (hematoxylin and eosin [stain]).

Courtesy of Madhu Dahiya, M.D., Department of Pathology, Loyola University Medical Center and Stritch School of Medicine, Maywood, IL.

(Figure 50-2). This architecture has been referred to as "lobular" and has also been used to describe pyogenic granuloma and epithelioid hemangioma. The *sine qua non* of capillary hemangiomas is the presence a proliferating phase and an involuting phase.

Cavernous Hemangioma. Cavernous (deep) hemangiomas are less common than capillary (superficial) hemangiomas. They are generally larger, less well circumscribed, and more likely to involve deep structures, such as solid organs (e.g., liver). Grossly, they appear as indistinct purplish-blue nodules or masses in the skin (Figure 50-3). Histologically, they appear as massively engorged capillary hemangiomas (Figure 50-4), but unlike capillary hemangiomas, cavernous hemangiomas tend not to involute or do so more slowly and incompletely. They are also more likely to cause local tissue destruction.

Many cavernous hemangiomas are discovered incidentally on imaging studies. Both computed tomography (CT) and magnetic resonance (MR) imaging show an enhancing heterogeneous mass resulting from fibrous, vascular and fat components. There may be erosion of adjacent bones. The most characteristic imaging findings, however, are *phleboliths*, which are small rounded calcifications or ring calcifications of venous walls or thrombi. Phleboliths are found in up to one-third of cavernous hemangiomas (Figures 50-5 and 50-6).[15] Complex hemangiomas with thrombus, hemosiderin, and hyalinization may resemble neoplasms.

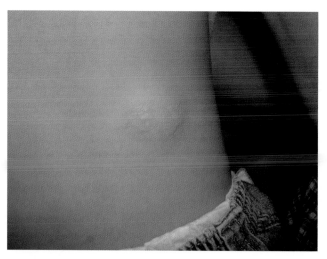

● **FIGURE 50-3.** Combined hemangioma with resolution of superficial component, revealing deep (cavernous) component.

Pyogenic Granuloma. See next section.

Pediatric Hemangiomas. Hemangioma of infancy (HOI) is the most common soft tissue tumor in the pediatric population, occurring in nearly 10% of Caucasian infants. Although the etiology and pathophysiology of hemangiomas remains unclear (see above), a number of risk factors have been identified (Table 50-4). Of those affected, 20% have multiple lesions.[16] The vast majority of HOI occur sporadically, although familial autosomal dominant cases have been reported.[17]

Most HOI are superficial (capillary type). Many are not evident at birth, in contrast to VM, but become noticeable within the first few days or months of life. HOI can involve nearly any organ, but most are cutaneous on the head and

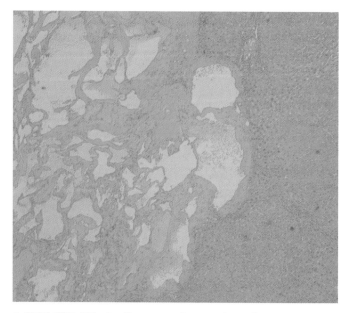

● **FIGURE 50-4.** Cavernous hemangioma (hematoxylin and eosin [stain]).

Courtesy Madhu of Dahiya, M.D., Department of Pathology, Loyola University Medical Center and Stritch School of Medicine, Maywood, IL.

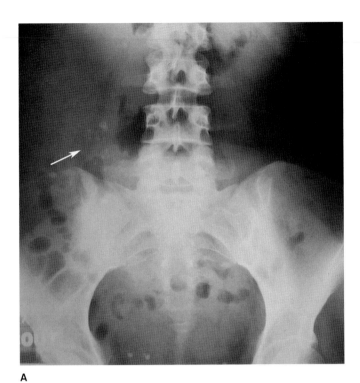

A

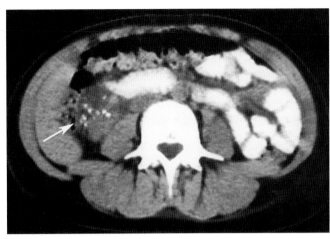

B

● **FIGURE 50-5.** Retroperitoneal hemangioma or KH with phleboliths. (A) Abdominal radiograph shows cluster of calcified phleboliths (*arrow*). (B) CT shows heterogeneous lesion containing phleboliths (*arrow*). Retroperitoneal hemangiomas are rare, but round and circular calcifications in masses anywhere in the body suggest vascular lesions.

neck (Figure 50-1A and 50-1B) (Table 50-2). Superficial hemangiomas appear as red papules, nodules, or plaques. Deep tissue hemangiomas often have a bluish hue (Figure 50-3).

Hemangiomas are characterized by a phase of proliferation followed by phase of involution and regression. They typically grow to maximal size by age 6 to 18 months and their growth is disproportionate to that of the infant. With

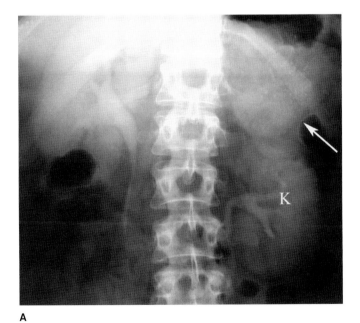

A

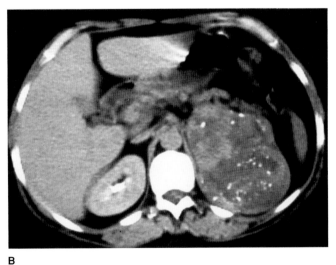

B

● **FIGURE 50-6.** Adrenal hemangioma. (A) Radiograph shows left shows left kidney (K) displaced caudally by suprarenal mass (*arrow*) with small irregular calcifications. (B) CT shows the large heterogeneous adrenal hemangioma containing multiple phleboliths. These multiple small well-defined phleboliths shown by CT are typical findings in hemangiomas and other vascular tumors.

TABLE 50-4. Risk Factors: Infantile Hemangiomas

Caucasian race
Female gender (5:1 female to male)
Advanced maternal age (>35 y)
Preterm infants
Low birth weight
Multiple gestations
Placenta previa
Preeclampsia

few exceptions, they range in size from a few millimeters to several centimeters in diameter. Most will spontaneously involute. As a general rule, approximately 10% involute per year after 1 year of age. By 7 years of age, 75% to 90% will have involuted. However, even when a lesion fully involutes and regresses, a residual hypopigmented scar with redundant skin is evident in 50% of cases. The risk of scarring increases with larger combined lesions, and with lesions of the nose, ear, lip, or breast.

Congenital Hemangiomas. Congenital hemangiomas are rare and of two types: Rapidly involuting congenital hemangioma (RICH) and noninvoluting congenital hemangioma (NICH).[18] RICH is similar to HOI but is fully developed at birth, lacks female preponderance, and pursues a course of rapid involution. Imaging studies can aid in making a diagnosis and differentiating this tumor from other entities, but occasionally biopsy is necessary. Accurate diagnosis of RICH is important in order to avoid unnecessary interventional therapy for this rapidly regressing lesion. NICH is so called because it is fully formed at birth and never involutes. Enjolras et al.[19] published a series of 53 patients and found that all NICH lesions were single, averaged 5 cm in size, and more than 40% were on the head and neck.

Hemangiomatosis. Most hemangiomas are single and cutaneous, but 20% of patients will have more than one lesion.[16] Hemangiomatosis is a syndrome that mostly affects neonates and is defined by the presence of multiple small hemangiomas (≥5 lesions).[13,20] Most cases are confined to the skin. Sometimes, hundreds of lesions are present and envelop an entire extremity (Figure 50-7).

A more severe variant can result in significant morbidity and rarely mortality because of systemic involvement.[21,22] In order of decreasing frequency, the liver, GI tract, brain, and lung may be affected. Hepatomegaly, congestive heart failure (CHF) and anemia appear early in severely affected infants, and death may result from heart failure. Despite its potentially aggressive nature, there are no reports of hemangiomatosis progressing to malignancy, and it remains a benign lesion that is often histologically identical to other common manifestations of hemangioma. Ultrasound

(US) is a useful imaging modality for screening infants with more than five cutaneous hemangiomas for visceral lesions. Tumors in patients with hemangiomatosis recur in 90% of cases, so treatment should be as conservative as possible.[22]

Syndromes. Aside from hemangiomatosis, there are several other rare clinical syndromes associated with hemangiomas (Table 50-5).[13] *Gorham disease* (vanishing bone disease) is a syndrome of massive osteolysis that can occur with hemangiomatosis. *Maffucci syndrome* is a nonhereditary mesodermal dysplasia that manifests with multiple cavernous hemangiomas and enchondromas, most of which affect the phalanges and long bones (Figure 50-8). Patients with *blue rubber bleb nevus syndrome (Bean syndrome)*, *Peutz-Jeghers syndrome*, and *Klippel-Trenaunay-Weber syndrome* may have multiple bowel hemangiomas that bleed and cause iron-deficient anemia. *PHACE syndrome* affects multiple organ systems and is discussed separately (see below). The *Kasabach-Merritt syndrome* (KMS) is a consumptive coagulopathy associated with specific hemangiomas, especially KH and tufted angioma (see below). Contrary to reports in older literature, KMS is rarely, if ever, associated with infantile hemangioma.

Complications and Regionally Important Lesions. Most hemangiomas are asymptomatic. However, lesions affecting the face often cause psychosocial distress (Figure 50-1A and 50-1B). An additional 10% of pediatric hemangiomas will result in structural, coagulopathic, or metabolic complications (Table 50-6).

PSYCHOLOGIC ISSUES. Psychosocial distress, both for the patient and the family, is the most common complication of pediatric hemangiomas. Much has been published on this topic.[14,16,23,24] These issues are best dealt with by educating the parents and patient as to the natural course of the disease, explaining the treatment plans, and discussing reasonable expectations. Frequent and regular office follow-up is often necessary. Contact with other families through support groups and via the Internet may also be helpful.

ULCERATION AND BLEEDING. Ulceration and bleeding are common complications of rapidly proliferating cutaneous hemangiomas and those located in areas of friction and pressure, such as the intertriginous areas.[25] These lesions are generally painful, susceptible to secondary infection and often result in larger residual scaring and discoloration.

SOFT TISSUE LESIONS. Soft tissue hemangiomas may present as a mass, with pain and discomfort, or as an incidental finding on an imaging study. Functional impairment may arise when a hemangioma interferes with a vital structure. Physical examination findings are often subtle. Generally, there is no discoloration of the overlying skin. The size of the lesion cannot be reliably assessed by palpation. Thrills and bruits are rarely present. Therefore, imaging studies (e.g.,

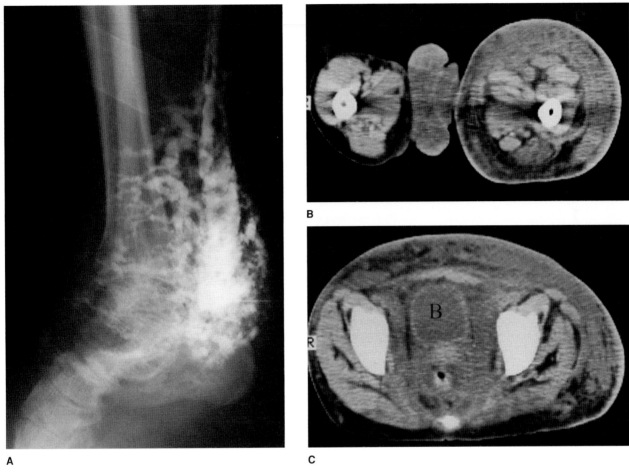

A

B

C

● **FIGURE 50-7.** Hemangiomatosis. (A) Angiogram shows a large angiomatous lesion of the left ankle. (B) CT shows markedly enlarged left thigh with subcutaneous angiomatous tissue. (C) Pelvic CT shows angiomatous subcutaneous tissue of left body wall and within pelvis displacing B: bladder. All organs can be involved in addition to soft tissue and bones. The prognosis is largely determined by the presence and extent of visceral involvement.

plain films, CT, MR, US, angiography) are especially useful in establishing the diagnosis (Figures 50-9 to 50-12). Biopsy should be performed if there is uncertainty regarding the diagnosis, particularly if there is a question of malignancy.

SKELETAL LESIONS. Hemangiomas are the most common benign vascular tumor of bone in children and adults, but constitute only 1% of bone tumors.[26,27] Most skeletal hemangiomas occur in the vertebrae (Figure 50-13) and skull (Figure 50-14) and are asymptomatic. Most of these tumors are discovered incidentally on routine imaging tests where they have a characteristic appearance. Appendicular skeletal lesions (Figure 50-15) are much less common, difficult to diagnose on imaging studies, and more likely to present with pain, swelling, or pathologic fracture.[28]

PERIORBITAL LESIONS. Periorbital hemangiomas are among the most complicated lesions, as the visible portion often represents only the tip of the iceberg (Figure 50-1A). Periorbital hemangiomas can compromise visual axis maturation, resulting in a range of functional disabilities.[29,30] Patients may present with exophthalmos, proptosis, astigmatism,

ptosis, strabismus, or visual impairment. MR is useful to assess the extent of the lesion and potential compromise to vital structures. Vision may be compromised by even small lesions so early pediatric ophthalmologic consultation is crucial.

UPPER AIRWAY LESIONS. Hoarseness or stridor in an infant patient of 6 to 12 weeks of age may herald a subglottic hemangioma.[31] Patients at highest risk for this complication have hemangiomas affecting the "beard" region of the face, which corresponds to the cranial nerve V3 trigeminal distribution (preauricular, anterior neck, chin, and lower lip). Early consultation with ENT is advisable. Bronchoscopy may be necessary to establish the diagnosis and/or treat the lesion.

PHACE SYNDROME. The PHACE syndrome (Online Mendelian Inheritance in Man [OMIM] No. 606519) describes patients with: (1) **P**osterior fossa malformation; (2) **H**emangioma; (3) **A**rterial abnormalities (including coarctation of the **A**orta); (4) **C**ardiac defects; and (5) **E**ye abnormalities (Figure 50-16).[32-34] It is thought to be caused

TABLE 50-5. Clinical Syndromes Associated with Vascular Tumors

	Description
Hemangiomatosis	Benign, but potentially aggressive syndrome of multiple cutaneous hemangiomas; sometimes involving other organs (liver, GI tract, brain, lung)
Gorham disease (vanishing bone disease)	Extremely rare syndrome of massive osteolysis that can occur with hemangiomatosis
Maffucci syndrome	Dyschondroplasia with multiple cavernous hemangiomas. Twenty-percent develop malignant tumors, especially chondrosarcoma; rarely AS
Blue rubber bleb nevus syndrome (Bean syndrome)	Autosomal dominant. Cavernous hemangiomas of the skin, GI tract, and other viscera
Peutz-Jeghers syndrome	Autosomal dominant. Multiple GI hemangiomas and hamartomatous polyps. Melanotic mucosal and cutaneous pigmentation around the lips, oral mucosa, face, genitalia and palms; increased risk of various carcinomas
Klippel-trenaunay-weber syndrome	Nonhereditary, sporadic disorder characterized by soft tissue and bony hypertrophy, varicose veins, and cutaneous portwine stain of the lower extremities; occasional GI involvement
PHACE syndrome	(1) **P**osterior fossa malformation; (2) **H**emangiomas; (3) **A**rterial abnormalities and coarctation of the **A**orta; (4) **C**ardiac defects; and (5) **E**ye abnormalities
Kasabach-Merritt syndrome	Consumptive coagulopathy (thrombocytopenia and DIC) associated with KH, tufted angioma and (rarely) AS
Stewart-Treves syndrome	AS of the breast following radical mastectomy. Associated with chronic lymphedema
Kettle's syndrome	AS of the lower extremities in patients with melanoma following inguinal lymphadenectomy. Associated with chronic lymphedema

by an unknown embryonic insult that occurs during the first trimester of gestation. However, a strong female predominance exists, suggesting X-linked inheritance, but no familial cases have been reported.

Infants with PHACE syndrome present a spectrum of anomalies and disease severity. The diagnosis should be considered in any infant presenting with a large plaque-like lesion on the face. The vascular lesion, which is a true hemangioma, can be confused with the port wine stain (a VM) associated with the Sturge-Weber syndrome. Affected patients require an extensive work-up and consultation with a dermatologist, ophthalmologist, neurologist, cardiologist, and radiologist familiar with the syndrome.

MR of the head and neck should be considered to evaluate for posterior fossa abnormalities (e.g., the Dandy-Walker complex, cerebellar hypoplasia, and abnormalities of the vermis). Cerebral vascular compromise and stroke can result from compression of the carotid arteries or circle of Willis by hemangioma.[35–37] Carotid and vertebral anomalies are best evaluated by MR angiography or traditional (invasive) angiography with digital subtraction. The aortic arch can be evaluated by CT angiography, MR angiography, or more invasively by angiography. Transthoracic echocardiography should be performed to evaluate for congenital heart disease, such as atrial septal defect, or ventricular septal defect.

VISCERAL LESIONS. In the general population, most visceral hemangiomas occur in the absence of cutaneous hemangiomas. However, in the pediatric population, the presence of large or multiple (≥ 5) cutaneous hemangiomas is a significant risk factor for the presence of visceral (especially hepatic) and brain hemangiomas. US is an effective noninvasive and relatively inexpensive method for screening the abdomen. In patients younger than 5 months of age, US may also be used to screen for the presence of brain hemangiomas.

The liver is the most common site of visceral hemangiomas (affecting 5% of the general population), and hemangioma is the most common benign hepatic tumor. Most liver hemangiomas are without clinical significance and are discovered incidentally during abdominal imaging studies (Figures 50-17 and 50-18). Most liver hemangiomas have characteristic imaging findings on CT, MR, and US (Figure 50-19A to 50-19D). Angiography is rarely used to establish the diagnosis, but classically shows highly vascular lesions with parallel arterial feeders and late venous stain. Technetium-99 m-labeled red blood cell (RBC) nuclear imaging can also be helpful when the diagnosis is in doubt based on other imaging studies (Figure 50-19E and 50-19F).[38]

When significant arterial–venous shunting occurs within a liver hemangioma, high-output CHF may result. Massive liver hemangiomas sometimes compress adjacent structures, such as renal veins and the inferior vena cava (IVC), causing abdominal compartment syndrome. In very rare instances, liver hemangiomas can cause a consumptive hypothyroidism as a result of high expression of the thyroid hormone inactivating enzyme type-3 iodothyronine deiodinase (D3).[39]

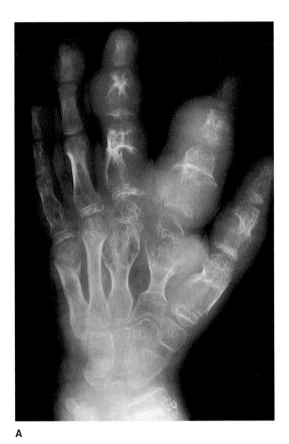 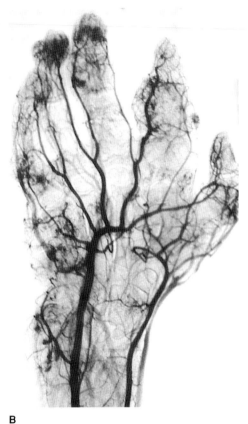

A   B

● **FIGURE 50-8.** Maffucci syndrome (enchondromatosis with hemangiomas). (A) Hand radiograph shows extensive bone and soft tissue deformities caused by enchondromas. (B) Arteriogram shows numerous soft tissue hemangiomas. Lesions are unilateral in one-half of patients. The hands are the most common site of involvement. Malignant transformation as high as 20% has been reported, usually after 40 years of age and most often chondrosarcoma, but many other neoplasms, including AS, also occur.

The presence of iron-deficient anemia or bowel obstruction in the pediatric population should prompt the consideration of gastrointestinal (GI) hemangioma. GI hemangiomas may present focally within the bowel wall, diffusely as intestinal hemangiomatosis, or as an extrinsic abdominal or pelvic cavernous hemangioma with direct invasion of the GI tract.[40] In these cases, a gastroenterology consult is warranted. The diagnosis may be established with endoscopy, tomographic imaging of the abdomen and pelvis (e.g., CT, MR), or angiography. GI hemangiomas are often associated with clinical syndromes (Table 50-5) and, when encountered, should raise the possibility of blue rubber bleb nevus syndrome (Bean syndrome), Klippel-Trenaunay-Weber syndrome, or Peutz-Jeghers syndrome.[41]

Congestive Heart Failure. High-output CHF as a result of arteriovenous (AV) shunting is an occasional complication of hemangiomas. In these cases, the offending lesion(s) is most often hepatic (see above). These patients should be evaluated by a cardiologist. An initial evaluation should include an electrocardiogram (ECG), an echocardiogram, a chest X-ray and basic laboratory work. Cardiac catheterization is often unnecessary in patients younger than 30 years of age, but may be useful in establishing the severity of the shunt. The liver, and potentially other viscera, should be evaluated for hemangioma by imaging studies (US, CT, MR, nuclear).

LUMBOSACRAL SPINE LESIONS. Hemangiomas affecting the lumbosacral region are of special significance (Figure 50-20). Their presence is associated with occult spinal

---

TABLE 50-6. Complications of Hemangiomas
Cosmetic
Psychosocial
Ulceration and bleeding
Persistent soft tissue deformity
Skeletal deformity and/or pain
Ophthalmologic complications
Upper airway obstruction
Cerebral vasculopathy and stroke (PHACE syndrome)
Spinal dysraphism
Genitourinary abnormalities
High-output CHF
Consumptive coagulopathy (KMS)

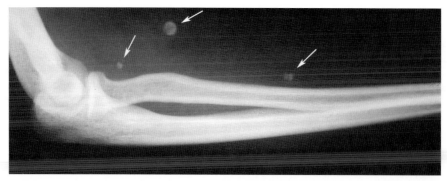

● **FIGURE 50-9.** Hemangioma of forearm. Round and circular (*arrows*) calcifications of this soft tissue mass are highly suggestive of vascular lesion.

dysraphism. Lesions that are macular and telangiectatic are of greatest concern. Deviation of the supragluteal cleft is another diagnostic clue to the presence of this complication. Genital or renal anomalies may accompany these lesions. The lumbosacral spine can often be sufficiently imaged by US in infants younger than 4 months. MR of the lumbar spine and pelvis should be performed in older patients.[42–44] Consider obtaining consultations with a neurologist, neurosurgeon, and urologist.

Adult Presentations and Considerations. Most hemangiomas present during infancy. However, diagnosis in adults is not uncommon. Whereas HOI tend to be superficial and visible, hemangiomas diagnosed in adulthood tend to be deep and subclinical. With the exception of pyogenic granulomas, de novo cutaneous hemangiomas are vanishingly rare in adults. Indeed, most hemangiomas diagnosed in adults are found incidentally during imaging studies.

It is unusual for an adult to complain of functional impairment as a result of a hemangioma. Adults with symptomatic hemangiomas tend to have vague or nonspecific symptoms, such as pain or discomfort with an insidious onset and chronic duration. Pregnancy and hormonal therapy can increase the size of an already existing hemangioma and make it more likely to become symptomatic.

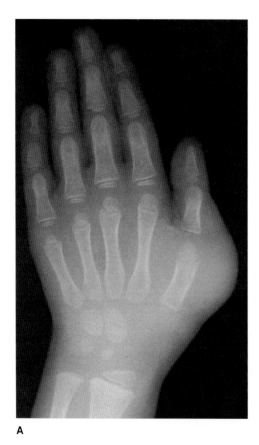

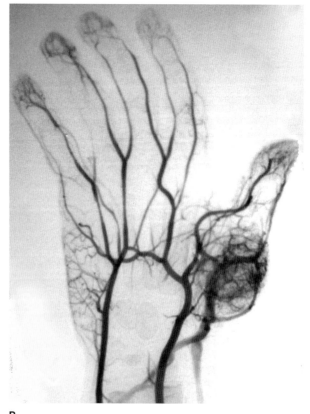

A   **B**

● **FIGURE 50-10.** Hemangioma of thumb. (A) Radiograph shows soft tissue mass adjacent to thumb. (B) Angiogram shows hypervascularity and stain of mass.

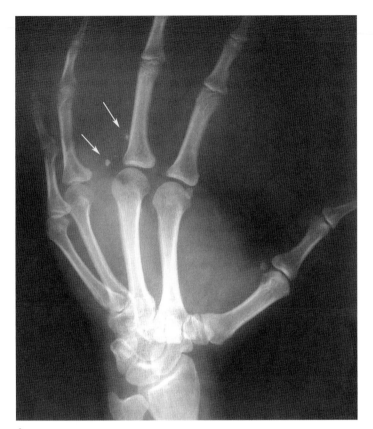

A

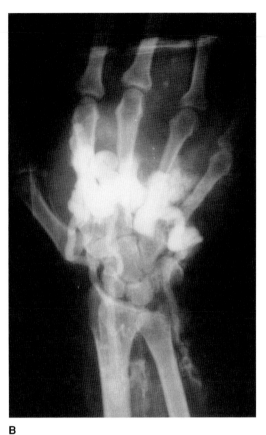

B

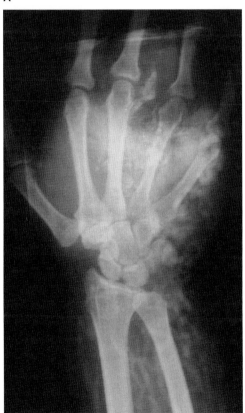

C

● **FIGURE 50-11.** Hemangioma of hand. (A) Radiograph shows metacarpals and phalanges displaced by soft tissue mass with phleboliths (*arrows*). (B) Arteriogram early image shows large abnormal vessels. (C) Arteriogram late image shows persistent faint vascular opacification. Phleboliths suggest a primary vascular lesion, and lack of early venous fillings favors a hemangioma rather than an AV malformation.

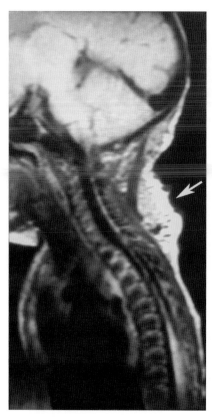

● FIGURE 50-12. Soft tissue hemangioma of the neck (*arrow*) shown by sagittal T2-weighted MR image.

Isolated liver hemangiomas are the most prevalent, with 5% of the population being affected. Women, especially with a history of multiparity, are affected more often than men (5:1), and tend to present at a younger age and with larger tumors. Hemangiomas affecting the digestive tract are less prevalent, but should be considered in the differential diagnosis of young adult patients presenting with iron-deficient anemia. GI hemangiomas affect women and men equally and tend to present in the third decade of life.[45] They may be focal or present as intestinal hemangiomatosis[40]

The skeleton is the second most prevalent anatomic location for hemangiomas in adults. Yet, skeletal hemangiomas are relatively rare, constituting approximately 1% bone tumors.[13,26,27] As in children, most occur in the vertebrae (Figure 50-13) and calvaria (Figure 50-14) and rarely in the appendicular skeleton (Figure 50-15). Histologically, they can be capillary or cavernous. They are diagnosed in all age groups, including the elderly, and affect men and women equally.[28]

Intramuscular and other soft tissue hemangiomas are occasionally seen in adults (Figures 50-9 to 50-11). They can easily be confused with malignant tumors, and differentiation from angiosarcoma (AS) is vital. Intramuscular cavernous hemangiomas are more easily distinguished as benign, but are sometimes misdiagnosed as lipomas.

Work-Up. Patients with hemangiomas most often present with an obvious cutaneous lesion seen early during infancy.

Other presentations are less straightforward. Many specific aspects of the work-up have been described in the preceding section: "Complications and Regionally Important Lesions." Here we describe a general approach to the work-up of a patient with suspected hemangioma.

Establishing the correct diagnosis and determining the extent of disease is predicated on taking a careful history and performing a thorough physical examination. When evaluating a patient with a known or suspected hemangioma, it is important to establish the course of the lesions (i.e., proliferation and involution). Further, any complications should be documented along with what prior work-up has already been performed (e.g., imaging studies, biopsy), as well as prior treatments and the response to those treatments. An understanding of the patient's other past medical history, birth history, maternal pregnancy history, and a review of systems (including psychologic concerns) are imperative.

The physical examination should be comprehensive in addition to a thorough examination of the skin. Skin findings should document lesion location, size, morphology, and presence of ulceration, bleeding, or secondary infection. Petechiae, purpura, and ecchymoses are indicative of a bleeding diasthesis such as KMS. It may be helpful to obtain serial photographs to monitor the patient's clinical course. Other major organs and organ systems should also be evaluated for involvement such as evidence of airway obstruction, CHF, visceral complications, neurologic deficits, or skeletal abnormalities.

A high index of suspicion for deep tissue involvement may warrant evaluation, such as imaging studies. Laboratory tests are unnecessary in the work-up of the vast majority of patients with hemangiomas, but should be obtained if there is evidence of a bleeding diathesis or metabolic derangement. If there is any suspicion of malignancy, biopsy is necessary.

Hemangiomas are small and uncomplicated in 90% of patients. However, physicians who encounter these patients should have a low threshold for consulting a dermatologist. Further work-up with imaging tests, other specialty consultations and, occasionally, biopsy may be warranted if the diagnosis is in question, the patient has complications, or therapeutic interventions are being considered.

Management. Most hemangiomas are small, cutaneous, and asymptomatic and require no treatment. In these cases, close follow-up is advisable in order to ensure that the patient remains asymptomatic and free of complications. Medical therapy and, occasionally, surgical resection or embolic therapy, are required to treat complicated hemangiomas. A multidisciplinary approach is often necessary.

The goals of treatment are not only the prevention of potential complications, such as loss of function, disfigurement, bleeding, infection and pain, but also to address the inherent psychosocial distress that often affects patients and their families. Although it is a potentially difficult conversation, patients and families should be made aware of the potential for unpredictability and the extremely

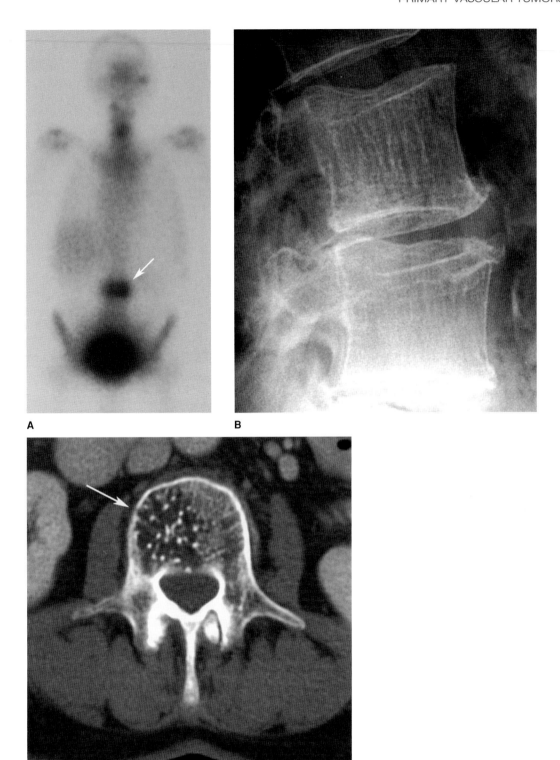

● **FIGURE 50-13.** Hemangioma of lumbar vertebra. (A) Bone scan shows nonspecific uptake in lumbar vertebra (*arrow*). (B) Lateral radiograph shows characteristic vertical bony striations. (C) CT shows vertical striations in cross section as characteristic dots within the low attenuation lesion (*arrow*) in right side of vertebral body. While the bone scan is nonspecific, the characteristic radiographic and CT findings are easily recognized.

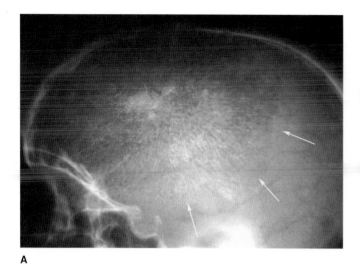

A

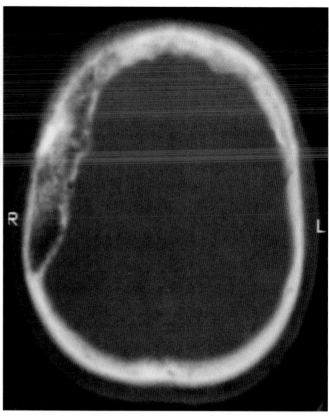

R   L

B

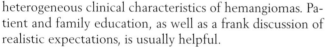

● **FIGURE 50-14.** Hemangioma of calvaria. (A) Lateral skull radiograph shows characteristic stellate trabecular pattern (*arrows*). (B) CT shows expansile lesion (*arrow*) with intact inner and outer table and abnormal diploic space trabeculae. Calvarial hemangiomas have a stellate "sunburst" appearance as a result of periosteal spicules that radiate from their center.

heterogeneous clinical characteristics of hemangiomas. Patient and family education, as well as a frank discussion of realistic expectations, is usually helpful.

Generalized guidelines for the management of hemangiomas of infancy have been published by the American Academy of Dermatology.[14] In practice, treatment of hemangiomas must be individualized according to various factors, such as the age of the patient, rate of proliferation/involution, location of the lesion, size of the lesion, and the potential for complications. Most lesions are primarily cutaneous and therefore best managed by dermatologists. Hemangiomas that are most likely to require intervention include periorbital lesions, lesions affecting the upper airway, ulcerated lesions, very large or rapidly expanding lesions, large hepatic lesions, and lesions that cause significant disfigurement.[46] The appropriate consulting specialties should be involved early in the management of these patients in order to establish questionable diagnoses, institute therapy and prevent complications.

Chemotherapy. The first-line chemotherapy for complicated hemangiomas is high-dose systemic corticosteroid (2–3 mg/kg/d for 3–12 months during the proliferative phase). The physician should be aware of the significant potential for side effects, which are especially considerable in the pediatric population. Intralesional corticosteroids (e.g., triamcinolone acetonide) and topical corticosteroids have been used effectively for small superficial lesions

with less risk of adrenal suppression and other major side effects.[47]

Following its successful use in the treatment of HIV patients with Kaposi's sarcoma (KS), the recombinant cytokine interferon alpha 2b (IFN-α 2b) was found to be useful in the treatment of pediatric hemangiomas. IFN-α 2b has subsequently become an established second-line therapy for corticosteroid-refractory hemangiomas. The mechanism of IFN-α 2b is antiangiogenesis. Despite its efficacy, the use of IFN-α 2b is limited by its transient, but often poorly-tolerated side effects including fever, malaise, neutropenia, and transaminitis. Severe neurotoxicity including spastic diplegia and demyelination, has also been reported.[48]

Vincristine has also been used successfully in the treatment of corticosteroid-refractory hemangiomas, particularly in the setting of KMS.[49,50] The mechanism of action is apoptosis of hemangioma tumor cells. Its use is limited by its long list of significant side effects, including peripheral neuropathy, constipation, jaw pain, leukopenia, and anemia. Furthermore, it must be must be administered under the supervision of a hematologist/oncologist and via a central line.

Ulceration and Bleeding. Ulceration and bleeding caused by hemangiomas should be treated with direct pressure and local wound care with topical antibiotics (e.g., metronidazole gel plus mupirocin), barrier creams, nonstick

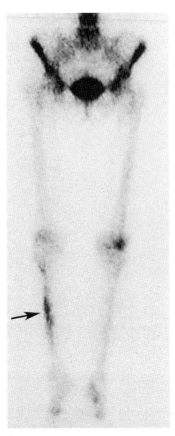
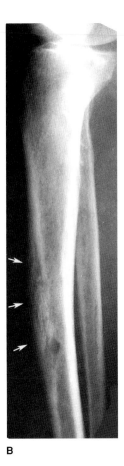

A   **B**

● **FIGURE 50-15.** Hemangioma of tibia. (A) Bone scan shows nonspecific focal tibial uptake (*arrow*). (B) Radiographs show focal tibial abnormality (*arrows*). Hemangiomas of the calvaria and vertebra have characteristic appearances but long bone lesions are rare and have varied, nonspecific bone manifestations.

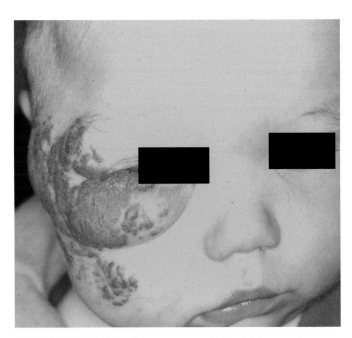

● **FIGURE 50-16.** A large segmental facial hemangioma, as seen in the PHACE syndrome.

dressings, and topical corticosteroids.[25,51] Becaplermin, a recombinant platelet-derived growth factor, has been successfully used in difficult cases (which is counterintuitive because it promotes angiogenesis).[52] Analgesia with oral acetaminophen and topical analgesics (e.g., lidocaine hydrochloride ointment) may also be useful. In refractory cases, surgical resection may be necessary. But since the resultant scar from the surgical resection of a hemangioma is often worse than the result of its spontaneous involution, surgery is best avoided for purely cosmetic reasons.

Intramuscular Lesions. The treatment of intramuscular hemangiomas is surgical excision. In large or complex lesions, presurgical transcatheter arterial embolization has been successfully used.[53] Intramuscular hemangiomas have never been reported to metastasize, but local recurrence rates are high (18%–50%), so one must be judicious when deciding which lesions should be resected.[13,54]

Skeletal Lesions. Treatment of skeletal hemangiomas is necessary only when there is severe functional compromise, such as vertebral hemangioma causing spinal cord compression or long bone hemangioma causing pathologic fracture. Consultation with an orthopedic surgeon is recommended. Treatment is either surgery or radiotherapy and the prognosis is favorable following either therapy.

Periorbital Lesions. Periorbital hemangiomas should be managed by an ophthalmologist experienced with these lesions. Potential therapies include patching the unaffected eye (to ensure use of the affected eye), medical therapy (e.g., corticosteroids), and surgical resection of the hemangioma.[29]

Upper Airway Lesions. Upper airway obstruction as a result of hemangioma should be treated promptly with systemic corticosteroids. Early evaluation by an otolaryngologist is reasonable, as tracheostomy and/or surgical resection of the hemangioma are occasionally necessary.[31] Laser ablation of upper airway hemangiomas has also been successful.[55]

Visceral Lesions. Large symptomatic visceral (e.g., hepatic) hemangiomas are usually responsive to chemotherapy. Refractory cases are traditionally surgically resected. More recently, selective arterial embolization has been successfully used, sometimes as a combined approach with surgery, to treat medically refractory and surgically difficult lesions.[56,57] However, results from embolization may be temporary and complications, such as abcess formation, have been reported.[58]

Congestive Heart Failure. High-output CHF caused by AV shunting in patients with large visceral (especially hepatic) hemangiomas is treated by correcting the shunt as soon as possible. Chemotherapy-induced tumor involution using corticosteroids is often the best initial approach.

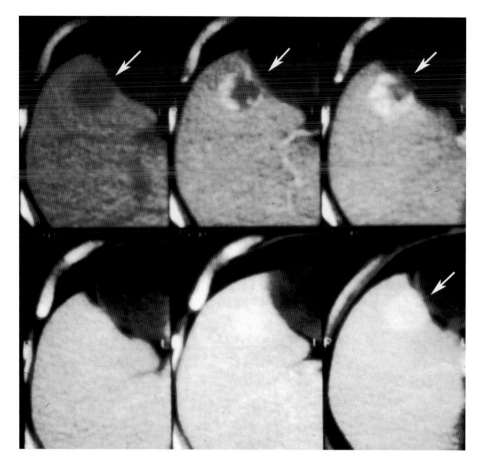

● **FIGURE 50-17.** Liver hemangioma; Single level CT before and after intravenous contrast material. Hemangioma (*arrow*) on 1st image prior to intravenous contrast material is low attenuation. Next five images after IV contrast injection show peripheral hypervascular foci that increase and then the hemangioma becomes isodense and finally hyperdense compared to the liver. Liver hemangiomas, incidental findings in 5% of the general population, must be distinguished from significant lesions. Well-defined focal collections of intravenous contrast material in peripheral slow flow sites of a hemangioma on CT, MR, nuclear medicine RBC study, and angiography are diagnostic. Uniform circumferential enhancement and delayed centripetal uniform enhancement are not.

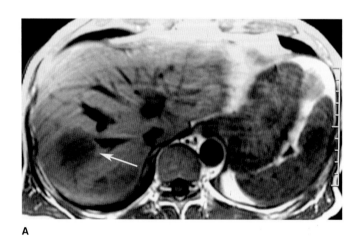

A

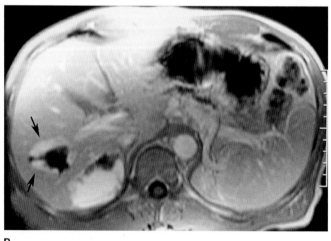

B

● **FIGURE 50-18.** Liver hemangioma; MR. (A) T1-weighted image shows focal low signal lesion (*arrow*). (B) T1-weighted image after IV contrast shows characteristic peripheral, discrete foci of intense enhancement (*arrows*).

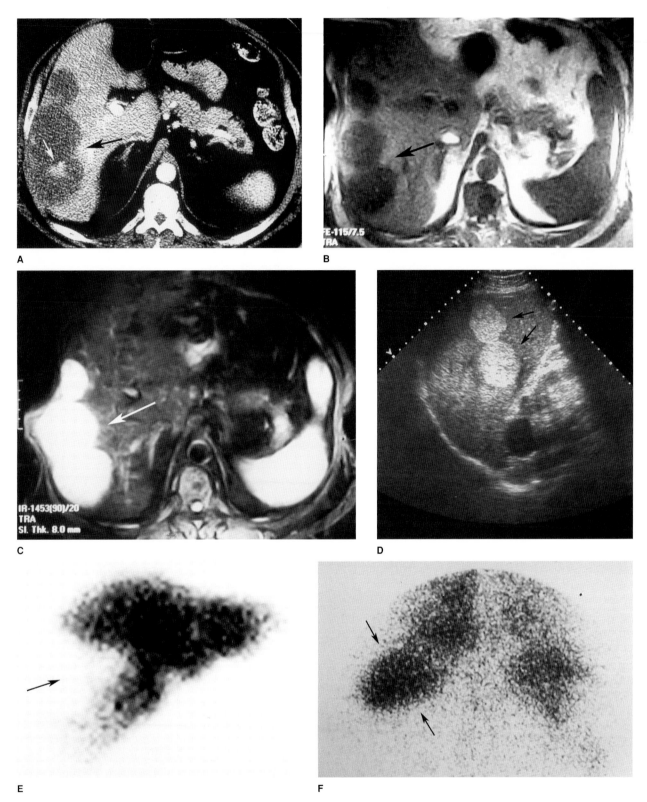

● **FIGURE 50-19.** Large liver hemangioma—CT, MR, US, liver spleen scan, and RBC spleen scan. (A) CT shows only a single site of dense enhancement (*white arrow*) in this large lobulated lesion (*black arrow*). (B) T1-weighted MR shows large lobulated low signal lesion. (C) T2-weighted MR shows characteristic uniform high signal of lesion. (D) US shows suggestive but nonspecific echogenicity of lesion (*arrows*). (E) Liver spleen scan shows large defect at site of lesion (*arrow*). (F) RBC scan shows diagnostic delayed uptake of lesion (*arrow*) Large liver hemangiomas may not show diagnostic imaging features because large vascular spaces do not accumulate enough contrast to show characteristic discrete focal peripheral enhancement. Small (<1 cm) hemangiomas show only uniform hypervascularity that is not diagnostic either.

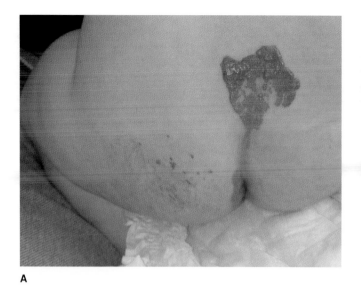

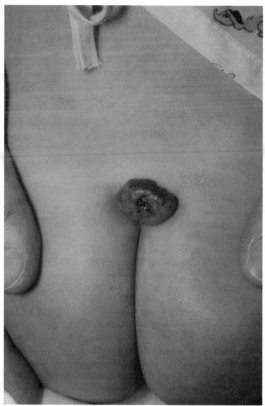

● **FIGURE 50-20.** (A) Lumbosacral hemangioma in an infant. (B) Ulcerated sacral hemangioma in an infant. Both of these infants were imaged and had spinal anomalies, the second required neurosurgic intervention.

B

However, in addition to the major common side effects associated with the use of corticosteroids, one should be alert to the potential for causing an acute decompensation from extra salt and water retention. In corticosteroid-refractory tumors, either IFN-α 2b or vincristine can be used. Hemangiomas refractory to medical therapy have been successfully treated with surgical resection and selective arterial embolization (described above). As in patients with low-output CHF, diuretics provide symptomatic improvement. However, in contrast to patients with low-output CHF, angiotensin-converting enzyme inhibitors (ACE-I) and angiotensin receptor blockers (ARB) are relatively contraindicated (the afterload is already low and the cardiac output is already high). The role of beta-blockers and digoxin is poorly defined.

Pyogenic Granuloma

Pyogenic granuloma (lobular capillary hemangioma or granulation tissue-type hemangioma) is a rare, benign vascular tumor. The misnomer originated because the lesion was once thought to be caused by pyogenic bacteria and was mistaken for granulation tissue. In fact, it is a form of capillary hemangioma. However, unlike other capillary hemangiomas, which most commonly affect infants, pyogenic granuloma affects all age groups, including the elderly, and affects males and females equally.

Grossly, pyogenic granuloma lesions are pedunculated and are characteristically red or purple and friable (Figure 50-21). They occur on either on mucosal surfaces (60%) or skin (40%) and are most common in the mouth, on the face, or on the fingers.[59–61] Histologically, they are similar to other capillary hemangiomas (Figure 50-22).

The lesions typically arise following minor trauma. Occasionally, multiple lesions arise simultaneously. The usual course of this benign tumor is a period of rapid growth over several weeks to a few months until reaching a maximum size of several millimeters to a few centimeters. Some lesions spontaneously involute, but most do not and require treatment. The recommended treatment is simple excision with linear closure, or superficial shave biopsy followed by light electrocautery. A minority of these lesions recur.[60,61]

Glomus Tumor

Glomus tumors are rare, benign vascular neoplasms of the glomus body. Glomus bodies are microscopic structures that modulate thermoregulation and consist of an AV anastomosis surrounded by a bundle of neurons. They are located in the deep dermis under the nailbeds in the lateral aspects of the digits and, to a lesser degree, in the palms, feet, and forearms. However, glomus tumors may also arise in the mediastinum, chest wall, and GI tract.[13,62–66] The majority are sporadic, but these tumors have been associated with neurofibromatosis (NF1).[67,68]

Most common in young adults, glomus tumors are equally prevalent in males and females. The typical clinical presentation of a glomus tumor is in a patient between

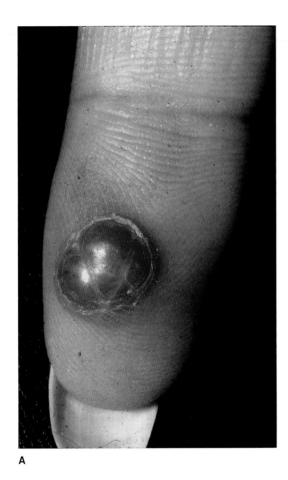

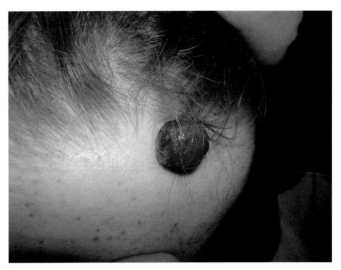

A

B

● **FIGURE 50-21.** Pyogenic granulomas. (A) Characteristic finger lesion. (B) Large scalp lesion.

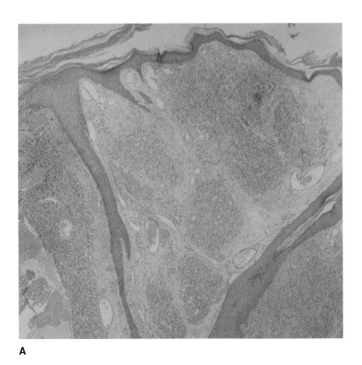

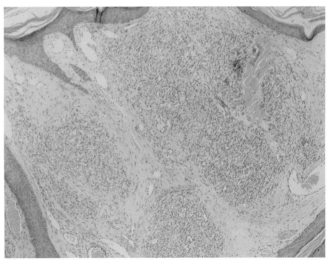

A

B

● **FIGURE 50-22.** Pyogenic granuloma (H&E). (A) Low power. (B) High power.

Courtesy of Madhu Dahiya, M.D., Department of Pathology, Loyola University Medical Center and Stritch School of Medicine, Maywood, IL.

20 and 40 years of age with a subungual finger lesion. The patient is likely to complain of paroxysms of exquisite pain, out of proportion to the size of the lesion. Triggers for pain crises include changes in temperature (especially cold) and tactile stimulation (even mild pressure). These subungual lesions are difficult to detect with the naked eye. But cutaneous lesions manifest as red-blue nodules (<1 cm) and are often readily apparent on physical examination.

More than 90% of glomus tumors are solitary[69] When multiple, the condition is known as *glomangiomatosis* (the glomoid analogue of hemangiomatosis). Unlike typical solitary glomus tumors, glomangiomas tends to occur in children. While they most often affect the hand and forearm, they usually spare the nail bed and are usually less tender. Glomangiomas may arise spontaneously or can be inherited in an autosomal dominant pattern with incomplete penetrance (gene localized to 1p21-22)[70,71]

A radiograph of a glomus tumor often reveals a small scalloped osteolytic defect in the terminal phalanx[72] (Figure 50-23A). MR is a more sensitive technique and can detect tiny, otherwise invisible lesions (Figure 50-23B and 50-23C).[73] MR shows heterogeneous signal intensity on both T1- and T2-weighted images. Glomus tumors appear as soft tissue masses with well-defined contours and feeding vessels that are sharply delineated after intravenous administration of gadolinium-based contrast material.[74]

Most glomus tumors are benign and can be cured by simple conservative excision. Approximately 10% of these lesions will recur.[75] There are no definitive medical therapies for glomus tumors.

Tufted Angioma

Tufted angioma is a very rare, benign cutaneous vascular tumor occuring mostly in children less than 5 years of age, but has been described in all age groups, including the elderly.[76] It is equally prevalent in both sexes. The etiology of this tumor is unclear and there are no known risk factors.

Most tufted angiomas occur on the upper body, especially upper trunk, neck, and shoulders. Grossly, these lesions are reddish-brown to purple macules or plaques, ranging from less than 1cm to several centimeters and are

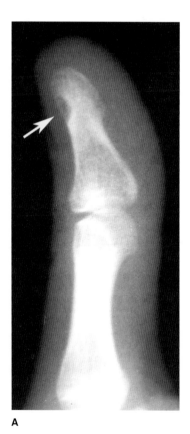
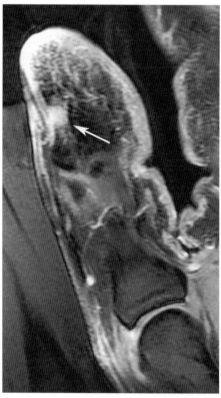

A   B

● **FIGURE 50-23.** Glomus tumor of distal phalanx index finger. (A) Radiograph of second patient shows nonspecific osteolytic defect (*arrow*) of distal phalanx. (B) Coronal post intravenous contrast MR shows high signal enhancement of lesion (*arrow*). These small tumors and are most often extraosseous in the fingertips and under the nail and produce episodic severe pain. Secondary bone involvement with a shallow erosion is usual, but more advanced deformity can mimic an aneurysmal bone cyst or enchondorma.

Courtesy of Laurie Lomasney, M.D., Department of Radiology, Loyola University Medical Center, Maywood, IL.

generally solitary. Sometimes there is a thick indurated border and central depression, a feature that has been likened to a doughnut. Tufted angiomas have a rubbery consistency and may be tender to palpation. Hyperhydrosis of the lesions and nearby skin occurs in 30% of patients.[77]

Histologically, tufted angioma is characterized by a lobular arrangement of densely packed "tufts" of capillaries that appear as "cannonballs" within the dermis. This microscopic appearance shares several features of capillary hemangiomas, KH, and KS. Indeed, some experts believe it represents the same, albeit more benign, disease process as KH (see below). The final diagnosis often rests on immunohistochemical staining.[13]

The natural course of tufted angioma is usually slow but with progressive spread over months to years with ultimate stabilization. Rarely lesions involve spontaneously or regress.[76] Most patients are asymptomatic, but some cases of tufted angioma have been associated with KMS.[78] If there is reason to suspect the lesion involves deep tissue, MR is useful in defining the extent of the lesion. However, deep lesions suggest the diagnosis of KH.

In most cases no treatment is necessary. Lesions may be surgically excised, but occasionally recur. In addition, cryosurgery, radiation therapy, and pulsed-dye laser therapy have all been described with varying degrees of success.[79–81] A role for chemotherapy is not well defined but there are case reports of response to corticosteroids[82] and IFN$_\alpha$ 2b.[83]

● INTERMEDIATE-GRADE NEOPLASMS

Kaposiform Hemangioendothelioma

KH is a rare intermediate-grade vascular neoplasm first described in 1991.[84] This lesion is exclusively in the pediatric population, with the vast majority of cases present during infancy. It is equally prevalent in both sexes. The etiology of KH is unclear and there are no known risk factors. However, the pathophysiology is thought to be similar to tufted angioma.

KH presents as a skin lesion 75% of the time and most are on the trunk and proximal extremities. The remaining cases arise in deep structures, including the retroperitoneum. The cutaneous appearance of KH is nondistinct. The lesion often presents as a small reddish-purple plaque or nodule or as an ill-defined purpuric mass. Typically, the lesion undergoes rapid proliferation and grows to a large size over ensuing months. Nevertheless, it generally remains a solitary lesion. Patients that have KH with the KMS (see below) may present with petechiae, purpura, or ecchymoses, indicative of the severe thrombocytopenia associated with this syndrome.

Histologically, KH has features of both capillary hemangioma and KS and is characterized by zones of fibrosis that contain dilated, thin-walled vessels surrounding nodules of closely packed spindle cells. These cells form small slit-like spaces filled with red cells in a pattern resembling KS (see

below).[85] Immunohistochemical staining suggests a lymphatic tissue origin.[13]

Unlike tufted angioma, KH often involves deep structures and imaging studies are usually necessary to evaluate the extent of the tumor. CT characteristically shows a heterogeneous mass, often containing phleboliths (Figure 50-5). Ill-defined margins that cross tissue planes are also common findings. MR is similarly useful in determining tumor size and involvement of surrounding structures.

The biologic behavior of KH is somewhere between a hemangioma and an angiosarcoma (see below); it is locally aggressive without metastases. Like tufted angioma, and in contrast to pediatric hemangiomas, KH does not spontaneously involute or regress. Most notably, KH is strongly associated with KMS.

Kasabach-Merritt Syndrome. KMS is a bleeding diathesis associated with vascular tumors, particularly KH. In fact, the link between KMS and KH is so strong that in retrospect, most cases of KMS have probably occurred in patients with KH, rather than other vascular tumors.[86,87] This includes the original description in 1940 of an infant with "giant capillary hemangioma."[88] The triad of KMS is: (1) a large primary vascular tumor; (2) microangiopathic anemia; and (3) thrombocytopenia. The characteristic severe thrombocytopenia results from platelet trapping within the tumor and disseminated intravascular coagulation (DIC).

The onset of KMS is heralded by rapid growth of the tumor. Often, the location of the tumor and the patient's tendency to bleed make biopsy a risky undertaking in the acute setting and the diagnosis of KH with KMS must be made clinically. In these cases, an imaging study, such as CT or MR, is essential. An initial laboratory work-up should include complete blood count with differential, fibrinogen, D-dimer, fibrin-split products, coagulation parameters, and urinary BFGF. The differential diagnosis for patients with KMS includes malignancy or other bone marrow disease, severe infection, and liver failure.

Treatment and Prognosis. The prognosis of patients with KH depends on the site of the tumor. Simple cutaneous lesions are rare but often curable with wide local excision. Most lesions are extensive and not amenable to complete resection. In these cases, selective arterial embolization has been an effective adjunct to surgery and/or chemotherapy.[89] Pharmacologic treatments include high-dose corticosteroids, IFN-α 2b, vincristine, cyclophosphamide, and actinomycin D.[90,91] The treatment for KMS is to eliminate the underlying tumor responsible for causing it. KMS is variably responsive to chemotherapy. Despite treatment, mortality caused by hemorrhage and infection ranges between 12% and 24%.[87,92,93]

Kaposi's Sarcoma

KS is an intermediate-grade vascular neoplasm first described by Moritz Kaposi[94] in 1872 at the University of

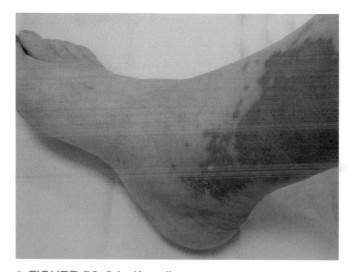

● **FIGURE 50-24.** Kaposi's sarcoma.

Courtesy of James Swan, M.D., Department of Medicine (Dermatology), Loyola University Medical Center and Stritch School of Medicine, Maywood, IL.

Vienna (Figure 50-24). There is some controversy among pathologists as to whether KS represents a differentiation of endothelial cells or lymphatic cells and whether KS represents a hyperplasia or a true neoplasm (Figure 50-25). Regardless, it has become clear in the past decade that KS is a human herpes virus 8 (HHV8)-induced disease that is strongly dependent on a patient's immune status.[95,96] There are four clinical forms of KS as follows.

Chronic KS. Ninety-percent of chronic KS occurs in elderly men, with a peak incidence in the sixth and seventh decades. It is most prevalent in Poland, Russia, Italy, and central equatorial Africa. In the United States it accounts for only 0.02% of cancers. A common presentation is the development multiple cutaneous lesions, usually on the distal aspect of a lower extremity. The lesion typically appears as a blue-red nodule accompanied by edema of the extremity. The lesions slowly grow proximally and then coalesce into plaques resembling pyogenic granuloma (see above). These lesions may ulcerate. Rarely, it occurs on an upper extremity or in a visceral organ. The chronic form of KS has a mortality rate of 10% to 20% and, in those who succumb to the disease, the median survival is 8 to 10 years after diagnosis.[13,97]

Lymphadenopathic (African or Endemic) KS. Quite the opposite of the chronic form, lymphadenopathic KS occurs primarily in young African children and has sparse cutaneous manifestations. These patients tend to have localized or generalized lymphadenopathy, most often involving the cervical, inguinal, and hilar lymph node chains. The course of this form is typically fulminant.

Transplant-Associated KS. This form of KS has been well described in renal transplant patients, occurring in less

than 1% of posttransplant patients in Western countries but in up to 4% of patients in Near East countries (Figure 50-24).[98,99] The mean time to onset of disease is 16 months posttransplant.[13] There are conflicting data as to whether the type of immunosuppression is related to development of the disease. The prognosis is generally favorable if the disease is purely cutaneous. Lowering the level of immunosuppression often yields a significant clinical improvement. However, when this form of KS involves other organs, it is generally fatal.[98]

AIDS-Associated KS. Acquired immunodeficiency syndrome (AIDS) is caused by human immunodeficiency virus 1 (HIV-1) and manifests as a profound immunodeficiency and susceptibility to opportunistic infections and various tumors.[100] Worldwide, approximately 30% of patients with AIDS develop KS[13] Interestingly, most of these cases occur in homosexual men. In other recognized risk groups (e.g., IV drug abusers, transfusion recipients) with AIDS, KS occurs in less than 5% of patients. This disparity is explained by the rates of coinfection with HHV8, the causative agent in KS. HHV8 seropositivity correlates highly with number of male homosexual partners and is probably sexually transmitted.[13] Among patients with AIDS, the mean age of onset of KS is 39 years. The first manifestation of KS in these patients is typically subtle skin findings, especially small, flat, pink macules that have a predilection for skin folds and the gingivae. These lesions coalesce and become blue-purple papules and then plaques that can affect any site on or in the body. Histologically, lesions involve most of dermis and subcutis and eventually form a characteristic nodular pattern (Figure 50-25). Prognosis is highly dependent on the immunologic state of the host and the stage of the disease. Treatment is with radiation therapy or chemotherapy (doxorubicin, bleomycin, and vincristine)[101] IFN-α 2b has also shown efficacy against KS.[13]

● MALIGNANT NEOPLASMS

Angiosarcoma

AS is a malignant neoplasm derived from endothelial cells. This malignant counterpart of hemangioma is rare with only 60 newly diagnosed cases per year in the United States, accounting for 1% to 2% of all soft tissue sarcomas.[102] The biologic behavior of AS is aggressive. It tends to be locally invasive and metastasizes to lymph nodes and distant sites. The prognosis is poor with 5-year survival rates averaging less than 20%.

AS affects all age groups but is most common in adults. With the exception of breast angiosarcoma, AS is more common in males than females. Primary lesions occur in the skin (Figure 50-26), soft tissue, viscera, bone or, very rarely, within large arteries (Figure 50-27).

The etiology of AS is unknown, but several risk factors have been identified (Table 50-7). Tumorigenesis of AS has been linked to mutations in the K-*ras*-2 gene[13] and

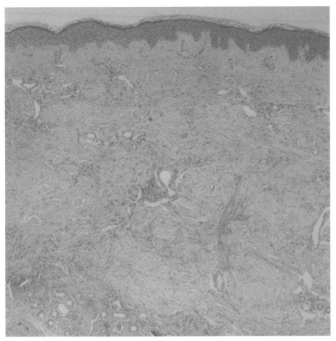

A

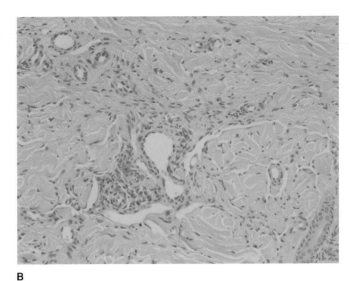

B

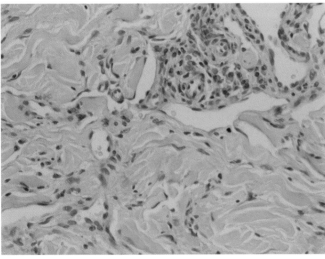

C

● **FIGURE 50-25.** Kaposi's sarcoma (H&E). (A) Low power. (B) Medium power. (C) High power.

Courtesy of Madhu Dahiya, M.D., Department of Pathology, Loyola University Medical Center and Stritch School of Medicine, Maywood, IL.

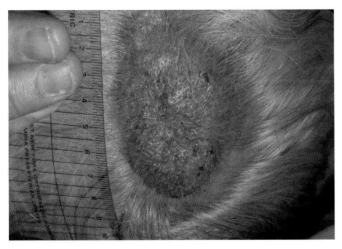

● **FIGURE 50-26.** AS of the scalp.

VEGF/VEGF-R.[103,104] Transformation of a benign tumor to an AS happens rarely, if ever. Descriptions of this phenomenon likely represent an incorrect initial diagnosis.[13] Likewise, reports of an association between AS and HHV8 are probably mistaken.[13,105,106]

Histologically, AS is characterized by irregular branching vascular channels in some areas and solid sheets of cells with increased mitotic figures and hyperchromicity in other areas (Figure 50-28). In its most differentiated form, AS resembles a hemangioma; in its most dedifferentiated form, it can be nearly indistinguishable from carcinoma or melanoma.[13] Immunohistochemical stains (e.g., von Willebrand factor, CD34, CD31, VEGFR-3) are used to confirm the diagnosis.[107–109]

Cutaneous AS Without Lymphedema. Cutaneous AS without lymphedema is the most common form of AS.[13]

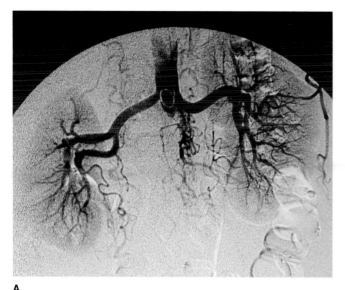

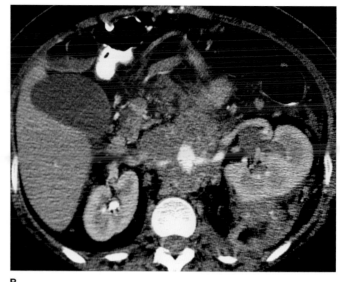

A   B

● **FIGURE 50-27.** Abdominal aortic AS. (A) Aortic angiogram shows complete infrarenal obstruction with collateral vessels. (B) CT shows 2 months later tumor encasement of aorta and renal arteries. These rare malignancies are seldom diagnosed preoperatively, have a poor prognosis, and usually mimic arteriosclerotic disease.

It affects primarily elderly patients. Most lesions develop in the sun-exposed skin of the head and neck, particularly scalp and forehead (Figure 50-26).[13] Grossly, these lesions appear as ill-defined ecchymoses with indurated borders. Extensive invasion into the dermis and deeper structures/fascia is common. Advanced lesions are raised, nodular, and sometimes ulcerated.[13] In 50% of cases there are multiple lesions. The most common sites of metastases are the cervical lymph nodes, lung, liver, and spleen.

Cutaneous AS has a poor prognosis.[110] The 5-year survival is as low as 12%, with most patients dying from direct complications of the tumor.[111,112] The most important prognostic factor is size of the initial lesion, with lesions less than 5 cm having a better prognosis.[102,111,112] Location of the tumor and gender do not impact the patient's prognosis.[113] Treatment is surgical excision and radiotherapy[102,111] Chemotherapy has not been shown to increase survival in cutaneous AS.

Cutaneous AS with Lymphedema. Chronic lymphedema is a risk factor for developing AS of the skin and soft tissue. "Immunologic privilege" of a lymphedematous region has been postulated as the mechanism of this association. Ninety percent of cases involve women following radical mastectomy for breast carcinoma (Stewart-Treves syndrome). However, other causes of chronic lymphedema resulting in AS have included inguinal lymphadenectomy in patients with melanoma (Kettles syndrome), congenital lymphedema, idiopathic lymphedema, traumatic lymphedema, and infectious lymphedema.

TABLE 50-7. Risk Factors for Angio Sarcoma

Sun exposure (cutaneous AS)
Chronic lymphedema
Ionizing radiation
Inherited diseases (e.g., neurofibromatosis, Klippel-Trénaunay syndrome, and Maffucci syndrome)
Thorotrast (thorium dioxide)
Arsenic (e.g., insecticides)
Vinyl chloride
Foreign bodies (e.g., Dacron grafts, plastic, metal, surgical sponges, bone wax)
AV fistula

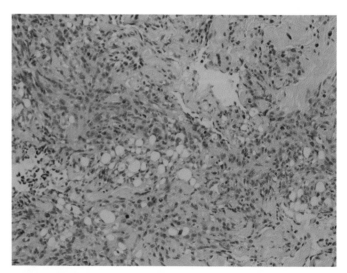

● **FIGURE 50-28.** Histopathology of cutaneous AS, high power (H&E).

Courtesy of Madhu Dahiya, M.D., Department of Pathology, Loyola University Medical Center and Stritch School of Medicine, Maywood, IL.

AS of the breast accounts for only 1 in 1700 to 2000 primary malignant breast tumors but is the most malignant form of breast cancer. Tumorigenesis of breast AS is related to chronic lymphedema and, independently, radiotherapy of prior breast carcinoma.[112,114–117] These lesions form in deep breast tissue. Grossly, they can appear as blue-red discoloration of the overlying skin, but classic signs of breast cancer (e.g., skin retraction, nipple discharge, axillary adenopathy) are absent. Metastases to the lung, pleura, chest wall, skin, and bone are common and cases of KMS have been described.[118,119] Treatment is simple mastectomy. Although there is a paucity of data, 2-year survival has been reported to be less than 10%.[13,120]

Even less is known about the biologic behavior of cutaneous AS in patients with lymphedema of the extremities. These patients also have a very poor prognosis. Anecdotally, long-term survivors underwent radical ablative surgery (either limb disarticulation or hindquarter or forequarter amputation).[121,122]

Visceral AS. Primary AS of the viscera is especially rare, representing less than 25% of cases.[13] These tumors can occur at any age and tend to be associated with an identifiable risk factor. One-third of cases are associated with an inherited disease, such as neurofibromatosis, Klippel-Trénaunay syndrome, or Maffucci syndrome. Other cases have strong associations with environmental exposure to various chemical carcinogens, foreign bodies, and radiation exposure.

Liver AS (Kupffer cell sarcoma) is strongly associated with prior exposure to thorium dioxide (Thorotrast), an IV contrast agent that was used for cerebral angiography from 1930 to 1953. Another strong association is exposure to arsenic-containing insecticides, as described in vineyard workers, and exposure to vinyl chloride, as described in certain factory workers.[123–125]

Many case reports have described an association between foreign bodies and AS.[126–129] Common materials such as steel, plastic, and Dacron grafts have been implicated. The meantime from introduction of the foreign body to the development of AS has been reported to average of approximately 10 years.

There are case reports of AS developing in the radiation field after radiotherapy for malignancies and even eczema. These cases are exceedingly rare. As previously described, radiotherapy of breast carcinoma has been associated with breast and chest wall AS. Additionally, radiotherapy for genitourinary malignancies such as cervical, ovarian, and endometrial cancers has been associated with the subsequent development of AS in the lower abdominal wall and retroperitoneum. Radiotherapy for Hodgkin's disease has been associated with AS in the lumbar spinal area. The mean interval between radiation therapy and the development of AS is 12 years.[112,114–117]

Large Vascular AS. Interestingly, angio sarcomas seem to have a predilection for nonfunctional AV fistulas of renal dialysis patients.[130–134] In five published reports, none of the patients had chronic lymphedema or any other previ-ously identifiable risk factor for AS. This complication is thought to be related to chronic immunosuppression, but it is unclear why the AV fistula site provides the substrate for AS. No viral etiology has been reliably established.

Rare cases of AS developing in large arteries, such as the abdominal aorta have also been described (Figure 50-27).[135] Some of these tumors arose at sites of prosthetic vascular grafts, specifically Dacron, but in most cases no foreign body or other risk factor could be established. The presentation of patients with large artery AS is variable and nonspecific. Most cases are mistaken for atherosclerotic occlusive disease. Indeed, aortic sarcomas mimic mural thrombus on CT and angiography in most reported cases.[135–139] Distant metastatic spread is common at the time of diagnosis and the prognosis is very poor. In patients with AS of the abdominal aorta without metastases, surgical resection resulted in 16.5% 3-year and 11.8% 5-year survival.[140]

Bone AS. Primary bone AS is rare, constituting far less than 1% of primary bone neoplasms. Any bone can be affected, but one-third of these tumors occur in the axial skeleton, and two-thirds in the appendicular skeleton. Multiple lesions in the same bone or same extremity are common. Radiographic assessment is the best initial study to localize and characterize these lesions.[141] AS lesions are osteolytic with variable margination. A distinctive pattern of soap bubble-like lesions may be seen along a length of the bone. Cortical destruction, extension into adjacent soft tissue, and pathologic fractures occur in 10% of patients. A skeletal survey is necessary to identify the extent of disease since many lesions are asymptomatic. Radionucleotide-tagged RBC scintigraphy may be similarly useful.[142] CT can also confirm the characteristics of the radiographic lesions and their multiplicity. MR reveals a nonspecific decreased or variable signal intensity in T1 and increased signal in T2. The lesions enhance with gadolinium. MR is most useful in characterizing extension into adjacent soft tissue.

As with other forms of AS, bone lesions tend to be aggressive with rapid local growth and early metastases. Prognosis depends on histologic grade. Radical ablative surgery and radiation therapy are mainstays of care. Neoadjuvant therapy in patients with high-grade or disseminated disease may result in clinical improvement.

Hemangiopericytoma

Hemangiopericytoma is a rare soft tissue tumor that is believed to arise from pericytes. Pericytes are cells that encircle the periphery of capillaries and venules.[143,144] There is considerable controversy as to whether these cells undergo malignant transformation or whether the entity called "hemangiopericytoma" represents a variety of other soft tissue tumors.[145] Regardless, pathologists do agree on various histologic and immunophenotypic diagnostic criteria for this vascular tumor and "hemangiopericytoma" remains the accepted terminology (Figure 50-29).[13] There is further debate within the pathology community as to what

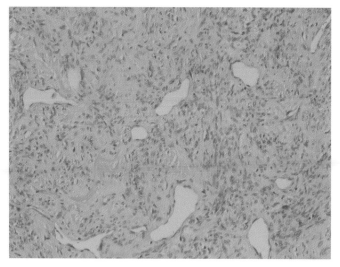

● **FIGURE 50-29.** Histopathology of hemangiopericytoma (H&E).

Courtesy of Madhu Dahiya, M.D., Department of Pathology, Loyola University Medical Center and Stritch School of Medicine, Maywood, IL.

constitutes a malignant hemangiopericytoma. Clinically, the biologic behavior of hemangiopericytoma depends largely on the age of its presentation. While it is relatively benign in most pediatric cases, especially in the congenital form, it is almost universally malignant in the adult population. For the purposes of this text, we define heman- giopericytoma as a malignant vascular tumor, as it has been classified elsewhere.[146]

Adult Hemangiopericytoma. Almost 90% of heman- giopericytomas occur in adults, with most of these oc- curring in the fifth to seventh decade of life. With the exception of one case report,[147] there is no evidence of inheritance. The incidence is equal in males and females. Hemangiopericytoma can arise in any part of the body, but most commonly present as a slowly enlarging painless mass in the soft tissues of the proximal lower extremity or pelvic retroperitoneum. Invasion of secondary sites, such as bone, is common with aggressive tumors. Because of its insidi- ous onset, the tumor may be quite large at the time eval- uation is sought. The average size at presentation is 4 to 8 cm in diameter, but tumors greater than 20 cm have been reported.[148]

Physical findings are nonspecific. Depending on its lo- cation, a solid, potentially tender, mass lesion may be pal- pated. As with other highly vascular lesions, elevated tem- perature of the overlying skin may be present and, rarely, a thrill or bruit may be appreciated. Retroperitoneal heman- giopericytomas may cause local swelling, lower extremity edema, or obstructive uropathy.

Occasionally, hemangiopericytomas manifest with para- neoplastic phenomena. Hypoglycemia may be a presenting sign due to expression of insulin-like growth factor (IGF) by some hemangiopericytomas.[149–151] More commonly

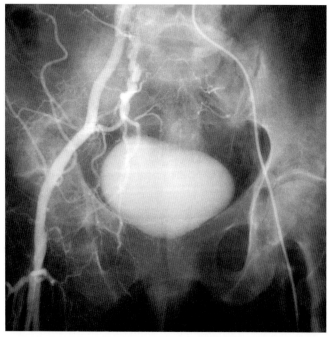

A

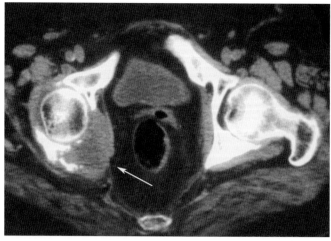

B

● **FIGURE 50-30.** Hemangiopericytoma in patient with osteomalacia. (A) Angiogram shows tumor vascularity from external and internal iliac arteries supplying osteolytic tumor of right acetabulum. Osteomalacia resolved after removal of tumor. (B) CT shows soft tissue mass (*arrow*) that invades and erodes acetabulum. Osteomalacia has been associated with many types of neoplasms, but vascular neoplasms are most common.

(yet still uncommon), patients may present with hypophosphatemia (oncogenic osteomalacia, ricketts).[152-156] Affected patients may complain of muscular weakness or have bone radiographs compatible with osteomalacia (Figure 50-30).

Radiographic findings of hemangiopericytoma are nonspecific. Speckled calcifications are occasionally seen. The tumor may be well circumscribed or have poorly defined borders and these radiologic features correlate with its histologic grade. The tumor may displace or invade surrounding structures. Bony lesions are usually lytic, sometimes with a honeycomb appearance. Osteomalacia may be present (as noted above). Angiography shows dense staining of the tumor vasculature with early venous drainage. Likewise, contrast-enhanced CT or MR images show marked enhancement and sometimes central necrosis that may distinguish hemangiopericytoma from other, less vascular, soft-tissue and bone tumors. MR images are isodense in T1 and have high signal intensity in T2.

Reports of metastasis vary from 10% to 60%.[13] A study from M.D. Anderson Cancer Center reported metastasis in 30% of patients and a 5-year survival of 71%. Better outcomes were associated with extremity lesions and worse outcomes were associated with retroperitoneal and meningeal lesions.[157]

The primary treatment for hemangiopericytoma, including its potential paraneoplastic manifestations, is radical ablative surgery with en bloc resection and a wide surgical margin. Amputation may be necessary to achieve a sufficiently wide margin. Preoperative arterial embolization may be helpful to reduce tumor size and intraoperative hemorrhage. In cases where there are surgically inaccessible lesions or there are multiple metastases, radiotherapy and multiple drug chemotherapy protocols may be used adjunctively.

Pediatric Hemangiopericytoma. In children, especially those less than 4 years of age, hemangiopericytoma is usually a benign, albeit sometimes aggressive, tumor. Infantile (congenital) hemangiopericytoma has different histologic characteristics than adult hemangiopericytoma. The tumor usually occurs in the subcutis or in the oral cavity.[158] Affected patients usually have solitary lesions, but rare instances of metastasis have been reported.[159] As with other primary vascular tumors, it has been reported to cause KMS.[160] When hemangiopericytoma occurs in older children, it tends to have a more aggressive course. Unlike adult hemangiopericytoma, pediatric lesions may be cured by less radical local excision or they may regress spontaneously.[161]

● CONCLUSION

In this chapter we have provided a general overview of the most common forms of vascular tumors in children and adults. Historically, there has been, and continues to be, much confusion regarding the classification of these vascular lesions. Despite different biologic behavior, vascular

tumors are often confused with VM. Primary vascular tumors constitute a group of neoplasms that are primarily derived from vascular elements, such as endothelial cells and pericytes. There are many different vascular tumors and their clinical significance varies widely depending on tumor type, age at presentation, location and extent of tumor burden. Aside from pediatric hemangiomas, primary vascular tumors are relatively rare and most physicians, outside a select few specialties, are unfamiliar with them. Their relative obscurity makes establishing the correct diagnosis difficult and they are commonly mistaken initially for more common diagnoses (Table 50-8). Nevertheless, primary vascular tumors arise in nearly every solid organ and, therefore, are encountered in every field of medicine and surgery.

TABLE 50-8. Differential Diagnosis of Vascular Tumors by Organ System

Cutaneous	**Peripheral and central**
Hemangioma	**nervous systems**
Vascular malformation	Hemangioblastoma
Tufted angioma	Paraganglioma
Glomus tumor	Hemangioma
Kaposiform	Glioma
hemangioendothelioma	Schwannoma
Kaposi sarcoma	Metastatic carcinoma
Cellulitis	**GI tract**
Basal or squamous	Hemangioma
cell carcinoma	Adenocarcinoma
Adrenal carcinoma	Myosarcoma
Nasal glioma	GIST
Myofibramatosis	AVM
Spindle and epithelioid	Ulcerative/erosive
(Spitz) nevus	disease
Dermoid cysts	Inflammatory bowel
Subcutaneous/soft tissue	disease
Hemangioma	**Liver**
Sarcoma	Hemangioma
Lipoma	Hepatocellular carcinoma
Chronic hematoma	Metastatic carcinoma
Skeletal	**Renal/adrenal**
Hemangioma	Hemangioma
Osteosarcoma	Wilm's tumor
Multiple myeloma	Renal cell carcinoma
Metastatic carcinoma	Adrenal cell
Hemangiopericytoma	adenocarcinoma
Osteomyelitis	Pheochromocytoma
Tuberculosis (Pott's	
disease)	
Paget's disease of the	
bone	
Osteoporosis/	
osteopenia	
Trauma	

GIST, gastrointestinal stromal tumor; AVM, arteriovenous malformation.

REFERENCES

1. Mulliken JB, Glowacki J. Hemangiomas and vascular malformations in infants and children: a classification based on endothelial characteristics. *Plast Reconstr Surg.* 1982;69(3):412-422.

2. Enjolras O, Mulliken JB. Vascular tumors and vascular malformations (new issues). *Adv Dermatol.* 1997;13:375-423.

3. Hand JL, Frieden IJ. Vascular birthmarks of infancy: resolving nosologic confusion. *Am J Med Genet.* 2002;108(4):257-264.

4. Barnes CM et al. Evidence by molecular profiling for a placental origin of infantile hemangioma. *Proc Natl Acad Sci U S A.* 2005;102(52):19097-19102.

5. North PE, Waner M, Brodsky MC. Are infantile hemangiomas of placental origin? *Ophthalmology.* 2002;109(4):633-634.

6. Haggstrom AN et al. Prospective study of infantile hemangiomas: demographic, prenatal, and perinatal characteristics. *J Pediatr.* 2007;150(3):291-294.

7. Bielenberg DR et al. Progressive growth of infantile cutaneous hemangiomas is directly correlated with hyperplasia and angiogenesis of adjacent epidermis and inversely correlated with expression of the endogenous angiogenesis inhibitor, IFN-beta. *Int J Oncol.* 1999;14(3):401-408.

8. Takahashi K et al. Cellular markers that distinguish the phases of hemangioma during infancy and childhood. *J Clin Invest.* 1994;93(6):2357-2364.

9. Tan ST et al. Cellular and extracellular markers of hemangioma. *Plast Reconstr Surg.* 2000;106(3):529-538.

10. Boye E et al. Clonality and altered behavior of endothelial cells from hemangiomas. *J Clin Invest.* 2001;107(6):745-752.

11. Walter JW et al. Somatic mutation of vascular endothelial growth factor receptors in juvenile hemangioma. *Genes Chromosomes Cancer.* 2002;33(3):295-303.

12. Ritter MR et al. Myeloid cells in infantile hemangioma. *Am J Pathol.* 2006;168(2):621-628.

13. Weiss SW, Goldblum JR. *Soft Tissue Tumors.* 4th ed. St. Louis, MO: Mosby; 2001:1622.

14. Frieden IJ et al. Guidelines of care for hemangiomas of infancy. American Academy of Dermatology Guidelines/Outcomes Committee. *J Am Acad Dermatol.* 1997;37(4):631-637.

15. Levine E, Wetzel LH, Neff JR. MR imaging and CT of extrahepatic cavernous hemangiomas. *AJR Am J Roentgenol.* 1986;147(6):1299-1304.

16. Drolet BA, Esterly NB, Frieden IJ. Hemangiomas in children. *N Engl J Med.* 1999;341(3):173-181.

17. Blei F et al. Familial segregation of hemangiomas and vascular malformations as an autosomal dominant trait. *Arch Dermatol.* 1998;134(6):718-722.

18. Mulliken JB, Enjolras O. Congenital hemangiomas and infantile hemangioma: missing links. *J Am Acad Dermatol.* 2004;50(6):875-882.

19. Enjolras O et al. Noninvoluting congenital hemangioma: a rare cutaneous vascular anomaly. *Plast Reconstr Surg.* 2001;107(7):1647-1654.

20. Lopriore E, Markhorst DG. Diffuse neonatal haemangiomatosis: new views on diagnostic criteria and prognosis. *Acta Paediatr.* 1999;88(1):93-97.

21. Golitz LE, Rudikoff J, O'Meara OP. Diffuse neonatal hemangiomatosis. *Pediatr Dermatol.* 1986;3(2):145-152.

22. Rao VK, Weiss SW. Angiomatosis of soft tissue. An analysis of the histologic features and clinical outcome in 51 cases. *Am J Surg Pathol.* 1992;16(8):764-771.

23. Metry DW, Hebert AA. Benign cutaneous vascular tumors of infancy: when to worry, what to do. *Arch Dermatol.* 2000;136(7):905-914.

24. Tanner JL, Dechert MP, Frieden IJ. Growing up with a facial hemangioma: parent and child coping and adaptation. *Pediatrics.* 1998;101(3, pt 1):446-452.

25. Kim HJ, Colombo M, Frieden IJ. Ulcerated hemangiomas: clinical characteristics and response to therapy. *J Am Acad Dermatol.* 2001;44(6):962-972.

26. Mulder JD. *Radiologic Atlas of Bone Tumors.* 2nd ed. Amsterdam, New York: Elsevier; 1993:xii, 749.

27. Unni KK. *Dahlin's Bone Tumors: General Aspects and Data on 11087 Cases.* 5th ed. Philadelphia, PA: Lippincott Williams & Wilkins; 1996:463.

28. Kaleem Z, Kyriakos M, Totty WG. Solitary skeletal hemangioma of the extremities. *Skeletal Radiol.* 2000;29(9):502-513.

29. Ceisler EJ, Santos L, Blei F. Periocular hemangiomas: what every physician should know. *Pediatr Dermatol.* 2004;21(1):1-9.

30. Yap EY, Bartley GB, Hohberger GG. Periocular capillary hemangioma: a review for pediatricians and family physicians. *Mayo Clin Proc.* 1998;73(8):753-759.

31. Orlow SJ, Isakoff MS, Blei F. Increased risk of symptomatic hemangiomas of the airway in association with cutaneous hemangiomas in a "beard" distribution. *J Pediatr.* 1997;131(4):643-646.

32. James PA, McGaughran J. Complete overlap of PHACE syndrome and sternal malformation-vascular dysplasia association. *Am J Med Genet.* 2002;110(1):78-84.

33. Metry DW et al. A prospective study of PHACE syndrome in infantile hemangiomas: demographic features, clinical findings, and complications. *Am J Med Genet A.* 2006;140(9):975-986.

34. Metry DW et al. A comparison of disease severity among affected male versus female patients with PHACE syndrome. *J Am Acad Dermatol.* 2008;58(1):81-87.

35. Bhattacharya JJ et al. PHACES syndrome: a review of eight previously unreported cases with late arterial occlusions. *Neuroradiology.* 2004;46(3):227-233.

36. Burrows PE et al. Cerebral vasculopathy and neurologic sequelae in infants with cervicofacial hemangioma: report of eight patients. *Radiology.* 1998;207(3):601-607.

37. Drolet BA et al. Early stroke and cerebral vasculopathy in children with facial hemangiomas and PHACE association. *Pediatrics.* 2006;117(3):959-964.

38. Miller JH. Technetium-99 m-labeled red blood cells in the evaluation of hemangiomas of the liver in infants and children. *J Nucl Med.* 1987;28(9):1412-1418.

39. Huang SA et al. A 21-year-old woman with consumptive hypothyroidism due to a vascular tumor expressing type 3 iodothyronine deiodinase. *J Clin Endocrinol Metab.* 2002;87(10):4457-4461.

40. Gentry R, Dockerty MB, Clagett OT. Vascular malformations and vascular tumors of the gastrointestinal tract. *Int Abstr Surg.* 1949;88:281-323.

41. Bandler M. Hemangiomas of the small intestine associated with mucocutaneous pigmentation. *Gastroenterology.* 1960;38:641-645.

42. Goldberg NS, Hebert AA, Esterly NB. Sacral hemangiomas and multiple congenital abnormalities. *Arch Dermatol.* 1986;122(6):684-687.

43. McAtee-Smith J et al. Skin lesions of the spinal axis and spinal dysraphism. Fifteen cases and a review of the literature. *Arch Pediatr Adolesc Med.* 1994;148(7):740-748.

44. Tubbs RS et al. Isolated flat capillary midline lumbosacral hemangiomas as indicators of occult spinal dysraphism. *J Neurosurg.* 2004;100(2 suppl Pediatr):86-89.

45. Ruiz AR Jr, Ginsberg AL. Giant mesenteric hemangioma with small intestinal involvement: an unusual cause of recurrent gastrointestinal bleed and review of gastrointestinal hemangiomas. *Dig Dis Sci.* 1999;44(12):2545-2551.

46. Dinehart SM, Kincannon J, Geronemus R. Hemangiomas: evaluation and treatment. *Dermatol Surg.* 2001;27(5):475-485.

47. Weiss AH. Adrenal suppression after corticosteroid injection of periocular hemangiomas. *Am J Ophthalmol.* 1989;107(5):518-522.

48. Ezekowitz RA, Mulliken JB, Folkman J. Interferon alfa-2 a therapy for life-threatening hemangiomas of infancy. *N Engl J Med.* 1992;326(22):1456-1463.

49. Fawcett SL et al. Vincristine as a treatment for a large haemangioma threatening vital functions. *Br J Plast Surg.* 2004;57(2):168-171.

50. Perez J, Pardo J, Gomez C. Vincristine–an effective treatment of corticoid-resistant life-threatening infantile hemangiomas. *Acta Oncol.* 2002;41(2):197-199.

51. Morelli JG et al. Treatment of ulcerated hemangiomas infancy. *Arch Pediatr Adolesc Med.* 1994;148(10):1104-1105.

52. Metz BJ et al. Response of ulcerated perineal hemangiomas of infancy to becaplermin gel, a recombinant human platelet-derived growth factor. *Arch Dermatol.* 2004;140(7):867-870.

53. Cohen AJ et al. Intramuscular hemangioma. *JAMA.* 1983;249(19):2680-2682.

54. Beham A, Fletcher CD. Intramuscular angioma: a clinicopathological analysis of 74 cases. *Histopathology.* 1991;18(1):53-59.

55. Rahbar R et al. The biology and management of subglottic hemangioma: past, present, future. *Laryngoscope.* 2004;114(11):1880-1891.

56. Srivastava DN et al. Transcatheter arterial embolization in the treatment of symptomatic cavernous hemangiomas of the liver: a prospective study. *Abdom Imaging.* 2001;26(5):510-514.

57. Vassiou K et al. Embolization of a giant hepatic hemangioma prior to urgent liver resection. Case report and review of the literature. *Cardiovasc Intervent Radiol.* 2007;30(4):800-802.

58. Pasqual E et al. Embolisation of arteriovenous intrahepatic fistulas associated with diffuse haemangiomatosis of the liver. Report of a case in an adult and review of the literature. *Chir Ital.* 2007;59(5):701-705.

59. Kerr DA. Granuloma pyogenicum. *Oral Surg Oral Med Oral Pathol.* 1951;4(2):158-176.

60. Bhaskar SN, Jacoway JR. Pyogenic granuloma—clinical features, incidence, histology, and result of treatment: report of 242 cases. *J Oral Surg.* 1966;24(5):391-398.

61. Mills SE, Cooper PH, Fechner RE. Lobular capillary hemangioma: the underlying lesion of pyogenic granuloma. A study of 73 cases from the oral and nasal mucous membranes. *Am J Surg Pathol.* 1980;4(5):470-479.

62. Apfelberg DB, Teasley JL. Unusual locations and manifestations of glomus tumors (glomangiomas). *Am J Surg.* 1968;116(1):62-64.

63. Brindley GV. Glomus tumor of the mediastinum. *J Thorac Surg.* 1949;18:417.

64. Appelman HD, Helwig EB. Glomus tumors of the stomach. *Cancer.* 1969;23(1):203-213.

65. Haque S, Modlin IM, West AB. Multiple glomus tumors of the stomach with intravascular spread. *Am J Surg Pathol.* 1992;16(3):291-299.

66. Barua R. Glomus tumor of the colon. First reported case. *Dis Colon Rectum.* 1988;31(2):138-140.

67. Okada O et al. A case of multiple subungual glomus tumors associated with neurofibromatosis type 1. *J Dermatol.* 1999;26(8):535-537.

68. Sawada S et al. Three cases of subungual glomus tumors with von Recklinghausen neurofibromatosis. *J Am Acad Dermatol.* 1995;32(2, pt 1):277-278.

69. Goodman TF, Abele DC. Multiple glomus tumors. A clinical and electron microscopic study. *Arch Dermatol.* 1971;103(1):11-23.

70. Conant MA, Wiesenfeld SL. Multiple glomus tumors of the skin. *Arch Dermatol.* 1971;103(5):481-485.

71. Boon LM et al. A gene for inherited cutaneous venous anomalies ("glomangiomas") localizes to chromosome 1p21-22. *Am J Hum Genet.* 1999;65(1):125-133.

72. Harris WS. Erosion of bone produced by glomus tumour. *Can Med Assoc J.* 1954;70(6):684-685.

73. Idy-Peretti I et al. Subungual glomus tumor: diagnosis based on high-resolution MR images. *AJR Am J Roentgenol.* 1992;159(6):1351.

74. Kneeland JB et al. High resolution MR imaging of glomus tumor. *J Comput Assist Tomogr.* 1987;11(2):351-352.

75. Tsuneyoshi M, Enjoji M. Glomus tumor: a clinicopathologic and electron microscopic study. *Cancer.* 1982;50(8):1601-1607.

76. Jones EW, Orkin M. Tufted angioma (angioblastoma). A benign progressive angioma, not to be confused with Kaposi's

sarcoma or low-grade angiosarcoma. *J Am Acad Dermatol.* 1989;20(2, pt 1):214-225.

77. Ban M, Kamiya H, Kitajima Y. Tufted angioma of adult onset, revealing abundant eccrine glands and central regression. *Dermatology.* 2000;201(1):68-70.

78. Enjolras O et al. Kasabach-Merritt syndrome on a congenital tufted angioma. *Ann Dermatol Venereol.* 1998;125(4):257-560.

79. Dewerdt S et al. Acquired tufted angioma in an adult: failure of pulsed dye laser therapy. *Ann Dermatol Venereol.* 1998;125(1):47-49.

80. Mahendran R et al. Response of childhood tufted angioma to the pulsed-dye laser. *J Am Acad Dermatol.* 2002;47(4):620-622.

81. Powell J. Update on hemangiomas and vascular malformations. *Curr Opin Pediatr.* 1999;11(5):457-463.

82. Munn SE, Jackson JE, Jones RR. Tufted haemangioma responding to high-dose systemic steroids: a case report and review of the literature. *Clin Exp Dermatol.* 1994;19(6):511-514.

83. Suarez SM, Pensler JM, Paller AS. Response of deep tufted angioma to interferon alfa. *J Am Acad Dermatol.* 1995;33(1):124-126.

84. Tsang WY, Chan JK. Kaposi-like infantile hemangioendothelioma. A distinctive vascular neoplasm of the retroperitoneum. *Am J Surg Pathol.* 1991;15(10):982-989.

85. Zukerberg LR, Nickoloff BJ, Weiss SW. Kaposiform hemangioendothelioma of infancy and childhood. An aggressive neoplasm associated with Kasabach-Merritt syndrome and lymphangiomatosis. *Am J Surg Pathol.* 1993;17(4):321-328.

86. Enjolras O et al. Infants with Kasabach-Merritt syndrome do not have "true" hemangiomas. *J Pediatr.* 1997;130(4):631-640.

87. Sarkar M et al. Thrombocytopenic coagulopathy (Kasabach-Merritt phenomenon) is associated with Kaposiform hemangioendothelioma and not with common infantile hemangioma. *Plast Reconstr Surg.* 1997;100(6):1377-1386.

88. Kasabach HH, Merritt KK. Capillary hemangioma with extensive purpura: report of a case. *Am J Dis Child.* 1940;59:1063.

89. Komiyama M et al. Endovascular treatment of huge cervicofacial hemangioma complicated by Kasabach-Merritt syndrome. *Pediatr Neurosurg.* 2000;33(1):26-30.

90. Deb G et al. Spindle cell (Kaposiform) hemangioendothelioma with Kasabach-Merritt syndrome in an infant: successful treatment with alpha-2 A interferon. *Med Pediatr Oncol.* 1997;28(5):358-361.

91. Hu B et al. Kasabach-Merritt syndrome-associated kaposiform hemangioendothelioma successfully treated with cyclophosphamide, vincristine, and actinomycin D. *J Pediatr Hematol Oncol.* 1998;20(6):567-569.

92. el-Dessouky M et al. Kasabach-Merritt syndrome. *J Pediatr Surg.* 1988;23(2):109-111.

93. Maceyko RF, Camisa C. Kasabach-Merritt syndrome. *Pediatr Dermatol.* 1991;8(2):133-136.

94. Kaposi M. Idiopathisches multiples pigmentsarkom der haut. *Arch Dermatol Syph.* 1872;4:265-273.

95. Chang Y et al. Identification of herpesvirus-like DNA sequences in AIDS-associated Kaposi's sarcoma. *Science.* 1994;266(5192):1865-1869.

96. Weiss RA et al. Human herpesvirus type 8 and Kaposi's sarcoma. *J Natl Cancer Inst Monogr.* 1998;(23):51-54.

97. O'Brien PH, Brasfield RD. Kaposi's sarcoma. *Cancer.* 1966;19(11):1497-1502.

98. Qunibi WY et al. Kaposi's sarcoma in renal transplant recipients: a report on 26 cases from a single institution. *Transplant Proc.* 1993;25(1, pt 2):1402-1405.

99. Shmueli D et al. The incidence of Kaposi sarcoma in renal transplant patients and its relation to immunosuppression. *Transplant Proc.* 1989;21(1, pt 3):3209-3210.

100. Fauci AS et al. NIH conference. The acquired immunodeficiency syndrome: an update. *Ann Intern Med.* 1985;102(6):800-813.

101. Krown SE. Acquired immunodeficiency syndrome-associated Kaposi's sarcoma. Biology and management. *Med Clin North Am.* 1997;81(2):471-494.

102. Mark RJ et al. Angiosarcoma. A report of 67 patients and a review of the literature. *Cancer.* 1996;77(11):2400-2406.

103. Brown LF et al. Strong expression of kinase insert domain-containing receptor, a vascular permeability factor/vascular endothelial growth factor receptor in AIDS-associated Kaposi's sarcoma and cutaneous angiosarcoma. *Am J Pathol.* 1996;148(4):1065-1074.

104. Hashimoto M et al. Expression of vascular endothelial growth factor and its receptor mRNA in angiosarcoma. *Lab Invest.* 1995;73(6):859-863.

105. Lasota J, Miettinen M. Absence of Kaposi's sarcoma-associated virus (human herpesvirus-8) sequences in angiosarcoma. *Virchows Arch.* 1999;434(1):51-56.

106. Lin BT et al. Absence of Kaposi's sarcoma-associated herpesvirus-like DNA sequences in malignant vascular tumors of the serous membranes. *Mod Pathol.* 1996;9(12):1143-1146.

107. Poblet E, Gonzalez-Palacios F, Jimenez FJ. Different immunoreactivity of endothelial markers in well and poorly differentiated areas of angiosarcomas. *Virchows Arch.* 1996;428(4-5):217-221.

108. Ramani P, Bradley NJ, Fletcher CD. QBEND/10, a new monoclonal antibody to endothelium: assessment of its diagnostic utility in paraffin sections. *Histopathology.* 1990;17(3):237-242.

109. Traweek ST et al. The human hematopoietic progenitor cell antigen (CD34) in vascular neoplasia. *Am J Clin Pathol.* 1991;96(1):25-31.

110. Holden CA, Wilson Jones E. Angiosarcoma of the face and scalp. *J R Soc Med.* 1985;78(suppl 11):30-31.

111. Holden CA, Spittle MF, Jones EW. Angiosarcoma of the face and scalp, prognosis and treatment. *Cancer.* 1987;59(5):1046-1057.

112. Maddox JC, Evans HL. Angiosarcoma of skin and soft tissue: a study of forty-four cases. *Cancer.* 1981;48(8):1907-1921.

113. Bardwil JM et al. Angiosarcomas of the head and neck region. *Am J Surg.* 1968;116(4):548-553.

114. Cafiero F et al. Radiation-associated angiosarcoma: diagnostic and therapeutic implications–two case reports and a review of the literature. *Cancer.* 1996;77(12):2496-2502.

115. Davies JD, Rees GJ, Mera SL. Angiosarcoma in irradiated post-mastectomy chest wall. *Histopathology.* 1983;7(6):947-956.

116. Marchal C et al. Nine breast angiosarcomas after conservative treatment for breast carcinoma: a survey from French Comprehensive Cancer Centers. *Int J Radiat Oncol Biol Phys.* 1999;44(1):113-119.

117. Parham D.M, Fisher C. Angiosarcomas of the breast developing post radiotherapy. *Histopathology.* 1997;31(2):189-195.

118. Bernathova M et al. Primary angiosarcoma of the breast associated Kasabach-Merritt syndrome during pregnancy. *Breast.* 2006;15(2):255-258.

119. Mazzocchi A et al. Kasabach-Merritt syndrome associated to angiosarcoma of the breast. A case report and review of the literature. *Tumori.* 1993;79(2):137-140.

120. Mc CB, Hogg L Jr. Angiosarcoma of the breast. *Cancer.* 1954; 7(3):586-594.

121. Sordillo PP et al. Lymphangiosarcoma. *Cancer.* 1981;48(7): 1674-1679.

122. Woodward AH, Ivins JC, Soule EH. Lymphangiosarcoma arising in chronic lymphedematous extremities. *Cancer.* 1972;30(2):562-572.

123. Alrenga DP. Primary angiosarcoma of the liver. Review article. *Int Surg.* 1975;60(4):198-203.

124. Makk L et al. Liver damage and angiosarcoma in vinyl chloride workers. A systematic detection program. *JAMA.* 1974;230(1):64-68.

125. Popper H et al. Development of hepatic angiosarcoma in man induced by vinyl chloride, thorotrast, and arsenic. Comparison with cases of unknown etiology. *Am J Pathol.* 1978;92(2):349-369.

126. Ben-Izhak O et al. Angiosarcoma of the colon developing in a capsule of a foreign body. Report of a case with associated hemorrhagic diathesis. *Am J Clin Pathol.* 1992;97(3):416-420.

127. Hayman J, Huygens H. Angiosarcoma developing around a foreign body. *J Clin Pathol.* 1983;36(5):515-518.

128. Jennings TA et al. Angiosarcoma associated with foreign body material. A report of three cases. *Cancer.* 1988; 62(11):2436-2444.

129. Weiss WM et al. Angiosarcoma at the site of a Dacron vascular prosthesis: a case report and literature review. *J Vasc Surg.* 1991;14(1):87-91.

130. Bessis D et al. Endothelin-secreting angiosarcoma occurring at the site of an arteriovenous fistula for haemodialysis in a renal transplant recipient. *Br J Dermatol.* 1998;138(2):361-363.

131. Byers RJ et al. Epithelioid angiosarcoma arising in an arteriovenous fistula. *Histopathology.* 1992;21(1):87-89.

132. Keane MM, Carney DN. Angiosarcoma arising from a defunctionalized arteriovenous fistula. *J Urol.* 1993;149(2): 364-365.

133. Medioni LD et al. Angiosarcoma arising from an arterio-venous fistula in a renal transplant recipient.

An unusual complication. *Ann Pathol.* 1996;16(3):200-202.

134. Wehrli BM et al. Epithelioid angiosarcoma arising in a surgically constructed arteriovenous fistula: a rare complication of chronic immunosuppression in the setting of renal transplantation. *Am J Surg Pathol.* 1998;22(9):1154-1159.

135. Brylka B, Demos TC, Pierce K. Primary angiosarcoma of the abdominal aorta: a case report and literature review (aortic angiosarcoma). *Abdom Imaging.* 2008. In press.

136. Abularrage CJ et al. Aortic angiosarcoma presenting as distal arterial embolization. *Ann Vasc Surg.* 2005;19(5):744-748.

137. Defawe OD et al. Primary sarcoma of an abdominal aortic aneurysm. *Abdom Imaging.* 2006;31(1):117-119.

138. Gittleman AM et al. Angiosarcoma of the aorta. *J Vasc Interv Radiol.* 2002;13(2, pt 1):214-215.

139. Hagspiel KD et al. Primary sarcoma of the distal abdominal aorta: CT angiography findings. *Abdom Imaging.* 2004;29(4):507-510.

140. Chiche L et al. Primary tumors of the thoracoabdominal aorta: surgical treatment of 5 patients and review of the literature. *Ann Vasc Surg.* 2003;17(4):354-364.

141. Lomasney LM et al. Multifocal vascular lesions of bone: imaging characteristics. *Skeletal Radiol.* 1996;25(3):255-261.

142. Joseph UA, Jhingran SG. Technetium-99 m labeled red blood cells in the evaluation of hemangiosarcoma. *Clin Nucl Med.* 1987;12(11):845-847.

143. Rouget C. Memoire sur le developpement, la structure, et proprietes physiologiques des capillaires sanguins et lymphatiques. *Arch Physiol Norm Pathol.* 1873;5:603.

144. Zimmermann KW. Der feinere Bau der Blutkapillaren. Z Anat Entwicklungsgesch. 1923;68:29.

145. Fletcher CD. Hemangiopericytoma—a dying breed? Reappraison of an "entity" and its varient: a hypothesis. *Curr Diagn Pathol.* 1994;1:19.

146. Kumar V, Abbas AK, Fausto N, eds. *Pathologic Basis of Disease.* 7th ed. Philadelphia, PA: Elsevier Saunders; 2005.

147. Plukker JT et al. Malignant hemangiopericytoma in three kindred members of one family. *Cancer.* 1988;61(4):841-844.

148. Morris P et al. Giant retroperitoneal pelvic hemangiopericytoma. *J Cardiovasc Surg (Torino).* 1991;32(6):778-782.

149. Simon R, Greene RC. Perirenal Hemangiopericytoma. A case associated with hypoglycemia. *JAMA.* 1964;189:155-156.

150. Paullada JJ et al. Hemangiopericytoma associated with hypoglycemia. Metabolic and electron microscopic studies of a case. *Am J Med.* 1968;44(6):990-999.

151. Pavelic K et al. The expression and role of insulin-like growth factor II in malignant hemangiopericytomas. *J Mol Med.* 1999;77(12):865-869.

152. Hanukoglu A et al. Surgically curable hypophosphatemic rickets. Diagnosis and management. *Clin Pediatr (Phila).* 1989;28(7):321-325.

153. Miyauchi A et al. Hemangiopericytoma-induced osteomalacia: tumor transplantation in nude mice causes

hypophosphatemia and tumor extracts inhibit renal 25-hydroxyvitamin D 1-hydroxylase activity. *J Clin Endocrinol Metab*. 1988;67(1):46-53.

154. Salassa RM, Jowsey J, Arnaud CD. Hypophosphatemic osteomalacia associated with "nonendocrine" tumors. *N Engl J Med*. 1970;283(2):65-70.

155. Shimada T et al. Cloning and characterization of FGF23 as a causative factor of tumor-induced osteomalacia. *Proc Natl Acad Sci U S A*. 2001;98(11):6500-6505.

156. Sweet RA et al. Vitamin D metabolite levels in oncogenic osteomalacia. *Ann Intern Med*. 1980;93(2):279-280.

157. Spitz FR et al. Hemangiopericytoma: a 20-year single-institution experience. *Ann Surg Oncol*. 1998;5(4):350-355.

158. Atkinson JB et al. Hemangiopericytoma in infants and children. A report of six patients. *Am J Surg*. 1984;148(3):372-374.

159. Jenkins JJ III. Congenital malignant hemangiopericytoma. *Pediatr Pathol*. 1987;7(1):119-122.

160. Chung KC, Weiss SW, Kuzon WM Jr. Multifocal congenital hemangiopericytomas associated with Kasabach-Merritt syndrome. *Br J Plast Surg*. 1995;48(4):240-242.

161. Chen KT, Kassel SH, Medrano VA. Congenital hemangiopericytoma. *J Surg Oncol*. 1986;31(2):127-129.

chapter 51

Contemporary Treatment of Congenital Vascular Malformations

Dirk A. Loose, MD

● INTRODUCTION

Vascular malformations, angiodysplasias represent a group of diseases, which is characterized by congenital vascular defects encountered in an enormous complexity and variety. In earlier times, these diseases could only be described[1-3] (Figure 51-1) and pathomorphology could not be clarified.

● DIAGNOSTICS

Since then various noninvasive and invasive diagnostic tools are available. It is mandatory that at first special diagnostic procedures have to be performed so that the different forms and types can be associated. Only after this identification a tactic of treatment can be worked out.

If we follow these principles, we will be able to reach the main basic diagnostic goals, i.e.,

1. definition of the predominantly involved vascular system,
2. fixation of the extent of the malformation and the involvement of adjacent structures, and
3. definition of the disturbed hemodynamics: local, regional, or systemic.

● CLASSIFICATION

The essential finding of the last decades was the clear differentiation of vascular anomalies in vascular tumors and vascular malformations. As there existed a discontent among the international specialists dealing with vascular malformations about the classification, in 1988 during the "7th International Workshop on Vascular Malformations" in Hamburg by a consensus conference, a classification was worked out concerning the species and anatomopathological form of the defects[4,4A,5] (see Table 51-1). These have two essential morphologic forms: truncular and exctratruncular.

● THERAPEUTIC TACTICS

A vascular surgical treatment of congenital vascular defects can be successful only if a strict indication for surgery is performed and if the basic principles of the therapeutic strategy are followed,[4,6,7,9] i.e.,

1. start in early childhood (at 3–7 years of age);
2. influence the pathophysiologic processes and abolish the hemodynamic disfunction;
3. adopt a harmonized individual therapy;
4. perform surgery radically without loss of function;
5. perform a stepwise surgical treatment;
6. perform a multidisciplinary therapy.

Within these therapeutic strategies, surgical and nonsurgical treatment can be achieved.[10] Nonsurgical methods have been proved true when surgery is not possible to perform or, when an operation is not yet possible to be performed.

The indication for a sole treatment by compression bandages as a result of a therapeutic frustration, as recommended by Baskerville et al,[11] cannot be accepted in the up-to-date knowledge and experiences.

The onset of surgery has a special importance in children with a vascular bone syndrome and limb length discrepancy.[12,13–18] Here the optimal occasion for surgery is the age between 3 and 7 years, because during this period a full compensation or partial

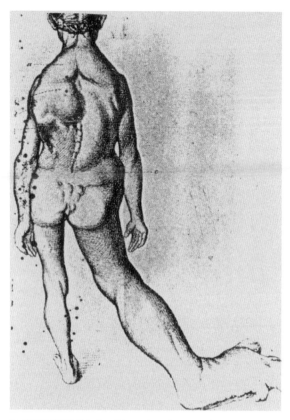

● **FIGURE 51-1.** Gigantism in combination with a vascular malformation of a right leg.

Reproduced, with permission, from Friedberg H. Riesenwuchs des rechten Beines. Virchows Arch. 1867;40:353.

compensation of the length discrepancy of the limbs can be expected.[19,20,21,21A,21B,21C,22] The consequence is that in the first place in such cases vascular surgery has to be considered to gain a reduction or even a removal of a length discrepancy. If later an *additional* treatment to correct the length discrepancy has to be performed, the following indications should be followed strictly:

1. Surgery only has to be performed in the affected limb,
2. when there is no indication for vascular surgery,

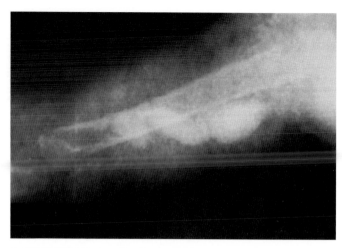

● **FIGURE 51-2.** Predominantly truncular arterial defect with an aneurysm of the brachial artery in a 7-month-old boy.

3. when in a severe discrepancy after vascular surgery the correction of the length is not sufficient,
4. after the end of growth (the temporary epiphysiodesis is excluded).

Recommendations for orthopedic surgery in order to gain a correction of the length discrepancy of the legs, as recommended by Servelle[23,24] or Ilizarow,[25] on the *not affected* leg have to be declined strictly.

● SURGICAL TREATMENT

Vascular surgical treatment is indicated for the five main types of peripheral vascular malformations which cause vascular insufficiency, cardiac overload and limb length discrepancy, disfiguration, and disfunction. The bases of this treatment are six different therapeutic strategies, which are linked to special indications and special techniques of surgery[7,13–15,21,21A,21B,21C,26–30]:

1. Reconstructive vascular surgery
2. Operations to remove the vascular defect
3. Operations to reduce the hemodynamic activity of the vascular defects

TABLE 51-1. Classification of Congenital Vascular Defects According to Their Species and Anatomic Form ("Hamburg Classification 1988")

	Anatomical Forms	
Species	*Truncular*	*Extratruncular*
Predominantly arterial defects	Aplasia or obstruction dilatation	Infiltrating limited
Predominantly venous defects	Aplasia or obstruction dilatation	Infiltrating limited
Predominantly lymphatic defects	Aplasia or obstruction dilatation	Infiltrating limited
Predominantly AV shunting defects	Deep AV fistulae superficial AV fistulae	Infiltrating limited
Combined vascular defects	Arterial and venous, (without AV-shunt)	
	Hemolymphatic (with or without AV-shunt)	Infiltrating hemolymphatic
		Limited hemolymphatic

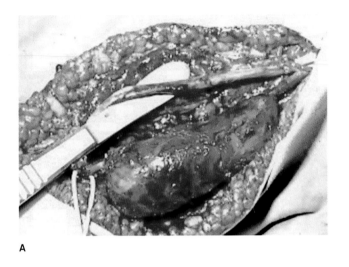

A

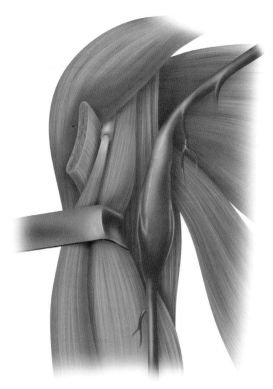

B

● FIGURE 51-3. Same case as Figure 51-2. (A) Site of the aneurysm of the brachial/axillary artery during surgery. (B) Sketch illustrating the finding during surgery.

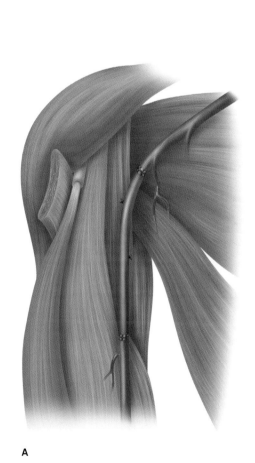

A

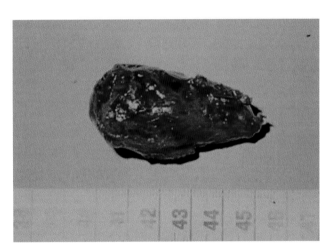

B

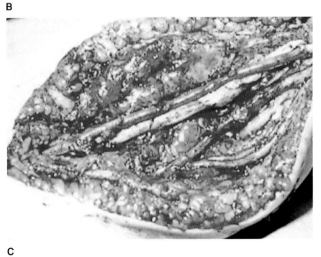

C

● FIGURE 51-4. Same case as Figure 51-2 and 51-3. (A) Sketch illustrating the surgical procedure of autologous venous interposition graft. (B) The resected aneurysm. (C) Surgical site after interposition graft.

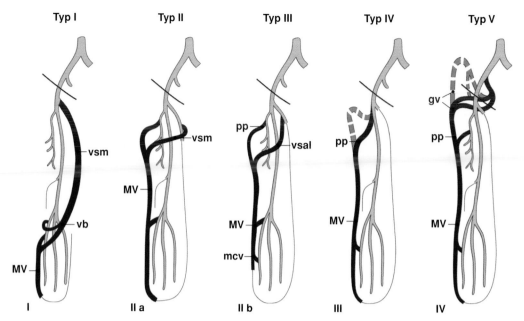

● **FIGURE 51-5.** Classification of the marginal veins concerning the types of the different segments as well as the types of the specific draining veins according to Weber[31].

4. Combined treatment
5. Unconventional surgical methods
6. Multidisciplinary treatment

Reconstructive Vascular Surgery

Reconstructive Vascular Surgery has to be performed following the rules of vascular surgery. These are quite rare cases in vascular malformations. Figures 51-2 to 51-4 demonstrate a typical clinical example.

Operations to Remove the Vascular Defect

In the venous circulation the marginal vein represents a main indication for the tactic of treatment, which is the operation to remove the vascular defect. The marginal vein is a dysplastic vein, which is localized at the lateral side of the thigh and shank region and it is formed already during the sixth week of the embryo. For the basics of treatment it is mandatory to know whether the principal veins are normal or hypoplastic.

Concerning the classification of the marginal veins, the types of the different segments as well as the types of draining veins were worked out by Weber[31] (Figure 51-5). This classification is useful and important for the tactics of any treatment of such lesions.

If the principal veins are normal, the marginal vein can be extirpated totally. It has, however, to be considered that this vein, as mentioned before, nearly always is accompanied by small AV fistulas, so that surgery cannot be performed in the same technique as stripping of varicose veins. That is why it has to be extirpated by several approaches (Figure 51-6). If, however, the principal veins are hypoplastic, the marginal

vein only is allowed to be extirpated stepwise: i.e., in several surgical sessions (Figure 51-7A and 51-7B). From the view of our experiences we recommend to start the resection at the peripheral region. By the stepwise extirpation of the epifascial venous components hypoplastic principal veins are able to adapt hemodynamically their calibre slowly[32] (Figure 51-7C and 51-7D).

On the contrary an embryonal vein is a special situation of a marginal vein, which means that there exists an aplasia of the principal veins (Figure 51-8). The surgical technique has to be absolutely different. The goal of the treatment is to reduce the venous hypertension provoked by multiple AV fistulas along the embryonal vein. The technique performed should be according to Belov I method[33]—the skeletonization of the embryonal vein, which includes the resection of arteriovenous fistulas by numerous incisions leaving the embryonal vein, i.e., the only existing draining vein intact (Figure 51-9).

The postoperative long follow up of 141 patients with a marginal vein and 20 patients with an embryonal vein was documented by a clinical and a subjective score. In 46 cases of a marginal vein the results were excellent, in 85 cases the results were good and in 20 cases the results were satisfying. In 20 patients with an embryonal vein, 16 patients showed up with good results and 4 patients with satisfying results.

Operations to Reduce the Hemodynamic Activity of the Vascular Defect

This type of surgery reduces the hemodynamic activity of the vascular defect and this tactic has its indication as well as in venous as in arterial defects. The skeletonization technique, recommended by Malan[34] and later also by Vollmar[35] (Figure 51-10), are techniques which have

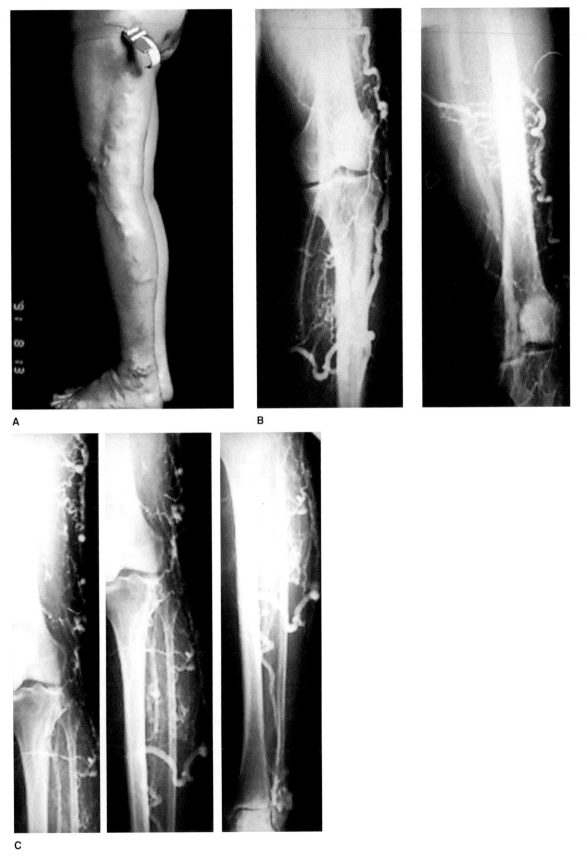

● **FIGURE 51-6.** (A) Clinical appearance of a marginal vein at the left leg of a patient. (B and C) Phlebographic documentation of this marginal vein demonstrating normal principal veins. *(continued)*

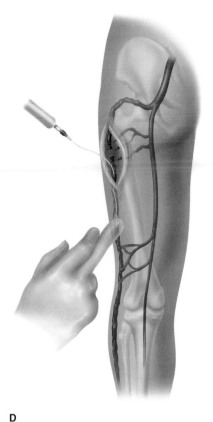

D

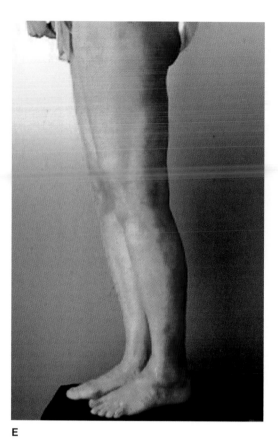

E

● **FIGURE 51-6.** *(Continued)* (D) Sketch demonstrating the technique of surgery type Loose I in such a marginal vein according to Loose and Funck.[32] (E) Clinical picture after surgery of this marginal vein.

been replaced successfully by transcatheter embolization of the diffuse extratruncular AV communications. Those arteriovenous malformations which cannot be occluded by catheter techniques can be reduced by vascular surgery: intraoperative ultrasonic Doppler identification and closure by sutures (technique Loose II)[21,21A,21B,21C] (Figure 51-11).

After the vascular sutures another control by ultrasonic Doppler is performed in order to prove the complete closure of the AV fistulas.

The Combined Therapy

In predominantly AV shunting defects the treatment of choice is the combined therapy. It consists not only of interventional occlusion of the vascular malformation by way of its feeding arteries with skeletonization and, if possible, excision, but also of further surgical and nonsurgical methods.

It does not consist of alternative or competitive techniques; rather, the nonsurgical and the surgical forms of treatment are complementary.

The indications of nonsurgical treatment include the following:

- Laser therapy—All persisting capillary AV lesions, where no feeder artery for embolization treatment is present.[36]

- Sclero therapy—Adjunctive treatment for superficial malformed veins.[37,38]

- Embolization therapy—The hypervascular lesions with AV shunting (dependent on the morphological form and site of the malformation).[31,39]

Before the combined treatment starts, the type of therapy must be planned.[40–42]

The main candidates for combined treatment are the extratruncular forms which are either infiltrating or limited. In both cases, combined surgical and nonsurgical treatment is indicated (Figure 51-12).

Unconventional Surgical Methods

These methods are applied in conventionally inoperable forms of vascular malformations. These inoperable forms are the extratruncular vascular defects that infiltrate the neighbouring tissues and organs, destroying their form and function in making their dissection and resection difficult, hazardous or even impossible.

Here are, for example, nine different techniques (see Table 51-2). Here is one example of the technique according to Belov IV[26] (Figures 51-13 and 51-14).

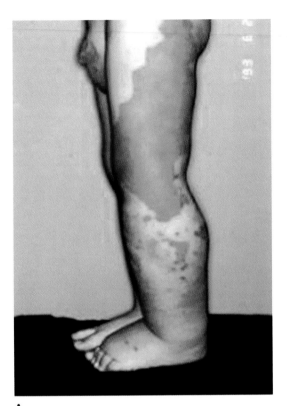
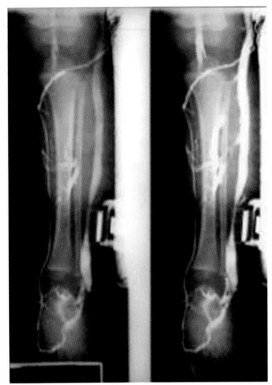

A

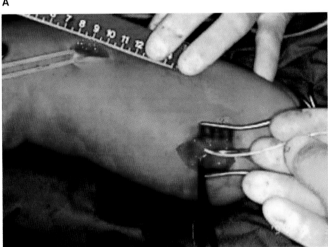

B

● **FIGURE 51-7.** (A) Clinical picture and phlebogram of a marginal vein with hypoplastic principal veins. (B) Site during surgery in the technique Loose I (see Figure 51-6). *(continued)*

Multidisciplinary Treatment

In many cases not only malformed vessels are involved but also the surrounding tissues. That is why an additional treatment by different specialists can be necessary (Figure 51-15).

Results. Within a multicentre study,[43] 1378 patients could be evaluated concerning the frequency of the applied surgical tactics. The following frequencies were documented:

Reconstructive operations: 118 cases
Operations to remove the vascular defects: 955 cases

Operations to reduce the hemodynamic activity of the defect: 51 cases
Combined treatment: 419 cases
Unconventional surgical methods: 242 cases
Multidisciplinary treatment: 107 cases

In this study, the long follow-up results of the different methods of treatment could also be evaluated by a subjective and an objective score. The results demonstrate that

- 15% had excellent results
- 42% had good results and
- in 34% an improvement could be achieved.

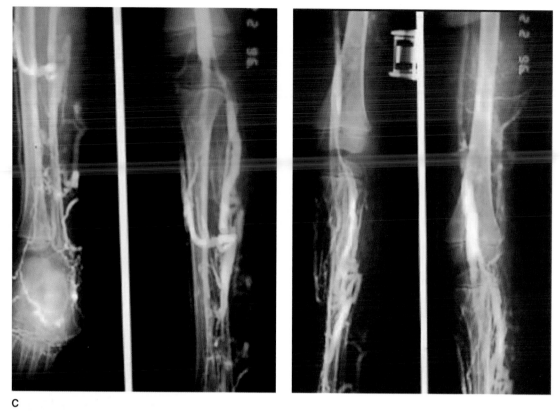

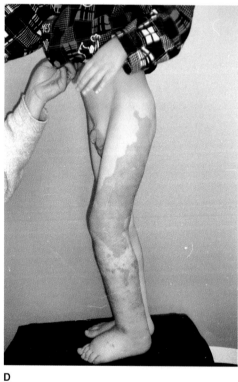

● **FIGURE 51-7.** *(Continued)* (C) Control phlebogram after surgery of a marginal vein with adaptation of the formerly hypoplastic principal veins. (D) Clinical picture of the leg after extirpation of the marginal vein by two steps of surgery.

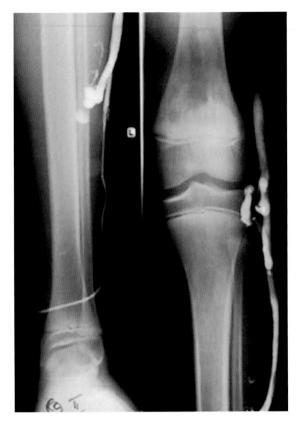
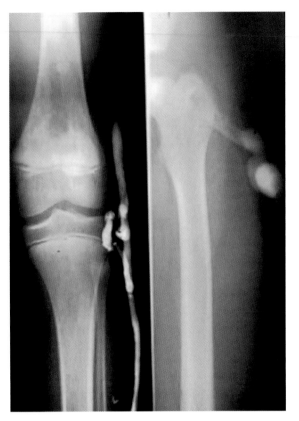
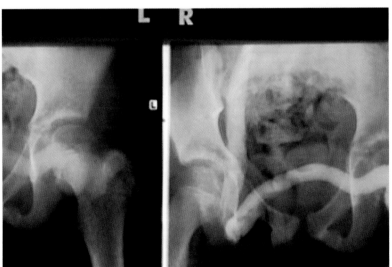

● FIGURE 51-8. Embryonal vein of the left leg of a 7-year-old girl with aplasia of all principal veins.

These results indicate that a positive result could be obtained in 91% of the cases. These numbers are proof that it is worthwhile to accept the challenge of diagnosis and treatment of vascular malformations.

● CONCLUSION

The modern surgical management of peripheral vascular malformations proves that the old, simple technique of an arterial ligature, removing only limited portions of vascular malformations by amputation must be completely abandoned. The treatment should conform to the indicated strategy, surgical tactics and operative methods as the therapeutic guidelines. The surgical technique must be individualized in each case and can often be unconventional, in accordance with the polymorphism and hemodynamic peculiarities of the vascular defect in each patient. Current surgical management in the framework of multidisciplinary surgical combined treatment should be performed in treatment centres for vascular malformations, directed by

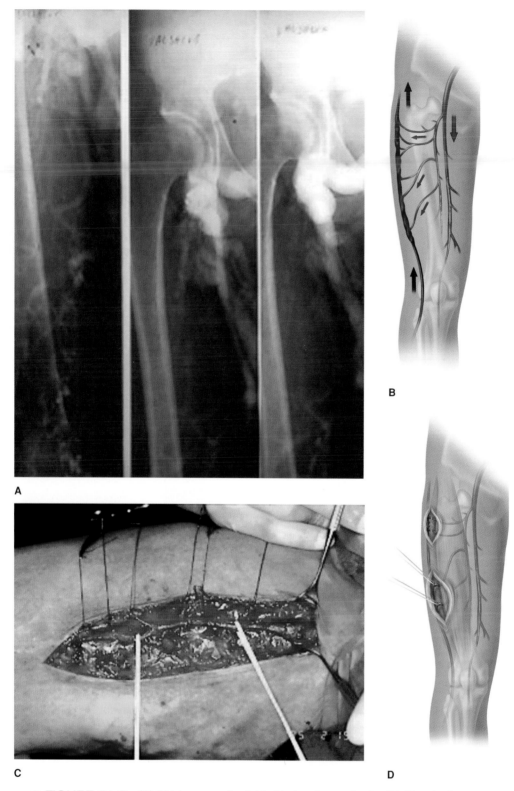

A

B

C

D

● **FIGURE 51-9.** (A) Phlebogram of a right-sided embryonal vein. (B) Sketch of an embryonal vein with several AV fistulas. (C) Site during surgery demonstrating AV fistulas of the embryonal vein. (D) Sketch of skeletonization of the embryonal vein.[33]

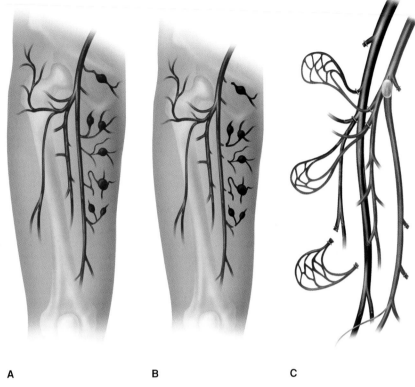

A   B   C

● **FIGURE 51-10.** Techniques of skeletonization of the afferent artery in AV malformations according to Malan[34] (A, B) and Vollmar[35] (C).

specialists in this congenital vascular pathology. A vascular surgeon and a radiologist are preferred and they should have brought knowledge of the indications, possibilities and limits of the different therapeutic methods.

Excellent preoperative planning and consecutive individual intraoperative considerations are the most important characteristics, which are expected from the vascular surgeon and the interventional radiologist dealing with vascular malformations.

Our experiences demonstrate that goodwill, patience, and specialized knowledge, combined with operative proficiency and therapeutic creativity and flexibility can produce satisfying long-term results in this very difficult and extremely challenging field of angiology.

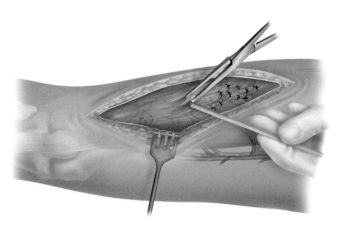

● **FIGURE 51-11.** Surgical technique of ultrasonic Doppler mapping followed by closing up AV fistulas by over-and-over stitching technique Loose II (1992).[41]

TABLE 51-2. Nine Unconventional Surgical Methods of Treatment

1. Belov I: Skeletonization of embryonal veins (1972)
2. Belov II: Restoration of deep venous drainage (1982)
3. Belov III: Sparing resection of extratruncular infiltrating vascular area (1989)
4. Belov IV: Segmental resection of infiltrating Vascular area (1992)
5. Loose I: Catheter technique for marginal vein resection (1995)
6. Loose II: Intraoperative Ultrasound mapping (1997)
7. Loose III: Intraoperative ceiling technique
8. Tasnadi I: Aspiration of malformations by ultrasound
9. Tasnadi II: Drainage of lymphatic malformation by Pudenz-Schulte shunt

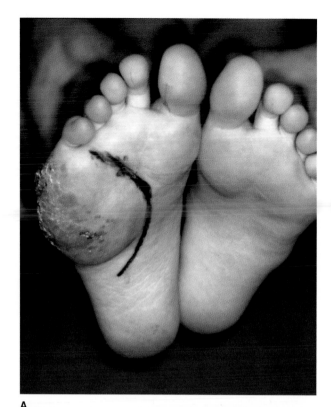

A

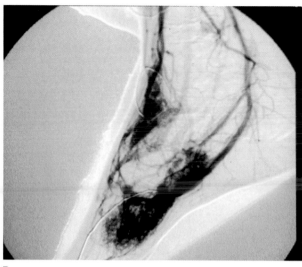

B

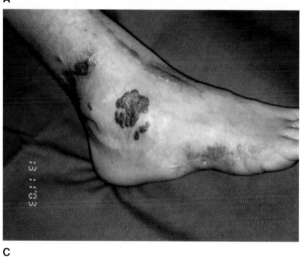

C

● **FIGURE 51-12.** Combined treatment in AV malformations. (A) Clinical picture of an AV malformation at the right foot of an 8-year-old girl. (B) Superselective arteriogram of the right foot with several nidus' of AV fistulas. (C) Clinical picture of the foot after catheter embolization and first step of surgery. In the technique Loose II (1992).[41]

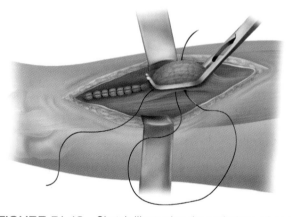

● **FIGURE 51-13.** Sketch illustrating the technique of partial resection of infiltrating malformations (Belov IV, 1992).[26]

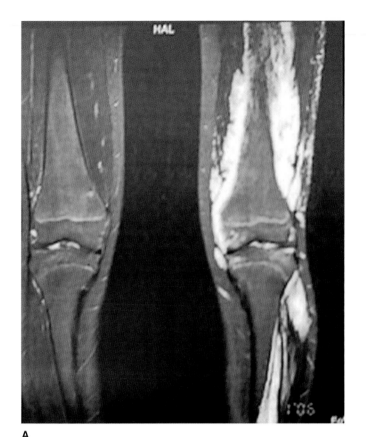

A

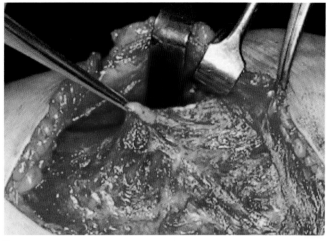

B

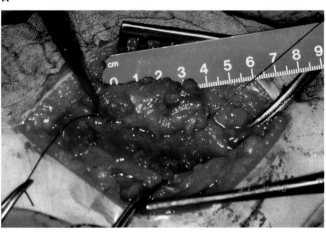

C

● FIGURE 51-14. (A) MRI of an infiltrating predominantly venous malformation in the vastus muscles of the left thigh. (B) Situs of the net like venous structures of the malformation during surgery. (C) Site after positioning of the Satinsky clamp and performing the suture (see also Figure 51-13).

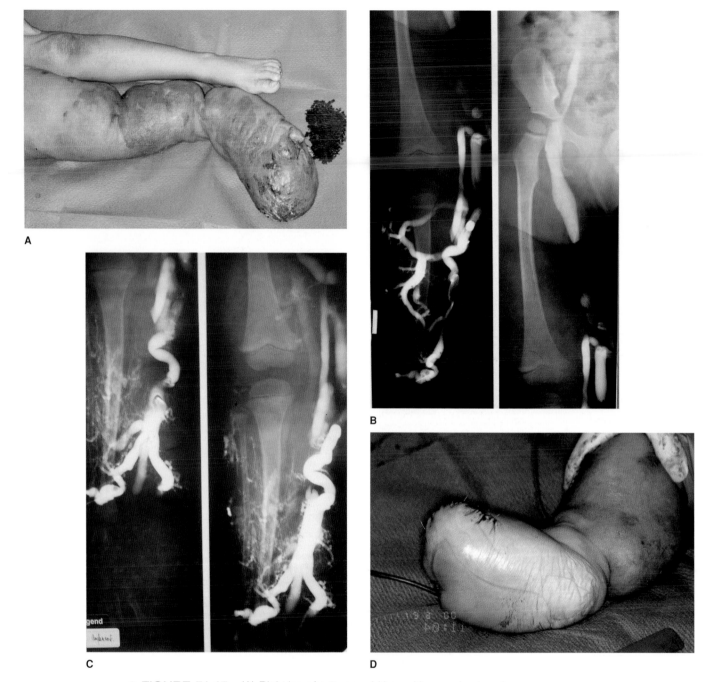

● **FIGURE 51-15.** (A) Right leg of a 5-year-old boy with a predominantly venous malformation and involvement of surrounding tissues. (B and C) Phlebogram demonstrating dysplastic principal and epifascial veins. (D) Aspect of the right foot after multidisciplinary treatment: vascular surgery and plastic surgery.

REFERENCES

1. Friedberg H. Riesenwuchs des rechten Beines. *Virchow Arch.* 1867;40:353.

2. Klippel M, Trenaunay I. Du naevus variqueux et ostéo-hypertrophique. *Arch Gén Méd.* 1900;3:641-672.

3. Weber FP. Angioma formation in connection with hypertrophy of limbs and hemihypertrophy. *Brit J Derm Syph.* 1907;19:231-235.

4. Belov ST, Loose DA, Weber J. (eds.) Vascular malformations. *Periodica Angiologica.* Vol 16. Hamburg: Einhorn-Presse, Reinbek; 1989:19-30.

4A. Belov ST, Loose DA, Mattassi R, Spatenka J, Tasnadi G, Wag Z. Therapeutical strategy, surgical tactics and operative techniques in congenital vascular defects (multicentre study). In: Strano A, Novo S, eds. *Advances in Vascular Pathology.* Vol 2. Amsterdam: Excerpta Medica; 1989:1355-1360.

5. Hulsmanns RFHJ. Congenital angiodysplastic syndromes associated with primary or secondary varicosis and/or phlebectasias. Scope on Phlebology and Lymphology; 1995; 2(1):8.

6. Belov ST. *Congenital Angiodysplasias and Their Surgical Treatment.* Sofia: Medicina I Fizkultura; 1971.

7. Belov ST. Late results of surgical treatment of congenital vascular defects. In: Maurer PC, Becker HM, Heidreich H, et al. eds. *What is new in Angiology? Trends and Controversies.* München: Zuckschwerdt; 1986;249-250.

8. Belov ST, Loose DA. Surgical treatment of congenital vascular defects. *Int Angiol.* 1990;9(3):175-182.

9. Rutherford RB. Congenital vascular malformations: diagnostic evaluation. In: Rutherford RB, Loose DA, eds. *Seminars in Vascular Surgery—Congenital Vascular Defects and Hemangiomas.* Vol 6. Philadelphia, PA: WB Saunders; 1993: 225-232.

10. Lee BB, Mattassi R, Loose DA, Yakes W, Tasnádi G, Kim HH. Consensus on controversial issues in contemporary diagnosis and management of congenital vascular malformation: Seoul communication. *Int J Angiol.* 2005;13:182-192.

11. Baskerville JS, Ackroyd M, Thomas L, Browze L. The Klippel-Trénaunay syndrome: clinical, radiological and haemodynamic features and management. *Br J Surg.* 1985; 72(3):232-236.

12. Belov St. Haemodynamic pathogenesis of vascular bone syndromes in congenital vascular defects. *Int Angiol.* 1990; 9(3):155-161.

13. Loose DA. Modern tactics and techniques in the treatment of angiodysplasias of the foot. *Chir del piede.* 2001;25: 1-17.

14. Loose DA. Sistemática del tratamiento quirúrgico de las malformaciones vasculares congénitas. *Patologia Vascular.* 2001;7(1):401-418.

15. Loose DA. Die chirurgiche Behandlung angeborener Gefässfehler (arteriell,venös,lymphatisch,arteriovenös und kombiniert). *Vasomed.* 2001;13(3):96-105.

16. Loose DA. Combined therapy in arteriovenous malformations—surgery and interventional radiology. *Przeglad Flebologiczuy.* 2005;13(2):137-144.

17. Loose DA, Wang Z. Surgical treatment in predominantly arterial defects. *Int Angiol.* 1990;9(3):183-188.

18. Loose DA, Hirsch-Gips N. Vascular bone syndrome with length discrepancy; Pathogenesis, treatment and results. Paper presented at: The 15th ISSVA Workshop; February 22-25, 2004; Wellington, New Zealand.

19. Belov ST. Correction of lower limbs length discrepancy in congenital vascular bone disease by vascular surgery performed during childhood. *Semin Vasc Surg.* 1993;6:245-651.

20. Loose DA. Angeborene Gefäßmalformationen. In: Alexander K, Hrsg. *Gefäßkrankheiten.* München: Urban und Schwarzenberg; 1994.

21. Loose DA. Malformaciones vasculares. Sistemática para el diagnósticó radiológico y la terapéutica. *Forum FL.* 1997; 2:101-108.

21A. Loose DA. Systematik, radiologische Diagnostik und Therapie vaskulärer Fehlbildungen. In: Hohenleutner U, Landthaler M, eds. *Operative Dermatologie im Kindes- und Jugendalter. Diagnostik und Therapie von Fehl- und Neubildungen.* Fortschritte der operativen und onkologischen Dermatologie, Band 12. Berlin, Wien: Blackwell Wissenschafts-Verlag; 1997.

21B. Loose DA. Therapie angeborener Gefäßmißbildungen. In: Görich J, Brams HJ, Sunder-Plasmann L, Götz HJ, eds. Interventionelle Radiologie, endovasculäre Chirurgie. "State-of-the-Art"-Symposium, Ulm. München: Zuckerschwerdt, 1997.

21C. Loose DA. Vascular Malformations.*Surgery.* 1997;15(2):39-43.

22. Tasnádi G. Postnatal development of the lower limb extremities in some forms of vascular malformations. Paper presented at: The 9th International Workshop for the Study of Vascular Anomalies; July 1-3,1992; Denver, CO.

23. Servelle M. Stase veineuse et croissance osseuse. *Bull Acad Nat Med.* 1948;132:471-474.

24. Servelle M. Klippel and Trénaunay's Syndrome. *Ann Surg.* 1985;201(3):365-373.

25. Ilizarow GA. *Transosseous Osteosynthesis. Theoretical and Clinical Aspects of the Regeneration and Growth of Tissue.* Berlin, Germany: Springer; 1991.

26. Belov ST. Operative-technical peculiarities in operations of congenital vascular defects. In: Balas P, ed. *Progress in Angiology.* Torino, Italy: Minerva Medica; 1992:379-382.

27. Belov ST. Vascular malformations and hemangiomas: surgical treatment. In: Chang JB, ed. *Textbook of Angiology.* New York: Springer 2000:1284-1293.

28. Loose DA. Röntgendiagnostik von venösen Dysplasien und ihre therapeutischen Konsequenzen. *Vasomed aktuell.* 1989;6(7):15-28.

29. Loose DA. Combined treatment of vascular malformations: Indications, methods and techniques. In: Chang JB, ed. *Textbook of Angiology.* New York, NY: Springer; 2000:1278ff.

30. Loose DA, Müller, E. Problems in surgery of congenital vascular malformations with Arterio-venous Shunts. In: De Castro Silva M, ed. *Atualização em Angiologia. Belo Horizonte.* Brasil; 1978;121-141.

31. Weber J. Embolisation von av-Malformationen. In: Loose DA, Weber J, eds. Angeborene Gefäßmißbildungen. Lüneburg: Nordlanddruck GmbH; 1997.

32. Loose DA, Funck I. Angeborene Venenfehler–Diagnostische und therapeutische Möglichkeiten. *Akt Chir.* 1995;30:329-340.

33. Belov ST. Congenital agenesis of the deep veins of the lower extremity: surgical treatment. *J Cardiovasc Surg.* 1972;13:594.

34. Malan E. Bases physiopathologiques du traitement chirurgical des fistules artérioveineuses congénitales. *Mén Acod Chir.* 1960;86:259.

35. Vollmar J. Rekonstruktive Gefäßchirurgie. Stuttgart, Germany: Thieme; 1967.

36. Philipp C, Poetke M, Berlien HP. Lasertherapie angeborener Gefäßfehlbildungen. In: Loose DA, Weber J, eds. Angeborene Gefäßmißbildungen. Lüneburg: Nordlanddruck GmbH; 1997:179-201.

37. van der Stricht J. The sclerosing therapy in congenital vascular defects. *Int Angiol.* 1990;9(3):224-227.

38. Cabrera J, Cabrera J Jr, Garcia-Olmedo MA, Redondo P. Treatment of venousmalformations with sclerosant in microfoam form. *Arch Dermatol.* 2003;139:1409-1416.

39. Rosen RJ, Riles TS, Berenstein A. Congenital vascular malformations. In: Rutherford RB, ed. *Vascular Sugery.* Philadelphia, PA: WB Saunders; 1995:1218-1232.

40. Mattassi R. Surgical treatment of congenital arteriovenous defects. *Int Angiol.* 1990;9(3):196-202.

41. Loose DA, Weber J. Indications and tactics for a combined treatment of congenital vascular defects. In: Balas P, ed. *Progress in Angiology* 1991. Torino, Italy: Edizione Minerva Medica; 1992:373-378.

42. Loose DA. Combined treatment of congenital vascular defects: indications and tactics. *Semin Vasc Surg.* 1993:6(4) 260-265.

43. Loose DA, Belov St, Mattassi R, Tasnádi G, Vaghi M, Rehder A. Chirurgische therapie von angiodysplasien: langzeitergebnisse von 1852 operationen. Symposium Medical, Berliner Med.Verlagsanstalt. 2000;10(12):29-30.

chapter 52

Arterial Complications in Transplantation

Roberto Gedaly, MD / *Salik Jahania, MD* / *Dinesh Ranjan, MD*

● INTRODUCTION

Heart, renal, hepatic, and pancreatic transplantations are being performed with increasing frequency, leading to a greater demand for knowledgeable evaluation of vascular complications involving these grafts. Arterial anomalies associated with implantation of these grafts and arterial complications following transplantation, both present unique anatomic and physiologic problems. Arterial and venous stenoses and occlusions, pseudoaneurysms, and arteriovenous fistulas may occur in this patient population. Here, we summarize the most common arterial complications that take place in transplant recipients with a discussion of how to approach these complications.

● ARTERIAL COMPLICATIONS IN RENAL TRANSPLANTATION

There is a wide spectrum of vascular complications that can occur with renal transplantation. Fortunately renal artery complications are not very common. The most frequent arterial problems seen are renal artery stenosis, renal artery thrombosis, dissection of the external, internal iliac or common iliac arteries, renal artery pseudoaneurysm, and renal transplant arteriovenous fistula.

While postrenal transplant hypertension is a common problem, renal artery stenosis should be considered in patients presenting with severe or intractable hypertension after renal transplantation. Transplant renal artery stenosis (TRAS) is important to identify because it is a correctable form of hypertension. Although it can present at any time, renal artery stenosis usually becomes evident between 3 months and 2 years posttransplant.[1]

Diagnosis of hemodynamically significant renal artery stenosis rests on a radiologic demonstration of ≥50% re-duction in renal artery diameter.[2] The rationale for this assumption is derived from experimental evidence that the stenosis needs to occlude at least 50% of the lumen before renal blood flow and perfusion pressure start to decrease and systemic blood pressure increase.[2] The risk factors for renal transplant artery stenosis include atherosclerotic disease of donor or recipient vessels, cytomegalovirus (CMV) infection, delayed allograft function, and rejection.[3-6] In a recent retrospective study of 29 recipients with stenosis and a case-control group of 58 patients, an increased risk of stenosis was significantly associated with CMV infection (41% versus 12%) and delayed graft function (48% versus 16%).[3]

Renal artery stenosis can present with short segment, long segment, unifocal, and multifocal involvement. The prevalence of anastomotic renal transplant artery stenosis can be difficult to assess because of discrepancy in the definition of hemodynamically significant lesions and the use of different diagnostic modalities. Renal artery stenosis occurs in 1% to 12% of the patients after transplantation.[7]

Persistent, uncontrolled hypertension, flash pulmonary edema, and an acute elevation in blood pressure are other common features of this disorder and should alert the clinician.[8,9]

Multiple techniques have been used to diagnose renal artery stenosis. Arteriography remains the procedure of choice for establishing the definitive diagnosis of renal artery stenosis after transplantation, but other noninvasive techniques such as duplex ultrasound (US), magnetic resonance (MR) angiography, and computed tomography (CT) angiography are increasingly utilized techniques to screen and/or diagnose transplant recipients for the presence of renovascular disease. It is essential to rule out renal parenchymal disease and usually a kidney biopsy is performed prior to angiography, since the presence of chronic renal allograft disease will decrease the likelihood of a successful response to correction of the stenosis and could be taken as a relative contraindication to intervention.[10,11]

Doppler ultrasonography is the preferred screening modality for stenosis of the transplanted renal artery in many centers. The presence of a peak systolic velocity of $\geq$2.5 m/s has a sensitivity and specificity of 100% and 95% respectively.[12] However, Doppler US has the caveat of being highly operator-dependent. Recently, other noninvasive procedures such as MR angiogram or CT angiogram are increasingly being used for screening in some centers.

In a small series, combined analysis using gadolinium-enhanced MRA and three-dimensional phase contrast postgadolinium had shown sensitivities and specificities close to 100% in detecting stenosis.[13] Spiral CT angiography has also been used as a noninvasive alternative to arteriography.[6,9]

Most interventional radiologist or cardiologist taking care of these problems use measurement of pressures during the diagnostic angiography and try to demonstrate a gradient through a kink or stricture.[14] In some instances, the diagnosis of TRAS even with angiography could be difficult, and some experts believe that kinks and strictures are significant if they create a gradient that ultimately will cause hypoperfusion of the graft, hypertension, and elevation of creatinine. In 2004, Chua et al. from St. George's Hospital in London described that kinks of the transplant artery cause velocity gradients on Doppler US, but some will have no intraarterial pressure gradient across the kink. This particular subgroup of patients may not benefit from any intervention. They concluded that kinks of the renal transplant artery with normal intraarterial pressures do not appear to progress and threaten renal graft function. In this study, satisfactory graft outcomes were seen after 5-year follow-up with conservative therapy alone.[14]

The management options available to correct stenosis of the transplant renal artery include angioplasty, with or without stenting, and surgery. The utilization of medical treatment will result sometimes in resolution of the hypertension episode but will not treat the perfusion problem to the transplanted kidney.

For many years, surgical correction had been the only treatment option for TRAS, with reported correction rates ranging from 63% to 92%.[15] The procedure, however, carries a significant risk of graft loss, urethral injury, reoperation, and mortality.[15]

In the last few years, percutaneous transluminal revascularization has gained large popularity as a relatively noninvasive approach to improve both blood pressure control and kidney perfusion and is now considered the treatment of choice for patients with renal artery stenosis. Initial technical success of Percutaneous Transluminal Angioplasty (PTA) in the treatment of TRAS has been reported to be greater than 80% although effectiveness is strongly depended on center experience and on the type of the lesion.[11,16–18] Long-term clinical success defined as either improvement in blood pressure control or sta-

bilization/improvement in renal function is reported to be 63% to 82% at 1 year,[11,17] with the restenosis rate after PTA to be in the range of 10% to 36%.[11,19,20] Endovascular stents have been used for the treatment of recurrent and/or ostial stenosis and in cases of suboptimal results with PTA. In addition, serious complications of PTA can be salvaged with stents. We found very few studies to date to assess the benefits of stent placement (TRAS). Stents have been used usually in the clinical scenario of recurrent or resistant TRAS,[21] but may be necessary after the initial angioplasty if the problem is at the level of the ostium (Figure 52-1A to 52-1C).

The extensive fibrosis and scarring around the transplanted kidney makes surgical correction of a transplant artery stenosis difficult. Surgery should therefore be considered in few cases where severe arteriosclerotic disease is present and percutaneous approach has failed. A risk of graft loss after surgical vascular reconstruction has been reported in as many as 20% of cases and recurrence rates ranging from 7% to 15% after surgical intervention.[22]

Thrombosis of the transplanted renal artery is a rare complication usually occurring immediately after transplantation. Posttransplant acute tubular necrosis (ATN) is responsible for approximately 90% of acute renal failure episodes occurring within the first few weeks following renal transplantation.[23] Most patients with ATN will eventually recover. ATN has to be distinguished from other causes of acute renal failure early after transplantation such as the renal artery thrombosis, hyperacute rejection, and obstruction of the urinary tract.[23] In the setting of renal artery thrombosis, conventional color Doppler US usually shows the absence of flow within the renal artery and graft. This can usually be confirmed by angiography. In some instances, hyperacute or severe acute rejection are associated with thrombosis of intrarenal branches and subsequent thrombosis of the main artery. Renal artery thrombosis can also be associated with technical problems, hypotension, hypercoagulable states, and atherosclerotic embolism. Renal infarction appears as a nonenhancing kidney with an enhancing capsule in the radioisotope renal scan. Thrombosis has been treated with percutaneous techniques using fibrinolytic agents or with surgical intervention with the intent of declotting the main renal artery, but the success rate is low and renal artery thrombosis usually results in loss of the renal allograft.

Iliac artery dissection can happen during dissection prior to actual implantation of the kidney or after reperfusion of the transplant kidney. Also dissection of the transplanted renal artery has been described.[24] Kidney transplant recipients have relatively higher incidence of peripheral vascular disease. Diabetes mellitus is the leading single cause of end-stage renal disease (ESRD). According to the 2002 Annual Data Report of the United States Renal Data System (US-RDS), 42% of non-Hispanic dialysis patients in the United States have ESRD caused by diabetes.[25] Hypertension is the second leading cause of ESRD in adults, accounting for 25% of the cases. These two diseases are common risk factors for peripheral vascular disease.[26,27] The presence

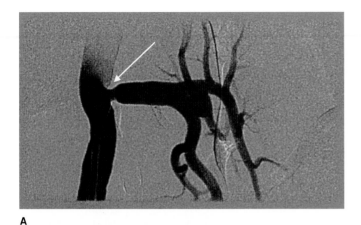

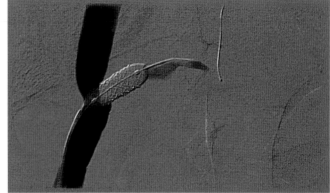

A

B

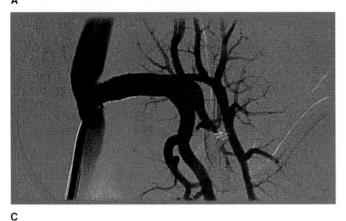

C

● **FIGURE 52-1.** Transplant renal artery stenosis. (A) Significant renal artery stenosis at the level of the anastomosis in a transplant recipient (arrow). (B) In the same patient, balloon dilatation of the strictures is being performed. The balloon is inflated across the stricture. (C) A stent has been placed in the same patient after the balloon dilatation and the stricture have been resolved.

of calcified and partially occlusive atheromatous plaque in these vessels makes intima fragile and prone to separate if not handle appropriately. Careful dissection of iliac vessels as well as appropriate selection of site for vascular clamps and the anastomosis is cructial (Figure 52-2A and 52-2B). In several cases, utilization of special atraumatic vascular clamps are necessary in order to avoid intimal injury. The consequences of dissection of the iliac vessel or the renal artery can be diverse and include ischemia to the transplanted kidney and/or to the ipsilateral lower extremity. Isolated dissection of the renal artery can also occur specially in the presence of extensive renal artery atherosclerosis and calcified plaques that are more often present in older and extended criteria donors.

Intrarenal arteriovenous fistulas and pseudoaneurysms are usually caused by trauma during percutaneous needle biopsy. They occur in 1% to 18% of renal biopsies.[28] Pseudoaneurysms can occur at the vascular anastomosis, biopsy sites, or in association with infection.[29] This diagnosis of pseudoaneurysm should be considered when a hypoechoic or complex mass is near the vascular anastomoses or within a graft after biopsy. Usually duplex shows a disorganized, pulsatile flow within a hypoechoic, or variably complex perivascular mass. Arteriovenous fistulas may form when an artery and vein are lacerated; pseudoaneurysms result when only the artery is lacerated. Small pseudoaneurysms may resolve spontaneously; if they do not, they can be successfully treated with percutaneous transcatheter em-

bolization. Seventy percent of all intrarenal arteriovenous fistulas and pseudoaneurysms close spontaneously with in 1 to 18 months.[28] They are usually asymptomatic but can manifest with hypertension and deterioration of renal function. Doppler US is the modality of choice for screening. Helical CT scan is a good alternative when US cannot define the nature of the lesion.

● **HEPATIC ARTERY PROBLEMS AFTER LIVER TRANSPLANTATION**

In order to be able to understand and treat arterial complications that occur in liver transplant recipients, one should have adequate knowledge of hepatic artery anatomy and its variants. The anatomy of the hepatic artery, and its anatomic variants, has been described in the literature starting with Haller in the eighteenth century, Tidemann in the nineteenth century and more recently by Flint and Michels in the twentieth century, 1930s, and 50s repetitively. An understanding of arterial anatomy is of importance in planning and performance of all surgical and radiologic procedures in the upper abdomen. Approximately 80% of the cases have the conventional anatomic configuration where the left and right hepatic arteries are the terminal branches of the main hepatic artery originating form the celiac axis[30–32] (Figure 52-3).

The left hepatic artery has its origin from the common hepatic artery trunk in most cases around 80% to 85% of

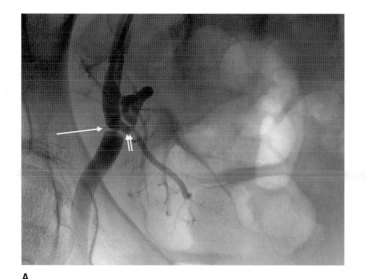

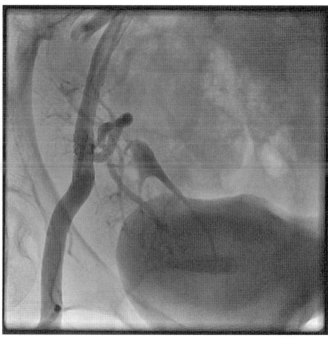

● **FIGURE 52-2.** (A) A lesion cause in the external iliac artery during the application of the vascular clamp (single arrow). The renal artery and the anastomosis showed no strictures (double arrow). (B) The stricture in the iliac artery was treated with balloon dilatation and stent placement.

cases, from the left gastric artery in approximately 15%, the splenic artery in approximately 1%, from the gastroduodenal artery in 1% and rarely directly from the aorta or the celiac axis or the superior mesenteric artery. The aberrant left hepatic artery runs in the lesser omentum, traversing forward and medially. The right hepatic artery has its origin from the main trunk of the common hepatic artery in approximately 75% of the cases, from the superior mesenteric in approximately 18%, gastroduodenal artery in 4%

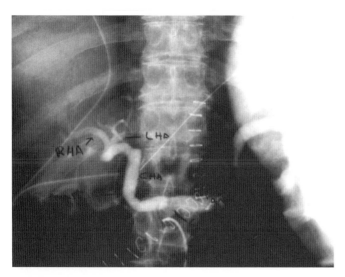

● **FIGURE 52-3.** An angiogram of a patient with normal arterial anatomy. The right and left hepatic arteries coming from common hepatic artery are visible.

to 6%, and rarely from the right gastric artery or the aorta. The anomalous right hepatic artery arising from the superior mesenteric or gastroduodenal artery runs a course to the right of the portal vein.[30,31]

These are the most common variations but other less common variants have been described such as celiac axis and the superior mesenteric artery with common origin and a completely replaced system with the absence of celiac axis and hepatic artery arising from the superior mesenteric artery.

Advances in the care of recipients of liver transplantation in conjunction with refinements in surgical technique have contributed to a current 1-year survival of 90% or better after transplantation.[33,34] Recently, the utilization of living donor liver transplantation and split livers has revolutionized the field of liver transplantation.[35,36] Living donor liver transplants are performed routinely in pediatric population.[37,38] The ethics and outcome of living donor liver transplants in the adult population is under extensive scrutiny.[39,40] The utilization of partial grafts have made the arterial reconstruction during transplantation even more challenging because of the utilization of smaller vessels such as segmental left or right hepatic arteries for reconstruction.

Hepatic artery thrombosis (HAT) is the most common vascular complication following liver transplantation, seen in 5% of adult and 9% to 18% of pediatric liver transplantation.[41,42] HAT is associated with a significant mortality of 20% to 60% and is the second leading cause of graft failure in the early postoperative period. This may present clinically in different ways: massive hepatic necrosis; biliary leak as a result of bile duct ischaemia and necrosis, or recurrent sepsis. In some patients, HAT can be asymptomatic and that is the rationale for the utilization of routine Doppler US after liver transplantation in some centers.[43] Associated risk factors include increased, cold, ischemic time of the donor liver, ABO blood type incompatibility, small donor or recipient vessels, complex arterial reconstructions, and acute rejection.[44,45] Delayed HAT, which may occur years after transplantation, is associated with chronic rejection and sepsis. US will enable detection of approximately 95% of patent hepatic arteries.[46] The absence of color or spectral Doppler flow, often with a "wall thump" in the US, necessitates further investigation. Advances in the CT and MR angiography now provide further noninvasive techniques for imaging of the hepatic artery.[47,48] However, arteriography remains the definitive investigation, particularly if surgery is being considered (Figure 52-4). Hepatic artery stenosis (HAS) occurs in 3% to 5% of transplant recipients,[49] most commonly developing at the site of the anastamosis and early in the postoperative period, although late development is well recognized. HAS is usually attributed to surgical technique, graft rejection, or microvascular injury. Causes include clamp injury, intimal trauma caused by perfusion catheters at the time of surgery, or disrupted vasa-vasorum leading to ischemia of the arterial ends. In duplex US, HAS produces an intrahepatic *tardus et parvus* waveform, defined as prolonged systolic acceleration time with an RI <0.5.[50,51] In the setting of markedly diminished hepatic artery flow, such as in severe hepatic edema, systemic hypotension, or high-grade HAS, or in a suboptimal duplex US study, perhaps limited by patient obesity or gross ascites, interpretation of intrahepatic tardus-parvus waveforms should be performed

with caution. In combination, these parameters have 85% to 97% sensitivity for detecting HAS.[50] Dodd et al.[50] found a sensitivity of 97% for significant hepatic artery complications (including thrombosis and stenosis) if one or more of the following Doppler US criteria were demonstrated: resistive index less than 0.5, acceleration time greater than 0.08 seconds, no flow in the main hepatic artery, or a peak hepatic artery velocity greater than 2 m/s. Spectral Doppler waveforms should be interpreted with caution in the intraoperative and immediate postoperative stage, as they may return to normal spontaneously. Clinically, it may lead to biliary ischemia, causing hepatic dysfunction and eventual hepatic failure. Treatment includes balloon angioplasty or retransplantation.

Celiac artery stenosis may be due to atheromatous disease or, in the younger patient, impingement by the diaphragmatic crura, or median arcuate ligament. The latter cause may be corrected surgically at the time of transplantation by dividing the muscular and fibrous bands of the diaphragm, allowing restoration of normal flow to the liver. If a celiac artery stenosis caused by atheromatous disease is severe, an aortohepatic interposition graft anastomosed to the recipient supraceliac or infrarenal aorta may be required to ensure adequate arterial supply to the implant.[52,53]

Hepatic artery pseudoaneurysm following transplantation is an uncommon complication, seen in less than 1% of cases.[54,55] They can be treated percutaneously or with revascularization. However, where stenosis is suspected, arteriography is required to confirm the diagnosis. Intrahepatic pseudoaneurysms typically arise as a result of percutaneous needle biopsy, whereas those in an extrahepatic location are often caused by a defect at the arterial anastamosis or infection. Further investigation with dual phase CT scan and arteriography, however, are often required.[56] Although embolization may occlude the pseudoaneurysm, surgical reconstruction, or retransplantation is usually required.[54]

● ARTERIAL COMPLICATIONS AFTER PANCREAS TRANSPLANTATION

Pancreatic transplantation is increasingly used for the treatment of type 1 diabetes mellitus. It is commonly performed in conjunction with kidney transplantation. The pancreas is placed intraperitoneal into the pelvis and the donor splenic and superior mesenteric arteries that come with the allograft are anastomosed to the recipient's iliac artery via a Y-graft consisting of the donor's common, internal, and external iliac arteries.[57] Technically, the pancreas transplantation could be performed in several different ways. It is important to understand the technical aspects of this transplant in order to be able to recognize, diagnose, and treat vascular complications. Usually, the arterial anastomosis is done using the donor iliac artery Y-graft to the recipient's iliac artery (Figure 52-5). The outflow can be restored by anastomosing the transplant pancreas portal vein into the recipient's iliac vein (systemic drainage) or the recipient's superior mesenteric vein (portal drainage). The last part of this operation includes the duodenal drainage that could

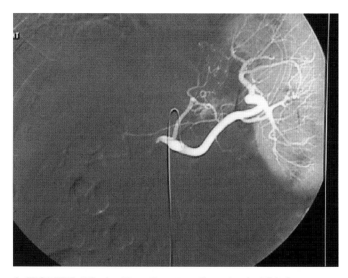

● **FIGURE 52-4.** Hepatic artery thrombosis. This is an angiogram of a patient who presented with elevated liver function tests in which Doppler ultrasound did not show hepatic arterial flow. This shows that splenic artery and its branches and left gastric artery are open. The common hepatic artery cannot be visualized making the diagnosis of hepatic artery thrombosis.

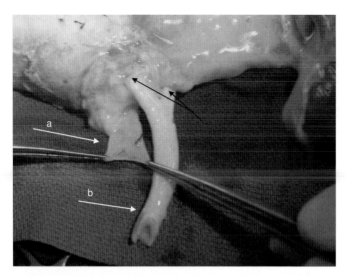

● **FIGURE 52-5.** Part of a pancreas allograft showing the portal vein, which is the outflow of the graft (arrow a). The superior mesenteric artery and the splenic artery (black arrows) were anastomosed to the Y-graft of external and internal iliac arteries from the donor (arrow b).

be accomplished by anastomosing the transplant duodenum to the recipient's bladder or small bowel. Vascular thrombosis is a common complication of pancreatic transplantation and is still considered the leading cause of nonimmunologic graft failure.[58] The underlying mechanisms of graft thrombosis are poorly understood. Proposed etiologic factors include traumatic donor procurement, prolonged cold ischemic time, potential thrombogenicity of some of the immunosuppressants, kinking or compression at the venous or arterial anastomosis, and intraglandular microthrombi.[59] Both arterial and venous thrombosis can occur and, if not detected early, necessitate transplant pancreatectomy. Thrombosis is second only to acute rejection in abnormalities leading to pancreas allograft removal.

The frequency of graft thrombosis reportedly varies from 13% to 20%.[58,60,61] Arterial and/or venous graft thrombosis can be a primary event or in association with other pathophysiologic processes. These processes included rejection, infection, or inflammation diagnosed by means of histopathologic examination and cultures.

Other vascular complications, including anastomotic bleeding, stenosis, pseudoaneurysms, and arteriovenous fistulas, have also been described. Vascular anastomotic leaks and arteriovenous fistulas can be because of surgical complications but can also be related to biopsy, inflammation, or infection. Massive gastrointestinal hemorrhage related to arterial-graft duodenal fistulas has been also described as one of the vascular complications after pancreas transplantation and is a rare cause of gastrointestinal bleeding. Coil embolization at the time of the angiography once the diagnosis is established is the preferred initial treatment to stop the bleeding. In some cases graft pancreatectomy may be necessary.[62]

Scintigraphy, abdominal and pelvic CT scan, US, Doppler imaging, and angiography have been utilized to assess vascular complications of pancreatic transplantation. Noninvasive studies, including duplex sonography, CT scan, and MR imaging, reduce the need for diagnostic angiography and serve to direct angiographic and surgical intervention.[60]

Sonography is typically the primary technique used to evaluate patients with graft dysfunction. However, detailed assessment of the complex vasculature of pancreatic allografts can be difficult and sometimes impossible with sonography. Because MR contrast agents are only minimally nephrotoxic, the use of 3-D contrast-enhanced MR angiography has been explored in this setting and occasionally preoperatively for the assessment of the pelvic arteries, and the successful use of this technique for the evaluation of these patients has been reported in several small series. The typical appearance of acute thrombosis on contrast-enhanced MR angiography is that of a very dark hypointense filling defect occluding the arterial lumen, with or without a trailing edge. MR angiography can also detect other arterial problems such as stenoses and kinks. Invasive pressure measurements may be needed to determine the hemodynamic relevance of these kinks and stenoses, and they can be treated endovascularly with PTA or stent placement.[60] Pseudoaneurysms and arteriovenous fistulas occur uncommonally. They can be related to the procurement technique of the allograft, namely, the blind ligation of mesenteric vessels along the inferior border of the pancreas. More frequently these are mycotic pseudoaneurysms in the setting of graft infection. Both surgical and endovascular interventions have been successfully utilized for these complications.

● PERIPHERAL AND ALLOGRAFT CORONARY ARTERIAL DISEASE AFTER CARDIAC TRANSPLANTATION

The incidence of end-stage heart failure continues to increase every year in the United States. With the increasing survival of baby boomers into seventh and eighth decades of life, and better management of ischemic cardiomyopathy, more patients are now diagnosed with NYHA class III and class IV heart failure than ever before. It is estimated that the health care cost of heart failure to CMS is greater than $15 billion annually. Heart transplantation remains the most definitive treatment option for patients with advanced end-stage heart failure, and survival rates continue to increase because of advances in surveillance and management of rejection and infection, but transplant related vasculopathy remains the Achilles' heal of long-term survival.

There is a well recognized correlation between presence of coronary artery disease and peripheral vascular disease. Newman et al.[63] have demonstrated a 33% incidence of angina and congestive heart failure in patients with an ankle-brachial index (ABI) of <0.8. Follow-up studies of patients with intermittent claudication have demonstrated a 10-year decrease in life expectancy, predominantly caused by premature cardiovascular disease.[64]

The incidence of clinically significant peripheral arterial disease (PAD) in cardiac transplant recipients has been reported by various authors and is generally felt to be 10% to 13%, which appears to be higher than the incidence in age-matched population. It has generally been recognized that cardiac transplant recipients whose indication for transplantation was ischemic cardiomyopathy and specially those who had a strong history of tobacco abuse have a higher tendency to develop significant PAD posttransplantation Erdoes et al. reported on a series of 239 consecutive patients who underwent heart transplants between 1990 and 1993 and were followed for a mean period of 3.2 years.[65]

These patients underwent prospective, serial, peripheral, and vascular studies including carotid artery duplex studies, peripheral arterial doppler derived ankle brachial indices, as well as abdominal US examinations as part of the routine annual evaluations posttransplant. These findings were compared with the patients screening studies which were performed prior to transplantation. The working hypothesis tested by the authors was the correlation between the adverse effects of immuosuppressive medications on lipoprotein metabolism as well as the presence of well known risk factors for PAD in this patient population, and a high incidence of PAD in the posttransplant period. In their experience, the incidence of development of significant PAD was 10% over the period of follow-up, and this included carotid stenosis, abdominal aortic aneurysm, aortoiliac occlusive disease, femoropopliteal occlusive disease, and renal artery stenosis. The authors concluded that the most important risk factors for development of PAD after heart transplant were diagnosis of ischemic cardiomyopathy and a history of smoking.

Other risk factors that have been implicated in the development of PAD in the posttransplant period include hypercholesterolemia, hypertriglyceridemia, uncontrolled hypertension, as well as diabetes mellitus. The association between use of calcineurin inhibitors such as cyclosporine and Prograf as well as prednisone on development of hyperlipidemia and hypertension is well known.[66] It is also clearly established that PAD and coronary artery disease (CAD) often come bundled together.[67] Furthermore, the use of high-dose steroids exacerbates hyperglycemia and often leads to potentiation of the secondary complications of diabetes mellitus including vasculopathy and arteriosclerosis, both of which play a role in development of worsening hypertension, renal artery stenosis, thus creating a milieu conducive to the development of accelerated PAD.

Several investigators have attempted to delineate the in vivo effects of calcineurin inhibitors on vasomotor properties of arteries in animal models. It has been postulated that cyclosporine may lead to increased tendency to develop hypertension by altering the vasomotor function of smooth muscles in arteries by affecting the secretion of endothelial-derived Nitric Oxide (eNO). Berkenboom et al. evaluated the endothelial function of internal mammary artery in several patient populations including normal controls, patients with CAD, recipients of cardiac allografts, and patients with both CAD and PAD.[68] They studied the response of the internal mammary arteries in these patients to escalating doses of acetylcholine, by measuring the diameter of the vessels by quantitative angiography. They concluded that peripheral arteries of recipients of cardiac allografts show a dysfunction of endothelial function, which was reversible in the face of infusion of an endothelial-derived Nitric Oxide donor such as L-arginine. The authors were also able to demonstrate an elevated level of endothelin in patients with the most severe PAD, which is a potent vascontrictor. Elevated concentration of endothelin has been linked to the administration of calcineurin inhibitors such as cyclosporine[69] as well as hypercholesterolemia.[70]

● POSTHEART TRANSPLANT ALLOGRAFT CORONARY ARTERY DISEASE

The most important factor that currently determines long-term survival after heart transplantation is allograft coronary artery disease (ACAD).[71]

This phenomenon is recognized as the leading cause of death after the first year postheart transplant, whereas opportunistic infections with viruses and fungi and acute allograft rejection are the leading causes of death within the first year. Interestingly, these two causes of early mortality (infection and rejection) also play an important role in the multifactorial milieu that eventually is felt to lead to the development of ACAD. The earliest animal models of heart transplants revealed presence of ACAD. This form of atherosclerosis was noted to progress with time regardless of presence or incidence of acute allograft rejection. First clinically recognized cases of ACAD were reported in pathologic specimens of diseased heart transplant recipients in early 1970s.[72] These specimens were noted to have extensive disease in coronary arteries of donor hearts, which during life did not reveal angiographically significant disease.

Incidence

In several series, up to 50% of heart transplant recipients are reported to have angiographically identifiable ACAD within 5 years of receiving the allograft.[73]

It is felt that in some patients with multiple risk factors, ACAD may begin as early as few weeks posttransplantation and progress at an accelerated pace leading to eventual allograft failure.

Etiology

ACAD is felt to be multifactorial, like native vessel CAD, with the addition of some factors which are peculiar to the transplant recipient population. A broad generalization of risk factors would categorize them into immune and nonimmune related. Among the immune-related risk factors are incidence and severity of acute cellular and humoral rejection episodes, presence of elevated panel reactive antibodies prior to transplantation, and donor-specific cross-match, all of which are interrelated. Nonimmune risk factors include increasing donor age, hyperlipidemia, and

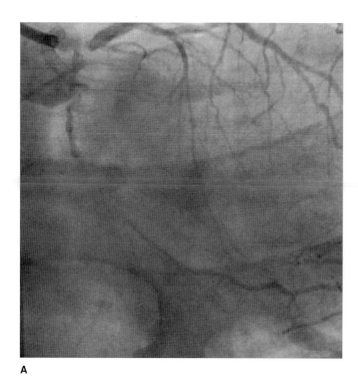

A

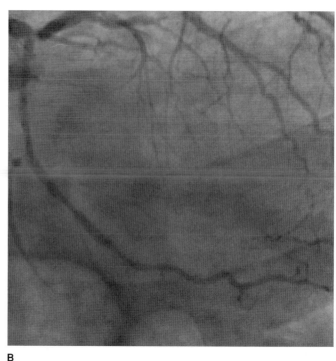

B

● **FIGURE 52-6.** (A) Coronary angiogram showing ACAD in transplanted heart. (B) Same patient after PTCA.

CMV infections. This is often further complicated by the development of de novo diabetic neuropathy and small vessel vasculopathy in vasa vasorum and vasa nervosum.[74]

Pathology

The pathologic lesion of ACAD is characterized by diffuse, concentric, and intimal hyperplasia distributed throughout the coronary tree extending more into distal end arteries. On electron microscopy, the typical lesions show infiltration by smooth muscle fibers along with macrophages.

Clinical Manifestation

Clinical manifestation of ACAD is often confusing and complicated by the fact that the cardiac allograft is autonomically denervated and traditional angina is not a presentation in most cardiac allograft recipients.[75] As such most cardiac ischemia in heart transplant recipients is silent. Because of these reasons, advanced ACAD often goes unrecognized and undertreated leading to the observation that patients often first present with symptoms of heart failure, ventricular arrhythmias, and sudden death.[76]

Diagnosis

The gold standard for diagnoses of ACAD currently is contrast angiography, performed as part of annual surveillance along with two-dimensional echocardiography, and right ventricular septum endomyocardial biopsies by most transplant programs. The caveat here is the observation that conventional angiography is both insensitive in detecting early changes of ACAD and underestimates the overall luminal decrease. This is because of the peculiar nature of ACAD, which is more concentric and generalized as opposed to native atherosclerotic coronary disease which appears as discrete lesions in larger epicardial vessels.[77] Electrocardiogram and cardiac enzyme leak are used as routine screening tools even in the absence of symptoms of chest pain due to cardiac denervation.

Because of under appreciation of the extent of ACAD by angiography some centers employ intravascular ultrasound (IVUS) to better complement the quantification of the extent of ACAD achieved with angiography alone.[78] Transthoracic two-dimensional echocardiography is performed at least annually to detect any regional wall motion abnormalities that may indicate presence of clinically significant vessel narrowing. In patients who can not tolerate the intravenous contrast load required for conventional angiography, dobutamine stress echocardiography has been used as a screening tool to detect clinically significant vessel ACAD. The role of multidetector, cardiac CT scanning in surveillance and management of ACAD remains to be well.[79]

Treatment and Prevention

The only effective long-term solution to advanced and clinically significant ACAD is retransplantation because of the fact that the disease mostly involves all large and small vessels diffusely with characteristic paucity of small collateral vessels. While retransplantation resets the clock on development of ACAD, the survival after retransplantation is substantially less than after primary heart transplantation, with one study reporting a 38% survival at 1-year for patients retransplanted within the first 6 months after primary heart transplantation.[80] However, this study reported on patients retransplanted for several reasons including acute rejection, more recent studies following results of retransplantation specifically for ACAD have reported better outcomes with up to 69% survival at 1 year.[81] ACAD in its most advanced form is seldom amenable to percutaneous coronary intervention (PCI) or surgical revascularization, although percutaneous coronary intervention[82] and coronary artery bypass-graft have been performed in those patients who have suitable targets[83,84] (Figure 52-6A and 52-6B).

The best medical practices are aimed at prevention and stabilization of the progression of ACAD. Dietary modification, smoking cessation, prevention, and prompt treatment of acute cellular rejection and opportunistic infections specially CMV, control of hypertension specially with calcium channel blockers, weight loss, strict control of hyperglycemia, and administration of HMG-CoA reductase inhibitors for cholesterol reduction, form the backbone of

preventive therapy. In those patients who show signs of humoral rejection, the use of high-dose steroids, plasmapheresis, and in advanced cases radiotherapy to lymphatic beds has been effective in halting the progress of ACAD which many investigators feel represents a chronic form of rejection, akin to bronchiolitis obliterans in lung transplant recipients.

Although conditional half-life after heart transplantation now is estimated 10 years, the most important limitation is development of ACAD. Advances in prevention and medical management, as well as revascularization procedures have not had an appreciable impact on the incidence or progression of ACAD. A better understanding of the factors contributing to development and progression of this phenomenon can further enhance the benefit to society from this invaluable medical resource. It is quite possible that progression of peripheral vascular disease in patients who are recipients of heart transplantation merely is a continuum of disease and natural progression of preexisting atherosclerosis.

REFERENCES

1. Bruno S, Remuzzi G, Ruggenenti P. Transplant renal artery stenosis. *J Am Soc Nephrol.* 2004;15(1):134-141.

2. Imanishi M, Akabane S, Takamiya M, et al. Critical degree of renal arterial stenosis that causes hypertension in dogs. *Angiology.* 1992;43(10):833-842.

3. Audard V, Matignon M, Hemery F, et al. Risk factors and long-term outcome of transplant renal artery stenosis in adult recipients after treatment by percutaneous transluminal angioplasty. *Am J Transplant.* 2006;6(1):95-99.

4. Pouria S, State OI, Wong W, et al. CMV infection is associated with transplant renal artery stenosis. *QJM.* 1998;91(3):185-189.

5. Fernandez-Najera JE, Beltrán S, Aparicio M, et al. Transplant renal artery stenosis: association with acute vascular rejection. *Transplant Proc.* 2006;38(8):2404-2405.

6. Humar A, Matas AJ. Surgical complications after kidney transplantation. *Semin Dial.* 2005;18(6):505-510.

7. Finlay DE, Letourneau JG, Longley DG. Assessment of vascular complications of renal, hepatic, and pancreatic transplantation. *Radiographics.* 1992;12(5):981-996.

8. Voiculescu A, Schmitz M, Hollenbeck M, et al. Management of arterial stenosis affecting kidney graft perfusion: a single-centre study in 53 patients. *Am J Transplant.* 2005;5(7):1731-1738.

9. Kobayashi K, Censullo ML, Rossman LL, Kyriakides PN, Kahan BD, Cohen AM. Interventional radiologic management of renal transplant dysfunction: indications, limitations, and technical considerations. *Radiographics.* 2007;27(4):1109-1130.

10. Sayegh M, Lazarus JM, eds. Renal parenchymal disease and hypertension. In: Cooke J, ed. *Current Management of Hypertension and Vascular Disease.* Philadelphia, PA: Decker; 1992:76.

11. Sankari BR, Geisinger M, Zelch M, et al. Post-transplant renal artery stenosis: impact of therapy on long-term kidney function and blood pressure control. *J Urol.* 1996;155(6):1860-1864.

12. O'Neill WC, Baumgarten DA. Ultrasonography in renal transplantation. *Am J Kidney Dis.* 2002;39(4):663-678.

13. Johnson DB, Lerner CA, Prince MR, et al. Gadolinium-enhanced magnetic resonance angiography of renal transplants. *Magn Reson Imaging.* 1997;15(1):13-20.

14. Chua GC, Snowden S, Patel U. Kinks of the transplant renal artery without accompanying intraarterial pressure gradient do not require correction: five-year outcome study. *Cardiovasc Intervent Radiol.* 2004;27(6):643-650.

15. Fervenza FC, Lafayette RA, Alfrey EJ, Petersen J. Renal artery stenosis in kidney transplants. *Am J Kidney Dis.* 1998;31(1):142-148.

16. Wong W, Fynn SP, Higgins RM, et al. Transplant renal artery stenosis in 77 patients–does it have an immunological cause? *Transplantation.* 1996;61(2):215-219.

17. Patel NH, Jindal RM, Wilkin T, et al. Renal arterial stenosis in renal allografts: retrospective study of predisposing factors and outcome after percutaneous transluminal angioplasty. *Radiology.* 2001;219(3):663-667.

18. Grossman RA, Naji A, Perloff LJ, et al. Percutaneous transluminal angioplasty treatment of renal transplant artery stenosis. *Transplantation.* 1982;34(6):339-343.

19. Raynaud A, Bedrossian J, Remy P, Brisset JM, Angel CY, Gaux JC. Percutaneous transluminal angioplasty of renal transplant arterial stenoses. *AJR Am J Roentgenol.* 1986;146(4):853-857.

20. Fauchald P, Vatne K, Paulsen D, et al. Long-term clinical results of percutaneous transluminal angioplasty in transplant

renal artery stenosis. *Nephrol Dial Transplant.* 1992;7(3):256-259.

21. Sierre SD, Raynaud AC, Carreres T, Sapoval MR, Beyssen BM, Gaux JC. Treatment of recurrent transplant renal artery stenosis with metallic stents. *J Vasc Interv Radiol.* 1998;9(4):639-644.

22. Merkus JW, Huysmans FT, Hoitsma AJ, Buskens FG, Skotnicki SH, Koene RA. Renal allograft artery stenosis: results of medical treatment and intervention. A retrospective analysis. *Transpl Int.* 1993;6(2):111-115.

23. Rao KV, Kjellstrand CM. Post transplant acute renal failure: a review. *Clin Exp Dial Apheresis.* 1983;7(1-2):127-143.

24. Takahashi M, Humke U, Girndt M, Kramann B, Uder M. Early posttransplantation renal allograft perfusion failure due to dissection: diagnosis and interventional treatment. *AJR Am J Roentgenol.* 2003;180(3):759-763.

25. Collins AJ, Roberts TL, St Peter WL, Chen SC, Ebben J, Constantini E. United States Renal Data System assessment of the impact of the National Kidney Foundation-Dialysis Outcomes Quality Initiative guidelines. *Am J Kidney Dis.* 2002;39(4):784-795.

26. Diehm C, Kareem S, Lawall H. Epidemiology of peripheral arterial disease. *Vasa.* 2004;33(4):183-189.

27. Gey DC, Lesho EP, Manngold J. Management of peripheral arterial disease. *Am Fam Physician.* 2004;69(3):525-532.

28. Sebastia C, Quiroga S, Boyé R, Cantarell C, Fernandez-Planas M, Alvarez A. Helical CT in renal transplantation: normal findings and early and late complications. *Radiographics.* 2001;21(5):1103-1117.

29. Nguan CY, Luke PP. Renal artery pseudoaneurysm of infectious etiology: a life-threatening complication after renal transplantation. *Urology.* 2006;68(3):668-669.

30. Koops A, Wojciechowski B, Broering DC, Adam G, Krupski-Berdien G. Anatomic variations of the hepatic arteries in 604 selective celiac and superior mesenteric angiographies. *Surg Radiol Anat.* 2004;26(3):239-244.

31. Gruttadauria S, Foglieni CS, Doria C, Luca A, Lauro A, Marino IR. The hepatic artery in liver transplantation and surgery: vascular anomalies in 701 cases. *Clin Transplant.* 2001;15(5):359-363.

32. Hiatt JR, Gabbay J, Busuttil RW. Surgical anatomy of the hepatic arteries in 1000 cases. *Ann Surg.* 1994;220(1):50-52.

33. Ramirez CB, Doria C, di Francesco F, Iaria M, Kang Y, Marino IR. Basiliximab induction in adult liver transplant recipients with 93% rejection-free patient and graft survival at 24 months. *Transplant Proc.* 2006;38(10):3633-3635.

34. United States Department of Health and Human Services: HRSA/OPTN-SRTR Annual Report. Table 1.12b One Year Unadjusted Patient Survival by Organ and Year of Transplant, 1996 to 2005. http://www.ustransplant.org/annual_reports/current/112b_dh.htm.

35. Marcos A, Ham JM, Fisher RA, Olzinski AT, Posner MP. Surgical management of anatomical variations of the right lobe in living donor liver transplantation. *Ann Surg.* 2000;231(6):824-831.

36. Marcos A. Split-liver transplantation for adult recipients. *Liver Transpl.* 2000;6(6):707-709.

37. Ueda M, Oike F, Ogura Y, et al. Long-term outcomes of 600 living donor liver transplants for pediatric patients at a single center. *Liver Transpl.* 2006;12(9):1326-1336.

38. Goss JA, Shackleton CR, McDiarmid SV, et al. Long-term results of pediatric liver transplantation: an analysis of 569 transplants. *Ann Surg.* 1998;228(3):411-420.

39. Eghtesad B, Jain AB, Fung JJ. Living donor liver transplantation: ethics and safety. *Transplant Proc.* 2003;35(1):51-52.

40. Kim DG, Na SE, Chung ES, Moon IS, Lee MD, Kim IC. Donor safety in living donor liver transplantation using the right lobe. *Transplant Proc.* 2003;35(1):53-54.

41. Silva MA, Jambulingam PS, Gunson BK, et al. Hepatic artery thrombosis following orthotopic liver transplantation: a 10-year experience from a single centre in the United Kingdom. *Liver Transpl.* 2006;12(1):146-151.

42. Karani J, Heaton N. Imaging in liver transplantation. *Clin Radiol.* 1998;53(5):317-322.

43. Sheiner PA, Varma CV, Guarrera JV, et al. Selective revascularization of hepatic artery thromboses after liver transplantation improves patient and graft survival. *Transplantation.* 1997;64(9):1295-1299.

44. Oh CK, Pelletier SJ, Sawyer RG, et al. Uni- and multivariate analysis of risk factors for early and late hepatic artery thrombosis after liver transplantation. *Transplantation.* 2001;71(6):767-772.

45. Vivarelli M, Cucchetti A, La Barba G, et al. Ischemic arterial complications after liver transplantation in the adult: multivariate analysis of risk factors. *Arch Surg.* 2004;139(10):1069-1074.

46. Sidhu PS, Shaw AS, Ellis SM, Karani JB, Ryan SM. Microbubble ultrasound contrast in the assessment of hepatic artery patency following liver transplantation: role in reducing frequency of hepatic artery arteriography. *Eur Radiol.* 2004;14(1):21-30.

47. Katyal S, Oliver JH III, Buck DG, Federle MP. Detection of vascular complications after liver transplantation: early experience in multislice CT angiography with volume rendering. *AJR Am J Roentgenol.* 2000;175(6):1735-1739.

48. Glockner JF, Forauer AR, Solomon H, Varma CR, Perman WH. Three-dimensional gadolinium-enhanced MR angiography of vascular complications after liver transplantation. *AJR Am J Roentgenol.* 2000;174(5):1447-1453.

49. Abbasoglu O, Levy MF, Vodapally MS, et al. Hepatic artery stenosis after liver transplantation–incidence, presentation, treatment, and long term outcome. *Transplantation.* 1997;63(2):250-255.

50. Dodd GD III, Memel DS, Zajko AB, Baron RL, Santaguida LA. Hepatic artery stenosis and thrombosis in transplant recipients: doppler diagnosis with resistive index and systolic acceleration time. *Radiology.* 1994;192(3):657-661.

51. Sidhu PS, Ellis SM, Karani JB, Ryan SM. Hepatic artery stenosis following liver transplantation: significance of the tardus parvus waveform and the role of microbubble contrast media in the detection of a focal stenosis. *Clin Radiol.* 2002;57(9):789-799.

52. Del Gaudio M, Grazi GL, Ercolani G, et al. Outcome of hepatic artery reconstruction in liver transplantation with an iliac arterial interposition graft. *Clin Transplant.* 2005;19(3):399-405.

53. Zamboni F, Franchello A, Ricchiuti A, Fop F, Rizzetto M, Salizzoni M. Use of arterial conduit as an alternative technique in arterial revascularization during orthotopic liver transplantation. *Dig Liver Dis*. 2002;34(2):122-126.

54. Marshall MM, Muiesan P, Srinivasan P, et al. Hepatic artery pseudoaneurysms following liver transplantation: incidence, presenting features and management. *Clin Radiol*. 2001;56(7):579-587.

55. Johnston T, Jeon H, Gedaly R, Ranjan D. Importance of local infection in hepatic artery pseudoaneurysms. *Liver Transpl*. 2008;14(3):388.

56. Tobben PJ, Zajko AB, Sumkin JH, et al. Pseudoaneurysms complicating organ transplantation: roles of CT, duplex sonography, and angiography. *Radiology*. 1988;169(1):65-70.

57. Galazka Z, Grochowiecki T, Nazarewski S, et al. A solution to organ shortage: vascular reconstructions for pancreas transplantation. *Transplant Proc*. 2006;38(1):273-275.

58. Troppmann C, Gruessner AC, Benedetti E, et al. Vascular graft thrombosis after pancreatic transplantation: univariate and multivariate operative and nonoperative risk factor analysis. *J Am Coll Surg*. 1996;182(4):285-316.

59. Soon-Shiong P, White G, DeMayo E, Koyle M, Danovitch G. Mechanical obstruction of the portal vein as a cause of vascular thrombosis after pancreatic transplantation in humans. *Transplant Proc*. 1988;20(5):1059-1061.

60. Snider JF, Hunter DW, Kuni CC, Castaneda-Zuniga WR, Letourneau JG. Pancreatic transplantation: radiologic evaluation of vascular complications. *Radiology*. 1991;178(3):749-753.

61. Reddy KS, Stratta RJ, Shokouh-Amiri MH, Alloway R, Egidi MF, Gaber AO. Surgical complications after pancreas transplantation with portal-enteric drainage. *J Am Coll Surg*. 1999;189(3):305-313.

62. Lopez NM, Jeon H, Ranjan D, Johnston TD. Atypical etiology of massive gastrointestinal bleeding: arterio-enteric fistula following enteric drained pancreas transplant. *Am Surg*. 2004;70(6):529-532.

63. Newman AB, Siscovick DS, Manolio TA, et al. Ankle-arm index as a marker of atherosclerosis in the Cardiovascular Health Study. Cardiovascular Heart Study (CHS) Collaborative Research Group. *Circulation*. 1993;88(3):837-845.

64. Smith GD, Shipley MJ, Rose G. Intermittent claudication, heart disease risk factors, and mortality. The Whitehall Study. *Circulation*. 1990;82(6):1925-1931.

65. Erdoes LS, Hunter GC, Venerus BJ, et al. Prospective evaluation of peripheral vascular disease in heart transplant recipients. *J Vasc Surg*. 1995;22(4):434-440; discussion 440-442.

66. Tse KC, Lam MF, Yip PS, Li FK, Lai KN, Chan TM. A long-term study on hyperlipidemia in stable renal transplant recipients. *Clin Transplant*. 2004;18(3):274-280.

67. Sukhija R, Aronow WS, Yalamanchili K, Peterson SJ, Frishman WH, Babu S. Association of ankle-brachial index with severity of angiographic coronary artery disease in patients with peripheral arterial disease and coronary artery disease. *Cardiology*. 2005;103(3):158-160.

68. Berkenboom G, Crasset V, Giot C, Unger P, Vachiery JL, LeClerc JL. Endothelial function of internal mammary artery in patients with coronary artery disease and in cardiac transplant recipients. *Am Heart J*. 1998;135(3):488-494.

69. Kon V, Sugiura M, Inagami T, Harvie BR, Ichikawa I, Hoover RL. Role of endothelin in cyclosporine-induced glomerular dysfunction. *Kidney Int*. 1990;37(6):1487-1491.

70. Horio T, Kohno M, Murakawa K, et al. Increased plasma immunoreactive endothelin-1 concentration in hypercholesterolemic rats. *Atherosclerosis*. 1991;89(2-3):239-246.

71. Gao SZ, Schroeder JS, Alderman EL, et al. Prevalence of accelerated coronary artery disease in heart transplant survivors. Comparison of cyclosporine and azathioprine regimens. *Circulation*. 1989;80(5, pt 2): III100-III105.

72. Mason JW, Strefling A. Small vessel disease of the heart resulting in myocardial necrosis and death despite angiographically normal coronary arteries. *Am J Cardiol*. 1979;44(1):171-176.

73. Schroeder JS, Gao SZ, Hunt SA, Stinson EB. Accelerated graft coronary artery disease: diagnosis and prevention. *J Heart Lung Transplant*. 1992;11(4, pt 2):S258-S265.

74. Benedini S, Fiocchi R, Battezzati A, et al. Energy metabolism in diabetic and nondiabetic heart transplant recipients. *Diabetes Care*. 2002;25(3):530-536.

75. Aranda JM Jr, Hill J. Cardiac transplant vasculopathy. *Chest*. 2000;118(6):1792-1800.

76. Uretsky BF, Kormos RL, Zerbe TR, et al. Cardiac events after heart transplantation: incidence and predictive value of coronary arteriography. *J Heart Lung Transplant*. 1992;11(3, pt 2):S45-S51.

77. Pinney SP, Mancini D. Cardiac allograft vasculopathy: advances in understanding its pathophysiology, prevention, and treatment. *Curr Opin Cardiol*. 2004;19(2):170-176.

78. Rickenbacher PR, Kemna MS, Pinto FJ, et al. Coronary artery intimal thickening in the transplanted heart. An in vivo intracoronary untrasound study of immunologic and metabolic risk factors. *Transplantation*. 1996;61(1):46-53.

79. Lazem F, Barbir M, Banner N, Ludman P, Mitchell A, Yacoub M. Coronary calcification detected by ultrafast computed tomography is a predictor of cardiac events in heart transplant recipients. *Transplant Proc*. 1997;29(1-2):572-575.

80. Hosenpud JD, Novick RJ, Breen TJ, Keck B, Daily P. The Registry of the International Society for Heart and Lung Transplantation: twelfth official report-1995. *J Heart Lung Transplant*. 1995;14(5):805-815.

81. Smith JA, Ribakove GH, Hunt SA, et al. Heart retransplantation: the 25-year experience at a single institution. *J Heart Lung Transplant*. 1995;14(5):832-839.

82. Sharifi M, Siraj Y, O'Donnell J, Pompili VJ. Coronary angioplasty and stenting in orthotopic heart transplants: a fruitful act or a futile attempt? *Angiology*. 2000;51(10):809-815.

83. Patel NC, Patel NU, Loulmet DF, McCabe JC, Subramanian VA. Emergency conversion to cardiopulmonary bypass during attempted off-pump revascularization results in increased morbidity and mortality. *J Thorac Cardiovasc Surg*. 2004;128(5):655-661.

84. Dieter RS, Gauthier GM, Nanjundappa A, Wolff MR. Angioplasty versus stenting for cardiac allograft vasculopathy. *Therapy*. 2006;3:517-520.

85. Bossaller C, Försterman U, Hertel R, Olbricht C, Reschke V, Fleck E. Ciclosporin A inhibits endothelium-dependent vasodilation and vascular prostacyclin production. *Eur J Pharmacol*. 1989;165:165-169.

chapter 53

Diagnosis and Management of Perioperative Ischemic Stroke

Michael J. Schneck, MD / *Simona Velicu, MD*

● INTRODUCTION

Acute stroke is the abrupt onset, within seconds to hours, of neurologic deficits resulting from occlusion or rupture of arteries or veins that supply the central nervous system (CNS). By convention, this is a clinical definition and the radiologic–pathologic correlation is infarction. Acute strokes are classified as either hemorrhagic (15%–20%) or ischemic (80%–85%).[1] Of the hemorrhagic strokes, intracerebral hemorrhage is three times more common than subarachnoid hemorrhage. Additionally, transient ischemic attacks are temporary episodes of focal neurologic deficits to the brain or retina followed by complete recovery. Also, by convention, the definition of transient ischemia attack (TIA) encompasses full recovery without imaging evidence of infarction, within 24 hours. Most TIAs last for 5 to 20 minutes and events with persistent deficits for several hours are often associated with infarction. As such, a new definition for TIA suggested that the time window for TIA be reduced to less than 6 hours.[2] Awareness of these definitions is important in perioperative cerebrovascular disease as the goal of all acute stroke therapies is to recognize stroke symptoms, as well as differentiate strokes, and TIA from other acute, focal, neurologic, perioperative deficits such as focal seizures or complicated migraine, and ultimately, through rapid and aggressive interventions, convert all putative strokes into TIAs.

"Time is brain" as regards the treatment of acute ischemic stroke.[3] Jeffrey Saver quantified the ongoing damage in an acute stroke and calculated that each minute during an acute stroke, 1.9 million neurons and 14 billion synapses are lost. Furthermore, for those patients with a large vessel (i.e., carotid, middle cerebral [MCA], or basilar artery occlusion) acute ischemic stroke, 120 million neurons, 830 billion synapses, and 714 km (447 miles) of myelinated fibers are lost each hour. Thus, rapid diagnostic evaluation and intervention, whenever possible, is critical regardless of whether the patient presents from home or has an in-hospital stroke. The challenge, however, for the patient in the perioperative period is recognition of an event. Whereas acute stroke in hospitalized patients potentially offers a greater likelihood of treatment, as there is no delay in arrival to the hospital, determining the onset of stroke symptoms in the perioperative period may be difficult, as the timing of onset may be hard to define because of patient sedation, pharmacologic paralysis, or a delirious state.[4] Additionally, while time of arrival to hospital is not an issue, patients who are stable and transferred out of the postoperative care unit or intensive care unit may not be seen as frequently by nursing staff and thus the time window for intervention may be lost. Finally, surgery is typically an absolute exclusion criterion for intravenous (IV) thrombolysis and alternate acute interventions may not always be possible.[1]

● FREQUENCY AND DISTRIBUTION OF STROKE

The incidence of stroke in the perioperative period is low. In one series, clinic strokes occurred in 3.6% of cases within 9 days following surgery though the frequency of acute infarct, as diagnosed by CT scan or MRI, was only 2.5%.[5] In this series, 74% of stroke patients were diagnosed on the day of surgery, and 91% within the first 3 postoperative days. The authors reported that the stroke distribution was predominantly in the anterior circulation with 78% of acute infarcts located in the MCA distribution and 7% in the anterior cerebral artery distribution. However, there were more posterior circulation infarcts than otherwise would be predicted with 28% in the posterior cerebral artery distribution, 28% specifically in the cerebellum, reflecting with 36% of strokes occurring in multiple vascular territories probably as a result of cardiac embolism. Differences in cerebral distribution between infarct types were statistically significant with embolic strokes occurring in the right hemisphere in 34% of patients, left in 20%, vertebrobasilar in 19%, multiple in 26%, while watershed strokes occurred in the right hemisphere in 19%, left in 28%, vertebrobasilar in 0%, and multiple distributions 53% ($p < 0.0001$). This reflects the relative preservation of blood flow to the brainstem in the context of hypotension.

The risk of stroke after noncardiac procedures is low with the risk being significantly higher in cardiac and vascular (especially aortic and cervico-cerebral) procedures.[6,7] The most recent data indicate that strokes in surgical patients have the highest incidence in those undergoing cardiovascular-related procedures (1%–9%) followed by head and neck surgery (5%), vascular surgery (1%–3%), and lastly general surgical procedures (0.1%–0.7%).[6–9] Very important differences exist with respect to the type of cardiovascular procedure. Combined cardiac/valvular/aortic procedures have the highest associated risk as opposed to coronary artery bypass grafting (CABG) alone. Salazar et al.[5] found a 3.6% incidence of clinical stroke in a prospective study involving a population of 5971 patients undergoing various isolated or combined cardiac and valvular and/or carotid procedures, performed between 1992 and 1997. Combined CABG and carotid endarterectomy (CEA) procedures were associated with the highest incidence (17.3%), followed by CABG/valve (6.7%), aortic (4.2%), CABG (3.2%, $p < 0.0001$), and valvular (2.8%) procedures. Dacey et al. reported a 1.61% incidence of perioperative stroke in 33 062 patients undergoing CABG alone between 1992 and 2001.[10] Valvular surgery alone has a risk of between 5% and 9%.[7,9,11] CEA alone has a postoperative risk of 6% in symptomatic patients and 2% in asymptomatic patients.[12] However, review of studies encompassing simultaneous CEA-CABG totaling 1923 subject with a combination either symptomatic or symptomatic carotid artery stenosis and stable or unstable coronary disease (CAD) noted that an average perioperative complication rate of 3.0% stroke (range 0%–9%), 2.2% myocardial infarction (MI) (range 0%–6%), and 4.7% death (range 2.6%–8.9%).[12] Three studies reported long-term survival and the 5- to 6-year survival among 492 subjects ranged between 73% and 91%. In the only study with more than 50 subjects where CEA preceded the CABG, 257 patients with stable coronary artery disease were studied and the perioperative stroke rate was 1.9%, for MI 4.7%, and for death 1.6% though the data was observational and retrospective. Thus, the death rate for combined CEA-CABG is higher but the overall complication rates did not appear significantly increased in this instance compared to CEA alone.[9–12] Furthermore, while the risk of stroke is increased in both general surgical patients and those undergoing cardiovascular procedures in the context of greater than 50% cervical

carotid artery stenosis, there was no association with increasing stenosis and stroke risk.[6] Because of the risk of stroke from general surgical procedures related to carotid stenosis is estimated at 3.6% and the risk of stroke from surgery on an asymptomatic carotid artery stenosis is variably estimated at 2% to 3%, prophylactic CEA or carotid stenting cannot be supported at this time.[6]

● PATHOETIOLOGY AND RISK FACTORS FOR PERIOPERATIVE STROKE

Perioperative ischemic strokes are generally classified by pathophysiologic mechanism into cardio-embolic, atheroembolic, atherothrombotic, hypoperfusion (watershed), and hypercoaguable/other strokes. Most of the perioperative strokes are cardio- or atheroembolic and hemorrhagic stroke are much less common. Atherothrombotic (In situ thrombus) strokes, while common in de novo cerebra ischemia, are much less common in the perioperative period.[7–13] Salazar et al.[5] reported that out of 151 patients with acute infarction diagnosed on brain imaging, 71% had a pure embolic stroke, 12% had a watershed (border) zone infarct, with a mixed pattern (embolic + watershed) being present in 12%. By contrast, a Johns Hopkins series of 98 cardiac surgery patients identified with an acute clinical stroke found that 48% of patients had bilateral watershed infarcts on MRI.[14] Fat or air emboli are additional rare causes of stroke as are hyperextension or flexion injuries to the posterior circulation.

About half of all strokes occur within the first day following surgery and are typically because of manipulation of vessels or debris from cardiac surgery, whereas a large proportion of delayed stroke is typically related to atrial fibrillation.[13,15,17] Hypotension is typically not a cause of stroke in the perioperative period even in patients with severe large vessel cervicocerebral atherosclerosis (i.e., extracranial carotid stenosis or vertebrobasilar stenosis). While patients with carotid artery stenosis are at higher risk for perioperative stroke, especially in the context of cardiac surgery, most of the strokes are not directly referable to the stenotic artery suggesting that the carotid disease is simply a surrogate marker for athero-embolism from the heart or aorta during manipulation of the heart or great vessels.[17] In one series, postoperative strokes in watershed areas as a result of hypoperfusion occurred in less than 10% of cases following coronary artery bypass graft surgery (CABG).[16]

Several authors have enumerated a number of distinct preoperative, intraoperative, and postoperative risk factors for stroke.[6–9] Risk factors for perioperative stroke include age, metabolic syndrome risk factors of hypertension, diabetes, hyperlipidemia or obesity, renal failure, aortic or cervico-cerebral atherosclerosis, and a history of arrhythmias. Intraoperative factors include type of surgery and duration of surgery, duration of cardiac bypass cardiac and aortic cross-clamping (for cardiac surgery patients), intraoperative hypotension, intraoperative hypertension, and transient arrhythmias. There is some debate about the comparative benefit of regional versus general anesthesia in decreasing stroke risk.[7–18] In general, volatile anesthetic agents, barbiturates, and propofol reduce ischemic neurologic injury and may have a neuroprotectant effect and the main issue related to general anesthesia is the induced hypotension that may occur with these agents.[19] Postoperative risk factors include hyperglycemia, dehydration or blood loss, heart failure or myocardial ischemia or low cardiac ejection fraction, or cardiac arrhythmias.[6–8,20]

Dacey et al.[10] found that in a population of 35 733 patients undergoing isolated CABG, the characteristics of the patients who suffered stroke were age (mean value 70.7 years versus 65.4, $p < 0.001$), ejection fraction (49.7% versus 52.9%, $p < 0.001$), diabetes (42.4% versus 30.5%, $p < 0.001$), renal failure or creatinine >2 mg/dL (8.4% versus 3.2%, $p < 0.001$), and priority of surgery. A preoperative risk prediction model was developed by Charlesworth et al.[21] based on the same population from New England of 33 062 consecutive patients undergoing isolated CABG. This risk prediction, model developed by the Northern New England Cardiovascular Disease Study Group to predict the risk of stroke after CABG, notes the relative weigh of the variables of age, elective versus urgent surgery, female sex, ejection fraction less than 40%, diabetes mellitus, creatinine greater than two and history of prior stroke or TIA, or prior history of peripheral vascular procedures.

A second cohort of 16 184 patients was also analyzed in terms of risk factors for developing stroke.[15] Regression analysis led to the identification of several independent risk factors for stroke. The highest odds ratio of 3.55 was seen with documented cerebrovascular disease including neurologic deficits lasting less than 24 hours, less than 3 weeks, and those lasting longer than 3 weeks or causing death. Other significant risk factor included endocarditis, documented peripheral vascular disease, diabetes mellitus, hypertension, prior cardiac surgery, urgency of surgery, cardiopulmonary bypass (CPB) time longer than 2 hours, and hemofiltration intraoperatively. The incidence of stroke in these patients was 16.8% as compared to a reported 7% to 13% frequency in prior studies.[11,22]

Particularly in cardiac surgery, ischemic strokes that occur early in the postoperative period are generally attributed to the use of cardiopulmonary bypass and the consequent release of atherosclerotic fragments from the heart/aorta/carotid arteries, while strokes that occur late in the postoperative period can have several causative mechanisms: atrial fibrillation, myocardial infarct, coagulopathy, bed rest, the perioperative withholding of antiplatelet, and/or anticoagulant agents. Cerebral microembolism, resulting from either application of coronary bypass or the early manipulation of the aorta during cardiac surgery whether on- or off-pump, is considered to be among the primary early pathophysiologic mechanisms of perioperative stroke post-CABG.[23,24] The nature of the microemboli can be either gaseous (introduced shortly after aortic arch cannulation) or solid (released during mechanical manipulation of the aorta). Other possible mechanisms for cerebral ischemia facilitated by coronary bypass include the replacement of pulsatile cerebral blood flow (CBF) to a nonpulsatile type which has been associated with the development of diffuse brain edema.[25]

Paroxysmal atrial fibrillation is a very important cause of perioperative stroke.[6,7,9,26,27] In particular, atrial fibrillation is a common late complication among postoperative cardiac patients, most typically between the second and fourth postoperative days. Atrial fibrillation may occur in upward of 50% of patients following cardiac surgery though the means for detecting, diagnosing, treating, and preventing this condition are highly variable. The present recommendations include IV heparin for high-risk patients (those with history of TIA or stroke) who develop postoperative atrial fibrillation and oral anticoagulation for at least 30 days following reversion to sinus rhythm with indefinite anticoagulation for patients in persistent atrial fibrillation or for those with a postoperative atrial fibrillation related stroke.[26]

● THERAPEUTIC DECISIONS RELATED TO PERIOPERATIVE STROKE

Guidelines for the risk of perioperative MI and timing of surgery post-MI are well-delineated.[28] Clinical data regarding timing of surgery poststroke is limited, however. Delaying elective surgery following stroke is mainly based on theoretical grounds.[8] Following an ischemic stroke, autoregulation of CBF is impaired and while the duration of that impairment is unclear, disruptions in CBF may last from days to weeks. Additionally, following a stroke there are a number of inflammatory changes that increase the risk for worsening or extension of cerebral infarction or increasing the susceptibility to hemorrhagic reperfusion injury. The process whereby a cerebral infarct scars down typically occurs over several weeks to months depending, to a very real extent, on the size of the infarct. As such, a minimum of 4 to 6 weeks delay for elective and major surgeries seems appropriate, assuming delay is feasible, and especially for larger infarcts.

The largest risk factor for perioperative stroke is a history of stroke. Prior history of stroke or TIA conveys a stroke risk of up to 2.9% in general surgical procedures where the overall risk is just 0.2%.[8] In patients who undergo CABG there is a similar increased risk with a stroke risk of up to 8.5% with a prior history of stroke or TIA, as compared to an overall risk of stroke in CABG patients of 1% to 2% without a prior history of stroke or TIA.[8] Carotid disease is particularly a marker of generalized atherosclerotic vascular disease with less than half of the risk attributable to carotid artery stenosis in patients undergoing CABG specifically attributable to the ipsilateral carotid artery.[17] In trying to minimize risk, those patients with symptomatic carotid stenosis 70% should undergo a carotid procedure (CEA or CAS) prior to elective cardiac and noncardiac surgeries. The indications for carotid procedures prior to surgery for patients with asymptomatic carotid artery disease are less clear. The perioperative risk of symptomatic basilar or vertebral artery disease may be as high as 6% though the data is even more obscure for patients with asymptomatic disease or remote strokes attributable to the posterior circulation or intracranial circulation.[8]

One underconsidered problem with substituting a CAS for CEA as a prophylactic procedure is that CAS necessitates the use of combination antiplatelet therapy with clopidogrel and aspirin. However, there is a preponderant body of evidence that shows that cessation of any antithrombotic therapy for surgical procedures may actually increase the risk of stroke or heart attack. The risk of MI or death, for example, is doubled within the first 90 days following discontinuation of clopidogrel, prescribed for acute coronary syndromes and numerous small case series have reported an increased risk of stroke following cessation of even aspirin in the immediate preoperative period.[29,30] Because cessation of antiplatelet and anticoagulant medications, prescribed for primary or secondary prevention of stroke or other cardiovascular disease significantly increases the risk of perioperative stroke and myocardial infarction, serious consideration should be given to whether antithrombotic therapies really need to be completely discontinued. For minor procedures, the risk of bleeding may be outweighed by the risk of stroke or MI even in the context of anticoagulation. For major procedures, early resumption of antithrombotic therapy, at the very least substituting aspirin for clopidogrel or warfarin if necessary, may at least reduce the risk of perioperative cerebral or cardiac ischemia.

Despite aggressive interventions, perioperative stroke remains among the most devastating postoperative complications and is associated with significantly increased morbidity and mortality.[5,10,15] Early stroke findings are associated with delays in postoperative awakening and prolonged hospitalization.[5,15] Furthermore long-term survival is marked diminished.[5,10] Disability predictors, as measured by the modified Rankin Score at long-term follow-up, are the presence of a watershed infarct ($p < 0.0001$), age ($p < 0.0001$), peripheral vascular disease ($p = 0.049$), history of prior stroke ($p = 0.023$), and postoperative length of stay ($p < 0.0001$).[5] As such stroke prevention measures such as continuation of antithrombotic therapies, risk factor reduction, and careful risk assessment are of paramount importance.

When, however, a suspected acute ischemic stroke is identified in the postoperative period, the interventional options are, as noted previously, limited (Table 53-1). Intravenous thrombolysis is associated with a noninsignificant risk of systemic bleeding especially in the context of recent surgery. Thus, in the pivotal National Institutes of Neurological Disorders and Stroke (NINDS) study of IV tissue plasminogen activator (TPA) for acute ischemic stroke, major surgery within 14 days of stroke onset was (and remains) an absolute contraindication for thrombolysis.[1,31] Whether patients who undergo minor procedures such as endoscopy, dental procedures, or muscle and skin biopsies can routinely receive IV TPA remains to be determined. In the absence of intra-arterial (IA) thrombolytic therapies, these patients might be candidates for IV TPA, albeit with a higher risk of bleeding complications (see Table 53-1).[32]

However, if an interventional team is available, and the time of onset of stroke can be determined, patients who have undergone a surgical procedure may potentially be a candidate for IA endovascular mechanical or pharmacologic thrombolysis. For very high-risk patients, even IA pharmacologic thrombolysis may be contraindicated and in those patients mechanical IA thrombolysis alone may be used (see Table 53-1).

IA pharmacologic thrombolysis was first shown as conceptually useful in the Prolyse in Acute Cerebral

TABLE 53-1. Guidelines for Thrombolytic Treatment Options for Selected Patients Who Have Perioperative Acute Ischemic Stroke (33)

	IV Thrombolysis <3 Hours	IA Thrombolysis <6 Hours	Mechanical Thrombolysis <8 Hours
Low-risk Surgery Muscle biopsy Digit amputation Skin grafting Arthroscopy Endoscopy Dental procedures	*	Yes	Yes
Medium-risk Surgery GI/colonic surgery CABG CEA/stenting	No	Yes	Yes
High-risk Surgery Craniotomy Transplant surgery	No	Yes	Yes

*In selected patients when IA and mechanical thrombolysis are unavailable.

Thromboembolism II (PROACT-II) trial that showed 66% recanalization of the MCA for those patients treated with prourokinase as compared to 18% recanalization of the MCA in the control group.[33] Forty percent of the patients in the treatment group achieved functional independence versus 25% of the control group at 90 days ($p = 0.04$). However 10% of the treated patients sustained a symptomatic intracranial hemorrhage as compared with 2% in the control group ($p = 0.06$). As such, pro-urokinase was not approved by the United States Food and Drug Administration (FDA) but has served as a proof of concept for IA thrombolysis. IA thrombolysis using TPA or urokinase has been used in acute ischemic stroke for patients who are not eligible for IV TPA including patients with stroke in the 3 to 6 hours window for anterior circulation stroke (and with an even longer time window for posterior circulation stroke) especially for those patients who would otherwise be ineligible because of recent surgery.[32]

Additionally, a recent development has been the adoption of mechanical IA endovascular thrombo-embolectomy. The advantage of this approach is that it presumably decreases the risk of hemorrhagic conversion seen with pharmacologic thrombolysis and IA mechanical thromboembolectomy can be done in patients with elevated INR or who are at very high risk in the postoperative period (see Table 53-1). At present the only approved IA, mechanical, thrombo-embolectomy device approved in the United States is the Mechanical Embolus Removal in Cerebral Ischemia (MERCI®) catheter.[34,35] The MERCI trial reported recanalization rates of 46% using the device which was better than the 18% recanalization rate seen in the PROACT-II historical control group.[34] However, overall mortality was higher in the MERCI study (44% versus 25% for the PROACT-II control group) and randomized comparisons with either pharmacologic IV or IA thrombolysis are not yet available. However, a second single arm registry trial, the multi-MERCI trial, showed similar recanalization rates using an improved version of the MERCI device.[35] Fifty-four percent (60/111) patients had successful recanalization using the device alone and 69% (70/111) had recanalization of an occluded intracranial artery using device along with adjunctive IA TPA. Again however, mortality remained high with a 31% mortality rate at 90 days and only 34.3% of the patients achieved reasonable functional independence (modified Rankin Scale ≤2 at 90 days). The Interventional Management of Stroke (IMS III) Trial is a randomized, open-label, multicenter study underway comparing combined IV and IA treatment approach to restoring blood flow to the brain to the current standard FDA-approved treatment approach of giving IV rt-PA alone with a goal enrollment of 900 subjects with moderate to severe ischemic stroke within 3 hours of stroke onset.[36]

Pending additional data, mechanical thrombo-embolectomy remains an option for eligible postoperative ischemic

---

TABLE 53-2. Approach to Arterial Hypertension in Acute Ischemic Stroke

1. If patient is eligible for treatment with IV rtPA or IA pharmacologic or mechanical thrombolysis, one can bring down the pressure prior to thrombolysis; otherwise see Item 3
   - If blood pressure level = systolic >185 mm Hg or diastolic >110 mm Hg
     I. Labetalol 10–20 mg IV over 1–2 min, may repeat ×1; or
     II. Nicardipine infusion, 5 mg/h, titrate up by 2.5 mg/h at 5- to 15-min intervals, maximum dose 15 mg/h; when desired blood pressure attained, reduce to 3 mg/h. (continuous nicardipine drip is possibly more easily titrated rapidly than bolus labetolol)
     III. If blood pressure does not decline and remains >185/110 mm Hg, do not treat with thrombolytic therapy.
2. Management of blood pressure during and after treatment IV rtPA or IA pharmacologic or mechanical thrombolysis
   - Monitor blood pressure every 15 min during treatment and then for another 2 h, then every 30 min for 6 h, and then every hour for the remainder of the 24-hour period
   - Goal blood pressure level: systolic ≤180 mm Hg and diastolic <105 mm Hg
     I. If systolic >180–230 mm Hg or diastolic >105
        Nicardipine infusion, 5 mg/h, titrate up to desired effect by increasing 2.5 mg/h every 5 min to maximum of 15 mg/h or
        Labetalol 5 to 10 mg IV over 1–2 min, may repeat every 10–20 min, maximum dose of 300 mg; or Labetalol 10 mg IV followed by an infusion at 2–8 mg/min
        If no response to beta-blockers or nicardipine can then consider nitroprusside.
3. If patient is not a candidate for IV or IA thrombolysis, there is no data to define the levels of elevated blood pressure requiring emergent treatment poststroke and acutely (in the first 12–24 h); there is no urgency to treat elevated blood pressures. Current AHA/ASA recommendations suggest parenteral drugs be used only if the systolic blood pressure is greater than 220 mm Hg or the mean arterial pressure is greater then 130 mm Hg. Recommended agents include labetalol, nicardipine, or IV enalapril. (Oral agents can be considered, but only if the patient has passed a formal swallowing evaluation or has a nasogastric tube in place; parenteral agents have the advantage of shorter onset of action and duration/lack of overshoot.)

stroke patients. In the absence of other effective treatments for acute ischemic stroke that are not associated with the high intracranial hemorrhage rates of IV or IA thrombolysis, supportive measures including prevention of medical and neurologic complications poststroke, avoiding relative hypotension poststroke (see Table 53-2), and prevention of early stroke recurrence remains the mainstay of stroke management in postoperative patients.[1]

REFERENCES

1. Adams HP Jr, del Zoppo G, Alberts MJ, et al. Guidelines for the early management of adults with ischemic stroke. *Stroke.* 2007;38:1655-1711.

2. Albers GW, Caplan LR, Easton JD, et al. Transient Ischaemic attack—proposal for a new definition. *New Engl J Med.* 2002;347:1713-1716.

3. Saver JL. Time is brain-quantified. *Stroke.* 2006;37:263-266.

4. Castil PR, Miller DA, Meschia JF. Choice of neuroimaging in acute stroke management. *Neurol Clin.* 2006;24:807-820.

5. Salazar et al., 2001.

6. Bernstein RA. Risk of stroke from general surgical procedures in stroke patients. *Neurol Clin.* 2006;24:777-782.

7. Selim M. Perioperative stroke. *N Engl J Med.* 2007;356:706-713.

8. Blacker DJ, Kelly D, Flemming MD, Link MJ, Brown RD Jr. The preoperative cerebrovascular consultation: common cerebrovascular consultations before general or cardiac surgery. *Mayo Clin Proc.* 2004;79:223-229.

9. Dafer RM. Risk estimates of stroke after coronary artery bypass graft and carotid endarterectomy. *Neurol Clin.* 2006;24:795-906.

10. Dacey LJ, Likosky DS, Leavitt BJ, et. al. Perioperative stroke and long-term survival after coronary bypass graft surgery. *Ann Thor Surg.* 2005;79:532-537.

11. Shaw PJ, Bates D, Cartlidge NEF. An analysis of factors predisposing to neurological injury in patients undergoing coronary bypass operations. *Q J Med.* 1989;72:633-646.

12. Chaturvedi S, Bruno A, Feasby T, et al. Carotid endarterectomy—an evidence-based review: report of the Therapeutics and Technology Assessment Subcommittee of the American Academy of Neurology. *Neurology.* 2005;65(6):794-801.

13. Limburg M, Wijdicks EF, Li H. Ischemic stroke after surgical procedures: clinical features, neuroimaging and risk factors. *Neurology.* 1998;50:895-902.

14. Gottesman RF, Sherman PM, Grega MA, et al. Watershed strokes after cardiac surgery-diagnosis, etiology and outcome. *Stroke.* 2006;2306-2311.

15. Bucerius J, Gummert JF, Borger MA, et al. Stroke after cardiac surgery: a risk factor analysis of 16184 consecutive adult patients. *Ann Thor Surg.* 2003;75:472-478.

16. Likosky, 2008.

17. Naylor AR, Mehta Z, Rothwell PM, Bell PR. Carotid artery disease and stroke during coronary artery bypass: a critical review of the literature. *Eur J Vasc Endovasc Surg.* 2002;23:283-294.

18. Kettler RE. Perioperative stroke (letter). *New Engl J Med.* 2007;7:2325-2326.

19. Jellish WS. Anesthetic issues and perioperative blood pressure management in patients who have cerebrovascular diseases undergoing surgical procedures. *Neurol Clin.* 2006;24:647-659.

20. McGirt MJ, Woodworth GF, Brooke BS, et al. Hyperglycemia independently increases the risk of perioperative stroke, myocardial infarction and death after carotid endarterectomy. *Neurosurgery.* 2006;58(6):1066-1073.

21. Charlesworth DC, Likosky DS, Marrin CAS, et al. Development and validation of a prediction model for strokes after coronary artery bypass grafting. *Ann Thorac Surg.* 2003;76:436-443.

22. Rorich MB, Furlan AJ. Risk at cardiac surgery in patients with prior stroke. *Neurology.* 1990;40:835-837.

23. Lund C, Hol PK, Lundblad R, et al. Comparison of cerebral embolization during off-pump and on-pump coronary artery bypass surgery. *Ann Thor Surg.* 2003;76:765-770.

24. Kapetanakis EI, Sotiris CS, Dullum MKC, et al. The impact of aortic manipulation on neurologic outcomes after coronary artery bypass surgery: a risk-adjusted study. *Ann Thorc Surg.* 2004;78:1564-1571.

25. Anderson RE, Li TQ, Hindmarsh T, Settergren G, Vaage J. Increased extracellular brain water after CABG is avoided by off-pump surgery. *J Cardiothorac Vasc Anesthesia.* 1999;13:698-702.

26. Epstein AE, Alexander JC, Gutterman DD, Maisel W, Wheaton JM. Anticoagulation: American College of Chest Physicians guidelines for the prevention and management of postoperative atrial fibrillation after cardiac surgery. *Chest.* 2005;128(suppl 2):24S-27S.

27. Lahtinen J, Biancari F, Salmela E, et al. Postoperative atrial fibrillation is a major cause of stroke after on-pump coronary artery bypass surgery. *Ann Thor Surg.* 2004;77:1241-1244.

28. Fleisher LA, Beckman JA, Kenneth A, Brown KA, et al. ACC/AHA 2007 Guidelines on perioperative cardiovascular evaluation and care for noncardiac surgery. *Circulation.* 2007;116:e418–e499.

29. Ho et al., 2007.

30. Armstrong MJ, Schneck MJ, Biller J. Discontinuation of perioperative antiplatelet and anticoagulant therapy in stroke patients. *Neurol Clin.* (Preoperative and Perioperative Issues in Cerebrovascular Disease) 2006;24:607-630.

31. National Institutes of Neurological Disorders and Stroke rt-PA Stroke Study Group. Tissue plasminogen activator for acute ischemic stroke. *N Engl J Med.* 1995;333:1581-1587.

32. Mullen MT, McGarvey ML, Kasner SE. Safety and efficacy of thrombolytic therapy in postoperative cerebral infarctions. *Neurol Clin.* (Preoperative and Perioperative Issues in Cerebrovascular Disease) 2006;24:783-794.

33. Furlan A, Higashida R, Wechsler L, et al. Intra-arterial prourokinase for acute ischemic stroke. The PROACT II

study: a randomized controlled trial. Prolyse in acute cerebral thromboembolism. *JAMA*. 1999;282(21):2003-2011.

34. Smith WS, Sung G, Starkman S, et al. Safety and efficacy of mechanical embolectomy in acute ischemic stroke: results of the MERCI trial. *Stroke*. 2005;36:1432-1438.

35. Smith, 2007.

36. Broderick, 2008.

37. Broderick JP. Interventional Management of Stroke-III (IMS) trial. NIH/NINDS study number U 01 NS052220. www.ims3.org.

38. Smith WS. Safety of mechanical thrombectomy and intravenous tissue plasminogen activator in acute ischemic stroke. Results of the multi Mechanical Embolus Removal in Cerebral Ischemia (MERCI) trial, part I. *AJNR Am J Neuroradiol*. 2006;27(6):1177-1182.

39. Ho PM, Peterson ED, Wang L, et al. Incidence of death and acute myocardial infarction associated with stopping clopidogrel after acute coronary syndrome. *JAMA*. 2008;299(5):532-539.

Index

Page numbers followed by *f* or *t* indicate figures or tables, respectively